Brief Contents *Continued*

GET CONNECTED

To Content Updates, Study Tools, and More!

FREE CD • SIMON • INSIDE

Meet SIMON   Your free online website companion

sign on at:

http://www.wbsaunders.com/SIMON/Black/medsurg

what you'll receive:

Whether you're a student or an instructor, you'll find information just for you. Things like:
- Content Updates   ● Links to Related Publications
- Author Information . . . and more

plus:

WebLinks

Access hundreds of active websites keyed specifically to the content of this book. The WebLinks are continually updated, with new ones added as they develop.

Free Study and Tutorial CD-ROM

with every copy of Black's *Medical-Surgical Nursing Clinical Management for Positive Outcomes, 6th Edition*

With a Strong Emphasis on Clinical and Functional Relevance, this Valuable CD-ROM Features:

- Detailed discussions for the "Thinking Critically" questions found in the book provide examples of appropriate answers.
- 10 case studies from the text—plus 2 bonus case studies—are presented with discussions for each of the questions as well as 7 to 10 multiple choice questions for further review. Answers include rationales for incorrect answers. Finally, a nursing care plan based on the case study pulls it all together.
- Over **700** NCLEX review questions provide you with an opportunity for review before exams and for additional review before your licensure exam.

W.B. SAUNDERS COMPANY

Medical-Surgical Nursing

CLINICAL MANAGEMENT for POSITIVE OUTCOMES

VOLUME 2

6th EDITION

Joyce M. Black, PhD, RN, CPSN, CCCN, CWCN
Assistant Professor
College of Nursing
University of Nebraska Medical Center
Omaha, Nebraska

Jane Hokanson Hawks, DNSc, MSN, RN, C
Associate Professor of Nursing
Midland Lutheran College
Fremont, Nebraska

Annabelle M. Keene, MSN, RN, C
Bellevue Public Schools
Bellevue, Nebraska
Formerly, Associate Professor
College of Saint Mary
Omaha, Nebraska

W.B. SAUNDERS COMPANY
An Imprint of Elsevier Science
Philadelphia   London   New York   St. Louis   Sydney   Toronto

W.B. SAUNDERS COMPANY
An Imprint of Elsevier Science

The Curtis Center
Independence Square West
Philadelphia, Pennsylvania 19106

NOTICE

Library of Congress Cataloging-in-Publication Data

Medical-surgical nursing: clinical management for positive outcomes / edited by Joyce M. Black, Jane Hokanson Hawks, Annabelle Keene.—6th ed.

    p.;   cm.

    Includes bibliographical references and index.

    ISBN 0–7216–8198–0 (single volume)

    ISBN 0–7216–8197–2 (2 vol set)

    1. Nursing. 2. Surgical nursing. 3. Psychophysiology.   I. Black, Joyce M.   II. Hawks, Jane Hokanson.   III. Keene, Annabelle.
    [DNLM: 1. Nursing Care. 2. Perioperative Nursing.   WY 150 M489365 2001]

RT41.L87 2001
610.73—dc21

                                            99–089356

Vice-President and Nursing Editorial Director: Sally Schrefer

Executive Editor: Thomas Eoyang

Production Managers: Linda Garber, Natalie Ware

Developmental Editor: Victoria Legnini

Manuscript Editor: Carol J. Robins

Illustration Coordinator: Rita Martello

Design Coordinator: Karen O'Keefe Owens

There are several people at the University of Nebraska who seemingly never tire of my questions on how to explain or teach something more clearly. Thank you, Drs. Janet Cuddigan, Louise LaFramboise, and Barbara Manz. I also appreciate the countless students and patients who taught me the value of caring and teaching. I appreciate the expertise of the contributors to this text. And I thank my family for their ongoing understanding of the considerable strain on my time and energy.

J. M. B.

I want to thank my family, parents, and nursing friends from my doctoral and master's programs; my colleagues at Midland Lutheran College, Fremont, Nebraska; and my peers from the Iowa Nurses' Association and Society of Urologic Nurses and Associates (SUNA) who helped me with words of encouragement and support.

J. H. H.

To Chuck, Alice, and Clair. Words cannot express my thanks for your support of my projects, including this book. May you have similar support to pursue your dreams.

A. M. K.

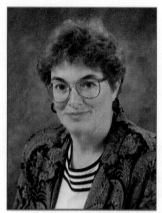

At the time of publication of the fifth edition, **Joyce M. Black, PhD, RN, CPSN, CCCN, CWCN,** was a Nursing Specialist with the Adult Health and Illness Department of the University of Nebraska Medical Center (UNMC). In December 1999 she received her Doctorate from the University of Nebraska College of Nursing. Her dissertation research focused on patient, wound, treatment, and health care system risk factors affecting the rate of pressure ulcer healing. Since graduation, she has returned to her position as Assistant Professor at UNMC, where she teaches medical-surgical nursing. She received her Master's degree from UNMC and her undergraduate degrees from Winona State University in Winona, Minnesota, and Rochester Community College in Rochester, Minnesota.

Dr. Black has also had several years of experience as a medical-surgical nurse at Saint Mary's Hospital, which is affiliated with the Mayo Clinic in Rochester, Minnesota. Her practice has included critical care, burns, respiratory disorders, orthopedics, and plastic surgery. She is certified by the American Society of Plastic and Reconstructive Surgical Nurses and Wound, Ostomy, and Continence Nurses, and she serves as editor of *Plastic Surgical Nursing.* Her area of research concerns pressure ulcers.

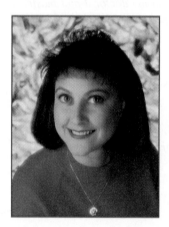

Jane Hokanson Hawks, DNSc, RN, C, is an Associate Professor of Nursing at Midland Lutheran College, Fremont, Nebraska. She teaches sophomore students in medical-surgical nursing and senior students in advanced medical-surgical nursing and nursing management. Dr. Hawks received her Doctorate of Nursing Science in collegiate nursing education from Widener University in Chester, Pennsylvania; her Master of Science degree in Nursing in medical-surgical nursing and nursing administration from UNMC in Omaha, Nebraska; and her Bachelor of Science degree in Nursing from St. Olaf College in Northfield, Minnesota.

Dr. Hawks has worked in and taught medical-surgical nursing for more than 22 years. She has practiced in a variety of areas, including critical care, renal transplantation, orthopedics, general surgery, and urology. She serves as the editor of *Urologic Nursing.* Her areas of research include empowerment and alcoholism. She and her colleagues developed the NANDA nursing diagnosis Altered Family Process: Alcoholism.

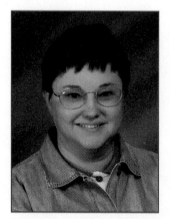

Annabelle M. Keene, MSN, RN, C, is a School Nurse with Bellevue Public Schools in Bellevue, Nebraska. She directs the health offices of several school buildings (approximately 2000 students and staff) and is certified by the State of Nebraska as a school nurse for grades K through 12. She also is a data analysis consultant for nursing graduate students who are studying nurses' perceptions of ethical problems across various specialty areas. Ms. Keene received her Master's degree from UNMC and her B.S.N. from Cornell University–New York Hospital School of Nursing, New York, New York.

Anne Keene has worked in and taught medical-surgical nursing for more than 25 years. She has been a staff nurse, a head nurse, a staff development instructor, and a nursing instructor in a multitude of clinical areas. She has been Assistant Professor at the University of Nebraska College of Nursing, teaching health assessment and medical-surgical nursing to undergraduate students. Anne also has been Associate Professor at the College of Saint Mary, Omaha, Nebraska, teaching in the undergraduate program. Ms. Keene is certified in medical-surgical nursing by the American Nurses Credentialing Center.

Contributors

Mary A. Allen, MS, RN
Clinical Trials Specialist, National Institute of Allergy and Infectious Diseases, National Institutes of Health, Bethesda, Maryland

Chris Stewart Amidei, MSN, RN, CNRN, CCRN
Clinical Nurse Specialist, University of Chicago, Chicago, Illinois

Helen Andrews, RN, BSN
Care Manager, Alegent Health Bergan Mercy Medical Center, Omaha, Nebraska

Jane Allen Austgen, RN, BSN, CRNH
Hospice Nurse Care Manager, Alegent Health Home Care & Hospice, Omaha, Nebraska

Susan Baker, DNS, RN
Instructor, Indiana University School of Nursing, Indianapolis, Indiana

Patricia McCallig Bates, BSN, CURN
Clinical Urology Nurse, Urology Department, Kaiser-Permanente, Portland, Oregon

Deborah L. Bayliss, MS, RN
Community Nurse Care Manager, Poudre Valley Health System, Fort Collins, Colorado

Francie Bernier, BSN, RN, C
Clinical Consultant for Continence Care, Independent Urologic/Urogynecologic Clinical Consultant, Specialist in Continence Care, Leesburg, Virginia

Deborah S. Bjerstedt, MSN, RN, CS, FNP
Family Nurse Practitioner, Allina Medical Group, Shoreview, St. Paul, Minnesota

Hilary S. Blackwood, MSN, RN
Clinician III, Surgical Nutrition Support Services, University of Virginia Health System, Charlottesville, Virginia

Meg Blair, BA, BSN, MSN
Assistant Professor, Nebraska Methodist College of Nursing and Allied Health; Staff Nurse, Emergency Department, St. Joseph's Hospital, Omaha, Nebraska

R. B. Boley, PhD
Professor (Ret.), Biology Department, University of Texas at Arlington, Arlington, Texas

Cynthia A. Bolin, RN
Program Coordinator, Congestive Heart Failure Management Center, St. Luke's Hospital, St. Louis, Missouri

Shawnda Braun, RN
Case Manager, Allied Health Alternatives, Inc., Faribault, Minnesota

Sarah Jo Brown, PhD, RN
Principal and Consultant, Practice-Research Integrations, Norwich, Vermont

Terri Sellin Brown, BSN, RN
School Nurse, Omaha Public Schools, Omaha, Nebraska

Mary Vorder Bruegge
Clinician IV, Nerancy Neuro ICU, University of Virginia Health System, Charlottesville, Virginia

Candace Cantwell, RD
Clinical Dietitian, Clinical Nutrition Support Services, University of Pennsylvania Health System, Philadelphia, Pennsylvania

Robert G. Carroll, PhD
Professor of Physiology, Brody School of Medicine, East Carolina University, Greenville, North Carolina

Bernice B. Christopher, BSN, RN
Keystone Mercy Health Plan, Philadelphia, Pennsylvania

Linda K. Clarke, MS, RN, CORLN
Head and Neck Nurse Specialist, Greater Baltimore Medical Center, Towson, Maryland

Marsha E. Cloud, BSN, RN
Clinician II, Surgical Services, University of Virginia Health System, Charlottesville, Virginia

Linda Carman Copel, PhD, RN, CS, DAPA, ACFE, CGP, CFLE
Associate Professor, Villanova University, Villanova, Pennsylvania; Psychotherapist, Private Practice, Ardmore, Pennsylvania

Pamela Cornwell, MA, RN
Manager, Intensive and Intermediate Care Units, Shriners Hospitals for Children, Northern California, Sacramento, California

Sherill Nones Cronin, PhD, RN, C
Professor of Nursing, Bellarmine College; Nurse Researcher, Jewish Hospital, Louisville, Kentucky

Janice Z. Cuzzell, MA, RN
Vice President, Island Home Care, Inc., Savannah, Georgia

Jean Elizabeth DeMartinis, PhD, APRN, FNP-C
Assistant Professor and Director of the Masters in Cardiac Health and Rehabilitation CNS/ANP Program, Creighton University School of Nursing, Omaha, Nebraska

Kaye M. Dietrich, MS, RN, C
Consultant, Kiel, Wisconsin

Peggy Doheny, PhD, MSN, RN
Associate Professor, Kent State University College of Nursing, Kent, Ohio

Rebecca M. Dudley, RN
Staff Nurse, Fairview Lakes HomeCaring & Hospice, Chisago City, Minnesota

Kimberly Elgin, BSN, RN
Clinician III, Clinical Manager, Surgical Services, University of Virginia Health System, Charlottesville, Virginia

Charlotte Eliopoulos, PhD, MPH, RN, C
President, Health Education Network, Glen Arm, Maryland

James A. Fain, PhD, RN, FAAN
Associate Professor and Director, PhD Nursing Program, University of Massachusetts Graduate School of Nursing, Worcester, Massachusetts

Kathryn Fiandt, DNS, ARNP
Associate Professor, University of Nebraska College of Nursing; Coordinator, Family Nurse Practitioner Program, University of Nebraska Medical Center; Clinical Director, Family Health Care Center, Omaha, Nebraska

Mary L. Fisher, PhD, RN, CNAA
Associate Professor, Nursing Administration, Indiana University School of Nursing, Indianapolis, Indiana

Susan Flannigan, MPH, RN, ANP
Adult Nurse Practitioner, Fairview Lakes Medical Center, Chisago City, Minnesota

Ann K. Frantz, BSN, RN
Independent Health Care Consultant, Pontiac, Michigan

Anne Marie Johnson Fredrichs, MSN, RN, CPNP
Research Coordinator, Nebraska Foundation for Spinal Research, Omaha, Nebraska

Peggy Gerard, DNSc, RN
Professor, School of Nursing, Purdue University, Calumet, Hammond, Indiana

Nancy Girard, PhD, MSN, RN
Associate Professor and Chair, Acute Nursing Care Department, University of Texas Medical School at San Antonio, School of Nursing, San Antonio, Texas

Elizabeth W. Good, MSN, RN, C
Clinician III, Urology Care Coordinator, Surgical Services, University of Virginia Health System, Charlottesville, Virginia

Michelle Goodman, MS, RN, OCN
Assistant Professor of Nursing, Rush University College of Nursing; Oncology Clinical Nurse Specialist, Section of Medical Oncology, Rush Cancer Institute, Rush Presbyterian–St. Luke's Medical Center, Chicago, Illinois

Lisa A. Gorski, MS, RN
Clinical Nurse Specialist, Covenant Home Health and Hospice, Milwaukee, Wisconsin

Maribeth Guzzo, MSN, RN, CRNP
Nurse Practitioner, Division of Cardiology, the Hospital of the University of Pennsylvania, Philadelphia, Pennsylvania

Sheila A. Haas, PhD, RN
Dean and Professor, Loyola University of Chicago Marcella Niehoff School of Nursing, Chicago, Illinois

Diana P. Hackbarth, PhD, RN
Professor, Department of Community, Mental Health, and Administrative Nursing, Loyola University of Chicago Marcella Niehoff School of Nursing, Chicago, Illinois

Linda R. Haddick, MSN, RN
Clinical Nurse Specialist, Alegent Health Home Care & Hospice, Omaha, Nebraska

Margie Hansen, PhD, RN
Clinical Associate Professor, Family Nurse Practitioner Program, University of North Dakota College of Nursing, Grand Forks, North Dakota

Karen A. Hanson, MS, RN, CNP
Urology Nurse Practitioner, Mayo Clinic, Rochester, Minnesota

Tammi G. Hardiman, BSN, RN
Nurse Consultant, Community Services Quality Assurance, Department of Social and Health Services, State of Washington, Arlington, Washington

Jeannine Mueller Harmon, MSN, RN, FNP, CS
Family Nurse Practitioner, Metropolitan State University, St. Paul, Minnesota

Debra E. Heidrich, MSN, RN, AOCN, CHPN
Nursing Consultant, West Chester, Ohio

Esther A. Hellman, PhD, RN
Assistant Professor, Creighton University School of Nursing, Omaha, Nebraska

Beverley E. Holland, PhD, MSN, ARNP
Associate Professor, Lansing School of Nursing, Bellarmine College, Louisville, Kentucky

Rhonda Holloway, BSN, RN, MBA, NP
Women's Wellness Center, Lone Tree, Colorado

Roberta Jorgensen, BSN
Gastrointestinal Nurse Coordinator, Mayo Clinic, Rochester, Minnesota

Juanita Fogel Keck, DNS, BSN
Associate Professor, Indiana University School of Nursing, Indianapolis, Indiana

Catherine A. Kernich, MSN, RN
Clinical Faculty, Frances Payne Bolton School of Nursing, Case Western Reserve University; Director, Ambulatory Practice, Department of Medicine; University Faculty Services, University Hospitals Health Systems, Cleveland, Ohio

Helene J. Krouse, PhD, ARNP, CORLN
Associate Professor of Nursing, University of Florida College of Nursing, Gainesville, Florida

Kim K. Kuebler, MN, RN, ANP-CS
Adjunct Faculty, College of Nursing and Health Sciences, Saginaw Valley State University, University Center, Michigan; Adult Nurse Practitioner, Oncology/Palliative Care, Private Practice, Adjuvant Therapies, Inc., Lake, Michigan

Joanie J. Kush, MS, RN
Director of Hospice, Visiting Nurse Association of Omaha, Omaha, Nebraska

Louise Nelson LaFramboise, PhD, RN
Assistant Professor, University of Nebraska College of Nursing, Omaha, Nebraska

Joan Lappe, PhD, RN
Associate Professor, Creighton University Schools of Nursing and Medicine, Omaha, Nebraska

Anne Larson, PhD, MS, BA, RN, C
Associate Professor of Nursing, Midland Lutheran College, Fremont, Nebraska

Joyce Larson-Presswalla, PhD, RN
President, "Culture Counts," Marketing Coordinator, James A. Haley Veterans Hospital, Tampa, Florida

Cindi Leo-Gofta, BSN, RN
Operations Director, Resource and Referral/Business Development, Alegent Health Home Care & Hospice, Omaha, Nebraska

James Higgy Lerner, RN, LAc
Private practice of acupuncture, traditional Oriental medicine, and biofeedback, Chico, California

Cindy Ludwig, MS, RN
Nurse Manager, Providence Saint Joseph Medical Center, Burbank, California

Cyndy Hunt Luzinski, MS, RN
Community Nurse Case Manager, Poudre Valley Health System, Fort Collins, Colorado

Donna W. Markey, MSN, RN, ACNP-CS
Clinician IV, Surgical Services, University of Virginia Health System, Charlottesville, Virginia

Karen S. Martin, MSN, RN, FAAN
Health Care Consultant, Martin Associates, Omaha, Nebraska

Cynthia McCurren, PhD, MSN
Associate Professor, University of Louisville School of Nursing; Nurse Researcher, University of Louisville Hospital, Louisville, Kentucky

James McLean, BSN, RN, WOCN
Enterostomal Therapist, Fort Worth, Texas

Norma D. McNair, MSN, RN, CCRN, CNRN, CS
Assistant Clinical Professor, University of California, Los Angeles, School of Nursing; Clinical Nurse III, Liver Transplant and Surgical Subspecialties, Intensive Care Unit, UCLA Medical Center, Los Angeles, California

Mary E. McQuinn, RPT
Physical Therapist, Visiting Nurse Association of Omaha, Omaha, Nebraska

Colette H. McVaney, BSN, RN
Lead Nurse, Geriatric Clinic, Nebraska Health System, Omaha, Nebraska

Patricia Meier, MA, BSN, RN, AOCN
Nurse Manager, Shady Grove Adventist Hospital, Rockville, Maryland

Stephanie Mellon-Reppen, MSN, RN, ACNP, OCN
Acute Care Nurse Practitioner and Oncology Certified Nurse, Section of Bone Marrow Transplant and Cell Therapy, Rush Presbyterian–St. Luke's Medical Center, Chicago, Illinois

Melanie Minton, BSN, RN, MBA, CNRN
Lead Adjunct Faculty, Le Tourneau University; Nurse Specialist, Nursing Support and Patient Education, The Methodist Hospital, Houston, Texas

Kim Miracle, MSN, RN, C
Clinical Nurse Specialist, Outcomes Manager, Jewish Hospital, Louisville, Kentucky

Anita E. Molzahn, PhD, MN
Professor, School of Nursing, and Dean, Faculty of Human and Social Development, University of Victoria, Victoria, British Columbia, Canada

Bernadette K. Mruz, RN
Clinical Manager, Visiting Nurse Association of Omaha, Omaha, Nebraska

Elizabeth A. Murphy-Blake, MSEd, MS, RN, ARNP
Assistant Professor of Nursing, Midland Lutheran College, Fremont, Nebraska

Pamela J. Nelson, MS, RN
Assistant Professor of Nursing, Bethel College, St. Paul, Minnesota

Noreen Heer Nicol, MS, RN, FNP
Clinical Senior Instructor, University of Colorado School of Nursing; Director of Nursing, Dermatology Clinical Specialist and Nurse Practitioner, National Jewish Medical and Research Center, Denver, Colorado

Cheryl Noetscher, MS, RN
Director of Case Management, Crouse Hospital and Community–General Hospital, Syracuse, New York

Janice D. Nunnelee, PhD, RN, CS/ANP, CRN
Clinical Associate Professor of Nursing, University of Missouri–St. Louis. Adult Nurse Practitioner, Vascular Nurse Practitioner, Unity Medical Group, St. Louis, Missouri

Barbara B. Ott, PhD, RN, CCRN
Associate Professor, Villanova University College of Nursing, Villanova, Pennsylvania

Arlene L. Polaski, MEd, MSN, RN
Program Director (Ret.), York Technical College/University of South Carolina Lancaster Cooperative Program in Associate Degree Nursing, Rock Hill, South Carolina

Kathleen Popelka, DNSc, CFNP
Family Nurse Practitioner, Women's Veterans Coordinator, Veterans Administration Medical Center, Omaha, Nebraska

David Porta, PhD
Associate Professor, Bellarmine University; Adjunct Faculty, University of Louisville School of Medicine, Louisville, Kentucky

Kathleen Rea, BSN, RN
Clinician III, Clinical Manager, Surgical Services, University of Virginia Health System, Charlottesville, Virginia

Marlene Reimer, PhD, RN, CNN(C)
Associate Dean, Research and Graduate Programs, University of Calgary Faculty of Nursing, Calgary, Canada

Roxanne Rivard, BSN, RN, CWOCN
Enterostomal Therapy Nurse, Fairview Lakes, HomeCaring & Hospice, Chisago City, Minnesota

Dottie Roberts, MSN, MACI, RN, C, ONC, CNS
Medical-Surgical Clinical Nurse Specialist, Penrose–St. Francis Health Services, Colorado Springs, Colorado

Helen Murdock Rogers, BS, MS, DNSc
Associate Professor, Adult Health, Research, and Physical
Assessment, Department of Nursing, Worcester State College;
Community Nurse, University of Massachusetts, Memorial
Home Health, Worcester, Massachusetts

Amy Perrin Ross, MSN, RN, CNRN
Neuroscience Program Coordinator, Loyola University Medical
Center, Maywood, Illinois

Vicki M. Ross, MSN, RN
Nurse Clinician, Nutritional Support Services, Truman Medical
Center, Kansas City, Missouri

Pamela K. Schaid, MA, RN
Administrator, Seasons Hospice, Rochester, Minnesota

Nancy J. Scheet, MSN, RN
Compliance Officer, Visiting Nurse Association of Omaha,
Omaha, Nebraska

Linda Ludy Scott, MS, CFNP
Nurse Practitioner, National Institute of Allergy and Infectious
Diseases, Laboratory of Allergic Diseases, National Institutes of
Health, Bethesda, Maryland

Carol Sedlak, PhD, MSN, RN
Assistant Professor, Kent State University College of Nursing,
Kent, Ohio

Judy Selfridge-Thomas, MSN, RN, CEN, FNP
Nurse Practitioner, Department of Emergency Medicine, St.
Mary Medical Center, Long Beach, California; General Partner,
Selfridge, Sparger, Shea and Associates, Ventura and Orange
Counties, California

Carol Sharkey, MSN, PhD
Associate Professor, Department of Nursing, Regis University,
Denver, Colorado

Sandra Sharma, PhD, ARNP, CS
James A. Haley Veterans Hospital, Tampa, Florida

Suzanne Shaw, BSN, RN
Director, Walls Regional Hospital Home Health, Cleburne, Texas

Nancy Shoemaker, MS, RN, CS-P
Nursing Program Consultant, State of Maryland, Department of
Public Safety and Correctional Services, Jessup, Maryland

Mary Sieggreen, MSN, RN, CS, NP, CUN
Assistant Professor, Wayne State University; Clinical Nurse
Specialist/Nurse Practitioner, Vascular Surgery, Harper Hospital,
Detroit Medical Center, Detroit, Michigan

Pamela Singh, CS, MSN, RN, FNP
Family Nurse Practitioner, San Diego, California

Dianne Smolen, PhD, MSN, RN, C
Associate Professor and Director of Continuing Nursing
Education, Medical College of Ohio School of Nursing, Toledo,
Ohio

Debra A. Solomon, MSN, RN, FNP-C
Clinical Coordinator, Fairview Lakes HomeCaring & Hospice,
Chisago City, Minnesota

Kimberly Stallo, BSN, RN, CETN
Wound, Ostomy, and Continence Nurse, Fort Worth, Texas

Mary M. Stasiak, MA, BSN, RN, PHN
Case Manager, Allied Health Alternatives, Inc., Rochester,
Minnesota

Eleanor M. Stockbridge, MS, CRRN, FNP
Community Nurse Case Manager, Poudre Valley Health System,
Fort Collins, Colorado

Nancy Evans Stoner, MSN, RN, CNSN
Education Manager, Clinical Nutrition Support Services,
University of Pennsylvania Health System, Philadelphia,
Pennsylvania

Linda J. Svatora, OTR/L, MBA
Occupational Therapist, Visiting Nurse Association of Omaha,
Omaha, Nebraska

Janice Tazbir, MS
Assistant Professor, Purdue University Calumet, Hammond,
Indiana

Jill E. Timm, BAN, RN, PHN
Public Health Nurse II, Washington County Department of
Public Health and Environment, Stillwater, Minnesota

Peter J. Ungvarski, MS, RN, FAAN, ACRN
Clinical Associate Professor, City University of New York,
Hunter College–Bellevue School of Nursing; Clinical Nurse
Specialist, HIV/AIDS, and Clinical Director, AIDS Services, The
Visiting Nurse Service of New York, New York, New York

Linda A. Vader, BS, RN, CRNO
Head Nurse, W. K. Kellogg Eye Center, University of
Michigan, Ann Arbor, Michigan

Amy Verst, MSN, RN, CPNP, ATC
Assistant Professor, Bellarmine College; Pediatric Nurse
Practitioner, Jefferson County Health Department, Louisville,
Kentucky

Bernadette White, MSN, RN
Assistant Professor, Creighton University School of Nursing,
Omaha, Nebraska

Connie White-Williams, MSN, RN, FNP
Affiliate Faculty and Cardiothoracic Transplant Coordinator,
University of Alabama, Birmingham, Alabama

Gail F. Wilkerson, MSN, RN, CS
Disease Management Specialist, Heart Failure, Group Health
Plan, St. Louis, Missouri

Linda Yoder, MSN, MBA, PhD
Colonel, United States Army Nurse Corps, McDonald Army
Community Hospital, Fort Eustis, Virginia

Nancy York, MSN, RN
Assistant Professor of Nursing, Bellarmine College, Lansing
School of Nursing, Louisville, Kentucky

Bridget A. Young, BSN, RN, MBA
Vice President of Clinical Services, Visiting Nurse Association
of Omaha, Omaha, Nebraska

Reviewers

Jan Anderson, MSN, RN, CNS
Assistant Director, ADN Program, Santa Barbara City College, Santa Barbara, California

Linda J. Becker, MSN, RN, C
Department Chair, St. Clair County Community College, Port Huron, Michigan

Barbara J. Benz, MS
Roswell Park Cancer Institute, Buffalo, New York

Veronica K. Casey, MA, RN, C
Assistant Professor, Norwalk Community-Technical College, Norwalk, Connecticut

Joy Churchill, MSN, RN
Northern Kentucky University, Highland Heights, Kentucky

Betty R. Ferrell, PhD, RN, FAAN
City of Hope National Medical Center, Duarte, California

Kay Fitterer, MA, RN
Central Lakes College, Brainerd, Minnesota

Gloria J. Green, PhD, MSN, RN
Southeast Missouri State University, Cape Girardeau, Missouri

Angie B. Greer, MSN, RN, CS
Henderson State University, Arkadelphia, Arkansas

Joyce Harris, MA, RN
Director, Butler County Program of Practical Nursing Education, Hamilton, Ohio

JoAnn Romanzi Herne, MS, RNC, FNP-CS
Student Health Supervisor, Crouse Hospital School of Nursing, Syracuse, New York

Robin Higley, MSN
Fairview Hospital, Cleveland, Ohio

Sheilagh Helen Hunt, BA, RN
Certificate in Palliative Care and Thanatology; Professor, Fanshawe College, London, Ontario, Canada

Mary Jane Jones, MN, RN
Associate Professor, Henderson Community College, Henderson, Kentucky

Elizabeth A. Kassel, MSN, RN
Assistant Professor, Syracuse University, Crouse Hospital School of Nursing, University Hospital, Syracuse, New York

Anne Larson, PhD, RN, C
Associate Professor, Midland Lutheran College, Fremont, Nebraska

Suzanne K. Marnocha, MSN, RN, CCRN
Assistant Professor, University of Wisconsin, Oshkosh, Oshkosh, Wisconsin

Jeanette A. McNeill, DrPH, RN, AOCN
Associate Professor/Department Chair, School of Nursing, University of Texas, Houston, Houston, Texas

Captain John J. Melvin, BSN, RN, CCRN
Brooke Army Medical Center, Fort Sam Houston, Texas

Christine C. Mihal, MS, RN, CS
Lecturer, Fairleigh Dickinson University, Teaneck, New Jersey

Carla Mueller, MS, RN
Associate Professor, Department of Nursing, University of Saint Francis, Fort Wayne, Indiana

Elizabeth A. O'Connor, MSN, RNCS, FWP, CCRN
Montana State University at Bozeman, College of Nursing, Great Falls, Montana

Netha O'Meara, MS, RN, CNS
Former Director of Associate Degree Nursing, Wharton County Junior College, Wharton, Texas

Kay B. O'Neal, MSN, RN
El Centro Community College, Dallas, Texas

Molly R. Parker, MHR, BSed, RN
Practical Nursing Program Director, Green Country Area Vocational-Technical School, Okmulgee, Oklahoma

Diana Reding, MS, RN
El Centro College, Parkland Hospital, Dallas, Texas

Lisa Anderson Shaw, DrPH, MSN, MA, RN, CS
Clinical Instructor, Medical/Surgical Nursing, University of Illinois at Chicago College of Nursing; Clinical Ethics Consultant, University of Illinois at Chicago Medical Center, Chicago, Illinois

Beth Ann Stevenson, MSN, RN, CS
School Nurse, Columbus Public Schools; Nurse Clinician, Ohio Department of Health, Columbus, Ohio

Martha Summers, MSN, C-FNP
West Virginia University, Morgantown, West Virginia

Janice M. Thompson, PhD, MSN, RN, C
Associate Professor, Quinnipiac College, Hamden, Connecticut

Lieutenant Michael Welker, BSN, RN, AN
Brooke Army Medical Center, Fort Sam Houston, Texas

Charlene A. Winters, DNSc, RNCS
Montana State University, Missoula, Montana

Preface

It is our conviction that a book is not a static document. Certainly, a book—bound and printed—portrays health care at a given moment in time. The sixth edition of *Medical-Surgical Nursing* is our best attempt to provide instructors and students with a guide to delivering safe and appropriate nursing care. To that end, we see this book as a "work in progress." Future editions will continue to improve, and we appreciate your comments, questions, and corrections to guide our ongoing work. We can improve only with your input. We also realize that educators and students must share in the task of bringing the book to life.

PHILOSOPHY AND APPROACH

This text grows out of the belief that nurses and physicians do not compete with each other but instead collaborate to reach certain outcomes in cooperation with the client and family. Nonetheless, nursing and medicine are separate disciplines. Consequently, in this text nursing and medical content are not intermingled. However, because nursing and medicine are collaborative efforts, it is often difficult for nursing students to understand one without having an understanding of the other. We therefore present thorough coverage of both nursing management and medical management.

With the increased emphasis on outcomes in health care, we have organized client care under the heading of Outcome Management. Several headings appear under this heading, including: Medical Management, Nursing Management of the Medical Client, Surgical Management, and Nursing Management of the Surgical Client, as appropriate.

In this text, we use the nursing process to describe nursing management but we do not apply the nursing process to every disorder. Instead, we have designated the nursing process for major or prototypical disorders. Within the presentation of the nursing process for those disorders, we have developed nursing diagnoses and collaborative problems, as appropriate, with their own outcomes and interventions. Collaborative problems define those client problems that are not resolvable through independent nursing actions; they are potential complications that may develop because of a disorder, a surgical procedure, or a nonsurgical treatment. Collaborative problems complete the picture of nursing care and eliminate the need to force-fit every client problem into the framework of nursing diagnosis. We have written Outcomes and Intervention sections for *each* identified nursing diagnosis and collaborative problem because we have found, from our teaching experience, that students cannot easily pull apart lists of diagnoses, followed by lists of outcomes and interventions, and rebuild them into care plans.

ORGANIZATION

This edition is organized from simple to complex and from common to uncommon disorders. The early portion of the text focuses on care of clients usually assigned to beginning students. The book then progresses to address care of clients with more complex disorders, which are more commonly taught in upper division classes.

Another change in organization is the use of separate chapters for complex disorders, such as renal failure, the need for transplantation, AIDS/HIV, respiratory failure, myocardial infarction, and central nervous system trauma. These disorders are complex and more commonly addressed in upper division course work. We also separate some other material on fluids and electrolytes, stroke, immune disorders, and nutrition to provide adequate coverage and to differentiate major concepts for these disorders.

The sixth edition is divided into 17 units. The first three units are devoted to content that is applicable to all medical-surgical clients. The material in this first portion of the book will guide the student in learning to provide comprehensive care regardless of the specific diagnosis or problem. Concepts that span medical-surgical practice, such as health promotion, care delivery settings, pain, perioperative care, and oncology, are found in this portion of the book. The remainder of the text is divided into common responses to health disorders. Most of these units begin with a review of anatomy and physiology, followed by a chapter on health and diagnostic assessment; thereafter, one or more "Nursing Care" chapters present the nursing care of clients with specific disorders.

Unit 2 presents an overview of nursing and health care today. Chapter 4 describes the "stakeholders" in health care delivery, because medical-surgical nurses (not just managers) in all areas of practice must be increasingly aware of how health care is financed. Because the practice of medical-surgical nursing is not confined to certain areas, more material has been added to this edition on nursing care and philosophy in various care settings. Chapters 5 through 8 address nursing care in ambulatory, acute, home health, and long-term care settings.

Unit 3 covers health assessment, physical examination, and diagnostic testing. The format for health assessment and physical examination that is introduced in Chapters 9 and 10 is carried through in the Assessment chapters for each body system. This structure helps the student to become familiar with one form of thorough assessment and then to apply it in a focused way for clients with specific disorders.

Unit 4 looks at concepts that are common to many medical-surgical clients. Fluid and electrolyte disorders have been separated into two chapters. Other chapters address acid-base disorders, the surgical experience, wound healing, infectious disorders, cancer, psychosocial and mental health concerns, and sleep and sensory disorders, including new material on fatigue and pain. New to this edition is a chapter on end-of-life concerns (Chapter 22). Material on substance abuse has been moved forward into the introductory material because of the increasing numbers of people with substance abuse problems. Chapter 24 discusses the effects of substance abuse on major body systems. It also identifies populations at risk for substance abuse and presents strategies for care.

Units 5 through 16 focus on management of clients with specific disorders. Each unit begins with a structure and function overview of the pertinent body systems as well as a nursing assessment chapter. The structure and function overview has been shortened and redesigned, with more artwork added for each body system.

Discussion of specific disorders generally includes headings for Etiology, Pathophysiology, Clinical Manifestations, and Outcome Management. Because more and more nursing care is being directed toward health promotion, in this edition we have added content focusing on health promotion, health maintenance, and health restoration to the Risk Factors and Etiology topics in chapters on disorders. To emphasize the importance of understanding pathophysiology and its relationship to treatment of a disorder, we have incorporated headings in the management sections that will help the student see the relationship between the pathophysiologic changes and specific strategies to promote positive outcomes in nursing management. The term "clinical manifestations" has been selected to encompass signs and symptoms along with diagnostic findings. The term "manifestations" replaces "signs and symptoms" in all chapters except one; in Chapter 22, "end-of-life symptom management" is the preferred term.

The major content areas for Units 5 through 16 are mobility disorders (Unit 5); nutritional disorders, including ingestive and digestive disorders as well as a new chapter on malnutrition (Unit 6); elimination disorders, including urinary and intestinal problems (Unit 7); sexuality and reproductive disorders (Unit 8); metabolic disorders (Unit 9); integumentary disorders (Unit 10); circulatory disorders (Unit 11); cardiac disorders (Unit 12); oxygenation disorders (Unit 13); sensory disorders (Unit 14); cognitive and perceptual disorders (Unit 15); and protective disorders (Unit 16).

Unit 17 presents care of clients with multisystem disorders. A new chapter, Chapter 79, covers care of the client with HIV infection and AIDS. Chapter 80, also new, looks at organ donation issues, the transplantation process, quality of life issues, and specific interventions for clients requiring organ transplantation. Shock and multisystem disorders are discussed in Chapter 81. Chapter 82 examines the basic concepts of triage, ethical issues, and maintaining the chain of custody of medicolegal evidence. The chapter organizes emergency conditions by various nursing diagnoses identified and treated.

SPECIAL FEATURES

Bridging the gap between classroom instruction and clinical nursing care is difficult. We find that students often think, "I learned that for a test last year," and question how the material is relevant to the clinical situations that they face today. To address those questions, Joyce Black has devised a method of clinical teaching in which the pathophysiology of a disorder is presented graphically and is then overlaid with corresponding clinical manifestations and treatments. The overlays allow students to visualize how changes in pathophysiology lead to certain

manifestations and how a particular treatment is designed to block the progression of the pathophysiologic changes into the development of clinical manifestations. Underlying this teaching method is the assumption that it is easier to "transfer" material if you can visualize the links among pathophysiology, clinical manifestations, and interventions. The fifth edition incorporated this teaching method in special features called **Pathophysiology/Treatment Algorithms (PTAs).** These features are presented on such topics as "Understanding Asthma and Its Treatment." A new PTA on Cushing's disease has been added because of the positive response to the PTAs from the fifth edition.

As another way to help students, particularly at the upper level, to integrate material that they have learned in many courses over the span of a number of years, we have retained all six **Case Studies** from the fifth edition and have added four new ones. The Case Studies, some of which are illustrated, present complex client scenarios that are typical of the situations that students will encounter in clinical practice. Following each scenario is a series of questions for students to consider. The discussions for these questions are included on the CD-ROM packaged with the text.

More and more, students are recognizing the importance of providing quality nursing care to clients with backgrounds different from their own. To help them, this edition includes **Diversity in Health Care** boxes about such topics as "Cultural Perspectives on Pain," "Cultural Aspects of Death and Dying," and "Cultural Influences on Nutrition."

The increased use of alternative and complementary therapies by clients affects their health care management. A new feature, **Alternative Therapies,** has been added to help the student understand what complementary therapies may be used by their clients and the impact that these treatments might have on prescribed therapy ordered by the health care provider. Although many of the alternative therapies are not scientifically supported, they are widely endorsed and should be considered as part of the nursing assessment.

Client Education Guides are presented throughout the text. This important feature helps nurses teach clients how to collaborate in their own care and are worded in client-centered language.

Unlicensed assistive personnel continue to provide direct client care in hospitals. We also recognize that few nursing students have had the opportunity to learn how to delegate care safely. In this edition, we have added 10 additional **Management and Delegation** features, for a total of 19. These discuss assessments and interventions that can, under certain circumstances, be delegated to assistive personnel. They also provide guidance about how to decide whether a particular aspect of care is safe to delegate, and they emphasize that in all cases the responsibility for client care, analysis of client data, and the safety of the client rests squarely on the nurse.

Case management is another area of ongoing change in hospital nursing, and one of the hallmarks of case management is the use of clinical pathways. Two features in this revision highlight the importance of this content area. The first is Case Management. This feature, written by a practicing case manager, presents key coordination and anticipatory issues under consistent headings of "Assess," "Advocate," and "Prevent Readmission," thus linking nursing care with patient-focused case management. Many textbooks now incorporate clinical pathways. In this book we have gone a step further by including a group of **Clinical Pathway Guides** (or CareMap) that have been carefully selected by two experts in case management as among the best in use today. We have included portions of the clinical pathway and a guide to orient the student to the value and important components of each pathway.

The growing use of standardized language in nursing has been addressed by including a list of appropriate **Nursing Outcomes Classification (NOC)** labels at the start of each nursing management chapter. The outcomes chosen include those that may apply to clients with any of the conditions presented within the chapter.

Critical Monitoring features highlight for the student those clinical manifestations that must be reported to the physician without delay. **Care Plans** summarize the nursing diagnoses, outcomes, interventions and rationales, and evaluation criteria for selected disorders.

We have found that students often struggle with how to record normal assessment findings. This edition again includes **Physical Assessment Findings in the Healthy Adult** features, which serve both to remind students of the relevant normal findings for each body system and to demonstrate how to chart those findings with clinical precision.

Bridging the distance from the theoretical to the practical, and from the hospital to the home, is essential in nursing today. To that end, we have asked practicing home care nurses to write new **Bridge to Home Health Care** features for this edition. These features provide practical suggestions on the ever more critical skill of adapting medical-surgical care to the home.

Nursing research is providing evidence to guide practice decisions for all nurses. No longer can just one study be summarized and included in a chapter. We have examined nursing research findings and have incorporated them into the discussion of nursing care. A new feature has been designed to help the student gain a sense of the "state of the science" in selected areas of practice. The **Bridge to Evidence-Based Practice** features examine an integrative review of research evidence for a specific topic by identifying the research questions, studies examined, findings of the studies, limitations, and application to practice. These features appear at the end of units in which the content is related.

Another feature, the **Bridge to Critical Care,** highlights common treatment modalities and assessments performed in critical care. Rather than attempt to discuss all of critical care nursing in these features, we have tried to impart through them a basic understanding of hospital-based critical care treatments as they are used in inpatient care. Some examples are the use of pulmonary pressure monitors, ventilators, and arterial lines.

The prevalence of many diseases in older adults and the special needs of older adults prompted retention of sections called **Modifications for Elderly Clients** for many disorders. Because it is often difficult to differentiate normal manifestations of aging from pathologic conditions in the elderly, we have also included content on normal aging for each body system.

Because of the growing importance of being able to

"think critically" as a nurse, we have concluded each nursing care chapter in the book with a series of **Thinking Critically** exercises. Each of these exercises presents a typical client scenario and poses several questions about what actions to take. To give the student clues about how to think through these clinical problems, each exercise includes one or more *Factors to Consider*. On the enclosed CD-ROM, we provide a brief discussion of each of these exercises. Because there is no one right answer to a *Thinking Critically* question, these are *discussions* rather than hard-and-fast *answers*.

SUPPLEMENT PACKAGE

Student Study CD-ROM

Packaged with each copy of the text, this new feature provides students with a wealth of study materials. All of the Case Studies from the text, plus two *bonus* Case Studies, are presented with the corresponding questions and a discussion for each question. Each Case Study also provides 7 to 10 multiple choice questions for further review and presents a nursing care plan in summary. The Thinking Critically questions, with discussions written by the authors, are also included. Students will also benefit from the more than 700 NCLEX-style test questions included for study and review. Icons throughout the text provide reminders for students to refer to the CD-ROM.

Study Guide

The *Study Guide* is designed to improve understanding of each chapter of the textbook. Learning objectives are provided to help the student focus on critical content in each chapter. In addition, *Study Guide* chapters include the following sections, as appropriate:

- Learning the Language
- Critical Thinking: Understanding Rationales
- Thinking Clinically: Knowing What to Do and Why
- Client Education: Knowing What to Teach and Why
- Putting It All Together
- Diagnostic Tests: Knowing Why You Do What You Do
- At-a-Glance Worksheets

Instructor's Electronic Resource

The *Instructor's Electronic Resource* (IER) is designed to help faculty develop lectures, assignments, and clinical assignments based on the content of the textbook and is free to textbook adopters. The IER is a CD-ROM composed of four components:

- A 2000 multiple-choice question test bank in the ExaMaster format
- Image Collection of approximately 200 illustrations from the text
- NEW! LectureView composed of more than 1000 Powerpoint slides
- Instructor's Manual

ExaMaster, a computer test bank, provides approximately 2000 NCLEX-style questions from which instructors can automatically or manually generate examinations. Provided for each question is the correct answer, the rationale for the correct answer, the cognitive level according to Bloom's taxonomy, and the corresponding learning objective in the *Study Guide* and *Instructor's Manual*. These questions are also available to textbook adopters in printed form.

Approximately 300 color illustrations from the text are available through the **Image Collection** and provide exciting visual aids to help the instructor with classroom presentations.

LectureView presents more than 1000 Powerpoint slides organized by each unit of the text. These slides provide instructors with ready-made lectures and are an effective teaching tool.

The **Instructor's Manual** repeats the Learning Objectives from the Student Study Guide and includes Facilitating Student Learning ideas and Critical Points to Emphasize summaries.

SIMON WEB SITE

The SIMON Web site provides instructors and students who are using this textbook with several tools to enhance teaching and learning. It acts as an "Internet"-based ancillary that includes Web links that connect the content of each chapter to numerous Web sites. These linkages are updated during the life of the book so that the content is always current. The Web site also provides content updates, ethics challenges, and other relevant and helpful material.
(http://www.wbsaunders.com/SIMON/Black/medsurg/)

ACKNOWLEDGMENTS

We have been asked several times, "Isn't a revision a lot less work than a new book?" You would think so, but it's amazing—a revision is no less work than a new book.

A project of this size certainly could not be accomplished without the collaboration of many people. First and foremost, we recognize the importance of the clinical expertise of our many contributing authors, which enables us to present a new edition that continues to be the "gold standard" for textbooks of medical-surgical nursing. We would also like to thank the special feature contributors and to acknowledge Anne Larson for her contribution of the Case Studies.

There are also many people at W. B. Saunders Company who have made this monumental task a "do-able" task. Thank you, Thomas Eoyang, former Editorial Manager, Nursing Books, for your ongoing encouragement, help, and support. Thank you, Terri Ward, former Developmental Editor, and Victoria Legnini, Developmental Editor; without your help and day-to-day management, we would still be behind on the deadlines. Your organization made this project move well. Thank you, Ceil Roberts and Rita Martello, for your meticulous coordination of a massive art program. Thank you, Observatory Group, for your stunning new full-color illustrations. Thank you, Karen O'Keefe Owens, Designer, for your fresh, appealing, full-color design. Thank you, Carol J. Robins, Manuscript Editor, for finding just the right words when we could not, for coordinating the work of other copy editors, and for fielding countless changes, additions, and deletions with unfailing grace. Thank you, Linda Garber and Natalie Ware, Production Managers, for keeping the book on schedule against overwhelming odds. Thank you, Fran Murphy, for coordinating the peer reviews of the book, and Adrienne Simon for handling the countless administrative tasks associated with the publication of the book. Thank you, Barbara Nelson Cullen, Executive Editor, for developing and producing the book's supplement package.

Finally, we want to thank *you*—educators and students—for allowing us to join you in the teaching and learning of medical-surgical nursing. We trust that you will find the sixth edition of *Medical-Surgical Nursing: Clinical Management for Positive Outcomes* a valuable asset.

JOYCE M. BLACK
JANE HOKANSON HAWKS
ANNABELLE M. KEENE

Contents

UNIT 3

UNIT
4

UNIT 5

UNIT 6

UNIT
7

UNIT

8

UNIT

11

UNIT
12

UNIT 13

UNIT
16

UNIT
17

Anatomy and Physiology Review
The Integumentary System
Robert G. Carroll

The integument, or skin makes up 15% to 20% of body weight. Intact skin is the body's primary defense system. It protects us from invasion by organisms, helps regulate body temperature, manufactures vitamins, and provides our external appearance. Skin has three primary layers (i.e., (*epidermis,* or outer layer; the *dermis,* or inner layer; and the *hypodermis,* or subcutaneous layer) as well as epidermal appendages (i.e., eccrine glands, apocrine glands, sebaceous glands, hair follicles, and nails).

The skin is the most prominent organ containing *epithelium,* which is composed of cells that provide a continuous barrier between the body contents and the outside environment. Epithelial cells also cover the gastrointestinal (GI) tract, pulmonary airways and alveoli, renal tubules and the urinary system, and the ducts that empty onto the surface of the skin (lumen) of the GI and respiratory systems. Epithelial cells allow selective transport of ions, nutrients, and metabolic wastes and have a permeability to water that is partially regulated. Epithelial cells are joined to each other through tight junctions and express different populations of protein transporters on the apical side (generally facing a lumen) and the basolateral (facing the blood, or serosal) side. The functional significance of epithelial transport is covered in the GI and renal chapters (see Units 6 and 7).

STRUCTURE OF THE INTEGUMENTARY SYSTEM

EPIDERMIS

The epidermis is the thin, stratified outer skin layer that is in direct contact with the external environment (Fig. U10–1). The thickness of the epidermis ranges from 0.04 mm on the eyelids to 1.6 mm on the palms and soles. *Desmosomes* (points of intercellular attachment that are vital for cell-to-cell adhesion) are found in the epidermis. *Keratinocytes,* the principal cells of the epidermis, produce *keratin* in a complex process. The cells begin in the basal cell layer and change constantly, moving upward through the epidermis. On the surface, they are sloughed off or lost by abrasion. Thus, the epidermis constantly regenerates itself, providing a tough keratinized barrier.

Skin color reflects both the production of pigment granules *(melanin)* by melanocytes and, in light-skinned people, the presence of blood *(hemoglobin).* Skin color reflects a combination of four basic colors:

- Exogenously formed carotenoids (yellow)
- Melanin (brown)
- Oxygenated hemoglobin in arterioles and capillaries (red)
- Reduced hemoglobin in venules (blue)

Melanin plays the largest role in skin color; it is produced in the epidermis and in corresponding layers of the hair follicle. Although melanin is not produced in the dermis, it can be deposited in the dermis from the epidermis through various processes (such as inflammation).

Melanosomes are granules in melanocytes that synthesize melanin. Skin color differences result from the size and quantity of melanosomes as well as from the rate of melanin production. In natives of equatorial Africa, there is an increase in the size and number of melanosomes (not melanocytes) as well as increased melanin production. The melanosomes are large, discrete, and dispersed. In natives of northern Europe, the melanosomes are small and aggregated, producing less melanin. Sun exposure initially increases the size and functional activity of both melanocytes and melanosomes. With chronic sun exposure, there is an increase in concentration of melanocytes as well as in size and functional activity. The presence of melanin limits the penetration of sun rays into the skin and protects against sunburn and development of ultraviolet light–induced skin carcinomas.

Epidermal Appendages

Epidermal appendages are downgrowths of epidermis into the dermis and consist of eccrine glands, apocrine units, sebaceous glands, hair, and nails.

GLANDS

Eccrine glands produce sweat and play an important role in thermoregulation. They are found throughout the skin except on the vermilion border (junction of the pink area of the lip with the surrounding skin), the ears, nail bed, glans penis, and labia minora. They are more numerous on the palms, soles, forehead, and axillae. Sweat is similar to plasma but is more dilute. Eccrine gland secretion is stimulated by heat as well as by exercise and emotional stress. Eccrine glands exit the body independently of the hair shaft (see Fig. U10–1).

Apocrine glands occur primarily in the axillae, breast areolae, anogenital area, ear canals, and eyelids. In lower-order animals, apocrine secretions function as sexual attractants (pheromones), and the apocrine secretion musk is used as a perfume base. The role, if any, in humans is not established. Mediated by adrenergic innervation, apocrine glands secrete a milky substance that becomes odoriferous when altered by skin surface bacteria. These glands do not function until puberty, and they require a high output of sex hormone for activity.

Sebaceous glands are found throughout the skin except on the palms and soles and are most abundant on the face, scalp, upper back, and chest. They are associated with hair follicles that open onto the skin surface, where *sebum* (a mixture of sebaceous gland-produced lipids and epidermal cell-derived lipids) is released. Sebum has a lubricating function and bactericidal activity. Androgen is responsible for sebaceous gland development. In utero

UNIT 10

Integumentary Disorders

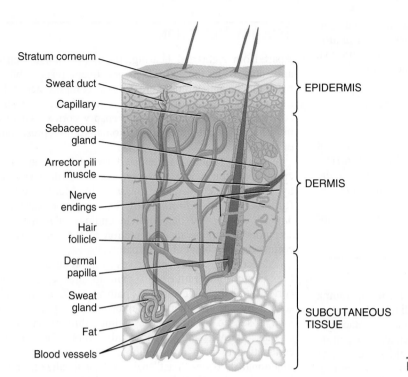

Stratum corneum
Sweat duct
Capillary
EPIDERMIS
Sebaceous gland
Arrector pili muscle
Nerve endings
DERMIS
Hair follicle
Dermal papilla
Sweat gland
Fat
SUBCUTANEOUS TISSUE
Blood vessels

FIGURE U10–1 Structure of the skin.

androgen causes neonatal acne; after puberty, sebum production can cause acne in adolescents.

HAIR AND NAILS

Hair is a nonviable protein end-product found on all skin surfaces except the palms and soles. Each hair follicle functions as an independent unit and goes through intermittent stages of development. Hair develops from the mitotic activity of the hair bulb. The rate of hair growth varies in different parts of the body. In a typical adult scalp, 85% to 90% of hairs are in an *anagen* (growth) phase. The remainder are in a *telogen* (rest) phase. About 50 to 100 hairs are lost each day. As a rule, the growing phase of hair on the eyebrows, trunk, and extremities does not exceed 6 months. Its resting phase is 3 to 4 months.

Hair form (straight or curly) depends on the shape of the hair in cross-section. Straight hair has a round cross-section; curly hair has an oval or ribbon-like cross-section. Curved follicles also affect the curliness of hair. Melanocytes in the bulb determine hair color. Hair follicles usually occur with sebaceous glands, and together they form a pilosebaceous unit. *Arrector pili* muscles of the dermis attach to hair follicles and elevate the hairs when body temperature falls, producing "goose bumps."

Nails are horny scales of epidermis. The nail matrix is the source of specialized, nonkeratinized cells. They differentiate into keratinized cells, which make up the nail protein. The matrix for nail formation is located in the proximal nail bed. It grows forward from the nail fold to cover the nail bed. Fingernails grow about 0.1 mm/day; complete reproduction takes 100 to 150 days. Toenails grow one third as fast as fingernails do. A damaged nail matrix, which may result from trauma or aggressive manicuring, produces a distorted nail. Nails are also sensitive to physiologic changes; for instance, they grow more slowly in cold weather and during periods of illness.

Nails and hair consist of keratinized and, therefore, "dead" cells. The ingestion of gelatin has not been shown to increase nail growth or strength.

DERMIS

The dermis, a dense layer of tissue beneath the epidermis, gives the skin most of its substance and structure. It varies from 1 to 4 mm in thickness and is thickest over the back. The dermis contains fibroblasts, macrophages, mast cells, and lymphocytes, which promote wound healing. The skin's lymphatic, vascular, and nerve supplies, which maintain equilibrium in the skin, are in the dermis.

The dermis is divided into two parts: papillary and reticular. The papillary dermis, which contains increased amounts of collagen, blood vessels, sweat glands, and elastin, is in contact with the epidermis. The *reticular* dermis also contains collagen but with increased amounts of mature elastic tissue. The dermis houses many specialized cells, blood vessels, and nerves.

The epidermis and dermis meet at the *dermoepidermal junction.* This area contains wave-like projections from the dermis called *papillae,* which correspond to reciprocal structures in the epidermis. The *subepidermal basement membrane zone* is a semipermeable filter that permits fluid exchange of components such as nutrients, metabolites, and waste products.

HYPODERMIS

The *subcutaneous layer* is a specialized layer of connective tissue. It is sometimes called the *adipose layer* because of its fat content. This layer is absent in some sites such as the eyelids, scrotum, areola, and tibia. Age, heredity, and many other factors influence the thickness of the subcutaneous layer. Subcutaneous fat is generally thickest on the back and buttocks, giving shape and contour over the bone. This layer functions as insulation from extremes of hot and cold, as a cushion to trauma, and as a source of energy and hormone metabolism.

FUNCTION OF THE INTEGUMENTARY SYSTEM

The skin is a morphologically complex structure that serves several functions essential to life. The skin differs anatomically and physiologically in various areas of the body. Functions of the skin include protection, maintenance of homeostasis, thermoregulation, sensory reception, vitamin synthesis, and processing of antigenic substances.

PROTECTION

The skin protects the body against many forms of trauma (e.g., mechanical, thermal, chemical, radiant). The intact tough epidermal layer is a mechanical barrier. Bacteria, foreign matter, other organisms, and chemicals penetrate it with difficulty. The oily and slightly acid secretions of its sebaceous glands protect the body further by limiting the growth of many organisms. The thickened skin of the palms and soles provides additional covering to absorb the constant use of or trauma to these areas.

HOMEOSTASIS

Skin forms a barrier that prevents excessive loss of water and electrolytes from the internal environment and also prevents the subcutaneous tissues from drying out. The effectiveness of this impermeable membrane is readily recognized when one observes the extreme loss of fluids that occurs with damage to the skin, as with burns and other injuries. Insensible loss of water and electrolytes occurs only through pores in this effective barrier.

THERMOREGULATION

The skin, under normal conditions, adjusts heat loss to balance metabolic heat production. The rate of heat loss depends primarily on the surface temperature of the skin, which is in turn a function of the skin's blood flow. The blood flow of the skin varies in response to changes in the body's core temperature and to changes in temperature of the external environment. Generally, the vessels dilate during warm temperatures and constrict during cold. The hypothalamus is partly responsible for regulating skin blood flow, particularly to the extremities, the face, ears, and the tip of the nose. Maintenance of the thermal balance allows the internal temperature of the body to remain at approximately 37° C (98.6° F).

Under severe heat stress, increased cutaneous blood flow is inadequate to dissipate the thermal load. Eccrine glands produce sweat, and cooling is enhanced by fluid evaporation from the skin. Eccrine gland innervation is unique, in that these sympathetic cholinergic nerves use acetylcholine (rather than norepinephrine) as the neurotransmitter. Sweating contributes significantly to the body's capacity for thermoregulation.

SENSORY RECEPTION

Apart from sight and hearing, the major human sensory apparatus is in the skin. Sensory fibers responsible for pain, touch, and temperature form a complex network in the dermis. This information is transmitted to the spinal cord and relayed to the somatosensory cortex, where the information is integrated into a somatotopic representation of the body.

The skin contains specialized receptors to detect discriminative touch and pressure. *Touch* (flutter) is sensed by Meissner's corpuscles; *pressure,* by Merkel cells and Ruffini endings; *vibration,* by Pacinian corpuscles; and *hair movement,* by hair follicle endings. Together these receptors communicate information to the somatosensory cortex via the dorsal column pathways.

A second grouping of nerves communicates information about temperature and pain to the somatosensory cortex via the anterolateral pathways. *Temperature* is sensed by specific thermoreceptors in the epidermis, and *pain* is sensed by free nerve endings throughout the epidermal, dermal, and hypodermal layers. The speed of conduction of pain information to the cortex results in a functional division. "Fast" pain is well localized, and has a short latency. "Slow" pain is more diffuse, has a longer latency, and is more difficult to endure.

The density of receptors determines the sensitivity of the skin. For example, two-point discrimination is most acute on the skin of the fingers and face, where the highest density of touch receptors occurs. In contrast, the skin on the back has a low density of touch receptors and the ability to localize touch is therefore reduced.

VITAMIN D PRODUCTION

The epidermis is involved in synthesis of vitamin D. In the presence of sunlight or ultraviolet radiation, a sterol found on the malpighian cells is converted to form cholecalciferol (vitamin D_3). Vitamin D_3 assists in the absorption of calcium and phosphate from ingested foods.

PROCESSING OF ANTIGENIC SUBSTANCES

Langerhans cells are scattered among the keratinocytes located primarily in the epidermis; however, they can also be seen in the dermis. These cells originate in the bone marrow and migrate to the epidermis. Langerhans cells play a role in the cell-mediated immune responses of the skin through antigen presentation.

Cells in both the epidermis and dermis of the skin are important in the immune function. Skin is now recognized not only as a physical barrier but also as a participant in immunologically mediated defense against various antigens. These specialized cells include Langerhans cells and keratinocytes located in the epidermis and lymphocytes located in the dermis. An antigen entering immunologically competent skin is likely to encounter a coordinated response of Langerhans and T cells to neutralize its effect. An antigen entering diseased skin can induce and elicit immune responses. These reactions may be involved in the pathogenesis of many inflammatory skin diseases.

DERMATOLOGIC CARE

As the largest and most visible organ of the body, the skin plays a major role in our physical and mental health and protects us from an array of natural and man-made attacks. Yet, the skin is rarely taken as seriously as other organ systems, such as the heart and the lung. In both outpatient and inpatient practice settings, as a nurse you have a unique opportunity to affect a client's dermatologic care. You can teach clients to appreciate the skin's important role and to recognize that some skin conditions are indeed life-threatening. For example, forecasts have indicated that by the year 2000, as many as 1 in 75 Americans would be afflicted by malignant melanoma, an often fatal skin cancer. In the United States today, one person dies every hour from skin cancer. Also, burn injuries continue, despite advances in fireproofing homes and clothes. Pressure ulcers, a serious alteration in skin integrity, poses a growing concern as the elderly population increases and may result in 60,000 deaths per year.

APPEARANCE AND SELF-ESTEEM

Skin is integral to self-image and self-esteem. Each client's unique appearance is established through the skin. The skin was once thought to reflect the normal "aging process" and how that aging process affected the genetic skin types we inherit. We now know that skin type more likely reflects the cumulative amount of sun exposure over a lifetime. It is hoped that with education, untanned skin will once again be viewed as attractive and healthy. Cosmetic surgery should not be considered a procedure for vanity but a procedure to enhance self-esteem.

Today's society has a long-standing prejudice that needs to be dispelled regarding impaired skin. Historically, skin diseases were perceived as divine punishment for being spiritually and physically "unclean." Subtle punishment for skin diseases still exists because of ignorance. For example, a woman with atopic dermatitis may sit isolated and shunned in a waiting room because others view eczematous lesions as contagious. A waitress may be encouraged to work in the back of the kitchen so that customers will not notice the healed burn scars on her hands and body. Vitiligo, loss of pigment in the skin, is sometimes mislabeled "white leprosy," and so on. Clients who have visible chronic skin problems often withdraw from social situations and have altered interpersonal relationships and increased social isolation. When these clients seek professional care for skin problems, psychosocial as well as physical concerns need to be met.

Another function of skin, hair, and nails is to provide an outward appearance or *cosmetic adornment*. The appearance of our skin, hair, and nails is crucial to our psychosocial well-being and can affect our experiences positively or negatively. Skin disorders are often a major cause of a morbidity because we live in a beauty-conscious society. Health care providers must be acutely aware of the role of the skin in a person's self-esteem and ability to function in relationships.

EFFECTS OF AGING

The skin undergoes numerous changes that a person can see and feel throughout the life span. Many of these changes are natural, unchangeable, and harmless. Some may be bothersome or painful and are treated until there is an acceptable resolution or acceptance of the condition. Other skin changes may go unnoticed or not be bothersome because they are slow-growing, such as senile keratosis. Table U10–1 lists some age-associated changes.

Adolescence

During puberty, hormone secretion stimulates the maturation of hair follicles, sebaceous glands, and apocrine and eccrine units in certain body areas. Hair follicles on the face (males), pubic region, and axillae activate to produce coarse terminal hairs. Normal changes may bother teen-

TABLE U10–1	COMMON SKIN CHANGES ASSOCIATED WITH AGING
Skin Change	**Description**
ADOLESCENCE	
Folliculitis	Hair follicle inflammation
Acne	Inflammation of pilosebaceous follicle
Increased perspiration	Response to heat, emotional stress, exercise
Apocrine secretion	Related to sex hormone activity
Skin irritation	Often caused by overuse of over-the-counter skin products
Pigmented nevi	Benign cluster melanocyte-like cells
ADULTHOOD	
Melasma	Blotchy hyperpigmentation
Alopecia	Baldness (hormonal and genetic factors)
Excessive facial or body hair	Androgen-related problem in women
Actinic keratosis	Slightly raised, red papules (premalignant)
Sebaceous cyst	Enclosed cyst in dermis (potentially infectious)
Acrochordon	Small, flesh-colored papule
OLDER ADULTHOOD	
Xerosis	Dry skin (decreased natural oils and sweat)
Wrinkling	Natural change affected by many factors (e.g., loss of elasticity and subcutaneous fat, sun exposure, gravity, cigarette smoking)
Skin tears	Epidermal thinning; seen most in clients using oral corticosteroids
Senile lentigenes	Black or brown flat lesions ("liver spots")
Seborrheic keratosis	Harmless raised black or brown spots or wart-like growths
Cherry angiomas	Dilated blood vessels that form loops

agers, but caution adolescents about the potential for irritating the skin with excessive use of over-the-counter products.

New nevi can appear after adolescence. At any age, raised, pigmented lesions that bleed or change in color or size should be assessed by a physician to determine whether they require only minor care or removal because of early malignant changes.

Adulthood

Temporary *hormonal changes* account for some adult skin changes. Pregnancy and birth control pills may alter hormonal status and thus change skin structures that are hormonally linked. Pregnancy may cause changes in hair growth patterns and a temporary thinning of hair after pregnancy.

Heredity and exposure to environmental factors, such as sun, tobacco, alcohol, and chemicals, play a major role in many of the skin changes that occur in adults. Some lesions (i.e., seborrheic keratosis and acrochordons) may be removed for cosmetic reasons, if desired, or if physically irritating. Actinic keratoses (because of their premalignant status) and sebaceous cysts (because of their infectious potential) need to be assessed and may be removed.

Older Adulthood

The skin of older people reflects the cumulative influence of environmental insults, decreased circulation, and diminished function of various skin structures. As the stratum corneum becomes thinner, the skin reacts more readily to minor changes in humidity, temperature, and other irritants. The skin also becomes more transparent. Hair loss is often noticeable on the trunk, pubic area, axillae, and limbs. Loss of pigment causes gray hair. Nails become brittle and may yellow or thicken. Skin may be leathery from overexposure to ultraviolet light. There is no known treatment for past overexposure; protection from ultraviolet light is the only preventive measure.

CONCLUSIONS

The skin is the largest and most visible organ of the body. Anatomically, the skin is divided into (1) the epidermis (outer layer), (2) the dermis (inner layer), and (3) the hypodermis (subcutaneous layer). The skin serves many functions. It is the first line of defense against many forms of trauma. Skin maintains body temperature, prevents water loss, and provides sensations of touch, temperature, and pain. Skin also produces vitamin D and recognizes antigens. Finally, healthy skin is aesthetically pleasing.

BIBLIOGRAPHY

1. Arndt, K. A., et al. (1996). *Cutaneous medicine and surgery.* Philadelphia: W. B. Saunders.
2. Freedburg, I., et al. (Ed.). (1998). *Fitzpatricks' dermatology in general medicine.* New York: McGraw-Hill.
4. Pogue, S. (1995). Vitamin D synthesis in the elderly. *Dermatology Nursing, 1*(2), 103–105.
5. Silverthorn, D. (1998). *Human physiology.* Upper Saddle River, NJ: Prentice Hall.

Assessment of the Integumentary System

Noreen Heer Nicol

A thorough health history assists in diagnosis of integumentary disorders, such as occupationally related contact dermatitis, or in revealing psychosocial aspects of disease processes. The medication history is important because side effects of certain medications can cause skin changes. The physical examination can confirm integumentary disorders as well as reveal disorders that the client may have omitted during the history.

HISTORY

The history includes questions about the current manifestations, past health history (including medications and allergies), family health history, psychosocial history (including occupational and travel history), and a review of systems.

■ CURRENT HEALTH

Chief Complaint

The most common problems related to the integument are itching (pruritus), dryness, rashes, lesions, ecchymoses (small hemorrhagic patches), lumps, and masses. Ask about changes in the skin, hair, and nails that may be related to the chief complaint. Sample questions that elicit pertinent information related to the presenting dermatologic problem are listed in Table 48–1.

Symptom Analysis

Conduct a symptom analysis, including the factors noted in Table 48–1. Sexual history may also be important if the differential diagnosis includes a sexually transmitted disease (STD) (see Chapter 37).

■ PAST HEALTH HISTORY

Various systemic diseases are characterized by cutaneous manifestations. Does the client have other systemic disorders relevant to the skin (i.e., immunologic, endocrine, collagen, vascular, renal, or hepatic conditions)? Ask about recent exposure to ticks, other insects, or infectious or childhood diseases, and find out about the vaccination status. Previous trauma and surgical intervention may ex-

plain unusual lesions or their location. A history of past allergic reactions to foods or medications is important for avoiding inadvertent reaction through readministration.

Medications

Note prescription and over-the-counter medications that the client is currently taking or has recently finished. Sensitivity to antibiotics or other drugs in the form of a drug rash may not occur until the end of a routine course of therapy. Photosensitizing drugs (e.g., phenothiazides, tetracyclines, diuretics, sulfonamides) may cause a sunburn-like rash in areas of sun exposure. Topical preparations may include preservatives or active ingredients that are known sensitizers. The most commonly encountered are neomycin, benzocaine, and diphenhydramine hydrochloride. Oral corticosteroids (e.g., prednisone), if used at high doses or routinely, can cause acne breakouts, thinning of skin, stretch marks, and many other systemic side effects.

Ask about self-treatment with herbal remedies. Aloe vera (*A. barbadensis, A. ferox, A. africana, A. spicata*) is used for relief of eczema and psoriasis, and to promote wound healing. Chamomile (*Matricaria recutita, Chamaemelum nobile*), comfrey (*Symphytum officinale*), evening primrose (*Oenothera biennis*), and gotu kola (*Centella asiatica*) have similar uses.

Allergies

Ask the client about allergies to medications and foods. Does the ingestion of certain foods cause itching, burning, or eruption of rashes? Fresh fruits that have been treated with pesticides or preservatives may also be problematic, as may prepared foods containing preservatives.

There is a difference between allergy and irritation. *Allergy* is an immunologic response that happens consistently with exposure. *Irritation* can occur unpredictably. Inquire about substances that may cause local skin irritation or lesions on direct contact, such as textiles or metals. Wool is irritating to most people. Jewelry containing nickel may cause skin discoloration, irritation, rash, or other problems in people who are sensitive to this metal.

TABLE 48–1	DERMATOLOGIC ASSESSMENT HISTORY: SAMPLE QUESTIONS
Information Needed	**Questions**
Chief complaint	"Please tell me what brings you here today."
Definition of problem (onset, location)	"Tell me more about the problem. Where did it start? Have you noticed this problem before?"
Duration	"When did it start? Does it come and go? Has it changed? Has it become better or worse?"
Accompanying manifestations	"Did you have any feelings—such as fatigue, nausea, skin tightness, skin burning—before this problem started? Does it itch?"
Evolution of lesion or eruption	"How does it feel now? Are you experiencing any discomfort? Do you feel tenderness, tightness? Does clothing irritate your skin? Do you have any problems sleeping? Does it limit any of your activities? Has it interfered with your normal daily routine?"
Aggravating and relieving factors	"Have you noticed whether the problem worsens after any of these activities: eating particular foods? Using cosmetics? Using soaps? Wearing clothing? Do changes in temperature or climate affect the problem? Does it worsen or improve with changes in season? Are you more comfortable when warm or when cool?"
Medical intervention	"Did you see a physician about this? Were you told what the problem was? Was any treatment recommended? Did it help?"
Self-treatment	"What have you tried to do on your own to get relief? What did you use? What over-the-counter medications or home remedies have you tried? What do you do yourself that helps the problem?"
Compliance and treatment factors	"How often were you able to apply or take prescribed medication? Were you able to complete prescribed treatment? How did you use the medication? (e.g., How did you apply it? How did you take it? For how long? Why did you stop?)"

■ FAMILY HEALTH HISTORY

A family health history helps determine genetic predisposition to skin disorders as well as predisposition to parasitic or other conditions related to the family's lifestyle and living environment. Many dermatologic disorders or systemic disorders with a dermatologic presentation are passed on genetically. Genetically transmitted dermatologic conditions include alopecia (loss of patches of hair), ichthyosis (thickened, scaly skin), atopic dermatitis, and psoriasis. Systemic diseases with dermatologic manifestations include diabetes mellitus, blood dyscrasia, and collagen-vascular diseases (e.g., lupus erythematosus). Other diseases, such as scabies, are likely to be passed on to family members because of close and frequent exposure.

■ PSYCHOSOCIAL HISTORY

Psychosocial factors that influence dermatologic disorders often play a large role, particularly in long-term and chronic processes. Skin disease can greatly affect lifestyle and self-image. Cultural and familial influences in caring for a particular disorder may conflict with prescribed therapies. Misconceptions about skin problems (e.g., acne lesions can be scrubbed away) need to be determined and corrected. Visually or physically disabling chronic skin diseases have been associated with chronic unemployment, poor mental health, and even suicide. Assess the sexual history, which can help alert to or explain the presence of tissue trauma or lesions caused by STDs (see Chapter 37).

Do not overlook socioeconomic factors. Compliance with outlined therapies and return for follow-up care are influenced by social expectations and ability to pay for medications or treatments. When recommending therapies or medications, consider the impact on the client's day-to-day routine as well as the type of prescription insurance plan. Many topical therapies—whether or not they are covered by insurance—are expensive, and expense is a factor that affects compliance.

Occupation and Travel

Occupational history is important because a large number of skin problems are caused or worsened by exposure to irritants and chemicals in the home and work environment. Learn what substances the client comes in contact with and to what extent. For example, chronic flaring of hand eczema may be caused by use of certain glues and glazes in a hobby project, total body rash by chemical mists penetrating nonprotective gear at the work site, or hand rash by latex glove allergies.[14, 19]

The travel history can be helpful, especially if it includes hiking or exposure to outdoor agents that result in dermatologic disorders, such as poison ivy, poison sumac, or poison oak or Lyme disease.

Habits

Inquire about the client's habits. Determine the frequency of hygiene practices, the products used (e.g., soaps, lotions, abrasives), and whether cosmetics are used. Record the products used, including brand names. Inquire whether there have been any changes in clothing or bedding, and discuss how these items are cleaned. Review the client's diet history for intake of sufficient nutrients, such as water, protein, dietary fat, and vitamins A, D, E, and C. Also, ask about exercise and sleep patterns, which affect circulation, nourishment, and repair of the skin.

Does the client engage in recreational activities that involve prolonged exposure to the sun, unusual cold, or other conditions that may damage the integument? For example, does the client visit tanning salons? More than 1 million persons use tanning salons each day, and federal regulation of salons is limited. Advise clients that exposure leads to premature aging, increased risk of skin cancer, risk of corneal burns if eye guards are not worn, exacerbation of photosensitivity disorders, and increased development of lentigines ("liver spots").[18]

■ REVIEW OF SYSTEMS

Obtain a complete history of the skin. Specifically, ask about past problems with unusual itching, dryness, lesions, rashes, lumps, ecchymoses, and masses. Has the client had problems with moles or other lesions, especially if they have undergone changes in size, shape, or color? A more complete list of questions for the review of systems appears in Chapter 9, Box 9–2.

PHYSICAL EXAMINATION

Examine the skin as thoroughly as any other body organ. This procedure cannot be done properly in the hall or at a quick glance, which the dermatologist or the nurse is often requested to do. Use inspection, palpation, and olfaction to assess hair, nails, and skin. Effective assessment requires knowledge, awareness, and practice in describing skin of individuals of all ages and different lifestyles and in recognizing normal and abnormal skin changes. The Physical Assessment Findings in the Healthy Adult feature describes normal conditions of the integumentary system.

PHYSICAL ASSESSMENT FINDINGS IN THE HEALTHY ADULT

Integumentary System

Inspection

Skin. Even skin tones, darker on exposed areas of face, neck, arms, and lower legs; lighter on trunk and back. Small tan freckles scattered over face and arms. Scars, striae absent.

Hair and Scalp. Hair evenly distributed over scalp. Clean, without nits or lice. No dandruff, scaling, or scalp lesions. Axillae and legs probably shaved; pubic hair distributed as inverted triangle from symphysis pubis to perineum (female). Pubic hair distributed in diamond pattern from below umbilicus to perineum (male).

Nails. Regular, smooth, oval shape. Pink nail beds. Cuticles manicured, clean. Nail bed angle 160 degrees (no clubbing).

Palpation

Skin. Warm, well hydrated, smooth, elastic, nontender. No lesions, masses, or lumps.

Hair and Scalp. Hair non-oily, even textured, resilient. Scalp smooth, intact, nontender.

Nails. Firm without tenderness or bogginess. Rapid blanch response.

■ TERMINOLOGY

The terms used in dermatology have been referred to as a "foreign language" and have been known to inhibit use of the correct terminology for skin disorders by health care providers. Use of standard terminology often leads to differential diagnosis. This section clarifies some commonly used dermatologic terms and should assist the reader in recognizing and describing skin disorders. Table 48–2 is a glossary of commonly used dermatologic terms.

■ TYPES OF LESIONS

Examination and making the correct diagnosis of skin disorders depend on identifying skin lesions or changes. Two major types of lesions are distinguished: *primary* and *secondary* lesions.

The primary lesion is the first lesion to appear on the skin and has a visually recognizable structure. Figure 48–1 depicts 10 primary lesions: macule, papule, plaque, nodule, tumor, wheal, vesicle, bulla, cyst, and pustule. Frequently, the health care provider does not see a primary lesion and must depend on the client's description of "how it looked when it first appeared."

When a primary lesion undergoes changes, it becomes a secondary lesion. These alterations, brought about by the client or by the client's environment, often occur in the epidermal layer. The changes may result from many factors, including scratching, rubbing, medication, natural disease progression, or processes of involution and healing. Figure 48–2 presents nine secondary lesions: scale, crust, erosion, deep ulcer, scar, lichenification, excoriation, fissure, and atrophy.

■ EXAMINATION ENVIRONMENT

The best setting for conducting a dermatologic assessment is a well-lit, private room with moderate temperature and neutral, white, or cream-colored walls. Excessive warmth can produce changes in skin color (e.g., redness) by causing vasodilation. Colored walls can affect normal skin hue (color). For a complete examination, ask the client to undress and provide a gown. Explain that all skin surfaces will be examined. Avoid unnecessary exposure during the examination. Have warm hands to avoid stimulation of the skin and to add to the overall comfort of the client.

■ DEPTH OF EXAMINATION

The examination is systematic and as complete as appropriate. A total-body skin examination involves assessment of the hair, scalp, nails, mucous membranes, and skin, including the axillae, areas in skinfolds, external genitalia, webs between toes and fingers, palms of hands, and soles of feet. Begin at the head, and proceed to the toes. General changes can alter total-body skin color (e.g., jaundice, cyanosis, pallor), thickness, turgor, temperature, and vascularity (e.g., purpura, petechiae). General findings can suggest systemic disease and may require complete physical examination and appropriate evaluation. The diagnosis of skin disorders is accomplished by careful observation and evaluation of individual lesions. This discussion is limited to assessment of hair, scalp, nails, and skin lesions.

Table 48-2	GLOSSARY OF DERMATOLOGIC TERMS
Actinic	Pertaining to ultraviolet light (UVL)
Amelanotic	Without pigment
Circinate (pronounced *sir-sin-ate*)	Circular
Circumscribed	Limited to a certain area by sharply defined border
Coalesce	To merge one with another
Comedo	Plug in a skin duct containing keratin (open, blackhead; closed, whitehead)
Cytotoxic	Toxic to cells
Dermatome	Area of skin supplied by a single dorsal nerve root
Dermatophyte	Fungus that enters the skin's surface, causing infection
Desquamation	Scaling, peeling of epidermis
Discoid	Coin-like
Eczematous	General term for disease process characterized by scaling, weeping, crusting, and inflammation
Erythema	Redness
Exacerbation	Worsening of disease state
Exfoliative	Shedding of skin in fairly large quantities
Folliculitis	Hair follicle inflammation
Guttate	Small, water drop–sized lesions, usually widespread
Hives	Spontaneously occurring wheals
Hyperkeratosis	Thickening of stratum corneum, usually from repeated pressure or friction
Hyperpigmentation	Increased or excessive skin pigmentation (melanin) causing an area of skin to be darker than surrounding areas
Hypopigmentation	Decreased pigmentation
Indurated	Hard (tissue)
Intertrigo	Irritation of body areas with opposing skinfolds that are subject to friction
Lesion	Detectable change from normal skin structure
Maceration	Tissue softening or disintegration from excessive moisture
Milia	Small, white papules
Perioral	Around the mouth
Periungual	Under the nail plate
Pigmentation	Degree of skin or mucous membrane color
Plantar	Pertaining to sole of the foot
Polymorphic	Existing in many forms
Pruritus	Itching
Punctate	Pinpoint or dot-shaped
Sclerosis	Hardening or induration of skin
Sebum	Lipid excretion produced by sebaceous glands
Tautness	Degree of skin tightness
Texture	Tactile or visual skin characteristics (e.g., coarseness, dryness)
Ultraviolet light (UVL)	Electromagnetic radiation from the sun (wavelengths 4–400 nm)
Urticaria	Wheals (hives)
Verruca	Lesion characterized by surface roughness (e.g., wart)
Wheal	Lesion found in hives

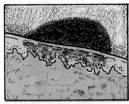

MACULE: Skin color change without elevation, i.e., flat (e.g., freckles or petechia). Described as a "patch" if greater than 1 cm (e.g., vitiligo).

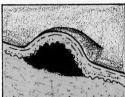

PAPULE: Elevated, solid lesion of less than 1 cm, varying in color (e.g., warts or elevated nevus).

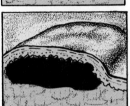

PLAQUE: Raised, flat lesion formed from merging papules or nodules.

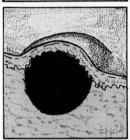

NODULE: Larger than a papule. Raised solid lesion extending deeper into the dermis.

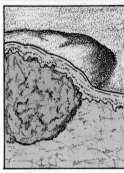

TUMOR: Larger than a nodule. Elevated firm lesion that may or may not be easily demarcated.

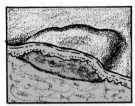

WHEAL (hive): Fleeting skin elevation that is irregularly shaped because of edema (e.g., mosquito bite or urticaria).

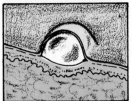

VESICLE (blister): Elevated, sharply defined lesion containing serous fluid. Usually less than 1 cm (e.g., blister, chickenpox, or herpes simplex).

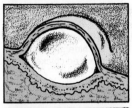

BULLA (plural, *bullae*): Large, elevated, fluid-filled lesion greater than 1 cm (e.g., second-degree burn).

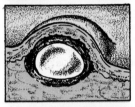

CYST: Elevated, thick-walled lesion containing fluid or semisolid matter.

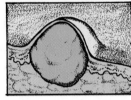

PUSTULE: Elevated lesion less than 1 cm containing purulent material. Lesions larger than 1 cm are described as boils, abscesses, or furuncles (e.g., acne, or impetigo).

FIGURE 48-1 Primary lesions: visually recognizable structural changes in the skin that have specific characteristics.

Although you may examine the client's integument over the complete body surface at one time, this is usually not done in the screening examination. Instead, integument assessment is integrated as each body region is examined. For the purpose of discussion, however, assessment of the integument is presented as a separate body system. Significant or abnormal findings are commonly reported as part of each regional assessment rather than separately.

■ INSPECTION AND PALPATION

Hair and Scalp

Examine *hair distribution* patterns for symmetry and distribution according to age and sexual development. Fine hair covers much of the body and is the same color as scalp hair. Increased distribution occurs normally in the axillae and pubic area. Having excess body hair is known as *hirsutism.*

Inspect the hair and scalp under good light. Wear gloves if you suspect lesions or infestation with lice. Inspect and palpate the hair for distribution, thickness, texture, lubrication, and signs of infestation or infection. Because natural hair color varies greatly, ask the client whether hair dye is used, as it alters texture. Hair should be resilient and distributed evenly over the scalp. Individual hair shafts can range from thin and fine to thick and coarse; the shape of hair fibers can be straight, curly, or wavy. Texture and lubrication are affected by the type of hair care products used (e.g., harsh shampoo, curling irons, or hair dryers) as well as by a protein-deficient diet or health problems, such as febrile illness, all of which tend to leave hair dry and brittle. Hair loss or thinning *(alopecia)* can result from genetic predisposition to bald-

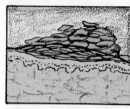

SCALE: Dried fragments of sloughed epidermal cells, irregular in shape and size and white, tan, yellow, or silver in color (e.g., dandruff, dry skin, or psoriasis).

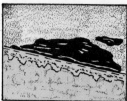

CRUST: Dried serum, sebum, blood, or pus on skin surface producing a temporary barrier to the environment (e.g., impetigo).

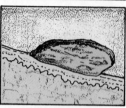

EROSION: A moist, demarcated, depressed area due to loss of partial- or full-thickness epidermis. Basal layer of epidermis remains intact (e.g., ruptured chickenpox vesicle).

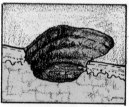

ULCER: Irregularly shaped, exudative, depressed lesion in which entire epidermis and upper layer of dermis are lost. Results from trauma and tissue destruction (e.g., stasis ulcer).

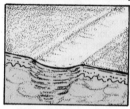

SCAR: Mark left on skin after healing. Replacement of destroyed tissue by fibrous tissue.

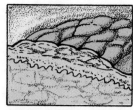

LICHENIFICATION: Epidermal thickening resulting in elevated plaque with accentuated skin markings. Usually results from repeated injury through rubbing or scratching (e.g., chronic atopic dermatitis).

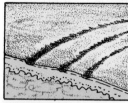

EXCORIATION: Superficial, linear abrasion of epidermis. Visible sign of itching caused by rubbing or scratching (e.g., atopic dermatitis).

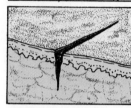

FISSURE: Deep linear split through epidermis into dermis (e.g., tinea pedis).

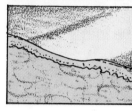

ATROPHY: Wasting of epidermis in which skin appears thin and transparent, or of dermis in which there is a depressed area (e.g., arterial insufficiency).

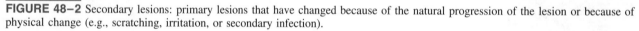

FIGURE 48–2 Secondary lesions: primary lesions that have changed because of the natural progression of the lesion or because of physical change (e.g., scratching, irritation, or secondary infection).

ness or a health problem, such as recent chemotherapy or a thyroid disorder.

Inspect and palpate the *scalp* for lesions, excoriations (from scratching), lumps, or bruises, which should be absent. Examine hair shafts for the presence of nits, which are the eggs of the human head louse *(Pediculus humanus capitis)* and appear as particles of oval dandruff. Adult lice often bite the scalp behind the ears and along the back of the neck, which results in pustular lesions. It may be difficult to see adult lice on the scalp; they are very small (1 to 2 mm) and have gray-white bodies.

If you see lesions, describe them and ask the client about recent trauma or injury to the head. If the client has not already provided information during the health history interview, conduct a symptom analysis.

Nails

Inspect the client's nails for color, shape, texture, integrity, and thickness (Table 48–3). The nails reflect the client's overall health, indicating nutrition and respiratory status.

COLOR AND SHAPE

The nail plate is usually transparent and colorless and, when viewed from the side, has a convex shape. The vascular bed underlying the nail plate gives the nail its color. The color is pink in white clients and darker in dark-skinned clients. A hemoglobin deficiency is seen in the nail bed as pallor, and decreased arterial circulation appears as cyanosis.

Perform a *blanch test* by palpating the nail beds to assess capillary refill. Press the nail bed firmly for 5 seconds, then quickly release while observing the rate of color return to the nail bed. Color should return within 3 to 5 seconds in healthy individuals. Document results of the blanch test as "rapid" or "sluggish" capillary refill. When palpated, the nail bed feels firm with no softness (i.e., bogginess) or tenderness.

TEXTURE

Texture should be smooth; healthy nails are of uniform thickness with no signs of dryness, softness, brittleness, splitting, peeling, ridges, or pitting. The *angle* formed between the nail plate and posterior nailfold is approximately

TABLE 48–3	ASSESSING THE NAILS	
Assessment Finding	**Description**	**Causes**
Normal nail	Nail shape is convex, and nail plate angle is approximately 160°	
Beau's line	Horizontal depression in nail plate; depressions can occur singly or in multiples	Nail growth is disturbed temporarily; related to systemic illness (e.g., infection) or direct injury to the nail root
Splinter hemorrhages	Linear (vertical) red or brown streaks in the nail bed	Minor trauma to the nail bed; subacute bacterial endocarditis; trichinosis
Paronychia	Inflammation of the skinfold at the nail margin	Trauma; skin infection at the nail base
Spoon shape	Nail shape is concave as the nail curves upward from the nail bed	Use of strong detergents; iron deficiency anemia; syphilis
Clubbing	Increased angle between nail plate and nail base	Long-standing hypoxia

160 degrees without separation (see Table 48–3). Changes in nail shape and nail bed angle can indicate health problems. Clubbing of the nails refers to an increase of more than 160 degrees in the angle between the nail plate and nail base. The base of a clubbed nail is spongy and soft on palpation. These changes result from hypoxia (diminished tissue oxygenation). Nail clubbing commonly occurs in clients with congenital heart defects or chronic lung disease.

INTEGRITY

The tissue surrounding the nail should appear intact without signs of inflammation, jagged edges (hangnail), or dryness. Inferior or lateral nailfold inflammation is a sign of paronychia (i.e., nailfold infection). If these abnormalities are noted, ask the client about nail care habits such as biting or cutting cuticles.

THICKNESS

While examining the fingers and toes, you may note common abnormalities such as calluses or corns. A *callus* is a flat, painless thickening of a circumscribed area of skin. Calluses usually occur on the hands and feet. A *corn* is a horny induration and thickening of the skin caused by friction and pressure and is often painful.

Skin

COLOR

Assess overall skin color during the health history interview. Conduct a more thorough assessment as you proceed through the remainder of the physical examination. Observe the client's face and visible skin surfaces for color tones, which should be congruent with the stated race. Abnormal findings include pallor (paleness), a flushed or ruddy complexion, cyanosis (blue cast), jaundice (yellow cast), and areas of irregular pigmentation. Normal variation occurs from one region of the body to another, particularly in areas protected from the sun and exposure by clothing; these areas are lighter. Overall color should be uniform. Skin tone may range over a variety of colors including light ivory to deep brown or blue-black, yellow to olive, or light pink to dark, ruddy pink.

Areas that are less pigmented reveal abnormal findings more readily than more heavily pigmented surfaces. For example, *pallor* is best seen in the buccal (mouth) mucosa, especially in clients with dark skin. *Cyanosis* is evident more readily in less pigmented areas, such as the nail beds, lips, and palms. *Jaundice* sharply contrasts with the white of the sclera, especially in dark-skinned clients who have more carotene deposits. Jaundice is best assessed in dark-skinned clients by inspecting color changes in the hard palate.

Examine local areas of color change closely. *Hyperpigmentation* describes areas of increased pigmentation; *hypopigmentation* describes areas of decreased pigmentation. Skin color also results from the circulation; an increased blood supply may lead to the redness of inflammation *(rubor)*, whereas extreme pallor may be a result of anemia or impeded arterial circulation to the area.

MOISTURE

Moisture refers to the skin's hydration level in terms of both wetness and oiliness. Overall skin moisture in healthy individuals can be described as well hydrated. Skin moisture often reflects ambient temperature and humidity levels. Moistness usually occurs in intertriginous areas (where skin touches skin), such as the axillae and groin. Skin that feels overly moist and cool (i.e., clammy) or overly dry, scaling, or cracked is abnormal.

TEMPERATURE

Assess temperature with the dorsum of the hand. The skin should feel uniformly warm because it reflects circulation. Compare areas of hypothermia or hyperthermia with the same areas on the opposite side. See Figure 48–3.

TEXTURE

Palpate *texture* by stroking the skin lightly with the fingertips. The skin should feel smooth, soft, and resilient. There should be no areas of lumps or unusual thickening or thinning (atrophy).

TURGOR

Turgor, a reflection of the skin's elasticity and hydration status, is measured by the time needed for the skin and underlying tissue to return to their original contour after being "pinched up." Lightly pinch the skin over the forearm between the thumb and index finger, then release it.

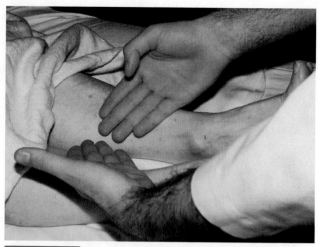

FIGURE 48–3 Assessing skin temperature. (Courtesy of Mary Sieggreen.)

If the skin remains elevated (i.e., tented) for more than 3 seconds, turgor is decreased. Skin with normal turgor is mobile and elastic and should return to baseline contour within 3 seconds. Turgor decreases with age as the skin loses elasticity. Assessment of turgor is discussed in Chapter 10.

EDEMA

Palpate for *edema* (fluid retention), particularly if areas of taut, shiny skin are noted. Edema refers to a collection of fluid in underlying tissues that separate the skin's surface from pigmented and vascular layers, which results in a blanched appearance. It is an abnormal finding. Palpate edematous areas for consistency, temperature, shape (i.e., extent), tenderness, and mobility. Assess and describe edematous areas using the technique described in Chapter 51. Areas examined for edema include those over the sacrum (especially in bedridden clients), the feet, the ankles, and the shins (over the tibia).

TENDERNESS

Tenderness is an abnormal finding and is elicited with palpation. No areas of tenderness should be found in a healthy, uninjured client.

ODOR

The skin should be free of pungent odors. Odors, when noted, are usually present in the axillae and skinfolds or in open wounds and are related to the presence of bacteria on the skin, inadequate hygiene, or infection. Assess odor in open wounds after cleansing the wound, since odor can be related to the drainage itself or to the type of dressing used (e.g., hydrocolloid).

LESIONS

Inspect the skin for detectable lesions. Assess and describe lesions in an orderly fashion: location, distribution, size, arrangement, color, configuration, secondary changes, and presence of drainage. Palpate skin lesions to determine the characteristics of contour (e.g., flat, raised, or depressed), size (using a measuring device), consistency (e.g., firm, soft), mobility, and tenderness. Lesions can be mobile or immobile (fixed to underlying tissue). Photographing lesions of concern is an excellent way to document changes over time.

LOCATION, DISTRIBUTION, AND SIZE. *Location* is described in reference to anatomic landmarks. Measure the lesions for *size* to help classify their type (e.g., macule, papule). If multiple lesions are present, the *distribution pattern* can be helpful in determining the diagnosis. Note the extent of the lesions. Lesions can be (1) localized (confined to a specific area), (2) regional, or (3) generalized (present over a large surface). Compare sides bilaterally to determine whether lesions are symmetrical or asymmetrical. Another commonly noted distribution is on sun-exposed areas. Certain diseases feature a classic lesion distribution; for example, lesions of herpes zoster follow along a nerve root dermatome. Table 48–4 presents common configurations and distributions. Figure 48–4 depicts the locations of common skin disorders found during physical examination.

ARRANGEMENT. The *arrangement* refers to the pattern of nearby lesions. Two of the typical patterns are "linear" and "satellite," which can also be helpful in confirming diagnosis. Linear lesions appear in a straight line (e.g., in scabies). Satellite lesions appear as small peripheral lesions around a central larger lesion (e.g., in diaper candidiasis).

COLOR. Skin lesions are found in a wide variety of colors; they may be skin-colored, brown, red, yellow, tan, or blue. Color can be influenced by many factors, including the client's normal skin hue, which may make accurate description difficult. Slight color changes can best be assessed in areas having the least amount of natural pigmentation and those with superficial capillary beds (i.e., buccal membrane of the mouth, mucosa, lips, nail beds,

TABLE 48–4	TERMINOLOGY FOR SKIN LESION CONFIGURATION AND DISTRIBUTION
	Description
CONFIGURATION*	
Annular	Ring-shaped
Iris	Concentric rings, "bull's eyes"
Gyrate	Spiral-shaped
Linear	Forming a line
Nummular	Coin-like
Polymorphous	Occurring in several forms
Punctate	Marked by points or dots
Serpiginous	Snake-like
DISTRIBUTION†	
Solitary	Single lesion
Satellite	Single lesion occurring in close proximity to but separate from a large group of lesions
Grouped	Clustered
Confluent	Merged together
Diffuse	Widely distributed
Discrete	Separate from other lesions
Generalized	Diffusely distributed
Localized	Limited, clearly defined
Symmetrical	Bilaterally distributed
Asymmetrical	Unilaterally distributed
Zosteriform	Band-like distribution of lesions along a dermatome

*Position of lesions relative to other lesions.
†Grouping, or pattern, of lesions over entire skin surface.

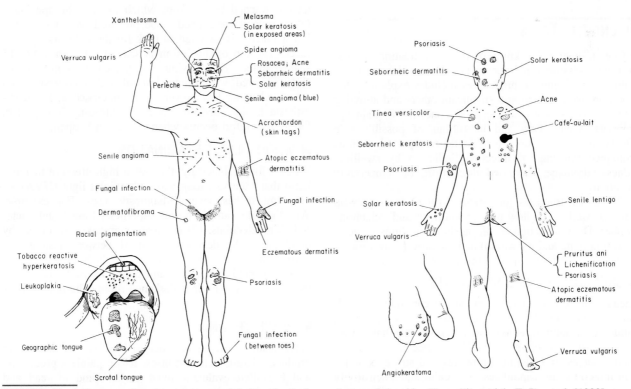

FIGURE 48–4 Common disorders encountered during physical examinaton of the skin. (From Fitzpatrick, T. B., et al. [1993]. *Dermatology in general medicine* [4th ed]. New York: McGraw-Hill.)

ocular conjunctiva, palms, and soles). These areas are especially important in assessing darkly pigmented skin.

CONFIGURATION. The term configuration refers to the shape or the outline of the lesion. Most lesions are circular. The term *nummular* is used for a circular lesion that is the size of a large coin (i.e., nummular eczema). *Annular* describes lesions with an active ring-shaped border and some central clearing (e.g., granuloma annulare). Table 48–4 shows other configurations that may be found during assessment.

■ SKIN SELF-EXAMINATION

Although it is crucial that all health care providers learn to perform an accurate and complete assessment of the skin, it is more important to teach every individual how to do a skin self-examination. Routine self-examination greatly lowers individual risk for severe skin disorders, such as skin cancer. Teach clients to examine their entire bodies to look for any changes in the skin or their moles or skin lesions. See the Client Education Guide in Chapter 49.

Danger signals to look for are the *ABCDs* of melanoma:

A = *Asymmetry*: one half unlike the other half;
B = *Border*: irregular, scalloped, or poorly circumscribed border;
C = *Color*: varied from one area to another, shades of two colors, or changing colors;
D = *Diameter*: larger than 6 mm as a rule (diameter of a No. 2 pencil eraser).

Also see the Physical Assessment Findings in the Healthy Adult feature in this chapter. Encourage clients to visit their health care provider for further evaluation of any suspicious-looking lesions.

DIAGNOSTIC TESTS

Before a diagnostic skin procedure (or treatment), perform an assessment and document findings. Nursing intervention for diagnostic procedures includes explaining the procedure to the client and significant others and allowing them to ask questions and express concerns. Explain appropriate wound care and indications of possible side effects and complications that should be reported, such as prolonged bleeding or infection (indicated by swelling, redness, drainage, increased discomfort, or temperature elevation).

Provide instructions (preferably written) for follow-up care as well as follow-up appointment and telephone number. Documentation of diagnostic procedures (exactly what was done and by whom) and the specific location of the lesion must be completed by appropriate personnel.

■ SKIN CULTURE AND SENSITIVITY

Bacterial infections of the skin can be confirmed by culture. Because of the cost and delay in getting results, culture is usually reserved for infections that have been nonresponsive to routine care. Clients who have had frequent courses of systemic antibiotics and still experience skin infections are candidates for a culture and sensitivity test to determine which antibiotic is indicated for treatment.

■ POTASSIUM HYDROXIDE EXAMINATION AND FUNGAL CULTURE

Fungal infection of skin, hair, or nails may be confirmed by microscopic identification or culture of scrapings from the area or both. Any area of scaly dermatitis may be scraped for this test. Typical sites are the scalp, intertriginous areas (between the toes, axillae, groin, under or between the breasts, abdominal folds), and the nailfold.

Fine scales from the edge of the site are scraped with a No. 15 scalpel blade or the edge of a glass slide onto a second glass slide. A drop of 10% to 20% potassium hydroxide is added to the scale, and a coverslip is placed over the specimen. Gentle pressure is applied to the coverslip to flatten the scales. The slide may be gently heated to dissolve the keratin or the cells more quickly. The scrapings are examined under the microscope. For a culture, scrapings from a suspicious lesion are implanted in the appropriate culture medium. For a nail culture, an altered, dystrophic nail is snipped and implanted in the medium. Debris from the nail's subungual area is less suitable for culture.

■ TZANCK'S SMEAR

Tzanck's smear is used for microscopic assessment of fluids and cells from vesicles or bullae. The presence of multinucleated giant cells establishes a diagnosis of viral infection, such as herpes simplex or herpes zoster infection. An intact, recently evolved vesicle's top is removed, and its base is scraped with a scalpel or small curet. The debris is smeared onto a labeled slide and sent for cytologic assessment.

■ SCABIES SCRAPING

The most difficult part of the test for scabies is selecting an unscratched lesion from which to take the specimen. Often several areas need to be prepared. When visible, a linear burrow is sampled to look for the mite, its eggs, or feces. The top of the lesion is shaved off with a No. 15 scalpel blade. The shavings are placed on a microscope slide, covered with immersion oil and a coverslip, and examined under low power on the microscope. Local anesthesia is not necessary, and fine bleeding is expected. Some discomfort occurs when the lesion is opened.

■ WOOD'S LIGHT EXAMINATION

Wood's light ("black light") uses a high-pressure mercury lamp that transmits long-wave ultraviolet light (UVA), or 360 nm; it has several diagnostic uses. For example, Wood's light can (1) detect superficial fungal and bacterial skin infections, (2) delineate pigmentary disorders by highlighting the degree of contrast between lesions and normal skin color, and (3) accentuate the contrast between hypopigmented and totally amelanotic areas. Wood's light examination is done in a darkened room. The procedure is painless.

■ PATCH TESTING

Patch testing is done in order to identify substances that produce allergic skin responses. It is a painless procedure, and a skilled evaluator must be on hand to read and interpret the results. Patch testing is often done to differentiate between an *irritant* contact dermatitis and an *aller-*

gic contact dermatitis. Small amounts of various substances or allergens are applied to the skin using a commercially prepared tape containing the allergens, or allergens are placed on aluminum discs on a special tape. The client and significant others need to understand that whereas potential allergic substances (allergens) can produce inflammatory skin reactions, compounds of low concentration are used to prevent possible excessive irritation.

Patch testing should not be performed if acute dermatitis is present; the potential allergen may worsen the dermatitis.

The tape must be worn for 48 hours without disturbing the patches; then it is removed. Interpretations are made at 48, 72, and 96 hours and sometimes at 1 week. An eczematous response at the test site with erythema, papules, or small vesicles indicates a positive reaction and confirms an allergic contact sensitivity to the substance on the disc.

■ BIOPSY

Skin biopsy refers to removal of a skin tissue specimen for histologic (cellular microscopic) assessment. There are three types: shave, dermal punch, and surgical excision. In all three procedures, local anesthesia is used. Small-gauge (26- to 30-gauge) needles are recommended to limit trauma to the skin.

Depending on the size and location of the biopsy specimen and the skill of the practitioner, the procedure is usually quick and almost painless. The most common source of pain is the initial administration of local anesthetic. The specimen is placed in a preservative such as formalin solution, properly identified, and sent for pathologic assessment. Use clean or sterile technique, as appropriate, to dress or cover the biopsy site.

PROCEDURES
SHAVE BIOPSY
A shave biopsy is performed to obtain tissue for analysis from possibly malignant epidermal growths except potential melanoma (Fig. 48–5A). After skin cleaning and infiltration of local anesthesia, tissue is removed with a lateral motion by use of a scalpel with a No. 15 blade. Alternatively, a specimen can be obtained by snipping with curved tissue scissors. Tissue removed includes the epidermis and upper portions of the dermal layers.

Hemostasis of the biopsy site is obtained by applying pressure, by using ferric subsulfate (Monsel's solution) or aluminum chloride solution, or by instituting electrodesiccation (cautery).

PUNCH BIOPSY
For a dermal punch biopsy, a circular instrument with a sharp cutting edge is used to remove a specimen of skin

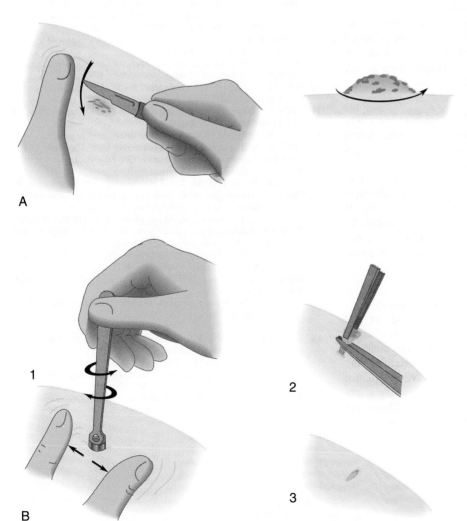

FIGURE 48–5 Skin biopsies. *A, Shave* biopsy. A tissue specimen is obtained by use of a scalpel (No. 15 blade) in a horizontal-lateral motion. *B, Punch* biopsy. A tissue specimen is obtained with the instrument pressed down firmly on the skin. The specimen is freed from surrounding tissue by a rotary back-and-forth cutting motion. The specimen base is severed with tissue scissors.

A

B

1

2

3

that includes epidermal, dermal, and subcutaneous tissue. This method is used to obtain a biopsy specimen of a well-developed, mature lesion (Fig. 48–5*B*). An appropriate-sized punch is chosen (from 2 to 6 mm). The skin site is cleaned, and a local anesthetic is injected. Skin surrounding the lesion is stretched taut, and the punch is pressed firmly downward into the skin site. The instrument is rotated back and forth in a cutting motion that frees the specimen from surrounding tissue. The specimen is then gently grasped with a tissue forceps or needle, and its base is severed with scissors or a scalpel blade.

Depending on the size of the specimen, hemostasis can be achieved with pressure or application of Monsel's solution or aluminum chloride solution. The oval defect may be closed with a 4-0 or 5-0 silk or nylon suture to produce a linear scar. Sutures are removed after about 7 to 14 days (with facial biopsies, 3 to 5 days).

SURGICAL EXCISION BIOPSY

The surgical excision biopsy is used (1) when it is necessary to excise a lesion completely (e.g., when full skin thickness is needed), (2) when a lesion's borders are indistinct from surrounding skin, or (3) when there is a recurrent or aggressive cancer, such as malignant melanoma. The site is cleansed, the excisional lines are marked with a gentian violet pen, and local anesthetic is administered. The lesion is excised with a scalpel by means of a variety of surgical techniques; a commonly used technique is an elliptical incision.

Hemostasis is achieved with pressure and ligation (suturing closed) of superficial vessels. The incision is closed with sutures. The suture site is rinsed with saline-dampened gauze. A pressure dressing of sterile nonadhering gauze is applied and taped in place.

PREPROCEDURE CARE

Depending on the size of the excision, instruct the client to avoid the use of aspirin and products containing aspirin for 48 hours before the biopsy to avoid a prolonged postprocedure bleeding time. If the client is taking anticoagulants (e.g., heparin or warfarin), notify the physician. Review the client's medical history for systemic disorders such as liver malfunction, which affects clotting time. If the client has a history of cardiac valve replacement, be sure that prophylactic antibiotics are prescribed. The client should eat a light meal before the procedure to avoid syncope (fainting).

POSTPROCEDURE CARE

After the procedure, cover the majority of biopsy sites with an antibiotic ointment and a clean bandage or dry dressing unless ordered otherwise. Many nonadhesive types of dressings are available and may be preferable for clients who have fragile or sensitive skin. Remind the client that follow-up assessment is necessary, and plan a follow-up appointment for suture removal. Tell the client how and when biopsy results will be reported. Remember that individuals have different levels of anxiety about the biopsy results, depending on the anticipated possible outcome (e.g., melanoma versus wart).

CONCLUSIONS

Although the skin is the largest organ in the body, it is often taken for granted. The skin protects us from the sun and many dangerous elements and helps fight diseases and infections. The top layers of healthy skin have the ability to regenerate and repair themselves every 3 to 4 weeks. Skin must be handled with care to maintain its many functions.

BIBLIOGRAPHY

1. Arnold, H. L., Odom, R. B., & James, W. D. (1990). *Andrew's diseases of the skin* (8th ed.). Philadelphia: W. B. Saunders.
2. Bates, B. (1995). *A guide to physical examination* (6th ed.). Philadelphia: J. B. Lippincott.
3. Burrage, R., et al. (1991). Physical assessment. An overview with sections on the skin, eye, ear, nose and neck. In W. Chenitz, et al. (Eds.), *Clinical gerontological nursing*. Philadelphia: W. B. Saunders.
4. Callen, J. P. (1995). *Current practice in dermatology*. Philadelphia: W. B. Saunders.
5. Dellasega, C., & Burgunder, C. (1991). Perioperative nursing care for the elderly surgical patient. *Todays OR Nurse, 13*(6), 12–17.
6. Dermatology Nurses' Association. (1998). *Dermatology nursing essentials: A core curriculum*. Pitman, NJ: Anthony J. Jannetti.
7. Fitzpatrick, T. B., & Eisen, T. B. (1992). *Dermatology in general medicine* (4th ed.). Hightstown, NJ: McGraw-Hill.
8. Fitzpatrick, T. B., et al. (1997). *Color atlas and synopsis of clinical dermatology*. New York: McGraw-Hill.
9. Habif, T. (1996). *Clinical dermatology: A color guide to diagnosis and therapy* (3rd ed.). St. Louis: Mosby–Year Book.
10. Hill, M. J. (1994). Skin disorders. In *Mosby's clinical nursing series*. St. Louis: Mosby–Year Book.
11. Jarvis, C. (2000). *Physical examination and health assessment* (3rd ed.). Philadelphia: W. B. Saunders.
12. Nicol, N. H. (1998). Alteration in the integument in children. In J. McCance & S. Huetner (Eds.), *Pathophysiology: The biologic basics for disease in adults and children* (3rd ed.). St. Louis: Mosby–Year Book.
13. Nicol, N. H., & Hill, M. J. (1994). Altered skin integrity. In R. Foster, M. Hunsberger, & C. Betz (Eds.), *Family-centered nursing care of children* (2nd ed.). Philadelphia: W. B. Saunders.
14. Nicol, N. H., Ruszkowski, A. M., & Moore, J. A. (1995, February). Contact dermatitis and the role of patch testing in its diagnosis and management. *Dermatology Nursing, Supplement*, 5–10.
15. Pogue, S. (1992). Nursing assessment of the elderly for dermatologic procedures. *Dermatology Nursing, 4*(1), 15–23.
16. Pogue, S. (1995). Vitamin D synthesis in the elderly. *Dermatology Nursing, 7*(2), 103–105.
17. Rudy, S. (1991). From conception to birth: The development of the skin and nursing implications. *Dermatology Nursing, 3*(6), 381–392.
18. Sinni-McKeehen, B. (1995). Health effects and regulation of tanning salons. *Dermatology Nursing, 7*(5), 307–312.
19. Truscott, W., & Roley, L. (1995). Glove-associated reactions: Addressing an increasing concern. *Dermatology Nursing, 7*(5), 283–292.
20. Weston, W. L., Lane, A. T., & Morelli, J. G. (1996). *Color textbook of pediatric dermatology* (2nd ed.). St. Louis: Mosby–Year Book.

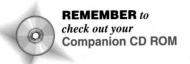

REMEMBER *to*
check out your
Companion CD ROM

CHAPTER

49

Management of Clients with Integumentary Disorders

Noreen Heer Nicol
Joyce M. Black

NURSING OUTCOMES CLASSIFICATION (NOC)
for Nursing Diagnoses—Clients with Integumentary Disorders

Altered Tissue Perfusion: Peripheral
Sensory Function: Cutaneous
Tissue Perfusion: Peripheral
Anxiety
Aggression Control
Anxiety Control
Coping
Impulse Control
Self-Mutilation Restraint
Social Interaction Skills
Body Image Disturbances
Body Image
Grief Resolution
Psychosocial Adjustment: Life Change
Self-Esteem
Chronic Low Self-Esteem
Self-Esteem
Fear
Fear Control

Impaired Skin Integrity
Tissue Integrity: Skin and Mucous
  Membranes
Wound Healing: Primary Intention
Wound Healing: Secondary Intention
Pain
Comfort Level
Pain Control
Pain: Disruptive Effects
Pain Level
Risk for Infection
Immobility Consequences: Physiologic
Immune Status
Immunization Behavior
Knowledge: Infection Control
Risk Control
Risk Detection
Risk for Impaired Skin Integrity
Immobility Consequences: Physiologic

Nutritional Status
Nutritional Status: Biochemical Measures
Physical Aging Status
Risk Detection
Tissue Integrity: Skin and Mucous
  Membranes
Wound Healing: Primary Intention
Wound Healing: Secondary Intention
Sleep Pattern Disturbance
Anxiety Control
Rest
Sleep
Well-Being
Ineffective Management of Therapeutic
Regimen: Individual
Compliance Behavior
Knowledge Treatment Regimen
Participation: Health Care Decisions
Treatment Behavior: Illness and Injury

The skin is the largest and most visible organ of the body. Thus, disorders of the skin offer the nurse an opportunity to provide care that makes a noticeable and rewarding difference to clients. Five primary dermatologic therapies—topical medications, wound dressings, soaks and wet wraps, skin lubricants, and ultraviolet light (UVL) therapy—are reviewed in this chapter. These therapies are the most common interventions provided by nurses for a variety of dermatologic conditions.

TOPICAL MEDICATIONS

■ TOPICAL THERAPY

The skin's large surface area allows the absorption, penetration, and permeation of topically applied preparations.

The factors that determine how well these processes occur include the client's age, the size of the affected region, the condition of the stratum corneum, the cutaneous blood supply, and the medication vehicle (the word *vehicle* is used here to mean the substance containing the medication or the form in which the medication is delivered).

Topical therapy can be used to:

- Restore hydration
- Alleviate clinical manifestations
- Reduce inflammation
- Protect the skin
- Reduce scale and callus
- Clean and debride
- Eradicate causative organisms

Topical medications are chosen both for the action of the active ingredients (which are delivered directly to the skin surface) and for the vehicle. Topical medications have many different actions and cover a large spectrum of drug categories, including anti-infective, corticosteroid, and antipruritic (Table 49–1).

■ TOPICAL VEHICLES

Examples of various topical medication vehicles (Table 49–2) are ointments, creams, gels, aerosols, lotions, solutions, and powders. Ointments are more occlusive and therefore provide better delivery of the medication by preventing water loss from the skin. However, in some cases, especially under conditions of excessive heat or humidity, this occlusion may result in increased itching or skin infection; in such cases, creams may be better tolerated. Although creams spread more easily than ointments,

they are less occlusive, leading to increased skin drying in some people. Sprays and lotions are available for use on the scalp and other hairy areas. The various ingredients used to formulate the different bases may be irritating to the skin, and care must be taken in recommending any product.

Both the active ingredient and the vehicle must be appropriate for the condition being treated. For acute dermatosis (i.e., weeping, blistering lesions), an aqueous (water-based) compound provides a drying effect. A greasy vehicle has the opposite effect; it promotes lubrication and occlusion and helps treat the dryness and scaling caused by chronic dermatosis. Differences in skin permeability also influence the effectiveness of topical medications. For example, absorption is increased in inflamed skin. Depending on the medication and the specific condition, topical medication may be applied to localized lesions or to larger skin

TABLE 49–1	NURSING IMPLICATIONS FOR MEDICATIONS USED TO TREAT SKIN DISORDERS		
Class (Example)	**Assessing Therapeutic Responses**	**Assessing Adverse Responses**	**Nursing Implications**
Corticosteroids Triamcinolone (Kenalog)	Inflamed areas should become less red, painful, and swollen	Assess for thinning of skin and delayed healing	Apply evenly over skin Use with caution in clients with systemic bacterial, fungal, or viral infections May be applied to hydrated skin to increase penetration
Antipruritics *Wet Dressings* Potassium permanganate 1:4000–1:16,000) Aluminum acetate Burow's solution (1:10–1:40) Boric acid (1 tbsp in 1 L of water) Normal saline (2 tsp salt in 1 L of water) Magnesium sulfate (8 tsp in 1 L of water)	Pruritic areas should become less "itchy," and evidence of scratching should decrease	Assess for allergy or contact sensitivity to substances	Use in bathtub for full body immersion or on dressings for local use Use caution in tub bathing; solutions are slippery Protect linens from stains when wet dressings are used
Topical Lotions Calamine lotion			Apply frequently unless solution contains anesthetic agents; then apply as directed
Anti-infectives Bacitracin and polymyxin B (Polysporin)	Reduce or eliminate bacterial infection	Superinfection Allergic reaction	Remove adherent crust before applying Apply 1–4 times/day
Nystatin (Mycostatin)	Reduce or eliminate fungal infection	Nausea, vomiting, diarrhea	Requires twice-daily application for 2–3 wk
Lindane (Kwell)	Eradicate scabies and pediculosis	Vomiting, restlessness, ataxia, seizures Observe for reinfestation	Treat webs of fingers and toes Avoid eyes Full course of treatment must be completed
Benzoyl peroxide	Decreased number of anaerobic bacteria and free fatty acids in sebaceous follicles	Extreme dryness, redness, or scaling	Apply once or twice daily after washing Apply sparingly Improvement should occur in 2 weeks

TABLE 49–2	TOPICAL MEDICATION VEHICLES			
Category	**Examples**	**Action**	**Use**	**Nursing Implications**
Powders	Talc, cornstarch	Leaves a film of powder May absorb fluid	Intertriginous dermatitis	Dry surface before applying to prevent caking; reapply often
Lotions				
Suspension-based	Calamine lotion	Leaves a thin film of powder as water evaporates	Pruritus	Shake lotions well before applying Observe for overdrying of skin Apply in long, even strokes along direction of hair growth
Solutions	Salicylic acid	Leaves a film of powder as alcohol base evaporates	Warts, acne	Shake well before applying; observe for skin overdrying and drying and tightness of skin due to alcohol Apply as for suspension
Aerosols	Triamcinolone acetonide aerosol	Leaves a thin film after alcohol evaporates	Pruritus, when direct application is painful	Shake well before applying; prevent inhalation by turning client's face to the side
Gels	Fluocinonide gel	Promotes drying of the skin	Eczema Pruritic rash	Observe for skin drying; avoid application to open skin areas
Creams	Hydrocortisone cream Eucerin	Leaves medication on skin after evaporation	Pruritus Eczema	Apply in thin layer along direction of hair growth Use during daytime Reapply often because perspiration or drainage may remove preparation
Ointments	Hydrocortisone ointment			
Water-in-oil	—	Lubricates skin	Xerosis Dermatitis	Removable with soap and water
Absorbent	Aquaphor	Lubricates skin	Xerosis, dermatitis	Difficult to remove; may feel greasy
Water-repellent	Petrolatum	Promotes absorption of water and medication	Xerosis, dermatitis	Retains heat, difficult to remove; observe for maceration; avoid use in hair-bearing areas

surfaces. When increased absorption of the medication is needed, topical medication may be prescribed for application under an occlusive dressing (Table 49–3). Ointments, creams, and gels have greatly increased absorption if they are applied to skin that is wet.

■ TOPICAL CORTICOSTEROIDS

Corticosteroids are among the most commonly used topical medications for treatment of a variety of dermatologic conditions. Corticosteroids can also be injected directly

TABLE 49–3	OCCLUSIVE DRESSINGS FOR INCREASED ABSORPTION OF MEDICATION
Purpose/Desired Effect	**Nursing Implications**
Produces airtight barrier, usually with plastic film Enhances absorption of topically applied medication (e.g., corticosteroids, keratolytics) by preventing evaporation Increases stratum corneum rehydration Softens hyperkeratotic areas by moisture retention	Clean skin site of debris and "old" medication before applying prescribed topical medication Apply topical medication while skin is still damp Apply plastic film (e.g., Saran wrap) snugly Use plastic bags for feet, polyethylene gloves for hands, plastic shower cap for scalp Press air out; seal borders with paper tape Leave dressing intact for 2–12 hr (as prescribed); then remove and gently cleanse the site Observe and document complications—maceration, oozing, signs of secondary fungal or bacterial infection, folliculitis With prolonged use in conjunction with topical corticosteroids, striae, nonhealing ulcerations, telangiectases, erythema, and skin atrophy may develop

into the lesion or given systemically. Attempts to diagnose the condition before any corticosteroid use are important because the effects of the medication can mask or change the clinical manifestations. Topical corticosteroids reduce inflammation by relieving itching, by reducing blood flow via vasoconstriction, which reduces redness of the skin from capillary dilation (erythema), and by interfering with the action of inflammatory cells.

A large selection of topical steroids, ranging in potency from low to high, is available today. Low-potency topical steroids are now available in over-the-counter (OTC) formulations (e.g., hydrocortisone, 0.5% or 1.0%) and in prescription strength (e.g., desonide, alclometasone). Generally, low-potency steroids are safe to use for longer periods of time and even on thin-skinned areas like the face, groin, or axilla. Prolonged use should still be monitored. Medium-potency (e.g., triamcinolone, fluocinolone) to high-potency (e.g., halcinonide, fluocinonide) corticosteroids should be used with caution and for short periods of time and not on the face, groin, or axilla. High-potency or superhigh-potency (e.g., betamethasone dipropionate, clobestasol) steroids should be reserved for use on very acute or resistant dermatoses (e.g., contact dermatitis) or areas with thick plaque such as in psoriasis.

Clients should know the strength of the topical steroid they are taking and its potential side effects. The lowest-potency corticosteroid that is effective should be used. Side effects are more likely with prolonged use of medium-potency to high-potency topical corticosteroids. The most common side effect is skin atrophy, which presents as thin, shiny skin with increased prominence of blood vessels, telangiectases, easy bruising, and striae.

Clients must clearly understand how, when, and where to use topical steroids. Properly applying the medication evenly and sparingly once or twice daily to the affected areas can eliminate many potential problems. It is rarely helpful to apply the topical corticosteroid more than twice a day. More frequent application increases the chance of side effects, makes the therapy more costly, and does not usually increase effectiveness. As the skin disorder resolves, the frequency of use may be changed or a less potent topical corticosteroid prescribed. The condition can recur if treatment is stopped abruptly. When the skin disease disappears or comes under good control, a tar preparation, moisturizer, or other topical preparation may be substituted for the topical steroid.

WOUND DRESSINGS

Application of wound dressings allows control of the affected skin's environment and remains important in the treatment of wounds, ulcers, and recalcitrant dermatitis. Historically, the primary role of wound dressings has been protection. Today, the role of dressings is to create an environment that promotes healing (see Table 49–3). Dressings limit the exposure of injured skin to dirt, mechanical trauma, and irritants. Ulcers and denuded skin heal more quickly when kept damp by an occlusive or semi-occlusive dressing because regenerating epithelium migrates more easily across a moist surface. These wounds are also less painful when kept damp, and absorption of topical medications is enhanced.

The clinician is challenged to understand the properties of the hundreds of wound care dressings on the market. Wound dressing materials include film, hydrocolloid, hydrogel, foam, alginates, and gauze, among others (see Table 49–3).

■ UNNA BOOT

The Unna boot, a dressing designed to be removed only by medical personnel at a later clinical visit, can be extremely useful for treatment of stasis ulcers in clients who have venous insufficiency or in whom there is a concern about compliance, scratching, or even self-injury. The Unna boot is a fixed, protective dressing applied to the foot and ankle that stimulates granulation tissue and restores epithelial growth. It is made from dressing materials impregnated with zinc oxide paste, glycerin, and gelatin, which harden into a cast-like "boot" after application. The "boot" protects the skin from mechanical injury, promoting venous return.

Before application, the damaged skin surface is gently irrigated with warm saline to remove previous medication and debris. The damaged skin area is then measured and assessed. Prescribed topical agents (i.e., antibiotic ointments) may be applied. Next, starting at the dorsum of the foot, the dressing is applied. It is wrapped obliquely over the heel and up the calf. The greatest pressure is applied at the ankle and over the lower third of the leg. The boot ends just below the popliteal space. A layer of tube gauze is applied over the dressing. For additional support, an elastic bandage is secured appropriately with tape. The Unna boot is usually removed weekly so that damaged skin can be assessed and normal skin cleaned.

Ideally, with all wound dressings, the area of damaged skin decreases, granulation tissue forms, and signs of inflammation are reduced. Treatment may continue for weeks until improvement occurs. Instruct the client and family numbers to keep the dressing intact and to notify the primary health care provider if there is excessive drainage or localized pain (signs of infection). Routine follow-up examination is very important in wound care.

SOAKS AND WET WRAPS

Soaks serve several purposes. Moisture softens dry epidermis, which aids in removal of crusts. Removal of cellular skin debris promotes healing and improves absorption of topical medication. The risk of infection is reduced by removal of necrotic tissue and occlusive crusts. Cooling also results from the gradual evaporation of water and has an anti-inflammatory effect, thus relieving itching (pruritus).

Soaks can be accomplished by either soaking the affected area or bathing for 15 to 20 minutes in warm—not hot—tap water. The agent added to the soaks is the least important aspect of this therapy. Addition of substances such as colloidal oatmeal (Aveeno) or starch to the bath water may be soothing for some people but does nothing to increase water absorption. Coal tar preparations (Balnetar, T/Derm) have an anti-inflammatory effect and can be helpful in some eczematous and psoriatic conditions. Aluminum acetate (Burow solution), aluminum sulfate and calcium acetate (Domeboro), and povidone-iodine (Betadine) are also effective antibacterial substances; however, they have drying effects. Bath oils are not recommended because they give the client a false sense of lubrication and make the bathtub very slippery.

After bathing, clients should remove excess water by gently patting the skin with a soft towel. Then they should immediately apply the recommended occlusive substance. Immediate application of this substance to damp skin is the most important detail, because if the occlusive barrier is not provided within 3 to 5 minutes, evaporation begins to occur.

Wet wraps used immediately after soaking and occlusion can optimize hydration and topical therapy; this also promotes cooling of the skin. Wet wraps and occlusion can be applied in various ways. The location and severity of lesions often determine the choices. Total-body wet wraps can be accomplished by putting on wet pajamas or wet long underwear followed by dry pajamas or a dry or plastic sweat suit. The hands and feet can be covered with wet tube socks or wet cotton gloves followed by dry tube socks. Any extremity or the trunk can be covered with wet rolled (e.g., Kerlix) gauze and occluded with elastic bandages or by pieces of tube sock, wet followed by dry. The face can be wrapped with two layers of wet Kerlix gauze, followed by two layers of dry Kerlix gauze held in place with elasticized netting or other tubular dressings; holes are cut out for the eyes, nose, and mouth (Fig. 49–1). If the dressing becomes dry, it should be rewetted before removal because debridement by the wet-to-dry method produces tissue damage and pain. Gentle debridement usually still occurs if dressings are removed when damp.

Skin Lubricants

Agents to hydrate the skin play an important role in many xerotic, pruritic, and inflammatory skin disorders. Measures to prevent skin dryness include elimination of

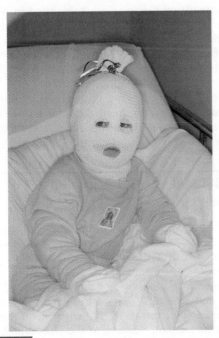

FIGURE 49–1 Wet wraps applied to the entire body.

irritating or drying compounds, which may include *soaps* and *solvents,* and use of *cleansing agents* and *moisturizers.* Moisturizers may be classified as follows:

1. *Occlusive* preparations are extremely effective when applied to damp skin because they prevent evaporative water loss and replace oils in the stratum corneum. The primary means of correcting dryness is to add water to the skin by bathing and then apply an occlusive substance to retain the absorbed water. To seal in the water, use occlusives such as white petrolatum (Vaseline) or petrolatum with mineral oil and wool wax alcohol (Aquaphor ointment). Occlusives are greasy and may be cosmetically unacceptable to some people.

2. *Emollients* contain fatty acids, oil, and other agents that soften and soothe the skin. There are many emollients available in the form of creams and lotions. Creams contain less water than lotions and therefore evaporate less quickly and provide more skin hydration. Clients often prefer these cosmetically pleasing products because they can be rubbed into the skin without leaving a greasy residue. Although the chemicals in these lotions provide benefit, the water loss continues. Lotions and creams may be irritating and drying because of the evaporative property of water and the substances used as preservatives, solubilizers, and fragrances.

3. If emollient products are not successful, more potent agents may be necessary. *Humectants* are substances such as urea (Aquacare 10%, Carmol 20% to 40%) that attract and hold water, which results in transepidermal water migration, and they have a concentration-dependent desquamation action. Ammonium lactate (Lactydrin) is also an effective keratolytic which moisturizes and thickens the stratum corneum. The alpha-hydroxy acids (AHAs) have become extremely popular and effective additives; these hold moisture and reduce the rough scale that creates the sensation of dryness. The AHAs are naturally derived organic acids and include citric acid, glycolic acid, malic acid, and tartaric acid. Many of the AHAs have been used for years; the industry has invested in reformulating and promoting these products. Also popular with clients are additives such as aloe, vitamin E, jojoba, elastin, and collagen; however, no scientific evidence has shown that these substances have special, intrinsic properties beyond their minimal lubricating effects. Clients should be taught the basic principles of hydration and moisturization to avoid spending unnecessarily high prices for any needed products.

Ultraviolet Light Therapy

Artificially reproduced forms of ultraviolet light (UVL) are used therapeutically with topical or systemic photosensitizing drugs to cause desquamation (shedding or peeling of the epidermis). UVL also temporarily suppresses mitosis of the basal cell layer by inhibiting deoxyribonucleic acid (DNA) mitosis. Ultraviolet A (UVA) light and ultraviolet B (UVB) light are used to treat diseases responsive to UVL, such as psoriasis, vitiligo, cutaneous T-cell lymphoma, uremic pruritus, and chronic eczematous eruptions. At present, three treatment modalities involve UVL: (1) UVA; (2) UVB, in the Goeckerman or modified Goeckerman regimen; and (3) photochemotherapy, or PUVA (psoralen plus UVA). Many of these regimens are given two or three times a week initially, and the frequency is then decreased to two to four times per month.

Obtain a complete history and physical examination in every client before initiation of any UVL therapy. Record the highlights of the client's history; take care to include the complete medication history, because the client may be taking one or more of the many photosensitizing drugs (e.g., thiazide diuretics, tetracyclines). Ask clients specifically about previous herpes simplex infections, which can be stimulated by UVL. Pre-treatment assessment includes identifying solar energy–induced skin malignancies, cataracts, or lupus erythematosus and any additional photosensitive skin changes. Clients with a history of basal cell or squamous cell epithelioma are at risk for additional neoplastic changes with this treatment. Thus, potential benefit is weighed against potential risk.

A complete ophthalmologic examination before treatment begins is important and should be performed yearly during long-term treatment. A history of cataract formation is a potential contraindication to PUVA therapy. Clients who exhibit early cataract changes need extra photoprotective measures (e.g., the complete occlusion provided by goggles or PUVA glasses) and more frequent ophthalmologic assessments (every 3 to 6 months). The skin changes of lupus erythematosus are worsened by sun exposure, and phototherapy is thus contraindicated. Before therapy is initiated, an antinuclear antibody (ANA) test should rule out this condition when suspected.

Be aware that because treatments to the face and genitalia add to the cumulative effects of UVL, minimal exposure is indicated. Periodic assessments must be done throughout the course of therapy for signs of actinic damage (e.g., severe wrinkling, "tissue paper" transparency) or cutaneous malignancy. After completion of therapy, clients must be observed for potential side effects including dry skin, pruritus, and potential delayed (36 to 48 hours after exposure) phototoxic reaction (erythema, vesicles, and pain). All phototherapy should be administered by qualified and well-trained dermatologic personnel. Use of home UVL equipment and tanning salons should be considered only when the client has no access to qualified dermatologic personnel. Numerous risks are associated with home and salon therapy.

■ ULTRAVIOLET B THERAPY

UVB therapy requires no oral medications and is usually the first-line UVL therapy used before progression to PUVA. Types of UVB therapy include (1) plain UVB treatment, (2) UVB with topical tar and topical anthralin, the *Ingram method,* and (3) UVB with topical tar, referred to as the Goeckerman treatment or regimen.

One of the most common types of UVB therapy is the *Goeckerman regimen* and variants of it. The photosensitizing, keratoplastic, and antipruritic properties of topical tar preparations are used in conjunction with UVL in UVB wavelengths. This method is often used to treat psoriasis vulgaris and atopic dermatitis. The regimen includes a therapeutic tar emulsion bath, followed by an application of topical tar medication (e.g., crude coal tar in petrolatum). Several hours later, a specific dose of UVL is administered to the skin surface. If the skin condition is severe, hospitalization or daily care in an ambulatory or day care setting may be necessary for this treatment. Outpatient phototherapy, combined with treatment baths and tar applications at home, can be helpful for clients with less severe involvement.

■ PHOTOCHEMOTHERAPY

Photochemotherapy (PUVA) combines oral or topical 8-methoxypsoralen with UVA. PUVA is used to treat severe, unresponsive forms of psoriasis, atopic dermatitis, cutaneous T-cell lymphoma, and alopecia areata or vitiligo. The potent systemic photosensitizing medications used in PUVA increase skin sensitivity to long-wave UVL (UVA). In conjunction with exposure to artificially reproduced forms of UVA light, these medications induce repigmentation (melanin production) in vitiligo and have an antimitotic effect in psoriasis and cutaneous T-cell lymphoma.

Dosage is determined by body weight. The medication is taken orally with food to minimize nausea 1 to 2 hours before UVL irradiation. Topical medication is used to treat localized sites and for clients in whom systemic administration is contraindicated (such as clients with liver or renal disease).

The skin must be protected from ambient UVL irradiation before and for 8 hours after taking the photosensitizing medication. The client should (1) wear protective clothing, such as long sleeves, (2) apply sunscreen to exposed skin, (3) minimize natural skin exposure, and (4) wear dark green or brown plastic sunglasses that can screen both UVA and UVB to protect the eyes for 48 hours after taking the medication.

■ COMBINATION THERAPIES

Many combination therapies are being used in phototherapy units across the United States. These include PUVA with various topical medications, PUVA with retinoid therapy (RE-PUVA), PUVA with methotrexate, PUVA with cyclosporine, PUVA with UVB therapy, UVB therapy with retinoids, and UVB with methotrexate. The purpose of combination therapy is to accelerate clearing of lesions and to reduce the total cumulative dose of UVL. These therapies should be administered according to protocol and by highly qualified dermatologic personnel.

PSYCHOSOCIAL ASPECTS OF SKIN DISORDERS

Anger, frustration, and anxiety are commonly experienced by clients with skin disorders, which often exacerbates the condition. Clients with skin disease are more likely to respond to stress, frustration, embarrassment, or any emotionally upsetting event with itching and scratching. Excitability and arousal of the central nervous system from an emotional upset can intensify the vasomotor and sweat responses in the skin, leading to the *itch-scratch-itch cy-*

cle (see Pruritus). In some instances, scratching is used as an expression of anger, because typically it will get an immediate response from those nearby. The added dimension of family hostility, rejection, and guilt can damage the family structure.

Learning about the acute or chronic nature of the given disorder, the exacerbating factors, and the management measures that can control it is important for both the client and family members. Maintaining a healthy outlook is important. Counseling and other psychosocial interventions are often helpful in dealing with the frustrations of skin disease, especially for adolescents and young adults, who may consider the lesions disfiguring.

The educational needs of people affected by skin disease are vast. Health care providers need to consistently provide information that includes detailed skin care plans, general disease information, and availability of client-ori-ented support organizations as well as updates on encouraging research results. Clients tend to forget or confuse the important skin care recommendations without written instructions. Clearly outlining the skin care recommendations orally and in writing is essential for good outcomes.

The accompanying Client Education Guide provides information about skin self-examination. Nurses play the major role in providing this important aspect of care. Adequate time and client teaching materials are needed to provide education effectively. Be resourceful in obtaining or writing educational materials and instruction sheets. Client education pamphlets are available through a variety of sources, including the many dermatologically oriented client support groups and professional dermatology agencies such as the Dermatology Nurses' Association and the American Academy of Dermatology.

CLIENT EDUCATION GUIDE

Skin Self-Examination

You will need a bright light; a full-length mirror; a hand mirror; two chairs or stools; a blow dryer; body maps; and a pencil.

A. Examine your face—especially the nose, lips, mouth, and ears—front and back. Use one or both mirrors to get a clear view.

B. Thoroughly inspect your scalp, using a blow dryer and mirror to expose each section to view. Get a friend or family member to help, if you can.

C. Check your hands carefully: palms and backs, between the fingers, and under the fingernails. Continue up the wrists to examine both the front and back of your forearms.

D. Standing in front of the full-length mirror, begin at the elbows and scan all sides of your upper arms. Do not forget the underarms.

E. Next, focus on the neck, chest, and torso. Women should lift breasts to view the underside.

F. With your back to the full-length mirror, use the hand mirror to inspect the back of your neck, shoulders, upper back, and any part of the back of your upper arms you could not view previously.

G. Still using both mirrors, scan your lower back, buttocks, and backs of both legs.

H. Sit down; prop each leg in turn on the other stool or chair. Use the hand mirror to examine the genitals. Check front and sides of both legs, thigh to shin; ankles; and tops of feet, between toes, and under toenails. Examine soles of the feet and the heels.

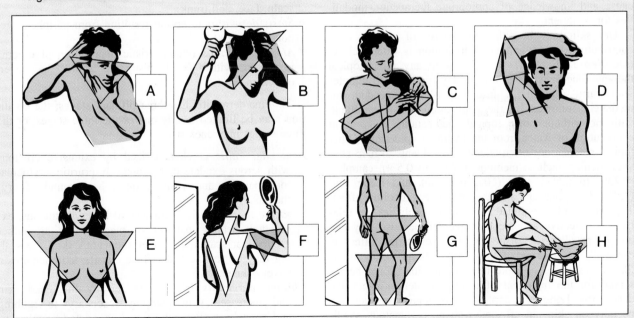

From The Skin Cancer Foundation (1992). *Skin cancer. If you can spot it, you can stop it.* New York: Author.

COMMON SKIN DISORDERS

PRURITUS

Pruritus (itching), one of the most common manifestations of skin problems, is a symptom, not a disease. It has been defined as an unpleasant skin sensation, resulting in a strong desire to scratch, localized to or generalized over a body area. Pruritus can lead to damage if scratching injures the skin's protective barrier, with possible resultant infection and scarring. Relieving this symptom, especially for chronically ill clients, is a nursing challenge because of its common occurrence and the major effect it may have on quality of life.

Pruritus can be a secondary clinical manifestation of conditions ranging from dry skin to cancer. Systemic diseases that can cause generalized and severe pruritus include chickenpox, liver failure, diabetes mellitus, uremia, drug hypersensitivity reaction, intestinal parasites, leukemia, and lymphoma.

Stimulation of itching can be initiated by almost any chemical or physical substance, especially if skin is damaged. Once the itch sensation is established, the client has an almost uncontrollable urge to scratch. Scratching leads to further skin damage and increased inflammation. Pruritus therefore worsens, and the urge to scratch is also intensified. Thus, the itch-scratch-itch cycle develops. To minimize skin trauma caused by scratching, clients should keep fingernails short.

The client usually volunteers subjective reports of the degree and location of itching. Listen carefully to the client's description of the severity and location of pruritus, and seek information about how pruritus interferes with activities of daily living. Objective signs include excoriations and other secondary skin changes such as lichenification. Document all assessment findings.

Appropriate management of itching requires a complete assessment that attempts to discover the underlying cause and knowledge of appropriate therapeutic modalities for treatment.

Dry skin may be either the source of pruritus or a contributing factor, and good hydration is often helpful (see Xerotic Eczema), in addition to any other topical therapy. One bath or shower per day for 15 to 20 minutes with warm water and a mild soap is recommended, immediately followed by the application of an emollient, with or without other topical medications, to prevent evaporation of water from the hydrated epidermis. Other topical medications often added to emollients to help alleviate itching include menthol (0.25% to 0.5%), camphor (0.25% to 0.5%), urea (10% to 20%), and lactic acid (12%). Camphor and menthol produce a cooling effect. Topically applied antihistamines and anesthetics are relatively ineffective and are best avoided because they can be potent allergic sensitizers. The sensitizing effect is especially pronounced if these products are used on inflamed skin. Use of topical corticosteroids should be reserved for the treatment of a specific steroid-responsive dermatosis. Long-term application of topical steroids, especially on skin not affected with an eczematous condition, may result in thinning of the skin, striae, telangiectases, and easy bruising.

Systemic antihistaminic agents are most helpful in disorders in which histamine is the principal mediator but may be of benefit through a sedative or even placebo effect. A trial of a histamine$_1$ (H$_1$) blocker (hydroxyzine, diphenhydramine, chlorpheniramine) is appropriate either on a regular schedule or as indicated for itching. Tricyclic antidepressants (TCAs) (doxepin HCl, amitriptyline HCl) have a high binding capacity for H$_1$ receptors and may be helpful in clients who would benefit from their antidepressant as well as antipruritic effect.

Older clients may have difficulty in following through with frequent bathing or showering because of decreased mobility. In such clients, when hydration cannot precede the application of moisturizers, more frequent application and use of more hydrating products may be needed. In addition, elderly people may have difficulty applying the needed topical agents properly, and assistive personnel may be required to ensure proper therapy. Antihistaminics should be administered carefully, with use of small doses initially, because many older people have a very low tolerance of these agents and may experience severe drowsiness, especially at the initiation of therapy.

ECZEMATOUS DISORDERS

Eczema is not a specific disease. *Dermatitis* and eczema are terms that may be used interchangeably to describe a group of disorders with a characteristic clinical appearance. Some examples of eczema or dermatitis are:

- *Allergic contact dermatitis* (eruptions from allergy to poison ivy, sumac, or oak or a proven allergen)
- *Irritant dermatitis* (eruption from direct contact with irritating substances such as cosmetics, chemicals, dyes, or detergents)
- *Nummular eczema* (appearance of coin-shaped, oozing, crusting patches)
- *Seborrheic dermatitis* (yellowish pink scaling of the scalp, face, and trunk)
- *Stasis dermatitis* (eruption resulting from peripheral venous disorders)
- *Atopic dermatitis* (characteristic distribution of eczema in persons with a family history of asthma, hay fever, or eczema)

Eczema/dermatitis has three primary stages; the condition may be limited to any one of the three stages, or the three stages may coexist.

Acute dermatitis is characterized by extensive erosions with serous exudate or by intensely pruritic, erythematous papules and vesicles on a background of erythema.

Subacute dermatitis is characterized by erythematous, excoriated, scaling papules or plaques that are either grouped or scattered over erythematous skin; the scaling may be so fine and diffuse that the skin acquires a silvery sheen.

Chronic dermatitis is characterized by thickened skin and increased skin marking secondary to rubbing and scratching (lichenification); excoriated papules, fibrotic papules, and nodules (prurigo nodularis); and postinflammatory hyperpigmentation and hypopigmentation.

■ ATOPIC DERMATITIS

Atopic dermatitis is a common, chronic, relapsing, pruritic type of eczema. The word "atopic" refers to a group of three associated allergic disorders: asthma, allergic rhinitis (hay fever), and atopic dermatitis.

Etiology

According to several studies, 75% to 80% of clients with atopic dermatitis have a personal or family history of asthma, hay fever, eczema, or food allergies. Atopic dermatitis is a common disorder, affecting 10% to 20% of children in the United States. The cause is unknown.

Pathophysiology

It is clear that an immune dysfunction exists in clients with atopic dermatitis, but whether the dysfunction is the cause or the effect of the disorder is still unclear. Altered $CD4^+$ T-helper cells produce interleukins which stimulate IgE. Mast cells release histamine and tumor necrosis factor (TNF). Compared with normal skin, the dry skin of atopic dermatitis has reduced water-binding capacity, higher rate of transepidermal water loss, and decreased water content.[73] Water loss leads to further drying and cracking of the skin, which leads to more itching. Rubbing and scratching of itchy skin are responsible for many of the changes seen in the skin.

Clinical Manifestations

Atopic dermatitis begins in many clients during infancy. The dermatitis is usually of acute onset, with a red, oozing, crusting rash. Over time, the skin tends to show the chronic form of dermatitis, with thickened dry texture, brownish-gray color, and scales. The rash tends to become localized to the large folds of the extremities as the client becomes older (Fig. 49–2). It is found mainly on elbow bends, the backs of the knees, the neck, the eyelids, and the backs of the hands and feet. Hand and foot dermatitis becomes a significant problem in some adults.

Pruritus is the major clinical manifestation of atopic

ALTERNATIVE THERAPY

Integumentary Disorders

The management of skin disorders is often difficult. Nutritional and herbal approaches to the treatment of skin problems have been shown to be effective for some disorders, often with fewer side effects than with conventional methods.

In a general article on atopic dermatitis, commonly known as eczema, naturopathic physician Michael Murray touches on a number of possible causes and treatments of this chronic condition.[4] He cites evidence that food allergies may be the culprit, at least in some people. Commonly, milk, eggs, and peanuts may be the offending foods. Food allergy tests using a small sample of blood, such as the enzyme-linked immunosorbent assay (ELISA) and immunoglobulin E (IgE) and IgG tests, are now available. These tests expose the blood sample to food antigens to determine reactivity to foods. Controversial but of interest, breast-feeding of infants may be preventive for atopic dermatitis and allergies in general. Breast-fed infants who developed eczema due to food allergy experienced relief of manifestations when the mothers refrained from eating specific foods.

Another nutritional issue is the ratio of omega-3 to omega-6 fatty acids in the diet. This ratio appears to be lower in people who have eczema. Supplementation with fish and/or flaxseed oils or consumption of coldwater fish may therefore be of benefit in the treatment of eczema.

Chinese herbs have long been used in Asian countries for the treatment of skin diseases. A landmark study done in England showed the effectiveness of Chinese herbs in treating atopic dermatitis.[5] This study was undertaken after dermatologists were impressed by the results seen in their patients who were also under the care of a Chinese herbalist. Participants in the study who received the active herbal formula reported decreases in the number of lesions and itching as well as improved sleep.

A traditional Australian plant remedy, tea tree oil (from *Melaleuca alternifolia*), has been shown to be effective in the treatment of acne.[1] In a single-blind, randomized study, topical tea tree oil was compared with topical benzoyl peroxide (both in a 5% solution). Although both treatments produced significant improvement after three months of daily application, the frequency of side effects such as dryness, burning, and skin redness was 44% with the tea tree oil and 79% with benzoyl peroxide.

A topical mixture of the essential plant oils of thyme, rosemary, lavender, and cedarwood, in a carrier of jojoba and grapeseed oils, was found to have significant effect in the treatment of alopecia areata.[3] This treatment was called "aromatherapy" in the study because such oils are commonly used in aromatherapy, but topical use of the preparation might be better regarded as a medicinal herbal application. Forty-four per cent of the subjects in the essential oil treatment group improved, compared with 15% of those in the placebo group.

In a 1998 published report from Taiwan,[2] acupuncture was stated to be effective in the treatment of urticaria (hives). Although the authors noted a lack of controlled studies in this area, they proposed that the improvement frequently observed clinically with use of this modality warrants consideration of acupuncture in the treatment of both acute and chronic urticaria.

References

1. Bassett, I. B., Pannowitz, D. L., & Barnetson, R. St. C. (1990). A comparative study of tea-tree oil versus benzoyl peroxide in the treatment of acne. *Medical Journal of Australia, 153,* 455–458.
2. Chen, C. J., & Yu, H. S. (1998). Acupuncture treatment of urticaria. *Archives of Dermatology, 134,* 1397–1399.
3. Hay, I. C., Jamieson, S. R. N., & Ormerod, A. D. (1998). Randomized trial of aromatherapy: Successful treatment for alopecia areata. *Archives of Dermatology, 134,* 1349–1352.
4. Murray, M. T. (1999). Atopic dermatitis (eczema). *Natural Medicine Journal, 2*(4), 1–6.
5. Sheehan, M. P., et al. (1998). Efficacy of traditional Chinese herbal therapy in adult atopic dermatitis. *Lancet, 340,* 13–17.

James Higgy Lerner, RN, LAc, *Private practice of acupuncture, traditional Oriental medicine, and feedback*

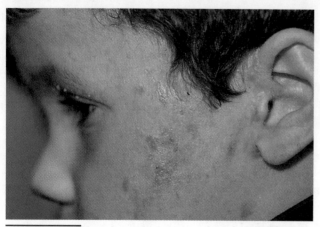

FIGURE 49–2 Atopic dermatitis. Intense pruritus leading to scratching and open lesions.

dermatitis and causes the greatest morbidity. The condition may be mild and self-limiting, or it may be intense, provoking scratching that results in severely excoriated lesions, infection, and scarring.

Complications

Clients with atopic dermatitis tend to experience viral, bacterial, and fungal skin infections. It is not clear whether these cutaneous infections arise secondary to a disruption of normal barrier function or are due to reduced local immunity. The most common viral infection is herpes simplex, which tends to spread locally or become generalized. Honey-colored crusting, extensive serous weeping, folliculitis, pyoderma, and furunculosis indicate bacterial infection, usually secondary to *Staphylococcus aureus* in clients with atopic dermatitis. Clients with atopic dermatitis are frequently heavily colonized with *S. aureus.* Superficial fungal infections may also appear more frequently.

Outcome Management

The goal of therapy is to break the inflammatory cycle that causes excess drying and cracking as well as the itching and scratching.[34] The health care team's understanding of each client's disease pattern and the discovery and reduction of exacerbating factors are crucial to effective management of this chronic disorder.

◼ Medical Management

LUBRICATE THE SKIN
Hydration is the key to management but is often difficult to achieve. Management begins with daily skin care that hydrates and lubricates the skin. Soaks followed by application of occlusive substances are usually prescribed (see Soaks and Wet Wraps).

REMOVE ALLERGENS
Allergens, food, aeroallergens, and emotional stresses may be inciting factors in this disorder. Clients should avoid exposure to substances for which there is a positive result on allergy testing and which are suspected to precipitate dermatitis. Stringent restrictions on lifestyle and activities are unjustified. Air conditioning may help reduce aeroallergen exposure at home and in the workplace. It is important to identify and eliminate triggers that cause the atopic dermatitis to flare. Many of these triggering factors are the same irritants that contribute to generalized pruritus (see Pruritus).

Dietary management of atopic dermatitis has continued to be controversial. Food allergies in the causation of atopic dermatitis seem to be more significant in certain populations of young children and infants. The most common allergens appear to be eggs, cow's milk, soy, wheat, nuts, and fish. Known allergens are avoided. People with food allergies must be taught to read labels. Care must be taken to avoid malnutrition when any type of restrictive diet is used.

Occlusives, emollients, topical corticosteroids, and tar preparations all can be employed in various combinations to control atopic dermatitis. The use of topical steroids is an important component of therapy for eczema (see Topical Corticosteroids). These preparations are best absorbed into hydrated skin or by using wet wraps and occlusion. Topical agents containing chemicals or drugs with the potential to cause skin eruptions are avoided.

Systemic medications may include antibiotics and antihistaminics. The use of a systemic corticosteroid is rarely warranted in atopic dermatitis. Some clients view the systemic use of steroids as a "quick cure" and find these agents much easier to use than hydration and topical therapy. Systemic corticosteroids should be avoided in this chronic, non–life-threatening disorder. Although there may be dramatic improvement with their use, the recurrence of dermatitis after their discontinuation is equally dramatic. The side effects of long-term systemic steroid use are both unpleasant and dangerous.

If a short-term course of oral steroid therapy is given, it is important to taper the dosage as the drug is discontinued. Intensified skin care should also be instituted during the taper to suppress flaring of the dermatitis.

Various therapeutic approaches are becoming available. Results are promising with the use of the new immune response modifier tacrolimus for therapy of moderate to severe atopic dermatitis as well as with the use of cyclosporine and other experimental modalities. Clients with severe, recalcitrant disease should be made aware of research advances and encouraged to participate in trials, when possible, to give them a sense of hope.

◼ Nursing Management of the Medical Client

Assess the client with atopic dermatitis for bathing habits, use of moisturizers, medication regimen, exposure to known allergens, environmental exposure, and history of skin eruptions. Nursing management of the client with atopic dermatitis is presented in the accompanying Care Plan.

◼ Modifications for Elderly Clients

Dermatitis is a common skin disorder in the elderly population. It may be caused by venous insufficiency, allergens, irritants, or underlying malignancy such as leukemia or lymphoma. Because older adults often take many medications, the potential for dermatitis from drug-drug interactions is increased. The fragility of the skin as a result of the flattened epidermal-dermal junction and loss of dermis should be considered in planning any form of treatment.

■ THE CLIENT WITH ATOPIC DERMATITIS

Nursing Diagnosis. Impaired Skin Integrity related to skin dryness

Outcomes. The client will maintain skin that has good hydration and reduced inflammation, as evidenced by:

- Verbalizing increased skin comfort
- Decreased flaking and scaling
- Decreased redness
- Decreased excoriations from scratching
- Healing of previous areas of breakdown

Interventions

1. Bathe the client at least once every day, soaking for 15 to 20 minutes. Immediately upon leaving the bath, apply an appropriate emollient or prescribed topical agent. Bathe more often when clinical manifestations increase.
2. Use warm water.

3. Use superfatted soaps (e.g., Dove or Basis) or soaps for sensitive skin (e.g., Oil of Olay, Eucerin, Neutrogena, Vanicream, Aveeno, Oilatum, Cetaphil). Avoid bubble baths.
4. Apply occlusive topical emollient (e.g., Aquaphor ointment, cream (Eucerin) or lotion, Vanicream, Cetaphil cream or lotion) or prescribed topical preparation two or three times per day.

Rationales

1. Soaking saturates the stratum corneum. Application of an occlusive moisturizer 2 to 4 minutes after the bath is critical for preventing evaporation of water from the hydrated epidermis.
2. Hot water causes vasodilation, which may increase pruritus.
3. The use of drying soap may compound the problem. Superfatted soaps are less alkaline and less drying to the skin. "Sensitive skin" formulas are usually fragrance-free.

4. Ointments and creams seal in water and thereby hydrate the skin. The particular emollient selected depends mostly on client preference and whether the ingredients in the base are irritants.

Evaluation. Outcomes should be met in 48 to 96 hours, depending on severity of eczema, frequency of baths, and adequate application of appropriate occlusive topical agent. Evaluate skin as often as possible.

Collaborative Problem. Alteration in Comfort related to pruritus

Outcomes. The client will experience a decrease in pruritus, as evidenced by:

- Decrease in observed and reported scratching
- Decreased excoriations from scratching
- Decreased restlessness during sleep
- Verbalizing increased skin comfort

Interventions

1. Explain the itching symptom as it relates to cause (i.e., dryness of the skin) and the principles of the selected therapy (i.e., hydration) and the itch-scratch-itch cycle.
2. Wash all new clothes before wearing for removal of formaldehyde and other chemicals, and avoid use of fabric softeners.
3. Change to a milder detergent, and add a second rinse cycle to ensure removal of soap.

4. Wear open-weave, loose-fitting, cotton-blend clothing. Avoid overdressing, rough or wool fabrics, and tightly woven fabrics.
5. Work and sleep in comfortable surroundings with a fairly constant temperature (68° to 75° F) and humidity level (45% to 55%). Air conditioning in the home, particularly the bedroom, may be beneficial.
6. Keep fingernails short, smooth, and clean.
7. Appropriate use of oral antihistamines may reduce itching to some degree.

8. Use sunscreen on a regular basis.
9. Immediately after swimming, take a shower or bath, washing with a mild soap from head to toe, and then apply an appropriate moisturizer.

Rationales

1. Understanding the physiologic or psychological process and principles of itching and its treatment increases cooperation.
2. Pruritus is often precipitated by irritant or allergic effects of certain chemicals or components of fabric softeners.

3. Residual laundry detergent in clothing may be irritating. The actual laundry soap that is used is not the key; rather, all soap is rinsed out so that an irritant effect is avoided.
4. Light cotton-blend clothing allows air circulation and minimizes perspiration, which intensifies itching.

5. Extremes of temperature cause pruritus frequently secondary to vasodilation and increased cutaneous blood flow. In addition to providing a cooler environment, air conditioning decreases aeroallergen exposure.
6. Trimmed nails prevent damage and infection to the skin.
7. Histamine is one of the best-known itch mediators. The sedating antihistaminics also provide relief through tranquilizing effects.
8. Sunburn may cause flare of dermatitis.
9. Residual chlorine or bromine on the skin after swimming in a pool may be irritating.

Care Plan continued on following page

Evaluation. Outcomes may not be achieved for days or weeks after eczema has been brought under control. Itching can become a learned behavioral response brought on by many factors, which may need to be modified through counseling, oral medications, and maintenance of good skin care.

Nursing Diagnosis. Risk for Infection related to skin excoriation or decreased resistance to cutaneous viral, fungal, and staphylococcal organisms

Outcomes. The client will be free of infectious lesions, as evidenced by absence of pustules, exudate, or crusting.

Interventions	Rationales
1. Explain to the client the signs of infection, and be sure the client understands that the presence of these signs indicates need for medical intervention.	1. Infections are a potentially serious complication of disorders of open skin.
2. Ensure that the client understands the importance of not self-treating with leftover medication at home.	2. Leftover medications may be outdated and may be inappropriate treatment. Medications can become contaminated, leading to infection, or may lose their potency.
3. Emphasize the importance of taking the antibiotic on schedule over the entire course.	3. The entire course of medication will completely eradicate the infectious organism.

Evaluation. Outcomes are usually achieved with 7 to 10 days of oral antibiotic therapy. However, some clients require an extended course for complete clearing. Evaluation should be done no later than at 7 days after initiation of therapy.

Nursing Diagnosis. Body Image Disturbance related to skin lesions and/or response of significant others to appearance

Outcomes. The client will exhibit a positive self-concept, as evidenced by engaging in social activities, expressing feelings of importance and self-worth, and enjoying interpersonal interactions.

Interventions	Rationales
1. Encourage the client to teach others that eczema is not contagious unless the lesions are severely infected.	1. Eczema can be mistaken for impetigo or as an indication of uncleanliness, causing social isolation.
2. Encourage the client and significant others to share feelings with one another and professional counselors, as needed, regarding the client's appearance and the chronic nature of eczema.	2. Unidentified fears and concerns may hinder interpersonal relationships.
3. Reinforce the client's sense of identity and personal competence. Encourage self-management of eczema and the understanding that controlling scratching will greatly reduce lesions.	3. Allowing the client to determine the need for various treatment modalities, such as when to initiate wet wraps or minor alterations in topical therapy, promotes a positive self-concept.

Evaluation. Outcomes are totally dependent on the degree of negative self-concept, chronicity of this process, and the degree to which eczema can be controlled. Depending on the age and motivation of the client, outcomes can be reached in weeks, months, years, or—unfortunately for a small few—never. Professional intervention should be facilitated early.

■ XEROTIC ECZEMA

Xerotic (dry) skin is dehydrated. Xerotic eczema may present as erythematous, scaling, and finely cracked skin. Xerosis occurs in patches and may involve any skin surface. It is common in the elderly population. If xerosis is severe, the skin is tight, itchy, and painful. Water loss causes xerotic chapping. The problem may be accentuated by use of drying skin cleansers, soaps, disinfectants, and solvents and infrequent use of moisturizers. Environmental factors play a large role, especially those that increase water loss in the stratum corneum. Any factors that decrease the relative humidity exacerbate this condition, such as cold or dry winter air, especially in artificially heated rooms.

Management includes hydration and moisturizing the skin plus avoiding irritating factors. Teaching the client correct daily skin care is essential to treating this condition. See the earlier discussion on soaks and wet wraps and skin lubricants.

■ STASIS DERMATITIS

Stasis dermatitis is characterized by the development of areas of very dry skin and sometimes shallow ulcers on the lower legs, primarily as a result of venous insufficiency. The process of dermatitis begins with edema of the leg due to slowed venous return. The client commonly has a history of varicose veins or deep vein thrombosis. As the venous stasis continues, the tissue becomes hypoxic from stagnant blood supply. As the blood pools, hemoglobin is released from the red blood cell and is deposited in the tissues, causing brown stains on the skin. Fluids escape into the interstitial space, and edema develops. This poorly nourished tissue begins to undergo necrosis.

Clinical manifestations include itching, a feeling of heaviness in the legs, brown-stained skin, and open shallow lesions (Fig. 49–3). Dilated veins may be obvious. The lesions are very slow to heal because of the lack of oxygenated blood.

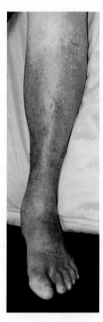

FIGURE 49-3 Stasis dermatitis. Note the dark, stained, shiny skin on the leg as well as the absence of hair.

Improvement of venous return in the legs is needed. This can be accomplished with leg elevation, wearing support hose or elastic wraps daily, and refraining from crossing the legs. Clients should be instructed to raise the legs periodically during the day, especially if their occupation requires standing still for long periods of time (e.g., cashier). Walking instead of standing or performing calf exercises while standing is encouraged to increase circulation. In addition, it is beneficial to raise the foot of the bed with two-by-four blocks or books.

Stasis ulcers are treated with moisture-retentive dressings and gradient pressure wraps. Unna boots can be used. Skin grafts may be required to heal large ulcers.

■ CONTACT DERMATITIS

Contact dermatitis is an inflammatory response of the skin to chemical or physical allergens. *Irritant contact dermatitis* is due to exposure to a chemical or physical irritant (cleaning product, fragrance, or topical skin care product), not to an immune-mediated response. Clinical manifestations range from mild erythema to vesicles to ulceration (Fig. 49-4).

Allergic contact dermatitis is a delayed hypersensitivity reaction resulting from contact with an allergen. This reaction is an immune-mediated response by previously sensitized lymphocytes to a specific allergen. Common examples are poison ivy, nickel sensitivity, and formaldehyde allergy. Clinical manifestations begin at the site of exposure with itching, stinging, erythema, and edema, which may extend to involve more distant sites. Manifestations may develop within an hour of contact or as late as 7 to 14 days after contact. With even brief contact of the irritant with the skin, an allergic response is possible. For example, contact with poison ivy may have happened quickly and the evident irritant washed off. However, areas of dermatitis may continue to appear for many days following the initial exposure.

Management begins with identification of the causative agent. First, question the client about recent exposure to chemicals, metals, and the like. Patch testing is done to attempt to determine the specific agent. Pain and itching may be controlled with topical medication or wet dressings (see earlier). Antihistaminic agents and topical or systemic steroids may be required. Each patch in a standardized test panel (T.R.U.E. test [thin-layer, rapid-use epicutaneous test]) contains a substance that is known to be a common cause of allergic contact dermatitis. When these tests elicit a positive reaction, much can be done to teach the client about what to avoid (see Chapter 48).

■ INTERTRIGO

Intertrigo is a superficial inflammatory dermatitis that occurs between two apposed (touching) skin surfaces. Adequate ventilation, friction, heat, and moisture buildup result in erythema and maceration, itching, and burning. Erosions and fissures with erythema and secondary bacterial or *Candida albicans* infection may occur. Whenever candidiasis is present, a careful evaluation is indicated. In an otherwise healthy person, candidiasis is a self-limiting disease that responds well to topical antifungal therapy; however, it can be the presenting sign of underlying systemic disease affecting the endocrine system (e.g., diabetes) or the immune system (e.g., immunodeficiency syndromes). Intertrigo is common in hot, humid weather in neck creases, axillae, antecubital fossae, the perineum, finger and toe webs, and abdominal skinfolds and beneath the breasts, particularly in obese clients. One of the most common causes of intertrigo is contamination with body fluids, as occurs in urinary incontinence.

The treatment of intertrigo is to eliminate maceration by promoting drying and to aerate the body skinfolds. For mobile clients, review environmental changes that promote drying of the body folds, such as wearing loose-fitting cotton-blend clothing or periodic removal of clothing to dry off. Instruct clients to avoid tight-fitting clothing such as jeans and activities that promote sweating. Care recommendations are very dependent on the degree of involvement and the overall condition of the skin. If the skin is still intact, recommendations include washing the area gently with tap water twice daily and

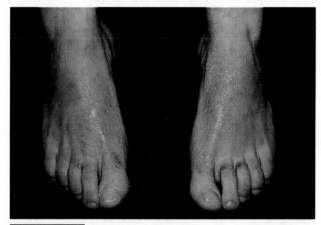

FIGURE 49-4 Contact dermatitis. Note the distinct line of erythema.

then rinsing and drying the area, followed by liberal application of a talc-containing powder or a cellulose-containing powder (e.g., Zeasorb) for extra absorption. Never use cornstarch because it encourages *C. albicans* overgrowth.

If inflammation is present, a low-potency topical corticosteroid in a nonocclusive vehicle (e.g., hydrocortisone 1.0% or 2.5% cream or lotion) or a combination steroid-antibiotic-antifungal agent (Vytone 1%) may initially be helpful, but long-term use should be avoided. Apply cool, wet soaks with tap water or Burows solution three to four times daily for removal of exudate if secondary infection is present. Applying folded gauze or clean cotton handkerchiefs in skinfolds promotes healing by keeping skin surfaces apart.

■ PSORIASIS VULGARIS

Psoriasis vulgaris is a chronic, recurrent, erythematous, inflammatory disorder involving keratin synthesis. Pruritus can be severe. Psoriasis occurs in both genders, usually commencing in early adulthood. The Latin *vulgaris* (from *vulgus* "the public") means "common." The cause of psoriasis vulgaris is unknown. However, alterations in cyclic nucleotides and possible immunologic abnormalities have been noted. Genetic predisposition is also possible.

Pathophysiology

Rapidly proliferating epidermal cells which do not mature form small, scaly patches of skin that develop into erythematous, dry, scaling patches of various sizes. The course of psoriasis vulgaris is prolonged and unpredictable. Anxiety and stress often precede flares. Exacerbations and remissions are common. The condition usually recurs at intervals and lasts for increasingly longer periods. Spontaneous clearing is uncommon. Clients with psoriasis have greater than normal numbers of staphylococci in colonized plaques. Psoriatic clients who are seropositive for human immunodeficiency virus (HIV) are at high risk of HIV infection from self-inoculation.

Clinical Manifestations

Psoriatic patches are covered with silvery white scales. The eruptions (usually in a symmetrical distribution) commonly occur on the scalp, elbows, knees, and sacral regions (Fig. 49–5). Lesions may develop at the site of a previous injury, which is known as Koebner's phenomenon. A generalized eruption may occur with severe psoriasis vulgaris. In a rare form of psoriasis, known as pustular psoriasis, generalized, sterile cutaneous pustules are produced. Severe systemic involvement can be fatal. About 15% to 20% of clients with psoriasis have psoriatic arthritis, which primarily affects the distal joints and may be deforming. Nail dystrophies and pitting occur in about 30% to 50% of clients.

Outcome Management

The goals of medical management of psoriasis are to control the rate of epidermal cell turnover and to monitor for complications of therapy.

■ Medical Management

REDUCE RATE OF EPIDERMAL CELL TURNOVER

Mild psoriasis may be treated locally with natural sunlight or topical therapy, including tar preparations and topical corticosteroids (see Topical Corticosteroids) or intralesional corticosteroids. Injecting small, dilute amounts of corticosteroids (e.g., triamcinolone acetonide) into or just beneath a lesion gives a high drug concentration at the injection site. Keratolytic agents (e.g., salicylic acid) may remove scale and allow greater penetration of topical agents. Anthralin reduces mitotic action in the cell and is an effective topical agent for treatment of psoriasis with widespread discrete lesions consisting primarily of thick plaques.

Scalp care in psoriasis consists of removing scales and treating inflammation. Tar shampoos with keratolytic agents, followed by topical corticosteroid lotions, are useful. Use of steroids under occlusion (under dressings) is often necessary to enhance percutaneous absorption; on the scalp, a plastic shower cap can be used for this purpose. There is no consistently effective treatment of psoriatic involvement of the nails. Usually, the scalp and nails improve with remission of psoriasis on the body surface.

Antimetabolites (e.g., methotrexate) in small doses are useful for inhibiting deoxyribonucleic acid (DNA) synthesis. Methotrexate is a folic acid antagonist used to treat psoriasis that is unresponsive to all topical therapies; it is reserved for the most severe cases.

Systemic treatment is sometimes prescribed for widespread psoriasis. The vitamin A derivative etretinate (Tegison) has been shown to be useful in pustular and erythrodermic psoriasis but less so in chronic plaque-type psoriasis. The mode of action may involve the correction of abnormal polyamine metabolism or leukocyte migration.

MONITOR FOR COMPLICATIONS

Potential localized side effects of corticosteroids include atrophy, hypopigmentation, infection, and, rarely, ulceration. The side effects of etretinate are similar to those of the oral retinoid isotretinoin (see Acne Vulgaris later). Because of the teratogenicity of the drug and its extremely long half-life, its use in women of childbearing age is contraindicated. Widespread involvement may require whole-body irradiation with UVL (see earlier).

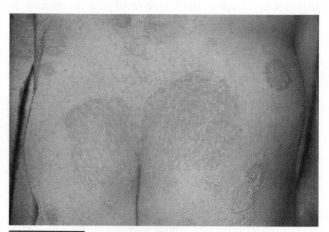

FIGURE 49–5 Plaque psoriasis of the buttocks.

Methotrexate is potentially toxic to the renal, hepatic, and hematopoietic systems. Thus, baseline assessment (e.g., blood chemistry, complete blood count, liver biopsy) is important before this medication is started. During treatment, periodic assessments are needed, including re-biopsy of the liver. If any serious side effects develop, such as bone marrow depression (decreased white blood cell count and platelet count) or gastrointestinal tract bleeding, treatment is discontinued. To limit potential liver damage, advise the client not to consume alcohol throughout therapy. Because methotrexate may cause chromosomal abnormalities, effective birth control methods are important for both women and men before and during treatment. Nausea, the most common side effect, can be limited by taking methotrexate with food or with prophylactic antiemetics.

■ Nursing Management of the Medical Client

Although the physician orders the medical regimen for the client, the nurse and the physician collaborate in the ongoing assessment of the client's response to treatment and the development of new lesions.

There are various methods of application of topical medications. With all methods, it is important to apply medication only to the affected lesions, avoiding contact with normal surrounding skin. The client should wash the hands immediately after application. The medication must be left on for the prescribed period of time and then removed by showering or bathing.

Anthralin products have the potential to stain fabric, hair, skin, nails, furniture, and bathroom fixtures. To avoid excessive staining, it is recommended that the medication be carefully applied and that as much medication as possible be removed with a tissue or a previously stained towel before bathing.

■ Self-Care

Your role in client self-care centers on teaching the client about the UVL treatments and medications. Assist the client in coping with an altered self-concept. The appearance of skin lesions may make the client feel "dirty" or untouchable. In addition, the smell of the tar preparations and the stain may add to the psychological reaction. Because open lesions are at high risk for secondary infection, the client should be taught to keep the creams or ointments on and to keep the area clean and dry.

To keep psoriasis in remission, the client needs to control the causative factors. Adequate rest, nutrition, and exercise promote health. Stress should be minimized, and illness and infection should be treated early.

■ ACNE VULGARIS

Acne is a common, self-limiting, multifactorial disorder. One in four clients affected has disease of sufficient severity for them to seek professional treatment. Potential facial disfigurement is a major concern. Acne requires active treatment for control until it spontaneously resolves.

Etiology

The exact cause of acne is unknown. The principal etiologic factors are abnormal keratinization of the follicular epithelium, excessive sebum production, proliferation of *Propionibacterium acnes,* and inflammation secondary to the action of extracellular inflammatory products produced by *P. acnes.* There is no scientific evidence that consumption of chocolate, nuts, or fatty foods affects acne. It is important to take time to dispel this popular misconception about foods, because frequently guilt related to "eating the wrong foods" causes major family confrontations. However, exacerbations coinciding with the menstrual cycle result from hormonal activity. Heat, humidity, and excessive perspiration also have a role in worsening of acne.

Clinical Manifestations

The types of acne lesions are comedones (open and closed), pustules, papules, and nodules (Fig. 49–6). A closed *comedone,* or whitehead, is a noninflamed lesion that develops as the follicle enlarges, with retention of horny cells. Open comedones, or blackheads, result from the continuing accumulation of horny cells and sebum, which dilate the follicles. Inflammation does not usually occur in comedones unless they are self-manipulated. *Pustules* and *papules* result as the inflammatory process progresses. With papules, the level of involvement of the dermis is deeper than it is with pustules. *Nodules* result from total disintegration of a comedone with subsequent collapse of the follicle. Nodules are the hallmark of serious acne, and deep scarring may result. Aggressive management is always indicated with nodular acne.

Outcome Management

■ Medical Management

Treatment depends on the severity of acne. There is no convincing evidence that dietary management, use of abrasive scrubs, or oral vitamin A has any beneficial effects on the management of acne. Some people with acne may notice an improvement in the summer months as a result of additional UVL exposure. Clients should be instructed to use products labeled noncomedogenic and cosmetics that are water-based, because contact with oily or oil-based products is known to exacerbate acne.

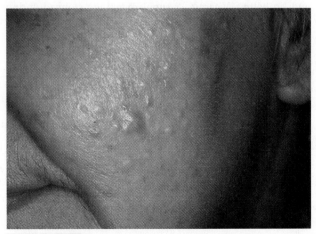

FIGURE 49–6 Acne. (From Cullen, J. P., et al. [1993]. *Color atlas of dermatology.* Philadelphia: W. B. Saunders.)

To prevent scarring, it is important to suppress inflammation. See Table 49–1 for a listing of acne medications. Benzoyl peroxide (a component of Desquam, Benzagel, Persa-Gel, Panoxyl) in 5% and 10% concentrations has a potent antimicrobial effect. The agent reduces the size and number of comedones present and may inhibit sebum secretion. Topical antibiotics (clindamycin and erythromycin) are also used. Topical retinoid products such as tretinoin (Retin-A, Avita) and adapalene (Differin) are two of the most effective comedolytic agents, used alone or in combination with benzoyl peroxide. The irritant effects sometimes limit the usefulness of these agents. Clients should receive written instructions regarding use of topical retinoids.

With failure of response to topical agents, the addition of oral antibiotics (tetracycline or erythromycin) should be considered. Tetracycline or erythromycin administered over an extended period (e.g., several months) suppresses *P. acnes* and decreases inflammation. However, long-term administration of systemic antibiotics can lead to monilial vaginitis and gastrointestinal disorders, and clients should be informed how to monitor for these problems and what interventions to use. Improvement may not be apparent for 4 to 6 weeks.

Hormone therapy may be indicated for severe cystic acne. Medication containing estrogens suppresses sebaceous gland activity. Estrogenic therapy requires treatment through a minimum of three to four menstrual cycles.

In severe cystic acne resistant to standard management, isotretinoin (Accutane) is used to inhibit inflammation. Dosage is determined by body weight. The drug is taken in divided daily doses for several months. Isotretinoin produces many side effects, necessitating frequent follow-up visits and laboratory evaluations. Adverse effects include elevated triglycerides, skin dryness, cheilitis (lip inflammation), and eye discomfort (i.e., dryness, burning). Isotretinoin is a teratogen; thus, women of childbearing age should use an effective contraceptive for at least 1 month before starting this medication and should have a pregnancy screening test 2 weeks before treatment. This drug should not be used in women without strict and adequate contraception throughout the course of therapy and for a determined period after therapy. Reinforce the fact that close medical follow-up is needed and that dry skin and cheilitis can be controlled by use of emollients and lip balms. Vitamin A supplements are stopped during this treatment.

Explain the mechanism of acne and the treatment plan, and set therapeutic goals. The client should understand that improvement is not usually seen for 4 to 8 weeks and that therapy is usually required for months to years to achieve control. Assess the client's skin care practices. Reinforce compliance with topical or systemic therapy regimens and appropriate skin-cleansing methods, with special emphasis on gentle washing technique and use of appropriate topical agents. Note areas of self-induced skin damage, and emphasize to the client the importance of refraining from squeezing, pricking, or picking at lesions.

■ ACNE ROSACEA

Acne rosacea is a chronic inflammatory eruption characterized by erythema, papules, pustules, and telangiectases.

It occurs on the face, especially the cheeks and over the bridge of the nose. Unlike with acne vulgaris, comedones are generally not seen. The onset is insidious, usually between 30 and 50 years of age, and women are affected more frequently than men. It is more common in fair-skinned people with a history of easy facial flushing. Precipitating factors that appear to make the flushing worse include tea, coffee, alcohol (especially wine), caffeine-containing products, sunlight, extremes of hot and cold, spicy foods, and emotional stress.

Sebaceous hyperplasia of the nose (rhinophyma) often develops after many years of chronic acne rosacea. This condition results from chronic inflammation with an increase in the amount of connective tissue and may be mistaken for an indication of excessive alcohol consumption. Ocular changes such as eyelid inflammation and conjunctivitis may occur.

Outcome Management

Avoidance of the stimuli that trigger acne rosacea may be sufficient for management of mild forms of the disorder. Instruct clients to avoid factors that provoke facial vasodilation, such as caffeine, excessive sunlight, alcohol (especially wine), temperature extremes, hot liquids, and spicy foods. Systemic antibiotics used to be the mainstay of therapy. Antibiotics are given in small, usually tapered doses for long periods. Remind the client that improvement with systemic antibiotics occurs gradually.

Topical metronidazole (MetroGel) is the drug of choice for treatment of acne rosacea. A thin layer is applied twice daily with usually only minimal problems of dryness or burning. Relapse is common in clients who discontinue therapy.

SKIN TEARS

Skin tears are wounds resulting from the separation of epidermis from the underlying connective tissue, creating a flap. The most common sites for skin tears, in order of frequency, are the forearm, hand, elbow, and upper arm.

Etiology

Most often, the actual cause of the skin tear is unknown. When known, causes typically are trauma such as falls and injury from wheelchair handles or brakes or injury that incurred during transfer to a chair. Even though the actual skin damage is minor, families and residents are disturbed by presence of skin tears, perceiving the injury as resulting from abuse. Skin tears are most common in older adults as a result of a thinning of the epidermis, a flattening of the dermal-epidermal junction, and reduced adhesion of the dermis to the epidermis.[28]

Outcome Management

Before choosing a dressing, determine whether the edges of the tear can be approximated or the flap can be replaced to cover the wound. Gently irrigate excess blood from the site with normal saline. If possible, replace the flap to approximate the wound edges, and affix the edges to the skin with wound closure strips (Steri-Strips). Protect the site from further damage and drying by applying rolled gauze. Do not apply tape to the skin, and do not cover the wound with a transparent dressing.

For tears with small to moderate losses of epidermal tissue, irrigate the wound as described earlier. Replace any flaps of epidermis, and secure as noted. Cover the open wound with nonocclusive, moisture-retentive dressing, such as petrolatum-impregnated gauze or opaque foam dressing. Past management techniques for this type of wound included the use of transparent film dressings. Although these dressings appear to provide needed skin protection, they have important drawbacks such as maceration of tissue related to the increased heat and moisture and the additional skin trauma incurred upon removal.

For tears with complete loss of epidermal tissue, use the same technique for cleansing as described previously, cover the wound with opaque foam dressing or petrolatum (Vaseline)-impregnated gauze, and wrap with rolled gauze to secure.

Prevention is important. Use protective gloves on the client's hands and soft armrests on wheelchairs, and train caregivers for proper transfer techniques (e.g., use of transfer belts). Less frequent bathing and use of emollient soap also help to prevent skin dryness. Daily assessment by unlicensed assistive personnel is critical to identify lesions early (see Management and Delegation).

PRESSURE ULCERS

A pressure ulcer is any lesion on the skin caused by unrelieved pressure resulting in damage to underlying tissue. Pressure ulcers occur commonly in areas subject to high pressure from body weight on bony prominences. Pressure ulcers have also been called "bed sores" and "decubitus ulcers." The word *decubitus* comes from the Latin *decumbere,* to lie down. The ulcers were so named because they are common in bedridden clients.

Etiology and Risk Factors

Pressure ulcers develop when soft tissue (skin, subcutaneous tissue, and muscle) are compressed between a bony prominence and a firm surface for a prolonged period of time. Therefore, immobility is a major risk factor. In bedridden or chair-bound clients, infrequent turning and repositioning or lack of padding between surfaces that touch (e.g., knees) is a common cause. The length of time of exposure to pressure before skin breakdown varies among clients; in very debilitated clients, permanent tissue damage can result in less than 2 hours. Cognitive or sensory impairments also increase risk because the client cannot recognize the need to turn or move.

Protein-calorie malnutrition is a major risk factor. Malnourished clients have poor skin integrity, and their skin

---

MANAGEMENT AND DELEGATION

Skin Inspection

Unlicensed assistive personnel frequently are in the position to observe the skin of clients as they assist with various activities of daily living and provide assistance with personal hygiene. Be sure to fully delineate their role in identifying and reporting skin abnormalities. Reportable findings are listed as follows.

- *Bruising or a change in skin color.* Ecchymosis, erythema, jaundice, and pallor may indicate a serious disease process or acute tissue injury. Identification of these changes in skin color by unlicensed assistive personnel should be immediately reported to you for thorough assessment and intervention. Redness overlying bony structures may indicate prolonged or undue pressure. Unlicensed assistive personnel should ensure pressure relief by assisting the client with frequent position changes.
- *Lumps.* Assess any skin lesion or growth in further detail.
- *Dry, scaling, or cracked skin.* Dry skin may indicate dehydration or other integumentary disorders. You may delegate the application of over-the-counter lotions to unlicensed assistive personnel if the skin is not broken. Some clients may need specific lubricants or medications prescribed by a physician; therefore, have any findings of dry skin reported to you.
- *Skin that feels excessively moist and cool or excessively warm.* It is appropriate for unlicensed assistive personnel to cover clients with extra bedding if they feel cool or to offer cool compresses for warm skin

(see Chapter 27). Localized areas of warmth may indicate underlying processes that need your prompt attention. Clearly communicate that any of these findings should be immediately reported to you for prompt assessment and intervention.
- *Any break in the skin with drainage or bleeding.* You may delegate the application of sterile gauze to the surface of the skin to unlicensed assistive personnel for the purpose of containing drainage (see Chapter 15). Skin tears should be treated with nonsticky dressings. Assess such skin abnormalities promptly after identification by unlicensed assistive personnel.
- *Taught and/or shiny skin.* This finding may indicate fluid shifting from the intravascular space. Such skin is prone to breakdown and infection. Employ proactive measures to prevent any undue pressure or damage to the skin. Assess the area carefully, and report any unknown disorders or significant change to a physician. Elevate the area to decrease swelling.
- *Client complaints of itching or tenderness:* Instruct unlicensed assistive personnel identifying such client complaints to communicate these findings to you promptly. Assess the client for potential allergic reaction, an underlying tissue pathologic process, or the need for additional analgesics.
- *Rashes.* New rashes or other skin eruptions sometimes suggest allergic reactions. Instruct that such findings be reported to you promptly.

Remember, you are ultimately responsible for thorough, ongoing assessment and evaluation of integument.

Kimberly Elgin, BSN, RN, *Clinician III, Clinical Manager, Surgical Services, University of Virginia Health System, Charlottesville, Virginia*

is damaged easily. In addition, incontinence, friction, and skin shearing can also lead to breakdown.

The reported incidence (number of new cases per year) of pressure ulcers in acute care facilities ranges from 2.7% to 29.5%. The prevalence (number of cases at one point in time) in acute care settings ranges from 3.5% to 29.5%. Several populations are at increased risk. Quadriplegic clients, older adults with femoral fractures, and clients in critical care facilities have the highest risk. Prevention of pressure ulcers begins with identifying the client at risk. Risk factors for alteration in skin integrity can be determined by assessing sensory perception, moisture, activity, mobility, nutrition, friction, and shear.

Pathophysiology

Continuous pressure on soft tissues between bony prominences and hard surfaces compresses capillaries and occludes blood flow. If the pressure is relieved, a brief period of rebound capillary dilation (called reactive hyperemia) occurs, and there is no tissue damage. If pressure is not relieved, microthrombi form in capillaries and completely occlude blood flow. A blister may form initially if there has been damage only to superficial tissues. Damage to underlying tissues creates a necrotic area of tissue. The necrotic tissue undergoes the process of inflammation as the body tries to get rid of it and ready the tissue for healing.

Healing occurs through secondary intention. Granulation tissue fills the base of the wound. Contraction of the ulcer edges closes the wound. Eventually, epithelial cells cover the wound. Stage III and IV pressure ulcers often require debridement and surgery to close the wound. Scar tissue predominates in ulcers healed without surgery.

Clinical Manifestations

The clinical manifestations of pressure ulcers have been described in four stages (Fig. 49–7). Ulcers most commonly occur on the sacrum, heel, greater trochanter (Fig. 49–8), and ischial tuberosities. The ulcer may or may not be covered with devitalized tissue, which can be yellow, white, brown, or black. Ulcers covered with devitalized tissue cannot be staged accurately until it is excised.

With pressure ulcers, few additional diagnostic assessments are required. Sometimes osteomyelitis is present in deep wounds. Bone scans are used for confirming this problem. If malnutrition is suspected as a cause, serum protein, albumin, or prealbumin levels may be monitored.

Outcome Management

▄▄ Medical Management

Management of the client with a pressure ulcer begins with a complete history and physical examination. There are many causes of delayed wound healing, and delayed healing of pressure ulcers may be the result of other health problems. The goal of medical management is to heal the wound by relieving the pressure over the lesion or decreasing tissue load, cleaning and dressing the wound, and improving nutrition. In addition, the ulcer is monitored for healing, and the client is monitored for complications.

MANAGE TISSUE LOAD

The term *tissue load* refers to the distribution of pressure, friction, and shear on the tissues. Interventions are designed to decrease tissue load and thereby decrease pressure. Special low-pressure beds may be required for clients with multiple pressure ulcers. Heels should be elevated from the bed by placing pillows under the calf or using pressure reduction boots.

PROVIDE ULCER CARE

Moist, devitalized tissue supports bacterial growth. Therefore, devitalized tissue must be removed from the ulcer. Several forms of debridement can be used depending on the client's goals and needs for healing. *Sharp debridement* is the use of a scalpel to excise devitalized tissue (eschar). This technique works best for a thick, adherent eschar. *Mechanical debridement* is the use of wet-to-dry dressings, hydrotherapy, wound irrigation, and dextranomers to soften and remove devitalized tissues. *Enzymatic debridement* is the use of topical debriding agents, such as collagenase, to remove necrotic tissues. Finally, *autolytic debridement* involves the use of synthetic dressings to cover an ulcer, allowing enzymes in the wound bed to digest the devitalized tissues. This form of debridement is the slowest and is usually reserved for clients who cannot tolerate the other forms. Heel ulcers are not debrided unless they are clearly infected. All forms of debridement (except autolytic) are painful; the client should be given analgesics before beginning.

MONITOR HEALING

If the ulcer does not heal within 2 weeks despite adequate nutrition, pressure reduction, daily cleaning, and use of appropriate dressings, the ulcer may be infected. An infected pressure ulcer looks like any other infected wound, with foul-smelling drainage, increasing size, increasing pain in the wound, and fever or elevation in white blood cell count. Older clients do not invariably demonstrate all of the signs of infection and are at risk for development of confusion; therefore, vigilance in assessing the ulcer for changes is critical. If infection is suspected, a 2-week trial of topical antibiotics is considered. Swab cultures are not appropriate for diagnosis of infection in the ulcer. All pressure ulcers are colonized (covered with surface bacteria), and a swab culture will grow only organisms that colonize the surface. Use a quantitative culture for suspected infection. Systemic antibiotics are used when the infection cannot be controlled locally or for systemic infection (manifested by fever or positive blood cultures).

Many conditions are associated with delays in healing. Diabetes, paralysis, and arterial diseases require close assessment because of increased risk of infection. Urine and bowel incontinence lead to skin excoriation and can contaminate open wounds.

IMPROVE NUTRITION

The association of malnutrition with pressure ulcer formation and delayed healing is quite clear. In fact, many clinicians believe that pressure ulcers are a specific indicator of malnutrition. If the client's serum albumin concentration is less than 3.5 g/dl, if the total lymphocyte count is less than 1800/mm^3, or if the client is not eating or is at a body weight that is less than 80% of ideal, consider nutritional supplementation. If the client has no

Stage I

Epidermis

Dermis

Subcutaneous fat

Muscle

Bone

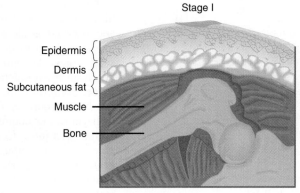

Non-blanching erythema
of intact skin; the heralding
lesion of skin ulceration

Stage II

Epidermis

Dermis

Subcutaneous fat

Muscle

Bone

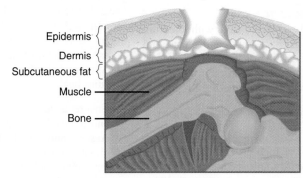

Partial-thickness skin loss
involving epidermis and/or
dermis. The ulcer is superficial
and presents clinically as an
abrasion, blister, or shallow
crater.

Stage III

Epidermis

Dermis

Subcutaneous fat

Muscle

Bone

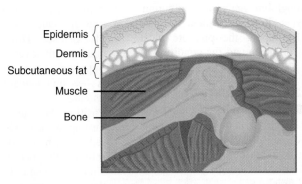

Full-thickness skin loss
involving damage or necrosis
of subcutaneous tissue, which
may extend down to, but not
through, the underlying fascia.
The ulcer presents clinically as
a deep crater with or without
undermining of adjacent tissue.

Stage IV

Epidermis

Dermis

Subcutaneous fat

Muscle

Bone

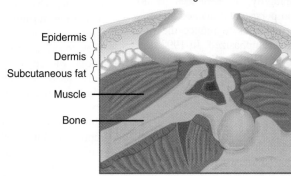

Full-thickness skin loss with
extensive destruction, tissue
necrosis, or damage to muscle,
bone, or supporting structures
(e.g., tendon, joint capsule, etc.)

FIGURE 49–7 Stages of pressure ulcers.

gastrointestinal disorders, feed oral supplements, or give tube feeding. Some clinicians use the phrase "if the gut works, use it" to summarize this recommendation. If the client has gastrointestinal problems, consider total paren-teral nutrition. These more aggressive forms of feeding must be compatible with the client's wishes. Monitor nu-tritional status (as described previously) every 3 months. Body weight should be assessed every 1 to 4 weeks.

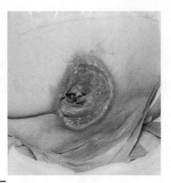

FIGURE 49–8 A stage IV pressure ulcer on the sacrum. The center of the ulcer contains necrotic tissue.

MONITOR FOR COMPLICATIONS

Many complications have been associated with pressure ulcers, including osteomyelitis, bacteremia and sepsis, and cellulitis. Amyloidosis, endocarditis, heterotopic bone formation, septic arthritis, and formation of a fistula from the ulcer to the perineum are rare but have been reported.

■ Nursing Management of the Medical Client

ASSESSMENT

The assessment of the client at high risk for development of pressure ulcers should identify any specific risk factors. The Braden Scale (Fig. 49–9) is an assessment tool that evaluates risk. This scale has been developed to assist the nurse in predicting which clients are at greatest risk. Assess laboratory data on hemoglobin, hematocrit, albumin, total protein, and lymphocytes. Risk assessment must be ongoing. Note objective data about the pressure ulcer (i.e., size, depth, or stage of drainage and the condition of periulcer tissue).

DIAGNOSIS, OUTCOMES, INTERVENTION

Risk for Impaired Skin Integrity. Clients who score between 12 and 16 on the Braden risk assessment scale are considered at risk for pressure ulcers. Scores below 12 indicate a high risk. This nursing diagnosis is written as *Risk for Impaired Skin Integrity related to malnutrition and unrelieved pressure.*

Outcomes. The client will experience a reduction in the risk of impairment of skin integrity, as evidenced by no actual tissue breakdown and no persistent reddened areas.

Interventions. Preventive measures to reduce the risk of pressure ulcers cannot be overemphasized. In 1992, the U.S. Department of Health and Human Services developed guidelines for prediction and prevention of pressure ulcers in adults[9] (Box 49–1).

EVALUATION

Outcomes should be met in 24 to 48 hours. Recall that skin integrity can be impaired in just 2 hours. Therefore, several hours are needed to determine whether skin injury occurred prior to risk reduction measures.

Impaired Skin Integrity. Use this diagnosis to describe an actual pressure ulcer. State the diagnosis as *Impaired Skin Integrity related to pressure ulcer secondary to prolonged immobility, malnutrition, and unrelieved pressure.*

Outcomes. The client will experience healing of the ulcer, as evidenced by development of granulation tissue and decreasing ulcer size. Do not use lower stages of pressure ulcers to describe healing. For example, do not state a stage IV will heal to a stage III. The body does not heal by regeneration of tissue but, rather, by scar tissue. For terminal clients, outcomes such as healing may not be appropriate. For these clients, outcomes of pain management or comfort may be more appropriate.

Interventions. Consistency in the nursing care provided is an important aspect of interventions directed at achieving wound healing. It is important to develop scientific protocols in ulcer care and to use them consistently. It is also important to give one protocol time to work before changing to another.

In 1994, the Agency for Health Care Policy and Research (AHCPR) established guidelines for pressure ulcer treatment.[8] The guidelines are summarized here. If your practice routinely involves nursing care of clients with pressure ulcers, obtaining the actual AHCPR document is recommended. See also Chapter 16 for information on wound healing.

- Ensure adequate dietary intake to prevent malnutrition and delayed healing.
- Assess nutritional status at least every 3 months in clients at risk for malnutrition, such as those in long-term care facilities. Clients in acute care settings need nutritional assessment weekly.
- Provide oral supplementation, tube feeding, or hyperalimentation to achieve positive nitrogen balance. For many clients, the decision not to eat is an important one that can give a sense of control over some aspect of existence. However, pressure ulcers cannot heal in clients with severe malnutrition.
- Supplement the diet with vitamins and minerals.
- Assess and manage pain associated with the ulcer and its care.
- Position the client to stay off the ulcer. If there is no turning surface without a pressure ulcer, use a pressure reduction bed and continue to turn the client. Do not rely on the bed exclusively to move the client. The client still needs to be repositioned. You cannot assess the skin if you cannot see it.
- Use positioning devices to hold the client in various positions. Do not use doughnut-type devices. Establish a written turning schedule, and post it according to agency policy.
- Elevate heels off the bed by using pillows or foam boots. Fleece heel covers do not relieve pressure, but they can reduce friction.
- Maintain the head of the bed at the lowest elevation consistent with the client's medical condition. If the client must have the head elevated to prevent aspiration, reposition into a 30-degree lateral position. Use a seat cushion in the chair, and assess for sacral ulcers daily. For dyspneic clients, position erect and assess for sacral and ischial ulcers daily.
- Use support surfaces for clients with multiple ulcers and for those who are not able to keep off the ulcer surface. Begin with a dynamic surface or mattress overlay. Progress to low-air-loss beds or air-fluidized beds (Fig. 49–10) if the ulcer does not heal.

RISK PREDICTORS FOR SKIN BREAKDOWN

Patient's Name _____

Evaluator's Name _____

	1	2	3	4
SENSORY PERCEPTION ability to respond to discomfort	**1. Completely limited:** Unresponsive to painful stimuli, either because of state of unconsciousness or severe sensory impairment, which limits ability to feel pain over most of body surface	**2. Very limited:** Responds only to painful stimuli (but not verbal commands) by opening eyes or flexing extremities. Cannot communicate discomfort verbally, OR has a sensory impairment which limits the ability to feel pain or discomfort over one half of body surface	**3. Slightly limited:** Responds to verbal commands by opening eyes and obeying some commands, but cannot always communicate discomfort or need to be turned, OR has some sensory impairment which limits ability to feel pain or discomfort in one or two extremities.	**4. No impairment:** Responds to verbal commands by obeying. Can communicate needs accurately. Has no sensory deficit which would limit ability to feel pain or discomfort
MOISTURE degree to which skin is exposed to moisture	**1. Very Moist:** Skin is kept moist almost constantly by perspiration and urine. Dampness is detected every time patient is moved or turned. Linen must be changed more than one time each shift	**2. Occasionally Moist:** Skin is frequently, but not always kept moist, linen must be changed two to three times every 24 hours	**3. Rarely Moist:** Skin is rarely moist more than three to four times a week, but linen does require changing at that time	**4. Never Moist:** Perspiration and incontinence are never a problem linen changed at routine intervals only
ACTIVITY degree of physical activity	**1. Bedfast:** Confined to bed	**2. Chairfast:** Ability to walk severely impaired or nonexistent and must be assisted into chair or wheelchair. Is confined to chair or wheelchair when not in bed	**3. Walks occasionally:** Walks occasionally during day, but for very short distances, with or without assistance. Spends majority of each shift in bed or chair	**4. Walks frequently:** Walks a moderate distance at least once every 1 to 2 hours during waking hours
MOBILITY ability to change and control body position	**1. Completely Immobile:** Unable to make even slight changes in position without assistance	**2. Very limited:** Makes occasional slight changes in position without help but unable to make frequent or significant changes in position independently	**3. Slightly limited:** Makes frequent though slight changes in position without assistance but unable to make or maintain major changes in position independently	**4. No limitations:** Makes major and frequent changes in position without assistance
NUTRITION usual food intake pattern	**1. Very Poor:** Never eats a complete meal. Rarely eats more than 1/3 of any food offered. Intake of protein is negligible. Takes even fluids poorly. Does not take a liquid dietary supplement, OR is NPO and/or maintained on clear liquids or IV for more than 5 days	**2. Probably Inadequate:** Rarely eats a complete meal and generally eats only about one half of any food offered. Protein intake is poor. Occasionally will take a liquid dietary supplement, OR receiving less than optimum amount of liquid diet or tube feeding	**3. Adequate:** Eats over half of most meals. Eats moderate amount of protein four to two times daily. Occasionally will refuse a meal. Will usually take a dietary supplement if offered OR is on a tube feeding or TPN regimen which probably meets most of nutritional needs	**4. Excellent:** Eats most of every meal. Never refuses a meal. Frequently eats between meals. Does not require a dietary supplementation
FRICTION AND SHEAR	**1. Problem:** Requires moderate to maximum assistance in moving. Complete lifting without sliding against sheets is impossible. Frequently slides down in bed or chair, requiring frequent repositioning with maximum assistance. Either spasticity, contractures or agitation leads to almost constant friction	**2. Potential Problem:** Moves feebly independently or requires minimum assistance. Skin probably slides against bedsheets or chair to some extent when movement occurs. Maintains relatively good position in chair or bed most of time but occasionally slides down	**3. No Apparent Problem:** Moves in bed and in chair independently and has sufficient muscle strength to lift up completely during move. Maintains good position in bed or chair at all times	

Key: 16, minimum risk; 13–14, moderate risk; 12 or less, high risk;
NPO, nothing by mouth; IV, intravenously; TPN, total parenteral nutrition.

FIGURE 49–9 The Braden Scale for evaluation of risk of pressure ulcers. (Courtesy of Barbara Braden and Nancy Bergstrom. Copyright 1988.)

BOX 49–1 Prevention of Pressure Ulcers

- Perform a systematic skin inspection for all clients at risk at least once a day, with particular attention paid to the bony prominences.
- Document results of skin inspection.
- Cleanse the skin at the time of soiling and at routine intervals. The frequency of skin cleaning should be individualized according to need and client preference.
- Avoid hot water; use a mild cleaning agent that minimizes irritation and dryness of the skin. During the cleaning process, take care to minimize the force and friction applied to the skin.
- Minimize environmental factors leading to skin drying, such as low humidity (<40%) and exposure to cold. Treat dry skin with moisturizers.
- Avoid massage over bony prominences, which may be harmful.
- Minimize skin exposure to moisture from incontinence, perspiration, or wound drainage. When these sources of moisture cannot be controlled, apply underpads or briefs that are made of materials that absorb moisture and present a quick-drying surface to the skin. Topical agents that act as barriers to moisture can also be used.
- Minimize skin injury due to friction and shear forces through proper positioning, transferring, and turning techniques. In addition, help reduce friction injuries by the use of lubricants (e.g., cornstarch and creams), protective films (e.g., transparent film dressings and skin sealants), protective dressings (e.g., hydrocolloids), and protective padding.
- When apparently well-nourished clients do not have an adequate dietary intake of protein or calories, caregivers should first attempt to discover the factors compromising intake and offer support with eating. Other nutritional supplements or support may be needed. If dietary intake remains inadequate and if consistent with overall goals of therapy, consider more aggressive nutritional intervention (enteral or parenteral feedings).
- For nutritionally compromised clients, implement a plan of nutritional support or supplementation that meets individual needs and is consistent with the overall goals of therapy.

- If the potential exists for improving the client's mobility and activity status, institute rehabilitation efforts if these measures are consistent with the overall goals of therapy. Maintaining current activity level, mobility, and range of motion is an appropriate goal for most clients.
- Use a written schedule for systematically turning and repositioning the client.
- For clients in bed, use pillows to keep bony prominences (such as knees or ankles) from direct contact with one another.
- For clients in bed who are completely immobile, the care plan should include the use of devices that totally relieve pressure on the heels, most commonly by raising the heels off the bed. Do not use doughnut-type devices; they tend to cause pressure ulcers, not prevent them.
- When the side-lying position is used in bed, avoid positioning the client directly on the trochanter.
- Maintain the head of the bed at the lowest degree of elevation consistent with medical conditions and other restrictions. Limit the amount of time during which the head of the bed is elevated.
- Use a lifting device (trapeze, bed linen) to move, rather than drag, clients in bed who cannot assist during transfers and position changes.
- Place at risk clients on a pressure-reducing device, such as a foam, static air, alternating air, or water mattress.
- Ensure that any person at risk for a pressure ulcer avoids uninterrupted sitting in chair or wheelchair. The client should be repositioned, with appropriate shifts of the points under pressure, at least every hour. Teach clients who are able to shift their weight every 15 minutes.
- For chair-bound clients, select a pressure-reducing device, such as one made of foam, air, or a combination of these. Do not use a doughnut-type device.
- When positioning chair-bound clients, consider postural alignment, distribution of weight, balance and stability, and pressure relief.
- Provide a written plan for the use of positioning devices and schedules to help chair-bound clients.

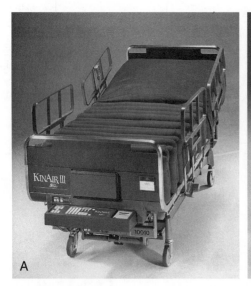

A

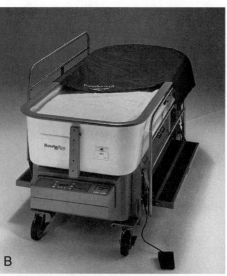

B

FIGURE 49–10 Pressure reduction surfaces. *A*, KinAir beds provide controlled air suspension to redistribute body weight away from bony prominences. *B*, FluidAir beds use air flow and bead fluidization. Both of these beds are covered with Gore-Tex fabric, which resists tearing. This fabric is also waterproof and acts as a barrier against bacteria. (Courtesy of Kinetic Concepts, Inc., San Antonio, TX.)

- Check for bottoming out beneath the mattress (Fig. 49–11). Place your hand between the mattress and the bed. If you feel less than an inch between the client's body and the mattress surface, the support is not adequate.
- Prevent moisture from coming in contact with the client's skin.
- Use support cushions for the wheelchair-bound client or for any client who prefers to sit.
- Teach wheelchair-bound clients to reposition themselves every 15 minutes.
- Debride the ulcer of devitalized tissue. Medicate for pain before debriding the ulcer.
- Clean the wound with normal saline. Avoid antiseptics on the wound bed.
- Use irrigation to clean the wound. Safe pressure ranges from 4 to 15 pounds per square inch. A 35-ml syringe with a 19-gauge angiocatheter is a good device for irrigation.
- Once the ulcer is free of devitalized tissue, apply dressings that keep the wound bed moist and the surrounding skin dry. Do not use occlusive dressings on ulcers that may be infected.
- Follow body substance isolation precautions; use clean gloves and clean dressings for wound care.

Reducing the risk of pressure ulcer development and identifying early signs of pressure ulcers are frequently delegated to unlicensed personnel (see the Management and Delegation feature). Case managers often assist in managing care between facilities. When preparing for discharge to home, case managers assist with advocating

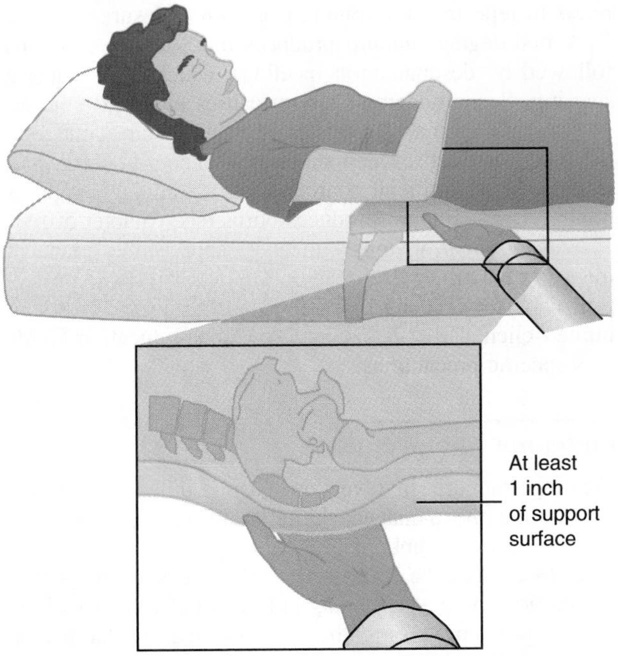

FIGURE 49–11 Assessment of pressure relief ("bottoming out"). Slide your hand (palm up and fingers flat) under the support surface, just under the pressure point. Do not flex your fingers. With adequate support, there will be at least 1 inch of uncompressed support surface between your hand and the client's body. (Modified from Gaymar Industries, Inc., Orchard Park, NY.)

and preventing readmission (see the Case Management feature).

EVALUATION

As the wound heals, assess the degree of outcome attainment every 3 to 4 days. Allow 2 weeks before changing the plan of care, unless the ulcer is deteriorating.

■ Self-Care

The clients at high risk for development of pressure ulcers should be referred to a home health agency before discharge from the acute care facility so that devices to reduce pressure can be obtained for home use. The family and the client need to understand the importance of frequent turning. A client who is wheelchair-bound and has arm function should be taught to lift the body, using the arms, off the chair twice every hour for repositioning. A client who is incontinent needs to wear protective pads to absorb the urine or stool and should be assessed often. The U.S. Department of Health and Human Services has developed a "patient guide" for preventing and treating pressure ulcers.[8, 9]

If the client is going home with an unhealed ulcer, the client and one or more family members must be taught

---

MANAGEMENT AND DELEGATION

Care of Clients with Pressure Ulcers

When working with unlicensed assistive personnel in the care of clients with pressure ulcers, help them to keep the following points in mind:

- Report any areas of skin redness that do not disappear after pressure relief.
- Report any development of foul odor or drainage from pressure ulcers.
- Reposition the client *at least* every 2 hours. Even a small shift in the client's body weight may be sufficient, but it must be done every 2 hours at a minimum.
- *Do not position the client on the ulcer.* If an ulcer is on the client's trunk, use a dynamic or overlay mattress. However, the use of these support surfaces does not eliminate the need for turning.
- If the client is wheelchair-bound, ensure that the padding provides adequate pressure relief by checking for "bottoming out."
- Keep all pressure off the client's heels. Use small pillows or foam padding to prevent direct contact.
- Keep the head of the bed at the lowest elevation to reduce shear and friction on the skin of the client's lower back.
- Keep the client's skin dry.

Be aware that even though you have delegated the skin care of these clients, you are still accountable for their skin condition. Assess the entire skin surface every day. Ask for help in turning the client so that you can see the client's heels and sacrum. Use an assessment guide such as the Braden Scale to determine the risk of further ulceration.

Donna W. Markey, MSN, RN, ACNP-CS, *Clinician IV, Surgical Services, University of Virginia Health System, Charlottesville, Virginia*

The Client with Impaired Skin Integrity

Impaired skin integrity, caused by breakdown, stasis, or iatrogenic conditions, is responsible for the expenditure of millions of health care dollars per year. When skin integrity is compromised, long lengths of stay and time-consuming, complex treatments are the result. The human costs—in terms of pain and suffering, infection, surgical procedures (amputation, debridement, grafting), and death—are even more staggering. Case management calls for primary prevention of skin breakdown and meticulous care and client education when skin integrity is impaired.

Advocate

It is much easier to prevent skin breakdown than to heal it after it occurs. Turning or ambulation schedules as well as good nutrition and hydration are often neglected in place of more complex nursing interventions, but they are just as important. When skin breakdown is present, be sensitive to the client's privacy needs and embarrassment resulting from the site of the problem or from the necessity of several caregivers to assist with treatment. Manage pain, allowing time for the analgesic to take effect before performing treatments or applying dressings. Sometimes skin breakdown occurs when clients can no longer care for themselves or do not realize the care needed. Help to realistically assess the client's needs after discharge from the facility, including the ability to return home.

Prevent Readmission

During hospitalization, the client may have benefited from use of a special low-pressure mattress or bed, special wound dressings, or ambulation and turning schedules. Surgical debridement or grafting may have facilitated wound healing. The fragile tissue can easily be damaged if conditions causing skin breakdown are able to reoccur.

Special beds, mattresses, or other equipment, such as a lifting device, may be useful as the client returns home. Make referrals for these devices (e.g., air-fluidized bed) and home nursing visits, aide support, physical therapy, and meal services as appropriate. Make sure that caregivers can manage the expected treatments and know how to use body mechanics and lifting devices.

Emphasize nutrition and hydration, and teach tube feeding or total parenteral nutrition techniques. Make sure that the client and caregivers are aware of hygiene and care for incontinence and know how to summon emergency assistance.

Cheryl Noetscher, RN, MS, Director of Case Management, Crouse Hospital and Community–General Hospital, Syracuse, New York

wound care, wound assessment, and in some cases the administration of intravenous (IV) antibiotics. Teach these interventions before the day of discharge, so that return demonstrations can be used to evaluate learning. In addition, procurement of equipment is often necessary, which takes time. Community nurses need to be involved early in the planning for the discharge of the client with an ulcer. The Bridge to Home Health Care describes ways to help the client and family manage pressure ulcers.

▬ Surgical Management

Surgical repair is frequently performed on stage III and stage IV ulcers (see Fig. 49–7), on ulcers over 2 cm in diameter, and in clients who can tolerate surgery. In stage III ulcers, undamaged tissue near the wound is rotated to cover the ulcer. In stage IV ulcers, musculocutaneous flaps are often used (see later).

PRECANCEROUS CHANGES IN THE SKIN

Precursors to cancer of the skin include damage from recurrent skin trauma and various skin lesions. In order to understand the role of prevention of skin cancer, these precursor conditions are discussed first.

■ SUNBURN

Pathophysiology

Sunburn is an acute inflammatory skin response that occurs as a reaction to excessive exposure to sunlight. Dermatopathologic changes include the production of epidermal cells that exhibit cytoplasmic and nuclear changes. These changes are cumulative over the life span and lead to an increased incidence of skin cancer. *Photodamage* refers to repeated skin trauma from sun exposure.

A first-degree sunburn produces mild, tender erythema followed by desquamation (peeling), which heals without scarring. Second-degree sunburn causes more extreme erythema and edema, and blistering results from damage to the epidermal cells. Deep sunburn is uncommon unless it is induced by artificial sources such as tanning lamps or booths. Deep sunburn produces burns (see Chapter 50).

Prevention is obviously the best approach to management of sunburn. Client teaching emphasizing sun protection should never be omitted when caring for the sunburned client. The accompanying Client Education Guide lists specific precautions.

Outcome Management

Treating sunburn involves decreasing inflammation and rehydrating the damaged skin. For localized, *superficial, partial-thickness* sunburn, use cool tap water soaks for 20 minutes or until the skin is cool. This measure limits skin destruction, prevents edema, and potentially reduces blisters. Tepid tap water baths are indicated for large sunburned areas. After a bath or soak, apply water-based emollients, preferably refrigerated for an additional cooling effect. Emollients should also be applied throughout the day to soothe the skin and relieve dryness. Lotions or foams containing camphor and menthol (e.g., Sarna) can also be beneficial. Avoid the use of OTC remedies containing local anesthetics—such as benzocaine, dibucaine

BRIDGE TO HOME HEALTH CARE

Managing Pressure Ulcers

For the client with pressure ulcers, a smooth transition from hospital to home care requires planning, preparation, and communication. For example, it may take a home health nurse several days to obtain special wound care supplies or pressure relief devices not ordinarily stocked by the home health agency. If a pressure relief bed or mattress overlay is required, the agency then contacts a durable medical equipment company and arranges delivery at a predetermined time. To facilitate the transition from hospital care, the home health agency should be notified of the referral before the client's discharge from the hospital and should receive specific instructions per physician orders for wound cleansing, dressing materials, and frequency of dressing changes. In addition, sending a day's supplies home with the client helps to minimize disruption in the wound treatment regimen.

Clients who are eligible for Medicare and have stage IV or draining, infected pressure ulcers may initially require daily skilled nursing visits. However, as the infection is treated and drainage subsides, the frequency of skilled nursing visits is usually decreased and the family member or informal caregiver is taught to perform the dressing change. Caregivers should participate in or at least observe dressing change procedures in the hospital, and should receive information about turning and other aspects of care. The earlier the caregiver is introduced to prevention and treatment goals, the faster the client can reach the desired clinical outcome. Hospital nurses can significantly enhance the continuity of care by coordinating educational efforts with the home health agency. The home health nurse should obtain copies of any teaching materials distributed in the hospital. Older adults are often fearful of leaving the security of an inpatient setting; therefore, reinforcing familiar teaching materials and wound care procedures helps to ensure a more seamless transition from inpatient to outpatient management.

Maintaining equipment and supplies is more difficult in the home than in inpatient settings. Estimate the needed amount of skin and wound care supplies, and arrange for delivery in a timely manner. Establish an intercommunication sheet in the home that flags a change in wound care orders for other members of the health care team. Leave specific directions for product use, especially when more than one product is being used. *Normal saline* can be made by using the following recipe: mix 8 teaspoons of salt in 1 gallon of bottled or boiled water. Do not use water from an outdoor well.

Adapting the home environment to meet the needs of the client and family members or other caregivers requires creativity and skill. Note the conditions under which the client spends prolonged periods of time. Any firm, unyielding surface can contribute to development of a pressure ulcer in unusual body areas. Sitting on ridged, corded edges of chairs or stools or a firm toilet seat for extended periods can restrict blood flow, leading to pressure ulcer development.

The limitations of older clients and their older caregivers pose additional changes. For example, it may not be possible for a debilitated client to be turned as often as needed during the night to relieve pressure over bony prominences. Frequent turning schedules usually result in increased anxiety and sleep deprivation for older caregivers. Accurately assessing the client's risk category and using an effective pressure-relieving mattress overlay can help to reduce the physical demands for caregivers and increase the possibility that the client can receive needed care and remain at home.

Janice Z. Cuzzell, MA, RN, *Vice-President, Island Health Care, Inc., Savannah, Georgia*

(Nupercaine), or lidocaine (Xylocaine)—because they are rarely effective and have the potential to induce contact sensitivity.

For *partial-thickness* sunburn, apply continuous cool, normal saline soaks or soaking baths to reduce oozing and edema. Aspirate very large blisters, and apply sterile dressings. Avoid debridement unless there is evidence of secondary bacterial infection. Silver sulfadiazine may be prescribed.

Prostaglandin inhibitors (nonsteroidal anti-inflammatory drugs [NSAIDs]) may be used to reduce erythema and inflammation in adults. Topical corticosteroids may be prescribed to be used sparingly in nonocclusive vehicles (i.e., lotion, spray, gel) for their vasoconstrictive effects. Systemic corticosteroids are prescribed only for clients with very extensive, painful burns, but their use has declined because they seem to offer little efficacy when given in a reasonable dose range.

■ ACTINIC KERATOSIS

Actinic keratosis, the most common epithelial precancerous lesion in white people, is caused by sun exposure. It affects nearly 100% of older white adults. There is a small but definite risk of malignant degeneration and subsequent metastatic potential in neglected lesions.

Actinic keratosis most frequently occurs in areas of chronic, usually high-intensity sun exposure including the face, the tops of the ears, the back of the neck, the forearms, and the backs of the hands.

The clinical appearance of actinic keratoses can be quite varied. The typical lesion is an irregularly shaped, flat, slightly erythematous macule or papule with indistinct borders and an overlying hard keratotic scale or horn. In some cases, the erythema or the horn may be absent. This scale can be periodically shed or peeled off, but then it regrows. The lesion varies in size from a pinhead to several centimeters across and is often more easily palpated than observed. Single lesions may be seen, but more often they appear in groups on a background of sun-damaged skin.

Outcome Management

The goals of medical management are to eradicate the lesion and to educate the client how to reduce risk and recognize early skin changes.

CLIENT EDUCATION GUIDE

Simple Guidelines to Help Protect You from the Damaging Rays of the Sun

1. Minimize sun exposure during the hours of 10 AM to 2 PM (11 AM to 3 PM Daylight Saving Time), when the sun is strongest. Try to plan your outdoor activities for the early morning or late afternoon.
2. Wear a hat, long-sleeved shirt, and long pants when out in the sun. Choose tightly woven materials for greater protection from the sun's rays.
3. Apply a sunscreen before every exposure to the sun and reapply frequently and liberally—at least every 2 hours—as long as you stay in the sun. The sunscreen should always be reapplied after swimming or perspiring heavily, because products differ in degree of water resistance. Sunscreens with an SPF (sun protection factor) of 15 or more printed on the label are recommended.
4. Use a sunscreen during high-altitude activities such as mountain climbing and skiing. At high altitudes, where there is less atmosphere to absorb the sun's rays, your risk of burning is greater. The sun is also stronger near the equator, where the sun's rays strike the earth most directly.
5. Do not forget to use your sunscreen on overcast days. The sun's rays are as damaging to your skin on cloudy, hazy days as they are on sunny days.
6. If you are at high risk for skin cancer (if you work outdoors, are fair-skinned, or have already had skin cancer), apply sunscreen daily.

7. Photosensitivity—an increased sensitivity to sun exposure—is a possible side effect of certain medications, drugs and cosmetics, and birth control pills. Consult your physician or pharmacist before going out in the sun if you are using any such products. You may need to take extra precautions.
8. If you develop an allergic reaction to your sunscreen, change sunscreens. One of the many products on the market today should be right for you.
9. Beware of reflective surfaces! Sand, snow, concrete, and water can reflect more than half of the sun's rays onto your skin. Sitting in the shade does not guarantee protection from sunburn.
10. Avoid tanning parlors. The ultraviolet light emitted by tanning booths causes sunburn and premature aging and increases your risk of developing skin cancer.
11. Keep young children out of the sun. Begin using sunscreens on children at 6 months of age, and then allow sun exposure with moderation.
12. Teach children sun protection early. Sun damage occurs with each unprotected sun exposure and accumulates over the course of a lifetime.

From The Skin Cancer Foundation, New York.

ERADICATE THE LESION

Topical application of 5-fluorouracil (5-FU) (Efudex), a topical antimetabolite, is at present one of the best approaches to treatment of widespread actinic damage, with multiple lesions. The advantage of 5-FU is that large areas of widespread disease can be treated at the same time. Use of 5-FU not only removes the majority of premalignant and superficial malignant lesions that can be seen but also uncovers and destroys clinically undetectable lesions of this type. However, the major disadvantage is the therapeutic inflammatory response that often accompanies successful treatment. This response sequence is erythema usually followed by vesiculation, erosion, ulcerations, necrosis, and epithelialization.

The medication should be applied twice daily with a gloved hand, carefully avoiding eyes, nose, mouth, and scrotum. A porous gauze dressing may be applied over the medication for cosmetic reasons without increase in reaction. However, occlusive dressing should be avoided because of increased inflammatory response. Medication should be continued until the inflammatory response reaches the erosion, necrosis, and ulceration stage, at which time the medication should be stopped. The usual duration of therapy is 2 to 4 weeks; by then, the client may experience extreme discomfort requiring pain medication. At the time 5-FU is stopped, topical corticosteroid creams may be applied to reduce inflammation and provide the client with additional pain relief. Complete healing of the lesions may not be evident for 1 to 2 months after cessation of therapy.

■ Surgical Management

CRYOTHERAPY

Cryotherapy using liquid nitrogen is the most common treatment for single lesions or for small numbers of actinic keratoses. Liquid nitrogen is usually applied with a cotton-tipped applicator or spraying device (Fig. 49–12A). No local anesthetic is required but the freezing process is associated with a small amount of discomfort, which may linger afterward. Intermittent application of a warm, damp wash cloth to the site may bring relief. Freezing frequently results in inflammation with blister formation, and blister care should be reviewed with the client. Care must be taken to avoid overfreezing the site, which may result in scarring. Cryotherapy is cost-effective and easy to perform and has minimal side effects.

ELECTRODESICCATION AND CURETTAGE

Electrodesiccation produces superficial destruction through generation of radiofreqency waves that cause a very hot spark to arc onto the lesion. The procedure is usually done using local anesthesia (Fig. 49–12B). The tissue is destroyed by mechanical disruption of cells and heat. The tissue is removed by scraping or scooping with a loop-shaped instrument called a curet (Fig. 49–12C). This method provides tissue for histologic diagnosis if needed. The curetted areas usually heal quickly with adequate wound care. The wound site should be kept moist with a nonsensitizing topical antibiotic ointment such as bacitracin.

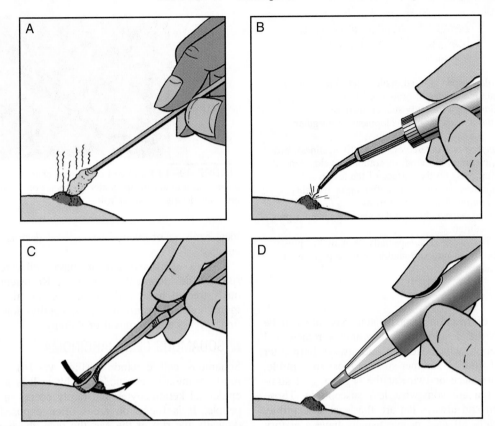

FIGURE 49–12 Methods for destroying skin lesions. *A,* Cryotherapy. Liquid nitrogen is applied with a saturated cotton-tipped applicator directly to the lesion or sprayed on. This causes tissue destruction by freezing. *B,* Electrodesiccation. Tissue is destroyed by heat from an electrical current; note the gloved hand. *C,* Curettage. A curet (cutting instrument) removes tissue by scraping or scooping; note gloved hand. *D,* The laser removes tissue by vaporizing it.

LASER EXCISION

Laser uses light energy to vaporize lesions (Fig. 49–12*D*). Depending upon the wave length of the light, various portions of the cell are heated. Tissue is not available for histologic examination. Local anesthesia is used.

SHAVE OR EXCISIONAL BIOPSY

Shave (excisional) biopsy is indicated for lesions that are large or have other characteristics of a cutaneous malignancy (induration, erythema, erosion). It is often difficult to distinguish a large actinic keratosis from a squamous cell carcinoma without histologic diagnosis. Biopsy should also be done on lesions that persist after adequate treatment with 5-FU. Local anesthesia is used for the biopsy procedure and allows electrodesiccation to be done painlessly after biopsy. Excisional biopsy requires primary closure of the site and may be a more extensive procedure than the lesion warrants; however, it ensures removal of the entire growth (see Chapter 48, Fig. 48–4).

SKIN CANCER

Skin cancer is the most common cancer in the United States, and the number of new skin cancers and the number of skin cancer deaths are increasing at alarming rates. Skin cancer is a malignant condition caused by uncontrolled growth and spread of abnormal cells in a specific layer of the skin. The several different kinds of skin cancer are distinguished by the types of cells involved. The three most common types are (1) basal cell carcinoma, (2) squamous cell carcinoma, and (3) malignant melanoma. More than 90% of all skin cancers fall into the first two classifications. Both basal cell carcinoma and squamous cell carcinoma are slow-growing tumors with a cure rate of 95% or greater after early treatment.

Etiology and Risk Factors

The cause of skin cancer is well known. Prolonged or intermittent, repeated exposure to UVL radiation from the sun, especially when it results in sunburn and blistering, plays a key role in the induction of skin cancer, especially malignant melanoma. The majority of all non-melanoma skin cancers occur on parts of the body unprotected by clothing (face, neck, forearms, and backs of hands) and in people who have received considerable exposure to sunlight. All people are at risk of skin cancer regardless of skin tone and hair color; however, some are at much greater risk than others. In general, people with red, blond, or light brown hair with light complexions or freckles, many of Celtic or Scandinavian origin, are most susceptible; blacks and Asians are least susceptible.

All clients should be taught to look for new moles or lesions and to evaluate them for danger signs of cancer. Danger signals in moles (pigmented nevi) are presented in Box 49–2. Suspicious lesions should be examined by a physician.

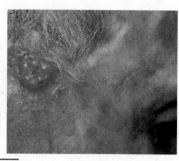

FIGURE 49–13 Basal cell carcinoma characterized by rolled edges and a crater in the center of the lesion. Scars are from previous destruction of skin lesions.

The pattern of reaction to acute sun exposure can be correlated with the development of actinic keratosis and skin cancer. People who never tan and always burn after 1 to 2 hours of midday summer sun are most susceptible. People who burn once or twice at the beginning of summer and then tan are somewhat less susceptible. Those who never burn and always tan are the least susceptible. The most severely affected people usually have a history of long-term occupational (farmers, construction workers, surveyors, sailors) or recreational (swimmers, skiers, surfers, sunbathers) sun exposure.

Clinical Manifestations
■ BASAL CELL CARCINOMA

Basal cell carcinoma, the most common form of skin cancer, is a malignant epithelial tumor of the skin that arises from the basal cells in the epidermis. The tumor is usually painless and slow-growing, generally appearing on sun-exposed skin of the face, ears, head, neck, or hands. Occasionally, basal cell carcinoma may appear on the trunk, especially the upper back and chest. The majority of cases are caused by chronic overexposure to UVL radiation, and only a few cases can be linked to arsenic, burns, scars, exposure to radiation, or genetic predisposition. Clinical and histologic findings are used to identify the tumor.

The most common clinical presentation of basal cell carcinoma is the nodular lesion (Fig. 49–13). This is a dome-shaped papule with a well-defined border having a classic "pearly" texture. Basal cell carcinoma has this flesh-colored "pearly" or shiny appearance because it does not keratinize. Telangiectatic vessels frequently overlie the lesion. As the lesion enlarges, the center may flatten or ulcerate; however, the border is still raised, giving a "rolled-edge" appearance.

Although basal cell carcinomas almost never metastasize, they can be locally destructive and invasive through tissue. This is particularly true on the face, where a lesion can invade deep structures with resultant loss of an eye or ear or the nose. If untreated, the tumor can invade through bone and brain. If the tumor is identified and treated early, local excision or even nonexcisional destruction is usually curative.

Clients who have had one basal cell carcinoma are at risk for development of another. Recurrences of previously treated basal cell carcinomas are also possible but more unusual; recurrence is generally noted within the first 2 years after removal or therapy.

■ SQUAMOUS CELL CARCINOMA

Squamous cell carcinoma (Fig. 49–14) is the second most common skin cancer in whites. It is a tumor of the epidermal keratinocytes and rarely occurs in dark-skinned people. It is found on areas often exposed to the sun, typically the rim of the ear, the face, the lips and mouth, and the backs of the hands.

Squamous cell carcinoma is more difficult to characterize than basal cell carcinoma. The tumor is poorly marginated; the edge often blends into surrounding sun-damaged skin. Squamous cell carcinoma may present as an ulcer, a flat red area, a cutaneous horn, an indurated plaque, or a hyperkeratotic papule or nodule. Often it presents as a red- to skin-colored papule surmounted by varying amounts of scale.

The lesions grow more rapidly than does basal cell carcinoma. These tumors are potentially dangerous because they may infiltrate surrounding structures and metastasize to lymph nodes, with a fatal outcome.

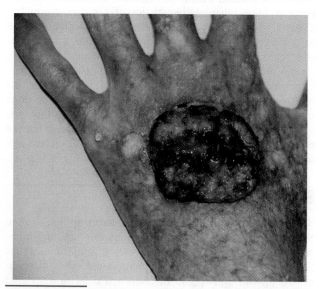

FIGURE 49–14 Squamous cell carcinoma on the hand.

■ MALIGNANT MELANOMA

Malignant melanoma (Figs. 49–15 and 49–16) is a cancer of melanocytes; it is the deadliest form of skin cancer. The incidence of and death rate from melanoma are rising worldwide. In countries populated with fair-skinned white people, the incidence of melanoma and the mortality rate have risen by 7% to 15% per year, more than doubling during the 1990s. Whites have 10 times the incidence of blacks.

Exposure to UVL continues to be one of the most important causes of malignant melanoma. However, melanoma can appear anywhere on the body, not just on sun-exposed areas. Most malignant melanomas appear to be associated with the intensity rather than the duration of sunlight exposure, in contrast to basal cell and squamous cell carcinomas. Melanoma tends to be observed more often in whites who have had a history of blistering sunburns or a family history of melanoma or atypical moles. The suspicion of melanoma is based on history as well as the clinical appearance.

Clinical Manifestations

The cardinal clinical manifestation of melanoma is a change in a skin lesion observed over a period of months. If a lesion grows so fast that it doubles in size in 10 days, it is usually an inflammation. If a lesion changes so slowly that neither the client nor family is sure of a change, it is usually benign. Changes that may signal melanoma include doubling size in 3 to 8 months, change in diameter, bleeding, itching, ulceration, a change in color, or development of a palpable lymph node.

Melanomas usually have the following features: (1) various shades of brown, black, or blue within one lesion, (2) an irregular raised surface, (3) an irregular perimeter, (4) ulceration of the surface, and (5) crusting. Four types of melanoma are presented in Table 49–4. The tumor can metastasize, usually to the brain, lungs, bones, liver, and skin, and is ultimately fatal. The prognosis with melanoma has become more predictable. Clinically, metastatic melanoma is universally fatal. Prognosis and mortality for melanoma that is not clinically metastatic at presentation depend on the depth of the lesion at the time of excision.

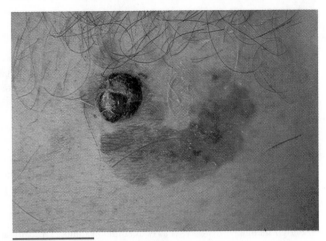

FIGURE 49–16 Nodular melanoma.

The more superficial or "thin" the tumor, the better the prognosis.

Outcome Management

■ Medical Management

Medical management begins with a high level of suspicion for any type of skin cancer but specifically for melanoma. The need for early detection cannot be overemphasized. Any indication, whether it is a confirmed risk factor or a suspicious lesion, is adequate reason for referral. The most exciting medical development in the treatment of melanoma is the creation and testing of therapeutic vaccines. A variety of vaccines targeting melanoma cell antigens are in the clinical trial phase.

■ Surgical Management

Treatment of all skin cancers requires removal of the lesion. The margins of the resected specimen must be free of tumor to a specified distance (depending on the type of skin cancer) to guarantee full removal.

A special surgical technique primarily used for the removal of skin malignancies such as basal cell carcinoma and squamous cell carcinoma is *Mohs' surgery*, which is also indicated for primary lesions in areas in which preservation of normal skin is necessary (e.g., eyelids, pinna, nasolabial folds). The technique involves a series of excisions with careful microscopic tissue assessment to "map" the presence or absence of malignant cells within each specimen. The procedure may be lengthy. After all tumor tissue is removed, the wound is closed with sutures or with a flap or allowed to close by secondary intention.

Basal cell carcinomas and squamous cell carcinomas can also be excised and the surgical wound closed primarily (with skin edges sewn together) or with a skin flap. The advantage of this technique is that it requires much less time, and the scar is controllable as a fine line. The tumor is completely excised with adequate margins of tumor-free tissue. If there is doubt about adequacy of margins, the specimen is sent for pathologic diagnosis (by frozen section technique).

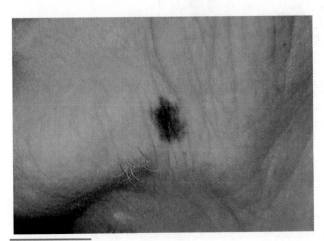

FIGURE 49–15 Superficial spreading melanoma.

TABLE 49–4	TYPES OF MELANOMA	
Tumor Type	**General Information**	**Clinical Manifestations**
Superficial spreading melanoma (SSM)	The most common form of melanoma; slowly changing lesion with more rapid growth just before diagnosis	Deeply pigmented area contained within a brown nevus (freckle); usually flat and asymmetrical; as lesion grows, color changes may occur, ranging from jet black to dark blue to pale gray or white; looks lacy; lesions may have areas of no color; usually 2 cm wide
Nodular melanoma (NM)	Second most common form of melanoma; more aggressive tumor than SSM, with shorter clinical onset time	Common on the trunk, head, and neck; usually 1–2 cm in diameter; frequently begin in normal skin, rather than in a pre-existing lesion; dark and more uniform in color; may resemble a blood blister or hemangioma; dome-shaped with sharp borders
Lentigo maligna melanoma (LMM)	Fairly uncommon tumor; typically appears on the face of white women; usually has been present for long period of time (5–15 yr)	Generally a large, flat lesion that looks like a stain on the skin; typically tan with various shades of brown; metastasis less common
Acral lentiginous melanoma (ALM)	Commonly occurs on palms and soles; more common in dark-skinned people; usually occurs in older adults; may evolve over a few months to years	Large lesion, about 3 cm in diameter; resembles LMM (a tan or brown flat lesion on the palm or sole); can be misdiagnosed as a corn; ulceration is common; likely to metastasize

The treatment of malignant melanoma is wide local excision. Surgical excision begins with biopsy to determine the stage of the cancer. Biopsies are performed whenever a benign nature of the lesion is uncertain. Excisional biopsy is the removal of the lesion and a narrow margin of normal-appearing tissue. This tissue is examined, and the melanoma is staged (Fig. 49–17).

Surgeons differ on the timing of the definitive surgery. Some surgeons excise the lesion after frozen section examination while the client is still on the operating table.

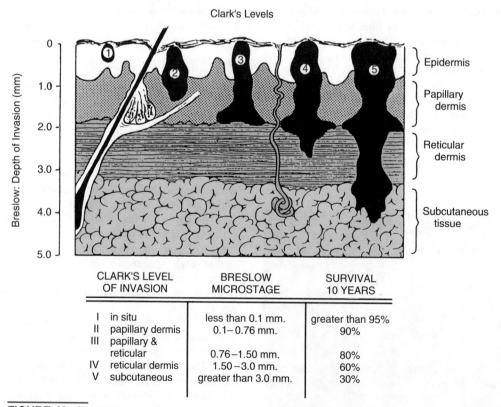

CLARK'S LEVEL OF INVASION		BRESLOW MICROSTAGE	SURVIVAL 10 YEARS
I	in situ	less than 0.1 mm.	greater than 95%
II	papillary dermis	0.1–0.76 mm.	90%
III	papillary & reticular	0.76–1.50 mm.	80%
IV	reticular dermis	1.50–3.0 mm.	60%
V	subcutaneous	greater than 3.0 mm.	30%

FIGURE 49–17 The combination of Clark's level of invasion and Breslow's depth of invasion allows prediction of 10-year survival in melanoma. (From Eisenbaum, S. L., & Black, J. M. [1988]. Melanoma. *Plastic Surgical Nursing, 8*, 42–47.)

Other surgeons wait for the results of permanent section pathologic diagnosis and then proceed with definitive treatment. The final excision is usually completed within 1 week of biopsy. Although there is a theoretical risk of tumor spread during biopsy, there is no convincing evidence that waiting 1 to even 6 weeks after biopsy jeopardizes the outcome. In fact, sometimes the delay gives the client time to prepare for surgery, both physically and psychologically.

The tumor is excised with a 1- to 3-cm margin of normal-appearing tissue. The margin width is based on the type of melanoma. The surgical wound is closed either primarily or with grafts or flaps.

Most clients with metastatic melanoma live less than 1 year. There is no cure today for metastatic melanoma, but some of the new developments in clinical trials may change currently accepted treatments. A treatment plan is formulated on the basis of several factors: site of the tumor, number of metastases, rate of tumor growth, previous treatments, response to treatment, and the age, general health, and desires of the client. Some treatments include surgery to remove metastatic lesions, radiation therapy, chemotherapy, and local hyperthermia. Of course, the client can opt for no further treatment.

CUTANEOUS T-CELL LYMPHOMA (MYCOSIS FUNGOIDES)

Cutaneous T-cell lymphoma (CTCL), or mycosis fungoides, is a malignant disease involving the T helper cells. Malignant T cells in the blood migrate to the skin, where they have an affinity for the epidermis. The malignant cells continue to grow and change, eventually moving into the dermis. The cause is not known, and the course is unpredictable, varying with the type of presentation.

The three distinct clinical presentations are patch, plaque, and tumor. Clinical manifestations include eversion of the eyelids and hyperkeratosis of the palms and soles, often with fissuring. Finally, the plaques form tumors that ultimately ulcerate. Tumors can also develop spontaneously in previously unaffected areas, and eventual visceral or organ involvement ensues. This disease is often described as a slow-growing but highly disfiguring debilitating cancer. Clients often feel desperate by the time diagnosis is confirmed, which adds to the psychological difficulties. The tumor presentation carries the worst prognosis, with a survival period of 3 years or less.

CTCL is extremely difficult to diagnose and is often misdiagnosed. In its early stages, CTCL can clinically mimic eczematous processes. The initial erythematous papules resemble those in other eczematous conditions, including psoriasis and atopic dermatitis. The original eruptions of CTCL may be either transitory or of prolonged duration and sometimes are pruritic.

Outcome Management

Control of pruritus is essential at all stages and is accomplished by rehydration of the skin, various dry skin therapies (see Xerotic Eczema), topical corticosteroids, and PUVA therapy (see Ultraviolet Light Therapy). Prevention of secondary infections is important. Nitrogen mustard and other chemotherapy agents are administered topically. Daily application of chemotherapeutic agents often constitutes the initial treatment. Photophoresis, a treatment involving the removal of small amounts of blood that is irradiated and then returned to the body, is used frequently in more advanced stages. Total-body electron beam therapy with or without adjuvant chemotherapy is an aggressive approach often used.

The primary systemic drug was formerly intravenous methotrexate. With advances in treatment, newer drugs have replaced methotrexate: one is denileukin diftitox (Ontak) used primarily in the treatment of persistent or recurrent CTCL. This agent has produced sustained regression of the tumors, in some cases for longer than 2 years. Unfortunately, fatalities remain extremely high in this disease as a result of progression to systemic involvement.

KAPOSI'S SARCOMA

Kaposi's sarcoma is a vascular malignancy that presents as a skin disorder. It has a long history. Kaposi's sarcoma used to be a skin disease seen predominantly in 50- to 60-year-old men in Central or Eastern Europe. It was also seen, although less frequently, in blacks and the immunosuppressed (e.g., renal transplant recipients). In the past two decades, Kaposi's sarcoma has been seen more often in clients with acquired immunodeficiency syndrome (AIDS).

Etiology and Risk Factors

The cause of Kaposi's sarcoma is not known, although infection with HIV and herpesvirus have been suggested as cofactors in its development. It is considered to be due to a failure in the immune system, perhaps as a result of frequent or overwhelming infections. The lesions begin in the mid-dermis and extend upward into the epidermis.

The client history must include specific details of the sexual history when lesions of this type are present. All known risk factors for AIDS should be identified, such as homosexual activity, intravenous (IV) drug use, and multiple sexual partners.

Clinical Manifestations

The lesions of Kaposi's sarcoma begin as red, dark blue, or purple macules on the lower legs that coalesce into larger plaques (Fig. 49–18). These large plaques frequently ulcerate or open and drain. The lesions spread by metastasis through the upper body and then to the face and oral mucosa. Lesions of the lymph nodes, gastrointestinal tract, and lungs develop in about 75% of clients. Clients also report pain and itching in the lesions; as Kaposi's sarcoma progresses, the legs become edematous.

The diagnosis of Kaposi's sarcoma is confirmed by skin biopsy. A high index of suspicion should exist for those clients with immunosuppression.

Outcome Management

Local lesions can be excised or treated with intralesional chemotherapy. Systemic lesions are treated with a combination of interferon-alpha, cytotoxic agents, and radiation therapy. In general, response to treatment is poor. A complete discussion of AIDS may be found in Chapter 79.

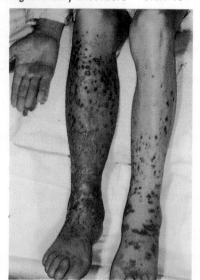

FIGURE 49–18 Kaposi's sarcoma.

Nursing interventions include obtaining informed consent for HIV testing and addressing the client's questions and concerns. Client education should include guidelines for safe sex and giving clients the addresses and telephone numbers of appropriate local and national resource groups.

BULLOUS DISORDERS: PEMPHIGUS

Pemphigus is a chronic disorder that results in the development of blisters (*bullae*). It is fairly uncommon in the general population, but the incidence is increased in Jewish and Mediterranean peoples. There are several types: pemphigus vulgaris, pemphigus foliaceus, and pemphigus erythematosus. This discussion focuses on pemphigus vulgaris, the most common type.

Pemphigus is an autoimmune disease caused by circulating immunoglobulin G (IgG) autoantibodies. These autoantibodies react with the intracellular cement—the substance that holds epidermal cells together. The reaction causes intraepidermal bulla (blister) formation and acantholysis (loss of cohesion between epidermal cells).

Clinical manifestations include flaccid bullae that rupture easily, emitting a foul-smelling drainage and leaving crusted, denuded skin. Nikolsky's sign is the result when the epidermis can be rubbed off by slight friction or injury; this sign is a hallmark of pemphigus. Even slight pressure on an intact blister may cause it to spread to adjacent skin. The lesions are common on the face, back, chest, groin, and umbilicus.

Outcome Management

Management includes large doses of steroids and immunosuppressives. Plasmapheresis has been of some benefit in the treatment of pemphigus. If a large proportion of the skin is denuded, management is similar to that for a burn-injured client. The client is at increased risk for infection, fluid and electrolyte imbalance, and stress response complications (i.e., stress ulcers, body system fail-

ure). In addition, nursing management focuses on self-concept and pain management. Potassium permanganate baths may be used to reduce the risk of infection, control the odor of the drainage, and ease the pain.

INFECTIOUS DISORDERS

Several organisms lead to skin infections and infestations. Common skin infections are described in Table 49–5. A few are discussed in detail here.

■ ERYSIPELAS AND CELLULITIS

Erysipelas is an acute, superficial, rapidly spreading inflammation of the dermis and lymphatics. The usual causative agent is beta-hemolytic group A streptococci. The organism enters tissue via an abrasion, bite, trauma, or wound. Fever and leukocytosis (elevated white blood cell count) are present. The initial lesion is small, elevated, and bright red. The involved area spreads peripherally to become a plaque with sharp, indurated borders. Lesions are most common on the face and extremities. Recurrence in the same area is common, possibly because of underlying lymphatic obstruction.

Cellulitis is a skin infection extending into the deeper dermis and subcutaneous fat that results in deep, red erythema without sharp borders that spreads widely through tissue spaces (see Fig. 49–19). The skin is erythematous, edematous, tender, and sometimes nodular. *Streptococcus pyogenes* is the usual cause of this infection; however, other pathogens may be responsible. Lymphangitis may occur; if cellulitis is untreated, gangrene, metastatic abscesses, and sepsis result.

At increased risk for erysipelas and cellulitis are older adults and clients with lowered resistance from diabetes, malnutrition, steroid therapy, or the presence of wounds or ulcers. Other predisposing factors include the presence of edema and of other cutaneous inflammation or wounds (e.g., tinea, eczema, burns, trauma). There is a tendency for recurrence, especially at sites of lymphatic obstruction.

Erysipelas and cellulitis are treated by either oral or IV antibiotics that are effective against both streptococci and *Staphylococcus aureus*. Before antibiotics are administered, a wound specimen for culture and sensitivity testing should be obtained, although culture rarely yields the causative organism. Soaks may reduce edema and inflammation. The enzymes that facilitate a rapid spread of infection also seem to produce other significant manifestations such as high fever, tachycardia, confusion, and hypotension; appropriate interventions should be undertaken if these occur. Monitor the client's temperature and administer prescribed antipyretic medication. Prevent cross-contamination by teaching the client proper hand-washing technique and careful handling of soiled linen, clothing, dressings, and so forth. Universal precautions should be used as appropriate. Close follow-up evaluation is necessary.

■ HERPES ZOSTER (SHINGLES)

Herpes zoster (Fig. 49–20), or shingles, is an infection caused by the reactivation of the varicella virus in clients who have had chickenpox. Although zoster is much less

TABLE 49-5	COMMON SKIN INFECTIONS AND INFESTATIONS	
Disease with Causative Organism	**Clinical Manifestations**	**Management**
PARASITIC		
Scabies: *Sarcoptes scabiei*	Multiple straight or wavy thread-like lines beneath the skin, itching	Application of a scabicide with re-treatment in 1 wk to kill residual eggs. All clothing and linen should be washed and dried in hot cycles or dry cleaned.
Lice: *Pediculus humanus, Phthirus pubis*	Intense itching; scratch marks may be evident	Application of pediculicides. For *head lice,* the shampoo should be worked into dry hair until it is saturated. A fine-toothed comb should be used to remove dead lice and nits. Brushes and combs should be washed in pediculicide also. For *body lice,* a pediculicide lotion is applied to involved body areas. Clothing should be washed and dried in hot cycles or dry cleaned. Other items can be stored in plastic bags for 30–35 days. Family members, close contacts, and sexual partners should be treated, too.
BACTERIAL		
Impetigo: group A streptococci, staphylococci	Pruritic vesicle or pustule that breaks and leaves a thick honey-colored crust	Antibiotics given until culture results available include erythromycin or dicloxacillin. Mupirocin preferable to oral antibiotics when lesions limited to small, localized area. Teach control of contagion; infection is contagious as long as skin lesions are present. Thorough hand-washing, separate laundry for client's linens, separate washing of client's dishes.
Folliculitis, furuncles, carbuncles: *Staphylococcus aureus*	White pustules on forehead, chest, upper back, neck, thighs, groin, and axillae; furuncles are deeper inflamed nodules; carbuncles are interconnected furuncles and often rupture, expelling purulent, foul-smelling thick drainage	Localized folliculitis is treated with warm compresses, gentle washing, and topical antibiotics. Furuncles are treated as for folliculitis with incision and drainage (I&D) to avoid rupture. Carbuncles are treated with systemic antibiotics and I&D. Instruct client to use disposable razors to avoid reinfection. Reduce spread of infection by careful hand-washing and separate laundry of linens.
FUNGAL		
Candidiasis: *Candida albicans*	Appearance depends on location; in the *mouth,* infection is called thrush and appears as white plaques with an underlying red base with fissures on corners of the mouth; *skin* lesions are pruritic, red, and moist with eroded scales, commonly found in the axilla and gluteal, perianal, and interdigital folds; *vaginal* thrush causes intense itching and a cheesy drainage	Eliminate or control predisposing factors such as antibiotics (which alter the flora), malnutrition, diabetes, immunosuppression, pregnancy, or use of birth control pills. Use topical antifungal powders and creams. Keep the skin dry, the environment cool.
Tinea: variety of dermatophytes (tinea corporis, on body; tinea capitis, on scalp; tinea cruris, jock itch; tinea pedis, athlete's foot)	Tinea corporis: round red macules and papules with scales—lesions have advancing borders and healing centers; tinea capitis: patchy hair loss, inflammation, scales, and folliculitis; tinea cruris: red lesions with raised borders; tinea pedis: scaling, maceration, pain, and vesicles	Infection is controlled with antifungal solutions and creams. Acute lesions may require wet dressings, keratolytic agents, or both to remove the scales. Client is taught to reduce risk by thoroughly drying after a bath or shower, wearing absorbent underwear and socks, applying talc to intertriginous areas, and wearing open shoes during warm weather.

Table continued on following page

TABLE 49–5	COMMON SKIN INFECTIONS AND INFESTATIONS *Continued*	
Disease with Causative Organism	**Clinical Manifestations**	**Management**
VIRAL		
Herpes simplex: herpes simplex virus	Vesicles preceded by sensation of itching or burning; clear exudate from vesicles, followed by crusting; common to the nose, lips, cheeks, ears, and genitalia	No cure is available. Treatment includes pain relief and topical anesthetics. Acyclovir, an antiviral drug, may decrease viral shedding and hasten healing. Avoiding the sun and using sunscreens reduce recurrent lesions on the lips. Reduce contagiousness by frequent hand-washing, not picking at lesions, avoiding sexual intercourse and kissing while lesions are active, and not sharing lipsticks. Try to identify (and avoid or control) personal triggers for lesions.
Warts: human papillomavirus	Rough, fresh, or gray-colored skin protrusion	Numerous therapies, some with over-the-counter medication. May require electrodesiccation or cryosurgery. Intralesional injections of cytotoxic drugs may also be used. No treatment also an acceptable option.

communicable than varicella, people who have not had chickenpox are at risk after exposure to a person with herpes zoster. An increased incidence of herpes zoster is seen in clients with lymphoma, leukemia, or AIDS, probably because of their decreased immunologic response.

Diagnostic tests may not be necessary because of the specific characteristics of herpes zoster; however, a Tzanck test demonstrates multinucleated giant cells (see Chapter 48), and a viral culture also is helpful.

Clinical Manifestations

The primary lesion of zoster is a vesicle. The classic presentation is grouped vesicles on an erythematous base along a dermatome. The vesicles appear 1 to 2 days after onset of pain and itching at the site. Occasionally, only papules appear and not vesicles. Because they follow nerve pathways, the lesions do not cross the body's midline; however, rarely, the nerves of both sides may be involved. Herpes zoster lesions evolve into ulcers on the superficial mucous membrane.

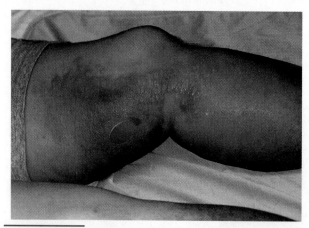

FIGURE 49–19 Cellulitis in a client with long-standing diabetes and stasis dermatitis.

The eruption generally clears in about 2 weeks, unless the period between the pain and the eruption is longer than 2 days. In such cases, a prolonged convalescence may be expected. Residual pain, called postherpetic neuralgia, and itching are the major complications with herpes zoster. The pain may be constant or intermittent and may range from light burning to a deep visceral sensation. The duration of the pain can be weeks or months to years. Unfortunately, in older clients, the pain generally lasts months to years. Another potential complication is loss of sight when herpes zoster involves the facial or acoustic nerve. Involvement of the ophthalmic branch of the facial nerve requires close medical attention to avoid ocular damage.

Outcome Management

Treatment for herpes zoster is administration of antiviral medications such as acyclovir (Zovirax), given in large doses orally or smaller doses intravenously five times daily. Newer antiviral agents (Valtrex) have more convenient dosing schedules. Antivirals, when started early in the course of the disease, reduce acute pain and also accelerate healing of the lesions. Studies now suggest that early oral antiviral therapy may assist in reducing postherpetic neuralgia. Analgesics and sedatives are prescribed for pain relief.

Topical therapy is primarily symptomatic: applications of cool compresses, use of cooling antipruritic preparations (see Table 49–1), and measures to prevent secondary infection. If pain is present, the client's normal pain tolerance and current pain level must be assessed. Systemic analgesics are usually required, and occasionally narcotics; however, in chronic pain, use of these agents raises the possibility of addiction. Assess the effectiveness and side effects of prescribed analgesics. Because postherpetic neuralgia can last a long time, the client and significant others need continued intervention and support. Chronic pain management may include the use of tricyclic antidepressants, phenothiazines, and other

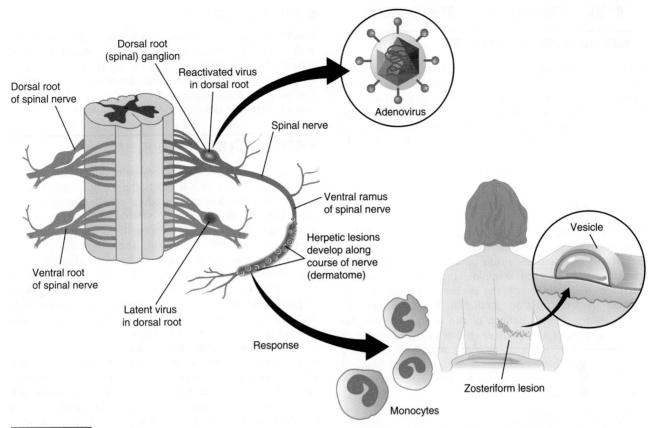

FIGURE 49–20 Pathophysiology of herpes zoster. The dormant herpes virus is reactivated causing vesicular lesions along the dermatome.

local physical modalities such as electrical stimulating units.

PLASTIC SURGERY AND OTHER COSMETIC/RESTORATIVE PROCEDURES

Plastic surgery is the surgical subspecialty that concentrates on the restoration of function and form to body structures damaged by trauma, transformed by the aging process, changed by disease processes (such as skin cancer), or malformed as a result of congenital defects. Plastic surgery can be divided into two major areas: (1) aesthetic (cosmetic) and (2) reconstructive.

Aesthetic plastic surgery improves physical features that are already within "normal" range. It is performed for changes that result from aging, to alter inherited features, or because of a client's personal desire. Clients seeking aesthetic surgery are so dissatisfied with the appearance of one or more body parts that they are willing to undergo surgery. Because aesthetic surgery is considered "cosmetic," it is not covered by insurance; clients pay out of pocket. Most clients are enthusiastic and happy because the surgery is a culmination of a personal desire that they may have held for a long time. In contrast, other clients may or may not have social support for their decision. The client may feel vain, embarrassed, or guilty about taking health care away from "people who really need it." Become sensitive to these feelings in the client, and be comfortable with a person's normal desires to feel good about the way he or she looks.

Reconstructive surgery attempts to restore a more normal appearance or function in a person who has an abnormal body part or in whom a body part is missing. The abnormality may be a result of injury or disease, it may be congenital, or it may be the cause of other medical problems. People undergoing reconstructive surgery are typically motivated to try to gain increased function of body parts and to improve their appearance. Although they may hope that plastic surgery will make them "normal," they usually know this may be unrealistic. Such clients are often struggling with diverse emotions: hope for a future without disease recurrence, eagerness to see final surgical results, anxiety over the surgery itself and impending postoperative pain, and weariness of the illness. The client having reconstructive surgery does have the advantage of social approval. Inasmuch as such a client is seen as a victim, society, as represented by either individuals or institutions, often provides treatment or makes appeals for payment of the operations.

Because of the significant impact of plastic surgery procedures on body image and self-esteem, psychological care is imperative. Plastic surgery is not only an operation on the skin; it reaches into the psyche of the person undergoing the surgery.

BASIC PRINCIPLES OF PLASTIC SURGERY

ACHIEVING MINIMAL SCARRING

Minimal postoperative scarring is the hallmark of successful plastic surgery. It is important to understand that no surgery can be done without creating a scar. Plastic surgery is conducted to minimize scars, so at times it seems that surgery can be done without scars. The quality of scarring is affected by many variables, such as the client's age, general health, skin type, and healing ability. Surgical technique and the quality of wound care also affect the healing process.

■ SKIN LINES

In every person, the skin has normal lines and folds. Incisions made perpendicular to these lines result in more obvious scars. Incisions made parallel to the lines heal camouflaged by natural skinfolds. Incisions can also be hidden in the scalp or by the eyebrow or concealed by clothing. A long incision parallel to these lines is less visible than a shorter incision placed at right angles. No amount of care in suturing can ensure an aesthetic scar if the incision is positioned at right angles or obliquely relative to the lines of minimal tension. Skinfolds and wrinkles become more pronounced with age, further obscuring incision lines.

■ ELLIPTICAL INCISIONS

When excising a lesion, the surgeon designs the incision lines to be longer than the lesion (Fig. 49–21). The resulting defect is elliptical, and the skin edges can be approximated easily. When the defect is round, tissues bunch at the ends of the incision, resulting in "dog ears."

■ SUTURING TECHNIQUES

To heal with minimal scarring, the edges of the skin incision must be approximated precisely, without undue tension. Each suture puncture represents a miniature wound, and scar tissue forms at the site of each puncture. Suture lines must be kept clean; otherwise, stitch abscesses may develop, increasing scarring. Sutures removed within 7 days leave no discernible suture marks or "tracks." Unfortunately, the skin on some areas of the body (e.g., the back) is thick and slower to heal, so that sutures must remain in place for a longer period of time. It is difficult to achieve fine scarring in these areas.

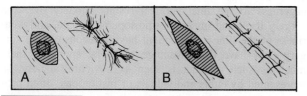

FIGURE 49–21 Elliptical excisions are used to reduce the scar. The *shaded area* shows the area of tissue removed with each lesion. *A,* If the ellipse is too short, puckers ("dog ears") form at the ends of the incision. This creates an unsightly scar. *B,* The correct length of elliptical incision for minimal scarring. (Redrawn from Grabb, W., & Smith, J. [1979]. *Plastic surgery* [3rd ed]. Boston: Little, Brown.)

■ OTHER VARIABLES

Blacks, people of Mediterranean origin, and other people with dark skin tend to have more noticeable scars. Wounds located in areas in which the tissue moves as it heals (e.g., over joints) are also more prone to scarring. The skin of malnourished clients heals slowly, and the wounds may also develop more obvious scars.

SELECTING CLIENTS

The success of a plastic surgery procedure is determined by the degree to which it meets the client's expectations. A surgical procedure may produce excellent technical results, but the client may not consider it a success if the results do not conform to expectations about a specific appearance or level of function. Therefore, it is essential that the surgeon and the nurse understand what the client expects and that the client have a realistic view of what can and cannot be accomplished by surgery. Most plastic surgery procedures are not emergencies, and ample time is available to ascertain that the client is physically and psychologically prepared for surgery.

Because most procedures affect appearance, clients make a considerable emotional commitment when they elect to have plastic surgery. It is important to determine client characteristics that may indicate lack of satisfaction with a result. In addition to being in good physical health, the client must be psychologically healthy. Assessing the client's motivation is essential. Plastic surgery neither cures a person's underlying emotional problems nor alleviates major stress. An external change does not make a happy, well-adjusted person out of a person who is unhappy, poorly adjusted, or excessively stressed. Clients who expect plastic surgery to do so are poor candidates for plastic surgery. Nurses help to identify appropriate candidates for surgery. In most situations, the client feels that the physician is too busy and talks more openly to the nurse about the desires for the surgical outcome.[27]

■ UNDERSTANDING MOTIVATIONS FOR SURGERY

The desire to be attractive or beautiful is present in people of all cultures, but the perception of what is attractive varies. Adorning the body with paints or scars dates from ancient times to the present (e.g., lipstick, nail polish, tattoos). Some people decorate the body by wearing objects in their noses, ear lobes, or lips. Western society pressures people to continue to look young (perhaps by exercise) and to combat the normal physical changes of aging (perhaps by plastic surgery). For many years, people were limited to highlighting their positive features with make-up and clothing.

The importance of physical appearance varies from person to person; however, it is an integral part of the sense of self. The desire to want to physically resemble one's peers reasonably closely — for instance, to have acceptably "normal" facial features — is a normal desire. Clients' physical aspects are consistent with their idea of who they are as people. Trauma, disease states, congenital deformities, or multi-stage reconstruction procedures can result in alterations in appearance that have an impact on self-esteem and body image. Physical appearance carries significant meaning to overall quality of life for both men and women and should be considered throughout all phases of treatment.

A significant portion of any deformity rests in the client's perception of the abnormality. Perceptions develop in part from body image. Body image describes a person's perception of his or her body—how the person *thinks* he or she looks, rather than an objective assessment of the person's characteristics. Body image is a factor in determining self-image, self-concept, and self-esteem. People with a positive body image display more confidence and interact more easily with others. Body image changes continually, depending on individual expectations and feedback from others.

A person with a physical deformity, real or perceived, can have a severely damaged body image. Even the usual processes of aging can be detrimental to body image. A self-perception of "getting old" can impair self-confidence, affect behavior, and interfere with interactions in society. Body image is an important factor in the nursing assessment of the client having plastic surgery.

The client's ability to cope with a temporary or permanent or a perceived or actual disfigurement is also assessed. Assess the client's coping mechanisms. Some coping mechanisms may be effective; others may be ineffective. Men may have more difficulty expressing their feelings about their appearance than that typically noted in women. Listen to the client, be alert for positive and negative self-statements, and note the degree of anxi-

ety and fear. Evaluate the client's willingness or unwillingness to touch or look at involved body areas and the client's comfort with being near other people.

Techniques for working with clients who have alterations in body image are presented in Box 49–3.

■ DETERMINING REALISTIC EXPECTATIONS

A client who understands what is and what is not a possible surgical outcome is said to have realistic expectations. Determining a client's expectations is a crucial first step before any surgery is performed. Most clients with conditions requiring plastic surgery have some degree of deformity. The deformity can be *actual,* that is, objectively observable by others (e.g., a missing breast or a deviated septum), or it can be *perceived*—that is, the client is aware of the deformity, but it may not be noticeable to other people (e.g., fine facial wrinkling indicative of aging). It is important to clearly understand what the client sees and wants changed.

Clients with realistic expectations understand that facial rejuvenating surgery cannot stop the clock. A face lift (rhytidectomy) cannot make a 65-year-old woman look like a 40-year-old. Realistic expectations are the realization that appearance will be improved, but aging continues.

Obviously, a face lift cannot get an unfaithful spouse to return home. Expectations can be very private and may be hidden from the physician and the nurse during interviews. Clients with documented or suspected psychiatric illness may or may not be candidates for plastic surgery. A consultation with the psychiatrist or psychologist who

---

BOX 49–3   Supporting the Client Who Has a Changed Body Image

Many clients undergoing plastic surgery experience some form of body image alteration. Clients may experience body image changes before surgery due to disease or injury. They may also have problems after surgery from edema, bruising, or less than desired results. Try to anticipate these problems and work with the client as soon as possible to facilitate needed adjustments. You may want to work with the nursing diagnosis of *Risk for Body Image Disturbance* or *Self-Esteem Disturbance related to perceived or actual disfigurement and changes in self-concept.* The expected outcome must be tailored to the client but may include improved self-image with incorporation of the changed body part into the body image, as evidenced by effective coping and appropriate use of defense mechanisms; verbalizing feelings comfortably and appropriately; expressing satisfaction with the changed body image; having the ability to openly verbalize feelings; making positive statements about self; having a normal level of anxiety and normal fears; comfortably looking at self in mirror and/or touching the deformed body area, healed surgical site, or other scars; being able to be with others comfortably; and having no indications of depression.

Some interventions that you may find effective with clients who are experiencing body image disturbances include the following:

- Continue to assess apparent self-concept, coping methods, defense mechanisms, degree of anxiety, and fears frequently.
- Assist the client to explore and express feelings; do not use phrases such as "I know how you feel." These empty phrases build barriers to communication, whereas statements

such as "you are angry" or "you seem depressed," for example, identify the feeling.
- Be sensitive to the client's feelings and needs.
- Acknowledge the client's feelings.
- Present reality; building false hope is detrimental (reality need not be brutal, however).
- Healing is unpredictable; refer questions about healing to the surgeon.
- Do not force the client to view or touch himself or herself; gently assist the client to look at and touch the deformity or healed surgical site (help incorporate it into the client's self-concept and body image).
- Encourage the client to begin meeting in public to begin desensitization to the reactions of others, such as by taking walks in halls; desensitization begins in safe environments and proceeds to new situations, prepare the client for stares and remarks.
- Discuss others' reaction to the client; support grief reactions.
- If the client has a facial deformity, prepare visitors and family members before they see the client.
- Look for vocal expression or hand gestures in cases of facial disfigurement; facial expression may be limited in clients with extensive facial scars or skin grafts.
- Refer the client and family to local support groups, such as About Face.
- Assist the client with techniques to camouflage scars; licensed aestheticians can assist with make-up choices and techniques.

is providing treatment for the client is necessary before any operation is undertaken.

The realistic client understands that plastic surgery does not occur as depicted in films: the bandages do not come off the next day, leaving the client perfectly healed and changed into a new person. Bruising can last for 2 weeks, and swelling can persist for 6 months.

Realistic clients understand that some scarring is inevitable, but that the scars are to be hidden in normal skinfolds and will therefore be less noticeable. Help clients to understand that any incision results in the formation of scar tissue. It is essential that the client have a realistic expectation of the location and extent of scarring that will result from the surgical procedure. Remind the client that a scar matures over a long period of time. Some scars take as long as several years to achieve their final appearance.

Explain that postoperative activities must be curtailed temporarily. Clients who are very athletic and refuse to remain inactive during healing and workaholics who refuse to take time off from work, present potential management problems. Preoperative teaching includes helping the client develop realistic postoperative expectations. Explain how the surgery will affect usual routines. Thorough planning ensures minimum disruption in routines. Preoperative teaching must include information about restrictions on activity, the location and extent of scars, and the clinical manifestations of possible complications. Including family members in the teaching process promotes an effective support system for the client.

The ideal candidate would have support from relatives and significant others. Family members may react negatively, regarding the surgery as a waste of time, a waste of money, or an expression of vanity, creating unnecessary stress during surgery. With short hospital stays, the family has taken over the caregiver role by providing postoperative care, which was in the past provided by nurses. The client may feel hesitant to rely on nonsupportive family members or may fear a negative postoperative result. You have the unique opportunity to serve as the facilitator of positive interaction between the family and the client.

Finally, the ideal candidate for surgery is healthy. Disorders such as hypertension and diabetes increase risk, but they do not prevent the client from having surgery. Alcohol and tobacco use should be stopped before surgery is undertaken. Nutritional impairments are identified and corrected before surgery. Other diagnostic assessments vary with specific procedures or with specific pre-existing medical problems.

■ DOCUMENTATION THROUGH PHOTOGRAPHY

Photographs are used extensively in plastic surgery. Document the client's condition before any surgical intervention. Once changes have been made in appearance, it is very difficult to remember the details of the original appearance; photographic documentation provides an accurate record.

In office settings, nurses commonly photograph the client before and after surgery. By protecting the client's privacy and explaining the importance of photographic documentation, you can make a photography session much less uncomfortable and embarrassing. The client must give written permission for photographs to be taken, especially if they are to be used for teaching purposes in addition to documentation for the medical record. Specific and standardized positions are used. Consistent positioning is crucial for comparison of preoperative and postoperative views.

FACIAL REJUVENATING SURGERY

In childhood, skin is very elastic and is supported at maximum distention by adipose tissue ("baby fat"). During aging, the skin loses elasticity and the subcutaneous fat diminishes and changes character. Skinfolds and wrinkles become increasingly noticeable. The tissue around the eyes and jaw line sags, producing a drooping, tired, weary, or worried expression. The rate of skin change varies among people. Weight loss, sun exposure, genetic tendencies, and alcohol and tobacco use affect the speed and character of the changes.

Habitual exposure to the sun leads to several alterations in the skin. Many of the cutaneous changes once attributed to normal aging are in large measure due to chronic exposure to sunlight. Skin exposed to sunlight (natural sun and sun lamps) develops a chronic state of inflammation, which in its final stages leads to disintegration of the support matrix of elastin and collagen.

RHYTIDECTOMY (FACE LIFT)

A rhytidectomy *(face lift)* consists of removal of the larger skin wrinkles and folds from the face and neck. The ideal candidate for the procedure has large wrinkles or sagging facial skin. Fine circumoral wrinkles cannot be removed with a face lift. Physical manifestations of aging occur throughout the body but are most obvious to others on the face. Rhytidectomy may restore a more youthful appearance to the face (perhaps from 5 to 10 years younger) by removing wrinkled skin from the forehead and around the eyes and mouth (Fig. 49–22). Rhytidectomy does not result in removal of all of the wrinkles of the face. Clients may require acid peeling for fine wrinkles (see following).

Rhytidectomy is usually performed on an outpatient basis with the client under general anesthesia, or using local anesthesia with intravenous (IV) sedation. Incisions are made from the temple along the ear and out into the hair-bearing scalp behind the ear (Fig. 49–23). Through the incisions, excess facial skin is undermined and pulled back toward the ear. *Undermining* is a surgical technique in which the skin is separated from underlying structures. Most clients elect to have additional procedures done, such as tightening of the underlying fascia or facial suction lipectomy. Further adjuncts to face lift include brow lift, blepharoplasty (eyelid revision), mentoplasty (chin revision), and, occasionally, rhinoplasty (nose revision). On completion of the operation, facial compression dressings are applied.

■ Nursing Management

Postoperatively, the client is placed in the Fowler position to reduce the risk of edema. Cold compresses can also be used to reduce swelling and bleeding. Suction drains are used to eliminate dead space and remove wound drainage.

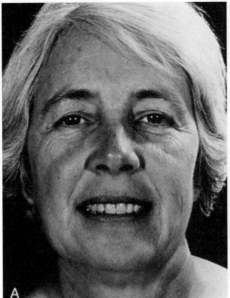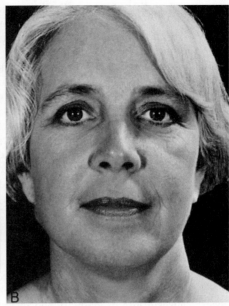

FIGURE 49–22 Before (*A*) and after (*B*) a face lift (rhytidectomy) and blepharoplasty.

Drains are removed in 24 to 48 hours, when drainage has subsided. Facial movement (talking and chewing) should be limited. Localized increases in blood pressure should be avoided by keeping the head elevated; any prescribed antihypertensive medications should also be resumed. Coughing also increases blood pressure and should be avoided (by not operating on clients with colds) or treated if it occurs after surgery.

Use antiemetics to reduce nausea and vomiting. Vomiting increases blood pressure and the risk of bleeding. Pain is minimal and can usually be managed with oral analgesics.

Complications

Complications associated with a face lift include hematoma, hair and skin loss, and nerve injury. Hematomas are caused by the resumption of bleeding in small vessels after the wound is closed. Large hematomas can cause tissue necrosis and must be surgically removed. Hematoma formation occurs most often in people who smoke or have pre-existing hypertension. Postoperative nausea and vomiting can also increase bleeding and hematoma formation. Hair loss is presumably due to altered circulation to hair follicles. The hair almost always grows back. Skin loss occasionally develops behind the ear, perhaps as a result of swelling or hematoma. Such a wound is allowed to heal by secondary intention and does not result in a very large scar. Nerve damage causing facial paralysis is a rare but devastating complication. Occasionally, facial paralysis results from nerve compression by a suture. When facial paralysis is observed, immediate surgical exploration to correct the problem and to prevent permanent damage is necessary.

FIGURE 49–23 Face lift (rhytidectomy) and blepharoplasty. Face lifts enable removal of large wrinkles and folds of skin from the face and neck. *A,* Area in pink shows amount of tissue that is undermined (lifted from the fascial connection) and moved during a face lift. For the face lift, the incision lines go around the ear and into the hair-bearing scalp; other incisions may also be used. Note also the incision line beneath the eyelid for the blepharoplasty, which enables removal of excess eyelid tissue. *B,* The postoperative near-final result, with tightened facial skin and neck folds.

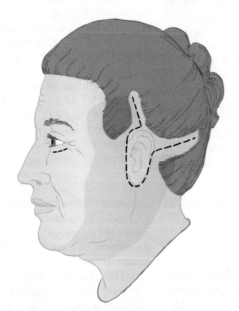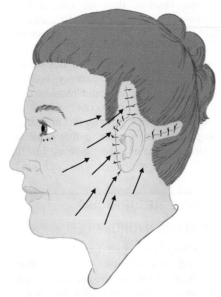

A Before face lift and blepharoplasty

B After face lift and blepharoplasty

Assess the client for complications, and instruct the family and client in how to recognize reportable changes in condition. Hematoma development is first noted as increasing facial asymmetry associated with pain or tightness on one side of the face. Increasing drainage and changes in facial sensation should also be reported.

Teach the client to keep the head of the bed elevated for 1 week to minimize edema and to rest the face for 1 week to achieve fine scars (minimize talking, and limit chewing by eating a soft diet). The surgeon usually removes dressings the morning after rhytidectomy. The face and hair may then be gently washed. Dandruff shampoo is avoided. Creams or cosmetics should not be applied to the suture line until healing is complete.

BLEPHAROPLASTY

Blepharoplasty is the surgical removal of excess skin and periorbital fat from the upper or lower eyelid. The aging process causes a loss of elasticity and relaxation of eyelid skin. Excess eyelid tissue in young and middle-aged people may be an inherited characteristic, may reflect an allergic reaction, or may be the result of cardiovascular or thyroid disease. Complete medical assessment is essential to rule out physical causes of excess eyelid skin. Most blepharoplasties are considered aesthetic operations, but if eyelid tissue obstructs vision, blepharoplasty is medically indicated.

Blepharoplasty is usually performed on an outpatient basis. General or local anesthesia with sedation can be used. Wide elliptical incisions are made on the upper eyelids. The excised wedge of excess tissue is lifted off, and herniated fat is removed. A lower-lid blepharoplasty incision is placed ⅛ inch below the edge of the eyelid.

Rapid, uneventful recovery is typical. Blepharoplasty can be performed alone or with rhytidectomy (face lift). Complications from blepharoplasty are rare.

Assess preoperative near and distant vision in each eye by asking the person to read from a book and from something in the distance while one eye is covered. These baseline data are crucial to assess postoperative visual changes. An ophthalmologic examination is indicated before surgery if vision problems are noted.

After blepharoplasty, the head is elevated to reduce edema. Iced normal saline compresses are applied to the eyes as prescribed. Activity is limited for 1 week to reduce blood pressure elevations that often lead to increased edema and ecchymosis (bruising). Normally, severe pain is not experienced after blepharoplasty. An itching sensation, similar to that associated with dry eyes, is usually experienced as a result of slight corneal swelling. This can be prevented with cold wet dressings.

FACIAL RESURFACING
■ ALPHA-HYDROXY PEELS

Alpha-hydroxy acids (AHAs) are a group of naturally occurring fruit acids that cause epidermolysis and detachment of keratinocytes of the superficial skin. AHAs can be used to remove acne scars, keratoses, warts, and superficial layers of skin. The best candidates for AHA peels are thin-skinned women with a fair complexion and fine facial wrinkling. Trained nurses perform the peel procedure.

The skin is prepared for the peel with a 2-week skin care regimen consisting of a facial wash and application of daytime treatment lotion and nighttime cream. The actual peel begins with the application of a pre-peel solution. Skin that will not be peeled is protected. For the peel, a thin layer of acid is applied to the face for a few minutes, and then it is neutralized. Care after the peel includes application of skin moisturizers, gentle cleansing, use of sunscreen, and avoidance of abrasive agents.

■ TRICHLOROACETIC ACID PEELS

Trichloroacetic acid (TCA) is generally used when a medium-depth peel is required. TCA is indicated for clients with moderate actinic damage or for clients with pigment changes.

The skin is prepared with a 2-week regimen of tretinoin (Retin-A) or glycolic acid in combination with a bleaching agent. If clients are taking estrogen, they should stop its use for 2 weeks before the peel. The choice of skin preparation can affect the depth of the peel. TCA is applied to the face for a few minutes until the skin "frosts." TCA does not need to be neutralized. Care after the peel includes application of skin moisturizers, use of hydrocortisone to reduce edema and erythema, gentle cleansing, and use of sunscreen. The client often resumes the pre-peel skin regimen after the peel. Hyperpigmentation is the most common complication.

■ LASER RESURFACING

Laser treatment of skin wrinkles is becoming the preferred method of facial resurfacing. The wound produced is shallow because the energy is absorbed very superficially. An ultra-pulse laser is used.

Laser irradiation is quite painful. Some clients can tolerate the procedure with anesthesia provided by local sedation or through the use of topical anesthetics such as eutectic mixture of local anesthetic (EMLA). The cream is applied 1 to 2 hours before the procedure and covered with an occlusive wrap (cellophane works well). However, most clients need nerve blocks and local infiltration with a local anesthetic agent.

Laser treatments result in skin injury similar to a second-degree burn. Postoperative edema is significant, especially if the periorbital area has been treated. The edema can be reduced somewhat with ice packs and oral corticosteroids for 48 hours. Some clients also experience a burn sensation for 12 to 18 hours after treatment.

In 2 to 4 days, the residual tissue separates and sloughs off. Wound care after that time usually consists of hydrogel dressings. These dressings keep the wound bed moist and occluded, which promotes epithelialization and reduces pain. Hydrogel dressings are used for about 48 hours; after that time, thin layers of antibacterial ointment or petrolatum are applied. Neither product is without problems—contact dermatitis can develop from antibacterials, and acne-like lesions can develop from petrolatum.[40]

The skin reepithelializes in about 5 to 10 days, depending on the depth of the injury. Varying degrees of erythema can remain, but clients can effectively cover the erythema with make-up that has a green foundation color.

Milia can form and may require tretinoin or they can be manually expressed. Sun-blocking agents are a must, as hyperpigmentation can develop.

■ DERMABRASION

Dermabrasion is a process of sanding the surface layers of skin on cheeks and forehead with an electric rotating brush to smooth out pitting and surface blemishes. This operation is the preferred treatment for depressed acne scars and other deep scars. Local anesthesia with sedation is used. The abraded surfaces are covered with antibiotic ointment and gauze. After removal of the gauze, the facial skin weeps serous fluid for 5 to 7 days. Once the weeping stops and new skin has appeared, the client can apply make-up to camouflage the redness. The redness fades over the following 6 weeks.

■ COLLAGEN INJECTION

Collagen is sometimes injected to fill in small wrinkles or depressed blemishes in the skin. The client's reaction to collagen is tested before treatment, because some people experience induration (hard, raised area) and swelling at the injection site. Clients with autoimmune disorders are not candidates for collagen injection.

After collagen injections, the face should not be washed and face cream or make-up should not be applied for 3 to 4 hours. Normal skin care can then continue. Exposure to strong sunlight, alcohol consumption, and excessive exercise can cause mild swelling and should be avoided as prescribed (e.g., for a week).

RHINOPLASTY

Rhinoplasty is the surgical correction of nasal deformities. This procedure is frequently performed as an outpatient procedure using either local anesthesia and sedation or general anesthesia. Incisions are made inside the nose. The surgical plan is individualized and may include reshaping the bony dorsum of the nose, the tip of the nose, and/or the cartilage along the nares (nostrils). The nasal bones may be fractured to achieve the desired result. After surgery, the inside of the nose may be packed and an external splint applied.

Preoperative nursing care focuses on teaching the client to breathe through the mouth after surgery and to not touch the nose. Postoperatively, assess for bleeding. While the client is sleepy from the anesthesia, excessive swallowing may be the only sign of bleeding. Examine the back of the throat with a flashlight to look for blood. Some bleeding is normal down the back of the throat and on the nasal packs and dressings. The nurse promptly reports excessive bleeding to the surgeon. The head of the bed is kept elevated to control postoperative edema. Nasal packing can be very uncomfortable. Pain management is important and can usually be achieved with oral analgesics (e.g., codeine, acetaminophen). Aspirin is avoided for 1 week before and 3 weeks after surgery. Postoperative care is discussed in the Client Education Guide.

BODY-CONTOURING SURGERY (LIPECTOMY)

Body-contouring surgical procedures (lipectomy) remove excess fatty tissue, skin folds, or subcutaneous fat from

---

CLIENT EDUCATION GUIDE

Postoperative Care After Rhinoplasty

After the procedure, follow these instructions:

1. Sleep with the head of the bed elevated for 1 week.
2. Do not remove the external splints or nasal packing.
3. Do not blow the nose. Sneeze only through an open mouth.
4. Continue a soft diet for 2 days.
5. After nasal packs are removed, avoid decongestant nasal sprays because they cause vasoconstriction and decrease the blood supply needed for healing.
6. After nasal packs and splints are removed, the nose will remain swollen and bruised for a while. Wait 12 months before judging the final results of the procedure.

---

various body parts, including the abdomen, thighs, arms, and buttocks. Generally, obesity is best treated by diet and exercise before any body-contouring surgery is performed. In exceptional cases, the client may become highly motivated to follow a weight-reducing diet *after* such surgery. In still other cases, despite an appropriate diet and exercise regimen, there may be no reduction in the size of fat deposits in certain areas of the body. Fat distribution is based on sex, heredity, and corticosteroid use. It is generally accepted that rapid growth of fat cells occurs during childhood. It is also accepted that few new fat cells are made during adult life. Fat cells deposited during childhood are very resistant and their number does not dwindle during dieting. Surgical removal then becomes an option. As with all surgery, careful preoperative assessment is necessary to determine whether the client's expectations are realistic.

SUCTION-ASSISTED LIPECTOMY

Suction-assisted lipectomy, or liposuction, is a technique used (1) to aspirate fatty tissue from areas of the body resistant to diet and exercise (lipodystrophy), (2) to contour flaps, and (3) to remove lipomas (benign fatty tumors). It is also used adjunctively with other plastic surgery procedures to create better contour and to enhance the aesthetic result.

A blunt, hollow cannula is inserted through a very small incision (Fig. 49–24). The cannula, attached to a powerful suction machine, is passed back and forth through the subcutaneous tissue, sucking up adipose tissue and creating a series of tunnels. The blunt tip pushes aside nerves and blood vessels. Precise surgical technique avoids ridges and dimpling on the surface as fatty tissue is suctioned away. Compression dressings or elastic compression garments may be used to help collapse the tunnels, thereby preventing fluid collection (hematoma and seroma); to maintain the desired body contour; and to promote healing. Tumescent technique involves the additional use of large volumes of dilute lidocaine and epinephrine. These medications promote vasoconstriction to minimize bleeding and provide postoperative analgesia. Ultrasonic lipectomy is the use of ultrasound to ease the removal of fat.[1, 2]

Complications of liposuction include hematoma, skin necrosis, infection, and undesirable scars or skin dimpling. If large volumes of fat were removed, the client can also develop hypovolemia. Pulmonary embolism has also been reported.

After liposuction, assess the client for hypovolemia and electrolyte imbalance (manifested by syncope, dizziness, and abnormal blood values). If drains are used, monitor the quantity and quality of drainage. Ice is effective in managing postoperative pain. Dressings usually remain in place for at least 24 hours. Nurses must ensure that dressings remain smooth and uniform; otherwise, contour irregularities can result. Sometimes the client wears a compression garment for several weeks postoperatively.

Clients may gradually resume normal activity except for strenuous exercise. It may be 4 to 6 weeks before the client works up to the preoperative level of exercise. Resuming activity too rapidly may result in soreness and swelling. Bruising is common after liposuction and may take weeks to disappear completely.

Many clients expect the results of liposuction to be immediate. Usually up to 6 months is required for final results to be apparent after edema subsides and subcutaneous tissue heals. Reinforce that results may not be apparent for 6 months following surgery. This period of time is required for complete resolution of edema and reconnection of soft tissues.

ABDOMINOPLASTY

Abdominoplasty is the removal of excess abdominal skin and fat and the repair and tightening of separated abdominal muscles. An incision is made across the lower abdomen, and tissue is undermined to the costal margin. The excess skin and fatty tissue are excised and recontoured. The umbilical stalk is detached and reattached once the overlying skin is in its proper position.

During abdominoplasty, the surgeon repairs diastasis (lateral separation of the rectus abdominis muscles) and/or umbilical hernia. Indications for abdominoplasty include abdominal skin flaccidity (e.g., after multiple pregnancies or major weight loss) and marked striae from pregnancy. An indwelling urinary catheter and surgical drains are inserted, and sequential compression devices are applied at the end of the surgical procedure.

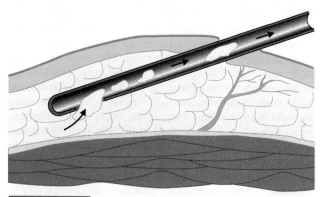

FIGURE 49–24 Suction-assisted lipectomy. To prevent extraction of subdermal fat, the surgeon directs the opening of the suction cannula toward the muscle fascia.

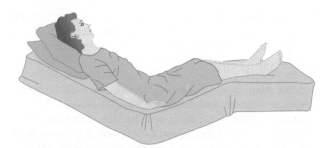

FIGURE 49–25 Position the client after abdominoplasty in a modified semi-Fowler position, with the knees bent, to reduce strain on the incision line.

Preoperative nursing care includes informing the client that drains and a urinary catheter will be in place after surgery, that a blood transfusion may be required, and that an IV infusion is continued until a diet is tolerated. After surgery, inspect the incision line for signs of pallor and/or lack of capillary refill. The operative site can swell, with resulting impairment of capillary blood supply. Smoking is prohibited, because nicotine further restricts blood flow to the skin. Tension on the suture line must be minimized; therefore, the client must lie in a contouring position (Fig. 49–25).

The client also needs to walk in a "hunched-over" position until the swelling decreases and abdominal skin relaxes. Teach the client postoperative pain management techniques. Abdominoplasty is an abdominal operation and produces significant postoperative discomfort. Adequate analgesia and other pain-relieving measures are essential. Reinforce to unlicensed personnel that these clients require usual postoperative care (see the Management and Delegation feature).

PANNICULECTOMY

In people who have experienced major weight loss, excess loose skin and subcutaneous tissue may develop over

---

MANAGEMENT AND DELEGATION

Care of Clients Recovering from Plastic Surgery

When unlicensed assistive personnel are caring for clients after plastic surgery, reinforce the need for adequate pain management and routine postoperative care. It is not uncommon for these clients to feel uncomfortable about asking for pain medications and for nursing assistance. Some people have the notion that surgery "for vanity" should hurt a little. This is a dangerous philosophy and should not be condoned. Any incision hurts, and these clients do not differ in their need for pain control. Likewise, routine vital signs, pulmonary care, monitoring intake and output, and encouraging ambulation are routine aspects of postoperative nursing care. Withholding care is not an acceptable manner of providing care.

Donna W. Markey, MSN, RN, ACNP-CS, *Clinician IV, Surgical Services, University of Virginia Health System, Charlottesville, Virginia*

the abdomen, thighs, and arms. This tissue may hang in large folds, and laxity is greater in older people who have lost skin elasticity. Panniculectomy, the removal of excess folds of tissue, usually requires more than one operation. The surgery is lengthy, and there is risk of major blood loss. As much as 10 pounds of redundant tissue has been surgically removed during one of these operations.

Clearly, this operation is not for the cure of the client's obesity, but it can offer some positive gains in self-esteem and reduction in health-related problems.

Postoperative care is usually focused on reducing stress on the long suture lines. For example, place the client in the Fowler position after abdominal panniculectomy. Monitor the suture lines closely for signs of non-healing. Fatty tissue is poorly perfused, and the client may have pre-existing diet-induced malnutrition. During the healing phase, the client needs to consume adequate amounts of protein and carbohydrate to heal.

RECONSTRUCTIVE PLASTIC SURGERY

One of the greatest challenges in plastic surgery is the reconstruction of deformities. In planning reconstruction, it is important to consider the following questions:

- *What tissue is missing?* Is bone, muscle, subcutaneous tissue, or skin missing? If only skin is missing (e.g., burns), skin grafts are used for reconstruction. People with large pressure sores may be missing muscle, subcutaneous tissue, and skin, and a rotation flap containing all of these tissues may be used to repair the defect. Facial trauma may result in loss of bone as well as of other tissues, and vascularized bone may be used in reconstruction.
- *Where is tissue available?* Some small defects have adequate tissue for repair nearby. This is ideal, because the tissue can be lifted from its base and rotated into the defect. Nearby tissue has the same color, thickness, and hair-bearing tendencies, contributing to a more natural appearance. If the tissue needed is not nearby, it may be moved from its location and attached to the defect by microscopic anastomosis (i.e., suturing small vessels and nerves with the aid of a microscope). Reconstruction with this technique is called *free flap reconstruction.*
- *What deficit might result from moving donor tissue?* Obviously, a person does not want a larger defect in the donor site than in the area being reconstructed! For example, a toe is often used to reconstruct a missing finger, but it is unlikely that a person would give up a finger to rebuild a toe.
- *What is the simplest method to achieve the desired results?* The simplest method to close any wound is simple suturing. More complex methods are used if adequate tissue is not available for primary closure or if a greater defect would result from simple suturing (e.g., a defect on the cheek could be closed by suturing, but this approach might pull the eyelid down into ectropion as it healed). Another method of closing a wound is to use a flap of nearby tissue and to rotate it onto the wound, maintaining the flap's own blood supply. Skin grafting is the third choice for reconstruction. The most complex form of wound closure is the free flap of skin, subcutaneous tissue, and, as indicated, muscle or bone.

RECONSTRUCTIVE MODALITIES

■ SKIN GRAFTS

A graft is tissue (e.g., skin, bone, nerve, or vessel) that is harvested without a blood supply from a donor site. It is transferred to a recipient site, where it develops a new blood supply. For the tissue to remain viable, or to *take,* a healthy vascular supply must be present at the recipient site.

Skin grafts are used extensively to resurface exposed surfaces. The grafts vary in thickness from very thin split-thickness skin grafts (STSGs), which contain epidermis and a very thin layer of dermis, to full-thickness grafts (FTSGs), which contain epidermis and all of the dermis. Thinner grafts are more likely to contract during healing, but they are also more likely to develop adequate blood supply. FTSGs are used in areas in which contraction would limit function, such as on the hand or over joints. FTSGs leave a full-thickness defect in the donor site that must be closed, either primarily or with an STSG.

Skin grafts can be expanded to cover a greater surface area by use of meshing techniques. Meshing the graft, achieved by cutting small slits in it, allows the skin to be expanded (like an accordion). Meshed skin grafts are used when there is little uninjured skin to use as a donor site (e.g., a major burn).

BANKING SKIN
Skin grafts can be removed or harvested during one surgical procedure and stored for application later, when a wound is clean or when an earlier graft has failed. Banked skin is folded in a dermis-to-dermis fashion, to preserve moisture, and then wrapped in moist saline gauze. The gauze with skin is placed into a dressing impregnated with ointment (such as petrolatum gauze); this is put into a bottle, which creates an airtight environment. Banked skin can be stored at 4° C for 10 to 21 days. Later, the skin graft can be placed on the wound without the need for another operation.

SKIN GRAFT SURVIVAL
A skin graft requires enough blood in its recipient site for survival. Capillary buds must revascularize the graft before the cells die. Blood supply that supports the growth of granulation tissue is usually adequate to support a skin graft. Good contact between the graft and the recipient bed is also critical. A thin fibrin network develops almost immediately after placement and serves as a temporary glue of sorts to hold the graft in place. Skin grafts require about 7 to 10 days to adhere and longer to mature.

Several factors reduce contact and thereby reduce skin graft survival. Collections of fluid between the graft and bed, improper tension on the graft, and movement of the graft on the bed are three common problems that lead to graft failure. Blood, serum, and purulent material may separate the graft from the bed. This collection prevents revascularization of the graft. A hematoma only 0.5 mm in diameter delays the time for revascularization by 12 hours. A 5-mm-thick hematoma delays revascularization by 120 hours. At body temperature, the skin graft cannot survive for the additional time, and necrosis begins.

Proper tension on the skin graft is crucial once the skin graft has been sutured in place. If tension is insufficient, wrinkles develop that will never revascularize because they are not in contact with the recipient bed. If the skin graft is too tight, it is stretched like a drumhead above the recesses of the wound, where the blood supply exists.

Movement between the graft and the bed shears capillary buds from the bed, which prevents revascularization. When skin grafts are applied to extremities, the adjacent joints are splinted to prevent movement. Tie-over dressings are commonly used to prevent the graft from moving.

HEALED SKIN GRAFTS

Skin grafts tend to carry their natural color. Grafts from the clavicle are a blush (pink) shade, whereas grafts from below the clavicle take on a yellow or brownish hue. Sweat gland, hair-bearing, and sebaceous features occur only in thick STSGs and FTSGs. Nerves regenerate from the edges of the graft, and in the absence of dense scarring, sensation parallels that of nearby skin. If the skin graft regains sensation, it is fairly durable. Grafted skin will usually grow in a manner parallel to that of the rest of the body.

Meshed skin grafts heal with a pebbled appearance. Therefore, they are only used on body areas normally covered by clothing.

■ Nursing Management

Skin graft recipient sites are covered with dressings, which should not be altered for at least 72 hours. Assess the site, and document pain, bleeding through the dressings, and adjacent skin color and temperature.

The donor site is usually covered with a hydrophilic dressing, such as hydrocolloid gel. Because clients have more pain in the donor site than in the grafted site, it is important to keep the open area covered.

It is imperative to keep a skin-grafted extremity elevated. If the graft is on the chest or back, be certain that it is anchored well and that the client is positioned off the grafted site. Avoid moving the grafted part. After the dressings are removed, continue to assess the skin graft for healing. The skin graft should become pink throughout (a graft with viability assured by a healthy pink color is called a *take*). Blisters (small blebs of serum) can also shear the skin graft from the underlying wound.

Document the presence of blisters and report this finding to the surgeon. Blisters under a skin graft sometimes need to be drained. When prescribed, this is accomplished by inserting a small (25-gauge) sterile needle into the blister and letting the fluid run out onto a sterile dressing or a cotton-tipped applicator. Rolling fluid to the edges of the skin graft is not advised, because it shears the graft from the capillaries in the bed en route. A standing order (as needed [prn]) may be given for this intervention. Large accumulations may require surgical removal.

■ FLAPS

Flaps are areas of tissue raised from one area of the body without being completely detached, so that the blood supply is intact; the flap is transferred (e.g., by rotation) to adjacent areas. Flaps of tissue can also be transferred to distant areas, where a blood supply is reestablished; these are called *free flaps* and are discussed later on. Local flaps are rotated or advanced to reconstruct an adjacent defect (see Fig. 49–26). An important consideration with the use of flaps is the preservation of the nutrient blood

vessels. The tissue attachment containing these vessels is sometimes called the *pedicle,* because in the past, flaps were moved from site to site with a visible portion of tissue that "carried" the flap to the recipient site. This style of flap can be seen in the deltopectoral flaps used to repair neck resection tissue loss. Flaps are also used to cover extensive wounds from pressure ulcers and long-standing defects from osteomyelitis.

The skin of the flap, after transfer, maintains its original color and texture. This is why skin from the head and neck is used to reconstruct facial defects. If, for example, abdominal skin were used for facial reconstruction, it would be bulky and would increase in size if the patient gained weight, because the graft would respond just as if it were still in the abdomen.

Hair growth and sebaceous secretion remain the same as they were in the donor area. Sensation and sweating are lost immediately after transfer and usually return sometime between 6 weeks and 3 years later. These functions reappear as superficial nerves regrow into the tissues; therefore, the sensation and sweating capacity match those of recipient site tissues.

MUSCULOCUTANEOUS FLAPS

Flaps comprising both muscle and skin are called *musculocutaneous flaps.* They are commonly used to fill in defects where muscle is missing or where muscle can provide ample blood flow to heal osteomyelitis. These flaps are named by the muscle of origin. For example, large trochanteric pressure ulcers can be repaired with tensor fasciae latae flaps, named for the tensor fasciae latae muscle of the lateral thigh. Intrathoracic muscle flaps used for chest wall reconstruction include serratus anterior, latissimus dorsi, and pectoralis muscles.

Tissue defects of the leg can also be managed with muscle flaps and skin grafting or with musculocutaneous flaps. Attempts are made to salvage all extremities unless nerve or vascular damage is irreparable, in which case amputation is preferred. It is common to treat less severe tissue loss in compound lower leg fractures with local rotation muscle flaps if possible. The use of these flaps has been overshadowed in recent years by the excitement over microvascular techniques, but definite indications exist for use of these local muscle flaps.

Care of the client after a flap reconstruction centers on maintaining perfusion and reducing tissue injury to the flap. You may choose to design your nursing care under the nursing diagnosis of *Risk for Altered Peripheral Tissue Perfusion related to tissue transfer.*

The outcome is that the client will maintain adequate peripheral tissue perfusion, as evidenced by usual color of skin, no pallor or cyanosis, warm and dry skin, blanching (capillary refill) in 3 to 5 seconds, no edema or blebs, intact incisions, and controllable pain.

The flap is monitored for color, capillary refill, and dermal bleeding. Look for pallor, coolness, decreased capillary refill, or dark dermal blood on lancing (see the Critical Monitoring feature) (lancing may not be allowed in some settings). It takes a fair amount of experience in clinical assessment of flaps to predict early flap demise using these subjective methods. Findings can vary because of oxygen content of the blood, capillary dilation, blood flow, and skin pigmentation. Therefore, in complex flaps, temperature and Doppler monitors are used to mon-

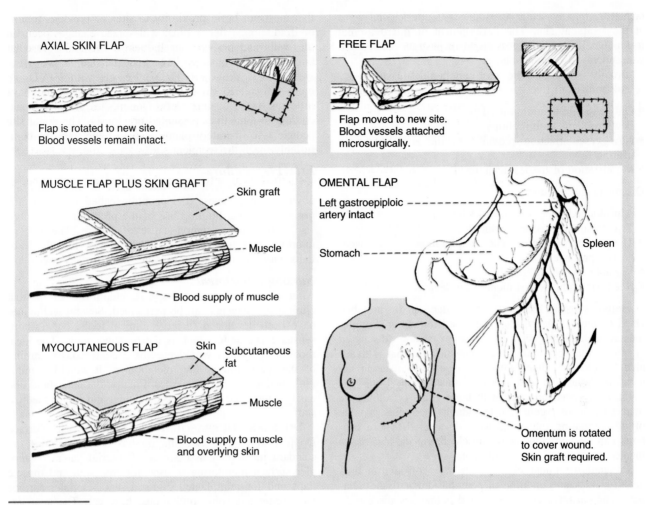

FIGURE 49-26 Common flaps.

itor circulation. The extremity is usually elevated to improve venous return as long as elevation does not interfere with arterial flow.

Protecting the blood supply to a flap is a primary nursing responsibility. Nursing interventions are designed to avoid factors that can jeopardize blood flow. Position the client so that the flap is relaxed and elevated. Gravity promotes edema and venous congestion, both of which impede blood flow. Interventions to increase venous return include elevating the involved body part and applying elastic stockings or wraps as prescribed. Tension on the flap can stretch or kink the feeding blood vessels, reducing the flow of blood to the tissues. A blood clot can restrict blood flow. The first sign of compromised blood flow is pallor.

Know the location of the pedicle that carries blood vessels to the flap. Most of the time the pedicle is buried, and little can be done to harm it. Some exceptions exist, though. When skin flaps are used, such as the deltopectoral flap, the pedicle is visible. Tracheostomy ties should not be tied tightly around the flap; otherwise, circulation to the distal portions will be compromised. When the breast is reconstructed after mastectomy with a latissimus dorsi flap, the pedicle is located in the ipsilateral axilla. The client cannot lie on the ipsilateral side.

Hydrate the client well, if prescribed, to help perfuse the flap. Maintain any postoperative splints to prevent tension on vessels. Limit the use of caffeine by the client and prohibit the use of nicotine by the client and by visitors.

Problems due to impaired arterial supply are apparent early after surgery. Altered perfusion due to venous obstruction may not be evident for a few hours.

FREE FLAPS

Free flaps are harvested from one area of the body to reconstruct a defect in a distant area. The donor tissue (skin, muscle, bone, or a combination of these) is detached from its blood supply at the donor site and reat-

---

CRITICAL MONITORING

Musculocutaneous Reconstruction

Report the following findings immediately:

- Development of coolness in the flap
- Development of duskiness or pallor in the flap
- Slowing of capillary refill in the flap
- Loss of pulses (palpable or detected by Doppler) in the flap
- Increasing pain in the flap

tached by microvascular anastomosis to arteries and veins at the recipient site. The development of microvascular techniques has made it possible to reconstruct defects that were previously untreatable.

Box 49–4 includes the most common donor sites.

Advantages to free flap reconstruction are as follows:

- Only a single operation needed
- Few problems with mobility
- New vascularization provided to the area to aid in healing
- Mobilization of tissues maximized

Disadvantages include:

- A prolonged operation (6 to 24 hours)
- Two separate incisions required
- The necessity of immediate reexploration of any vascular compromise
- Variable donor site mobility
- Need for sophisticated monitoring devices

Before surgical reconstruction, a flap can be prefabricated to build exactly what is needed for repair. Supplemental techniques, such as tissue expansion (discussed later on), may be used to augment the skin that is available for closure. Other advances have been made in the areas of bone and soft tissue reconstruction. Bone has traditionally been replaced with bone grafts or alloplastic materials. More recently, osteoinductive proteins capable of differentiating into bone were discovered. These proteins can be combined with muscle flaps, and the tissue then is transformed into useful bone.

Preoperative client characteristics to consider include health status and condition of potential donor tissue. Diabetes and cardiovascular, renal, and pulmonary disease do not present absolute contraindications, but these diseases do increase risk of flap failure. The vessels used for a flap must not be in proximity to sites of previous trauma or irradiation. After trauma, widespread changes occur in the walls and perivascular tissues of the major vascular bundles. These changes have been labeled as *post-traumatic vessel disease* (PTVD). Vessels with PTVD are more difficult to dissect, are easily damaged, and have little resistance against clots. Donor sites are chosen according to guidelines presented previously. The donor site pedicle is deliberately planned so that the flap can comfortably reach the recipient site.

Free Flap Failure

When all goes well, the advantages of free flaps are obvious. Nevertheless, the phantom called *free flap failure* looms large, limiting use of the procedure. Thrombosis is the most common cause of failure. The rate of microvascular thrombosis is 3.7%; almost two thirds of flaps with thrombosis are salvageable by timely revisions.

Nursing Assessment

After surgery, the free flap site is seldom dressed, so that clinical assessments can be performed. Several techniques have been developed in large clinical trials, but no consensus exists as to which is the best technique. The ideal monitoring system would provide a continuous recording of flap perfusion or flap metabolism. It should monitor both visible and buried tissues. Finally, the data should be easily interpreted by nursing personnel and junior medical staff.

DOPPLER ULTRASOUND EXAMINATION. Surface Doppler ultrasound examination has become almost the standard method of assessment of arterial patency. Doppler surface monitoring is used for free skin and muscle flaps and for reimplanted digits. Use of Doppler surface monitoring has some limitations, however. The axial artery must be located superficially, and sometimes venous obstruction still produces an arterial "hum." If venous obstruction is suspected, compression of the flap will produce a louder "hum." Implanted Doppler probes are also available and are in use in some centers.

TRANSCUTANEOUS OXYGEN DETERMINATION. Determination of tissue oxygen tension ($PtCO_2$) constitutes the simplest technique for monitoring perfusion. Absolute $PtCO_2$ greater than 20 mm Hg seems to suggest adequate perfusion. Sudden falls of $PtCO_2$ below 20 mm Hg that do not respond to the administration of oxygen suggest arterial occlusion. As in other forms of monitoring, trends in data, rather than absolute values, should be monitored. Implantable probes have been developed for oxygen monitoring also.

TISSUE pH. Measurement of tissue pH has been shown to be a more reliable index of perfusion than tissue oxygen. Arterial occlusion produces a rapid fall in tissue pH (0.66 pH unit per hour in laboratory animals, compared with a fall of only 0.27 pH unit per hour with venous occlusion).

PULSE OXIMETRY. Pulse oximetry is a good monitor for viability of digital free flaps or reimplanted digits. Digits remain viable if the oxygen saturation remains above 95%. Loss of pulsatile flow is indicative of arterial occlusion; a decrease in saturation to 85% indicates venous obstruction.

MUSCLE CONTRACTILITY. Ischemic muscles lose their contractility, and free muscle transfers can therefore

---

BOX 49–4	Common Donor Sites for Free Flaps

- *Temporalis fascia,* a thin conforming flap, is used to cover the dorsum of the foot or hand.
- *Radial forearm,* a flap of skin and fascia, can be used for reconstruction of intraoral and extraoral defects; it can be combined with portions of the radius if bony reconstruction is needed.
- *Lateral forearm,* a flap of skin and fascia, is used to cover body areas that demand thicker skin, such as weight-bearing surfaces.
- *Omentum,* the fatty drape over the anterior abdomen, can be transplanted into spaces that require pliability, such as the frontal sinuses or chest wounds.
- *Latissimus dorsi,* a large flap muscle with a skin segment, has a long pedicle and is useful for large bulky defects; it is the "workhorse" of flap reconstruction and is common for facial, chest, and breast reconstruction.
- *Rectus abdominis,* midline abdominal muscle and skin, has a long pedicle and is used for defects that require bulk.
- *Gracilis,* a skin and muscle flap with a short pedicle, is used to reconstruct defects of the distal tibia, ankle, and heel, and for facial reanimation.
- *Serratus anterior,* an easily sculpted flap, provides bulk and protects lower extremity defects.

be monitored by the continuing ability of the muscle to contract in response to electrical stimulation. Nerve stimulators are used to irritate the nerve every 15 minutes, and the response is recorded. A decrease in amplitude of the evoked potential is indicative of ischemia.

PHOTOPLETHYSMOGRAPHY. Photoplethysmography is commonly used to monitor several types of free flaps, because it is noninvasive and reliable. Infrared light from a light-emitting diode penetrates about 3 mm below the surface of the skin. Some of the light is reflected back to a photoelectric cell. Pulsatile changes in flow alter the proportion of light reflected back. Waveforms are monitored for changes. The waveforms can also be transmitted by telephone to remote stations for interpretation.

CLINICAL ASSESSMENT. Postoperative monitoring of free flaps used to be based solely on clinical assessment, which relied heavily on the experience of the nurse. In the 1990s, the monitors just described were used. It is interesting to note that some surgeons have abandoned external monitoring devices and are once more relying solely on the nurse's judgment. Most centers use a flow sheet to document color, texture, and temperature of the flap, as well as Doppler pulses and drainage from wound drains. Other postoperative care includes maintaining adequate hydration, keeping the client warm, managing pain, and allowing only the appropriate activities. Clients may express some concern with the decision to salvage a body part and/or may fear that the flap will fail and amputation will be required. The nurse needs to be supportive of the decision for surgery and allow time for expression of fears.

Long-Term Results

The ability to obtain soft-tissue coverage and limb salvage of a massively traumatized lower limb approaches 95%. A true measure of the adequacy of reconstruction, however, is whether the client can use the limb. A study was completed to examine the functional outcomes of 70 leg salvage procedures. The functional demands on the lower limb are great and include strength, stability, motion, and balance. Functional analysis of tibial shaft injuries revealed marked limb shortening and decreased ambulation and mobility. Most clients require some sort of ambulatory-assist devices. Clients requiring free flaps or foot resurfacing did not have limb shortening, and all of them could wear shoes.

■ IMPLANTS

Implant material can be used to augment or replace tissue in all parts of the body. Facial structures (including the nose, chin, ears, orbital floor, and malar complex), breasts, bones and joints, and genitalia are often augmented or reconstructed with implant material. Polymers such as medical-grade silicone are used most frequently in plastic surgical procedures. Silicone prostheses can be very soft (breast prostheses), flexible (finger and toe joints), or rigid (bones and joints). Stainless steel, cobalt-chromium alloy (Vitallium), and titanium plates, screws, and wire are used to approximate, replace, and stabilize bone fragments (Fig. 49–27). Injectable collagen can be used to fill out skin depressions and fine wrinkles. Material for implants must be biocompatible and not rejected by body tissues. It must not cause severe foreign body

reaction or infection. Implants must be noncarcinogenic, nontoxic, nonallergenic, and sterile.

Postoperatively, assessment and intervention focus on preventing displacement of the implant, ensuring adequate blood flow to the operative site, and preventing infection. Infection is a serious complication that can necessitate removal of the implant. Changes in temperature and local changes (e.g., drainage, increasing edema, hyperemia, increasing skin temperature) may indicate a developing infection or implant rejection. Excellent wound care is imperative. Teach the client to recognize the clinical manifestations of infection so that treatment can be initiated quickly. Implants themselves are not painful, but the surgical procedure causes mild to moderate pain. Pain not relieved with analgesics must be investigated.

■ SKIN EXPANSION

Skin expansion is a technique used to increase the amount of local tissue available to reconstruct a defect. An inflatable silicone balloon is placed under the skin or muscle flap adjacent to a defect. The expander is inflated sequentially over several weeks or months to stretch the overlying tissue. When tissue is sufficient to resurface the adjacent defect, the balloon is removed and the flap is contoured (shaped) and advanced to cover the defect.

The process of skin expansion involves an extended period of time, commitment, and significant, although temporary, disfigurement. It is essential that the client be motivated, well prepared for the experience, and able to comply with the treatment regimen. The client must be able to make additional trips to the physician's office where the expander will be inflated under sterile conditions. Each expander has an injection site into which a sterile needle is inserted percutaneously. Saline is injected slowly until the tissue is very tight over the expander.

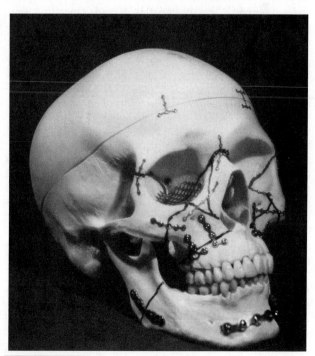

FIGURE 49–27 Titanium plates and screws used to treat facial fractures.

Sometimes a small amount of saline needs to be withdrawn to reduce discomfort. The tightness may be uncomfortable for several hours, but it subsides as the tissue begins to expand.

Teach the client to keep the incision and the injection site clean and dry to prevent infection. Make sure that the client understands that pressure on the expander compromises blood flow and can cause tissue breakdown. Infection may require that the expander be removed altogether. If dehiscence of the incision line occurs, exposing the expander, the treatment need not necessarily be aborted. Fluid can be removed from the expander to relieve the tension. When the incision has healed sufficiently, expansion can begin again.

In most cases, the client can camouflage the expander with clothing. The clothing must be loose so that no pressure is placed on the expander. Advise the client to sleep in a position that protects the expander from pressure. When the expander is placed in an exposed area, such as the neck or scalp, the client must be able to cope with the temporary physical inconvenience and insult to body image.

Nurses are instrumental in assisting the client in disguising the deformity caused by the expander. For example, when one breast is being expanded before reconstruction, the other breast will not match in size or shape. Assist the client in padding the other side of the bra to reduce obvious asymmetry.

■ LASERS

The laser (*l*ight *a*mplification by *s*timulated *e*mission of *r*adiation) is a coagulating, vaporizing, and cutting instrument. A precise beam of laser light is directed onto tissue. The light is converted into heat energy that is absorbed by the cells. The heat vaporizes the cells. The advantages of laser surgery include precision and accuracy of cell destruction, reduced bleeding and swelling, and, sometimes, less postoperative pain. Operating time may be longer, but tissue damage is less, and the postoperative infection rate is lower.

Laser light can be of different colors and wavelengths. Each is absorbed differently depending on cell pigment and water content. The carbon dioxide (CO_2) laser is primarily a cutting and vaporizing tool. Its energy is absorbed by the water in cells, so it penetrates tissue only superficially. The CO_2 laser is used primarily to excise or vaporize lesions such as warts, keloids, and vascular lesions. Argon, copper vapor, and pulsed-dye laser energy are preferentially absorbed by hemoglobin and are used primarily for coagulation. These types of lasers are used to treat birthmarks (e.g., port-wine stain), superficial vascular lesions, and pigmented lesions.

Laser energy generates intense heat, and clients experience a burning sensation or a pin-prick sensation. The tissue reaction can be similar to that of a second-degree burn with blistering. Ointment applied to the affected area for 2 to 4 weeks keeps the tissue moist until healing is complete. It is also essential that the area treated with laser energy be protected from sun exposure for several weeks.

Laser treatment to remove large pigmented lesions may require many operations. A single application may address only a small portion of the lesion, and the results are appreciated slowly as the site heals. Clients must be prepared for the length of time required and the inconvenience of multiple procedures.

REPAIR OF TRAUMATIC INJURIES

FACIAL INJURIES

Injuries to the face are a common result of automobile accidents and physical violence. Although they may be serious, facial injuries are seldom fatal. Proper management helps to avoid sensory impairment and permanent disability and can minimize disfigurement.

■ LACERATIONS

Facial lacerations can range from very small injuries (0.50 cm) that can be repaired using local anesthesia to extensive lacerations with soft tissue injury that require repair with the client under general anesthesia. Before closure, wounds are cleansed of debris and devitalized tissue.

Facial lacerations and facial soft tissue injuries are usually distressing to the injured client and family. Although it is important to remain optimistic about the outcome and reduce anxiety, it is also essential to provide accurate information. Explain that a scar forms with any injury. Scar revision can be performed later.

Excellent wound care, including cleansing and applying prescribed topical antibiotics, promotes the healing of facial abrasions and lacerations. A client who is receiving nothing by mouth (i.e., is on *nil per os* [NPO] status) and has dried blood in the mouth needs frequent oral care. If oral tissue contains sutures, the mouth is simply rinsed with saline. Oral care *must* be performed, however. With severe facial trauma, soft toothbrushes suffice for oral care. Use of oral irrigation devices (e.g., Water Pik) may further damage such injuries and is usually contraindicated. The nurse takes measures to prevent aspiration during oral care.

Teach the client and family members to keep facial incision lines clean and to apply a prescribed topical antibiotic. Skin incisions must not get wet (e.g., in the shower), because moisture allows bacteria to enter the wound along the sutures. Infected incisions tend to produce more scar tissue. (Wound care is also discussed in Chapter 16.)

■ FACIAL FRACTURES

Fractures can occur in the individual bones of the face: the nasal bones, orbit, malar prominence, mandible, or maxilla. Le Fort fractures are facial fractures with specific patterns (Fig. 49–28); they are classified as follows:

Le Fort I: transverse fracture of the alveolar process separating the upper dental arch from the maxilla
Le Fort II: fracture of the midface, maxilla, and orbits
Le Fort III: fracture of the orbits that leads to craniofacial dissociation

The client with facial fractures has often been involved in an automobile accident or an assault or has suffered a sports injury. Pain, improper bite (malocclusion), swelling, bruising, diplopia (double vision), facial asymmetry,

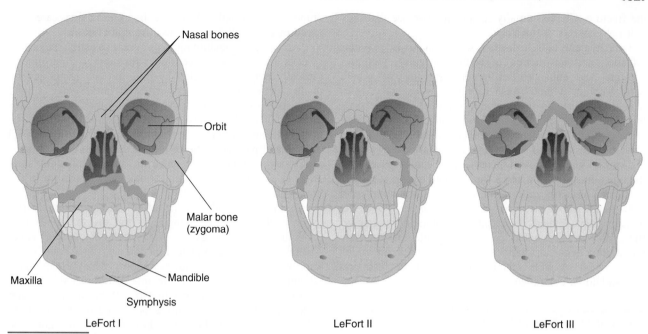

FIGURE 49–28 Le Fort fractures.

enophthalmos (sunken eye), and exophthalmos (bulging eye) are clinical manifestations of facial fractures. Diagnostic assessment includes x-ray studies. Life-threatening problems (e.g., airway obstruction, hemorrhage, or cervical spine injury) that may accompany facial trauma must be managed immediately. Repair of facial fractures can be delayed for up to 3 weeks and still achieve good results.

Like all fractures, facial fractures must be reduced, stabilized, and immobilized to ensure proper healing. Methods vary according to the location of the fractures. Nasal fractures are reduced and then splinted or stabilized with nasal packing and immobilized with an external nasal splint, which usually remains in place for at least 1 week.

Fractures of the mandible and maxilla and Le Fort fractures can be reduced and stabilized with intermaxillary fixation (wiring the upper and lower jaws together in occlusion) using arch bars. The jaws usually remain wired for 4 to 6 weeks. When small plates and screws are used to stabilize bone fragments, intermaxillary fixation may not be necessary.

Blowout fractures of the orbit can involve trapping of orbital structures between bone fragments, which may result in diplopia or enophthalmos. The integrity of the orbital floor is reestablished surgically, and the fracture fragments are stabilized with wire or small plates and screws. Implant material or bone graft may be used to complete the reconstruction. Malar (cheekbone) fractures may produce facial asymmetry. These fractures may also be stabilized with wire or small plates with screws. Malar implants may be necessary to reestablish facial symmetry.

Assesses airway patency and breath sounds every 2 hours (more often if bleeding is present). Suction equipment is present at the bedside. Teach the client to breathe through the nose. Trying to open the mouth may dislocate the fracture. When the client has intermaxillary wiring,

wire cutters should be in the client's possession at all times. If airway problems develop that cannot be managed with suction, the wires should be cut. The nurse and the client need to be informed about which wires should be cut. Two wires are usually present on each side of the mouth, and they are the only wires that attach the top and bottom teeth. Do not try to cut off the bands attached to the teeth.

Facial edema and ecchymoses may be present. The head of the bed is elevated. Artificial tears may be needed if the client's ability to blink is decreased as a result of swelling, injury, or nerve damage.

Assess the client for diplopia and blurred vision. When these disorders are present, the nurse assists the client during ambulation to prevent injury.

The client continues a liquified diet until the wires are removed. Without adequate nutrition, clients can lose 10 to 20 pounds during convalescence. Instruct the client how to "blenderize" food and to maintain an adequate balance of carbohydrates, fat, protein, and calories. Milkshakes can be made with a wide variety of foods. High-calorie food supplements can augment the regular diet, and liquid multivitamins may be useful. Alcoholic and carbonated beverages can cause nausea and can fizz and foam in the back of the throat, leading to airway problems; they are to be avoided.

Assess the client for clear rhinorrhea or otorrhea. Rhinorrhea or otorrhea may indicate leaking cerebrospinal fluid (CSF), which must be reported to the physician. With CSF leakage, the potential exists for development of meningitis. To assess for rhinorrhea or otorrhea, inspect the bed linens; CSF dries in concentric, halo-like rings and does not crust.

Initially, you and the client must establish a means of communication. Although talking is possible through clenched teeth, hand signals or writing may be most effective initially. Trying to open the mouth may dislocate the fracture. Clients initially require reassurance that they will not choke or suffocate.

Oral hygiene aids in healing of oral wounds, prevents infection and destruction of teeth and gums, increases comfort, and enhances self-esteem. Rinsing the mouth with water or a mouthwash followed by use of an oral irrigation device on low pressure removes particles from the front of the mouth while the tissues are still tender. Once the initial swelling and tenderness subside, the teeth must be brushed and the mouth rinsed after every meal and at bedtime. Pieces of paraffin wax can be placed on the open ends of the wires if they irritate buccal surfaces.

Before discharge, the client and family members need to be taught about the wires, diet, and oral care. Once the incisions have healed, the client can resume normal activities. However, as noted previously, while the jaws are wired, the client must carry a wire cutter and know which wires to cut. A well-balanced blenderized diet and oral care should be continued.

TRAUMATIC AMPUTATIONS

Immediate care of a person who has sustained a traumatic amputation, like that of any other injured person, focuses on life-saving activities (see Chapter 82). Hemorrhage is controlled with direct pressure on the bleeding points. Tourniquets and cautery are not used because they may damage surrounding tissue, so that reimplantation becomes impossible. All amputated parts, including small pieces of tissue, are sent to the health care facility with the injured person. As soon as possible, these parts are (1) rinsed with sterile normal saline, (2) wrapped in sterile wet gauze, (3) sealed in a watertight bag, and (4) placed on ice. Cooling the amputated part reduces metabolism, increasing the time the part can survive without blood. For example, an amputated finger can survive for 18 hours if effectively cooled. Although the part is rinsed with normal saline, it is never stored in normal saline or on dry ice, or frozen, which causes extensive cellular damage.

Reimplantation surgery is performed using a regional block or with the client under general anesthesia. An operating microscope guides the surgical reattachment of arteries, veins, tendons, and nerves. With severe injuries, such an operation may take 12 to 18 hours. After surgery, incisions are dressed, the extremity is immobilized with casts or splints, and the entire extremity is elevated.

After reimplantation, the client requires careful, frequent nursing assessment (every 15 minutes) including documentation of the reimplanted part's color, temperature, and capillary refill. Arterial or venous blood flow in the reimplanted part may become blocked; if the problem is not immediately corrected surgically, the part will die. Toes and fingertips are usually left uncovered for assessment. Doppler assessments help monitor pulses in the part. Temperature probes are often placed on the extremity. The surgeon usually states the ideal temperature range for reimplantations. A temperature decrease of 2° C or more in an hour or a decline to 32° C (89.6° F) demands immediate attention and is promptly reported to the surgeon. Aspirin is usually prescribed to reduce blood-clotting tendencies. A temperature of 34° to 36° C (93.2° to 96.5° F) is considered excellent for a reimplanted finger. Because anesthesia

time is prolonged (18 to 24 hours), nursing care also focuses on monitoring recovery from anesthesia.

An active rehabilitation program usually begins 2 weeks after injury and continues for months. Joint motion initially may be restricted by pins through joints and by bulky dressings. Because peripheral nerves take a long time to regenerate, protective sensation may be absent for months. The client must be careful to avoid injuring the part. Rehabilitation is accomplished through prescribed active and passive range-of-motion exercises several times each day. A final indication of the success of reimplantation is return of sensory and motor nerve function in the reimplanted part.

Psychosocial adjustment after reimplantation varies with each person. Grieving over the loss of appearance and function of the extremity (the reimplanted part never achieves normal complete function and appearance) is a normal reaction that requires support. Many clients have dreams about their injury. Dreams that depict the tragedy again are normal. Dreams that depict harm of a greater magnitude than was actually experienced by the client are abnormal, and the client who has such dreams should be counseled by a psychologist. Praise and encouragement during rehabilitation are very helpful.[4]

Teach the client to avoid activities and substances that cause vasoconstriction (which precipitates necrosis) for 2 weeks after surgery (e.g., tobacco, nicotine, cocaine, amphetamines). Exposure to air conditioning is also harmful. Advise the client to avoid cold and chilling (such as by wearing extra clothing and having the car prewarmed before entering to prevent vasoconstriction).

NAIL DISORDERS

Disorders of the nail can indicate any of several dermatologic processes. Potential causes include an infection of the nail (e.g, paronychia), a fungal infection of the nail (e.g., onychomycosis), a dermatologic disease with prominent nail changes (e.g., psoriasis), or pigmentary abnormalities of the nail (as in melanoma).

Unguis incarnatus (ingrown nail) is one of the most common nail conditions and is caused by improper nail trimming and by wearing tight or ill-fitting shoes. It primarily involves the great toe. A painful, warm inflammatory reaction results from excessive lateral growth of the nail into the nailfold. The nail acts as a foreign body, promoting granulation tissue. Decrease inflammation with warm soaks for 20 minutes several times a day. If the problem is minor, lifting the lateral portion of the nail by inserting a cotton wick prevents contact with the nailfold. Sometimes, the involved segment of the nailfold needs to be excised.

Paronychia, or infection around the nail, is characterized by red, shiny skin often associated with painful swelling. These infections frequently result from trauma, picking at the nail, or disorders such as dermatitis. Often these sites become secondarily infected with bacteria or fungi, which later involve the nail. As with ingrown toenail, warm soaks three or more times a day may reduce pressure and pain; however, incision and drainage of inflamed sites is frequently required. Samples for appropriate cultures of the purulent material and the nail should be obtained.

Onychomycosis refers to any fungal infection of the nail, whether due to dermatophytes or candidiasis. Prescribed topical or systemic antibiotic or antifungal therapy, with emphasis for compliance is important. Unfortunately, even with good compliance, recurrence of fungal infections in nails is frequent.

Clients should understand the importance of reducing trauma and irritation to involved nails by (1) trimming nails straight across to reduce further trauma, (2) avoiding overmanicuring or self-induced trauma, (3) limiting harsh chemical irritants such as abrasive cleansers and drying nail products, and (4) keeping the nails dry.

CONCLUSIONS

Skin disorders range from those that are a mere nuisance (such as dry skin) to life-threatening disorders (such as melanoma). Nurses frequently manage skin disorders independently; therefore, a thorough knowledge of the use of topical medications and therapies is crucial. Because much of the needed skin care is provided by the client or a family member, the nurse must use excellent teaching skills to convey the necessary self-care information.

THINKING CRITICALLY

1. **You are caring for an older woman who has had a stroke that left her with residual paralysis on the left side. She also has a pressure ulcer on the left trochanter, in part because she lies on her left side all the time. While caring for her on Monday, you convince her to sit in a chair and to lie on her right side. When you care for her again on Thursday, the ulcer is twice as large and deeper. She refuses to turn to the right and says: "I like lying on my left side." What can you do to help this client?**

Factors to Consider. What pressure reduction methods should be instituted? Is there any harm in lying on a pressure ulcer? Why might she be at increased risk because of malnutrition?

2. **The client is a 72-year-old white man who had undergone a wide excisional biopsy on his forearm to rule out squamous cell carcinoma. The next day the client calls the office complaining of pain at the surgery site. What additional questions need to be asked? What potential interventions might be necessary?**

Factors to Consider. What clinical manifestations would indicate an infection is present? Is age a factor in wound healing?

3. **The client is an otherwise healthy 41-year-old woman who presented to the clinic with a week-long history of intensely itchy, erythematous red lesions under her breasts. The rash appears to be spreading, and the centers of some of the lesions are seen to contain tiny pustules. In addition, the woman complains of a 12-pound weight loss over the past 6 months despite always feeling hungry and thirsty. She denies any medical problems and reports that she does not currently take systemic or topical medications.**

Factors to Consider. What is the common cause of intertriginous dermatitis? What diagnostic study can determine the cause of the problem? What endocrine disorder is suggested by the history of skin rash, thirst, and weight loss?

BIBLIOGRAPHY

1. Ablaza, V., Jones, M. R., & Gingrass, M. K. (1998). Ultrasound assisted lipoplasty: Part 1. An overview for nurses. *Plastic Surgical Nursing, 18*(1), 25–32.
2. Ablaza, V., Jones, M. R., & Gingrass, M. K. (1998). Ultrasound assisted lipoplasty: Part 2. Clinical management. *Plastic Surgical Nursing, 18*(1), 16–25.
3. American Society of Reconstructive Surgical Nurses. (1996). *Core curriculum for plastic and reconstructive surgical nurses* (2nd ed). Pitman, NJ: Author.
4. Anderson, K., & Maksud, D. (1994). Psychological adjustments to reconstructive surgery. *Nursing Clinics of North America, 29*(4), 711–724.
5. Anderson, L. G., & Leroux, C. (1996). Routine surgery, routine patients? Never. *Plastic Surgical Nursing, 16*(1), 41–42.
6. Anderson, S. V. (1998). Laser resurfacing: A survey of pre- and post-procedural care. *Plastic Surgical Nursing, 18*(4), 229–234.
7. Bergstrom, N., & Braden, B. (1987). The Braden scale for predicting pressure sore risk. *Nursing Research, 36*(4), 205–210.
8. Bergstrom, N., et al. (1994). *Treatment of pressure ulcers: Clinical practice guideline No. 15.* Rockville, MD: U.S. Department of Health and Human Services, Public Health Service, Agency for Health Care Policy and Research. AHCPR Pub. No. 95-0652.
9. Bergstrom, N., et al. (1992). *Pressure ulcers in adults: prediction and prevention.* Rockville, MD: U.S. Department of Health and Human Services, Public Health Service, Agency for Health Care Policy and Research. AHCPR Publ. No. 95-0050.
10. Black, J. (1996). Surgical options for wound healing. *Critical Care Nursing Clinics, 8*(2), 169–182.
11. Black, S. (1995). Venous stasis ulcers: A review. *Ostomy/Wound Management, 41*(8), 20–32.
12. Bondville, J. (1994). Pain-free harvesting of skin grafts with EMLA. *Plastic Surgical Nursing, 14*(4), 231–233.
13. Bueller, H. A., & Bernhard, J. D. (1998). Review of pruritus therapy. *Dermatology Nursing, 10*(2), 101–107.
14. Burris, L. M., & Roenigk, H. (1997). Chemical peel as a treatment for skin damage from excessive sun exposure. *Dermatology Nursing, 9*(2), 99–104.
15. Camisa, C., & Warner, M. (1998). Treatment of pemphigus. *Dermatology Nursing, 10*(2), 115–118, 123–131.
16. Clamon, J., & Netscher, D. (1994). General principles of flap reconstruction: Goals for aesthetic and functional outcomes. *Plastic Surgical Nursing, 14*(1), 9–14.
17. Dermatology Nurses' Association. (1996). *Phototherapy administration guidelines for nurse phototherapists and phototechnicians.* Pitman, NJ: Author.
18. Fitzpatrick, T. B. (1996). *Dermatology in general medicine* (5th ed). New York: McGraw-Hill.
19. Formica, K., & Alster, T. S. (1998). Complications for cutaneous laser resurfacing: A nursing guide. *Dermatology Nursing, 10*(5), 353–356.
20. Frankel, E. (1995). Psoriasis. *Journal of the American Academy of Nurse Practitioners, 7*(5), 237–240.
21. Fraser, M., Goldstein, A., & Tucker, M. (1997). The genetics of melanoma. *Seminars in Oncology Nursing, 13*(2), 108–114.
22. Gregory, R. (1997). Laser blepharoplasty. *Plastic Surgical Nursing, 17*(3), 129–133, 151–153.
23. Hinojosa, R. (1995). Postoperative nausea and vomiting: How nurses can help. *Plastic Surgical Nursing, 15*(2), 85–88.
24. Hinojosa, R. (1996). Anxiety of elective surgical patients' family members: Relationship between anxiety levels, family characteristics. *Plastic Surgical Nursing, 16*(1), 43–45.
25. Licata, A. G. (1998). High-dose adjuvant interferon therapy for melanoma. *Dermatology Nursing, 10*(5), 334–336.

26. Lusis, S. (1994). Nursing management of the elderly surgical patient. *Plastic Surgical Nursing, 14*(3), 139–146.

27. Maksud, D., & Cogwell-Anderson, R. (1995). Psychological dimensions of aesthetic surgery: Essentials for nurses. *Plastic Surgical Nursing, 15*(3), 137–144.

28. Malone, M., et al. (1991). The epidemiology of skin tears in the institutionalized elderly. *Journal of the American Geriatric Society, 39*, 591–595.

29. McClelland, P. (1997). New treatment options for psoriasis. *Dermatology Nursing, 9*(5), 295–306.

30. McClelland, P., et al. (1997). Psoralen photochemotherapy. *Dermatology Nursing, 9*(6), 403–417.

31. Mendez-Eastman, S. (1998). Negative pressure wound therapy. *Plastic Surgical Nursing, 18*(1), 27–29, 32–37.

32. Morgan, P., et al. (1997). UVB therapy: dermatology nursing considerations. *Dermatology Nursing, 9*(5), 309–321.

33. Morton, D., & Barth, A. (1996). Vaccine therapy for malignant melanoma. *CA: A Cancer Journal for Clinicians, 46*(4), 225–244.

34. Nicol, N. H., & Boguniewicz, M. (1999). Understanding and treating atopic dermatitis. *Nurse Practitioner Forum 10(2),* 48–55.

35. Nicol, N. H., Ruszkowski, A., & Moore, J. A. (1995, February). Contact dermatitis and the role of patch testing in its diagnosis and management. *Dermatology Nursing* (Suppl.), 5–10.

36. Payne, R., & Martin, M. (1990). The epidemiology and management of skin tears in older adults. *Ostomy/Wound Management, 26,* 26–27.

37. Pochi, P. E., et al. (1991). Report on the Consensus Conference on Acne Classification. *Journal of the American Academy of Dermatology, 24*(3), 495–500.

38. Salisbury, C. C., & Kaye, B. (1998). Complications of rhytidectomy. *Plastic Surgical Nursing, 18*(2), 71–77, 89.

39. Sams, V. M., & Lynch, P. (1990). *Principles and practice of dermatology.* New York: Churchill Livingstone.

40. Seckel, B. R., & Watson, L. (1997). Complications of laser resurfacing. *Plastic Surgical Nursing, 17*(3), 138–143, 151–153, 161.

41. Smith, P., Black, J., & Black, S. (1999). Infected pressure ulcers in the long-term care facility. *Infection Control and Hospital Epidemiology, 20*(5), 358–361.

42. Spencer, K. W. (1994). Selection and preoperative preparation of plastic surgery patients. *Nursing Clinics of North America, 29*(4), 697–710.

43. Springer, R. (1996). Rhytidectomy: From consultation to recovery. *Plastic Surgical Nursing, 16*(1), 27–30.

44. Springer, R. (1996). Liposuction: An overview. *Plastic Surgical Nursing, 16*(4), 215–224.

45. Strohl, R. A. (1998). Cutaneous manifestations of malignant disease. *Dermatology Nursing, 10*(1), 23–25.

46. Taylor, C. R. (1998). Photosensitivity: Classification, diagnosis, and treatment. *Dermatology Nursing, 10*(5), 323–330.

47. Urist, M. (1996). Surgical management of primary cutaneous melanoma. *CA: A Cancer Journal for Clinicians, 46*(4), 217–224.

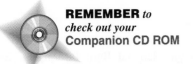

CHAPTER 50

Management of Clients with Burn Injury

Pamela Cornwell

NURSING OUTCOMES CLASSIFICATION (NOC)
for Nursing Diagnoses—Clients with Burns

Altered Nutrition: Less Than Body Requirements
Nutritional Status
Nutritional Status: Food and Fluid Intake
Nutritional Status: Nutrient Intake
Altered Tissue Perfusion: Peripheral
Sensory Function: Cutaneous
Tissue Integrity: Skin and Mucous Membranes
Tissue Perfusion: Peripheral
Altered Tissue Perfusion: Renal
Electrolyte and Acid-Base Balance
Fluid Balance
Hydration
Urinary Elimination
Vital Signs Status
Fluid Volume Deficit
Electrolyte and Acid-Base Balance
Fluid Balance
Hydration
Nutritional Status: Food and Fluid Intake
Hypothermia
Thermoregulation
Impaired Gas Exchange
Electrolyte and Acid-Base Balance
Respiratory Status Gas Exchange

Respiratory Status: Ventilation
Tissue Perfusion: Pulmonary
Impaired Physical Mobility
Ambulation: Walking
Ambulation: Wheelchair
Body Positioning: Self-Initiated
Joint Movement: Active
Mobility Level
Transfer Performance
Impaired Skin Integrity
Tissue Integrity: Skin and Mucous Membranes
Wound Healing: Primary Intention
Wound Healing: Secondary Intention
Impaired Tissue Integrity
Tissue Integrity: Skin and Mucous Membranes
Ineffective Airway Clearance
Aspiration Control
Respiratory Status: Airway Patency
Respiratory Status: Gas Exchange
Respiratory Status: Ventilation
Ineffective Family Coping: Compromised
Family Coping
Family Normalization

Knowledge Deficit
Knowledge: Health Resources
Knowledge: Illness Care
Knowledge: Infection Control
Knowledge: Medication
Knowledge: Personal Safety
Knowledge: Prescribed Activity
Knowledge: Treatment Procedures
Knowledge: Treatment Regimen
Pain
Comfort Level
Pain Control
Pain: Disruptive Effects
Pain Level
Risk for Infection
Immobility Consequences: Physiologic
Immune Status
Knowledge: Infection Control
Treatment Behavior: Illness or Injury
Self-Esteem Disturbance
Self-Esteem
Body Image
Hope
Mood Equilibrium

Injuries that result from direct contact with or exposure to any thermal, chemical, or radiation source are termed *burns.* Burn injuries occur when energy from a heat source is transferred to the tissues of the body. The depth of injury is related to the temperature and the duration of exposure or contact.

Burn care has improved in recent decades, resulting in a lower mortality rate for victims of burn injuries.[2, 71] Dedicated burn centers have been established in which multidisciplinary burn team members work together to care for the burn client and family. Advances in prehospital and inpatient care have contributed to survival. However, despite these advances, many people are still injured and die each year from burns. In the United States, 1.2 million people suffer burn injuries each year, resulting in 60,000 hospitalizations and 6000 deaths annually.[60]

Etiology

Burn injuries are categorized according to the mechanism of injury.

THERMAL BURNS
Thermal burns are caused by exposure to or contact with flame, hot liquids, semiliquids (e.g., steam), semisolids (e.g., tar), or hot objects. Specific examples of thermal burns are those sustained in residential fires, explosive automobile accidents, scald injuries, clothing ignition, and ignition of poorly stored flammable liquids.

CHEMICAL BURNS

Chemical burns are caused by tissue contact with strong acids, alkalis, or organic compounds. The concentration, volume, and type of chemical, as well as the duration of contact, determine the severity of a chemical injury. Chemical burns can result from contact with certain household cleaning agents and various chemicals used in industry, agriculture, and the military. Between 33,000 and 63,000 chemicals in use today have been recognized as hazardous and capable of causing chemical injuries.[77] Chemical injuries to the eyes and inhalation of chemical fumes are particularly serious.

ELECTRICAL BURNS

Electrical burn injuries are caused by heat that is generated by the electrical energy as it passes through the body.[26] Electrical injuries can result from contact with exposed or faulty electrical wiring or high-voltage power lines. People struck by lightning also sustain electrical injury.

The extent of injury is influenced by the duration of contact, the intensity of the current (voltage), the type of current (direct or alternating), the pathway of the current, and the resistance of the tissues as the electrical current passes through the body. Contact with electrical current of greater than 40 volts is potentially dangerous; however, current of greater than 1000 volts is considered to be high-voltage current and is associated with extensive tissue damage.[23]

RADIATION BURNS

Radiation burns are the least common type of burn injury and are caused by exposure to a radioactive source. These types of injuries have been associated with nuclear radiation accidents, the use of ionizing radiation in industry, and therapeutic irradiation. Sunburn, from prolonged exposure to ultraviolet rays (solar radiation), is also considered to be a type of radiation burn.

The amount of radioactive energy received after exposure depends on the distance the person is from the source of the radiation, the strength of the radiation source, the duration of exposure, the extent of body surface area exposed, and the amount of shielding between the source and the person. An acute localized radiation injury appears similar to a cutaneous thermal injury and is characterized by skin erythema, edema, and pain. In contrast, whole-body radiation exposure causes systemic symptoms (radiation sickness) that are dose-dependent.[52]

INHALATION INJURY

Exposure to asphyxiants and smoke commonly occurs with flame injuries, particularly if the victim was trapped in an enclosed, smoke-filled space (e.g., in a residential fire). Victims who die at the scene of the fire usually do so as a result of hypoxia and carbon monoxide poisoning.[18]

The pulmonary pathophysiologic changes that occur with inhalation injury are multifactorial and relate to the severity and type of smoke or gases inhaled. Exposure to asphyxiants, smoke poisoning, and direct thermal (heat) injury to lung tissue constitute the three facets of an inhalation injury. However, not all of these injury components may be present in the client suffering from an inhalation injury.[14, 70]

Risk Factors

Data collected from the National Burn Information Exchange reveal that 75% of all burn injuries result from the actions of the victim, with many of these injuries occurring in the home environment. Most at risk to suffer serious burn injuries are young children, older adults, and people with mental or physical limitations.[8]

Contact with scalding liquids is the leading cause of burn injury.[18] Toddlers (children 2 to 4 years of age) suffer more scald injuries than any other age group. Scald injuries are frequently the result of mishaps in the performance of everyday tasks such as bathing and cooking. Overturned coffeepots, cooking pans spilling hot liquid and grease, overheated foods, liquids cooked in microwave ovens, and hot tap water have been identified as specific causes.[68] In an effort to reduce the incidence of scald injuries the Consumer Products Safety Commission and Underwriters Laboratory has recommended that the maximum temperature on the thermostats of hot water heaters be lowered and that a warning label identifying the potential for injury be affixed to hot water heaters. Legislation requiring public buildings to lower water temperature to 120° F (48.8° C) has proved successful in reducing scald injuries.[59] In addition, a thermostatic control system (anti-scald device) has been developed that, when installed at the faucet or shower head, shuts off the flow of water when the temperature rises above a predetermined temperature, typically 119° F (48.3° C).

Direct contact with flame in the young adult (17 to 25 years of age) is the second leading cause of burn injury.[18] Frequently seen flame injuries in this category are burns to the hands and face that result from an explosion of flammable liquid, known as flash burns. Actions such as using gasoline to start or accelerate a fire and priming a carburetor on an automobile or boat can result in flash explosions.

Clothing ignition during routine meal preparation has also been cited as a leading cause of burn injury, particularly in the elderly population.[68] Synthetic fabrics are especially dangerous, as they melt and adhere to the skin, causing prolonged contact with the heat. Another age group at risk for clothing ignition is the pediatric population. During the early 1970s, the fatality rate among young children burned from ignition of sleepwear was significant. In 1975 it was mandated that children's sleepwear, sizes 0 to 6X, pass a standard flame test. This action significantly lowered mortality associated with children's clothing ignition.[65] The mandate for sleepwear to pass a flame test has since been repealed, and testing will no longer be required. This decision may add significantly to the risk of serious burn injury in the young. See Box 50–1 for burn injury prevention in the home.

Structural fires account for only 5% of burn-related hospital admissions; however, they are responsible for the greatest number of burn-related deaths.[18] Approximately 30% of all burn-related deaths are a result of structural fires,[14] seemingly from the associated smoke inhalation.[16, 70] Ignition from cigarettes is the nation's largest single cause of all fire deaths.[5, 9] Approximately 10% of residential fire deaths are caused by children playing with matches or other ignition sources.[59] Additionally, faulty chimneys, flue vents, fixed heating units, fireplaces, central heating systems, wood-burning stoves, ignition of wood-shingled roofs, as well as human error, all have been implicated.

Of primary importance in reducing injuries and deaths from residential fires is the presence of a working smoke detector and fire extinguisher. It has been estimated that the risk of dying in a residential fire is reduced 50% when an operating smoke detector is in place.[5]

Pathophysiology

The pathophysiologic changes that occur following a cutaneous burn injury depend on the extent or size of the burn. For smaller burns, the body's response to injury is localized to the burned area. However, with more extensive burns (i.e., involving 25% or more of the total body surface area [TBSA]), the body's response to injury is systemic and proportional to the extent of the injury.[64] The clinical manifestations of burn trauma evolve in dramatic fashion over the postinjury clinical course. Extensive burn injuries affect all major systems of the body. The systemic response to burn injury is typically biphasic, characterized by early hypofunction followed later by hyperfunction of each of the organ systems.

DIRECT INJURY TO THE SKIN

With direct injury to the skin, heat from an external source is conducted to the skin, where it denatures (devitalizes) the cells. The amount of damage is dependent upon the length of exposure to the heat and the temperature. At sustained temperatures of 40° to 44° C (104° F to 111.2° F), various cellular enzyme systems and cellular systems fail. The sodium-potassium pump fails, which leads to cellular edema. As the temperature rises to 44° C, cell necrosis occurs. In addition, free radicals are produced, increasing cell damage. The processes of cellular damage continue until the heat source is withdrawn and cooling processes return the cell temperature to a tolerable range.

Protein destruction occurs in tissues destroyed by heat. The directly damaged skin is coagulated and fully destroyed. This area of burned tissue is called the *zone of coagulation* (Fig. 50–1) and represents the area of direct heat injury. In surrounding skin, which has been exposed to heat, the tissue is edematous and has impaired blood flow. This middle zone is called the *zone of stasis* and consists of skin that initially is viable but may also eventually die from ischemia. The outer ring of tissue injury is called the *zone of hyperemia* and consists of tissue that is inflamed and vasodilated.

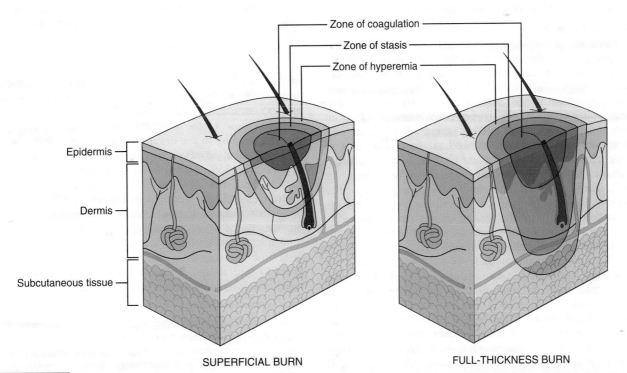

FIGURE 50–1 Zone of tissue injury. The zone of coagulation is the center of the burn wound and represents actual tissue damage. The zone of stasis is the surrounding area and represents areas of potential tissue loss. The outer ring is the zone of hyperemia and is unburned tissue that is inflamed.

Some types of burn create unique patterns of injury. In electrical injuries, heat is generated as the electricity travels through the body, resulting in internal tissue damage.[29] The concept of "the tip of the iceberg" is helpful to understand these injuries. For instance, only a very small percentage of total injury from an electrical burn can be seen from the body's surface. Cutaneous burn injuries may appear negligible, but muscle and soft tissue damage may be extensive, particularly with high-voltage electrical injuries. The voltage, type of current (direct or alternating), contact site, and duration of contact are important considerations because they may affect morbidity. Electricity seeks ground as it exits the body; en route, it creates heat and may pass though vital organs. Alternating current (AC) is more dangerous than direct current (DC). AC is often associated with cardiopulmonary arrest, ventricular fibrillation, tetanic muscle contractions, and long bone or vertebral compression fracture. The risk of acute renal failure is noteworthy in clients following an electrical injury. Hemoglobin, released from heat-damaged erythrocytes together with myoglobin, the protein that supplies muscles with oxygen, is released in significant quantities into the blood stream after deep burn injuries involving muscle damage. These substances pass through the glomeruli and are excreted in urine. However, these materials may precipitate and obstruct the renal tubules, causing renal damage unless a brisk urine output is maintained.[64] In addition, victims of electrical injuries may have fallen from the point of electrical contact and sustained associated injuries. Cataract formation is also associated with high-voltage electrical injury, especially in cases in which contact points are on the head or neck. In chemical burns, systemic toxic effects may result from cutaneous absorption of the offending agent. Organ failure and even death have resulted from prolonged contact with and absorption of different chemicals.

FLUID SHIFTS

Immediately following a burn injury, vasoactive substances (catecholamines, histamine, serotonin, leukotrienes, kinins, and prostaglandins) are released from the injured tissues.[34, 60] These substances initiate changes in capillary integrity, allowing plasma to seep into surrounding tissues (Fig. 50–2). Direct damage to vessels from heat further increases capillary permeability, which permits sodium ions to enter the cell and potassium ions to exit. The overall effect of these changes is creation of an osmotic gradient, which leads to increases in intercellular and interstitial fluid and further depletes intravascular fluid volumes. The vasoactive substances exert their effects both locally (in the area of injury) and systemically. The burn-injured client's hemodynamic balance, metabolism, and immune status are altered.

The body responds initially by shunting blood toward the brain and heart and away from all other body organs. Prolonged lack of blood flow to these other organs is detrimental. The degree of damage that results depends on the basal needs of the body organ. Some organs can survive for only a few hours without nutrient blood supply. The lack of renal blood flow decreases glomerular filtration rate, leading to oliguria (low urine output).[64] If fluid resuscitation is delayed or inadequate, hypovolemia progresses, and acute renal failure may occur. However, with adequate fluid resuscitation and a rise in cardiac

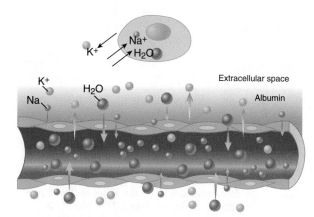

Fluid and electrolyte shift during burn shock

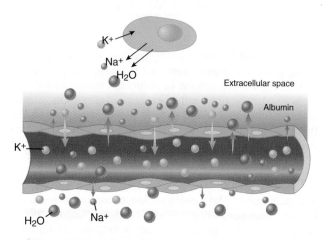

Fluid and electrolyte shift after burn shock

FIGURE 50–2 Changes in capillary permeability allow plasma to seep into interstitial spaces. In addition, the sodium pump fails and sodium remains in the cell. There is a corresponding rise in serum potassium.

output, renal blood flow will return to normal. After resuscitation, the body begins to reabsorb the edema fluid and to eliminate it through diuresis.

Blood flow to the mesenteric bed is also diminished initially, leading to the development of intestinal ileus and gastrointestinal dysfunction in clients with burns of greater than 25% TBSA.[59] With the reduction in blood flow to the gastric mucosa, ischemic changes to the upper gastrointestinal tract occur, which slows production of the protective mucous lining, resulting in small, superficial erosions to the stomach and duodenum. If the gastrointestinal tract is left untreated and unprotected by antacids or histamine H_2-receptor antagonists, the erosions can progress to ulcerations—called Curling's ulcers in burn injured clients—and gastrointestinal bleeding.

PULMONARY SYSTEM

Minute ventilation is often normal or slightly decreased early after a burn injury. Following fluid resuscitation, a rise in minute ventilation—manifested by hyperventilation—may occur especially if the client is fearful, anxious, or in pain. This hyperventilation is the result of an increase in both respiratory rate and tidal volume and appears to be the result of the hypermetabolism that is seen after burn injury. It typically peaks in the second postinjury week and then gradually returns to normal as the burn wound heals or is closed by grafting.[59]

Pulmonary vascular resistance may increase slightly, and lung compliance may decrease. The changes in lung compliance cause a proportionate increase in the work of breathing; however, these changes are typically small, and in the absence of any pulmonary parenchymal (tissue) damage, they require no specialized treatment.

INHALATION INJURY. Exposure to asphyxiants is the most common cause of early mortality from inhalation injury.[18] Carbon monoxide (CO), a common asphyxiant, is produced when organic substances (e.g., wood or coal) burn. It is a colorless, odorless, and tasteless gas that has an affinity for the body's hemoglobin that is 200 times greater than that of oxygen. With inhalation of CO, the oxygen molecules are displaced, and CO binds to hemoglobin to form carboxyhemoglobin (COHb). Tissue hypoxia occurs from an overall decrease in the blood's oxygen-delivering capability.

Direct heat injury to the upper airway results from inhalation of the air heated by fire. The heat immediately produces injury to the airway, which results in edema, erythema, and ulceration. Thermal burns to the lower airways of the pulmonary system are rare because of the protective reflex closure of the glottis and the ability of the respiratory tract to exchange heat effectively. However, thermal burns to the lower airways can occur with the inhalation of steam or explosive gases or with aspiration of scalding liquids.

Smoke poisoning results from the inhalation of the by-products of combustion: noxious chemicals and particulate matter. The pulmonary response includes a localized inflammatory reaction, a decrease in bronchial ciliary action, and a decrease in alveolar surfactant. Mucosal edema occurs in the smaller airways. After several hours, sloughing of the tracheobronchial epithelium may occur, and hemorrhagic tracheobronchitis may develop. Adult respiratory distress syndrome may follow.[18]

MYOCARDIAL DEPRESSION

Some research investigators have suggested that a myocardial depressant factor exists and circulates in the early postinjury period. More recently, a combination of inflammatory mediators and hormones has been suggested as the cause of myocardial depression occurring after the injury.[6]

ALTERED SKIN INTEGRITY

The burn wound itself exhibits pathophysiologic changes caused by disruption of the skin and alterations to the tissue beneath the surface. The skin, nerve endings, sweat glands, and hair follicles injured by burn lose normal functioning. Most important, the skin's barrier function is lost. Intact skin normally keeps bacteria from entering the body and body fluids from seeping out, controls evaporation, and maintains body warmth. With destruction of the skin in burn injury, mechanisms for maintaining normal body temperature can be altered, the risk of infection from invasion of bacteria increases, and evaporative water loss increases.[31] Depending upon the depth of the injury, nerve endings either become exposed, resulting in pain and discomfort until wound closure, or are damaged, leaving the innervated area insensate, with potential for permanent impairment of ability to sense touch, pressure, and pain.

IMMUNOSUPPRESSION

Immune system function is depressed following burn injury. Depression of lymphocyte activity, a decrease in immunoglobulin production, suppression of complement activity, and an alteration in neutrophil and macrophage functioning are evident following extensive burn injuries.[53] In addition, the burn injury disrupts the body's primary barrier to infection, the skin. Together these changes result in an increased risk of infection and life-threatening sepsis.

PSYCHOLOGICAL RESPONSE

Numerous psychological and emotional responses to burn injuries have been identified, ranging from fear to psychosis.[7] A victim's response is influenced by age, personality, cultural and ethnic background, the extent and location of the injury, and the resulting impact on body image. In addition, separation from family and friends during hospitalization and the change in the client's normal role and responsibilities affect the reaction to burn trauma. Four stages in the psychosocial response to burn trauma have been described: (1) impact, (2) retreat or withdrawal, (3) acknowledgment, and (4) the reconstructive period.[37]

Clinical Manifestations

DEGREE OF INJURY

Depending on the skin layers damaged, burn wounds are termed either partial-thickness burns or full-thickness burns. Burn wounds are also classified as first-, second-, third-, or fourth-degree burns. Partial-thickness burns involve injury to the epidermis and portions of the dermis (Fig. 50–3). *First-degree* partial-thickness burns are superficial and painful and appear red. They heal on their own by epidermal cell regeneration within about 3 to 7 days. Sunburn is a good example of a first-degree partial-thickness burn. *Second-degree* partial-thickness burns appear wet or blistered and are extremely painful but can heal on their own (that is, without skin grafting) if they are small and do not become infected.

Third-degree full-thickness burns are characterized by damage throughout the dermis (Figs. 50–4 and 50–5). A

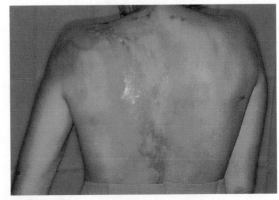

FIGURE 50–3 Partial-thickness burn injury (second-degree burn).

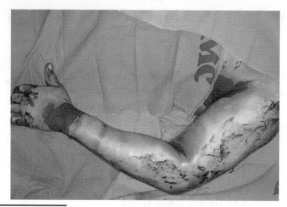

FIGURE 50–4 Full-thickness burn injury (third-degree burn).

full-thickness burn appears dry and may be black, brown, white, or ivory. The denatured skin is called eschar (pronounced "ĕs-car"). The burned tissue is painless as a result of damage to the nerve endings; however, the surrounding skin is painful. Unless the area is very small (the size of a half-dollar), the full-thickness burn must be skin-grafted to heal. The appearance of the burn relative to the depth of injury is described in Figure 50–6.

Fourth-degree full-thickness burns involve skin, fat, muscle, and sometimes bone. The skin appears charred or may be completely burned away. Areas of a fourth-degree burn require extensive surgical debridement and grafting. Amputations are common in these deep injuries.

In addition to altered physical appearance, the loss of skin leads to other problems. Hypothermia results from loss of body heat through the burn wound and is characterized by a core body temperature below 98.6° F. Hypothermia is extremely harmful because it leads to shiver-

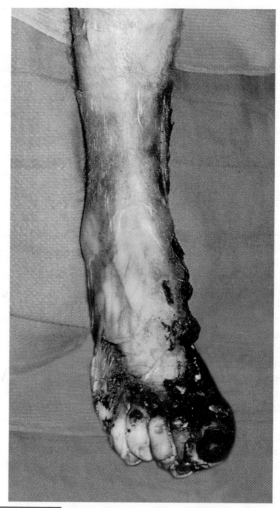

FIGURE 50–5 Full-thickness burn injury (fourth-degree burn).

		WOUND APPEARANCE	WOUND SENSATION	COURSE OF HEALING
EPIDERMIS Sweat duct Capillary	**PARTIAL-THICKNESS BURN** — 1st-degree	Epidermis remains intact and without blisters. Erythema; skin blanches with pressure.	Painful	Discomfort lasts 48–72 hours. Desquamation in 3–7 days
Sebaceous gland Nerve endings DERMIS Hair follicle	2nd-degree	Wet, shiny, weeping surface Blisters Wound blanches with pressure.	Painful Very sensitive to touch, air currents	Superficial partial-thickness burn heals in < 21 days. Deep partial-thickness burn requires > 21 days for healing. Healing rates vary with burn depth and presence/absence of infection.
Sweat gland Fat Blood vessels	**FULL-THICKNESS BURN** — 3rd-degree	Color variable (i.e., deep red, white, black, brown) Surface dry Thrombosed vessels visible No blanching	Insensate (↓ pinprick sensation)	Autografting required for healing
Bone	4th-degree	Color variable Charring visible in deepest areas Extremity movement limited	Insensate	Amputation of extremities likely Autografting required for healing

FIGURE 50–6 Burn injury classification according to depth of injury.

ing, which in turn increases oxygen consumption and caloric demands.

The evaporative water loss through the burn contributes to the client's diminished fluid volume and compromised hydration status. Evaporative losses not compensated for by fluid replacement will be evidenced by a low blood pressure, decreased urine output, dry mucous membranes, and poor skin turgor.

FLUID AND ELECTROLYTE IMBALANCE

Hyponatremia, hypernatremia, and hyperkalemia are common electrolyte abnormalities that affect the burn-injured client at different points in the recovery process. Extensive burns (greater than 25% TBSA) result in generalized body edema affecting both burned and nonburned tissues and in a decrease in circulating intravascular blood volume (Fig. 50–7).[18, 60, 65] Hematocrit levels are elevated in the first 24 hours after injury, demonstrating hemoconcentration from the loss of intravascular fluid. In addition, evaporative fluid losses through the burn wound are 4 to 20 times greater than normal and remain elevated until

TABLE 50–1	CLINICAL MANIFESTATIONS OF CARBON MONOXIDE (CO) POISONING
CO Level (%)	**Clinical Manifestations**
5–10	Impaired visual acuity
11–20	Flushing, headache
21–30	Nausea, impaired dexterity
31–40	Vomiting, dizziness, syncope
41–50	Tachypnea, tachycardia
>50	Coma, death

Adapted from Cioffi, W. G., & Rue, L. W. (1991). Diagnosis and treatment of inhalation injuries. *Critical Care Clinics of North America, 3*(2), 195.

complete wound closure is obtained. The result is a decrease in organ perfusion. If the intravascular space is not replenished with intravenous (IV) fluids, hypovolemic (burn) shock and, ultimately, death ensue for the victim of an extensive burn.[2, 18, 20, 34, 46, 74]

Urine output for the adult client receiving insufficient fluid replacement following a major burn injury will diminish to less than 0.5 ml/kg of body weight. Physical findings of the urine sample will demonstrate dehydration, characterized by dark amber, concentrated urine and elevated specific gravity. Laboratory tests reveal elevated blood urea nitrogen (BUN) levels until the client has been adequately hydrated.

Manifestations of decreased gastrointestinal motility following major burn injuries include the absence of bowel sounds, stool, or flatus; nausea and vomiting; and abdominal distention. After adequate fluid resuscitation, gastrointestinal motility returns, signaled by a return of hunger/appetite, bowel sounds, flatus, and stool production.

At approximately 18 to 36 hours after burn injury, capillary membrane integrity begins to be restored. The initial rise in hematocrit seen early after injury falls to below normal by the third or fourth day after injury owing to red blood cell loss and damage incurred at the time of injury. Over the ensuing days and weeks, the body begins to reabsorb the edema fluid, and the excess fluid is excreted via diuresis (see Fig. 50–7).

ALTERATIONS IN RESPIRATION

The client may exhibit tachypnea following the burn injury. Arterial blood gas analysis may demonstrate a relatively normal arterial partial pressure of oxygen (PaO_2), with oxygen saturation lower than expected relative to the PO_2. Diagnosis is made by measuring the COHb level in the blood. The clinical manifestations of acute CO poisoning are directly related to the level of COHb saturation and relative degree of tissue hypoxia (Table 50–1). The onset of clinical manifestations will typically not occur until COHb levels reach 15%. Initial signs and symptoms are related to decreased cerebral tissue oxygenation and are neurologic in nature. The neurologic problems caused by CO exposure can lead to progressive and permanent cerebral dysfunction.

Thermal burns to the upper airways (mouth, nasopharynx, and larynx) characteristically appear erythematous

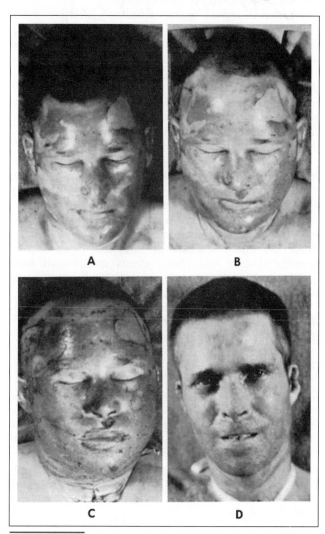

FIGURE 50–7 Edema formation after a burn injury to the face and neck. Edema worsens over the first 24 to 48 hours after burn injury. *A,* At 3 hours after burn. *B,* At 8 hours after the burn. *C,* At 24 hours after burn, when edema has typically maximized. *D,* Complete healing after 40 days. (From Artz, C. P., et al. [1979]. *Burns: A team approach.* Philadelphia: W. B. Saunders.)

and edematous, with mucosal blisters or ulcerations. Increasing mucosal edema can lead to upper airway obstruction, typically between the first 24 and 48 hours after injury. Clinical manifestations, including stridor, dyspnea, increased work of breathing, and eventually cyanosis, may be noted when critical narrowing of the airway is present.[14, 38, 57]

Physical findings on admission indicative of smoke exposure include soot on the face and nares, facial burns, soot in the sputum, coughing, and wheezing. The manifestations of tracheobronchitis typically do not present until 24 to 48 hours after injury. Early signs consist of bronchospasm evidenced as wheezing and bronchorrhea. Lung compliance is decreased, causing an increased work of breathing. Impaired clearance of secretions accentuates the problem. Normally, ventilation and perfusion are matched by equal volumes of air and blood on the alveolar-capillary level. The client with smoke inhalation exhibits pathophysiologic changes that reduce alveolar ventilation, causing a ventilation-perfusion (V-Q) mismatch, which in turn impairs gas exchange.[19, 42]

DECREASED CARDIAC OUTPUT

Following a major burn injury, heart rate and peripheral vascular resistance increase in response to the release of catecholamines and to the relative hypovolemia, but initial cardiac output falls (hypofunction).[10] At approximately 24 hours after burn injury in clients receiving adequate fluid resuscitation, cardiac output returns to normal and then increases (2 to 2.5 times normal) to meet the hypermetabolic needs of the body (hyperfunction). This change in cardiac output occurs even before circulating intravascular volume levels are restored to normal. Arterial blood pressure is normal or slightly elevated unless severe hypovolemia exists. The decreased cardiac output seen initially after burn injury is evidenced by a decreased blood pressure, decreased urine output, weak peripheral pulses, and if monitored via a pulmonary artery catheter, a cardiac output below 4 L/min, cardiac index of less than 2.5 L/min, and systemic vascular resistance of less than 900 dyne-sec/cm.[5, 18]

PAIN RESPONSES

The client experiences substantial pain as a result of the burn wound and exposed nerve endings from lack of skin integrity.[42, 43] Burn victims typically describe two types of pain resulting from their injury: background pain and procedural pain. Background pain is experienced when the client is at rest or engages in non–procedure-related activities, such as shifting position in bed, or with chest or abdominal wall movements that occur with deep breathing or coughing. Background pain is described as continuous in nature and low in intensity, typically lasting for the duration of the clinical course.[17] Procedural pain is experienced during the performance of therapeutic measures commonly used in burn care. Nearly 52% of clients report moderate to severe pain during burn wound debridement.[19] Procedural pain is described as acute and high in intensity. Clinical responses to pain may include an increase in blood pressure, heart rate, and respiratory rate and dilated pupils, rigid muscle tone, and guarded positioning.

ALTERED LEVEL OF CONSCIOUSNESS

Rarely do burn-injured clients suffer neurologic damage.

The client with a major burn injury is most often awake and alert on admission to the hospital. If agitation develops in the immediate postinjury period, the client may be suffering from hypoxemia or hypovolemia and needs further assessment for identifying the origin of these changes. When an alteration in level of consciousness is present, it is most often related to neurologic trauma (e.g., fall, motor vehicle accident), impaired perfusion to the brain, hypoxemia (as from a closed-space fire), inhalation injury (as from exposure to asphyxiates or other toxic materials from the fire), electrical burn injury, or the effects of drugs present in the body at the time of injury.

Clients with associated head trauma may have scalp lacerations, swelling, tenderness, or ecchymosis. Level of consciousness may fluctuate between intervals of lucidity followed by rapid deterioration. Pupils may be of unequal size. Neurologic manifestations may include headache, dizziness, memory loss, confusion or loss of consciousness, disorientation, visual changes, hallucinations, combativeness, and coma.

PSYCHOLOGICAL ALTERATIONS

The period of *impact* begins immediately after injury and is characterized by shock, disbelief, and feelings of being overwhelmed. The client and family members may be aware of what is happening but may be coping with the situation poorly. During this period, families of critically ill clients have a need for assurance, proximity to the injured person, and information. Specifically, families want to know how the client is being treated, specific facts about the client's progress, and why certain procedures are being done.

Retreat is characterized by repression, withdrawal, denial, and suppression. Although seemingly destructive, these coping strategies may be protective in that they allow the client to maintain an intact psyche.

The third phase, *acknowledgment,* begins when the client accepts the injury and the resultant change in body image. Mourning of actual or perceived losses may be apparent. During this phase, clients may benefit from meeting with other burn-injured clients in one-on-one contact or group support meetings.

The final phase, the *reconstructive period,* begins when the client and family accept the limitations imposed by the injury and begin to plan realistically for the future.

Outcome Management

The burn client undergoes a wide range of physiologic and metabolic changes in response to the burn injury. To accomplish the best outcomes, it is essential to have a clear understanding of the pathophysiologic process and the necessary treatment modifications needed over the entire course of burn treatment. Three distinct periods or phases of treatment can be defined in the care of the seriously burned client: the emergent, the acute, and the rehabilitation phases.

EMERGENT PHASE

The emergent phase of burn injury consists of the time between the initial injury and 36 to 48 hours after injury. This phase ends when fluid resuscitation is complete.

During this phase, life-threatening airway and breathing problems are of major concern. It is also characterized by the development of hypovolemia which results as capillaries leak fluid from the intravascular spaces into the interstitial spaces, causing edema. Although the fluid remains in the body, it is unable to contribute to maintaining adequate circulation, because it is no longer in the vascular space. The burn itself, except for initial assessment of severity and depth and, in certain cases, a procedure (escharotomy) performed to restore perfusion to areas exhibiting circulatory compromise, is of less immediate concern. The adequacy of initial treatment of pulmonary and circulatory abnormalities sets the stage for subsequent management. Any early management error will lead to a dramatic increase in morbidity and mortality during the subsequent injury phases.

Management of the burn client begins at the scene of the accident. The first step should be removing the victim from the area of immediate danger, followed by stopping the burning process. Basic life support measures should be implemented during transport of the client to the hospital.

■ Medical Management in the Emergent Phase of Burn Injury

ASSESS BURN SEVERITY

The American Burn Association has published a severity classification schedule for burn injuries (see Table 50–2). These guidelines are intended to assist the clinician in determining injury severity for the burn client. This classification schedule separates injuries into major, moderate, and minor categories. Clients with major burns are usually transferred to a specialized burn care facility after local emergency treatment has been provided. Clients with moderate burns can usually be managed on an inpatient basis at the receiving hospital. Clients with minor burns usually receive initial care in the emergency department and are then discharged for follow-up care on an outpatient basis.

The severity of a burn injury is classified according to the risk of mortality and the risk of cosmetic or functional disability.[3] Several factors influence injury severity.

BURN DEPTH. The deeper the burn wound, the more serious the injury. Deep partial-thickness and full-thickness burns are more likely to become infected, have more profound systemic effects, and are more frequently associated with contractures.

BURN SIZE. The size of a burn (percentage of injured skin, excluding first-degree burns) is determined by one of two techniques: (1) the rule of 9s and (2) an age-specific burn diagram or chart.[45, 61] Burn size is expressed as a percentage of TBSA. The *rule of 9s* was introduced in the late 1940s as a quick assessment tool for estimating burn size. The basis of the rule is that the body is divided into anatomic sections, each of which represents 9%, or a multiple of 9%, of the TBSA (Fig. 50–8). This method is easy and requires no diagrams to determine the percentage of TBSA injured. Therefore, it is frequently used in emergency departments, where initial triage occurs. A *burn diagram* charts the percentages for body segments according to age and provides a more accurate estimate of burn size (Fig. 50–9). It should be noted that the extent of burn injury is most accurate after initial debridement and should therefore be verified again at that time.

BURN LOCATION. With burns of the head, neck, and chest, associated pulmonary complications are frequent. When burns involve the face, associated injuries often include corneal abrasions. Burns of the ears are prone to auricular chondritis and are susceptible to infection and further loss of tissue. Management of burns of the hands and joints often requires intense physical and occupational therapy, with the potential for major loss of work time and for permanent physical and vocational disability. Burns involving the perineal area are prone to infection owing to autocontamination by urine and feces. Circumferential burns of extremities may produce a tourniquet-like effect, leading to distal vascular compromise. Circumferential thorax burns may lead to inadequate chest wall expansion and pulmonary insufficiency.

AGE. The client's age affects the severity and outcome of the burn. Mortality rates are higher for children younger than 4 years, particularly in newborns and infants up to 1 year of age, and for clients older than 65 years.[5, 18, 68] High mortality and morbidity rates in the older burn-injured client result from the combination of age-related functional impairments (slower reaction time, impaired judgment, and decreased mobility), living alone, environmental hazards, and significant preburn morbidity. Compounding this vulnerability to burn injury is the thinning of the skin and atrophy of skin appendages that occur with aging.

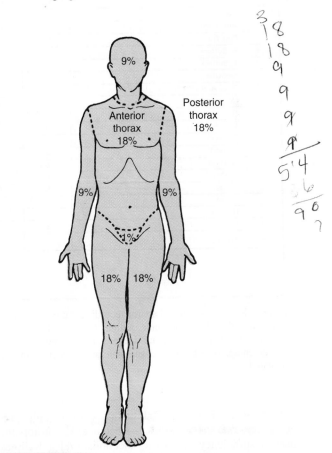

FIGURE 50–8 The rule of 9s provides a quick method for estimating the extent of a burn injury in the adult.

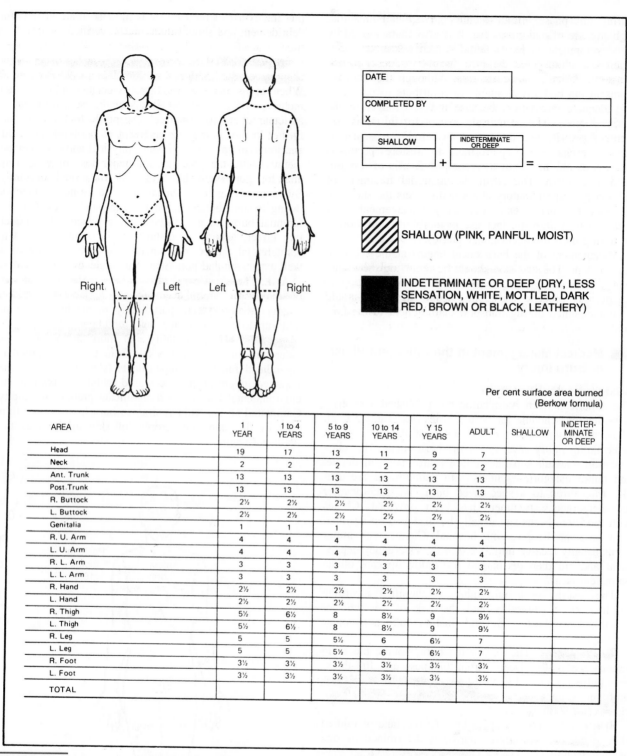

DATE

COMPLETED BY
X

| SHALLOW | + | INDETERMINATE OR DEEP | = _____ |

Right Left   Left Right

▨ SHALLOW (PINK, PAINFUL, MOIST)

■ INDETERMINATE OR DEEP (DRY, LESS SENSATION, WHITE, MOTTLED, DARK RED, BROWN OR BLACK, LEATHERY)

Per cent surface area burned
(Berkow formula)

AREA	1 YEAR	1 to 4 YEARS	5 to 9 YEARS	10 to 14 YEARS	Y 15 YEARS	ADULT	SHALLOW	INDETER- MINATE OR DEEP
Head	19	17	13	11	9	7		
Neck	2	2	2	2	2	2		
Ant. Trunk	13	13	13	13	13	13		
Post.Trunk	13	13	13	13	13	13		
R. Buttock	2½	2½	2½	2½	2½	2½		
L. Buttock	2½	2½	2½	2½	2½	2½		
Genitalia	1	1	1	1	1	1		
R. U. Arm	4	4	4	4	4	4		
L. U. Arm	4	4	4	4	4	4		
R. L. Arm	3	3	3	3	3	3		
L. L. Arm	3	3	3	3	3	3		
R. Hand	2½	2½	2½	2½	2½	2½		
L. Hand	2½	2½	2½	2½	2½	2½		
R. Thigh	5½	6½	8	8½	9	9½		
L. Thigh	5½	6½	8	8½	9	9½		
R. Leg	5	5	5½	6	6½	7		
L. Leg	5	5	5½	6	6½	7		
R. Foot	3½	3½	3½	3½	3½	3½		
L. Foot	3½	3½	3½	3½	3½	3½		
TOTAL								

FIGURE 50–9 A sample chart for recording the extent and depth of a burn injury using the Berkow formula. To estimate burn extent using this chart, the nurse outlines the injured areas, excluding first-degree burns. Shallow (second-degree) burns are designated by parallel lines, and deeper (third-degree and fourth-degree) burns are designated by shading in the appropriate areas. The percentage of each injured anatomic area is then estimated using the age-specific table. Total body surface area burn is then calculated.

GENERAL HEALTH. Debilitating cardiac, pulmonary, endocrine, and renal disease—specifically, cardiopulmonary insufficiency, diabetes, alcoholism-related disease, and renal failure—have been observed to influence the client's response to injury and treatment.[58] The mortality rate for clients with pre-existing cardiac disorders is 3.5 to 4 times higher than that for burn-injured clients without cardiac disorders. Alcoholic clients with burn injury have a threefold increase in mortality rate over that of nonalcoholic clients with burns. In addition, alcoholic clients who survive their burn injury have longer hospital stays and more complications. The increased morbidity among clients with burn injury who are alcoholics may be related to impaired immune function. Obese clients with burn injury are also at increased risk owing to cardiopulmonary complications.

MECHANISM OF INJURY. The mechanism of injury is another factor used to determine the severity of injury. In general, special attention to this aspect of the injury is required for any electrical or chemical burn injury or any burn associated with inhalation injury. The client, people at the scene of the injury, and emergency medical personnel may have important information that could help in determining the severity of the burn. Useful information includes the time of injury, the level of the client's consciousness at the scene, whether the injury occurred in an enclosed or open space, the presence of associated trauma, and the specific mechanism of injury. If the victim has suffered a chemical burn, knowledge of the offending agent, its concentration, the duration of exposure, and whether irrigation was initiated at the scene is useful. For victims of electrical injuries, knowledge of the electrical source, type of current, and the current voltage is useful in determining the extent of the injury. Information concerning the client's past medical history as well as his or her general health should be obtained. Specifically, information regarding cardiac, pulmonary, endocrine, or renal disease should be obtained because it may have implications for treatment. Known allergies should also be identified, as should any current medication regimen.

TREAT MINOR BURNS

Care of the client with minor burn injuries is frequently provided on an ambulatory or outpatient basis. In making the decision about whether to manage a client as an outpatient, the seriousness of the injury must first be assessed. As outlined in Table 50–2, a minor burn injury in the adult is generally considered to be less than 15% TBSA in clients younger than 40 years of age or 10% TBSA in clients older than 40 years, without a risk of cosmetic or functional impairment or disability.[3] In addition, the client's or caregiver's ability to perform wound care in the home environment must be considered. Medical care of the minor burn includes wound evaluation and initial care, tetanus immunization, and pain management. While providing initial wound care, the nurse is responsible for teaching home wound care and the clinical manifestations of infection that necessitate further medical care. Other teaching needs include the need to perform active range of motion (ROM) exercises to maintain normal joint function and to decrease edema formation. The need for any follow-up evaluations or treatments should be confirmed with the client at this time.

TREAT MAJOR BURNS

The medical goals for burn care depend on the phase of care. Initial goals are saving life, maintaining and protecting the airway, and restoring hemodynamic stability. Later goals are replacement of missing skin, promoting healing, and assessing and correcting complications.

MONITOR AIRWAY AND BREATHING. The adequacy of the airway and breathing should take prime importance during the emergent phase of burn injury.[11, 21, 30, 39, 45, 54]

The oropharynx should be inspected for evidence of erythema, blisters, or ulcerations, and the need for endotracheal intubation should be considered. If inhalation injury is suspected, administration of 100% oxygen via a tight-fitting facemask continues until COHb levels fall below 15%.[18] Hyperbaric oxygen is also considered with any exposure to CO. If breathing appears to be compromised by tight circumferential trunk burns, bilateral escharotomies of the trunk may be necessary to relieve ventilatory compromise.

PREVENT BURN SHOCK. In adults with burn injuries affecting more than 15% TBSA, IV fluid resuscitation is generally required.[2, 46] Two peripheral large-bore IV lines placed through nonburned skin, proximal to any extremity burns, is recommended. IV lines may be placed through burned skin if necessary; however, these lines should be secured with a suture. For clients with extensive burns or limited peripheral IV access sites, cannulation of a central vein (subclavian, internal or external jugular, or femoral) by a physician may be necessary.

TABLE 50–2	AMERICAN BURN ASSOCIATION SEVERITY CLASSIFICATION FOR BURN INJURIES

MAJOR BURN INJURY

25% TBSA burn in adults <40 yr of age
20% TBSA burn in adults >40 yr of age
20% TBSA burn in children <10 yr of age

or

Burns involving the face, eyes, ears, hands, feet, and perineum likely to result in functional or cosmetic disability

or

High-voltage electrical burn injury

or

All burn injuries with concomitant inhalation injury or major trauma

MODERATE BURN INJURY

15%–25% TBSA burn in adults <40 yr of age
10%–20% TBSA burn in adults >40 yr of age
10%–20% TBSA burn in children <10 yr of age

with

Less than 10% TBSA full-thickness burn without cosmetic or functional risk to the face, eyes, ears, hands, feet, or perineum

MINOR BURN INJURY

<15% TBSA burn in adults <40 yr of age
<10% TBSA burn in adults >40 yr of age
<10% TBSA burn in children <10 yr of age

with

<2% TBSA full-thickness burn and no cosmetic or functional risk to the face, eyes, ears, hands, feet, or perineum

TBSA, total body surface area.
Adapted from American Burn Association. (1984). Guidelines for service standards and severity classification in the treatment of burn injury. *American College of Surgeons Bulletin*, 69(10), 24–28.

Fluid resuscitation is used to minimize the deleterious effects of the fluid shifts. The goal of fluid resuscitation is to maintain vital organ perfusion while avoiding the complication of inadequate or excessive fluids. Several formulas used to calculate fluid requirements are listed in Table 50–3. In the calculation of fluid infusion rates, the time of injury, not the time at which fluid resuscitation was initiated, serves as time zero. Thus, if a burned client is delayed 2 hours in reaching an emergency department, those 2 hours must be considered in any calculation of needed fluid.

Although each formula is different, fluid management during the first 24 hours after burn injury generally includes the infusion of balanced salt solution, typically lactated Ringer's solution. The exact amount of fluid is based on the client's weight and the extent of injury. Other factors to be considered include the presence of an inhalation injury, a delay in initiation of resuscitation, and deep tissue damage. These factors tend to increase the amount of IV fluid required for adequate resuscitation above the calculated amount.[18] With the exception of the Evans and Brooke formulas, colloid-containing solutions are not given during this period because of the changes in capillary integrity that allow leakage of protein-rich fluid (e.g., albumin) into the interstitial space, resulting in the formation of additional edematous fluid. During the second 24 hours after burn injury, colloid-containing solutions are administered, along with 5% dextrose and water in varying amounts. It is important to remember that all resuscitation formulas are only guides and that fluid resuscitation volumes should be adjusted according to the client's physiologic response. Adequacy of fluid resuscitation is based upon urine output when hemodynamic monitoring is not used.[20] An indwelling urethral catheter connected to a closed drainage system should be placed to measure hourly urine production and to guide IV fluid replacement.

Vital signs are used to provide a baseline of information as well as additional data for determining the adequacy of fluid resuscitation. Baseline laboratory studies should include blood glucose, BUN, serum creatinine, serum electrolytes, and hematocrit levels. Arterial blood gas and COHb levels should also be obtained, particularly if an inhalation injury is suspected. A chest x-ray film should be obtained for all clients with extensive burns or inhalation injury. Other laboratory tests in addition to the radiographic study should be performed in all clients with associated trauma, as indicated. Depending on the circumstance of the injury, an alcohol and/or drug screen may be appropriate. Continuous electrocardiographic (ECG) monitoring should be initiated in all clients with major burn injuries, particularly those who have suffered a high-voltage electrical injury or who have a history of cardiac ischemia.

PREVENT ASPIRATION. Many burn centers advocate the placement of a nasogastric tube for management of unresponsive clients and clients with burns of 20% to 25% TBSA or more, to prevent emesis and reduce the risk of aspiration. Gastrointestinal dysfunction results from the intestinal ileus that develops almost universally in clients during the early post–burn injury period.[54] All oral fluids should be restricted at this time.

TABLE 50–3   **FLUID RESUSCITATION FORMULAS USED IN BURN CARE**

Formula Name	First 24 Hours			Second 24 Hours		
	Electrolyte-Containing Solution	Colloid-Containing Solution	Dextrose in Water	Electrolyte-Containing Solution	Colloid-Containing Solution	Dextrose in Water
Evans	Normal saline 1 ml/kg/% burn	1 ml/kg/% burn	2000 ml	½ of first 24-hr requirement	½ of first 24-hr requirement	2000 ml
Brooke	Lactated Ringer's 1.5 ml/kg/% burn	0.5 ml/kg/% burn	2000 ml	½–¾ of first 24-hr requirement	½–¾ of first 24-hr requirement	2000 ml
Modified Brooke	Lactated Ringer's 2 ml/kg/% burn	None	None	None	0.3–0.5 ml/kg/% burn	Titrate to maintain urine output
Parkland	Lactated Ringer's 4 ml/kg/% burn	None	None	None	0.3–0.5 ml/kg/% burn	Titrate to maintain urine output
Hypertonic saline solution	Fluid containing 250 mEq of sodium/L to maintain hourly urine output of 70 ml in adults	None	None	Same solution to maintain hourly urine output of 30 ml in adults	None	None

Adapted from Rue, L. W., & Cioffi, W. G., Jr. (1991). Resuscitation of thermally injured patients. *Critical Care Nursing Clinics of North America 3*(2), 185; and Wachtel, T. L., & Fortune, J. B. (1983). Fluid resuscitation for burn shock. In T. L. Wachtel et al. (Eds.), *Current topics in burn care* (p. 44). Rockville, MD: Aspen Publishers.

MINIMIZE PAIN. Pain management for the patient with a moderate or major burn is achieved through the administration of IV narcotic agents, typically morphine sulfate. In the adult, small doses are given and repeated in 5- to 10-minute intervals until pain appears to be under control. The intramuscular and subcutaneous routes are *not* used during this phase because absorption from the soft tissues is unreliable during the emergent period, when peripheral perfusion is sporadic. The oral route for pain medication administration is not used owing to the likelihood of gastrointestinal dysfunction.

Clients presenting to emergency departments with minor burn injuries often are initially given small doses of IV narcotics (e.g., morphine sulfate). Oral analgesic agents are then prescribed for outpatient use.

WOUND CARE

STOP THE BURNING PROCESS. All burn wound care begins at the scene of the injury. Flame and scald burns should be cooled by submerging small burns in cool water until the sensation of burning stops. Major burn victims should have an initial "wet down" at the scene to stop the burning process, but not be submerged in water. Smoldering clothing should be carefully removed, and the client should be covered with a blanket to preserve body heat. Ideally, treatment of chemical burn wounds also begins at the scene of the injury. All clothing should be promptly removed; any chemical powder should be brushed off the skin. Wet chemical burns should be irrigated continuously with copious amounts of water,[13] for at least 20 minutes. Neutralizing agents are not recommended because the neutralizing reaction causes heat, which results in further tissue damage.

For chemical eye injuries, irrigate the eyes with a gentle stream of normal saline, flushing both the injured eye and the conjunctiva. It is recommended to irrigate the eyes from the inner canthus outward, to avoid washing any chemicals down the tear duct or toward the other eye.

Electrical burn care also includes stopping the burning process. It is important to remember to shut off any power source before approaching the victim. Early care is directed at assessment of the entire person, owing to the potential path of the electricity through the body (e.g., dysrhythmias, fractures).

IMMEDIATE CARE. If transfer to a burn center will be accomplished within 12 hours of injury, wound care should consist of covering the wound with sterile towels and placing clean dry sheets and blankets over the client. Unless transport time to the receiving medical facility is prolonged, debridement and application of topical antimicrobial agents are unnecessary. Definitive wound care begins following inpatient admission to the hospital.[30]

Wound care for burns consists of cleansing, debridement, removal of any damaging agents (e.g., chemicals, tar), and application of an appropriate topical agent and a dressing. Burn wounds should be washed with a mild soap and rinsed thoroughly with warm water.[4] Loose, nonviable tissue should be carefully trimmed away, and any hair should be shaved to within a 1-inch margin around the burn wound.[12]

The removal of tar or asphalt is easily accomplished with the use of a citrus-petroleum product such as Medi-

sol (Orange-Sol, Inc. Chandler, Ariz.) or with mineral oil and a petroleum-based antibiotic ointment such as bacitracin or polymyxin-neomycin-bacitracin (Neosporin).

Clients with minor burns are generally taught wound care and discharged home with instructions to continue wound care twice daily and return to the outpatient clinic or their private physician for follow-up assessment and care.

PREVENT TETANUS. Burns, even minor ones, are tetanus-prone wounds. The current protocol for tetanus immunization in clients with minor burns is the same as in clients with any other type of trauma.[54] Clients who have been previously immunized against tetanus, but not within the past 5 years, should receive a tetanus toxoid booster. For clients who have not been immunized, tetanus immune globulin (a passive immunizing agent) and the first of a series of active immunizations with tetanus toxoid should be administered.

PREVENT TISSUE ISCHEMIA

Circumferential burns of the extremities may compromise circulation in the affected limb.[31] Elevating injured extremities above the level of the heart and active exercise help to reduce dependent edema formation. However, circulatory compromise may still occur. Therefore, frequent assessment of distal extremity perfusion is necessary. Doppler flowmeter assessment of the palmar arch vessels (for the upper extremity) and the posterior tibial artery (for the lower extremity) provides the most precise indication of peripheral perfusion and should be performed regularly during the resuscitation period. The absence of flow or the progressive diminution of the Doppler flowmeter signal intensity is an indication that perfusion is impaired.

An escharotomy is the appropriate treatment for circulatory compromise due to constricting, circumferential burns.[18, 49] A midlateral or midmedial incision of the involved extremity is made from the most proximal to the most distal extent of the full-thickness burn. The depth of the incision is limited to the eschar. It is generally performed at the bedside without local or general anesthesia, because full-thickness burns are insensate. However, viable tissue beneath the escharotomy may bleed if cut, and then the client may feel pain. Bleeding can be controlled with pressure, suture ligation, or electrocautery. Pain control is achieved with IV narcotic administration. After escharotomy, the burn wound can be dressed with topical antimicrobial creams and gauze dressings.

If adequate tissue perfusion does not return following escharotomy, a fasciotomy may be necessary. This procedure, in which the fascia is incised, is performed in the operating room with the client under general anesthesia. A fasciotomy is usually necessary only in injuries caused by high-voltage electricity or those with concomitant crush injury (Fig. 50–10).

TRANSPORT TO A BURN FACILITY

Consideration of transfer to a specialized burn care facility is appropriate for all clients with major burn injuries (see Table 50–2). Prompt contact with the receiving burn center is important to facilitate a smooth transfer. All copies of medical records, which should include all fluids and medications given, hourly urine output values, and vital signs, must accompany the client.[20] The client's burn

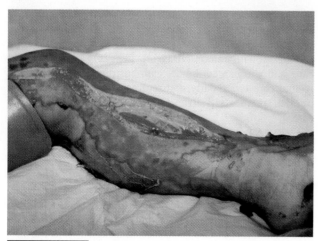

FIGURE 50–10 Escharotomy. Incision is made through the constricting burn eschar to permit expansion of the underlying subcutaneous tissues as edema forms.

wounds should simply be covered with a sterile sheet and blankets. The burn center will perform a complete assessment of the wounds; therefore, it is best if topical care has not been initiated.

■ Nursing Management of the Medical Client in the Emergent Phase of Burn Care

ASSESSMENT

Because the body's immediate physiologic responses to burn injury can either be life-threatening or lead to significant morbidity, prudent nursing assessment during the emergent phase of burn injury is crucial.

DIAGNOSIS, OUTCOMES, INTERVENTIONS

Impaired Gas Exchange. Effective gas exchange may become impaired when clients have experienced smoke inhalation because of tracheobronchial swelling, the presence of carbonaceous debris in the airway, or CO poisoning.

Outcomes. Adequate gas exchange will be evidenced by a PaO_2 of greater than 90 mm Hg; oxygen saturation (SaO_2) of greater than 95%, arterial partial pressure of carbon dioxide ($PaCO_2$) of 35 to 45 mm Hg; respiratory rate of 16 to 24 breaths/min with a normal pattern and depth; and clear bilateral breath sounds.

Interventions. The client must be frequently assessed for signs of respiratory distress such as restlessness, confusion, labored breathing, tachypnea, dyspnea, diminished or adventitious breath sounds, tachycardia, decrease in PaO_2 and SaO_2, and cyanosis. Monitor SaO_2 continuously in clients with major burns during the emergent phase of burn injury. Draw and monitor arterial blood gas and COHb levels per physician order. Report changes in the client's condition immediately.

Instruct the client on the use of the incentive spirometer to encourage deep breathing every 2 hours. Elevate the head of the bed to facilitate lung expansion and to reduce facial edema.

Ineffective Airway Clearance. Because of the occurrence of airway epidermal sloughing, increase in secretions, inflammation and swelling of the nasopharyngeal mucous membranes from smoke irritation, and depressed ciliary action from inhalation injury, the client becomes at risk for ineffective airway clearance.

Outcomes. Clients will have an effective airway clearance, as evidenced by clear bilateral breath sounds, clear to white pulmonary secretions, effective mobilization of pulmonary secretions, and unlabored respiration with a respiratory rate of 16 to 24 breaths/min.

Interventions. A thorough pulmonary assessment should be performed every 1 to 2 hours during the first 24 hours after injury, and every 2 to 4 hours the second 24 hours after injury, evaluating breath sounds, rate and depth of respirations, and level of consciousness. Be alert to a declining respiratory status as evidenced by crackles, rhonchi, stridor, labored breathing, dyspnea, tachypnea, restlessness, or a decreasing level of consciousness. Report significant findings promptly. Have the client turn, cough, and deep-breathe every 1 to 2 hours for 24 hours and then every 2 to 4 hours. Place an oral suctioning device within the client's reach for independent use. Perform endotracheal or nasotracheal suction as needed. Assess and document the character and amount of secretions.

Fluid Volume Deficit. The client with a major burn injury is at risk for hypovolemia, most significantly during the first 36 hours after burn injury. The fluid volume deficit is directly related to the increased capillary leakage and fluid shift from the intravascular to the interstitial space after the burn insult.

Outcomes. The client will have improved fluid balance, as evidenced by a urine output of 0.5 to 1.0 ml/kg/hr, clear sensorium, pulse rate less than 120 beats per minute (BPM), absence of dysrhythmias, adequate amplitude of peripheral pulses (2+ or better) and blood pressure within the expected range for age and medical history.

Interventions. Assess the client for signs of hypovolemia every hour for 36 hours, including tachycardia, decreased blood pressure, decreased amplitude of peripheral pulses, urine output of less than 0.5 ml/kg/hr, thirst, and dry mucous membranes. Report significant findings.

Carefully monitor and document intake and output, administering fluid therapy as prescribed; titrate the infusion every hour to maintain urine output between 0.5 and 1.0 ml/kg/hr. Large volumes of fluid may be required to produce adequate urine volumes.

Monitor serum electrolyte and hematocrit values. Hyponatremia, hyperkalemia, and elevated hematocrit levels are common findings during the emergent phase. As the circulation is restored, levels should return to normal values.

Altered Tissue Perfusion: Renal. Clients who have suffered deep burn and tissue injury, such as in electrical injury or crush injuries, and those in whom adequate fluid resuscitation has not been achieved are at risk for renal failure. Myoglobin and hemoglobin released from the damaged muscles and red blood cells that precipitate in the renal tubules can create acute tubular necrosis.

Outcomes. The client with evidence of deep tissue injury will maintain a urinary output of 75 to 100 ml/hr, or 1 ml/kg/hr, or higher, until the pigment load has decreased.

Interventions. Monitor and document hourly output and urine color. A dark brown or red color is indicative of the presence of hemochromagens. Send urine samples for myoglobin or hemoglobin assay per physician order to provide quantitative information for documentation of the client's condition. Ensure that the catheter is patent, as the tubing may become plugged with hemochromagens. Administer IV fluids per physician orders. Hemochromagens must be flushed from the body; therefore, the rate of fluid administration is based on maintaining an hourly urine output of 1 ml/kg/hr or greater.

Altered Tissue Perfusion: Peripheral.
The client may exhibit altered peripheral tissue perfusion as a result of constricting circumferential burns.

Outcomes. The client will have adequate peripheral perfusion, as evidenced by the presence of pulses on palpation or Doppler flowmeter assessment, capillary refill time for unburned skin of less than 2 seconds, absence of numbness or tingling, and absence of increased pain with active ROM exercises.

Interventions. Remove all constricting jewelry and clothing, because constricting items may compromise circulation as edema formation ensues. Limit the use of the blood pressure cuff on the affected extremity, as the cuff can reduce arterial inflow and venous return. Elevate the burned extremity above the level of the heart to promote venous return and to prevent excessive dependent edema formation.

Monitor arterial pulses by palpation or with the use of an ultrasonic flow detector (Doppler flowmeter) hourly for up to 72 hours after burn injury. Pulses will diminish with circulation impairments. Assess capillary refill of unburned skin on the affected extremity; capillary refill will be prolonged with impaired circulation. Encourage ROM exercises, and assess the level of pain associated with efforts. Increasing pain with movement is a result of tissue ischemia. When pain is not present, increased movement of the affected area will promote venous return and assist in decreasing edema.

If tissue perfusion is threatened, anticipate and prepare the client for an escharotomy. Once the underlying tissue edema has exceeded the expansion ability of the burned skin, an escharotomy will be needed to restore perfusion. After the procedure is complete, recheck for restoration of circulation by assessing pulses, color, movement, and sensation of the affected extremity. Anticipate some bleeding after escharotomy, as the tissue beneath the eschar bleeds. Bleeding can be controlled by electrocautery or suturing by the physician. Continue to observe and assess the extremity after the procedure.

Risk for Infection.
The burn-injured client faces an increased risk for infection related to inadequate primary and secondary defenses resulting from traumatized tissue, bacterial proliferation in burn wounds, and an immunocompromised status.

Outcomes. The client will remain free from significant burn wound microbial invasion, as evidenced by quantitative wound cultures containing less than 100,000 colony-forming units (CFUs)/g. In addition, core body temperature will be maintained between 99.6° and 101.0° F (37.5° C to 38.3° C); there will be no swelling, redness, or purulence present at IV line insertion sites; and results of blood, urine, and sputum cultures will be negative.

Interventions. Tetanus prophylaxis should be administered per physician order, as the anaerobic environment beneath eschar is ideal for tetanus organism growth. Intramuscular or IV antibiotic therapy is not used because the area of potential infection is avascular and would not be reached by antibiotics. Antimicrobial agents are used to deter the growth of bacteria on the surface of the wound.

It is essential to maintain infection control techniques at all times during the client's hospitalization to prevent cross-contamination. Ensure aseptic technique when administering care to burned areas and performing invasive techniques. Enforce strict hand-washing, and instruct family members or significant others on infection control measures.

When wound care is performed, it is important to debride the wound of loose, nonviable tissue, which serves as a medium for bacterial growth. Hair within and around a wound should be shaved (with the exception of eyebrows and eyelashes), as hair is contaminated and also prevents adherence of the burn cream. Apply a topical therapeutic agent (an antimicrobial) and loose gauze dressings.

Impaired Physical Mobility.
The client's mobility during the emergent phase of burn injury is impaired by tissue edema, pain, and dressings.

Outcomes. The outcomes related to physical mobility are measured throughout the hospitalization and recovery process. The long-term outcome goal is return of the client to maximum independence in performance of activities of daily living (ADL) with minimum disability and disfigurement. Although this outcome will be demonstrated long after the emergent phase, it is important to initiate care on the day of admission and to follow through continually throughout hospitalization.

Interventions. Encourage the client to participate in self-care and ROM exercises at the earliest time possible. The time of the emergency department visit is not too soon to help motivate the client and to overcome fear and dependence related to the injury. Additionally, during early postinjury fluid shifts, increasing movement helps to improve circulation and decrease edema. Consult with occupational and physical therapists for initial assessment and follow-up care throughout the hospitalization.

Ineffective Family Coping: Compromised.
Because of the urgent and critical nature of the injury, the client and family are at risk for ineffective coping skills.

Outcomes. Family members and significant others will have accurate information about the immediate status of the client, as evidenced by their ability to verbalize an understanding of the client's injury and treatment goals. Support services will be provided as needed.

Interventions. It is important to prepare family members or significant others for their first visit with the client after injury. Provide a simple explanation of procedures and equipment, communicate the extent of the burn, and describe changes in the client's appearance. For impending client transfer, provide family members or significant others with support services to assist with travel arrangements. Providing support at this time will help to reduce their anxiety during the client's transfer. Families of clients remaining in the facility should be provided with information that meets their basic needs (e.g., information about lodging, location of cafeteria, parking).

ACUTE PHASE

The acute phase of recovery following a major burn begins when the patient is hemodynamically stable, capillary integrity is restored, and diuresis has begun. This is generally 48 to 72 hours after the time of injury. Many of the same principles of care outlined for the emergent phase apply to the acute phase; however, more emphasis is placed on restorative therapies. The acute phase continues until wound closure is achieved.

▰ Medical Management in the Acute Phase of Burn Injury

PREVENT INFECTION

Infection control is a major component of burn management. An infection control policy is necessary for managing burn-injured clients to control the transmission of microorganisms that can lead to infection or colonization.[23, 75] Universal precautions should be followed in caring for all clients with burn injuries; however, specific infection control practices and isolation techniques exist for all burn centers. These practices include the use of gloves, caps, masks, shoe covers, scrub clothes, and plastic aprons. Strict hand-washing is stressed to reduce the incidence of cross-contamination between clients and is the single most important means of preventing the spread of infection. Staff and visitors are generally prevented from client contact if they have any skin, gastrointestinal, or respiratory tract infections. See Box 50–2 for basic infection control strategies. All visitors as well as healthcare providers from other departments should be oriented to established infection control practices before their first contact with the burn-injured client.

PROVIDE METABOLIC SUPPORT

Maintenance of adequate nutrition during the acute phase of burn care is essential in promoting wound healing and preventing infection.[36, 78] Basal metabolic rates may be 40% to 100% higher than normal levels, depending on the extent, of the burn. This response is thought to be the

---

TABLE 50–4	ENERGY CALCULATION FORMULAS USED FOR THE BURN-INJURED ADULT
Formula/Author Name	**Formula for Daily Caloric Expenditure Estimate**
Curreri	(25 kcal/kg body weight) + (40 kcal × % TBSA burn)
Modified Harris-Benedict	RMR × activity factor × injury factor
U.S. Army Institute of Surgical Research	[Age- and gender-specific BMR × (0.89142 + 0.01335 × % TBSA burn) × m² × 24 × activity factor]

TBSA, total body surface area; RMR, resting metabolic rate; BMR, basal metabolic rate.

---

result of a resetting of the homeostatic "thermostat" of the hypothalamic-pituitary-adrenal axis, leading to an increase in heat production. Metabolic rates decrease as wound coverage is achieved.

Aggressive nutritional support is required to meet the increased energy requirements necessary to promote healing and to prevent the untoward effects of catabolism.[22, 62] Several different formulas (Table 50–4) are currently used to estimate energy requirements by factoring different indices: weight, gender, age, extent of burn, and amount of activity. Additional support is generally indicated for the burn-injured client with any of the following: 30% or greater TBSA burn, clinical course requiring multiple operations, need for mechanical ventilatory support, compromised mental status, and poor preinjury nutritional state. Methods for delivering nutritional support include oral intake, enteral tube feedings, peripheral parenteral nutrition, and total parenteral nutrition, which may be used alone or in combination. The preferred feeding route is oral or enteral[44]; however, the decision of how to best meet the client's nutritional needs should be individualized. Typically, parenteral nutrition is reserved for clients with a prolonged ileus or for those in whom enteral feedings fail to meet nutritional needs.[27]

MINIMIZE PAIN

Pain continues to be a significant problem throughout the client's hospitalization. During the acute phase of injury, an attempt is made to find the right combination of medications and interventions to minimize the discomfort and pain associated with the injury. As in the emergent phase, the most common approach to pain control is with the use of pharmacologic agents. However, in addition to the narcotics used during the emergent phase, other modalities may be utilized during the acute phase of burn injury to help alleviate the client's pain. Patient-controlled analgesia devices, inhalation analgesics such as nitrous oxide, oral analgesic "pain cocktails," and narcotic agonist-antagonist agents may be beneficial during the acute phase of burn injury.[32, 42] Nonsteroidal anti-inflammatory agents (NSAIDs) are also prescribed for the treatment of mild to moderate pain. When NSAIDs are used, extra precautions must be taken to prevent gastric ulceration.

Nonpharmacologic modalities used to treat burn-related

BOX 50–2 Basic Principles of Infection Control

1. Thorough hand-washing should be done before and after each contact with the burn-injured client.
2. Protective garb (aprons or gowns) should be donned before each contact and promptly discarded after leaving the bedside or room.
3. Gloves should be changed when they become contaminated with secretions or fluids from one anatomic site before contact with another site.
4. Equipment, materials, and surfaces are considered contaminated for the individual client and should be properly decontaminated before use with another client.

From Weber, J. M., & Tompkins, D. M. (1993). Improving survival: Infection control and burns. *AACN Clinical Issues in Critical Care Nursing* 4(2), 418–419.

pain include hypnosis, guided imagery, art and play therapy, relaxation techniques, distraction, biofeedback, and music therapy. These modalities have been found to be effective in decreasing anxiety, thereby decreasing the perception of pain. They are often used as adjunctive therapies to the pharmacologic treatment of burn pain.[43]

PROVIDE WOUND CARE

Care of the burn wound is ultimately aimed at promoting wound healing. Daily wound care involves cleansing, debridement of eschar (devitalized tissue), and dressing of the wound.[12]

WOUND CLEANSING. The practice of hydrotherapy remains a mainstay of burn treatment plans for cleansing the wounds.[66] This is accomplished by immersion, showering, or spraying (Fig. 50–11). A hydrotherapy session of 30 minutes or less is optimal for clients with acute burns. Longer time periods may increase sodium loss (water is hypotonic) through the burn wound and may promote heat loss, pain, and stress. During hydrotherapy, the wounds are gently washed using any one of a variety of solutions. Care should be taken to minimize bleeding and to maintain body temperature during this procedure. To prevent cross contamination between clients, single-use plastic hydrotherapy tub liners are available. Clients excluded from hydrotherapy are generally those who are hemodynamically unstable and those with new skin grafts. If hydrotherapy is not used, wounds are washed and rinsed while the client is in bed, before the application of antimicrobial agents.

DEBRIDEMENT. Burn wound debridement involves the removal of the eschar. This serves to promote wound healing by preventing bacterial proliferation in and under the eschar.[75] Debridement of the burn wound is accomplished through mechanical, enzymatic, or surgical means.

Mechanical debridement can be accomplished with careful use of scissors and forceps to lift and trim away loose eschar. Hydrotherapy softens and loosens eschar so that it is more easily removed. Wet-to-dry dressing

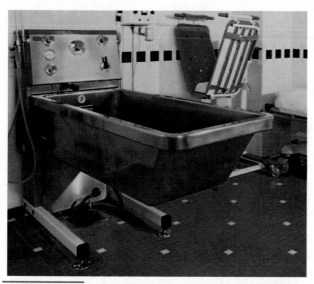

FIGURE 50–11 A low-boy whirlpool tank is used for immersion hydrotherapy treatment of burn wounds. (Courtesy of Shriners Hospitals for Children of Northern California.)

changes are another effective means of mechanical debridement. Coarse gauze dressings are saturated with a prescribed solution, wrung out until the dressing is slightly moist, and applied to the wound. The dressing is left in place to dry. Typically 6 to 8 hours later the gauze is carefully removed from the wound, mechanically lifting drainage, exudate, and loose necrotic tissue that has dried on to the gauze. Mechanical debridement of the burn wound can be extremely painful; therefore, effective pain management is paramount.

Enzymatic debridement involves the application of commercially prepared proteolytic and fibrinolytic topical enzymes to the burn wound, which facilitates eschar removal. These agents require a moist environment to be effective and are applied directly to the burn wound. Enzymatic debridement is not widely practiced, as several serious side effects are associated with use of these agents.[47] As the enzyme digests necrotic tissue, it also opens up thrombosed blood vessels. This causes some oozing of blood from the blood vessels and creates a site for bacteria to enter the bloodstream. Bacteremia, pain, and bleeding can occur; therefore, if enzymatic debridement is used, the client should be assessed for complications continuously throughout the course of treatment. The use of enzymatic debridement agents is contraindicated for wounds communicating with major body cavities, and for wounds with exposed nerves or nervous tissue.

Surgical debridement of the burn wound involves excision of the eschar and coverage of the wound. Early surgical excision begins during the first week after injury, once the client is hemodynamically stable. Advantages of early excision include early mobilization, reduction of pain (which is otherwise experienced with repeated dressing changes), early wound closure (which reduces the potential for wound infection), and reduced length of hospitalization.[33, 76] A disadvantage of early excision is the risk of excising viable tissue that may heal with time.

Two techniques of surgical debridement are currently used.[50] In *tangential* excision, very thin layers of eschar are sequentially shaved until viable tissue is reached. *Fascial* excision involves removing the burn tissue and underlying fat down to fascia. This technique is frequently used for debridement of very deep burns.

TOPICAL ANTIMICROBIAL TREATMENT. Deep partial-thickness or full-thickness burn wounds are treated initially with topical antimicrobial agents.[73] These agents are applied once or twice daily following cleansing, debridement, and inspection of the wound. The nurse assesses for eschar separation, the presence of granulation tissue or reepithelialization, and signs of infection. The most commonly used topical antimicrobial agents are listed in Table 50–5. Although no single agent is used universally, many burn centers choose silver sulfadiazine cream as the initial topical agent.[31]

Burn wounds are treated using either an open or a closed dressing technique. For the *open method,* the antimicrobial cream is applied with a gloved hand (Fig. 50–12) and the wound is left open to the air without gauze dressings. The cream is reapplied as needed, although formal reapplication is necessary every 12 hours in keeping with the duration of activity of the agent. The

| TABLE 50–5 | TOPICAL ANTIMICROBIAL AGENTS USED IN BURN CARE | | | |

Agent	Antimicrobial Spectrum	Application	Side Effects	Nursing Considerations
WATER-BASED CREAMS				
1% silver sulfadiazine	Broad spectrum; effective against some fungi and yeast	2× daily, 1/16-inch thickness Gauze dressing not required	Transient leukopenia typically appearing after 2 or 3 days of treatment Macular rash	Do not store in warm environment (e.g., warm client room)
Mafenide acetate	Broad spectrum; little antifungal activity	2× daily, 1/16-inch thickness Gauze dressing not required	Hyperchloremic metabolic acidosis from bicarbonate diuresis due to the inhibition of carbonic anhydrase Pain/burning sensation on application to superficial burns Maculopapular rash	Assess for side effects Assess adequacy of pain management; if pain and discomfort continue, consider other topical treatments Use cautiously in clients with acute renal failure
SOLUTIONS				
5% mafenide acetate	Broad spectrum	Gauze dressing required, moistened with solution for application to the wound	Pain on application Pruritus Rash Fungal colonization	Assess for side effects Assess adequacy of pain management
0.5% silver nitrate	Broad spectrum; effective against *Candida* species	Multiple layers of gauze dressing required, moistened with solution for application to the wound	Hyponatremia Hypochloremia Hypokalemia Hypocalcemia	Check serum electrolytes daily Penetrates eschar poorly Remoisten dressings every 2 hours to avoid wound desiccation Protect the environment; stains everything a blackish-brown color
PETROLEUM-BASED OINTMENTS				
Polymyxin B	Gram-negative organisms	Apply as needed in a thin layer; gauze dressing not used unless clothing protection is needed	Hypersensitivity (rash)	Assess for side effects
Neomycin sulfate	Predominantly gram-negative organisms		Overgrowth of nonsusceptible organisms including fungi	
Bacitracin	Predominantly gram-positive organisms			

advantages of the open method include increased visualization of the wound, greater freedom for mobility and joint motion, and simplicity in wound care. The disadvantages include an increased chance of hypothermia from exposure.

In the *closed method* of wound care, gauze dressing is impregnated with antimicrobial cream and applied to the wound. To prevent circulatory compromise in extremity burns, the gauze should be wrapped from the most distal portion of the extremity in a proximal direction. The advantages of the closed method are decreases in evaporative fluid and heat loss from the wound surface. In addition, gauze dressings may aid in debridement. The disadvantages of gauze dressings are mobility limitations and a potential decrease in effectiveness of ROM exer-

cises. Wound assessment is also limited to the times at which dressing changes are performed.

Temporary wound coverings (skin substitutes) are frequently used as a kind of wound "dressing." Table 50–6 outlines the most common biologic, biosynthetic, and synthetic wound coverings available. These products are temporary wound coverings, and each has specific indications.[25, 63, 67] The character of the wound (depth of injury, amount of exudate, location of the wound on the body, and phase of recovery) and treatment goals are considered in choosing the most appropriate wound covering.

MAXIMIZE FUNCTION. Maintenance of optimal physical functioning in the client with a burn injury is a challenge for the entire team. Nurses work closely with occupational and physical therapists to identify the reha-

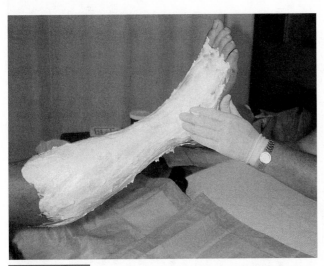

FIGURE 50–12 Silver sulfadiazine, a common antimicrobial cream used in burn care, is applied to the burn wound using a sterile, gloved hand. (Courtesy of the University of Washington Burn Center, Harborview Medical Center, Seattle.)

bilitative needs of the burn-injured client. An individualized program of splinting, positioning, exercise, ambulation, performance of ADL, and pressure therapy should be implemented in the acute phase of recovery to maximize functional recovery and cosmetic outcome. Therapeutic goals at this stage in recovery are to prevent early contracture formation and to maintain soft tissue length.

Wound contracture and hypertrophic scarring are two major problems for the burn-injured client.[72] Wound contractures are typically more severe with extensive burns. Areas seemingly predisposed to contracture are the hands, head and neck, and axilla.[71] Measures used to prevent and treat wound contractures include therapeutic positioning, ROM exercises, splinting, and client/family education.

Table 50–7 lists corrective and therapeutic techniques for positioning clients with specific areas of burn injury during periods of inactivity or immobilization. Allowing the burn-injured client to assume a position of comfort most often contributes to contracture formation. Therefore, proper positioning, both in and out of bed, should be maintained for the burn-injured client. These techniques place affected body parts in positions that are in opposition to positions of potential contracture or deformity. The natural tendency with healing and immobility is for muscles and joints to contract into a shortened, flexed position. Thus, for example, to reduce the risk of neck contractures, the use of pillows—which place the neck in flexion—is not allowed.

Active ROM exercises are prescribed early in the acute phase of recovery to promote resolution of edema and to maintain strength and joint function. In addition, ADL can be effective in maintaining function and ROM. Ambulation also maintains strength and ROM of the lower extremities and should begin as soon as the client is physiologically stable. Passive ROM and stretching exercises should be included as part of the daily treatment plan if the client is unable to perform active ROM exercises.

Splints are used to maintain proper joint position and to prevent or correct contractures.[28] Two types of splints are frequently used. A *static splint* immobilizes the joint. Static splints do not replace exercise and are frequently applied for periods of immobilization or during sleeping hours or are used for clients who cannot maintain proper positioning. In contrast, *dynamic splints* exercise the affected joint. Care must be taken to ensure that all splints fit properly and do not apply excessive pressure, which may lead to further tissue or nerve damage.[73]

PROVIDE PSYCHOLOGICAL SUPPORT

The longest period of adjustment occurs during the acute phase. The burn-injured adult may demonstrate a variety of emotional and psychological responses. Anxiety and fearfulness related to potential disfigurement and perceived changes in role and identity plague the client during this time period. Depression, withdrawal, and regression may result.[7]

The client may begin discussing the burn injury or accident, recounting significant events and searching for the meaning of what has happened.[1] Allowing the expression of these worries and validating that they are "normal" are essential in providing support. Staff members need to actively listen and to allow the client to talk about the accident. Detailed and repetitious recounting of the injury is useful in desensitizing clients to the horror of what has happened and in decreasing nightmares.[7]

Clients who have little information about specific treatment procedures, potential associated discomfort or pain, and available resources or options for pain management typically react with anxiety and a heightened pain response. Providing the client with information about what will occur during a particular procedure or what is expected over the course of recovery is a concept known as providing preparatory information. This technique is a psychologically based method that has proved successful in reducing pain and anxiety during certain procedures.[1, 7] To enhance the client's sense of personal control, teaching should include education about various coping mechanisms and the use of nonpharmacologic methods for pain control.

Involving clients in their own care helps them to feel some control over the situation at hand. Clients can be encouraged to participate in wound care (e.g., bathing, simple debridement, dressing application) and physical therapy (e.g., active versus passive ROM exercises, application of splints and pressure garments). These interventions have been found to be effective in supporting the client's psychological needs.[43]

■ Nursing Management of the Medical Patient in the Acute Phase of Burn Injury

Impaired Gas Exchange. Note that the consequences of smoke inhalation may not be fully appreciated until the acute phase of burn care. The decreased ciliary action in the airways leads to a high risk for infection (which usually is not manifested until day 3 or 4 after the burn injury); that is demonstrated first by tracheobronchitis and followed by bronchopneumonia.

Outcomes. The client will have improved gas exchange, as evidenced by unlabored respirations, a respiratory rate of 16 to 24 breaths/min, PaO_2 of greater than 90

TABLE 50–6　TEMPORARY WOUND COVERINGS USED IN BURN CARE

Category/Examples	Description	Indications	Nursing Considerations
Biologic			
Amnion	Amniotic membranes collected from human placentas	To protect partial-thickness burns	Cover dressing is changed every 48 hours with amnion
Allograft homograft	Donated human cadaver skin harvested within 24 hours after death	To protect granulation tissue prior to autograft application To debride exudative wounds To cover excised wounds and test for receptivity prior to autograft application To cover and protect meshed autografts	Observe for wound exudate and signs of infection that may be indicative of a wound infection beneath the allograft/xenograft
Xenograft heterograft	Porcine skin is harvested after slaughter, then cryopreserved or lyophilized for storage	To promote healing of clean, superficial partial-thickness wounds	Xenograft over granulation tissue is changed every 2–5 days For superficial wounds, ensure that the wound is clean and well rinsed; apply xenograft with slight overlapping of edges to allow for shrinkage; trim away xenograft when skin beneath it has healed
Biosynthetic			
Biobrane (Bertek Pharmaceuticals, Morgantown, WV)	Nylon fabric bonded to a silicone rubber membrane containing collagenous porcine peptides	Donor site dressing Protective cover over meshed autografts To promote healing of clean superficial partial-thickness wounds	Secure to the surrounding intact skin by staples, skin closure strips, tape, or sutures and then wrap with a gauze dressing; this outer dressing can be removed by 48 hours to check for adherence of the Biobrane; once adherence has occurred, the tape, sutures, and staples can be removed; the Biobrane can then be left exposed to the air New and healing donor sites of the legs require support during ambulation; the figure eight elastic (Ace) bandage wrapping technique is recommended to minimize trauma to newly formed capillaries Assess for infection beneath the fabric and at wound periphery
Integra (Integra Life Sciences, Plainsboro, NJ)	Bilaminate substitute composed of collagen (dermal analog) and a Silastic covering (epidermal analog) The dermal analog is allowed to incorporate into the wound, becoming permanent	For application to excised wounds	The Silastic portion is removed after 2–3 days, providing a wound bed for placement of a very thin split-thickness skin graft Assess for infection Protect the site from mechanical shearing forces
Calcium alginates (Curasorb, Kendall Co, Mansfield, MA; Kalginate, DeRoyal Textiles, Camden, SC)	Dressing material derived from brown seaweeds (alginate) and calcium/sodium salts	Donor site dressing To promote healing of superficial partial-thickness wounds (contraindicated in full-thickness wounds)	To apply, irrigate wound with a physiologic solution, apply calcium alginate dressing to the wound, cover with an absorptive dressing The entire dressing should be changed when the outer dressing is saturated with drainage
Transparent films (Bioclusive, Johnson & Johnson, Arlington, TX; Op-Site, Smith & Nephew, Memphis, TN)	Hypoallergenic film dressing that is occlusive, waterproof, and permeable to moisture vapor	Donor site dressing To promote healing of clean, small, superficial partial-thickness wounds	Use a margin of intact skin around the entire wound or donor site to adequately secure the dressing Assess for pooling exudate; if significant exudate forms that threatens the integrity of the closed dressing, drain the exudate aseptically with a small gauge needle and syringe; seal hole with a film patch
Non-adhering gauze (Aquaphor gauze, Beiersdorf Inc. Norwalk, CT; Xeroform gauze, Sherwood Medical, St. Louis)	Fine-mesh gauze impregnated with ointment	Donor site dressing To cover meshed autografts To cover fragile, newly healed epithelium	Dressing material over donor site should remain intact until healed beneath (10–14 days) New and healing donor sites of the legs require support during ambulation; the figure eight (Ace) wrapping technique is recommended to minimize trauma to newly formed capillaries

TABLE 50–7	THERAPEUTIC POSITIONING FOR THE BURN-INJURED CLIENT	
Burned Area	**Therapeutic Position**	**Positioning Techniques**
Neck		
Anterior	Extension	No pillow Small towel roll beneath shoulders to promote neck extension
Circumferential	Neutral toward extension	No pillow
Posterior or asymmetrical	Neutral	No pillow
Shoulder/axilla	Arm abduction to 90–110 degrees	Splinting Arms positioned away from the body and supported on arm troughs
Elbow	Arm extension	Elbow splint Elbows positioned in extension with slight bend at the elbow (no more than 10 degrees of elbow flexion) Arms supported on arm troughs with the forearm in slight pronation
Hand		
Wrist	Wrist extension	Hand splint
MCP	MCP flexion at 90 degrees	Hand splint
PIP/DIP	PIP/DIP extension	Hand splint
Thumb	Thumb abduction	Hand splint with thumb abduction
Finger web spaces	Finger abduction	Web spacers of foam, silicone products, or custom-fitted pressure garments to decrease webbing formation
Hip	Hip extension	Supine with the head of bed flat and legs extended Trochanter roll to maintain neutral hip rotation (toes should be pointing toward the ceiling) Prone positioning
Knee	Knee extension	Supine with knees extended (toes should be pointing toward the ceiling) Prone positioning with feet extended over the end of the mattress Sitting in chair with legs extended and elevated Knee splint
Ankle	Neutral	Padded footboard Ankle positioning devices (avoid heel cord tightening)—provide heel protection to prevent pressure sore development

MCP, metacarpal interphalangeal joint(s); PIP/DIP, proximal/distal interphalangeal joint(s).

mm Hg, PaCO$_2$ of 35 to 45 mm Hg, SaO$_2$ greater than 95%, and clear bilateral breath sounds.

Interventions. Interventions continue unchanged from the emergent phase of injury. Comprehensive respiratory assessment and preventive pulmonary toilet should be performed every 2 hours.

Ineffective Airway Clearance. Upper airway and facial edema caused by heat-induced tissue and mucosal damage begins to resolve between 2 and 4 days after injury with superficial burns. Full-thickness injuries, however, resolve more slowly, making ineffective airway clearance a problem that may last well into the acute phase of treatment.

Outcomes. The client will have effective airway clearance, as evidenced by clear bilateral breath sounds, clear to white pulmonary secretions, effective mobilization of pulmonary secretions, and unlabored breathing.

Interventions. Continue interventions begun in the emergent phase of treatment. Pulmonary toilet including turning/coughing/deep breathing, use of an incentive spirometer every 2 to 4 hours while the client is awake, and endotracheal suctioning as needed will facilitate clearance of secretions and sputum. Leave an oral suctioning device within the client's reach for independent use.

Hypothermia. Clients remain at risk for loss of body heat through burn injuries until wound closure is complete. During dressing changes, clients are especially at risk for becoming hypothermic.

Outcomes. The client will maintain a core body temperature between 99.6° and 101.0° F (37.5° and 38.3° C).

Interventions. To help prevent the loss of heat from open wounds that occurs as a result of evaporation, limit hydrotherapy treatment sessions to 30 minutes or less with water temperatures of 98° to 102° F (36.6° C to 38.8° C). Cover the client with sterile sheets after the hydrotherapy session, exposing only limited areas of body surface during topical agent–dressing application. Provide heat lamps or heat shields and increase the ambient temperature in the treatment room and/or in the client's room if the client exhibits subnormal temperatures.

Risk for Infection. During the acute phase of injury, infection remains an ongoing risk owing to inadequate primary and secondary defenses secondary to traumatized tissue, bacterial proliferation in the burn wound, presence of invasive lines or urinary catheters, and an immunocompromised status.[24]

Outcomes. The client will have no significant burn wound microbial invasion, as evidenced by quantitative wound cultures containing less than 100,000 CFUs/g. In addition, the client will maintain core body temperature at 99.6° to 101° F; will demonstrate evidence of no swelling, redness, or purulence at invasive line insertion sites; and will have negative results on blood, urine, and sputum cultures.

Interventions. Continue to follow infection control policy for burn-injured clients in an effort to prevent cross-contamination. Assess for clinical signs of infection in the burn wound: discoloration of wounds (e.g., brown, black, or hemorrhagic); drainage; odor; delayed healing; or spongy eschar. As in the emergent phase, provide meticulous wound care in an aseptic fashion, cleaning and rinsing the wound, and debriding loose nonviable tissue to discourage bacterial growth. Apply a topical antimicrobial agent to the wound to decrease the risk for local wound infection. Continue to shave or cut body hair around wound margins until wound closure.

Observe for clinical indicators of sepsis: headache, chills, anorexia, nausea, changes in vital signs, hyperglycemia and glycosuria, paralytic ileus, and confusion, restlessness, or hallucinations. Assess for signs of infection at the catheter insertion site. Obtain cultures per physician order, and administer antibiotics and antipyretics as prescribed.

Impaired Tissue Integrity. Remember that stress ulcers can occur at any time after a burn injury. The assessment and preventive treatment started in the emergent phase of injury should continue until wound coverage is completed.[40]

Outcomes. The client will exhibit no signs of gastrointestinal bleeding and will maintain gastric pH above 5.

Interventions. Monitor and document gastric pH values and heme content every 2 hours while the client's nasogastric tube is in place. Administer antacids and/or H_2 blockers per physician order to reduce the gastric acid content, as high acid levels may lead to bleeding. Monitor stools for occult blood.

Altered Nutrition: Less Than Body Requirements. The burn-injured client must maintain adequate protein and caloric intake to meet metabolic demands for wound healing.

Outcomes. The client will have adequate nutrition, as evidenced by maintenance of 85% to 90% of preburn weight and healing of burn wounds, donor sites, and skin grafts.

Interventions. Caloric needs are based upon preburn weight. Obtain a daily weight to assess whether caloric needs are being met and to provide documentation for staff to follow trends. Assess eating habits and patterns, and identify food preferences and food allergies. Order meals high in calories and proteins. Encourage family members or significant others to bring favorite foods from home. Provide nutritious supplements between meals.

Document daily caloric intake, and consult with the dietitian to perform a nutritional assessment. Consider other methods to meet caloric needs such as tube feeding or total parenteral feeding, as oral feeding may not provide adequate calories for healing.

Performing oral hygiene during each nursing shift and as needed helps to prevent stomatitis and enhance appetite. Provide an a esthetically pleasing environment, which is conducive to eating. Schedule treatments to provide for uninterrupted meal times. Allow a period of rest before meal times if the client has endured a painful procedure or treatment, because pain will decrease appetite.

Pain. The client can be expected to experience a significant amount of pain during the acute burn phase. The pain experienced during this phase of recovery is directly associated with the burn wound and donor sites, wound care procedures, and ROM exercises.

Outcomes. The client will verbalize a level of acceptable pain control.

Interventions. Continue to frequently assess for pain, and administer appropriate narcotic and anxiolytics. Time the administration of medications so that the client receives the benefit of the drug's peak performance during painful procedures, and evaluate the effectiveness of interventions as initiated during the emergent burn phase.

During the acute phase, nonpharmacologic interventions should be initiated to enhance medication effects and to assist in controlling pain. Explore the benefits of relaxation techniques, guided imagery, music therapy, distraction, and biofeedback.

Impaired Physical Mobility. Impaired physical mobility during the acute phase of burn treatment is related to pain, the presence of dressings and splints, surgical procedures, and wound contractures.

Outcomes. The client will maintain soft tissue length, as evidenced by maintaining ROM without signs of early contracture formation.

Interventions. The main interventions during the acute phase of injury are splinting, positioning, and ROM exercises. Collaboration with physical and occupational therapists is essential for guidance in an individualized program for each client.

Optimal positioning of the client involves continuing use of anticontracture positions. Maintaining burned areas in a position of physiologic function by either splinting or positioning will help to prevent or reduce contracture development.

Encourage the client to participate in ADL, to ambulate, and to spend time sitting up in a chair. These activities will not only improve mobility but also assist in moving the client toward independence.

Self-Esteem Disturbance. During the acute burn phase, the client recognizes the extent of injury and realizes that his or her body is changed forever. Depression, grief, fear, and anxiety confront the client.

Outcomes. The client will acknowledge body changes and demonstrate movement toward incorporating these changes into the self-concept. The client will not exhibit maladaptive responses such as severe depression.

Interventions. The client should be expected to experience emotional lability in progress through recovery. Staff members should provide an accepting atmosphere for the client, although the client should be assisted to exercise control over any destructive behaviors. Family members or significant others should be involved in care as much as possible to demonstrate continued support for the client. Staff members should be available to provide information about the appearance of burns and grafts and to explain changes that can be expected over time (up to 1 year). Providing information helps to reduce misconceptions and can give hope that the painful procedures can produce good results.

Ineffective Family Coping Skills. Recognize that families often imagine that the survival of the family unit is threatened following a member's injury. Normal coping mechanisms become overwhelmed.

Outcomes. Family members will demonstrate coping strategies, as evidenced by verbalizing realistic expectations for client outcomes, expressing knowledge of the goals of treatment regimen, interacting appropriately with the client, and demonstrating decreased emotional stress.

Interventions. Once beyond the emergent phase, it will be important to provide the family members or significant others with information about what to expect for the burn-injured client in the future. It is helpful to provide families with daily updates regarding changes in the client's condition. This assists in maintaining realistic perceptions of the client's progress. Assist the family in finding ways to nurture the client and to participate in some aspects of care. These measures not only assure the client of the family's love and acceptance but also allow family members or significant others to regain some feelings of control. It may also be useful to introduce the family members to the local burn support group. Burn survivors and their families can provide emotional support and validation and also can reinforce the concept that it is possible to survive burns and live acceptable happy lives.

■ Surgical Management in the Acute Phase of Burn Injury

Definitive wound care for full-thickness burns is accomplished by *autografting,* the surgical removal of a superficial layer of the client's own unburned skin, which is subsequently grafted to the excised or clean and granulating burn wound. Because the epidermis is split (in layers) rather than taken in full, these grafts are referred to as *split-thickness grafts.* This procedure is performed in the operating room while the client is under general anesthesia. Autografts can be applied either as a *sheet* (*sheet graft*) or in a meshed form (*meshed graft*).

A sheet autograft is applied to the excised wound bed without alteration in its integrity. Sheet autografts are frequently used to graft burns in visible areas.

In contrast, a meshed autograft contains many little slits that allow for expansion of the donor skin. Meshing permits coverage of larger areas of irregularly shaped wounds and allows for drainage from a bleeding wound bed. When healed, the meshed pattern of the autograft remains visible. Therefore, meshed grafts are used on hidden body areas. When a thicker layer of skin is removed, consisting of the epidermis and the dermis, this is referred to as a *full-thickness graft.* For all autografts, the area of the body from which the skin was removed is referred to as the donor site (Fig. 50–13).

Graft adherence is dependent on the formation of a fibrin bond between the recipient bed and the graft.[50] There are no vascular connections between the graft and the wound bed immediately after surgery. The graft is held in place only by weak fibrin bonds and is nourished by the diffusion of serum from the wound bed. The graft begins to stabilize after 3 days as a fibrovascular and collagen network form and provide durability to the graft. A bleeding wound bed, hematoma formation, or shearing of the graft will disrupt formation of this bond between graft and bed. Care must be taken during the postoperative period to assess for bleeding, remove accumulated serum beneath sheet grafts (as described next in the discussion on nursing management of the surgical client), and prevent unwanted movement and shearing of autografts.[49]

Various types of dressings are used to cover donor sites, depending on the size, location, and condition of adjacent skin or tissue.[35] However, despite the differences in dressings, the donor site wound requires the same meticulous care as for other partial-thickness wounds, to expedite healing and prevent infection. If the donor site becomes infected, the dressing should be gently removed or soaked off. The wound can then be thoroughly cleansed and an antimicrobial agent applied. Once the donor site has healed, lubricating lotions can be applied to soften the area and reduce itching. Donor sites can be reused after they are healed.

Cultured *epithelial autografting* is a technique for closure of massive burn wounds.[49, 51] The process of autolo-

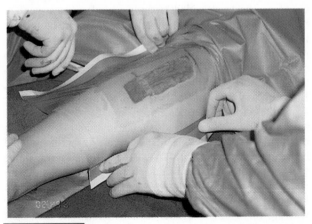

FIGURE 50–13 Harvesting donor skin from the lateral portion of the client's thigh.

gous epithelial cell growth begins with taking a full-thickness skin specimen from an uninjured body site. This specimen is sent to a specialized laboratory for culture and growth. Typically, in 3 to 4 weeks, several sheets of cultured epithelial autografts are ready for application. In the operating room, the cultured epithelial autograft sheets are carefully applied to an excised and non-bleeding wound bed and are secured in place with staples. Dressings are applied and moistened with an antibiotic solution shown to be nontoxic to the cultured epithelial autografts.

Reports demonstrating the success of cultured epithelial autografts in the treatment of massive burn wounds have been limited. Both early and late cultured epithelial autograft loss due to mechanical shearing, nutritional imbalance, infection, or an autoimmune response have been reported.[69]

▬ Nursing Management of the Surgical Client in the Acute Phase of Burn Injury

PREOPERATIVE CARE
Routine care of clients undergoing surgery is discussed in Chapter 15. Specific preoperative care of the client scheduled for debridement includes providing information about areas to be debrided and plans for pain control. Debridement cases are usually considered contaminated in the operating room and are often done at the end of the surgical list; therefore, clients may wait for many hours before undergoing the scheduled procedure. Specific orders for medications to be given or withheld, and the time to begin *nil per os* (NPO) (i.e., nothing by month) status should be obtained.

Before skin grafting, clients need information on the type of skin graft to be used, the location of the donor site, the postoperative plans for pain control, and the need for immobility and elevation of the graft site. Fears over scarring should be addressed; in general, scarring cannot be predicted because scar tissue requires a full year to mature. Both debridement and grafting can be multiple procedures, and clients may become anxious over repeated surgical procedures. Severe anxiety should be communicated to the surgeon and anesthesia personnel.

POSTOPERATIVE CARE
Routine postoperative care is discussed in Chapter 15. Care specific to debrided wounds includes assessment of bleeding and pain control. Many clients report more pain in donor sites (owing to exposed nerve endings) than in recipient sites. Skin-grafted sites must be immobilized to promote adherence of the graft to the wound bed. Various techniques are used, including suture, tape, and dressings. Blebs of serum should be removed from graft sites using a small needle and cotton-tipped applicator. Skin-grafted sites are elevated to prevent edema, in which the swelling of edematous tissue will lift the graft from the wound bed. Bed rest may be prescribed for up to 10 days. If the graft is on the legs, a schedule of progressive leg dependency is used. For example, the client can position the legs hanging down ("dangling") while sitting in a chair or walking for 5 minutes, then for 10 minutes the next day, and so on. The graft site is inspected for rubor and edema after each episode.

REHABILITATION PHASE

The rehabilitation phase of recovery represents the final phase of burn care and encompasses the time from wound closure to discharge and beyond. In order for the best outcomes to be achieved, caregivers must understand the consequences of burn injury, and treatment for rehabilitation must begin from the day of injury. Rehabilitation should overlap the acute care phase and last well beyond the acute inpatient hospitalization. Ultimately, a burn rehabilitation program is designed for maximal functional and emotional recovery. Measures to promote wound healing, to prevent or minimize deformities and hypertrophic scarring, to increase physical strength and function, to promote emotional support, and to provide education are a part of the ongoing rehabilitation phase.

See the Bridge to Home Health Care: Managing After Burns.

▬ Medical Management in the Rehabilitation Phase of Burn Injury

MINIMIZE FUNCTIONAL LOSS
Early wound excision helps to minimize short-term and long-term functional loss by removing the nonpliable eschar and eliminating wound pain.[49] A skin graft, although more elastic than eschar, still does not have normal elasticity, and wound stiffness will still be present, which must be counterbalanced with aggressive therapy and splinting.

Exercise, splinting, and positioning continue through all phases of burn injury; however, it is during this phase that the importance of these efforts becomes paramount. These measures are crucial to the client's progression to optimal functional independence.[73]

Hypertrophic scarring, which results from an overabundant deposition of collagen in the healed burn wound, can be minimized with the use of massage and pressure therapy.[56] Constant pressure applied to healing burn wounds has been found to reduce the scarring process. Several commercially available products provide the constant, even pressure required. Although hypertrophic scarring usually does not peak until several months after the injury, it is important to plan ahead before the onset of loss of function. By the rehabilitation phase of injury, the client should be measured for custom-fitted anti–burn scar support garments for any area that did not heal within 3 weeks of injury[56] (Fig. 50–14).

PROVIDE PSYCHOSOCIAL SUPPORT
In this, the last phase of burn injury, during which the wounds are almost healed and specific plans are made for hospital discharge, the client must face numerous issues and overcome many concerns.[55] Self-image issues, pain, physical limitations, and fear of rejection represent only a few of the issues the client must deal with as discharge nears.[7] During this time, it is important to maintain good communication with the client. It is beneficial to the client for the staff to encourage independence and carry the message that survivors can find ways to achieve whatever goals they set for themselves. Pain control and anxiety prevention continue to require assessment and medical management as needed.[41] Psychosocial assistance for the client and family members or significant others should carry through from admission to discharge.

BRIDGE TO HOME HEALTH CARE

Managing After Burns

When admitting the burn-injured client to home health services, remember that each case is unique and involves detailed treatment instructions. Include the client's and family members' responses to the client's discharge from the hospital and to the client's being home in the nursing assessment. If clients require assistance with activities of daily living (ADL), they will need a primary caregiver to provide both emotional support and direct care. This person is a critical member of the health care delivery team.

Work with the client and the primary caregiver to set up a place in the home for dressing changes and storage of needed dressing materials that limits the possibility of contamination. This area should be comfortable and relaxing and off-limits to family pets. If possible, select a room that clients do not use for other activities, especially sleeping, so that they do not associate these activities with pain from dressing changes. The dressing materials and an up-to-date wound care plan can be neatly organized and stored in a sealed plastic box or plastic bag. Supplies should be ordered on a weekly basis in quantities that can be used for one dressing change. In some agencies, prepackaged wound care kits provide an excellent method of infection control and reduce the amount of waste significantly.

Although dressing changes and physical therapy can be painful experiences for the client, both are essential for recovery. Identify ways to decrease the pain or the length of time for which pain will occur. Work with the physical therapist, the client, and the family to determine the best schedule for these activities. Consider scheduling joint visits if this would improve the care given to the client. Instruct a family member to give prescribed pain medications 1 hour before the scheduled dressing change to provide the best relief for the client. While changing dressings, use soft music or relaxation techniques, and involve the client and family as much as possible. These strategies offer a sense of control and can decrease the client's perception of pain.

Unless mechanical debridement of the wound is necessary, the dressings should not stick to the wound bed. Avoid removing dried-on dressings because they cause unnecessary pain. If the dressings are sticking, soak them off with normal saline, or after obtaining the physician's approval, remove them in the shower. Collaborate with the primary physician or a wound care nurse to obtain an appropriate moisture-retentive dressing, to reduce or eliminate pain with dressing changes.

Rehabilitation of people who have suffered burn injury involves more than dressing changes and physical therapy. It is also important to consider the psychological stress of the initial injury, scarring, and surgical procedures and other treatments as well as the financial burden from loss of work time and the lengthy recovery period. Evaluate the need of the client and family members for referrals to local agencies that offer social, counseling, financial, and spiritual services as well as support groups. Such services may be essential in order for clients and their families to cope with the traumatic life event that a major burn injury with its sequelae represents.

Roxanne Rivard, RN, BSN, CWOCN, *Enterostomal Therapy Nurse, Fairview Lakes HomeCaring and Hospice, Chisago City, Minnesota*

Nursing Management of the Medical Client in the Rehabilitation Phase of Burn Injury

Impaired Physical Mobility. During the rehabilitation phase of burn injury, the client's physical mobility and ability to provide self-care are impaired by the presence of dressings, pain, scarring, contracture, and muscle atrophy.

Outcomes. The client will have improved physical mobility, as evidenced by maximum independence in performance of ADL, with minimum disability and disfigurement.

Interventions. The physical and occupational therapy consultations initiated in the early phases of burn injury are especially important for continued treatment in the rehabilitation phase as the client works toward functional independence. Typically, the therapist provides an individualized rehabilitation schedule as well as needed assistive devices for the client.

Motivate the client to participate in self-care activity such as brushing teeth and self-feeding, as this increased activity will not only improve mobility but also lessen dependence. Provide assistive devices furnished by therapy consultants to assist the client with any limitations. Expect tasks to take longer when the client works independently. Allow adequate time for the client to complete the undertaking. Self-confidence will be gained with independent functioning regardless of the time spent.

Encourage active ROM every 2 to 4 hours while the client is awake unless contraindicated because of a recent grafting procedure. Increased activity prevents muscle atrophy, tendon adherence, joint stiffness, and capsular tightness. Help the client to ambulate, to promote muscle strength and cardiopulmonary reserve. Provide passive exercise and stretching if the client is unable to actively participate (e.g., if the client is comatose or paralyzed).

Wrap donor sites on both burned and unburned legs with elastic bandage wraps (Ace bandages), using a figure-eight technique, before placing the limbs in a dependent position. The support will decrease capillary venous stasis, which impairs wound healing. Explain the rationale for activities to the client and family members, as understanding improves compliance. Avoid the position of comfort, and maintain burned areas in the position of physiologic function, within the client's limit of endurance. Continue to follow the splinting and positioning regimen recommended in the therapy consultation.

Pain. Pain experienced during the rehabilitation phase of burn injury is typically associated with wound care and therapeutic activity, particularly ROM exercises.

Outcomes. The client will have an acceptable level of comfort, as evidenced by verbalizing relief or control of pain or discomfort and actively participating in care.

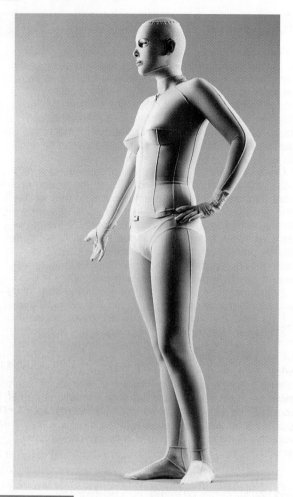

FIGURE 50–14 The model is wearing custom-fitted anti-scar support garment. When worn 23 hours a day, this garment is effective in providing pressure over healing burn wounds. Pressure therapy helps to minimize the development of hypertrophic scarring. (Courtesy of Medical Z Corporation, San Antonio.)

Interventions. Formulate a plan for controlling the client's pain based on an assessment of the client's response to pain and documentation of previous successful treatment regimens. As in the earlier phases of injury, allow adequate time for the onset of the medication for maximum benefits of the medication (5 to 10 minutes for the IV route; 45 minutes for the oral route). Nonpharmacologic methods of pain control, such as relaxation techniques, music therapy, guided imagery, distraction, and hypnosis, may improve the client's comfort, even if such methods were not successful in early phases of injury. As described earlier, effective communication assists in decreasing the client's anxiety. In preparation for impending discharge, the client should at some point during the rehabilitation phase progress to analgesia given only by the oral route.

Self-Esteem Disturbance. The client is at risk for self-esteem disturbances related to threatened or actual change in body image, physical loss, and loss of role responsibilities.

Outcomes. The client will develop improved self-esteem, as evidenced by making social contact with oth-

ers outside the immediate family, developing effective coping mechanisms throughout the stages of recovery, and verbalizing feelings about self-concept.

Interventions. Allowing time for two-way communication with the client is especially important during this phase of injury. Provide an atmosphere of acceptance as the client tries various coping strategies to deal with the injury. Provide honest and accurate information about the client's projected appearance in an effort to reduce misconceptions that he or she may have.

Assess the need for limit-setting for maladaptive behavior. Consult with burn team members to establish such limits and to formulate a treatment plan for such behaviors; explain limit-setting to family members or significant others and assist them to maintain the same limits. Promote the client's self-confidence by providing information about the progress made, and support the client's role in care and treatment, providing encouragement and positive reinforcement.

Encourage family members to interact with the client, as this encouragement facilitates societal reintegration. During this phase of recovery, encourage the client to interact with others outside the facility. Use of a family day pass during this time is useful. Help to prepare the client for social interaction after discharge by discussing potential situations and how the client might deal with them. Such preparation provides rehearsal of events and reduces anxiety.

Impaired Skin Integrity. The expectation is that by the time the client reaches the rehabilitation phase of burn injury, the majority of wounds will be either healed or grafted. The new skin over areas of donor site, graft, and healed burn is characteristically very thin, with disrupted oil glands. The skin therefore is fragile; it becomes very dry and shears or cracks easily; and it is prone to infection.

Outcomes. The client will have intact skin with no evidence of infection, breakdown, or blistering.

Interventions. Daily wound and skin care should continue throughout hospitalization. Clean burned areas, grafts, and donor sites daily with a mild soap (without fragrance) and water. Rinse thoroughly to remove the soap. After cleaning, the healed skin should be lubricated with a nonirritating, alcohol-free moisturizer. Itching associated with dry skin can be minimized with application of the moisturizer at least 3 times a day. Avoid any shearing of tissue with dressings, clothing, or splints.

Knowledge Deficit. The burn-injured client or a family member or significant other must have knowledge of important treatment modalities that need continuation after discharge from the hospital.

Outcomes. The client or a family member or significant other will verbalize knowledge and demonstrate techniques that facilitate continued wound healing and limb mobility.

Interventions. Demonstrate and discuss the following skin care interventions with the client and appropriate family member or significant other: daily skin and wound care and dressing instructions if any; lubrication of grafts, donor sites, and healed burn wounds using an alcohol-free skin moisturizer at least 3 times daily; wearing pressure dressings or garments for 23 hours daily; and complete avoidance of direct sunlight for 1 year after injury owing to increased sensitivity to ultraviolet rays.

Review current medications and the dosage, precautions, and potential side effects. Discuss nutritional needs and the benefits of diets with adequate protein and calories.

Provide information on support groups or peers and counseling as needed for adjustment to life outside the hospital setting. Stress the need for follow-up care, and provide appointment dates and times if these have been established.

CONCLUSIONS

Nursing care of the burn-injured client is both complex and challenging. The psychological and physical trauma sustained following a burn injury can be devastating for both the victim and family members or significant others. Having a thorough understanding of the pathophysiologic changes that occur after a burn, knowing what to expect clinically as a result of the injury, and becoming familiar with the standards of care will guide nursing care to promote positive patient outcomes. As a key member of the burn team, you are responsible for an individualized plan of care that reflects the client's changing needs during progression through the different phases of recovery. Priority issues and care change as the client moves from the critical emergent phase into and, ultimately, through the rehabilitation period.

THINKING CRITICALLY

1. **You are working on the night shift in your hospital's burn center and receive a call that a client is in transport via ambulance to your unit. He will be a direct admission and bypass the emergency department. The telephone report reveals that the client was found unconscious on the floor of the bedroom. He is covered with soot and has obvious burns on his face, arms and torso. An intravenous line of lactated Ringer's solution was started and is running wide open. Oxygen is being administered via face mask. On admission, the client is received lying in the supine position on a gurney. He is restless, confused, and combative. He appears anxious and in pain. The eyebrows, eyelashes and hair are singed. There is soot in the nares and mouth and on the tongue. His voice is raspy, and he is coughing up thick black sputum. Breath sounds with scattered crackles; oxygen saturation, 75%. Face mask is in place but was disconnected from oxygen tank while the client was being moved onto the burn center gurney.**

   Heart rate is 142 BPM, with sinus tachycardia. Respiratory rate is 40 breaths/min and labored. Blood pressure is 144/88; temperature is 35° C. Bowel sounds are absent. There is thick, white leathery eschar on the chest, neck, left and right arm, and hands. The skin of the face and back are pink, moist, and blistered. The body from the waist to the feet is unburned. An IV line is infusing the LR right saphenous vein.

Weight, 85 kg. What priorities should be set for the client's care? What interventions should be undertaken?

Factors to Consider. What is the client's respiratory status? Do the physical examination and history provided by the ambulance crew give you any clues to his respiratory status? What should you consider when administering pain medication or anxiolytics to this client? What is the client's fluid volume status? How will you monitor adequate fluid resuscitation?

2. **It is now 7 days after the injury, and the client has just returned to the unit after receiving grafts on the chest, neck, bilateral arms, hands, and axillae. Donor skin was taken circumferentially from both thighs. What assessments should you perform? What interventions should be undertaken?**

Factors to Consider. What factors disrupt graft adherence? What can you do to help prevent contracture formation?

3. **It is now 2 months since the client was injured, and the team begins to discuss discharge plans. The client tells you that he does not want to go home and does not want to talk any more about discharge. What can you do to help the client?**

Factors to Consider. What concerns might a burn survivor face upon discharge from the hospital? What professional resources might be helpful in addressing this situation? What lay resources might be helpful?

REFERENCES

1. Adcock, R., Boeve, S., & Patterson, D. (1998). Psychological and emotional recovery. In G. J. Carrougher (Ed.), *Burn care and therapy* (pp. 329–347). St. Louis: Mosby–Year Book.
2. Ahrns, K. S., & Harkins, D. R. (1999). Initial resuscitation after burn injury: Therapies, strategies, and controversies. *AACN Clinical Issues in Critical Care Nursing, 10*(1), 46–60.
3. American Burn Association. (1984). Guidelines for service standards and severity classification in the treatment of burn injuries. *Bulletin of the American College of Surgeons, 69*(10), 24–28.
4. Atkinson, A. (1998). Nursing burn wounds on general wards. *Nursing Standard, 12*(1), 58–65.
5. Barillo, D. J., & Goode, R. (1996). Fire fatality study: Demographics of fire victims. *Burns, 22*(2), 85–88.
6. Barton, R. G., & Saffle, J. R. (1997). Resuscitation of thermally injured patients with oxygen transport criteria as goals of therapy. *Journal of Burn Care and Rehabilitation, 18*(1), 1–9.
7. Blakeney, P., & Meyer, W. (1996). Psychosocial recovery of burned patients and reintegration into society. In D. N. Herndon (Ed.), *Total burn care* (pp. 556–563). London: W. B. Saunders.
8. Brigham, P. A., & McLoughlin, E. (1996). Burn incidence and medical care in the United States: Estimates, trends, and data sources. *Journal of Burn Care and Rehabilitation, 17*(2), 95–107.
9. Brigham, P. A., & McGuire, A. (1995). Progress towards a safe cigarette. *Journal of Public Health Policy, 16*(4), 433–439.
10. Carleton, S. C., Tomassoni, A. J., & Alexander, J. K. (1995). The cardiovascular effects of environmental traumas: Cardiac problems associated with burns. *Cardiology Clinics, 13*(2), 257–262.
11. Carrougher, G. J. (1999). Inhalation injury. *AACN Clinical Issues in Critical Care Nursing, 10*(1), 367–376.
12. Carrougher, G. J. (1998). Burn wound assessment and topical treatment. In G. J. Carrougher (Ed.), *Burn care and therapy* (pp. 133–159). St. Louis: Mosby–Year Book.
13. Cartotto, R. C., et al. (1996). Chemical burns. *Canadian Journal of Surgery, 39*(3), 205–220.

14. Cioffi, W. G. (1998) Inhalation injury. In G. J. Carrougher (Ed.), *Burn care and therapy* (pp. 35–59). St. Louis: Mosby–Year Book.

15. Cusick, J. M., & Grant, E. J. (1997). Children's sleepwear: Realization of the Consumer Product Safety Commission's flammability standards. *Journal of Burn Care and Rehabilitation, 18*(5), 469–474.

16. Darling, G. E., et al. (1996). Pulmonary complications in inhalation injuries with associated cutaneous burn. *Journal of Trauma Injury, 40*(1), 83–89.

17. Davis, S. T., & Sheely-Adolphson, P. (1997). Psychosocial interventions: Pharmacologic and psychologic modalities. *Nursing Clinics of North America, 32*(2), 331–340.

18. Demling, R. H. (1998). *Burn trauma.* New York: Thieme.

19. Everett, J. J. (1994). Pain assessment from patients with burns and their nurses. *Journal of Burn Care and Rehabilitation, 15*(2), 194–198.

20. Gordon, M., & Goodwin, C. (1997). Initial assessment, management and stabilization. *Nursing Clinics of North America, 32*(2), 237–248.

21. Gordon, M., & Winfree, J. (1998). Fluid resuscitation after a major burn. In G. J. Carrougher (Ed.), *Burn care and therapy* (pp. 107–126). St. Louis: Mosby–Year Book.

22. Gottschlich, M., & Jenkins, M. (1998). Metabolic consequences and nutritional needs. In G. J. Carrougher (Ed.), *Burn care and therapy* (pp. 213–226). St. Louis: Mosby–Year Book.

23. Greenfield, E., & McManus, A. (1997). Infectious complications. Prevention strategies for their control. *Nursing Clinics of North America, 32*(2), 297–308.

24. Harris, B., & Gelfand, J. (1995). The immune response to trauma. *Seminars in Pediatric Surgery, 4*(2), 77–81.

25. Hansbrough, J., & Franco, E. (1998). Skin replacements. *Clinics in Plastic Surgery, 25*(3), 407–423.

26. Heimbach, D., Mann, R., & Engrav, L. (1996). Evolution of the burn wound. Management decisions. In D. N. Herndon (Ed.), *Total burn care* (pp. 81–97). London: W. B. Saunders.

27. Hildreth, M., & Gottschlich, M. (1996). Nutritional support of the burned patient. In D. N. Herndon (Ed.), *Total burn care* (pp. 237–245). London: W. B. Saunders.

28. Hurren, J. S. (1995). Rehabilitation of the burned patient: James Laing memorial essay for 1993. *Burns, 21*(2), 116–126.

29. Jain, S., & Bandi, V. (1999). Electrical and lightning injuries. *Critical Care Clinics, 15*(2), 319–329.

30. Jordan, B., & Barillo, D. (1998). Prehospital care and transport. In G. J. Carrougher (Ed.), *Burn care and therapy* (pp. 61–88). St. Louis: Mosby–Year Book.

31. Jordan, B., & Harrington, D. (1997). Management of the burn wound. *Nursing Clinics of North America, 32*(2), 251–270.

32. Kealey, G. P. (1995). Pharmacologic management of background pain in burn victims. *Journal of Burn Care and Rehabilitation, 16*(3), 358–362.

33. Kirn, D S., & Luce, E. A. (1997). Early excision and grafting versus conservative management of burns in the elderly. *Plastic and Reconstructive Surgery, 9,* 1013–1017.

34. Kramer, G., & Nguyen, T. (1996). Pathophysiology of burn shock and burn edema. In D. N. Herndon (Ed.), *Total burn care* (pp. 44–52). London: W. B. Saunders.

35. Ladin, D. (1998). Understanding dressings. *Clinics in Plastic Surgery, 25*(3), 433–440.

36. LeBoucher, J., & Cynober, L. (1997). Protein metabolism and therapy in burn injury. *Annals of Nutrition and Metabolism, 41,* 69–82.

37. Lee, J. (1970). Emotional reactions to trauma. *Nursing Clinics of North America, 5*(4), 577–587.

38. Lee-Chiong, T. (1999). Smoke inhalation injury. When to suspect and how to treat. *Postgraduate Medicine, 105*(2), 55–62.

39. Lim, J., Rehmar, S., & Elmore, P. (1998). Rapid response: Care of burn victims. *AAOHN Journal, 46*(4), 169–178.

40. Linares, H. A. (1996). The burn problem: A pathologist's perspective. In D. N. Herndon (Ed.), *Total burn care* (p. 372). London: W. B. Saunders.

41. Malenfant, A., et al. (1998). Tactile, thermal and pain sensibility in burned patients with and without chronic pain and paresthesia problems. *Pain, 77,* 241–251.

42. Marvin, J. (1998). Management of pain and anxiety. In G. J. Carrougher (Ed.), *Burn care and therapy* (pp. 167–179). St. Louis: Mosby–Year Book.

43. Marvin, J., et al. (1996). Pain response and pain control. In D. N. Herndon (Ed.), *Total burn care* (pp. 529–544). London: W. B. Saunders.

44. Mayes, T. (1997). Enteral nutrition for the burnpatient. *Nutrition in Clinical Practice, 12*(1), S43–S45.

45. Mlcak, R., Dimick, A., & Micak, G. (1996). Prehospital management, transport and emergency care. In D. N. Herndon (Ed.), *Total burn care* (pp. 33–43). London: W. B. Saunders.

46. Monafo, W. (1996). Initial management of burns. *New England Journal of Medicine, 335*(21), 1581–1586.

47. Monafo, W. (1996). Wound care. In D. N. Herndon (Ed.), *Total burn care* (pp. 88–97). London: W. B. Saunders.

48. Moritz, A. R. (1945). The effect of inhaled heat on the air passages and lung: An experimental investigation. *American Journal of Pathology, 21*(2), 311–332.

49. Mozingo, D. (1998). Surgical management. In G. J. Carrougher (Ed.), *Burn care and therapy* (pp. 233–246). St. Louis: Mosby–Year Book.

50. Muller, M., et al. (1996). Modern treatment of a burn wound. In D. N. Herndon (Ed.), *Total Burn Care* (pp. 136–147). London: W. B. Saunders.

51. Munster, A. (1996). Cultured skin for massive burns. *Ann Surg, 224*(3), 372–377.

52. Nenot, J. C. (1990) Medical and surgical management for localized radiation burns. *Journal of Radiation Biology, 57*(4), 783–795.

53. Nguyen, T., et al. (1995). Current treatment of severely burned patients. *Annals of Surgery, 223*(1), 14–25.

54. Oman, K., & Reilly, E. (1998), Initial assessment and care in the emergency department. In G. J. Carrougher (Ed.), *Burn care and therapy* (pp. 89–101). St. Louis: Mosby–Year Book.

55. Partridge, J., & Robinson, E. (1995). Psychologic and social aspects of burns. *Burns, 21*(6), 453–457. Patino, O., et al. (1998) Massage in hypertrophic scars. *Journal of Burn Care and Rehabilitation, 20*(3), 268–271.

56. Pessina, M., & Ellis, S. (1997). Rehabilitation. *Nursing Clinics of North America, 32*(2), 365–373.

57. Pruitt, B., & Cioffi, W. (1995). Diagnosis and treatment of smoke inhalation. *Journal of Intensive Care Medicine, 10*(3), 117–127.

58. Pruitt, B., & Goodwin, C. (1995). Thermal injury. In J. H. Davis & G. F. Sheldon (Eds.), *Clinical surgery.* St. Louis: Mosby–Year Book.

59. Pruitt, B., & Mason, A. (1996). Epidemiological, demographic and outcome characteristics of burn injury. In D. N. Herndon (Ed.), *Total burn care* (pp. 5–15). London: W. B. Saunders.

60. Ramzy, P., Barret, J., & Herndon, D. (1999). Thermal injury. *Critical Care Clinics, 15*(2), 333–352.

61. Richard, R. (1998). Assessment and diagnosis of burn wounds. *Advances in Wound Care, 12*(9), 468–471.

62. Rodriguez, D. (1996). Nutrition in patients with severe burns: State of the art. *Journal of Burn Care and Rehabilitation, 17*(1), 62–70.

63. Rose, J. K., et al. (1997). Allograft is superior to topical antimicrobial therapy in the treatment of partial-thickness scald burns in children. *Journal of Burn Care and Rehabilitation, 18*(4), 338–341.

64. Rutan, R. (1998). Physiologic response to cutaneous burn injury. In G. J. Carrougher (Ed.), *Burn care and therapy* (pp. 1–28). St. Louis: Mosby–Year Book.

65. Sakurai, H., Traber, L., & Traber, D. (1998). Altered systemic organ blood flow after combined injury with burn and smoke inhalation. *Shock, 3*(5), 369–374.

66. Shankowsky, H. A., Callioux, L. S., & Tredget, E. E. (1994). North America survey of hydrotherapy in modern burn care. *Journal of Burn Care and Rehabilitation, 15*(2), 143–146.

67. Smith, D. (1995). Use of Biobrane in wound management. *Journal of Burn Care and Rehabilitation, 16*(3), 317–320.

68. Thompkins, R. M., & Carrougher, G. J. (1998). Burn prevention. In G. J. Carrougher (Ed.), *Burn care and therapy* (pp. 497–522). St. Louis: Mosby–Year Book.

69. Tompkins, R., and Burke, J. (1996). Alternative wound coverings. In D. N. Herndon (Ed.), *Total burn care* (pp. 164–183). London: W. B. Saunders.

70. Traber, D., & Polland, V. (1996). Pathophysiology of inhalation injury. In D. N. Herndon (Ed.), *Total burn care* (pp. 175–183). London: W. B. Saunders.

71. Ward, C. G. (1998). What's new in burns? *Journal of the American College of Surgery, 186*(2), 123–126.

72. Ward, R. S (1998). Physical rehabilitation. In G. J. Carrougher (Ed.), *Burn care and therapy* (pp. 293–320). St. Louis: Mosby–Year Book.

73. Ward, R. S., & Saffle, J. R. (1995). Topical agents in burn and wound care. *Physical Therapy, 75*(6), 526–538.

74. Warden, G. D. (1996). Fluid resuscitation and early management. In D. N. Herndon (Ed.), *Total burn care* (pp. 53–60). London: W. B. Saunders.

75. Weber, J. (1998). Epidemiology of infections and strategies for control. In G. J. Carrougher (Ed.), *Burn care and therapy* (pp. 185–206). St. Louis: Mosby–Year Book.

76. Williams, W., & Phillips, L. (1996). Pathophysioiogy of the burn wound. In D. N. Herndon (Ed.), *Total burn care* (pp. 63–70). London: W. B. Saunders.

77. Winfree, J., & Barillo, D. (1997). Nonthermal injuries. *Nursing Clinics of North America, 32*(2), 275–294.

78. Wolfe, R. (1996). Metabolic responses to burn injury: Nutritional implications. In D. N. Herndon (Ed.), *Total burn care* (pp. 217–222). London: W. B. Saunders.

UNIT
11

Circulatory Disorders

Anatomy and Physiology Review
The Circulatory System
Robert G. Carroll

The vascular system is a vast network of vessels through which blood circulates in the body. The major functions of the cardiovascular system—delivery of nutrients to tissues and removal of metabolic wastes—are accomplished in the capillaries. Blood leaving the ventricles is distributed through arteries and arterioles, in progressively smaller branches to the capillaries (a *divergent* pattern, like a river to a delta). Blood leaving the capillaries follows progressively larger venules and veins on its way back to the atria (a *convergent* pattern, like tributaries flowing into a river).

The anatomic arrangement of blood vessels allows regulation of blood flow at the individual tissue level, so that blood flow delivery can be proportional to the tissue's metabolic needs. Because the volume of blood flowing from the arteries to the capillaries is a major determinant of blood pressure, the blood pressure control systems also include control of arteriolar diameter by the sympathetic nervous system and circulating hormones.

STRUCTURES OF THE VASCULAR SYSTEM

Two series of blood vessels—the systemic and the pulmonary circulations—distribute blood to the capillaries and return blood to the heart. Blood exiting the left ventricle enters the *systemic circulation,* passing progressively through the aorta, arteries, arterioles, capillaries, venules, veins, and finally the vena cava before entering the right atrium (Fig. U11–1). For the *pulmonary circulation,* blood flows from the right ventricle into the pulmonary artery, then passes through arterioles, pulmonary capillaries, and venules, before returning to the pulmonary vein and the left atrium.

GENERAL BLOOD VESSEL STRUCTURE

The anatomic division of blood vessels into arteries, arterioles, capillaries, venules, and veins is based on the presence of up to three histologic layers (Fig. U11–2).

1. The *tunica intima* (innermost layer) consists of endothelial cells that separate the blood from the extravascular spaces. The tightness of the junctions between the endothelial cells varies among tissues. For example, the very tight junctions of cerebral capillaries restrict movement of some drugs to brain cells (the blood-brain barrier). In contrast, the endothelial cell holes and relatively loose junctions in the liver and spleen allow easy transit between the blood and tissue spaces in those organs. The endothelium generates substances such as endothelial-derived relaxing factor (EDRF, or nitric oxide), allowing nitroglycerin, friction, and stress to cause vasodilation. Damage to the endothelium may allow blood to enter the middle layer of a blood vessel, creating an aneurysm.

2. The *tunica media* (middle layer) consists of elastic connective tissue and smooth muscle cells. Particularly in the aorta and large arteries, the elastic tissue contributes to the shape of the arterial pressure pulse. The amount of smooth muscle contraction regulates the diameter of the vessel and causes a change in blood flow and blood pressure. Smooth muscle is normally partially contracted because of sympathetic nerve activity. Smooth muscle contraction can also be regulated by circulating hormones and (in the smaller vessels) by tissue metabolic factors.

3. The *tunica adventitia* (outermost layer) consists of a relatively thin layer of connective tissue providing shape for the blood vessels. This layer also houses the vasa vasorum, the small arteries and veins that provide nutrients to the cells of the blood vessel.

VASCULAR SEGMENTS

Arteries

Arteries, particularly the aorta, have an extensive elastic tissue layer that accounts for the difference between arterial pressure (120/80 mm Hg) and left ventricular pressure (120/10 mm Hg). The elastic tissue stretches during ventricular ejection, storing energy. When the aortic valve closes and ventricular ejection stops, recoil of the elastic tissue slows the fall of arterial pressure during the interval until the next period of ventricular ejection. The efficiency of the elastic tissue decreases with age and with atherosclerosis, contributing to the rise in systolic arterial blood pressure usually seen in older adults.

Arterioles (5 to 100 μm in diameter) contain a high proportion of vascular smooth muscle. The degree of contraction of this muscle is regulated by background activity of the autonomic nervous system, primarily the sympathetic nerves. In addition, circulating hormones such as epinephrine, norepinephrine, and angiotensin can also cause smooth muscle contraction.

Capillary Beds

Capillary beds include the small arterioles and venules, and the vessels connecting them (see *Inset,* Fig. U11–1). The smooth muscle of these small arterioles is contracted by sympathetic nerves, but local factors become increasingly important as the diameter of the vessel decreases. The *precapillary sphincters* (the last band of smooth muscle before the capillaries) respond only to local factors. Blood passes from the arterioles into capillaries (5 to 10 μm in diameter). The capillary diameter approaches that

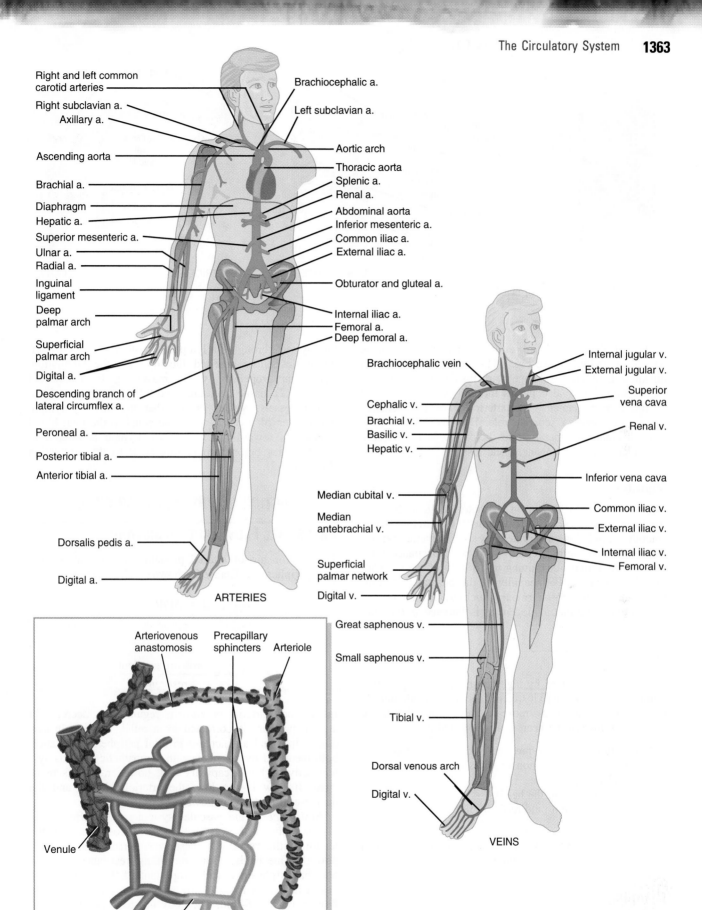

Right and left common carotid arteries

Right subclavian a.

Axillary a.

Ascending aorta

Brachial a.

Diaphragm

Hepatic a.

Superior mesenteric a.

Ulnar a.

Radial a.

Inguinal ligament

Deep palmar arch

Superficial palmar arch

Digital a.

Descending branch of lateral circumflex a.

Peroneal a.

Posterior tibial a.

Anterior tibial a.

Dorsalis pedis a.

Digital a.

Brachiocephalic a.

Left subclavian a.

Aortic arch

Thoracic aorta

Splenic a.

Renal a.

Abdominal aorta

Inferior mesenteric a.

Common iliac a.

External iliac a.

Obturator and gluteal a.

Internal iliac a.

Femoral a.

Deep femoral a.

ARTERIES

Brachiocephalic vein

Cephalic v.

Brachial v.

Basilic v.

Hepatic v.

Median cubital v.

Median antebrachial v.

Superficial palmar network

Digital v.

Internal jugular v.

External jugular v.

Superior vena cava

Renal v.

Inferior vena cava

Common iliac v.

External iliac v.

Internal iliac v.

Femoral v.

Great saphenous v.

Small saphenous v.

Tibial v.

Dorsal venous arch

Digital v.

VEINS

Arteriovenous anastomosis

Precapillary sphincters

Arteriole

Venule

True capillaries

FIGURE U11–1 Major systemic arteries and veins. *Inset,* Capillary network.

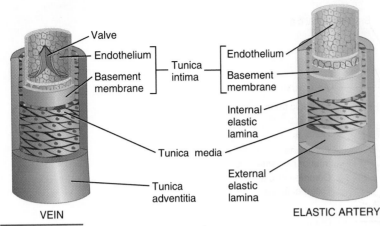
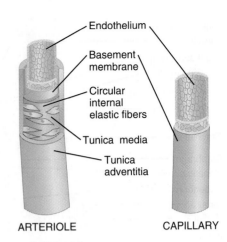

FIGURE U11–2 Structure of blood vessels.

of the red blood cell (7 μm in diameter). Capillaries have only a tunica intima (see Fig. U11–2), and the small wall thickness facilitates exchange by diffusion. In tissues such as the skin, blood also passes through *metarterioles* (10 to 100 μm in diameter). Metarterioles are not exchange vessels but serve a separate role. Decreased blood flow through cutaneous metarterioles helps the body conserve heat; increased flow enhances heat loss.

Venules

Venules (10 to 100 μm in diameter) collect drainage from the capillaries in a convergent flow pattern. Venule smooth muscle is innervated by sympathetic nerves. Along with the veins, venules serve as capacitance (volume storage) areas, containing up to 75% of the circulating blood volume. Permeability of the postcapillary venules is regulated by hormones such as histamine and bradykinin. Note that angiogenesis is initiated in the venules.

Veins

Veins are characterized by high volume and low pressure. Sympathetic nerve activity constricts the smooth muscle of the veins and helps move blood toward the heart. Blood flow toward the heart is also assisted by:

- A drop in intrathoracic pressure during respiration
- Extravascular compression of veins in exercising skeletal muscle,
- Gravity (for veins in the head)
- Valves that insure a unidirectional flow

Damage to venous valves can cause swellings, such as varicose veins, and lack of leg muscle movement can lead to venous stasis and clotting.

Lymphatics

Lymphatics are a network of endothelial tubes that merge to form two large systems that enter the vena cava. Terminal lymphatics lack tight junctions, allowing large proteins (and metastasizing cancer cells) to enter the circulatory system through the lymphatic system. In the GI tract, lymphatics allow digested fats to enter the circulation. Lymph is propelled by (1) massaging from adjacent muscle, (2) tissue pressure, and (3) contraction of the lymph vessels. Valves ensure that the flow of lymph, which over 24 hours is a volume equal to the total blood volume, is toward the vena cava. Lymph is filtered in lymph nodes before progressing back to the circulation (Fig. U11–3).

FUNCTION OF THE VASCULAR SYSTEM

PRESSURE, FLOW, AND RESISTANCE

The relationship of arterial pressure, cardiac output, and total peripheral resistance is shown by the equation

$$Q = \Delta P/R$$

or

$$\text{flow} = \frac{\text{pressure gradient}}{\text{resistance}}$$

In the body, arterial *pressure* is regulated. A decrease in arterial pressure is corrected by a reflex increase in cardiac output and an increase in total peripheral resistance, both mediated by an increase in sympathetic nervous system activity. For a capillary bed, however, *flow* is regulated. If flow is too low, the arteriole dilates and the decrease in resistance allows flow to increase.

Resistance in the vascular system can be affected by (1) the radius of the vessel, (2) fluid viscosity, and (3) the length of the vessel. Of these, vessel radius is the most powerful mechanism for controlling resistance and the one that is physiologically important. If the radius of the vessel decreases to ½ of the starting value, resistance to flow increases 16-fold. The body utilizes vascular smooth muscle to alter the diameter of arteries and arterioles and, therefore, to regulate both pressure and flow. Occasionally, changes in blood viscosity can alter resistance, particularly when the hematocrit is increased (polycythemia)

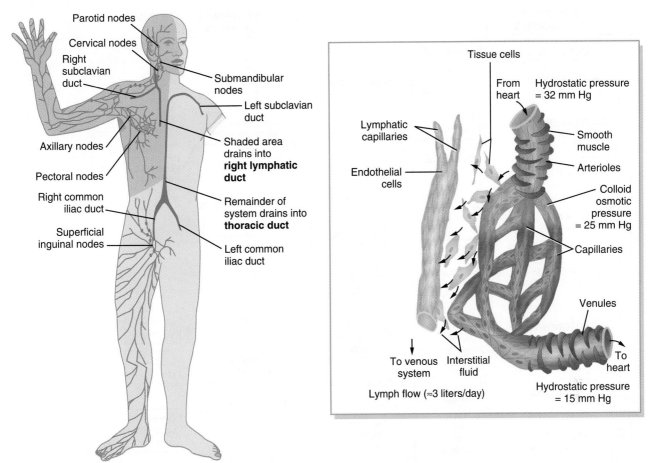

FIGURE U11–3 Major lymphatic vessels and drainage. *Inset,* Fluid exchange at the capillary bed. The primary driving force to move fluids from the capillary is *hydrostatic pressure.* The primary pulling force to bring fluids back into the vessel is *colloid osmotic pressure* from the proteins in the capillary fluids (e.g., albumin). The hydrostatic pressure at the arterial end of the capillary is 32 mm Hg. As the fluid moves through the capillary, the pressure falls. Because proteins do not move across the capillary endothelium, colloid osmotic pressure is constant at 25 mm Hg. Thus, at the arterial end the hydrostatic pressure is greater than the colloid osmotic pressure, and fluids then move into interstitial spaces. The opposite is true at the venous end where pressure falls to 15 mm Hg. The hydrostatic pressure is lower than the colloid osmotic pressure, and fluids thus return to the capillary. There is a net loss of fluids out of the capillary (~3 L/day). This fluid is absorbed by the lymphatic system and is returned to circulation at the lymphatic duct.

or decreased (anemia). Resistance increases as viscosity increases and decreases as viscosity decreases.

CAPILLARY EXCHANGE

Exchange of nutrients and wastes between the blood and the tissues is the primary purpose of the cardiovascular system. The movement of nutrients from the blood to the tissue and removal of metabolic wastes are driven by diffusion, filtration, and pinocytosis.

Diffusion

Diffusion is quantitatively the most important process. The rate of diffusion is enhanced by (1) increasing the surface area available for exchange, (2) increasing the concentration gradient, and (3) decreasing the distance that a compound must travel. In tissues such as exercising

skeletal muscle, an increase in the number of perfused capillaries enhances the delivery of nutrients to the tissues.

Filtration

Fluid movement across the capillary depends on the balance of the hydrostatic pressure gradient (which favors filtration) and the oncotic pressure gradient from plasma proteins (which favors reabsorption) (Fig. U11–4). The net force favors filtration at the arteriolar end of the capillary bed, and reabsorption at the venular end of the capillary bed. In most capillary beds, the volume filtered is slightly greater than the volume absorbed, and the excess fluid is removed from the tissue spaces by the lymph vessels. *Edema* (accumulation of fluid in the tissue spaces) occurs because of (1) increased filtration, (2) decreased reabsorption, or (3) impaired lymph drainage.

CAUSES OF HYPOTENSION
LEADING TO SHOCK

FACTORS DETERMINING SYSTEMIC
ARTERIAL PRESSURE

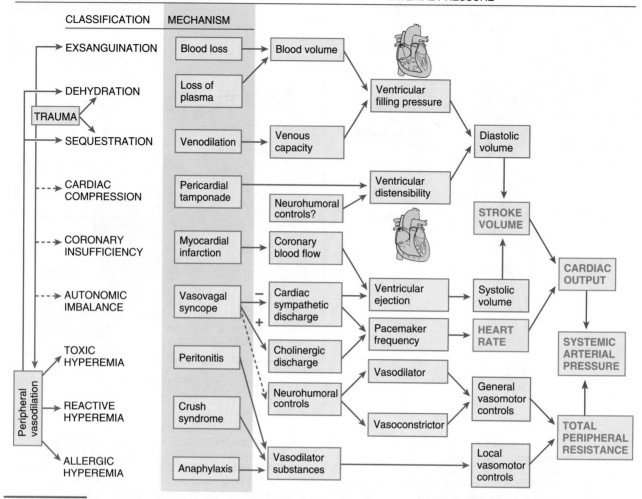

FIGURE U11-4 Control of arterial pressure. Arterial blood pressure is controlled by several factors. *Right,* Blood pressure is controlled by two major factors: cardiac output and total peripheral vascular resistance. Cardiac output is also a function of two factors: stroke volume and heart rate. Reading the diagram from the right, you will find the factors that govern each step. Each bifurcation represents possible compensatory mechanisms. *Far left,* Disorders that can lead to shock. These factors are extremes of the various control mechanisms. (Modified from Rushmer, R. F. [1976]. Cardiovascular dynamics [p. 207]. Philadelphia: W. B. Saunders.)

Pinocytosis

Pinocytosis is the movement of vesicles, especially from outside the cell to inside the cell. Pinocytosis is thought to be important only as a route for large proteins to cross the capillary wall.

CARDIOVASCULAR CONTROL

Much like the power and water supply systems in a city, the distribution of blood flow in the body depends on a sufficient driving pressure (arterial pressure), allowing the end users (capillary beds) to determine how much of the resource to utilize. Cardiovascular control is best described in terms of (1) regulation of arterial pressure and (2) local regulation of tissue blood flow.

■ REGULATION OF ARTERIAL PRESSURE

The normal arterial pressure is maintained by a negative feedback mechanism called the *baroreceptor reflex.* Pres-

sure-sensitive nerve endings in the aortic arch and carotid sinus monitor arterial pressure. This information is transmitted to the cardiovascular centers of the medulla, where it is integrated with other sensory information. The cardiovascular centers then adjust the activity of the sympathetic and parasympathetic nervous systems. Parasympathetic nerves help slow the heart rate; sympathetic nerves can increase heart rate, increase cardiac contractility, constrict the veins (to decrease venous capacity, thus increasing venous return), and constrict the arterioles (to increase total peripheral resistance and, therefore, arterial pressure). The relationships among all of these events in controlling arterial pressure are shown in Figure U11-4. Thus, a decrease in blood pressure activates the sympathetic nervous system, increasing cardiac output (heart rate, venoconstriction for venous return, and cardiac contractility) and increasing peripheral resistance to trap blood within the arteries.

Baroreceptor control of blood pressure is augmented by volume-sensitive receptors in the low-pressure atria and veins, which control renal fluid balance, and endocrine vasoconstrictor agents such as angiotensin II, antidiuretic hormone (ADH), and norepinephrine. Chronic regulation of blood pressure depends on the volume of blood in the system and, ultimately, is tied to renal regulation of body fluid balance.

■ LOCAL REGULATION OF BLOOD FLOW

If arterial pressure is sufficient, tissues can regulate their blood flow to match their metabolic needs. If blood flow is inadequate, metabolites such as carbon dioxide, adenosine, potassium, and acids accumulate, acting as vasodilators of the arteriolar smooth muscle only of that local area. The resulting increase in blood flow washes out the metabolites and diminishes the vasodilator stimulus. This control system allows tissue blood flow to increase as tissue metabolic activity increases and accounts for the period of increased blood flow that follows a period of occlusion. In the long term, inadequate blood flow to a tissue can cause the growth of new capillaries, again matching blood flow to the tissue's metabolic needs. Blood flow to tissues such as the brain and myocardium is dominated by local control.

At the other extreme of regulation, cutaneous blood flow responds primarily to neural control. Because skin blood flow is tied to thermoregulation rather than nutrition, metabolic control is poorly developed. Other vascular beds, such as the kidney and the splanchnic circulation, respond both to sympathetic control and to local control. During increased sympathetic activity, blood flow to these tissues is decreased and is shunted to the brain and the myocardium.

CARDIOVASCULAR ADJUSTMENT TO EXERCISE

Cardiovascular control must balance the need for a steady arterial blood pressure against the ability to respond to a physiologic challenge. Exercise, which increases skeletal muscle consumption of oxygen and other nutrients, requires a marked increase in both cardiac output and skeletal muscle blood flow. The increase in cardiac output results from a cerebral cortical stimulation of the medullary cardiovascular center and activation of the sympathetic nervous system. The increased cardiac output requires an increased venous return, accomplished both by the vasodilation of the skeletal muscle beds and by a sympathetic-mediated venoconstriction. In rhythmic activity such as running, compression of the veins by the contracting skeletal muscle along with the negative intrathoracic pressure from breathing assists the flow of blood toward the heart.

The increased cardiac output is preferentially directed to the exercising muscles (including the heart). Local factors in the exercising muscles cause a vasodilation of those vascular beds. The sympathetic activity constricts the arteriolar smooth muscle of the nonexercising vascular beds, such as the gastrointestinal tract, the kidney, and the nonworking muscles. Cerebral blood flow remains unchanged because that vascular bed is regulated primarily by local control. Cutaneous blood flow may be diminished initially but increases as the heat generated by the exercising muscles raises body core temperature, and cutaneous vasodilation helps to cool the body.

CONCLUSIONS

The vascular system is a series of vessels that transport blood to the capillary exchange vessels. In the capillaries, nutrients pass to the tissues and wastes pass into the blood for transport to excretory organs. Blood pressure regulation by the baroreceptor reflex ensures that arterial pressure remains sufficient to propel blood toward the tissues. Tissue blood flow is controlled by the metabolic needs of the tissues, and it increases when tissue metabolism increases.

BIBLIOGRAPHY

1. Berne, R., and Levy, M. (1998). *Physiology (4th ed.).* St. Louis: Mosby–Year Book.
2. Gartner, L., and Kiatt, J. (1997). *Color textbook of histology.* Philadelphia: W. B. Saunders.
3. Guyton, A., and Hall, J. (1996). *Textbook of medical physiology (9th ed.).* Philadelphia: W. B. Saunders.
4. Silverthorn, D. (1998). *Human physiology.* Saddle River, NJ: Prentice Hall.

CHAPTER

51

Assessment of the Vascular System

Mary Sieggreen

Peripheral vascular disease is common among elderly and diabetic clients. It is characterized by disturbances of blood flow through the peripheral vessels. These disturbances eventually damage tissues as a result of ischemia, excessive accumulation of waste and fluid, or both. Damage can be due to any disorder that narrows, obstructs, or injures blood vessels, thus impeding blood flow. Without intervention, damage may progress to the point of tissue or organ death. Assessment of the peripheral vascular system includes data collection through the health history, physical examination, and diagnostic tests when indicated.

HISTORY

When assessing the client, note risk factors for atherosclerosis (see Chapter 52), diabetes (see Chapter 45), and cardiac (see Chapters 55 and 58) as well as arterial, venous (see Chapter 53), and lymphatic disorders. Some clients are reluctant to mention what they believe to be minor symptoms. Consequently, perform a careful assessment, ask specific questions skillfully, and be alert for information that may indicate early manifestations of insidious conditions.

■ BIOGRAPHICAL AND DEMOGRAPHIC DATA

Biographical data include the client's age. Atherosclerosis (hardening of the arteries) is more prevalent in older people. Venous disease, although also more prevalent in the elderly, may be identified in younger people. Ask about occupation, and clarify whether the occupation increases the risk for vascular disease. If the client is retired, ask about the previous employment history.

■ CURRENT HEALTH

Ask about frequency and duration of clinical manifestations that may indicate a vascular disorder. The following section describes the typical chief complaints of clients who have arterial and venous disorders.

Chief Complaint

ARTERIAL DISORDERS

In arterial insufficiency of the lower extremities, the chief complaint is often cramping leg pain in the calf muscles during ambulation that disappears with 1 to 2 minutes of rest. The pain is called *intermittent claudication*. The pain occurs in the muscle group distal to the diseased artery (see Chapter 53).

Intermittent claudication results from inadequate tissue oxygenation (*ischemia*) due to arterial stenosis, usually secondary to atherosclerosis. It is a pathologic process similar to angina. Claudication is predictable and reproducible; this means that (1) the client can walk the same distance each time before pain occurs and (2) the pain occurs each time that this distance is walked.

As an artery becomes more stenosed, the pain may become more severe. When clients report distal forefoot burning, numbness or tingling, pain at rest, or pain that awakens them during the night (*rest pain*), urgent attention is needed. This pain is related to arterial disease and exacerbated by decreased cardiac output during sleep. The relative leg elevation while in a supine position decreases blood flow through stenosed arteries. Pain is relieved when the client stands because gravity pulls the blood toward the feet. Even during non-sleep hours, elevation of the legs decreases blood flow and increases pain. Clients may report that they sleep upright with the legs dependent (below heart level) to control pain.

Ask about precipitating factors, duration and persistence of the discomfort, the manner of its onset, and associated manifestations. Document the activity required to cause pain. The extent of disease involvement can be gauged by the distance the client is able to walk without pain, or *claudication distance*. For example, one client may be able to walk only one block before experiencing pain, whereas another may be able to walk six blocks.

Disorders of the aorta and iliac vessels can lead to impotence. If a male client has aortoiliac disease, ask about problems with penile erection. Sexuality may be a sensitive issue; ask questions carefully to elicit areas of concern or problems (see Chapters 9 and 37).

VENOUS DISORDERS

Chronic venous disease has an insidious onset. Many clients do not recall any precipitating event. There may be a positive family history for venous disease, a job history involving many hours of standing in one place, or multiple pregnancies. Obesity may be a factor. In contrast to the pain in arterial disorders, pain in chronic venous disease has a slow onset and is not associated with exercise or rest. Clients may also have varicose veins and a history of phlebitis. In these clients, the leg veins have been subjected to increased pressure and return of venous blood has been obstructed. Vein walls are compliant and distend with increased pressure. Valves become incompetent because the distended wall prevents the valve leaflets from meeting each other when they close. An *incompetent vein* allows the column of blood to flow backward, increasing the hydrostatic pressure in the venous end of the capillary. This increase in pressure against the vein wall moves fluid from the intravascular to the interstitial space, causing edema. As the process continues, blood flow slows and tissues become hypoxic (lacking in oxygen). The client may report a feeling of heaviness in the legs or nighttime cramping. Exercise and elevation generally relieve the discomfort and swelling because venous return of blood is improved.

In more severe forms of chronic venous disorders, lower extremity edema may be the initial complaint. Edema worsens toward the end of the day and diminishes after nighttime leg elevation. Pitting edema (see discussion of edema) may be seen at first, but as the edema becomes more chronic, tissue sclerosis develops and the tissue becomes more difficult to compress.

Initial skin changes noted with chronic venous disorders may include erythema (redness), followed in the late stages by lipodermatosclerosis (brawny, thick, darkly pigmented skin). The skin becomes dry and flaky, which leads to itching and scratching. Continued irritation results in stasis dermatitis, and the skin eventually ulcerates. Ulcers develop in the lower third of the leg, most commonly above the medial malleolus, where venous pressure is highest and there are more perforator veins than elsewhere in the leg. Chronic venous edema and sclerotic subcutaneous tissue may compress the lymph vessels.

Lymphatic disorders also lead to edema. If the lymphatic obstruction is prolonged, edematous tissue becomes fibrotic and almost impossible to compress. Chapter 74 describes the assessment of the lymphatic system.

Symptom Analysis

Vascular disease may be arterial, venous, or lymphatic. Table 51–1 compares the clinical manifestations of arterial and venous disorders in the lower extremities.

The client who has venous disease may report chronic aching pain in the legs when they are in a dependent position. Chronic venous insufficiency produces the following manifestations:

- Edema
- Dependent cyanosis
- Brown discoloration of the skin at the ankle
- Ulcers
- Pruritus

Skin temperature remains normal or slightly elevated and pulses are present, although they may be difficult to palpate through the edema.

Chronic arterial insufficiency produces the following manifestations:

- Decrease or absence of arterial pulses
- Thin, shiny, hairless skin
- Thick, ridged toenails
- Cool skin temperature
- Pain with ambulation (claudication)
- Pain with leg elevation, or at night (rest pain)

The skin is pale when the legs are elevated above heart level and dusky red after they are placed in a dependent position (*dependent rubor*). Edema is not usually present in pure arterial insufficiency. There may be ulcers from trauma, over pressure points, or on the tips of toes.

■ PAST HEALTH HISTORY

Note any history of vascular impairment. Inquire about changes that indicate vasospastic disorders, such as changes in color or temperature of digits. Ask specifically whether the client has a history of hypertension, diabetes, stroke, transient ischemic attacks (TIAs), changes in vision, pain in legs during activity, leg cramps, phlebitis, venous or arterial blood clots, pulmonary emboli, edema, varicose veins, leg ulcers, or extremities that are cold,

TABLE 51–1	CLINICAL MANIFESTATIONS IN LOWER EXTREMITY DISORDERS	
Manifestation	**Arterial Disorder**	**Venous Disorder**
Pain	Intermittent claudication. Rest pain may be present, or pain may worsen with elevation	Aching, heaviness Exercise and elevation decrease pain Nocturnal cramping Heaviness in the legs at the end of day
Skin	Absence of hair in chronic condition. Thin, shiny skin Thick toenails if fungal infection present	Brown discoloration Normal toenails
Color	Pale with dependent rubor	Brown discoloration. Dependent cyanosis
Temperature	Cool	No change, or may be warmer than unaffected areas
Sensation	Decreased; tingling, numbness may be present	Pruritus may be present
Pulses	Decreased to absent	Present, but may be difficult to palpate if edema is present
Edema	May be present but usually absent	Present, worse at end of day, improved with elevation
Muscle mass	Reduced in chronic disease	Unaffected in pure venous disease
Ulcers	Small, painful ulcers on pressure points, points of trauma, between toes, or distal most point, especially lateral malleolus and toes	Broad, shallow, slightly painful ulcers of the ankle and lower leg. Surrounding skin is brown, fibrotic

pale, or blue. Question any previous history of frostbite, which increases risk of vasospasm. Visual changes and TIAs may indicate carotid artery disease. Ask about any past medical tests, operations, or treatments involving the vascular system and about any previous treatment for diabetes mellitus, collagen disorders, or hypertension.

In addition, note medications that the client takes, including over-the-counter drugs and herbal remedies. Some medications increase risk for vascular disorders (e.g., birth control pills.

Herbal remedies used to self-treat peripheral vascular disorders include those for hypertension, varicose veins, atherosclerosis, and vascular spasm. Herbs with antihypertensive action include garlic (*Allium sativum*), hawthorn (*Crataegus oxyacantha*), kudzu (*Pueraria lobata*), nettle (*Urtica dioica*), onion (*Allium cepa*), purslane (*Portulaca oleracea*), reishi mushroom (*Ganoderma lucidum*), and valerian (*Valeriana officinalis*). Garlic is also thought to be preventive for atherosclerosis. *Ginkgo biloba* is used for varicose veins, obliterative arterial disease of the lower extremities, and intermittent claudication. Horse chestnut (*Aesculus hippocastanum*) is used for varicose veins and phlebitis, and valerian is used as an antispasmodic. Antihypertensive spices include basil, black pepper, fennel, and tarragon.

Note allergies, especially to iodine. Iodine is found in contrast agents used in diagnostic testing for vascular disorders.

■ FAMILY HEALTH HISTORY

The family health history helps to determine risk factors and provides clues about reported and observed manifestations. Note any family history of diabetes, hypertension, coronary artery disease, collagen diseases, and peripheral vascular disease.

■ PSYCHOSOCIAL HISTORY

Record the occupational history. If the client's occupation is unfamiliar to you, ask questions about the number of hours spent in various positions or activities (e.g., standing, prolonged sitting, walking, using vibrating machinery). In addition, some occupations involve contact with chemicals or are associated with cold or wet environments; note these also.

Find out whether or not the client smokes or has ever used any tobacco products. Ask about the use of prescription and over-the-counter nicotine products. Nicotine in any form is a potent vasoconstrictor.

Determine the client's nutrient and fluid intake (see Chapters 12 and 28). Ask about the usual intake of protein and calories. Also ask about sodium, cholesterol, and fat intake.

Assess the client's activity, rest, and sleep habits. Assess the extent to which clinical manifestations interfere with activities of daily living. Obtaining information about the frequency and duration of manifestations, precipitating activities, and their influence on daily life enables determination of disease severity. Assessment of the client's stress level, emotional state, and coping mechanisms (including the use of tobacco products, alcohol, or recreational drugs) is important.

Remain sensitive to the emotional effect of peripheral vascular disorders. Clients who have visible lesions may be embarrassed. Clients may have concern about the inability to perform self-care and about changes in role and sexual performance. Fear of amputation or functional loss may be significant.

■ REVIEW OF SYSTEMS

Review each body system as it relates to peripheral vascular disorders. Inquire about headaches, dizziness, TIAs, stroke, visual disturbances, hypertension, diabetes, pulmonary emboli, phlebitis, blood clots, leg pain or cramps, varicose veins, leg or foot ulcers, and cold hands or feet. Also see Chapter 9 for additional information about the review of systems.

PHYSICAL EXAMINATION

Physical examination of the vascular system involves inspection, palpation, and auscultation. Before starting the physical examination, prepare the environment. Natural lighting is the best because it allows assessment of subtleties in skin color. Warm the room to minimize cutaneous vasoconstriction. A quiet room is helpful for auscultating the low-pitched sounds commonly found in blood vessels. Clients who are free of vascular disorders display characteristics such as those described in the feature Physical Assessment in the Healthy Adult.

■ INSPECTION

Observe the extremities, noting skin color, hair distribution, nail beds and capillary refill, presence of muscle atrophy or edema, venous pattern, and ulcers. These are reviewed in detail next. Compare one side with the other. Begin with the head and upper extremities, and proceed toward the legs and feet.

Skin Color

A range of normal skin color is noted among people. Localized areas of cyanosis, rubor, or pallor are easily

---

PHYSICAL ASSESSMENT FINDINGS IN THE HEALTHY ADULT

Peripheral Vascular System

Inspection

Extremities of even contour, without edema. Even hair distribution; symmetrical venous pattern. Varicosities, skin lesions, and ulcers absent. Capillaries refill in less than 3 seconds on blanching.

Palpation

Extremities warm and dry without areas of localized heat or tenderness. Pulses (temporal, carotid, brachial, radial, ulnar, femoral, popliteal, posterior tibial, dorsalis pedis) are bilaterally equal and regular. No aneurysmal dilation of aorta.

Auscultation

Blood pressures equal in the upper extremities. Orthostatic hypotension absent. No bruits.

noticed in a person with fair skin (Fig. 51–1) but are more difficult to see in a person with darker skin tones (Fig. 51–2). For all clients, changes in skin color are best assessed by comparison with the contralateral limb. Ischemic pallor may be detected by comparing the palms of the hands, the soles of the feet, or the nail beds. Clients with arterial disorders may have pale extremities and cyanotic (blue-tinged) or red extremities with venous disorders.

Hair Distribution

Lack of hair growth may indicate chronically inadequate circulation to an area. This sign must be correlated with other signs of arterial insufficiency. It is not a valid indicator of acute arterial insufficiency.

Capillary Refill

Capillary refill time is an evaluation of peripheral perfusion and cardiac output. This assessment is usually com-

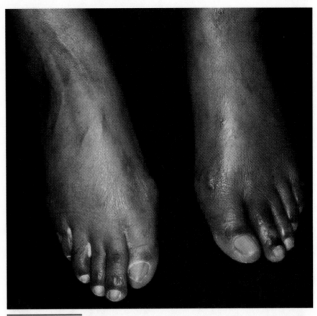

FIGURE 51–2 Dependent rubor in dark skin in the client's left foot has a reddish hue when compared to the unaffected right foot.

pleted while pulses are assessed. Depress the nail bed or the pad of the toe or finger until it blanches (becomes pale) (Fig. 51–3). Release pressure on the blanched area, and note the length of time for usual skin color to return. Capillaries usually refill in a fraction of a second, but "normal" times range up to 3 seconds for color return. With diminished blood flow, the return to the baseline color is delayed and a refill time of more than 3 seconds is sometimes called "sluggish." Note whether the room in which you are conducting the test is cold, because external temperatures can delay capillary refill.

Muscle Atrophy

There can be many reasons for muscle atrophy in an extremity. If atrophy is noted, it may represent long-standing arterial insufficiency. Measure the muscle circumference, and compare it with that of the muscle on the opposite side.

Edema

To assess edema of the leg, push with your thumb on the skin over the client's foot or tibia for 5 seconds. If the skin is edematous, an indentation or pit will remain (thus the term *pitting edema*). Edema is often graded; however, scales used to grade edema are not universal. Because there is no established standard, it is most accurate to describe the edema as *present* or *absent, pitting* or *non-pitting* (Fig. 51–4).

Edema resulting from cardiac disease is generally bilateral and occurs in dependent areas (in the legs of a client who is ambulatory and the sacrum of a client who is bedridden). Unilateral edema is usually caused by oc-

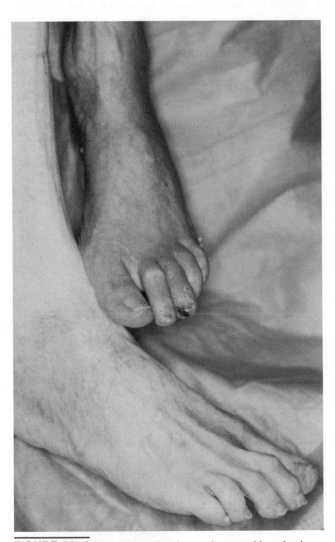

FIGURE 51–1 Dependent rubor is noted as a ruddy color in severe arterial insufficiency in this white client's left leg just minutes before amputation. (Note area of ulceration and necrosis on the third toe.)

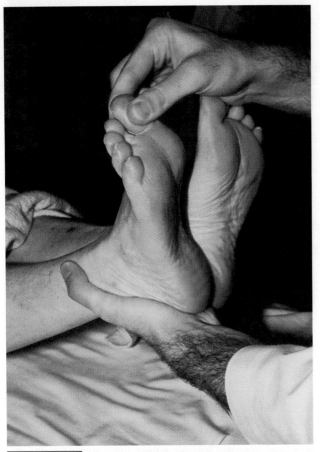

FIGURE 51–3 Determine capillary refill time by compressing the great toe and then releasing pressure. Count the number of seconds required for color to return to the skin.

clusion of a deep vein. Long-standing edema destroys the structure of the skin and the subcutaneous tissue and is easily recognized from its fibrotic appearance and firm texture.

Venous Pattern

Varicosities may indicate superficial or deep venous insufficiency. Note the presence, location, and distribution of *telangiectasias,* or "spider veins."

Ulcers

Note the presence of skin lesions or scar tissue (indicating healed ulcers); fissures of the feet and ulcers of the ankles and heels may be signs of arterial insufficiency. Tissue necrosis (see Fig. 51–1) and gangrene may be present with severe arterial disease. Examine between the toes for moist ulcers penetrating into the web spaces (Fig. 51–5).

Note the presence of other lesions, such as *angiomas* (benign tumors of blood and lymph vessels) and *petechiae* (small, purplish spots on the skin from several causes, including hemorrhage).

Additional Inspections

If arterial or venous disease is suspected but not confirmed, additional assessments can be performed, such as elevation pallor and Trendelenburg's test.

ELEVATION PALLOR

If arterial insufficiency is suspected, perform the test for elevation pallor. Because leg elevation can cause pain, perform this test only when needed. Note the degree of pallor at rest, and use the test only to determine the severity of ischemia. Perform the test as follows:

1. Elevate the legs 30 cm (12 inches) (Fig. 51–6). Pallor occurring within 60 seconds indicates arterial insufficiency.
2. Have the client dangle the legs from the side of the bed or examination table. Normally, the color returns within 10 seconds. Severe arterial insufficiency causes an exaggerated color change of dependent rubor.

FIGURE 51–4 To assess peripheral edema, press a finger into the skin over the client's tibia. Note the presence, depth, and persistence of any resulting depression. Use descriptive terms to record your findings.

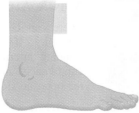

No edema

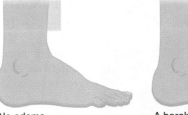

A barely detectable depression accompanied by normal foot and leg contours

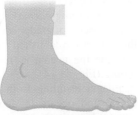

A deeper depression (less than 5 mm) accompanied by normal foot and leg contours

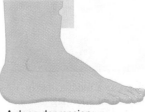

A deep depression (5 to 10 mm) accompanied by foot and leg swelling

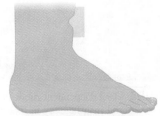

An even deeper depression (more than 1 cm) accompanied by severe foot and leg swelling

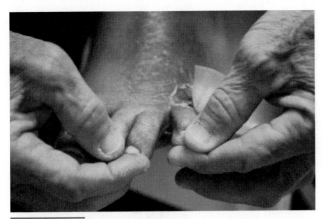

FIGURE 51–5 Carefully examine the web spaces for ulcers or maceration when assessing the foot.

TRENDELENBURG'S TEST

Intended to help detect abnormal venous filling time, Trendelenburg's test reveals valvular incompetence of the deep veins. Superficial varicose veins are easy to recognize. They appear as dilated, tortuous (twisted) veins. This test helps confirm leg vein valve competence. This noninvasive assessment maneuver may be performed by nurses who possess advanced assessment skills, as follows:

1. Have client lie down with the leg elevated until the veins empty.
2. Apply a tourniquet at midthigh snugly enough to occlude the superficial veins.
3. With the tourniquet in place, help the client stand.
4. Note the time required for the veins to fill from below. Veins usually fill in about 30 seconds.
5. After 60 seconds, release the tourniquet. Normally, when the tourniquet is released, no further blood fills the veins. Additional blood flowing into the vein from above indicates that a valve is incompetent and has allowed back-flow of blood.

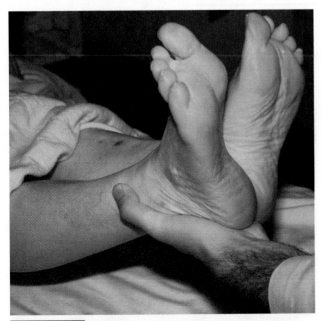

FIGURE 51–6 Assess for elevation pallor if arterial insufficiency is suspected.

■ PALPATION

Temperature

Palpate the arms and legs with the dorsal surface of your hand, and note the temperature (see Chapter 48, Fig. 48–3). Temperature should be similar in both contralateral limbs. Vasoconstriction produces cold, pale skin. Bilateral vasoconstriction may be caused by smoking, environmental temperature, anxiety, or generalized arterial disease. Unilateral or localized arterial vasoconstriction indicates arterial disease. Venous disorders may cause an increase in local skin temperature.

Pulses

Palpate pulses by placing the first three fingers of your dominant hand along the length of the selected artery. Apply gentle pressure against the artery, followed by a gradual release. Palpate temporal, carotid, brachial, radial, and ulnar pulses (upper extremities), and femoral, popliteal, posterior tibial, and dorsalis pedis pulses (lower extremities), as shown in Figure 51–7. Palpate pulses bilaterally and simultaneously, except for the carotid pulse (Fig. 51–8). Palpate carotid pulses separately to avoid stimulation of the carotid sinus, which may produce bradycardia or sinus arrest. Assess the ulnar pulse during Allen's test, as described later.

Palpate the abdominal aortic pulse by placing the palm of your hand over the upper abdomen just beneath the sternum while the client is supine. Use gentle pressure to push the abdomen downward. When you feel the aortic pulse, cup your fingers and thumb together to determine the width of the aorta (Fig. 51–9). You can use both hands if the client is large. When using both hands, place the lateral side of your right hand just left of the midline of the abdomen. Palpate using gentle pressure on the side of the aorta. Then place your left hand to the right of the abdominal midline. Estimate the width of the aorta as it pulsates toward your hands. In very obese clients, you may not be able to feel the aorta.

Always note the rhythm, amplitude, and symmetry of pulses. Compare peripheral pulses on the two sides for rate, rhythm, and quality. There are no standard numerical grades or rating scales for pulses. It is most accurate to describe the pulse as *palpable* (or present), *diminished* (weak), *absent,* or *aneurysmal* (easily palpable, bounding).

Note whether a pulse feels unequal on the two sides. The dorsalis pedis pulse is congenitally absent in approximately 10% to 17% of the normal adult population. The posterior tibial pulse is absent congenitally in 9% of the black adult population of the United States. In the elderly, dorsalis pedis and posterior tibial pulses may be more difficult to palpate. If they are found, mark the site with a pen to facilitate later examinations. Clients who have arterial grafts may have palpable pulses along the length of the graft.

If there is any question about the presence of a specific pulse, position your hand below the pulse you are seeking; then attempt to palpate the client's pulse again. This position will reduce the chance of mistaking your pulse for that of the client by establishing the difference between the two pulses.

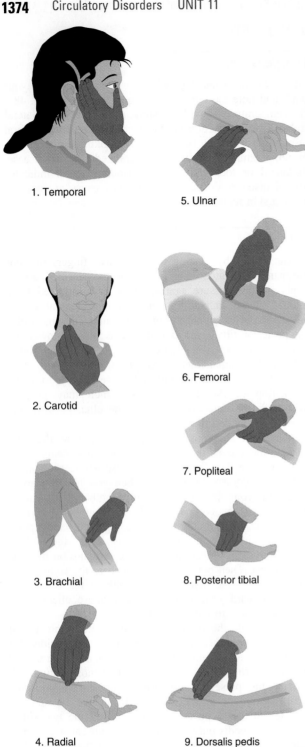

1. Temporal

5. Ulnar

2. Carotid

6. Femoral

3. Brachial

7. Popliteal

4. Radial

8. Posterior tibial

9. Dorsalis pedis

FIGURE 51–7 Assess pulses bilaterally from head to toe, comparing one side to the other for amplitude, rhythm, and symmetry. To prevent possible carotid sinus massage, do not palpate carotid pulses simultaneously. The carotid sinus is nerve tissue, located in the wall of the carotid artery, that helps regulate blood pressure. Massaging over this area may cause sinus bradycardia or syncope.

Allen's Test

Blood flow to the hand is supplied by both the ulnar and the radial arteries, which join at the volar arch in the palm. Allen's test is used to assess the patency of the

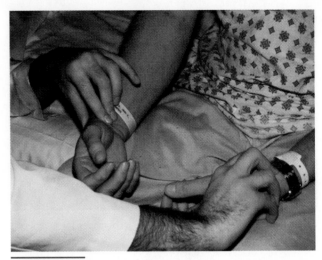

FIGURE 51–8 Palpating radial pulses.

radial and ulnar arteries distal to the wrist. It is commonly performed before arterial blood samples are drawn for analysis (see Chapter 14) or before an arterial line is inserted (see Chapter 55). Perform Allen's test as follows:

1. Ask the client to make a tight fist while you compress the radial and ulnar arteries.
2. Have the client open the hand, which should be pale and mottled.
3. Release the pressure on the radial artery while continuing to compress the ulnar artery. If the client's hand regains full color within about 6 seconds, the radial artery has normal patency.
4. Repeat steps 1 to 3, this time releasing the pressure on the ulnar artery to assess its patency.

If the client's hand remains pale during either portion of the test, the artery being tested may be occluded. Allen's test is shown in Chapter 59, Figure 59–14.

Homans' Sign

The test for Homans' sign involves gently compressing the gastrocnemius muscle of the calf and asking the client whether this maneuver causes pain or tenderness. The test

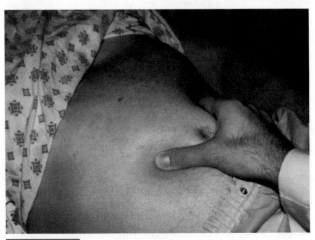

FIGURE 51–9 Palpate the abdomen for aortic aneurysm.

can also be performed by quickly dorsiflexing the foot (pointing the toes downward); calf pain that occurs with this maneuver is a positive finding of Homans' sign.

Homans' sign is unreliable, however. Studies indicate that only about 35% of people with deep venous thrombosis (DVT) have a positive response to Homans' test. Superficial phlebitis, Achilles' tendinitis, and plantar muscle injury can also elicit a positive Homans' sign. Therefore, 50% of the people who display a positive response to Homans' test do not have DVT. Doppler studies (see later discussion) are more accurate and should be used to confirm the diagnosis.

■ AUSCULTATION

Limb Blood Pressure

The measurement of arterial blood pressure is the most commonly performed noninvasive test of cardiac and vascular function. It may be the best single indicator of arterial perfusion. Arterial stenosis or occlusion produces regional hypotension. Arterial blood pressure is measured with a sphygmomanometer and a properly fitting cuff. For an accurate reading, place the cuff on the client's arm at the level of the heart; it should be wide enough to transmit pressure to the center of the arm and long enough to encircle the arm firmly. Auscultate the blood pressure in both arms. A few points' difference between readings is normal. A difference of 20 mm Hg between extremity readings may indicate aortic dissection or subclavian artery stenosis. Document asymmetrical readings. All subsequent blood pressure measurements should be performed on the arm with the higher reading. Measure blood pressure while the client is in supine, sitting, and standing positions when possible, and document the position of the client and the site used for each reading. Note *orthostatic* (positional) changes in blood pressure.

Auscultate over the carotid artery, aorta, and renal, femoral, and popliteal arteries to assess for the presence of bruits. A *bruit* is a "whooshing" sound that may be soft or loud; it results from turbulent blood flow from vessel wall irregularities. The presence of a bruit indicates some arterial narrowing. These arterial sounds are best heard with the bell of the stethoscope.

DIAGNOSTIC TESTS

■ NONINVASIVE VASCULAR LABORATORY TECHNIQUES

Noninvasive diagnostic techniques have assumed an increasingly important role in the management of vascular disorders. Noninvasive diagnostic tests provide reliable, objective data that can be used to evaluate the extent of vascular disease. Variables include blood flow velocity, blood flow abnormality, and some measure of functional limitations.

Doppler Ultrasonography

Hand-held Doppler ultrasonographic instruments permit assessment of arterial disease through (1) evaluation of audible arterial signals or (2) measurement of limb blood pressures (Fig. 51–10). Doppler ultrasonography is sim-

ple and inexpensive, but the technique may not detect minor disease, and it is less accurate than duplex scanning (see later). There is no special client preparation for this test.

Brightness-mode (*B-mode*) ultrasound refers to the creation of a two-dimensional image from ultrasound waves. It can be used to assess a vessel's size and compressibility, flow patterns, the presence or absence of thrombus, and valve function.

Ankle-Brachial Index

The ankle-brachial index (ABI) is a commonly used parameter for overall evaluation of extremity status. There is no special preparation for this test.

The client assumes a supine position, and a regular arm blood pressure cuff is applied to the leg above the malleolus. Doppler probes are used to identify the systolic end-point at both the dorsalis pedis and the posterior tibial sites (see Fig. 51–7). The higher of the two pressures is used as the indication of ankle blood pressure status. This number is then divided by the higher of the two brachial systolic artery pressures by means of the following formula:

$$\text{Ankle-brachial index} = \frac{\text{higher systolic ankle pressure}}{\text{higher systolic brachial pressure}}$$

A systolic ankle pressure of 60 mm Hg with a systolic brachial pressure of 120 mm Hg yields an ABI of 0.5. In normal circulation, ankle pressure is the same as or higher than the brachial pressure. Thus, an ABI of 1 or more is considered a normal finding; the client with an ABI of 0.5 to 0.8 typically experiences claudication, and the client with an ABI of 0.4 or less typically experiences rest pain.

In the presence of diabetes, the ABI is artificially elevated because of calcification, which prevents vessel wall compression. A toe-brachial index (TBI) is more reliable in clients who have diabetes (see Fig. 51–10).

Ultrasonic Duplex Scanning

Ultrasonic duplex scanners are used to (1) localize vascular obstruction, (2) evaluate the degree of stenosis, and (3) determine the presence or absence of vascular reflux (backward flow). This anatomic and physiologic test eval-

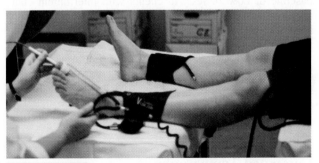

FIGURE 51–10 A Doppler probe is used to check toe pressures in the client with diabetes. Ankle pressures may be erroneously high because of calcification in the vessel wall.

uates the hemodynamic effects of arterial lesions. It is also the most sensitive and specific noninvasive modality for detecting DVT. Both an ultrasound image of the vessel and a Doppler audible signal and waveform are provided. The visual ultrasound data allow more specific localization of stenosis than simple pressure or waveform techniques. No special client preparation is required.

Air Plethysmography

Air plethysmography (APG) uses a pneumatic plethysmograph to measure volume changes in the legs. Venous reflux, venous obstruction, calf muscle pump function, and venous volume can be measured. A large cuff is applied to the client's calf, and a known volume of air is instilled to calibrate the cuff. Venous volume, ejection fraction, and residual volume fractions are then measured.

Impedance Plethysmography

Impedance plethysmography (IPG) and photoplethysmography (PPG) are also used to measure venous blood volume changes in the extremities. During the procedure, electrodes from a plethysmograph are applied to a limb along with a pressure cuff. As pressure is increased, electrical resistance is increased; thus, the quality of venous blood flow is demonstrated.

Inform the client about the purpose of the procedure. Explain that a technique similar to blood pressure measurement will be used. The client must be able to assume a supine position with the involved extremity elevated above the level of the heart.

Exercise Testing

Exercise or stress testing provides an objective measurement of the severity of intermittent claudication. It suggests the extent to which intermittent claudication interferes with the client's lifestyle. The most commonly used method for stress testing is the *treadmill exercise test*. This test is similar to that used for clients who have had a myocardial infarction, except that walking speed is usually 1.5 to 2 miles per hour (mph) with a grade elevation of 10% to 20% and a time limit of 5 minutes. A client who can walk 5 minutes is considered mildly symptomatic; a walking time of 1 minute represents severe disease.

Performance on the treadmill test is also gauged by measurement of ankle systolic pressure. In asymptomatic clients, the time required for return to pre-exercise ankle pressure is usually less than 3 minutes with a drop from baseline of 20% or less. In clients with intermittent claudication, recovery time is longer; ankle pressure is usually less than 50 mm Hg, and may be unrecordable during recovery.

The client undergoing stress testing should wear loose-fitting clothes and comfortable walking shoes. Explain the procedure so that the client knows what to expect. Inform the client that exercise will be stopped at the maximal level of exertion or when clinical manifestations become disabling.

Computed Tomography

Computed tomography (CT) provides a cross-section of vessel walls and other structures. CT scans can be used in the diagnosis of abdominal aortic aneurysms and postoperative complications, such as graft infection, graft occlusion, hemorrhage, and abscess. Chapter 11 covers client preparation during CT.

Magnetic Resonance Imaging

Magnetic resonance imaging (MRI) is used to detect tissue changes, such as tumors, aneurysms, and DVT, in the pelvic iliac veins and leg veins (see Chapter 11). Blood flow in an extremity is evaluated, with the limb to be examined placed in a cradle-like support in a flow cylinder.

In the future, MRI techniques likely will supply much of the information that today is available only with invasive angiography. Although MRI does not require ionizing radiation or injection into the arterial system, the expense and time necessary limit its use for routine screening and follow-up.

Magnetic Resonance Angiography

Magnetic resonance angiography (MRA) uses magnetic imaging techniques to access blood vessels. The advantage of this technique is that the images are not obscured by bone, bowel gas, fat, or vascular calcification. The vessel anatomy is displayed as a three-dimensional angiogram. MRA can be used to measure blood flow volume and blood viscosity. It is a noninvasive modality. The disadvantages are its limited availability, its cost, and the need for the client to hold still during the procedure. MRA cannot be used for people who have cardiac pacemakers or intracranial aneurysm clips.

■ INVASIVE TECHNIQUES

Angiography

Contrast angiography is the most invasive of the diagnostic procedures for arterial disorders and poses the greatest risk for the client. It is frequently performed before a vascular operation and can be used intraoperatively to evaluate the results of an operation.

PROCEDURE

The procedure involves injecting a contrast agent into the arterial system and performing radiographic studies. Angiography is performed in an interventional laboratory or a special procedures room in the radiology department. The procedure is performed under sterile conditions. Local anesthesia is given at the injection site, and a catheter is placed percutaneously. After injection of a contrast agent through the catheter, fluoroscopy may be performed. Serial pictures of the dye movement are taken by cameras positioned over the study field (see Chapter 11).

PREPROCEDURE CARE

Explain the procedure, and obtain an informed consent. The client is given nothing by mouth (NPO) for 2 to 6 hours before the procedure. A mild sedative may be used.

POSTPROCEDURE CARE

Nursing care after angiography usually involves routine postprocedural orders, including the following:

1. Frequent assessment of vital signs and neurologic function and distal pulse checks, with particular attention to the extremity that has been punctured.
2. Assessment of the puncture site for hematoma (bruising) and of the appearance of the extremity distal to the puncture site.
3. Bed rest for 6 to 8 hours, with the punctured extremity kept in straight alignment if the transfemoral approach was used. Use of the transaxillary approach does not require postprocedure bed rest.
4. Continuous intravenous (IV) hydration for 6 to 8 hours to assist with contrast excretion. Encourage oral fluid intake.
5. Assessment of blood urea nitrogen (BUN) and creatinine levels the next day.
6. Resumption of preprocedure diet and medications. If the client was receiving heparin, its administration may not be resumed until sealing of the puncture site has been confirmed.

Also assess motor and sensory function, especially if the client has undergone catheter insertion at the axillary site. Bleeding can compress the brachial plexus, resulting in permanent neurologic deficits. Report changes in neurologic function of the upper extremity immediately because they require emergency attention from the physician.

Pain at the injection site is fairly common and can usually be managed with mild analgesics. Severe pain or pain distal to the puncture site requires further assessment of peripheral pulses, neurovascular assessment, and palpation for masses, which may indicate a hematoma. Notify the physician of abnormal assessment data.

Complications of angiography, in addition to allergic reaction to the contrast medium, include thrombi, vessel wall perforation, emboli, renal failure, and pseudoaneurysm. *Pseudoaneurysm* is a significant complication and may extend the inpatient stay. A pseudoaneurysm is caused by blood leaking outside the vessel wall but within a contained area adjacent to the artery. There is a persistent communication between the artery and the fluid mass. Pseudoaneurysms generally result from arterial trauma (after arterial puncture). They provide a site for potential infection, can be a source of emboli, or may cause intravascular thrombosis. Pseudoaneurysms can become enlarged, compress an adjacent structure, and even rupture, although rupture is rare.

Venography

Venography, performed in a manner similar to that for angiography, is used to examine the venous system. Venograms can be used to detect DVT and other abnormalities, such as incompetent valves. This diagnostic test is performed less frequently than in the past. Newer, noninvasive vascular laboratory studies pose less risk, are more accurate, and provide functional information.

PROCEDURE

For an *ascending* venogram, dye is injected into a vein in the foot to record patency of the veins. A *descending* venogram involves injecting a contrast agent into the femoral vein at the groin to evaluate vein reflux and valve incompetence.

PREPROCEDURE CARE

Document the presence and quality of peripheral pulses before the procedure. The client is usually given clear liquids for 3 to 4 hours before the procedure to help maintain adequate hydration. (See the earlier discussion of angiography and Chapter 11 for information about client preparation, informed consent, and use of contrast medium.)

POSTPROCEDURE CARE

After the procedure, a pressure dressing is placed on the injection site. The client should remain at bed rest for 2 hours after the procedure if the femoral vein was punctured. Monitor pulses distal to the site for the next 4 to 6 hours. Continue IV fluids for 8 to 24 hours after the procedure to help promote dye excretion. Assess fluid balance: observe for signs of fluid overload (also see Chapter 12). When the client returns to the nursing unit, monitor vital signs, palpate pulses, and observe the insertion site frequently for bleeding or hematoma formation.

Vascular Endoscopy (Angioscopy)

Vascular endoscopy permits imaging of intra-arterial disease with the use of fiberoptic technology. Images are in color and in three dimensions. Equipment consists of a flexible fiberoptic angioscope, a light source, an irrigation system, a camera, a video recorder, and a monitor. The major advantage of angioscopy is the internal visualization of the vessel lumen. This enables identification of thrombus (blood clot), plaque, hemorrhage, ulceration, or embolus (clot that has broken off from a thrombus and lodged in a more distal artery). Angioscopes can be used to remove debris from vessels and to check the integrity of an anastomosis (suture line that connects a vessel grafted to a native vessel) from within a vessel. They may also be used to remove venous valves in preparation for use of the vein as a bypass graft.

Complications of vascular endoscopy are rare but may include intimal damage, vessel spasm, thrombosis or embolism, perforation, fluid overload, and infection. Postprocedure care is similar to that for clients who have undergone angiography.

Intravascular Ultrasonography

Intravascular ultrasonography provides information about the atherosclerotic intima beneath the luminal surface. It can thus determine the thickness of the arterial wall and can distinguish thrombus and calcium from vascular tissue, allowing more exact removal of lesions. One current limiting factor is the need for specialized interpretation of the scans.

CONCLUSIONS

Vascular assessment requires inspection, palpation, and auscultation skills. Knowledge of anatomy is critical for correct performance of assessments. Diagnostic modalities can range from simple noninvasive tests to complex, sophisticated, invasive technology. A clear understanding of the indications for diagnostic tests and interpretation of the findings assists the clinical decision-making.

BIBLIOGRAPHY

1. Baker, J. D. (1991). Assessment of peripheral arterial occlusive disease. *Critical Care Nursing Clinics of North America, 3*(3), 493–498.
2. Barnes, R. W. (1991). Noninvasive diagnostic assessment of peripheral vascular disease. *Circulation, 83*(suppl. I), I-20–I-27.
3. Bright, L. D., & Georgi, S. (1992). Peripheral vascular disease: Is it arterial or venous? *American Journal of Nursing, 92*(9), 34–43.
4. Fahey, V. (1999). *Vascular nursing* (3rd ed.). Philadelphia: W. B. Saunders.
5. Herbert, L. M. (1997). *Caring for the vascular patient.* New York: Churchill Livingstone.
6. Kerstein, M. D., & White, J. V. (1995). *Alternatives to open vascular surgery.* Philadelpia: J. B. Lippincott.
7. Moore, W. S. (Ed). (1998). *Vascular surgery: A comprehensive review.* Philadelphia: W. B. Saunders.
8. Rutherford, R. B. (Ed). (2000). *Vascular surgery* (5th ed.). Philadelphia: W. B. Saunders.
9. Sloan, H., & Wills, E. M. (1999). Ankle-brachial index: Calculating your patient's vascular risks. *Nursing, 99*(10), 58–59.

REMEMBER *to* *check out your* **Companion CD ROM**

C H A P T E R

52

Clients with Hypertensive Disorders: Promoting Positive Outcomes

Jean Elizabeth DeMartinis

HYPERTENSION

Arterial hypertension, simply put, is high blood pressure. It is defined as a persistent elevation of the systolic blood pressure at a level of 140 mm Hg or higher and of diastolic pressure at a level of 90 mm Hg or higher. The National Institute of Health's Sixth Report of the Joint National Committee on Detection, Evaluation, and Treatment of High Blood Pressure (JNC VI) and the Centers for Disease Control and Prevention (CDC) publications *Healthy People 2000* and *Healthy People 2010* have documented the advances made over the last few decades regarding prevention, detection, and treatment of hypertension.[16, 25] Members of the public have become more knowledgeable about high blood pressure, are more likely to visit a health care provider for hypertension, and are more likely to follow medical advice. The use of increasingly effective antihypertensive agents has also dramatically reduced the mortality rate associated with hypertension. The percentage of people receiving treatment for their hypertension has increased from 31% to 55%, and of those with controlled hypertension, from 10% to 29%.

Ultimately, the combined effects of these measures have contributed to a 60% decline in stroke and a 53% decline in coronary artery disease mortality.[13] These impressive gains have been seen across all age groups, in both men and women, and in special populations.

However, the JNC VI and *Healthy People 2010* reports also document some disturbing current trends. After years of decline, the mortality rates for coronary heart disease and stroke leveled off and have begun to rise again. Hypertension prevalence is on the rise, and control rates are decreasing. Arterial hypertension affects approximately 50 million persons—1 in 4—in the United States, with the highest rates of occurrence among the elderly, African Americans, less educated, and poorer people. It is estimated that only 25% of all people with hypertension have blood pressure controlled at a target level below 140/90 mm Hg. Lack of client compliance and providers' continued ignorance of the need to prescribe and manage holistic treatment protocols are cited as the two major factors that have contributed to this abysmal decline in improvement in client outcomes toward identification and control of their hypertension.[9, 11, 16, 25]

Coronary events such as a "heart attack" are still the most common result of hypertension.[30] Increased blood pressure level is related to increased severity of atherosclerosis, stroke, nephropathy, peripheral vascular disease, aortic aneurysms, and heart failure. Nearly all people with heart failure have antecedent hypertension. If hypertension is left untreated, nearly half of hypertensive clients will die of heart disease, a third will die of stroke, and the remaining 10% to 15% will die of renal failure.[16] Hypertension is also a "silent factor" in the etiology of many deaths attributed to stroke or heart attacks.[25, 26]

These disturbing trends indicate the need for renewed vigor in the battle against hypertension.[23] Hypertension-related morbidity and mortality will not decrease until providers appreciate the need for changes in existing treatment protocols that support a comprehensive holistic management plan, and that are based on quantifiable client outcomes. The *Healthy People 2000/2010* guidelines are prevention-focused, and the JNC VI guidelines are also now primarily prevention-focused and strongly recommend the use of nonpharmaceutical as well as pharmaceutical measures to prevent and treat hypertension.[16, 25] Nurses are faced with a profound urgency to enhance public and professional education toward this end and to translate the results of research into improved practice.[30] An ambitious, but nevertheless feasible, goal is the diagnosis and treatment of hypertension in all affected people in the United States.

Types of Hypertensive Disease, Etiology, and Severity

Hypertension is characterized by type, cause, and severity (Box 52–1).[2, 10–12, 17, 23, 24] People with hypertensive disease have either combined systolic and diastolic elevations in pressure or isolated systolic pressure elevation alone. The blood pressure remains elevated and continues to rise over time because of a persistent and progressive increase in peripheral arterial resistance. The persistent rise in arterial resistance is due to inappropriate renal retention of salt and water and/or abnormalities of or within the vessel wall. The severity of the condition directly relates to the number and magnitude of risk factors present, the length of time for which these risk factors have been present, and the presence of accompanying disease states.

Epidemiology and Risk Factors

Primary *(essential)* hypertension constitutes more than 90% of all cases of hypertension. Fewer than 5% to 8% of adult hypertensive clients have secondary hypertension. However, hypertension, regardless of type, results from an array of genetic and environmental factors. The following text discusses the major nonmodifiable and modifiable risk factors that contribute to the development of hypertension. There is necessarily some overlap between categories.[2, 10, 12, 16, 24]

Secondary hypertension is an elevation in blood pressure from an identifiable disease, such as renal failure. *Malignant* hypertension, or persistent severe hypertension, is a sustained elevation in blood pressure combined with end-organ damage.

NONMODIFIABLE RISK FACTORS

FAMILY HISTORY. Hypertension is thought to be polygenic and multifactorial—that is, in any person with a family history of hypertension, several genes may interact with each other and the environment to cause the blood pressure to elevate over time. The genetic predisposition that makes certain families more susceptible to hypertension may be related to an elevation in intracellular sodium levels and to lowered potassium-to-sodium ratios. This is found more often in blacks. Clients with parents who have hypertension are at greater risk for hypertension at a younger age.

AGE. Primary hypertension typically appears between the ages of 30 and 50 years. The incidence of hypertension increases with age; 50% to 60% of clients older than 60 years have a blood pressure over 140/90 mm Hg.

BOX 52–1 **Types of Hypertension**

Primary hypertension—also known as *essential* or idiopathic hypertension. The etiology is a multifactorial, with no identifiable cause, but several interacting homeostatic forces are generally involved concomitantly. Most cases of combined systolic and diastolic elevation fall into this category. Severity of sequelae increases as the blood pressure, both systolic and diastolic, increases.

Secondary hypertension—results from an identifiable cause. Various specific disease states or problems are responsible for the elevation in blood pressure (see Box 52–2), and underlying causes may be correctable. Therefore, it is important to isolate the root of the problem so that the most appropriate treatment regimen can be prescribed. Severity depends on underlying causes, personal and environmental factors, and duration of concurrent disease states.

"White coat hypertension"—defined as hypertension in people who are actually normotensive except when their blood pressure is measured by a health care professional. An intermittent vasovagal response accounts for the transient elevation in blood pressure. Differentiation between this diagnosis and essential or secondary hypertension is crucial so that the latter can be treated effectively. Treating this false hypertension produces significant hypotension and severe deleterious sequelae. However, the converse is also true; essential or secondary hypertension disguised as "white coat" hypertension and left undiagnosed and untreated can have ominous consequences over time.

Isolated systolic hypertension (ISH)—occurs when the systolic blood pressure is 140 mm Hg or higher but the diastolic blood pressure remains less than 90 mm Hg. It is thought to emerge because of increased cardiac output or atherosclerosis-induced changes in blood vessel compliance or both in older adults. The likelihood of development of ISH increases with advancing age, as does the severity of ISN.

Malignant hypertension—persistent *severe* hypertension characterized by a diastolic blood pressure above 110 to 120 mm Hg. It results when hypertension is left untreated or is unresponsive to treatment and becomes a truly severe emergency condition as the pressure continues to rise unchecked.

However, epidemiologic studies have shown a poorer prognosis in clients whose hypertension began at a young age. Isolated systolic hypertension occurs primarily in people older than 50 years, with almost 24% of all people affected by age 80 years. Among older adults, systolic blood pressure readings are a better predictor of possible future events such as coronary heart disease, stroke, heart failure, and renal disease than are diastolic blood pressure readings.

GENDER. The overall incidence of hypertension is higher in men than in women until about age 55 years. Between the ages of 55 and 74 years, the risk in men and that in women are almost equal; then, after age 74 years, women are at greater risk. Men are also at greater risk for cardiovascular morbidity and mortality. The reasons are not clear.

ETHNICITY. Mortality statistics indicate that the death rate for adults with hypertension is lowest for white women at 4.7%; white men have the next lowest rate at 6.3%, and black men have the next lowest at 22.5%; the death rate is highest for black women at 29.3%. The reason for the increased prevalence of hypertension among blacks is unclear, but the increase has been attributed to lower renin levels, greater sensitivity to vasopressin, higher salt intake, and greater environmental stress.

MODIFIABLE RISK FACTORS

STRESS. Because stress is a matter of perception, people's interpretations of events are what create most stressors and stress responses. Environmental factors or events, personality characteristics, and physiologic phenomena may either cause or set the stage for the mobilization of the stress response. Stressors such as noise, infection, inflammation, pain, decreased oxygen supply, heat, cold, trauma, prolonged exertion, responses to life events, obesity, old age, drugs, disease, surgery, and medical treatment can elicit the stress response. These noxious stimuli are perceived by a person as a threat or capable of causing harm, and subsequently a psychophysiologic "fight-or-flight" response is initiated in the body.

Stress increases peripheral vascular resistance and cardiac output and stimulates sympathetic nervous system activity. Over time, hypertension can develop. Chronic stress, when unable to be stopped, will aggravate existing physical and emotional instability, further exacerbating the response. Should stress arousal be excessive or prolonged, target organ dysfunction or disease will result. A report from the American Institute of Stress estimates that 60% to 90% of all primary care visits involve stress-related complaints.[3]

OBESITY. Obesity, especially in the upper body (giving an "apple" shape), with increased amounts of fat about the midriff, waist, and abdomen, is associated with subsequent development of hypertension. However, people who are overweight but who carry most of their excess weight in the buttocks, hips, and thighs (giving a "pear" shape) are at far less risk for development of hypertension secondary to increased weight alone.

NUTRIENTS. Sodium consumption can be an important factor in the development of essential hypertension. A high-salt diet may induce excessive release of natriuretic hormone, which may indirectly increase blood pressure. Sodium loading also stimulates vasopressor mechanisms within the central nervous system (CNS). Studies also show that low dietary intake of calcium, potassium, and magnesium can contribute to the development of hypertension.

SUBSTANCE ABUSE. Cigarette smoking, heavy alcohol consumption, and some illicit drug use all are risk factors for hypertension. The nicotine in cigarette smoke and drugs such as cocaine cause an immediate rise in blood pressure that is dose-dependent; however, *habitual* use of these substances has been implicated in increased incidence of hypertension over time. The incidence of hypertension is also higher among people who drink more than 3 ounces of ethanol per day. The impact of caffeine is controversial. Caffeine raises blood pressure acutely but does not have sustained effects.

Pathophysiology

PRIMARY (ESSENTIAL) HYPERTENSION

The exact pathologic underpinnings of primary hypertension remain to be established. Any factor producing an alteration in peripheral vascular resistance, heart rate, or stroke volume affects systemic arterial blood pressure. Four control systems play a major role in maintaining blood pressure[12]: (1) the arterial baroreceptor and chemoreceptors system, (2) regulation of body fluid volume, (3) the renin-angiotensin system, and (4) vascular autoregulation. Hypotheses derived to explain the onset of primary hypertension in people at risk propose that a defect or malfunction must exist in some or all of these systems. Probably no single defect causes essential hypertension in all affected people.

Arterial baroreceptors and chemoreceptors work reflexively to control blood pressure (Fig. 52–1). Baroreceptors, major stretch receptors, are found in the carotid sinus, aorta, and wall of the left ventricle. They monitor the level of arterial pressure and counteract rises through vasodilatation and slowing of the heart rate via the vagus nerve. Chemoreceptors, located in the medulla and carotid and aortic bodies, are sensitive to changes in concentrations of oxygen, carbon dioxide, and hydrogen ions (pH) in the blood. A decrease in arterial oxygen concentration or pH causes a reflexive rise in pressure, whereas an increase in carbon dioxide concentration causes a decrease in blood pressure. The major reflex response is to changes in oxygen saturation, and effects of changes in pH and carbon dioxide are minor.

The role of the arterial baroreceptors and chemoreceptors in hypertension is not well understood. The stretch receptors may become desensitized because they must continue to "reset" as prolonged, sustained increases in pressure continue. Chemoreceptor autoregulation may be altered as blood volume rises, and sympathetic overstimulation becomes apparent.

Changes in fluid volume affect systemic arterial pressure. Thus, an abnormality in the transport of sodium in the renal tubules may cause essential hypertension. When sodium and water are in excess, total blood volume increases, thereby increasing blood pressure. In functional kidneys, a rise in pressure leads to diuresis. Pathologic changes that alter the pressure threshold at which kidneys excrete salt and water alter systemic blood pressure. In addition, the overproduction of sodium-retaining hormones has been implicated in hypertension.

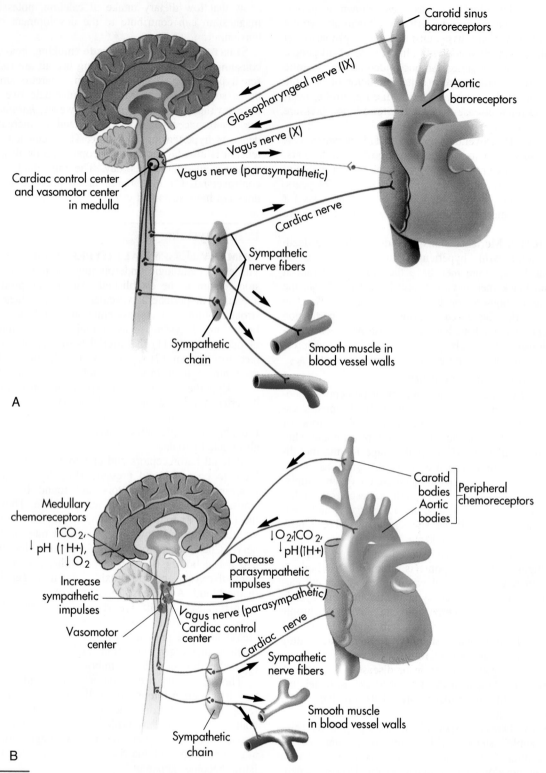

FIGURE 52–1 Baroreceptor and chemoreceptor reflex control of blood pressure. *A,* Baroreceptor reflexes. Baroreceptors located in the carotid sinuses and aortic arch detect changes in blood pressure. The heart rate can be decreased by the parasympathetic system; the heart rate and stroke volume can be increased by the sympathetic system. The sympathetic system also can constrict or dilate blood vessels. *B,* Chemoreceptor reflexes. Chemoreceptors located in the medulla oblongata and in the carotid and aortic bodies detect changes in blood oxygen, carbon dioxide, or pH. In response, the vasomotor center can cause vasoconstriction or dilation of blood vessels by the sympathetic system, and the cardioregulatory center can cause changes in the pumping activity of the heart through the parasympathetic and sympathetic systems. (From Seeley, R. R., Stephens, T. D., & Tate, P. [1995]. *Anatomy and physiology* [3rd ed.]. St. Louis: Mosby–Year Book.)

Renin and angiotensin play a role in blood pressure regulation. Renin is an enzyme produced by the kidney that catalyzes a plasma protein substrate to split off angiotensin I, which is removed by a converting enzyme to the lung to form angiotensin II and then angiotensin III (Fig. 52–2). Angiotensin II and III act as vasoconstrictors and also stimulate aldosterone release. With increased sympathetic nervous system activity, angiotensin II and III also seem to inhibit sodium excretion, which results in elevated blood pressure. Increased renin secretion has been investigated as a cause of increased peripheral vascular resistance in primary hypertension. Hypertension may also develop from deficiencies in vasodilator substances, such as prostaglandins, from congenital abnormalities in resistance vessels (arterioles), or from defects in neuroendocrine secretion.

SECONDARY HYPERTENSION

Many renal, vascular, neurologic, endocrine, and drug- and food-induced problems that directly or indirectly negatively affect the kidneys can result in serious insult to these organs that interferes with sodium excretion, renal perfusion, or the renin-angiotensin-aldosterone mecha-

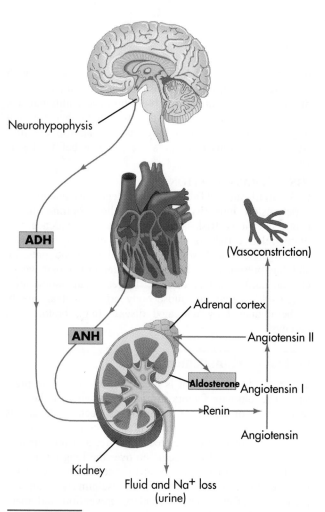

FIGURE 52–2 Renin-angiotensin-aldosterone regulation of blood pressure. (From Thibodeau, G. A., Patton, K. T. (1999). *Anatomy and physiology: A student survival guide.* St. Louis: Mosby.

nism, leading to an elevation in blood pressure over time (Box 52–2).

Chronic renal disease, mainly chronic glomerulonephritis and renal artery stenosis, is the most common cause of secondary hypertension. Also, the adrenal glands cause secondary hypertension as a result of primary excesses of aldosterone, cortisol, and catecholamines. Primary aldosteronism usually arises from solitary benign adenomas of the adrenal cortex that release excess aldosterone. Excess aldosterone causes renal retention of sodium and water, expands blood volume, and elevates blood pressure. Pheochromocytoma, a small tumor of the adrenal medulla, can cause dramatic hypertension because of the release of excessive amounts of epinephrine and norepinephrine. Other adrenocortical problems can result in excess production of cortisol (Cushing's syndrome). Clients with Cushing's syndrome have an 80% risk for development of hypertension. Cortisol increases blood pressure by increasing renal sodium retention, angiotensin II levels, and vascular reactivity to norepinephrine. Chronic stress induces prolonged elevated blood levels of catecholamines, certain hormones, and cortisol.

VESSEL CHANGES

Early in the course of development of hypertension, there may be no obvious pathologic changes in the blood vessels and organs other than intermittent elevations of blood pressure (*labile* hypertension). Slowly, widespread pathologic changes take place in both the large and small blood vessels and in the heart, kidneys, and brain.[12]

The large vessels, such as the aorta, coronary arteries, basilar artery to the brain, and peripheral vessels in the limbs, become sclerotic, tortuous, and weak. Their lumina narrow, with resultant decreased blood flow to the heart, brain, and lower extremities. As the damage continues, large vessels may become occluded or may hemorrhage, causing infarction of the tissue supplied by the vessel that has suddenly been robbed of its blood supply.

Small vessel damage, equally dangerous, causes structural changes in the heart, kidneys, and brain. Elevated diastolic blood pressure damages the intimal lining of the small vessels. Because of intimal damage, fibrin accumulates in the vessels, local edema develops, and intravascular clotting may occur. The net results of these changes are (1) a decreased blood supply to the tissues of the heart, brain, kidneys, and retina; (2) progressive functional impairment of these organs; and (3) finally, as a consequence of the chronic ischemia, infarction of the tissue supplied by these vessels, originating in much the same way as with occlusion of the large vessels.

Clinical Manifestations

In the early stages of development of hypertension, there are no clinical manifestations overt to clients or practitioners. Eventually, the blood pressure will rise, but early on, no clinical manifestations are present to alert the client of the problem. If elevated blood pressure is not caught during a routine screening, clients are still unaware that they have an elevated pressure and therefore do not seek health care for diagnosis of the cause and management of the condition. If the condition is left un-

---

BOX 52–2   Causes of Secondary Hypertension

Renal disorders

Renal parenchymal disease
  Acute glomerulonephritis
  Chronic nephritis
  Polycystic disease
  Connective tissue diseases
  Diabetic nephropathy
  Hydronephrosis
Renal artery stenosis
Renin-producing tumors

Endocrine disorders

Acromegaly
Hypothyroidism
Hyperthyroidism
Adrenal disorders
  Cortical
    Cushing's syndrome
    Primary aldosteronism
  Medullary
    Pancreatitis
    Pheochromocytoma

Neurologic disorders

Increased intracranial pressure
  Brain tumor
  Encephalitis
Sleep apnea
Autonomic dysreflexia

Medications

Oral contraceptives
Glucocorticoids
Mineralocorticoids
Cyclosporine
Erythropoietin
Monoamine oxidase (MAO) inhibitors
Tricyclic antidepressants
Cocaine use
Amphetamine use

Tyramine-containing foods

Aged cheeses (especially cheddar)
Chicken liver
Yeast extract
Beer, wine

Acute stress

Psychogenic hyperventilation
Hypoglycemia
Burns
Alcohol withdrawal

Vascular disorders

Arteriosclerosis
Coarctation of the aorta
Sickle cell crisis
Increased intravascular volume

Pregnancy-induced hypertension

---

diagnosed, the blood pressure will continue to rise, clinical manifestations will become apparent, and clients will eventually report to a provider's office with complaints of persistent headaches, fatigue, dizziness, palpitations, flushing, blurred or double vision, or epistaxis.[11, 16, 18, 23, 24]

Assessment of the client with hypertension involves the following three main objectives:

- To determine the extent of target organ involvement
- To ascertain the presence of other cardiovascular risk factors
- To identify the type of hypertension (primary or secondary)

Clinicians can obtain information relevant to these areas from the history, physical examination, and laboratory studies (Box 52–3).[21] The diagnosis of hypertension is made when, after the seated client has been allowed to rest for at least 5 minutes, the average of two or more readings separated by at least 2 minutes is 140 mm Hg or higher for the systolic blood pressure and 90 mm Hg or higher for the diastolic pressure. Follow-up examinations are scheduled to diagnose or rule out the presence of hypertension (see Table 52–1), unless first-visit measurement averages fall into either stage 2 or stage 3 or the client is in risk group C (see later). In such cases, the client is diagnosed with hypertension on the basis of the first-visit measurements, and a temporary management plan is implemented to bring the blood pressure down immediately or in a short time. However, careful differentiation of primary from secondary causes of the high blood pressure must precede any long-term management plan.

Hypertension is classified into stages 1 through 3 according to the blood pressure readings (see Table 52–2). It is important to identify "high-normal" values as well, because this range of blood pressures is associated with an increased risk of hypertension. Clients with high-normal pressures, particularly those who have additional risk factors, should be informed that full-blown hypertension may be imminent unless they institute appropriate lifestyle modifications to address the problem before it gets worse.

RISK STRATIFICATION

Risk stratification (Table 52–3) categorizes clients with hypertension into risk groups to allow optimal therapeutic decisions. Risk is based on outcome evidence outlining relative risk for morbidity and mortality in clients with hypertension based on the level of blood pressure and the presence or absence of target organ damage or clinical cardiovascular disease. Target organs, sometimes called *end organs,* are those body organs that are likely to be damaged by untreated disease (e.g., brain, eyes, kidneys).

Outcome Management

The goal of management is to control arterial blood pressure. The ultimate factors in evaluating whether the correct choice of treatment regimen has been made are as follows: the desired, "control" blood pressure is reached, treatment choices are tolerated and safe, and the client is willing to commit to the regimen over the long term.

The most pronounced positive client outcomes have resulted from a systematic, multidisciplinary team approach for primary and secondary prevention and management of hypertension using diverse qualified health care professionals.[11, 24–26, 29, 30] Multidisciplinary teams can provide the most comprehensive, cost-effective care of clients with a multitude of prevention and management

BOX 52-3   Assessment of the Client with Hypertension

History

Note the following points when interviewing the hypertensive client:

- Family history of hypertension, diabetes mellitus, cardiovascular disease, hyperlipidemia, or renal disease, smoking, stress, obesity, or sedentary lifestyle
- Previous documentation of high blood pressure, including age at onset, level of elevation, and currently prescribed medical regimen
- History of all prescribed and over-the-counter medications and the client's exact compliance with taking the medications—*Note:* Medications that may either raise blood pressure or interfere with the effectiveness of antihypertensive medications include oral contraceptives, steroids, nonsteroidal anti-inflammatory drugs, nasal decongestants, appetite suppressants, cyclosporine, tricyclic antidepressants, monoamine oxidase inhibitors, and erythropoietin
- History of any disease or trauma to target organs
- Results and side effects of previous antihypertensive therapy
- Clinical manifestations of cardiovascular disorders, such as angina, dyspnea, or claudication
- History of or recent weight gain, exercise activities, sodium intake, fat intake, alcohol use, and smoking
- Psychosocial and environmental factors (e.g., emotional stress, cultural food practices, economic status) that may influence blood pressure control

Physical Examination

Physical assessment should include accurate determination of blood pressure as well as evaluation of target organs.

- Vital signs and weight
- Blood pressure—because blood pressure is variable and can be affected by multiple factors, it should be measured so that readings are representative of the client's usual level; the following techniques are strongly recommended:

  - The client should be seated with the arm bared, supported, and positioned at heart level. The client should not have smoked tobacco or ingested caffeine within the previous 30 minutes.
  - Measurement should begin after at least 5 minutes of quiet rest. The client's back should be supported, and both feet should be flat on the floor with the legs uncrossed. The client should not speak while the blood pressure is being monitored.

- Use of the appropriate cuff size will ensure an accurate measurement. The rubber bladder should encircle at least 80% of the limb being measured. The bladder's width should be one-third to one-half the circumference of the limb. Several sizes of cuffs (e.g., child, adult, large adult) should be available.
- Measurements should be taken with a mercury sphygmomanometer, a recently calibrated aneroid manometer, or a validated electronic device.
- Postural blood pressures should be measured and recorded according to position and arm used, including lying, sitting, and standing measurements from both arms.

  - Both systolic and diastolic blood pressures should be recorded. The disappearance of sound (phase V) should be used for the diastolic reading.
  - Two or more readings should be averaged. If the first two readings differ by more than 5 mm Hg, additional readings should be obtained.

- Funduscopic examination for retinal arteriolar narrowing, hemorrhages, exudates, and papilledema
- Examination of the neck for distended veins, carotid bruits, and enlarged thyroid
- Auscultation of the heart for increased heart rate, dysrhythmias, enlargement, precordial impulses, murmurs, and S3 and S4 heart sounds
- Examination of the abdomen for bruits, aortic dilation, and enlarged kidneys
- Examination of extremities for diminished or absent peripheral pulses, edema, and bilateral inequality of pulses
- Neurologic evaluation for signs of cerebral thrombosis or hemorrhage

Laboratory Studies

Studies used in the routine evaluation of hypertension include a complete blood count, urinalysis, determinations of serum potassium and sodium levels, fasting blood glucose level, serum cholesterol level, blood urea nitrogen and serum creatinine levels, electrocardiogram, and chest radiography. These tests provide useful information in determining the severity of vascular disease, the extent of target organ damage, and the possible causes of hypertension. Clients with potential for secondary hypertension may need more extensive studies.

---

needs, including those related to the prevention, diagnosis, and management of hypertension.

Long-term compliance/adherence has emerged as the most essential element in reducing morbidity and mortality associated with hypertension.[9] However, poor compliance with or adherence to antihypertensive therapy persists as one of the most frustrating blocks to effective therapeutic management. More than two thirds of clients with hypertension do not have adequate control of their blood pressure because of poor compliance or adherence. The reasons vary; the client may choose not to have the initial prescription filled, may successfully initiate therapy only to abandon it after a few weeks or months, or may comply with only part of the regimen and thus fail to achieve optimal control.

NORMALIZING ARTERIAL PRESSURE

The outcome goal of prevention and management of hypertension is to restore the elevated blood pressure to as normal a level as possible using lifestyle modification alone or in combination with drug therapy in order to prevent morbidity and mortality associated with the sequelae of hypertension. The objective is to achieve and maintain arterial blood pressure below 140/90 mm Hg, or

TABLE 52-1	FOLLOW-UP CRITERIA FOR FIRST-OCCASION MEASUREMENT OF BLOOD PRESSURE

Initial Screening Blood Pressure (mm Hg)*		Follow-up Recommended†
Systolic	*Diastolic*	
<130	<85	Recheck in 2 yr
130–139	85–89	Recheck in 1 yr‡
140–159	90–99	Confirm within 2 mo‡
160–179	100–109	Evaluate or refer to care within 1 mo
≥180	≥110	Evaluate or refer to care immediately or within 1 wk, depending on clinical situation

*If the systolic and diastolic categories are different, follow recommendation for the shorter follow-up time.
†The scheduling of follow-up visits should be modified by reliable information about past blood pressure, other cardiovascular risk factors, or target organ disease.
‡Encourage lifestyle modifications.
From the Joint National Committee. (1997). The sixth report of the Joint National Committee on the Detection, Evaluation, and Treatment of Hypertension. *Archives of Internal Medicine, 157,* 2418.

TABLE 52-2	CLASSIFICATION OF BLOOD PRESSURE IN ADULTS 18 YEARS OF AGE AND OLDER*

Category	Blood Pressure (mm Hg)	
	Systolic	*Diastolic*
Normal	<130	<85
High-normal	130–139	85–89
Hypertension		
Stage 1: mild	140–159	90–99
Stage 2: moderate	160–179	100–109
Stage 3: severe	≥180	≥110

*Not taking antihypertensive medications and not acutely ill. When systolic and diastolic pressures fall into different categories, the higher category should be selected to classify the client's blood pressure status. For example, 170/96 would be classified as stage 2, and 178/112 would be classified as stage 3.
From the Joint National Committee. (1997). The sixth report of the Joint National Committee on the Detection, Evaluation, and Treatment of Hypertension. *Archives of Internal Medicine, 157,* 2417.

as near to that goal as possible, while controlling modifiable risk factors for cardiovascular disease.[11, 16, 25, 26, 30]

Lifestyle Modifications

Strong research evidence has conclusively illustrated that lifestyle modifications are effective in lowering blood pressure and reducing cardiovascular risk factors at little overall cost and with minimal risk. Lifestyle modifications are widely advocated to prevent high blood pressure. They are suggested as definitive therapy for some clients, at least for the first 6 to 12 months after initial diagnosis.

Lifestyle modification is also strongly encouraged as adjunctive therapy for all clients with hypertension who are also receiving pharmacologic therapy. Positive adjustments in lifestyle alone may completely normalize the blood pressure for an extended period of time or indefinitely. When lifestyle management alone is not entirely successful in normalizing pressure, continued healthy lifestyle practices can reduce the number and dosage of antihypertensive medications needed to manage the condition.

Weight Reduction

Excess body weight, exhibited by a body mass index (BMI)—weight in kilograms divided by height in meters squared—of 27 or greater, correlates closely with elevated blood pressure. Also, excess body fat accumulated in the torso with a waist circumference of 34 inches or greater for women and 39 inches or more for men has

TABLE 52-3	RISK STRATIFICATION AND TREATMENT IN CLIENTS WITH HIGH BLOOD PRESSURE

Blood Pressure	Treatment*		
	Risk Group A *No Risk Factors,* *No TOD/CCD*	*Risk Group B* *At Least 1 Risk Factor,* *Not Including Diabetes;* *No TOD/CCD*	*Risk Group C* *TOD/CCD ± Diabetes,* *± Other Risk Factors*
High-normal: 130–139/85–89	Lifestyle modification	Lifestyle modification	Drug therapy†
Stage 1: 140–159/90–99	Lifestyle modification (up to 12 mo)	Lifestyle modification‡ (up to 6 mo)	Drug therapy
Stages 2 and 3: ≥160/≥100	Drug therapy	Drug therapy	Drug therapy

*Lifestyle modification should be adjunctive therapy in all clients receiving pharmacologic therapy.
†For clients with heart failure, renal insufficiency, or diabetes.
‡For clients with multiple risk factors, clinicians should consider drug therapy as initial treatment plus lifestyle modifications.
TOD/CCD, target organ disease/clinicial cardiovascular disease.
Modified from the Joint National Committee. (1997). The sixth report of the Joint National Committee on the Detection, Evaluation, and Treatment of Hypertension. *Archives of Internal Medicine, 157,* 2419.

also been associated with increased risk for hypertension. For many people with hypertension whose body weight is more than 10% over ideal, weight reduction of as little as 10 pounds can lower blood pressure. Weight reduction also enhances effectiveness of antihypertensive medications. Therefore, reassess the client's blood pressure during weight loss, and make appropriate changes in pharmacologic interventions as needed.

Sodium Restriction

An estimated 40% of people with hypertension are sodium-sensitive. A moderate restriction of sodium intake to 2.3 g of sodium, or 6 g of salt, can be used to lower blood pressure in some cases of stage I hypertension. The amount of medication otherwise needed may be decreased if sodium intake is lowered. In addition, this moderate sodium restriction may reduce the degree of potassium depletion that often accompanies diuretic therapy.

Dietary Fat Modification

Modification of dietary intake of fat by decreasing the fraction of saturated fat and increasing that of polyunsaturated fat has little, if any, effect on decreasing blood pressure but can decrease the cholesterol level significantly. Because dyslipidemia is a major risk factor in the development of coronary artery disease, diet therapy aimed at reducing lipids is an important adjunct to any total dietary regimen. In addition to the usual recommendations for sensible eating following the Food Pyramid (see Chapter 3), the Dietary Approaches to Stop Hypertension (DASH) diet (Table 52-4) which is rich in fruits, vegetables, nuts, and low-fat dairy foods with reduced saturated and total fats, should be recommended for clients who need a more structured, fat-limited, dietary intervention.

Exercise

A regular program of aerobic exercise adequate to achieve at least a moderate level of physical fitness facilitates cardiovascular conditioning and can aid the obese hypertensive client in weight reduction and reduce the risk for cardiovascular disease and all-cause mortality. Blood pressure can be reduced with moderate-intensity (as low as 40% to 60% of maximum oxygen consumption) physical activity, such as a brisk walk (about 2.5 to 3 miles per hour) for 30 to 45 minutes most days of the week.

Weight training using *light* weights is a positive addition to any exercise regimen. However, lifting *heavy* weights may be harmful, because blood pressure rises, sometimes to very high levels, with the vasovagal response that occurs during an intense isometric muscle contraction. Advise hypertensive clients to initiate exercise programs gradually, slowly increasing intensity and duration of activity as the body adjusts and becomes more conditioned with ongoing professional surveillance.

Alcohol Restriction

The consumption of more than 1 ounce of alcohol per day is associated with a higher prevalence of hypertension, poor adherence to antihypertensive therapy, and, occasionally, refractory hypertension. Carefully assess alcohol intake. Advise clients who do drink to do so in moderation (i.e., no more than 1 ounce of ethanol per day for men and 0.5 ounce for women). There is 1 ounce

(30 ml) of ethanol in 2 ounces (60 ml) of 100-proof whiskey, in 10 ounces (300 ml) of wine, or in 24 ounces (720 ml) of beer.

Caffeine Restriction

Although acute ingestion of caffeine may raise blood pressure, chronic moderate caffeine ingestion appears to have no significant effect on blood pressure. Therefore, caffeine restriction is not necessary unless cardiac response or other excessive sensitivity to caffeine is present.

Relaxation Techniques

A variety of relaxation therapies, including transcendental meditation, yoga, biofeedback, progressive muscle relaxation, and psychotherapy, reduce blood pressure in hypertensive clients at least transiently. Although each modality has its advocates, none has been conclusively shown to be either practical for the majority of hypertensive clients or effective in maintaining a significant long-term effect.[3, 20]

Smoking Cessation

Although smoking has not been statistically linked to the development of hypertension, nicotine definitely increases heart rate and produces peripheral vasoconstriction, which does raise arterial blood pressure for a short time during smoking and afterward. Smoking cessation is strongly recommended, however, to reduce the client's risk for cancer, pulmonary disease, and cardiovascular disease. Smokers appear to have a higher frequency of malignant hypertension and subarachnoid hemorrhage. In addition, risk reduction brought about by antihypertensive therapy may not be as great in smokers as in nonsmokers.

Potassium Supplementation

The high ratio of sodium to potassium in the modern diet has been held responsible for the development of hypertension. However, even though potassium supplements may lower blood pressure, they are too costly and potentially too hazardous for routine use. A reduction in consumption of high-sodium, low-potassium processed foods with an increase in consumption of low-sodium, high-potassium natural foods may be all that is needed for maximum benefits.

Pharmacologic Intervention

Considerable debate continues regarding the appropriate time and circumstances for the initiation of pharmacologic management of hypertension. Although antihypertensive agents are known to be effective in decreasing cardiovascular morbidity and mortality associated with hypertension, clinicians sometimes question whether the benefit of immediate initiation of medication therapy, particularly in mildly hypertensive clients, outweighs the risks in terms of untoward effects of the drugs and other inconveniences. Other clinicians prefer to recommend lifestyle modification, as indicated in the previous section, and to add drug therapy as needed.

In any event, once a decision has been made to use pharmacologic intervention, any one of several drugs can be used.[6, 8, 11, 14, 15, 19, 24, 28, 30] Table 52-5 outlines the major antihypertensive agents.

Antihypertensive medications can be classified into the following categories: diuretics, alpha- and beta-adrenergic antagonists, alpha$_2$-agonists, vasodilators, calcium antago-

Text continued on page 1391

TABLE 52–4 **DIETARY APPROACHES TO STOP HYPERTENSION (DASH) DIET**

The DASH eating plan shown below is based on 2000 calories a day. Depending on your caloric needs your number of daily servings in a food group may vary from those listed. This eating plan is from the "Dietary Approaches to Stop Hypertension" (DASH) clinical study supported by the National Institutes of Health. The DASH combination diet lowered blood pressure and so may help prevent and control high blood pressure.

Food Group	Daily Servings (No.)	Serving Size	Examples	Significance of Each Food Group to DASH Diet Pattern
Grains and grain products	7–8	1 slice bread; ½ cup dry cereal; ½ cup cooked rice, pasta, or cereal*	Whole wheat breads, English muffin, pita bread, bagel, cereals and fiber, grits, oatmeal	Major source of energy and fiber
Vegetables	4–5	1 cup raw, leafy vegetable; ½ cup cooked vegetable; 6 oz vegetable juice	Tomatoes, potatoes, carrots, peas, squash, broccoli, turnip greens, collards, kale, spinach, artichokes, beans, sweet potatoes	Rich sources of potassium, magnesium, and fiber
Fruits	4–5	6 oz fruit juice, 1 medium fruit; ¼ cup dried fruit; ½ cup fresh, frozen, or canned fruit	Apricots, bananas, dates, grapes, oranges, orange juice, grapefruit, grapefruit juice, mangoes, melons, peaches, pineapples, prunes, raisins, strawberries, tangerines	Important sources of potassium, magnesium, and fiber
Low fat or nonfat dairy foods	2–3	8 oz milk; 1 cup yogurt; 1.5 oz cheese	Skim or 1% milk, skim or low-fat buttermilk, nonfat or low-fat yogurt, part skim mozzarella cheese, nonfat cheese	Major sources of calcium and protein
Meats, poultry, fish	2 or less	3 oz cooked meats, poultry, or fish	Select only lean; trim away visible fats; broil, roast, or boil, instead of frying; remove skin from poultry	Rich sources of protein and magnesium
Nuts, seeds, and legumes	4–5/wk	1.5 oz or ⅓ cup nuts; ½ oz or 2 tbsp seeds; ½ cup cooked dry beans	Almonds, filberts, mixed nuts, peanuts, walnuts, sunflower seeds, kidney beans, lentils and peas	Rich sources of energy, magnesium, potassium, protein, and fiber
Fats and oils†	2–3	1 tsp soft margarine; 1 tbsp low-fat mayonnaise; 2 tbsp light salad dressing; 1 tsp vegetable oil	Soft margarine, low-fat mayonnaise, light salad dressing Vegetable oil (such as olive, corn, canola, or safflower)	Besides considering the fats added to foods, choose foods that contain less fats
Sweets	5/wk	1 tbsp sugar; 1 tbsp jelly or jam; ½ oz jelly beans; 8 oz lemonade	Maple syrup, sugar, jelly, jam, fruit-flavored gelatin, jelly beans, hard candy, fruit punch, sorbet ices	Sweets should be low in fat

*Serving sizes vary between ½ and 1¼ cups. Check the nutrition label.
†Fat content changes per serving size of fats and oil, for example, 1 tbsp regular salad dressing equals 1 serving, 1 tbsp low-fat dressing equals ½ serving, 1 tbsp fat-free dressing equals zero servings.
Modified from Kolasa, K. M. (1999). Dietary Approaches to Stop Hypertension (DASH) in clinical practice: A primary care experience. *Clinical Cardiology, 22*(7 suppl), III-16–22.

TABLE 52–5   MEDICATIONS USED TO TREAT HYPERTENSION

Drug Class with Example(s)	Action	Therapeutic Outcome	Adverse Outcomes	Dose
Thiazide and Related Diuretics Hydrochlorothiazide (Hydro-DIURIL)	Promote renal excretion of water, sodium, potassium, and hydrogen	Lower BP, diuresis, weight loss Generally a first-line agent	Hypotension, dehydration, hypokalemia	12.5–50 mg/d daily to twice daily Administer in AM These drugs potentiate other antihypertensive medications; monitor BP closely
Loop Diuretics Bumetanide (Bumex) Furosemide (Lasix)	Inhibits absorption of sodium and chloride from ascending loop of Henle, causing excretion of water, sodium, potassium, chloride, magnesium, and calcium	Lower BP, reduce edema First-line agent in clients with renal failure	Hypotension, dehydration, hypokalemia Drugs decrease effect of antidiabetic agents	Lasix: 20–40 mg q 6–8 h initially Bumex: 0.5–4 mg Maintenance dose given daily or twice daily Administer last dose in early evening Monitor BP and positional BP, daily weight, I&O Closely monitor potassium levels
Potassium-Sparing Diuretics Amiloride hydrochloride (Midamor) Spironolactone (Aldactone)	Competes with aldosterone for receptor sites in distal renal tubules, increasing sodium and chloride excretion	Management of edema associated with hyperaldosteronism Weak diuretics	Hyperkalemia, dehydration, impotence	Daily to twice-daily dosing Amiloride: 5–10 mg daily Spironolactone: 25–100 mg
Selective Beta Blocker Metoprolol (Lopressor)	Selective inhibitor of beta$_1$-adrenergic receptors; no effect on beta$_2$ receptors	Decreased BP, decreased heart rate May be less effective in treating black clients and the elderly	Hypoglycemia in diabetics, with masking of clinical manifestations except for diaphoresis, dizziness, fatigue	50–300 mg bid Monitor I&O, BP, daily weight
Nonselective Beta Blocker Propranolol (Inderal)	Nonselective inhibitor of beta$_1$- and beta$_2$-adrenergic receptors	Decreased BP, decreased heart rate, decreased myocardial oxygen demand	Bronchial constriction Hypoglycemia in diabetics (as for metoprolol above), dizziness, fatigue, insomnia	Daily to twice-daily dosing 40–480 mg/day Monitor I&O, BP, daily weight Avoid using in clients with asthma
Peripheral-Acting Adrenergic Antagonist Guanadrel (Hylorel)	Deplete the brain and peripheral nerve tissues of norepinephrine, decreasing peripheral vascular resistance	Decreased heart rate and standing BP	Depression, weight gain, bradycardia, postural hypotension (due to loss of norepinephrine) GI upset	Daily or twice-daily dosing 10–75 mg/day Often used in combination with other diuretics or beta-blockers Concurrent use of digitalis or quinidine may potentiate dysrhythmias
Centrally Acting Alpha$_2$ Agonists Clonidine (Catapres) Methyldopa (Aldomet)	Suppress sympathetic nervous system Action potentiated by alcohol, sedatives, propranolol	Decreased BP Bradycardia	Xerostomia, dizziness, headache, fatigue, GI disturbances	Clonidine 0.1 mg bid Methyldopa 250 mg bid–tid Used only for severe hypertension or renin-dependent hypertension Monitor BP closely Monitor for bradycardia Chewing gum or hard candy may relieve dry mouth

Table continued on following page

TABLE 52–5 | **MEDICATIONS USED TO TREAT HYPERTENSION** *Continued*

Drug Class with Example(s)	Action	Therapeutic Outcome	Adverse Outcomes	Dose
Calcium Channel Blockers Diltiazem (Cardizem SR or CD) Verapamil (Calan SR) Nifedipine (Procardia XL)	Blocks entry of calcium into smooth muscle channels in arterioles Used for cardioprotective effects with angina, atrial fibrillation, diabetes	Vasodilation Decreased peripheral vascular resistance Reduce heart rate, slow ventricular conduction, depress contractility	Hypotension Bradycardia from heart block Nocturia	Daily dosing Diltiazem 120–360 mg/day or bid Verapamil 80–120 mg tid **Short-acting forms, particularly nifedipine, should no longer be used because of increased risk of MI and mortality after MI**
Angiotensin-Converting Enzyme (ACE) Inhibitors Captopril (Capoten) Enalapril (Vasotec) Fosinopril (Monopril)	Inhibit the conversion of angiotensin I to angiotensin II, thereby preventing release of renin	Reduces peripheral vascular resistance without changing cardiac output	Digitalis toxicity Hyperkalemia Ticklish, dry cough Renal damage	5–40 mg (qid to tid) Do not administer with antacids Monitor potassium levels, urine protein, leukocyte counts
Alpha₁-Receptor Blockers Doxazosin (Cardura) Prazosin (Minipress)	Competitively inhibits postsynaptic receptors	Vasodilation, decreased peripheral vascular resistance	Orthostatic hypotension, with loss of consciousness especially with first dose	Given 1–4 times daily Doxazosin: 1 mg up to qid Prazosin: 2–30 mg bid–tid Monitor BP closely Titrate dose based on standing BP Teach clients to move slowly to prevent orthostasis
Alpha/Beta-Blocker Labetalol (Normodyne)	Same as for alpha/beta-blockers	Same as for alpha/beta-blockers	Same as for alpha/beta-blockers	May be more effective in black clients than a beta-blocker alone
Vasodilator Hydralazine (Apresoline)	Direct vasodilation of arterioles, no effect on veins	Decreased peripheral vascular resistance	Orthostatic hypotension, palpitations, tachycardia, flushing, headache	10–70 mg 4 times daily Monitor positional BP closely, especially when drug given IV Headache responds to acetaminophen and ice compresses

BP, blood pressure; GI, gastrointestinal; I&O, intake and output (fluid); MI, myocardial infarction.

nists, and angiotensin-converting enzyme (ACE) inhibitors. If therapy is chosen carefully, more than half of mild hypertension cases can be controlled with a single drug, and more than 90% should be controlled with no more than two drugs. Cultural aspects of antihypertensive medications are discussed in the Diversity in Health Care feature.

PROVIDER RESPONSIBILITIES
Stepped-Care Therapy
The goal of antihypertensive therapy is to control blood pressure with a minimum of side effects. The stepped-care approach is prescribed as treatment for hypertension (Box 52–4). Prevention-based healthy lifestyle change

with the addition of pharmacologic therapy as indicated is the preferred treatment regimen. An individualized approach to prescription of lifestyle management and drug therapy is used, taking into consideration demographic concerns, concomitant diseases or therapies, and the client's perceived quality of life within the confines of the treatment regimen.

If more than one drug is necessary, several combination therapies have proved effective. For example, the combination of a diuretic with a beta-adrenergic blocker or other adrenergic inhibitor has been effective in both blacks and whites, in contrast to the responses to the individual drugs, whereas blacks respond less well to

---

DIVERSITY IN HEALTH CARE

Ethnopharmacology and Hypertension

Ethnopharmacology

How medications are metabolized varies not only in relation to a person's age, gender, body composition, and size but also with ethnicity[3]; these factors, therefore, must be considered in any treatment regimen. The variation in metabolism is called drug polymorphism and is influenced by several ethnicity-related factors. In this regard, Kudzma[3] has identified environmental, cultural, and genetic factors.

Environmental factors affect the assimilation and half-life of a medication and include diet, smoking, and alcohol use. Cultural factors include (1) values and beliefs, which can influence adherence to a medication regimen, (2) reporting or nonreporting of manifestations, and (3) use of herbal and homeopathic remedies. Some people may doubt the need for medication when manifestations ease or disappear, and some may be unwilling to accept the use of particular routes of medication. In addition, religious beliefs may dictate fasting periods, which may affect medication absorption.[5]

Genetic factors determine medication metabolism in terms of genetic polymorphism, because each person's inherited genes affect liver metabolism. Some people are slow or poor metabolizers, whereas others are rapid or extensive metabolizers. An estimated 9% of whites and 32% of Asians are slow metabolizers.[5] In rapid metabolizers, a drug is more efficient but may sometimes be metabolized so quickly that full benefit is not realized. In slow metabolizers, a drug is less effective and greater drug toxicity may be experienced.[3] The speed of metabolism is an important issue in determining the appropriate dose of medication for a client and has been examined in some studies of ethnic groups, although more studies across a variety of groups need to be done.

Hypertension

Hypertension, as well as some other related conditions such as stroke, has been connected to cultural, economic, social, and political factors that have had a negative impact upon the health of African Americans in large urban areas.[4] Davis and Curley[1] have described African Americans as having the poorest health of all ethnic groups in the United States, as measured by certain indicators. Giger and Davidhizar[2] note that the incidence of

hypertension has been reported to be significantly higher in African Americans than in white Americans. In addition, the age at onset of hypertension is younger and the level of severity is higher.

Because the incidence of hypertension is higher among blacks than among whites, many studies have been conducted to investigate the effectiveness of commonly prescribed medications among blacks. What has not yet been clearly determined is whether genetics, the pathophysiology of hypertension, or some other factor is responsible for the results. Kudzma[3] reported that most of the major classes of antihypertensive drugs—diuretic agents, angiotensin-converting enzyme (ACE) inhibitors, beta-blockers, and calcium-channel blockers—are found to be effective in blacks. However, if only one drug is used, blacks appear to respond better to diuretics than to ACE inhibitors or beta-blockers. Also, lower doses are required for some drugs in blacks than in whites.

In general, become aware that drug metabolism differs across ethnic groups for a variety of reasons and that certain medications may be more effective for some groups than for others. In addition to considering the differences that may occur in treatment response, consider the many factors that may have contributed to certain conditions occurring in higher frequencies in some groups. Such factors include diet, socioeconomic status, habits, beliefs and norms, and access to and acceptability of preventive care. Try to improve the health outcomes of clients by monitoring their responses to medication, communicating pertinent information to physicians, and assisting clients in modifying the impact of the multiple factors, both internal and external, affecting them.

References

1. Davis, C. M., & Curley, C. M. (1999). Disparities of health in African Americans. *Nursing Clinics of North America, 34*(2), 345–357.
2. Giger, J. N., & Davidhizar, R. E. (1999). *Transcultural nursing: Assessment and intervention* (3rd ed.). St. Louis: Mosby.
3. Kudzma, E. C. (1999). Culturally competent drug administration. *American Journal of Nursing, 99*(8), 46–51.
4. Leininger, M. (1995). *Transcultural nursing: Concepts, theories, research and practices.* New York: McGraw-Hill.
5. Pavlovich-Davis, S. (1999). Drug of choice? Medicinal effects vary widely, depending on ethnicity and culture. *Nursing Spectrum,* Oct. 4, 18–19.

Sandra Sharma, PhD, ARNP, CS, *James A. Haley Veterans Hospital, Tampa, Florida*

BOX 52–4   Stepped-Care Approach to Management of Hypertension

Step 1:   Implement lifestyle modifications.
Weight reduction
Moderation of alcohol intake
Regular aerobic physical activity
Reduction of sodium intake with maintenance of adequate intake of potassium, calcium, and magnesium
Decreased intake of saturated fats and cholesterol
Smoking cessation

If there is inadequate blood pressure control, move to step 2.

Step 2:   Continue lifestyle modifications and make initial pharmacologic selection; diuretics or beta-blockers are recommended because of studies that demonstrate reduced morbidity and mortality. If co-morbid conditions exist, evidence supports the use of other drugs as first-line therapy.

■ Start with lowest therapeutic dose of a long-acting drug given once daily, then titrate dose.
■ Low-dose combination drugs may be appropriate.

If there is inadequate blood pressure control, move to step 3.

Step 3:   Increase drug dose.
　　　OR
　　　Substitute another drug if no response or side effects become apparent.
　　　OR
　　　Add second drug from a different class or a diuretic if not already used, particularly if there is an inadequate response but initial drug well tolerated and at maximum dose.

If there is inadequate blood pressure control, move to step 4.

Step 4:   Add second or third drug if not already prescribed; continue to add medications from other classes; consider referral to a hypertensive specialist.

From the Joint National Committee. (1997). The sixth report of the Joint National Committee on the Detection, Evaluation, and Treatment of Hypertension. *Archives of Internal Medicine, 157,* 2430.

beta-adrenergic blockers alone or as first-line treatment. The combination of a diuretic with an ACE inhibitor or a calcium-channel blocker has additive effects on blood pressure.

Finally, combination drugs can be less expensive than the individual drugs, and the need for only one drug may improve compliance in a client who does not like "taking so many pills."

Follow-up Care: Step-Down Therapy

Reducing the number and amounts of antihypertensive medications should be considered once a client's blood pressure has been controlled effectively for at least 1 year. Medication dosages must be decreased slowly and progressively until the lowest effective dosages are reached and maintained. Step-down methods are most often successful in clients who are also participating in healthy lifestyle change interventions. Lifestyle change habits should be established and can be regulated to provide the most appropriate and practical regimen for each client. Regular follow-up evaluation is essential if drug therapy has been completely stopped, because blood pressure can rise again over time, especially if positive lifestyle change practices have been neglected or also stopped.

■ Nursing Management

ASSESSMENT

The many sequelae of untreated hypertension can be prevented, or the severity of such problems reduced, if hypertension is well managed. Client education and understanding are crucial to successful management.

Ineffective Management of Therapeutic Regimen (Individual). Use the nursing diagnosis *Ineffective Management of Therapeutic Regimen (Individual)* to identify the learning needs of the newly diagnosed hypertensive client. The diagnosis can be written *Risk for Ineffective Management of Therapeutic Regimen (Individual) related to a new diagnosis, no previous learning about the disease process, potential consequences, the rationale for intervention, and proper administration of prescribed medications.*

Outcomes. The client and significant others will demonstrate knowledge required for self-care, as evidenced by (1) describing hypertension and its associated risk factors; (2) discussing the importance of lifelong medical follow-up; (3) listing the prescribed medications, including drug name, rationale for use, dosage, frequency, potential side effects, and measures to minimize side effects; and (4) demonstrating proper blood pressure measurement technique for home blood pressure monitoring.

Interventions. Because of the chronicity of hypertension and its dangerous complications, clients with hypertension need clear, practical, and realistic learning guidelines. Guidelines should include information concerning hypertension and its management. Use written materials with clear illustrations for teaching the client with newly diagnosed hypertension about the condition. Teach the client to measure blood pressure at home at least once a week and to record the findings in a diary.

Inform clients of their blood pressure reading, and advise them of the need for periodic remeasurement. When working with most clients, the examiner should refer to hypertension as *high blood pressure* to help avoid confusion associated with the term *hypertension.* Many clients unfamiliar with medical terms may believe that hypertension denotes a state of being "hypertense"—that is, being worried or agitated. For these clients, the term *high blood pressure* more accurately conveys the nature of the health problem.

Altered Nutrition: More Than Body Requirements. Dietary adjustments can reduce the severity of hypertension and in some cases reduce the need for medication. Client teaching about and assessment of needed changes constitute an important aspect of nursing care. Write the diagnosis as *Altered Nutrition: More Than Body Requirements related to high sodium, fat, and total calorie intake.*

Outcomes. The client will demonstrate knowledge of and adherence to the nutritional regimen, as evidenced by describing specific dietary modifications including sodium, fat, and calorie restrictions and their rationales (see the three Client Education Guides to these topics), by reduction in levels of urine sodium and blood cholesterol, and by losing weight.

Interventions. The two most important aspects of dietary intervention for hypertension are weight reduction (for overweight clients) and mild to moderate sodium restriction. Therefore, advise the client with hypertension to eat a diet low in salt, calories, cholesterol, and saturated fat. Discuss the prescribed diet with the household members who prepare food. If possible, enlist the aid of a dietitian to provide detailed dietary instructions. Before dietary intervention begins, assess the client's patterns of food intake, lifestyle, food preferences, and ethnic, social, cultural, and financial influences. A highly individualized approach to dietary counseling is crucial to compliance and adherence.

Restrict Sodium. Sodium is a hidden ingredient in many processed foods, beverages (including water from certain sources), and over-the-counter drugs (particularly antacids, cough remedies, and laxatives). It cannot be seen and is often not tasted. The average adult daily intake of salt is 5 to 15 g, but the therapeutic effects of sodium reduction on blood pressure do not occur until salt intake is reduced to equal to or below 6 g/day. Low-salt diets can be very difficult to adhere to, at least initially. Reassure the client that dietary adherence becomes easier as the palate adjusts to decreased salt over a period of several weeks to months. After the client becomes fully accustomed to the low-salt diet, unsalted foods usually cease to taste bland. The Client Education Guide on low-salt diets presents guidelines for teaching clients about sodium reduction.

Reduce Fat and Cholesterol. Hypertension and high serum cholesterol (>250 mg/dl) are linked as risk factors in the development of coronary artery disease. The level

---

CLIENT EDUCATION GUIDE

Low-Fat, Low-Cholesterol Diet

Client Instructions

Avoid foods high in saturated fats and cholesterol:

Use margarine and vegetable oils instead of butter.
Avoid gravies, creams, and cheese sauces.
Avoid fried foods; instead, eat broiled, baked, or boiled foods
Use skim or low-fat milk and milk products.
Choose lean cuts of meat. Trim off all visible fat. Remove all poultry skin.
Use a wire rack when roasting, broiling, or baking meats so that the fat can drip off.
Keep in mind that poultry, fish, and veal have a relatively low fat content. Chicken and turkey breasts are the leanest poultry available. Avoid duck and goose. Haddock, cod, and water-packed tuna are the leanest fish available.
Use pans with a nonstick coating when cooking to reduce the need for oil or shortening.
Prepare meat stews, soups, and gravies in advance and chill them until the fat hardens. Then skim off the fat.
Eat no more than three egg yolks per week. Egg whites are low in cholesterol, as are many egg substitutes.
Limit your intake of organ meats and shellfish.

---

of serum cholesterol is partly determined by the consumption of cholesterol, saturated and polyunsaturated fats, and total calories. Cholesterol is contained in animal fats and dairy products. Saturated fats occur predominantly in animal fats and tropical oils (e.g., coconut and palm oils). Unsaturated fats predominate in most plant-derived fats. Polyunsaturated fats occur predominantly in vegetable and seed oils. A diet low in saturated fats and high in polyunsaturated fats is beneficial in reducing blood pressure. (See DASH diet, Table 52–4.) The Client Education Guide on low-fat, low-cholesterol diets also provides guidelines for teaching clients about fat and cholesterol reduction.

Reduce Calories and Weight. Not all clients with hypertension need to lose weight. As discussed previously, only people with a BMI of greater than 27 should consider the need to lose weight. Ideally, the rate of weight loss should be no more than 0.5 kg (about a pound) a week. Advise the average adult with hypertension to reduce caloric intake by at least 250 calories per day. Caution the client to avoid over-the-counter appetite suppressants because these preparations often contain sympathomimetic agents, which elevate blood pressure. The Client Education Guide on calorie-restricted diets provides advice on regulating caloric intake.

Altered Health Maintenance. Exercise is like dietary management: A regular exercise program can lower blood pressure in hypertensive clients. This diagnosis can be written as *Altered Health Maintenance related to a lack of regular exercise regimen.*

Outcomes. The client will begin and maintain an appropriate exercise program, as evidenced by self-report, demonstration of ability to monitor heart rate during exercise, sensation of reduced physical and emotional stress, and reduced blood pressure.

CLIENT EDUCATION GUIDE

Low-Sodium Diet

Client Instructions

Avoid foods high in sodium:

Read labels of foods carefully for "sodium," "Na⁺," "salt," "NaCl," "bicarbonate of soda," and "MSG" because these are all sources of sodium. If these words appear in the first four to five ingredients listed on the package, avoid the food item.
Avoid common commercial preparations that are high in sodium, including baking powder, baking soda, monosodium glutamate, meat tenderizer, and soy sauce.
Avoid canned, boxed, and some frozen foods to which sodium has been added. (Frozen fruits and vegetables are okay.)
Avoid canned, smoked, pickled, or cured meat and fish products. (Canned tuna in water is okay.) Pickled or preserved vegetables always contain salt.
Be aware that not all dietetic foods are sodium-free; read the labels before purchasing and using.
In restaurants, choose foods that are baked, broiled, boiled, or roasted and without salted gravies or juices. Avoid soups and salted or cheesy dressings. Carry your own salt substitute if desired. Be aware that "fast foods" also tend to be high in sodium.

CLIENT EDUCATION GUIDE

Calorie-Restriction Diet

Client Instructions

To regulate your caloric intake:

Never eat when you are doing something else, such as watching television or reading. Chew properly and slowly, and always sit down to eat.

Begin each meal with raw vegetables or salad.

Do not eat more than one slice of bread at a time. Except for a piece of toast with breakfast or a sandwich at lunch, do not eat bread with meals. Do not put butter or margarine on bread.

Stop eating when you feel not quite full. (A feeling of satiety will usually occur about 20 minutes after eating.)

Never wait until you are very hungry before you eat. Eat low-calorie, between-meal snacks if necessary.

Eat something before going to parties. Avoid high-calorie party snacks such as potato and corn chips and peanuts, almonds, and other nuts.

Drink only low-calorie beverages, such as coffee or tea (decaffeinated). Avoid adding sugar to them, although nonfat milk may be added. Do not quench your thirst with milk; use water.

Drink one to two glasses of water before drinking an alcoholic beverage. Alcoholic beverages are high in calories (7 kcal/ml).

Avoid sugar; use artificial sweeteners instead.

To appease an irresistible urge to eat something sweet, take $\frac{1}{5}$ teaspoon of sugar or a tiny bite from a chewy candy. Leave the sugar on your tongue for as long as possible. Doing this even up to six times a day will provide fewer calories than a piece of cake or several cookies.

Intervention. Exercise programs can heighten the client's sense of well-being, provide an outlet for emotional tensions, and raise the levels of high-density lipoproteins (HDLs) relative to total blood cholesterol. Elevated HDL levels are associated with a decreased risk of cardiovascular morbidity and mortality. Instruct the client, however, to avoid heavy weight-lifting, isometric exercises, and other activities inappropriate to the client's physical limitations. A modest but consistent exercise program provides greater benefits than those obtainable with spurts of strenuous activity mixed with periods of inactivity. A gradually increasing program of aerobic activity such as walking, jogging, or swimming can thus be recommended.

Current recommendations include aerobic exercise of an intensity aimed at maintaining 45% to 75% of maximal heart rate for 20 to 30 minutes, three times a week, depending on age and the coexistence of other co-morbid conditions. Maximal heart rate is calculated by subtracting the client's age from 220. Before advising and initiating an exercise prescription for your client, a qualified specialist must conduct a careful performance evaluation.

Risk for Noncompliance. Many aspects of hypertension management set the stage for noncompliance. Several factors related to specific drug use, including side effects, interference with lifestyle, cost, and inconvenience of physician visits and taking prescribed medications,

play an important role in noncompliance. Assess the reasons for noncompliance, and then state the diagnosis as *Risk for Noncompliance related to a lack of understanding about the seriousness of high blood pressure, cost of therapy, side effects of medications, complexity of management,* or *multiple changes in lifestyle.*

Outcomes. The client will actively participate in creating a treatment plan, describing the underlying causes of hypertension and self-care strategies, adhering to scheduled follow-up appointments, describing the actions and side effects of current medications, and expressing commitment to and self-responsibility for controlling hypertension.

Intervention. The greatest problem in the management of chronic hypertension involves the client's lack of adherence to nonpharmacologic and pharmacologic interventions. An estimated 40% to 60% of clients with hypertension fail to comply with prescribed therapy. There are several reasons why hypertensive clients do not follow prescribed regimens:

1. The asymptomatic nature of the disease tends to minimize the perceived seriousness of the problem and importance of intervention.
2. Therapeutic regimens often demand difficult lifestyle changes, such as low-sodium diets, weight loss, and smoking cessation.
3. Many hypertensive agents produce annoying side effects, and clients who require antihypertensive medication may consider the intervention worse than the disease.
4. The high cost of medications and the inconvenience of obtaining health care also contribute to noncompliance.

Nursing interventions for promoting compliance with the antihypertensive treatment regimen include individualizing care, ensuring adequate follow-up, communicating often with the client, and teaching the client and family. Compliance usually improves dramatically when the client understands the causative factors underlying hypertension as well as the consequences of inadequate intervention and health maintenance.

EVALUATION

Medications can bring blood pressure down quickly. The remainder of interventions, such as stress management, exercise, and smoking cessation, are more difficult to implement and maintain. Expect the client to struggle with compliance with all of the necessary changes. Ask specific questions in a nonjudgmental manner. As needed, recommend involvement in various self-help groups, such as smoking cessation groups.

■ Modifications for Elderly Clients

Hypertension is one of the most prevalent cardiovascular diseases among older adults, and because of their advanced age, these clients are more likely to suffer from end organ damage secondary to chronically elevated pressure.[10, 22] Blood pressure readings in older adults show greater variability from one measurement to the next than seen in younger clients; therefore, the diagnosis is made after several readings. Recent research findings indicate a need to treat hypertension in elderly people, regardless of whether both the systolic *and* diastolic pressures are involved or there is evidence of only isolated systolic hypertension. Older adults are more likely to experience adverse reactions to antihypertensive drugs and are monitored closely for evidence of such reactions; they are given detailed advice on the specifics of their medication regimens; and the clinical course of the disease is carefully followed.

The ultimate goal of antihypertensive therapy in older adults is not to try to lower the pressure to "normal" values but, rather, to lower the pressure gradually to a level sufficient to eliminate target organ damage and to minimize the risk of hypoperfusion. "Start low and go slow" is the principle followed for prescribing medications to the older adult. Too rapid a reduction in blood pressure in elderly clients, particularly those with chronic hypertension, may produce cerebral hypoperfusion manifested by decreased mental status, weakness, and dizziness. These changes may appear at measured blood pressures still above the upper limit of normal.

HYPERTENSIVE CRISES: URGENCY VERSUS EMERGENCY [11, 16, 18, 22, 25]

Elevated blood pressure alone, in the absence of clinical manifestations or new or progressive target organ damage, rarely requires *emergency* therapy. In most cases, the hypertensive crisis really constitutes a hypertensive *urgency,* in which severe elevation in blood pressure has been reached but there is mild or no acute target organ damage. Hypertensive urgencies include cases in which it is desirable to reduce blood pressure within a few hours to 24 hours.

However, *malignant hypertension,* a seldom-used term today, constitutes a true medical emergency and is currently referred to as *persistent severe hypertension.* The seriousness of the crisis correlates not so much with the level of blood pressure elevation as with the extent of target organ damage. Without treatment, persistent severe hypertension results in a 90% mortality rate within 1 year secondary to renal or heart failure, cerebrovascular accident, myocardial infarction, or aortic dissection. The most common cause of persistent severe hypertension is untreated hypertension. Other causes include eclampsia, dissecting aortic aneurysm, pyelonephritis, sudden catecholamine release (as from a pheochromocytoma), drug or toxic substance ingestion or exposure, and food and drug interactions (e.g., between a monoamine oxidase inhibitor [MAO] and aged cheese).

Clinical manifestations include those of hypertensive encephalopathy evidenced by restlessness, changes in level of consciousness (e.g., confusion, somnolence, lethargy, memory defects, coma, seizures), blurred vision, dizziness, headache, nausea, and vomiting. Assessment may also reveal renal insufficiency, proteinuria, hematuria, urinary sediment casts, hemolytic anemia, left ventricular failure, and pulmonary edema. Severe headache may be occipital or anterior in location, is steady and throbbing in quality, and is often worse in the morning. Visual blurring, reduced visual acuity, and even blindness can occur. Acute renal failure, rapid vascular deterioration, and stroke can also develop.

Outcome Management

True hypertensive emergencies are uncommon but do occur occasionally; in such cases, immediate blood pressure reduction is imperative to prevent or limit target organ damage. The usual initial treatment is parenteral administration of appropriate pharmacologic agents in an emergency department or an intensive care unit. Conversely, hypertensive urgencies can be managed in a hospital or clinic setting with *oral* doses of drugs with relatively fast onset of action. Oral and parenteral drugs currently used for hypertensive urgencies and emergencies are listed in Table 52–6. Although sublingual administration of nifedipine had been widely used for this purpose, it is no longer considered appropriate therapy because of several reports of severe adverse effects from its use.

The initial goal of therapy in hypertensive crisis is to reduce mean arterial pressure by no more than 25% within the first minutes to 2 hours. Then reduction in blood pressure toward 160/100 mm Hg is accomplished over the next 2 to 6 hours. Blood pressure is monitored frequently (every 5 to 15 minutes depending on the drug and route of administration used), and medications are titrated to manage the course of blood pressure reduction. It is essential to avoid excessive falls in blood pressure, which can precipitate renal, cerebral, or coronary ischemia. Consequently, restoration of normal blood pressure must be done slowly and with care. Once the client is out of immediate danger, oral medications are adjusted while vital signs are monitored continuously, and changes in drug therapy regimens are made if necessary.

COMMUNITY SCREENING AND SELF-CARE
Public Health Initiative
Research showing the importance of normalized blood pressure for clients' optimum health led to the introduction by the National Heart, Lung and Blood Institute (NHLBI) of the National High Blood Pressure Education Program (NHBPEP) in 1972.[25] The NHBPEP is the first large-scale public outreach and education campaign to reduce high blood pressure. Its promotion of the detection, treatment, and control of high blood pressure has been credited with influencing the dramatic increase in the public's understanding of hypertension and its role in heart attacks and strokes.

However, the prevention and treatment of hypertension continues to represent a major public health concern for the United States.[16, 25] Prevention of hypertension and early discovery of new cases depend on a broader national public health effort. With guidance from the *Healthy People 2000/2010* initiatives, this national effort has begun. In addition to the diligent work of the NHBPEP, government support is increasing, and nationwide attention and assistance from business and industry, labor organizations, health care institutions, voluntary associations, and local communities are also on the rise. Revised goals of the national public health plan are as follows:

- To prevent the rise of blood pressure with age
- To decrease the existing prevalence of hypertension
- To increase hypertension awareness and detection
- To improve control of hypertension
- To reduce cardiovascular risks

TABLE 52–6 PHARMACOLOGIC TREATMENT FOR HYPERTENSIVE URGENCIES AND EMERGENCIES

Drug Class with Example(s) and Dosage	Monitoring*	Comments/Nursing Considerations
HYPERTENSIVE URGENCIES		
ACE Inhibitors Captopril (Capoten)—first-line agent 25 mg PO; may repeat in 30 min Enalapril (Vasotec)—second-line agent 5 mg PO, may repeat in 30 min	BP should be checked at 15-min intervals over first hour, at 30-min intervals over second hour, then hourly	Very effective first-line therapy in hypertensive *urgency* with diastolic BP >110 mm Hg when client has no end-organ problems and oral treatment over several hours is indicated.
Centrally Acting Alpha$_2$ Agonist Clonidine (Catapres) 0.1–0.2 mg loading dose, followed by 0.1 mg every 20 min to 1 h up to 0.7–0.8 mg total	Monitor level of consciousness BP should be checked at 15-min intervals over first hour, at 30-min intervals over second hour, and then hourly	Effective second-line treatment of hypertensive urgency. Sedation is a common side effect. After 8 h, clonidine dosing may begin again if necessary.
Adrenergic Inhibitor Labetalol is the most commonly used agent in this group—see under Hypertensive Emergencies for discussion Oral dose determined per client situation.	BP should be checked at 15-min intervals over first hour, at 30-min intervals over second hour, and then hourly	Effective second-line treatment of hypertensive urgency. Be particularly watchful for the development of heart block—adrenergic blockade of normal cardiac conduction.
Calcium Antagonists/Calcium Channel Blockers Diltiazem (Cardizem) and verapamil (Calan) are drugs of choice in this category but are currently used cautiously; therapy must be completely individualized	Monitor pulse closely BP should be checked at 15-min intervals over first hour, at 30-min intervals over second hour, and then hourly	May be effective and efficient choice if BP elevation is secondary to a tachyarrhythmia. Be particularly watchful for the development of heart block—adrenergic blockade of normal cardiac conduction. Sublingual nifedipine or any fast-acting form of nifedipine is now **contraindicated** in the treatment of hypertensive emergency.
HYPERTENSIVE EMERGENCIES (Drugs listed in order of rapidity of action, with most rapid listed first)		
Vasodilators Sodium nitroprusside (Nipride) 0.25–10 μg/kg/min as IV infusion† (maximal dose for 10 min only) Fenoldopam mesylate 0.1–0.3 μg/kg/min IV infusion Nitroglycerin 5–100 μg/min as IV infusion Nicardipine hydrochloride 5–15 mg/h IV Hydralazine hydrochloride 10–20 mg IV 10–50 mg IM Enalaprilat 1.25–5 mg q 6 h IV	For all of these drugs: careful and continuous monitoring of IV lines and blood pressure is essential Monitor for too rapid a fall in BP or increase in pulse Monitor for side effects; most cause GI disturbance in varying degrees such as nausea/vomiting, tachycardia, headache, flushing, sweating—all secondary to increased vasodilation IV use of these drugs restricted to hospital emergency room and intensive care settings; drug titration continued until normotensive status prevails and persists	Nipride, fenoldopam, and nicardipine are most commonly used in hypertensive emergencies, with certain precautions to indicate which drug to use in a given situation. Nitroglycerin is drug of choice when coronary ischemia is also present (may use with extreme caution in combination with sodium nitroprusside). Enalaprilat may be most effective with acute left ventricular failure; however, it must be avoided in acute myocardial infarction.
Adrenergic Inhibitors Esmolol hydrochloride 250–500 μg/kg/min for 1 min, then 50–100 μg/kg/min for 4 min; may repeat sequence Phentolamine 5–15 mg IV Labetalol hydrochloride 20–80 mg IV bolus q 10 min 0.5–2.0 mg/min IV infusion	In addition to foregoing outcome and monitoring considerations, be particularly watchful for development of heart block—adrenergic blockade of normal cardiac conduction	Labetalol is the only one of this group that is commonly used for most hypertensive emergencies, except in acute heart failure. All of these drugs may be used in combination with vasodilators to increase effectiveness. Esmolol and phentolamine are reserved for specific underlying causes of increased blood pressure (i.e., aortic dissection and catecholamine excess, respectively).

*See Table 52–5 for drug actions and therapeutic outcomes.
ACE: angiotensin-converting enzyme; BP, blood pressure.

- To increase the recognition of the importance of controlled isolated systolic hypertension
- To improve recognition of the importance of the persistence and damage from high-normal blood pressures
- To reduce ethnic, socioeconomic, and regional variations in hypertension
- To improve opportunities for treatment
- To enhance community programs

Managed Care and Community Screening

Because high blood pressure is very common, its management requires a major commitment from clinicians and managed care organizations. Managed care programs offer the opportunity for a coordinated systematic, multifactorial, multidisciplinary approach to care. Nurse-managed clinics offer attractive opportunities to improve adherence and outcomes.

Hypertensive clients usually find out about their condition through incidental screening in health care facilities or through organized community screening in public settings (e.g., shopping malls, schools, the workplace). Nurses are actively involved in both approaches. About 80% of Americans come into contact with some aspect of the health care system at least once a year (e.g., in a health care provider's office, clinic, or hospital). Each encounter with the health care system presents an opportunity for incidental blood pressure screening. Blood pressure measurement should be a routine procedure at every initial encounter with a health care practitioner and annually thereafter.

Organized community screening programs help assess the remaining 20% of Americans not in contact with any part of the health care system.[29] Such programs identify not only clients with untreated hypertension but also those who have discontinued intervention or whose hypertension is not adequately controlled by current intervention. In addition, screening programs provide an opportunity to educate the public. It is particularly important to screen members of high-risk "target groups," such as black and elderly populations. Community services need to keep target groups in mind when choosing the setting for blood pressure screenings. Practitioners who take blood pressure readings need to inform clients in writing of their blood pressure and its significance and, if necessary, the importance of follow-up evaluation. Culturally and linguistically appropriate counseling by health care providers is important to those efforts.

Self-Measurement of Blood Pressure

Measurement of blood pressure outside a health care provider's office can provide valuable information for initial evaluation and subsequent follow-up of people with hypertension. Most drug, medical supply, and grocery stores provide standardized blood pressure monitors that their customers can use at no cost. These monitoring stations are generally located near the pharmacy or medical supplies department. Such stores also usually carry a variety of self-measurement blood pressure devices for home use. Choosing a monitoring device may be confusing for some people; however, several models of accurate and appropriate electronic or aneroid-type sphygmomanometers are available. Most insurance packages cover the cost of a home blood pressure unit, and these devices are generally easy to use.

Manual and electronic arm and wrist cuffs are the most accurate. Finger monitors are available but have proved inaccurate in standardized testing. Periodically, the accuracy of the instrument used in the home should be checked by comparing home readings with those obtained in the health care provider's office, at a "health fair," or in a community nursing clinic.

SYNCOPE

Syncope (fainting) is defined as generalized muscle weakness and inability to stand erect accompanied by loss of consciousness. It is a good measure of cardiovascular status because it may indicate decreased cardiac output, fluid volume deficits, or defects in cerebral tissue perfusion.

Syncope is a common occurrence when a person tries to stand after being bedridden for a time. This form of syncope, called *postural hypotension,* can be seen in clients attempting to ambulate the first few times after surgery, in clients who have been on prolonged bed rest, and clients who have dysrhythmias. When a person quickly moves to a standing position, blood normally pools in the lower legs. The arterial pressure receptors in the aortic arch detect the fall in cardiac output that occurs with the lack of venous return, and they increase sympathetic tone to compress arterioles to improve venous return.[5] If the sympathetic response is not adequate or is blocked by medication, the person becomes dizzy because of the decreased cerebral perfusion. All medications taken to reduce blood pressure have the potential to cause orthostatic hypotension or postural hypotension—some more than others, such as potent diuretics, alpha$_1$-receptor blockers, and vasodilators.

When a client reports dizziness or is at risk of syncope because of medication use or prolonged bed rest, assess fluid volume status and check the pulse for irregularities. If syncope develops, it can usually be managed by having the client move slowly to a sitting position and rest a moment before standing. If the client becomes dizzy, instruct him or her to breathe deeply and to keep both eyes open. Syncope should resolve within moments. If it is prolonged, place the client supine, use leg exercises to improve venous return, and wait until the blood pressure returns to a normotensive state. Confused clients who do not wait for syncope to resolve before walking are at risk for falls. Bed alarms may be needed.

CONCLUSIONS

New coalitions between health care providers and individual communities are forming to focus on the prevention and management of hypertension throughout all stages of life. Support from the community and greater use of technology such as the Internet will play an increasingly greater role in promoting long-term adherence to lifestyle and pharmacologic regimens. Achieving long-term control of blood pressure risk factors requires that the same interest and attention given to initial evaluation and treatment decisions also be given to long-term management issues.

THINKING CRITICALLY

A 50-year-old obese black man presents to your clinic with persistent elevated blood pressure. He has

had hypertension for 7 months. Despite attempts at lifestyle management, his blood pressure continued to rise. He was started on a regimen of antihypertensive medication 1 month ago. He has returned to the clinic today for a follow-up visit. His blood pressure is higher than it was initially. What might explain his continued elevated blood pressure?

Factors to Consider. What other history and physical examination data should you obtain in order to more effectively analyze this case? When and how long should lifestyle modifications alone be encouraged? How long does it take for various medications to be effective? What diseases worsen hypertension? What psychosocial factors affect compliance with or adherence to a treatment regimen? What modifications in the pharmacologic treatment plan, if any, would be most appropriate at this time?

BIBLIOGRAPHY

1. Patient education. Understanding hypertension. (1999). *Nurse Practitioner: American Journal of Primary Health Care, 24*(5), 38.
2. Ambler, S. K., & Brown, R. D. (1999). Genetic determinants of blood pressure regulation. *Journal of Cardiovascular Nursing, 13*(4), 59–77.
3. Benson, H., & Friedman, R. (1996). Harnessing the power of the placebo effect and renaming it "remembered wellness." *Annual Review of Medicine, 47,* 193–199.
4. Bushnell, K. L., & Smith, L. A. (1998). Hypertension clinical outcomes in a nurse practitioner managed care setting. *Seminars in Nursing Management, 6*(3), 155–160.
5. Engstrom, J. W., & Aminoff, M. J. (1997). Evaluation and treatment of orthostatic hypotension. *American Family Physician, 56,* 1378–1384.
6. Fagan, T. C. (1995). Calcium antagonists and mortality: Another case of the need for clinical judgment. *Archives of Internal Medicine, 155,* 2145.
7. Kolasa, K. M. (1999). Dietary Approaches to Stop Hypertension (DASH) in clinical practice: A primary care experience. *Clinical Cardiology, 22*(7 suppl.), III16–III22.
8. Kuncl, N., & Nelson, K. M. (1997). Antihypertensive drugs: Balancing risks and benefits. *Nursing, 27*(8), 46–49.
9. Kyngas, H., & Lahdenpera, T. (1999). Compliance of patients with hypertension and associated factors. *Journal of Advanced Nursing, 29*(4), 832–839.
10. Lever, A. F., & Ramsey, L. E. (1995). Treatment of hypertension in the elderly. *Current Science, 13,* 571–579.
11. Mancia, G., & Grassi, G. (1998). Antihypertensive treatment: Past, present and future. *Journal of Hypertension, Supplement, 16*(1), S1–S7.
12. McCance, K. L. (1998). Structure and function of the cardiovascular and lymphatic systems. In K. L. McCance & S. E. Huether (Eds.), *Pathophysiology: The biologic basis for disease in adults and children* (pp. 968–1023). St. Louis: Mosby–Year Book.
13. McPaul, K. (1999). New hypertension guidelines: Commentary. *AAOHN Journal, 47*(3), 114–116.
14. Michels, K. B., et al. (1998). Prospective study of calcium-channel blocker use, cardiovascular disease, and total mortality among hypertensive women. The Nurses' Health Study. *Circulation, 97,* 1540–1548.
15. Moser, M. (1998). Why are physicians not prescribing diuretics more frequently in the management of hypertension? *Journal of the American Medical Association, 279*(22), 1813–1816.
16. National High Blood Pressure Education Program, National Institutes of Health, National Heart, Lung and Blood Institute. (1997). *The Sixth Report of the Joint National Committee on Detection, Evaluation, and Treatment of High Blood Pressure* (NIH Publication No. 98-4080). Bethesda, MD: U.S. Government Printing Office.
17. Pinkowish, M. D. (1995). What is white-coat hypertension? *Patient Care, 23*(2), 15.
18. Porsche, R. (1995). Hypertension: Diagnosis, acute antihypertension therapy, and long-term management. *AACN Clinical Issues, 6,* 515–525.
19. Psaty, B. M., et al. (1997). Health outcomes associated with antihypertensive therapies used as first-line agents. A systematic review and meta-analysis. *Journal of the American Medical Association, 277,* 739–745.
20. Schneider, R. H., et al. (1995). A randomized controlled trial of stress reduction for hypertension in older African Americans. *Hypertension, 26,* 820–827.
21. Seidel, H. M., et al. (1999). *Mosby's guide to physical examination* (4th ed.). St. Louis: Mosby.
22. Sullivan, J. A. (1998). Hypertension in the elderly: Don't treat too quickly! *Journal of Emergency Nursing, 24*(1), 20–26.
23. Tobin, L. J. (1999). Evaluating mild to moderate hypertension. *Nurse Practitioner, 24*(5), 22, 25–26, 29–30.
24. Uphold, C. R., & Graham, M. V. (1998). *Clinical guidelines in family practice* (3rd ed.). Gainesville, FL: Barmarrae Books.
25. U.S. Department of Health and Human Services. (2000). *Healthy People 2010: National health promotion and disease prevention objectives.* Washington, DC: Public Health Service.
26. U.S. Department of Health and Human Services. (1995). *Clinical practice guideline number 17: Cardiac rehabilitation.* (AHCPR Pub. No. 96-0672). Rockville, MD: Author.
27. Van Wissen, K., Litchfield, M., Maling, T. (1998). Living with high blood pressure. *Journal of Advanced Nursing, 27*(3), 567–574.
28. Vantrimpont, P., et al. (1997). Additive beneficial effects of beta-blockers to angiotensin-converting enzyme inhibitors in the Survival and Ventricular Enlargement (SAVE) study. *Journal of American College of Cardiology, 29,* 229–236.
29. Wang, C., & Abbott, L. J. (1998). Development of a community-based diabetes and hypertension preventive program. *Public Health Nursing, 15*(6), 406–414.
30. Weber, M. (1999). Guidelines for assessing outcomes of antihypertensive treatment. *American Journal of Cardiology, 84*(2A), 2K–4K.

REMEMBER *to*
check out your
Companion CD ROM

CHAPTER

53

Management of Clients with Vascular Disorders

Janice D. Nunnelee

NURSING OUTCOMES CLASSIFICATION (NOC)
for Nursing Diagnoses—Clients with Vascular Disorders

Altered Tissue Perfusion
Pain Level
Tissue Perfusion: Cardiac
Tissue Perfusion: Pulmonary
Vital Signs Status
Anxiety
Anxiety Control
Coping
Delayed Surgical Recovery
Endurance
Infection Status
Self-Care: Activities of Daily Living (ADL)
Wound Healing: Primary Intention
Wound Healing: Secondary Intention
Health Seeking Behaviors
Adherence Behaviors
Health Beliefs
Health Promoting Behavior
Health Seeking Behavior
Knowledge: Health Promotion
Knowledge: Health Resources
Impaired Gas Exchange
Electrolyte and Acid-Base Balance
Respiratory Status: Gas Exchange

Respiratory Status: Ventilation
Tissue Perfusion: Pulmonary
Impaired Physical Mobility
Ambulation: Walking
Body Positioning: Self-Initiated
Immobility Consequences: Physiologic
Mobility Level
Transfer Performance
Knowledge Deficit
Knowledge Deficit: Disease Process
Knowledge Deficit: Health Behaviors
Knowledge Deficit: Health Resources
Knowledge: Medication
Knowledge Deficit: Illness
Knowledge: Prescribed Activity
Knowledge Deficit: Treatment
    Procedure(s)
Knowledge: Treatment Regimen
Pain
Comfort Level
Pain Control
Pain: Disruptive Effects
Pain Level

Risk for Activity Intolerance
Coping
Health Beliefs: Perceived Control
Mood Equilibrium
Nutritional Status: Energy
Symptom Control
Symptom Severity
Risk for Fluid Volume Deficit
Bowel Elimination
Electrolyte and Acid-Base Balance
Fluid Balance
Hydration
Nutritional Status: Food and Fluid Intake
Urinary Elimination
Risk for Impaired Skin Integrity
Immobility Consequences: Physiologic
Nutritional Status
Physical Aging Status
Risk Control
Risk Detection
Tissue Integrity: Skin and Mucous
    Membranes
Tissue Perfusion: Peripheral

PERIPHERAL ARTERY DISORDERS

Peripheral vascular disease encompasses three systems: the arterial, the venous, and the lymphatic. Peripheral arterial occlusive disorders involve narrowing of the arterial lumen or damage to the endothelial lining. Narrowing can be partial (stenosis) or complete (occlusion). The clinical manifestations and management may differ, depending on the client's needs and the degree of occlusion. Additionally, the manifestations of chronic disease differ considerably from those of acute arterial disease.

Etiology and Risk Factors

Peripheral arterial occlusive diseases are caused primarily by atherosclerosis. Other causes include embolism, throm-

bosis, trauma, vasospasm, inflammation, and autoimmunity. Obesity is a risk factor for arterial disorders. The cause of some disorders remains unknown. Most of the pathologic changes that occur in peripheral arterial occlusive disease are caused by atherosclerosis. Atherosclerosis is considered in detail in Chapter 56.

Pathophysiology

The peripheral arterial system delivers oxygen-rich blood to the peripheral vascular beds. Any alteration in blood flow disrupts the balance between oxygen supply and demand. Prolonged reduction in blood flow or the presence of large areas of decreased perfusion initiates vasodilation and promotes the development of collateral arterial pathways and utilization of anaerobic pathways for oxygen demands to be met. These compensatory mechanisms are designed to bring in new blood supplies but are limited in effectiveness. Vasodilation has a limited effect because arteries that are deprived of oxygen quickly become maximally dilated. Collateral vessels needed to improve blood supply develop slowly over time. Cellular anaerobic metabolism tries to meet the basic requirements, but the waste products of lactic acid and pyruvic acid build up quickly, are extremely toxic, and are excreted slowly. Significant increases in these two acids can lead to acidosis.

As the compensatory mechanisms prove inadequate to meet peripheral arterial needs, and without other intervention, the eventual result is pain. The pain is analogous to anginal pain and is called *intermittent claudication,* which occurs when a muscle is forced to contract without an adequate blood supply to meet the metabolic needs of exercise. It is a specific manifestation of peripheral arterial disease and results from muscular hypoxia and metabolite accumulation. Any muscle can claudicate, including muscles in the arms, legs, jaw, or anywhere that decreased arterial supply exists. This section primarily focuses on lower extremity disease.

The physiologic effect of any given stenosis is variable because it is determined not only by the degree of narrowing but also by the number of collateral vessels that have developed. The lower limbs are more susceptible to arterial occlusive disorders and atherosclerosis than the upper limbs because of the natural collateral system in the upper extremities. The most common locations of stenosis supplying a lower extremity are the aortoiliac bifurcation and the femoral bifurcation (Fig. 53–1). In general, stenoses occur at bifurcations in arteries.

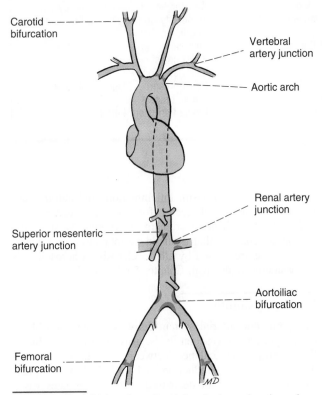

Carotid bifurcation

Vertebral artery junction

Aortic arch

Renal artery junction

Superior mesenteric artery junction

Aortoiliac bifurcation

Femoral bifurcation

FIGURE 53–1 Major sites of peripheral atherosclerotic occlusive disease.

Clinical Manifestations

The most important manifestations of chronic arterial occlusive disease are *intermittent claudication* and *rest pain.* The client typically complains of pain described as tightening pressure in the calves or buttocks or a sharp, cramp-like or burning sensation that occurs during walking and disappears with rest. The pain is reproducible and not positional. It always occurs in a muscle distal to the stenosis or occlusion.

Intermittent claudication is influenced by the speed and incline of the walk, conditions that increase the demand for oxygen by muscles of the legs. The more rapid the speed or the greater the incline, the faster claudication occurs. The client's exercise tolerance generally decreases over time; episodes of claudication occur with less exertion. Claudication response is constant, reproducible, and not positional. *Reproducible* means that the client who walks the same distance at the same speed and incline has manifestations at the same distance each time. The client who cannot walk the length of a house because of leg pain one day but can walk indefinitely the next day does not have intermittent claudication.

Another hallmark of chronic arterial insufficiency is a dusky, purplish discoloration of the foot and leg when the foot is placed in a dependent position. This *dependent rubor* changes to white pallor when the leg is elevated.

Clinical manifestations of chronic arterial occlusion may not appear for 20 to 40 years. Claudication, usually insidious in onset, generally occurs in men, although the incidence rises in women after menopause. Usually, claudication strikes males in their 50s or 60s. Nearly half of clients who experience claudication also have associated severe coronary artery disease.

As the disease progresses, clinical manifestations become more severe. The development of pain at rest, usually occurring at night when the client lies supine, indicates limb-threatening disease. Usually described as a dull, deep pain in the toes or forefoot, this sensation awakens clients from sleep and may cause them to hang the foot over the side of the bed or to get up and walk around for relief. Clients may start to sleep in a chair with their legs dependent. Placing the leg in a dependent position provides increased gravitation supply of blood. This often results in a moderate degree of lower extremity edema. The affected foot usually demonstrates dependent rubor.

Manifestations of cutaneous arterial insufficiency are nonspecific. Their presence in combination with claudication, however, indicates advanced disease. Skin and subcutaneous tissues require little blood flow for maintenance of normal nutrition. Coldness of feet is an unreliable sign, but a sudden onset of coldness suggests acute arterial insufficiency or occlusion. Other objective data associated with arterial insufficiency include weak or absent peripheral pulses, dependent rubor and pallor with elevation, hypertrophied toenails, tissue atrophy, ulceration, and gangrene (Fig. 53–2). Paresthesias with exertion indicate ischemia of the peripheral nerves because of the phenomenon of *arterial steal.* This phenomenon occurs as arterioles of the muscles are maximally dilated because of hypoxia. To meet muscular metabolic needs, these arterioles steal from cutaneous and peripheral nerve vessels,

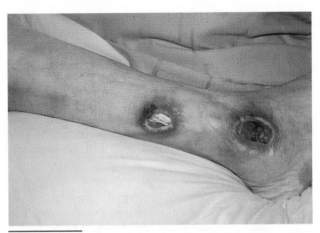

FIGURE 53–2 Arterial ulcers of the lateral malleolus and distal lateral portion of the leg. Note round, smooth shape.

which results in coldness and a "pins and needles" sensation.

Lower extremity pain may also appear in several other disorders unrelated to arterial disease. Other conditions that cause a similar type of pain include arthritis, lumbar disc protrusion, neuritis, and muscle cramps. However, the pain of other conditions is not consistent or replicable. The pain of arthritis, disc protrusion, and neuritis may also be positional.

Aortoiliac disorders are a form of chronic arterial occlusive disease characterized by aortoiliac stenosis and occlusion. These disorders result in clinical manifestations in the legs (Fig. 53–3). Assessment reveals hip, thigh, and buttock claudication with absent or diminished femoral and distal pulses. In males, impotence is also part of the syndrome known as Leriche's syndrome. Dependent rubor is common when aortoiliac and femoropopliteal disorders are combined.

A femoropopliteal disorder refers to an occlusion in the chief arteries of the proximal leg or thigh. The most common manifestation of superficial femoral artery and popliteal disease is calf claudication, which may improve, stay the same, or potentially progress to rest pain. Popliteal artery disease and stenosis in the anterior or posterior tibial artery results in claudication in the distal leg and foot.

Diagnostic evaluation of the lower extremity includes both noninvasive and invasive techniques. Techniques range from simple measurement of ankle/brachial index (ABI) to the use of magnetic resonance imaging (MRI) to measure arterial blood flow. Recording of an ABI provides information at the bedside. Segmental Doppler systolic blood pressure and pulse waveform analysis provide more objective information about the level and severity of occlusive disease. Treadmill examination, a form of lower extremity stress testing, measures the fall of arterial pressure with ambulation and the rapidity with which it returns to baseline. Color flow imaging visualizes the blood flow in the vessels and records pressures within the vessel. It is possible that imaging may replace arteriography in the future.

Arteriography is the definitive examination when surgery is being considered. It reveals the lumen of the blood vessels. It is not a measurement of actual blood flow, as the noninvasive assessment is, but instead shows the outline of the contrast media within the lumen. Because of the contrast media, there are many potential complications. Computed tomography (CT) angiography, sometimes called spiral CT, is in its infancy but may replace conventional angiography.

Outcome Management

The goals of management are to reduce the risk of progressive arterial disease, promote arterial flow, and reverse the disease that is present. Important outcomes include improving the quality of life if no other intervention is possible. Specialists in the field exist in both the medical and advanced nursing practice realm. Medical management is appropriate for clients with intermittent claudication and non-limb-threatening ischemia. Additionally, medical management may be the only course of action in the client with multiple morbidities who is a poor surgical risk.

▬ Medical Management

RISK REDUCTION

WEIGHT REDUCTION. Clients are advised and counseled to reduce body weight by following a low-fat, low-

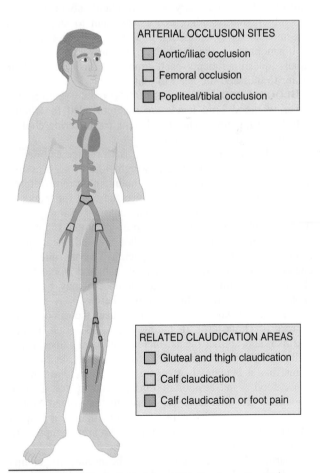

ARTERIAL OCCLUSION SITES
- Aortic/iliac occlusion
- Femoral occlusion
- Popliteal/tibial occlusion

RELATED CLAUDICATION AREAS
- Gluteal and thigh claudication
- Calf claudication
- Calf claudication or foot pain

FIGURE 53–3 Occlusion of the arterial system at any given location leads to a specific portion of claudication in distal tissues.

cholesterol diet containing more fruits and vegetables. There is no evidence that any special diet alters the course of atherosclerosis once it has appeared. Small studies claim that rigid diets reverse atherosclerosis, but no major body of data exists to support this hypothesis.

EXERCISE. A prescribed moderate program of exercise and rest helps increase collateral circulation and improve conditioning. Several studies have shown that clients involved in an exercise program generally feel better and can slowly improve their walking distance. Clients are instructed to walk every day, provided that no skin ulcerations are present. The exercise program should begin judiciously and progress gradually until the client has substantially lengthened walking distances. For obese and chronically ill clients, an exercise program should be (1) individually tailored to the client's abilities, goals, interests, and resources and (2) written with specific instructions.[20] Most clients can significantly increase their walking distance, and many can avoid surgery if they exercise regularly and stop smoking.

SMOKING CESSATION. Cigarette smoking influences vascular disability. Nicotine is a potent vasoconstrictor. Clients who stop smoking improve their treadmill walking distance. Smoking cessation is extremely difficult, because nicotine is a highly addictive chemical. Social support, especially of friends and family members, seems to be an important factor in assisting smokers to quit. Pharmacologic measures may be instituted by the primary care provider if necessary. Educate clients about the dangers of cigarette smoke, encourage them to stop, act as role models for nonsmoking, and support policies to prohibit smoking in the workplace. Primary care providers should question clients each time they visit about their desire to quit and the need to quit.

BLOOD LIPID LEVEL REDUCTION. Interventions for lowering blood lipid levels are recommended for clients with hyperlipidemia. The initial steps for lowering cholesterol involve dietary intervention.

For obese clients, the first goal is to reduce calories to achieve ideal body weight. If weight loss is seen as improbable, the client should try to maintain current weight.

The next major step is to reduce the total fat intake in the diet to 30% or less of total calories. Saturated fat intake should be reduced. The most common sources of saturated fat in the American diet are red meat, fried foods, and dairy products, especially whole milk and cheese. Increasing the quantity of fish and poultry and changing to skim milk and nonfat cheese may be sufficient to meet saturated fat recommendations.

The third major goal is to reduce the amount of sources of cholesterol, including egg yolks, organ meats, shellfish, and animal meats. Increasing dietary fiber, especially soluble fiber, such as that found in oats, lentils, and beans, has a beneficial effect on lipid levels. Fast foods, snack foods, and restaurant dining account for a large amount of the increased fat intake in the United States. Dietary counseling by a registered dietitian is a helpful intervention for clients and families who are attempting to change eating habits.

Pharmacologic intervention may be needed for clients with high levels of hyperlipidemia and for those whose dietary changes have been less than successful. The major drug groups include nicotinic acid, fibrin acid derivatives,

bile acid resins, meglutol (hydroxymethylglutaryl), coenzyme A (CoA) reductase inhibitors, and probucol. These medications have varying degrees of effectiveness, and each produces important side effects. Guidelines have changed over the past few years, with intervention encouraged when the low-density lipoproteins (LDLs) reach 160 in a client with no risk factors and 130 (with levels of 100 recommended) in diabetic clients or when clients have two or more risk factors. Controversy exists over treatment in younger clients with high LDLs or triglycerides.

PROMOTE ARTERIAL FLOW

Vasodilators were popular in the remote past, although no convincing studies ever supported their use. Pentoxifylline (e.g., Trental) was introduced and shown to be somewhat effective in increasing walking distance in combination with conditioning exercise. Pentoxifylline is reported to reduce blood viscosity and enhance oxygen delivery to the muscle of the affected limb. The major side effect is gastrointestinal upset, which may be avoided by taking the medication with meals. A new drug, cilostazol (Pletal), helps to increase walking distance with or without exercise. Ongoing trials will give evidence to its efficacy.

In severe cases of arterial insufficiency, the physician may order that the reverse Trendelenburg position be used. The head of the client's bed should be elevated on 6-inch blocks (either constructed, or use steady books such as encyclopedias) so that blood from the heart flows more easily, via gravity, to the extremities when the client sleeps or rests.

▪ Nursing Management of the Medical Client

ASSESSMENT

The history should include an account of arterial problems, surgery, medications, and ulcerations. Because of the chronic nature of the problem, a psychosocial assessment is warranted. Feelings of powerlessness may exist. Some clients are not aware of chest pain, shortness of breath, or fatigue because their attention is focused on leg discomfort. Question them carefully about these discomforts. Medical or surgical intervention may reduce pain and thus improve walking ability.

The physical examination should include peripheral pulses, ABI, assessment of quality of arterial flow with a hand-held Doppler, notations of skin color, assessment of skin integrity (including the presence of ulcers, darkened areas of skin, tinea pedis, thickened nails), capillary refill (≤ 3 seconds is normal), and the presence of venous filling when the foot is dependent.

DIAGNOSIS, OUTCOMES, INTERVENTIONS

Altered Tissue Perfusion. The ideal nursing diagnosis for clients with arterial disorders is *Altered Peripheral Tissue Perfusion*. Write the diagnosis as *Altered Peripheral Tissue Perfusion related to interruption of blood flow secondary to arterial occlusion.*

Outcomes. The client will maintain adequate peripheral tissue perfusion in affected extremities, as evidenced by warm, dry skin with normal peripheral pulse, color, temperature, motor and sensory function, and capillary filling.

Interventions

Promote Arterial Flow. For safe positioning of a client with peripheral vascular disease, first learn whether the disorder is arterial or venous in nature. Because blood flows to dependent parts of the body (i.e., parts lower than the heart), position clients with arterial disease so that blood flows toward the legs and feet. In milder cases, clients can benefit from sitting for periods of time with their feet flat on the floor. If the reverse Trendelenburg position is used, assess for dependent edema. Remind clients with arterial insufficiency to avoid raising their feet above heart level unless the physician has specifically prescribed this as an exercise. Authorities vary in their opinion as to the best position for enhancing arterial flow to the feet.

Prevent Vasoconstriction. Explain the dangers of smoking to the client who uses tobacco. Encourage the client to stop smoking completely. The client who realizes that smoking literally threatens life and limbs may develop sufficient motivation to quit. Help the client locate therapy groups or biofeedback training. Do not recommend the use of nicotine patches. Patches provide continuous administration of nicotine and can cause continuous vasospasm.

Encourage the client to avoid stressful situations and to try to relax, both mentally and physically. Counseling services may be indicated for nervous, high-strung clients. Offer information regarding stress reduction classes. Remember to involve significant others.

Prevent the client from becoming chilled. Clients should wear protective clothing in layers during cold weather, warm cars before entering them, and follow winter driving precautions.

Risk for Impaired Skin Integrity. Because of altered peripheral tissue perfusion, the client is at risk of arterial ulceration and skin infection. Write the diagnosis as *Risk for Impaired Skin Integrity related to decreased peripheral circulation.* If the client has an arterial ulcer, this diagnosis can still be used for the remaining intact skin.

Outcomes. The client will maintain intact skin surfaces, with healed skin surfaces, freedom from signs of infection, and signs of wound healing.

Interventions. Prevent injury to the extremities, particularly the feet. Excellent foot care should be an integral part of the daily routine of clients with peripheral vascular disorders, because prevention is easier to initiate and maintain than is correction (see the Client Education Guide on foot care).

CLIENT EDUCATION GUIDE

Foot Care

Client Instructions

Daily Hygiene

Do not soak your feet; use mild soap and a washcloth to clean them.
Dry well between your toes.
Check water temperature with a bath thermometer or your elbow, not your toes, to prevent burns; 32.2° to 35° C (90° to 95° F) is safe.
Gently rub corns or calluses. Avoid cutting, digging, or using harsh commercial products.

Daily Inspection and Lubrication

Use good lighting.
Put on your glasses or contacts, if you wear them.
Promptly report ulcerations, redness, calluses, blisters, or cracking of the skin on the feet or thickening of the nails to the physician.
Rub soothing lotions or lanolin on your hands, feet, legs, and arms to prevent dryness.
Do not use lotion on sores or between your toes.
Do not use perfumed lotions.
Dust your feet lightly with cornstarch if they sweat.

Care of Toenails

Use clippers, not scissors or razor blades.
Cut straight across the nail.
Do not perform "bathroom surgery."
If your eyesight is poor or if you are unable to reach your toes, find qualified assistance.
Place lamb's wool between overlapping toes.

Proper Footwear

Never go barefoot, not even at the beach or at home.
Avoid high heels and shoes with pointed toes.

Make sure nothing is in your shoes before putting them on your feet.
Avoid tight socks and shoes.
Wear cotton socks for absorbency. Change your socks daily.
Alternate several pairs of comfortable, firm, well-made shoes during the week.
Avoid shoes that cause your feet to perspire (for example, canvas shoes and rubber boots).
Make sure that your shoes and slippers fit well and are sturdy enough to prevent foot injury.

Safety

Avoid sunburn.
Avoid scratching insect bites on your legs to prevent creating open lesions.
Do not use heating pads.
Wear adequate foot protection on cold days.
Turn on the lights before entering a dark hallway or room.
Avoid sitting with your legs crossed.
Use a cane or walker, if indicated.
When in doubt, ask for help. Have telephone numbers of people who can assist you at hand.

Activity

Walking is good, but get your physician's permission before beginning a regular program.
Do not walk if you have open ulcerations.
Walk until pain begins, stop and rest, then begin again.
Elevate your feet if they swell.
Find a nurse and a physician who will get to know you and your foot problems and will take the time to talk with you when you need help.

Pain. Intermittent claudication is caused by ischemia. The diagnosis can be written *Pain related to inadequate arterial blood supply to the legs.*

Outcomes. The client will experience increased comfort, as evidenced by self-report and demonstrated knowledge of pain relief measures, both pharmacologic and nonpharmacologic.

Interventions. The pain of ischemia is usually chronic, continuous, and difficult to relieve. Arterial leg ulcers are exquisitely painful. Because of pain, clients with arterial disorders are often depressed and irritable. Pain limits their activities, disturbs their sleep, saps their energy, and has a demoralizing emotional effect. Thus, pain must be relieved if the client is to rest and improve.

Help clients assess and plan ways of correcting the position of their beds at home. The head of the bed can be elevated to promote blood flow to the legs. Remind the client with arterial insufficiency to:

- Avoid standing in one position for more than a few minutes
- Avoid crossing the legs at the knees
- Seek the most comfortable position
- Watch for and report edema

Any measure that increases circulation to the extremities helps alleviate ischemic pain. Although pain also can be subdued by analgesics, interventions that augment circulation are best. For more information on pain control, see Chapter 23. When strong analgesics such as morphine are necessary around the clock, the client may require amputation. Amputation can improve the quality of life by diminishing pain and improving mobility with a prosthesis.

Risk for Activity Intolerance. The client's pain (intermittent claudication) may greatly deter activity. This common diagnosis is written as *Risk for Activity Intolerance related to leg pain after walking.*

Outcomes. The client will develop appropriate levels of activity free from pain and excess fatigue, as evidenced by normal vital signs, absence of pain, and verbalized understanding of the benefits of gradual increase in activity and exercise.

Interventions. When assisting the client with a walking program, assert that *pain* should be the guide for the amount of activity to be undertaken. Intermittent claudication signals that the muscles and tissues of the legs are not receiving enough oxygen. Before the client begins a walking program, take a careful history and perform a physical assessment. Establish a cardiopulmonary profile, and carefully examine the client's feet and legs to locate open ulcerations or anatomic deformities. The client should have sturdy shoes to prevent foot trauma.

Although exercise helps most clients with vascular disorders, some clients must not exercise, such as clients with leg ulcers, pain at rest, cellulitis, deep vein thrombosis (DVT, unless the client is receiving low-molecular-weight heparin), or gangrene. Exercise and activity increase the metabolic needs of tissues and, consequently, tissue requirements for oxygenated blood. Thus, clients with tissue breakdown or necrosis must remain for a period on complete bed rest. Even minimal activity raises the oxygen requirements of the tissues above those that damaged arteries can provide.

Knowledge Deficit. The nursing diagnosis *Knowledge Deficit* can be used as a guide to teaching the client about a walking program. State the diagnosis as *Knowledge Deficit related to walking program as evidenced by no previous experience.*

Outcomes. The client will follow a progressive walking program.

Interventions. Remind clients that at first it may be painful to walk any distance and they may need to stop frequently to rest. They should walk through the pain as much as possible without causing undue distress. Encourage them to walk in enclosed shopping malls in the winter for safety from falls on icy pavement and to avoid vasoconstriction from the cold outdoors. In the summer, malls help to avoid heat exhaustion or stress on other comorbidities. It is important to emphasize that small increments of exercise increase are not dramatic but are evidence of improvement. Even improvements that enable clients to shop in the grocery store is a cause for celebration.

Health-Seeking Behaviors. Health-conscious clients may request information about self-improvement and interventions to reduce the severity of manifestations. Write the diagnosis as *Health Seeking Behaviors related to lack of knowledge about the role of exercise, weight reduction, and smoking cessation in management of arterial disease.*

Outcomes. The client will begin and maintain the chosen health promotion program, as evidenced by demonstrated knowledge of the specific activities of the program, regular evaluation of goals against performance, and verbalized feelings of increased well-being.

Interventions. Instruct the client in areas of concern or interest (see the nonpharmacologic intervention methods described earlier). Refer the client to groups in the community if available. The client with intermittent claudication caused by arterial disease should be routinely reexamined at least every 3 months for progression of the disease. Use the information in the Alternative Therapies feature to teach clients about other treatments.

EVALUATION

Arterial disorders are chronic, and you should not expect to see reversal of the problems. Write outcomes that allow for time and client adjustments.

Modifications for Elderly Clients

Age-related changes and impairments of physiologic function concomitant with arterial disease affect the nursing diagnoses of *Activity Intolerance* (possibly increased), *Altered Peripheral Tissue Perfusion* (possibly reduced), and *Pain.* Recognition of pain may be complicated by physical or cognitive impairments, ongoing drug therapy, and psychosocial factors (e.g., depression or social isolation). Additionally, sight reduction and flexibility limitations may prevent or decrease self-care. Diminished sight may increase risks for falls or other injury, which may be disastrous in the client with impaired circulation.

Surgical Management

ENDOVASCULAR INTERVENTIONS

Endovascular interventional therapies use angioscopy, intraluminal ultrasonography, balloon angioplasty, laser,

ALTERNATIVE THERAPY

Vascular Disorders

A number of natural therapies may be useful in the treatment of vascular problems. During the 1940s and 1950s, researchers found that vitamin E can be useful in the treatment of intermittent claudication, with a number of randomized, double-blind trials supporting the use of vitamin E. Dosages from the most successful studies were 400 to 800 mg/day, with effects becoming apparent generally after 3 months. However, recent studies indicate doses above 400 mg/day increase the risk of intracranial bleeding, especially if used with aspirin. Interestingly, vitamin E use "was associated with marked decreases in the rate of leg amputation and even overall mortality, in addition to decreasing claudication."[2] No further trials of vitamin E in treating intermittent claudication have been conducted since the 1970s, perhaps because of the resistance in the medical community to nutritional, nonpharmaceutical therapies.

A number of herbs have been studied for their circulatory effects. Ginkgo biloba has been found minimally effective for intermittent claudication as well as for decreased cerebral circulation leading to reduced function. Manifestations can include decreased memory, vertigo, tinnitus, and mood swings with anxiety.[4] One study of ginkgo use in clients with mild to moderate cognitive impairment found improvements in a number of parameters as well as significant decreases in diastolic blood pressure in those receiving a low (40 mg three times a day) daily dose of ginkgo.[5] Optimal dosage may need to be determined by further research.

In the treatment of chronic venous insufficiency, horse-chestnut seed extract (HCSE, *Aesculus hippocastanum*) may be superior to placebo, equivalent to a reference medication, and therapeutically equivalent to compression stocking therapy.[3] German health authorities have approved HCSE for the treatment of chronic venous insufficiency as well as for pain and heaviness in the legs and varicose veins. Gastrointestinal side effects may occur but are uncommon.[4]

Garlic has been studied for its effects on arteriosclerosis and lipids with varying results. The amount of fresh garlic a person would need to eat for a therapeutic dosage is quite high and likely to cause gastric upset. Garlic preparations vary widely in terms of their active constituents. In one study of garlic powder versus a placebo in people with advanced plaque buildup in the arteries beneficial effects were noted from the powder. All subjects had at least one additional risk factor for heart disease, such as hypertension, diabetes, or a smoking history. Whereas subjects on placebo experienced an increase of plaque volume over 48 months, those taking garlic experienced plaque reductions.[1]

Caution must be exercised and clients taking anticoagulants should be advised regarding the use of certain vitamins and herbs, including garlic, ginkgo, and vitamin E. Although natural, these substances can obviously have potent therapeutic activity. This may in part be due to anticoagulant effects, which may potentiate the action of blood-thinning drugs. Health practitioners should be aware of the use of such substances so that any interactions can be monitored safely. Not enough controlled research is available to make definite predictions.

References

1. Kosielny, J. et al. (1999). The antiatherosclerotic effect of Allium sativum. *Atherosclerosis, 144,* 237–249.
2. Goodwin, J. S., & Tangum, M. R. (1998). Battling quackery: Attitudes about micronutrient supplements in American academic medicine. *Archives of Internal Medicine, 158,* 2187–2191.
3. Pittler, M. H., & Ernst, E. (1998). Horse-chestnut seed extract for chronic venous insufficiency: A criteria-based systematic review. *Archives of Dermatology, 134,* 1356–1360.
4. Tyler, V. E. (1994). *Herbs of choice: The therapeutic use of phytomedicinals.* Binghamton, NY: Pharmaceutical Products Press.
5. Winther, K. (1998). Effects of ginkgo biloba extract on cognitive function and blood pressure in elderly subjects. *Current Therapeutic Research, 59,* 881–888.

James Higgy Lerner, RN, LAc, *Private practice of acupuncture, traditional Oriental medicine, and biofeedback*

mechanical atherectomy, thrombolytic therapy, and stents to treat vascular disorders. The goal is to operate from within the artery to remove partial or total blockages. Most of the procedures can be performed in the radiology department or in cardiac catheterization laboratories. Benefits of endovascular interventions include use of a small puncture wound for access rather than a long incision and minimal postoperative care. Complications from long-duration (>3 hours) general anesthetics are reduced and the client is quickly ambulatory. Obvious cost reduction occurs.

PERCUTANEOUS TRANSLUMINAL ANGIOPLASTY. Percutaneous transluminal angioplasty (PTA), or balloon angioplasty, is a procedure in which a catheter with a distal inflatable balloon is used to dilate stenotic vessels mechanically. Angioplasty stretches the artery, thereby enlarging the lumen. Observation of a segment of an arterial wall that has undergone PTA reveals rupture of the plaque at its thinnest place, stretching of the artery wall away from the plaque, and rupture of the media with the lumen of the artery being maintained by the adventi-

tia. The enlarged vessel's new dimensions are maintained by the hydrostatic pressure of the increased luminal blood flow.

PREPROCEDURAL CARE

Assess and document peripheral pulse quality. Use a pen to mark the location of pulses on the foot to guide later assessments. Note color, skin temperature of the feet, and level of rest pain. Document the location and characteristics of any open lesions. Teach clients about the procedure and any sensations they will feel.

PTA has been used successfully, in varying degrees, for the treatment of hemodynamically significant stenoses in the coronary, aortic, iliac, femoral, popliteal, tibial, mesenteric, and renal circulations as well as for stenoses in arteriovenous dialysis shunts. Current practice also is to place a stent in the area that was treated with angioplasty to reduce the recurrence of stenosis. Several types of stents have been developed, including flexible, rigid, balloon-expandable, and self-expanding varieties. After a stent has been in place for about 8 months, it becomes covered by a thin neointimal layer. After the procedure, clients are given aspirin to reduce the risk of occlusion.

Complications of balloon angioplasty include bleeding, hematoma and thrombus formation at the insertion site, perforation, and dissection of the artery. Reocclusion that occurs over a longer period of time is caused by accelerated cell growth of the intima (intimal hyperplasia), which occurs in response to injury to the vessel.

POSTPROCEDURAL CARE

Nursing care is similar to that for routine diagnostic arteriography (Chapter 11). Major concerns are acute reocclusion and bleeding. Clients are given heparin as an anticoagulant during the procedure; thus, the arterial puncture site requires frequent assessment for swelling, bleeding, ecchymosis, or hematoma formation. Peripheral pulses are usually assessed every 15 to 30 minutes during the first hour following the procedure, then hourly for the next 4 to 8 hours. Report clinical manifestations of circulatory compromise immediately (e.g., sudden change in limb color or temperature, increasing muscle discomfort, pain at rest, and motor or sensory paresthesias). Long-term aspirin administration is prescribed after angioplasty to prevent occlusion.

THROMBOLYTIC THERAPY. Thrombolytic therapy is an important aspect of management of extensive venous or arterial thrombosis. Streptokinase and urokinase are used to treat acute arterial emboli and arterial graft occlusion. Contraindications to therapy include surgery within the past 10 days (e.g., arteriogram, lumbar puncture, paracentesis), recent trauma (e.g., cardiopulmonary resuscitation), renal or liver biopsy, and pregnancy. Renal function must be adequate because of the amount of contrast material given during thrombolytic therapy.

Thrombolytic agents are administered through a peripheral vein or through an intra-arterial catheter. A test dose is given; if it is determined to be safe, it is followed by a loading dose and then by continuous infusion. The agents have a half-life of 16 to 18 minutes. Activated partial thromboplastin times (aPTT), fibrinogen levels, or both may be monitored to be certain that the thrombolytic system has been activated. Major adverse reactions include hemorrhage, allergic reactions, and fever.

Nursing management is related to the stage of fibrinolytic therapy: preinfusion, intrainfusion, and postinfusion. Prior to infusion, the client is monitored closely (usually in intensive care). Baseline values are obtained for aPTT, prothrombin time (PT), thrombin time, platelet count, hematocrit, and white blood cell (WBC) count. Because of the risk of hemorrhage, if data reveal a bleeding disorder, the physician is notified. A history of recent streptococcal infection may diminish the drug's effects. Baseline pulses and assessments are performed in each extremity with Doppler ultrasonography if needed.

During infusion, vital signs, pulses, skin color, movement, and sensation are assessed frequently. Assess for clinical manifestations of bleeding and hematoma formation. If bleeding occurs apply direct pressure, stop the infusion, and notify the physician. Bleeding is usually from the gastrointestinal or genitourinary tract or is intramuscular, intracerebral, or retroperitoneal. Intracerebral bleeding presents as pain in the head or neck, changes in

cognition, or loss of motor function. Retroperitoneal bleeding presents as back or flank pain.

No intramuscular injections are given for 24 hours after infusion, and any medications that have bleeding as a side effect are used with caution. There is also a chance that a partially lysed thrombus will embolize. After infusion, pressure is continued on the puncture site. The involved extremity is positioned in straight alignment to facilitate perfusion. The client's leg remains immobile. Heparin therapy in low doses is also begun. Streptokinase is administered from glass bottles because it is inactivated by plastic containers. Administration is regulated by a volume-control pump.

ARTERIAL BYPASS

Arterial obstruction can be reconstructed with bypass operations. Clients are selected for surgery after a careful history and physical and diagnostic assessments, including arteriography. Arteriography provides a necessary road map to indicate the level of obstruction, because it is essential to reconstruct the arterial inflow to the legs before correcting the outflow. This process prevents newly placed bypass grafts from becoming thrombosed because of inadequate blood supply to the graft. During the operation, the surgeon assesses inflow, and a distal site is chosen for outflow after it is ascertained that inflow to the femoral system is adequate.

Improvements in vascular surgery have provided outstanding examples of long-term limb salvage in clients who in the past would have required amputation. Revascularization should be the first option considered in clients with critical limb ischemia. This recommendation is based on observations that previous revascularization does not raise the level of amputation, mortality rates for amputation are at least as high as those for arterial bypass, and there is no difference in cost between amputation and successful bypass surgery.

Various locations along the arterial system can be reconstructed as follows. Femoral artery bypass grafting or axillofemoral reconstruction (Fig. 53–4) is used if the aortoiliac segment is obstructed. The operative mortality rate is 1%. The patency rates of aortofemoral grafts are 80% to 90% at 5 years.

Axillofemoral grafting is reserved for clients who have increased operative risk, usually because of their cardiopulmonary status or the presence of intra-abdominal infection. The graft begins at the axillary artery and travels subcutaneously along the lateral chest wall to the femoral artery. It may then be combined with a femorofemoral graft to revascularize both extremities. Axillofemoral grafts have a higher incidence of occlusion than aortofemoral grafts and carry a mortality rate of 4% to 5%, but the necessary anesthesia time is greatly reduced. The patency rates are 60% to 70% at 5 years, in part because thrombi are easily removed from axillofemoral grafts.

The femoral artery can be bypassed with grafts anastomosed (surgically connected) to any one of three lower leg arteries (posterior tibial, anterior tibial, or peroneal artery). The success of bypass grafts of the legs depends largely on what material is used for grafting. The client's own saphenous vein remains the most successful grafting material used today. Seventy-five per cent of saphenous vein grafts are patent after 5 years; in contrast, only 12%

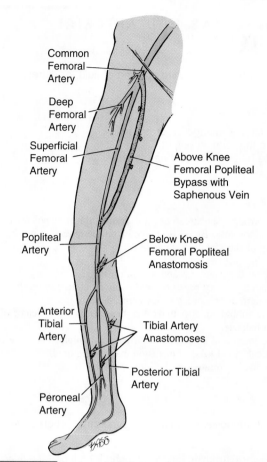

FIGURE 53–4 Femoral artery bypass grafts. The anastomosis can be to any one of three tibial arteries. (From Fahey, V. A. [1994]. *Vascular nursing*. Philadelphia: W. B. Saunders.)

of synthetic material (polytetrafluoroethylene [PTFE]) is patent after the same length of time. (Gore-Tex is a common brand name for PTFE.) Unfortunately, the client's own saphenous vein is not always large enough or long enough for the surgery, or it may have been removed during another operation. In these cases, PTFE is used. In situ grafts can also be used for reconstruction. In situ grafting permits the client's own vein to be used for a bypass of the artery. A section of vein is anastomosed proximally and distally, and the valves are disabled. The vein then acts as an artery.

Anticoagulant medications (e.g., heparin) are used in clients who have had previously thrombosed femoral bypass grafts. Low-molecular-weight heparin may be safer, with fewer bleeding side effects and rare occurrences of heparin-induced thrombocytopenia. It is also possible to treat some clients with fibrinolytics; however, these agents are seldom used immediately after surgery because of the potential for bleeding. Three drugs—streptokinase, urokinase, and tissue plasminogen activator (TPA)—are in current clinical use. All three drugs convert the client's plasminogen to the active molecule plasmin, which instigates fibrinolysis. The client is eventually given warfarin sodium based on the International Normalized Ratio (INR). Dextran is sometimes used to improve blood flow in the microcirculation but is only recommended in complex cases. Medications that decrease platelet aggregation

(aspirin, clopidogrel [Plavix] are also used to increase the length of graft patency. Some authors recommend the use of anticoagulants in clients who have never had an occluded graft, including clients with poor outflow, complicated procedures, or a small-caliber graft. Broad-spectrum antibiotics are used before and after surgery.

■ Nursing Management of the Surgical Client

PREOPERATIVE CARE

Preoperatively, obtain baseline vital signs and document the character of peripheral pulses, comparing one side with the other. Know exactly which pulses are palpable and which pulses can be assessed only with Doppler. Mark with ink the sites where peripheral pulses can be palpated to assist with postoperative assessment.

Before surgery, it is common to begin administration of intravenous (IV) fluids, insert a urinary catheter, and weigh the client. Just before surgery, arterial and central venous pressure (CVP) lines may be inserted. In addition, broad-spectrum antibiotics normally are prescribed for 48 hours preoperatively. All infections (e.g., tooth abscesses, urinary tract and respiratory infections) must be resolved, especially if the surgeon plans to use a synthetic graft. Adequate circulating blood volume must be maintained to permit good perfusion throughout the period of arterial repair.

As with any preoperative assessment, perform careful cardiac and pulmonary evaluations. Even though the incision for a femoral artery bypass is peripheral and major complications are infrequent, the client probably has other manifestations of atherosclerosis (such as heart and kidney disease) that may complicate the surgery. If the operation is not an emergency, malnutrition can be reversed and open wounds can be cleaned. The client should have a complete medical evaluation, and hypertension should be controlled. If the blood pressure is outside normal parameters, or well above the client's normal value, report it to the surgeon or anesthesia department.

The client and family are taught the various procedures involved and are offered psychological support. First assess the client's readiness and desire to learn about the surgery. The importance of maintaining the medication routine is to be stressed with appropriate guidance from the physician or anesthesia department.

POSTOPERATIVE CARE

The client is placed on bed rest for the evening after surgery, with the leg flat in bed. The leg is wrapped with light dressings or a vascular boot. Boots are commonly used in clients who had a loss of sensation prior to surgery or who are at risk for pressure ulcers. Elastic wraps are not used if vein grafts have been used for reconstruction. Leg swelling is common after revascularization resulting from the reperfusion of ischemic muscles and surgical dissection around lymphatic drainage systems in the leg. If edema worsens when the client's leg is dependent, elastic wraps can be used. Edema usually resolves within 4 to 8 weeks, especially with ambulation.

Oxygen saturation monitors may also be used to measure tissue perfusion. Daily aspirin is usually required after surgery. Incisions are carefully monitored for clinical manifestations of infection. The Care Plan describes the remainder of nursing care of the client after bypass surgery.

POSTOPERATIVE CARE OF THE CLIENT WHO HAS HAD ARTERIAL BYPASS SURGERY OF THE LOWER EXTREMITY

Nursing Diagnosis. Risk for Fluid Volume Deficit related to hemorrhage, hematoma, third spacing of fluid, or diuresis from contrast given during angiography

Outcomes. The client will maintain adequate vascular fluid volume, as evidenced by:

- Hemodynamic stability
- Urine output ≥30 ml/hr
- Warm, dry skin
- Being alert, awake

- No excess drainage on dressings
- Intake that equals output
- Stable hemoglobin and hematocrit

Interventions

1. Observe the client for an increase in pulse, decrease in blood pressure, anxiety, restlessness, pallor, cyanosis, thirst, oliguria, clammy skin, venous collapse, and decreasing level of consciousness.
2. Check the client's dressings for excessive drainage.
3. Assess the client's pulmonary artery pressures and cardiac output if parameters are available.
4. Check the client's daily weights; monitor intake and output closely.
5. Check hematocrit and hemoglobin values and notify the physician if they are abnormal.
6. Check the client's creatinine level after angiography.

Rationales

1. Hemorrhagic shock can develop from surgical or postoperative blood loss. Blood is shunted from peripheral stores because of the effect of epinephrine.
2. Incision drainage first appears on dressings.
3. Pulmonary artery pressures and cardiac output parameters are reliable indicators of hemodynamic stability.
4. Intake should equal output. Weight is a reliable indicator of fluid balance.
5. Hematocrit and hemoglobin normally fall slightly because of surgical blood loss. Transfusion may be required.
6. Contrast is excreted by the kidneys.

Evaluation. This outcome should be attainable within 24 hours.

Nursing Diagnosis. Risk for Altered Tissue Perfusion related to graft thrombosis, compartment syndrome, progressive arterial disease, or inadequate anticoagulation

Outcomes. The client will maintain adequate tissue perfusion to the lower extremities, as evidenced by full pedal pulses, intact sensory and motor function, and minimal swelling.

Interventions

1. Check the client's pedal pulses every hour for 24 hours, then every shift, unless otherwise ordered. Obtain Doppler pressures per doctor's orders.
2. Check the sensory and motor function of the client's extremities.
3. Check the client's leg for hematoma or severe swelling.
4. Monitor creatine phosphokinase levels when appropriate.
5. Observe for a change in color and the presence of red blood cells in the client's urine.
6. Avoid raising the knee section of the gatch bed and placing pillows under the client's knees.

Rationales

1. Pedal pulses indicate graft patency.

2. Compartment syndrome may develop because of bleeding.
3. Severe swelling may impede the flow through the graft.
4. Enzymes are released from ischemic muscle.
5. These manifestations may be caused by a release of myoglobin secondary to muscle ischemia.
6. Pressure may increase the risk of thrombosis.

Evaluation. Outcomes related to tissue perfusion should be met within 48 hours.

Nursing Diagnosis. Risk for Impaired Skin Integrity related to altered circulation, altered nutritional state, infection, and multiple surgical procedures

Outcomes. The client will maintain adequate skin integrity.

Interventions

1. Inspect the client's lower extremities on daily basis.

2. Provide proper skin care using lanolin-based creams.
3. Protect the client's lower extremities from trauma.

4. Use sheepskin, a bed cradle, or heel protectors when appropriate.
5. Check the sensory and motor function of the client's extremities.
6. Avoid using tape on the skin below the client's knee.

Rationales

1. Early detection of ulceration will improve the chances of healing
2. Soft skin does not crack open.
3. Tissue perfusion is decreased and injured sites heal poorly.
4. These devices are used to protect the skin from breakdown.

5. Compartment syndrome may develop because of bleeding or edema.
6. Tape burns from tape removal may be slow to heal.

Interventions

1. Monitor the client's nutritional status and albumin level. Obtain a dietitian's consultation, if necessary.
2. Observe strict aseptic technique during dressing changes.
3. Monitor the client for low-grade fever, elevated white blood cell count, any drainage from the wound, and graft exposure at each shift.
4. If ordered, apply Ace bandages below the knee to the affected extremity when the client is out of bed.
5. Instruct client to inspect feet and incisions daily. (See Foot Care Guide.)

6. Assess for presence of footdrop.

Rationales

1. Malnutrition is the most common cause of delayed healing.

2. Aseptic technique reduces risk of infection.
3. These are clinical manifestations of wound infection.

4. Edema, although normal after surgery, can inhibit wound healing.
5. Circulation to the legs and feet is impaired from arteriosclerosis. Daily assessment and proper care can lead to early intervention.
6. Nerve injury due to ischemia can lead to footdrop.

Evaluation. Expect the wound to heal slowly over 10 days if arteriosclerosis is extensive.

Nursing Diagnosis. Impaired Physical Mobility related to a surgical procedure, pain, or nerve injury secondary to ischemia

Outcomes. The client will maintain intact motor function, avoid potential complications of immobility, and demonstrate use of adaptive devices to increase mobility.

Interventions

1. Assess the causative factors for immobility and the client's range of motion and ability to ambulate.
2. Encourage progressive ambulation and range of motion while the client is in bed.
3. Request a physical therapy consult when appropriate.
4. Encourage independence in the client's activities of daily living.

Rationales

1. Mobility can be facilitated once the cause is known.

2. These activities promote venous return and muscle strength.

3. Assistive devices may be necessary for ambulation.
4. Independence improves both physical and psychological recovery

Evaluation. Outcomes related to mobility may require several days, depending on initial physical status.

Nursing Diagnosis. Pain related to surgical incision

Outcomes. The client verbalizes and demonstrates an increased level of comfort.

Interventions

1. Assess the client's level of pain: type, duration, and location.

2. Provide comfort measures and means of distraction.
3. Medicate with prescribed analgesics as needed.
4. Evaluate the effectiveness of pain medication after each administration.

Rationales

1. This assessment provides baseline data to evaluate the effectiveness of treatment.
2. Distraction is a nonpharmacologic method of pain management.
3. Adequate pain management promotes healing.
4. This evaluation allows the adequacy of analgesics to be determined.

Evaluation. Acute pain should subside over 48 to 72 hours.

Adapted from Fahey, V. A. (1994). *Vascular nursing.* Philadelphia, W. B. Saunders.

COMPLICATIONS

Bleeding may develop along the suture line and can indicate a disruption in the suture line, pseudoaneurysm formation, or a slipped ligature (suture). For these problems, additional surgery is required. Reclotting of the graft is also possible. Peripheral tissue perfusion is monitored, and noninvasive follow-up studies are performed to assess patency.

Infection is not a common complication after bypass surgery, but it can occur, especially when synthetic grafting material is used. Because infection in a synthetic graft necessitates its removal, infection often results in the loss of a limb. Poorly nourished clients appear to be at highest risk for infection and delayed healing.

Compartment syndrome may also develop from swelling around the fascial compartments of the leg. In addition to loss of sensation and function, muscle cells can die and release myoglobin, which can cause acute tubular necrosis in the kidney. The manifestations of compartment syndrome include pain out of proportion to the surgery, a tense swollen leg and pain with muscle stretching, and decreased sensation. A change involving any of these manifestations or change in the color of the urine to rusty brown should be reported immediately.

Self-Care

Most clients are discharged home. Because activity was limited by claudication before surgery, the client needs to begin regular permissible exercise, including climbing stairs and going out of doors. Explain that swelling of the operative leg is normal. Elastic wraps can be used when the client is ambulating, but they should not be worn continuously.

AMPUTATION

Amputation is the oldest operation, existing before recorded history. Early amputations were done as punishment for crime. Today's amputations are used to treat injuries, cancer, overwhelming limb gangrene, and limb-threatening arterial disease or rest pain. Amputation is common, with nearly 2 million people in the United States having undergone the procedure. Unlike many other forms of surgery, such as removal of a body organ, amputation is followed by a replacement with a prosthetic device that can restore a reasonable degree of function. However, the surgical loss is visible, and therefore amputation has an emotional component that does not exist in the same manner following removal of many other body organs.

For many years, amputation was performed with an apology and often a sense of failure. More recently, there has been increasing media attention featuring amputees who have "overcome their handicap" and are back in mainstream society. There are organizations of amputee skiers, golfers, and runners. Publicity has removed much of the old stigma.

Clients with peripheral vascular disease are the most frequent candidates for amputation of the lower extremities. Diabetes mellitus is a major cause of arterial occlusion and has been associated with more than 55% of major amputations in clients with lower extremity occlusive disease. Traumatic injuries are also a common cause of amputation, especially in younger clients.

PREOPERATIVE ASSESSMENT

Usual preoperative assessment is performed (see Chapter 15). In addition, a rehabilitation team designs an individualized care plan focusing on the whole client rather than on a diseased or missing limb. Before amputation, the surgeon and rehabilitative team should consider the client's physical condition and attitude toward amputation and the type and level of amputation required.

PHYSICAL CONDITION. The following physical conditions may predicate the rehabilitation potential of clients: age, ability to become ambulatory or remain ambulatory, comprehension level, willingness to participate in a rehabilitation program, and pre-existing conditions (e.g., chronic and progressive mental deterioration, advancing neurologic problems, chronic obstructive pulmonary disease, or cardiac disease with heart failure or angina). Ideally, clients should attain independent function with the use of a prosthesis.

TYPE OF AMPUTATION PERFORMED. There are two types of amputation procedures: the *open,* or guillotine, amputation and the *closed,* or "flap," amputation. The major indication for guillotine amputation is infection. In open amputation, the surgeon does not close the stump with a skin flap immediately but leaves it open, allowing the wound to drain freely. Antibiotics are used. Once the infection is completely eradicated, the client undergoes another operation for stump closure.

During a "flap" amputation, the surgeon closes or covers the stump with a flap of skin sutured over the end of the stump. This type of amputation is performed when there is no evidence of infection and, consequently, no need for open drainage. However, the surgeon may insert small drains (e.g., Jackson-Pratt drain) to promote wound healing.

LEVEL OF AMPUTATION REQUIRED. The level of amputation for any extremity should be as distal as possible (Fig. 53–5). Arteriography is used to guide the decision about the level of amputation. Clients with below-knee amputations (even bilateral) more successfully achieve independent function with a prosthesis than do those with above-knee amputations.

CLIENT'S GENERAL ATTITUDE TOWARD AMPUTATION. Attitude toward amputation depends, to a large degree, on the client's age and maturity. Young clients may resist amputation, even though it might greatly improve function. For some, the thought of amputation dramatically conflicts with their ideal self-image. Conversely, some clients who suffer from the pain of chronic ischemia may welcome amputation. These clients are more concerned with removing the source of their pain than with altering their body image or function.

Diagnostic assessments include the usual preoperative blood studies and x-rays. In addition, arteriography may be done to determine the level of blood flow in the extremity. Doppler studies are used to measure blood flow velocity, and transcutaneous tissue oxygen levels may also be measured (see Chapter 51). These studies assist with determining the level of amputation most likely to heal.

PREOPERATIVE CARE
ASSESSMENT

Perform the usual preoperative assessments (see Chapter 15). In addition, assess the peripheral vascular system thoroughly, palpate pulses, and assess the skin temperature, sensation, and capillary refill in both extremities to serve as a baseline for comparison. If the nails have hypertrophied, assess the skin of the toe as a measure of capillary refill. If the client is diabetic, assess blood glucose levels and follow orders for sliding scale insulin to maintain normal glycemic levels.

DIAGNOSIS, OUTCOMES, INTERVENTIONS

Anxiety. Clients may fear amputation because it destroys a familiar body image, imposes physical and social limitations, and temporarily upsets their personal lifestyle. Such fears and anxiety must be resolved preoperatively to ensure successful postoperative recovery. Depending on the reason for the amputation, fear may lead the client to experience anticipatory grief. State this nursing diagnosis as *Anxiety related to impending loss of limb, change in mobility, pain, changes in body image, fear about feelings after amputation.* Other nursing diagnoses may also be appropriate, such as *Ineffective Individual Coping, Self Esteem Disturbance,* or *Body Image Disturbance.*

Outcomes. The client will openly discuss feelings and express reduced anxiety before surgery.

Interventions. Establish open, honest communication. Allow free expression of fears and negative feelings about the loss of a limb. Ask significant others how they feel about the amputation and how they perceive the

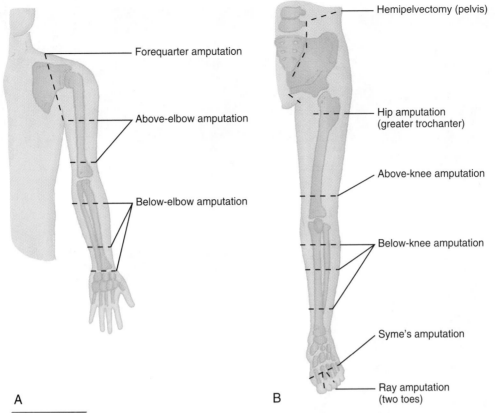

FIGURE 53-5 Common sites of amputation: *A,* upper extremity; *B,* lower extremity.

client to be responding. The social worker or psychologist may need to be involved if the client is responding poorly.

The client may also be anxious about unknown consequences and sensations after the amputation. Provide and reinforce information. Most clients feel less anxious when they know what to expect on awakening from surgery. Prepare the client for *phantom limb sensation* (see later discussion). Most clients with new amputations experience the peculiar sensation that their missing limb is still present. This phantom limb sensation may or may not be painful.

Delayed Surgical Recovery. For clients who require amputation on an emergent basis, the usual preoperative care to stabilize health conditions cannot occur. The need for emergent surgery can create a risk for delayed recovery. State this nursing diagnosis as *Delayed Surgical Recovery related to pre-existing health conditions.*

Outcomes. The risk for delayed surgical recovery will be minimized.

Interventions. Clients with diabetes mellitus are a high-risk surgical group and require careful preoperative assessment of their metabolic status. Blood glucose is normalized with blood testing four times a day and sliding scale insulin. Clients with ulcerated legs or osteomyelitis may be treated with wound packing, antibiotics, and leg elevation with bed rest. Malnourished clients are nourished with foods high in protein or tube-feeding. They also may benefit from vitamin and mineral supplements. Severely anemic clients may require iron prepara-

tions and blood transfusions. Dehydrated clients should receive preoperative IV fluids to restore fluid balance.

Pain. The client may experience very severe to moderate pain before surgery. The nursing diagnosis of *Pain related to ischemia of the limb* is used.

Outcomes. The client will be comfortable, as evidenced by statements of reduced pain, use of unchanging doses of narcotics (e.g., pain is controlled without increasing dosage), ability to move about comfortably, and ability to sleep or rest.

Interventions. Administer prescribed analgesics as necessary to relieve pain. Intervene with supportive measures. For example, use footboards and cradles to avoid pressure on injured or ischemic limbs. Keep ischemic limbs warm with wraps.

Knowledge Deficit. The diagnosis can be written as *Knowledge deficit related to expectations after surgery.*

Outcomes. The client will express an understanding of the usual postoperative regimens.

Interventions. Clients want to know what to expect after surgery and what will be expected of them by health care professionals. Emphasize that the client is the most important member of the rehabilitation team. To achieve independence, teach the client about

- Exercising legs and arms several times a day
- Strictly limiting weight-bearing (for leg amputations) until instructed otherwise
- Learning the intricacies of stump and prosthesis care
- Mastering the use of the prosthesis.

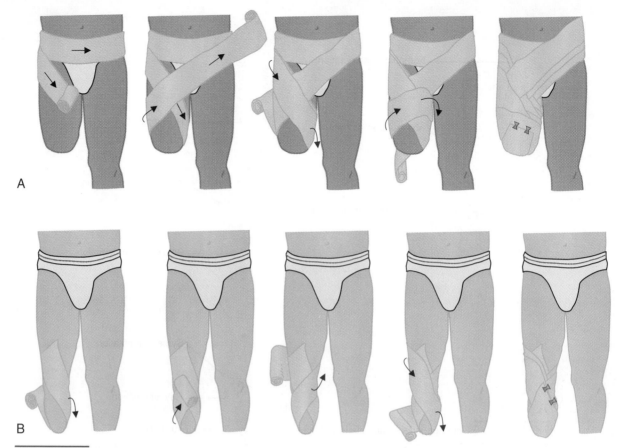

FIGURE 53–6 Common methods of stump wrapping. *A,* For an above-knee stump, two bandages are required. *B,* For a below-knee stump, one bandage is usually sufficient.

POSTOPERATIVE CARE

After the operation is completed, the surgeon applies a dressing on the incision (such as silk or Telfa bandage) and places a small amount of fluffed gauze over the end of the stump. A rigid dressing (usually a cast) is applied, distributing pressure evenly over the end of the stump. The cast protects the stump from injury and reduces swelling by gently compressing the tissues. The socket of the distal end of the cast connects to a pylon, an adjustable rigid support, the proximal end of which attaches to the below-knee socket or to the knee unit of an above-knee prosthesis. The distal end connects to a foot-ankle assembly. The rigid dressing is usually changed three to four times before application of a permanent prosthesis. Cast changes are necessary because the stump tends to shrink as it heals and, consequently, is no longer adequately compressed by the original cast.

Edema is controlled by elevating the stump for the first 24 hours after surgery. The stump then is placed flat on the bed to reduce hip contracture. Edema is also controlled by stump wrapping techniques. In below-knee amputations, the knee is immobilized to eliminate joint flexion. A trapeze and frame are attached over the bed to assist the client to develop upper arm and shoulder strength.

PHANTOM LIMB SENSATION

Phantom sensations are feelings that the amputated part is still present. Although these sensations are often referred to as *phantom pain,* not all of the sensations are painful.

The client may describe sensations of warmth, cold, itching, or pain, especially in amputated fingers or toes. Phantom sensations are caused by intact peripheral nerves proximal to the amputation site that carried messages between the brain and the now amputated part. These sensations are normal, and the client should be prepared for them. Phantom sensations often are felt immediately after surgery and gradually decrease over the next 2 years.

Phantom pain is a form of central pain. The client reports actual pain that is usually burning, cramping, squeezing, or shooting in nature. Phantom pain is less well understood than phantom sensations and may occur in a large percentage of clients. Although it is thought to be caused by a combination of physiologic and psychological components, no research has identified a link between phantom pain and any clinical psychological disorder. Phantom pain occurs most often in clients who have had pain in the limb before the amputation. Interventions that may reduce phantom pain include range-of-motion exercises, visual imaging, and other interventions for chronic pain (see Chapter 23).

REHABILITATION

Fit the Prosthesis. For clients with a below-knee amputation, the patellar tendon–bearing limb prosthesis is the most common choice. The interior of the prosthesis contacts all surfaces of the stump, and weight-bearing is on several areas. Clients with an above knee amputation are fitted with either a quadrilateral socket or an ischial containment prosthesis. Weight is borne on the ischial tuberosity and soft tissues of the proximal stump, respectively.

Prostheses for the upper extremity consist of a hook or hand device, a harness to supply force to the hand, and a socket for attachment. The client coping with an upper extremity amputation must be highly motivated to master the prosthesis and to achieve independence. For successful rehabilitation, the client must integrate the prosthetic arm and hand into the total body image.

Cosmetic prostheses are primarily used to enhance self-esteem and to make reentry into society minus a limb more tolerable for clients who are not candidates for a functioning prosthesis. Because the construction of cosmetic prostheses does not allow weight-bearing, caution the client never to attempt transfers or ambulation with a cosmetic prosthesis.

Immediate prosthetic fitting is not always possible. However, anyone with a new amputation who can walk should receive a temporary prosthesis as soon as possible after surgery. When a conventional delayed prosthesis fit-

ting is anticipated, the client returns from surgery with the stump dressed and covered with elastic bandages or stump socks (Fig. 53–6). When the sutures are removed 2 to 3 weeks after surgery, the surgeon or prosthetist fits the client with a provisional temporary prosthesis made of plaster of Paris or plastic. A permanent prosthesis is fitted once the stump is healed and molded (Fig. 53–7).

Provide Gait Training. Physical mobility is compromised for the client who has just experienced an amputation. Amputating a limb displaces the center of gravity, normally located just below the umbilicus. A client coping with an amputation must relearn balance because the prosthesis, however similar, is not an exact replica in weight and movement of the lost limb. Adapting to a change in the center of gravity occurs slowly but progressively until the conscious effort of maintaining balance comes under unconscious control. Physically, the client increases strength and endurance with regularly scheduled exercise, controls weight-bearing until the wound completely heals, and practices ambulating with the new prosthesis until a skillful, automatic gait is developed. Physi-

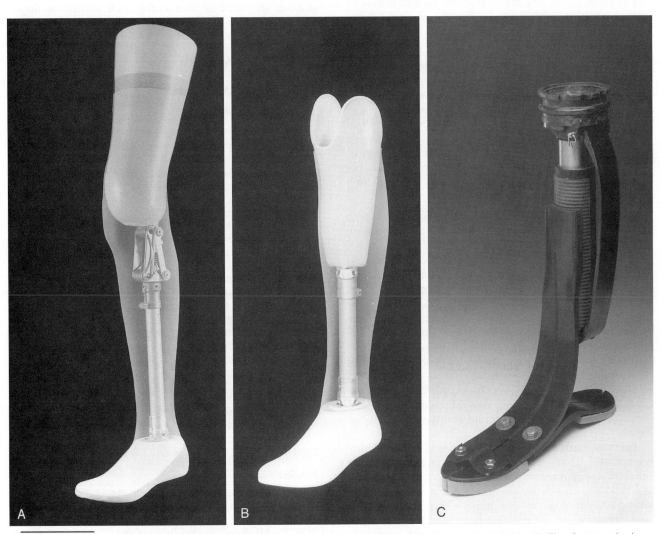

FIGURE 53–7 Permanent lower-extremity prostheses. *A,* Above-knee prosthesis. *B,* Below-knee prosthesis. *C,* Flex-foot prosthesis, which connects to the distal end of the pylon of an above-knee or below-knee prosthesis and provides increased flexibility for people who want to be more active than they are able to be with a traditional foot-ankle assembly. (*A* and *B,* Courtesy of Otto Bock Orthopedic Industry, Inc., Minneapolis. *C,* Courtesy of Flex Foot, Inc., Mission Viejo, CA.)

cal therapists usually work with the client twice daily for strengthening and gait training.

When the prosthesis is not worn (e.g., during the night), turning also requires a readaptation in body balance. Consequently, the client may need assistance while turning until the new center of gravity is comfortable.

DIAGNOSIS, OUTCOMES, INTERVENTIONS

After an amputation, the usual postoperative care is given. Look for bleeding or oozing. Outline the drainage, including the time on the temporary prosthesis or soft dressing. If drains are placed in the wound, carefully monitor the amount and type of drainage.

Postoperative management of acute pain is essential. Acute surgical pain management is similar to other postoperative techniques. To prevent increased pain, handle the stump carefully when assessing the site or drainage beneath the stump or dressings.

Because of pre-existing conditions such as diabetes, open infected wounds, and decreased perfusion, the client remains at high risk for infection. Broad-spectrum antibiotics are usually prescribed for several days after surgery until there is an indication that the wound is healing. Monitor the client and the wound for manifestations of wound infection, which usually develop about 72 hours after surgery.

Pain. Following amputation, phantom limb sensation is often present. State this diagnosis as either *Pain related to phantom sensation in amputated limb* or *Anxiety related to phantom sensation in amputated limb*.

Outcomes. The client will express an understanding of the sensations present and recognize that they are normal and usually diminish in time.

Interventions. Emphasize that phantom sensation is usual and, more important, subsides in time. It is not helpful to correct clients by telling them that the limb cannot be hurting because it is absent.

Ineffective Individual Coping. For clients with some chronic disorders, such as diabetes, the amputation may signal further losses in their battle. These clients may express anger openly or covertly. Many clients express depression after amputation. Clients may cry easily, eat little, sleep poorly or sleep more, or avoid interactions with others. Depression is a common reaction to the fear that they will never walk again, and therefore early ambulation is therapeutic. State the nursing diagnosis as *Ineffective Individual Coping related to a reaction or response to change in body image, or fear over loss of independence.*

Outcomes. The client openly verbalizes fears about changes in body image and loss of independence and begins to speak optimistically and realistically about the future.

Interventions. Listen to the client, and confront misconceptions about the rehabilitation. If possible, arrange for the client to meet with an amputee.

The client may express concerns that it will be impossible to return to a previous lifestyle, including job, leisure activities, or intimate relationships. With advancements in prosthetic devices, many clients can have both functional and aesthetic prosthetic devices.

Some clients feel the use of the word "stump" is distasteful and report feeling as if they are part of a tree.

Use of other terms may be controversial, however, if such words encourage or support denial of the problem. Some rehabilitation specialists use the term "residual limb" instead.

Knowledge Deficit. Clients require information and time to learn all the new information about the care of the stump and the prosthesis. Use the nursing diagnosis *Knowledge deficit related to gait training, care of the stump, and care of the prosthesis.*

Outcomes. The client will express and demonstrate ability to don and doff the prosthesis and to inspect the stump for abrasions.

Interventions. The Client Education Guide: Stump and Prosthesis Care suggests ways for clients with a lower limb amputation to care for their stump and prosthesis in the health care facility or at home.

■ Self-Care

When making discharge plans for the client with a new amputation (and probably a prosthesis), consider the client's ambulatory level and the tasks with which the client may need help. Frequently, by the time clients with amputations are aware of their changed circumstances, they

---

CLIENT EDUCATION GUIDE

Stump and Prosthesis Care

Client Instructions

Stump Care

Inspect the stump daily for redness, blistering, or abrasions.

Use a mirror to examine all sides and aspects of the stump. Skin breakdown on the stump is extremely serious because it interferes with prosthesis training and may prolong hospitalization and recovery. If you have diabetes mellitus, you are particularly susceptible to skin complications, because changes in sensation may obliterate your awareness of stump pain.

Perform meticulous daily hygiene. Wash the stump with a mild soap, then carefully rinse and dry it. Apply nothing to the stump after it is bathed. Alcohol dries and cracks the skin, whereas oils and creams soften the skin too much for safe prosthesis use.

Wear woolen stump socks over the stump for cleanliness and comfort. Wash woolen socks in cool water and mild soap to prevent shrinkage. To prevent stretching, wash socks gently. Dry stump socks flat on a towel. Replace torn socks; mending creates wrinkles that irritate the skin.

Put on the prosthesis immediately when arising and keep it on all day (once the wound has healed completely) to reduce stump swelling.

Continue prescribed exercises to prevent weakness.

Prosthesis Care

Remove sweat and dirt from the prosthesis socket daily by wiping the inside of the socket with a damp soapy cloth. To remove the soap, use a clean damp cloth. Dry the prosthesis socket thoroughly.

Never attempt to adjust or mechanically alter the prosthesis. If problems develop, consult the prosthetist.

Schedule a yearly appointment with the prosthetist.

are at home, alone, and without the informed and professional advice that can prepare them for their altered lives. Schedule home visits from community health care nurses until such clients have adjusted to their new situation and feel reasonably comfortable and confident in their ability to provide self-care.

TRAUMATIC AMPUTATION

Not all amputations are planned. Some clients suffer traumatic loss of a limb due to farm machinery accidents, chain saw accidents, and automobile accidents. Sometimes the amputated limb can be replanted because usually both the client and the limb were healthy up to the time of injury. It is important to properly store and transport the amputated limb prior to replantation. The limb should be wrapped in a cloth and placed in a plastic bag and then on ice. The limb or digit should not come in contact with ice or water to prevent direct tissue damage. No promises should be made to the client about the ability to successfully replant an amputated limb prior to an evaluation by the replantation surgery team. People whose limbs are amputated because of trauma have not had time before surgery to grieve the loss or adjust to their perceived alterations in body image. They may express sadness or anger or may show a strong determination not to let the amputation alter their ability to function.

Outcomes after replantation vary with the complexity of repair required and the amount of tissue replanted. Months of rehabilitation are required, and the peripheral nerve repairs itself very slowly.

ACUTE ARTERIAL OCCLUSION

Etiology and Pathophysiology

Acute occlusion of a limb's main artery may be caused by trauma, embolism, or thrombosis and may occur in a healthy or diseased artery; about 90% occur in the lower limbs. In arterial embolism, the wall of the artery is often healthy; the obstruction in the artery arises most frequently from a thrombus within the heart. Causes include atrial fibrillation, myocardial infarction, prosthetic heart valves, and rheumatic heart disease. Sometimes portions of a blood clot, such as platelet emboli that form at points of turbulence and then lodge at a bifurcation, can initiate a thrombus. Atheromatous emboli sometimes block small arteries. In the lower extremity, more than half the emboli lodge in either the superficial femoral or the popliteal artery. Other noncardiac sources of emboli are laminated clots in an abdominal aortic aneurysm or peripheral aneurysm, and up to 20% are from an unidentified source. Most of these emboli lodge in the lower extremities, and about 15% travel to the arms. Arterial thrombosis is usually superimposed on atherosclerosis and consequently develops in a damaged vessel. However, coagulopathy from heparin-induced thrombocytopenia, inherited coagulation disorders, disseminated intravascular coagulation, or polycythemia vera may also occur.

The circulatory changes that follow arterial occlusion and that predict the outcome are complex and depend on various factors. Acute occlusion produces a fall in mean and pulse pressures in the distal arteries and a decrease in tissue perfusion and oxygenation. In a normal artery, blood flow is restored by collateral channels; with acute emboli, collateral vessels have not had time to develop.

It is important to differentiate between *arterial thrombosis* and *arterial embolism.* Acute arterial thrombosis is usually caused by arterial obstruction from a blood clot that forms in an artery that has been damaged by atherosclerosis. Arterial thrombosis may also develop in an arterial aneurysm, especially an aneurysm that has formed in the popliteal artery. Arterial emboli form in the terminal end of an artery and lead to distinct areas of necrotic tissue.

Clinical Manifestations

The classic manifestations of acute ischemia caused by peripheral thrombus or embolism, which are known as the *six P's,* are shown in Box 53–1. Muscle necrosis may start as early as 2 to 3 hours after occlusion. Paresthesias indicate advanced damage. Complete paralysis with stiffness of muscles and joints (rigor mortis) indicates irreversible damage. The leg must be amputated to prevent systemic reaction to the products of massive muscle destruction and systemic sepsis.

Outcome Management

Surgery is required to correct arterial embolism. Arterial emboli can be removed by an embolectomy.

Surgery for thrombosis usually involves an arterial reconstructive procedure for revascularization of the leg. If the decision is made to remove the occluding embolus or thrombus, surgery should be performed as quickly as possible, generally with the client under local anesthesia. If hours have elapsed since the occlusion occurred, the viability of the limb determines whether embolectomy should be attempted.

If surgery is not performed immediately, anticoagulants are used to reduce the risk of further occlusion. Heparin is usually continued for a minimum of 2 to 7 days, after which a change to an oral anticoagulant may be made. The prevailing practice is to treat all clients who have a definite source of embolism and who have satisfactorily recovered from the acute episode of occlusion with long-term anticoagulant therapy. Fibrinolytic agents may also be used to dissolve a thrombus or embolus (see Chapter 58).

While decisions about surgery are being made, put the

BOX 53–1   Clinical Manifestations of Acute Arterial Occlusion: The Six P's

1. *Pain* or loss of sensory nerves secondary to ischemia
2. *Pulselessness*
3. *Poikilothermia* (coldness)
4. *Pallor* caused by empty superficial veins and no capillary filling; pallor can progress to a mottled, cyanotic, cadaverous, cold leg
5. *Paresthesias* and loss of position sense; the client cannot detect pressure or sense a pinprick; the client cannot tell whether toes are flexed or extended
6. *Paralysis*

client to bed in a comfortable, warm room. Protect the limb from pressure and other trauma, and keep it at room temperature, neither warm nor chilled. The best position for the limb is level or slightly dependent.

ARTERIAL ULCERS

Areas of an ischemic foot subjected to local pressure or minor trauma may undergo skin breakdown. The usual sites of arterial ulcers are the medial and lateral metatarsal heads and the tip of the heel. The ulcers are very painful, which distinguishes them from venous stasis ulcers. Arterial ulcers also have a sharp edge and a pale base and often are surrounded by atrophic tissue (see Fig. 53–7). In contrast, venous stasis ulcers are irregular and have a red healthy base (see later).

Once an ulcer develops, it tends to heal poorly if at all (especially in diabetic clients). Without adequate blood flow, the damaged tissues do not receive needed oxygen, nutrients, antibodies, and leukocytes, and the process of tissue damage continues. Eventually, the client may be forced to undergo limb amputation.

Although skin grafting may ultimately be required to cover the site of arterial ischemic leg ulcers (once the ulcerated area is free from infection and granulation tissue is evident), intervention for the skin lesion does not cure the underlying disease. For most ulcers, revascularization is required for healing. Arterial bypass surgery improves circulation when the client has an aortoiliac or femoropopliteal occlusion. For this surgery to be successful, however, the arteries in the leg must be healthy enough to carry sufficient blood to the foot once the block has been removed or bypassed.

General intervention involves keeping the area of ulceration clean and free from pressure and irritation. Bed rest reduces the oxygen needs of the impaired tissues. Whirlpool treatments provide debridement. If surgical debridement is necessary, a qualified health care provider should perform this procedure. After revascularization, if the ulcer bed is clean and granulating, healing is enhanced with damp normal saline dressings or a moist occlusive dressing, such as DuoDerm.

ANEURYSMS

An aneurysm is a permanent localized dilation (50% increase in size) of an artery. Once formed, an aneurysm tends to enlarge gradually; this, along with the thrombus that develops within the aneurysm, leads to the usual complications: rupture, pressure on surrounding structures, thrombosis, and distal embolization. Atherosclerotic aneurysms occur about 10 times more often in men than in women and, for the most part, after age 50 years. There is a hereditary tendency for abdominal aortic aneurysms, with a 25% increase in the rate among first-degree relatives (male).

The most common cause of arterial aneurysms is atherosclerosis. Less common causes include congenital defects of the arterial wall (e.g., Marfan's syndrome), trauma (both blunt and penetrating types), infection (including syphilis), polyarteritis, and hereditary abnormalities of connective tissue. Hypertension seems to enhance aneurysm formation.

A combination of factors, such as "wear and tear," impaired nutrition, and inherited elastin insufficiency, results in weakening of the arterial wall over time, which leads to tortuosity (twisted), dilation, and aneurysm formation in atherosclerotic arteries. The most common sites of arteriosclerotic aneurysms are the thoracic and abdominal aorta, the iliac arteries, and the femoral and popliteal arteries.

CLASSIFICATION

Aneurysms may be classified according to the following characteristics:

1. *Location.* Aneurysms are designated as being either *venous* or *arterial.* They are also described according to the specific vessel in which they develop (e.g., aortic, iliac artery) and, more precisely, the exact area of the vessel that they affect (e.g., thoracic aorta, abdominal aorta).
2. *Etiology.* Aneurysms can be classified according to the cause, such as atherosclerotic aneurysm, mycotic aneurysm (caused by bacterial infection), anastomotic graft aneurysm, or syphilitic (luetic) aneurysm.
3. *Gross Appearance.* Classification of aneurysms is sometimes based on their shape, anatomic features, and size. *Fusiform* aneurysms are localized, rather uniform dilations of an artery; the term *saccular* is used to describe an outpouching of an artery at a point at which the medial coat is thinned (Fig. 53–8). A *dissecting* aneurysm occurs as the hematoma in the arterial wall forms a localized enlargement of the involved artery, separating the layers of the arterial wall. A dissecting aneurysm may be either acute or chronic. A *pseudoaneurysm,* or false aneurysm, results from the development of a sac around a hematoma that maintains a communication with the lumen of an artery whose wall has been ruptured or penetrated.

ABDOMINAL AORTIC ANEURYSMS

Abdominal aortic aneurysms (Fig. 53–9A) occur about four times more often than thoracic aneurysms. The natural course of an untreated abdominal aortic aneurysm is to expand and rupture. The aorta is under greater stress than the rest of the arterial system because of its large diameter and its exposure to high pressure during each systolic ejection of blood. Abdominal aneurysms may extend into the iliac arteries. When the aneurysm reaches about 5 cm in diameter, it can usually be palpated, except in the obese client. An abdominal aneurysm measuring 6 cm or more in diameter has a 20% chance of rupturing in 1 year.

Most abdominal aneurysms are asymptomatic; discovery is usually made on physical or x-ray examination of the abdomen or lower spine for other reasons. Smaller aneurysms and aneurysms in obese clients may be more difficult to confirm. The most common clinical manifestation is the client's awareness of a pulsating mass in the abdomen, with or without pain, followed by abdominal pain and back pain. Groin pain and flank pain may be experienced because of increasing pressure on other structures. Sometimes mottling of the extremities or distal em-

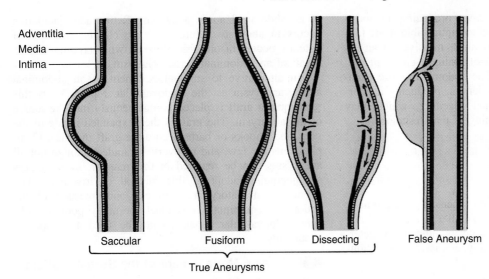

Adventitia
Media
Intima

Saccular   Fusiform   Dissecting   False Aneurysm

True Aneurysms

FIGURE 53–8 Classification of aneurysms. In a true aneurysm, layers of the vessel wall dilate in one of the following ways: *saccular*, a unilateral outpouching; *fusiform*, a bilateral outpouching; or *dissecting*, a bilateral outpouching in which layers of the vessel wall separate, with creation of a cavity. In a false aneurysm, the wall ruptures, and a blood clot is retained in an outpouching of tissue, or there is a connection between a vein and an artery which does not close.

boli in the feet can alert the clinician to a source in the abdomen.

Ultrasonography and CT are the most accurate diagnostic tools. Abdominal aortography is not essential for making the diagnosis but helps identify circulatory anomalies important at the time of resection. Therefore, angiography is not performed until surgery is contemplated.

The most frequent complication is rupture, which occurs most often in aneurysms 5 cm or more in diameter. The abdominal aneurysm may rupture in the following body areas:

- Into the peritoneal cavity (usually with fatal results)
- Into the mesentery

- Behind the peritoneum (the most common type of rupture with the best prognosis)
- Into the inferior vena cava (resulting in shock and heart failure from massive arteriovenous fistula)
- Into the duodenum or rectum (causing severe gastrointestinal hemorrhage)

Ruptured abdominal aortic aneurysm presents with a triad of manifestations, including:

- Abdominal pain combined with intense back and flank pain and possible scrotal pain
- A pulsating abdominal mass or a rigid abdomen from the hemorrhage
- Shock, with systolic blood pressure below 100 mm Hg and apical pulse rate greater than 100 per minute

Other manifestations include syncope; ecchymosis in the flank and perianal area; severe sudden pain in the abdomen, paravertebral area, or flank; lightheadedness; and nausea with sudden hypotension. In addition, the red blood cell (RBC) count falls and the WBC count rises. These are also the signs of a ruptured postoperative abdominal bypass graft.

After the initial retroperitoneal rupture, the blood may be walled off in the retroperitoneal space, or tamponaded, for a period. If the ruptured abdominal aortic aneurysm can be identified during this phase, the client has a much greater chance of survival. Once the aorta ruptures anteriorly into the peritoneal cavity, death is almost certain because there are no structures in the abdomen to wall off the bleeding, such as the retroperitoneal space. Rupture occurring more than an hour away from medical care severely decreases the chances of survival.

Surgery is the only intervention for clients with ruptured abdominal aortic aneurysm. New surgical and grafting techniques and faster methods for transport (e.g., helicopters) now permit rapid resection of ruptured abdominal aortic aneurysm and sometimes save the client's life. Even with new advances in surgery, the operative mortality rate for repair of ruptured abdominal aneurysm may be as high as 35%.

About 4% of all ruptured abdominal aortic aneurysms

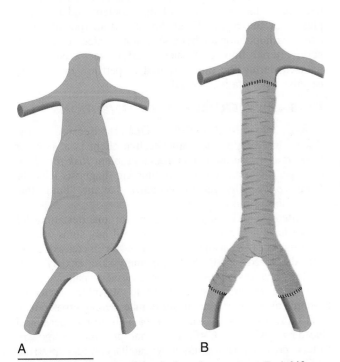

A   B

FIGURE 53–9 *A,* An abdominal aortic aneurysm. *B,* A bifurcated synthetic graft in place.

rupture into the inferior vena cava, producing an aorto-caval fistula. Manifestations include intractable heart failure because of the right-to-left shift, massive lower extremity edema, acute abdominal pain, ascites, pleural effusions, and hepatomegaly. The abdominal aortic aneurysm may rupture into the duodenum, producing an aortoenteric fistula. Gastrointestinal bleeding, which may progress to shock, is the beginning of manifestations.

Outcome Management

Medical Management

Surgery is usually not performed when an asymptomatic abdominal aortic aneurysm is smaller than 4 to 5 cm. Every 6 months, an ultrasonography is indicated to determine any change in size. Antihypertensive medications are usually prescribed if indicated.

Surgical Management

Surgical management of an aneurysm may be performed as either an emergency or an elective procedure. Elective resection and graft replacement carry a surgical mortality of less than 5%; emergency surgical treatment after the aneurysm has ruptured is associated with a much higher mortality rate.

The surgical technique involves exposing the aneurysm, applying clamps just above and below the aneurysm, opening the aneurysm, and placing a polyester (Dacron) graft within the aneurysm. The aneurysm sac is then wrapped around the graft to protect it (see Fig. 53–9B). Excision of an abdominal aneurysm is done through a midline incision that extends from the xiphoid process to the symphysis pubis.

Abdominal aortic aneurysm repair is considered a major operation, and many specific postoperative complications can develop. Complications after abdominal aortic aneurysm repair are generally caused by underlying coronary artery disease and chronic obstructive pulmonary disease (COPD). These conditions decrease the excretion of the anesthetic, increase the risk of postoperative atelectasis, and decrease the client's tolerance of hemodynamic changes from blood loss and fluid shifts.

One of the most serious complications is acute myocardial infarction. To reduce the risk of this complication, many clients undergo coronary artery bypass grafting (CABG) before aneurysm repair.

Prerenal failure can develop for several reasons. The kidney can sustain ischemia from decreased aortic blood flow, decreased cardiac output, emboli, inadequate hydration, or the need for clamps on the aorta above the renal arteries during surgery.

Emboli can also develop and lodge in the arteries of the lower extremities or mesentery. Clinical manifestations include those of acute occlusion in the leg. Bowel necrosis is exhibited as fever, leukocytosis, ileus, diarrhea, and abdominal pain.

The spinal cord can also become ischemic, resulting in paraplegia, rectal and urinary incontinence, or loss of pain and temperature sensation. Spinal cord ischemia tends to occur more commonly when an abdominal aortic aneurysm has ruptured.

Changes in sexual function may also occur after repair

of an abdominal aortic aneurysm. Retrograde ejaculation occurs in about two thirds of male clients, and loss of potency occurs in one third of men who have undergone repair of an abdominal aortic aneurysm.

An alternative to surgical treatment of an abdominal aortic aneurysm is the endovascular repair. With this technique, a graft is placed percutaneously into the lumen of the aneurysm. The graft is then expanded inside of the sac. Small hooks or barbs secure the graft in place. Complications are few, and recovery is rapid. Although not all aneurysms can be repaired in this manner, more centers are becoming adept at this method of treatment. The client is ambulatory and can eat, and invasion of the abdomen is minimal. It is ideal for many poor-risk clients. Endovascular repair cannot be used for ruptured aneurysms.

Nursing Management of the Surgical Client

PREOPERATIVE CARE

Abdominal aortic surgery is major surgery and lasts approximately 4 hours. During the hours under anesthesia, the client is at high risk for pulmonary and cardiac complications. Preoperative assessment must include detection of concurrent coronary artery disease and cerebrovascular disease. Assess all peripheral pulses for baseline comparison postoperatively. If dissection or rupture occurs, the client may receive IV fluids (often in large volumes) for maintenance of tissue perfusion.

For endovascular repair, the procedure is much shorter. Standard evaluation must occur because the potential for an open repair of the aneurysm still exists.

POSTOPERATIVE CARE
ASSESSMENT

A very comprehensive postoperative assessment of the client after open surgical repair of an abdominal aortic aneurysm is essential. Potential complications are many, because of the seriousness of the problem and the complexity of the repair. Even though extracorporeal perfusion (cardiopulmonary bypass) is not needed for the surgery, arterial flow to tissues distal to the aneurysm is reduced during the time required to perform the surgery because the aorta is clamped.

DIAGNOSIS, OUTCOMES, INTERVENTIONS

Risk for Fluid Volume Deficit. Because of the risk of bleeding at the graft site, the client is at risk for hemorrhage. Use the collaborative problem *Risk for Hemorrhage.* You can also use the nursing diagnosis *Risk for Fluid Volume Deficit,* but recognize that the "fluid" that can be lost is blood.

Outcomes. The nurse monitors for manifestations of hemorrhage and notifies the physician if any signs occur.

Interventions. Monitor the client for increased pulse rate, decreased blood pressure, clammy skin, anxiety, restlessness, decreasing levels of consciousness, pallor, cyanosis, thirst, oliguria less than 30 to 50 ml/hr, increased abdominal girth, increased chest tube output greater than 100 ml/hr for 3 hours, and back pain (from retroperitoneal bleeding). Monitor CVP, left atrial pressure, pulmonary artery pressure, and pulmonary capillary wedge pressure (PCWP) continuously. Assess for changes indicating hypovolemia. Report any of these manifestations immediately.

Impaired Gas Exchange. The large abdominal incision impairs deep inspiration and usually reduces effective coughing. Write the diagnosis as *Impaired Gas Exchange related to ineffective cough secondary to pain from large incision.*

Outcomes. The client will demonstrate improved gas exchange, as evidenced by oxygen saturation or PaO_2 greater than 95%, increasing effectiveness in coughing, and clearing of lung sounds.

Interventions. Monitor settings on the ventilator to ensure that the client is adequately oxygenated. Assess lung sounds every 1 to 2 hours, and report any adventitious sounds. Monitor oxygen saturation continuously, and report any desaturation. After extubation, assist with coughing by using incentive spirometry, provide splinting pillows before coughing, encourage ambulation, and provide adequate analgesia to promote coughing with severe pain.

Altered Tissue Perfusion. During the operation, the aorta is clamped to stop bleeding while the graft is placed. During that time, peripheral tissues are not perfused. The graft site can also become occluded with thrombus. In addition, the client often has pre-existing arterial disease. Write the diagnosis as *Altered Peripheral Tissue Perfusion related to temporary decrease in blood supply.*

Outcomes. The client will maintain adequate tissue perfusion, as evidenced by pedal pulses, warm feet, capillary refill of less than 5 seconds, absence of numbness or tingling, and dorsiflexion and plantiflexion of both feet equally.

Interventions. Assess dorsalis pedis and posterior tibial pulses every hour for 24 hours. Report changes in pulse quality or absent pulses; assess with Doppler imaging if needed. Assess dorsiflexion and plantiflexion and sensation (needles and pins sensation) every hour for 24 hours. Inspect lower extremities for mottling, cyanosis, coolness, or numbness every 4 hours.

Pain. Abdominal aortic aneurysm repair necessitates a long incision. Write this common postoperative diagnosis as *Pain related to surgical incision.*

Outcomes. The client will experience increased comfort, as evidenced by self-report of decreasing levels of pain, use of decreasing amounts of narcotic analgesics for pain control, and ambulating and coughing without extreme pain.

Ischemia of the Bowel. Extensive aortic procedures that involve clamping the mesenteric vessels can result in ischemic colitis. In addition, the inferior mesenteric artery can embolize. The lack of blood supply may lead to ischemia and ileus. This diagnosis is a collaborative problem.

Outcomes. The nurse will monitor the client for abdominal distention, diarrhea, severe abdominal pain, sudden elevations in WBC count, and bowel sounds.

Interventions. Maintain accurate intake and output, and analyze data hourly for 24 hours. Notify the physician if output falls below 30 to 50 ml/hr. Assess urine specific gravity and daily weight. Monitor blood urea nitrogen (BUN) and creatinine levels. Assess bowel sounds every 4 hours. The client should have nothing by mouth. Provide oral care every 2 to 4 hours. Provide routine nasogastric (NG) tube care, and assess nares for tissue impairment. Perform guaiac tests of NG drainage every 4 hours or if bleeding is suspected (i.e., drainage has dark, coffee-ground appearance or is bright red).

▉ Self-Care

Most clients who require abdominal aortic aneurysm repair have significant degrees of arterial disease. Many of the postoperative instructions should address care of clients with arterial disorders (see earlier). Review all medications to be used to be certain that the client understands their purpose, scheduling, and side effects. Explain incision care and manifestations of infection.

The client should ambulate as tolerated, including climbing stairs and walking outdoors. If leg swelling develops, the leg should be wrapped in elastic bandages or support stockings should be used. Activities that involve lifting heavy objects, usually more than 15 to 20 pounds, are not permitted for 6 to 12 weeks postoperatively. Activities that involve pushing, pulling, or straining may also be restricted. Driving may also be restricted because of postoperative weakness and decreased response time.

Clients can resume sexual activity as soon as they can walk without shortness of breath (e.g., two flights of stairs), usually in 4 to 6 weeks. The risk of impotence in male clients should be discussed before discharge. Causes vary from pre-existing aortoiliac disease or diabetes to side effects from aortic cross-clamping. Referral may be appropriate if the client is amenable.

AORTIC DISSECTION

Aortic dissection, the longitudinal splitting of the medial (muscular) layer of the aorta by blood flowing through it, is the most common catastrophe involving the aorta. Dissection occurs following a tear in the intima, or inner lining, of the aorta, which allows blood to dissect between it and the medial layer. As the dissection progresses, blood flow through the arterial branches of the aorta becomes blocked and blood flow to the organs served by these branches is reduced. Aortic dissections occur more often in men between ages 50 and 70 years, most of whom are hypertensive. Aortic dissections differ from *aneurysms,* in that a false lumen is formed by separation of the intima from the medial layers of the aorta. An aneurysm is a dilation of the entire aortic wall.

Etiology and Classification

The exact cause of dissection is not known. The medial layer of the aorta can become necrotic and thereby lose strength. Marfan's syndrome (a hereditary condition of connective tissue that predisposes it to aneurysm formation) is associated with a high incidence of dissection. Blunt trauma to the chest wall, such as impact on the steering wheel during a car accident, can also lead to tearing of the aorta.

Dissections are classified by the anatomic location and time of occurrence:

• Type I—the most common and most lethal form—starts above the aortic valve and extends to the iliac bifurcation, traversing the entire aorta.

- Type II is confined to the ascending aorta and proximal transverse arch and is most often seen in conjunction with Marfan's syndrome.
- Type III dissections begin just distal to the left subclavian artery and extend to the iliac bifurcation; they carry the best prognosis and are usually treated medically.

Dissections are also classified as *acute* (occurring during the preceding 2 weeks) and chronic (persisting more than 2 weeks). If dissections are untreated, 50% of clients die within the first 48 hours, 60% to 70% within the first week, and 90% within 3 months after dissection.

Clinical Manifestations

Abrupt, excruciating pain is the most common presenting manifestation in clients with aortic dissection. Clients describe the pain as "ripping" or knife-like tearing sensations that radiate to the back, abdomen, extremities, or anterior part of the chest. Hypertension is a common finding, although the client looks "shocky," is sweating profusely, is severely apprehensive, and has diminished peripheral pulses. Other manifestations of decreased perfusion include unequal pulses, different blood pressures in the arms, paraplegia or hemiplegia, decreased urine output or hematuria, mental status changes, and chest pain. A murmur of aortic regurgitation can be heard if the dissection proceeds proximally.

Chest x-ray studies reveal a widened mediastinum and sometimes fractured ribs. Echocardiography can be used to determine the size, shape, and location of the tear. Laboratory tests during emergency settings are usually not helpful except for hemoglobin and hematocrit assays to calculate blood loss and transfusion needs. If the client's condition is stable, aortography can be used to determine the extent of the dissection.

Complications

Cardiac tamponade can develop in the presence of dissection of the ascending aortic arch. This life-threatening complication occurs when blood escapes from the area of dissection into the pericardial sac. Clients have pulsus paradoxus, muffled heart sounds, narrowed pulse pressure, and distended neck veins. Pulsus paradoxus occurs when beats are weaker in amplitude during inspiration and are stronger with expiration. Blood pressure readings decrease more than 10 mm Hg during inspiration and increase with expiration.

Because the dissection decreases blood supply to many vital organs, ischemic changes in many organs can occur. The spinal cord, kidneys, and abdominal organs are most commonly affected. Ischemia of the spinal cord can lead to manifestations ranging from weakness to paralysis. Renal ischemia can lead to oliguria. Ileus is the most common sign of decreased bowel perfusion.

Management

Emergency management is directed at lowering the blood pressure to decrease the force of the blood tearing the aorta. Potent vasodilators, such as trimethaphan and nitroprusside, are used to quickly reduce blood pressure. Beta-

blockers can also be used to decrease myocardial contractility.

If the client's condition is stable, the goals are to reduce pain, initiate blood transfusion (as needed), and manage heart failure (as needed). Pain levels are used as a guide for needed treatment. Pain subsides when the dissection stabilizes.

Surgery is warranted for clients whose condition is unstable, who have severe heart failure, who have a leaking aneurysm, or whose arteries to major organs are occluded. During surgery, the torn area is resected and repaired with synthetic graft materials. The operation is similar to that for repair of an abdominal aortic aneurysm.

Nursing care is directed at reducing blood pressure. The client is kept on bed rest in a semi-Fowler position. Unnecessary environmental stresses (e.g., noise) should be minimized. Narcotics are administered to reduce pain; tranquilizers may also be needed. If the client is receiving potent antihypertensive agents, monitor blood pressure continuously with an arterial line. Usually, the desired parameters for blood pressure are maintained by titrating the vasodilators. Observe the client often for signs of further tearing or rupture. Monitor peripheral pulses, level of anxiety, level of pain, and pulse pressure, and check for pulsus paradoxus.

If the client is being managed medically, explain the need for antihypertensive agents and beta-blocker drugs. The client and family should understand that if pain recurs, they should return immediately to the emergency room.

■ THORACIC AORTIC ANEURYSMS

Aneurysms of the thoracic aorta appear most often in hypertensive men between ages 40 and 70 years. The aneurysms can develop in any portion of the aorta (ascending, transverse, or descending) and are the most common aneurysms to dissect. The thoracic aorta is relatively out of the reach of physical examinations unless the aorta becomes large enough to be palpable above the clavicle. Therefore, the aneurysm is usually asymptomatic early. If the mass presses on other structures in the chest, various manifestations develop. Respiratory manifestations are a result of compression of the trachea or bronchus and can include cough, dyspnea, and hemoptysis. Respiratory arrest can develop, and pressure on the recurrent laryngeal nerve can lead to hoarseness. Dysphagia can result from pressure on the esophagus. Swelling of upper extremity and head can ensue from superior vena cava obstruction. Aortic valve insufficiency can occur if the aneurysm is located in the ascending aorta. The aneurysm can be seen on a chest x-ray and an angiogram.

The client with a ruptured aneurysm reports intense chest pain; hemoglobin is decreased, and hemodynamic instability develops. The pain is described as a ripping sensation up or down the aorta and is more intense when the client lies supine. The pain is usually substernal but may be noted in the back, lower back, shoulders, or abdomen. Increased pain intensity usually indicates rapid enlargement or imminent rupture and is a sign of extreme peril. Unless fortuitous tamponade develops in local tissue, death ensues rapidly. Surgical repair and postoperative management are the same as that for abdominal aortic aneurysm.

RAYNAUD'S SYNDROME

Raynaud's syndrome, a condition in which the small arteries and arterioles constrict in response to various stimuli, can be classified as *vasospastic* or *obstructive*. Manifestations of vasospastic Raynaud's syndrome can be induced by cold, nicotine, caffeine, and stress. Obstructive Raynaud's syndrome is often found in association with autoimmune disorders such as systemic lupus erythematosus, scleroderma, or rheumatoid arthritis.

Raynaud's syndrome may be a benign primary disorder (formerly, *Raynaud's disease*) or secondary to another disease or underlying cause (formerly, *Raynaud's phenomenon*). Manifestations of both types are the same.

Clinical Manifestations

Raynaud's syndrome causes classic color changes in the hands. Exposure to causative stimuli leads to spasm of the digital arteries, which results in pallor. The resulting tissue hypoxia causes the arteries to dilate slightly. Because the fingers carry mainly deoxygenated hemoglobin, they look cyanotic (bluish). Finally, rubor (redness) develops when arterial spasms stop completely.

Criteria for the diagnosis of primary Raynaud's disease include

- Manifestations for at least 2 years
- Intermittent attacks of pallor or cyanosis of the digits from exposure to cold or emotional stimuli
- Bilateral or symmetrical involvement
- No evidence of occlusive disease in the digital arteries or of any systemic disease that might be the cause of the changes
- Gangrene, which (when it occurs) is limited to the skin of the tips of the digits

Noninvasive blood flow studies to determine finger pressures both pre-cold and post-cold challenges may be necessary. Occasionally, the presence of vasospasm during examination makes the use of cold challenge unnecessary.

Outcome Management

Conservative measures are helpful for most clients. These measures include keeping hands and feet warm and dry, protecting all parts of the body from cold exposure to prevent reflex sympathetic vasoconstriction of the digits, and cessation of tobacco use. Biofeedback has helped some clients.

Medication is used when the vasospastic attacks interfere with the client's ability to work or to perform activities of daily living. Medications are used to induce smooth muscle relaxation, to relieve spasm, and to increase arterial flow. Calcium antagonists, such as nifedipine and verapamil, are the drugs of choice because they can decrease the frequency, duration, and intensity of vasospastic attacks. Other categories of drugs used in treatment include alpha-adrenergic receptor blockers and agents that interfere with sympathetic nerve activity (sympatholytic drugs). Medications may be necessary only during the winter months. People who rarely go out in the cold weather may take medications prophylactically 1 to 2 hours before exposure to cold.

Because the manifestations of Raynaud's syndrome may be alarming, reassure the client that the condition is unlikely to lead to a serious disability. Advise the client to stay warm by wearing wool gloves and turtleneck sweaters, turning up the thermostat at home if necessary, and staying out of drafts. Advise the client to warm up a cold car before driving. Body core heating is important to prevent chilling and the shunting of blood from the extremities to the trunk. Encourage clients to limit their intake of caffeine or chocolate. They must stop smoking to control the disease. Stress can also bring on vasospasm, and stress management workshops and biofeedback programs may prove beneficial. Teach the client about any prescribed medications.

THROMBOANGIITIS OBLITERANS (BUERGER'S DISEASE)

Thromboangiitis obliterans is a vasculitis of small and medium-sized veins and arteries in the extremities of young adults. The disease process starts distally and progresses cephalad, involving both upper and lower extremities. The cause remains unknown. The most commonly affected clients are young men who smoke heavily. Many clients have a hypersensitivity reaction to intradermal injection of tobacco products. Therefore, the probable etiologic mechanism is an exaggerated autoimmune reaction.

Clinical Manifestations

Pain is the outstanding clinical manifestation. Digital ulcerations and pain may result from ischemia. The pain may be accompanied by manifestations of ischemia, such as color or temperature changes in the fingers. Cold sensitivity, with color changes and pain, may be another early manifestation. Various types of lower extremity paresthesias may occur. Claudication-type pain is common with pain in the arch of the foot. Pulsations in the posterior tibial and dorsalis pedis arteries are weak or absent. In advanced cases, the extremities may be abnormally red or cyanotic, particularly when they are dependent.

Ulceration and gangrene are common complications and may occur early in the course of the disease. These lesions can appear spontaneously from migratory superficial thrombophlebitis but can also occur after trauma. Gangrene usually occurs in one extremity at a time. Edema of the legs is fairly common in advanced cases. Changes may appear in the nails and skin, and segmental thrombophlebitis affects the smaller veins in about 40% of clients.

Outcome Management

The goals of management include arresting progress of the disease, producing vasodilation, relieving pain, and providing emotional support.

The primary diagnostic study is leg arteriography. Biopsy may also be in order; inflammatory lesions are usually noted.

The need for smoking cessation must be clearly and unequivocally conveyed to the client and family. Provide information about programs to promote abstinence from tobacco. Because of vasoconstriction, teach the client to avoid exposure to cold.

For clients with rest pain and ischemic lesions, adequate pain control is essential. Vasodilation by calcium-channel blockers may be helpful in a few cases. Regional sympathetic ganglionectomy also produces vasodilation and may be recommended. In the past, it was the only method of treatment but is rarely used today. Ulcerations need wound care to facilitate healing. Amputation should be deferred until conservative interventions have failed. Thromboangiitis is usually not life-threatening; however, it does result in disability from pain and amputation.

■ PERIPHERAL ANEURYSMS

Peripheral aneurysms are found more commonly in the lower extremities than in the upper extremities, most commonly in the popliteal space. Popliteal aneurysms cause ischemic manifestations in the lower limbs, and pulses are easily palpable. Although the client may be aware of an enlarged area behind the knee, discomfort is seldom present. Peripheral aneurysm is differentiated from other swellings by the presence of expansile pulsation. Thrombosis may occur and may result in severe ischemia with gangrene and loss of the limb. Popliteal artery aneurysms may also become entrapped, with marked flexion of the knee, or may embolize to the feet.

Bypass operations are the only satisfactory intervention for aneurysms of the popliteal artery and must be performed before emboli develop. Results are excellent in uncomplicated cases.

SUBCLAVIAN STEAL SYNDROME

Subclavian steal syndrome produces arm ischemia arising from subclavian artery blockage. The arm is perfused from the vertebral artery as blood is taken from the brain to supply the arm. The most prevalent physical finding is a significant difference in blood pressure of the right and left arms (20 mm Hg or more). Other manifestations include dizziness and syncope when the arm is exercised. Arm paresthesias and bruit in the supraclavicular fossa are present. The client may not be symptomatic, and no intervention is necessary.

Intervention is surgical, by carotid-subclavian bypass, transluminal dilation of the subclavian artery, or endarterectomy of the subclavian artery.

THORACIC OUTLET SYNDROMES

Thoracic outlet syndromes are a group of disorders that produce symptoms affecting the neck, shoulder, and upper extremities by compression or mechanical irritation of the brachial plexus, subclavian artery, or subclavian vein as these structures pass through the thoracic outlet.

Aching or throbbing pain and paresthesias of the neck and upper limb are the most prominent clinical manifestations. In more than half of the clients, the manifestations appear to follow a hyperextension injury to the neck or upper back. Intervention is usually nonsurgical and involves physical therapy. The syndrome has sometimes been treated by surgical removal of the first rib, but this intervention is controversial.

Arterial thoracic outlet syndromes result from chronic compression of the subclavian artery. This leads to the formation of intimal and mural thrombus and, eventually, to peripheral embolization. Arterial thoracic outlet syndrome is more serious because it frequently results in severe ischemia of the upper extremity. Diagnosis is made by arteriography; treatment involves surgical excision of the anatomic abnormality and removal of the emboli.

Venous thoracic outlet syndrome is caused by external compression of the axillosubclavian vein that results in thrombosis. The primary symptoms are sudden swelling, pain, and cyanosis of the upper extremity. Management is conservative and may involve arm elevation and anticoagulation, thrombectomy, or thrombolytic therapy.

VENOUS DISORDERS

Venous disorders can be *acute* (e.g., thromboembolism) and *chronic*. Chronic venous disorders can be further separated into varicose vein formation and chronic venous insufficiency. Acute venous disorders are discussed first.

ACUTE VENOUS DISORDERS

Acute venous disorders are caused by thrombus (clot) formation, which obstructs venous flow. Blockage may occur in the superficial veins, the deep veins, or both.

Superficial thrombophlebitis is usually an easily diagnosed condition and may be iatrogenic, resulting from IV catheters or instillation of caustic chemicals. Deep vein thrombosis (DVT) is thrombophlebitis of the deep veins. DVT is a common disorder, affecting more women than men and adults more than children. It is particularly common among hospitalized clients. Around one third of clients older than 40 years who have had either major surgery or an acute myocardial infarction have DVT, and clients with cancer or a family history of clotting disorders are at high risk.

Etiology and Risk Factors

Thrombus formation is usually attributed to Virchow's triad: (1) venous stasis, (2) hypercoagulability, and (3) injury to the venous wall. At least two of the three preceding conditions must be present for thrombus formation.

Venous stasis is usually caused by immobilization or absence of the calf muscle pump. Other etiologic factors are age over 40 years, surgery, immobility, prolonged travel, stroke, obesity, pregnancy, paralysis, and heart disease, such as heart failure, myocardial infarction, or cardiomyopathy.

Hypercoagulability often accompanies malignant neoplasms (especially visceral and ovarian tumors). Dehydration and blood dyscrasias may raise the platelet count, decrease fibrinolysis, increase the clotting factors, or increase blood viscosity. Oral contraceptives and hematologic disorders may also increase blood coagulability.

Conditions that may cause vein wall trauma are IV injections, fractures and dislocations, severe blows to an area, chemical injury from sclerosing agents, contrast x-rays, certain antibiotics (such as chlortetracycline), and thromboangiitis obliterans (Buerger's disease). The resulting damage to the vein wall attracts platelets, and blood debris accumulates. Platelets do not stick to an intact endothelium. This injury, in combination with low blood flow and a hypercoagulable state, results in thrombus formation.

There are many risk factors for the development of venous thrombosis (Box 53–2). Untreated immobile clients with DVT are at lower risk for pulmonary embolism than clients who are ambulatory. Thus, the risk of pulmonary embolism is often underestimated after hospital discharge in clients who have "low-risk" surgery. Presumably, hospitalized clients are treated prophylactically with antiembolism stockings and anticoagulants. Clients discharged to their homes seldom receive this prophylaxis.

Pathophysiology

Usually, venous return is aided by the calf muscle pump. When the legs are inactive or the pump is ineffective, blood pools by gravity in the veins (Fig. 53–10). Thrombus development is a local process. It begins by platelet adherence to the endothelium. Several factors promote platelet aggregation, including thrombin, fibrin, activated factor X, and catecholamines. In addition, where the platelets adhere to collagen, adenosine diphosphate (ADP) is released. ADP is also released from the damaged tissues and disrupted platelets. ADP produces platelet aggregation that results in a platelet plug.

Deep vein thrombi vary from 1 mm in diameter to long tubular masses filling main veins. Small thrombi are found commonly in the pocket of deep vein valves. As thrombi become larger in diameter and length, they obstruct the veins. The resulting inflammatory process can destroy the valves of the veins; thus, venous insufficiency and postphlebitic syndrome are initiated.

Newly formed thrombi may become pulmonary emboli. Probably 24 to 48 hours after formation, thrombi undergo lysis or become organized and adhere to the vessel wall. Lysis diminishes the risk of embolization.

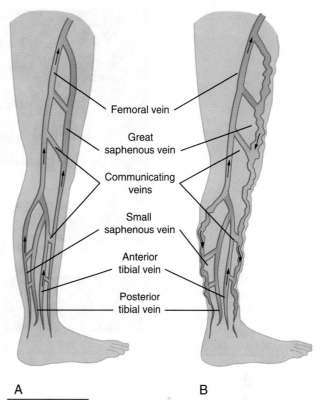

A   **B**

FIGURE 53–10 Venous return from the legs. *A,* Normal flow. *B,* Varicosities and retrograde venous flow.

If a thrombus occludes a major vein (e.g., femoral, vena cava, axillary), venous pressure and volume rise distally. Conversely, if a thrombus occludes a deep small vein (e.g., tibial, popliteal), collateral venous channels usually relieve the increased venous pressure and volume.

Pulmonary emboli, most of which start as thrombi in the large deep veins of the legs, are an acute and potentially lethal complication of DVT. Pulmonary embolism is discussed in Chapter 61.

Prevention

Prevention is geared toward reversing the three risk factors by promoting venous stasis, treating hypercoagulability, and reducing risk of injury to the venous wall.

Venous stasis is improved by any activity that causes the leg muscles to contract. Passive or active contraction, such as leg exercises and ambulation, promote venous return. Passive leg muscle contraction occurs by using sequential intermittent pneumatic compression (IPC) devices (Fig. 53–11). Use of these devices is initiated at the time of many operations and continues until the client is ambulatory. The leggings or boots are attached by polyethylene tubing to an electric pump attached to the foot of the bed. Air is pumped sequentially into three chambers (ankle, calf, and thigh) at a pressure of 45 to 60 mm Hg for 15 to 20 seconds. The compression is followed by deflation and a 45-second resting period. IPC is clinically effective in reducing the incidence of DVT and is also a good alternative for clients who cannot tolerate any anticoagulation therapy. These devices should not be used in clients with known DVT. Other

---

BOX 53–2   **Common Conditions Associated with Venous Thrombosis and Thromboembolism**

Age above 40 years
Surgery requiring more than 30 minutes of general, spinal, or epidural anesthesia
Venous stasis (bed rest, prolonged travel, stroke)
Previous deep vein thrombosis
Cardiac disease (heart failure, myocardial infarction, cardiomyopathy)
Pregnancy
Trauma, especially of the lower extremities
Estrogen therapy or oral contraceptives
Malignancy
Obesity
Family history of clotting disorders

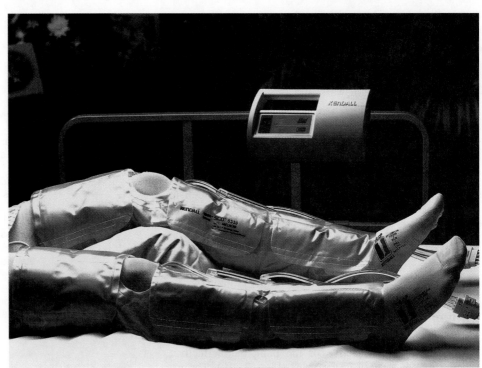

FIGURE 53–11 Pneumatic compression devices, such as the Kendall sequential compression device, are commonly used to prevent deep vein thrombosis in high-risk clients. (Courtesy of Kendall Company, Mansfield, MA.)

methods of promoting venous return include elevating the foot of the bed, applying compression stockings, using motorized foot devices, and providing passive range-of-motion exercises. Encouraging postoperative deep-breathing exercises promotes thoracic pull that is due to negative thoracic pressure on venous stores in the legs.

Pharmacologic prevention directed at reducing the hypercoagulability includes warfarin, platelet antiaggregation agents (aspirin being the most common), heparin, and dextran. Other methods to reduce coagulation include preventing the venous blood from pooling. Avoid using pillows under the client's knees postoperatively. Teach the client to avoid sitting or standing in one position for prolonged periods.

Measures to prevent injury to the vein wall include the avoidance of infiltration during intravenous therapy, pressure on the calf veins during prolonged surgery, and trauma to veins in procedures requiring prolonged positioning (delivery, colonoscopy). In addition, access ports should be used in clients requiring multiple IV sticks.

Clinical Manifestations

Clinical manifestations of superficial thrombophlebitis include redness (rubor), induration (tumor), warmth (calor), and tenderness (dolor) along a cord following the course of the involved vein. Discomfort may be relieved by application of heat. Activity should be encouraged, and a supportive wrap or stocking should be applied.

The clinical manifestations of DVT are less distinctive; about 50% of clients are asymptomatic. The most common clinical manifestation is unilateral swelling distal to the site. Other clinical manifestations include pain, redness or warmth of the leg, dilated veins, and low-grade fever. Unfortunately, the first clinical manifestation may

be pulmonary embolism. Clients may have thrombi in both legs even though the manifestations are unilateral, but this is more common in the client with cancer.

Homans' sign—discomfort in the upper calf during forced dorsiflexion of the foot—is commonly assessed during physical examination. Unfortunately, it is not reliable. It is present in fewer than a third of clients with documented DVT. In addition, more than 50% of clients with a positive Homans sign do not have venous thrombosis.

Venous duplex scanning has become the primary diagnostic test of DVT because it allows visualization of the vein, which provides an extremely reliable diagnosis of venous thrombus. Venography, previously the gold standard of diagnosis, results in exposure to contrast and is seldom used.

The Doppler ultrasonographic flowmeter determines blood flow in the larger blood vessels and the patency of vessels. Reliability of the test is directly related to the skill of the examiner; its accuracy is affected by an inability to detect partially or totally occluded veins, inaccessibility of deep pelvic and thigh veins, and inability to distinguish collateral circulation from that in native veins.

The D-dimer test is being used more frequently in evaluation of DVT. The D-dimer is a product of fibrin degradation and is indicative of fibrinolysis that occurs with thrombosis. The use of the D-dimer, a risk assessment score, and duplex imaging appear to be excellent at predicting and diagnosing DVT in asymptomatic people.

Plethysmography of the venous system is seldom used; however, these studies may be found in client records. In the past, the test was performed by recording volume changes in a limb during venous filling and emptying. Impedance plethysmography measures maximal venous filling capacity by applying a pneumatic cuff at thigh level and then recording the rate of venous emptying after cuff release.

Outcome Management

■ Medical Management

The goals of medical management are to detect the thrombus early, prevent extension or embolization of the thrombus, and prevent further thrombus formation.

Superficial thrombophlebitis can be managed with local measures, such as warm packs and elevation of the extremity. Ambulation is encouraged. Sometimes anti-inflammatory medications are required. Encourage clients to be seen in follow-up, because an extension of a superficial phlebitis can result in DVT.

ANTICOAGULATION

Anticoagulant therapy is based on the premise that the initiation or extension of thrombi can be prevented by inhibiting the synthesis of clotting factors or by accelerating their inactivation.

HEPARIN. Heparin is the drug of choice for the treatment of thromboembolic disease. Unfractionated heparin prevents the activation of clotting factor IX and inhibits the action of thrombin in forming fibrin threads. The primary anticoagulant effect is from the binding on antithrombin III. Heparin has a 4-hour half-life and, in the event of bleeding, is stopped immediately. The specific antidote to heparin is protamine sulfate, which neutralizes the effects of heparin immediately and lasts for 2 hours. Unfortunately, an excessive dose of protamine may actually prolong clotting.

Heparin is contraindicated in any conditions of bleeding or disorders that increase the risk of bleeding, including severe hypertension, cerebrovascular hemorrhage, active gastrointestinal ulceration, recent neurosurgery, and overt bleeding from the gastrointestinal, genitourinary, or respiratory tract.

Low-molecular-weight (LMW) heparin is a variant of heparin. Its primary action is from inactivation of factor Xa; advantages include decreased bleeding complications, subcutaneous (not IV) route, no need for laboratory testing, and ability of the client to be ambulatory. The anticoagulants heparin and warfarin do not induce thrombolysis, but they effectively prevent clot extension. The use of LMW heparin allows the client to ambulate, to go home, and to treat the DVT with an injectable medication. LMW heparin therapy is still followed by 3 to 6 months of warfarin therapy.

WARFARIN. Warfarin (Coumadin) inhibits hepatic synthesis of the vitamin K–dependent clotting factors. The effect of the warfarin is determined by measurement of the INR. The therapeutic level for DVT is an International Normalized Ratio (INR) of 2.0 to 3.0. The antidote for the warfarin derivatives is vitamin K (Mephyton). The warfarin derivatives require 24 to 48 hours to eliminate the vitamin K–dependent factors. Therefore, anticoagulation can include both medications. Heparin, which is fast-acting, is used initially with warfarin and discontinued when the warfarin begins to take effect. Anticoagulation therapy is usually continued about 3 to 6 months after an acute venous thrombosis and after pulmonary embolism.

FIBRINOLYTIC AGENTS. Fibrinolytic medications (e.g., streptokinase and urokinase) dissolve thrombi by stimulating the conversion of plasminogen to plasmin, an enzyme that decomposes fibrin (see Chapter 58).

■ Nursing Management of the Medical Client

Goals of nursing management are to prevent existing thrombi from becoming emboli and to prevent new thrombi from forming. Nurses also closely monitor the effect of anticoagulant medications.

ELEVATE THE CLIENT'S LEGS

Elevation of the legs above the level of the heart facilitates blood flow by the force of gravity. The increase of blood flow prevents venous stasis and the formation of new thrombi. Elevation of the legs also decreases venous pressure, which in turn relieves edema and pain. Elevate the foot of the bed 6 inches (Trendelenburg's position), with a slight knee bend to prevent popliteal pressure. The veins of the legs should be level with the right atrium. The head of the bed may be raised to facilitate eating and bathing.

Various forms of elastic support are used to promote venous return. Elastic bandages are advantageous for clients with large or misshapen legs. Apply elastic wraps snugly from toe to groin. Include the heel with wrapping. Rewrap the legs every 4 to 8 hours. If compression stockings are prescribed, they must be fitted correctly and removed for a short time every day.

RELIEVE DISCOMFORT

Elevation of the extremity and application of warm packs usually relieve discomfort. Some clients need a mild sedative or analgesic.

MONITOR ANTICOAGULANT THERAPY

Most physicians use an algorithm to adjust the dose of heparin based on the client's partial thromboplastin time (PTT) levels. Blood is sampled every 4 to 8 hours for PTT or INR, and the dose is adjusted accordingly. Use of warfarin therapy requires that PT or INR be monitored on a regular basis. LMW heparin therapy requires no testing. When invasive studies are necessary (e.g., arterial blood gas analyses), apply pressure for 30 minutes to the puncture site.

Bleeding can occur in any client receiving anticoagulation therapy. Observe the client observed for the following:

- Bleeding, evidenced by pink-tinged or frank blood in the urine, tarry or frank blood in the stool, and bleeding after brushing the teeth
- Subcutaneous bruising
- Flank pain

MONITOR THE CLIENT FOR DEVELOPMENT OF PULMONARY EMBOLISM

Pulmonary embolism is an acute and potentially lethal complication of DVT. Chest pain is the most common clinical manifestation of pulmonary embolism, but it is not diagnostic of the condition. The pain most often associated with pulmonary embolism is pleuritic. Pleuritic pain is caused by an inflammatory reaction of the lung parenchyma or by pulmonary infarction or ischemia caused by obstruction of small pulmonary arterial branches. Pleuritic chest pain is typically sudden in onset and is worsened by breathing.

Hemoptysis occurs in about 30% of clients. The presence of hemoptysis indicates that pulmonary infarction or atelectasis has produced alveolar hemorrhage. Other clinical manifestations may include cough, diaphoresis, dyspnea, and apprehension. Because of the seriousness of pulmonary embolism, promptly notify the physician of these clinical manifestations. Document the lack of manifestations of pulmonary embolism in the medical record to provide evidence of monitoring for the condition. Pulmonary embolism is discussed in Chapter 61.

Surgical Management

Surgical treatment of thrombophlebitis is directed against pulmonary embolism by filtering blood flow from the lower extremities and pelvis through a filter inserted into the inferior vena cava. In the past the direct removal of venous thrombi was recommended; now this procedure is rarely performed because of the high incidence of recurrent postoperative thrombosis. Excision of the pulmonary emboli from the lung can also be performed, but this procedure is also rare.

VENA CAVA FILTERS (UMBRELLA)

A filter is inserted in the vena cava to trap large emboli. Devices include those that look like umbrellas and those that are a complex web of threads (bird's nest) to stop the emboli. The surgeon can insert these devices, using local anesthesia, by threading the device through the femoral or jugular vein. Indications for surgery include the presence of a large thrombus or the presence of "showers" of emboli. A rare complication of this technique is the migration of the filter into the iliac vein, renal vein, right atrium, right ventricle, or pulmonary artery. Another complication includes complete obstruction of the filter. This results in back pain and swelling of the lower extremities.

Self-Care

Prevention is key in DVT. Therefore, teach clients about the risk factors of DVT and how to avoid them. Continue to explain medications being taken, actions, doses, timing, adverse effects, and the importance of monitoring coagulation status. Begin teaching on the first day of heparinization, and discuss the need for anticoagulants. Clients need to know who to contact and how to reach a health care provider in the event that problems develop. Inform the client about the monitoring required while they are receiving anticoagulants. Some clients may be apprehensive about being up and about while they have DVT, when past practice has been recommend bed rest. Reassure clients about the change in practice.

CHRONIC VENOUS DISORDERS

■ VARICOSE VEINS

Varicose veins are permanently distended and develop because of the loss of valvular competence. Faulty valves elevate venous pressure, causing distention and tortuosity of the superficial veins. The greater and lesser saphenous veins and perforator veins in the ankle are common sites of varicosities.

Primary varicose veins often result from a congenital or familial predisposition that leads to loss of elasticity of the vein wall. *Secondary* varicosities occur when trauma, obstruction, DVT, or inflammation causes damage to valves.

Varicose veins affect many adults 24 million Americans. Prevalence increases with age and peaks in people between their 40s and 50s. Varicose veins are more common in women; however, the sex ratio decreases with advancing age and almost disappears in clients older than 70 years. Prolonged standing has been implicated as a cause, but epidemiologic studies have not demonstrated an association between standing at work and an increased incidence of varicose veins.

Clients often complain of aching, a feeling of heaviness, itching, moderate swelling, and, frequently, the unsightly appearance of their legs. Severity of discomfort is difficult to assess and does not seem related to the size of varicosities. A superficial inflammation may occasionally develop along the path of the varicose vein. To assess for varicose veins, carefully examine both of the client's legs in good lighting. Varicosities appear as dilated, tortuous skin veins (Fig. 53–12).

Outcome Management

Medical Management

In the early stages of varicosity, the goals are to reduce venous pooling, prevent complications, and improve comfort levels. The simplest form of treatment is the applica-

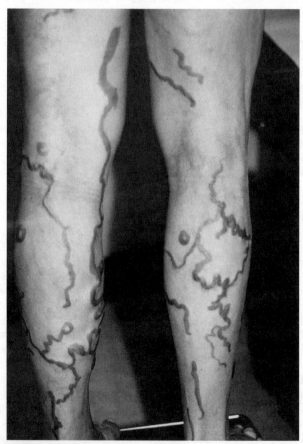

FIGURE 53–12 Varicose veins marked with a pen on the legs. Note the tortuous pattern.

tion of below-knee compression stockings or elastic wraps. These stockings are designed to exert the greatest amount of pressure over the ankle. Teach the client to avoid standing still in one position for extended periods.

Surgical Management

SCLEROTHERAPY

Sclerotherapy is the injection of an agent into the varicose vein that damages the vein and endothelium, causing an aseptic thrombosis that closes the vein. Application of pressure causes the vein walls to grow together. Sclerotherapy is usually performed for cosmetic reasons but may also relieve the discomfort of both short segments of varicosities and spider veins. It is most effective in closing small, residual varicosities after surgical intervention for varicose veins. (Sclerotherapy is contraindicated before such surgery, because it makes vein stripping more difficult.) Within minutes after injection, elastic compression and active walking should commence. Elastic support is worn for 1 to 3 weeks, morning to night.

VEIN LIGATION AND STRIPPING

Surgical management of varicose veins consists of ligation (tying off) of the greater saphenous vein with its tributaries at the saphenofemoral junction, combined with removal of the saphenous vein (stripping) and ligation of incompetent perforator veins. Removal of the vein is performed through multiple, short incisions. An incision is made at the ankle over the saphenous vein, and a nylon wire is threaded up the vein to the groin. The wire is brought out through the groin and capped, and the wire and vein are then pulled out through the ankle incision. If the perforator veins alone are ligated, ligation may be done through multiple, small endoscopic incisions.

Elastic compression bandages are applied from foot to groin. The client is rarely hospitalized overnight. Complications are infrequent and include bleeding, infection, and nerve damage. Hemorrhage most commonly occurs at the surgical wound site in the groin. Bleeding comes primarily from the stripped canal. The risk of serious bleeding can be decreased by carefully wrapping the leg from foot to groin and by applying compression, especially to the upper thigh and groin. Some discoloration with bruising along the stripped tract is normal. Saphenous nerve damage may occur. In the distal third of the leg, the saphenous nerve runs close to the saphenous vein. Thus, the risk of nerve injury increases when the distal part of the vein is involved. DVT, embolism, and infection are rare following varicose vein surgery, especially if postoperative precautions (e.g., bandaging, movement, exercise) are taken.

Some clients only require tying off of the junction of the saphenous and the femoral vein at the groin. This involves one short incision, often local anesthesia, and no hospital stay. Postoperative care is the same.

Nursing Management of the Surgical Client

Provide routine postoperative assessment and care. Specific care includes maintaining firm elastic pressure over the whole limb, reducing the risk of thrombophlebitis by promoting regular movement and exercise of the legs, and improving venous return by elevating the foot of the bed 6 to 9 inches so that the legs are above the heart level when the client is in bed. The client ambulates for short periods, starting immediately after surgery. Clients should walk rather than stand or sit. After ambulation, elevate the client's legs again.

CHRONIC VENOUS INSUFFICIENCY

Chronic venous insufficiency, a group of disorders resulting from faulty venous valves, is also known as *postphlebitic syndrome*. It follows most severe cases of DVT but may take as long as 5 to 10 years to develop; however, about 20% of clients with chronic venous insufficiency have no history of DVT.

Within 5 years of a known DVT, almost 50% of clients develop chronic induration and stasis dermatitis, and 20% suffer from venous stasis ulcer. Therefore, clients with a history of DVT must be monitored periodically for life. Alert these clients to observe for the slightest skin changes. Once the skin is broken and a venous ulcer develops, the client faces a frustrating chronic problem. Venous stasis ulcers do not heal well.

Chronic venous insufficiency results from dysfunctional valves that reduce venous return, which thus increases venous pressure and causes venous stasis. Skin ulcerations also occur. Because existing valves are destroyed, venous blood flow is bidirectional, resulting in inefficient venous outflow. The net effect of this change is that the weight of the venous blood column from the right atrium is transmitted along the full length of the veins. Very high venous pressure is exerted at the ankle, and the venules become the final pathway for the highest venous pressure. It is hypothesized that the abnormal capillaries lead to extravasation of RBCs, activation of endothelial cells, and WBC trapping. The end result is capillary thrombosis.

Chronic venous insufficiency is marked by chronically swollen limbs; thick, coarse, brownish skin around the ankles (the "gaiter" area); venous stasis ulceration; and itchy, scaly skin (Fig. 53–13).

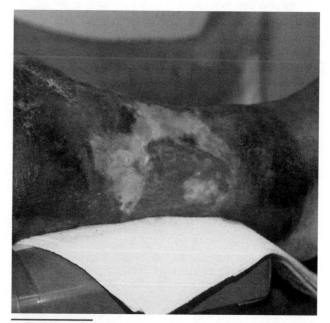

FIGURE 53–13 Severe post-phlebitic syndrome with liposclerosis and scars from healed ulcers.

Management

Goals of management are to increase venous blood return and to decrease venous pressure. Antigravity measures increase blood return to the heart and include elevating the client's legs above the heart level and avoiding prolonged standing or sitting. Advise the client to avoid:

- Crossing the legs
- Sitting in chairs that are too high to allow the feet to touch the floor or that are too deep (and press on the popliteal area)
- Wearing garters or tightly rolled socks or stockings
- Garments that exert pressure above the legs (e.g., tight girdles)

Encourage the client to sleep with the foot of the bed elevated 6 inches. At least one third of every 24 hours should be spent with the feet and legs elevated above the heart.

The Bridge to Home Health Care feature describes how increased venous pressure on the tissues of the leg can be counteracted by the compression of elastic support hose. Ideally, this support should just balance the increased venous pressure. Thus, hose should be fitted individually to the client's legs. Measurements of the ankle and calf circumference and from 1 inch below the knee or 1 inch below the groin to the bottom of the foot are usually taken. Measure after the client has been recumbent and leg edema is minimal. Stockings that extend above the knee often bind the popliteal space and act as a tourniquet, especially when the knee is bent. Knee-length elastic stockings are preferable. Elastic wraps are often preferable for clients who have periods of leg swelling. Apply the elastic wrap using a graded technique, placing more tension on the lower leg. The problem with elastic wraps is that most of them only maintain their elastic properties for a few washings, and clients tend to use them long past their effective compression. Additionally, wraps often are not used properly and do not exert adequate compression. See the Alternative Therapy chart earlier for information about nontraditional therapies.

After thrombosis of a deep calf vein, clients should wear elastic support for at least 3 to 6 months and probably for life. Elastic support compresses the superficial veins when the client walks, and blood flow in the larger veins is increased while venous pressure is kept to a minimum. Standing and sitting are not allowed for long periods during the acute phase because they increase the hydrostatic pressure in the capillaries, which pro-

---

BRIDGE TO HOME HEALTH CARE

Managing Peripheral Vascular Disease

Many clients who are referred to home health agencies or clinics that serve older people have peripheral vascular disease. Consider what you can do to help clients prevent further complications through assessment and evaluation, blood pressure monitoring, health education, and reporting changes in your clients' status to their physicians.

Assessment

Inspect clients for temperature variations; color changes in the skin; dorsal and ankle foot pulses; extremity size comparisons; shiny, taunt, hairless, or blistered skin; diminished toenail growth and color change; pain with palpation, dependent position, or weight-bearing; and skin breakdown and ulcerations. As part of the assessment, measure the calves, ankles, and feet correctly, as the involved areas of edema indicate. Use a monofilament (thin plastic filament) test for sensation and dorsiflexion and plantiflexion of the great toe (proprioception), especially for diabetic clients. The loss of touch sensation may require special foot protection. The loss of proprioception of the foot (position perception) indicates the need to discourage or stop driving. For many clients, this news is very traumatic. You may want to discuss this safety recommendation with a family member or significant other. Be prepared to problem-solve transportation alternatives.

Use the correct cuff size when monitoring the blood pressure. You may need to travel with a child, adult, and large cuff or have all sizes in the clinics. For consistency, document the cuff size and position. Discuss the benefits of self-monitoring devices with clients. Because clients may have decreased hand strength or arthritis, they may have difficulty pumping the bulb of a partially automatic cuff. Fully automatic, one-button devices are reasonably accurate and may be better options. When your clients have checkups, suggest that they take their blood pressure equipment along and compare their readings with those obtained at the clinic. Instruct them to record and share their list of self-recorded measurements with you and their physician, a strategy that is helpful for blood pressure management.

Education

Health education is an essential component of the care you provide. It is important for clients to avoid smoking, wearing constrictive clothing, and applying excessive heat to their extremities. Clients need information about elevating their legs and performing daily foot hygiene. They may be able to reduce lower extremity edema by wearing properly fitted antiembolic hose or compression socks (Siguaris or TEDS); home health clients need physicians' orders. Before ready-made compression socks are bought, measure the heel to knee or heel to thigh and the largest calf circumference; the cost ranges from $8 to $15. Before purchasing custom-ordered antiembolic socks, clients need a prescription and are measured by a supply company; these socks cost up to several hundred dollars. Clients need to exercise caution when using compression socks. Most ready-made ones lose significant compression after 6 to 12 months and need to be replaced. When possible, use the "open toe" design to prevent excess pressure on the toes, especially with diabetic clients. The nylon content in these socks causes moisture retention and leads to skin maceration in clients who have poor circulation. The socks should not be worn around the clock.

Deborah S. Bjerstedt, RNCS, MSN, FNP, *Family Nurse Practitioner, Allina Medical Clinic-Shoreview, St. Paul, Minnesota*

motes edema. Encourage walking and exercises in bed to decrease venous pressure and to promote blood flow.

■ VENOUS STASIS ULCERATION

Venous stasis ulceration is the end stage of chronic venous insufficiency. Prolonged venous pressure prevents nutrient blood flow, depriving cells of needed oxygen, glucose, and other substances. Skin of the lower legs ulcerates (*stasis ulcer*) because it occurs as a result of stasis of blood and is characteristically located in the malleolar area (Fig. 53–14).

Outcome Management

Management of venous stasis ulceration includes leg elevation, wound care, moist dressings, and support stockings. Gravity is the major enemy of venous stasis disease. Clients should rest with their legs elevated 6 inches. Regular walking is encouraged.

When ulcers are present, specimens are often obtained for culture for clients with painful, odorous, or weeping wounds to rule out infection. Antibiotics may be required to treat infection or cellulitis. Local wound care is essential by a health care provider familiar with the disease process. For some ulcers, debridement of eschar is necessary; for others, protection is needed. Techniques of wound care are addressed in Chapter 17.

Hydrocolloid dressings are used to protect new epithelium. Protect granulation tissue with wet-to-moist saline dressings, petroleum jelly (Vaseline) gauze, or moist occlusive dressings. Almost all ointments, creams, powders, and local antibiotics are harmful to healing tissue. They contribute to skin sensitivity problems, which complicate healing. To clean the ulcer, use sterile normal saline. The surrounding skin is probably dry and scaly. Gently clean the area and apply a lanolin-containing lotion (e.g.,

Eucerin, Alpha-Keri) every day. Avoid lotions containing alcohol and perfumes because they dry and irritate the skin. Solutions such as povidone-iodine (Betadine) are often used to control infection, but any solution other than normal saline retards healing.

No topical treatment is adequate without compression. Stockings are the easiest to apply, but soiling may be a problem. In addition, stockings do not fit abnormally shaped legs or those clients with dressings over the ulcer. Elastic wraps may provide one alternative because they can be adjusted for size. Elastic wraps must be wrapped with the most tension at the foot and ankle and rewrapped twice daily.

An *Unna boot* is a popular form of bandage impregnated with calamine, zinc oxide, and glycerin. When wrapped snugly around the leg, it provides excellent compression during ambulation and applies minimal pressure during limb elevation. An Unna boot is a permeable dressing that can be applied directly over skin ulcers, thereby allowing drainage of exudate. It creates a moist and warm interface between the ulcerated skin and the bandage. It can be changed on a weekly or biweekly basis, which clients wear without interruption, and thereby improves compliance. The Unna boot has been shown to achieve healing rates of 70%.

Disadvantages include allergy, skin irritation, discomfort, difficulty in bathing, and pain while one is changing the boot.

Skin grafting is rarely necessary to achieve healing. Surgery to remove incompetent varicose veins or incompetent perforator veins may also be necessary.

LYMPHATIC DISORDERS

LYMPHEDEMA

Lymphedema is swelling caused by impaired transcapillary fluid transport and transportation of lymph. Failure of lymph transport allows the plasma proteins in the interstitial fluid to accumulate. The increase in interstitial colloid osmotic pressure encourages fluid accumulation. The osmotic pressure is reduced by drawing water into interstitial areas. In addition, as the lymph channels dilate, valves become incompetent. The fluid seeks new pathways through the tissues, which causes inflammation, lymphatic thrombosis, and, eventually, fibrosis. Lymphedemas are best classified into primary and secondary forms.

Primary lymphedema may be classified according to age at onset: congenital (present at birth), praecox (before age 35), or tarda (after age 35). Congenital and familial lymphedema is also called Milroy's disease. It is inherited as an autosomal dominant trait.

Secondary lymphedema occurs because of some damage or obstruction to the lymph system by another disease process or by a procedure: trauma, neoplasms (primary or metastatic), filariasis, inflammation, surgical excision, or high doses of radiation. Postoperative lymphedema is usually seen after surgical excision of axillary, inguinal, or iliac nodes. These operations are usually performed as a prophylactic or therapeutic treatment for metastatic tumor. For example, lymphedema of the arm is encountered after

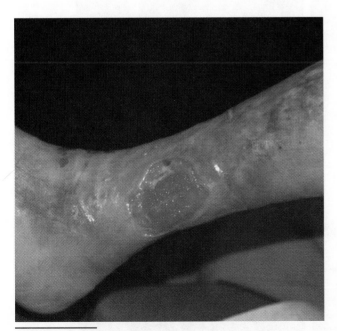

FIGURE 53–14 Venous stasis ulcers usually develop in the lower outer leg, appear irregular, and have a beefy-red base.

mastectomy (see Fig. 53–15A) Radiation in moderate amounts does not appear to damage the lymph vessels. However, heavy radiation for a particularly resistant tumor usually leads to lymphatic obstruction.

Of the primary forms, lymphedema praecox encompasses the largest group of clients; it peaks in the teenage years and is more common in females than in males. The edema usually appears spontaneously and without known cause (Fig. 53–15B).

Filariasis, caused by the filarial nematode *Wuchereria bancrofti* (and others), is one of the most common diseases in undeveloped nations; it is transmitted by mosquitoes from human to human. The living embryos (microfilariae) of the adult worms are found in the bloodstream. The larvae migrate to the lymphatics, where they mature into adult worms. Adult worms in the lymph nodes and lymphatics lead to obstruction, lymphedema, and elephantiasis.

Lymphedema secondary to neoplasms in the lymph nodes is common. The malignant disease may be primary (lymphoma or Hodgkin's disease) or metastatic from another site.

Clinical Manifestations

Primary lymphedema presents as bilateral mild edema of ankles and legs in women at puberty or shortly after puberty, unilateral edema of the entire leg in men and women (see Fig. 53–14), or bilateral edema present at birth or early age. The skin of clients with congenital lymphedema contains vesicles (blisters) filled with lymph. A dull, heavy sensation is present, but actual pain is absent. Elevation of the limb and rest in bed cause a reduction but not disappearance of the sensation. Smooth skin becomes roughened; the edema is nonpitting. Acute lymphangitis and cellulitis are infrequent. Ulceration of the skin does not occur. However, the limb becomes greatly enlarged, uncomfortable, and unsightly (Fig. 53–16). Lymphedema can be diagnosed with isotopic lymphography, lymphangiography, and phlebography.

Outcome Management

There is no known cure for lymphedema once the swelling appears. The goal of treatment is to remove as much fluid as possible from the affected extremity and to maintain a normal appearance.

Physical therapy for arm or leg lymphedema involves mechanical or manual squeezing of the tissue in order to press the stagnant lymphatic fluid to the proximal part of the limb. This is followed by specific active and passive exercises to transport the lymph farther into the lymphatic system and finally into the bloodstream. Many pneumatic pumping devices for intermittent compression are available. Diuretics may also be prescribed. Elastic stockings or sleeves are used to maintain the effects of the pneumatic pump.

To reduce the swelling, the extremity is elevated above the right atrium. Pneumatic pumps may be used to reduce the extremity size. If pumps are used, teach the client how to apply the device, the frequency of application, and the reasons for its use. When stockings are used, ascertain that the stockings fit and do not gather behind the knee. Activity such as walking, rather than sitting or standing, should be promoted. For bedridden clients, teach bed exercises to promote venous and lymphatic return and to maintain muscle strength.

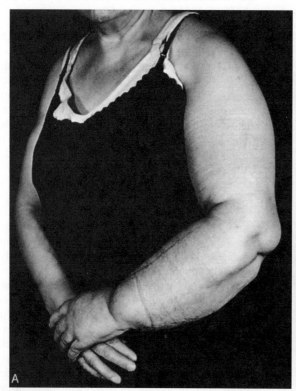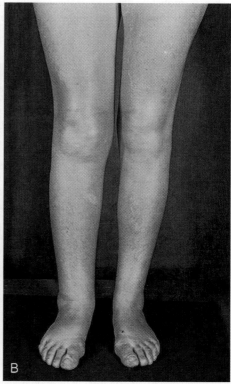

FIGURE 53–15 Types of lymphedema. *A,* Secondary lymphedema of the arm following mastectomy. *B,* Primary lymphedema.

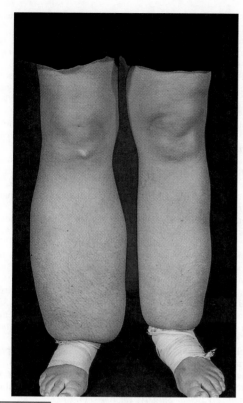

FIGURE 53–16 Severe lymphedema. The client's feet were bandaged so that shoes could be worn.

The client with lymphedema is at high risk for infection. The affected extremity is monitored for clinical manifestations of infection such as redness, warmth, and pain. Meticulous skin care is given to the extremity using mild soaps and lotions. Nails are kept trimmed.

Clients with lymphedema may suffer from disturbances in self-concept because of the visibility of their deformity. Encourage the client to discuss these feelings and help the client understand that such feelings are normal. Variations in clothing style may be suggested to disguise the deformity. When caring for clients with lymph disorders, remember that these clients must cope with difficult, chronic diseases. Take time to give emotional support to the client and the family. Emphasize the possible need for lifelong follow-up.

When lymphedematous limbs are massively swollen to the point that compression devices or stockings are no longer beneficial, surgery may be required. The most common surgical procedure for lymphedema is excision, in which all skin, subcutaneous tissue, and deep fascia in the leg are removed. The leg is covered with skin grafts. Scarring is evident, and the cosmetic appearance may not be acceptable to all clients. Another form of surgery, removal of the bulk of edematous tissues, is not curative, but the final appearance may be more acceptable.

CONCLUSIONS

Clients with vascular diseases can challenge a broad range of the nurse's capability and skill, from monitoring a client with rupture of an abdominal aortic aneurysm in an intensive care unit, to performing and teaching meticulous foot care, to educating and counseling a client to make significant lifestyle changes. Vascular diseases involve a broad spectrum of arterial, venous, and lymphatic problems.

Nursing care for clients with arterial disorders centers on promoting circulation and adequate tissue perfusion, protecting against skin breakdown and injury, managing pain, and encouraging positive lifestyle changes. Limb amputation requires particularly sensitive assessment, teaching, and counseling skills.

Nursing care for clients with venous disorders focuses on monitoring therapeutic regimens such as thrombolytic therapy, controlling and preventing thrombus formation, and promoting circulation by increasing venous blood return and decreasing venous pressure. Nursing care for lymphedema is palliative. The unique nursing care needs of clients with vascular disorders along with the exploding knowledge base that nurses need to command led to the growth of vascular nursing as a recognized area of specialty practice. The Society for Vascular Nursing was founded in 1982 and is an international organization with the *Journal of Vascular Nursing* as its scientific voice.

THINKING CRITICALLY

1. **A male client is admitted to the hospital for the care of leg ulcers. He is homeless and usually wanders the streets, sleeping on external heating grates in the sidewalk. He has large, irregularly shaped ulcers covered with thick, yellow, devitalized tissue. The ulcers are weeping, and his stockings have adhered to the ulcers. What type of ulcers are present? What type of wound care does he need? How can he continue to do wound care after discharge?**

Factors to Consider. How would you distinguish arterial from venous ulcers? Is it important to remove the devitalized tissue? If so, how? How does the client's lifestyle influence his recovery?

2. **A middle-aged man enters the emergency department with complaints of a painful leg. The pain began about 3 hours earlier after he noted a very rapid heartbeat. You note that his leg and foot are cold and white. What may have happened? What other factors need to be addressed in relation to to his leg? What are the possible treatments available? What might his post-hospital instructions include?**

Factors to Consider. How do you determine the acuteness of the tissue insult? What are the potential outcomes if you delay treatment? What might be the source of emboli, and how can this be assessed?

BIBLIOGRAPHY

1. Adams, S. (1999). Evaluation and conservative management of chronic lower extremity arterial disease. *Clinical Excellence for Nurse Practitioners, 3*(2), 88–96.
2. Anderson, L. (1999). Ischemic venous thrombosis: Its hidden agenda. *Journal of Vascular Nursing, 17*(1), 1–5.

3. Aster, R. (1995). Heparin induced thrombocytopenia and thrombosis. *New England Journal of Medicine, 332,* 1330–1335.

4. Blebea, J., et al. (1999). Deep venous thrombosis after percutaneous insertion of vena caval filters. *Journal of Vascular Surgery, 30*(5), 821–829.

5. Bradbury, A., et al. (1994). Recurrent varicose veins: Assessment of the sapheno-femoral junction. *British Journal of Surgery, 1,* 373–375.

6. Braun, C., Colucci, A., & Patterson, R. (1999). Components of an optimal exercise program for the treatment of clients with claudication. *Journal of Vascular Nursing, 17*(2), 32–36.

7. Clagget, G., & Krupski, W. (1995). Antithrombotic therapy in peripheral arterial occlusive disease. *Chest, 108*(4), 431S–443S.

8. Defraigne, J., Vazquez, C., & Limet, R. (1999). Systematic review of randomized controlled trials of aspirin and oral anticoagulants in the prevention of graft occlusion and ischemic events after infrainguinal bypass. *Journal of Vascular Surgery, 30*(4), 701–709.

9. Ekers, M., & Hirsch, A. (1999). Vascular medicine and vascular rehabilitation. In V. Fahey (Ed.), *Vascular nursing* (3rd ed., pp. 188–211). Philadelphia: W. B. Saunders.

10. Executive Committee, Nicolaides, A. (chair), American Venous Forum. (1996). Classification and grading of chronic venous disease in the lower limbs: A consensus statement. In P. Gloviczki & J. S. T. Yao (Eds.), *Handbook of venous disorders* (pp. 652–660). London: Springer-Verlag.

11. Fahey, V. (1995). Heparin induced thrombocytopenia. *Journal of Vascular Nursing, 13,* 112–116.

12. Gardner, A., & Poehlman, E. (1995). Exercise rehabilitation programs for the treatment of claudication pain: A meta-analysis. *Journal of the American Medical Association, 274*(12), 975–980.

12a. Gardner, A. W. (1996). The effect of cigarette smoking on exercise capacity in clients with intermittent claudication. *Vascular Medicine, 1*(3), 181–186.

13. Gross, K. (1999). Ultrasonographic diagnosis and guided compression repair of fenoral artery pseudoaneurysm: An update for the vascular nurse. *Journal of Vascular Nursing, 17*(3), 59–64.

14. Haraldur, B., et al. Iliofemoral deep venous thrombosis: Safety and efficacy outcome during 5 years of catheter directed thrombolytic therapy. *Journal of Vascular and Interventional Radiology, 8,* 405–418.

15. Hirsch, A., et al. (1997). The role of tobacco cessation, anti-platelet and lipid lowering therapies in the treatment of peripheral arterial disease. *Vascular Medicine, 2,* 243–251.

16. Johnson, M. (1997). Treatment and prevention of varicose veins. *Journal of Vascular Nursing, 15*(3), 97–103.

17. Katzenschlager, R., et al. (1995). Incidence of pseudoaneurysm after diagnostic and therapeutic angiography. *Radiology, 195,* 463–466.

18. Kowallak, D., & DePalma, R. (1999). A new approach to an old and vexing problem: Subfascial endoscopic perforator surgery. *Journal of Vascular Nursing, 17*(3), 65–70.

19. Kramer, S. (1999). Effect of providone-iodine on wound healing: A review. *Journal of Vascular Nursing, 17*(1), 17–23.

20. Kurgan, A., & Nunnelee, J. (1995). Upper extremity venous thrombosis. *Journal of Vascular Nursing, 13*(1), 21–23.

21. Lawrence, P., et al. (1999). The epidemiology of surgically repaired aneurysms in the United States. *Journal of Vascular Surgery, 30*(4), 632–640.

22. Lennox, A., et al. (1999). Combination of a clinical risk assessment score and rapid whole blood D-dimer testing in the diagnosis of deep vein thrombosis in symptomatic clients. *Journal of Vascular Surgery, 30*(5), 794–804.

23. Lensing, A., et al. (1995). Treatment of deep venous thrombosis with low molecular weight heparins—a meta-analysis. *Archives of Internal Medicine, 155,* 601–607.

24. Liem, T., & Silver, D. (1997). Options for anticoagulation. In A. Whittimore, D. Bandyk, & J. Cronnenwett (Eds.), *Advances in vascular surgery* (pp. 201–221.) St. Louis: Mosby–Year Book.

25. Lombardo, K. (1997). Endovascular grafting of abdominal aortic aneurysms. *Journal of Vascular Nursing, 15*(3), 83–87.

26. Moore, W., & Rutherford, R. (1996). Transfemoral endovascular repair of abdominal aortic aneurysm: Results of the North American EVT phase 1 trial. *Journal of Vascular Surgery, 23,* 543–553.

27. Nunnelee, J. (1997). Low molecular weight heparin. *Journal of Vascular Nursing, 15,* 94–96.

28. Nunnelee, J. (1999). Medications used in vascular clients. In V. Fahey (Ed.), *Vascular nursing* (3rd ed., pp. 159–174). Philadelphia: W. B. Saunders.

29. Nunnelee, J., & Kurgan, A. (1993). Interruption of the inferior vena cava for venous thromboembolic disease. *Journal of Vascular Nursing, 11*(3), 80–82.

30. Racelis, M. (1995). Vascular medicine: An alternative approach to arterial disease. *Journal of Vascular Nursing, 13*(3), 69–74.

31. Regensteiner, J., Steiner, J., & Hiatt, W. (1996). Exercise training improves functional status in clients with peripheral arterial disease. *Journal of Vascular Surgery, 23,* 104–115.

32. Sasso, C., et al. (1999). Vascular procedures. In L. Morgan & J. Nunnelee (Eds.), *Core curriculum for radiologic nursing* (pp. 319–368). Oak Brook, IL: American Radiological Nurses Association.

33. Schaefer, A. (1996). Low molecular weight heparin: An opportunity for home treatment of venous thrombosis. *New England Journal of Medicine, 334,* 724–725.

34. Sutton, K., et al. (1999). Contrast media. In L. Morgan & J. Nunnelee (Eds.), *Core curriculum for radiologic nursing* (pp. 5–56). Oak Brook, IL: American Radiological Nurses Association.

35. Twardowski, P., & Green, D. (1999). Thrombotic disorders in vascular clients. In V. Fahey (Ed.), *Vascular nursing* (3rd ed., pp. 175–187). Philadelphia W. B. Saunders.

36. Weitz, J., et al. (1996). Diagnosis and treatment of chronic arterial insufficiency of the lower extremities: A critical review. *Circulation, 94*(11), 3026–3049.

37. Zheng, Z., et al. (1997). Associations of ankle-brachial index with clinical coronary heart disease, stroke and preclinical carotid and popliteal atherosclerosis: The Atherosclerosis Risk in Communities (ARIC) Study. *Atherosclerosis, 131*(1) 115–125.

UNIT
12

Cardiac Disorders

Anatomy and Physiology Review:
The Heart
Robert G. Carroll

The human heart, through rhythmic contraction, provides the pressure necessary to propel blood through the body. Blood flow is essential to deliver nutrients to the tissues of the body and to transport metabolic wastes, including heat, to removal sites. Presence of an arterial pulse, caused by the beating of the heart, is appropriately designated as a vital sign.

The heart weighs about 300 g and is located within the mediastinum; it is cone-shaped and tilted forward and to the left. Because of its orientation during fetal development, the apex of the heart (tip of the cone) is at its bottom and lies left of the midline. The base is at the top, where the great vessels enter the heart, and lies posterior to the sternum. The heart consists of four chambers: two smaller atria at the top (the base) of the heart, and two larger ventricles at the apex. A band of fibrous tissue separates the atria from the ventricles and seats the four cardiac valves. A muscular septum separates the right from left atrium, and the right from left ventricle. Table U12–1 describes the basic structures and their functions.

Functionally, the heart is actually two pumps working simultaneously (Fig. U12–1). The right atrium and right ventricle generate the pressure to propel the oxygen-poor blood through the pulmonic circulation; the left atrium and left ventricle propel oxygen-rich blood to the remainder of the body through the systemic circulation. At rest, each side of the heart pumps approximately 5000 ml (5 liters) of blood per minute *(cardiac output)*. This is accomplished by a contraction frequency *(heart rate)* of 72 beats per minute (BPM), with each contraction ejecting a volume of 70 ml *(stroke volume)* into the arterial system. Cardiac output can increase five-fold during exercise as a result of increases in both heart rate and stroke volume.

TABLE U12–1	THE HEART: ITS STRUCTURE AND FUNCTIONS
Structure	**Function**
Pericardium	Two-layered sac that encases and protects the heart
Atrium	Upper, receiving chambers of the heart
Right atrium	Receives deoxygenated systemic blood via superior and inferior vena cava; blood passes to right ventricle
Left atrium	Receives oxygenated blood from the lungs. Blood passes to the left ventricle.
Ventricles	Lower, pumping chambers of the heart
Right ventricle	Receives blood from atrium via the tricuspid valve; pumps it to the pulmonary circulation
Left ventricle	Receives blood from atrium via the bicuspid (mitral) valve; pumps it to the systemic circulation
Cardiac valves	Prevent backflow of blood
Tricuspid and bicuspid (mitral) valves	Prevent backflow from right ventricle to right atrium and from left ventricle to left atrium, respectively
Semilunar valves	Prevent backflow from pulmonary artery to right ventricle *(pulmonic semilunar)* and from aorta to left ventricle *(aortic semilunar)*
Coronary arteries (common pattern)	Provide blood supply to the heart
Right coronary artery	Perfuses right atrium, right ventricle, inferior portion of the left ventricle and posterior septal wall, SA node, and AV node
Left coronary artery:	
Left anterior descending artery	Supplies blood to anterior wall of left ventricle, anterior ventricular septum, and apex of left ventricle
Circumflex artery	Provides blood to left atrium, lateral and posterior surfaces of left ventricle, occasionally the posterior interventricular septum; also, sometimes supplies SA and AV nodes
SA node	"Pacemaker" node, initiates heartbeat by generating an electrical impulse
AV node	Normal pathway for impulses originating in the atria to be conducted to ventricles; can be a secondary pacemaker
Bundle of His, bundle branches, Purkinje's fibers	Rapidly transmit cardiac action potentials to enable synchronous contraction of ventricles

AV, atrioventricular; SA, sinoatrial.

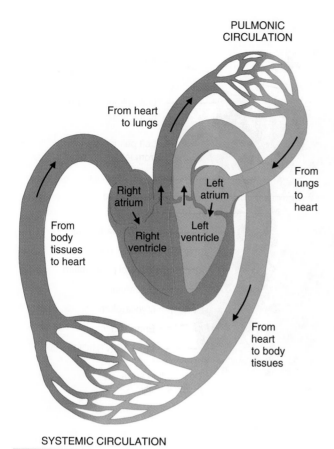

PULMONIC
CIRCULATION

From heart
to lungs

Right
atrium

Left
atrium

From
lungs
to
heart

From
body
tissues
to heart

Right
ventricle

Left
ventricle

From
heart
to body
tissues

SYSTEMIC CIRCULATION

FIGURE U12–1 Functions of the heart. In the peripheral capillaries, blood oxygen is exchanged for carbon dioxide. The deoxygenated blood returns to the right atrium and right ventricle to be pumped into the lungs, where carbon dioxide is exchanged for oxygen. Oxygenated blood from the lungs enters the left atrium and left ventricle of the heart to be pumped once again into the systemic circulation.

STRUCTURE OF THE HEART

LAYERS OF THE HEART

The heart consists of three distinct layers of tissue: endocardium, myocardium, and epicardium (Fig. U12–2, inset). The *endocardium* (innermost layer) consists of thin endothelial tissue lining the inner chambers and the heart valves. The *myocardium* (middle layer) consists of striated muscle fibers forming interlaced bundles and is the actual contracting muscle of the heart. The *epicardium* or *visceral pericardium* covers the outer surface of the heart. It closely adheres to the heart and to the first several centimeters of the pulmonary artery and aorta.

The visceral pericardium is encased by the *parietal pericardium,* a tough, loose-fitting, fibrous outer membrane that is attached anteriorly to the lower half of the sternum, posteriorly to the thoracic vertebrae, and inferiorly to the diaphragm. Between the visceral pericardium and the parietal pericardium is the *pericardial space,* which holds 5 to 20 ml of pericardial fluid. This fluid lubricates the pericardial surfaces as they slide over each other when the heart beats. Excessive fluid accumulation in the pericardial space can diminish the filling of the ventricles *(cardiac tamponade).*

CHAMBERS OF THE HEART

The heart consists of four chambers: two upper collecting chambers *(atria)* and two lower pumping chambers *(ventricles)* (see Fig. U12–2). Muscular walls *(septa)* separate the chambers of the right side from those of the left side. The *right atrium* receives deoxygenated blood from the body. The blood moves to the *right ventricle,* which pumps it to the lungs against low resistance. The *left atrium* receives oxygenated blood from the lungs. The blood flows into the *left ventricle* (the heart's largest, most muscular chamber), which pumps it against high resistance into the systemic circulation.

CARDIAC VALVES

The cardiac valves are delicate, flexible structures that consist of endothelium covered by fibrous tissue. They permit only unidirectional blood flow through the heart. The valves open and close passively, depending on pressure gradients in the cardiac chambers (Fig. U12–3). "Leaky" valves that do not seal when closed are called *regurgitant* or *insufficient.* "Stiff" valves that cannot open completely are called *stenotic.*

Cardiac valves are of two types: (1) atrioventricular (AV) and (2) semilunar (see Table U12–1). *Atrioventricular valves* lie between the atria and ventricles. The *tricuspid valve,* on the right side, is composed of three leaflets. The *mitral (bicuspid)* valve, on the left, is composed of two. Attached to the edges of the AV valves are strong, fibrous filaments called *chordae tendineae,* which arise from papillary muscles on the ventricular walls. The papillary muscles and chordae tendineae work together to prevent the AV valves from bulging back into the atria during ventricular contraction (systole).

The *semilunar valves* consist of three cup-like cusps that open during ventricular contraction and close to prevent backflow of blood into the ventricles during relaxation (diastole). Unlike the AV valves, the semilunar valves open during ventricular contraction The *pulmonic semilunar valve* (right ventricle to pulmonary artery) and the *aortic semilunar valve* (left ventricle to aorta) do not have papillary muscles.

CARDIAC BLOOD SUPPLY

The heart muscle requires a rich oxygen supply to meet its own metabolic needs. The *coronary arteries* (right and left) branch off the aorta just above the aortic valve, encircle the heart, and penetrate the myocardium (Fig. U12–4). Coronary vessel distribution can vary greatly, but the pattern described in Table U12–1 is the most common.

Contraction of the muscle of the left ventricle generates enough extravascular pressure to occlude the coronary blood vessels and prevent blood flow to the muscle of the heart during ventricular systole. Thus, 75% of the coronary artery blood flow occurs during diastole, when the heart is relaxed and resistance is low.[1] For adequate blood flow through the coronary arteries, the diastolic blood pressure must be at least 60 mm Hg. Coronary blood flow increases with increased heart work load (i.e.,

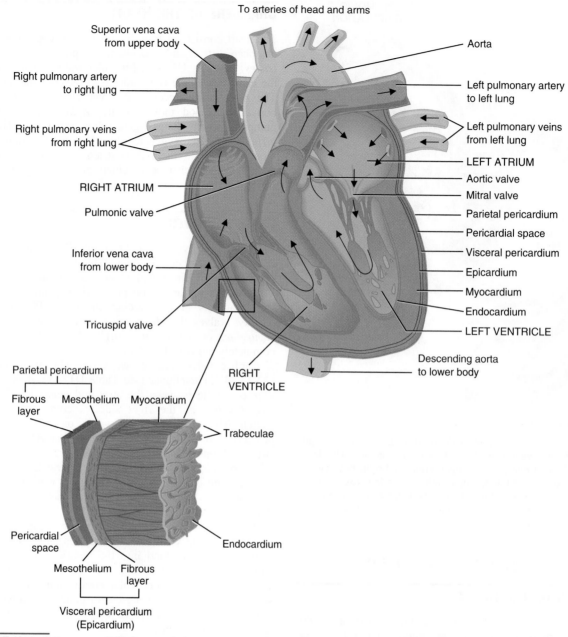

To arteries of head and arms

Superior vena cava
from upper body

Aorta

Right pulmonary artery
to right lung

Left pulmonary artery
to left lung

Right pulmonary veins
from right lung

Left pulmonary veins
from left lung

LEFT ATRIUM

RIGHT ATRIUM

Aortic valve

Pulmonic valve

Mitral valve

Parietal pericardium

Pericardial space

Visceral pericardium

Inferior vena cava
from lower body

Epicardium

Myocardium

Endocardium

Tricuspid valve

LEFT VENTRICLE

Descending aorta
to lower body

RIGHT
VENTRICLE

Parietal pericardium

Fibrous
layer

Mesothelium

Myocardium

Trabeculae

Pericardial
space

Endocardium

Mesothelium Fibrous
layer

Visceral pericardium
(Epicardium)

FIGURE U12–2 Structure of the heart and circulation of blood through the heart. Blood entering the left atrium from the right and left pulmonary veins flows into the left ventricle. The left ventricle pumps blood into the systemic circulation through the aorta. From the systemic circulation, blood returns to the right atrium through the superior and inferior venae cavae. From there, the right ventricle pumps blood into the lungs through the right and left pulmonary arteries. *Inset,* The pericardium and layers of the heart.

exercise). The coronary veins return blood from most of the myocardium to the coronary sinus of the right atrium. Some areas, particularly on the right side of the heart, drain directly into the cardiac chambers.

FUNCTIONS OF THE HEART

ELECTROPHYSIOLOGIC PROPERTIES

The electrophysiologic properties of cardiac muscle regulate the heart rate and rhythm. These properties include excitability, automaticity, contractility, refractoriness, and conductivity.

Excitability

The ability of cardiac muscle cells to depolarize in response to a stimulus—*excitability*—is influenced by hormones, electrolytes, nutrition, oxygen supply, medications, infection, and autonomic nerve activity.

In myocardial cells, as in other types of muscle and neurons, differences in intracellular and extracellular ion concentrations create electrical and concentration gradients for ionic movement across the semipermeable cell membrane. At rest, the inside of a myocardial cell is more negative than the outside. This *resting membrane potential* results primarily from the differences in concen-

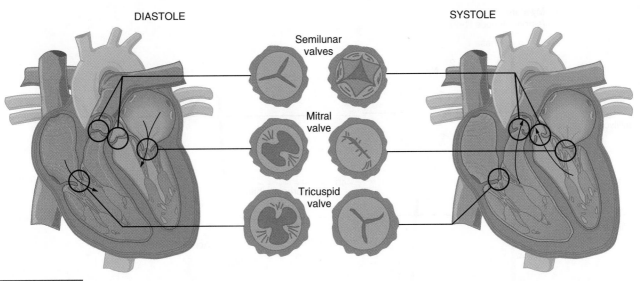

DIASTOLE

SYSTOLE

Semilunar valves

Mitral valve

Tricuspid valve

FIGURE U12–3 Valves of the heart. The semilunar, mitral, and tricuspid valves are shown as they appear during diastole, or ventricular filling *(left)* and during systole, or ventricular emptying *(right)*.

trations of potassium (K^+) and sodium (Na^+). Although both ions are present on either side of the cell membrane, potassium has a greater intracellular concentration and sodium has a greater extracellular concentration. Selective channels can increase membrane permeability for specific ions, allowing the ion to move down the electrochemical gradient and to alter the resting membrane potential.

When the cardiac cell is stimulated to a certain threshold, a sequence of ion permeability changes cause a dra-

matic change in the transmembrane potential, this is known as an *action potential* (Fig. U12–5A). The action potential consists of depolarization and repolarization phases. The electrocardiogram (ECG) reflects currents generated by the depolarization and repolarization of regions of the heart.

Depolarization is caused by an increase in cell membrane permeability to sodium. The cell returns to its resting (relaxed) state during *repolarization*. Sodium permeability drops sharply, and potassium permeability in-

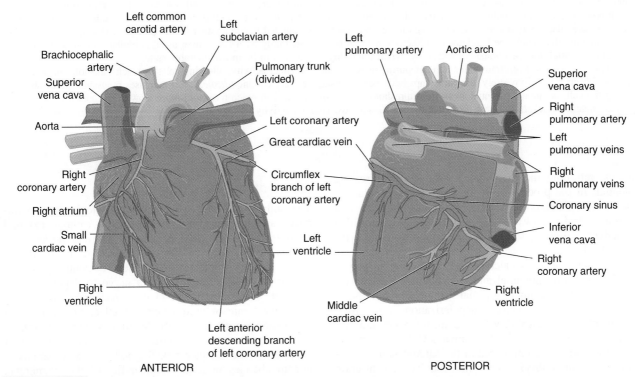

Left common carotid artery

Left subclavian artery

Brachiocephalic artery

Superior vena cava

Aorta

Right coronary artery

Right atrium

Small cardiac vein

Right ventricle

Pulmonary trunk (divided)

Left coronary artery

Great cardiac vein

Circumflex branch of left coronary artery

Left ventricle

Left anterior descending branch of left coronary artery

ANTERIOR

Left pulmonary artery

Aortic arch

Superior vena cava

Right pulmonary artery

Left pulmonary veins

Right pulmonary veins

Coronary sinus

Inferior vena cava

Right coronary artery

Right ventricle

Middle cardiac vein

POSTERIOR

FIGURE U12–4 The coronary arteries. The right and left coronary arteries branch off the aorta just above the aortic valve; they normally supply the myocardium with oxygenated blood.

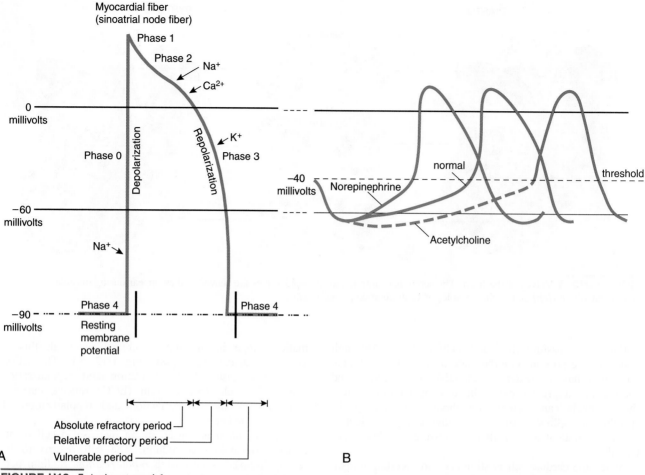

FIGURE U12-5 Action potential.

A, The action potential of cardiac cells has five phases: *Phase 0:* Sodium permeability increases through fast sodium channels, and cell depolarization (contraction) begins. *Phase 1:* The fast sodium channels close. *Phase 2:* Some sodium and calcium permeability remains through slow Na^+/Ca^{2+} channels. *Phase 3:* Potassium permeability increases in the cell. *Phase 4:* The cell returns to its resting potential, sodium is pumped out of the cell, and potassium is pumped into the cell through the cell's sodium-potassium pump. In all cardiac cells, a period occurs during which the cells cannot be stimulated to fire another action potential. During the end of the action potential, the membrane is relatively refractory and can be reexcited only by a larger than usual stimulus. Immediately after the action potential, the membrane has transitory hyperexcitability and is said to be in a vulnerable state.

B, The sympathetic neurotransmitter norepinephrine increases slow channel activity, allowing cells to reach threshold more rapidly (increased heart rate). Conversely, the parasympathetic neurotransmitter acetylcholine *(dashed line)* increases potassium permeability, moving the cell membrane potential away from threshold, and causes the cell to reach threshold more slowly (decreased heart rate). Calcium channel blockers slow the heart rate by decreasing slow channel activity.

creases, returning the membrane to the negative resting potential. In the process of depolarization and repolarization, small amounts of sodium leak into the cell and potassium leaks outward. The cell compensates for this by actively pumping sodium back out and potassium inward (Na-K ATPase).

Other ions, such as calcium and chloride, also play a role in the action potential and the contraction it causes. For the heart, calcium is especially important because it initiates contraction. During depolarization, myocardial cell membrane permeability to calcium increases and calcium moves into the cell. This inward Ca^{2+} triggers the release of more calcium stored in the sarcoplasmic reticulum (see Contractility). As the intracellular concentration of calcium increases, calcium reacts with contractile elements and myocardial muscle fibers contract.

Automaticity (Rhythmicity)

The ability of cardiac pacemaker cells to initiate an impulse spontaneously and repetitively, without external neurohormonal control, is known as *automaticity,* or *rhythmicity.* Given the proper conditions, the heart can continue to beat outside of the body. In contrast, skeletal muscle must be stimulated by a nerve to depolarize and contract. The sinoatrial (SA) node pacemaker cells have the highest rate of automaticity of all cardiac cells. The conduction tissue area with the highest automaticity, or rate of spontaneous depolarization, assumes the role of pacemaker (see Chapter 57). SA node cell automaticity is due to changes in ionic permeability of the membrane. Even at rest, a decreasing potassium permeability and increasing slow channel permeability (for Na^+ and Ca^{2+}

ions) move the cell membrane potential more positively towards threshold voltage. When threshold is reached, the cell initiates an action potential. Norepinephrine and acetylcholine cause heart rate to increase and decrease, respectively (Fig. U12–5B). The rate of spontaneous depolarization can also be affected by other hormones, body temperature, drugs, and disease.

Contractility

The heart muscle is composed of long, narrow cells or fibers. Cardiac muscle fibers, like striated skeletal muscle, contain myofibrils, Z bands, sarcomeres, sarcolemmas, sarcoplasm, and sarcoplasmic reticulum. Contraction results from the same sliding filament mechanism described for skeletal muscle (see Unit 5 review).

The action potential initiates the muscle contraction by releasing calcium through the T tubules of the cell membrane. The calcium reaches the sarcoplasmic reticulum, causing additional calcium release. The intracellular calcium diffuses to myofibrils, where it binds with troponin. When the actin filaments become activated by calcium, the heads of the cross-bridges from the myosin filaments immediately become attracted to the active sites of the actin. Contraction then occurs by power stroke repetition. After contraction, free calcium ions are actively pumped back into the sarcoplasmic reticulum, and muscle relaxation begins.

One important difference between cardiac and skeletal muscle is that cardiac muscle needs extracellular calcium. All of the calcium involved in skeletal muscle comes from the sarcoplasmic reticulum. In cardiac muscle, however, extracellular calcium enters through the T tubules and triggers release of more calcium from the sarcoplasmic reticulum. Because of this, calcium channel blockers can alter contraction of the heart, but not the contraction of skeletal muscle.

Refractoriness

Refractoriness is the heart's inability to respond to a new stimulus while still in a state of depolarization from an earlier stimulus. Refractoriness develops when the sodium channels of the cardiac cell membrane become inactivated and unexcitable during an action potential. Thus, the heart muscle does not respond to restimulation, preventing the possibility of tetanic contractions that are seen in skeletal muscle.

Refractoriness occurs in two periods (see Fig. U12–5A). The *absolute refractory period* occurs during depolarization and the first part of repolarization. During this period, cardiac cells do not respond to any stimuli, however strong. The *relative refractory period* occurs in the final stages of repolarization; refractoriness diminishes and a stronger-than-normal stimulus can excite the heart muscle to contract. At the end of the refractory period, there is a transient hyperexcitability *(vulnerable period)*. The sodium channels are reset and the cardiac cells can again conduct action potentials.

Normally, the ventricles have an absolute refractory period of 0.25 to 0.3 seconds, which approximates the duration of the action potential. The relative refractory period for the ventricles lasts about 0.05 seconds. The atria have a refractory period of about 0.15 seconds, and

they can therefore contract rhythmically much more quickly than the ventricles. The duration of the action potential and the refractory period are not fixed, however; both can shorten as heart rate increases.

Conductivity

Conductivity is the ability of heart muscle fibers to propagate electrical impulses along and across cell membranes. The heart muscle must conduct the action potential from its origin throughout the heart both rapidly and smoothly so that the atria and ventricles contract as a unit. Intercalated disks join adjacent myocardial cells, allowing the action potential to travel over the entire muscle mass (Fig. U12–6). However, the fibrous band of tissue that separates the atria and ventricles lacks intercalated disks. Thus, the atria are isolated electrically from the ventricles except for the only normal conduction pathway, the atrioventricular node. The conduction system consists of the following major parts:

- Sinoatrial (SA) node
- AV node
- Bundle of His and bundle branches
- Purkinje fibers

The *SA node,* or *pacemaker,* is located at the junction of the superior vena cava and right atrium. Under normal circumstances, the SA node initiates electrical impulses (heartbeats) approximately 60 to 100 times per minute but it can adjust its rate. Three internodal and one interatrial tract carry the wave of depolarization through the right atrium to the AV node and to the left atrium, respectively.[2] The sympathetic and parasympathetic nervous systems regulate the SA node. Any myocardial tissue that generates impulses at a higher rate than the SA node can become an abnormal pacemaker.

The (AV) node, or *AV junction,* is located in the lower aspect of the atrial septum. The AV node can be a secondary cardiac pacemaker, but it normally receives electrical impulses from the SA node and is the only pathway for conducting impulses from the atria to the ventricles. Within the AV node, the impulse is delayed 0.07 second while the atria contract. This delay enables atrial contraction to be completed before the ventricles contract.

The common *bundle of His* in the interventricular septum is relatively short, branching into right and left segments. The *right bundle branch* (RBB) courses down the right side of the interventricular septum. The *left bundle branch* (LBB) bifurcates into anterior and posterior fascicles, both of which extend into the left ventricle. The right and left bundle branches terminate in Purkinje fibers.

Purkinje fibers are a diffuse network of conducting strands beneath the ventricular endocardium; they rapidly spread the wave of depolarization through the ventricles. Activation of the ventricles begins in the septum and then moves from the apex of the heart upward. Within the ventricular walls, depolarization proceeds from endocardium to epicardium. Repolarization occurs in each cell and does not involve the conduction system. Repolarization occurs in reverse order, so that the last cells to depolarize are the first to repolarize. The action potentials of Purkinje fibers have the longest duration, and their

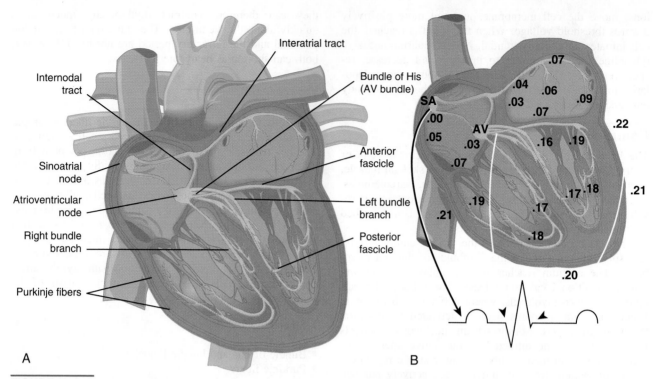

FIGURE U12–6 *A,* The cardiac conduction system. *B,* Transmission of the cardiac impulse through the heart, showing the time of appearance (in fractions of a second) of the impulse in different parts of the heart. (*B,* After Guyton, A. C., & Hall, J. E. [1996]. *Textbook of medical physiology* [9th ed.]. Philadelphia: W. B. Saunders).

repolarization is occasionally seen as a U wave of the ECG.

CARDIAC CYCLE

One cardiac cycle (Fig. U12–7) is equivalent to one complete heartbeat. The sequence of events in the cardiac cycle is divided into two parts: ventricular *systole* (contraction) and ventricular *diastole* (relaxation). The cardiac cycle normally begins with the spontaneous depolarization of the pacemaker cells of the SA node and ends following the filling of the relaxed ventricles.

Atrial Systole

Depolarization of the SA node spreads through the atria, both cell to cell and using the internodal and interatrial pathways. Depolarization of the atrial cells (P wave of the ECG) allows calcium entry, followed by contraction and pressure generation (a wave of the venous pressure tracing). Contraction of the atria propels a small amount of blood into the ventricles.

Ventricular Systole

Following a delay at the AV node, the wave of depolarization enters the ventricles, where it is rapidly spread by the bundle branches and Purkinje fibers (QRS complex of the ECG). Following depolarization, calcium enters, initiating contraction of the ventricle. In the *isovolumic contraction phase,* the ventricles begin to contract, closing the AV valves and building up pressure within the ventricles. As the AV valves close, the first heart sound (S_1) is

heard. Because the aortic and pulmonic valves remain closed at this point, no blood leaves the ventricle. The *ejection phase* begins when pressure in the ventricles exceeds the aortic and pulmonic pressures. The semilunar valves open, and the ventricles pump blood into the systemic and pulmonary circulations.

Ventricular Diastole

In early diastole, as the ventricles begin to relax, aortic and pulmonic pressures exceed ventricular pressures, and the semilunar valves close. The valve closure causes the second heart sound (S_2). The AV valves remain closed, and no blood moves in or out of the ventricles. This is called *isovolumic relaxation.* As the ventricles continue to relax, pressure in the ventricles falls below that of the atria, the AV valves open, allowing blood which has been pooling in the atria to flow into the ventricles (*ventricular filling*). When the ventricles have filled passively, the cardiac cycle is ready to begin again.

Extra Heart Sounds

The ventricular wall must expand to accommodate rapid ventricular filling. If ventricular wall compliance is decreased (as in heart failure or valvular regurgitation), structures within the ventricular wall vibrate and a third heart sound (S_3) may be heard. An S_3 heart sound may be a normal finding in people younger than age 30 years. During the last phase of ventricular diastole, atrial contraction (atrial systole or atrial kick) occurs, contributing 5% to 30% more blood volume to the ventricles.

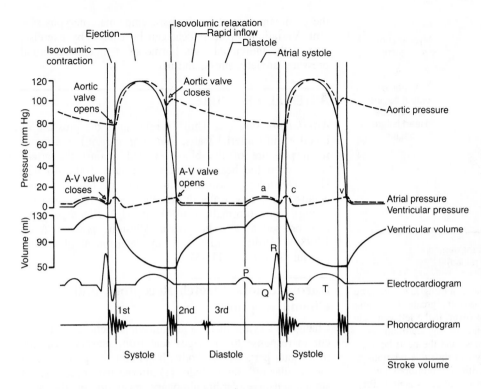

FIGURE U12–7 Changes that occur during the cardiac cycle in left atrial pressure, left ventricular pressure, aortic pressure, ventricular volume, the electrocardiogram, and the phonocardiogram. (From Guyton, A. C., & Hall, J. E. [1996]. *Textbook of medical physiology* [9th ed.]. Philadelphia: W. B. Saunders.)

A fourth heart sound (S_4) may be heard on atrial systole if resistance to active ventricular filling is present. This is not a normal finding. It may be a result of hypertrophy, disease, or injury of the ventricular wall.

CARDIAC OUTPUT AND CARDIAC INDEX

Cardiac output (CO) is the volume of blood ejected per minute by rhythmic ventricular contraction. At the end of ventricular diastole (and atrial kick), each ventricle contains approximately 140 ml of blood (end-diastolic volume [EDV]). Normally, during systole, the heart ejects approximately half of its EDV. The volume ejected with each contraction (heartbeat) of the ventricle is the stroke volume. Cardiac output can be calculated as

$$CO = [EDV - ESV] \times HR$$

where ESV is the end-systolic volume and HR is the heart rate.

Cardiac output averages between 4 and 8 L/min in adults. For a normal 150-pound (70-kg) adult at rest, cardiac output is 5 to 6 L/min. Adjustments in either stroke volume or heart rate can compensate for fluctuations in the other, or both can rise or fall.

Cardiac output is commonly measured by thermodilution with the use of a pulmonary artery (Swan-Ganz) catheter. Several other approaches can also be used, such as obtaining heart rate from an ECG and stroke volume through ventricular imaging techniques.

Clinicians compute the *cardiac index* (CI) from the cardiac output to compensate for individual differences in body size:

$$CI = \frac{cardiac\ output}{body\ surface\ area}$$

The normal cardiac index is 2.5 to 4.0 L/min/m².

Stroke volume has a major influence on cardiac output and is determined by (1) preload, (2) afterload, and (3) the contractile state of the heart.

Preload

Preload is the myocardial fiber length of the left ventricle at end diastole. It is determined by the EDV. The Frank-Starling law of the heart states that the greater the resting myocardial fiber length, or stretch, the greater its force of contraction. Preload therefore increases when increased EDV (e.g., from increased venous return) subjects myocardial fibers to greater stretch. The ventricles respond with a greater force of contraction, producing a larger stroke volume and increased cardiac output. This phenomenon, however, has limits (Fig. U12–8), such as the greatly distended ventricles characteristic of heart failure.[3]

Afterload

Afterload is the resistance to left ventricular ejection. More specifically, it is the amount of pressure required by the left ventricle to open the aortic valve during systole and to eject blood. Afterload directly relates to arterial blood pressure and the characteristics of the valves.[6] If arterial blood pressure is high, the heart must work harder to pump blood into the circulation. Stroke volume is inversely related to afterload. For example, if afterload increases because of peripheral vasoconstriction (which increases arterial blood pressure), myocardial fiber shortening is reduced and ejections are less effective. Then the ventricles cannot eject a normal stroke volume.

Contractile State

The contractile *(inotropic)* state refers to the vigor of contraction generated by the myocardium regardless of its

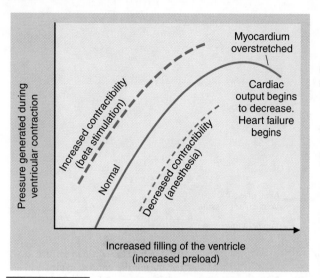

FIGURE U12–8 According to the Frank-Starling law, the more the left ventricle fills with blood (preload), the greater the quantity of blood ejected into the aorta. However, if the left ventricle fills to such an extent that it overdistends the myocardium *(arrow)*, cardiac output begins to decrease and the heart begins to fail. Agents that change contractility can shift this relationship. Norepinephrine increases contractility (+ inotrope) and improves cardiac performance; anesthesia decreases contractility (− inotrope) and impairs cardiac performance.

blood volume (preload). Unlike skeletal muscle, the myocardium can alter contractile velocity and, therefore, force. The rate of cross-bridge cycling in the myocardium is calcium-dependent, and agents that increase intracellular calcium thus increase contractile force. For example, sympathetic stimulation increases myocardial contractility and ventricular pressure, thereby ejecting blood more rapidly and increasing stroke volume. Metabolic abnormalities (e.g., hypoxemia) and metabolic acidosis decrease myocardial contractility, therefore reducing stroke volume (see Fig. U12–8).

Cardiac Pressures

With the use of a pulmonary artery pressure (Swan-Ganz) catheter, pressures in the right atrium, right ventricle, and pulmonary artery can be measured. Inflation of a balloon at the catheter tip allows measurement of pulmonary capillary wedge pressure (PCWP), an estimate of left atrial pressure. Assuming normal aortic valve function, arterial systolic pressure reflects left ventricular systolic pressure. These pressures are useful in determining factors that characterize cardiac performance, such as preload, afterload, volume, filling pressures, and resistance. Normal cardiac pressures are shown in Figure U12–9.

HEART RATE

The normal heart rate is 60 to 100 BPM. *Sinus tachycardia* is a rate of more than 100 BPM; *sinus bradycardia* is a rate of fewer than 60 BPM. (The *sinus* in these terms indicates that the impulse arose in the sinoatrial node, the normal pacemaker region of the heart.) The intrinsic heart rate is 90 BPM. At rest, the heart rate of 70 BPM reflects

the dominant control by the parasympathetic nervous system. Variations in heart beat can be caused by exercise, size of the individual, age, hormones, temperature, blood pressure, anxiety, stress, and pain.

ARTERIAL PRESSURE

Arterial pressure (see Unit 11 review) is the pressure of blood against arterial walls. *Systolic pressure* is the maximum pressure of the blood exerted against the artery walls when the heart contracts (normally 100–140 mm Hg). *Diastolic pressure* is the force of blood exerted against the artery walls during the heart's relaxation (or filling) phase (normally 60–90 mm Hg). *Blood pressure* is expressed as systolic pressure/diastolic pressure (e.g., 120/80). Cardiac output is a key determinant of arterial pressure (see Fig. U11–5).

Baroreceptors, Stretch Receptors, and Chemoreceptors

Changes in sympathetic and parasympathetic activity occur in response to messages sent from sensory receptors in various parts of the body. Important receptors in cardiovascular reflexes include: (1) arterial baroreceptors, (2) stretch-sensitive cardiopulmonary receptors of the atria and veins, and (3) chemoreceptors.

Baroreceptors (pressoreceptors) are stretch-sensitive nerve endings affected by changes in arterial blood pressure. They are located in the walls of the aortic arch and carotid sinuses. Increases in arterial pressure stimulate baroreceptors (Fig. U12–10), which send impulses to the medulla oblongata, resulting in heart rate and arterial pressure decreases (the vagal response). When arterial pressure decreases, baroreceptors receive less stretch and thus send fewer impulses to the medulla oblongata. Then sympathetic-mediated increase in heart rate and vasoconstriction occurs.

Cardiopulmonary stretch receptors are located in terminal sections of the vena cava and the atria. These receptors respond to length changes, which reflect circulatory volume status. When blood pressure decreases in the vena cava and the right atrium (e.g., hypovolemia), stretch receptors send fewer impulses than usual to the central nervous system (CNS). This process results in a sympathetic response, particularly to the kidney, to enhance salt and water retention. These changes also stimulate release of antidiuretic hormone (ADH) from the posterior pituitary. Hypervolemia produces the opposite effects.

Chemoreceptors, found in the aortic arch and carotid bodies, are primarily sensitive to increased carbon dioxide and decreased arterial pH (acidemia) and secondarily sensitive to hypoxemia. When these changes occur, chemoreceptors transmit impulses to the CNS to increase heart rate.

THE AUTONOMIC NERVOUS SYSTEM AND THE HEART

The autonomic nervous system (ANS) is the effector limb of the baroreceptor reflex, and plays an important role in regulating:

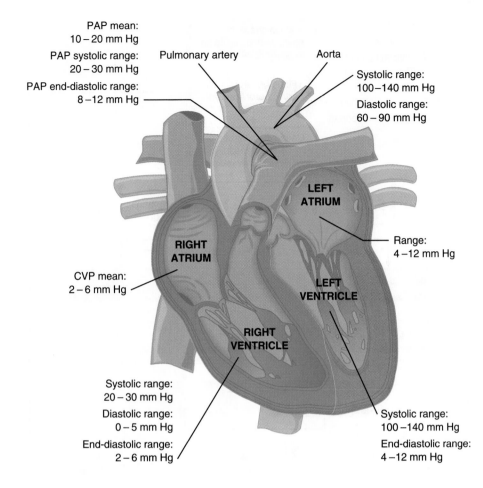

PAP mean:
10 – 20 mm Hg

PAP systolic range:
20 – 30 mm Hg

PAP end-diastolic range:
8 –12 mm Hg

Pulmonary artery

Aorta

Systolic range:
100 –140 mm Hg

Diastolic range:
60 – 90 mm Hg

LEFT ATRIUM

RIGHT ATRIUM

Range:
4 –12 mm Hg

CVP mean:
2 – 6 mm Hg

LEFT VENTRICLE

RIGHT VENTRICLE

Systolic range:
20 – 30 mm Hg

Diastolic range:
0 – 5 mm Hg

End-diastolic range:
2 – 6 mm Hg

Systolic range:
100 –140 mm Hg

End-diastolic range:
4 –12 mm Hg

FIGURE U12–9 Normal pressures in the cardiac chambers and associated major blood vessels. CVP, central venous pressure; PAP, pulmonary artery pressure.

- Heart rate (chronotropic effect)
- Myocardial contractility (inotropic effect)
- Conduction velocity at the AV node
- Peripheral vascular resistance (arteriole constriction and dilation)
- Venous return (venule and vein constriction and dilation)

The two subdivisions of the autonomic nervous system (sympathetic and parasympathetic) generally exert opposing influences and balance their activities to promote cardiovascular adaptation to internal and external demands. Autonomic nervous system responses are involuntary.

Parasympathetic nerves arise from the dorsal motor nucleus of the vagus nerve, located in the medulla oblongata. They innervate the SA node atria, AV node, and to a lesser extent the ventricles and Purkinje system. When stimulated, parasympathetic nerve endings release the neurotransmitter acetylcholine, which produces inhibitory effects by binding to muscarinic receptors. Parasympathetic stimulation decreases the rate of SA node firing, thus lowering heart rate; atrial conductivity lessens as well.

Sympathetic nerve fibers originate between the first and fifth thoracic vertebrae and terminate in all areas of the heart. With stimulation, the nerve endings release the neurotransmitter norepinephrine and produce the following effects: (1) increased heart rate, (2) increased conduction speed through the AV node, (3) increased atrial and ventricular contractility, and (4) peripheral vasoconstric-

tion, by bending to adrenergic receptors, activation of G proteins, and opening of ionic channels.

The sympathetic nervous system influences adrenal activity. The adrenal medulla responds to stimulation by secreting catecholamines (norepinephrine and epinephrine) into the circulation. Norepinephrine and epinephrine interact with adrenergic receptors found within cell membranes of the heart and blood vessels. The response to stimulation depends on the type and location of adrenergic receptors involved. The five types of receptors follow:

1. *Alpha$_1$-adrenergic receptors* are located in peripheral arteries and veins. When stimulated, alpha receptors produce a dramatic vasoconstrictive response.
2. *Alpha$_2$-adrenergic receptors* are located in several tissues. Their actions include contraction of some vascular smooth muscle, inhibition of lipolysis, inhibition of neurotransmission, and promotion of platelet aggregation.
3. *Beta$_1$-adrenergic receptors* are predominantly located in the heart. When stimulated, beta$_1$ receptors cause an increase in heart rate, AV node conduction, and myocardial contractility. This may result in increased cardiac output and blood pressure.
4. *Beta$_2$-adrenergic receptors* are found in the arterial and bronchial walls. Stimulation of beta$_2$ receptors causes smooth muscles to dilate, producing vasodilation of arterial vessels and bronchodilation.

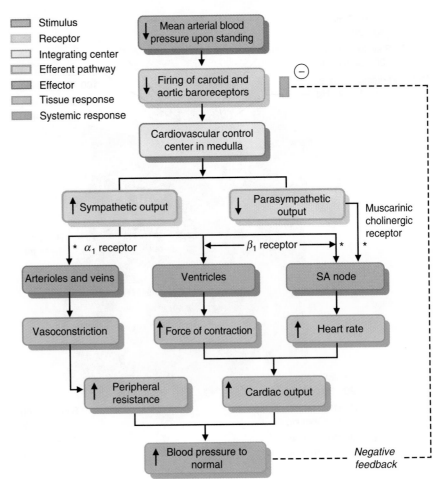

Stimulus
Receptor
Integrating center
Efferent pathway
Effector
Tissue response
Systemic response

FIGURE U12-10 Baroreceptor control of cardiac function. Baroreceptors sense changes in blood pressure and stimulate either a sympathetic nervous system response to constrict peripheral blood vessels or the parasympathetic system to relax blood vessels. These actions maintain blood pressure at a steady state. SA, sinoatrial. (Modified from Silverthorn D. *Human physiology,* 1988. Upper Saddle River, NJ: Prentice Hall.)

5. *Beta₃-adrenergic receptors* are found in adipose tissue, where they promote lipolysis. Indirectly, this may assist cardiac performance because the myocardium can utilize fatty acids as metabolic fuels. Currently, no direct cardiac role for beta₃ adrenoreceptors has been identified.

Hormonal and Other Influences

In addition to epinephrine and norepinephrine from the adrenal medulla, several other hormones regulate cardiac output indirectly by controlling body fluid volume (and thus venous pressure and venous return). The most important hormones include ADH and the renin-angiotensin-aldosterone mechanism.

Other factors also influence cardiac activity and blood pressure. For example, cerebral cortical input from anger, fear, pain, or excitement can augment the effects of the sympathetic nervous system.

EFFECTS OF AGING

At birth, the neonate ventricles are of equal size. However, the vascular changes associated with birth lead to a decrease in pulmonary vascular resistance and pressure and an increase in systemic vascular resistance and pressure. During childhood, the greater work of the left ventricle to eject its cardiac output into the high pressure systemic circulation causes a hypertrophy of the left ventricular muscle, which is characteristic of the adult heart. The heart muscle also undergoes changes with further aging that lead to dilation of the cardiac chambers and lessening of contractility. This has little effect on stroke volume, but it reduces cardiac reserve. Coronary arteries become thickened and rigid. These changes decrease the ability of the heart to respond to additional demands and increase the likelihood of coronary artery disease. Heart valves may thicken and become incompetent, resulting in a systolic ejection murmur.

CONCLUSIONS

Although the heart can be viewed simply as a pump, this remarkable, durable organ is much more than that. The heart is a continuously beating organ that never rests. It moves blood throughout the body to oxygenate cells for energy. It propels blood through its four chambers in one direction, from right to left. Left ventricular contraction moves blood into the arteries under high pressure. This pressure propels blood through the systemic circulation.

Heart disease remains the major cause of death and involves disorders both of structure and of function of the heart. These disorders are studied in the following chapters.

BIBLIOGRAPHY

1. Ahrens, T., & Taylor, L. (1992). *Hemodynamic waveform analysis.* Philadelphia: W. B. Saunders.
2. Berne, R. M., & Levy, M. N. (1998). *Physiology* (4th ed.). St. Louis: Mosby–Year Book.
3. Braunwald, E., et al. (Ed.). (1992). Normal and abnormal circulatory function. In *Heart disease: A textbook of cardiovascular medicine* (4th ed.). Philadelphia: W. B. Saunders.
4. Guyton, A. C., & Hall, J. E. (1996). *Textbook of medical physiology* (9th ed.). Philadelphia: W. B. Saunders.
5. Hurst, J. W. (1990). *The heart.* New York: McGraw-Hill.
6. Hurst, J. W., et al. (1988). *Atlas of the heart.* New York: McGraw-Hill.
7. Jarvis, C. (1999). *Physical examination and health assessment* (3rd ed.). Philadelphia: W. B. Saunders.
8. Silverthorn, D. (1998). *Human physiology.* Upper Saddle River, NJ: Prentice Hall.

54

Assessment of the Cardiac System

Kathleen Popelka

Cardiovascular disease (CVD) is the leading cause of illness and death in the United States, affecting more than one in five people. According to the National Center for Health Statistics (NCHS), if all forms of major CVD were eliminated, life expectancy would rise by almost 10 years. About one sixth of those who die of CVD are younger than 65 years of age.[3] CVD is not just a "man's disease." More than 52.6% of deaths in women are due to CVD. CVD has claimed the lives of more women than men (47.4%) since 1984—more than half a million women every year, or more than the next 16 causes of death combined.[3, 20] The gap between male and female CVD-related death widens as women approach menopause, lose the protective effect of estrogen, and have a continuously rising risk of heart disease and stroke with age.

The prevalence and complications of CVD have significant implications for nurses to utilize physical assessment skills. Assessment of the cardiovascular system incorporates data from history-taking, relating the information to the physical examination and diagnostic tests, and correlating it with the underlying pathophysiology.

HISTORY

The history of CVD is inseparable from the client's total health history. Important information may be overlooked unless previous illnesses, manifestations, habits, lifestyle, socioeconomic considerations, and family history are examined. Table 54–1 summarizes common risk factors for CVD. Significant cardiovascular data are obtained by assessment of the following areas.

■ RISK FACTOR ANALYSIS

During the interview, be alert for data indicating the presence of CVD. Note whether the client has ever had an illness or problem related to the heart or blood vessels, such as an enlarged heart, heart murmur, rheumatic heart, heart attack, or heart failure. When reviewing the demographic data, ask whether the client has not been accepted for the armed services or sports, not passed an insurance examination, or had a high rating on an insurance examination.

While conducting the symptom analysis and review of systems, note statements about the following: chest discomfort or pain; shortness of breath on exertion or while sleeping; ankle swelling; dizzy spells; fainting spells; palpitations or rapid heartbeats; unexplained fatigue; coughing at night; coughing up blood; and cramps or pain in the calves, thighs, or hips while walking that is relieved by rest.

Must the client sleep on more than one pillow to breathe comfortably at night? Does the client need to arise several times during the night to urinate? Does the client have tender or swollen calves or varicose veins? These questions screen for the presence of heart disease that is producing physiologic impairment.[11, 36] With the exclusion of chest pain and palpitations, the manifestations are all traceable to the secondary effects of heart disease on other organs, particularly the lungs, brain, kidneys, and blood vessels.

Tailor questions to the client, depending on the manifestations, prior illnesses, physical findings, and other information gathered in order to help determine possible causes. Of all the CVDs tracked by the American Heart Association (AHA), the following are considered to be major[3, 4]:

• Ischemic (coronary) heart disease (CHD)
• Hypertensive disease
• Rheumatic fever or rheumatic heart disease
• Cerebrovascular disease (stroke)

Classification of the functional severity of illness is also important. Although there is a rough correlation between severity of heart disease, manifestations, and client limitations, the pathophysiologic impairment does not always correlate closely with the manifestations. This lack of correlation is sometimes true even with far advanced heart disease. Diagnostic studies and the client's actual capacities and limitations warrant further investigation.

Ask about current activities and limitations. Do any activities bring on shortness of breath (SOB), chest discomfort, fatigue, or dizziness? How far can the client walk, run, and climb steps? Can the client complete housework, mow the lawn, participate in sports, shop, do a full day's work, or have sexual intercourse?[11, 36]

Evaluation of previous treatments, medications, and surgical and nonsurgical interventions provides a foundation for further therapeutic regimens. Ascertain whether the client understood and followed previously prescribed medical regimens. Clients are often said not to respond to therapy when, in reality, they do not take the medications

TABLE 54-1	RISK FACTOR ANALYSIS FOR CARDIOVASCULAR DISEASE	
Risk Factor	**High Risk**	**Highest Risk**
Sex and age	Women after menopause	Men older than 60
Family history of high blood pressure	Two blood relatives	Three or more blood relatives
Family history of heart attack	One relative, before age 60	Two relatives, before age 60
Family history of diabetes	One or more relatives with type 1 diabetes	One or more relatives with type 2 diabetes
Blood pressure† (degree of control somewhat modifiable)	Systolic: 160–200 mm Hg Diastolic: 90–110 mm Hg	Systolic: >200 mm Hg Diastolic: >110 mm Hg
Diabetes† (degree of control somewhat modifiable)	Type 1 diabetes uncontrolled or type 2 diabetes controlled	Type 2 diabetes uncontrolled
Weight*	30%–40% overweight	50% or more overweight
Cholesterol level†	240–280	Over 280
Serum triglycerides, fasting†	400–1000	Over 1000
Percentage of fat in diet†	30%–50%	Over 50%
Frequency of recreational exercise*	Minimal	No activity
Frequency of occupational exercise*	Minimal	Sedentary occupation
Cigarette smoking*	20–40 a day	Over 40 a day
Stress at home*	High	Extremely high
Stress at work†	High	Extremely high
Behavior pattern (especially men)†	Type A	Type A
Use of oral contraceptives (women)†	Younger than 40 and use oral contraceptives	Older than 40 and use oral contraceptives
Air pollution†	Moderate	High
Sleep patterns*	More than 8 hr sleep a night	4–6 hr sleep a night

*Modifiable risk factors.
†Possibly modifiable risk factors.

correctly. Diets are commonly not adhered to as prescribed. Confusion about the use, frequency, and amount of different medications or the expense is the cause of noncompliance and of the lack of expected improvement. Question the client's understanding of the illness so that appropriate education can be initiated, corrected, or reinforced.

■ BIOGRAPHICAL AND DEMOGRAPHIC DATA

Biographical and demographic data include name, age, sex, place of birth, race, marital status, occupation, and ethnic background. Alterations in health status may have caused changes in occupation and status within the family as the provider. There are known transcultural considerations regarding heart disease and stroke among culturally diverse individuals. Mortality from heart disease for Native Americans is twice as high as that for all Americans. Black men are nearly twice as likely to die from stroke as white men. Among American adults age 20 and older, the estimated prevalence of coronary heart disease is 7.2% for the general population, 7.5% for non-Hispanic whites, 6.9% for non-Hispanic blacks, and 5.6% for Mexican Americans.[3, 40]

■ CURRENT HEALTH

Documenting the progression of the first manifestations to the current complaints or problems helps organize the history and reveals the sequence of events that led the client to seek help.

Chief Complaint

Inquire about the chief complaint or complaints to establish priorities for intervention and to evaluate how well the client understands the presenting condition. Common

clinical manifestations of CVD are listed in Box 54–1.[20, 36] There may be more than one major manifestation. When this occurs, assess them in order of importance.

Symptom Analysis

Conduct a symptom analysis to evaluate and clarify the chief complaint. Chapter 9 describes symptom analysis. Following are the more common cardiac manifestations.

CHEST PAIN

Chest pain is one of the most important manifestations of cardiac disease. It may result from pulmonary, intestinal, gallbladder, and musculoskeletal disorders. *Angina pectoris* is the true symptom of coronary artery disease (CAD). Angina is caused by myocardium ischemia (hypoxia), an imbalance of oxygen supply and demand as the coronary arteries support myocardial tissue. Because chest pain is caused by a number of conditions, it is highly variable. Evaluate chest pain and its cause with a careful symptom analysis. Table 54–2 compares selected cardiac, pulmo-

---

BOX 54–1 Important Manifestations of Cardiac Disease

- Chest pain
- Irregularities of heart rhythm—palpitations
- Respiratory manifestations—dyspnea
- Syncope
- Fatigue
- Weight gain, dependent edema
- Cyanosis
- Hemoptysis

TABLE 54–2　DIFFERENTIAL ASSESSMENT OF CHEST PAIN

Condition	Location	Quality	Quantity	Timing	Aggravating and Relieving Factors	Associated Manifestations
Angina pectoris	Substernal or retrosternal region; radiates to neck, jaw, epigastrium, shoulders, arms (especially left)	Pressure, burning, squeezing, tight heaviness, indigestion	Moderate to severe	<10 min	Aggravated by exertion, cold, stress, or after meals; relieved by rest or nitroglycerin; atypical (Prinzmetal's) angina may be unrelated to activity and caused by coronary artery spasm	Sinus tachycardia, bradycardia, S_4, paradoxical split S_2 during pain episode
Coronary insufficiency	Same as angina	Same as angina	Increasingly severe	>10 min	Same as angina, with gradually decreasing tolerance for exertion	Same as angina
Myocardial infarction	Precordial, substernal; may radiate like angina	Heaviness, crushing pressure, burning, constriction	Severe, sometimes mild (in 30% of clients)	Sudden onset; lasting longer than 15 min	Unrelieved	Dyspnea, sweating, weakness, nausea, vomiting, severe anxiety
Pericarditis	Usually begins over sternum and may radiate to neck and down left upper extremity	Sharp, stabbing, knife-like	Moderate to severe	Lasts many hours to days	Aggravated by deep breathing, rotating chest or supine position; relieved by sitting up and leaning forward	Fever, infection, pericardial friction rub, syncope, dyspnea, orthopnea
Dissecting aortic aneurysm	Anterior chest; radiates to thoracic area of back; may be abdominal; pain shifts in chest	Tearing	Excruciating, tearing, knife-like	Sudden onset, lasts for hours	Unrelated to anything	Lower blood pressure in one arm, absent pulses, CVA, dyspnea, murmur of aortic insufficiency, pulsus paradoxus, stridor; myocardial infarction can occur
Mitral valve prolapse syndrome	Usually not substernal; sometimes radiates to the left arm, back, jaw	Stabbing, sharp, sticky quality, "kick"	Variable; generally mild but can become severe	Sudden, recurrent	Not related to exertion, not relieved by nitroglycerin or rest	Variable palpitations, dysrhythmias, dizziness, syncope, dyspnea, late systolic or pansystolic murmur
Pulmonary embolism (many pulmonary emboli do not produce chest pain)	Substernal, "anginal"	Deep, crushing; if pulmonary infarction, may be pleuritic	Can be absent, mild, or severe	Sudden onset; lasts minutes to < 1 hr	May be aggravated by breathing	Fever, tachypnea, tachycardia, hypotension, elevated jugular venous pressure, right ventricular lift, accentuated pulmonary valve (P_2) sound during S_2, occasional murmur of tricuspid insufficiency and right ventricular S_4; with infarction usually in the presence of heart failure; crackles, pleural rub, hemoptysis, clinical phlebitis present in minority of cases

Table continued on following page

TABLE 54–2 DIFFERENTIAL ASSESSMENT OF CHEST PAIN *Continued*

Condition	Location	Quality	Quantity	Timing	Aggravating and Relieving Factors	Associated Manifestations
Spontaneous pneumothorax	Unilateral	Sharp, well localized, stabbing	Moderate, severe	Sudden onset; lasts many hours	Painful breathing	Dyspnea, shock, tension pneumothorax
Pneumonia with pleurisy	Localized over area of consolidation	Sharp, grabbing aching	Variable	Sudden	Painful breathing	Dyspnea, cough, fever, hemoptysis, crackles, occasional pleural rub
Gastrointestinal disorders (esophageal reflux)	Lower substernal area, epigastric, right or left upper quadrant	Burning, colic-like aching, tightness, pressure	Moderate to severe	Waves, continuous radiation	Precipitated by recumbency, large meals, alcohol ingestion	Nausea, regurgitation, food intolerance, melena, hematemesis, jaundice
Musculoskeletal disorders	Variable	Aching	Variable	Short or long duration Prolonged period of time	History of muscle exertion, viral illness	Tender to pressure or movement
Neurologic disorders (herpes zoster)	Dermatomal in distribution	Aching constant burning, pins and needles, sharp	Moderate, severe	Unassociated with external events	Aggravated by systemic stress	Pain before rash, vesicles
Psychogenic states (depression, self-gain, or attention-seeking)	Usually localized to a point	Vague, burning, diffuse	Mild to moderate, disabling	Varies; usually very brief	Situational anger, depression, anxiety	Sighing, chest wall tenderness, fatigue, dyspnea, anorexia

CVA, cerebrovascular accident; P_2, pulmonic second sound; S_2, second heart sound; S_4, fourth heart sound.

Modified from Andreoli, K., et al. (1987). *Comprehensive cardiac care* (6th ed., pp. 54–55). St. Louis: Mosby–Year Book; Seller, R. H. (1996). *Differential diagnosis of common complaints* (3rd ed., pp. 57–68). Philadelphia: W. B. Saunders; and Hill, B., & Geraci, S. A. (1998). A diagnostic approach to chest pain based on history and ancillary evaluation. *Nurse Practitioner, 23*(2), 20–45.

nary, gastrointestinal, musculoskeletal, neurologic, and anxiety-related conditions in relation to chest pain.[20, 32, 36] Table 54–3 compares gender differences in manifestations associated with angina.[34]

TIMING. Note the time the pain begins and ends to determine the duration of discomfort. Several intermittent small episodes of chest pain are not considered as one long period of pain. Generally, the pain of myocardial infarction lasts longer than 30 minutes or until intervention is begun. Conversely, angina is usually relieved within 5 to 15 minutes by rest, with or without the use of vasodilator drugs such as nitroglycerin. Angina pectoris rarely lasts less than 1 minute or more than 15 minutes in the absence of myocardial infarction or persistent dysrhythmias (abnormal heart rhythms).[2]

QUALITY. Chest pain may be described as a "strange feeling," indigestion, a dull heavy pressure, burning, crushing, constricting, aching, stabbing, or tightness. Angina pectoris characteristically has a crescendo (gradually increasing) pattern at onset. Pain described as "shooting" or "stabbing" and reaching maximum intensity virtually instantaneously is often not angina but musculoskeletal or neural in origin.[2]

QUANTITY. To better quantify chest pain, ask the client to use a scale of 1 (least severe) to 10 (most severe). This recorded scale can then be used to compare future episodes of chest pain. For example, the client may report 10/10 for pain on admission and then report 3/10 for pain after administration of a vasodilating medication.

LOCATION. The site of discomfort provides additional information for determining its cause. Anginal pain is ordinarily retrosternal, felt slightly to the left of the midline or partly under the sternum. The chest pain of myo-cardial ischemia tends to radiate bilaterally across the chest into the arms, left greater than right, and into the neck and lower jaw. Occasionally, radiation to the back or occiput is noted. Chest pain may be diffuse, localized, or so minor that clients dismiss true ischemic pain or possible infarction. Painless or atypical presentation of myocardial infarction occurs in up to 30% of clients, particularly in diabetic and older clients.[2]

PRECIPITATING OR AGGRAVATING FACTORS. The pain may be associated with certain factors or conditions. Emotional or sexual excitement, temperature extremes, exertion, deep sleep, position changes, deep breathing, straining during bowel movements, or eating may trigger the onset of chest pain.

RELIEVING FACTORS. Anginal pain may be relieved by rest, nitroglycerin, oxygen, and a change in position. Chest pain that is not relieved by these interventions and lasts 20 minutes or longer highly suggests myocardial infarction.[2]

ASSOCIATED MANIFESTIONS. Ask the client whether other manifestations accompany the onset of chest pain, for example, anxiousness, shortness of breath, nausea, vomiting, diaphoresis (perspiration), vertigo, palpitations, or a feeling of impending doom. Pain associated with transmural Q-wave infarction is usually more severe and longer lasting than angina and is often associated with nausea, vomiting, and diaphoresis. Myocardial infarction is frequently accompanied by symptoms of sustained left ventricular dysfunction (*dyspnea* [labored breathing] and *orthopnea* [difficult breathing except in an upright position]) and evidence of autonomic nervous system hyperactivity (tachycardia, diaphoresis, bradycardia).[2]

IRREGULARITIES OF HEART RHYTHM— PALPITATIONS

The word "palpitation" is derived from the Latin *palpitare*, "to throb." *Palpitations* are uncomfortable sensations in the chest associated with a wide range of dysrhythmias (Box 54–2). They are common and do not necessarily indicate serious heart disease. A palpitation is a sensation of rapid heartbeats, skipping, irregularity, thumping, or pounding and may be accompanied by anxiousness.

Tachycardia (rapid heart rate), increased force of myocardial contraction (as can occur with ingestion of caffeine or with emotional or physical stress), or premature ventricular beats may cause palpitations. Any condition in which there is an increased stroke volume, as in aortic regurgitation, may be associated with a sensation of forceful contraction.

The onset and termination of palpitations are often abrupt. Question the client about (1) medications; (2) the frequency of palpitations, precipitating factors, and aggravating or relieving factors; and (3) any manifestations such as dizziness or shortness of breath associated with the onset of the palpitations. See Box 54–2 for common causes of palpitations.[2, 32]

RESPIRATORY MANIFESTATIONS—DYSPNEA

Dyspnea is defined as shortness of breath or labored breathing. Like chest pain, this common manifestation affects clients with cardiac and pulmonary disorders. *Acute dyspnea* may occur with a fever, exposure to high altitude, acute pulmonary edema, hyperventilation, anemia, pneumonia, pneumothorax, pulmonary emboli, and

TABLE 54–3	GENDER DIFFERENCES IN MANIFESTATIONS ASSOCIATED WITH ANGINA	
Rank in Frequency	Among Women	Among Men
1	Fatigue	Rest pain
2	Rest pain	Fatigue
3	Weakness	Shortness of breath
4	Shortness of breath	Weakness
5	Dizziness	Arm pain
6	Arm pain	Dizziness
7	Nausea	Sweating
8	Back pain	Neck pain
9	Lost of appetite	Nausea
10	Neck pain	Heartburn
11	Sweating	Palpitations
12	Heartburn	Throat pain
13	PND	Back pain
14	Palpitations	Loss of appetite
15	Jaw pain	Jaw pain
16	Throat pain	PND
17	Toothache	Toothache

PND, paroxysmal nocturnal dyspepsia.
From Penque, S., et al. (1998). Women and coronary artery disease: Relationship between descriptors of signs and symptoms and diagnostic and treatment course. *American Journal of Critical Care,* 7(3), 175–182.

BOX 54–2	Common Causes of Palpitations

Dysrhythmias

1. Bradyarrhythmias
   a. Heart block
   b. Sinus arrest
2. Extrasystoles
   a. Premature atrial contractions (PACs)
   b. Premature nodal contractions
   c. Premature ventricular contractions (PVCs)
3. Tachyarrhythmias
   a. Atrial fibrillation
   b. Atrial flutter
   c. Multifocal atrial tachycardia
   d. Paroxysmal supraventricular tachycardia
   e. Ventricular tachycardia

Other

1. Anemia
2. Anxiety states
3. Caffeine
4. Drugs
   a. Antidepressants
   b. Bronchodilators
   c. Digitalis
5. Fever
6. Hyperthyroidism
7. Hypoglycemia
8. Perimenopausal
9. Pheochromocytoma
10. Smoking
11. Thyrotoxicosis

airway obstruction. *Chronic dyspnea* also may occur in clients experiencing anxiety, depression, left ventricular heart failure, pulmonary disease, pleural effusion, asthma, obesity, poor physical fitness, and various psychosomatic conditions.

Although dyspnea can develop in any form of heart disease, it usually occurs with cardiac enlargement and other pathologic, cardiovascular, structural, and physiologic changes. Dyspnea develops when the left ventricle fails to function and the lungs become congested with fluid.[2]

There are several forms of dyspnea: exertional dyspnea, orthopnea, and paroxysmal nocturnal dyspnea.

Exertional Dyspnea. This is the most common form of cardiac-related dyspnea. Also known as *dyspnea on exertion* (DOE),[2] it occurs during mild to moderate exercise or activity and disappears with rest. If severe, exertional dyspnea can greatly limit activity tolerance. Ask the client to describe the degree of activity that typically precipitates the onset of dyspnea, for example, walking up one flight of stairs or walking to the mailbox. Noncardiac conditions such as obesity, poor physical conditioning, anemia, asthma, and obstructions of the nasal passages may also lead to dyspnea after mild exercise.

Orthopnea. Orthopnea (difficult breathing) results from an increase in hydrostatic pressure in the lungs when the person is lying flat and is relieved when the person assumes an upright or semivertical position. It consists of a cough and dyspnea in clients with left ventricular failure or mitral valve disease. Clients with orthopnea need to use two or more pillows when lying down. Clients with severe obstructive lung disease, especially acute asthma, also cannot lie flat comfortably.

Ask clients what actions they take to facilitate breathing. Do they sit up in a chair or dangle their feet at the bedside? What position do they sleep in? How many pillows do they sleep with? Record the degree of head elevation required to breathe. Orthopnea usually indicates a more serious compromise of the cardiovascular system than does exertional dyspnea.[2]

Paroxysmal Nocturnal Dyspnea. Paroxysmal nocturnal dyspnea (PND) is dyspnea during sleep that awakens the sleeper with a "terrifying breathing attack." It commonly occurs 2 to 3 hours after the person goes to bed and is relieved when the person assumes an upright position. The dyspnea usually does not recur after the client goes back to sleep. Episodes can be mild, or they can be severe with wheezing, coughing, gasping, and apprehension. Some episodes associated with severe left ventricular failure progress to pulmonary edema.[2]

Syncope

Syncope, or fainting, is a transient loss of consciousness related to inadequate cerebral perfusion. Certain cardiac disorders, especially cardiac dysrhythmias (irregular heart rhythms), can precipitate a sudden decrease in cardiac output. Valvular disorders may also lead to an adverse change in circulatory hemodynamics and cause syncope or vertigo. Clients who are susceptible to syncopal episodes (e.g., those with Stokes-Adams syndrome) should wear Medic-Alert bracelets to inform emergency health care providers.[2]

Fatigue

Easy fatigability on mild exertion is a frequent problem for clients experiencing cardiac disease; it is a common manifestation of decreased cardiac output. Progressive deterioration of activity tolerance results from the heart's inability to pump an effective volume of blood to meet the varying metabolic demands of the body. Fatigue, however, is not specific for cardiac problems. The most common causes of fatigue are anemia, anxiety, chronic diseases, depression, and thyroid dysfunction.

Weight Gain and Dependent Edema

As the heart fails, or the blood volume expands, fluid accumulates. A client may notice weight gain, shortness of breath, swelling of the lower extremities, or a combination of these. An increase in body weight of 3 pounds or more within 24 hours results from fluid rather than body mass changes. Body weight is a sensitive indicator of water and sodium retention and increases even before edema occurs. The client with heart failure has symmetrical edema of the lower extremities that worsens as the day progresses. Daily weight measurement is important for clients with cardiac problems. Changes in weight should be reported to the health care provider.[2]

Other Associated Manifestations

Cyanosis is a subtle bluish discoloration. Cyanosis from birth is associated with congenital heart lesions. *Differential cyanosis* is related to a right-to-left shunt through a patent ductus arteriosus (PDA). In right-to-left shunting resulting from pulmonary hypertension, blood in the pulmonary artery crosses the PDA, which is located below the carotid and left subclavian arteries; deoxygenated blood is pumped to the lower extremity, producing cyanosis in only that location. *Peripheral cyanosis* is due to increased oxygen extraction in states of low cardiac output and is seen in cooler areas of the body such as the nail beds and the outer surfaces of the lips.

Clubbing of the fingernails is seen in association with significant cardiopulmonary disease.[2]

Hemoptysis refers to coughing up of blood. A careful description of hemoptysis is essential because it can include clots of blood as well as blood-tinged sputum. Recurrent episodes of hemoptysis may result from mitral stenosis and pulmonary causes.[2]

■ PAST HEALTH HISTORY

Ask the client about the following areas.

Childhood and Infectious Diseases

In addition to the usual information about common childhood diseases and immunizations, ask about the client's experiences with rheumatic fever, scarlet fever, and severe streptococcal infections. These conditions are associated with structural mitral valve disease. Investigate known or corrected congenital anomalies (e.g, atrial or ventricular septal defect, persistent PDA, tetralogy of Fallot, Eisenmenger's syndrome).[2, 12, 38]

Immunizations

Clients with chronic conditions, such as cardiovascular disorders, should be vaccinated yearly against influenza. Indications for the pneumococcal polysaccharide vaccine are similar to those for the influenza vaccine. Revaccination is recommended every 6 to 10 years.[21]

Major Illnesses and Hospitalizations

Note conditions that influence the client's current cardiovascular performance, that is, diabetes mellitus, chronic obstructive lung disease, kidney disease, anemia, hypertension, stroke, gout, thrombophlebitis (vein inflammation associated with thrombus formation), collagen diseases, and bleeding disorders. Explore previous hospitalizations, surgical procedures, obstetric history, and outpatient interventions. Inquire about previous cardiovascular diagnostic studies, such as an electrocardiogram (ECG), exercise stress test, and echocardiogram. The results of such studies provide baseline data for comparative analysis when later studies are performed.[12, 38]

Medications

Evaluate the use of prescription medications, over-the-counter medications, herbs, and recreational drugs. Whenever possible, use brand names or simple descriptors instead of generic names. For example, ask clients whether they are currently taking "water pills," "heart pills," or "blood pressure" medications.

Numerous medications can affect the cardiovascular system. Ask specifically about the use of antihypertensives, diuretics, vasodilators (nitroglycerin), cardiotonic drugs (digoxin), anticoagulants, bronchodilators, contra-

ceptives, and steroids. Noncardiac medications can have profound secondary effects on cardiovascular performance. For example, tricyclic antidepressants and other psychotropic medications can potentiate dysrhythmias. Oral contraceptives increase the incidence of thrombophlebitis. Steroid use increases fluid retention and may cause hypertension. Various antineoplastic agents may be cardiotoxic, causing dysrhythmias and cardiomyopathy.

Discuss the use of recreational drugs. Cocaine toxicity is a major threat to the cardiovascular system. The systemic sympathomimetic effects of cocaine result in a "fight-or-flight" reaction that increases heart rate, contractility, blood glucose levels, and peripheral vasoconstriction. Cocaine can potentiate the effects of circulating catecholamines (epinephrine and norepinephrine), resulting in sudden death.

Finally, discuss the use of over-the-counter drugs such as aspirin, cold remedies, and vitamins. Note the dose and times of administration. Ask about use of herbal remedies. Herbs are used for cardiac disorders such as angina, dysrhythmias, and heart disease and for related disorders such as high blood pressure (BP) and peripheral vascular disease.[16, 42]

Antianginal herbs include angelica (*Angelica archangelica*), bilberry (*Vaccinium myrtillus*), evening primrose (*Oenothera biennis*), flaxseed (*Linum usitatissimum*), garlic (*Allium sativum*), ginger (*Zingiber officinale*), hawthorn (*Crataegus*), khella (*Ammi majus*), kudzu (*Pueraria lobata*), onion (*Allium cepa*), purslane (*Portulaca oleracea*), Sichuan lovage (*Ligusticum chuanxiong*), and willow (*Salix*). Some of these herbs are anticoagulants (e.g., evening primrose, garlic, Sichuan lovage, willow). Others are vasodilators (e.g., bilberry, hawthorn, khella, kudzu). Some have calcium-channel blocking action (e.g., angelica). Hawthorne, garlic, bilberry, evening primrose, and flaxseed can lower BP and cholesterol levels. Antioxidants include ginger and purslane.

Herbs known to have antidysrhythmic action include angelica, astragalus (*Astragalus*), barberry (*Berberis vulgaris*), canola (*Brassica*), cinchona (*Cinchona*), ginkgo (*Gingko biloba*), hawthorn, horehound (*Marrubium vulgare*), khella, motherwort (*Leonurus cardiaca*), purslane, reishi (*Ganoderma lucidum*), Scotch broom (*Cytisus scoparius*), and valerian (*Valeriana officinalis*).

Other herbs used for heart disease include chicory (*Cichorium intybus*), grape (*Vitis vinifera*), olive (*Olea europaea*), peanut (*Arachis hypogaea*), pigweed (*Amaranthus*), and rosemary (*Rosmarinus officinalis*). Chicory has digitalis-like properties. Red grape and olive products protect against heart attack. Pigweed is high in omega-3 fatty acids, preventing blood clots that can trigger a heart attack. Peanut and rosemary are antioxidants.

In addition to the types and names of the medications the client takes, ask how many pills and how often they are taken. Is the client currently taking these medications? Clients with cardiac disease occasionally stop taking prescribed medications because they (1) are taking too many pills, (2) are experiencing unwanted side effects, (3) believe that the problem has resolved, or (4) worry about the cost. A client may neglect to take prescribed diuretics because "it makes me go to the bathroom all the time." Clients receiving antihypertensive medications may stop taking them when their BP reaches a normal range because they perceive that the problem has resolved. Careful questioning can identify areas for client teaching.

Review for substance abuse including cigarette smoking and using alcohol or street drugs. Determine the pack-year history (number of cigarette packs smoked per day multiplied by the number of years smoked) of tobacco abuse and the history of alcohol consumption and dependence. If the client is not smoking currently, does he or she use a nicotine inhalation system or a nicotine transdermal product or chew nicotine gum or smokeless tobacco? All nicotine products have a vasoconstrictive effect on the heart and vessels.

Allergies

Note and describe any environmental, food, or drug allergies. Clearly document the manifestations of an allergic reaction, such as rashes, itching, or anaphylaxis (a sudden severe allergic reaction).

■ FAMILY HEALTH HISTORY

Ask about prolonged contact with a communicable disease or the effect of a family member's illness on the client. Specifically, inquire about a family history of heart disease, high BP, stroke, diabetes, or kidney disease. A detailed health history of the client's family can provide insight into possible genetic, environmental, and lifestyle conditions contributing to a cardiac condition. Note nonmodifiable cardiac risk factors such as heredity, age, sex, and race.

Genetic factors contribute to four traits that increase the incidence of atherosclerosis: hypertension, dyslipidemia, diabetes, and obesity. Modifiable risk factors, when corrected, significantly reduce the likelihood of a cardiac event. Modifying risk factors includes reducing stress, losing weight, reducing cholesterol levels, stopping tobacco abuse, and becoming more physically active.[3–6, 10, 17, 33, 35]

■ PSYCHOSOCIAL HISTORY

The psychosocial history includes data on lifestyle, household members, marital status, children, relationships with significant others, education, military service, religious beliefs (in relation to perceptions of health and treatment), the living environment, employment, and hobbies. Note

data that help identify support systems and coping mechanisms. Psychosocial data provide information about risk factors for the development of CVD (see Chapter 58). Background information can be used to formulate a plan to assist the client in making necessary lifestyle adaptations to promote health and lessen disease.

Occupation

Inquire about all occupations the client has had and the duration of each. The present occupation may be relevant to the significance of the disease; that is, coronary artery disease or dysrhythmias may be incompatible with continuing a career as an airline pilot or truck driver. The amount of perceived job-related stress may need to be evaluated; stress is a modifiable risk factor for CVD.

Geographical Location

Where one lives is significantly related to death caused by cardiac events. The American Heart Association categorizes age-adjusted death rates for total CVD, coronary heart disease, and stroke by state. See Box 54–3.

Environment

Ask the client about the following:

- The home, such as safety issues, type of dwelling (number of steps), state of repair, exits for fire, heating and cooling adequacy
- Mode of transportation
- Access to public transportation
- The neighborhood, in regard to noise, pollution, and violence
- Access to family and friends, grocery store, a pharmacy, laundry, church, and health care facilities

After a stroke or with deteriorating cardiac function and output, a client may need assistance or environmental adjustments to live safely and fully and meet daily needs.

Exercise

Ask about the type and amount of exercise routinely engaged in during an average week before and after the

---

BOX 54–3 **Death Rates from Total Cardiovascular Disease, United States (2000)**

Rate	State
300.7 to 339.4	Alaska, Arizona, Colorado, Hawaii, Idaho, Massachusetts, Minnesota, Montana, New Mexico, Oregon, Utah, Washington, Wyoming
345.2 to 366.7	California, Connecticut, Florida, Iowa, Kansas, Maine, Nebraska, New Hampshire, North Dakota, Rhode Island, South Dakota, Vermont, Wisconsin
368.3 to 409.8	Delaware, District of Columbia, Illinois, Maryland, Michigan, Nevada, New Jersey, North Carolina, Ohio, Pennsylvania, Texas, Virginia
411.4 to 480.0	Alabama, Arkansas, Georgia, Indiana, Kentucky, Louisiana, Mississippi, Missouri, New York, Oklahoma, South Carolina, Tennessee, West Virginia

Total cardiovascular diseases are defined here as ICD/9 390–459.
Reproduced with permission, American Heart Association World Wide Web Site www.americanheart.org, 2000. Copyright American Heart Association.
Source: National Center for Health Statistics (NCHS) compressed mortality file for the years 1994 to 1996. Age adjustments are based on the 2000 standards.

onset of current manifestations. Research confirms that a sedentary lifestyle potentiates the lethality of myocardial infarction, and it is considered a significant risk factor in the development of coronary artery disease.

Effective, routine *aerobic* exercise is thought to lower the likelihood of a coronary event. Aerobic exercise includes such activities as swimming, jogging, brisk walking, bicycling, and rowing.

To be beneficial, aerobic exercise should raise the heart rate from 50% to 100% of baseline (depending on age and prior physical conditioning) for at least 30 minutes three to five times a week. Along with general body conditioning, this form of exercise increases the heart's efficiency in using oxygen. Advise clients who are older than 40 years of age or who have a history of CVD to consult their physician before beginning an exercise program.[2, 3, 9]

Nutrition

Assess excess or deficit caloric intake and the client's approximate intake of foods high in sodium, cholesterol, saturated fat, and caffeine. Although these are common components of the average American diet, they have been linked to the development of atherosclerosis and hypertensive disease. Elevated serum cholesterol levels are associated with coronary artery disease. This correlation diminishes with age but still remains. Elevated serum triglyceride levels are positively related to the development of coronary artery disease, especially in women.

Examine not only daily food habits but also attitudes toward food and resistance to therapeutic alterations in diet. Cultural beliefs and economic status greatly affect food choices. Consider these factors before recommending dietary changes. Identify and include the primary food purchaser and preparer in dietary instruction.[2, 6, 10, 17, 24, 35]

Results from the Dietary Approaches to Stop Hypertension (DASH) study have established that a diet high in fruits, vegetables, and low-fat dairy products and low in cholesterol and total and saturated fat reduces BP significantly. These changes occurred in the absence of weight loss or fluid restriction. A subgroup analysis of that study suggested that although all groups benefited significantly in terms of systolic BP reduction, two subgroups gained the most from adopting these dietary changes in daily life.[37] The DASH diet resulted in (1) lower systolic BP in African Americans than in whites (6.8 versus 3.0 mm Hg) and (2) an even lower systolic BP in clients with hypertension than in those with high-normal BP (11.4 versus 3.4 mm Hg).[37]

Habits

If the client smokes, inquire about the duration of the smoking habit and the number of cigarettes smoked daily. Cigarette smoking increases the risk of coronary artery disease and worsens hypertension. Nicotine, a major ingredient in cigarettes, causes peripheral vasoconstriction, increasing resistance to left ventricular emptying and thus increasing the myocardial workload. Smoking increases the mortality rate of middle-aged clients with coronary artery disease and greatly potentiates the development of peripheral vascular disease. The death rate for coronary heart disease is 70% higher in cigarette smokers than in nonsmokers. Clients who stop smoking will, after several years, have a death rate from heart attack almost as low as that of people who never smoked.[3, 4]

Evidence that caffeine and alcohol ingestion increases the risk of atherosclerosis is inconclusive. Nevertheless, caffeine is a stimulant that, in excessive amounts, can increase heart rate and BP and contribute to palpitations, both of which can raise the myocardial workload and precipitate angina pectoris, heart failure, and some dysrhythmias. Therefore, assess caffeine intake and caution those with known heart disease to limit caffeine intake to the equivalent of two 8-oz cups of coffee per day.

Researchers state that only excessive alcohol intake has deleterious effects on the cardiovascular system and its performance. An intake of 100 g of pure (100%) alcohol may slightly increase BP and heart rate. This amount is approximately equal to three beers or one mixed drink. Alcoholism, in contrast, has been associated with the development of hypertension and damage to the heart muscle, leading to congestive cardiomyopathy. Ask about the client's approximate daily and weekly alcohol consumption (see Chapter 2). Keep in mind that the alcoholic client may lie about the type and amount consumed.

■ REVIEW OF SYSTEMS

Ask about past problems involving the cardiovascular system, including chest pain, palpitations, fatigue, edema, shortness of breath, orthopnea, wheezing, fainting (syncope), weight gain, heart murmurs, hypertension, paroxysmal nocturnal dyspnea, and history of rheumatic fever.

Cardiovascular problems also affect the pulmonary, renal, and neurologic systems. Ask about productive cough, decreased urination, dark or concentrated urine, edema of the legs, dizzy spells, and memory loss. Detailed questions for the review of systems may be found in Chapter 9, Box 9-2.

PHYSICAL EXAMINATION

The cardiac physical examination includes the following:

- A general inspection
- Assessment of BP, arterial pulses, and jugular venous pulse
- Percussion, palpation, and auscultation of the heart
- Evaluation for edema

The client is supine. Stand at the client's right side. The head of the bed or examination table may be elevated slightly for comfort. Proceed in logical fashion from head to foot. Necessary equipment includes a stethoscope with diaphragm and bell, a penlight, ruler, and an applicator stick. Ensure a woman's privacy by keeping her breasts draped. The female left breast overrides part of the area examined in a cardiac examination. Gently displace the breast upward, or ask the woman to hold it out of the way.[12, 37] See the accompanying Physical Assessment Findings in the Healthy Adult feature.

■ GENERAL APPEARANCE

Begin with inspection. Much may be learned through simple observation. Look at the client and consider the following:

- Does the client lie quietly, or is there restlessness or continual moving about?
- Can the client lie flat, or is only an upright, erect position tolerated?
- Does the facial expression reflect pain or obvious signs of respiratory distress?
- Are there signs of significant cyanosis or pallor?
- Can the client answer questions without dyspnea during the interview?

■ LEVEL OF CONSCIOUSNESS

Note the client's general *level of consciousness* (LOC). The level of consciousness reflects the adequacy of cerebral perfusion and oxygenation. Also assess whether the client manifests appropriate behavior for the surroundings:

- What is the client's affect?
- Are there obvious signs of anxiety, fear, depression, or anger?
- How does the client react to those in the immediate vicinity, including significant others?

Assessment of general appearance and level of consciousness provides an initial composite picture of the client and indicates the level of comfort and distress.

■ HEAD, NECK, NAILS, AND SKIN

When examining the head, pay particular attention to the eyes, ear lobes, lips, and buccal mucosa. Examine the eyes for *arcus senilis* (a light gray ring around the iris, possibly caused by cholesterol deposits) and *xanthelasma* (yellow raised plaques around the eyelids resulting from lipid deposits). Both findings are common in elderly clients but may indicate a predisposition to atherosclerosis.

Observe the skin and mucous membranes for abnormalities such as central or peripheral *cyanosis*. The presence of a bluish tinge or duskiness is indicative of central cyanosis, indicating poor arterial circulation. Central cyanosis indicates serious heart or lung disease in which hemoglobin is not fully saturated with oxygen. Peripheral cyanosis, seen in lips, ear lobes, and nail beds, suggests peripheral vasoconstriction.

Assess *capillary refill* (circulation) by putting slight pressure on a nail bed until it blanches (see Chapter 59). Quickly release the pressure. When circulation is adequate, nail color returns to baseline in less than 2 seconds. Always check capillary refill before using pulse oximetry; if capillary refill is abnormal, pulse oximetry findings are inaccurate.

Check fingers for *clubbing*, in which the distal tips of the fingers become bulbous and the angle between the base of the nail and the skin next to the cuticle increases from the normal 160 to 180 degrees or more (see Chapter 59). In addition, the nails feel soft and spongy. Finger clubbing is associated with pulmonary and cardiovascular disease. Splinter hemorrhages of the nail are classically associated with subacute bacterial endocarditis.

Assess *skin turgor* (elasticity) by lifting a fold of skin over the sternum or lower arms and releasing it (see Chapter 48). Normal skin immediately returns to the baseline position, but skin with decreased turgor stays pinched (tenting) for up to 30 seconds. Decreased skin turgor occurs with dehydration, volume depletion, rapid weight loss, and advanced age. The temperature of the skin may reflect cardiac disease. Severe anemia, beriberi, and thyrotoxicosis tend to make the skin warmer; intermittent claudication (leg pain related to peripheral vascular disease) is associated with coolness of the lower extremity compared with the upper extremity.[2, 12, 30, 38]

■ EDEMA

Edema occurs in right-sided heart failure when the excess intravascular volume begins to increase capillary hydrostatic pressure and force fluid into the interstitium.

Inspect dependent areas for edema. In the mobile client, edema is best seen in the feet, ankles, and lower legs. In the chair-ridden or bedridden client, edema may be palpated over the sacrum, abdomen, or scapula. Assess the severity of edema by pressing a thumb or finger carefully into the area. A depression that does not rapidly resume its original contour is noted as orthostatic, or pitting, edema. Because there is a wide discrepancy in edema grading scales, record the actual amount of time in seconds for the indentation to resolve (see Chapter 51).[2, 12, 38]

■ BLOOD PRESSURE

Measure BP in both arms initially to rule out dissecting aortic aneurysm, coarctation of the aorta, vascular obstruction, vascular outlet syndromes, and errors in measurement. If the arms are inaccessible, obtain pressures from the thighs and popliteal arteries or the calves and posterior tibial arteries. When pressures are difficult to auscultate, systolic pressures can be determined through palpation or by Doppler ultrasonography.

When recording measurements, note both systolic and diastolic pressures, for example, 120/70. The muffling of

Korotkoff's sounds may also be included and recorded as 120/80/70. The American Heart Association recommends recording the point at which the sound disappears (fifth Korotkoff sound) as the diastolic pressure in adults. Also, record the arm in which the measurement was taken and the client's position at the time of the reading.

Postural Blood Pressure

Perform a postural BP reading when an extracellular volume depletion or decreased vascular tone is suspected. Note the client's position at the time of the reading (Fig. 54–1).

Paradoxical Blood Pressure (Pulsus Paradoxus)

Pulsus paradoxus is an abnormal fall in systolic BP of more than 10 mm Hg during inspiration. It is frequently found in clients with pericardial tamponade, constrictive pericarditis (inflammation of the pericardial sac), and pulmonary hypertension.

Use a sphygmomanometer and stethoscope to assess for a paradoxical pulse over the brachial artery. Instruct the client to breathe normally. Inflate the cuff 20 mm Hg above the systolic BP. Slowly deflate the cuff (1 to 2 mm Hg/sec), and listen for Korotkoff's sounds to appear only during expiration. (Sounds are first heard during expiration and then during inspiration.) Continue deflating the cuff until Korotkoff's sounds are heard equally well during inspiration and expiration.

The paradoxical pressure is the difference between the BP when the sounds are first heard during expiration and the BP when the sounds are heard on both expiration and inspiration. Normally, this difference is less than 10 mm Hg. If the client is breathing normally and the systolic difference is greater than 10 mm Hg, cardiac compression, such as cardiac tamponade, may be present.

■ PULSE

Pulse characteristics can vary. If the pulse is irregular, assess for a pulse deficit by taking apical and radial

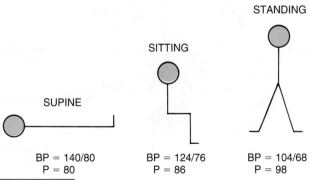

STANDING

SITTING

SUPINE

BP = 140/80
P = 80

BP = 124/76
P = 86

BP = 104/68
P = 98

FIGURE 54–1 Recording postural blood pressure (BP). After measuring the client's BP and pulse in the supine position, leave the BP cuff in place and help the client sit. Then measure the BP within 15 to 30 seconds. Help the client stand, and measure again. Postural hypotension is indicated by a BP drop of more than 10 to 15 mm Hg systolic pressure and more than 10 mm Hg diastolic pressure. Postural hypotension is typically accompanied by a 10% to 20% increase in heart rate (pulse).

pulses simultaneously, noting differences in rate. Peripheral pulse assessment is discussed in Chapter 51.

■ RESPIRATIONS

Note the rate, rhythm, depth, and quality of the breathing pattern. Variations in the respiratory rate and character may indicate heart failure or pulmonary edema. Auscultate the lungs for the presence of crackles, rhonchi (dry rattling), or other abnormal breath sounds (see Chapter 59). Severe left ventricular failure may produce pulmonary congestion and resultant frothy sputum with deep respiratory efforts.

■ HEAD AND NECK

Neck Veins

Neck vein distention can be used to estimate *central venous pressure* (CVP). The amount of distention reflects pressure and volume changes in the right atrium. The internal jugular veins, although more difficult to detect than the external jugular veins, are more reliable indicators of CVP. The external jugular vein engorges easily with only slight provocation, for example, by holding the breath, twisting the neck, and being constricted by clothing (except in weight lifters, football players, and professional speakers and singers, who have overdeveloped neck muscle tendons). The vessels are prominent and visible but soft and compressible.

A relaxed supine position with the head of the bed inclined between 15 and 30 degrees maximizes jugular vein prominence. Clients who have greatly increased right atrial pressure may require head elevation from 45 to 90 degrees. Support the client's head with a small pillow and avoid sharp neck flexion. Turn the client's head slightly away from you. Loosen or remove clothing that compresses the neck or upper thorax. Tangential (oblique) lighting enhances the veins' appearance. Observe both sides of the neck. The internal jugular vein lies deep to the sternocleidomastoid muscle and runs parallel along its length to the jaw and ear lobe (Fig. 54–2). Identify the pulsations of the internal jugular. Use the external jugular vein if the internal jugular is not visible.

Note the highest point at which the internal jugular pulses can be seen (the *meniscus*). The *sternal angle* (manubrial joint) is a reference point to measure the height of venous pulsation, approximately 4 to 5 cm above the center of the right atrium. Use a centimeter ruler to measure the vertical distance between the sternal angle and the point of highest venous pulsations. See Figure 54–3.

The value is usually less than 3 or 4 cm above the sternal angle when the head of the bed is elevated 30 to 40 degrees. Higher values indicate increased right atrial or right ventricular pressure, as seen in right ventricular failure, tricuspid regurgitation, and pericardial tamponade. Flat jugular veins in a supine client suggest extracellular volume depletion. Unilateral distention may indicate vessel obstruction on that side.

The timing and amplitude of the jugular vein pulsations may also be assessed to evaluate right-sided heart function, tricuspid valve performance, and the presence of certain dysrhythmias.[12, 30, 38]

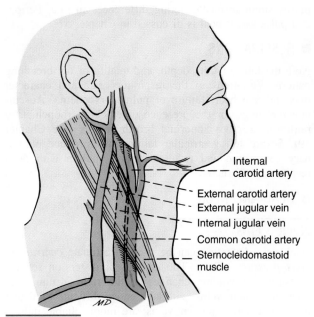

FIGURE 54-2 Location of the internal jugular vein.

Carotid Arteries

Carotid artery examination indicates the adequacy of stroke volume and the patency of the arteries. Using your finger tips, gently palpate the carotid arteries one side at a time. Check and compare the rate, rhythm, and amplitude of the pulses. Note whether a *bruit* (a blowing sound) is present by listening with the diaphragm of a stethoscope over the arteries while the client holds the breath. Tracheal breath sounds are heard while respiration is ongoing. A bruit generally indicates that the carotid artery has narrowed. Bruits typically result from atherosclerosis or radiation of sounds from an aortic valve murmur.

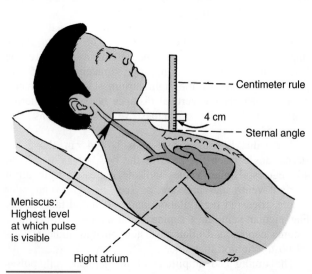

FIGURE 54-3 Estimation of jugular vein measurement to assess central venous pressure.

■ CHEST

Precordium

Perform inspection and palpation of the precordium together to determine the presence of normal and abnormal pulsations. Ideally, the client should be supine with the chest exposed. The left lateral position allows the heart to move closer to the chest wall, accentuating precordial movements and certain heart sounds. Good lighting and a warm, quiet environment are essential. Stand at the client's right side and observe the anterior chest for size, shape, symmetry of movement, and any evident pulsations. Record the location of pulsation in relation to the intercostal space and the midclavicular line. Confirm your observation with palpation. When palpating, use the fingers and palm of the hand.

The *point of maximum intensity* (PMI) or apical impulse is usually seen at the apex. The PMI is associated with left ventricular contraction and should appear at the fifth intercostal space medial to the left midclavicular line. It may be prominent in thin people and obscured in those who are obese or have large breasts. When palpated, the PMI is a single, faint, instantaneous tap beneath the fingers, no more than 2 cm in diameter. The left lateral recumbent position may enhance locating the PMI, but its position is displaced. With left ventricular enlargement and aneurysm, the PMI is more diffuse, sustained, and displaced downward and to the left of the midclavicular line.

Right ventricular enlargement can produce an abnormal pulsation that may be seen as a sustained thrust along the left sternal border. Termed *"heaves" or "lifts,"* these pulsations may be found with various disorders, such as valvular disease and pulmonary hypertension. *Thrills* represent turbulent blood flow through the heart, especially across abnormal heart valves. Use the heel or ulnar surface of the hand to palpate over each of the five cardiac landmarks (Fig. 54-4). Thrills are perceived as a rushing

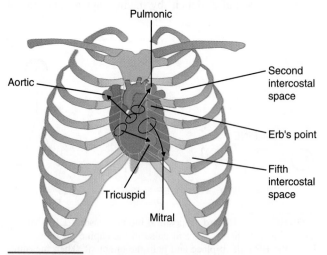

FIGURE 54-4 Precordial locations for cardiac palpation and auscultation of heart sounds. Closure of mitral and tricuspid valves produces the S_1 heart sound; closure of pulmonic and aortic (semilunar) valves produces the S_2 heart sound.

vibration, much like feeling the throat of a purring cat. Thrills are associated with significant heart murmurs. They may also be palpated over partially obstructed blood vessels.[12, 30, 38]

Heart Sounds

Auscultation of the precordium yields valuable information about normal or abnormal heart rate and rhythm, ventricular filling, and blood flow across heart valves. Assessment of heart sounds is a sophisticated skill, requiring study of heart sound characteristics and extensive clinical practice. To become skilled, you must be thoroughly familiar with normal cardiac sounds. With practice and experience, you will be able to detect abnormal heart sounds.

Discerning abnormal heart sounds is difficult even for skilled practitioners under ideal circumstances. The sensitivity of the human ear falls sharply when the frequency of sound vibrations is below 1000 Hz. Most cardiac murmurs and sounds are below that frequency. A reliable stethoscope is a must. Use the bell to hear low-pitched sounds and the diaphragm to hear high-pitched sounds. Always warm the chestpiece before placing it on the client's skin.

The environment is key to successful auscultation. The surroundings should be warm and quiet. An exposed chest is ideal, but prevent shivering, which can greatly distort heart sound transmission. Instruct the client to breathe through the nose while supine. The left lateral position may facilitate auscultation. An upright position, leaning forward and holding the breath after exhalation, helps when assessing early diastolic murmurs and pericardial friction rubs.

Always use a systematic approach when evaluating heart sounds. Methods vary. Develop your own routine to ensure a thorough assessment each time you perform cardiac auscultation.

Examination of heart sounds may progress from the base (right second intercostal space) of the heart to the apex or from the apex to the base. Whichever approach you use, pay special attention to each of the precordial locations diagrammed in Figure 54–4. Each area corresponds to a specific valvular outflow tract. Concentrate on one component of the cardiac cycle at a time, that is, the first heart sound (S_1), then the second heart sound (S_2), and so on. It is difficult to assess everything at one time. As many as three or four abnormalities may occur simultaneously. Listen to several complete cardiac cycles at each of the five precordial areas. Listen carefully, noting the quality (crisp or muffled), intensity (loud or soft), rhythm (irregular or regular), and presence of extra sounds (murmurs, gallops, rubs, or clicks). Repeat this process using the bell over each of the precordial areas.[7, 12, 30, 38]

NORMAL HEART SOUNDS

The *first heart sound (S_1)* is linked to closure of the mitral and tricuspid valves (atrioventricular [AV] valves). It marks the onset of systole (ventricular contraction). It is heard best with the diaphragm at the apex (the mitral valve area) and left lower sternal border (the tricuspid valve area). S_1 results from abrupt closure of the AV valves, which causes some blood turbulence and vibration

of structures within the ventricles. This vibration is transmitted across the chest wall as a heart sound. Phonetically, if both heart sounds are appreciated as "lub-dup," S_1 is "lub." Although closure of both mitral and tricuspid valves is heard as a single sound, the mitral valve closes a fraction of a second earlier.

The intensity of S_1 may vary in certain pathologic conditions. Diseased and stiffened AV valves (as seen in rheumatic heart disease) may augment S_1; rhythms of asynchrony between the atria and ventricles (as in atrial fibrillation and AV block) cause varying intensity of S_1. If you are not sure which sound is S_1, check the carotid artery for a pulsation or look for the upstroke of the R wave in the QRS complex (described later) on the ECG monitor.

The *second heart sound (S_2)* is related to closure of the pulmonic and aortic (semilunar) valves and is heard best with the diaphragm at the aortic area. Phonetically, it is the "dup" of the heart sounds. It signifies the end of systole and the onset of diastole (ventricular filling). At the base of the heart, normal S_2 is always louder than S_1, whereas both sounds are usually of nearly equal intensity at the left sternal border over Erb's point. Usually, S_1 is the louder of the two sounds at the apex and occurs just after or along with the carotid pulse.

Knowing the usual quality of sounds that occur over the precordium can help you to distinguish between S_1 and S_2 during rapid heart rates. Simultaneous palpation of the carotid pulse during auscultation also helps discriminate sounds. Carotid pulsation occurs with systole or S_1. Figure 54–5 shows the relationship of heart sounds to events during the cardiac cycle.

Physiologic (normal) *splitting of S_2* occurs during inspiration. Normal splitting results from delayed closure of the pulmonic valve. During S_2, both the aortic and pulmonic components of S_2 (A_2 and P_2) can be heard. Inspiration creates negative pressure within the thoracic cavity, "pulling" blood from the periphery into the right side of the heart. Because of this transient augmentation of venous return, right ventricular volume increases and emptying is delayed, delaying pulmonic valve closure. The "split-second heart sound" is best heard over the pulmonic and mitral areas. The two components of S_2 occur so close together that the pause between them produces a phonetic gap similar to the "pl" sound in the word "split." If a split S_2 is heard when the client is sitting or during expiration, it usually indicates right ventricular failure or other cardiac disease.[2, 7]

ABNORMAL HEART SOUNDS

Many abnormal heart sounds may indicate a serious heart disorder or change in cardiac function. You may not be able to label each abnormality, but with a thorough understanding of the normal sounds, you should be able to recognize various abnormal sounds and refer the problem to the physician.

PATHOLOGIC SPLITTING OF S_2

A wide splitting of S_2 may be heard during both inspiration and expiration, with an increase during inspiration. This form of splitting occurs in right bundle branch block and is related to delay in depolarization of the right ventricle and late closure of the pulmonic valve. Fixed split-

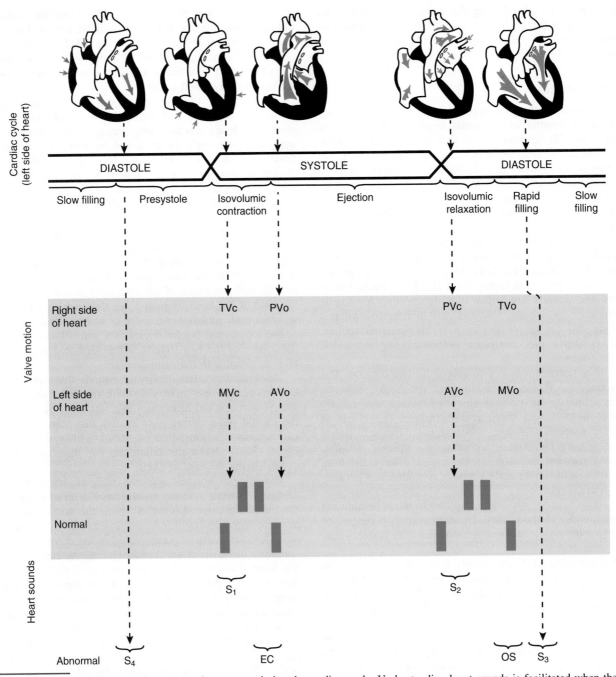

FIGURE 54–5 Relationship of heart sounds to events during the cardiac cycle. Understanding heart sounds is facilitated when they are correlated with cardiac cycle events and valvular movements. MVc, mitral valve closing; TVc, tricuspid valve closing; PVo, pulmonic valve opening; AVo, aortic valve opening; AVc, aortic valve closing; PVc, pulmonic valve closing; TVo, tricuspid valve opening; MVo, mitral valve opening; EC, ejection click; OS, opening snap.

ting is the hallmark of atrial septal defect. This form of S_2 split is continuous and does not vary with respirations. Fixed splitting occurs because the emptying of the right ventricle is prolonged. Paradoxical splitting results from a delay in closure of the aortic valve because of aortic stenosis, left bundle branch block, or patent ductus arteriosus. In paradoxical splitting, the S_2 split is heard during expiration rather than inspiration.[2, 7]

GALLOPS

Diastolic filling sounds or *gallops* (S_3 and S_4) occur during the two phases of ventricular filling. Sudden changes of inflow volume cause vibrations of the valves and ventricular supporting structures, producing low-pitched sounds that occur either early (S_3) or late (S_4) in diastole. Such sounds can originate in either side of the heart. These extra heart sounds create a triplet rhythm, acoustically mimicking a horse's gallop. For that reason, the term "gallop" is often used to denote these heart sounds.

A gallop sound that occurs in early diastole, during passive, rapid filling of the ventricles, is known as the *third heart sound (S_3)*. It is heard best with the bell at the apex and with the client in the left lateral recumbent position. An S_3 immediately follows S_2 and is a dull, low-pitched sound. An S_3 gallop is considered a normal finding in children and young adults. In adults older than 30 years of age, an S_3 is considered characteristic of left ventricular dysfunction.[2, 7]

Clinical conditions associated with an S_3 gallop are those that precipitate heart failure, such as myocardial infarction and valvular incompetence. Third heart sounds arising in the left ventricle are best heard at the apex, with the client on the left side. Right ventricular gallops are best detected along the left sternal border, with the client supine.

A *fourth heart sound,* or *S_4 gallop,* occurs in the later stage of diastole, during atrial contraction and active filling of the ventricles. This soft, low-pitched sound is heard immediately before S_1 and is also referred to as an atrial gallop. An atrial gallop is found most commonly in disorders involving increased stiffness of the ventricle, such as ventricular hypertrophy, ischemia, and fibrosis. These conditions are often associated with elevated diastolic ventricular pressures and a vigorous atrial contraction. The ventricles become resistant to filling, and the structures within the ventricles vibrate in response to the added blood input during the "atrial kick."

The presence of S_4 may result from myocardial infarction (transient S_4), hypertension, hypertrophy, fibrosis, cardiomyopathy, cor pulmonale, aortic stenosis, or pulmonic stenosis. S_4 is never heard in the absence of atrial contraction (i.e., atrial fibrillation). S_4 is heard best with the bell of the stethoscope at the apex, with the client in the supine, left lateral position.[2, 7]

QUADRUPLE RHYTHM

At times a quadruple rhythm is noted when both S_3 and S_4 are audible. Clients with this unusual heart sound often have tachycardia, which causes the diastolic filling sounds to fuse, forming a *summation gallop* that may be louder than S_1 or S_2. It can be heard best at the apex and resembles the sound of a galloping horse.

CLICKS

Clicks are extracardiac sounds that can be heard any time during the cardiac cycle in clients with aortic stenosis, valve prolapse, or prosthetic valves. There are three basic types of clicks[2, 7]:

1. *Click.* A *simple click* occurs during systole and is usually caused by a prolapsed mitral valve.
2. *Ejection sound.* An *ejection click* is a high-pitched sound heard in systole. It can be associated with either opening of the semilunar valves or prolapse (inversion) of the mitral valve. Ejection clicks heard during early systole usually result from sudden tensing of the aortic or pulmonic root at the peak of systolic ejection. They are often the result of high ventricular pressure generated in order to open a rigid, calcified aortic valve. Middle to late systolic clicks are more likely to be due to a benign form of mitral insufficiency (regurgitation). When a billowing mitral valve allows prolapse of the leaflets into the left atrium, a click can be heard as the chordae tendineae act as a tether and prohibit further leaflet excursion into the atria.
3. *Opening snap.* Valves normally open silently, but when they become calcified or rigid from disease,

greater pressure is required to force them open. When they do "pop" open, they produce a characteristic sound. Opening snaps occur with the opening of a stenotic mitral and (rarely) tricuspid valve. The resulting sound is brief, high-pitched, and of a snapping quality. It is heard early in diastole at the apex using a diaphragm.

PERICARDIAL FRICTION RUB

A pericardial friction rub is produced by inflammation of the pericardial sac (pericarditis). The roughened parietal and visceral layers of the pericardium rub against each other during cardiac motion. The sound has three components corresponding to cardiac activity: ventricular systole, ventricular diastole, and atrial systole.

A pericardial friction rub is best detected with the diaphragm at the apex and along the left sternal border. It may be accentuated when a person leans forward or lies prone and exhales. Friction rubs produce a sound that is described as "to and fro," scratchy, grating, rasping, and much like "squeaky leather." Friction rubs may be present during the first week after myocardial infarction or after open heart surgery. Differentiate a pericardial friction rub from a pleural friction rub by noting the timing of the rub in relation to breathing. Pleural friction rubs are heard during inspiration. Pericardial friction rubs are heard throughout the respiratory cycle.

MURMURS

Murmurs are heard as a consequence of turbulent blood flow through the heart and large vessels. Turbulent blood flow produces vibrations in the heart and great vessels that can be detected as a blowing or swooshing sound. Murmurs are caused by (1) increased rate or velocity of blood flow, (2) abnormal forward or backward flow across stenosed or incompetent valves, (3) flow into a dilated chamber, or (4) flow through an abnormal passage between heart chambers. Bruits are due to turbulence in vessels. Murmurs are best heard with the bell of the stethoscope when the client is in the left lateral recumbent position. Table 54–4 describes the characteristics of murmurs. Box 54–4 gives the scale for grading the loudness of murmurs.

Systolic murmurs, also called "benign" murmurs, are often caused by vigorous myocardial contraction or strong blood flow. They are common in children, adults younger than 50 years of age, and pregnant women. All diastolic murmurs are pathologic and are produced by mitral and tricuspid valve stenosis or aortic or pulmonic insufficiency.[2, 7, 12, 29, 38] Table 54–5 presents a comparison of selected heart murmurs.

Lungs

Because the cardiovascular and respiratory systems are intimately related, assessment of the cardiovascular system must include evaluation of the respiratory system. The respiratory assessment is covered in Chapter 59. Common respiratory findings related to CVD are as follows.

TACHYPNEA

Tachypnea, or rapid respirations, is often associated with pain and anxiety accompanying myocardial ischemic pain. Tachypnea is also a common compensatory mechanism in heart failure and pulmonary edema.

TABLE 54-4	CHARACTERISTICS OF MURMURS
Characteristic	**Description**
Location	Area where the murmur is best heard
Pitch	Classified as either high or low; describe quality as musical, harsh, blowing, or buzzing
Timing	Refers to whether the murmur occurs in systole or diastole. Systolic murmurs, unlike diastolic murmurs, are harmless
Place and duration	When the murmur occurs during the cardiac cycle: early, middle, or late. Holosystolic or pansystolic murmurs are heard during the entire systolic phase. An ejection murmur is best heard during midsystole
Loudness	Graded on a six-point scale from I (barely audible) to VI (audible without stethoscope)
Quality	A murmur's sound pattern. A *crescendo* starts low and grows louder; a *decrescendo* starts loud and gets softer; a *crescendo-decrescendo* starts softly, becomes loud, and then becomes soft again; *a plateau* is a consistent sound
Radiation	Sound migration to other parts of the body; for example, aortic murmurs often radiate to the carotid arteries, and mitral murmurs radiate to the axilla
Variations	Changes that occur with movement or interruption of normal respirations

From Alexander, R. W., et al. (Eds.). (1998). *Hurst's the heart* (9th ed.). New York: McGraw-Hill, and O'Hanlon-Nickols, T. (1997). The adult cardiovascular system. *American Journal of Nursing, 97*(12), 34–40.

CRACKLES

Crackles frequently signal left ventricular failure and usually occur just after the onset of an S_3 gallop. As pulmonary capillary pressure rises because of the backward pressure of left ventricular failure, fluid shifts into the intra-alveolar spaces and crackles can be auscultated. Crackles may also result from atelectasis (incomplete lung expansion) related to limited chest wall excursion during prolonged bed rest, chest splinting from pain, and the effects of sedatives and narcotics. Crackles are high-pitched, noncontinuous sounds. Crackles are best heard at the lung bases (because of gravitational effects on the fluid) during late inspiration.[2]

BLOOD-TINGED SPUTUM

Pink, frothy sputum may indicate acute pulmonary edema. This manifestation accompanies diffuse pulmonary crackles and denotes serious left ventricular failure. Frank hemoptysis may be associated with pulmonary embolus. A cough frequently occurs with hemoptysis.

CHEYNE-STOKES RESPIRATIONS

Cheyne-Stokes respirations are characterized by abnormal periods of deep breathing alternating with periods of apnea. They are a common finding in heart failure, anemia, and brain damage (from anoxic encephalopathy).

BOX 54-4	Grading of Heart Murmurs
Grade I	Faint; heard after listener has "tuned in"
Grade II	Faint murmur heard immediately
Grade III	Moderately loud, with accompanying thrill
Grade IV	Loud
Grade V	Very loud; heard only with the stethoscope
Grade VI	Very loud; heard without the stethoscope

■ ABDOMEN

Examination of the abdomen provides information regarding cardiac competence. Findings, however, are of less value than those of other examinations discussed in this section. Abdominal assessment is described in Chapters 28 and 42.

Inspection and Palpation

Inspection may reveal abdominal distention. Palpation may confirm the presence of *ascites* (fluid accumulation in the peritoneal cavity) and an enlarged liver. Both of these findings indicate liver failure, which can be a sequela (result) of chronic right ventricular failure. In addition, you may elicit a hepatojugular reflex in the client with right ventricular distention.

After assessing for jugular vein distention, apply mild pressure with one hand over the liver for 1 minute. An increase in jugular vein distention during and immediately after liver compression indicates chronically elevated right ventricular pressure.

Auscultation

Auscultation can yield the following clues about cardiovascular function. Decreased bowel tones may accompany potassium (K^+) depletion. Potassium depletion can complicate chronic diuretic use without sufficient potassium replacement. Increased bowel tones, indicative of hypermotility, may result from laxative use or may be a side effect of certain antiarrhythmic agents (such as quinidine). Loud bruits, heard with the bell just over or above the umbilicus, may indicate an aortic obstruction or aortic aneurysm (the latter can be detected by a palpable abdominal pulsation). Bruits heard over the upper midline or toward the back typically arise from renal arterial stenosis.

TABLE 54–5   **HEART MURMURS**

Type of Heart Sound	Origin	Preferred Method of Auscultation
Systolic murmurs Ejection type S_1 S_2	Systolic ejection murmurs are associated with forward blood flow during ventricular contraction across stenotic aortic or pulmonic valves	Use the stethoscope diaphragm. Ejection murmurs are typically of medium pitch and harsh quality and may be associated with early ejection click. Aortic ejection murmurs are best heard over aortic valve and radiate into the neck, down left sternal border, and occasionally to apex. May be accompanied by decreased S_2. Pulmonic ejection murmurs are heard best over pulmonic valve, and radiate toward left shoulder and left neck vessels. May be accompanied by a wide split S_2
Pansystolic regurgitant murmurs S_1 S_2	Pansystolic murmurs occur when blood regurgitates through incompetent mitral and tricuspid valves (AV valves) or ventricular septal defect as pressures rise during systole and blood seeks chambers of lower pressure. Damage to valve leaflets, papillary muscles, and chordae tendineae results in mitral valve insufficiency (blood regurgitates from left ventricle to left atrium) and tricuspid valve insufficiency (blood regurgitates from right ventricle to right atrium). Ventricular septal defect results in blood regurgitation from left ventricle to right ventricle	All regurgitant murmurs are high-pitched, and those of AV valve incompetence have blowing quality. Mitral regurgitant murmurs are heard at apex, radiate into left axilla, and may be accompanied by ejection click and signs of left ventricular failure. Tricuspid regurgitant murmurs are heard loudest over the tricuspid area and radiate into the sternum. Ventricular septal defects are usually loud, harsh, and heard best over left sternal border in fourth, fifth, and sixth intercostal spaces and radiate over the precordium but not the axilla
Early systolic murmurs S_1 S_2	Early systolic (innocent) murmurs are associated with high cardiac outputs, as blood flow velocity is increased across normal semilunar valves. Causes include anemia, tachycardia, thyrotoxicosis, and fever. Murmur disappears with correction of underlying condition. Normal variant in children	These are best heard with bell over base of heart or along lower left sternal border. Are usually no greater than grade II, are of medium pitch, and have blowing quality. Intensity may increase during inspiration with client in left recumbent position or with increased heart rates
Late systolic murmurs S_1 EC S_2	These imply mild mitral regurgitation as mitral valve balloons into left atrium late in ventricular systole	Best heard with diaphragm of stethoscope over apex and are often preceded by mid-systolic or late systolic ejection click
Diastolic murmurs Early diastolic murmur S_1 S_2 S_1	These (decrescendo murmurs) are usually caused by semilunar valve insufficiency, with regurgitation due to valvular deformity or dilation of valvular ring. Are heard immediately after S_2 and then diminish in intensity as pressure in aorta or pulmonary artery falls and ventricles fill	Heard best with diaphragm at base of heart while the client leans forward in deep expiration. Are high-pitched and blowing and radiate down left sternal border, perhaps to apex or down right sternal border. Accompanying signs of heart failure may be present
Diastolic filling rumbles 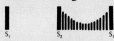 S_1 S_2 S_1	Caused as blood flows across stenotic AV valves (more often mitral). May also occur during augmented blood flow across normal AV valves. Murmur has two phases, becoming louder as the blood flow from the atrium to ventricle increases with passive ventricular filling just after AV valve opening and again during atrial contraction (presystole)	With the bell, this murmur is heard over only a small area at and just medial to the apex. Exercise and a left lateral position of the client increase the intensity of the sound. It is a low-pitched, rumbling sound often accompanied by an augmented S_1 and an opening snap

AV, atrioventricular.
Modified from Huang, S. L., et al. (1989). *Coronary care nursing* (2nd ed., p. 19). Philadelphia: W. B. Saunders; and Alexander, R. W., et al. (Eds.). (1998). *Hurst's the heart* (9th ed.) New York: McGraw-Hill.

DIAGNOSTIC TESTS

The four most common types of diagnostic procedures used in the diagnosis of CVD are:

- Laboratory tests
- Graphic procedures (e.g., ECG)
- Radiographic (x-ray) studies
- Hemodynamic studies

Nursing responsibilities in diagnostic testing include the following:

- Explaining the purpose and the procedure and answering any questions
- Witnessing signing of the consent form
- Scheduling the test
- Providing any necessary preliminary care (e.g., adjustments in medications and special diets)
- Promoting maximal emotional and physical comfort

After the procedure, review instructions for home care, returning to work, and general aftercare.

■ LABORATORY TESTS

Laboratory test data are used to (1) diagnose a variety of cardiovascular ailments (e.g., myocardial infarction), (2) screen people considered at risk for CVD, (3) determine baseline values, (4) identify concurrent disorders (e.g., diabetes mellitus, electrolyte imbalance) that may affect treatment, and (5) evaluate the effectiveness of intervention. Tests that are more commonly used to determine cardiovascular function and disease are discussed here.[31]

Prepare the client for the laboratory test by explaining the procedure. Determine whether the client should fast or refrain from intake of a particular substance before blood is drawn; if so, provide clear instructions. Determination of therapeutic levels of specific medications may require documenting the last time the drug was taken by the client to correlate with the laboratory value. Ask whether the client is taking any blood thinners such as warfarin sodium (Coumadin), which would require a longer time and pressure over the venipuncture site.

Handle blood samples carefully. Gently invert laboratory tubes to prevent clotting of specimens for a complete blood count (CBC). Avoid vigorous handling of specimens, which may lead to hemolysis and falsely elevated levels of intracellular ions, such as potassium and magnesium. Apply pressure to the puncture site until bleeding stops. Assess the site for hematoma formation.

Complete Blood Cell Count

The *red blood cell (RBC) count* or *erythrocyte count* is usually decreased in rheumatic fever and infective endocarditis. The count is usually increased in heart diseases characterized by inadequate tissue oxygenation, for example, right-to-left congenital shunts and heart conditions accompanied by obstructive lung disease.

Measuring the packed cell volume, or *hematocrit*, is the easiest way to ascertain the concentration of red blood cells in the blood. An elevated hematocrit can result from obstructive lung disease and conditions of vascular volume depletion with hemoconcentration (e.g., hypovolemic shock and excessive diuresis). Decreases in hematocrit and hemoglobin indicate anemia, which is commonly caused by hemorrhage, hemolysis (from prosthetic valves), and chronic disease states. Clients with anemia have a significant reduction in red blood cell mass and a decrease in oxygen-carrying capacity. Anemia can be manifest as angina or exacerbate heart failure and produce heart murmurs.

The *white blood cell (WBC) count* is elevated in infectious and inflammatory diseases of the heart (e.g., infective endocarditis and pericarditis). It is also elevated after myocardial infarction because large numbers of WBCs are necessary to dispose of the necrotic tissue resulting from the infarction.

Cardiac Enzymes

Enzymes are special proteins that catalyze chemical reactions in living cells. Cardiac enzymes are present in high concentrations in myocardial tissue. Tissue damage causes release of enzymes from their intracellular storage areas. For example, myocardial infarction causes cellular anoxia, which alters membrane permeability and causes spillage of enzymes into the surrounding tissue. This leakage of enzymes can be detected by rising plasma levels.

Myoglobin is a useful marker of myocardial necrosis that is rapidly released from the circulation within 1 to 2 hours of infarction. Its release allows very early detection, but its short half-life makes it less useful in clients who present several hours after onset. Measurement of myoglobin levels is not recommended if there is evidence of muscle damage, trauma, or renal failure because of the greater potential for false-positive test results in these circumstances.[28]

The enzymes most commonly used to detect myocardial infarction are *creatine kinase* (CK) and *lactic acid dehydrogenase* (LDH). Serum elevations of these two enzymes occur in sequence after myocardial insult. Because these enzymes are also found in other organs and tissues (e.g., skeletal muscle and liver), cardiac specificity must be determined by measuring isoenzyme activity. *Isoenzymes* are various forms of CK and LDH, identified by a process known as electrophoresis.

There are three isoenzymes of CK:

- CK-MM (skeletal muscle)
- CK-MB (myocardial muscle)
- CK-BB (brain)

Elevated CK-MB indicates myocardial damage. Plasma MB is significantly elevated within 6 to 8 hours of the onset of manifestations of myocardial infarction, maximal levels are reached between 14 and 36 hours, and levels return to normal after 48 to 72 hours. Samples should be taken immediately on admission and every 6 to 8 hours for the first 24 hours. Diagnosis of injury requires no fewer than two samples separated by at least 4 hours.

Of the five isoenzymes for LDH (numbered 1 to 5), only LDH_1 and LDH_2 are cardiac-specific. If the serum concentration of LDH_1 is higher than the concentration of LDH_2, the pattern is said to have "flipped," signifying myocardial necrosis. Eighty per cent of clients have elevations in LDH within 48 hours after myocardial infarction.

The use of *troponin* has led to increased specificity in the detection of myocardial infarction. Troponin has three components: I, C, and T. Troponin I modulates the contractile state, troponin C binds calcium, and troponin T binds I and C. Although troponin is present in all striated muscle, troponin components in cardiac muscle have different amino acid sequences. Therefore, antibodies against cardiac troponins I and T are very specific. Elevated levels of troponin I are as sensitive as CK-MB for the detection of myocardial injury. They correlate highly with the development of new areas of regional dysfunction determined by echocardiography and correlate in a linear fashion with the development of complications. Troponins are useful for diagnosis after 4 to 6 hours have elapsed. Once present, troponin I persists for 4 to 7 days.[15, 19, 28]

Because of their higher specificity for myocardial injury, troponins can be used to exclude myocardial infarction when CK-MB may be falsely positive, as in athletes, clients with skeletal trauma, and after direct-current (DC) cardioversion, or when CK totals may be high and MB missed, as in the postoperative state.

As well as indicating myocardial damage, elevations in serum cardiac enzymes can reveal the timing of the acute cardiac event (see Chapter 58).

Blood Coagulation Tests

Blood coagulation tests are used to examine the ability of blood to clot. Evaluate coagulation tests such as *prothrombin time* and *partial thromboplastin time* in people with a greater tendency to form thrombi (e.g., clients with atrial fibrillation, infective endocarditis, or prosthetic valves). Research has shown an increase in coagulation factors during and after a myocardial infarction. Therefore, the client is at greater risk for thrombophlebitis and extension of clots in the coronary artery. Chapter 74 discusses coagulation tests in detail.

Serum Lipids

Serum lipids play a major role in the development of atherosclerosis. They are composed of fatty substances that are insoluble in water. These lipids are derived from fats in the diet or synthesized in the liver. The lipid profile shows serum cholesterol, triglyceride, and lipoprotein levels and is used to assess the risk for development of coronary artery disease. Serum lipids are discussed in Chapter 51.

Serum Electrolytes

Fluid and electrolyte regulation may be affected by cardiovascular disorders. Electrolyte balance is also altered by certain medications. Chapters 12 and 13 describe fluids and electrolytes.

POTASSIUM. The serum potassium level decreases as a result of diuretic therapy, vomiting, diarrhea, and alkalosis. *Hypokalemia* (abnormally low potassium) increases cardiac electrical instability, the occurrence of ventricular dysrhythmias, and the risk of digitalis toxicity. A characteristic change on the ECG is a U wave. A high serum potassium level is usually associated with kidney and endocrine disorders. *Hyperkalemia* can lead to a tall T wave on the ECG, asystole, and ventricular dysrhythmias.

SODIUM. The serum sodium level reflects water balance and may decrease (i.e., *hyponatremia*, indicating water excess) with heart failure, stress, excessive intravenous (IV) infusion of hypotonic fluids, and vomiting. Extensive use of diuretics and severely restricted sodium intake also lower serum sodium.

CALCIUM. The serum calcium level decreases as a result of multiple transfusions of citrated blood, renal failure, alkalosis, and laxative and antacid abuse (phosphate excess). *Hypocalcemia* can lead to serious ventricular dysrhythmias, a prolonged QT interval, and cardiac arrest. *Hypercalcemia* occurs with thiazide diuretic use, acidosis, adrenal insufficiency, immobility, and vitamin D excess. Hypercalcemia shortens the QT interval and causes AV block, tachycardia, bradycardia, digitalis hypersensitivity, and cardiac arrest.

MAGNESIUM. Magnesium helps regulate intracellular metabolism, activates essential enzymes, and aids in the transport of sodium and potassium across the cell membrane. It plays a vital role in neuromuscular excitability.

Hypomagnesemia may result from prolonged use of diuretics, malnutrition, chronic alcoholism, severe diarrhea, and dehydration. Manifestations include mental apathy, facial tics, leg cramps, respiratory depression, and severe cardiac dysrhythmias, including ventricular tachycardia and fibrillation. *Hypermagnesemia* may develop in the client with chronic renal failure. Manifestations include profound muscle weakness, hyporeflexia, hypotension, and bradycardia with a prolonged PR interval and wide QRS complex.

PHOSPHORUS. Most extracellular phosphorus is present in the bone with calcium (85% of the body's total phosphorus). A small amount of phosphorus is found in intracellular fluid. There it helps regulate energy formation (adenosine triphosphate [ATP]) and maintain acid-base balance and neuromuscular excitability. Phosphate levels are inversely related to calcium levels as the kidneys retain or excrete one or the other. Interpret the two levels together.

Hypophosphatemia may result from hyperparathyroidism, diabetic ketoacidosis, prolonged use of IV dextrose infusions, or renal tubular acidosis. Manifestations of hypophosphatemia include bleeding, decreased WBC levels, muscular weakness (including respiratory muscles), and nausea and vomiting.

Hyperphosphatemia usually occurs in clients with chronic renal failure or skeletal disease (including healing fractures) and those undergoing chemotherapy. Manifestations are similar to those of hypocalcemia, with muscle tetany being the most common finding.

Blood Urea Nitrogen

Blood urea nitrogen (BUN) is an indicator of renal function, specifically the ability of the kidney to excrete urea and protein. It is elevated in kidney diseases, during water and saline depletion, and cardiac disorders that adversely affect renal circulation, for example, heart failure and cardiogenic shock.

Blood Glucose

Diabetes mellitus is a major risk factor for the development of atherosclerosis. In addition, the stress of an acute cardiac event can greatly elevate blood glucose, causing unstable *hyperglycemia* in clients with latent diabetes mellitus. For these reasons, blood glucose is routinely assessed in all clients with acute cardiovascular disorders.

■ ELECTROCARDIOGRAM

PROCEDURE

The ECG is an essential tool in evaluating the heart rhythm. Electrocardiography detects and amplifies the very small electrical potential changes between different points on the surface of the body as the myocardial cells depolarize and repolarize, causing the heart to contract. The same electrical impulses spread outward from the heart to the skin, where they can be detected by electrodes attached to the skin. The ECG displays the electrical action of the heart.

There are several types of ECGs: continuous monitoring, 12-lead, signal-averaged, and Holter monitored ECGs. Analysis of ECG waveforms allows identification of disorders of cardiac rate, rhythm, or conduction.

Electrocardiography is a common noninvasive test. It is performed for clients older than 40 years of age before surgery to detect any unknown heart disease and is frequently used for clients with known or suspected heart disease.

PREPROCEDURE CARE

Prepare the client for a 12-lead ECG or continuous monitoring. Explain that the test helps evaluate the heart's function by recording its electrical activity. The steps required for ECG monitoring are (1) attaching the electrodes to the client's skin, (2) connecting the electrodes to the monitor by a cable, and (3) adjusting the monitor to obtain a readable ECG. During the procedure, advise the client to lie still, breathe normally, and refrain from talking. Record the client's age, height, and weight, and note any cardiac medications being taken.[2]

POSTPROCEDURE CARE

After the procedure, disconnect the equipment. If using conductive gel, wipe the gel from the client's skin. If using conductive stickers, remove them unless serial ECG readings are to be done. If serial ECGs are ordered, leave the stickers in place to ensure consistent lead placement.

CONTINUOUS ELECTROCARDIOGRAM MONITORING

For the client who is undergoing continuous ECG monitoring, adjust the monitor by setting the alarms for desired high and low rates. Reassure the client that the equipment does not cause electrical shock or hurt. Clients receiving telemetry are monitored continuously with radiofrequency waves rather than by direct cable attachment. They can get up and move about their rooms or walk in the halls while their heart rhythm is monitored.

Attaching the Electrodes

Electrodes detect electrical impulses from the heart on the skin. Unless the signal is detected accurately, ECG monitoring has little value. The most common electrodes are disc-type or floating electrodes, which are separated from the skin by a spacer filled with conductive gel. The gel improves the signal by reducing local electrical interference on the skin. An adhesive ring surrounds the gel. Peel the paper backing off the pad and apply the electrode to the skin. Three electrodes are required for continuous ECG monitoring. Two of these detect the heart's activity; the third is an electrical ground.

Attach the electrodes to the lead wires before applying them to the chest wall. This process makes it unnecessary to apply pressure to the electrode, which could hurt the client and squeeze the gel outward, reducing contact.

Thorough skin preparation improves impulse conduction. Clean the areas where electrodes are to be applied. Wipe the skin with alcohol, and allow it to air-dry before applying the electrodes. If the client has a great deal of chest hair, clip the hair to improve contact.

Position the electrodes on the chest wall by selecting locations that will provide the clearest ECG waveforms. Two common positions are (1) the conventional position and (2) the modified chest lead position (Fig. 54–6). The lead II waveform (shown) is the most common rhythm strip lead. MCL$_1$ (shown), V$_1$, and V$_6$ are more helpful for detecting dysrhythmia. When close monitoring of ST

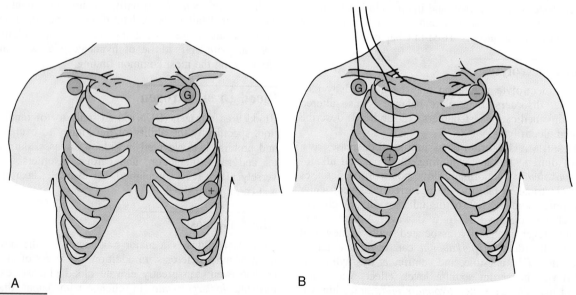

A   B

FIGURE 54–6 Common positions for continuous monitoring lead placement. Use lead II *(A)* or lead V$_1$ *(B)*. (From Phillips, R. E., & Feeney M. K. [1990]. *The cardiac rhythms. A systematic approach to interpretation* [3rd ed.]. Philadelphia: W. B. Saunders.).

1 second

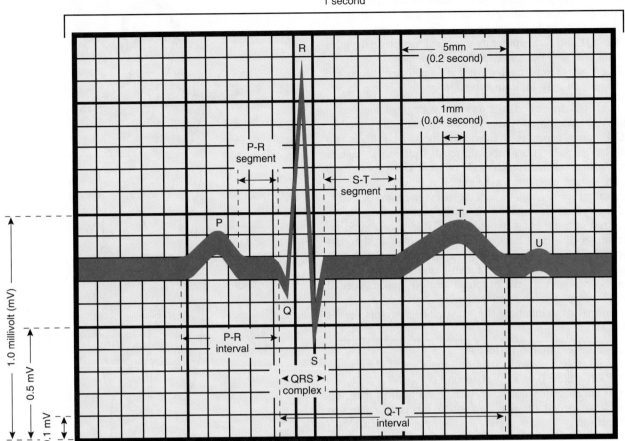

FIGURE 54–7 Normal electrocardiographic (ECG) pattern. The P wave represents depolarization of the atria to the ventricles. The QRS complex represents depolarization of the ventricles, and the T wave represents repolarization of the ventricles. The small U wave is sometimes seen following the T wave. Time and voltage lines of ECG paper: *vertically,* 1 mm = 0.1 mV; 5 mm = 0.5 mV; 10 mm = 1.0 mV; *horizontally,* one small box = 0.04 second; five small boxes = 0.20 second; 25 small boxes = 1 second.

segments is essential, such as after cardiac bypass surgery, thrombolytic therapy, or coronary angioplasty, the lead most closely associated with the area of involved heart muscle should be monitored. Change electrodes if the tracing is unclear, the electrodes become dry, or skin contact is lost. Electrodes should be routinely changed every 48 hours to avoid skin irritation and to ensure that electrode gel is sufficient for clear conduction.

Connecting the Monitor
The electrodes are connected to the monitor by lead wires, which are 12 to 18 inches long. One end snaps onto the electrode, and the other end is attached to a cable that is connected to the monitor. The cable has a receptacle for the attachment of each wire. The receptacle and lead wires are color coded to facilitate connection.

Adjusting the Monitor
The ECG pattern should be clear and distinct. If the pattern is not clear, recheck the first steps. Monitor adjustments depend on the brand of monitor in use. Refer to the operating instructions for assistance.

Setting the Alarms
Set alarm limits appropriately to signal any acute changes. Many monitors have default alarm settings. Verify these for each client. If there are no default settings or institutional standards, alarm limits should be set approxi-

mately 20 beats above and below the client's typical heart rate.

At times, false alarms may occur because of poor electrode contact or client movement. Occasionally, you may find that the alarm limits have been set far apart (e.g., 40 to 180 beats per minute [BPM]) or, worse, that the alarms have been turned off completely. This practice defeats the purpose of the alarm system and should never be adopted.

ELECTROCARDIOGRAM TRACINGS
When continuous ECG monitoring is used, assess the heart rhythm hourly. Log rhythm strips into the medical record routinely as well as when dysrhythmias are noted. Dysrhythmias are discussed in Chapter 57.

The impulse waves, recorded by the ECG machine on graph paper, are arbitrarily designated by the letters P, Q, R, S, and T. The QRS letters are generally referred to as the QRS complex. Figure 54–7 depicts the typical ECG pattern formed by these waves.

The components of the ECG are defined as follows:

- The P wave represents depolarization of the atria.
- The PR interval represents the time it takes for the impulse to spread from the atria to the ventricles.
- The QRS complex represents depolarization of the ventricles.

- The T wave represents repolarization of the ventricles.
- The ST segment indicates that ventricular depolarization is complete and repolarization is about to begin.
- The QT interval represents electrical systole and varies with age, sex, heart rate, and medications.
- The U wave is a small wave that sometimes follows the T wave. It may indicate hypokalemia.

An ECG tracing also shows the voltage of the waves and the duration of both the waves and the intervals. ECG graph paper is divided into horizontal lines and vertical lines, large squares and small squares. Voltage is represented on the vertical axis of the ECG paper. Each small square is 1 mm in height. Five small squares are equivalent to 5 mm, which is equivalent to 0.5 mV. Voltage yields information about the presence and degree of atrial or ventricular hypertrophy. Time is measured on the horizontal axis. Each small square signifies the passage of 0.04 second. Each large square indicates the passage of 0.20 second. By studying the duration of the waves and intervals, the examiner can diagnose abnormal impulse formation and conduction.

Normal time durations for waves and intervals are as follows:

- *P wave:* less than 0.11 second
- *PR interval:* 0.12 to 0.20 second (average, 0.16 second)
- *QRS complex:* 0.04 to 0.11 second
- *QT interval:* in women, up to 0.43 second; in men, up to 0.42 second (normal duration is inversely related to heart rate)

Because of its normal variation in configuration, more must be said about the QRS complex. The Q wave is always the first downward (negative) deflection of the complex. The R wave is always the first upward (positive) deflection. If there is a negative deflection (below the baseline) after an R wave, it is labeled an S wave. In most instances, a Q wave is not obvious on the ECG of the normal heart. The QRS complex may appear as a mostly positive or mostly negative deflection, depending on the recording electrode used.

ELECTROCARDIOGRAM VARIATIONS

The 12-Lead Electrocardiogram

Indications for a 12-lead ECG are listed in Box 54–5.

The standard ECG has a 12-lead system, offering 12 points of reference for recording the electrical activity of the heart. The 12-lead ECG can be conceptualized as 12

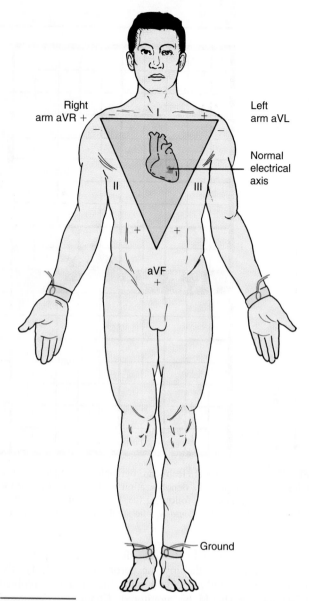

FIGURE 54–8 Standard positions for electrocardiogram leads. Bipolar limb leads are I, II, and III (Einthoven's triangle). Augmented unipolar limb leads: aVR (right arm), aVL (left arm), and aVF (left leg).

BOX 54–5	Indications for a 12-Lead Electrocardiogram

Dysrhythmias
Chest pain
Myocardial infarction
Heart rate determination
Chamber dilation or hypertrophy
Preoperative assessment
Pericarditis
Effect of medications (especially cardiac)
Effect of systemic disease on the heart (i.e., renal or pulmonary disease)
Effect of electrolyte disturbances (especially potassium)

---

different views of the heart, looking in both horizontal and vertical planes. The standard 12-lead ECG has six *limb* leads (used to view the heart in a frontal or vertical plane) and six *precordial* leads (used to view the heart in a horizontal plane).

The limb leads are composed of three *bipolar* leads (leads I, II, and III) and three *unipolar* leads (leads aVR, aVL, and aVF). The bipolar leads have two electrodes and measure the difference in electrical potential flowing through the heart between two extremities. The unipolar leads compare the electrical potential of a positive electrode, placed on one limb, and a negative pole within a central terminal that averages the potential of the other two limb leads.

Standard bipolar limb leads are called I, II, and III (Fig. 54–8):

- *Lead I* measures the difference in electrical potential between the left arm and right arm.
- *Lead II* measures the difference in potential between the left leg and right arm.
- *Lead III* measures the difference in potential between the left leg and left arm.

Augmented unipolar limb leads are as follows (see Fig. 54–8):

- aVR measures electrical potential between the center of the heart and the right arm.
- aVL measures electrical potential between the center of the heart and the left arm.
- aVF measures electrical potential between the center of the heart and the left leg.

The precordial leads (V_1, V_2, V_3, V_4, V_5, and V_6) provide six views of the heart from the anterior and left lateral vantage points. These unipolar leads compare the electrical potential between a positive electrode (in the six different chest locations) and a central, negative terminal that represents an average potential of the three standard limb leads (Fig. 54–9).

Together, the 12 leads permit multidirectional examination of the electrical events in the heart. The location of pathologic change within the heart, which alters electrical activity, can be pinpointed. Table 54–6 correlates the area of infarct with expected ECG changes and coronary artery lesion location. Views from the different leads are oriented to various surfaces of the myocardium:

- Leads I, aVL, V_5, and V_6 record electrical events occurring on the lateral surface of the left ventricle.
- Leads II, III, and aVF record electrical events occurring on the inferior surface of the left ventricle.
- Leads V_1 and V_2 record electrical events occurring on the surface of the right ventricle and anterior surface of the left ventricle.
- Leads V_3 and V_4 record electrical events occurring within the septal region of the left ventricle.

The placement of 12-lead electrodes is shown in Figures 54–8 and 54–9. Unbroken contact must be made

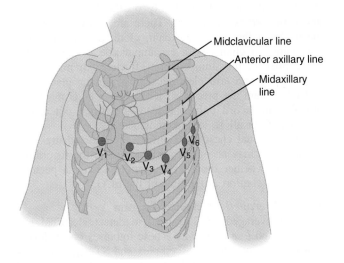

A

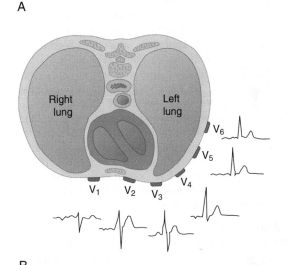

B

FIGURE 54–9 Placement of the chest (V) leads. *A*, Precordial (chest) lead placement. *B*, Normal electrocardiographic findings with corresponding chest leads to cross-section at the fourth rib level.

TABLE 54–6	CORONARY ARTERY LESION LOCATION, AREA OF INFARCT, AND ELECTROCARDIOGRAPHIC (ECG) CHANGES		
Coronary Artery	Area of Infarct	ECG Leads	Dysrhythmias
LAD	Anterior	V_{2-4}	RBBB, LAH, Mobitz type II, CHB
	Septal	V_{1-2}	
	Anteroseptal	V_{1-4}	
Circumflex	Lateral	I, aVL	Ventricular and possibly SA and AV node conduction disturbances
	Anterolateral	I, aVL, V_{5-6}	
	Inferolateral	aVF, II, III, V_{5-6}	
	Posterior	Reciprocal, V_{1-3}	
RCA	Inferior	II, III, aVF	SA node, AV node, and His bundle conduction disturbances
	Right ventricle	II, III, aVF, V_{4-6R}	

AV, atrioventricular, CHB, complete heart block; LAD, left anterior descending, LAH, left anterior hemiblock; RBBB, right bundle branch block; RCA, right coronary artery; SA, sinoatrial.

From Alspach, J. G. (Ed.) (1992). *Instructor's resource manual for the AACN core curriculum for critical care nursing*. Philadelphia: W. B. Saunders.

between the skin and the electrodes. To facilitate contact, the electrodes are placed firmly on the flat surface just above the wrists and ankles. There are many varieties of electrodes: adhesive back, foam, cloth, plastic, and suction cups. In clients with an amputation, the electrodes are applied to the stump of the affected extremity. Note that the leg and arm electrodes must remain attached in order to obtain the precordial leads. Some ECG machines are able to record only one lead at a time; others can record 3, 6, or all 12 leads simultaneously.

Note unusual chest deformities, respiratory distress, or tremors that may account for alterations in the recording. Also note whether the client experiences angina pectoris or chest discomfort at the time of the ECG.

Signal-Averaged Electrocardiogram

A signal-averaged ECG is used to detect electrical impulses called *late potentials*. These impulses occur during diastole late into the QRS complex and ST segment. This noninvasive test may be done at the bedside and is used to determine whether the client is susceptible to ventricular tachycardia that could result in sudden death. For a signal-averaged ECG, a computer is used to record and process low-level signals that are not detected by a traditional ECG. This technique allows detection of signals that might otherwise be masked by noise that conceals the small electrical events of the heart. Late potentials are multiphasic, low-amplitude, high-frequency spikes that appear after the terminal portion of the QRS complex and extend into the ST segment. They are thought to be generated by delayed activation in an abnormal area of the heart. The presence of late potentials in clients with normal sinus rhythm indicates a risk of ventricular tachycardia and sudden cardiac death.[2]

Holter Monitoring

When the client wears a portable Holter monitor, an ECG tracing may be recorded continuously for a day or longer on an outpatient basis, whereas a standard ECG is obtained in a relatively short time. Thus, Holter monitoring is used to detect dysrhythmias that may not appear on a routine ECG but occur when the client is ambulating at home or work. Holter monitoring is also useful in evaluating the effectiveness of antiarrhythmic or pacemaker therapy.[2] The monitoring system records at preset time intervals and when it senses an unusual event.

To prepare the client, place two to three electrodes on the chest and attach them to the telemetry unit. This unit is not much larger than a beeper and is worn in a sling about the chest or waist. Encourage the client to go about the usual daily activities and keep a written account of these activities along with any manifestations that develop. These data are used to document transient dysrhythmias and correlate the client's perceived symptoms with the underlying rhythm.

EXERCISE ELECTROCARDIOGRAM (STRESS TESTING)
PROCEDURE
Exercise testing defines the body's reaction to measured increases in acute exercise. Changes in heart rate, BP, respirations, and perceived level of exertion provide data for quantitative estimation of cardiovascular conditioning and function. The exercise testing may be used in con-

junction with myocardial radionuclide testing. Regardless of the technique used, the optimal exercise testing protocol lasts 6 to 12 minutes and is adjusted to the type of client being tested. The advantages of the exercise test are that it is easily performed, relatively inexpensive, and completely noninvasive.

Exercise testing may consist of single or multiple stages. A single-stage test is one in which the exercise workload is constant throughout. Multiple-stage testing involves increasing the exercise workload in increments until a desired point is reached. The incremental increases in workload may occur every 1 to 5 minutes. The duration of testing varies with the type of test being used and the client's tolerance.

There are two major modes of exercise used for stress testing:

1. *Bicycle ergometry* involves a device equipped with a wheel operated by pedals that can be adjusted to increase the resistance to pedaling (multistage testing). It can be used for arm cranking, foot pedaling, or both. Advantages are that this mode of exercise is relatively inexpensive and the equipment is portable. However, frequent recalibration is required and localized muscle group fatigue is often induced.
2. *Treadmill testing* is the most common mode of stress testing, especially when used in conjunction with thallium 201 imaging. The treadmill is a motorized device that has an adjustable conveyor belt able to reach speeds of 1 to 10 miles per hour. The conveyor belt can be adjusted from a horizontal position to a 20% gradient, allowing the client to walk or run on slopes of different angles.[2, 11]

PREPROCEDURE CARE
Before stress testing, inform the client of the purposes and risks of exercise testing and obtain a signed consent. Instruct the client not to eat or smoke for 2 to 3 hours before the test and to dress appropriately for exercise. No strenuous physical efforts should be made for at least 12 hours before testing. Most clients are allowed to take their usual medications; the physician orders otherwise.

Brief history-taking and physical examination are performed. Obtain a baseline resting ECG immediately before testing. A standing ECG and BP should be recorded to determine vasoregulatory abnormalities, particularly ST-segment depression. Prepare the skin for electrode placement as previously described. Secure electrodes to the chest with tape or a belt. Drape lead wires, cable, and BP cuff to allow maximal freedom of movement. See the Client Education Guide for further client instructions. During the exercise test, the client's BP (taken with an automatically inflating cuff) and ECG are closely monitored by a physician or appropriately trained person.

During the procedure, perform the following:

- Obtain baseline BP, heart rate, and rhythm strip.
- Observe the ECG monitor constantly for changes.
- Record the client's BP, heart rate, rhythm strip, and activity level and time at specified intervals.
- Monitor the client for chest pain, dysrhythmias, ST-segment changes, unexpected changes in BP, or other cardiac manifestations (extreme dyspnea, claudication, vertigo).

CLIENT EDUCATION GUIDE

Stress Testing

- Get sufficient rest the night before the test.
- Avoid eating a heavy meal just before the test, although it is advisable to eat a light meal 1 to 2 hours before the test.
- Avoid smoking, alcohol, and beverages containing caffeine during the day of testing.
- Wear nonconstrictive, comfortable clothing and rubber-soled, supportive shoes during testing. Only a loose-fitting, front-buttoning shirt (or blouse) should be worn. (Women should wear a brassiere.)
- Continue all usual medications unless specified otherwise by the physician. (An inquiry about this should be made to the physician.)
- After the test, rest and keep the physician informed of any lingering manifestations of cardiovascular distress (i.e., chest pain, shortness of breath, or dizziness).
- Avoid taking a hot shower for 1 to 2 hours after the test because it may potentiate hypotension, resulting in a fainting episode. If bathing is desired, use only tepid water.

A multilead monitoring system is most often used to provide maximal views of the heart wall. The examiner makes frequent observations throughout testing for untoward manifestations related to impaired cardiovascular performance. These include chest pain, ventricular dysrhythmia, extreme dyspnea, claudication (leg pain), vertigo, and a sudden drop in BP. Reasons for terminating the test are as follows:

1. Chest pain or fatigue
2. Greatly increased heart rate (age-related):
   a. 20 to 29 years: 170 BPM
   b. 30 to 39 years: 160 BPM
   c. 40 to 49 years: 150 BPM
   d. 50 to 59 years: 140 BPM
   e. 60 to 69 years: 130 BPM
3. Untoward manifestations of myocardial ischemia or heart failure
4. Failure of systolic BP to rise or a drop in BP (below resting levels)
5. Sudden development of bradycardia
6. Serious cardiac dysrhythmia
7. Severe hypertension
8. Severe dyspnea
9. ST-segment depression (greater than 2 to 4 mm)
10. Sudden loss of coordination (cerebral ischemia)

Because these manifestations occur with some frequency, an emergency cart containing cardiac drugs and resuscitation equipment is kept close at hand at all times. Clients rarely die because of this procedure, but some may need assistance with resuscitation from dysrhythmias.

A positive exercise test is one that must be terminated before the predicted maximal (or submaximal) limits have been achieved because of manifestations of cardiovascular intolerance. Generally, the earlier these manifestations appear, the more serious the disease. Alterations in the ST segment and T wave on the ECG during exercise and recovery are often considered diagnostic of coronary ar-

tery disease because these alterations reflect an imbalance between myocardial oxygen demand and supply. There is, however, controversy about what extent of ST-segment change constitutes an abnormal response to exercise. The most widely held position is that the stress test is positive when the configuration and magnitude of the ST segment fulfill any of the following criteria:

- A 1-mm flat (horizontal) ST-segment depression lasting for 0.08 second
- A 1-mm downsloping ST-segment depression lasting for 0.08 second (this has the highest predictive value)
- A 1.5- to 2.0-mm upsloping ST-segment depression lasting for 0.08 second (this characteristic alone does not constitute a positive response)

Although the exercise test is helpful as an adjunct diagnostic study for coronary artery disease, it can produce false-positive findings in some cases, especially in women. In some people, ST-segment alterations may occur during exercise even though coronary artery disease is not present. Hyperventilation, certain drugs, and electrolyte imbalances can produce false-positive readings. For this reason, a diagnosis cannot be based on exercise findings alone.

False-negative findings also occur, although with less frequency. Medications such as beta-blocking agents and nitrates can produce false-negative results. Another limitation of the study is that it is absolutely contraindicated for clients with various cardiovascular and noncardiac conditions. See Box 54–6 for contraindications to exercise testing.

Become familiar with the stress testing procedure to provide clear teaching guidelines to clients scheduled for exercise testing. Many clients have misconceptions and unnecessary fears. Although not painful, the procedure can produce great fatigue. Warn the client that this test

---

BOX 54–6   Contraindications to Exercise Testing

Acute Cardiovascular Disease

Acute myocardial infarction (usually avoided in clients less than 2 weeks after infarction)

Unstable angina pectoris
Heart failure
Pericarditis
Myocarditis
Endocarditis
Life-threatening dysrhythmias
Thrombophlebitis
Recent systemic embolism
Dissecting or enlarging aneurysm

Others

Severe diseases restricting mobility
Renal failure
Severe pulmonary disruptions
Orthopedic disorders affecting the spine or lower extremities
Neurologic impairment (e.g., stroke or paralysis)
Systemic infection
Left ventricular outflow obstruction (aortic stenosis, hypertension, or hypertrophic cardiomyopathy)

may trigger chest pain and dyspnea. Along with this warning, explain that the procedure is performed in a controlled environment under close nursing and medical attention. It is essential that the client arrive for the exercise testing appointment relaxed and well rested. Teaching guidelines for stress testing appear in the Client Education Guide.

POSTPROCEDURE CARE

After the procedure, assist the client to a chair, cart, or bed for recovery. Periodically monitor the client's BP, heart rate, and rhythm strip for a least 15 minutes after test completion or until the ECG returns to baseline.

■ ELECTROPHYSIOLOGIC STUDIES

The electrophysiologic study is an invasive method of recording intracardiac electrical activity. It is used to (1) shed light on the mechanisms of dysrhythmias, (2) differentiate between supraventricular and ventricular dysrhythmias, (3) evaluate sinoatrial (SA) or AV node dysfunction, (4) determine the need for a pacemaker, and (5) evaluate the effect of antiarrhythmic agents used to prevent the occurrence of tachycardias.

An electrophysiologic catheter has four electrodes at the distal tip that record or stimulate (pace). Under fluoroscopy, the catheter is threaded into the heart via the femoral, basilic, or subclavian vein. The catheter sites selected depend on the purpose of the examination. One catheter is placed at the bundle of His just beneath the AV node as a point of reference. An additional catheter is introduced high in the right atrium. If Wolff-Parkinson-White syndrome is suspected, a catheter may be placed in the coronary sinus. A catheter may also be placed in the right ventricle. During mapping of ventricular tachycardia, a catheter may be introduced into the left ventricle via an artery.

The purpose of the procedure is to reproduce any dysrhythmia so that its origin may be isolated. Ventricular tachycardia is induced by using programmed stimulation to fire an impulse at different times during the cardiac electrical cycle. If dysrhythmia is induced, the client's BP and hemodynamic responses are observed. It is possible to record simultaneously arterial pressure, surface ECGs, and ECGs from intracavitary catheters. The morphology and rate of the induced tachycardia are compared with those of the client's spontaneous ventricular tachycardia. Ventricular tachycardia is often terminated by rapid ventricular decremental pacing. If the tachycardia cannot be stimulated, IV isoproterenol may be infused to simulate stress or exercise, which may produce the tachycardia.

Antiarrhythmic drugs may be administered during the study to evaluate their effect. After the initial antiarrhythmic has been given, induction of ventricular tachycardia is attempted. If ventricular tachycardia is induced, the dosage may be increased or other drugs administered. The electrophysiologic studies are repeated in several days to determine the effectiveness of antiarrhythmic drug therapy.

Frequently, when the irritable focus has been identified (e.g., accessory pathway or bundle of His), ablation (destruction) may be performed. Ablation of the irritable focus may be accomplished by the use of radiofrequency waves, direct current, ethyl alcohol, or cryosurgery. Radiofrequency ablation is the most popular method because its effect may be localized, with less damage to surrounding tissue.

PREPROCEDURE AND POSTPROCEDURE CARE

Preprocedure and postprocedure nursing care of the client undergoing electrophysiologic studies is similar to that of the client undergoing cardiac catheterization. Because these studies attempt, under controlled circumstances, to induce potentially lethal dysrhythmias, it is imperative that emergency drugs, equipment, and a defibrillator be immediately accessible.

■ CARDIAC DIAGNOSTIC IMAGING

X-ray studies, magnetic resonance imaging (MRI), ultrasonography, and radioisotopes are discussed in Chapter 11. Use of these diagnostic tools to evaluate the heart is discussed next. See Chapter 11 for the preprocedure care and postprocedure care for each of these diagnostic examinations.

Chest X-ray Studies

Posteroanterior, lateral, and oblique chest x-ray films help to determine the size, silhouette, and position of the heart. For the acutely ill client, a portable anteroposterior x-ray study is performed at the bedside. Specific pathologic changes of the heart are difficult to determine with x-ray examination, but anatomic changes in the heart and pulmonary sequelae of various cardiac conditions can be seen. Assessed on x-ray film are valvular and pericardial calcifications; pulmonary congestion (from heart failure); pericardial effusion; and placement of central lines, endotracheal tubes, hemodynamic monitoring devices, and intra-aortic balloon catheters.

Magnetic Resonance Imaging

Although MRI is one of the most expensive noninvasive diagnostic options, a variety of information may be obtained in a single image. MRI provides the best information on chamber size, wall motion, valvular function, and great vessel blood flow. MRI is commonly used for examination of the aorta and detection of tumors or masses, cardiomyopathies, and pericardial disease. MRI can show the heart beating and the blood flowing in any direction. All standard quantitative functional indices can be obtained from a MRI study with the exception of transstenotic gradients.

Information obtained from MRI includes the following:

- Normal morphology and structural changes
- Wall thickness, chamber volumes, valve areas, vessel cross-sections, and extent, location, and size of lesions
- Global and regional biventricular function, including ejection fraction, stroke volume, and cardiac output
- Blood flow quantifications within vessels over the cardiac cycle
- Tissue characterization of paracardiac and intracardiac masses, pericardial effusions, and myocardial infarction

Positron Emission Tomography

The positron emission tomographic (PET) scanner is a diagnostic imaging tool that allows visualization of regional physiologic function and biochemical changes that often separate normal from diseased myocardium. Cellular metabolic information is obtained by mapping regional myocardial glucose metabolism. Combining information from the perfusion and metabolism images provides a thorough assessment of regional cardiac viability. For further discussion of PET, see Chapter 11.

The scanning procedure takes about 2 to 3 hours. An IV radiopharmaceutical, [^{13}N]-ammonia, is administered and a 20-minute blood flow image is begun. An IV injection of glucose follows. Localization of glucose in the myocardium takes about 40 minutes. Final uptake of the tracer is proportional to the glucose metabolic activity of myocardial cells and provides an excellent indication of regional tissue viability.

The following are clinical indications for PET scanner use:

- Detection of coronary artery disease
- Assessment of myocardial viability
- Assessment of progression of coronary artery stenosis
- Documentation of collateral coronary circulation
- Differentiation of ischemia from dilated cardiomyopathy

The terms "match" and "mismatch" describe the relationship between the perfusion and metabolism studies. A perfusion study showing poor blood flow and a metabolic study showing decreased glucose uptake of necrotic tissue are described as a *match*. A perfusion study that shows poor blood flow and a metabolic study that shows only stunned viable myocardium that has survived the initial insult are described as a *mismatch*.

Echocardiography

Echocardiography, a noninvasive diagnostic procedure based on the principles of ultrasonography, is used to evaluate structural and functional changes in a wide variety of heart ailments.

An echocardiogram is obtained by placing a transducer on several areas of the chest wall. Bursts of ultrasound waves are directed at the part of the heart under investigation. The echocardiogram records the structure and motion of that area in relation to its distance from the anterior chest wall (Fig. 54–10). An ECG is recorded simultaneously on the graph. Two-dimensional echocardiography generates a continuous picture of the beating

heart. These images are recorded on videotape for analysis.

Echocardiograms are used to help assess and diagnose pericardial effusion, cardiomyopathy, valvular disorders (including prosthetic valves), cardiac shunts, myocardial ischemia, chamber size, left ventricular function, ventricular aneurysms, and cardiac tumors (atrial myxoma). In addition, they are useful during heart biopsies because the physician can view the heart on a monitor while taking tissue samples.

Transesophageal Echocardiography

PROCEDURE

Transesophageal echocardiography (TEE) yields a higher quality picture of the heart than does regular echocardiography. It is especially useful for clients who have thickened lung tissue or thick chest walls or who are obese. The procedure may also be used intraoperatively, where conventional echocardiography is ineffective. Dobutamine stress testing is now being used in combination with TEE to evaluate clients with suspected coronary artery disease and to evaluate left ventricular wall motion.

This combination test involves inserting a flexible endoscope equipped with an ultrasonic transducer tip into the esophagus of a sedated client, administering dobutamine to mimic the effects of exercise (by increasing myocardial oxygen demand through stimulation of beta$_1$ receptors), and recording ultrasonic images of the heart's response. Because the probe is placed behind the heart, it allows the left atrium to be viewed. TEE allows clearer visualization of the heart and its structures and is most useful in diagnosis of cardiac masses, prosthetic valve function, aneurysm, and posterior effusions. The procedure lasts approximately 15 minutes to 1 hour.[1, 2, 14]

PREPROCEDURE CARE

Explain the procedure to the client. Obtain an informed consent. Assure the client that sedation will be used. The client should receive nothing by mouth for 6 to 8 hours before the procedure.

During the procedure, do the following. Administer sedation and topical anesthetic as ordered. If the client has a nasogastric tube in place, remove it before the esophageal scope is inserted. If dobutamine is used, the nurse is responsible for calculating the dose according to

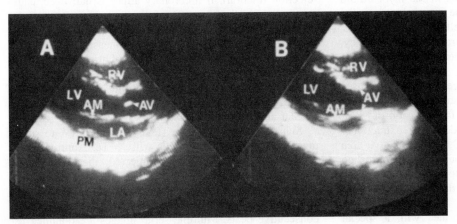

FIGURE 54–10 Long-axis, cross-sectional echocardiographic images of the left ventricle (LV), right ventricle (RV), mitral valve, aortic valve, and left atrium (LA) during diastole *(A)* and systole *(B)*. During diastole, the anterior (AM) and posterior (PM) mitral leaflets are apart and the aortic valve leaflets (AV) come together as a single echo in the midportion of the aorta *(A)*. With systole *(B)* the mitral leaflets come together and the aortic valve leaflets separate. (From Braunwald, E. [1992]. *Heart disease* [4th ed., p. 67]. Philadelphia: W. B. Saunders.)

the client's weight. To imitate the effects of increasing physical activity, the dose is slowly increased from a baseline infusion of 2.5 to 5 μg/kg/min and thereafter increased in increments of 5 to 10 μg/kg/min up to a maximum of 40 μg/kg/min. Each dose is infused for 5 minutes; images are captured during the final 2 minutes of the infusion. Monitor the client's vital signs, ECG, respiratory status, and pulse oximetry throughout the procedure.

POSTPROCEDURE CARE

After the procedure, closely monitor vital signs for 30 minutes and record the ECG every 10 minutes. Keep the client fasting until the gag reflex is fully restored. Instruct the client that there may be mild throat discomfort for a day or two and to report significant discomfort or hemoptysis to the physician immediately. Because of the sedation, advise the client not to drive or operate machinery for 24 hours.

Phonocardiography

Phonograms are recordings of audible vibrations from the heart and great vessels. Phonograms are used to assist in determining the timing of cardiac sounds and murmurs. Microphones are placed under elastic straps, usually at the base and apex of the heart. No preparation is required for this assessment.

Myocardial Scintigraphy

Myocardial function, motion, and perfusion may be studied by a method called scintigraphy, which involves IV injection of a radioactive isotope. As the isotope is absorbed by the blood cells of the heart muscle, photons are emitted. These photons are detected by an external gamma camera, which produces a radionuclide image. Because these nuclear imaging techniques are relatively noninvasive, they are frequently used diagnostic tools.

THALLIUM 201 SCINTIGRAPHY

Thallium 201 is the most widely used isotope for myocardial perfusion because of its short half-life (73 hours) and low total body radiation dose. Thallium 201 is a radioactive analog of potassium that is easily extracted by smooth skeletal and cardiac muscle fibers that have the potassium active transport system. Eighty-eight per cent of blood-borne ^{201}Tl is taken up on its first pass through the heart. The amount of ^{201}Tl found in the myocardium after an IV injection depends on the regional myocardial perfusion and the efficiency of cellular extraction. Regional perfusion is dependent on coronary artery patency. Areas of the myocardium that receive less blood flow also receive less thallium.

A high concentration of ^{201}Tl is present in well-perfused cells, and a lower concentration remains in the blood, setting up a concentration gradient for diffusion of ^{201}Tl. Infarcted or scarred myocardium does not extract any ^{201}Tl and shows up as "cold spots." If the defective area is ischemic, the cold spots fill in or become "warm" on the delayed images. Infarcts continue to appear cold with little or no perfusion of ^{201}Tl either during a stress test or with delayed images.

The perfusion scanning is performed with a special camera that is capable of showing the source of emitted low-energy photons on a screen. Each photon detected by the camera is recorded on film and a computer screen over a half-hour period. The computer refines and enhances the images and then provides quantitative information about the myocardial walls.

Thallium 201 imaging can be performed before or after an exercise ECG study or as a resting study only. Ischemic myocardium may be detected by a resting ^{201}Tl study. Two sets of images are taken 3 hours apart and compared. The ^{201}Tl stress test begins with a graded exercise protocol on a treadmill. The client receives a slow IV infusion of normal saline. The ECG is monitored continuously. About 1 minute before the peak of the stress test, ^{201}Tl is injected intravenously. The client should exercise for the last minute to ensure ^{201}Tl distribution to the heart during 85% maximum stress. The client then cools down and reclines on an examination table for the perfusion scan. Continuous imaging in a 180-degree arc over the chest is performed. The client then waits for 3 hours and returns for repeated films. Before the delayed images are obtained, the client receives additional ^{201}Tl by IV injection. The two sets of images are then carefully compared.

DIPYRIDAMOLE THALLIUM 201 TEST

This test may be used as an alternative to standard treadmill exercise when the client is not able to achieve a vigorous level of exercise. Dipyridamole serves as a pharmacologic stress agent. It is given IV to dilate the coronary arteries, which would normally dilate during the stress of exercise. Arteries that are narrowed as a result of coronary artery disease do not expand as much as normal arteries. Infusion of dipyridamole for 5 minutes is followed by injection of ^{201}Tl. Thallium 201 travels easily through normal arteries that have dilated and travels less freely through narrowed arteries. At 7 minutes, images are taken.

Any form of caffeine as well as medications for asthma, such as theophylline or aminophylline, should be omitted before this test. Aminophylline is an antagonist of dipyridamole and may be given slowly IV to reverse any adverse side effects.

TECHNETIUM 99m VENTRICULOGRAPHY (MULTIPLE GATED ACQUISITION SCANNING)

This test is used to study the motion of the left ventricular wall and measure the ventricle's ability to eject blood (ejection fraction). If a coronary artery is narrowed, causing ischemia, the segment of the myocardium it serves exhibits diminished wall motion or contractility. In addition, hemodynamic changes may be measured by observing the actual filling and emptying of the cardiac chambers. Changes in cardiac output as well as ejection fraction may be obtained. Multiple gated acquisition (MUGA) scans represent the blood pool within the ventricular and atrial chambers.

Stannous pyrophosphate (PYP) is given IV to allow tagging of the red blood cells with ^{99m}Tc. Approximately 20 minutes after the PYP is injected, the ^{99m}Tc is injected. A heart monitor is then attached, and images are begun.

MUGA scans use counts from any one of a number of consecutive beats. Multiple serial images are obtained using a gamma camera. The cardiac cycle is broken into intervals, with counts taken during these intervals for a number of beats. These counts are stored and then displayed in a weighted average picture.

If a stress study is to be performed, the client is put on a bicycle ergometer with a gamma camera positioned to project the right and left blood pools. The ECG is monitored continuously. Images are obtained at rest and during each stage of exercise.

FIRST-PASS CARDIAC STUDY
PROCEDURE
During a first-pass study, a single IV injection of ^{99m}Tc is administered and traced as it passes through the heart. Only the initial pass of the ^{99m}Tc through the cardiac chambers is recorded. Ejection fraction and information about ventricular wall motion are obtained. A first-pass study may be performed during exercise or rest.

PREPROCEDURE CARE
Before the procedure, ask female clients if they are or may be pregnant because these studies involve radiation exposure (although minimal). Explain the purpose of the procedure, and tell the client what to expect during the procedure. Explain that electrodes will be placed on the chest and an IV line will be inserted for administration of the radioisotope. Generally, total exposure to radiation during these scans is less than or equal to that of one chest x-ray study.

Instruct the client to wear walking shoes if exercise on the treadmill or bicycle is anticipated. Follow the diet protocol of the institution. Some tests may require fasting. A light meal is preferred if the scan is to be performed during exercise as it prevents nausea and stomach cramping during exercise and allows better uptake of the radioisotope. Instruct the client to avoid alcohol and smoking on the day of the procedure.

Check the physician's orders for omission of any medications. Usually, beta-blockers, calcium-channel blockers, and xanthines are prohibited before the procedure. Ensure that the client signs a consent form. During the procedure, ask the client to notify the nurse or technologist of any chest pain (ischemia).

POSTPROCEDURE CARE
After the procedure, again ask the client to report any chest pain. If the client must return for follow-up scanning, instruct the client to rest between studies.

Cardiac Catheterization

This complex procedure involves insertion of a catheter into the heart and surrounding vessels to obtain detailed information about the structure and performance of the heart, the valves, and the circulatory system. Specifically, cardiac catheterization is performed to:

- Confirm a diagnosis of heart disease and determine the extent to which the disease has affected the structure and function of the heart
- Determine congenital abnormalities
- Obtain a clear picture of cardiac anatomy before heart surgery
- Obtain pressures within the heart chambers and the great vessels (aorta and pulmonary artery [PA])

- Measure blood oxygen concentration, tension, and saturation within the heart chambers
- Determine cardiac output
- Perform angiography for better coronary artery visualization
- Obtain endocardial biopsy specimens
- Allow infusion of fibrinolytic agents directly into an occluded coronary artery in an attempt to restore coronary blood flow

Cardiac catheterization is usually performed in the controlled environment of a cardiac catheterization laboratory. Typically, only one side of the heart is catheterized, although it is sometimes necessary to insert the catheter into both sides of the heart. See Chapter 11 for discussions of the preprocedure and postprocedure nursing care and possible complications after cardiac catheterization.[1, 2, 39]

RIGHT-SIDED CATHETERIZATION
For right-sided cardiac catheterization, the physician inserts a sterile, radiopaque catheter through the antecubital or femoral vein. Under fluoroscopic guidance, the catheter is advanced slowly to the right atrium and right ventricle and is finally wedged in a small branch of the PA. The ECG is continuously monitored during the procedure. Premature ventricular contractions may occur as the catheter is being passed through the ventricles. The client may experience fluttering sensations or palpitations as the catheter passes through the heart. If they occur frequently, cardiac output falls and the physician may need to withdraw the catheter temporarily or order administration of lidocaine (an antiarrhythmic).

LEFT-SIDED CATHETERIZATION
This procedure is far more difficult to perform than right-sided catheterization. There are two major methods of catheter introduction. (1) The catheter can be passed retrograde (backward) from the brachial or femoral artery into the aorta and then to the left ventricle. (2) Rarely during right-sided catheterization, the middle or lower third of the atrial septum is punctured and the catheter is passed transseptally into the left atrium.

As the catheter is passed through the venous or arterial system and into various heart chambers, the desired studies are performed. The catheter has several end or side holes that allow blood withdrawal for oxygen analysis from the various cardiac chambers. Pressures can be obtained by attaching the catheter to a transducer with its connecting amplifier and recording device. Radiopaque contrast materials and indicator solutions can be injected via the catheter into the left ventricle to examine the mitral valve, the left ventricular outflow tract, wall motion and thickness, left ventricular end-diastolic volume, and ejection fraction.[7] The client may experience pain when contrast material is injected and the dye replaces blood flowing through the arteries. The lack of oxygenated blood causes regional cardiac hypoxia.

Angiography

Angiocardiography involves IV injection of contrast material into the heart during cardiac catheterization. Immediately after the injection, a series of x-ray films are taken that reveal the course of the contrast material as it circulates through the heart, lungs, and great vessels. (See Chapter 11, Fig. 11–7.)

Cineangiography is a technique in which moving pictures are taken during cardiac catheterization. The examiner can view the film at both rapid and slow speeds, permitting detailed and unlimited review of the study.

Coronary angiography involves injection of contrast material directly into the coronary arteries (via the coronary ostia) during cardiac catheterization. Table 54–7 outlines the various forms of angiocardiography. See Chapter 11 for preprocedure and postprocedure nursing care.

■ HEMODYNAMIC STUDIES

Hemodynamic status is assessed with four parameters: CVP, PA pressure, cardiac output, and intra-arterial pressure. Each parameter is obtained through an invasive procedure. Critical care nurses perform all of these studies routinely at the bedside. Hemodynamic studies provide a wealth of information reflecting the earliest changes in the circulatory system that are not yet clinically detectable.

Hemodynamic pressure monitoring provides information about blood volume, fluid balance, and how well the heart is pumping. Current technology allows measurement of right atrial pressure (CVP), PA pressures during systole and diastole (reflecting right and left ventricular pressures), and pulmonary capillary wedge pressure (PCWP) (an indirect indicator of left ventricular pressure).

The Pulmonary Artery Catheter

Development of the balloon-tipped, flow-directed catheter has enabled continuous direct monitoring of PA pressure (see Bridge to Critical Care).

The PA catheter has four lumina. The proximal lumen

terminates in the right atrium, allowing CVP measurement, fluid infusion, and venous access for blood samples. The distal lumen terminates in the PA and measures PA systolic pressure, PA diastolic pressure, PA mean pressure, and PCWP. A small, third lumen is used for inflation and deflation of the balloon. The fourth lumen is the thermistor port and permits measurement of cardiac output. In addition, some catheters have a fifth port for infusion of fluids and capabilities for cardiac pacing and measuring oxygen saturation of the blood.

INSERTING THE CATHETER

Insertion of a PA catheter involves risk for the client. The potential complications are PA infarction, pulmonary embolism, injury to the heart valves, and injury to the myocardium. In addition, while the catheter is in place, the heart valves are unable to close completely.

PA monitoring must be carried out in a critical care unit under careful scrutiny of an experienced nursing staff. Before insertion of the catheter, explain to the client that (1) the procedure may be uncomfortable but not painful, and (2) a local anesthetic will be given at the catheter insertion site. Support of the critically ill client at this time helps promote cooperation and lessen anxiety.

The physician inserts the PA flow-directed catheter at the bedside via percutaneous puncture of the brachial, subclavian, jugular, or femoral vein using sterile technique. The catheter is connected to a transducer and a fluid-filled pressure monitoring system. Pressure levels and fluctuations are monitored both graphically and by numerical display.

The inflated balloon follows the direction of blood flow through the right ventricle into the PA, where it finally wedges in the right or left branch of the PA. Clinicians can follow the path of the balloon by observing waveforms and pressure readings on the monitor (see Bridge to Critical Care).

When wedged, the catheter is "pointing" indirectly at the left end-diastolic pressure. Therefore, PCWP is the most accurate, although indirect, indicator of left ventricular end-diastolic pressure or left ventricular *preload* available at the bedside. The normal PCWP is 8 to 13 mm Hg. Elevations of PCWP (greater than 18 to 20 mm Hg) indicate increased left ventricular pressure, as seen in left ventricular failure, and may coincide with the onset of pulmonary congestion. Pressures climbing to more than 30 mm Hg generally herald the onset of pulmonary edema. Conversely, low PCWP suggests insufficient volume and pressure in the left ventricle, as seen in hypovolemic shock. Pressure changes commonly related to various cardiac conditions are shown in the Bridge to Critical Care.

Central Venous Pressure

Central venous pressure is the pressure within the superior vena cava. It reflects the pressure under which the blood is returned to the superior vena cava and right atrium. CVP is determined by vascular tone, blood volume, and the ability of the right side of the heart to receive and pump blood. When the tricuspid valve is open at the end of diastole, the atrium and ventricle are, in effect, one chamber. At this time, the CVP is equal to the pressure in the right ventricle and indicates right ven-

TABLE 54–7	MAJOR TYPES OF ANGIOCARDIOGRAPHY
Angiocardiography Procedure	**Method Employed**
Right-sided angio-cardiography	Contrast medium is injected into the right heart chambers and pulmonary artery by means of a catheter threaded up a vein and into the heart during cardiac catheterization
Left-sided angiocardiography	Contrast medium is injected into the left side of the heart through a transvenous catheter passed through the atrial septum during cardiac catheterization or via a catheter passed retrograde through an artery into the left heart
Selective coronary artery angiocardiography	Contrast medium is injected directly into the ostium of each coronary artery via a catheter that is placed retrograde through an artery into the aorta

BRIDGE TO CRITICAL CARE

Swan-Ganz Monitoring

Positioning the Swan-Ganz Catheter

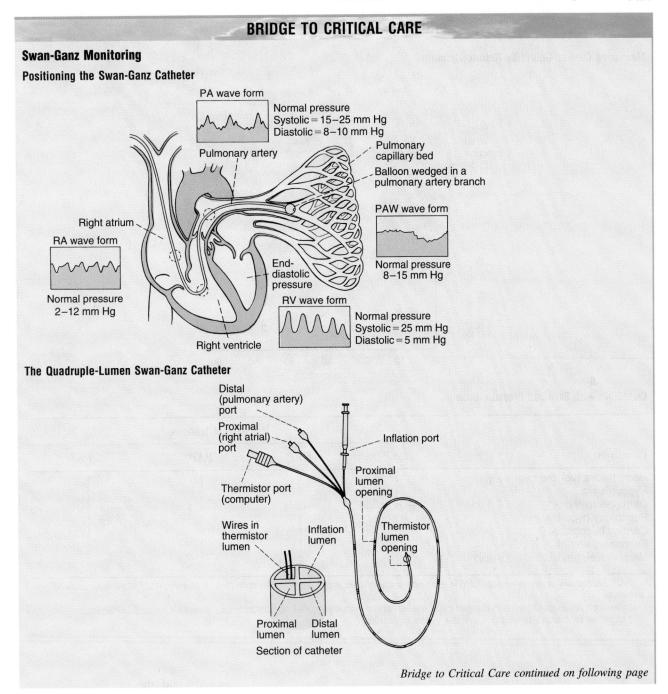

PA wave form

Normal pressure
Systolic = 15–25 mm Hg
Diastolic = 8–10 mm Hg

Pulmonary artery

Pulmonary capillary bed

Balloon wedged in a pulmonary artery branch

PAW wave form

Normal pressure
8–15 mm Hg

Right atrium

RA wave form

Normal pressure
2–12 mm Hg

End-diastolic pressure

RV wave form

Normal pressure
Systolic = 25 mm Hg
Diastolic = 5 mm Hg

Right ventricle

The Quadruple-Lumen Swan-Ganz Catheter

Distal (pulmonary artery) port

Proximal (right atrial) port

Inflation port

Proximal lumen opening

Thermistor port (computer)

Wires in thermistor lumen

Inflation lumen

Thermistor lumen opening

Proximal lumen

Distal lumen

Section of catheter

Bridge to Critical Care continued on following page

tricular function (Table 54–8). CVP can also be seen as a measurement of preload on the right side of the heart. Preload is the amount of blood presented to the heart or when the ventricle is full before the next ejection. Preload is the right ventricular end-diastolic pressure. (Preload is also discussed in Chapter 55.)

CVP can be measured with a central venous line placed in the superior vena cava or a balloon flotation catheter in the PA. Normal CVP pressure is 2 to 12 mm Hg. A drop in CVP pressure indicates a decrease in circulating volume, which may result from fluid imbalance, hemorrhage, or severe vasodilation and pooling of blood in the extremities with limited venous return. A rise in CVP indicates an increase in blood volume be-

cause of a sudden shift in fluid balance, excessive IV fluid infusion, renal failure, or sodium and water retention.

Accurate CVP measurement requires a baseline for the transducer position. The zero point on the transducer needs to be at the level of the right atrium. The right atrium is located at the midaxillary line at the fourth intercostal space when measured while the client is supine with the head of the bed elevated to no more than 45 degrees for the most accurate reading.

During measurement of CVP, the client should be relaxed. Straining, coughing, or any other activity that increases intrathoracic pressure can cause falsely high measurements. When measuring the CVP of a client with a

BRIDGE TO CRITICAL CARE *Continued*

Measuring Cardiac Output by Thermodilution

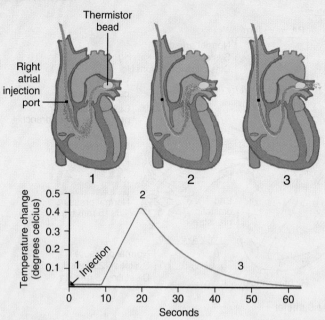

Conditions with Expected Pressure Changes

	Pressure Changes			
Condition	*RAP*	*RVP*	*PAP*	*PAWP*
Heart failure (volume overload)	↑	↑	↑	↑
Hypovolemia	↓	↓	↓	↓
Cardiogenic shock*	—or ↑	—or ↑	—or ↑	—or ↑ (diastolic)
Pulmonary hypertension				—or ↑
Cardiac tamponade	↑	↑	↑	↑ (diastolic)
Pulmonary emboli	↑	↑	↑	↑ (systolic)
Mitral valve stenosis/insufficiency†	↑	↑	↑	↑

PAP, pulmonary artery pressure; PAWP, pulmonary artery wedge pressure; RAP, right atrial pressure; RVP, right ventricular pressure.
*Pressure readings depend on the heart's ability to handle circulating volume. Chronic lung disease elevates all readings.
†Mitral valve disease produces unreliable pressure readings.

TABLE 54–8	INDICATIONS FOR CENTRAL VENOUS PRESSURE (CVP) AND HOW THEY MAY AFFECT THE READINGS	
To Assess	**↑ CVP (>11 cm H$_2$O)**	**↓ CVP (<3 cm H$_2$O)**
Right-sided heart hemodynamics	Right heart failure (including chronic heart failure, LVF) Constrictive pericarditis Cardiac tamponade Valvular stenosis Pulmonary hypertension	Early LVF
Blood volume	↑ Circulating volume	↓ Circulating volume
Vascular tone	Vasoconstriction Hypertension	Vasodilation, peripheral pooling Septic shock

LVF, left ventricular failure.
Modified from Huang, S. H., et al. (1989). *Coronary care nursing* (2nd ed., p. 101). Philadelphia: W. B. Saunders.

ventilator, take the readings at the point of end expiration for greatest accuracy.

Check the connections between the catheter and the attachments frequently to ensure that they are secure (in order to prevent air embolism). Change the dressing at the insertion site according to health care facility policy to prevent infection. In order to maintain patency of the system, a small amount of fluid is delivered under pressure at a constant rate of flow. This fluid may or may not be heparinized. Complications of the procedure include pneumothorax, phlebitis, air emboli, pulmonary emboli, fluid overload, dysrhythmia, sepsis, and microelectric shock.

Pulmonary Artery Pressure

The CVP is unsatisfactory for determining the status of left-sided heart function, especially in critically ill people, for example, those who are immediately recovering from cardiac surgery, have experienced myocardial infarction, have cardiomyopathy, or are in cardiogenic shock. Significant changes can occur in the left side of the heart and not be reflected for some time in the right side of the heart. Failure to detect such changes can lead to delayed or inappropriate intervention.

During diastole, blood flows freely from the PA through the pulmonary capillaries, left atrium, and open mitral valve to the left ventricle. Therefore, the pressure in the left ventricle at the end of diastole approximates the diastolic pressure in the PA, pulmonary capillaries, and left atrium.

Starling's principle indicates that the heart muscle contracts most effectively when under slight stretch. PA pressure measurements can assist in determining whether the ventricle is understretched (in need of fluids), overstretched (in need or diuretics), or appropriately stretched (at maximal function).

Cardiac Output Measurement

As detailed in the anatomy and physiology feature for the cardiac system, cardiac output is the amount of blood pumped out of the left ventricle into the arterial system every minute. That is, cardiac output is equal to the stroke volume (volume of blood pumped out with each beat) multiplied by the heart rate. If the stroke volume of the left ventricle is between 50 and 90 ml (average, 70 ml) and the heart rate is 80 BPM, the normal cardiac output of the left ventricle is approximately 4 to 8 L/min. Table 54–9 lists the conditions that change cardiac output. The cardiac output of the right ventricle is considered equal to that of the left because the right ventricle, although not as muscular as the left ventricle, pumps against less resistance.

Intra-arterial Pressure Monitoring

PROCEDURE

Systemic intra-arterial monitoring is a common method for obtaining BP measurements in the acutely ill client. This method provides continuous detection of arterial BP via an indwelling catheter. It is of greatest benefit for clients whose cuff BP measurements are undetectable or unreliable, such as those with low cardiac output, fluctuating hemodynamic status, and excessive peripheral vaso-

TABLE 54–9	CONDITIONS THAT CAUSE A CHANGE IN CARDIAC OUTPUT
Conditions That Decrease Cardiac Output	Conditions That Increase Cardiac Output
Acute heart failure	Hypoxia
Pericarditis with effusion	Hyperthyroidism
Old age	Excitement
Arterial hemorrhage	Exercise
Standing motionless, which decreases venous return to the heart	Food intake
Myxedema	Oral and intravenous fluid intake
Shock	Early stage of septic shock
Valvular heart disease	Pregnancy
Myocardial ischemia	
Dysrhythmias	
Paroxysmal atrial tachycardia (PAT)	
Atrial fibrillation	
Heart block	
Ventricular tachycardia	
Heat stroke	

constriction. Note that intra-arterial pressure readings are at least 10 mm Hg higher than cuff BP readings. The intra-arterial line simplifies obtaining blood samples for arterial blood gas and blood studies, minimizing the need for arterial or venous punctures. Major complications of intra-arterial monitoring include hemorrhage caused by loose connections of the monitoring system, hematoma at the insertion site, infection (local or systemic), and embolization of the artery that supplies the distal portion of the cannulated extremity.

The physician introduces a short, nonreactive polytetra-fluoroethylene (Teflon) catheter into an artery (radial, brachial, axillary, femoral, or dorsalis pedis) using sterile technique.

PREPROCEDURE CARE

Informed consent is required. Before catheter insertion, the adequacy of circulation in the selected extremity must be assessed. If the radial artery is chosen as the site for insertion, blood flow to the hand is evaluated with an Allen test to determine ulnar artery patency. Allen's test is described in Chapter 59. If ulnar artery obstruction is suspected, cannulation of the radial artery should not be attempted.

Besides accurate monitoring and recording of arterial pressure, nursing responsibilities focus on preventing complications of arterial cannulation. Do the following: Check all connections frequently to ensure that they remain tight and secure. Evaluate the cannulated extremity for neurovascular function every 2 hours. Assess color, temperature, capillary filling, and sensation distal to the site of cannulation. Check the insertion site for redness or signs of infection daily, and change dressing per institutional policy.

POSTPROCEDURE CARE

After removal of the arterial cannula, maintain firm constant pressure for 5 to 15 minutes over the site of the artery to prevent hematoma formation. Secure a pressure dressing over the site for 12 hours. Monitor for infection (increased redness, warmth, tenderness, and induration at the catheter insertion site, elevated temperature) and neurovascular compromise (pain, paresthesia [abnormal touch sensation], decreased pulse quality, pallor, coolness). Report these complications immediately to the physician.

CONCLUSIONS

Cardiovascular assessment can range from taking blood presssure to monitoring hemodynamic parameters. Learning how to perform adult cardiac assessment takes time and perseverance. Abnormal heart sounds are harder to interpret than normal heart sounds; be persistent and practice frequently. Even though invasive diagnostic tests are more prevalent, you need to be able to evaluate accurately the client's history, BP, and physical assessment. These data are just as important as the results of invasive studies if the nurse continues to assess the client effectively, provide primary preventive care, and monitor treatment. Assessment skills and nursing interventions can make a significant difference in the client's quality of life by preventing complications and improving outcomes.

BIBLIOGRAPHY

1. Aiello, S. (1997). Radiologic workup for angina. *American Journal of Nursing, 97*(12), 50.
2. Alexander, R. W., et al. (Eds.). (1998). *Hurst's the heart* (9th ed.). New York: McGraw-Hill.
3. American Heart Association. (1998). *Heart and stroke: Statistical update*. Dallas: Author.
4. American Heart Association. (1998). *HeartStyle*. Dallas: Author.
5. Arnold, E. (1997). The stress connection: Women and coronary artery disease. *Critical Care Nursing Clinics of North America, 9*(4), 565–575.
6. Carney, R. M., et al. (1998). New CAD risk factors: How useful? *Patient Care, 32*(11), 134–165.
7. Cheitlin, M., et al. (1998). The art of auscultation. *Patient Care, 32*(23), 35–48.
8. Colbath, J. D. (1997). Holistic health options for women. *Critical Care Nursing Clinics of North America, 9*(4), 589–599.
9. Cox, M. H., & DiNubile, N. A. (1997). Exercise for coronary artery disease: A cornerstone of comprehensive treatment. *Physician and Sportsmedicine, 25*(12), 27–35.
10. Eckel, R. H., & Krauss, R. M. (1998). American Heart Association call to action: Obesity is a major risk factor for coronary heart disease. *Circulation, 97*(21), 2099–2100.
11. Ellestad, M. H. (1997). Is the standard exercise ECG test obsolete? *Internal Medicine, 18*(11), 33–45.
12. Epstein, O., et al. (1997). *Clinical examination* (2nd ed.). Philadelphia: Mosby–Year Book.
13. Evanoski, C. A. M. (1997). Myocardial infarction: The number one killer of women. *Critical Care Nursing Clinics of North America, 9*(4), 489–496.
14. Frizzell, J. (1997). Transesophageal echocardiography. *American Journal of Nursing, 97*(9), 17–18.
15. Gasperetti, C. M. (1997). Recent development in the rapid diagnosis of acute chest pain syndromes. *Veterans Health System Journal, 2*(5), 51–55.
16. Glisson, J., et al. (1999). Review, critique, and guidelines for the use of herbs and homeopathy. *Nurse Practitioner, 24*(4), 44–67.
17. Hahn, R. A., et al. (1998). Cardiovascular risk factors and preventive practices among adults—United States, 1994: A behavioral risk factor atlas. *Morbidity and Mortality Weekly Report, 47*(SS–5), 35–69.
18. Halm, M. A., & Penque, S. (1999). Heart disease in women. *American Journal of Nursing, 99*(4), 26–31.
19. Hamm, C., et al. (1997). Emergency room triage of patients with acute chest pain by means of rapid testing for cardiac troponin T or troponin I. *New England Journal of Medicine, 337*(23), 1648–1688.
20. Hill, B., & Geraci, S. A. (1998). A diagnostic approach to chest pain based on history and ancillary evaluation. *Nurse Practitioner, 23*(4), 20–45.
21. Immunization Action Coalition. (August 1999). *Summary of recommendations for adult immunization*. St. Paul, MN: Author.
22. Jadin, R. L., & Margolis, K. (1998). Coronary artery disease in women: How customary expectations can interfere with interpretation of test results. *PostGraduate Medicine, 103*(3), 71–84.
23. JNC VI guidelines: Hypertension treatment shifts to total CV risk. (1997). American Heart Association 70th scientific sessions. *Geriatrics, 52*(12), 52–58.
24. Laurienzo, J. M. (1997). Detection of coronary artery disease in women. *Critical Care Nursing Clinics of North America, 9*(4), 469–475.
25. Meyer, N. (1999). Using physiologic and pharmacologic stress testing in the evaluation of coronary artery disease. *Nurse Practitioner, 24*(4), 70–82.
26. Miller, D. B. (1997). Secondary prevention for ischemic heart disease: Relative numbers needed to treat with different therapies. *Archives of Internal Medicine, 157*(18), 2045–2052.
26a. Miracle, V. A., & Sims, J. M. (1999). Making sense of the 12-lead ECG. *Nursing, 29*(7), 34–39.
27. Montes, P. (1997). Managing outpatient cardiac catheterization. *American Journal of Nursing, 97*(8), 34–37.
28. Murphy, M. J., & Berding, C. B. (1999). Use of measurements of myoglobin and cardiac troponins in the diagnosis of acute myocardial infarction. *Critical Care Nurse, 19*(1), 58–66.
29. Norman, E. M. (1997). Combining dobutamine stress testing and TEE. *American Journal of Nursing, 97*(7), 16HH and 16MM.
30. O'Hanlon-Nickols, T. (1997). The adult cardiovascular system. *American Journal of Nursing, 97*(12), 34–40.
31. Pagana, J. D., & Pagana, T. J. (1998). *Mosbys manual of diagnostic and laboratory tests*. St. Louis: Mosby.
32. Paul, S. (1997). Arrhythmias in women. *Critical Care Nursing Clinics of North America, 9*(4), 545–553.
33. Pennington, J. C., Tecce, M. A., & Segal, B. L. (1997). Heart protection: Controlling risk factors for cardiovascular disease. *Geriatrics, 52*(12), 40–50.
34. Penque, S., et al. (1998). Women and coronary artery disease: Relationship between descriptors of signs and symptoms and diagnostic and treatment course. *American Journal of Critical Care, 7*(3), 175–182.
35. Pinkowish, M. D. (1998). New CAD risk factors: Interesting, but how useful? *Patient Care, 32*(11), 134–165.
36. Seller, R. H. (1996). *Differential diagnosis of common complaints* (3rd ed.). Philadelphia: W. B. Saunders.
36a. Siomka, A. J. (2000). Demystifying cardiac markers. *American Journal of Nursing, 100*(1), 36–40.
37. Svetkey, L. P., et al. (1999). Effects of dietary patterns on blood pressure: Subgroup analysis of the Dietary Approaches to Stop Hypertension (DASH) randomized clinical trial. *Archives of Internal Medicine, 159*(3), 285–293.
38. Swartz, M. H. (1998). *Textbook of physical diagnosis: History and physical* (3rd ed.). Philadelphia: W. B. Saunders.
39. Tremko, L. A. (1997). Understanding diagnostic cardiac catheterization. *American Journal of Nursing, 97*(2), 16K–16R.
40. Trends in ischemic heart disease death rates for black and whites—United States, 1981–1995. (1998). *Morbidity and Mortality Weekly Report, 47*(44), 945–949.
41. Wingate, S. (1997). Cardiovascular anatomy and physiology in the female. *Critical Care Nursing Clinics of North America, 9*(4), 447–452.
42. Youngkin, E. Q., & Israel, D. S. (1996). A review and critique of common herbal alterative therapies. *Nurse Practitioner, 21*(10), 39–62.

CHAPTER 55

Management of Clients with Structural Cardiac Disorders

Barbara B. Ott

NURSING OUTCOMES CLASSIFICATION (NOC)
for Nursing Diagnoses—Clients with Structural Cardiac Disorders

Activity Intolerance	**Impaired Gas Exchange**	Neurological Status: Consciousness
Activity Tolerance	Respiratory Status: Ventilation	Tissue Perfusion: Cerebral
Endurance	Tissue Perfusion: Pulmonary	**Risk for Ineffective Airway Clearance**
Energy Conservation	Vital Signs Status	Aspiration Control
Altered Nutrition: Less Than Body	**Impaired Physical Mobility**	Respiratory Status: Airway Patency
Requirements	Ambulation: Walking	Respiratory Status: Ventilation
Nutritional Status: Food and Fluid	Joint Movement: Active	**Risk for Ineffective Management of**
Intake	Mobility Level	**Therapeutic Regimen: Individuals**
Decreased Cardiac Output	**Pain**	Compliance Behavior
Cardiac Pump Effectiveness	Comfort Level	Participation: Health Care Decisions
Circulation Status	Pain Control	**Risk for Infection**
Tissue Perfusion: Abdominal Organs	Pain: Disruptive Effects	Immune Status
Tissue Perfusion: Peripheral	**Risk for Altered Tissue Perfusion:**	Tissue Integrity: Skin and Mucous
Vital Signs Status	**Cerebral**	Membranes

Adequate tissue perfusion is essential to good health. Many disorders of the heart can cause inadequate tissue perfusion. Specifically, disorders that affect the structure of the heart may decrease the heart's pumping ability and thus may result in inadequate tissue perfusion.

INFECTIOUS DISORDERS

Bacteria and other microbes are found in abundance in our environment. The heart can become infected by these microbes, a process that prompts an inflammatory response. Involvement of the heart can be lethal during the acute stage or lead to structural damage.

RHEUMATIC FEVER

Rheumatic fever is a diffuse inflammatory disease. It is a delayed response to an infection by group A beta-hemolytic streptococci. Although this infection remains common, the incidence of rheumatic fever has declined dramatically to about 2 per 100,000 people in the United States. This decline is due to an emphasis on prevention. The incidence in developing countries is about 100 per 100,000 people.[7]

Etiology and Risk Factors

Rheumatic fever develops in only a relatively small percentage of people (3%), even after a virulent bout of streptococcal infection; there is, therefore, some evidence of host predisposition. Genetic links are less advanced and less widely performed than for other diseases such as cancer.[13] Once rheumatic fever is acquired, the person becomes more susceptible than the general population to recurrent infection. Poor hygiene, crowding, and poverty are risk factors for acute rheumatic fever. If appropriate antibiotic therapy for group A beta-hemolytic streptococcal infection is given within the first 9 days, rheumatic fever can usually be prevented.[7]

Prevention is the best treatment. The most effective measures against rheumatic fever are probably socioeconomic. In the affluent neighborhoods of Western cities, where there is spacious housing with no crowding, the incidence of rheumatic fever is low. Identification of high-risk persons is also important. Nurses can help to identify mitral valve prolapse (see later) early to prevent valvular disease. Nurses in community settings can identify those with beta-hemolytic streptococcal infections and refer clients for appropriate diagnosis and medical management.

Pathophysiology

Rheumatic fever initiates a diffuse, proliferative, and exudative inflammatory process. In rheumatic fever, the heart, joints, subcutaneous tissue, central nervous system (CNS), and skin are affected. Although the cellular disease process is not clear, the mechanism is probably an abnormal humoral and cell-mediated response to streptococcal cell membrane antigens. These antigens bind to receptors on the heart, other tissues, and joints, which begins the autoimmune response. The inflammatory process often produces permanent and severe heart damage.

Rheumatic fever produces *carditis* (inflammation of the heart). Carditis affects the pericardium, epicardium, myocardium, and endocardium. There may be Aschoff's bodies, minuscule nodules with localized fibrin deposits surrounded by areas of necrosis in the myocardium, which are due to the inflammation of rheumatic fever. Endocardial inflammation causes swelling of the valve leaflets, which leads to valve dysfunction and murmurs. Small bacterial vegetations form on the valve tissues. Rough eroded areas of the valves attract platelets, which adhere and form platelet-fibrin clumps that eventually cause scarring and shortening of the valve. The valves lose their elasticity, and cardiac function is impaired.

First, the damaged valve may become stenosed. This increases the cardiac workload, because higher pressure must be generated to propel blood through the narrow valve. Second, the valve leaflets may become so short that they cannot close securely. As a result, blood regurgitates (leaks backward) through the damaged valve into the chamber from which it was ejected. Both valvular stenosis and regurgitation eventually cause heart failure from the high workload (Table 55–1).

Complications of rheumatic fever include valvular disorders, cardiomegaly, and heart failure. These complications may be fatal.

Clinical Manifestations

The clinical manifestations of rheumatic fever are related to the inflammatory response and include fever, weakness, malaise, weight loss, anorexia, arthritis, carditis, subcutaneous nodules, erythema marginatum, chorea, abdominal pain.

Fever, with a temperature of 38° C (100.4° F) or higher, alternates with normal temperature. Weakness, malaise, weight loss, and anorexia probably develop as a result of fever, pain, and the general debilitation associated with serious illness.

Arthritis, a prominent finding, is painful and migratory. It most often affects the larger joints, such as the ankles, knees, elbows, shoulders, and wrists. The arthritis may or may not be symmetrical. If the client takes aspirin early in the course of the disease, arthritis manifestations may not be as apparent. Joint manifestations may last hours or days.

Carditis, one of the most common manifestations of rheumatic fever, is the most destructive consequence of this disease. Characteristics include a significant murmur, cardiomegaly, pericarditis that produces a significant friction rub, and heart failure. Chest pain due to pericardial inflammation may be present. Sometimes there is myocardial involvement that produces atrioventricular (AV) conduction defects or atrial fibrillation.

Subcutaneous nodules are small, painless, firm nodules that adhere loosely to the tendon sheaths, especially in knees, knuckles, and elbows. They are usually evident

TABLE 55–1	EFFECTS OF RHEUMATIC FEVER ON THE MYOCARDIUM, ENDOCARDIUM, AND PERICARDIUM		
Condition	**Characteristic Lesion**	**Cause of Lesion**	**Significance of Pathophysiologic Involvement**
Rheumatic myocarditis	Aschoff's bodies (minute nodules in connective tissue around small arteries in myocardium)	Formed by leukocytes that mass in inflamed tissues	Nodules may eventually become fibrotic. Damage from fibrosis may eventually damage arteries in myocardium. Myocarditis may cause temporary loss in contractile power of heart. Permanent damage rarely results.
Rheumatic endocarditis	Tiny vegetations resembling little beads form along line of closure of valve leaflets (primarily mitral and aortic valves)	Probably result from inflammation, ulceration, and erosion of valve leaflets	Progressive fibrosis, scarring, and calcification of valve leaflets result in valvular incompetence and stenosis
Pericarditis	Nonspecific lesions	Result from diffuse, nonspecific fibrinous or serofibrinous inflammatory reaction	May cause pericardial friction rub; usually no serious sequelae.

only during the first week or so and, generally, only in children.

Erythema marginatum is an unusual rash seen primarily on the trunk. The lesions are crescent-shaped and have clear centers. The rash is transitory and may change in appearance in minutes or hours.

Chorea, a CNS disorder, is manifested by sudden, irregular, aimless, involuntary movements. Chorea disappears without treatment and produces no permanent sequelae.

Abdominal pain, a common clinical manifestation, varies in site and severity. The pain may be related to engorgement of the liver.

No single diagnostic feature identifies rheumatic fever. Many of the common clinical manifestations are associated with other disorders as well as rheumatic fever. The Jones criteria were developed to assist in diagnosis (Box 55–1). The clinical manifestations of rheumatic fever may last 3 months.

A positive throat culture for group A beta-hemolytic streptococci can help to confirm the diagnosis. An elevated white blood cell (WBC) count, erythrocyte sedimentation rate (ESR), and C-reactive protein may indicate inflammation.

Outcome Management

▰ Medical Management

The goals of medical management include (1) eradicating infection, (2) maximizing cardiac output, and (3) promoting comfort.

> **BOX 55–1** **Guidelines for the Diagnosis of Initial Attack of Rheumatic Fever (Jones Criteria)***
>
> **Major Manifestations**
>
> 1. Carditis
> 2. Polyarthritis
> 3. Chorea
> 4. Erythema marginatum
> 5. Subcutaneous nodules
>
> **Minor Manifestations**
>
> 1. Clinical findings
>   a. Arthralgia
>   b. Fever
> 2. Laboratory findings
>   a. Elevated acute phase reactants
>   (1) Erythrocyte sedimentation rate
>   (2) C-reactive protein
>   b. Prolonged P-R interval
>
> **Supporting Evidence of Antecedent Group A Streptococcal Infection**
>
> 1. Positive throat culture or rapid streptococcal antigen test
> 2. Elevated or rising streptococcal antibody titer
>
> *If supported by evidence of preceding group A streptococcal infection, the presence of two major manifestations, or of one major and two minor manifestations, a high probability of acute rheumatic fever is indicated.
> Modified from Diagnosis of Rheumatic Fever—Special Writing Group (1992). *Journal of the American Medical Association, 268*(15), 2069–2073.

ERADICATE INFECTION

The first priority is to eradicate the streptococcal infection. Usually this can be accomplished with oral administration of penicillin. For penicillin-allergic clients, the physician usually prescribes erythromycin.

The client typically takes prophylactic agents for rheumatic fever for 5 years after the initial attack. After 5 years, recurrences are rare. Clients who have had rheumatic fever remain vulnerable to bacterial endocarditis. Therefore, in addition to the antibiotics they take to prevent rheumatic fever recurrence, they must be referred for evaluation for possible prophylactic medications before and after any surgical procedure or dental work. Specific evaluation for prophylaxis medication must be individualized according to recommendations by the American Heart Association.[6]

Careful monitoring for side effects of multiple cardiac drugs that may be prescribed for clients with valvular disease is essential.

MAXIMIZE CARDIAC OUTPUT

Corticosteroids are used to treat carditis, especially if heart failure is evident. If heart failure develops, treatment, including cardiac glycosides and diuretics, is effective.

PROMOTE COMFORT

Clients with arthritic manifestations obtain clinical relief with salicylates; however, because these drugs can result in a misdiagnosis, a firm diagnosis should be in place before administration of salicylates. Bed rest is usually prescribed to reduce cardiac effort until evidence of inflammation has subsided. For clients with rheumatic valvular heart disease, bacterial endocarditis prophylaxis may be necessary (see Infective Endocarditis).

▰ Nursing Management of the Medical Client

ASSESSMENT

Nursing assessment involves gathering baseline and ongoing subjective and objective data. Assess vital signs to reveal the presence of fever, tachycardia, and stability of blood pressure. Vital signs are also used as a measure of activity tolerance. Auscultate heart sounds for presence of a friction rub, and palpate peripheral pulses. A baseline electrocardiogram (ECG) is documented. Assess baseline nutritional and hydration data.

Assess psychosocial data on the client's feelings regarding restrictions of activity, support systems, coping strategies, level of discomfort, and knowledge (the client's and family's) concerning the nature of, and intervention for, rheumatic fever.

DIAGNOSIS, OUTCOMES, INTERVENTIONS

Activity Intolerance. A reduced cardiac reserve and enforced bed rest can quickly lead to activity intolerance. The nursing diagnosis statement would be *Activity Intolerance related to reduced cardiac reserve and enforced bed rest.*

Outcomes. The client will progress toward an optimal level of physical activity tolerance, based on underlying cardiovascular status and psychosocial readiness, as evidenced by ability to (1) pace activity, (2) verbalize improvement in fatigue, (3) express acceptance of any imposed activity restrictions, and (4) steadily increase activity level to include climbing one flight of stairs without chest pain or without ECG changes, while the heart rate remains under 90 BPM (beats per minute).

Interventions. Bed rest is important in the acute phase, because it reduces myocardial oxygen demand, and usually continues until the following criteria are met:

- Temperature remains normal without use of salicylates
- Resting pulse remains under 100 BPM
- ECG tracings show no signs of myocardial damage
- ESR returns to normal
- Pericardial friction rub is not present

Once ambulatory, the client must still be careful not to overdo. Assess the client's stamina and response to exercise to gauge the degree of gradual activity progression. Assess vital signs before and after exercise. After 3 to 5 minutes of rest, reassess vital signs. The client should reduce or discontinue activity if chest pain, vertigo, dyspnea, confusion, a drop in blood pressure, or an irregular pulse develops. The length of activity restriction depends on whether carditis develops and the extent of permanent heart damage. Restrictions may extend for months. In severe cases of rheumatic carditis, clients may be forced to undergo restrictions on a permanent basis. Encourage a gradual increase in activity within the limits of the client's condition.

The client experiencing chorea requires sedatives, bed rest, and protection from self-injury. A carefully planned and supervised activity schedule should be maintained and evaluated.

Pain. The inflammatory response in the joints can lead to pain. The nursing diagnosis statement would be *Pain related to the inflammatory response in the joints.*

Outcomes. The client will experience increased comfort, as evidenced by (1) reports of restful sleep and reduced discomfort, (2) expression of joint pain relief, (3) reduced use of pain medications, and (4) a relaxed body posture and calm facial expression.

Interventions. Obtain a clear description of the pain or discomfort. Identify the source of greatest discomfort as a focus for intervention. Administer analgesics as needed. Balance rest and activity according to the degree of pain and activity tolerance. Other pain interventions are discussed in Chapter 23.

Altered Nutrition: Less Than Body Requirements. Hypermetabolism seen with fever and inflammation and other factors in rheumatic fever can lead to protein calorie malnutrition. This diagnosis is stated as *Altered nutrition: Less Than Body Requirements, related to fever, inflammation, anorexia, and fatigue.*

Outcomes. The client will maintain or restore adequate nutritional balance, as evidenced by (1) resumption of body weight before the illness or no further weight loss, (2) consumption of 75% or more of each meal served, (3) normal serum albumin or prealbumin, and (4) a positive nitrogen balance.

Interventions. A high-protein, high-carbohydrate diet helps maintain adequate nutrition in the presence of fever and infection. Hypermetabolic states (fever and infection) can induce a catabolic state, thus delaying healing. Vitamin and mineral supplements may also benefit the client. Oral hygiene every 4 hours, small attractive meal serv-ings, and foods that are not overly rich, sweet, or greasy stimulate the appetite. Adequate fluid intake prevents dehydration resulting from fever. If the client shows signs of severe carditis or heart failure, sodium and fluids must be restricted. Daily weights can serve as an indication of nutritional and fluid status.

Risk for Ineffective Management of Therapeutic Regimen (Individuals). Following rheumatic fever, the client must follow a lifelong regimen to reduce risk of rheumatic heart disease. This diagnosis is stated as *Risk for Ineffective Management of Therapeutic Regimen (Individuals) related to a need for lifelong therapy.*

Outcomes. The client and family will demonstrate adequate knowledge of rheumatic fever and its cause, course, and therapy, as evidenced by the ability to accurately describe the causes and process of rheumatic fever, its clinical manifestations, its prevention, and the rationale for prescribed interventions.

Interventions. Today, streptococcal infections do not have to develop into rheumatic fever if the client seeks immediate assessment and begins antibiotics. Clients who have recovered from an episode of rheumatic fever may avoid subsequent attacks by taking prophylactic doses of antibiotics and observing good health practices. Because repeated attacks may lead to serious heart disease and permanent cardiac disability, it is important to emphasize means of avoiding subsequent attacks.

Instruct the client how to reduce exposure to streptococcal infection as follows:

1. Take good care of teeth and gums, and obtain prompt dental care for cavities and gingivitis. Prophylactic medication may be needed before invasive dental procedures, and individualized evaluation for prophylaxis medication is needed.[6]
2. Avoid people who have an upper respiratory infection or who have had a recent streptococcal infection.
3. Notify the physician if any of the manifestations of streptococcal sore throat (pharyngitis) develop. It is extremely important to begin antibiotic therapy promptly for any infection. The clinical manifestations include fever (102° to 104° F), chills, sore throat, and enlarged, painful lymph nodes. Advise clients who have had rheumatic fever that they must guard against infections for the rest of their lives to avoid development of heart disease.

EVALUATION

Rheumatic fever is treated over 10 days. Expect activity tolerance to improve once fever and pain are controlled. Altered nutrition may require more than 2 weeks to show improvement, depending on the severity of anorexia and the fever.

INFECTIVE ENDOCARDITIS

Endocarditis is an inflammatory process of the endocardium, especially the valves. This disorder was once lethal, but morbidity and mortality have been greatly reduced with the use of antibiotics and advanced diagnostic procedures.

In the past, many different terms and classifications were used to describe infective endocarditis. You may still see these terms used or find them in old medical records. Some are defined here.

- *Subacute bacterial endocarditis* (SBE): develops gradually over several weeks or months; usually caused by organisms of low virulence, such as *Streptococcus viridans,* which has a limited ability to infect other tissues
- *Acute bacterial endocarditis:* develops over days or weeks with an erratic course and earlier development of complications; commonly caused by *Staphylococcus aureus,* which is capable of infecting other body tissues
- *Native valve endocarditis:* an infection of a previously normal or damaged valve
- *Prosthetic valve endocarditis:* an infection of a prosthetic valve
- *Nonbacterial thrombotic endocarditis:* caused by sterile thrombotic lesions (often aggregates of platelets), which may develop in people with cancer or other chronic diseases

Changes in the population at risk are altering the classic picture of endocarditis. The incidence is continuing to rise. Each year, about 15,000 to 20,000 new cases are appearing. Infective endocarditis is now the fourth leading cause of life-threatening infectious disease syndromes.[3] The median age of clients has increased from 30 to 40 years in the early antibiotic era to 47 to 64 years in recent decades.[12] Fewer clients are being seen with the classic physical signs of advanced endocarditis, such as Osler's nodes, finger clubbing, or Roth's spots (see Clinical Manifestations). The proportion of cases due to streptococci has fallen slightly. The proportion of cases caused by gram-negative bacilli, fungi, and other unusual microbes is increasing.

The changes are traced to several notable alterations in the population. The increased incidence of endocarditis caused by yeasts and fungi is attributable to the increased number of persons with valve prostheses, to the increased number of persons using intravenous (IV) drugs, and rising use of long-term antimicrobial therapy or immunosuppression.

The decreased incidence of rheumatic fever results in a lower incidence of endocarditis, whereas the number of children surviving congenital heart disease results in an increased incidence. The growing elderly population also leads to an increase in the number of endocarditis episodes.

Etiology and Risk Factors

Common infecting organisms include staphylococci (*S. aureus, S. faecalis, S. epidermidis*), streptococci, *Escherichia coli,* gram-negative organisms (*Klebsiella, Pseudomonas, Serratia marcescens*) and fungi (*Candida, Aspergillus*). These organisms enter the body through the oral cavity after dental procedures, mouth or tooth abscesses, oral irrigations, or oral irritations from dental floss or bridgework. The upper respiratory tract is another port of entry following surgery, intubations, or infections. Direct exposure of the bloodstream to organisms can occur with prolonged IV catheters, hemodialysis catheters, and IV drug use. Procedures involving the gastrointestinal and genitourinary tracts (e.g., barium enemas, sigmoidoscopy, colonoscopy, percutaneous liver biopsy, catheterization, urethrotomy, prostatectomy, cystoscopy) have been associated with infective endocarditis.

Reproductive conditions have also been linked (e.g., delivery of a newborn, abortion, intrauterine devices, pelvic inflammatory diseases). Defective heart valves causing changes in blood flow and pressures encourage the proliferation of vegetations. Open heart surgery to replace damaged valves increases the risk of endocarditis. Fortunately, coronary artery bypass grafting (CABG), one of the most frequently performed surgical procedures in the United States, carries a low risk of infective endocarditis because the endocardium is not invaded during the operation.

Circulating microorganisms in the bloodstream attach to the endocardial surface and multiply. Usually the multiplication of these organisms requires a rough or abnormal endocardium. IV drug abusers may be injecting particulate matter into the bloodstream, with damage to the previously normal endocardium that allows the organism to adhere, thereby initiating acute bacterial endocarditis.

Pathophysiology

Microorganisms enter the bloodstream in many ways. Once the colonization process begins on the endothelium, replication occurs and bacterial colonies form within layers of platelets and fibrin. As the colonies become entangled within the tight layers of fibrin and platelets, the colony becomes less and less vulnerable to the body's defense mechanisms. The bacteria stimulate the humoral immune system to produce nonspecific antibodies, but the bacteria are protected by the fibrin-platelet aggregation. It is not uncommon for these vegetations to form clots that travel to other organs, forming abscesses. The vegetations can severely damage heart valves by perforating and deforming the valve leaflets (Fig. 55–1). Extensions of the

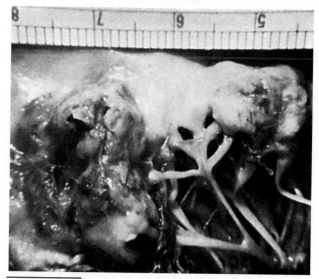

FIGURE 55–1 Vegetations of the heart valves resulting from infective endocarditis. Large vegetations were present on the leaflets of the mitral valve. (From Braunwald, E. [1992]. *Heart disease: A textbook of cardiovascular medicine* [4th ed.] Philadelphia: W. B. Saunders.)

bacteria may invade the aorta or pericardium. The amount of damage depends on the type and virulence of the organisms causing the infection.

There are many possible complications. Heart failure may develop as a result of structural valvular damage. Arterial emboli can occur from the vegetation. Systemic embolization occurs in 30% of clients with left-sided infective endocarditis. Common infarction sites are the kidney, spleen, and brain. Pulmonary embolus is associated with right-sided infective endocarditis. Emboli can also travel to the brain and produce myriad manifestations. Occasionally, immune complex glomerulonephritis will develop. Renal function usually returns to normal after the infection has been controlled.

Clinical Manifestations

Clinical manifestations of infective endocarditis include those related to the infectious process, embolization, and the immune response.

Clinical manifestations related to the infection include fever, chills alternating with sweats, malaise, weakness, anorexia, weight loss, pallor, backache, and splenomegaly.[24] Clients may report feeling as if they have the flu with headaches and musculoskeletal aching. In acute infection, clients appear very ill. Fever, chills, and prostration are so severe that hospital admission is usually necessary within a few days.

Cardiac murmurs eventually develop, but they may be absent in the early stages of infection. In clients with preexisting valvular disease, new murmurs may be heard. Heart failure may develop suddenly in either acute or subacute endocarditis. Mechanical complications include perforation of a valve leaflet, rupture of one of the chordae tendineae, or development of a functional stenosis from obstruction of blood flow by large vegetations.

Embolization occurs in about 30% of clients with infective carditis. Clinical manifestations related to embolization can occur in any part of the body. They are presented here in order from head to toe:

- Stroke, transient ischemic attacks, aphasia, or ataxia
- Loss of vision from embolization to the brain or retinal artery
- Petechiae on the neck, conjunctiva, chest, abdomen and mouth
- Roth's spots—a white or yellow center surrounded by a bright-red, irregular halo seen by ophthalmoscope
- Myocardial infarction, which may develop as a result of coronary artery embolism
- Pulmonary embolus
- Splinter hemorrhages, which look like tiny splinters under the nail
- Osler's nodes—painful, erythematous, pea-sized nodules on tips of the fingers and toes resulting from inflammation around a small, infected embolus
- Finger clubbing, although less common today, may occur in clients with long-standing infective endocarditis; pathogenesis remains unclear
- Janeway's lesions—flat, small, nontender red spots on the palms of the hands and the soles of the feet
- Evidence of an immunologic reaction to infection, including arthralgia, proteinuria, hematuria, casts, and acidosis

Because the clinical manifestations of endocarditis are numerous and often nonspecific, several modalities are employed for differential medical diagnosis. Blood cultures for bacteria, fungus, and yeast are the most important diagnostic tests. Blood cultures should be obtained for all clients with both fever and heart murmur. ECGs should be done on admission to the hospital and repeated during the hospital stay. Although a negative ECG does not rule out endocarditis, transesophageal echocardiography can be useful in arriving at a diagnosis. A chest x-ray study is useful in identifying early heart failure. A complete blood count (CBC) and other routine diagnostic procedures are also helpful.

Outcome Management

▉ Medical Management

The chief aims of management are to eradicate the infecting organism and to treat complications. The advent of antimicrobial therapy has changed this infection from one that was almost always fatal to one that is rarely fatal. The choice of antibiotic depends on the organism involved. Penicillin and streptomycin are commonly used. Therapy is usually administered by the IV route and continued for 4 to 6 weeks. Drug administration is usually begun in the hospital but is occasionally continued at home with extensive discharge planning and education.

Occasionally, after the infection is under control (negative blood cultures, absence of fever, and normal WBC count), it may be necessary for the client to undergo heart valve replacement for reversal of newly developed heart failure. Complications that could have developed as a result of the infecting organism warrant careful evaluation.

▉ Nursing Management of the Medical Client

Nursing assessment focuses on gathering data about the client's hemodynamic stability (particularly the presence of a new heart murmur and embolic complications), level of comfort, coping ability, support from significant others, and potential for self-care.

Administer IV antibiotics as prescribed. Antibiotics relieve much discomfort within a few days. Treat fever, when present, with rest, cooling measures, forced fluids, and sometimes salicylates. As with most infectious processes, encourage the client to eat a nutritious diet, drink sufficient fluids, and rest mentally and physically.

The client may need to be hospitalized for 2 to 6 weeks if home care is not an option. Do not enforce complete bed rest unless fever or signs of heart damage develop. Auscultate the heart every 8 hours for heart murmurs. Assess for rapid pulse, easy fatigability, dyspnea, restlessness, signs of heart failure, and embolic manifestations. Document these manifestations if they occur, and report them to the physician.

When the client's condition improves, plan and implement a progressive activity schedule and a teaching plan (see the Client Education Guide: Infective Carditis) As activity increases, monitor the client's physical response to exercise. For example, assess blood pressure, heart rate, diaphoresis, vertigo, and weakness.

Infective Endocarditis

1. Continue taking your intravenous antibiotics with the help of a family member after you leave the hospital.
2. Follow your doctor's advice about gradually resuming activities. A month of convalescence at home is typical.
3. Tell your physician and dentist about having had infective endocarditis. If you are going to have surgery or extensive dental work, be sure you take a full course of antibiotics first.
4. Floss every day, and brush with a soft toothbrush. Consult your dentist before using water-jet cleaning devices because these devices may cause gums to bleed and may put you at risk for infection.
5. Monitor yourself for manifestations of infective endocarditis. Take your temperature every day for the next month; and keep a record of your readings. Report any fever, chills, malaise, loss of appetite, weight loss, or increased fatigue to your physician.

■ Self-Care

The trend toward early hospital discharge has changed the course of treatment for clients with infective endocarditis. IV therapy may now be routinely given in the home. Clients who are alert, cooperative, and reasonably stable and who want to return home may be allowed to do so. Typically, the nurse, pharmacist, and physician teach the techniques of self-administered IV antibiotics. Before discharge, the client must demonstrate the knowledge and technique required. The physician's office or home health care nurses often monitor the client's progress.

Home IV antibiotic therapy offers many benefits. It is less costly than hospital care, motivates clients to become active participants in their own care, reestablishes a more normal lifestyle, and promotes a sense of control that aids in psychosocial and physiologic recovery. To be effective, this program calls for exceptional communication and cooperation between health care team members and the client.

MYOCARDITIS

Myocarditis is an inflammation of the myocardial wall. It can be caused by almost any bacterial, viral, or parasitic organism as well as by radiation, toxic agents such as lead, and drugs such as lithium and cocaine. Myocarditis affects people of all ages and may be acute or chronic. An immunodeficient person is at greater risk for myocarditis. Frequently, the inflammation is not limited to the myocardium but extends to the pericardium, with production of an associated pericarditis. The incidence is not possible to ascertain[17] and varies with the client's age and with various etiologic agents.

Etiology

In the United States, most cases of myocarditis are due to viral infections. Viruses associated with this disorder include coxsackieviruses A and B, mumps, influenza virus serotypes A and B, rubella virus, measles virus, adenoviruses, echoviruses, cytomegalovirus, and Epstein-Barr virus.

Other causes include bacterial infections from diphtheria, typhoid fever, staphylococci, pneumococci, tetanus, and tuberculosis. Myocarditis can also be caused by hypersensitivity immune reactions seen with acute rheumatic fever and postcardiotomy syndrome, toxins and chemicals such as alcohol, large doses of radiation therapy to the chest for the treatment of malignancy, and parasitic infections, including Chagas' disease and toxoplasmosis.

Pathophysiology

Myocardial damage from acute myocarditis is usually the result of the direct invasion or the toxic effects of the microorganism in cardiac myocytes. This can cause an alteration in cellular energy systems and cellular damage. Endomyocardial biopsies are used in diagnosis of the viral infection.[17]

Usually, myocarditis involves both ventricles. If myocardial contractility is impaired, ventricular diastolic pressures and volumes may be elevated in order to maintain stroke volume. Disruptions leading to cardiac dysrhythmias can decrease cardiac output.

Clinical Manifestations

Clinical manifestations vary widely, and there may be no clinical manifestations at all. The health history may reveal a recent upper respiratory infection, a viral pharyngitis, or tonsillitis. The most frequent manifestations, however, are fatigue, dyspnea, palpitations, and chest pain. The client often experiences chest pain as a mild continuous pressure or soreness in the chest. Thus, the chest pain of myocarditis can be distinguished from the effort-induced pain of angina pectoris. Tachycardia, if present, may be disproportionate to the degree of fever, exertion, or illness. Dysrhythmias can also occur, sometimes producing a fatal circulatory collapse. There may be a pericardial friction rub if the client has pericarditis.

In most cases, myocarditis is self-limiting and uncomplicated. If myocardial involvement becomes extensive or prolonged, myofibril degeneration can produce heart failure, with pulmonary congestion, dyspnea, neck vein distention, peripheral edema, and cardiomegaly. Recurrent myocarditis can produce cardiomyopathy. Possible complications include heart failure, dilated cardiomyopathy, and sudden death from lethal dysrhythmias or rupture of a myocardial aneurysm.

The chest x-ray may show an enlarged cardiac silhouette due to ventricular enlargement or pericardial effusion. Blood tests may show a moderate leukocytosis and elevated cardiac enzymes. Echocardiography is helpful in determining heart chamber size and ventricular functioning. Gallium scan shows regional wall abnormalities, dilated ventricles, and hypokinesis of the left ventricle. ECG abnormalities and elevated serum levels of cardiac enzymes are helpful in the diagnosis. The ECG may show a bundle branch block or complete AV heart block, ST-segment elevation, or T-wave flattening.

Outcome Management

Clients with acute myocarditis are usually admitted to the hospital for observation. Clients with pericardial effusion, dysrhythmias, heart failure, or hypotension are usually admitted to the intensive care unit (ICU). Medical management begins with specific therapy for the underlying infection. Bed rest is suggested to decrease cardiac work. Supplemental oxygen may be prescribed for clients with low cardiac output or dysrhythmias. Immunosuppressive therapy had been previously considered helpful, but new research does not support this therapy.[11, 27] Antipyretic agents are helpful for the fever and its hemodynamic effects, which result in increased myocardial workload. Clients who remain at home may use Holter monitoring, which provides continuous surveillance of the client's heart rhythm.

The outlook for clients with myocarditis is generally good. Although most clients recover rapidly, some have recurrent or chronic myocarditis and some become very ill and die.

Nursing management for the client experiencing myocarditis is essentially the same as that provided to clients with infective endocarditis and rheumatic fever. Review those sections within this chapter.

Teaching begins when acute manifestations have subsided and the client has demonstrated physical and emotional readiness. Teach clients how to monitor their pulse rate and rhythm. Instruct them to report any sudden changes in heart rate, rhythm, or palpitations immediately. Encourage family members to take cardiopulmonary resuscitation (CPR) training, which can be obtained from such groups as the local fire department, the American Red Cross, or the American Heart Association. Educating family members about CPR can enhance their sense of preparedness for an emergency.

Because the myocardial infectious process resolves slowly and late complications can occur, advise clients to continue self-monitoring and to schedule clinical follow-up appointments, even after apparent recovery.

The potential of lethal dysrhythmias may frighten the client and significant others. The client who is experiencing extreme anxiety, fear, and ineffective coping may manifest insomnia, tearfulness, somatic complaints, inability to problem-solve, and agitation. Determine with the client (and family) the specific focus of anxiety. Clarify any misconceptions that arise. Speak slowly and calmly, and focus on the present situation, giving feedback about current reality. Encourage the use of relaxation techniques to help allay stress. Schedule activities around periods of undisturbed sleep.

PERICARDITIS

Pericarditis may be either acute or chronic (*recurrent*). It is not known why pericarditis may be an acute illness in some clients and recurrent in others. Chronic pericarditis (*constrictive* pericarditis) is present when a fibrotic, thickened, and adherent pericardium restricts diastolic filling of the heart. This process eventually results in cardiac failure.

■ ACUTE PERICARDITIS

Pathophysiology

Acute pericarditis is a syndrome resulting from inflammation of the parietal and visceral pericardium. Because of the proximity of the pericardium to the pleura, lungs,

sternum, diaphragm, and myocardium, pericarditis may be a consequence of a number of inflammatory or infectious processes (Box 55–2). Acute pericarditis is usually viral (idiopathic) in origin.

Agents or processes causing pericardial inflammation create an exudate of fibrin, WBCs, and endothelial cells. The exudate covers the pericardium and causes further inflammation of the surrounding pleura and tissues. The fibrinous exudate may localize to one region of the heart or may be generalized. Acute pericarditis may be either *dry* (fibrinous) or *exudative*. Under normal conditions, the pericardial sac contains about 50 ml of clear, serous-like fluid. Volumes from 100 to 3000 ml of serofibrinous exudate can accumulate with pericarditis. The exudate accumulates in the pericardial sac, causing cardiac tamponade that restricts cardiac filling and emptying. Without prompt treatment, shock and death can result from decreased cardiac output.

Dry pericarditis can occur after a common viral infection, myocardial infarction, tuberculosis, bacteremia, or renal failure. Delicate adhesions form within the pericardial space along with serous fibrin deposition, hemorrhage, and calcification. Adhesions may eventually obliterate the pericardial sac. Inflammation of the pericardium frequently penetrates the myocardium to some degree, which produces myopericarditis.

Clinical Manifestations

The most characteristic subjective clinical manifestation of pericarditis is chest pain. The nature of this pain varies with the client. Sometimes the pain is similar to that of

---

BOX 55–2 **Causes of Pericarditis**

Infections
  Viral: coxsackie, influenza
  Bacterial: tuberculosis, staphylococcus, streptococcus, meningococcus, pneumococcus
  Parasitic
  Fungal
Myocardial injury
  Myocardial infarction (Dressler's syndrome)
  Cardiac trauma: blunt or penetrating
  Post cardiac surgery
  Hypersensitivity
Collagen diseases
  Rheumatic fever
  Scleroderma
  Systemic lupus erythematosus
  Rheumatoid arthritis
Drug reaction
  Procainamide
  Methysergide
  Hydralazine
Radiation therapy
Cobalt therapy
Metabolic disorders
  Uremia
  Myxedema
Chronic anemia
Neoplasm: lymphoma
Aortic dissection

myocardial infarction; at other times, it mimics the pain of pleurisy. The pain is exacerbated with respiration and rotating the trunk but usually does not radiate to the arms. Sitting up often relieves the pain.

Pericardial *friction rub* is a classic objective manifestation of acute pericarditis. The rub is produced by inflamed, roughened pericardial layers that create friction as their surfaces rub together during heart movement. Auscultation over the precordium reveals a scratchy, leathery, or creaky sound that is heard anywhere over the precordium but most frequently at the third intercostal space left of the sternal border. The rub is best heard with the diaphragm of the stethoscope and with the client holding his or her breath. In some clients, the sound is best heard with the client sitting up. Pericardial friction rubs vary in intensity from hour to hour and from day to day.

Fever is another common finding in clients with pericarditis. The temperature may rise to 39.4° C (103° F). Chills, malaise, joint pain, anorexia, nausea, and weight loss accompany the fever. Dyspnea and chest pain can potentiate anxiety. An increase in heart rate usually corresponds to the degree of fever and anxiety.

The ECG may indicate bradycardia or atrial fibrillation. The ECG frequently shows a decrease in the amplitude of the QRS complex and changes in the ST-segment elevation in leads I, II, aVF, and V_4 to V_6 and inversion of the T wave.[15] Laboratory studies show an elevated ESR and may show an elevated WBC count. Cardiac enzymes are usually normal but may be elevated.

Outcome Management

When the cause of acute pericarditis is known, treatment of the cause can be planned accordingly. If no causal agent is known, symptomatic intervention for acute dry pericarditis is provided. Pain and fever, usually self-limited, may be eased by aspirin given in maximally tolerated doses. The physician may prescribe a nonsteroidal anti-inflammatory drug (NSAID). Stronger analgesia, such as morphine sulfate, may be necessary if chest pain becomes severe.

If acute pericarditis is present after a myocardial infarction, reassure the client that the pain experienced with pericarditis is not to be associated with another infarction. If the client becomes anxious, thinking that this pain might be that of another infarction, oxygen demand increases and myocardial ischemia may develop.

The focus of nursing care related to pericarditis is the same as that described for the other inflammatory cardiac diseases discussed in this chapter. Nursing assessment of the client with pericarditis also includes scrutiny for the presence of pericardial tamponade (pulsus paradoxus, distended neck veins). Vigilant assessment is necessary. Provide reassurance concerning the temporary nature of the disease.

■ ACUTE PERICARDITIS WITH EFFUSION

Acute pericarditis with effusion results when fluid accumulates within the pericardial sac. Rapid or excessive fluid accumulations may compress the heart and reduce ventricular filling and cardiac output. When fluid accumulates slowly, the fibrous pericardium is better able to stretch and accommodate its presence. Clients can tolerate 1 to 2 L of fluid without an increase in intrapericardial

pressure if accumulation is slow. However, the normal unstretched pericardial sac can accommodate the rapid addition of only 80 to 200 ml of fluid without a decrease in cardiac output.

Pericardial effusion may be asymptomatic. If dry pericarditis precedes the condition, the friction rub may disappear. Fever may develop. Heart sounds may be muffled because the pericardial fluid accumulates between the stethoscope and the heart valves and chambers quieting the heart sounds.

Pulsus paradoxus can be present. If the client has normal breathing and a systolic difference of greater than 10 mm Hg, evaluation for cardiac compression and possibly cardiac tamponade should be performed.[15]

Echocardiography is the most accurate technique for evaluating pericardial effusion.[15] The test is sensitive enough to detect as little as 20 ml of pericardial fluid. Pericardiocentesis is not indicated unless there is evidence of cardiac compression caused by cardiac tamponade (see next). If pericardial effusion is present, an enlarged cardiac silhouette is seen on the chest radiograph.

Care of the client with pericardial effusion is similar to the plan of intervention for dry pericarditis. Bed rest, analgesia, and proper positioning can help alleviate symptoms. Psychological support is very important.

■ CHRONIC CONSTRICTIVE PERICARDITIS

Chronic constrictive pericarditis is a chronic inflammatory condition in which the pericardium changes into a thick, fibrous band of tissue. This tissue encircles, encases, and compresses the heart, preventing proper ventricular filling and emptying. Cardiac failure eventually results from this slow compression.

This condition usually begins with an episode of acute pericarditis characterized by fibrin deposition, often with pericardial effusion. In most cases, the visceral and parietal layers become completely fused. The heavily fibrosed pericardium restricts diastolic filling in all chambers and decreases systolic ejection.

Clinical manifestations include right ventricular failure first, followed by decreased cardiac output manifesting as fatigue on exertion, dyspnea, leg edema, ascites, low pulse pressure, distended neck veins, and delayed capillary refill time.[18]

Constrictive pericarditis is a progressive disease without spontaneous reversal of manifestations. Relatively few clients survive for many years with minor symptoms. Most of these clients become progressively more disabled over time.

Treatment is both surgical and medical. Medical treatment includes digitalis, diuretics, and sodium restriction to relieve manifestations of right ventricular failure. Surgical intervention involves the excision of the damaged pericardium (pericardiectomy) and should be performed early in the course of the disease.

■ CARDIAC TAMPONADE

Cardiac tamponade is a life-threatening complication caused by accumulation of fluid in the pericardium. This fluid, which can be blood, pus, or air in the pericardial sac, accumulates fast enough and in sufficient quantity to compress the heart and restrict blood flow in and out of the ventricles. *This is a cardiac emergency!*

Large or rapidly accumulating effusions raise the intrapericardial pressure to a point at which venous blood cannot flow into the heart, which decreases ventricular filling. As a result, venous pressure rises and cardiac output and arterial blood pressure fall. A narrowing pulse pressure signals cardiac tamponade. The heart attempts to compensate by beating rapidly (tachycardia), but tachycardia cannot sustain cardiac output for very long. Prompt intervention is necessary to prevent shock and death.

In the client with cardiac tamponade, assessment reveals hypotension, tachycardia, jugular venous distention, cyanosis of lips and nails, dyspnea, muffled heart sounds, diaphoresis, and paradoxical pulse (a decrease in systolic arterial pulsation exceeding 10 mm Hg, during inspiration). The client may be comfortable and quiet one minute and then very restless with a feeling of impending doom. Clients may panic when fluid accumulates rapidly. Slowly developing tamponade is characterized by manifestations resembling those of heart failure: nonspecific ECG changes, decreased voltage, and visualization of fluid in the pericardial sac on echocardiogram (see Critical Monitoring: Cardiac Tamponade).

Immediate intervention is required. The emergency intervention of choice is pericardiocentesis, a procedure in which fluid or air is aspirated from the pericardial sac (Fig. 55–2). This procedure relieves pressure on the heart, thereby improving cardiac function and perhaps saving the client's life. Pericardiocentesis is now performed with a soft catheter, which is resulting in fewer cardiac lacerations.[15]

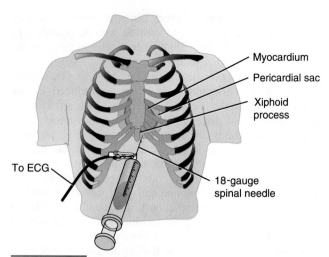

FIGURE 55–2 Pericardiocentesis. ECG, electrocardiogram.

Four conditions seem to increase the risk for its development:

- Chronic ingestion of excessive amounts of alcohol
- Pregnancy
- Systemic hypertension
- Various infections

Table 55–2 compares diagnostic data for the three types of idiopathic cardiomyopathy. These forms of cardiomyopathy are described separately.

■ DILATED CARDIOMYOPATHY

Pathophysiology

Dilated (congestive) cardiomyopathy is the most common form. Usually, both the left and right ventricles dilate, the myocardial fibers degenerate, and fibrotic tissue replaces viable tissue. Severe dilation of the heart occurs, but reduced contractility results in decreased stroke volume, low cardiac output, and a compensatory increase in heart rate. These changes eventually lead to heart failure accompanied by lethal ventricular dysrhythmias. The combined problem of ventricular dilation and ineffective myocardial contractility also increases the risk of blood pooling within the heart and subsequent clot formation. Many clients (75%) with idiopathic dilated cardiomyopathy die within 5 years after the onset of manifestations.[27]

Some forms of dilated cardiomyopathy are idiopathic. Other etiologic mechanisms include viral myocarditis, infections, metabolic problems, toxins, pregnancy, neuromuscular disorders, connective tissue disorders and genetic predisposition (20% of cases). Dilated cardiomyopathy associated with pregnancy can disappear. There may be spontaneous rapid improvement in some women and early fatality in others.

Clinical Manifestations

Clinical manifestations usually develop gradually. Fatigue and weakness are common. Chest pain may be present and may be associated with ischemic heart disease. Right-

CARDIOMYOPATHY

Cardiomyopathy (Fig. 55–3) is a heart muscle disorder of unknown cause (idiopathic). The three major classes are:

- Dilated (congestive)
- Hypertrophic (also called hypertrophic subaortic stenosis)
- Restrictive

CRITICAL MONITORING

Cardiac Tamponade

Report the following manifestations of cardiac tamponade immediately!

Elevated venous pressure (increased central venous pressure)
Distended neck veins
Kussmaul's sign (distended neck veins on inspiration)
Hypotension
Narrowed pulse pressure
Tachycardia
Dyspnea
Restlessness, anxiety
Cyanosis of lips and nails
Diaphoresis
Muffled heart sounds
Pulsus paradoxus
Decreased friction rub
Decreased QRS voltage and electrical alternans

SYSTOLE   DIASTOLE

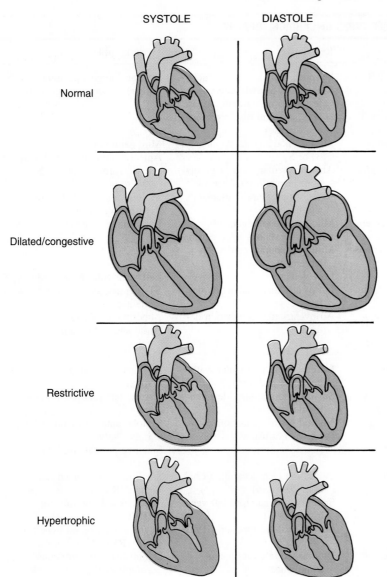

Normal

Dilated/congestive

Restrictive

Hypertrophic

FIGURE 55–3 The three types of cardiomyopathy.

sided heart failure is a late and ominous sign. Systemic blood pressure is usually normal or low. Heart failure develops steadily and is seen as dyspnea, orthopnea, tachycardia, palpitations, peripheral edema, enlargement of jugular veins, and liver engorgement.

An S_4 gallop often precedes the development of heart failure, and an S_3 gallop generally occurs with heart failure. If the heart rate is rapid, both S_4 and S_3 may fuse to form a summation gallop sound. There may be a systolic murmur of mitral or tricuspid insufficiency, because ventricular dilation prevents sufficient closure of those valves. Gallop sounds and regurgitant murmurs may be intensified by an isometric hand grip exercise because of the increase it causes on systemic vascular resistance. Pulmonary crackles become audible as failure progresses.

Diagnostic tests, including ECG, cardiac biopsy, echocardiography, chest x-ray, and blood chemistries, are useful for diagnosis. ECG findings include sinus tachycardia, ventricular dysrhythmias, ST-segment changes, and left bundle branch block.

Outcome Management

Treatment is similar to that for heart failure. Inotropic agents are used to enhance myocardial contractility and to unload the heart. Nitroglycerin as a vasodilator can be used to decrease preload and afterload. Diuretics and sodium-restricted diets are used to decrease pulmonary congestion and to reduce fluid overload. Anticoagulants may help prevent clots and emboli. Antidysrhythmic agents may help suppress ventricular irritability. In appropriate candidates, the implantation of the automatic internal cardiac defibrillator may be used to prevent sudden cardiac death[27] (see Chapter 57).

Rest improves cardiac function and reduces heart size. Most clients experience severe activity intolerance during the later stages of the disease, which automatically limits their activities. However, during the earlier stages, most clients find it difficult to accept rigidly imposed restrictions on activity. Clients should avoid poorly tolerated activities. Advise clients that physical and emotional stress exacerbate the disease. Because alcohol depresses

TABLE 55–2	DIAGNOSTIC DATA FOR THE THREE TYPES OF CARDIOMYOPATHY		
	Dilated	**Restrictive**	**Hypertrophic**
Manifestations	Heart failure, particularly left-sided Fatigue and weakness Systemic or pulmonary emboli	Dyspnea, fatigue Right-sided heart failure manifestations of systemic disease (e.g., amyloidosis, iron storage disease)	Dyspnea, angina pectoris Fatigue, syncope, palpitations
Physical examination	Moderate to severe cardiomegaly: S_3 and S_4 Atrioventricular valve regurgitation, especially mitral	Mild to moderate cardiomegaly: S_3 or S_4 Atrioventricular valve regurgitation; inspiratory increase in venous pressure (Kussmaul's sign)	Mild cardiomegaly Apical systolic thrill and heave; brisk carotid upstroke S_4 common Systolic murmur that increases with a Valsalva maneuver
Chest x-ray	Moderate-to-marked cardiac enlargement, especially left ventricular pulmonary venous hypertension	Mild cardiac enlargement Pulmonary venous hypertension Mild to moderate cardiac enlargement	Left atrial enlargement
Electrocardiogram	Sinus tachycardia Atrial and ventricular dysrhythmias ST-segment and T-wave abnormalities Intraventricular conduction defects	Low voltage Intraventricular conduction defects Atrioventricular conduction defects	Left ventricular hypertrophy ST-segment and T-wave abnormalities Abnormal Q waves Atrial and ventricular dysrhythmias
Echocardiogram	Left ventricular dilation and dysfunction Abnormal diastolic mitral valve motion secondary to abnormal compliance and filling pressures	Increased left ventricular wall thickness and mass Small or normal-sized left ventricular cavity Normal systolic function Pericardial effusion	Asymmetrical septal hypertrophy Narrow left ventricular outflow tract Systolic anterior motion of the mitral valve Small or normal-sized left ventricle
Radionuclide studies	Left ventricular dilation and dysfunction (RVG)	Infiltration of myocardium (thallium 201 scan) Small or normal-sized left ventricle (RVG) Normal systolic function (RVG)	Small or normal-sized left ventricle (RVG) Vigorous systolic function (RVG) Asymmetrical septal hypertrophy (RVG ^{201}Tl scan)
Cardiac catheterization	Left ventricular enlargement and dysfunction Mitral/tricuspid regurgitation Elevated left-sided and often right-sided filling pressures Diminished cardiac output	Diminished left ventricular compliance Square root sign in ventricular pressure recordings Preserved systolic function Elevated left-sided and right-sided filling pressures	Diminished left ventricular compliance Mitral regurgitation Vigorous systolic function Dynamic left ventricular outflow gradient

RVG, radionuclide ventriculogram.
From Braunwald, E. (1997). *Heart disease: A textbook of cardiovascular medicine* (5th ed.). Philadelphia: W. B. Saunders.

myocardial contractility, the client should abstain from drinking alcoholic beverages.

Only transplantation and specific vasodilator therapy (hydralazine plus nitrates) have resulted in prolonged life.[27] Heart transplantation shows a 5-year survival of greater than 70% in appropriately selected clients.[27]

■ HYPERTROPHIC CARDIOMYOPATHY

Pathophysiology

Hypertrophic cardiomyopathy (sometimes called *asymmetrical septal hypertrophy*) is disproportionate thickening of the interventricular septum, compared with the free wall of the ventricle. This overgrowth leads to wall rigidity

and thereby increases resistance to blood flow from the left atrium. There is also obstruction of left ventricular outflow. Although this disease is also known as idiopathic hypertrophic subaortic stenosis, many clients do not have the obstructive or stenotic component of the disease. Therefore, it is more accurate to use the term *hypertrophic cardiomyopathy* to describe this disease.

Hypertrophic cardiomyopathy appears to be a genetically transmitted disease (~50% of cases). It can also be idiopathic, caused by hypertension or hypoparathyroidism. It appears most often in young adults, both men and women.

In its severest form, the left ventricular wall reaches tremendous dimensions and encroaches on the left ventricular chamber, which becomes small and elongated. Septal hypertrophy may obstruct the left ventricular outflow tract during systole. Frequently, there is diastolic dysfunction in the form of stiffness of the left ventricle during diastolic filling. This stiffness raises left ventricular end-diastolic pressure, which eventually results in elevation of left atrial, pulmonary venous, and pulmonary capillary pressures.

Clinical Manifestations

Clients with hypertrophic cardiomyopathy most commonly present with clinical manifestations in late adolescence or early adulthood, but clinical manifestations may appear at any age. Many clients with hypertrophic cardiomyopathy are asymptomatic and can lead long lives. Interestingly, they often have relatives with incapacitating manifestations of the disease. Sadly, sudden death is frequently the first clinical manifestation of the disease in asymptomatic clients. Sudden death appears more often in younger clients and, if the presence of the disease is known, may be avoided by elimination of strenuous exercise.

The most common manifestation is dyspnea. Dyspnea is due to the high pulmonary pressures produced by the elevated left ventricular end-diastolic pressure. Angina pectoris, fatigue, and syncope are also common clinical manifestations. Cardiac dysrhythmias are frequently present. Palpitations, paroxysmal nocturnal dyspnea, and frank heart failure are less common. Many clients complain of dizzy spells. Exertion tends to worsen most manifestations.

Physical examination may be normal in asymptomatic clients. The appearance of a fourth heart sound may be the only sign of the disease. An increase in the intensity of the heart murmur usually suggests progression of the condition. ECG, chest film, echocardiogram, and radionuclide scanning are very useful in the diagnosis.[27]

Management

The goals of intervention for hypertrophic cardiomyopathy are to reduce ventricular contractility and to relieve left ventricular outflow obstruction. Beta-adrenergic blocking agents, such as propranolol, and calcium channel blockers provide the mainstay of medical intervention. These medications reduce myocardial contractility. With decreased vigor of ventricular contraction, outflow obstruction diminishes. Beta-adrenergic blockade also reduces the heart rate (which further reduces myocardial workload) and prevents dysrhythmias.

Medications that decrease preload (e.g., nitrates, diuretics, morphine) and that increase contractility (e.g., isoproterenol, dopamine, digitalis) are to be avoided. Anticoagulants are used if the client is in atrial fibrillation. The client is at risk for endocarditis and should follow the prophylactic care for that condition.

■ RESTRICTIVE CARDIOMYOPATHY

Pathophysiology

Restrictive cardiomyopathy, the least common form, is characterized by excessively rigid ventricular walls. This rigidity impairs filling during diastole; however, contractility with systole is usually normal. Any infiltrative process of the heart that results in fibrosis and thickening can cause restrictive cardiomyopathy. The most frequently associated disease is amyloidosis (deposition of eosinophilic fibrous protein in the heart). Other disorders include glycogen storage disease, hemochromatosis, and sarcoidosis.

Fibrotic infiltrations into the myocardium, endocardium, and subendocardium cause the ventricles to lose their ability to stretch. Filling pressures increase, and cardiac output falls. Eventually, cardiac failure and mild ventricular hypertrophy occur.

Restrictive cardiomyopathy causes decreased cardiac output. As cardiac output falls and intraventricular pressures rise, manifestations of heart failure appear. The earliest manifestations may include exercise intolerance, fatigue, and shortness of breath, followed by neck vein distention, peripheral edema, and ascites. In severe or end-stage disease, the clinical manifestations of restrictive cardiomyopathy are indistinguishable from those of chronic constrictive pericarditis (see preceding discussion of pericarditis). Cardiac murmurs are usually minimal or absent. The manifestations progress rapidly producing a high mortality.[27]

Outcome Management

At present there are no specific interventions for restrictive cardiomyopathy. Intervention aims at diminishing heart failure. A pacemaker, diuretics, vasodilators, and salt restriction may help accomplish this goal.[27] Digitalis may help in some forms of restrictive cardiomyopathy.

Death attributable to dysrhythmia may occur suddenly, or a more progressive course may be followed by eventual, intractable heart failure. The prognosis largely depends on the underlying cause. Unfortunately, intervention rarely brings about long-term improvement.

■ Surgical Management for Cardiomyopathy

Surgical intervention for hypertrophic cardiomyopathy may become necessary if medical management is ineffective. Several surgical procedures have been developed to reduce the outflow gradient. The most popular surgical treatment involves an incision into the ventricular septum with or without resection of part of the septum.

The excision of fibrotic endocardium is successful in a limited number of clients with restrictive cardiomyopathy. Recent advances in surgical treatment have shown some success. Surgery has been effective for some dysrhythmias. Cardiac transplantation is becoming increasingly common for the treatment of dilated cardiomyopathy. Valve replacement may also be required, but it is not commonly performed.

■ Nursing Management

The management of the client with cardiomyopathy is outlined in the Care Plan. In addition, clients who are acutely or chronically ill with cardiomyopathy require strong psychosocial support. The uncertain and serious consequences of the disease create fear and anxiety. The chronic nature of the disorder can deplete coping resources, leaving those afflicted with feelings of helpless-

▪ THE CLIENT WITH CARDIOMYOPATHY

Collaborative Problem. Risk for Heart Failure related to mechanical dysfunction of the heart

Outcomes. Monitor the client for the following clinical manifestations of heart failure:

- Peripheral edema
- Pulmonary edema
- Decreased renal perfusion
- Decreased CO
- Diaphoresis
- Dyspnea, orthopnea
- Anxiety
- Frothy, pink sputum

Interventions

1. Assess the client every 4 to 8 hours for:

- Neck vein distention
- Peripheral edema
- Altered lung sounds
- Dyspnea or orthopnea
- Tachycardia
- Hypotension
- Confusion
- Urine output > 30 ml/hr

2. Monitor BUN, bilirubin, liver enzymes, and creatinine.
3. Monitor fluid balance every 8 to 24 hours, and record daily weights.

Rationales

1. These assessments can help detect early signs of heart failure; as the heart muscle fails to pump effectively, falling cardiac output stimulates the adrenergic system and the renin-angiotensin-aldosterone system. These changes lead to tachycardia and oliguria. Increased preload and afterload lead to neck and vein distention, peripheral edema, altered lung sounds, dyspnea, and orthopnea. Hypoxia may lead to confusion.

2. Laboratory results can indicate liver congestion.
3. Clients are given potent diuretics to reduce pulmonary and peripheral edema. Accurate assessment of fluid balance and weight assist in determining effectiveness of treatment.

Evaluation. Heart failure will remain an active problem. Some clients will show improvement after diuresis. Others may have such severe cardiomyopathy that the goal is to have no further deterioration.

Nursing Diagnosis. Decreased Cardiac Output related to alterations in cardiac structure and function

Outcomes. The client will demonstrate improved cardiac output, as evidenced by:

- Clear lung sounds
- Vital signs WNL
- Warm, dry skin
- Normal sinus rhythm
- Absence of S_3 or S_4
- Urine output > 30 ml/hr
- Decreased peripheral edema, neck vein distention, and ascites

Interventions

1. Monitor for clinical manifestations of decreasing CO.

2. Encourage bed rest during acute phase; limit self-care.

3. Avoid Valsalva's maneuver (with hypertrophic cardiomyopathy).
4. Observe and record dysrhythmias every 4 to 8 hours.
5. Monitor intake and output every 1 to 8 hours.
6. Restrict IV and oral fluids as ordered.
7. Administer unloading and inotropic agents.

8. Administer calcium antagonists as ordered.

9. In hypertrophic cardiomyopathy, avoid nitrates, beta-adrenergic agents, and cardiac glycosides.
10. Hemodynamic monitoring: monitor arterial pressure, RAP, PAP, PCWP, CO/I every 2 to 4 hours as indicated.

Rationales

1. Early detection of decreasing CO improves treatment options.
2. Rest decreases oxygen consumption and demand on myocardium.
3. Valsalva's maneuver impedes venous return and impairs outflow.
4. Dysrhythmias may further impair CO.
5. Fluid retention may occur with decreased CO and CHF.
6. This restriction decreases the amount of circulating fluids.
7. These agents are used to improve ejection, reduce preload, and improve contractility.
8. These agents are used to decrease LV outflow obstruction and to increase LV compliance to improve ventricular filling.
9. These agents increase contractility and increase obstruction.
10. These monitor the degree of heart failure and the response to therapy.

Evaluation. Like heart failure, decreased cardiac output will remain an active problem. Degree of outcome attainment varies greatly.

■

Outcomes. The client will show an improved activity tolerance, as evidenced by:

- Demonstrating a progression of activity appropriate to the disorder
- Showing a willingness to combine rest and activity
- Demonstrating minimal change in pulse or BP during activities
- Having pulse, respirations, and BP return to normal range within 3 minutes of the activity
- Accepting any imposed restrictions

Interventions	Rationales
1. Assess the tolerance to activities in bed before ambulating	1. This assessment provides a baseline to plan activity.
2. During activity, monitor pulse, respiration, color, and ECG.	2. Changes in vital signs, skin color, and ECG are evidence of orthostatic changes and the ability of the diseased myocardium to meet oxygen demand with exercise.
3. Discontinue activity if chest pain, dyspnea, cyanosis, dizziness, hypotension, sustained tachycardia, or dysrhythmias develop.	3. These manifestations are evidence of myocardial hypoxia.
4. Monitor pulse, respirations, and BP 3 minutes after activity.	4. These measures aid in evaluating tolerance of activity.
5. Explore which sedentary activities client may enjoy.	5. Sedentary activities may provide diversion if activity is not permitted; sedentary activities do not place a demand on the diseased myocardium.

Evaluation. If the cardiomyopathy is severe, plan to achieve only small increments in activity tolerance. This problem will remain active, since the condition is not curable.

BP, blood pressure; BUN, blood urea nitrogen; CO, cardiac output; CO/I, cardiac output/cardiac index; ECG, electrocardiogram; IV, intravenous; LV, left ventricular; PAP, pulmonary artery pressure; PCWP, pulmonary capillary wedge pressure; RAP, right atrial pressure; WNL, within normal limits.

---

ness and hopelessness. As physical capabilities diminish, feelings of inadequacy, frustration, and poor self-esteem grow. Clients may become irritable, angry, withdrawn, or dependent.

Even though the prognosis is often poor, you can help clients who suffer from this debilitating disorder to maintain hope and dignity. Encouragement, a caring touch, a listening ear, and attainable goals can promote a high quality of life. Create an environment in which clients can openly express concerns and acknowledge fears. Acceptance, empathy, and kindness can help clients with cardiomyopathies adopt more successful coping strategies.

■ Self-Care

With hypertrophic cardiomyopathy, syncope or sudden death may follow physical exertion. Therefore, warn the client with hypertrophic cardiomyopathy to avoid strenuous physical exercise such as running or active competitive sports. In addition, encourage household members to learn CPR. Although chest pain often accompanies this disease, nitroglycerin can worsen obstruction. Instead, clinicians treat chest pain with reduced activity and beta-blocking agents.

Hypertrophic cardiomyopathy predisposes the client to the risk of infective endocarditis. Advise clients with this cardiomyopathy to check with their physician about taking prophylactic antibiotics before and after dental and surgical procedures as American Heart Association Guidelines have changed.[6]

All clients with cardiomyopathy need clear, honest education concerning the disease and its cause and intervention. Both you and the client must be watchful for un-

toward effects of therapy. Clients with restrictive cardiomyopathy are especially vulnerable to the toxic effects of digitalis (see Chapter 56).

VALVULAR HEART DISEASE

Valvular dysfunction occurs when the heart valves cannot fully open or fully close. A stenosed valve may impede the flow of blood from one chamber to the next; an insufficient (incompetent) valve may allow blood to regurgitate (flow backward) (Fig. 55–4). The aortic and mitral valves become dysfunctional more often than the pulmonary and tricuspid valves. This change occurs because the left side of the heart is a system of higher pressures; the right side of the heart is exposed to the lower pressures in the pulmonary circulation.

Valvular heart disease remains fairly common in the United States even though the incidence is steadily decreasing as the incidence of rheumatic fever decreases. Mitral valve prolapse syndrome is one of the most common cardiac abnormalities; as much as 5% of the population is affected, with women affected more than men.[16]

MITRAL VALVE DISEASE

Disorders of the mitral valve obstruct the flow of blood from the atrium to the ventricle (stenosis) or allow blood to leak back from ventricle to atrium (regurgitation). *Mitral stenosis* is a block in blood flow resulting from an abnormality of the mitral valve leaflets that prevents proper opening of the valve during diastole. This disorder

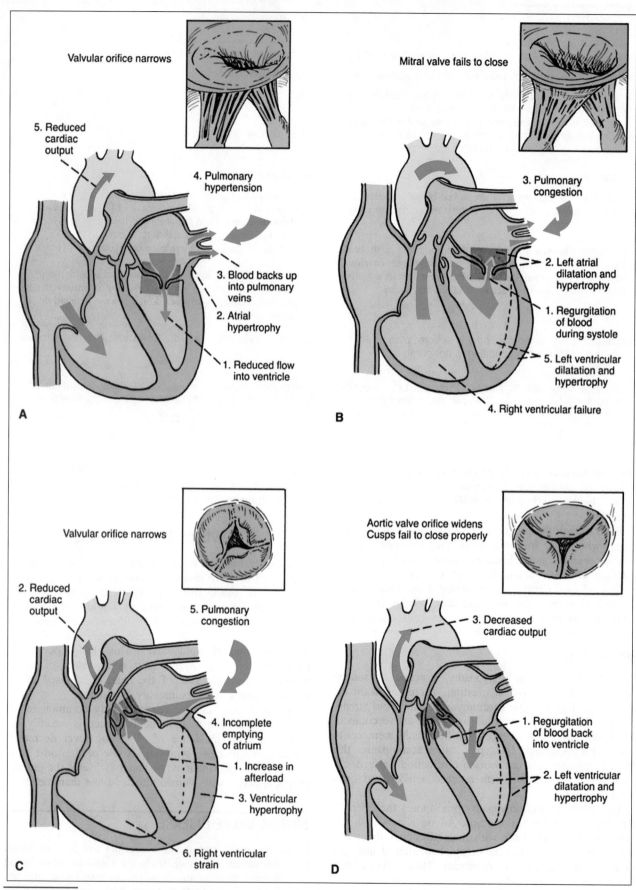

FIGURE 55–4 Dysfunctions of the cardiac valves. *A*, Mitral stenosis. *B*, Mitral regurgitation. *C*, Aortic stenosis. *D*, Aortic regurgitation.

causes overwork for the left atrium. *Mitral regurgitation* occurs when blood from the left ventricle is ejected back into the left atrium during systole because of abnormalities in the mitral valve. This disorder results in overwork for the left atrium and left ventricle. Regurgitation of the mitral valve sometimes occurs with mitral stenosis.

In *mitral valve prolapse* (see later), one or both of the valve leaflets bulge into the left atrium during ventricular systole. Various names have been given to the disorder: late apical systolic murmur, Barlow's syndrome, and floppy mitral valve syndrome. Usually a benign disorder, it may progress to a stage of pronounced regurgitation and ventricular dilation. Although it is often an isolated abnormality, this syndrome is associated with a number of other conditions, such as endocarditis, myocarditis, atherosclerosis, systemic lupus erythematosus, muscular dystrophy, acromegaly, and cardiac sarcoidosis. In addition, there may be a genetic component.

Etiology and Risk Factors

Factors leading to the development of acquired valvular disease include acute rheumatic fever, infectious endocarditis, and connective tissue abnormalities. Rheumatic heart disease, the most common cause of valvular heart disease, is preventable. Community health nurses working in health care centers or schools can often detect people with beta-hemolytic streptococcal infections (the precursor to rheumatic heart disease). Refer these clients for appropriate diagnosis and intervention.

Pathophysiology

Acquired valvular dysfunction is usually caused by inflammation of the endocardium due to acute rheumatic fever or infectious endocarditis. The inflammation causes the valve leaflets and chordae tendineae to become fibrous. The chordae tendineae shorten, which narrows the outflow tract.

In the client with valvular stenosis, the valve orifice narrows, and the valve leaflets (cusps) may become fused or thickened in such a way that the valve cannot open freely. With valvular insufficiency, scarring and retraction of the valve leaflets result in incomplete closure. Either problem increases the heart workload. Valvular stenosis subjects the chamber behind the stenotic valve to greater stress (e.g., the left ventricle in aortic stenosis). This is because the heart must generate more pressure to force blood through the narrowed opening. In the client with valvular insufficiency, the chambers in front and behind the valve are taxed.

For a time, the heart may be able to compensate for the additional strain through dilation and eventual hypertrophy. If valvular damage worsens, however, without intervention the heart eventually fails.

MITRAL STENOSIS

As the valves become calcified and immobile, the valvular orifice narrows, which prevents normal passage of blood from the left atrium to the left ventricle. The valve orifice normally is 4 to 6 cm². When the orifice is mildly stenosed, it is reduced to 2 cm². This mild stenosis allows blood to flow from the left atrium to the left ventricle only if increased pressure is generated.

The obstruction of blood flow across the mitral valve during diastolic filling creates a pressure gradient between the left atrium and the left ventricle of approximately 20 mm Hg in critical stenosis.[4] Therefore, the pressure in the left atrium is elevated to approximately 25 mm Hg. The elevated left atrial pressure, in turn, raises the pulmonary venous and pulmonary capillary pressures. The left atrium hypertrophies to accommodate the increase in pressure and volume, and the right ventricle hypertrophies because of the chronic pulmonary hypertension. Right ventricular failure can result, and inadequate filling of the left ventricle (preload) can result in reduced cardiac output[4] (Fig. 55–4A).

MITRAL REGURGITATION

Mitral regurgitation occurs during systole. During the systole, much pressure is generated within the left ventricle. The blood in the left ventricle is ejected forward into the aorta and also backward into the left atrium through the mitral valve that is not completely closed. The backward flow of blood causes left atrial and left ventricular enlargement. The left atrium responds to the large volume of blood it is receiving during systole, causing dilation and hypertrophy. The left ventricle responds to the large amount of blood lost to the left atrium by pumping harder to preserve cardiac output. This causes hypertrophy of the left ventricle and, eventually, left ventricular failure (Fig. 55–4B).

Over time, the increase in blood to the left atrium causes a rise in left atrial pressure. This pressure is reflected backward into the pulmonary venous and arterial system. With continued high pressures, right-sided heart failure can develop.

MITRAL VALVE PROLAPSE

In the client with mitral valve prolapse, the anterior and posterior cusps of the mitral valve billow upward into the atrium during systolic contraction (Fig. 55–5). The chordae tendineae can be lengthened, which allows the valve cusps to stretch upward. The cusps may be enlarged and thickened. If blood leaks backward into the atrium during systole, mitral regurgitation is present.

Clinical Manifestations

The clinical manifestations of valvular heart disease may appear gradually or suddenly.

MITRAL STENOSIS

On auscultation, a loud first heart sound and then an opening snap that ushers in a low-pitched, rumbling diastolic murmur is heard. The opening snap is best heard at the apex with the diaphragm of the stethoscope. The diastolic murmur is best heard at the apex using the bell of the stethoscope while the client is in a left lateral recumbent position.

Atrial fibrillation is a common finding in clients with mitral stenosis. During episodes of atrial fibrillation, the pulse becomes irregular and faint and the blood pressure often drops. In some cases of mitral stenosis, systemic embolization is present. Ineffective atrial contractions allow some stagnation of blood in the left atrium and encourage the formation of mural thrombi. These thrombi easily break away and travel as emboli throughout the arterial system, causing tissue infarction.

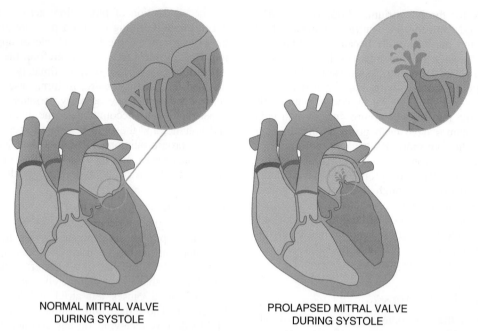

NORMAL MITRAL VALVE
DURING SYSTOLE

PROLAPSED MITRAL VALVE
DURING SYSTOLE

FIGURE 55–5 Mitral valve prolapse. The main figure shows a normal mitral valve; the *inset* shows a prolapsed mitral valve. Prolapse permits the valve leaflets to billow back into the atrium during left ventricular systole. The billowing causes the leaflets to part slightly, permitting regurgitation of blood into the atrium.

MITRAL REGURGITATION

Clients with mitral regurgitation may be asymptomatic, but if cardiac output falls, manifestations will develop. When cardiac output falls, fatigue and dyspnea are the first manifestations. Clinical manifestations gradually increase to include orthopnea, paroxysmal nocturnal dyspnea, and peripheral edema. Pulmonary manifestations are less severe than in mitral stenosis because changes in the mean pulmonary capillary pressure are less exaggerated. However, when the right side of the heart is affected, the manifestations are the same as in mitral stenosis.

Auscultation reveals a blowing, high-pitched systolic murmur with radiation to the left axilla, heard best at the apex. The first heart sound may be diminished, and often a splitting of the second sound will be heard. Severe regurgitation is associated with a third heart sound (S_3).

Vital signs are usually normal unless mitral regurgitation is severe. Atrial fibrillation is common in clients with this condition; however, emboli and hemoptysis occur far less often than in mitral stenosis.

MITRAL VALVE PROLAPSE

It is not uncommon for many clients with mitral valve prolapse to be completely asymptomatic. In a healthy client, a physical examination may reveal a regurgitant murmur or a midsystolic click on auscultation. Manifestations, if present, may include tachycardia, lightheadedness, syncope, fatigue, weakness, dyspnea, chest discomfort, anxiety, and palpitations related to dysrhythmias.[4] Manifestations may be vague. Minimal morbidity and mortality are associated with mitral valve prolapse. Clinically, clients have no physical limitations.

Various diagnostic assessments are used to detect valvular lesions or structural heart changes. These studies include echocardiography, chest radiography, stress tests and cardiac catheterization.[4]

Outcome Management

The goals of medical management are to maintain cardiac output and activity tolerance. When cardiac output falls or the client is unable to tolerate simple activities, the valve can be surgically replaced.

MITRAL STENOSIS

Improvement of manifestations may be achieved with oral diuretics and a sodium-restricted diet. Digitalis is useful in clients with atrial fibrillation for slowing the ventricular heart rate. Beta-blockers may decrease the heart rate and, therefore, increase exercise tolerance. Anticoagulants are helpful in these clients. A client with untreated mitral stenosis can progress from having mild disability to severe disability in about 3 years.[4]

MITRAL REGURGITATION

The client should restrict physical activities that produce fatigue and dyspnea. Reducing sodium intake and promoting sodium excretion with diuretics can lessen the work of the heart. Nitrates, digitalis and angiotensin-converting enzyme (ACE) inhibitors have brought about hemodynamic improvement and symptomatic relief in clients with chronic mitral regurgitation.[4]

MITRAL VALVE PROLAPSE

Treatment of mitral valve prolapse depends on the manifestations. Beta-blockers are helpful in relieving syncope, palpitations, and chest pain. For preventing infective endocarditis, the client may receive antibiotics prophylactically before any invasive procedures.

AORTIC VALVE DISEASE

Aortic valve disease is far less common than mitral valve disease but often occurs in conjunction with mitral valve disease. Aortic stenosis obstructs the forward flow of blood during systole from the left ventricle into the aorta and systemic circulation. This obstruction to flow creates a resistance to ejection and increased pressure in the left ventricle. *Aortic regurgitation* (aortic insufficiency) allows blood to leak back from the aorta into the left ventricle. During systole, blood that is ejected into the aorta reenters the left ventricle. To maintain normal pressures, the left ventricle hypertrophies. Both aortic stenosis and regurgitation overwork the left ventricle.

Etiology and Risk Factors

Aortic stenosis can be caused by several congenital defects of the aortic valve and by two degenerative processes: (1) calcification of the valve in older adults and (2) retraction and stiffening of the valve from rheumatic fever. As the population in the United States ages, the incidence of aortic stenosis from calcification has been rising.[4]

Aortic regurgitation is most often a result of infectious disorders such as rheumatic fever, syphilis, and infective endocarditis. Connective tissue disorders can also lead to aortic regurgitation.

Pathophysiology

AORTIC STENOSIS

In the client with aortic stenosis, the orifice of the aortic valve becomes narrowed, which causes a decrease in the blood flow from the left ventricle into the aorta. The pressure within the left ventricle rises as the blood is ejected through the narrowed opening. A pressure gradient develops between the left ventricle and the aorta. The elevated pressure in the left ventricle during systole causes the ventricle to hypertrophy. Dilation of the left ventricle occurs over time when there is a deterioration of the contractility of the hypertrophied muscle. Eventually, dilation and hypertrophy of the left ventricle are unable to maintain adequate cardiac output, resulting in elevated left ventricular end-diastolic pressure, decreased cardiac output, and increased pulmonary hypertension (Fig. 55–4C).

AORTIC REGURGITATION

Aortic regurgitation is a diastolic event in which blood that is propelled forward into the aorta regurgitates back into the left ventricle through an incompetent valve. This causes abnormal filling and a volume overload of the left ventricle. The magnitude of the overload depends on the severity of the incompetence. However, a small incompetent area can result in significant aortic regurgitation over time.

Because the left ventricle receives blood from both the atrium and the systemic circulation, aortic regurgitation gradually increases left ventricular end-diastolic volume. Left ventricular stroke volume is increased to produce an effective forward-moving volume into the systemic circulation. There is a compensatory dilation of the left ventricle but minimal increase in left ventricular end-diastolic pressure.[4] The compensatory mechanisms of dilation and hypertrophy help to maintain an adequate cardiac output. As the condition progresses and the contractile state of the myocardium declines, however, cardiac output falls (Fig. 55–5D).

Clinical Manifestations

AORTIC STENOSIS

Clinical manifestations of aortic stenosis tend to occur gradually and late in the course of the disease. There is usually a long latent period in which the client is asymptomatic. Manifestations begin to appear as the obstruction and ventricular pressure increase to critical levels. Angina pectoris (chest pain) is a frequent finding in approximately 60% of clients. The character of the angina is similar to that in clients with coronary artery disease, and pain is commonly brought on by exertion and relieved by rest. Myocardial oxygen consumption is higher in clients with aortic stenosis because of the hypertrophy of the left ventricle, and this probably accounts for the angina.

Syncope, another common clinical manifestation, also occurs during exertion because of a fixed cardiac output and an increased demand.[4] Syncope at rest may be due to dysrhythmias. Exertional dyspnea, paroxysmal nocturnal dyspnea, and pulmonary edema occur with increasing pulmonary venous hypertension attributable to left ventricular failure. In severe aortic stenosis, additional manifestations may include palpitations, fatigue, and visual disturbances.

On auscultation, the systolic murmur may be associated with a diminished second heart sound and an early ejection click. A systolic thrill is present over the aortic areas.

AORTIC REGURGITATION

Clients with chronic severe aortic regurgitation may be asymptomatic for a long time. During this time, the left ventricle gradually enlarges. Clients may complain of an uncomfortable awareness of the heartbeat and palpitations. These manifestations are due to the large left ventricular stroke volume with rapid diastolic runoff. This is also apparent with prominent pulsations in the neck and even head-bobbing with each heartbeat. Sinus tachycardia or premature ventricular contractions may make palpitations more pronounced.

On physical examination, systolic blood pressure may be due to the large stroke volume and a decreased diastolic blood pressure due to the regurgitation and distal runoff. Carotid artery pulsations may be exaggerated. The arterial pulse pressure widens, and palpable pulse amplitude increases. This may be noted as a sudden sharp pulse, followed by a swift collapse of the diastolic pulse (Corrigan's or water-hammer pulse). Auscultation reveals a soft, high-pitched, blowing decrescendo diastolic murmur heard best at the second right intercostal space and radiating to the left sternal border.

Outcome Management

■ Medical Management

The goals of medical management are to maintain or improve cardiac function and activity tolerance. When the client reaches maximum benefit from medications, surgery may be warranted.

AORTIC STENOSIS

Noninvasive assessment of clients with Doppler echocardiography should be performed. Advise clients with known or suspected critical obstruction of the aortic valve to avoid vigorous physical activity. Clients with mild obstruction may continue exercise if it is tolerated.

Prophylactic antibiotics may be given on an individual basis for invasive medical or dental procedures for prevention of infective endocarditis. Digitalis and diuretics that are usually used for ventricular failure must be used with caution.[4] Beta-blockers are not usually ordered because they can depress myocardial function and induce left ventricular failure. Cardiac dysrhythmias should be treated pharmacologically.

AORTIC REGURGITATION

Medical intervention for aortic regurgitation is the same as for aortic stenosis: relief of manifestations of heart failure and prevention of infection in the already deformed aortic cusps.

TRICUSPID VALVE DISEASE

Tricuspid stenosis, or *regurgitation*, usually develops from rheumatic fever or in combination with other structural disorders of the heart.[4] Because the tricuspid valve is on the right side of the heart, the major hemodynamic alterations are decreased cardiac output and increased right atrial pressure. The inability of the right atrium to propel blood across the stenosed valve may account for these changes. With *tricuspid regurgitation*, although pressure in the right atrium is elevated, it is due to regurgitation of the blood volume in the right ventricle back into the right atrium during systole.

Clinical manifestations of tricuspid stenosis are dyspnea and fatigue, pulsations in the neck, and peripheral edema. Physical assessment reveals prominent waves in the neck veins as the atrium vigorously contracts against the stenotic valve. A diastolic murmur is heard best along the left lower sternal border. The murmur increases with inspiration. The ECG reveals tall, tented P waves in leads II, III, and aV. Tricuspid insufficiency causes hepatic congestion and peripheral edema. Often atrial fibrillation is present, and jugular waves are evident. The murmur is holosystolic along the left sternal border.

Tricuspid stenosis usually responds well to diuretics and digitalis therapy. If the leaflets are severely stenotic, surgery may be required.

PULMONIC VALVE DISEASE

Abnormalities of the *pulmonic valve* are usually congenital defects. Few lesions develop after birth. Pulmonary hypertension, caused by mitral stenosis, pulmonary emboli, or chronic lung disease, can precipitate functional pulmonary regurgitation. Pulmonic stenosis and regurgitation lead to a decrease in cardiac output because blood does not reach the left side of the heart in adequate supply for metabolic demands. Pulmonic regurgitation may lead to dyspnea and fatigue. The murmur is a high-pitched diastolic blow along the left sternal border. There are no significant changes in the ECG.

Pulmonic stenosis causes similar clinical manifestations, but the murmur is often a crescendo-decrescendo type. Right-sided heart failure can also develop.

Intervention focuses on ameliorating the underlying cause and right-sided heart failure.

Outcome Management

Nursing Management of the Medical Client

Nursing assessment should address the type, severity, and progress of the valvular disorder; presence of fatigue; clinical manifestations of heart failure; heart rhythm (including ECG); vital signs; auscultation and palpation of the heart; the client's support systems; and the degree of knowledge that the client and family have concerning the nature of and intervention in the disorder.

The main focus of nursing intervention in valvular heart disease is to help the client maintain a normal cardiac output, thereby preventing manifestations of heart failure, venous congestion, and inadequate tissue perfusion. To evaluate the effectiveness of therapeutic interventions, perform ongoing hemodynamic assessment. Monitor vital signs closely every 1 to 4 hours. A decrease in cardiac output is manifested in a compensatory rise in heart rate, a drop in blood pressure, or a decrease in urinary output. Carefully auscultate the chest every 4 hours to identify the presence of abnormal breath sounds (crackles, rhonchi) or heart gallops (S_3, S_4).

Self-Care

Clients with valvular heart disease require lifelong management. With a sincere desire to understand and accept each client's response to chronic illness, you can help these clients adapt to difficult lifestyle changes and achieve a positive sense of well-being.

Clients may find it difficult to cope physically and psychosocially after hospital discharge. The chronicity of valvular heart disease and its potential complications can create an atmosphere of uncertainty, fear, and frustration. Take time to help the client identify support people, personal strengths, and coping strategies. Assess how the client handles frustration or anger and which activities are particularly relaxing. Address the client's fears and misconceptions. In some instances, counseling referrals may help. Stress the importance of follow-up physical examinations and intervention.

Before discharge, prepare detailed teaching material for the client and family concerning the therapeutic regimen, the disease process, factors contributing to manifestations, and the rationale for intervention. Give information concerning prescribed medications. Medications frequently prescribed include digoxin, quinidine, diuretics, beta-blockers, potassium supplements, anticoagulants, and sometimes prophylactic antibiotics. Explain their rationale, dosages, side effects, and special considerations in their use.

Review exercise prescriptions with the client. Clients with aortic stenosis often require activity restrictions. The client should demonstrate ability to pace activity, verbalize improvement in fatigue, and accept activity restrictions.

Address dietary restrictions, and plan interdisciplinary follow-up. Make sure the client knows whom to call when questions arise.

Surgical Management

When conservative medical intervention fails to improve hemodynamic status in valvular disorders, surgical intervention is indicated. Mitral valve repair is becoming more common because it carries relatively few complications, good long-term survival, and low hospital mortality.[24] Additionally, long-term anticoagulant therapy is not needed.[14]

Surgical intervention should be considered for aortic stenosis when the pressure gradient is greater than 50 mm Hg or the valve orifice is less than 0.8 cm[2]. The prognosis for clients with symptomatic aortic stenosis is poor without surgical intervention. The incidence of sudden death rises once myocardial failure develops. Surgical replacement of the incompetent valve provides the only effective long-term intervention for aortic regurgitation. A high percentage of clients with aortic regurgitation and aortic stenosis show striking clinical improvement with valve replacement.[4]

CONGENITAL DISORDERS

Congenital heart disorders result from faulty development of cardiac structures in utero. Congenital disorders include septal defects, vessel stenosis, abnormally positioned vessels, and patency of the ductus arteriosus. Advances in the medical and surgical treatment of people with congenital heart disease have assisted an ever-growing number of clients to survive into adulthood. As this number grows, medical and nursing support has grown also.

With today's available treatments, about 85% of children with congenital heart disease will survive into adulthood.[8] Therefore, we can expect to see more adults with congenital defects in the future.[19] Each congenital defect brings its own morbidity and mortality statistics; in general, however, people with the less complex defects will have a longer survival than those with more complex defects (the course for such defects is still uncertain).

Operations may be palliative or corrective. Most adult clients today underwent their surgical procedures many years ago during the developmental phase of these interventions. Their course would probably be quite different from that followed today. Many refinements in surgical techniques continue to be developed so that clinical outcomes vary significantly.

Many people with a congenital heart defect have remained asymptomatic; others have had varying levels of functional ability. Clients may have both residual problems (those not corrected or improved at the time of the surgical repair) and sequelae (results of the surgery).[19] Common lifelong problems include the risk of infective endocarditis in clients with artificial valves or with suture repair of an atrial septal defect. It is not uncommon for a client with a repaired coarctation of the aorta to find that the aorta has gradually become narrowed again. In such cases, hypertension may develop. Clients who as children underwent repair for cyanotic defects tend to experience sequelae and complications in adulthood.[19] There may be some degree of exercise intolerance that can be better managed after proper stress testing.

Dysrhythmias frequently present a lifelong complication. Clients who have had intraventricular repairs may present with ventricular dysrhythmias or complete heart block. A 24-hour Holter monitor and stress testing may help evaluate the client's tolerance for activity.

Many people who have had surgical procedures as infants and children had to have repeated operations as they "outgrew" their repairs or prosthetic devices. Our growing geriatric population also may be experiencing unknown late consequences of congenital heart disease or surgical repair. It is important to encourage these people to participate in long-term follow-up.

Your role as a nurse who is caring for the adult with congenital heart disease varies with the setting. However, you play an integral role in helping these clients achieve optimal health and functioning. Nursing assessment, intervention, education, and follow-up are directed toward improving functional levels, managing medications, psychosocial adjustment, and preventing complications.

CARDIAC SURGERY

Cardiac surgery is performed when the probability of survival with a useful life is greater with surgical treatment than with nonsurgical treatment. The first heart surgery, performed in 1923 by Cutler and Levine,[43] was a repair of a stenosed mitral valve. Since that time, heart surgery has been revolutionized by the development of open heart techniques that allow surgeons to visualize the heart directly while they explore, cut, repair, and sew. Further advances include minimally invasive open heart surgery. These improved operating conditions have enabled today's surgeons to replace diseased valves with prosthetic valves, to repair severe congenital lesions, and to perform heart transplantation procedures. Today, under ideal conditions, the hospital mortality rate associated with cardiac surgery should be approaching zero. However, reporting the results of cardiac surgery by hospital mortality alone (as is frequently done in the popular press) is not sufficient. The preoperative condition of the client's heart and other body systems greatly influences the results of cardiac surgery. The identification of incremental risk factors should continue to improve results.

TYPES OF HEART SURGERY

There are three types of cardiac surgery:

1. *Reparative* procedures are likely to produce cure or excellent and prolonged improvement. Examples: closure of a patent ductus arteriosus, atrial septal defect, and ventricular septal defect; repair of mitral stenosis; and simple repair of tetralogy of Fallot.
2. *Reconstructive* procedures are more complex. They are not always curative, and reoperation may be needed. Examples: coronary artery bypass grafting (CABG) and reconstruction of an incompetent mitral, tricuspid, or aortic valve.
3. *Substitutional* procedures are not usually curative because of the preoperative condition of the client. Examples: valve replacement, cardiac replacement by transplantation, ventricular replacement or assistance, and cardiac replacement by mechanical devices.

■ VALVULAR SURGERY

The repair or replacement of cardiac valves with acquired stenosis or incompetence is not considered curative, but the results are generally good and long-lasting. Cure is usually unattainable because of the preoperative condition of the heart or other body systems. Indications for surgery include the following:

1. Progressive impairment of cardiac function due to scarring and thickening of the valve with either impaired narrowing of the valvular opening (stenosis), or incomplete closure (insufficiency, regurgitation)

2. Gradual enlargement of the heart with manifestations of decreased activity, shortness of breath, and heart failure.

3. Surgical therapy for mitral valve stenosis, which can include valve repair. Valve repair can be accomplished if the preoperative assessment indicates that the valve is pliable. If the valve is not pliable, valve replacement is necessary. In clients with mitral regurgitation, valve reconstruction or annuloplasty may be done. This may include the use of a flexible ring that is sewn into the valve for stabilization. Aortic stenosis may be surgically treated with valve replacement or balloon aortic valvuloplasty. In the valvuloplasty procedure, a catheter with a balloon is used to dilate the valve orifice (Fig. 55–6). Surgery for the client with aortic regurgitation is not always the treatment of choice but may be considered.

Artificial cardiac valves are continuing to show improvements in design, safety, function, and durability. Mechanical and tissue prosthetic valves are available. The type of valve prosthesis used is based on a number of considerations. The surgeon primarily considers (1) the client's tolerance of anticoagulation and (2) the durability of the valve.

Clients with mechanical valves require continuous anticoagulation therapy for the remainder of their lives. Therefore, if the client has a preoperative history of bleeding or noncompliance with pharmacologic regimens, the surgeon may decide to use a tissue valve. The overall advantages and disadvantages of tissue and mechanical valves are almost equal. Mechanical valves are very durable, but anticoagulant therapy is necesssary; no anticoagulation therapy is needed for tissue valves, but they are less durable. Some physicians recommend mechanical valves in clients younger than 65 or 70 years of age and tissue valves in clients 70 years or older.[4] Artificial valves are shown in Figure 55–7.

Potential complications of heart valves include a risk of thrombus formation, especially in mechanical valves. Newer types of heart valves have shown reduced rates of thrombosis. Most clients require long-term anticoagulation therapy. The major drawback with tissue valves is durability. The leaflets of these valves may degenerate or calcify or may develop structural abnormalities. Mitral valves tend to fail usually because of the higher stress on the valve. The rate of tissue valve failure is 2% to 5% for the first 6 years, with the rate accelerating thereafter. Almost every client with a tissue valve will require replacement eventually.[4]

Management of the client after heart surgery is discussed later in this section.

■ HEART TRANSPLANTATION

Cardiac transplantation is now a standard and effective treatment for clients with end-stage cardiac disease. Formerly, widespread application of heart transplantation depended on the development of improved immunosuppressive therapy. The use of cyclosporine has resulted in superior results. Later favorable results resulted from the rapidly accumulating experience.

In 1998, 2389 hearts were transplanted in the United States. The number of clients who died while on the waiting list was 773, and 4167 clients remained on the list at the end of 1998.[25] As of 1999, 85% of heart transplant clients survived 1 year and 76% survived 3 years.[25] Heart transplant recipients who die following the

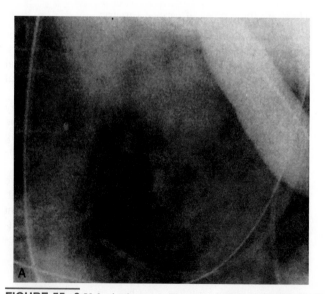
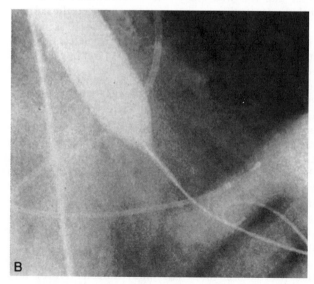

FIGURE 55–6 Valvuloplasty. *A*, The valvuloplasty balloon is inflated across the aortic valve. Note the indentation ("waist") in the balloon. *B*, The valvuloplasty balloon inflated across the aortic valve after dilation. Note the disappearance of the indentation seen in *A*. (From Barden, C., et al. [1990]. Balloon aortic valvuloplasty: Nursing care implications. *Critical Care Nurse, 10*[6], 26.)

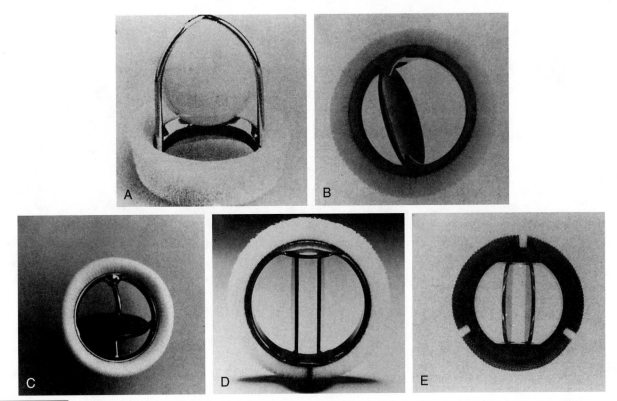

FIGURE 55–7 Prosthetic heart valves. *A,* Starr-Edwards cage and ball valve with a cloth sewing ring and bare struts. *B,* Omniscience valve. *C,* Medtronic-Hall valve. *D,* St. Jude valve. *E,* Carbomedics bileaflet valve. (From Braunwald, E. [1997]. *Heart disease: A textbook of cardiovascular medicine* [5th ed., p. 1062]. Philadelphia: W. B. Saunders.)

procedure usually do so within the first 30 days postoperatively. Clients at greatest risk are those who deteriorate rapidly before the transplant procedure. Infection, cardiac failure, or rejection is usually the cause of death.

Potential candidates must be evaluated and screened. Their cardiac status is evaluated to determine the need for the heart transplant. The candidates are also evaluated for underlying conditions that predispose to an unfavorable outcome. Selection criteria for heart transplantation are shown in Box 55–3.

The current *orthotopic* technique retains a large portion of the right and left atrium in the recipient and implants the donor heart to the atria (Fig. 55–8). Cardiopulmonary bypass is used during the operation (see later). Temporary pacemaker wires and chest drainage catheters are inserted.

Another type of procedure, the *heterotopic* technique, is performed only rarely. The donor heart is placed parallel to the recipient's heart (Fig. 55–9). The right side of the client's heart can continue to function while the dysfunctional left side of the heart is bypassed.

Recognition and treatment of rejection are the most difficult tasks in heart transplantation. The most reliable technique for assessing organ rejection is the endomyocardial biopsy, which enables identification of the diffuse interstitial infiltrate associated with rejection.

Drug therapy is adjusted to give the maximum amount of immunosuppression with the minimum amount of side effects. This is a very individualistic regimen. There is a higher risk of acute rejection soon after transplantation that decreases dramatically after 3 months. Immunosuppression treatment relies on several drugs: cyclosporine,

prednisone, methylprednisolone, and azathioprine (Table 55–3). Even with this intensive regimen, 84% of heart transplant recipients experience at least one episode of rejection during the first 3 months.

For these rejection episodes, pulse therapy with methylprednisolone is used. High doses are given for 3 consecutive days, then gradually reduced over the next 2 weeks. Because of the side effects of increased steroid therapy, the client must be monitored carefully for infec-

---

BOX 55–3   Selection Criteria for Heart Transplantation

- End-stage heart disease
- Current medical management is unsuccessful
- New York Heart Association class III or IV
- Prognosis of less than 1 year to live
- Under 65 years of age
- Nonsmoker
- No drug or alcohol abuse
- Client is well motivated and will follow postoperative instructions and medications
- No underlying condition that would limit survival:

  - Systemic infection
  - Irreversible hepatic insufficiency
  - Irreversible renal insufficiency
  - Cancer
  - Active peptic ulcer
  - Recent pulmonary embolus
  - Irreversible pulmonary insufficiency

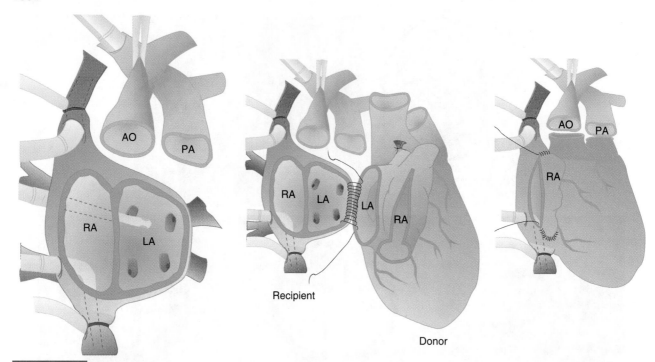

FIGURE 55–8 Orthotopic technique of heart transplantation. AO, aorta; PA, pulmonary artery; RA, right atrium; LA, left atrium.

tions. If the steroid therapy has not been successful in reversing the rejection, other, more aggressive therapy is begun. Equine antithymocyte globulin or OKT3 monoclonal antibody therapy may be used. Some clients have persistent recurrent rejection episodes, which may be treated with total lymphoid irradiation. In the long term, survival and rehabilitation can be expected in most recipients.

■ ASSISTED CIRCULATION AND MECHANICAL HEARTS

Cardiac failure leads to multisystem organ failure if it is not reversed. Sometimes, despite maximal therapy, the failing heart cannot adequately respond to therapy. If, for various reasons, cardiac transplantation is not an immediate option, other therapies are sought. It is in these cases that assisted circulation devices or mechanical hearts seem to be the only option (see Intra-aortic balloon counterpulsation). Other modalities being used in practice include ventricular assist devices, implantable left ventricular assist systems, and orthotopic biventricular replacement prostheses (artificial hearts). Many of these devices offer a bridge to transplantation when the client's heart is failing and a donor heart is not readily available. These devices can maintain a client until transplantation can be performed. The total artificial heart is available only as a bridge to transplantation. Research is continuing on a device that will be suitable for long-term outpatient use.[20]

■ OPEN HEART SURGERY

Cardiopulmonary bypass is used during cardiac surgery to divert the client's unoxygenated blood and to return re-oxygenated blood to the client's circulation. This technique, called extracorporeal circulation (ECC), is accomplished with a pump oxygenator (heart-lung machine). Diversion of the client's blood allows the surgeon to visualize the heart directly during the operation. The pump oxygenator, more than any other device, has made sophisticated open heart surgery possible (Fig. 55–10). It is used to:

- Divert circulation from the heart and lungs, providing the surgeon with a bloodless operative field
- Perform all gas exchange functions for the body while the client's cardiopulmonary system is at rest
- Filter, rewarm, or cool the blood

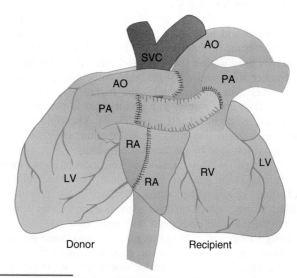

FIGURE 55–9 Heterotopic technique of heart transplantation. AO, aorta; PA, pulmonary artery; RA, right atrium; RV, right ventricle; LV, left ventricle; SVC, superior vena cava.

TABLE 55-3	IMMUNOSUPPRESSIVE PROTOCOL FOR HEART TRANSPLANTATION	
Medication	**Early Postoperative**	**Late Postoperative**
Cyclosporine	6–10 mg/kg/day PO* *or* 0.5–2 mg/kg/day IV	3–6 mg/kg/day PO
or		
Tacrolimus	0.15–0.30 mg/kg/day PO	0.15–0.30 mg/kg/day PO
Methyprednisolone	500 mg IV after cardiopulmonary bypass	125 mg q 8 hr × 3 doses
Prednisone	1 mg/kg/day PO tapered to 0.4 mg/kg	0.1–0.2 mg/kg/day PO
Azathioprine	2 mg/kg/day PO†	1–2 mg/kg/day PO

* Not given if preoperative serum creatinine is greater than 1.5 mg/dl, given IV instead.
† Not given if white blood cell count is below 4000 mm².
PO, orally.
From Braunwald, E. (1997). *Heart disease: A textbook of cardiovascular medicine* (5th ed.). Philadelphia: W. B. Saunders.

• Circulate oxygenated, filtered blood back into the arterial system

Although the pump oxygenator is considered safe, there are some risks; for instance, the pump can crush and destroy blood cells, sludging of cells can lead to thrombus formation, or air emboli can form. Other complications related to ECC are shock, hemorrhage, fluid overload, hemolysis, and kidney or lung damage.

Outcome Management

Medical Management Before Cardiac Surgery

Preoperative laboratory tests include urine tests and blood electrolyte, enzyme, and coagulation studies. Important diagnostic studies that provide valuable information about cardiac status include the ECG, echocardiogram, vectorcardiogram, chest x-ray films, and cardiac catheterization.

Any physiologic imbalance or problem in cardiac or respiratory status is corrected when possible by means of rest, diet, medication, or other appropriate therapy. Physiologic baselines should be established for postoperative comparison of vital signs, weight, and laboratory values.

Preparation for surgery in general is discussed in Chapter 15. For the client undergoing the stress of heart surgery, special preparation and instruction are needed.

ASSESSMENT

The client undergoing heart surgery has probably experienced cardiopulmonary clinical manifestations for months or years. Data to collect during the initial assessment include the following:

• The primary cardiovascular problem requiring surgical correction and its duration
• The purpose of the surgery and the risk involved stated in the client's own words
• Past cardiopulmonary illnesses that may predispose the client to postoperative complications (e.g., bacterial endocarditis, pulmonary embolus, allergy, abnormal bleeding)
• The degree of cardiac impairment (e.g., does the client have manifestations when at rest or only during exertion?)
• The types of medications, herbal or natural substances, and interventions that the client has received or is currently receiving (e.g., digitalis, quinidine, oxygen)

Note the client's psychological readiness for surgery and his or her reaction to the need for heart surgery. The client may initially experience shock and grief over the impending surgery. Chief concerns may be helplessness and fear of disability or death.

The psychological preparation of the cardiac surgery client is very important. Many hospitals throughout the United States have extensive preoperative education programs that greatly reduce client and family anxiety. Such a program should include a thorough explanation of the preoperative, intraoperative, and postoperative procedures. Also helpful is the introduction of the client to involved health care team members and the health care facility environment. Box 55-4 provides a list of topics for education. Your institution probably has written material for you to use.

Allow clients to tell you in their own words about their heart problem and the surgery. Correct any misconceptions, using pictures and a model of the heart. Clients tend to ask the greatest number of questions about what will happen to them in the recovery room and intensive care unit (ICU).

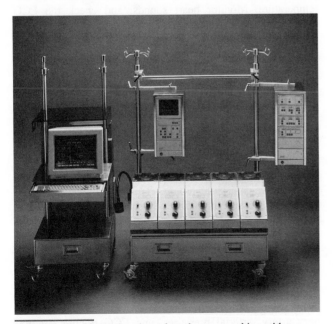

FIGURE 55-10 Stöckert heart-lung bypass machine with a computer-aided perfusion system—a type of pump-oxygenator, or heart-lung bypass machine. Machines like this are used during open heart surgery to circulate oxygenated blood while the heart is unable to pump. (Courtesy of Sorin Biomedical, Irvine, CA.)

| BOX 55-4 | Guidelines to Preparing the Client Undergoing Cardiac Surgery |

Plan teaching well in advance of the surgical date, if possible. By the time of surgery, the client should be prepared by the following:

1. Describe the surgical procedure:
   a. All steps, including heart-lung machine
   b. Review of anatomy and physiology of heart and valves
   c. Brief definition of unfamiliar technical terms
   d. Length of time in surgery and approximate time of first visit by family
   e. Giving the client pictures of the heart and involved valve for future reference
2. Describe the intensive care unit (ICU) environment and monitoring equipment:
   a. Cardiac monitor and alarm
   b. Endotracheal (ET) tube and projected length of time with ET tube in place
   c. Mechanical ventilator and alarm
   d. Suctioning procedure
   e. Arterial line and automatic blood pressure cuff
   f. Any limitation on visits from family
   g. Chest tubes or mediastinal tubes
   h. Nasogastric tube and length of NPO (nothing by mouth) status
   i. Urinary catheter
   j. High noise level in ICU
   k. Multiple intravenous lines and fluids
3. Describe preoperative preparation:
   a. Showering with antimicrobial soap
   b. Shaving of chest, abdomen, neck, and groin
   c. Special cardiac studies: echocardiogram, electrocardiogram, cardiac catheterization
4. Describe comfort measures:
   a. Pain relief
   b. Turning, range-of-motion exercises
   c. Out of bed next morning
   d. Medication for sleep, if needed

Explain that they will awaken from anesthesia with a chest tube in place. Discuss the ventilator that will assist the client's breathing for the first 8 to 24 hours. Remind clients that during this time they will be unable to talk. Explain that an IV line for fluid or blood will be inserted in an arm and that various equipment that continuously monitors vital signs will be attached to their skin.

Answer questions concerning the necessity of using blood products. Use these facts to respond to concerns about transfusion. Blood transfusions postoperatively are used only as needed; blood is screened carefully, and there is little risk of contracting acquired immunodeficiency syndrome (AIDS). Family members can be screened for possible donation of blood. Emphasize that although the client will experience pain, the pain will be swiftly relieved by medication and comfort measures.

Finally, explain that the client will be awakened frequently in the ICU for vital nursing assessments and interventions. Give examples of scheduled activities: vital signs every 15 minutes; temperature every 2 hours; frequent turning, coughing, and deep breathing; blood drawn for tests every morning.

Clients also need information concerning discharge from the ICU and health care facility. Explain the average length of stay in the ICU, the room to which the client will return from the ICU, the average length of stay in the health care facility, and the diet and activities permitted once the client returns home. Be general in the discussion. Remember, many unforeseen events can arise and greatly alter the postoperative course.

Give verbal and written information concerning health care facility services, rules, and regulations; visiting hours; the chaplain's name and visiting hours (if appropriate); and names of clinical nurse-specialists and other health care professionals who can be contacted for information.

Most clients benefit from a tour of the recovery room and ICU. If they are not physically able to participate in a tour, audiovisual material is helpful.

Familiarize the client with the equipment that will be used in the ICU (e.g., chest drainage tubes, oxygen apparatus, ventilators, cardiac monitors, IV setups). Reassure the client that lights and alarm noises are part of the critical care environment and are not indicators that something is wrong.

■ Nursing Care Before Cardiac Surgery

Preparation the evening before and the day of surgery is essentially the same as the preparation of clients for any thoracic surgery (see Chapter 62). The client may take several showers with an antimicrobial soap; skin preparation (shaving) for a thoracotomy is performed in the operating room. If the surgeon plans a CABG, the legs may also be prepared in the operating room (see Chapter 15).

■ Nursing Management After Cardiac Surgery
ASSESSMENT

The most reliable measures of cardiovascular function and tissue perfusion are the vital signs, including arterial blood pressure, pulses, venous and left heart filling pressures, and temperature. Monitor heart sounds, and check the ECG continuously as appropriate. Stabilization of vital signs after heart surgery usually indicates adequate cardiovascular function. Conversely, severe deviations indicate a complication such as hemorrhage, shock, cardiac tamponade, or infection. The normal ranges for each vital sign after cardiac surgery and the meaning of deviations follow.

ARTERIAL BLOOD PRESSURE. For an accurate blood pressure reading postoperatively, an 18- or 20-gauge polytetrafluoroethylene (Teflon) catheter is inserted into an artery (usually the radial artery) and attached to a strain-gauge transducer via stiff connecting tubing called pressure transmission tubing. This is connected to an electronic pressure monitor and oscilloscope. The monitor provides numerical pressure readings and produces a continuous tracing of the arterial pressure wave form (see Bridge to Critical Care). The arterial line is usually irrigated (continuously or at intervals) with heparinized water or saline. The arterial line is sometimes used as a route for obtaining blood for laboratory studies.

Most pressure monitors are able to monitor the pulmonary artery, arterial pressures, and ECG tracing simultaneously. This capability assists in determining the possible effect of surgery on hemodynamic status and cardiac output and demonstrates the effect of a dysrhythmia or change in body temperature on cardiac output.

In general, the physician will request that the blood pressure be maintained between 20 mm Hg above and 20 mm Hg below the baseline blood pressure. Frequently, this is a mean arterial pressure of 70 mm Hg or above. After mitral and aortic valve surgery, clients may tolerate a low systolic blood pressure of 90 mm Hg without difficulty. After coronary artery surgery, clients may not tolerate systolic blood pressure drops of more than 10 mm Hg below preoperative baseline because the myocardium may not be adequately perfused. Maintaining a sufficient diastolic blood pressure is also important because the myocardium receives 70% of its blood supply during this phase of the cardiac cycle. Careful assessment and monitoring of the client's hemodynamic status are essential.

Hypertension is also dangerous in a client who has undergone a CABG procedure because high blood pressure may cause the new graft to break loose or leak. Vasoactive medications (e.g., vasodilators such as nifedipine, nitroprusside, phentolamine, labetalol) can be used to improve cardiac function.

PULSES. Check radial pulse for rate, rhythm, and volume. A rapid radial pulse may indicate dysrhythmia, shock, fear, fever, hypoxia, heart failure, or hemorrhage. A slow radial pulse may indicate heart block or severe anoxia. Check the apical radial pulse for a pulse deficit, which may indicate atrial fibrillation, a frequent complication of mitral stenosis.

Assess peripheral pulses. Absence of pedal pulses may indicate the presence of peripheral emboli blocking a blood vessel in the extremity. Report this finding immediately to the surgeon. If pulses are absent, assess all pulses in the extremity and check the lower extremities for coldness, pallor, or cyanosis.

VENOUS AND LEFT-HEART FILLING PRESSURES. The central venous and pulmonary artery pressures are usually monitored postoperatively. A pressure higher than normal may be acceptable after open heart surgery, because a heart that has been diseased and then subjected to surgical trauma is weak and needs a higher filling pressure to strengthen the force of myocardial contraction and to maintain an adequate cardiac output. Therefore, the surgeon usually specifies values for venous and pulmonary artery pressures that address this problem.

If a pulmonary artery catheter is in place, a pulmonary artery wedge pressure (PAWP) can be obtained and cardiac output measured by the thermodilution method. The PAWP is a reflection of the left atrial filling pressure. (See Bridge to Critical Care, Chapter 57, which covers the Swan-Ganz catheter and these measurements.)

Causes of abnormally elevated central venous pressure (CVP) and left heart filling pressure include hypervolemia and ineffective myocardial contractions. Abnormally decreased CVP and left heart filling pressure result from hypovolemia.

BODY TEMPERATURE. Initially, the client has a low temperature of 35° to 36° C (95° to 96.8° F) because of hypothermia induced during surgery. With careful warming in a heating blanket, the client's temperature may become normal within 4 hours. Be aware that the blood pressure may drop as body temperature rises as a result of vasodilation.

The temperature may rise 1° to 1.5° C (2° or 3° F) above normal during the first or second day postoperatively and may remain elevated for 3 to 4 days. Treat this elevation with acetaminophen suppositories as prescribed and with minimal bed covering. For persistent elevations, apply ice bags or use a hypothermia blanket if prescribed.

Report abnormal findings, such as an elevated temperature to 38.5° C (101° F) or higher or an elevation that persists for more than 4 or 5 days. Abnormal temperature elevation may result from infection, dehydration, hemolysis due to transfusion reaction, or atelectasis. The untoward effects of the elevated temperature include increased metabolic demands (which increase the work of the heart), dehydration, and hypovolemia.

Abnormally low temperatures ranging from 34.4° C (94° F) to 36° C (96.8° F) result from shock or cardiac decompensation. The physician may order a warming blanket to increase temperature. Rectal, oral, or tympanic temperature readings are the most accurate.

RESPIRATIONS. To assess respiratory function, prevent respiratory complications, and provide appropriate intervention, closely monitor the rate and depth of respirations, the presence of dyspnea, and the presence of wheezing.

Make certain the ventilator is set at a rate that adequately ventilates the client and delivers an appropriate tidal volume and oxygen percentage. A conscious client may initiate respirations in addition to those delivered by the ventilator (usually the assist light will come on). Adjust the rate, tidal volume, and oxygen level to ensure adequate ventilation of the lungs and oxygenation of the blood. Adjustments are usually determined by arterial blood gas (ABG) analysis and the assessments by the physician and the nurse.

Assessment of depth of respiration may reveal shallow respirations, which may be due to pain. Give a narcotic if vital signs are stable.

Assessment of dyspnea may reveal that the client is "fighting" the ventilator (breathing against instead of with the machine), which can lead to inadequate ventilation. The client may feel short of breath. Airway obstruction (possibly due to excessive secretions), pain, fear, anoxia, acidosis, hemorrhage, and improper placement of the tube may cause difficulty in breathing and must be investigated immediately. The physician usually orders ABG studies and a chest film. The ventilator settings may need adjustment, and the client may require sedation (see Bridge to Critical Care for ventilators, Chapter 63). While the client is on the ventilator, make sure the ventilator alarms are functioning. Never turn off the alarms, not even during suctioning.

Wheezing results from pulmonary edema, bronchospasm, or airway obstruction. It may be treated with bronchodilators.

Assess the amount of pulmonary secretion. Is it copious or scant?

Assess the color of sputum. Sputum is normally white and translucent. Yellow suggests infection and represents the presence of WBCs. Green represents old retained secretions with the breakdown of WBCs. Green and foul-smelling secretions usually suggest *Pseudomonas* infection. Red denotes fresh blood. Streaking with red suggests upper airway or tracheal bleeding. Brown represents old blood residue.

Assess for accompanying signs of retained secretions, such as apprehension, perspiration, rapid pulse, dyspnea, cyanosis, and gurgling respirations.

Assessment of respiration in the pre-extubation period involves drawing blood for ABG analysis and obtaining respiratory values, including inspiratory effort and tidal volume. The client is ready for extubation if these values are within normal limits.

Respiratory assessment in the postextubation period begins with careful assessment of clinical manifestations of respiratory distress. Check the rate, depth, and character of respirations frequently. Note the client's skin color and vital signs; changes may indicate inadequate ventilation and the need for reintubation. Perform ABG analysis to determine whether the client is breathing adequately after extubation.

HEART SOUNDS. For the first 2 days postoperatively, assess heart sounds at least every 4 hours. Pericardial rubs are commonly caused by the irritation and inflammation from surgery. A new murmur may indicate valve problems. Notify the physician if one develops. A gallop probably indicates hypervolemia. See discussion of cardiovascular assessment in Chapter 54.

ELECTROCARDIOGRAM TRACINGS. Monitor the electrical activity of the client's heart continuously for at least 3 or 4 days after surgery. Observe carefully for abnormal ECG tracings; heart block, ventricular tachycardia, and atrial fibrillation commonly complicate open heart surgery. The physician requests 12-lead ECGs preoperatively, immediately postoperatively, and before discharge to observe for signs of perioperative infarction.

Most dysrhythmias can be treated effectively with antidysrhythmic medications. Clients with certain life-threatening dysrhythmias require defibrillation or cardioversion (see Chapter 57).

During surgery, the surgeon may implant atrial or ventricular pacing wires. These small wires lead from the myocardium through the chest wall. They can be connected to an external pacemaker and are used to treat bradycardia or heart block. These wires should always be insulated. When connecting them to a pacemaker, wear rubber gloves. Microshocks to these wires may result in atrial or ventricular fibrillation. Atrial pacing wires can also be connected to the chest leads of an ECG machine for differential diagnosis of atrial dysrhythmias.

CHEST DRAINAGE. The surgeon inserts chest tubes to drain air and fluid from the pleural cavity, thereby allowing the lungs to respond after surgery. Chest tubes that drain the pericardial sac are called *mediastinal tubes*.

Measure and observe chest drainage by collecting drainage in a calibrated cylinder (most hospitals use disposable chest drainage setups that are clearly calibrated). Measure findings and record hourly. Up to 100 ml of drainage may be lost during the first hour postoperatively as a result of reexpansion of the lungs, which forces drainage through the chest tube. Approximately 500 ml of drainage occurs over the first 24 hours. Large gushes of drainage are sometimes expelled when the client coughs or turns. Usually dark red during the early postoperative phase, the drainage gradually becomes more serous as time passes. Chest tubes are described in Chapter 62.

Bloody mediastinal drainage that is collected from the chest tubes can be transfused back into the client *(autotransfusion)*. This transfused blood has the advantage of not originating at the blood bank. There is reduced risk of infection or disease to the client and less cost when the client's own blood is used. The bloody drainage is infused via filtered IV tubing. Some manufacturers produce disposable chest drainage systems that have this autotransfusion capability.

FLUID BALANCE. Carefully measure and record intake and output. Obtain daily weights to determine accurately whether the client is retaining fluids within tissues or losing excessive fluid rapidly. Significant fluctuations in weight act as a guide to fluid replacement.

RENAL FUNCTION. Measure urine volume hourly for the first 8 to 12 hours after surgery. The client almost always has an indwelling urinary catheter. Normal urine output is greater than 30 ml/hr except during the night, when it is lower. Urine may be bloody as a result of hemolysis of erythrocytes during ECC.

Assess the urine 24-hour specific gravity. The normal value is 1.015 to 1.020. Specific gravity may rise because of oliguria or the presence of red blood cells. Lowered specific gravity results from overhydration or inability of kidney tubules to filter waste products.

ELECTROLYTE BALANCE. Daily electrolyte studies are performed to determine blood levels of sodium, potassium, and chloride. The physician replaces electrolytes parenterally if the values are deficient. If diuretics are given to reduce volume overload, monitor potassium closely and replace as prescribed. The heart may be particularly sensitive to hypokalemia (low potassium level) soon after surgery. Obtain hematocrit, hemoglobin, and prothrombin time daily to determine extent of blood loss or hemorrhage, and check ABG values daily to determine the pH and partial pressures of arterial carbon dioxide ($PaCO_2$) and oxygen (PaO_2) (see Chapter 14).

NEUROLOGIC RESPONSE. After heart surgery, carefully observe the client's level of consciousness, pupil size and reaction, orientation, and ability to move extremities.

The client should awaken within 1 to 2 hours after surgery. Not awakening may result from embolization of air, calcium, fat, or thrombotic particles to the brain. Slow return to consciousness (over 2 to 4 days) may result from a diffuse neurologic deficit due to poor cerebral capillary perfusion during ECC.

Check pupils hourly during the early postoperative period for size, equality in size, and reaction to light. Pupils dilate when blood contains excess carbon dioxide.

Disorientation and restlessness may indicate anoxia or embolization to the brain. Also, fatigue or fear can produce mental confusion.

Hemiplegia (inability to move an extremity) or extreme weakness of an extremity may indicate embolization to the motor area of the brain.

After cardiac surgery, clients may become disoriented, delusional, and psychotic. Severe depression is not uncommon. Causes of confusion, hallucinations, and psychotic behavior include:

- Isolation in the ICU
- Sensory deprivation
- Lack of rest and sleep over an extended period

- Fear and anxiety
- An impersonal environment if care providers are preoccupied with monitors and machines
- Desynchronization of circadian rhythm (ICUs are active and well lighted 24 hours a day).

Causes of postoperative depression include fatigue and debility after surgery along with resumption of responsibilities.[53]

DIAGNOSIS, OUTCOMES, INTERVENTION

Risk for Decreased Cardiac Output. Heart failure, metabolic acidosis, weakening of the left ventricle, dysrhythmias, and cardiac tamponade can decrease cardiac output. State this diagnosis as *Risk for Decreased Cardiac Output related to (appropriate cause).*

Outcomes. The client will have improved cardiovascular function, as evidenced by adequate tissue perfusion, stabilization of vital signs, clear lung sounds on auscultation, stable body weight, adequate urine output (30 ml/hr or greater), no reported or observed dyspnea or orthopnea, regular heart sounds without S_3 or S_4, and decreased or absent peripheral edema (blood pressure within 20 mm Hg of baseline values).

Interventions. Interventions for a failing heart muscle often involve administration of inotropic agents (e.g., dopamine, dobutamine), which increase cardiac contractility. Administer inotropic agents cautiously because they also increase the work of the heart and its need for oxygen.

Complications resulting from persistent hypotension are cerebral ischemia, renal shutdown, myocardial infarction, and shock. To correct these complications, the surgeon may use a mechanical device to support the failing heart if medications are unsuccessful.

The intra-aortic balloon pump (IABP) is a counterpulsation device that supports the failing heart by increasing coronary artery perfusion during diastole and reducing afterload. It consists of a sausage-shaped balloon catheter that is passed through the femoral artery and positioned in the descending thoracic aorta just distal to the subclavian artery. The catheter is attached to a power console that inflates and deflates the balloon in time with the heart.

The balloon is inflated during diastole; blood is pushed back into the aorta, and coronary artery perfusion is improved.

The balloon is deflated during systole; resistance is decreased, and the workload of the heart is thus reduced (see Bridge to Critical Care). The timing of the balloon inflations and deflations is critical. A nurse educated in the use of the balloon pump is assigned to care for the client. Monitoring the effects of the pumping on the client's vital signs requires special skills.

Risk for Ineffective Airway Clearance. Retained secretions are common after open heart surgery. State the diagnosis as *Risk for Ineffective Airway Clearance related to retained secretions.* Also consider using the diagnosis of *Impaired Gas Exchange* if the client has marginal levels of oxygen saturation.

Outcomes. The client will exhibit improved airway clearance, as evidenced by clear lung sounds, afebrile state, strong nonproductive cough, and ABG values within normal limits.

Interventions. Turn and suction the intubated client frequently. Monitor the client's response to suctioning, noting changes in heart rhythm, restlessness, or pallor. Suctioning is seldom indicated routinely and is done when the secretions can be heard in the endotracheal tube. Today, most clients are extubated within hours of surgery. Skilled nursing care to promote pulmonary hygiene is crucial. Help the nonintubated client to turn, take deep breaths, and cough every 1 to 2 hours; suction the trachea if the temperature rises to above 38.5° C (101° F) and the client is coughing ineffectively.

After the endotracheal tube is removed, the client can wear a high-humidity oxygen mask to aid in loosening secretions; chest physiotherapy may also be used. In rare cases, bronchoscopy may be indicated for removal of secretions. Complications of retained secretions include atelectasis, pneumonia, and subsequent inadequate oxygenation of the tissues. Monitor oxygen saturation continuously.

Risk for Hemorrhage. State the collaborative problem as *Hemorrhage related to surgical trauma or slipped ligature (suture).*

Outcomes. Collaborative problems are monitored only by the nurse. Therefore, the expected outcome addresses your actions, not the client's goals. The nurse will monitor the client for amounts of drainage that exceed 2 ml/kg of body weight per hour or a sustained period of bleeding through the chest tube.

Interventions. If bleeding is noted, notify the physician because the client may need to be returned to the operating room for repair of the bleeding sites. Replace blood by transfusion as prescribed. The chest drainage may be autotransfused back into the client from the chest drainage system through an IV line. The use of blood transfusions has decreased dramatically since the onset of human immunodeficiency virus (HIV) infection. However, sometimes it is necessary to replace blood lost during surgery. If the client's hematocrit is adequate, albumin or high-molecular-weight plasma expanders, such as hetastarch, may be prescribed in place of blood.

Risk for Cardiac Tamponade. Occlusion in the pericardial drainage system can lead to cardiac tamponade. State this collaborative problem as *Risk for Cardiac Tamponade related to occlusion of the pericardial drainage system.*

Outcomes. The nurse will monitor the client for sudden cessation of chest drainage with an increase in venous pressure, pulsus paradoxus, dyspnea, oliguria, distant or inaudible heart sounds, or lowered left atrial pressure.

Interventions. Gently milk the chest tube to express clots that may be blocking drainage. Do not pull vigorously on the tube or strip the tube by creating negative pressure in it. If clots cannot be removed by gentle milking of the tube, the physician may need to declot the tube using a long catheter with an inflatable balloon on the end. The client may need to be returned to the operating room or may need a pericardial tap for removal of fluid.

Risk for Renal Failure. State this collaborative problem as *Risk for Renal Failure related to* (add specific risk). Hypovolemia, decreased cardiac output, or hemolysis of erythrocytes during cardiopulmonary bypass can result in acute renal failure.

Outcomes. The nurse will monitor the client's urinary output, expecting output greater than 30 ml/hr. Also mon-

Intra-aortic Balloon Pumping–Counterpulsation Device

When the left ventricle fails to support adequate circulation and perfusion, an intra-aortic balloon pumping (IABP) device can be used to augment coronary artery filling and decrease left ventricular workload. A polyethylene balloon is inserted via the femoral artery into the descending thoracic aorta distal to the left subclavian artery and connected to an external pneumatic pumping system. The pump inflates the balloon with helium or carbon dioxide during diastole, and deflates it during systole. The inflation-deflation cycle is triggered by the client's ECG, specifically by the R wave, which signals the beginning of systole. Balloon inflation during diastole augments coronary artery filling. Systolic balloon deflation decreases afterload.

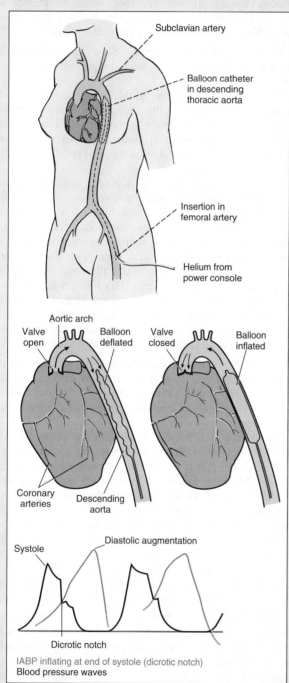

Subclavian artery

Balloon catheter in descending thoracic aorta

Insertion in femoral artery

Helium from power console

Aortic arch

Valve open — Balloon deflated

Valve closed — Balloon inflated

Coronary arteries — Descending aorta

Systole — Diastolic augmentation

Dicrotic notch

IABP inflating at end of systole (dicrotic notch)
Blood pressure waves

The IABP device is used in clients with cardiogenic shock, septic shock, acute anterior myocardial infarction (MI), complications following MI, angioplasty with MI, ventricular dysrhythmias with ischemia, left ventricular failure, unstable angina refractory to medications, and low cardiac output after surgery.

Guidelines for Management

1. Select an ECG lead that optimizes the R wave.
2. Time the IABP device using an arterial waveform.
3. Monitor perfusion in the extremity with IABP.
4. Monitor perfusion in arms (catheter can occlude subclavian artery)
5. Monitor arterial pressures (which should improve).
6. Monitor urine output (the catheter can occlude the renal artery).
7. Keep the affected limb straight to prevent dislodgment of the catheter.
8. Monitor for balloon rupture and misplacement (loss of augmentation, wrinkled appearance in safety chamber, blood in tubing).
9. Monitor for bleeding resulting from anticoagulant use.
10. Monitor for aortic dissection (acute back, retroperitoneal, testicular or chest pain, decreased pulses, variations in blood pressure between arms, decreased cardiac output, tachycardia, decreased filling pressures, decreased hemoglobin, decreased hematocrit).
11. Monitor skin integrity on the sacrum, the coccyx and the heels.
12. Do not elevate the head of the bed above 15 degrees.
13. Clarify or reinforce the client's and family's understanding of the IABP device.

Complications

Dissection of the femoral or iliac artery or aorta
Bleeding
Plaque dislodgment, which can cause embolization
Balloon rupture
Arterial occlusion with limb ischemia or neuropathy
Mechanical destruction of red blood cells
Inability to wean from the IABP device
Hematoma at the insertion site
Mesenteric/renal ischemia (catheter too low)
Arm ischemia (catheter too high)

Weaning

The ratio of IABP-assisted beats to unassisted beats is decreased from 1:1 to 1:2 based on the following parameters:

- Heart rate < 110 BPM
- No dysrhythmias
- Mean arterial pressure > 70 mm Hg without vasopressors
- Pulmonary arterial wedge pressure < 18 mm Hg
- Cardiac index > 2.5
- Capillary refill > 3 sec
- Urine output > 0.5 ml/kg/min
- SvO_2 between 70% and 80%

BPM, beats per minute; ECG, electrocardiogram.

itor laboratory values for blood urea nitrogen (BUN), creatinine, and potassium.

Interventions. A client with decreased urine output may be treated with extra fluids (sometimes called a *fluid challenge*) if dehydration is the probable etiologic factor. Other interventions may include correcting shock or low output failure and administering a diuretic (e.g., furosemide) via the IV route. If renal failure occurs, peritoneal dialysis or hemodialysis should be instituted.

During the course of surgery, the client typically receives 3 to 4 L of extra fluid. Often this fluid accumulates as edema and does not greatly increase the vascular volume. However, this additional fluid does place the client at high risk for circulatory overload. For this reason, IV fluids are administered judiciously for the first 3 days postoperatively to prevent overwork of the heart. Typically, 500 to 700 ml/m^2 body surface over 24 hours, including oral intake (normal surface area is 1.5–2.0 m^2), is given. Administer sodium-containing fluids cautiously to prevent circulatory overload and heart failure.

Risk for Paralytic Ileus. Sympathetic responses leading to shunting of blood from the gastrointestinal tract during surgery, side effects of anesthesia and narcotics, and immobility lead to paralytic ileus. State this collaborative problem as *Risk for Paralytic Ileus related to (appropriate cause* [all may apply in this case]).

Outcomes. The nurse will monitor the client for clinical manifestations of ileus, as evidenced by hypoactive or absent bowel sounds, abdominal distention, nausea, vomiting, lack of appetite, and no passing of flatus.

Interventions. Give sips of water 4 hours after extubation if the client is fully responsive and not nauseated. The client may have clear liquids next, followed by solid foods. Watch for signs of abdominal distention and paralytic ileus (see Chapter 15). If either condition develops, stop oral fluids and notify the physician.

Risk for Pain. Sternal and leg incisions cause intense pain after surgery. Express this common diagnosis as *Risk for Pain related to sternal and leg incision.*

Outcomes. The client will experience increased comfort, as evidenced by normal heart rate, absence of restlessness, normal respiratory rate, verbalization of increased comfort, decreasing use of narcotics, and periods of rest.

Interventions. Give narcotic analgesics for pain postoperatively as ordered. Avoid overmedicating a client who is recovering from hypothermia because narcotic metabolism is slowed and the medication may not be excreted. Attempt to relieve the pain and restlessness with comfort measures before administering a narcotic. Most clients have more pain in the legs than in the sternum.

Risk for Altered Tissue Perfusion. The surgical procedure, hemodynamic stability, electrolyte imbalances, hypoxia, medications, and several other potential problems can lead to impaired cerebral circulation. Use this nursing diagnosis early after surgery. Later, if confusion develops, use *Risk for Injury or Acute Confusion* as the best diagnosis.

Outcomes. The client will demonstrate adequate cerebral tissue perfusion, as evidenced by continuous progress toward an alert level of consciousness.

Interventions. To prevent mental confusion, undue fear, anxiety, and tension, always address the client by name and introduce yourself by name. Take an interest in the client. Do not ignore the client while working with

monitors and equipment. Place a calendar and clock at the bedside to orient the client to date and time of day. Position the cardiac monitor so that it is out of the client's view. Many clients become nervous watching their own heart action.

Schedule the day so that periods of nursing intervention alternate with periods of rest and relaxation. Encourage the client to freely discuss fears and anxieties. Prepare significant others for changes in the client's sensorium after surgery. Before visiting times, warn visitors if the client is hallucinating or is severely depressed so that they know what to expect. Explain all interventions to the client, and allow time for questions.

Risk for Impaired Physical Mobility. Prolonged bed rest after surgery and a weakened condition before surgery lead to impaired physical mobility. State this diagnosis as *Impaired Physical Mobility related to prolonged bed rest or weakened condition before surgery (or both).*

Outcomes. The client will demonstrate postoperative mobility, as evidenced by having mobility that is equal to or greater than preoperative mobility.

Interventions. Prolonged periods of bed rest after heart surgery (or any surgery) may cause weakness, pooling of respiratory secretions, atelectasis, thrombophlebitis, osteoporosis, urinary retention, renal calculi, and a negative nitrogen balance. Planned activity is the most important single factor in preventing the complications of bed rest. The type and amount of activity allowed for each client depend on the type of surgery and the client's general postoperative condition.

If the client is hemodynamically stable, turn him or her from side to side at intervals for pressure relief. Perform passive exercises and leg flexion every 2 hours to prevent thrombosis of lower extremities.

The day after surgery, the client usually dangles the legs over the side of the bed for a short period. That evening or on postoperative day 2, the client usually sits in a chair for a brief time. On day 3 to 5, the client begins to ambulate in the room and up and down the hallway. By day 8 to 10, the client is usually fully ambulatory. Cardiac monitors are used to evaluate the client's response to increasing activity.

It usually takes 8 to 10 weeks for clients to fully regain strength after surgery. On discharge home, the client gradually increases activity until moderate walks and climbing stairs do not cause undue fatigue. The client usually returns to work 2 months after surgery.

Risk for Transplant Rejection. Recall that the body's normal response to foreign protein is to recognize and destroy it. Rejection of the transplanted heart is a common concern. State this collaborative problem as *Risk for Transplant Rejection related to immune response after surgery.*

Outcomes. The nurse will monitor the client for clinical manifestations of rejection, as evidenced by decreases in oxygenation, fever, malaise, anxiety, and infiltrates on chest film.

Interventions. Rejection and infection are the most common complications of cardiac transplantation. The prevention of rejection with immunosuppression is continually being examined (see immunosuppressive protocol, Table 55–3). Cyclosporine has been helpful in preventing rejection, but it is toxic. Renal failure, hypertension, liver toxic effects, and neurologic disturbances are not uncommon.

Risk for Infection. The loss of primary defenses and use of immunosuppressive agents in transplant recipients makes these clients excellent candidates for infection. State this common nursing diagnosis as *Risk for Infection related to loss of primary defenses (skin incision) and use of immunosuppression.*

Outcomes. The client will be free from clinical manifestations of infection, as evidenced by remaining afebrile and having WBC levels within normal limits, no malaise, and no abnormal heart sounds.

Interventions. Infection remains the major cause of death in the early postoperative period as well as a major cause of death after 1 year in heart transplant recipients. Clients are treated prophylactically with antibiotics. Non-healing sternal wounds are treated promptly. Myocutaneous flaps may be required (see Chapter 49).

EVALUATION

Clients who have open heart surgery for coronary bypass may have a leg incision from a saphenous vein graft. These long incisions can be slow to heal, in part due to decreased peripheral circulation. Delayed leg wound healing is a common problem. Wounds are usually cleaned twice daily with povidone-iodine and redressed.

The degree of expected outcome attainment should be examined frequently. Some of the problems discussed in the care of the client after heart surgery require prompt treatment (e.g., dysrhythmias); others can be evaluated over longer periods of time.

■ Self-Care

At home, the client's activity level will continue to increase. It takes approximately 6 weeks postoperatively for the sternum to heal. During that time, advise the client to lift nothing heavier than 5 pounds. Also, the client must refrain from driving, which may strain the incision. As the client gets into and out of bed or a chair, the arms should not bear weight; the arms are used only for balance. Teach the client and significant others to inspect the incision daily. Care of the incision may include swabbing with povidone-iodine and applying dry dressings over oozing areas.

In some cities, exercise rehabilitation programs have been developed for clients who have had heart attacks or heart surgery. These programs involve supervised, closely monitored exercise sessions and teaching. It is important for the partner or significant other to understand how much activity is desired, since many partners who mean well allow the client to assume a "sick role" once home and ultimately delay healing and recovery. See Bridge to Home Health Care.

BRIDGE TO HOME HEALTH CARE

Recovery After Heart Surgery

Following cardiac surgery, your role as a nurse is to assess for the early onset of complications; teach clients, their families, and their informal caregivers to identify problems; and evaluate recovery progress during each visit. It is also important that you encourage clients to reduce their risks and adopt a healthier lifestyle in relation to smoking, hypertension, hyperlipidemia, inactivity, and stress.

Cardiac dysrhythmias, such as atrial fibrillation, often occur after surgery and can be identified during your nursing assessment by a portable electrocardiogram (ECG) monitor. Auscultate heart tones to assess for a pericardial rub; it may not be present until 2 weeks after surgery and can be safely managed with anti-inflammatory medications. Instruct clients to weigh themselves daily and to report gains of 2 pounds in 24 hours or 5 pounds in a week. Such weight gain may indicate heart failure.

Assess pulmonary status to detect early evidence of pneumonia. Evaluate incentive spirometry measurements; decreasing lung volumes indicate early pneumonia or an enlarging pleural effusion. Instruct clients to use their incentive spirometers a minimum of 10 times each day until presurgical lung volume returns. Typically, the goal is to increase lung volume by 200 ml every other day.

Incisions remain red and tender for 2 to 3 weeks but should not demonstrate discolored drainage, increased edema, or heat at the site. Instruct clients to take a daily shower, pat their incisions dry, and keep them open to air unless drainage occurs. If you remove staples or sutures, apply Steri-strips over the incisions. If the Steri-strips do not fall off in the shower, they can be removed within 2 weeks.

Even though clients usually have a poor appetite for

the first 4 to 6 weeks after surgery, they need to eat a diet that promotes healing; the diet should be 300 to 500 kilocalories (kcal) above their basal metabolic rate. Clients, their family members, and informal caregivers are often concerned about limiting fats during the recovery period. However, anorexic clients need to limit only sodium and caffeine until their incisions heal. Encourage a high fiber intake to prevent constipation. Most clients will be ready to begin the American Heart Association Step 2 diet 3 to 4 weeks after surgery.

Urge clients to take their prescribed pain medication to promote comfort, to enable them to perform their deep-breathing exercises, and to foster restful sleep. Clients should use several pillows to obtain a comfortable position and to minimize pain. Women should wear a supportive brassiere to decrease sternal stress. Instruct clients to use stretching and range-of-motion exercises to reduce left shoulder discomfort, which results from positioning during surgery. Transient postoperative depression is common. Instruct clients that the "blues" may occur between 2 and 6 weeks after hospital discharge and should subside in a few weeks.

Typical recovery instructions include increasing low level activity, such as walking, by 2 minutes each day until the client is able to tolerate 20 minutes of sustained activity. Clients are instructed not to lift anything heavier than 5 pounds, and driving is generally restricted for 1 month per physician's order. Clients, young and old, want to know when they can safely resume sexual relations. When the client can tolerate climbing two flights of stairs, sexual activity is safe. Clients are instructed to assume passive positions that will not stress the sternum for the first few months after surgery.

Ann K. Frantz, RN, BSN, Independent Health Care Consultant, Pontiac, Michigan

Low-sodium and low-cholesterol diets are often prescribed for clients after cardiac surgery. For the client to be able to comply with dietary instruction, the diet must be carefully planned (see Chapter 56).

Teach the client or significant other to check the pulse daily for rate and regularity and to call the physician if the resting heart rate rises by more than 20 beats per minute or a new irregularity is present. The client can also use heart rate to monitor responses to exercise. Authorities usually recommend a rise of not more than 20 BPM for the immediate postoperative period.

Make sure the client knows how and when to schedule follow-up appointments. Instruct the client to report the following to the primary health care provider:

- Manifestations of infection, including fever, and increased redness, tenderness, or swelling of incisions
- Palpitations, tachycardia, or irregular pulse (if normally regular)
- Dizziness or increased fatigue
- Sudden weight gain or peripheral edema
- Shortness of breath

Modifications for Elderly Clients

Older clients commonly have many other disorders that interfere with or delay their ability to respond to the hemodynamic changes of surgery and recovery. The elderly client is also at risk for skin breakdown and renal impairment. Fluids must be closely titrated because of the possibility of a pre-existent heart disorder.

CONCLUSIONS

The client with a cardiac disorder frequently has activity intolerance, decreased cardiac output, and ineffective coping due to the seriousness of the disorder. Nurses must be skilled in the physical and psychosocial aspects of disease when providing care.

THINKING CRITICALLY

1. **A 45-year-old man arrives in the emergency department after an automobile accident. Initially, he does not complain about himself, but then he is more concerned about his daughter, who was injured in the accident. Neither the child nor the client were wearing seat belts when their car was struck from behind. While sitting at his daughter's bedside in the emergency department, the client becomes more and more anxious; his respiratory rate increases, and he becomes restless. The vital signs reveal a blood pressure of 88/72, pulse of 118, and respirations of 28. What other assessments are needed to rule out cardiac tamponade? What intervention will relieve pressure on the heart and improve cardiac function?**

Factors to Consider. What are the clinical manifestations of cardiac tamponade? How is cardiac output affected by cardiac tamponade?

2. **The client is a 60-year-old man with dilated cardiomyopathy. His prognosis is very poor. He is** able to tolerate only minimal amounts of activity: using the bedside commode, feeding himself, and shaving himself in bed. Today, he continues to be short of breath but seems particularly withdrawn. Repeated physical assessment to identify cardiovascular status shows no change in assessment findings. He continues to take his medications at the proper dosages. His physician thinks these medications are at their maximal levels. Repeated psychosocial assessment would show that the client is withdrawn because he is anxious that he will become physically worse, hospitalized, and placed on a ventilator again. He does not wish to be placed on a ventilator. He was terrified the last time and sees no purpose in just prolonging his dying. What nursing actions might help your client?

Factors to Consider. What are the clinical manifestations of cardiomyopathy? What are the psychological considerations for the client's care?

3. **A 52-year-old man with a lengthy history of mitral valve prolapse is recovering from kidney transplantation surgery. This is his fourth postoperative day, and he and his spouse are asking questions about care at home. What priorities for client education should be established?**

Factors to Consider. What complication is associated with mitral valve prolapse? How does the medication regimen following transplantation surgery further place the client at risk?

BIBLIOGRAPHY

1. Alexander, R. W., Schlant, R. C., & Fuster, V. (1998). *Hurst's the heart* (9th ed.). New York: McGraw-Hill.
2. Bates, B. (1995). *A guide to physical examination and history taking.* Philadelphia: J. B. Lippincott.
3. Bayer, A.S., et al. (1998). AHA Scientific Statement: Diagnosis and management of infective endocarditis and its complications. *Circulation, 98,* 2936–2948.
4. Braunwald, E. (1997). Valvular heart disease. In E. Braunwald (Ed.), *Heart disease* (pp. 1007–1076). Philadelphia: W. B. Saunders.
5. Carpenito, L. J. (1995). *Nursing diagnosis.* Philadelphia: J. B. Lippincott.
6. Dajani, A.S. (1997). Prevention of bacterial endocarditis: Recommendations by the American Heart Association. *Journal of the American Medical Association, 277*(22), 1794–1801.
7. Dajani, A. S. (1997). Rheumatic fever. In E. Braunwald (Ed.), *Heart disease* (pp. 1769–1775). Philadelphia: W. B. Saunders.
8. Findlow, D., & Doyle, E. (1997). Congenital heart disease in adults. *British Journal of Anesthesia, 78,* 416–430.
9. Futterman, L. G., & Lemberg, L. (1995). New indications for dual chamber pacing: Hypertrophic and dilated cardiomyopathy. *American Journal of Critical Care, 4*(1), 82–87.
10. Halm, M. A. (1996). Acute gastrointestinal complications after cardiac surgery. *American Journal of Critical Care, 5*(2), 109–117.
11. Kawai, C. (1999). From myocarditis to cardiomyopathy: Mechanisms of inflammation and cell death. *Circulation, 99*(8), 1091–1100.
12. Karchmer, A. W. (1997). Infective endocarditis. In E. Braunwald (Ed.), *Heart disease* (pp. 1077–1104). Philadelphia: W. B. Saunders.
13. Lashley, F. R. (1999). Genetic testing, screening, and counseling issues in cardiovascular disease. *Journal of Cardiovascular Nursing, 13*(4), 110–126.

14. Lawrie, G. M. (1998). Mitral valve repair vs. replacement. *Cardiology Clinics, 16*(3), 437–448.

15. Lorell, B. H. (1997). Pericardial Diseases. In E. Braunwald (Ed.), *Heart disease* (pp. 1478–1534). Philadelphia: W. B. Saunders.

16. McLachlan, J., Reddy, P., & Ratts, T. E. (1998). Mitral valve prolapse: A common diagnosis in women. *Journal of the Louisiana State Medical Society, 150,* 92–96.

17. Micevski, V. (1999). The use of molecular technologies for the detection of enteroviral ribonucleic acid in myocarditis. *Journal of Cardiovascular Nursing, 13*(4), 78–90.

18. Myers, R. B.,& Spodick, D. H. (1999). Constrictive pericarditis: Clinical and pathophysiologic characteristics. *American Heart Journal, 138,* 219–232.

19. Perloff, J. K. (1997). Congenital heart disease in adults. In E. Braunwald (Ed.), *Heart disease* (pp. 963–987). Philadelphia: W. B. Saunders.

20. Richenbacher, W. E., & Pierce, W. S. (1997). Assisted circulation and the mechanical heart. In E. Braunwald (Ed.), *Heart disease* (pp. 534–547). Philadelphia: W. B. Saunders.

21. Riddle, M. M., Dunstan, J. L., & Castanis, J. L. (1996). A rapid recovery program for cardiac surgery patients. *American Journal of Critical Care, 5*(2), 152–159.

22. Simpson, T., & Lee, E. R. (1996). Individual factors that influence sleep after cardiac surgery. *American Journal of Critical Care, 5*(3), 182–189.

23. Simpson, T., Lee, E. R., & Cameron, C. (1996). Patients' perceptions of environmental factors that disturb sleep after cardiac surgery. *American Journal of Critical Care, 5*(3), 173–181.

24. Sparacino, P. A. (1999). Cardiac infections: Medical and surgical therapies. *Journal of Cardiovascular Nursing, 13*(2), 49–65.

25. United Network of Organ Sharing (1999). Transplant patient data source. Available: *http://www.unos.org*

26. Wakowski, C. A., & Bierman, P. Q. (1995). Dual chamber pacing in patients with hypertrophic obstructive cardiomyopathy: A case study. *American Journal of Critical Care, 4*(2), 165–168.

27. Wynne, J., & Braunwald, E. (1997). The cardiomyopathies and myocarditides. In E. Braunwald (Ed.), *Heart disease* (pp. 1404–1463). Philadelphia: W. B. Saunders.

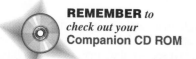

C H A P T E R

56

Management of Clients with Functional Cardiac Disorders

Peggy Gerard
Janice Tazbir

NURSING OUTCOMES CLASSIFICATION (NOC)
for Nursing Diagnoses—Clients with Functional Cardiac Disorders

Altered Tissue Perfusion
Sensory Function: Cutaneous
Tissue Perfusion: Peripheral
Tissue Perfusion: Pulmonary
Decreased Cardiac Output
Cardiac Pump Effectiveness
Circulation Status
Tissue Perfusion: Abdominal Organs
Vital Signs Status

Fluid Volume Excess
Electrolyte and Acid/Base Balance
Fluid Balance
Hydration
Impaired Gas Exchange
Electrolyte and Acid/Base Balance
Respiratory Status: Ventilation
Risk for Activity Intolerance
Activity Tolerance
Endurance

Energy Conservation
Self-Care: Activities of Daily Living
Self-Care: Instrumental Activities of Daily
Living
Risk for Anxiety
Anxiety Control
Coping
Risk for Impaired Skin Integrity
Tissue Integrity: Skin and Mucous
Membranes

Normal functioning of the heart is based on a balance between oxygen supply and oxygen demand. In order to function as an effective pump, the heart muscle must be adequately supplied with blood from the coronary arteries. In *coronary heart disease* (CHD), atherosclerosis develops in the coronary arteries, causing them to become narrowed or blocked. When a coronary artery is narrowed or blocked, blood flow to the area of the heart supplied by that artery is reduced. If the remaining blood flow is inadequate to meet the oxygen demand of the heart, the area may become ischemic and injured and myocardial infarction (MI) may result. In addition, the heart may fail to pump sufficient blood supply to the other organs and tissues in the body. Over time, changes resulting from CHD may lead to the development of chronic heart failure.

The term coronary heart disease, also called *coronary artery disease* or *ischemic heart disease,* refers to diseases of the heart that result from a decrease in blood supply to the heart muscle. This chapter reviews the risk factors, etiology, pathophysiology, clinical manifestations, and medical and nursing intervention for two major disorders of cardiac function: CHD and heart failure. The related conditions of angina pectoris and MI are discussed in Chapter 58.

CORONARY HEART DISEASE

CHD is the single largest killer of men and women in the United States and currently affects more than 12 million people.[7] Although these numbers seem high, the death rate from coronary heart disease decreased 24.2% from 1986 to 1996. Contributing to this decline in the death rate are factors such as improved technology for diagnosis and treatment, use of thrombolytic drugs in acute MI, improved interventional therapies and surgical techniques, and modification of risk factors in populations at risk.

Etiology and Risk Factors

CHD results from the development of obliterative atherosclerotic lesions within the coronary arteries that narrow or obstruct these vessels. Atherosclerosis is a disorder of lipid metabolism and underlies most causes of cardiovascular disease and death.

Although CHD claims more lives each year than any other disease, its causes are poorly understood. Clinical evidence suggests that many factors contribute to the onset of atherosclerosis. Risk factors that precipitate CHD can be presented in two categories: major risk factors and contributing risk factors (Box 56–1). Major risk factors are those that are significantly associated with the development of CHD. Contributing risk factors are those that are associated with the risk of cardiovascular disease but whose significance and prevalence have not been determined.

The more risk factors a person has, the greater the risk of CHD. Although risk factors influence the development of CHD in all people, the importance of selected risk factors may vary by gender and race. Overall, risk factors are found more frequently in lower socioeconomic and educational groups.[49] Although a few risk factors cannot be changed, a person may reduce the risk of CHD by controlling risk factors that can be modified by lifestyle or medication.

MAJOR NONMODIFIABLE RISK FACTORS

Heredity (Including Race)
Children whose parents had heart disease are at higher risk for CHD. This increased risk is related to genetic factors that contribute to four risk factors that increase the incidence of CHD:

- Hypertension
- Dyslipidemia
- Diabetes
- Obesity

For people ages 35 to 74 years, the age-adjusted death rate from CHD for African American women is 72% higher than that for white women. The prevalence of CHD is lowest among Mexican Americans.[6]

Increasing Age
Age influences both the risk and the severity of CHD. Symptomatic CHD appears predominantly in people older than 40 years of age, and four out of five people who die of CHD are age 65 years or older. However, angina and MI can occur in a person's 30s and even in one's 20s. At older ages, women who have heart attacks are twice as likely as men to die of the heart attack.[6]

Gender
CHD is the number one killer of both men and women. In 1996, mortality from CHD was almost equal for men and women. Although men are at higher risk for heart attacks at younger ages, the risk for women increases significantly at menopause, so that one of every three women in the United States 65 years of age and older has CHD.

Women who take oral contraceptives and who smoke or have high blood pressure are at greater risk for CHD. Women with an early menopause are also at higher risk than are women with a normal or late menopause.[6, 49]

Two lifestyle changes during the past two decades may be responsible for the increased incidence of CHD among women. More women (many with full responsibility for the household and children) have entered the work force, and more women have begun to smoke tobacco at an earlier age.

MAJOR MODIFIABLE RISK FACTORS
Smoking, hypertension, elevated serum cholesterol levels, physical inactivity, obesity, and diabetes mellitus constitute the other major risk factors. Their effect on CHD can be modified or reduced by treatment.

Smoking
Smokers are two times more likely to have a heart attack and to die from it than nonsmokers. Recent evidence suggests that nonsmokers who are exposed to second-hand tobacco smoke at home or work may also have a higher mortality rate from CHD. Smoking triples the risk of heart attack in women and doubles the risk of heart attack in men. Clients who smoke have two to four times the risk of sudden cardiac death.[6, 49]

Although the means by which smoking causes CHD remains unknown, the three substances thought to increase the prevalence of CHD are tar, nicotine, and carbon monoxide. Tar contains hydrocarbons and other carcinogenic substances. Nicotine increases the release of epinephrine and norepinephrine, which results in peripheral vasoconstriction, elevated blood pressure and heart rate, greater oxygen consumption, and increased likelihood of dysrhythmias. In addition, nicotine activates platelets and stimulates smooth muscle cell proliferation in the arterial walls. Carbon monoxide reduces the amount of blood available to the intima of the vessel wall and increases the permeability of the endothelium. Clients who quit smoking lose their increased risk in 3 to 5 years.[49]

Hypertension
High blood pressure afflicts nearly 50 million American adults and children. It increases the workload of the heart, thus causing the heart to enlarge and weaken over time. As blood pressure increases, the risk of a serious cardiovascular event also escalates. When hypertension is combined with other risk factors, such as obesity, smoking, high cholesterol levels, and diabetes, the risk of heart attack or stroke increases significantly.

Compared with whites, African Americans have hypertension at an earlier age and it is more severe at any age. Consequently, the rate of heart disease in African Americans is 1.5 times greater than that of whites. Although hypertension cannot always be prevented, it should be treated to lower the risk of CHD and premature death.[6, 7]

Elevated Serum Cholesterol Levels
The risk of CHD increases as blood cholesterol levels increase. The risk increases further when other risk fac-

---

BOX 56–1	**Risk Factors for Coronary Heart Disease**

Nonmodifiable Major Risk Factors
- Heredity, including race
- Age
- Gender

Modifiable Major Risk Factors
- Cigarette smoking
- Hypertension
- Elevated serum cholesterol
- Diabetes mellitus
- Physical inactivity
- Obesity

Contributing Risk Factors
- Stress
- Homocysteine level

tors are present. In adults, total cholesterol levels of 240 mg/dl are classified as "high" and levels ranging from 200 to 239 mg/dl are classified as "borderline-high." At young and middle ages, men have higher cholesterol levels. In women, cholesterol levels continue to increase up to about age 70.[49]

Cholesterol, a sterol found in animal tissue, circulates in the blood in combination with triglycerides and protein-bound phospholipids. This complex is called a *lipoprotein*. There are four basic groups of lipoproteins, all produced in the intestinal wall. Elevation of lipoproteins is called *hyperlipoproteinemia*. Elevation of lipids, a component of lipoproteins, is called *hyperlipidemia*. Lipoproteins and their functions are as follows:

- Chylomicrons primarily transport dietary triglycerides and cholesterol.
- Very-low-density lipoproteins (VLDLs) mainly transport triglycerides synthesized by the liver.
- Low-density lipoproteins (LDLs) have the highest concentration of cholesterol and transport endogenous cholesterol to body cells.
- High-density lipoproteins (HDLs) have the lowest concentration of cholesterol and transport endogenous cholesterol to body cells.

Recent investigations have documented how the presence of lipoproteins may predispose the body to CHD. People with high levels of HDL in proportion to LDL are at less risk for CHD than people with a low HDL:LDL ratio. High concentrations of HDL seem to protect against the development of CHD. Experts believe that the cholesterol in HDL, in contrast to that in LDL, does not become incorporated into the fatty plaques that develop in the lining of the artery wall.

The ratio of total cholesterol to HDL or of LDL to HDL is the best test for predicting the risk of CHD. Exercise and low-fat, low-cholesterol diets increase the amount of HDL in the blood. Current recommendations[21] for cholesterol and lipoproteins are:

- Total blood cholesterol < 200 mg/dl
- LDL < 160 if fewer than two other risk factors (<130 mg/dl if two or more risk factors)
- HDL > 35 mg/dl

Triglycerides are not an independent risk factor in men, but their significance in women is unknown. However, the combination of a high triglyceride level and a low HDL level seems to be a more important predictor of CHD in women than in men. The Consensus Panel Statement from the American Heart Association (AHA) recommends that triglyceride levels be below 200 mg/dl.[21]

In the average American diet, approximately 45% of the total calories come from fat. This level exeeds that recommended in the *AHA Step 1 Diet*. Dietary fat comes in many forms and disguises. A high intake of cholesterol and saturated fats is associated with the development of CHD, whereas a proportional intake of polyunsaturated and monounsaturated fats is linked with lower risk. The AHA Step 1 Diet contains no more than 30% of calories from fat, 55% from carbohydrate (at least half of which should be complex), and 15% from protein. When fat intake does not exceed 30% of total calories, the expected rise in triglycerides from a high carbohydrate diet is mini-mal. Saturated fats should account for no more than 10% of caloric intake.[7, 21]

Physical Inactivity

Twenty-five per cent of adults in the United States report no leisure-time physical activity even though regular aerobic exercise is important in preventing heart and blood vessel disease. The Framingham Study demonstrated an inverse relationship between exercise and the risk of CHD. Those who exercise reduce their risk of CHD because they have (1) higher HDL levels; (2) lower LDL cholesterol, triglyceride, and blood glucose levels; (3) greater insulin sensitivity; (4) lower blood pressure; and (5) lower body mass index.[9]

Obesity

Obesity places an extra burden on the heart, requiring the muscle to work harder to pump enough blood to support added tissue mass. In addition, obesity increases one's risk for CHD because it is often associated with elevated serum cholesterol and triglyceride levels, high blood pressure, and diabetes.

Distribution of body fat is also important. In older women, a waist-to-hip ratio of 0.8 or higher is one of the major risk factors for CHD. People can lower their heart disease risk by losing as little as 10 to 20 pounds.[6] However, an alternating pattern of weight gain and weight loss is associated with an increased risk for CHD.[49]

Diabetes

Diabetes frequently appears in middle-aged, overweight people. A fasting blood glucose level of more than 126 mg/dl or a routine blood glucose level of 180 mg/dl and glucosuria signals the presence of diabetes and represents an increased risk for CHD. Diabetes leads to early atherosclerosis and in women increases the risk of CHD by three-fold to seven-fold.[49]

CONTRIBUTING RISK FACTORS

Response to Stress

A person's response to stress may contribute to the development of CHD. Some researchers have reported a relationship between CHD risk and stress levels, health behaviors, and socioeconomic status. Stress appears to increase CHD risk through its effect on major risk factors. For example, people may respond to stress by overeating or by starting or increasing smoking. Stress is also associated with elevated blood pressure. Although stress is unavoidable in modern life, an excessive response to stress can be a health hazard. Significant stressors include major changes in residence, occupation, or socioeconomic status.

Homocysteine Levels

Researchers have reported that elevated levels of plasma homocysteine (an amino acid produced by the body) are associated with an increased risk of CHD. However, scientists do not know whether homocysteine directly or indirectly increases CHD risk because homocysteine levels are related to renal function, smoking, fibrinogen, and C-reactive protein. Elevated homocysteine levels can be reduced by treatment with folic acid, vitamin B_6, and vitamin B_{12}. Experts currently recommend that homocysteine levels be measured in people with a history of premature CHD, cerebrovascular accident, or both in the absence of other risk factors.[9]

Menopause

The incidence of CHD markedly increases among women after menopause. Before menopause, estrogen is thought to protect against CHD risk by raising HDL and lowering LDL levels. Epidemiologic studies have shown that the loss of natural estrogen as women age may be associated with increases in total and LDL cholesterol and a gradually increasing CHD risk. If menopause is caused by surgical removal of the uterus and ovaries, the risks of CHD and MI rise.

Estrogen replacement therapy (ERT) is currently recommended for women without a confirmed diagnosis of CHD who are not at high risk for breast cancer or thromboembolism. A large number of studies suggest that ERT substantially decreases the risk of coronary events and is associated with increases in HDL and decreases in LDL and fibrinogen levels.

Evidence regarding the role of ERT for women with diagnosed CHD is conflicting. Observational studies indicate that ERT is beneficial for women with diagnosed CHD; however, recent results from a large multicenter clinical trial show an increase in cardiovascular events after 1 year of treatment with estrogen and progesterone therapy but a decrease in cardiovascular events in years 4 and 5.[26] Additional research is being conducted in this area.[34]

Pathophysiology

There are three layers in the arterial wall:

1. The *intima*, a single layer of cells on the inner surface of the artery, normally provides an impermeable barrier to proteins in the blood.
2. The *media* (middle layer) is made up almost entirely of smooth muscle cells.
3. The *adventitia* consists mainly of smooth muscle cells, fibroblasts, and loose connective tissue.

Atherosclerosis primarily affects the intima of the arterial wall and normally takes years to develop. When clinical manifestations develop, atherosclerosis is usually well advanced.

PATHOGENESIS OF ATHEROSCLEROSIS

In the 1950s, pathologists proposed that atherosclerosis progressed through three developmental stages: the fatty streak, the fibrous plaque, and the complicated lesion. This classification system was commonly used until the late 1990's. In 1995, the AHA published a report that reclassified atherosclerosis into five phases, including six progressive types of lesions (Table 56–1).[46] *Phase I* is present in most people 30 years of age and younger and is characterized by lesions of types I through III that do not appreciably thicken the arterial wall or narrow the arterial lumen. Lesion types I and II, also called *early lesions*, occur primarily in infants and children but also may be present in adults.

Type I lesions are microscopic, occur most often near branches in the arteries, and consist of adaptive thickening of the smooth muscle and lipid-filled macrophages, called foam cells. Type I lesions progress and mature into *type II* lesions that consist of fatty streaks containing intracellular lipid droplets, clusters of foam cells, and smooth muscle cells.[16, 17]

Type III lesions, known as *intermediate* lesions, develop during one's 20s. These lesions appear as raised fatty streaks in which extracellular connective tissue, fibrils, and lipid deposits surround the smooth muscle cells. Type III lesions are also referred to as "pre-atheromas" because they form the bridge between early and advanced lesions. In phase I, the progression of lesions is predictable, characteristic, and uniform.[17, 46]

Phase II, characterized by type IV and V lesions, represents the development of vulnerable plaques that contain pools of extracellular lipids. The *type IV* lesion, also called an *atheroma,* is characterized by further changes in the intimal structure caused by the accumulation of large amounts of extracellular lipids and fibrous tissue localized into a lipid core. The lipid core thickens the artery wall but often does not narrow the lumen of the artery. The periphery of type IV lesions is vulnerable to rupture, which may lead to rapid progression to more severe lesions.

When new fibrous connective tissue forms a thin protective cap over the atheroma, the lesion is classified as *type V.* These lesions are further subdivided into types Va, Vb, and Vc. *Type Va* lesions contain irregularly stacked multiple layers of lipid cores separated by thick layers of fibrous connective tissue. These lesions may rapidly progress to a *type VI* lesion or may continue to develop into stenotic plaques that may eventually occlude the entire lumen of the artery.[16] A type V lesion that contains calcium in the lipid core and other parts of the lesion is referred to as type *Vb.* The absence of a lipid core, with minimal lipid deposition in other parts of the lesion, is characteristic of a type *Vc* lesion. Type *Vc* lesions are often seen in arteries in the legs.[17, 46]

Phase III is marked by the acute disruption of type IV and V lesions that causes thrombus formation and the development of a type VI lesion (*complicated*). If thrombus formation during phase III does not limit the flow of blood through the artery, these events are often asymptomatic. The net result of phase III is a rapid increase in plaque size that may result in stable angina. However, if the thrombus reduces or significantly blocks flow through the artery (*phase IV*), an acute coronary syndrome such as unstable angina, MI, or sudden cardiac death often results (see Chapter 58). Type VI lesions are characterized by a core containing extracellular lipids, tissue factor, collagen, platelets, thrombin, and fibrin. These lesions may also be associated with disruption of the plaque surface, hematoma or hemorrhage into the plaque, and thrombosis.[17, 46]

Phase V follows a phase III or IV event and occurs when the thrombus over the disrupted plaque begins to calcify (type Vb lesion) or fibrose (type Vc lesion), forming a chronic stenotic lesion. The phase V lesion often contains organizing thrombus from several earlier episodes of plaque disruption, ulceration, hemorrhage, and organization. As the phase V lesion progresses, it occludes a greater portion of the arterial lumen and eventually may lead to total occlusion. Phase V lesions are associated with chronic stable angina and are often accompanied by the development of collateral circulation.[17, 46]

Collateral circulation is the presence of more than one artery supplying a muscle. There is normally some collateral circulation in the coronary arteries, especially in

TABLE 56-1	PROGRESSION OF ATHEROSCLEROSIS, CLINICAL MANIFESTATIONS, AND ASSOCIATED LESIONS			
Phase of Coronary Heart Disease	Type and Characteristics	Earliest Onset	Clinical Manifestation	Illustration
Phase I	*Type I (initial lesion)* Isolated macrophage foam cells Intimal thickening located near bifurcations of artery	Infancy and childhood	Clinically silent	Intima / Media / Adventitia — Adaptive thickening (smooth muscle)
	Type II (fatty streak) No decrease in lumen Flat, fatty streaks Lipid accumulation with clusters of macrophage foam cells	Infancy and childhood	Clinically silent	Macrophage foam cells
	Type III (preatheroma) Raised fatty streaks Lipid-filled foam cells and smooth muscle cells	From third decade on	Clinically silent	Extracellular lipids
Phase II	*Type IV (atheroma)* Disturbed intimal structure with extracellular lipid and fibrous tissue in core Small to moderate decreases in lumen	From third decade on	Clinically silent	Core of extracelluar lipid
	Type Va (fibroatheroma) Lipid core with fibrotic layer Multiple lipid cores and fibrotic layers	From fourth decade on	Va is usually clinically silent, whereas Vb may be associated with chronic stable angina	Fibrous thickening
Phase III	*Type VI (complicated lesion)* Plaque rupture Mural thrombus with partial occlusion of lumen	From fourth decade on	Angina pectoris that is due to partial occlusion of vessel	Thrombus
Phase IV	*Type VI lesion* Same as above except greater degree of occlusion	From fourth decade on	Acute syndromes, unstable angina, myocardial infarction, sudden death	Fissure and hematoma

Table continued on following page

TABLE 56–1	PROGRESSION OF ATHEROSCLEROSIS, CLINICAL MANIFESTATIONS, AND ASSOCIATED LESIONS *Continued*			
Phase of Coronary Heart Disease	**Type and Characteristics**	**Earliest Onset**	**Clinical Manifestation**	**Illustration**
Phase V	*Type Vb-c* Complicated plaques from phase III become calcified (Vb) or fibrotic (Vc)	From fourth decade on	Stable angina	Organized thrombus covered over by fibrous or calcified tissue

older people. Collateral vessels develop when the blood flow through an artery progressively decreases and causes ischemia to the muscle. Extra blood vessels develop to meet metabolic demands of the muscle. The development of collateral circulation takes time. Therefore, an occlusion of a coronary artery in a younger person is more likely to be lethal because there are no collateral arteries present to supply the myocardium with blood.

For many years, researchers thought that the more obstructive lesions (types Vb and Vc) were responsible for most occlusions of the coronary arteries and acute coronary events. In contrast, more recent studies suggest that lesions that produce mild stenosis (types IV and Va) are more frequently associated with rapid progression to coronary occlusion. In fact, nearly 60% to 70% of all acute coronary syndromes occur in arteries with mild (< 50% stenosis) or moderate (50% to 70% stenosis) occlusion. It is thought that this occurs because less occlusive lesions are more vulnerable to plaque rupture and thrombosis.[44, 54] Plaque disruption is thought to result from external stresses on the vessel and internal changes that increase plaque fragility. Physical forces that exert external pressure on the atherosclerotic plaques such as blood and pulse pressures, heart contraction, vasospasm, and shear stress may trigger plaque rupture.[54] Internal factors, such as inflammation, may increase plaque vulnerability.

Systemic infections of *Chlamydia pneumoniae* and *Helicobacter pylori* have been linked to the development of atherosclerosis and are thought to contribute to plaque instability because they activate the inflammatory response. Treatment of these infections with antibiotics has been found to improve the prognosis after an acute coronary event.[22, 23] Researchers are investigating methods to detect vulnerable plaques and are evaluating the effectiveness of interventions designed to stabilize atherosclerotic plaques.

Clinical Manifestations

Atherosclerosis by itself does not necessarily produce subjective clinical manifestations. For manifestations to develop, there must be a critical deficit in the blood supply to the heart in proportion to the demands for oxygen and nutrients. In other words, a supply-and-demand imbalance must exist. When atherosclerosis progresses slowly, the collateral circulation that develops generally can meet the heart's demands. Thus, whether manifestations of CHD develop depends on the total blood supply to the myocardium (by way of the coronary arteries and collateral circulation) and not solely on the condition of the coronary arteries.

Rapid progression of atherosclerotic lesions (type VI) may cause ischemia and may result in the development of acute coronary syndromes of unstable angina, MI, and sudden cardiac death. Slow progression of atherosclerotic lesions (types Vb and Vc) is associated with stable coronary artery disease and the clinical manifestation of chronic stable angina. These lesions usually cause ischemia during periods when myocardial oxygen demand increases.[17] Angina, MI, and sudden cardiac death are discussed in Chapter 58.

Techniques to determine the extent of CHD and identify the affected vessels include the electrocardiogram (ECG), B-mode ultrasonography, Doppler flow studies, intravascular ultrasound, electron-beam computed tomography, and thallium, sestamibi, or echocardiographic stress tests (see Chapter 58).[46]

Outcome Management

■ Medical Management

The primary goals that guide the medical management of a client with CHD are reducing and controlling risk factors and restoring blood supply to the myocardium.

REDUCE RISK FACTORS

Prevention, rather than treatment, is the goal with regard to CHD. Modification of risk factors can significantly improve prognosis even after an acute coronary event.[17] Recent findings indicate that risk factor reduction may limit and even prevent the progression of CHD by increasing the stability of atherosclerotic plaques, decreasing thrombogenicity, and limiting external stress on the vessel. Consensus Panel Statements, revised in 1999, outline recommendations for primary prevention of CHD as well as comprehensive risk reduction for clients with diagnosed CHD.[6] For people without diagnosed CHD, the goal of medical treatment is to prevent the development of risk factors and clinical disease. Cessation of cigarette smoking, participating in regular exercise, and controlling blood pressure, diabetes, cholesterol levels, and weight can reduce the risk of CHD.[6]

Primary and secondary prevention goals are in place for all of the major risk factors. Ideally, primary prevention should begin with promoting healthy lifestyles in children. Primary care should include family-oriented risk factor education, review of family history, and risk factor modification. For clients with diagnosed CHD, the goals of prevention are to (1) reduce the incidence of subsequent coronary events, (2) decrease the need for treatments such as angioplasty and coronary artery bypass graft (CABG) surgery, (3) extend overall survival, and (4) improve quality of life.

People should stop smoking and avoid contact with secondary smoke. Health professionals should provide counseling, nicotine replacement, and referrals to smoking cessation programs for clients who smoke. Blood pressure should be measured at least every 2 years in adults, and clients should be encouraged to control blood pressure by maintaining ideal weight, exercising regularly, moderating alcohol intake, and following a moderately low sodium diet. Blood pressure should be below 140/90 (<130/85 for those with heart failure, diabetes, or renal insufficiency). Antihypertensive therapy should begin if blood pressure exceeds 140/90 after 6 months of lifestyle modification or if the initial blood pressure exceeds 160/100 (130/85 mm Hg for those with heart failure, diabetes, or renal insufficiency).[6, 9]

Total, LDL, and HDL cholesterol should be measured annually for adults older than 20 years of age. Primary prevention goals for cholesterol management are as follows:

- LDL < 160 mg/dl if no or one risk factor
- LDL < 130 mg/dl if two or more risk factors
- HDL > 35 mg/dl
- Triglycerides < 200 mg/dl

Secondary prevention goals for cholesterol management are:

- LDL < 100 mg/dl
- HDL > 35 mg/dl
- Triglycerides < 200 mg/dl

The AHA Step 1 Diet should be recommended for clients not meeting primary prevention goals, and the Step 2 Diet should be recommended for those with CHD who do not meet recommended goals. In addition, drug therapy is recommended for clients who do not meet recommended goals for cholesterol management.[9, 20, 28]

During routine physical examinations, health professionals should determine the client's activity level and participation in exercise. Clients should be encouraged to exercise three to four times weekly for 30 to 60 minutes and to increase their physical activity in daily life. An exercise test may be needed to guide an exercise prescription for clients with confirmed CHD.[6, 9]

Clients should be encouraged to maintain ideal body weight as indicated by a body mass index (BMI) between 21 and 25 kg/m² and a waist circumference less than 40 inches in men and 36 inches in women. Height, weight, BMI, and waist-to-hip ratio should be measured at each

visit. People with BMIs and waist circumferences higher than those recommended should be counseled regarding weight management and physical activity.[6, 9]

Fasting blood glucose should be maintained near normal levels in clients with diabetes mellitus. Hypoglycemic therapy should be used to achieve normal fasting plasma glucose, as indicated by hemoglobin A_{1c} (HbA_{1c}). Other risk factors should be treated aggressively.[6, 9]

ERT should be considered for all postmenopausal women without diagnosed CHD, particularly if they have multiple risk factors. However, the decision regarding therapy should be made by considering the risks for breast cancer, gallbladder disease, thromboembolic disease, and endometrial cancer.[6, 49] It has been reported that estrogen-progesterone therapy increases cardiovascular events in women with diagnosed CHD during the first year of treatment but decreases events in the fourth and fifth years. Consequently, initiating estrogen and progesterone therapy for women with confirmed CHD is not recommended. For women with CHD who have already been receiving ERT for more than 1 year, continuing therapy is recommended until the results of additional research are known.[34]

Additional management strategies are recommended for clients with diagnosed CHD. These include the use of antiplatelet therapies such as acetylsalicylic acid (aspirin), heparin, and low-molecular-weight heparin if not contraindicated.[6, 17] Aspirin reduces the risk of fatal or nonfatal MI by 71% during the acute phase, by 60% at 3 months, and by 52% at 2 years.[17] Adjunctive therapies, such as angiotensin-converting enzyme (ACE) inhibitors, beta-blockers, and nitrates, are also recommended.[6, 9, 17]

Glycoprotein IIb/IIIa receptor antagonists are the most recent pharmacologic treatment for secondary prevention of CHD. These drugs prevent platelet aggregation in acute coronary syndromes, and when combined with aspirin, they decrease the incidence of recurrent cardiac events.[17] The therapeutic effects, adverse responses, and nursing implications of pharmacologic agents used in the primary prevention of CHD are outlined in Table 56–2.

RESTORE BLOOD SUPPLY

For some clients, even aggressive management of risk factors fails to prevent coronary occlusion. Various techniques have been developed to open the vessels and restore blood flow through the coronary arteries. Collectively, these procedures—coronary angioplasty, intracoronary stent placement, and laser atherectomy—are called *interventional cardiology*.[12, 15]

Percutaneous Transluminal Coronary Angioplasty

Percutaneous transluminal coronary angioplasty (PTCA) is a technique in which a balloon-tipped catheter is inserted into a leg artery and threaded under x-ray guidance into a blocked coronary artery. The balloon is inflated several times to reshape the lumen by stretching it and flattening the atherosclerotic plaque against the arterial wall, thus opening the artery (Fig. 56–1). In 1996, more than 482,000 PTCA procedures were performed in the United States. The success rate (defined as >20% reduction in stenosis) was reported as 82%. PTCA is less invasive and less expensive than open heart surgery and therefore is an attractive alternative.[7]

Guidelines for selection of clients for PTCA are rap-

TABLE 56–2	PREVENTIVE PHARMACOTHERAPY IN CORONARY HEART DISEASE		
	Assessing Therapeutic Responses	Assessing Adverse Responses	Nursing Implications
Antiplatelet-aggregating agents			
Acetylsalicylic acid (ASA)	ASA blocks prostaglandin synthesis action, which prevents formation of the platelet-aggregating substance thromboxane A_2. The therapeutic response would be the absence or slowed formation of coronary artery disease.	Clients may experience heartburn, stomach pains, nausea and vomiting, rash, weakness, hemolytic anemia, and gastrointestinal (GI) ulceration. Overdose symptoms include tinnitus, headache, dizziness, confusion, and metabolic acidosis.	▪ Avoid use in clients with severe liver or renal disease. ▪ Monitor serum concentrations, renal function, hearing changes, skin inflammation, and abnormal bleeding. ▪ Administer with food or large quantities of water to decrease GI upset. ▪ Instruct clients to avoid concurrent use of over-the-counter products that contain ASA.
Antilipemic agents			
Simvastatin	It inhibits an enzyme, 3-hydroxy-3-methylglutaryl coenzyme A reductase, which is responsible for catalyzing an early step in the synthesis of cholesterol. Total cholesterol and low-density lipoprotein levels will decline.	Clients may experience headache, dizziness, abdominal cramps, constipation, diarrhea, flatus, heartburn, and rashes.	▪ Monitor plasma triglycerides, cholesterol, and liver function tests. ▪ Instruct clients to report any unexplained muscle pain or weakness. ▪ Administer with food. ▪ Advise clients that medication should be used along with diet restrictions.

Data from Armstrong, L. L. (Ed.). *The University of Chicago formulary of accepted drugs.* Hudson, OH: Lexi-Comp, Inc., 1998.

idly changing. Clients with no or mild manifestations to clients with unstable angina may be suitable candidates. PTCA may also be successful in single-vessel or multiple-vessel disease. However, balloon angioplasty is most successful in men who are younger than age 70 and have normal pumping ability; no more than two blocked arteries; and no history of diabetes, MI, or coronary artery bypass surgery.[12] One study indicated that clients with "type A" behavior, specifically hostility, carry an increased risk of restenosis after PTCA.[19] In addition to PTCA, new therapeutic devices for coronary application continue to evolve as alternatives to bypass surgery.

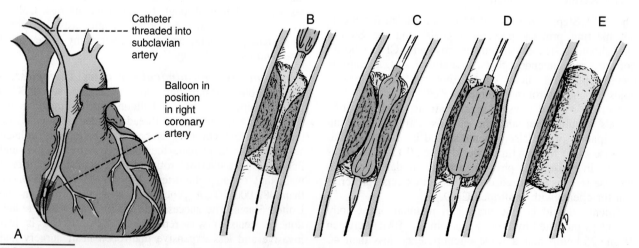

FIGURE 56–1 Percutaneous transluminal coronary angioplasty (PTCA). *A,* A balloon-tipped catheter positioned in a blocked artery. *B,* The balloon is centered. *C,* The balloon expands to compress the blockage (*D*). *E,* The artery is restored to its original diameter.

Directional Coronary Atherectomy

Atherectomy was designed to overcome two of the most significant complications of PTCA: restenosis and abrupt closure of the coronary artery.[15, 42] Restenosis occurs in 25% to 50% of clients within 2 to 6 months after PTCA, whereas abrupt closure resulting from plaque fracture, coronary artery dissection, localized thrombus, or coronary artery spasm occurs in 2% to 6% of clients after PTCA. Directional coronary atherectomy (DCA) reduces coronary stenosis by excising and removing atheromatous plaque. The DCA cutter consists of a catheter that contains a rigid cylindrical housing with a central rotating blade (Fig. 56–2). The blade shaves off the atherosclerotic material and deposits it in the nose cone of the housing for later histopathologic study. Because the spinning of the cutter can cause vibrations that irritate the vessel wall and cause coronary vasospasm, calcium-channel blockers are usually given before the procedure.[15]

DCA is very appropriate for lesions in medium to large coronary arteries located in the proximal or middle portions of the vessel. It is not recommended for use with tortuous vessels, distal lesions, or heavily calcified lesions. The large size of the catheter (10 or 11F) limits the usefulness of DCA in treating women. The use of DCA

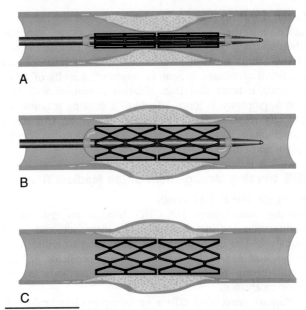

FIGURE 56–3 Placement of a coronary artery stent. *A,* The stent is positioned at the site of the lesion. *B,* The balloon is inflated, expanding the stent. The balloon is then deflated and removed. *C,* The implanted stent is left in place.

has decreased because of the increasing use of stents and reports that the results are not comparable to those of PTCA.[12] Complications of DCA include embolus formation, acute vessel occlusion, vessel perforation, and arterial spasm. After DCA, clients are given enteric-coated aspirin to prevent thrombosis.

Intracoronary Stents

Intracoronary stents were originally designed to reduce restenosis and abrupt closure of coronary vessels resulting from complications of coronary angioplasty. They are now used instead of PTCA to eliminate the risk of acute closure and to improve long-term patency.[15] There are several different stent designs, but most are balloon-expandable or self-expandable tubes that, when placed in a coronary artery, act as a mechanical scaffold to reopen the blocked artery (Fig. 56–3). Coronary stents are made of numerous materials, ranging from stainless steel to bioabsorbable compounds.

The procedure for placing a stent is similar to that for PTCA. Once the coronary lesion is identified by angiography, the balloon catheter bearing the stent is inserted into the coronary artery and the stent is positioned at the site of the occlusion. A major concern related to stent placement is the prevention of acute thrombosis, especially during the first several weeks after the procedure. During the initial recovery period, clients receive an antiplatelet, such as ticlopidine, and an anticoagulant. To prevent thrombosis, clients must take antiplatelet inhibitors over the long term. If anticoagulation is continued after discharge, clients are usually given warfarin for 6 weeks after the procedure. Long-term anticoagulation therapy is required only when optimal stent expansion is not achieved or when the resulting lumen diameter is less than 3 mm.[15] Complications include stent occlusion, bleeding secondary to anticoagulation, and coronary artery dissection.[12, 15]

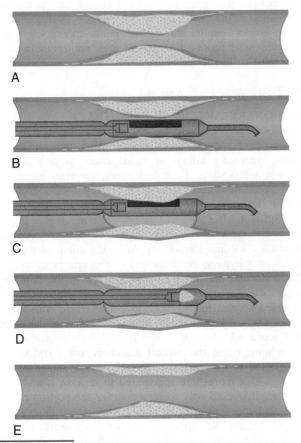

FIGURE 56–2 Atherectomy. *A,* Lesion. *B,* The catheter is advanced through the artery so that the cutting device is positioned over the lesion. *C,* The balloon on the device is inflated to stabilize the catheter. *D,* The cutting portion of the catheter is advanced, slicing away the lesion and trapping it in the cylindrical housing. The balloon is then deflated, and the catheter is removed. *E,* Result of the procedure.

Laser Ablation

Lasers are used with balloon angioplasty to vaporize atherosclerotic plaque. After the initial balloon angioplasty, a brief burst of laser radiation is administered and additional remaining plaque is removed. Results of clinical trials indicate that laser ablation combined with balloon angioplasty is more effective in treating lesions that typically respond poorly to angioplasty alone. Complications include coronary dissection, acute occlusion, perforation, and embolism.[12, 15]

■ Nursing Management of the Medical Client

REDUCE RISK FACTORS

Nursing management for CHD focuses on risk factor modification and includes risk assessment, screening, and education. The client's level of motivation to reduce cardiovascular risk factors is the primary predictor of success. Nursing researchers are studying methods to improve motivation.

Primary prevention efforts include providing health education on reducing risk factors for CHD. Encourage clients to reduce their risk by lowering dietary intake of fats and cholesterol, exercising, controlling diabetes and hypertension, keeping body weight near ideal levels, and ceasing smoking. The risk and incidence of CHD are so high that many clients are doing these activities on an ongoing basis. Reinforce these behaviors. Participate in risk factor screening for children and adults, and maintain a high index of suspicion for clients at increased risk for CHD. Teach stress reduction techniques, such as progressive muscle relaxation and guided imagery. Instruct postmenopausal women to discuss the need for estrogen replacement therapy (ERT) with their physician. Monitor blood pressure control in clients with diagnosed hypertension, and monitor HbA_{1c} levels in diabetic clients.

Nursing interventions for clients with diagnosed CHD include assessing their CHD risk and explaining diagnostic tests, when to seek treatment, clinical manifestations of complications, and the actions, dosages, and side effects of prescribed medications. Assess cardiovascular risk factors, and provide individualized education on risk reduction. Emphasize the importance of adopting risk-reduction behaviors and participating in cardiac rehabilitation to prevent recurrence or progression of CHD. Teach clients the clinical manifestations of angina and MI. Monitor therapeutic drug levels as appropriate. Emphasize the importance of keeping follow-up appointments with health care practitioners. Most important, instruct clients to seek prompt medical attention if symptoms of CHD return.

Many clients use forms of alternative therapies for self-treatment of heart disease. See the Alternative Therapy feature.

RESTORE BLOOD SUPPLY

Before interventional procedures, the client is usually given an antiplatelet medication, such as aspirin. The client is also given an anticoagulant (heparin) to prevent occlusion and calcium-channel blockers or nitrates to reduce coronary spasm during the procedure. After the procedure, the client may continue with this drug regimen to prevent reocclusion or arterial spasms.[15, 24]

The client's blood is also typed and crossmatched in the event that emergency CABG surgery is needed. A consent form is signed for the interventional procedure and surgery, if required, for spasm, perforation of the artery, or acute occlusion. Following interventional procedures, monitor the client for changes in vital signs, especially the quality and rhythm of pulse, and in the ECG. Report any indication of coronary ischemia to the physician. ST-segment monitoring is frequently used to detect ischemia. If the client complains of chest pain, obtain a 12-lead ECG immediately. Force fluids, orally or intravenously, to assist the body in excreting contrast, which causes diuresis and may cause acute tubular necrosis. Monitor the puncture site for hematoma, and palpate pulses to assess peripheral perfusion. Complications include bleeding and hematoma formation at the puncture site, acute MI resulting from perforation of an artery, refractory spasm, or occlusion. The physician may order bed rest for longer periods for clients undergoing stent placement and DCA because of the larger sheaths used to dilate the vessels in these procedures.

Nursing considerations specific to the care of the client with a coronary stent include close monitoring of anticoagulation status and ongoing assessment for bleeding. Until the sheath is removed, instruct the client to limit movement of the sheathed leg and keep the head of the bed below 30 degrees to prevent bleeding and hematoma formation at the site. Clients with coronary stents usually have longer hospital stays than clients undergoing other interventional procedures because their antithrombin therapy must be monitored closely.[47, 48]

■ Surgical Management

CORONARY ARTERY BYPASS GRAFT

CABG surgery involves the bypass of a blockage in one or more of the coronary arteries using the saphenous veins, mammary artery, or radial artery as conduits or replacement vessels. Prior to surgery, coronary angiography precisely locates lesions and points of narrowing within the coronary arteries.

During CABG surgery, the surgeon harvests a length of saphenous vein from the thigh. The heart is accessed through a median sternotomy. With the client on cardiopulmonary bypass, the distal end of the vein is sutured to the aorta and the proximal end is sewn to the coronary vessel distal to the blockage (Fig. 56–4). The veins are reversed so that their valves do not interfere with blood flow. The cardiopulmonary bypass machine is discussed in Chapter 57.

In some cases, the internal mammary artery (IMA) can be grafted to a coronary artery. The disadvantage of the IMA is that more time is required to remove it and it is shorter. It is used only to revascularize the portion of the myocardium supplied by the left anterior descending (LAD) artery. An advantage is that IMA grafts have a greater chance of remaining patent. Radial arteries have been used as an alternative to saphenous vein conduits and show excellent short-term and long-term patency rates.[52]

A new approach to CABG surgery, called minimally invasive direct CABG (MIDCABG) surgery, is being per-

ALTERNATIVE THERAPY

Cardiac Disorders

Cardiovascular disease has been shown to be largely related to lifestyle habits such as exercise, diet, and smoking. Unfortunately, although many people are aware of the importance of these factors, they are often ignored. New research continues to elucidate the effects of often simple lifestyle changes that can help prevent cardiac problems. An examination of fiber intake and coronary heart disease (CHD) among women in the Nurses' Health Study, a very large cohort study of female nurses followed for 10 years, found that high fiber intake from cereal sources reduced the risk of CHD.[11] Another study, looking again at the Nurses' Health Study as well as men in the Health Professionals' Follow-up Study, found a protective benefit from consumption of fruit and vegetables, particularly green leafy and cruciferous vegetables and citrus fruit and juice, for ischemic stroke.[3] The former study examined a cohort of nearly 70,000; the latter examined 113,000 people.

An intensive program of lifestyle changes pioneered by Dean Ornish has been shown to lead to regression of coronary atherosclerosis.[8] The lifestyle changes included a vegetarian diet limited to 10% fat intake, aerobic exercise, stress management, smoking cessation, and group psychosocial activity. Although some have debated the results achieved and whether other lifestyle modifications might be as successful, there is little doubt that lifestyle changes can be not only preventive but also therapeutic in managing clients with heart disease.[2, 4, 7]

CoEnzyme Q10 (CoQ10), or ubiquinone, is synthesized in all human cells and is also present in many foods. First isolated in 1957, CoQ10 was later produced in large quantities, and many studies demonstrated its therapeutic benefits in the treatment of heart problems.[9] CoQ10 has been helpful in treating angina, heart failure, and dysrhythmias and in preventing problems following heart surgery. It is thought that a deficiency of CoQ10 may be a factor in the development of heart disease in certain people. Certain medications may lower CoQ10 levels. Many cardiologists are now aware of the research on CoQ10, and laboratory tests are available to monitor its levels. CoQ10 has the potential to be an important adjunct in the treatment of a number of heart problems.

The nutrients magnesium, thiamine (vitamin B_1), and carnitine have all been found to have potentially positive effects in the management of heart failure. Interestingly, drugs such as diuretics, commonly used in treating heart failure, may lead to depletion of nutrients such as magnesium and thiamine. Many older adults, especially those on poorer diets, may have thiamine and other nutritional deficiencies that could have an impact on cardiovascular health.[5]

The leaves, berries, and flowering tops of the herb hawthorn (Crataegus monogyna) have been traditionally used for heart problems. Although hawthorn may improve cardiac output, decrease angina, and lower cholesterol,[6] the German Commission E has only approved the leaf with flowers for treatment of decreased cardiac output in patients with stage II of the New York Heart Association's classification for 1994.[1] Tyler[10] comments that although hawthorn is "devoid of side effects," it may be difficult to obtain adequate quality preparations of it, and he questions the wisdom of self-treatment for problems as serious as cardiac ones.

References

1. Blumenthal, M. (Ed.). (1998). *The complete German Commission E monographs: Therapeutic guide to herbal medicines.* Austin, TX: American Botanical Council.
2. Herbert, P. N. (1999). Effect of lifestyle changes on coronary heart disease. [Letter]. *Journal of the American Medical Association, 282,* 130.
3. Joshipura, K. J., et al. (1999). Fruit and vegetable intake in relation to risk of ischemic stroke. *Journal of the American Medical Association, 282,* 1233–1239.
4. Lear, S. A. (1999). Effect of lifestyle changes on coronary heart disease. [Letter]. *Journal of the American Medical Association, 282,* 131.
5. Murray, M. T. (1997). Natural support for congestive heart failure. *American Journal of Natural Medicine, 4*(5), 14–17.
6. Murray, M. T. (1999). Important considerations in angina. *Natural Medicine Journal, 2*(2), 1–8.
7. Miller, M. (1999). Effect of lifestyle changes on coronary heart disease. [Letter]. *Journal of the American Medical Association, 282,* 130.
8. Ornish, D. et al. (1998). Intensive lifestyle changes for reversal of coronary heart disease. *Journal of the American Medical Association, 280,* 2001–2007.
9. Sinatra, S. T. (1999). CoEnzyme Q10: A cardiologist's commentary. *Natural Medicine Journal 2*(2), 9–15.
10. Tyler, V. E. (1994). *Herbs of choice.* Binghamton, NY: Pharmaceutical Products Press.
11. Wolk, A., et al. (1998). Long-term intake of dietary fiber and decreased risk of coronary heart disease among women. *Journal of the American Medical Association, 281,* 1998–2000.

James Higgy Lerner, RN, LAc, *Private practice of acupuncture, traditional Oriental medicine, and biofeedback*

formed in many institutions. MIDCABG surgery is a less invasive approach for clients who need revascularization of the anterior coronary arteries. The internal mammary arteries are used as conduits, and the client does not have to be placed on cardiopulmonary bypass. MIDCABG surgery is less costly than traditional CABG surgery and is associated with fewer postoperative complications.[32]

Surgical methods only ease the manifestations. Surgery cannot halt the process of atherosclerosis, although it may prolong life in some cases. The surgical management of CHD in women is being studied. Data from several studies have reported that, compared with men, women have higher operative mortality rates, lower rates of graft patency, less frequent use of arterial conduits for grafting, more frequent reoperations, increased incidence of perioperative infarction and heart failure, and less long-term symptomatic relief.[49] However, a report from the Bypass Angioplasty Revascularization Investigation found better outcomes for women than men in nonemergent situations.[27] Scientists are continuing to conduct research in this area.

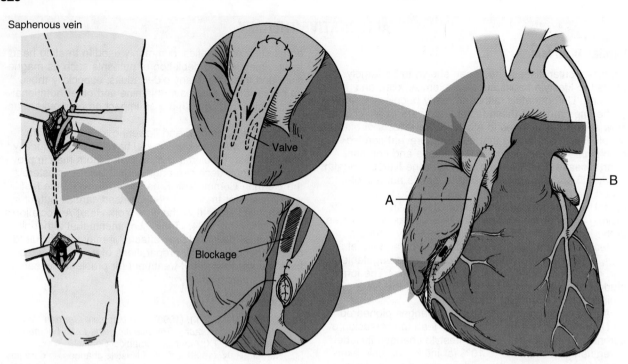

FIGURE 56-4 Coronary artery bypass grafting (CABG). *A,* A section of saphenous vein is harvested from the leg and anastomosed (upside down, because of its directional valves) to a coronary artery to bypass an area of occlusion on the right coronary artery. *B,* Bypass of the left coronary artery with mammary artery.

Possible complications of CABG surgery include:

- Postoperative bleeding
- Wound infection and dehiscence
- Intraoperative stroke
- MI
- Blood clots
- Multiple organ system failure
- Death

The development of calcium-channel blockers and non-surgical interventions such as PTCA, atherectomy, and stents have reduced the number of CABG surgical procedures being performed. Survival rates in CABG have not been significantly better than survival rates of medically treated clients. CABG nevertheless remains a common procedure, and because it can reduce angina in 80% to 90% of clients who do not respond to medical management, it will continue as an important intervention in the management of CHD. Benefits from CABG surgery also include prolongation of life, increased exercise tolerance, reduced need for medication, and ability to resume former activities.

TRANSMYOCARDIAL REVASCULARIZATION

A new procedure that is still experimental shows promise for clients with widespread atherosclerosis involving vessels that are too small and numerous for replacement or balloon catheterization. In transmyocardial revascularization (TMR), a high-powered laser is used to open up channels in the heart through a relatively small chest incision by punching holes in a fraction of a second in the beating heart. The laser beam is applied between heartbeats when the ventricle is filled with blood. The laser creates from 15 to 40 1-mm channels through the myocardium into the distal two thirds of the left ventricle.

The exact mechanism by which TMR works has not been established. However, scientists believe that the "controlled trauma" caused by creating the channels promotes vascular growth or angiogenesis. TMR should be used only for the most severely debilitated clients who are not helped by PTCA or CABG surgery. The procedure is estimated to cost $15,000, slightly more than angioplasty but much less than CABG. Sustained improvement has been seen up to 27 months after the operation.[4, 11]

◼ Modifications for Elderly Clients

More than half of all CABG procedures are performed on people older than 65 years of age, and 71% of them on men.[7] Older clients have a postoperative recovery similar to that for younger clients, but the pace is slower and they typically remain hospitalized an average of 2 to 4 days longer. They also have a higher mortality rate.

Postoperative complications that are more prevalent in older clients include dysrhythmias related to aged sinoatrial node cells, drug toxicity associated with impaired hepatic and renal perfusion, multiple drug interactions, and decreased physical stamina. These complications contribute to a 15-day mean length of hospital stay for clients older than age 80.

During the first and second weeks after discharge, depression, fatigue, incisional chest discomfort, dyspnea, and anorexia are common. By the fourth to fifth weeks, elderly clients report improved mood, comfort, and appetite. At 1 year, almost all (93%) are pleased with the outcome and improved quality of life.

■ Nursing Management of the Surgical Client

Many hospitals have initiated rapid recovery programs for cardiac surgery clients that reduce the hospital stay to 4 days. With rapid recovery programs, most of the client's recovery takes place in the home, with the client and family assuming primary responsibility for many aspects of care. Discharge planning begins at the time of admission, activity progression in the postoperative period is accelerated, and client and family education continues on a daily basis throughout hospitalization. Many hospitals have developed clinical pathways for CABG. Use the clinical pathway for your client to assist you in planning your clients' care (see Guide to Clinical Pathway: Coronary Bypass Grafting, p. 1529). In addition, a three-phase program of activity is implemented (see discussion that follows).

PHASE I (IN-HOSPITAL) REHABILITATION PROGRAMS

Most CABG clients participate in cardiac rehabilitation following surgery. Phase I begins immediately after the client returns from surgery. The goals of phase I inpatient rehabilitation are as follows:

- To prevent the negative effects of prolonged bed rest
- To assess the client's physiologic response to exercise
- To manage the psychosocial issues related to recovery from CABG surgery
- To educate the client and family concerning recovery and the adoption of risk reduction behaviors

While in the intensive care unit, the client is turned every 2 hours during the first several hours after surgery. Once extubated, the client gets up in a chair and ambulates in the room. After transfer to the intermediate care unit, the client continues to walk three or four times a day, increasing the distance walked each time.

Assess the client's blood pressure, heart rate, ECG, and oxygen saturation before, during, and after activity. Systolic blood pressure should not increase more than 20 mm Hg or decrease more than 10 to 15 mm Hg after exercise. Heart rate should not increase more than 20 beats per minute (BPM) above resting, and no significant dysrhythmias should occur. Activity levels will be reduced if clients have adverse physiologic responses (e.g., tachycardia, dysrhythmias, pain) to exercise. Clients are seated for all meals. Research has demonstrated that early mobilization improves cardiac function and benefits the client psychologically.[5]

Education for a healthier lifestyle is an important part of each phase of cardiac rehabilitation. The emphasis in phase I is on the identification and modification of reversible risk factors to prevent further deleterious cardiac events.

■ Self-Care

Before hospital discharge, instruct the client and family (or significant other) about medication actions and side effects, dietary restrictions, physical activity restrictions and progression, and wound care. Because it is not always possible to anticipate all of the problems clients may encounter the first few days at home, instruct the client whom to call when there is an emergency or when there are questions or concerns. If possible, introduce the client to the home health nurse who will be supervising home care. Following discharge, the home health care nurse provides additional education and counseling and assesses the client for complications.[32, 47, 53] In addition, instruct the client on how to assess response to exercise and activity.[40, 41]

Before discharge, a low-level symptom-limited exercise test may be performed to evaluate the client's ability to perform activities of daily living (ADL) and exercise. The test results are used to prescribe a safe and effective exercise program for the first few weeks at home and serve as a basis for the initial exercise prescription in phase II.[5]

PHASE II (OUTPATIENT EXERCISE TRAINING) REHABILITATION PROGRAMS

Outpatient (phase II) exercise training usually takes place in a facility that provides continuous ECG monitoring, emergency equipment, and medically supervised exercise. Outpatient treatment usually begins 10 to 14 days after discharge and requires physician referral. The goals of phase II are as follows:

- To restore clients to a desirable exercise capacity appropriate to their health status, lifestyle, and occupation
- To provide additional education and support to the client and family for adoption of risk-reduction behaviors
- To meet the psychosocial needs of clients and families, restore confidence, and minimize anxiety and depression
- To promote early identification of medical problems through close observation and monitoring of clients during exercise
- To assist clients in returning to occupational and leisure activities

Exercise therapy is conducted three times weekly for 2 to 3 months. The duration of the aerobic exercise session ranges from 20 to 40 minutes at an intensity of 70% to 85% of the baseline exercise heart rate. During each exercise session, blood pressure, heart rate, respiratory rate, and ECG are monitored before, during, and after exercise. Activity levels are increased gradually, based on the client's response. A nutritionist may counsel clients about proper diet, and a psychologist or social worker may counsel clients on stress management and adoption of other risk prevention behaviors.

At the end of the program, clients are given a symptom-limited exercise test and are reevaluated. Decisions regarding progression to a phase III or home program are based on the client's results of the stress test, ability to self-monitor his or her response to exercise, the client's stability, and psychological or emotional status. Periodic evaluations are scheduled so that activity progression and cardiopulmonary function can be assessed.[5, 50]

PHASE III (COMMUNITY) REHABILITATION PROGRAMS

Phase III programs are conducted in community settings, such as a "Y" or a health club. The goals of phase III are as follows:

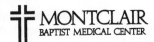

MONTCLAIR
BAPTIST MEDICAL CENTER

CABG/VALVE CAREMAP

(Addressograph)

	PRE-OP Date: _____	INITIAL Met	Not Met
General Safety:	Fall Precautions Bed Rails Up x 2 Bed in Preventive Mode		
Activity	As ordered.		
	Goal:	___	___
Dietary: Consult Date/Time Completed ____	NPO after midnight		
	Goal: _____ %	___	___
Respiratory: Consult Date/Time Completed ____	Spirometry teaching per respiratory therapy/nurse.		
	Goal: SaO2 > 90%. **Goal:** Performs correct Incentive Spirometry technique **Goal:** Clear, patent airway	___ ___ ___	___ ___ ___
Rehab: Consult Date/Time Completed ____			
	Goal:	___	___
Discharge Planning: Consult Date/Time Completed ____	Assess support system for post-hospital stay and notify social services if not adequate.		
	Goal: Adequate support system.	___	___
Nursing: Consult Date/Time Completed ____	Vital signs as ordered. B/P in both arms, height, actual weight, and SaO2 recorded on front of chart. Pre-op teaching by floor nurse and/or CCU nurse. Give patient/caregiver cardiac packet for "Open Heart Surgery Patient". Patient/Caregiver to review "Open Heart Surgery" video on patient education channel. Telemetry. Call MD if SaO2 < 90%. Do not continue Coumadin, Ticlid, Persantine, Plavix, or _____. Notify cardiologist, attending M.D., surgeon and surgeon's/physician's assistant of admission/surgery as appropriate. Request and obtain old records immediately and send old chart to surgery with patient. Antimicrobial scrub for a total of two (1 HS and 1 AM). Shave with electric surgical razor. Obtain appropriate Operative and Blood permits. Encourage patient/cargiver to verbalize and ask questions. Consult Pastoral Care. If emergency, beep on-call chaplain.		
	Goal: Patient/Caregiver verbalizes understanding of pre-op teaching. **Goal:** No symptomatic dysrhythmias.	___ ___	___ ___
Tests:	Labwork (If labwork done within 14 days, call lab to obtain results and do not repeat). CBC, S7, PT (only obtain PT if patient on Coumadin). EKG (if done within 3 months, call for report). CXR (If age > 70 or re-operation and not done within 6 months). Type and screen 2 units packed red cells. If patient is re-operation or HCT < 35, type and crossmatch 2 units of packed red cells.		
	Goal: Blood work WNL.	___	___

G-99-5179-2PG REV. 11/15/99

- To maintain and, if possible, increase exercise capacity
- To institute long-term follow-up of risk-reduction behavior change
- To encourage clients to take responsibility for continuing lifestyle changes

Exercise consists of walking, jogging, weight training, and recreational games. Clients are usually not monitored while exercising, although some facilities obtain exercise ECGs on a monthly basis. Clients are responsible for monitoring their own heart rate response to exercise, although blood pressure can be taken by program personnel if indicated.[5, 50]

HOME EXERCISE REHABILITATION PROGRAMS
For CABG clients, a home exercise program is usually prescribed in conjunction with or in place of the outpatient program. Clients are given detailed exercise instruc-

GUIDE TO CLINICAL PATHWAY

Coronary Bypass Grafting

Immediately following coronary bypass grafting (CABG) the client is in the intensive care unit (ICU). The focus of care in the ICU includes monitoring and treating hemodynamic instability and assessing respiratory status. Stays in the ICU have become very short, and many clients who were healthy before surgery are treated on "fast-track" programs to decrease their length of stay. This full care map projects a 5-day stay, with 1 day in the ICU.

Because postoperative fluid shifts increase pulmonary fluid accumulation and chest incisions create pain with deep breathing, the risk of pneumonia is great. The care map includes many interventions to promote lung aeration. Respiratory therapists assist with monitoring and care, including the use of percussion to loosen thick secretions. Use pillows to splint the incision. Ambulation is an important aspect of recovery; be certain that the client ambulates three times the second day after surgery. Administer medications as ordered for pain prior to ambulation, and monitor the client closely for dysrhythmias and desaturation during ambulation.

Many intravenous lines and tubes are discontinued on day 2. Before pulling the lines or tubes, be sure that the parameters needed (such as minimal chest tube output) are within established standards. On day 3, pacer wires are removed. In most facilities, a nurse must be certified to pull pacer wires.

Care of leg incisions varies by surgeon. Most clients report more pain in the leg than in the chest. Be prepared to explain that this is common and does not mean anything is wrong.

Discharge teaching begins on day 2. This information is an important component of full recovery. Many clients and their spouses are fearful of "doing something wrong" on discharge, and clients have been allowed to become dependent rather than independent. Work with the client and educate the family on the advantages and importance of activity to promote recovery.

The CareMap is reprinted with permission from Baptist Health System.

The CareMap shown is an excerpt of one that covers the Preoperative phase through phase III.

Helen Andrews, BSN, RN, *Care Manager, Alegent Health Bergan Mercy Medical Center, Omaha, Nebraska,* and **Linda R. Haddick, MSN, RN,** *Clinical Nurse Specialist, Alegent Health Home Care & Hospice, Omaha, Nebraska*

---

tions and are told to keep a log of heart rates, perceived exertion rates, exercise parameters, and any problems that may occur during the home program. Cardiac rehabilitation staff members or the client's physician should analyze the data and adjust the home exercise program if necessary. Once clients reach their optimal level of functional capacity, they are instructed to continue to exercise at least three times weekly so that cardiopulmonary exercise capacity can be maintained.[50]

HEART FAILURE

Despite aggressive medical and surgical treatment, CHD may eventually lead to the development of heart failure. Heart failure is a significant cardiac functional disorder that can result in reduced oxygen delivery to the body's organs and tissues. Heart failure affects approximately 4.8 million people in the United States, with 465,000 new cases diagnosed each year. In contrast to decreases in mortality rates associated with other cardiovascular diseases, the incidence of heart failure and the mortality associated with it have increased steadily since 1975.[7] Annually, about 250,000 clients die from direct or indirect consequences of heart failure, and the number of deaths that are due to heart failure has increased six-fold over the past 40 years.[7, 35]

Heart failure can affect both women and men, although it occurs more often in men, with a poorer prognosis.[38] There are also racial differences; at all ages, death rates are higher in African Americans than in non-Hispanic whites. Heart failure is primarily a disease of older adults, affecting 6% to 10% of those over 65 years of age. It is also the leading cause of hospitalization in older people.[7]

Heart failure is a physiologic state in which the heart cannot pump enough blood to meet the metabolic needs of the body (determined as oxygen consumption). Heart failure results from changes in systolic or diastolic function of the left ventricle. The heart fails when, because of intrinsic disease or structural defects, it cannot handle a normal blood volume or, in the absence of disease, cannot tolerate a sudden expansion in blood volume (e.g., during exercise). Heart failure is not a disease itself; instead, the term refers to a clinical syndrome characterized by manifestations of volume overload, inadequate tissue perfusion, and poor exercise tolerance. Whatever the cause, pump failure results in hypoperfusion of tissue, followed by pulmonary and systemic venous congestion. Because heart failure causes vascular congestion, it is often called *congestive heart failure,* although most cardiac specialists no longer use this term. Other terms used to denote heart failure include *cardiac decompensation, cardiac insufficiency,* and *ventricular failure.*[30]

Etiology and Risk Factors

The performance of the heart depends on four essential components:

- Contractility (inotropic state) of the muscle
- Preload (amount of blood in the ventricle at the end of diastole)
- Afterload (the pressure against which the left ventricle ejects)
- Heart rate

Table 56–3 defines the terms commonly used to describe cardiac function. Adverse changes in these determinants of myocardial performance ultimately cause the heart to fail. CHD is the primary cause of heart failure in two thirds of clients with decreased ventricular dysfunction.

TABLE 56-3	TERMS USED TO DESCRIBE CARDIAC FUNCTION
Term	**Function**
Afterload	Force that the ventricle must develop during systole in order to eject the stroke volume
Cardiac output	Stroke volume × heart rate
Inotropic state	A measure of contractility
Preload	Stretch of myocardial fibers at end-diastole
Stroke volume	The amount of blood ejected from the ventricle with each contraction

However, heart failure may also be caused by other disorders. The causes of heart failure can be divided into three subgroups[38]:

* Abnormal loading conditions
* Abnormal muscle function
* Conditions or diseases that limit ventricular filling

ABNORMAL LOADING CONDITIONS

Abnormal loading is associated with any condition that increases either the pressure or the volume load of the ventricle. The effect of increasing volume on the ventricle can be explained by the analogy that the heart muscle is like a stretched rubber band. When the rubber band is stretched, it contracts with more force. The heart muscle does the same. Venous return stretches the heart and improves contractility. When the rubber band is overstretched, it becomes limp and cannot contract. Likewise, when the heart is overloaded with blood, excessive stretch and decreased contraction occur. Overload develops because blood does not leave the ventricles during contraction. Therefore, cardiac workload increases in an effort to move blood.

Preload refers to the stretch of the ventricular myocardial fibers just before ventricular contraction. The load or stretch placed on the ventricular fibers corresponds to the end-diastolic ventricular volume and pressure. Preload is determined by the condition of the heart valves (especially the mitral valve), blood volume, ventricular wall compliance, and venous tone.

Table 56-4 lists conditions that increase preload. Increased preload usually increases contractility (more stretch on the rubber band) and stretch because of filling pressures from venous return and previous volume. Stretch and filling pressures may rise beyond the capabilities of the normally compliant heart. This increased preload lessens the force and efficiency of ventricular contraction. Cardiac output decreases. Under the strain of this load, the heart will fail.

Increased pressure load in the ventricle is related to *afterload,* the amount of tension the heart must generate to overcome systemic pressure and to allow adequate ventricular emptying. Thus, afterload indicates how hard the heart must pump to force blood into circulation. The tone of systemic arterioles, the elasticity of the aorta and large arteries, the size and thickness of the ventricle, the presence of aortic stenosis, and the viscosity of the blood all determine afterload. High peripheral vascular resistance and high blood pressure force the ventricle to work harder to eject blood (see Table 56-4). Subjected to prolonged high pressures, the ventricle eventually fails.[90]

ABNORMAL MUSCLE FUNCTION

Certain conditions interfere directly with myocardial contractility and affect the inherent contractility of cardiac muscle:

* MI
* Myocarditis, an inflammation of the myocardium associated with viral, bacterial, fungal, or parasitic diseases or toxic chemical injury
* Cardiomyopathy
* Ventricular aneurysm

Such disorders impair the contractile function of the myocardial fibrils, which reduces ventricular emptying and stroke volume.[38]

After an MI, some of the heart muscle is replaced by noncontracting scar tissue and the ventricles pump less efficiently. Some degree of heart failure, either chronic or transient, appears in more than half of clients after MI. Other conditions that affect the intrinsic condition of the heart muscle are listed in Table 56-4.

TABLE 56-4	ETIOLOGY OF HEART FAILURE	
Abnormal Loading Conditions	**Abnormal Muscle Function**	**Limited Ventricular Filling**
Conditions that increase preload		
Regurgitation of mitral or tricuspid valve	Myocardial infarction	Mitral or tricuspid stenosis
Hypervolemia	Myocarditis	Cardiac tamponade
Congenital defects (left-to-right shunts)	Cardiomyopathy	Constrictive pericarditis
Ventricular septal defect	Ventricular aneurysm	Hypertrophic obstructive cardiomyopathy
Atrial septal defect	Long-term alcohol consumption	
Patent ductus arteriosus	Coronary heart disease	
	Metabolic heart disease	
	Endocrine heart disease	
Conditions that increase afterload		
Hypertension, pulmonary or systemic		
Aortic or pulmonic stenosis		
High peripheral vascular resistance		

LIMITED VENTRICULAR FILLING. Certain conditions externally compress the heart, thereby limiting ventricular filling and myocardial contractility. Disorders that greatly restrict cardiac chamber filling and myocardial fiber stretch include *constrictive pericarditis,* an inflammatory and fibrotic process of the pericardial sac; and *cardiac tamponade,* which involves the accumulation of fluid or blood within the pericardial sac. Because the pericardium encloses all four heart chambers, compression of the heart both decreases diastolic relaxation, thereby elevating diastolic pressure, and hampers forward blood flow through the heart.[38] Other conditions that limit ventricular filling are listed in Table 56–4.

Some clients have pre-existing mild to moderate heart disease with no evidence of heart failure. In these clients, adequate cardiac output depends on functional compensatory mechanisms. When the heart undergoes undue stress, these compensatory mechanisms may prove inadequate and the heart fails. Careful assessment helps identify precipitating causes of the great increase in cardiac workload. Recognition of these factors allows prompt treatment and long-term prevention.[30] Precipitating factors are described next.

CONDITIONS THAT PRECIPITATE HEART FAILURE

Heart failure can be precipitated by conditions that increase cardiac and systemic oxygen demand, reduce the ability of the heart to contract, or increase the workload of the heart. Conditions that increase demand for oxygen delivery include physical or emotional stress, dysrhythmias (most notably tachycardia), infections, anemia, thyroid disorders, pregnancy, and Paget's disease. Thiamine deficiency can precipitate heart failure because it reduces myocardial contractility, causing tachycardia and ventricular dilation. Chronic pulmonary disease and volume overload can precipitate heart failure because they increase the workload of the heart.

Pathophysiology

The healthy heart can meet the demands for oxygen delivery through the use of cardiac reserve. Cardiac reserve is the heart's ability to increase output in response to stress. The normal heart can increase its output up to five times the resting level. The failing heart, even at rest, however, is pumping near its capacity and thus has lost much of its reserve. The compromised heart has a limited ability to respond to the body's needs for increased output in situations of stress.

When cardiac output is not sufficient to meet the metabolic needs of the body, compensatory mechanisms, including neurohormonal responses, become activated. These mechanisms initially help improve contraction and maintain integrity of the circulation but, if continued, lead to abnormal cardiac growth and reconfiguration (remodeling) of the heart. The compensatory responses to a decrease in cardiac output are ventricular dilation, increased sympathetic nervous system stimulation, and activation of the renin-angiotensin system.

VENTRICULAR DILATION

Ventricular dilation refers to lengthening of the muscle fibers that increases the volume in the heart chambers.

Dilation causes an increase in preload and thus cardiac output, because a stretched muscle contracts more forcefully (Starling's law). However, dilation has limits as a compensatory mechanism. Muscle fibers, if stretched beyond a certain point, become ineffective. Second, a dilated heart requires more oxygen. Thus, the dilated heart with a normal coronary blood flow can suffer from a lack of oxygen. Hypoxia of the heart further decreases the muscle's ability to contract.[35]

INCREASED SYMPATHETIC NERVOUS SYSTEM STIMULATION

Sympathetic activity produces venous and arteriolar constriction, tachycardia, and increased myocardial contractility, all of which work to increase cardiac output and improve delivery of oxygen and nutrients to tissues. However, this compensatory effect occurs at the cost of increasing peripheral vascular resistance (afterload) and myocardial workload. In addition, sympathetic stimulation reduces renal blood flow and stimulates the renin-angiotensin system.[35, 38]

STIMULATION OF THE RENIN-ANGIOTENSIN SYSTEM

When blood flow through the renal artery is decreased, the baroreceptor reflex is stimulated and renin is released into the bloodstream. Renin interacts with angiotensinogen to produce angiotensin I. When angiotensin I comes into contact with ACE, it is converted to angiotensin II, a potent vasoconstrictor. Angiotensin II increases arterial vasoconstriction, promotes release of norepinephrine from sympathetic nerve endings, and stimulates the adrenal medulla to secrete aldosterone, which enhances sodium and water absorption. Stimulation of the renin-angiotensin system causes plasma volume to expand and preload to increase.

Cardiac compensation exists when the initial compensatory mechanisms of ventricular dilation, sympathetic nervous system stimulation, and renin-angiotensin system stimulation succeed in maintaining an adequate cardiac output and oxygen delivery to the tissues in the presence of pathologic changes. Once cardiac output is restored, the body produces counterregulatory substances that restore cardiovascular homeostasis. If underlying pathologic changes are not corrected, prolonged activation of the compensatory mechanisms eventually leads to changes in the function of the myocardial cell and overexpression of the neurohormones. These processes are responsible for the transition from compensated to decompensated heart failure. At this point, manifestations of heart failure develop because the heart cannot maintain adequate circulation.[3, 35, 38]

When compensatory mechanisms fail, the amount of blood remaining in the left ventricle at the end of diastole increases. This increase in residual blood in turn decreases the ventricle's capacity to receive blood from the left atrium. The left atrium, having to work harder to eject blood, dilates and hypertrophies. It is unable to receive the full amount of incoming blood from the pulmonary veins, and left atrial pressure increases. This leads to pulmonary edema (Fig. 56–5).

The right ventricle, because of the increased pressure in the pulmonary vascular system, must now dilate and hypertrophy in order to meet its increased workload. It

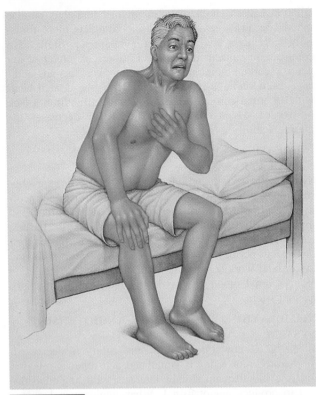

FIGURE 56–5 Appearance of a client with both right-sided and left-sided heart failure. (From *Mayo Clinic Health Letter* (1997), *15*:1–3. Mayo Foundation for Medical Education and Research, Rochester, MN. By permission of Mayo Foundation.)

too eventually fails. Engorgement of the venous system then extends backward to produce congestion in the gastrointestinal tract, liver, viscera, kidneys, legs, and sacrum, with edema as the main manifestation. Right ventricular failure (RVF) results. RVF usually follows left ventricular failure (LVF), although occasionally it may develop independently.

DECOMPENSATED HEART FAILURE

Remodeling

Several structural changes, known as remodeling, occur in the ventricle during decompensated heart failure. Remodeling is thought to result from hypertrophy of the myocardial cells and sustained activation of the neurohormonal compensatory systems. Recall that one of the initial compensatory responses to a decrease in cardiac output is dilation of the ventricle. This dilation increases cardiac output but also increases wall stress in the ventricle. To reduce wall stress, the myocardial cells hypertrophy, resulting in a thickening of the ventricular wall. According to Laplace's law, an increase in wall thickness reduces wall stress.

When used over time, these compensatory responses produce changes in the structure, function, and gene expression of the myocardial cell. Changes in the myocardial cells eventually increase failure by reducing myocardial contractility, increasing ventricular wall stress, and increasing oxygen demand. In addition to increasing myocardial dysfunction, the genetically abnormal myocytes die prematurely at an accelerated rate through the process of apoptosis (programmed cell death). Apoptosis

affects cells scattered throughout the myocardium and causes a further reduction in cardiac function.[2, 35, 38]

Sustained Neurohormonal Activation

Remodeling changes continue to increase wall stress and further stimulate neurohormonal activity. Long-term sympathetic activation exerts a direct toxic effect on the heart that promotes myocyte hypertrophy and apoptosis. Prolonged activation of the renin-angiotensin system also stimulates myocyte hypertrophy and myocardial fibrosis. This creates a self-perpetuating cycle of cell death and further hypertrophy.[2, 35, 38]

Clinical Manifestations

The manifestations of heart failure depend on the specific ventricle involved, the precipitating causes of failure, the degree of impairment, the rate of progression, the duration of the failure, and the client's underlying condition. Manifestations of pulmonary congestion and edema dominate the clinical picture of LVF. RVF is associated with signs of abdominal organ distention and peripheral edema.[30] Heart failure has been classified into several stages based on a client's functional ability and clinical manifestations (Box 56–2).

TYPES OF HEART FAILURE

Heart failure may be categorized as (1) LVF versus RVF, (2) backward versus forward, and (3) high-output versus low-output.[3]

Left Ventricular Versus Right Ventricular Failure

The theory of LVF versus RVF is based on the fact that fluid accumulates behind the chamber that fails first.

BOX 56–2 New York Heart Association Classification of Cardiovascular Disability

Class I

No limitation on physical activity. Ordinary physical activity does not cause undue fatigue, palpitation, dyspnea, or anginal pain.

Class II

Slight limitation of physical activity. Comfortable at rest, but ordinary physical activity results in fatigue, palpitation, dyspnea, or anginal pain.

Class III

Marked limitation of physical activity. Comfortable at rest, but less than ordinary physical activity causes fatigue, palpitation, dyspnea, or anginal pain.

Class IV

Unable to carry on any physical activity without discomfort. Symptoms of cardiac insufficiency or of the anginal syndrome may be present even at rest. If any physical activity is undertaken, discomfort is increased.

From Konstam, M., et al. (1994). *Heart failure: Evaluation and care of patients with left-ventricular systolic dysfunction. Clinical practice guideline No. 11* (AHCPR Pub. No. 94-0612). Rockville, MD: Agency for Health Care Policy and Research, Public Health Service, U.S. Department of Health and Human Services.

However, because the circulatory system is a closed circuit, impairments of one ventricle commonly progress to failure of the other. This is referred to as *ventricular interdependence*. Figure 56–6 depicts clinical manifestations that differentiate LVF from RVF.

Left Ventricular Failure

LVF causes either pulmonary congestion or a disturbance in the respiratory control mechanisms. These problems in turn precipitate respiratory distress. The degree of distress varies with the client's position, activity, and level of stress.

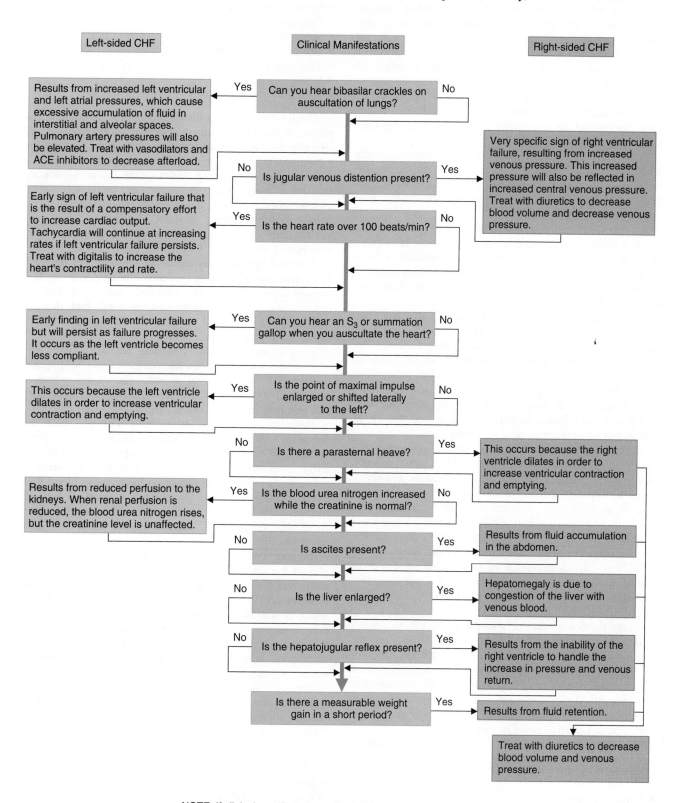

FIGURE 56–6 Clinical manifestations of left-sided and right-sided heart failure. CHF, congestive heart failure.

Dyspnea (difficult breathing) is a subjective problem and does not always correlate with the extent of heart failure. Because breathing is usually effortless at rest, the feeling of breathlessness can mean anything from an awareness of breathing to extreme distress. An apprehensive client with only moderate ventricular failure may be more aware of dyspnea than a client with advanced disease. To some degree, exertional dyspnea occurs in all clients. Therefore, elicit from the client a description of the degree of exertion that results in the sensation of breathlessness. The mechanism of dyspnea may be related to the decrease in the lung's air volume (vital capacity) as the air is displaced by blood or interstitial fluid. Pulmonary congestion can eventually reduce the vital capacity of the lungs to 1500 ml or less.

Cheyne-Stokes respirations sometimes occur in clients with severe forms of heart failure. Cheyne-Stokes respirations probably result from the prolonged circulation time between the pulmonary circulation and the central nervous system (CNS).

Cough is a common symptom of LVF. The cough, often hacking, may produce large amounts of frothy, blood-tinged sputum. The client coughs because a large amount of fluid is trapped in the pulmonary tree, irritating the lung mucosa. On auscultation, bilateral crackles may be heard.

Orthopnea is a more advanced stage of dyspnea. The client often assumes a "three-point position," sitting up with both hands on the knees and leaning forward. Orthopnea develops because the supine position increases the amount of blood returning from the lower extremities to the heart and lungs (preload). The client learns to avoid respiratory distress at night by supporting the head and thorax on pillows. In severe heart failure, the client may resort to sleeping upright in a chair.

Paroxysmal nocturnal dyspnea (PND) resembles the frightening sensation of suffocation. The client suddenly awakens with the feeling of severe suffocation and seeks relief by sitting upright or opening a window for a "breath of fresh air." Respirations may be labored and wheezing (*cardiac asthma*). PND represents an acute exacerbation of pulmonary congestion. It stems from a combination of increased venous return to the lungs during recumbency and suppression of the respiratory center to sensory input from the lungs during sleep. Once the client is upright, relief from the attack of PND may not occur for 30 minutes or longer.

Acute pulmonary edema, a medical emergency, usually results from LVF. In clients with severe cardiac decompensation, the capillary pressure within the lungs becomes so elevated that fluid is pushed from the circulating blood into the interstitium, then into the alveoli, bronchioles, and bronchi. The resulting pulmonary edema, if untreated, may cause death from suffocation. Clients with pulmonary edema literally drown in their own fluids.

The dramatic symptoms of acute pulmonary edema terrify the client and significant others. Typical manifestations include the following:

- Severe dyspnea
- Orthopnea
- Pallor
- Tachycardia
- Expectoration of large amounts of frothy, blood-tinged sputum
- Fear
- Wheezing
- Sweating
- Bubbling respirations
- Cyanosis
- Nasal flaring
- Use of accessory breathing muscles
- Tachypnea
- Vasoconstriction
- Hypoxia in arterial blood gas (ABG) findings

Cardiovascular signs also denote LVF. Inspecting and palpating the precordium may reveal an enlarged or left laterally displaced apical impulse. This occurs because the left ventricle dilates in an effort to augment ventricular contraction and emptying. Heart gallop (S_3 or S_4) sounds may be an early finding in heart failure as the left ventricle becomes less compliant and its walls vibrate in response to filling during diastole. The appearance of pulsus alternans (alternating strong and weak heartbeats) may also herald the onset of LVF.

Cerebral hypoxia may occur as a result of a decrease in cardiac output, causing inadequate brain perfusion. Depressed cerebral function can cause anxiety, irritability, restlessness, confusion, impaired memory, bad dreams, and insomnia. Impaired ventilation with resultant hypercapnia may also be a precipitant.

Fatigue and muscular weakness are often associated with LVF. Inadequate cardiac output leads to hypoxic tissue and slowed removal of metabolic wastes, which in turn cause the client to tire easily. Disturbances in sleep and rest patterns may worsen fatigue.

Renal changes can occur in both RVF and LVF but are more striking in LVF. Nocturia occurs early in heart failure. During the day, the client is upright, blood flow is away from the kidneys, and the formation of urine is reduced. At night, urine formation increases as blood flow to the kidneys improves. Nocturia may interfere with effective sleep patterns, which may contribute to fatigue. As cardiac output falls, decreased renal blood flow may result in oliguria, a late sign of heart failure.

In addition, if renal artery pressure falls, a lowered glomerular filtration rate (GFR) increases retention of sodium and water. In response to a continued reduction in renal blood flow, the renin-angiotensin-aldosterone mechanism is activated. Aldosterone, released from the adrenal cortex, promotes further retention of sodium and water by the renal tubule. This results in an expansion in blood volume of up to 30% and edema. As the sodium concentration in the extracellular fluid increases, so does the osmotic pressure of the plasma. The hypothalamus responds to the higher osmotic pressure by releasing antidiuretic hormone (ADH) from the posterior pituitary. This, in turn, promotes renal tubular reabsorption of water. However, aldosterone is more important than ADH in the production of edema.[30, 35]

Right Ventricular Failure

When right ventricle functioning decreases, peripheral edema and venous congestion of the organs develop. Liver enlargement (hepatomegaly) and abdominal pain occur as the liver becomes congested with venous blood.

If this occurs rapidly, stretching of the capsule surrounding the liver causes severe discomfort. The client may notice either a constant aching or a sharp pain in the right upper quadrant. In chronic heart failure, abdominal tenderness generally disappears.

In severe RVF, the lobules of the liver may become so congested with venous blood that they become anoxic. Anoxia leads to necrosis of the lobules. In long-standing heart failure, these necrotic areas may become fibrotic and then sclerotic. As a result, a condition called *cardiac cirrhosis* develops, manifested by ascites and jaundice.

In chronic heart failure, the increased workload of the heart and the extreme work of breathing increase the metabolic demands of the body. Anorexia, nausea, and bloating develop secondary to venous congestion of the gastrointestinal tract. The combination of increased metabolic needs and decreased caloric intake results in a marked wasting of tissue mass and cardiac cachexia.[35] Anorexia and nausea may also result from digitalis toxicity. This is a common problem because digitalis is usually prescribed for heart failure.[31]

Dependent edema is one of the early signs of RVF. Venous congestion in the peripheral vascular beds causes increased hydrostatic capillary pressure. Capillary hydrostatic pressure overwhelms the opposing pressure of plasma proteins, and fluid shifts out of the capillary beds and into the interstitial spaces, with resultant pitting edema. Edema is usually symmetrical and occurs in the dependent parts of the body, where venous pressure is highest. In ambulatory clients, edema begins in the feet and ankles and moves up the lower legs. It is most noticeable at the end of the day and often subsides after a night's rest. In the recumbent client, pitting edema may develop in the presacral area and, as it worsens, progress to the genital region and medial thighs. Concurrent jugular vein distention differentiates the edema of heart failure from that of lymphatic obstruction, cirrhosis, and hypoproteinemia.

Anasarca, a late sign in heart failure, is substantial and generalized edema. It can involve the upper extremities, genital area, and thoracic and abdominal walls. Cyanosis of the nail beds appears as venous congestion reduces peripheral blood flow.

Clients with heart failure often feel anxious, frightened, and depressed. Almost all clients realize that the heart is a vital organ and that when the heart begins to fail, health also fails. As the course of the disease progresses and manifestations worsen, the client may have an overwhelming fear of permanent disability and death. Clients express their fears in varying ways: nightmares, insomnia, acute anxiety, depression, or withdrawal from reality.

Backward Versus Forward Failure

The clinical presentation of heart failure arises from inadequate cardiac output, the pooling of blood behind the failing chamber, or both. *Backward* failure focuses on the ventricle's inability to eject completely, which increases ventricular filling pressures, causing venous and pulmonary congestion. *Forward* failure is a problem of inadequate perfusion. It results when reduced contractility produces a decrease in stroke volume and cardiac output. As cardiac output falls, blood flow to vital organs and peripheral tissues diminishes. This causes mental confusion, muscular weakness, and renal retention of sodium and water. Each of these types of failure is usually present to some degree in the client with heart failure.[3, 35]

High-Output Versus Low-Output Failure

High-output failure occurs when the heart, despite normal-output to high-output levels, is simply not able to meet the accelerated needs of the body. Causes include sepsis, Paget's disease, beriberi, anemia, thyrotoxicosis, arteriovenous fistula, and pregnancy.

Low-output failure occurs in most forms of heart disease, resulting in hypoperfusion of tissue cells. The underlying disorder is related not to increased metabolic needs of the tissues but to poor ventricular pumping action and a low cardiac output.

Acute Versus Chronic Heart Failure

The onset of heart failure may be *acute,* as when a client experiences an MI, or *gradual,* as in chronic heart failure. In chronic heart failure, there is a progression of compensatory events: a decrease in contractility, neurohormonal activation, increased preload and afterload, and finally cardiac remodeling.[3]

Diagnostic Findings

The diagnosis of heart failure rests primarily on presenting manifestations and pertinent data from the client's health history. Diagnostic studies assist in determining the underlying cause and the degree of heart failure. Such studies include an echocardiogram, chest x-ray, and ECG.[37]

The most useful diagnostic test is a two-dimensional (2-D) echocardiogram coupled with Doppler flow studies.[3] It provides information about cardiac chamber size and ventricular function and aids in assessing myocardial, valvular, congenital, endocardial, and pericardial heart disease. It allows the clinician to determine whether the dysfunction is systolic or diastolic.

In LVF, chest x-ray often depicts an enlarged cardiac silhouette, pulmonary and venous congestion, and interstitial edema. Interstitial edema on x-ray produces images called Kerley's B lines. Pleural effusions may develop and generally reflect biventricular failure.

ABG analysis is performed. Early heart failure with pulmonary edema may lead to respiratory alkalosis that is due to hyperventilation. As the disorder progresses and oxygenation becomes more impaired, acidosis develops. Pulse oximetry values show decreased oxygen levels.

Liver enzymes may reflect the degree of liver failure. Elevated blood urea nitrogen (BUN) and creatinine levels reflect decreased renal perfusion.

An ECG may give clues to the cause of LVF. Abnormalities in the ECG arise from the underlying cardiac disorder and from therapeutic agents. It may demonstrate evidence of a prior MI, dysrhythmias, or left ventricular dysfunction.

Outcome Management

▬ Medical Management

When clients experience acute heart failure, the body compensates in many ways. The short-term effects from these compensatory mechanisms are beneficial and directed toward restoration of normal cardiac output. If cardiac output continues to fall, however, these same compensatory mechanisms become counterproductive and lead to progressive deterioration in cardiac function.

The use of various drugs is typically the mode of therapy for the treatment of heart failure. However, mechanical devices may provide respite for the heart in acute failure. The most common devices are venoarterial bypass (see later) and counterpulsation (see Chapter 57). The goals of the management are to improve ventricular pump performance, reduce myocardial workload, and prevent further heart failure by affecting the process of cardiac remodeling.

IMPROVE VENTRICULAR PUMP PERFORMANCE

Oxygen

Administer oxygen in high concentrations by mask or cannula to relieve hypoxia and dyspnea and to improve oxygen–carbon dioxide exchange. For hypoxemia, the physician may order a partial rebreather mask with a flow rate of 8 to 10 L/min to deliver oxygen concentrations of 40% to 70%. A non-rebreathing mask can achieve higher oxygen concentrations. If these methods do not raise the arterial oxygen tension (PaO_2) above 60 mm Hg, the client may need intubation and ventilatory management. Intubation provides a route for removing secretions from the bronchi. If severe bronchospasm or bronchoconstriction occurs, bronchodilators are given. Monitor the client's heart rhythm because some bronchodilators also stimulate the myocardium and may lead to dysrhythmias.

Digoxin

Digoxin exerts a direct and beneficial effect on myocardial contraction in the failing heart. Improved cardiac output enhances kidney perfusion, which may create a mild diuresis of sodium and water. For a more complete discussion on digitalis, see Box 56–3.

Digoxin does not appear to have an effect on long-term mortality in clients with heart failure.[3] It is for clients who remain symptomatic despite ACE inhibitor and beta-blocker therapy. It is very effective in heart failure associated with low cardiac output caused by ischemic, rheumatic, hypertensive, or congenital heart disease. Digoxin therapy may also be initiated to control the ventricular response in atrial fibrillation, the most common dysrhythmia in heart failure. Digoxin is not given for heart failure associated with high cardiac output states, such as anemia and thyrotoxicosis. Digoxin is contraindicated in constrictive pericarditis or cardiac tamponade and should be used with caution in acute MI because it increases myocardial oxygen demand.

When administering digoxin, assess for signs of digoxin toxicity. Digoxin levels can become elevated as a result of medication interactions. The most common medications that increase digoxin levels are quinidine, verapamil, and amiodarone. Digoxin dosage may need to be reduced if the client is taking any of these medications.[29] Clients at risk for the toxic effects of digoxin are older people and those with advanced heart disease, severe dysrhythmias, or acute MI.

Digoxin toxicity occurs in approximately one in five clients and may present with systemic or cardiac manifestations (Box 56–3). Digoxin toxicity is more prevalent when the serum concentration is equal to or greater than 2 μg/L, serum potassium is less than 3 mEq/L, or serum magnesium is low. If any of these manifestations are present, notify the physician, withhold digoxin, and initiate interventions to abate the undesirable symptoms.

Digoxin toxicity may be a life-threatening condition. Carefully follow the guidelines in Box 56–3 to prevent toxicity.

Inotropes

Inotropic agents such as dopamine, dobutamine, and amrinone may be ordered for clients with severe low-output heart failure. These medications facilitate myocardial contractility and enhance stroke volume. Dopamine is a naturally occurring catecholamine with alpha-adrenergic, beta-adrenergic, and dopaminergic activity.

Dopamine, when given in small doses (<4 μg/kg/min), stimulates the dopaminergic receptors in the renal, mesenteric, cerebral, and coronary vascular beds, which causes vasodilatation. The primary result is an increase in renal blood flow, GFR, and sodium excretion. The alpha-adrenergic and beta-adrenergic receptors in the vasculature and myocardium are affected by moderate doses of dopamine (4 to 8 μg/kg/min). The results are increases in heart rate, stroke volume, and cardiac output. Alpha-adrenergic effects, such as intense vasoconstriction, dominate when dopamine is given in doses larger than 10 μg/kg/min.[48] Although dopamine may improve cardiac output, it may do so at the expense of the myocardium and renal blood flow. Tachycardia may increase myocardial oxygen demands and decrease myocardial oxygen supply, which may prove costly to the already ischemic myocardium.

Another inotropic agent, dobutamine, is a synthetic derivative of dopamine that produces strong beta-stimulatory effects within the myocardium; it increases heart rate, atrioventricular (AV) conduction, and myocardial contractility. Dobutamine is capable of increasing cardiac output without increasing myocardial oxygen demands or reducing coronary blood flow.

Amrinone is also used to increase cardiac output in severe heart failure. In addition to the positive inotropic effects, amrinone increases renal blood flow and GFR.

REDUCE MYOCARDIAL WORKLOAD

Positioning the Client

The client is placed in a high Fowler position or chair to reduce pulmonary venous congestion and to relieve the dyspnea. The legs are maintained in a dependent position as much as possible. Even though the legs are edematous, they should not be elevated. Elevating the legs increases venous return rapidly.

Reducing Preload

Diuretic therapy plays an integral part in the successful management of heart failure in clients with a predisposition for fluid retention. Diuretics enhance renal excretion of sodium and water, which reduces circulating blood volume, diminishes preload, and lessens systemic and pulmonary congestion. Table 56–5 describes the characteristics of a commonly used diuretic.

BOX 56-3 Cardiac Glycoside—Digoxin

Actions and Therapeutic Responses

Action: increases ventricular contractility (positive inotropic effect), increases ventricular emptying, slows conduction of impulses through the atrioventricular (AV) node and Purkinje's fibers, increases AV nodal refractory period, augments stroke volume, and increases cardiac output.

Therapeutic responses: slows heart rate and increases cardiac output.

Administration Guidelines and Rationales

Guidelines

1. Always take the client's apical pulse for 1 full minute before administration.
2. Withhold digoxin if heart rate is below 60 or newly irregular.
3. Check most recent digoxin and electrolyte levels before administration.

4. Intravenous (IV) administration must be given over 5 minutes.
5. Serum levels should be drawn at least 4 hours after an IV dose and 6 hours after an oral dose.

Rationales

1. Apical pulse for a full minute is the most reliable method for obtaining an accurate pulse rate.
2. Bradycardia or dysrhythmias may be indicative of digoxin toxicity.
3. The digoxin level must be below or within therapeutic range before administering. Hypokalemia increases myocardial sensitivity to digoxin.
4. Rapid IV administration may potentiate side effects.
5. To obtain accurate results in levels, they should be drawn after peak effect.

Pharmacokinetics

Onset: oral 1–2 hours, IV 5–30 minutes
Duration: 3–4 days in both forms
Peak effect: oral 2–8 hours, IV 1–4 hours
Absorption: upper small intestine

Excretion: renal
Half-life: 38–48 hours
Therapeutic plasma levels: 0.8–2.0 ng/ml
Toxic plasma levels: above 2.4 ng/ml

Drugs That May Increase or Decrease Serum Digitalis Concentrations

Increase

Amiodarone
Cyclosporine
Diltiazem
Diuretics
Erythromycin
Propantheline
Quinidine/quinine
Spironolactone
Tetracycline
Verapamil
Captopril

Decrease

Antacids
Cholestyramine
Colestipol
Kaolin-pectin
Metoclopramide
Neomycin
P-aminosalicylic acid
Rifampin
Sulfasalazine

Assessing Adverse Responses

The client may exhibit nausea, vomiting, abdominal pain, diarrhea, anorexia, sinus bradycardia, AV or sinoatrial (SA) block, dysrhythmias, drowsiness, fatigue, headache, lethargy, blurred vision, halos, green or yellow vision, or diplopia. disturbances, and confusion. Cardiac signs include ventricular tachycardia, premature ventricular contractions, bradycardia, AV block, ST depression, PR prolongation, and atrial and ventricular fibrillation.

Evidence of Digoxin Toxicity

Digoxin toxicity is manifested by a wide array of signs and symptoms and is often difficult to differentiate from effects of cardiac disease. Nausea and vomiting are the most common early indicators of toxicity. Other signs include anorexia, diarrhea, abdominal discomfort, headache, weakness, visual

Treatment of Toxicity

Discontinue digoxin administration. Digoxin immune Fab is administered intravenously. Each 40 mg binds approximately 0.6 mg of digoxin. Digoxin immune Fab causes hypokalemia; therefore, serum potassium levels must be obtained and replaced appropriately.

Data from Armstrong, L. L. (Ed.). *The University of Chicago Hospitals Formulary of Accepted Drugs.* Hudson, OH: Lexi-Comp, Inc., 1998.

TABLE 56–5   NURSING IMPLICATIONS FOR MEDICATIONS USED IN HEART FAILURE

Class (Example)	Assessing Therapeutic Responses	Assessing Adverse Responses	Nursing Implications
DECREASES MYOCARDIAL WORKLOAD			
Diuretic (furosemide)	The urine output should increase. The reduction in circulating volume decreases central venous pressures, pulmonary congestion, and peripheral edema. It may also decrease systemic blood pressure.	Clients may experience orthostatic hypotension, hypokalemia, electrolyte imbalance, blurred vision, headache, loss of appetite, hearing loss, and stomach cramps and pain.	Monitor electrolytes, intake and output, weight, blood pressure, and renal function. Intravenous (IV) administration should not exceed 0.5 mg/kg/min, and hearing loss is possible with high doses. Teach clients to rise slowly to avoid orthostatic hypotension.
Venous vasodilator (nitroglycerin)	Reducing peripheral resistance decreases blood pressure, and the reduction in preload may decrease the heart rate and pulmonary congestion. Vasodilatation of coronary vessels should keep clients free of anginal pain.	Clients may experience flushing, weakness, headache, postural hypotension, dizziness, and reflex tachycardia.	Monitor clients for hypotension. Ointment and patches should be rotated daily, and clients may need a nitrate-free interval to avoid tolerance. Avoid getting ointment on fingers. IV nitroglycerin should be in glass bottles with tubing specific for nitroglycerin. If a client is receiving continuous IV nitroglycerin, the blood pressure and heart rate should be continually monitored.
Vein and arteriole dilator (sodium nitroprusside)	The peripheral vasodilatation decreases the blood pressure. Decrease in afterload increases cardiac output by enhancing contractility.	Clients may experience hypotension, sweating, palpitations, restlessness, headache, nausea, and vomiting. Cyanide toxicity is possible in clients with decreased liver function, and thiocyanate toxicity is possible in clients with decreased kidney function or anyone who has prolonged use of nitroprusside. Signs of thiocyanate toxicity include psychoses, blurred vision, tinnitus, and seizures. Signs of cyanide toxicity include metabolic acidosis, tachycardia, decreased pulse and reflexes, and coma.	Solution must be mixed with 5% dextrose in water (D5W) and wrapped with opaque material to protect it from light. Blue color indicates almost complete degradation to cyanide. Constant blood pressure and heart rate monitoring is necessary. Monitor acid/base status, as acidosis can be the earliest indicator of cyanide toxicity. Monitor thiocyanate levels if infusion is for more than 3 days or the dose is more than 4 mg/kg/min.
Angiotensin-converting enzyme (ACE) inhibitor (captopril)	The decrease in afterload increases cardiac output by enhancing contractility. The neurohormonal effects include inhibition of ACE and vasodilatation and a decrease in systemic blood pressure.	Clients may experience oliguria, chest pain, palpitations, insomnia, dizziness, fatigue, nausea, vomiting, maculopapular rash, and cough.	Monitor blood pressure. Administer 1 hour before meals. Two weeks of therapy may be necessary before the full therapeutic effect is achieved. May increase blood urea nitrogen, creatinine, liver enzymes, and potassium levels. If given concurrently with digoxin, it may cause an increase in digoxin levels.

Drug			
Beta-adrenergic antagonist (atenolol)	The effects of blockade of beta-adrenergic receptors are seen clinically by decreased heart rate, blood pressure, and cardiac output. The neurohormonal response inhibits the sympathetic nervous system that causes vasodilatation and decreasing automaticity in the heart. Clinically, this decreases blood pressure and the heart rate and the incidence of dysrhythmias.	Clients may experience brochoconstriction, severe bradycardia, or hypotension. They may also experience atrioventricular conduction abnormalities, dizziness, confusion, constipation or diarrhea, and vomiting. Male clients may experience impotence.	Clients must be instructed not to stop taking medication abruptly because they may experience angina. The drug should not be given in clients with a history of bronchospastic pulmonary disease. If the client is diabetic, it may potentiate hypoglycemia. The nurse must monitor the heart rate, rhythm, and blood pressure frequently and assess pulmonary status for bronchoconstriction.

INCREASES PUMP PERFORMANCE

Drug			
Cardiac glycoside (digoxin)	The increased contractility increases cardiac output. Suppression of the atrioventricular node decreases the heart rate.	The client may experience nausea, vomiting, abdominal pain, diarrhea, anorexia, bradycardia, dysrhythmias, drowsiness, fatigue, and visual disturbances. Digoxin toxicity is a potentially fatal condition that must be assessed for whenever a client is on digoxin therapy.	Always take apical pulse for 1 minute and hold if the rate is under 60 or if the pulse is newly irregular. The most recent digoxin and electrolyte levels must be assessed prior to administration. IV doses should be given over 5 minutes. Serum levels should be drawn no sooner than 4 hours after an IV dose and 6 hours after an oral dose.
Inotrope (dobutamine)	The enhanced myocardial contractility increases cardiac output and may increase the heart rate and blood pressure.	Clients may experience anginal pain, increased heart rate, palpitations, premature ventricular beats, paresthesia, headache, nausea, and vomiting. Extravasation should be avoided; if present, treat with phentolamine.	Monitor the electrocardiogram and blood pressure continuously. Observe for hypertension and tachycardia. Use a central line for administration if possible. Observe the IV site frequently.
Inotrope (dopamine)	The enhanced myocardial contractility increases the systolic blood pressure, heart rate, and cardiac output. Improved circulation to renal vascular beds results in increased urine output in low to moderate doses.	The client may experience palpitations, cardiac dysrhythmias, tachycardia, vasoconstriction, or hypotension. Estravasation should be avoided; if present, treat with phentolamine.	Continuous monitoring of the blood pressure and heart rate is necessary. In higher doses, observe for decreases in urine output, cool extremities, and decreased pulses. The IV site must be monitored frequently to avoid extravasation. Central lines are preferred, especially in clients with occlusive vascular disease or diabetic endarteritis. The hemodynamic effects are dose dependent.

Data from Armstrong, L. L. (Ed.). *The University of Chicago Hospitals Formulary of Accepted Drugs.* Hudson, OH: Lexi-Comp, Inc., 1998.

Although they are effective, diuretics should be administered cautiously because of their side effect profile. Diuretics can produce mild to severe electrolyte imbalance. Hypokalemia, a particularly dangerous problem, potentiates digitalis toxicity and can cause myocardial weakness and cardiac dysrhythmias. Moreover, vigorous diuresis may produce hypovolemia and hypotension, jeopardizing cardiac output.

Reducing Afterload

Vasodilating agents have become an increasingly important intervention in clients with heart failure. Vasodilators vary in their mechanisms of action, which include:

- Direct dilation of veins
- Dilation of arterioles
- Combined action on veins and arterioles
- Inhibition of ACE

Closely assess the client receiving vasodilators, which can cause a rapid fall in blood pressure.

Venous dilators relax venous smooth muscle and increase the capacity of the systemic venous bed; blood is "trapped" in the veins, and venous return to the heart is decreased. This increased venous capacity reduces preload. Examples include nitroglycerin and isosorbide dinitrate.

Arteriolar dilators reduce systemic arteriolar tone, which decreases peripheral vascular resistance and afterload. Reduction in afterload reduces the left ventricular workload and increases cardiac output. Improved renal perfusion may initiate diuresis. Hydralazine is the most commonly used arterial dilator. Note that hydralazine may precipitate reflex tachycardia.

Combined venous and arteriolar dilators decrease both preload and afterload. Sodium nitroprusside helps manage severe heart failure. A potent vasodilator, sodium nitroprusside relaxes the smooth muscles of both veins and arterioles. It does not directly affect the heart muscle or heart rate.

ACE inhibitors suppress the renin-angiotensin-aldosterone system, blocking production of the potent vasoconstrictor angiotensin II. This results in an increase in renal blood flow and a decrease in renal vascular resistance, which enhances diuresis. They also lessen the effect of neurohormonal influences in heart failure. ACE inhibitors reduce remodeling changes in the hearts of animals and can increase client survival. One ACE inhibitor, captopril, improves hemodynamic status. All clients with left systolic heart failure should receive ACE inhibitors unless they cannot tolerate the drugs.

Beta-adrenergic antagonists (beta-blockers) are now used in clients with heart failure because they inhibit the effects of the sympathetic nervous system. They have been shown to increase clinical improvement[14] and to decrease mortality. These findings are apparent when clients are concurrently receiving ACE inhibitory therapy, suggesting that the combination of two agents that have inhibitory effects on two neurohormonal systems may have an additive effect.[3]

VENTRICULAR ASSIST DEVICES. For the past few decades, when conventional therapy such as medications and the intra-aortic balloon pump (IABP) became ineffective, there was little hope for the client with heart failure. Advances continue to be made in perfecting methods of mechanical ventricular support. The goal of mechanical circulatory support is to decompress the hypokinetic ventricle, decrease myocardial workload, reduce oxygen demands, and maintain adequate systemic perfusion to sustain end-organ function. In the client with heart failure, the two most common options are ventricular assist devices (VADs) as a bridge to transplantation and as permanent support.[43] VADs have the capability to support circulation, either partially or totally, until the heart recovers or is replaced. Devices may be right ventricular, left ventricular, or biventricular VADs. Complications of any VAD include bleeding, hemolysis, thromboembolism, infection, and multiorgan failure.[8, 26]

Traditionally, nonpulsatile pumps have been used as VADs. Difficulties with these devices include end-organ dysfunction, thromboembolic complications, and the need for full anticoagulation. Their use in clients with heart failure is diminishing because better technology is available. These pumps can be used for a relatively short period of approximately 10 days.

Pulsatile pumps are the newest, most advanced forms of mechanical support. Pulsatile flow decreases the amount of hemolysis, decreases thromboembolic episodes, and allows better perfusion to organs. They allow extended use with minimal anticoagulation.

External pulsatile VADs are utilized as a bridge to transplantation. They offer both short-term and long-term support. Cardiopulmonary bypass is not required for insertion. If the client is stable, they allow for mobility. Thromboembolism is the major concern with the external pulsatile devices.

Implantable VADs are currently approved as permanent devices to bridge over to transplantation. They were designed with larger clients in mind because these clients often have to wait the longest for a transplantation. The greatest advantage of the device is that it allows mobility for the client. It reduces the risk of infection, prevents muscle disuse, and prevents other systemic complications, such as pneumonia. Cardiopulmonary bypass is required to insert these devices. They are also more costly than the external pulsatile VADs.

Total artificial hearts provide complete control of the cardiovascular system and allow total mobility. Their use is limited in smaller people, because the device may not fit the client's small body. Complications include infection, thromboembolism, and the possibility of mechanical failure. Initially, total artificial hearts were limited to people awaiting transplantation. Currently, these devices are being used when there are contraindications to transplantation, such as advanced age.[39]

Extracorporeal membrane oxygenation (ECMO) systems are widely used for short-term hemodynamic stabilization. These devices remove blood from the inferior vena cava to a centrifugal pump that pumps the blood to an oxygenator. The oxygenated blood is returned to the client via the femoral artery. Long-term use (>48 hours) does not promote recovery. In addition, bleeding is a concern because anticoagulation therapy is needed.

As the number of people who require cardiac transplantation increases and the options for mechanical assist devices grow, the nurse needs to become more aware of these devices for clients with end-stage heart disease. Traditionally, clients were cared for in the intensive care unit (ICU), but today a critical care environment is not needed, except for those on ECMO, once the client is stabilized.

REDUCE FLUID RETENTION

Controlling sodium and water retention improves cardiac performance. Sodium restrictions are placed on the diet to prevent, control, or eliminate edema. Diets with 2 to 4 g of sodium are usually prescribed (Table 56–6).

From the use of some loop diuretics, potassium is lost via the kidneys, which can lead to dysrhythmias and electrolyte imbalances. Hypokalemia sensitizes the myocardium to digitalis and therefore predisposes the client to digitalis toxicity. Potassium supplements and adequate dietary potassium are important.

It is usually not necessary to restrict fluid intake in clients with mild or moderate heart failure. In more advanced cases, however, it is beneficial to limit water to 1000 ml/day (1 L/day). The reason is that excessive water intake tends to dilute the amount of sodium in body fluids and may produce a low-salt syndrome (*hyponatremia*). Hyponatremia is characterized by lethargy and weakness; it results more often from the combination of a restricted sodium diet, increased sodium loss during diuresis, and excessive water intake.

REDUCE STRESS AND RISK OF INJURY

In addition to improving ventricular pump performance and reducing myocardial workload, the client also needs to reduce physical and emotional stress. Sometimes clinicians overlook rest as an intervention to diminish the workload of the heart. The proper use of rest as the initial step in management offers many benefits. Rest can promote diuresis, slow the heart rate, and relieve dyspnea, all of which allow more conservative use of pharmacologic agents (e.g., ACE inhibitors, diuretics, beta-blockers).

Whether the physician prescribes complete, modified bed rest depends on the seriousness of the client's condition. The physician may prescribe a mild sedative or small doses of barbiturates and tranquilizers to promote rest and overcome problems of restlessness, insomnia, and anxiety.

The client may also be at risk for injury because of immobility. The client should be confined to bed only long enough to regain cardiac reserve but not so long as to promote complications of immobility. Give the client confined to bed rest specific guidelines to prevent the harmful effects of immobility. Clients should perform passive leg exercises several times daily to prevent venous stasis, which may lead to the formation of venous thrombi and pulmonary emboli. The physician may also initiate anticoagulant therapy to prevent these potentially deadly complications.[29]

■ Nursing Management of the Medical Client

The goals of nursing management for the client with heart failure are to:

- Monitor for reduced cardiac output
- Maintain adequate fluid balance
- Reduce myocardial workload
- Assess response to medical therapies
- Educate the client about self-care following discharge (see Bridge to Home Health Care, p. 1546)

Use Figure 56–6 to help differentiate right-sided from left-sided failure. Consider the psychosocial effect of heart failure on the client and family. Nursing diagnoses that may apply to the client with heart failure are discussed in the Care Plan.

TABLE 56–6	SODIUM CONTENT OF SELECTED FOODS
FOODS LOW IN SODIUM	
Dairy products	Skim milk, eggs, cottage cheese, cream cheese, ice cream
Meats*	Turkey, chicken, veal, lamb, liver, fresh fish, tuna packed in water (meats should be unprocessed)
Fruits and vegetables*	Any fresh or frozen food in this group
Beverages	Any juice (except tomato or V8 brand vegetable), coffee, tea, bottled water
Breads	Some breads and cereals
Seasonings	Garlic, onion, bay leaf, pepper, dill, nutmeg, rosemary, allspice, thyme, sage, caraway, cinnamon, almond and vanilla extract, fresh dried herbs
Fats	Margarine, oils, shortening, unsalted salad dressings
Desserts	Sherbet, fruit ice, gelatin, fruit drinks
Miscellaneous	Unbuttered, unsalted popcorn; unsalted nuts; vinegar
FOODS HIGH IN SODIUM	
Milk and dairy products	Aged, hard cheese; pasteurized, processed cheese; buttermilk
Meats	Sausage, frankfurters, ham, bacon, corned beef; all smoked, pickled, or cured meats; canned meats, salami, most luncheon meats, beef jerky; frozen "TV" dinners
Fruits and vegetables	Pickled or canned fruits and vegetables, olives, sauerkraut, pickles
Breads and cereals	Salted crackers, macaroni and cheese, pretzels, rye rolls, pizza, commercial pancake mixes
Beverages	Tomato juice, V8 vegetable juice, beef broth, bouillon
Fats	Commercial salad dressings, dips and party spreads, peanut butter
Seasonings	Garlic, celery, or onion salt; Accent, monosodium glutamate (MSG), meat tenderizer, soy sauce, ketchup, steak sauce, mustard, canned soup
Desserts	Fruit pies, doughnuts, cakes, commercial puddings
Miscellaneous	Baking soda, baking powder, salted popcorn, salted nuts, potato chips

* Food sources high in potassium.

Text continued on page 1546

■ THE CLIENT WITH HEART FAILURE

Nursing Diagnosis. Decreased Cardiac Output related to heart failure or dsyrhythmias or both.

Outcomes. The client will have an increase in cardiac output, as evidenced by regular cardiac rhythm, heart rate, blood pressure, respirations, and urine output within normal limits.

Interventions	Rationales
1. Assess blood pressure for hypotension or hypertension and respiratory rate for tachypnea q 1 hr (more or less frequently, depending on the client's stability).	1. Hypotension may indicate decreased cardiac output and may lead to a decrease in coronary artery perfusion. Hypertension may be caused by chronic vasoconstriction or may indicate fear or anxiety, and increased respiratoryl rate may indicate fatigue or increased pulmonary congestion.
2. Assess heart rate and rhythm q 1 hr for tachycardia or the presence of dysrhythmias.	2. Tachycardia can increase myocardial and oxygen demands and may be a compensatory mechanism related to the decreased cardiac output (increased heart rate to compensate for decrease in stroke volume). Ventricular enlargement decreases conduction of cardiac impulses and may lead to dysrhythmias. Dysrhythmias further compromise cardiac output by reducing ventricular filling time and myocardial contractility and by increasing myocardial oxygen demands. Common dysrhythmias include premature atrial contractions (PACs), premature ventricular contractions (PVCs), and paroxysmal atrial tachycardia (PAT). Ventricular dysrhythmias must be watched for because they can increase the chance of sudden death.
3. Document rhythm strips q 8 hr and if dysrhythmias occur. Measure and note rate, QRS, PR, and QT intervals and ST segment with each strip and note any deviations from baseline.	3. Documentation of rhythm confirms rhythm and gives a baseline for changes. Changes in the ST segment may indicate myocardial ischemia, which may be present because of decreased coronary artery perfusion.
4. Report dysrhythmias to the physician.	4. Dysrhythmias can decrease cardiac output and may lead to life-threatening dysrhythmias.
5. Auscultate heart rate q 2 hr for changes in heart sounds such as murmurs, S_3, or S_4.	5. Delayed filling time, incomplete ejection, and structural changes within the heart and fluid overload may cause abnormal heart sounds detected by auscultation. S_3 may indicate a noncompliant or stiff ventricle, and S_4 may indicate a weak, overdistended ventricle.
6. Monitor lung sounds q 2 hr for advantageous sounds such as crackles and for the presence of coughing.	6. Increased ventricular pressures are transmitted back to the pulmonary circulation, increasing pulmonary capillary hydrostatic pressure and exceeding oncotic pressure fluid moves within the alveolar septum, and are evidenced by the auscultation of crackles, increased shortness of breath, and sputum production. This indicates a further decrease in cardiac output and the possibility of the development of pulmonary edema. Coughing can be caused by the increased fluid in the lungs or by angiotensin-converting enzyme (ACE) inhibitors.
7. Monitor intake and output (I & O) and assess findings q 8 hr and as required (PRN). Note color and amount of urine q 2 hr and PRN.	7. If intake exceeds output, the patient is at risk for fluid overload and may not be able to clear fluids because of a decompensating heart. Dark, concentrated urine and oliguria may reflect a decrease in renal perfusion. Diuresis is expected in clients receiving diuretic therapy.
8. Assess for changes in mental status.	8. Change in mental status may indicate decreased cerebral perfusion or hypoxia.
9. Assess peripheral pulses for strength and quality and for pulsus alternans.	9. Decreased strength of peripheral pulses is often found in clients with decreased cardiac output, and a further decrease in pulses from baseline may indicate further cardiac failure. Pulsus alternans may be detected and indicates severe heart failure.
10. Administer prescribed medications and evaluate responses.	10. Prescribed medications are utilized to increase contractility and decrease preload or afterload, and their responses must be evaluated. Therapeutic levels must be monitored. Clients need to be monitored for potential side effects.
11. Encourage physical and psychological rest.	11. Increased physical or mental strain can increase myocardial and oxygen demands.
12. Encourage clients to eat small meals and rest afterward.	12. Larger meals increase myocardial workload and may cause vagal stimulation, which may lead to bradycardia.

■

Evaluation. Client's vital signs will be within normal parameters, and urine output will be normal.

Nursing Diagnosis. Fluid Volume Excess related to reduced glomerular filtration, decreased cardiac output, increased antidiuretic hormone (ADH) production, and sodium and water retention.

Outcomes. The client will demonstrate adequate fluid balance, as evidenced by output equal to or exceeding intake, clearing breath sounds, and decreasing edema.

Interventions	Rationales
1. Monitor I & O q 4 hr (more or less frequently depending on clients status).	1. I & O balance reflects fluid status.
2. Weigh clients daily.	2. Body weight is a sensitive indicator of fluid balance, and an increase indicates fluid volume excess.
3. Assess for presence of peripheral edema.	3. Heart failure causes venous congestion, resulting in increased capillary pressure. When hydrostatic pressure exceeds interstitial pressure, fluids leak out of the capillaries and present as edema in the legs, sacrum, and scrotum.
4. Assess for jugular vein distention, hepatomegaly, and abdominal pain.	4. Elevated volumes in the venae cavae occur as right atrium preload increase from inadequate emptying from right atrium and are transmitted to the jugular vein and present as distention; they can also be the cause of hepatomegaly, splenomegaly, and abdominal pain.
5. Low-sodium diet or fluid restriction.	5. Decreased systemic blood pressure can trigger renin, leading to a cascade of events that ends with stimulation of aldosterone, which causes increased renal tubular absorption of sodium. Low-sodium diet helps prevent increased sodium retention, which decreases water retention. Fluid restriction may be utilized to decrease fluid intake, hence decreasing fluid volume excess.
6. Auscultate breath sounds q 2 hr and PRN for the presence of crackles and monitor for sputum production.	6. When increased pulmonary capillary hydrostatic pressure exceeds oncotic pressure, fluid moves within the alveolar septum and is evidenced by the auscultation of crackles. Frothy, pink-tinged sputum is an indicator the client is developing the life-threatening complication of pulmonary edema.
7. Administer diuretic therapy as ordered and evaluate effectiveness of the therapy.	7. Diuretics are commonly prescribed to promote the diuresis of accumulated fluid. The nurse should expect an increase in urine output after the client receives diuretic therapy

Evaluation. The client has clear breath sounds, decrease in weight, equal or increased output in relationship to intake, and decreased peripheral edema.

Nursing Diagnosis. Impaired Gas Exchange related to fluid in alveoli.

Outcomes. The client will have improved gas exchange, as evidenced by decreased dyspnea, no cyanosis, normal arterial blood gases, and a decrease in pulmonary congestion upon auscultation.

Interventions	Rationales
1. Auscultate breath sounds q 2 hr.	1. Auscultation of crackles may indicate pulmonary congestion.
2. Encourage the client to turn, cough, and deep-breathe q 2 hr.	2. This will help facilitate oxygen delivery and clear the airways.
3. Administer oxygen if ordered.	3. Oxygen therapy will improve oxygenation by increasing the amount of oxygen available for delivery.
4. Assess respiratory rate and rhythm q 2 hr and PRN.	4. Increased respiratory rate indicates difficulty with oxygenation, and a decreased respiratory rate may indicate impending respiratory failure.
5. Assess for cyanosis q 4 hr and PRN.	5. Circumoral cyanosis or cyanosis to the finger tips or end of nose indicates hypoxia from lack of oxygen in peripheral tissues.

Care Plan continued on following page

6. Position the client to facilitate breathing and observe for paroxysmal nocturnal dyspnea.

6. Fowler position and orthopneic positioning facilitate diaphragmatic excursion. Paroxysmal nocturnal dyspnea may occur because as the client assumes a supine position, venous return to the heart is increased. This increase in return increases preload and will increase pulmonary capillary hydrostatic pressure and lead to pulmonary alveolar edema.

7. Monitor pulse oximetry.

7. A low SaO_2 reflects hypoxia.

8. Obtain arterial blood gases if ordered.

8. Arterial blood gases indicate whether the patient has hypoxia, acidosis, or both.

9. Administer diuretic therapy as ordered, and monitor for effectiveness.

9. Diuretics promote fluid loss in the alveoli as well as systemically.

Evaluation. The client has clear breath sounds, normal arterial blood gases, and saturation. Respiratory rate is normal.

Nursing Diagnosis. Altered Tissue Perfusion related to decreased cardiac output.

Outcomes. The client will have adequate tissue perfusion as evidenced by warm dry skin, peripheral pulses, and adequate urine output.

Intervention	Rationales
1. Note color and temperature of the skin q 4 hr.	1. Cool, pale skin is indicative of decreased peripheral tissue perfusion.
2. Monitor peripheral pulses q 4 hr.	2. Decreased pulses are indicative of decreased tissue perfusion from vasoconstriction of the vessels.
3. Provide a warm environment.	3. A warm environment promotes vasodilatation, which decreases preload and promotes tissue perfusion.
4. Encourage active range of motion.	4. Range of motion helps decrease venous pooling and promotes tissue perfusion.
5. Monitor urine output q 4 hr.	5. Decreased perfusion to the kidneys may result in oliguria.

Evaluation. The client has warm skin, adequate peripheral pulses, and normal urine output.

Nursing Diagnosis. Risk for Activity Intolerance related to decreased cardiac output.

Outcomes. The client will have improved levels of activity without dyspnea.

Interventions	Rationales
1. Space nursing activities.	1. Clustering activities increases myocardial demand and may cause extreme fatigue.
2. Schedule rest periods.	2. Rest periods help alleviate fatigue and decrease myocardial workload.
3. Monitor the client's response to activities.	3. Dyspnea, tachycardia, angina, diaphoresis, dysrhythmias, and hypotension are all indicative that the activity required more myocardial demand than the body was able to compensate for. Assess vital signs before and after an activity. The time it requires for the vital signs to return to baseline indicates the degree of cardiac deconditioning.
4. Increase activity as ordered or according to the rehabilitation nurse's direction.	4. Gradually and appropriately increasing physical activity may help the client gain cardiac conditioning and improve activity tolerance.
5. Instruct the client to avoid activities that increase cardiac workload.	5. Activities such as stair climbing, working with arms above the head, or sustained arm movement may cause extreme fatigue and demand more cardiac output than the body can supply.

Evaluation. The client will perform spaced activities without dyspnea and will gradually increase activity tolerance.

Nursing Diagnosis. Risk for Impaired Skin Integrity related to decreased tissue perfusion and activities.

Outcomes. The client will maintain intact skin.

■

Interventions

1. Reposition the client q 2 hr.

2. Provide a therapeutic mattress or bed while client is in bed.

3. Assess the skin, especially bony prominences, for redness, each shift, and as needed. Utilize protective devices if redness is noted.
4. Assist the client with morning care.

Rationales

1. Changing position frequently deters the formation of pressure ulcers by decreasing the amount of time of pressure on any given area.
2. Pressure reduction mattresses and beds are available to decrease the pressure on the sacrum when the client is in bed.
3. Redness is indicative of increased pressure to an area and is the first sign of breakdown. Risk areas include the sacrum, coccyx, heels, elbows, and back of the head.
4. Clients may have difficulty providing themselves with adequate skin care, and the nurse must ensure the skin is clean and has proper moisture.

Evaluation. The client has intact skin.

Nursing Diagnosis. Risk for anxiety related to decreased cardiac output, hypoxia, diagnosis of heart failure, and fear of death or debilitation.

Outcomes. The client will not exhibit signs of anxiety and will be able to express concerns.

Interventions

1. Provide a calm environment.
2. Explain in advance all procedures and routine regimens.

3. Encourage the client to ask questions.

4. Provide emotional support to clients and their significant others.

5. Encourage the client to utilize additional support systems.

Rationales

1. A calm environment decreases additional anxiety.
2. By providing information in advance, the client will not feel anxious about the routine care provided.
3. By encouraging the client to ask questions, the nurse is providing an open forum for discussion with the client.
4. Allowing clients and their support systems to vent fears and anxiety, the nurse assists them in decreasing anxiety.
5. Additional support people such as religious leaders, social workers, counselors, and clinical nurse specialists may increase the client's support system and decrease anxiety.

Evaluation: The client is calm, without apparent anxiety.

BRIDGE TO HOME HEALTH CARE

Managing Heart Failure

One third of all clients hospitalized for heart failure are readmitted within 90 days of discharge. Problems with self-monitoring techniques, medication, and diet are the primary reasons. Home health and outpatient care nurses can make a positive difference in readmission rates through nursing interventions.

Review clients' cardiovascular history, disease etiology, and medical management plan to guide your assessment. Auscultate the heart and lungs during each visit, and look for signs of fluid accumulation. Measure blood pressure with both the client sitting and standing. If blood pressure decreases significantly and the client experiences lightheadedness or dizziness, it may be necessary to adjust diuretic or vasoactive medications. Worsening cardiac status or drug toxicities can cause changes in pulse rate or rhythm.

Clients may experience unique manifestations such as fullness in their ears, increased urination at night, and chest heaviness. The client, family members, and informal caregivers need to be educated about the correlation between manifestations and clinical status. Evaluate changes in the prevalence and severity of manifestations. The assessment can include measuring intake and output, abdominal girth and lower extremities, and weight. Instruct clients to call you or their physicians if they lose or gain 2 to 3 pounds in 1 day or 5 to 7 pounds in 1 week. When manifestations are noted and cardiac decompensation is detected early, heart failure can be managed successfully in non-institutional, outpatient settings.

Use various techniques to help clients manage their medications. Write the medication schedule clearly, and suggest reminder systems such as pill boxes. Examine all pill bottles for the drug name, strength, expiration date, and available refills. Review brand versus generic labeling to minimize confusion and prevent drug administration errors. Simplify dosing frequencies; by limiting doses to twice a day (bid), three times a day (tid), or four times a day (qid), medication administration can be associated with daily routines such as meals and bedtime. Flexible dose times can promote drug tolerance and increase accurate administration. Discourage the use of over-the-counter medications because of the potential for drug interactions.

Limiting sodium intake to 2000 mg a day can help prevent fluid retention. Rarely do clients need to restrict fluid intake to less than 2000 ml/day. Evaluate the client's appetite, meal frequency, portion sizes, and food preferences, and provide appropriate health education. If possible, open cupboards and the refrigerator to gain insight into the client's eating patterns. Suggest a food diary to accurately assess intake. Teach clients, family members, and informal caregivers how to distinguish the sodium content of foods by reading food labels.

Because a client's functional status is often severely impaired, explain energy-conservation techniques before initiating limited mobility and aerobic routines. Even the most severely affected client may benefit from chair exercises, done while in a sitting position. Instruct clients to keep an activity log to demonstrate their progress toward activity goals. Clients should perceive their activities as only somewhat hard to do and should not participate in activities that worsen their manifestations or produce fatigue.

Clients who have chronic illnesses, including heart failure, often have feelings of depression. Consider whether clients need psychosocial and financial assistance. Antidepressant medications benefit some clients and improve their sense of well-being.

Cynthia A. Bolin, RN, Program Coordinator, Congestive Heart Failure Management Center, St. Luke's Hospital, St. Louis, Missouri

---

▪ Surgical Management for Heart Failure

HEART TRANSPLANTATION

When the heart is irreversibly damaged and no longer functions adequately and when the client is at risk of dying, cardiac transplantation and the use of an artificial heart to assist or replace the failing heart are measures of last resort. With the development of cyclosporine, and more recently FK-506 and mycophenolate mofetil, and with improvements in the procurement and preservation of donor hearts, cardiac transplantation has become an accepted therapeutic procedure. One-year survival rates after transplantation are greater than 85%. Although transplantation may not be appropriate for all clients, it may be the only option available to some. Heart transplantation is discussed in Chapter 57.

CARDIOMYOPLASTY

For clients with low cardiac output who are not candidates for cardiac transplantation, a procedure called *cardiomyoplasty* may support the failing heart. Initially developed in 1985, this procedure involves wrapping the latissimus dorsi muscle around the heart and electrostimulating it in synchrony with ventricular systole.

Immediate postoperative care is similar to that of any cardiac surgery client. Continuous cardiac and hemodynamic monitoring is initiated. Inotropic and vasopressor agents are administered to maintain cardiac output until the pulse generator is activated (within 2 to 3 weeks). Because the muscle flap obliterates the left upper lobe and can reduce vital capacity by as much as 20%, aggressive pulmonary hygiene and judicious pain management are essential to prevent atelectasis or pneumonia. In addition, an upper extremity exercise regimen is prescribed.

▪ Modifications for Elderly Clients

Heart failure is becoming increasingly a disorder of the very old. Cardiac decompensation can be triggered by seemingly minor illnesses and dietary indiscretions.[45] Medications commonly used by older people may have an impact on heart performance even though they pose little risk of interaction with cardiovascular medications. Nonsteroidal anti-inflammatory drugs (NSAIDs) tend to worsen heart disease because they promote sodium retention; tricyclic antidepressants (TCAs) and neuroleptic

CASE MANAGEMENT

Heart Failure

Heart failure is one of the most prevalent chronic diseases in the United States, causing millions of dollars of health care resources to be spent on hospitalizations and frequent readmissions. Without management and follow-up, clients tend to be readmitted repeatedly as they become more debilitated. Many case management programs have been initiated in an attempt to break the cycle of constant readmission. Through programs involving assessment, education, rehabilitation, and follow-up, clients have been able to have fewer manifestations and to return to a higher level of function. Moreover, scarce health care resources have been saved.

Assess

- What are the underlying causes of the heart failure (coronary artery disease, acute myocardial infarction, hypertension, valvular disease, cardiomyopathy, congenital heart disease, infections, dysrhythmias)?
- Are there co-morbid diseases that might worsen the condition (e.g., diabetes mellitus, renal disease, chronic obstructive pulmonary disease)?
- What are the warning manifestations for this client when an episode of heart failure is beginning?
- What did the client experience before this admission or readmission (shortness of breath, weight gain, cough, chest pain, fatigue, lower extremity or abdominal edema)?
- What does this client know about preventing an episode of heart failure, and what is your assessment of the client's ability to follow the care plan after discharge?

Advocate

A diagnosis of heart failure may be frightening; clients may think that "failure" means that the heart is not beating or that they will die. Carefully explain what "heart failure" means in terms the client can understand. Discuss care needs openly and honestly. This client may need assistance in making decisions regarding increased care or changes in residence. Caregivers, especially spouses, may need respite or assistance, but may be reluctant to ask for help.

Be alert for cognitive impairments or decreased mental function due to low oxygen saturation levels. Most clients take multiple medications, necessitating accurate administration and considerable cost. Does the client have financial concerns, or will lack of finances prevent obtaining medications?

Do environmental or safety issues in the home make it difficult for the client to manage, such as entry stairways or upstairs bedrooms? Be alert for manifestations of anxiety and stress in work or home situations that may exacerbate heart failure, and review safety measures if home oxygen therapy is to be used.

Prevent Readmission

Make sure that clients know about each medication they will be taking; help to create a schedule for them to follow at home.

Emphasize the need to manage hypertension and lipid levels. Discuss diet, sodium restrictions and weight gain. Clients may not be aware of the high sodium content in canned or prepared foods; in fact, they may use these products because of their easier preparation.

Find out if a scale is available at home; teach taking daily weights at the same time each day and how to keep a weight record.

Review the need for rest periods (sitting with legs elevated) and for some exercise. Evaluate the need for cardiac rehabilitation, referral for smoking cessation, or home care services.

Investigate the availability of telephone or home visitation follow-up through area hospitals or community or insurer disease management programs.

Finally, make sure the client knows about the manifestations needing immediate physician intervention, the need for follow-up visits with the primary physician, and how to obtain emergency assistance.

Cheryl Noetscher, RN, MS, Director of Case Management, Crouse Hospital and Community–General Hospital, Syracuse, New York

agents lead to orthostatic hypotension. Conversely, cardiac performance can affect the medication's action. The development of RVF can markedly increase the prothrombin time and thereby increase the action of anticoagulants.[45] See the Case Management feature on heart failure.

CONCLUSIONS

Disorders of cardiac function are the leading causes of death in the industrialized world. It is imperative that you fully understand the care of clients with heart disease to improve the outcomes and quality of life and to reduce morbidity and mortality. CHD is the precursor to several problems. Your role is to educate the client about risk reduction. Heart failure is a frequent end-point of cardiac disease. It is important to maximize cardiac output and reduce system demands on the heart.

THINKING CRITICALLY

1. **Your client is a 67-year-old man with newly diagnosed insulin-dependent diabetes in end-stage heart failure. The client was recently released from the hospital. You are to begin intravenous dobutamine therapy during this initial home visit. What assessment should be made prior to initiating dobutamine therapy? What other assessment interventions might be done?**

Factors to Consider. How does heart failure respond to the administration of dobutamine? What teaching or learning needs might be assessed in the client?

2. **A 70-year-old man is scheduled for a coronary artery bypass graft. What postoperative complications are most prevalent in older adults?**

Factors to Consider. How is CABG surgery accomplished? Why is CABG surgery a popular option?

BIBLIOGRAPHY

1. Abou-Awdi, N. L., & Samuels, W. L. (1995). Transmyocardial laser revascularization. *Seminars in Perioperative Nursing, 4,* 173–176.
2. Albert, N. (1994). Laser angioplasty and intracoronary stents: Going beyond the balloon. *AACN Clinical Issues in Critical Care Nursing, 5,* 15–20.
3. Albert, N. (1999). Heart failure: The physiologic basis for current therapeutic concepts. *Critical Care Nurse, 19*(suppl. 6), 2–13.
4. Allen, B., et al. (1999). Comparison of transmyocardial revascularization with medical therapy in patients with refractory angina. *New England Journal of Medicine, 341,* 1029–1036.
5. American Association of Cardiovascular and Pulmonary Rehabilitation. (1995). *Guidelines for cardiac rehabilitation programs.* Champaign, IL: Human Kinetics.
6. American Heart Association. (1999). *Scientific statement on prevention of cardiovascular diseases.* Dallas: Author.
7. American Heart Association. (1998). *1999 heart and stroke statistical update.* Dallas: Author.
8. Aregenziano, M., et al. (1997). The influence of infection on survival and successful transplantation in patients with left ventricular assist devices. *Journal of Heart and Lung Transplantation, 16,* 822–831.
9. Assmann, G., et al. (1999). Coronary heart disease: Reducing the risk. *Arteriosclerosis, Thrombosis, and Vascular Biology, 19,* 1819–1824.
10. Baig, M. K., et al. (1998). The pathophysiology of advanced heart failure. *Heart and Lung, 28,* 87–97.
11. Ballard, J. C., Wood, L. L., & Lansing, A. M. (1997). Transmyocardial revascularization: Criteria for selecting patients, treatment, and nursing care. *Critical Care Nurse, 17,* 42–49.
12. Bittl, J. A., & Thomas, P. (1996). Beyond the balloon. *Harvard Health Letter, 21,* 4.
13. Cheng, J. W. M., & Rovera, N. G. (1998). Infection and atherosclerosis: Focus on cytomegalovirus and *Chlamydia pneumoniae. Annals of Pharmacotherapy, 32,* 1310–1315.
14. Cohn, J., et al. (1997). The U.S. carvedilol heart failure study: Safety and efficacy of carvedilol in severe heart failure. *Journal of Cardiac Failure, 3,* 173–179.
15. Davis, C., et al. (1997). Vascular complications of coronary interventions. *Heart and Lung, 26,* 118.
16. Doering, L. V. (1999). Pathophysiology of acute coronary syndromes leading to acute myocardial infarction. *Journal of Cardiovascular Nursing, 13*(3), 1–20.
17. Fischer, A., Gutstein, D. E., & Fuster, V. (1999). Thrombosis and coagulation abnormalities in the acute coronary syndromes. *Cardiology Clinics, 17,* 283–294.
18. Futterman, L. G., & Lemberg, L. (1999). The use of antioxidants in retarding atherosclerosis: Fact or fiction. *American Journal of Critical Care, 8,* 130–133.
19. Goodman, M., et al. (1996). Hostility predicts restenosis after percutaneous transluminal coronary angioplasty. *Mayo Clinic Proceedings, 71,* 729–734.
20. Gotto, A. M. (1998). Assessing the benefits of lipid-lowering therapy. *American Journal of Cardiology, 82,* 2m–4m.
21. Grundy, S. M., et al. (1997). Guide to primary prevention of cardiovascular disease: A statement for healthcare professionals from the Task Force on Risk Reduction. *Circulation, 95,* 2329–2331.
22. Gurfinkel, E., et al. (1997). Randomized trial of roxithromycin in non–Q-wave coronary syndromes: ROXIS pilot study. *Lancet, 2,* 404–407.
23. Gutstein, D. E., & Fuster, V. (1998). Pathophysiologic bases for adjunctive therapies in the treatment and secondary prevention of acute myocardial infarction. *Clinical Cardiology, 21,* 161–168.
24. Homes, L. M., & Hollabaugh, S. K. (1997). Using continuous quality improvement process to improve the care of patients after angioplasty. *Critical Care Nurse, 17,* 56–65.
25. Horvath, K. A., et al. (1996). Transmyocardial laser revascularization: Operative techniques and clinical results at two years. *Journal of Thoracic and Cardiovascular Surgery, 111*(15), 1047–1053.
26. Hulley, S., et al., Heart and Estrogen/Progestin Replacement Study (HERS) Research Group. (1998). Randomized trial of estrogen plus progestin for secondary prevention of coronary heart disease in postmenopausal women. *Journal of the American Medical Association, 280,* 605–613.
27. Jacobs, A. K., et al. (1998). Better outcome for women compared with men undergoing coronary revascularization: A report from the Bypass Angioplasty Revascularization Investigation (BARI). *Circulation, 98,* 1279–1285.
28. Keller, K. B., & Lemberg, L. (1998). Therapy for hyperlipidemia when it is the only risk factor: Fact or fiction? *American Journal of Critical Care, 7,* 395–397.
29. Kinney, M. R. (1995). Assessment of quality of life in recovery settings. *Journal of Cardiovascular Nursing, 10,* 88–96.
30. Konstam, M., et al. (1994). *Heart failure: Evaluation and care of patients with left ventricular systolic dysfunction. Clinical practice guideline No. 11* (AHCPR Pub. No. 94-0612). Rockville, MD: Agency for Health Care Policy and Research, Public Health Service, U.S. Department of Health and Human Services.
31. Michael, K., & Parnell, K. J. (1998). Innovations in the pharmacologic management of heart failure. *AACN Clinical Issues, 9,* 172–191.
32. Mizell, J. L., Maglish, B. L., & Matheny, R. G. (1997). Minimally invasive direct coronary artery bypass graft surgery. *Critical Care Nurse, 17,* 46–55.
33. Moore, S. M. (1995). A comparison of women's and men's symptoms during home recovery after coronary artery bypass surgery. *Heart and Lung, 24,* 495–501.
34. Mosca, L., et al. (1999). Guide to preventive cardiology for women. *Circulation, 99,* 2480–2484.
35. Moser, D. K. (1998). Pathophysiology of heart failure update: The role of neurohormonal activation on the progression of heart failure. *AACN Clinical Issues, 9,* 157–171.
36. Packer, M. (1997). End of the oldest controversy in medicine: Are we ready to conclude the debate on digitalis? *New England Journal of Medicine, 336,* 575–576.
37. Packer, M., & Cohn, J. N. (1999). Consensus recommendations for the management of chronic heart failure. *American Journal of Cardiology, 83,* 1A–38A.
38. Piano, M., Bondmass, M., & Schwertz, D. (1998). The molecular and cellular pathophysiology of heart failure. *Heart and Lung, 27,* 3–19.
39. Poirier, V. (1997). The heartmate left ventricular assist system: Worldwide clinical results. *European Journal of Cardio-Thoracic Surgery, 11,* 539–544.
40. Redeker, N. S., et al. (1995). Women's patterns of activity over 6 months after coronary artery bypass surgery. *Heart and Lung, 24,* 502–511.
41. Riddle, M. M., Dunston, J. L., & Castanes, J. L. (1996). A rapid recovery program for cardiac surgery patients. *American Journal of Critical Care, 5,* 152–159.
42. Saatvedt, K., Dragsundm, M., & Nordstrandt, K. (1996). Transmyocardial laser revascularization and coronary artery bypass grafting. *Annals of Thoracic Surgery, 62*(1), 323–324.
43. Scherr, K., Jensen, L., & Koshal, A. (1999). Mechanical circulation as a bridge to cardiac transplantation: Toward the 21st century. *American Journal of Critical Care, 8,* 324–335.
44. Shah, P. K. (1996). Pathophysiology of plaque rupture and the concept of plaque stabilization. *Cardiology Clinics, 14*(1), 17–28.
45. Stanley, M. (1997). Current trends in the clinical management of an old enemy: Congestive heart failure in the elderly. *AACN Clinical Issues, 8,* 616–626.
46. Stary, H. C., et al. (1995). A definition of advanced types of atherosclerotic lesions and a histological classification of atherosclerosis. *Circulation, 92,* 1355–1374.
47. Strimike, C. L. (1995). Caring for a patient with an intracoronary stent. *American Journal of Nursing, 95,* 40–45.
48. Sulzbach, L. M., Hazard-Munro, B., & Hirshfield, J. (1995). A randomized clinical trial of the effect of bed position after PTCA. *American Journal of Critical Care, 4,* 221–226.
49. Wenger, N. K. (1998). Addressing coronary heart disease risk in women. *Cleveland Clinic Journal of Medicine, 65,* 464–469.
50. Wenger, N. K. (1999). Women, myocardial infarction, and coronary revascularization. *Cardiology in Review, 7,* 117–120.
51. Wenger, N. K., et al. (1995). *Cardiac rehabilitation as secondary prevention. Clinical practice guideline: Quick reference guide for clinicians, No. 17* (AHCPR Pub No. 96-0672). Rockville, MD:

Agency for Health Care Policy and Research, and the National Heart, Lung, and Blood Institute, Public Health Service, U.S. Department of Health and Human Services.

52. Wolff, C. A., Scott, C., & Banks, T. A. (1997). The radial artery: An exciting alternative conduit in coronary artery bypass surgery. *Critical Care Nurse, 17*, 34–39.

53. Zevola, D. R., et al. (1997). Clinical pathways and coronary artery bypass surgery. *Critical Care Nurse, 17*, 20–33.

54. Zhou, J., et al. (1999). Plaque pathology and coronary thrombosis in the pathogenesis of acute coronary syndromes. *Scandinavian Journal of Clinical and Laboratory Investigation, 59*(suppl. 230), 3–11.

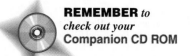

CHAPTER

Management of Clients with Dysrhythmias

Maribeth Guzzo

NURSING OUTCOMES CLASSIFICATION (NOC)
for Nursing Diagnoses — Clients with Dysrhythmias

Anxiety	**Decreased Cardiac Output**
Anxiety Control	Circulation Status
Coping	Vital Signs Status

The heart is endowed with a specialized system for generating rhythmic electrical impulses and for conducting these impulses rapidly throughout the heart to cause contraction of the heart muscle. When this system functions normally, the atria contract about one-sixth of a second ahead of the ventricles. This orderly electrical activity must precede contraction to provide adequate cardiac output for perfusion of all body organs and tissues.

The rhythmical and conduction systems of the heart are susceptible to damage by heart disease, especially by ischemia of the heart tissues resulting from decreased coronary artery blood flow. The consequence is often a bizarre heart rhythm or abnormal sequence of contraction through the heart chambers. The abnormal rhythms, called *dysrhythmias* (or arrhythmias), can severely decrease the heart's ability to pump effectively, even to the extent of causing death.

Before reading about dysrhythmias, you may want to review the electrical conduction system of the heart in the Unit 12 review and/or the electrocardiogram (ECG) in Chapter 54.

A *normal sinus rhythm* is a heart rhythm that begins in the sinoatrial (SA) node, is between 60 and 100 beats per minute (BPM), and has normal intervals and no aberrant or ectopic beats (Fig. 57–1). Characteristics of normal sinus rhythm are shown in Table 57–1.

DYSRHYTHMIAS

Dysrhythmias (abnormal heart rhythms) are common in people with cardiac disorders but also occur in people with normal hearts. Dysrhythmias are often detected because of associated manifestations of dizziness, palpitations, and syncope. Abnormalities in conduction are dangerous because of reduced cardiac output, which can lead to impaired cerebral perfusion. The most serious complication of a dysrhythmia is sudden death.[1, 9] Since seconds can literally make the difference between life and death for the person who is experiencing a serious dysrhythmia, evaluating responsiveness, quickly activating the emergency medical service (EMS), and initiating cardiopulmonary resuscitation (CPR) can determine the outcome.

Etiology and Risk Factors

Dysrhythmias result from disturbances in three major mechanisms: (1) automaticity, (2) conduction, and (3) problems with reentry of impulses.[6, 8, 32]

DISTURBANCES IN AUTOMATICITY

The term *automaticity* is used to describe alterations in the normal heart rates produced by various pacemaker cells in the myocardium. Recall that the SA node is the pacemaker of the heart because it possesses the highest level of automaticity. It normally produces a rhythm of 60 to 100 BPM. The SA node is regulated by the nervous system through the vagus nerve. Sympathetic stimulation increases the rate of firing; lack of sympathetic stimulation or vagal stimulation (which is parasympathetic) decreases the rate.

If the SA node fails to initiate an impulse, every other muscle cell in the myocardium can start the impulse. This fail-safe mechanism is crucial during heart disease. Latent pacemaker cells in the atrioventricular (AV) junction usually assume the role of pacemaker of the heart but at a slower rate (40 to 60 BPM). Such a pacemaker is called an "escape" pacemaker. If the AV junction cannot take over as the pacemaker because of disease, an escape pacemaker in the electrical conduction system below the AV junction (i.e., in the bundle branches or Purkinje

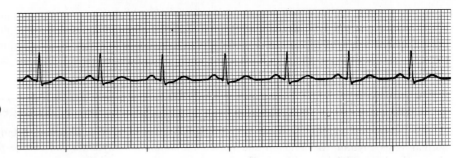

FIGURE 57-1 Normal sinus rhythm as seen on an electrocardiogram (ECG) strip. Note the regular R-R interval, a rate of 80 beats per minute, and a P-R interval of 0.16 second.

fibers) may take over at a still lower rate (<40 BPM). In general, the farther the escape pacemaker is from the SA node, the slower it generates electrical impulses.

These impulses can also occur prematurely—before the SA node would normally fire again. Premature impulses occur when the heart is ischemic, as with coronary artery disease. Myocardial infarction (MI) or heart failure is characterized by areas of calcification along different points in the heart as a normal variant or by irritation of the AV node, Purkinje system, or myocardium from drugs, nicotine, or caffeine.

Under a variety of circumstances, cardiac cells in any part of the heart, whether they are latent pacemaker cells or nonpacemaker myocardial cells, may take on the role of a pacemaker and start generating extraneous electrical impulses. When impulses begin from other sites, the sites are called "ectopic" pacemakers. For instance, if the SA node fails to fire, other sites in the atria can fire. If the atria do not initiate a beat, it can begin in the AV node; if the AV node does not initiate a beat, one can start in the ventricles. When an ectopic pacemaker initiates a beat, the appearance of the ECG differs from the way it looks with a normal sinus rhythm beat.

Each of these areas of myocardium (atria, AV node, ventricles) has its own intrinsic rate:

- Sinus node, 60 to 100 BPM
- Atria, 60 to 100 BPM
- AV node, 40 to 60 BPM
- Ventricles, 20 to 40 BPM

Latent pacemaker cells can also fire at increased rates beyond their inherent rate. When rates exceed these values, the rhythm is called "accelerated" and classified as a problem of "altered automaticity." For example, an accelerated junctional tachycardia can develop with a rate higher than 60 BPM (the inherent AV node rate). Abnormal automaticity is commonly caused by ischemia, hyperkalemia, hypocalcemia, hypoxia, increased catecholamine levels, digitalis toxicity, and administration of atropine. A rhythm faster than the intrinsic rate is called *tachycardia*. A rhythm slower than the intrinsic rate is called *bradycardia*. Therefore, sinus bradycardia is identified as a heart rate below 60 BPM and sinus tachycardia is defined as a heart rate above 100 BPM.

DISTURBANCES IN CONDUCTION

Conduction is the speed the impulse travels through the sinus node, AV node, and Purkinje fibers. Conduction may be either too rapid or too slow. Blocks that slow or stop an impulse can occur anywhere along the pathway. Blocks can result from ischemia of the tissues, scarring of

conduction pathways, compression of the AV bundle by scar tissue, inflammation of the AV node, extreme vagal stimulation of the heart, electrolyte imbalances, increased atrial preload, digitalis toxicity, beta-blocking agents, impaired cellular metabolism, MI (especially inferior), and valvular surgery.

Blocks result in ECG changes in appearance. Because the blocked impulse needs more time to travel to its destination, the wave is wider than normal. Disturbances in conduction can also lead to decreased cardiac output and life-threatening dysrhythmias.

REENTRY OF IMPULSES

Reentry is the activation of muscle for a second time by the same impulse. The waves of electrical impulse are not extinguished but persist because of a combination of slow conduction and blocks. Therefore, the conduction system is delayed or blocked (or both) in one or more segments while being transmitted normally through the rest of this system.

The problem occurs when some cells have been repolarized sufficiently so that they can prematurely depolarize again, producing ectopic beats and rhythms. Hyperkalemia and myocardial ischemia are the two most common causes of delay or block in the conduction system responsible for the reentry mechanism. The reentry mechanism can result in atrial fibrillation (AFib) and ventricular fibrillation (VFib).

RISK FACTORS

Understanding which client populations are at risk for development of abnormal heart rhythms can be useful in preventing and correcting these abnormalities. Myocardial

TABLE 57-1	CHARACTERISTICS OF NORMAL SINUS RHYTHMS
Rhythm	Regular, P–P intervals and R–R intervals may vary as much as 3 mm and still be considered regular
Rate	60–100 beats per minute
P waves	One P Wave preceding each QRS complex
P–R interval	0.12–0.20 second, consistent with each complex
QRS complex	0.04–0.10 second, consistent with each complex
Q–T interval	<0.40 second

ischemia, hypoxia, autonomic nervous system imbalances, lactic acidosis, electrolyte imbalances, drug toxicity, and hemodynamic abnormalities are risk factors for dysrhythmias.

Pathophysiology

The significance of all dysrhythmias is their effect on cardiac output and cerebral or vascular perfusion. During normal sinus rhythm, the atria fill and stretch the ventricles with about 30% more blood. This process is called the *atrial kick*. The extra stretch improves contractility of the ventricles and thereby increases cardiac output. When the impulse starts in the AV node or in the ventricles, atrial and ventricular contraction are no longer coordinated. Atrial kick is lost and cardiac output falls. For example, during contractions initiated in the ventricle the impulse begins in the ventricle and travels backward up the heart. As a result, the atria fill the ventricles while they are contracting or even afterward. Obviously, the efficiency of the heart as a pump is restricted during dysrhythmias and the clinical manifestations noted are due to changes in cardiac output.

Clinical Manifestations

The reduced cardiac output leads to clinical manifestations of dysrhythmias: palpitations, dizziness or syncope, pallor, diaphoresis, altered mentation (restlessness and agitation to lethargy and coma), hypotension, sluggish capillary refill, swelling of the extremities, and diminished urinary output. Palpitations, dizziness, and syncope are the clinical manifestations that are most effectively evaluated by ambulatory ECG monitoring. The client wears a portable ECG monitor and manually records (writes down) worrisome manifestations, and the correlation of manifestations to the heart rhythm can then be assessed. Shortness of breath, chest pain, and fatigue may also be caused by dysrhythmias. However, these manifestations are probably caused by other factors, such as myocardial ischemia and heart failure.

Depending upon the type of dysrhythmia, physical assessment findings may reveal (1) a heart rate below 50 or above 140 BPM; (2) an extremely irregular heart rhythm or pulse; (3) a first heart sound that varies in intensity; (4) sudden appearance of heart failure, shock, and angina pectoris; and (5) a slow, regular heart rate that does not change with activity or medications such as atropine or epinephrine.

Diagnostic findings include ECG abnormalities. The key to dysrhythmia interpretation is the analysis of the form and interrelations of the P wave, the P-R interval, and the QRS complex. The ECG should be analyzed with respect to its rate, rhythm, and site of the dominant pacemaker as well as the configuration of the P and QRS waves. Remember, any ECG findings should be correlated with clinical observations of the client; that is, "treat the client, not the monitor."

You will find it necessary to develop a method of analyzing ECG strips that allows you to consistently identify the rhythm demonstrated. The analysis of rhythms is one of two types: sight reading or paper analysis. Sight readers analyze ECGs by looking at the whole rhythm.

Much experience and continual, regular viewing of rhythm strips are required for this technique, which is of little use to the beginner. Health care providers with less experience need to develop a method of ECG analysis (Box 57-1).

Outcome Management

The goal of management is to control or ablate the dysrhythmia and reduce potential complications from it. The specific management of dysrhythmias depends on the type and on the client's response to it. All dysrhythmias can reduce cardiac output, which can cause a client to have no manifestations or to have many. Rhythm disturbances resulting in syncope, near-syncope, or sudden death warrant further evaluation. Ventricular dysrhythmias can be life-threatening, demanding immediate treatment. This chapter reviews dysrhythmias and their management, progressing from problems arising (1) in the atria, (2) in the AV junction, and (3) in the ventricles.

ATRIAL DYSRHYTHMIAS

DISTURBANCES IN AUTOMATICITY

SINUS TACHYCARDIA

Sinus tachycardia is characterized by a rapid, regular rhythm at a rate of 100 to 180 BPM with a normal P wave and QRS complex (Fig. 57-2A). It often occurs in response to an increase in sympathetic stimulation or decreased vagal (parasympathetic) stimulation. Causes include the following:

- Fever
- Emotional and physical stress
- Heart failure
- Fluid volume loss
- Hyperthyroidism
- Hypercalcemia
- Medications, including, atropine, nitrates, epinephrine, and isoproterenol
- Caffeine
- Nicotine
- Exercise

Most clients do not experience clinical manifestations except for occasional palpitations. However, the clinical manifestations depend on the heart rate and its effect on cardiac output. Between these quick beats, there is little time for ventricular filling and atrial contraction. Clients with underlying heart disease may not tolerate the increased myocardial workload and reduced coronary artery filling time that accompanies the increased heart rate. These clients may experience hypotension and angina pectoris (chest pain).

Management focuses on alleviating the underlying cause and reducing further demands on the heart. Medications such as digitalis, beta-adrenergic blocking agents (e.g., propranolol), and calcium channel blockers may be prescribed.[1, 23, 32] Bed rest is ordered to reduce metabolic demand. Oxygen may be prescribed to supply the myocardium adequately.

BOX 57-1   Electrocardiographic Interpretation of Dysrhythmias

There are seven basic steps to assist you in the identification of dysrhythmias. The electrocardiogram (ECG) should be studied in an *orderly* fashion as follows:

Step 1

Calculate the heart rate. The simplest method for obtaining the rate is to count the number of R waves in a 6-inch strip of the ECG tracing (which equals 6 seconds). Multiply this sum by 10 to get the rate per minute (BPM). Because the ECG paper is marked into 3-inch intervals (at the top margin), the approximate heart rate can be rapidly calculated.

Another method is to count the number of large squares between R waves. Find an R wave crossing a large square. Count the number of large squares until the next R wave. The approximate heart rate is

1 large square = 300 BPM
2 large squares = 150 BPM
3 large squares = 100 BPM
4 large squares = 75 BPM
5 large squares = 60 BPM
6 large squares = 50 BPM
7 large squares = 43 BPM
8 large squares = 37 BPM
9 large squares = 33 BPM
10 large squares = 30 BPM

Step 2

Measure the regularity (rhythm) of the R waves (ventricular rhythm). This can be done by gross observation or actual measurement of the intervals (R-R).

If the R waves occur at regular intervals (variance <0.12 second between beats), the ventricular rhythm is normal. When there are differences in R-R intervals (>0.12 second), the ventricular rhythm is said to be irregular. The division of ventricular rhythm into regular and irregular categories assists in identifying the mechanism of many dysrhythmias.

Note atrial regularity and measure the atrial rate. Measure the regularity (rhythm) of the P waves (P-P). Use the above method, but calculate the distance between the same point on two consecutive P waves.

Step 3

Examine the P waves. If P waves are present and precede each QRS complex, the heartbeat originates in the sinus node and a sinus rhythm exists. The absence of P waves or an abnormality in their position with respect to the QRS complex indicates that the impulse started outside the sinoatrial node and that an ectopic pacemaker is in command.

Step 4

Measure the P-R interval. Normally, this interval should be between 0.12 and 0.20 second. Prolongation or reduction of this interval beyond these limits indicates a defect in the conduction system between the atria and the ventricles.

Step 5

Measure the duration of the QRS complex. If the width between the onset of the Q wave and the completion of the S wave is greater than 0.12 second (three fine lines on the paper), an intraventricular conduction defect exists.

Step 6

Examine the ST segment. Normally, this segment is isoelectric, meaning it is neither elevated nor depressed because the positive and negative forces are equally balanced during this period. Elevation or depression of the ST segment indicates an abnormality in the onset of recovery of the ventricular muscle, usually because of injury (e.g., acute myocardial infarction).

Step 7

Examine the T wave. Normally, the T wave is upright and one-third the height of the QRS complex. Any condition that interferes with normal repolarization (e.g., myocardial ischemia) may cause the T waves to invert. An abnormally high serum potassium level causes the T wave to become very tall—sometimes the height of the QRS complex.

SINUS BRADYCARDIA

Sinus bradycardia occurs when the SA node fires at a rate of less than 60 times per minute. The P wave and QRS complex are normal (Fig. 57–2*B*). Sinus bradycardia may result from the following:

- Increased vagal (parasympathetic) tone, as occurs with Valsalva's maneuver (e.g., straining while moving bowels)
- Drugs (especially digitalis, propranolol, or verapamil)
- MI (most often inferior MI)
- Hyperkalemia
- Various diseases, such as hypothyroidism, myxedema, and obstructive jaundice

In some people, sinus bradycardia can be a normal condition. Athletes often have sinus bradycardia because their heart is an effective pump with a greater than normal stroke volume. Because cardiac output is the product of stroke volume and heart rate, the heart rate decreases, yet cardiac output is adequate.

Clients may be asymptomatic; when manifestations do develop, it is because cardiac output is decreased. Fatigue, hypotension, lightheadedness, syncope, shortness of breath, decreased level of consciousness, pulmonary congestion, or heart failure may develop. The slowed rate of SA discharge may allow junctional or ventricular pacemakers to take over, thereby producing ectopic beats.

The aim of management is to correct the underlying cause of sinus bradycardia, and the goal of intervention is to increase the heart rate just enough to relieve manifestations but not enough to cause tachycardia. The intervention sequence for treating symptomatic bradycardia is atropine, transcutaneous pacing if available, dopamine, epinephrine, and isoproterenol or insertion of a temporary transvenous pacemaker.[1, 23, 32]

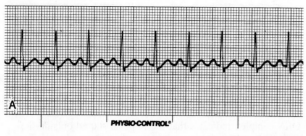

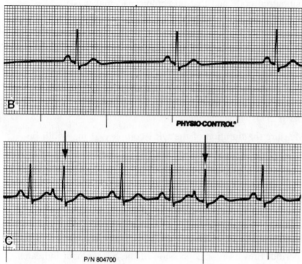

FIGURE 57–2 Atrial dysrhythmias. *A*, Sinus tachycardia—regular R-R interval, rate 125 beats per minute (BPM); P-R interval, 0.16 second. *B*, Sinus bradycardia—regular R-R interval, rate 40 BPM; P-R interval, 0.16. *C*, Premature atrial contractions. The second and fifth beat are premature atrial contractions (PACs). Note the difference in appearance of the P wave and the shortened R-R interval.

SINUS DYSRHYTHMIA

Sinus dysrhythmia is characterized by phasic changes in the automaticity of the SA node, which cause it to fire at varying speeds. The heart rate generally ranges between 60 and 100 BPM. The ECG shows a normal P wave, P-R interval, and QRS complex; the only abnormality is an irregular P-P interval.

Sinus dysrhythmia may develop from alterations in vagal tone and in response to delayed atrial filling with inhalation. During inspiration, venous return to the right atrium is delayed because of increased intrathoracic pressure. In quiet respiration, the heart rate can decrease about 5%; with deep respiration, the rate can decrease up to 30%.

Clients with sinus dysrhythmia do not usually require intervention other than alleviation of the underlying cause. Cardiac output is not affected.

PREMATURE ATRIAL CONTRACTIONS

Premature atrial contractions (PACs) are early beats arising from ectopic atrial foci, interrupting the normal rhythm. Commonly resulting from enhanced automaticity of the atrial muscle, PACs occur in both normal and diseased hearts. PACs are associated with valvular disease

and atrial chamber enlargement; they may also be seen with stress, fatigue, alcohol, smoking, coronary artery disease (CAD), cardiac ischemia, heart failure, cardioactive medications (digitalis, quinidine, procainamide), pulmonary congestion, and pulmonary hypertension. Frequent PACs may mark the onset of AFib or heart failure or may reflect electrolyte imbalances.

In clients with PACs, P waves are premature and differ from the normal sinus P wave in appearance, size, or shape (Fig. 57–2*C*). Premature beats from any ectopic focus can be palpated as skipped or irregular beats. The client who experiences numerous PACs may note palpitations, or "missed beats." PACs are usually benign; however, if the client has increasing numbers of "skipped beats" or feels palpitations often, the problem should be evaluated. Intervention usually focuses on correcting the underlying cause and may include administration of quinidine or procainamide.

DISTURBANCES IN CONDUCTION

SINOATRIAL NODE CONDUCTION DEFECTS

Under certain circumstances, the impulse from the SA node is either (1) not generated in the SA node *(SA arrest)* or (2) not conducted from the SA node *(sinus exit block)*. Causes of SA node conduction abnormalities include the following:

- Conditions that increase vagal tone
- Coronary artery disease
- MI
- Digitalis and calcium channel blocker toxicity
- Hypertensive disease
- Tissue hypoxia
- Scarring of intra-atrial pathways
- Electrolyte imbalances

During *SA arrest*, neither the atria nor the ventricles are stimulated, resulting in a pause in the rhythm. An entire PQRST complex will be missing for one or more cycles. After the pause of sinus arrest, a new pacemaker focus assumes the pacing responsibility. The new pacer paces the heart at its inherent rate, which is usually slower than the original SA node rate. The new pacer site is often another atrial focus, but the junction or ventricle can also assume pacing responsibility.

During *sinus exit block*, there is a conduction delay between the sinus node and the atrial muscle. Unlike the rhythm in SA arrest, the rhythm of SA node discharge in sinus exist block remains constant and uninterrupted. The ECG characteristically displays a normal sinus rhythm that is interrupted intermittently by pauses. This creates a pattern of pauses that, when measured, are multiples of the underlying P-P interval. Sinus arrest differs from SA exit block, in that the SA node at times does not fire at all. The result is the occurrence of pauses that are longer and not a multiple of the underlying P-P interval. These pauses are also frequently terminated by escape ectopic beats. Sinus arrest often is associated with a more serious prognosis.

The client usually remains asymptomatic, depending on the duration and frequency of the pauses; however, lengthy pauses can cause lightheadedness or syncope. Intervention is unnecessary unless the client becomes symptomatic and exhibits manifestations of decreased cardiac output. An irregular pulse can be palpated or auscultated. Clinicians can only infer impulse formation within the SA node from the appearance of P waves, which reflect atrial depolarization.

Intervention may include administration of a vagolytic (atropine) or a sympathomimetic (isoproterenol) agent to increase the rate of SA node firing. If pharmacologic measures fail, a pacemaker may be required. Finally, the physician must determine and treat the underlying cause of the dysrhythmia.[1, 23, 32]

REENTRY OF IMPULSES

PAROXYSMAL ATRIAL TACHYCARDIA

Paroxysmal atrial tachycardia (PAT) is the sudden onset and sudden termination of a rapid firing from an ectopic atrial pacemaker (Fig. 57–3A). PAT is due to the reentry phenomenon. This process allows (1) the atrial impulses to travel down less refractory conduction pathways to the bundle of His and (2) retrograde conduction through previously refractory parallel fibers. A circular circuit for rapid repetitive depolarizations results from these events.

PAT occasionally appears in clients with a normal heart but most commonly develops in clients with cardiac disease. Common cardiac problems precipitating PAT include the following:

- MI
- Cardiomyopathy
- Extreme emotions
- Caffeine ingestion
- Fatigue
- Smoking
- Excessive alcohol intake

Less common causes include rheumatic heart disease, valvular disease, pulmonary emboli, cor pulmonale, thyrotoxicosis, digitalis toxicity (PAT with block), and cardiac surgery.

Clinicians identify PAT by three or more consecutive atrial ectopic beats occurring at a rate greater than 150 BPM alternating with normal sinus rhythm. The P waves are usually upright, narrow, and peaked in lead II. At faster atrial rates, the P waves may become lost in the preceding T wave. The P-R intervals may be normal. However, rapid atrial rates may overcome the conduction limits of the AV node, causing varying degrees of AV block. Atrial tachycardia with 2:1 block (i.e., two P waves for every QRS complex) most often results from digitalis toxicity. The QRS complexes are usually normal, although aberrant ventricular conduction may occur at

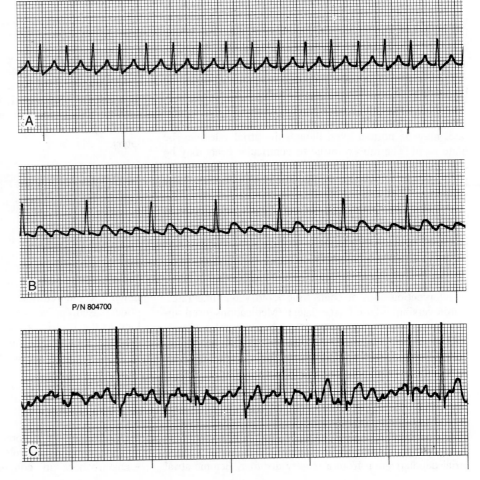

FIGURE 57–3 *A*, Paroxysmal atrial tachycardia (PAT). The rate is rapid, about 175 beats per minute (BPM). The P wave is not distinguishable, but the QRS complex is narrow, indicating that the impulse began above the atrioventricular node. *B*, Atrial flutter. Note the saw-toothed appearance of the P waves. There are three P waves for every QRS complex, indicating a 3:1 block. Atrial rate is 75 BPM. *C*, Atrial fibrillation is identifiable by a chaotic P wave, not one clear P wave, and an irregular R-R interval.

P/N 804700

very rapid atrial rates or when a conduction defect exists within the ventricle.

PAT decreases ventricular filling time and mean arterial pressure and also increases myocardial oxygen demand. Clients may report palpitations and lightheadedness.

Management varies with the severity of manifestations. Clients with extremely rapid heart rates or significant underlying cardiovascular disease may experience syncope and heart failure. In such instances, heart rate must be immediately reduced. Any maneuver that stimulates the vagus nerve can successfully terminate PAT or increase AV block. The vagus nerve can be stimulated by carotid sinus massage and Valsalva's maneuver (bearing down). Useful pharmacologic agents include adenosine, verapamil, and beta-blockers. Sedatives may also be used to reduce sympathetic stimulation. The physician may also employ cardioversion (see later) as an effective means of terminating PAT if medications and vagal stimulation are not effective.

Ablation procedures that destroy a part of the reentrant path are being more widely used (see later). Such procedures can result in a long-term cure in selected clients.[1, 6, 21, 23, 32]

ATRIAL FLUTTER

Atrial flutter is a dysrhythmia arising in an ectopic pacemaker or the site of a rapid reentry circuit in the atria, characterized by rapid "saw-toothed" atrial wave formations and usually by a slower, regular ventricular response. Atrial flutter differs from PAT, in that it produces a much more rapid atrial rate. The P waves are actually inverted or bidirectional, producing a "picket fence" or saw-toothed pattern of "flutter waves" (Fig. 57–3B). The atrial rate generally ranges from 220 to 350 BPM. The AV node cannot conduct all of the atrial impulses that bombard it; that is, the AV node blocks a 1:1 conduction. Therefore, the ventricular rate is always slower than the atrial rate. Thus, the pulse, which reflects the ventricular rate, may be normal even though the atrial rate may be quite rapid. The ratio of atrial to ventricular beats may be constant (2:1, 3:1, 4:1, and 7:1, and so forth) or may vary. A variable degree of block produces an irregular ventricular rhythm.

Atrial flutter most commonly occurs in association with organic diseases such as CAD, mitral valve disease, pulmonary embolus (PE), and hyperthyroidism. In addition, it may occur after cardiac surgery. The client may sense occasional palpitations and chest pain, especially when rapid ventricular rates exist.

Intervention aims at controlling rapid ventricular rates. Cardioversion is used (see later). Medications used include digitalis, quinidine, verapamil, propranolol, and procainamide, especially if cardioversion is not successful. Carotid sinus massage helps to slow the ventricular response temporarily so that flutter waves can be identified.[1, 23, 32]

ATRIAL FIBRILLATION

Atrial fibrillation (AFib) is characterized by rapid, chaotic atrial depolarization from a reentry disorder. Ectopic atrial foci produce impulses between 400 and 700 BPM. At extremely rapid rates, however, the entire atrium may not be able to recover from one depolarization wave before the next begins. This results in mechanical and electrical disorganization of the atria. As with atrial flutter, the AV node is bombarded with more impulses than it can conduct. Most of these impulses are blocked; however, as a result of the erratic atrial impulses, there is a very irregular ventricular rhythm. The ventricular rate ranges from 160 to 180 BPM.

Examination of the ECG reveals erratic or no identifiable P waves and underlying ventricular rhythm that appears to be irregular and undulating (Fig. 57–3C). Because of atrial disorganization, there is no "atrial kick." This loss of additional blood volume can decrease cardiac output by as much as 20% to 30%. With increasing ventricular rates, cardiac output falls even further and may result in angina pectoris, heart failure, and shock.

AFib may be associated with sick sinus syndrome, hypoxia, increased atrial pressure, pericarditis, and many other conditions. Clients may be asymptomatic, or they may note an irregular pulse and palpitations. The client may have a pulse deficit between apical and radial pulses.

Mural thrombi formation can severely complicate the condition. Blood pools in the "quivering" atria because of lack of adequate contraction of atrial muscle. This blood can clot, which increases the potential for cerebral and pulmonary vascular emboli. Most clients with sudden onset of AFib are given heparin as an anticoagulant to reduce risk of stroke and PE until the impulses are controlled.

Outcome Management

The initial treatment goal is to control the rate of impulses with administration of drugs such as diltiazem, verapamil, beta-blockers, or digoxin. Chemical cardioversion, usually after a period of anticoagulation therapy, can then be attempted with procainamide or quinidine. Electrical cardioversion is the third therapeutic option (see later).

ATRIOVENTRICULAR JUNCTIONAL DYSRHYTHMIAS

If the SA node fails to fire and an impulse is not initiated in other ectopic sites in the atria, the AV junction is the next pacemaker for the heart. An impulse begins in the junction and simultaneously spreads up to the atria and down into the ventricles. During junctional rhythms, there is decreased cardiac output resulting from a lack of atrial kick to the ventricles. Junctional rhythms are not dependable for a long-term cardiac pacemaker because the rate is slow and more irritable ectopic foci may fire, such as from the ventricles. Consider junctional rhythms to be a warning or forerunner of more serious dysrhythmias.

Two major types of dysrhythmias arise in the AV junction:

• Disturbances in automaticity, with the AV junctional tissue assuming the role of the pacemaker
• Disturbances in conduction, with the AV junction

blocking impulses journeying from the atria to the ventricles

Both types of dysrhythmias may result from ischemia or trauma in the area of the AV junction (i.e., after MI or cardiac surgery). Digitalis toxicity, quinidine toxicity, and hyperkalemia may also cause junctional dysrhythmias.

Junctional rhythms produce abnormal upward direction of impulse (e.g., in lead II the P waves are inverted), because the impulse is traveling through the atria in a direction opposite to that found in normal sinus rhythm. Also, the P-R interval shortens to less than 0.12 second. The impulse may spread through the atria at the same time that the ventricles are being activated by the AV junction. In this instance, the P wave would be buried in the QRS complex and not observed on the ECG. Also, the atria may contract after the ventricles. In this case, the P wave would follow the QRS complex. The QRS complex is normal if ventricular conduction is normal.

DISTURBANCES IN AUTOMATICITY

The major junctional dysrhythmias caused by changes in automaticity are (1) premature junctional contractions (PJCs), (2) junctional escape rhythm, and (3) junctional tachycardias. As with PACs, an ectopic focus in the AV junctional tissue may develop increased automaticity and discharge prematurely, initiating depolarization of the heart.

PREMATURE JUNCTIONAL CONTRACTIONS

A PJC is the single, early firing of a junctional ectopic focus (Fig. 57–4). PJCs are slower as a result of lower intrinsic rates. Usually, clients can tolerate junctional rhythms, although clients with severe forms of cardiac disease may not because of decreased cardiac output.

PAROXYSMAL JUNCTIONAL TACHYCARDIA

A junctional rhythm with a rate that exceeds 60 BPM is termed a *junctional tachycardia*. It usually stops and starts abruptly, thereby acquiring the name *paroxysmal junctional tachycardia*, or PJT. The usual rate is 140 to 220 BPM.

Causes of PJT include metabolic imbalances and increased sympathetic stimulation. Rapid ventricular rates can lead to left ventricular failure resulting from increased myocardial oxygen demand and decreased blood supply. PJT that cannot be distinguished from PAT on the ECG is called *supraventricular tachycardia* (SVT).

Management of rapid junctional rhythms begins with vagal stimulation such as carotid sinus massage. If clinical manifestations develop, treatment consists of pharmacologic agents and cardioversion. Common medications include propranolol, quinidine, and digitalis. Evaluation of digitalis intoxication and potassium levels may also be indicated.[1, 32]

DISTURBANCES IN CONDUCTION

AV block comprises the second group of disturbances arising in the area of the AV junction. Impulses passing through the AV junction are blocked to varying degrees. Therefore, the conduction of impulses from the atria to the ventricles slows or stops entirely, depending on the degree of the AV block. Normally the impulse coming from the SA node is delayed at the AV junction for less than 0.20 second before traveling on to the bundle of His. If the AV junction has been damaged by ischemia, rheumatic fever, or drug toxicity, impulses are delayed or completely blocked at the AV junction for abnormally long periods of time.

FIRST-DEGREE ATRIOVENTRICULAR BLOCK

First-degree AV block is a delay in passage of the impulse from atria to ventricles. This delay usually occurs at the level of the AV node. The rhythm is regular, and each P wave is followed by a QRS complex; however, the P-R interval is prolonged beyond the normal 0.20 second. The P-R interval usually remains constant (Fig. 57–5A). This characteristic is an important differentiation between first-degree AV block and the other AV blocks. This block is often associated with CAD, increased vagal tone, and congenital anomalies and may also result from digitalis administration.

First-degree AV block, existing alone as the only abnormal feature of a client's ECG, produces no clinical manifestations and requires no intervention. If the block is a result of digitalis, the medication may be discontinued. Because first-degree AV block can progress to a higher-degree AV block, the client requires observation and ECG monitoring.[1, 32]

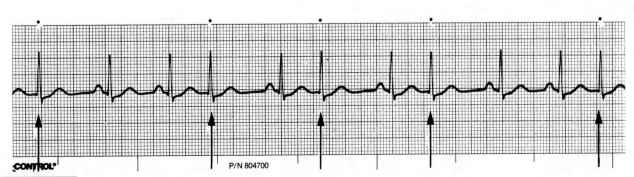

FIGURE 57–4 A premature junctional contraction. The beats marked with *arrows* are premature junctional contractions. Note the absence of a P wave but otherwise normal deflection, indicating that the impulse was initiated above the ventricles.

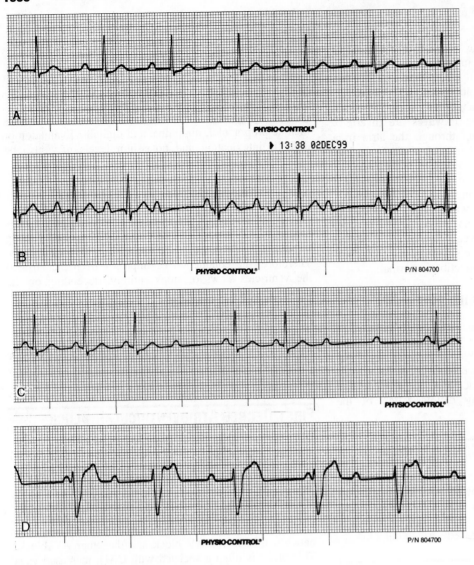

▶ 13:38 02DEC99

FIGURE 57–5 Junctional dysrhythmias. *A,* First-degree atrioventricular (AV) block. *B,* Second-degree AV block (Mobitz type I, Wenckebach phenomenon; note the regularly occurring P waves and the increasing P-R intervals). *C,* Second-degree AV block (Mobitz type II). *D,* Third-degree AV block (note variable P-R interval and lack of association of the P wave with the QRS complex).

SECOND-DEGREE ATRIOVENTRICULAR BLOCK

In a client with second-degree AV block, a more serious form of conduction delay in the heart, some impulses are conducted and others are blocked. Second-degree block results in intermittently dropped QRS complexes. Atrial depolarization continues without disturbance, and normal-appearing P waves occur at regular intervals. Second-degree AV block does not usually affect conduction through the ventricles, and QRS complexes appear normal in configuration. Second-degree AV block develops from CAD, digitalis toxicity, rheumatic fever, viral infections, and inferior wall MI.

Second-degree AV block is subdivided into two additional types: Mobitz type I (Wenckebach phenomenon) and Mobitz type II.

■ MOBITZ TYPE I BLOCK (WENCKEBACH PHENOMENON)

The Mobitz type I form of second-degree block is caused by an abnormally long refractory period. The level of block occurs at the AV node. On the ECG, the P-R interval gradually lengthens until a P wave is not con-

ducted (Fig. 57–5B). This is the mildest form of second-degree heart block. This dysrhythmia is due to increased vagal tone, digoxin administration or congenital anomalies.

Mobitz type I does not usually result in clinical manifestations because the ventricular rate is adequate; however, the client may have an irregular pulse. Vertigo, weakness, or other signs of low cardiac output may be experienced if the ventricular rate drops precipitously.

Intervention is not required as long as the ventricular rate remains adequate for perfusion. The client is assessed for progression to a higher (more serious) degree of block. Clinicians focus primarily on managing the underlying cause. Intervention, if needed, is similar to that described for Mobitz type II block.[1, 23, 32]

■ MOBITZ TYPE II BLOCK

Mobitz type II block occurs in the presence of a long absolute refractory period with little or no relative refractory period. The level of block is below the AV node, usually a consequence of a block within the His bundle system. The P waves are normal and are followed by normal QRS complexes at regular intervals, until suddenly a QRS complex is dropped (Fig. 57-5*C*). Mobitz type II blocks result from ischemia, digitalis, or quinidine toxicity or from anterior wall MI.

Mobitz type II, a more serious condition than Mobitz type I, may progress to third-degree AV block, especially in clients with an anterior wall MI. Clients with second-degree AV block require close ECG monitoring for possible progression to complete heart block.

Interventions include (1) administration of atropine and isoproterenol (which speed the rate of impulse conduction), (2) insertion of a temporary or permanent pacemaker, and (3) withholding cardiac depressant drugs (e.g., digitalis). Second-degree block, which occurs after MI, particularly an inferior MI, may be reversible as the injury of ischemia heals.[1, 23, 32]

THIRD-DEGREE ATRIOVENTRICULAR BLOCK

Third-degree AV block is the complete absence of conduction of the electrical impulses due to a block in the AV node, bundle of His, or bundle branches. Third-degree heart block is sometimes called *AV dissociation*, because the two halves of the heart are working independently of each other. The atria are paced by the SA node, but because the message is blocked, the ventricles are being paced by a ventricular ectopic pacemaker (Fig. 57-5*D*). The atrial rate is always equal to or faster than the ventricular in complete heart block. The ventricular rate is typically 40 to 60 BPM.

Other features of the ECG in third-degree heart block include (1) regular P-P intervals, (2) regular R-R intervals, (3) an absence of meaningful or consistent P-R intervals, and (4) normal-appearing P waves. The greatest danger inherent in third-degree AV block is ventricular standstill or asystole, characterized by the Stokes-Adams attack. If a focus in the ventricles does not initiate a heartbeat, asystole leads to immediate loss of consciousness and even death.

Third-degree AV block results from a variety of causes, including:

- Fibrotic or degenerative changes in the conduction system
- MI (especially anterior wall MI)
- Congenital anomalies
- Cardiac surgery
- Myocarditis
- Viral infections of the conduction system
- Drug toxicity (digitalis, beta blockers, calcium channel blockers)
- Trauma
- Cardiomyopathy
- Lyme disease

The slow ventricular rate leads to decreased cardiac output and circulatory impairment. Clients may experience hypotension, angina pectoris, and heart failure.

The major interventions in complete heart block are atropine, transcutaneous pacing, catecholamine infusions (dopamine or epinephrine), and transvenous pacemaker. If asystole develops, CPR is used until a pacemaker can be inserted. Isoproterenol is rarely indicated.[1, 23, 32]

DISTURBANCES IN CONDUCTION

BUNDLE BRANCH BLOCK

Bundle branch block indicates that conduction is impaired in one of the bundle branches (distal to the bundle of His) and thus the ventricles do not depolarize simultaneously. The abnormal conduction pathway through the ventricles is causing a wide or notched QRS complex. The defect may result from:

- Myocardial fibrosis
- Chronic CAD
- MI
- Cardiomyopathies
- Inflammation
- Pulmonary embolism
- Severe left ventricular hypertrophy
- Congenital anomalies

These disturbances of conduction through the ventricles result in either a right bundle branch block (RBBB) or a left bundle branch block (LBBB). Because of its association with left ventricular disease, LBBB carries a worse prognosis. The left bundle branch is composed of anterior and posterior fascicles (small bundles) of which one or both may be involved.

There is no specific intervention for this conduction defect. However, if RBBB exists along with block in one of the fascicles of the left bundle, the one remaining fascicle represents the only conduction pathway to the ventricles. Therefore, in this situation a pacemaker is required.[1, 31, 32]

VENTRICULAR DYSRHYTHMIAS

Ventricular dysrhythmias arise below the level of the AV junction. Like dysrhythmias in the atria or junction, dysrhythmias in the ventricles are caused by abnormalities of automaticity or conduction. Ventricular dysrhythmias are generally more serious and life-threatening than atrial or junctional dysrhythmias, because ventricular dysrhythmias more commonly develop in association with intrinsic heart disease. Also, ventricular dysrhythmias usually cause greater hemodynamic compromise (e.g., hypotension, heart failure, and shock). The independent contraction of the ventricles results in a reduced stroke volume and, therefore, a reduced cardiac output. Rapid ventricular rates prevent optimal filling of the ventricular chambers and reduce stroke volume even further. At rates of less than 40 contractions per minute, cardiac output is simply not sufficient to support the body's vital functions.

The ECG tracing of a client with ventricular dysrhythmias reveals wide and bizarre QRS complexes. Normally, impulses traverse the ventricles via the shortest, most efficient route. This normal pathway results in a narrow QRS complex. When an impulse originates in the ventricles, however, the impulse follows an abnormal pathway through the ventricular muscle tissue. This abnormality appears as a wide (>0.12 second) complex on the ECG.

DISTURBANCES IN AUTOMATICITY

Dysrhythmias due to problems in automaticity are characterized by ectopic impulses, which result from either myocardial irritability or the phenomenon of reentry. The four ventricular dysrhythmias due to automaticity are:

- Premature ventricular contractions (PVCs)
- Ventricular fibrillation (VFib)
- Ventricular tachycardia (VT)
- Torsades de pointes

PREMATURE VENTRICULAR CONTRACTIONS

PVCs, also called ventricular premature beats, are the most common of all dysrhythmias other than those of the sinus node. They are usually caused by the firing of an irritable pacemaker in the ventricle. PVCs result from enhanced ventricular automaticity or reentry. Factors promoting PVCs include:

- Myocardial hypoxia
- Hypokalemia
- Hypocalcemia
- Acidosis
- Alcohol
- Caffeine
- Nicotine
- CAD
- Heart failure
- Toxic agents (e.g., digitalis, tricyclic antidepressants)
- Exercise
- Hypermetabolic states
- Intracardiac catheters

PVCs produce easily recognized ECG changes. They occur earlier than the expected beat of the underlying rhythm and are usually followed by a compensatory pause. On the ECG, an unusually wide and bizarre QRS appears, interrupting the underlying rhythm (Fig. 57–6A).

Isolated PVCs are usually not treated. If the client becomes symptomatic because of decreased cardiac output, lidocaine or any of the other class I antidysrhythmics can be given to treat PVCs. In clients with acute MI, the development of PVCs indicates that the myocardium is ischemic; in such instances, ectopic foci become irritated and fire more often.

PVCs are dangerous when they are:

- Frequent (>6/min)
- Coupled with normal beats (bigeminy)
- Multiform (Fig. 57–6B)
- In pairs after every third beat (trigeminy) (Fig. 57–6C)
- A result of acute MI
- On the T wave (Fig. 57–6D)

Clinicians refer to "falling on the T wave" as the *R-on-T phenomenon*. The downward slope of the T wave is the most vulnerable period of the cardiac cycle. If the heart is stimulated at this time, it often cannot respond to the stimulus in an organized fashion because the muscle fibers are in various stages of repolarization. Therefore, PVCs that occur during this vulnerable period can precipitate the more life-threatening dysrhythmias of ventricular tachycardia (VTach) (Fig. 57–6E) and VFib.

Outcome Management

Management of dangerous PVCs involves administration of antidysrhythmic agents that have myocardial depressant actions. In acute situations, the clinician may administer class I and class II antidysrhythmic agents intravenously (IV), followed by a continuous IV drip. Table 57–2 describes a variety of antidysrhythmic agents.[1, 15, 17, 20, 22, 23, 32]

■ Nursing Management of the Medical Client
Assessment

Assess the client for clinical manifestations of decreased cardiac output. Monitor the ECG continuously for patterns of PVCs that indicate further deterioration (e.g., PVCs moving closer to the preceding T wave).

DIAGNOSIS, PLANNING, INTERVENTIONS

Decreased Cardiac Output. Dysrhythmias often lead to decreased ventricular filling due to rapid rate or from not being coordinated to allow for atrial kick. Express this common nursing diagnosis as *Decreased Cardiac Output related to decreased ventricular filling time secondary to (name the rhythm).*

Outcomes. The client will have an adequate cardiac output, as evidenced by (1) return of normal heart rate, rhythm, palpable pulse, and blood pressure to baseline levels; (2) return of level of consciousness to baseline value; (3) warm and dry skin; (4) clear lung sounds; (4) absence of S_3 or S_4; (5) absence of dysrhythmias; and (6) adequate urine output.

Interventions. Monitor heart rate and rhythm and vital signs continuously, aided by the computer when needed. Assess skin temperature, lung sounds, heart sounds, and peripheral pulses every 2 to 4 hours. Monitor laboratory studies, especially if an MI is suspected. Give antidysrhythmic medications according to orders. Use blood levels as a guide to dosage. Many medications, especially antidysrhythmics, can rise to toxic levels, especially if the client has a pre-existing liver, renal, or electrolyte disorder.

Maintain a quiet atmosphere, and administer analgesics to control pain. Stimulation can lead to increased levels of catecholamine release and may trigger tachycardias and increased oxygen demand.

Apply oxygen with nasal prongs to supplement serum levels. Hypoxia can lead to further myocardial ischemia and dysrhythmias.

If life-threatening dysrhythmias develop, many nurses are trained to use defibrillation for the client. Other emergency interventions include CPR, various medications, and preparation of the client for a transcutaneous or permanent pacemaker.

Anxiety. The risk of death from sudden onset of life-threatening dysrhythmias weighs heavily on most clients. Express this nursing diagnosis as *Anxiety related to fear about unknown outcome.*

Outcomes. The client will experience a reduced level of anxiety, as evidenced by (1) a report of feeling less anxious and not voicing feelings of helplessness or hopelessness, (2) increased ability to sleep and rest, (3) return of heart rate to baseline level, and (4) reduction of dyspnea.

Interventions. Identify the client's anxiety and assist the client in discussing sources of fear. Clarify miscon-

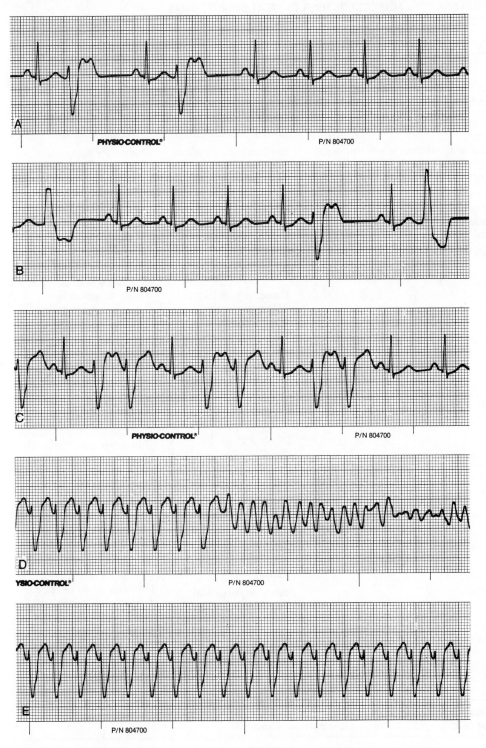

FIGURE 57–6 Ventricular dysrhythmias. *A*, Beats 2 and 4 are unifocal premature ventricular contractions (PVCs). *B*, Multifocal PVCs. *C*, Paired PVDs. *D*, R-on-T phenomenon, leading to ventricular fibrillation. *E*, Ventricular tachycardia.

ceptions. Commonly, the client or a member of the family has had a heart condition and the client's ability to cope may be directly influenced by that experience.

Explain the equipment present in the room. Most rooms are stocked with several types of equipment, and its presence does not always indicate the severity of the client's condition.

Remain with the client and tell the client and family what is happening now and what will be happening (e.g., blood will be drawn soon).

Finally, explore the usual coping methods with the cli-

ent. Positive coping methods are usually supported; discuss maladaptive coping mechanisms, and suggest substitutions. For example, smoking may be a common coping mechanism, but it is not permitted with cardiac disorders or in most hospitals. Therefore, if smoking is the client's coping mechanism when stressed, a substitute would need to be found, such as nicotine patches or chewing gum. Be aware that these patches actually can increase the levels of nicotine because they provide constant levels of the drug. Light smokers require less nicotine. Adjust the dose of the patch, beginning with the lowest levels.

Prototype	Actions	Evaluation of Therapeutic Effect	Evaluation of Adverse Effects	Nursing Considerations
		CLASS I ANTIDYSRHYTHMICS		
		Drugs with local anesthetic effects and membrane-stabilizing properties. Affect stroke velocity of phase 0. They are subdivided based on the magnitude of effects on phase 0, action potential duration, and effective refractory period		
		Type IA: Slowing of phase 0 upstroke (fast sodium channel). Prolongs action potential. Lengthens effective refractory period.		
Quinidine	Inhibits peripheral and myocardial alpha-adrenergic receptors Inhibits muscarinic receptors and causes a reflex increase in sympathetic tone Slows conduction Increases effective refractory period	Decreases reentrant activity Decreases ventricular and atrial dysrhythmias Decreases ventricular response to AFib and WPW	Evaluate patient for conduction delay and dysrhythmias Readdress therapy when: QRS widens >50%; QRS widens >20% with IVCD: QRS duration > 140 msecs and prolonged QT > 500 msecs Therapeutic blood quinidine levels 2.5 – 5.0 mg/ml	Monitor for hypotension because of alpha-adrenergic inhibition (especially with IV administration, although rarely used) Monitor for pro-dysrhythmic effects; measure Q–T interval and duration of QRS complex Monitor for sinus tachycardia (may be caused by increase in sympathetic tone) Watch for drug interactions: increased digoxin levels, increases anticoagulation for clients receiving warfarin (Coumadin) May cause GI upset; give with meals Decrease dose for decreased liver function, increased age
		Type IB: Effects similar to type IA. Slowing of phase 0 upstroke (fast sodium channel). Shortens action potential duration. Class IB agents act selectively on diseased or ischemic tissues.		
Lidocaine (Xylocaine)	Blocks fast sodium channel Shortens action potential Acts selectively on diseased or ischemic tissue	Suppression of dysrhythmia associated with cardiac surgery Suppression of VT	Half-life increases with >24 hour infusion Usually not associated with hemodynamic changes Rarely impairs nodal functions or conduction Watch for drowsiness, numbness, speech disturbances	After initial IV dose, drug is distributed rapidly and must be followed by an infusion to maintain therapeutic blood level Lidocaine levels increase when used in combination with beta-blockers and cimetidine Decreased dose for clients with liver disease Decreased dose for elderly clients
		Type IC: Powerful inhibition of the fast sodium channel, resulting in depression of the upstroke of the cardiac action potential. Inhibits His-Purkinje conduction (widens QRS). Shortens action potential duration.		
Propafenone (Rhythmol)	Blocks fast inward sodium channel Increases P–R and QRS intervals No effect on Q–T interval Mild beta-blocking properties Mild calcium channel–blocking properties	Suppression of ventricular tachyarrhythmias Suppression of SVT (including WPW) Suppression of AFib and atrial flutter	P–R/QRS prolongation Conduction block SA node inhibition Negative inotrope may exacerbate heart failure	Not used for clients with structural heart disease Drug interactions include increased serum digoxin levels and increased anticoagulation when taken with Coumadin Monitor for adverse effects when used in combination with other conduction-blocking drugs

Table continued on following page

| TABLE 57-2 | NURSING IMPLICATIONS FOR MEDICATIONS USED TO TREAT DYSRHYTHMIAS *Continued* |

Prototype	Actions	Evaluation of Therapeutic Effect	Evaluation of Adverse Effects	Nursing Considerations
CLASS II ANTIDYSRHYTHMICS				
Beta-adrenergic blocking agents. General myocardial depressants for both supraventricular and ventricular rhythm disturbances.				
Metoprolol (Lopressor)	Blocks sympathetic stimulation at the sinus node Reduced automaticity in Purkinje fibers	Suppression of inappropriate sinus tachycardia, paroxysmal atrial tachycardia, ventricular dysrhythmias and dysrhythmias of increased beta-adrenergic activity	Relatively safe Watch for bradycardia Can cause bronchospasm; contraindicated in bronchial asthma, bronchospasm, and COPD	Not recommended for clients with conduction defects Contraindicated in bronchial asthma
CLASS III ANTIDYSRHYTHMICS				
Act by lengthening action potential duration. Lengthen effective refractory period.				
Sotalol (Betapace)	Lengthens action potential duration Prolonged atrial and ventricular refractory periods Inhibits conduction along bypass tracts Mixed class II and III agent	Used for treatment of life threatening arrhythmia	May lengthen Q–T interval Q–T interval should not exceed 500 msec	Monitor vital signs and ECG closely Monitor Q–T interval Avoid inpatients with conduction defects
CLASS IV ANTIDYSRHYTHMICS				
Calcium-channel blockers				
Verapamil (Calan)	Blocks slow calcium channel; has slight nonspecific sympathetic depressant effect Increases relative refractory period through AV node Interferes with reentry of impulses at AV node	Used in controlling rapid ventricular response in AFib and atrial flutter Used for suppression of AV nodal reentry tachycardia	Hypotension, syncope, peripheral edema, constipation, bradycardia, AV blocks; may precipitate or worsen heart failure Watch P–R interval	Monitor vital signs and heart rhythm Monitor lung sounds and liver function tests Administer with food Monitor blood pressure and P–R interval
UNCLASSIFIED ANTIDYSRHYTHMICS				
Digoxin	Decreases AV node conduction to control ventricular response to AFib		Increases irritability and automaticity of ectopic sites in atria and ventricles	Given as rapid IV bolus to convert PSVT to NSR
Adenosine (Adenocard)	An endogenous nucleoside; decreases AV node conduction; interrupts AV reentry pathways			

AFib, atrial fibrillation; AV, atrioventricular; ECG, electrocardiogram; GI, gastrointestinal; IV, intravenous; IVCD, intraventricular conduction delay; NSR, normal sinus rhythm; PSVT, paroxysmal supraventricular tachycardia; PVCs, premature ventricular contractions; SA, sinoatrial; SVT, supraventricular tachycardia; VT, ventricular tachycardia; WPW, Wolff-Parkinson-White syndrome.

From Ophie, L. H., & Marcus, F. I. (1997). Antiarrhythmic drugs. In L. H. Ophie (Ed.), *Drugs for the heart* (4th ed.). Philadelphia: W. B. Saunders; and Zipes, D. P. (1997). Management of cardiac arrhythmias: Pharmacological, electrical and surgical techniques. In E. Braunwald (Ed.), *Heart disease* (5th ed.). Philadelphia: W. B. Saunders.

Data from Katzung, B. G. (1992). *Basic and clinical pharmacology* (5th ed.). Norwalk, CT: Appleton & Lange; Koda-Kimble, M. A., et al. (1992). *Handbook of applied therapeutics* (2nd ed.). Vancouver, WA: Applied Therapeutics.

EVALUATION

The degree of expected outcome attainment is assessed hourly (or more often) if the client has life-threatening dysrhythmias. Dysrhythmias are treated promptly and usually stop quickly once treatment is begun. Clients with recalcitrant dysrhythmias may require several medications. Anxiety can sometimes abate quickly but usually requires several days. Some clients remain anxious for their entire hospital stay.

VENTRICULAR FIBRILLATION

Ventricular fibrillation (VFib) is a life-threatening dysrhythmia characterized by extremely rapid, erratic impulse formation and conduction. This lethal dysrhythmia causes abrupt cessation of effective cardiac output. It usually results from severe myocardial damage, hypothermia, R-on-T phenomenon, hypoxia, contact with high-voltage electricity, electrolyte imbalance, or toxicity from quinidine, procainamide, or digitalis.

The ECG tracing displays bizarre, fibrillatory wave patterns, and it is impossible to identify P waves, QRS complexes, or T waves (Fig. 57–7A). VFib may be either coarse or fine. Untreated, the deflections become smaller and eventually all ventricular activity ceases. Death results within minutes without immediate intervention (i.e., defibrillation, CPR, and medications).

When VFib appears, the clinician must immediately initiate CPR until the defibrillator is engaged. Defibrillate up to three times if needed. Defibrillation can be performed by nurses who have advanced training (see Defib-

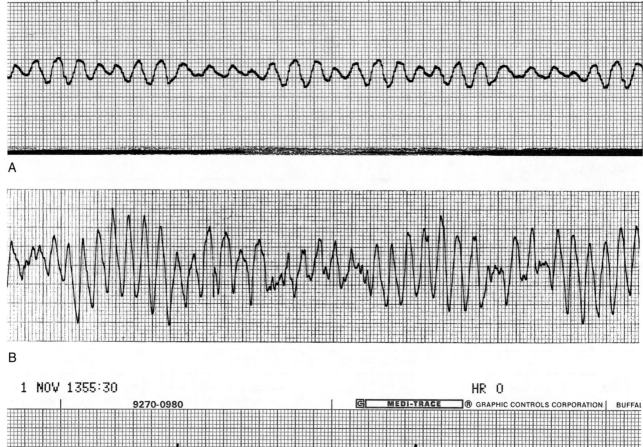

A

B

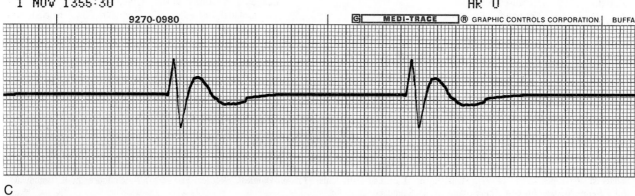

1 NOV 1355:30   HR 0

9270-0980   [G] **MEDI-TRACE** ® GRAPHIC CONTROLS CORPORATION | BUFFAL

C

FIGURE 57–7 *A,* Coarse ventricular fibrillation. *B,* Torsades de pointes. *C,* Ventricular asystole in a dying heart. (*B,* From Phillips, R. E., & Feeney, M. K. [1990]. *The cardiac rhythms: A systematic approach to interpretation.* [3rd ed., p. 393]. Philadelphia: W. B. Saunders.)

rillation later). A standard pattern of energy and current is used. Defibrillation begins with 200 joules (J); if not successful, it is advanced to 300 J, then to 360 J. With persistent VFib, epinephrine is given and the clinician defibrillates at 360 J. Other medications are alternated with defibrillation (lidocaine, bretylium, magnesium sulfate, sodium bicarbonate), depending on the client's cardiac rhythm and electrolyte and acid-base balance.[1, 23, 32]

VENTRICULAR ASYSTOLE

Ventricular asystole (cardiac standstill) represents the total absence of ventricular electrical activity (Fig. 57–7C). The client has no palpable pulse (no cardiac output), and a rhythm is absent if the client is monitored. The occurrence of sudden ventricular asystole in a conscious person results in faintness, followed within seconds by loss of consciousness, seizures, and apnea. If the dysrhythmia remains untreated, death ensues. Ventricular asystole must be treated immediately.

Cardiac standstill can occur as a primary event, or it may follow VFib or pulseless electrical activity. Asystole can occur also in clients with complete heart block (CHB) in whom there is no escape pacemaker. Possible causes include:

- Hypoxia
- Hyperkalemia and hypokalemia
- Pre-existing acidosis
- Drug overdose
- Hypothermia

The treatment of choice consists of CPR, epinephrine, atropine, transcutaneous pacing, and correction of the cause.[1, 23, 32]

PULSELESS ELECTRICAL ACTIVITY

Pulseless electrical activity represents the presence of some electrical activity in the heart, as seen on the monitor, other than VFib or VT; however, a pulse cannot be detected by palpation of any artery. Common causes include cardiac tamponade, massive pulmonary embolus, tension pneumothorax, and severe hypovolemia.

Rapid searching for the cause is imperative. Until the cause is located, CPR is initiated and fluid volume is restored.

REENTRY OF IMPULSES

VENTRICULAR TACHYCARDIA

Ventricular tachycardia (VTach or VT) is a life-threatening dysrhythmia that occurs when an irritable ectopic focus in the ventricles takes over as the pacemaker. It occurs in the presence of significant cardiac disease, such as in clients with CAD, cardiomyopathy, mitral valve prolapse, heart failure, acute MI with hypoxia and acidosis, and digitalis toxicity.

VT is characterized by rapidly occurring series of PVCs (three or more) with no normal beats in between (Fig. 57–12E). P waves are absent, and the P-R interval is absent. The QRS complex is wide (>0.12 second) and

bizarre. The ventricular rate ranges between 100 and 220 BPM, usually 130 to 170 BPM. The ventricular rhythm is slightly irregular. VT produces a very low cardiac output that can quickly lead to cerebral and myocardial ischemia. At any time, VT can develop into VFib. Clients with VT commonly express that they are experiencing feelings of impending death.

Sustained but hemodynamically stable VT is initially treated with antidysrhythmics (i.e., lidocaine, procainamide, or bretylium). Cardioversion may be required for conversion to sinus rhythm. VT that causes loss of consciousness must be terminated immediately with defibrillation. The physician may also order IV antidysrhythmic agents, usually lidocaine. Another drug gaining favor is magnesium sulfate, particularly if the client has low magnesium levels.[1, 19, 23, 32]

TORSADES DE POINTES

Torsades de pointes is a form of VT in which the QRS complexes appear to be constantly changing. Delayed repolarization of the ventricle is revealed as a prolonged Q-T interval and a broad flat T wave in the preceding sinus rhythm. The rhythm is regular or irregular with a ventricular rate of 150 to 300 BPM (Fig. 57–7B). The QRS complex is wide and bizarre.

Torsades de pointes is usually a result of drug toxicity (procainamide, quinidine, disopyramide) or electrolyte imbalances (hypokalemia or hypomagnesemia). Clinical manifestations begin with palpitations and syncope. This rhythm often precedes VFib and sudden death.

Torsades de pointes is treated only if the Q-T interval is prolonged with temporary overdrive ventricular or atrial pacing. Discontinuation of offending agents is also crucial. IV magnesium sulfate is considered the treatment of choice.[1, 19, 32]

PRE-EXCITATION SYNDROMES

Pre-excitation syndromes occur when part or all of the ventricle is reentered by a depolarization wave traveling down a congenital or acquired accessory conducting pathway between the atrium and ventricle.

An accessory pathway is abnormal conductile tissue connecting the atria and ventricle. Normally, the AV node is the only connection between the atria and ventricles and controls (blocks) rapid atrial rates that prevent rapid ventricular rates (e.g., AFib). When accessory pathways are present, there is nothing to block rapid atrial rates, and ventricular rates soar.

There are several types of disorders in this category, of which *Wolff-Parkinson-White syndrome* (WPW) appears most frequently. In clients with WPW, sudden attacks of very rapid supraventricular dysrhythmias suddenly develop. Most adults with WPW have normal hearts, but if the tachydysrhythmias occur persistently, myocardial fatigue and ventricular failure may result.

Clients with WPW do not require intervention unless they experience recurring tachydysrhythmias. In this instance, the physician may elect to use vagotonic maneuvers, cardioversion, adenosine, amiodarone (Cordarone), esmolol administration, or chemical, mechanical, or radiofrequency ablation. Ablation is an interventional procedure that destroys the accessory pathway.

Outcome Management

■ Medical Management of Life-Threatening Dysrhythmias

The goal of management is to immediately stop the dysrhythmia and restore normal sinus rhythm. Remember, because there is inadequate or no perfusion of blood during these dysrhythmias, CPR is performed. Finally, the cause of the dysrhythmia is identified and treated.

Life-threatening dysrhythmias can often be effectively managed with exogenously delivered currents of electricity. The most crucial element for survival after cardiac arrest is the time interval from collapse to care, especially defibrillation. With each passing minute, the chances of survival decline as much as 10%. Electrical intervention can (1) abruptly stop the heart's erratic electrical discharge or (2) resume the flow of electrical current where there is none. Methods of electrical therapy include defibrillation and cardioversion.

DEFIBRILLATION

The use of defibrillation delivers an electrical current (shock) of preset voltage to the heart through paddles placed on the chest wall (closed chest procedure). This current causes the entire myocardium to depolarize completely at the moment of shock, thus producing transient asystole and allowing the heart's intrinsic pacemakers to regain control. The amount of energy required to produce this effect is largely determined by the client's transthoracic impedance, or resistance to current flow. Because of this factor, the amount of energy that reaches the heart is less than the amount that the defibrillator is charged to deliver.[1, 15, 18]

The procedure is associated with potential hazards, particularly myocardial damage. The higher the amount of energy or frequency of the shocks, the greater the risk of injury. Advances in the equipment now allow measurement of transthoracic impedance. Once impedance is determined, the defibrillator automatically selects the amount of current needed that can restore rhythm and cardiac output. It is expected this mode of defibrillation will reduce the risk of complications.[1, 32]

The degree of transthoracic resistance depends on several variables:

1. *Energy level.* The higher the energy level selected, the more current follows.
2. *Number and frequency of shocks.* The more shocks administered and the shorter the time interval between them, the lower the transthoracic resistance.
3. *Ventilation phase.* Resistance is lower when shocks are delivered during exhalation, when there is less air (and therefore less diameter) in the lungs.
4. *Paddle size.* The larger the paddle, the lower the resistance.
5. *Chest size.* The smaller the distance between the defibrillator electrodes once they are in place, the lower the resistance.

6. *Paddle-skin interface material.* Conductive material between the skin and paddles reduces transthoracic impedance.
7. *Paddle pressure.* Applying firm pressure increases contact between the skin and the paddles, helping to overcome transthoracic resistance. Exert about 25 pounds of pressure on each paddle.
8. *Paddle placement.* Place one paddle on the upper chest, to the right of the sternum; place the other on the lower left chest, to the left of the nipple, with the center of the paddle in the midaxillary line.

If the client has a permanent pacemaker or an internal cardiac defibrillator, place the paddles at least 5 inches away from the generator to avoid damaging it. If a temporary pacing system is in use, disconnect the pacing lead from the pulse generator immediately before defibrillation and reconnect it after the shock.[1, 5, 7, 10, 11, 18]

Most defibrillators can be used to perform either *synchronized* cardioversion or *unsynchronized* cardioversion (commonly called defibrillation). Defibrillation is always indicated in VFib and is also used in VT when the client is unconscious and pulseless. Specially trained nurses, emergency medical technicians, and physicians perform this procedure in acute settings.

CARE BEFORE DEFIBRILLATION. Immediately before defibrillation, assess the client's responsiveness and do the following:

1. If the client is not responsive, activate the EMS system.
2. Call for the defibrillator.
3. Assess the client's airway, breathing, and circulation (ABCs). Open the airway. Look, listen, and feel.
4. If the client is not breathing, give two slow breaths.
5. Assess the client's circulation; if there is no pulse, start CPR.
6. Perform CPR until the defibrillator is in place.
7. Check the ECG to verify the presence of VFib or pulseless VT.
8. Check leads for any loose connections.
9. Remove any nitroglycerin patch.

On confirmation of the emergency, the code alarm is given over the health care facility intercom system or to their pagers to summon the emergency team (e.g., "Code 99, Dr. Blue"). In the meantime, CPR measures are started by the first person on the scene. The clinician turns on the defibrillator and sets it at 200 J. In the presence of VFib, the synchronous mode must not be used. Start an IV line, as needed, for administration of resuscitation medications. Intubation is completed with oxygen supplementation.

CARE DURING DEFIBRILLATION. When VFib develops, clinicians must attempt defibrillation at the earliest opportunity. The paddles are lubricated with electrode paste or conducting pads to enhance conduction and prevent burning of the skin. The paste should not extend beyond the paddles, and the paddles must lie flat against the body in order to avoid burns. The clinician places the paddles firmly against the chest. A transverse (anterolateral) position for paddle placement is used. One paddle is placed at the second intercostal space, at the right of the sternum, and the other paddle is positioned at the fifth intercostal space on the anterior axillary line (Fig. 57–8).

To ensure safe defibrillation, people who perform defibrillation must always announce when they are about to shock. The phrase "One. I'm clear. Two. You're clear. Three. All clear." is recommended. Because electricity is carried along metal devices and the client, all personnel, including the clinician administering the shock, must stand back from the bed. Open chest defibrillation occurs when electrical current is applied directly to the heart.

CARE AFTER DEFIBRILLATION. The clinician immediately assesses the ECG and pulse after defibrillation. If the first countershock is unsuccessful, immediate debrillation must be performed again at a higher energy level (300 and 360 J). Defibrillation may be applied up to three times (200, 300, 360 J), if needed, for persistent VFib or pulseless VT. Defibrillators are frequently equipped with paddles that can monitor the ECG, even immediately after defibrillation. Therefore, if the paddles are left in place after the shock has been delivered, the cardiac response can be quickly evaluated.

CPR should be continued if the three defibrillations have not been successful. A member of the health care team administers appropriate medications again before the next defibrillation attempt. A successful response is indicated by cessation of fibrillation, restoration of sinus rhythm, and palpation of a regular pulse. After successful defibrillation, continuous ECG monitoring is required. The client's vital signs and neurologic status must also be continuously assessed.

For clients with a pacemaker or an automatic implantable cardioverter-defibrillator (AICD), a programmer-ana-lyzer should be available to examine the system for damage and erroneous reprogramming after defibrillation. Continue to monitor for pacemaker malfunction for at least the next 24 hours.

In documenting the outcome of defibrillation, record the following points:

- Preprocedure rhythm
- Times and voltage of shocks delivered
- Postdefibrillation rhythm pattern
- Names, times of administration, and doses of administered medications
- Other hemodynamic data available before, during, and after defibrillation

TERMINATION OF RESUSCITATION. Generally, if an organized rhythm and pulse have not returned, the Advanced Cardiac Life Support team leader can cease efforts to resuscitate clients from confirmed and persistent asystole when the client has received successful endotracheal intubation, successful IV access, suitable basic CPR, and all rhythm-appropriate medications. Always consider any pre-existing problems that may make the client less responsive to defibrillation (acidosis, hypokalemia, hyperkalemia, hypoxia, hypovolemia), and treat them appropriately. In many cases, clients may have other, noncardiac, disorders that make resuscitation attempts futile.

The 1996 American Heart Association guidelines for emergency cardiac care do not state a specific time limit beyond which rescuers can never have a successful resuscitation. Cardiac arrests in special situations such as hypothermia, electrocution, and drug overdose present ex-

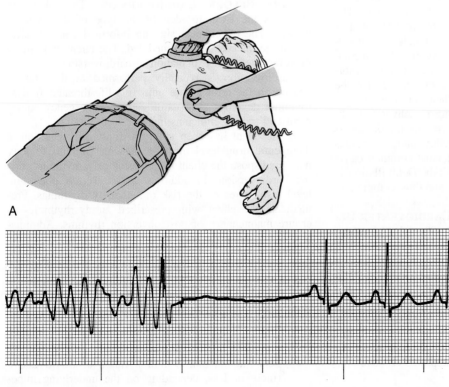

A

B

FIGURE 57–8 *A*, Anterolateral paddle placement for external countershock. External paddles are placed at the second right intercostal space and at the anterior axillary line in the fifth left intercostal space. *B*, Ventricular fibrillation converted to normal sinus rhythm.

ceptions to any rules. Special situations call for common sense and clinical judgment.[1, 23, 32]

Television portrayal of defibrillation and CPR contributes to many misconceptions about these treatments. One article discusses whether the information on television provides accurate information.[9] Three television shows were viewed (*ER, Chicago Hope,* and *Rescue 911).* The cause of the cardiac arrest, the demographics of the client, the underlying illness, and the outcomes were recorded. A total of 97 episodes of the three shows were reviewed. Of the 60 clients who received CPR, 46 (77%) survived the immediate cardiac arrest. Survival rates for CPR on these television programs are much higher than the highest rates reported in the literature. Most people resuscitated were children, teenagers, and young adults. In the hospital, cardiac arrest is most common in older adults. On television, most cardiac arrests have been caused by trauma; in reality, most cardiac arrests are due to heart disease. During the same episodes, 37 people died. In only eight of the situations in which people died was there any discussion about the use of CPR or reference to do-not-resuscitate orders.

Clients participate in discussions about their health care today more than ever before. Many people have few resources from which to hear about acute care. Consequently, images in the media strongly shape the public's belief about medical care, illness, and death. The portrayal of CPR and death on three popular programs has been misleading. Misrepresentation of CPR on television may lead people to misinterpret the outcomes seen there as real life. Nurses need to be able to clarify misconceptions.

OTHER FORMS OF DEFIBRILLATION

AUTOMATED EXTERNAL DEFIBRILLATOR. An automated external defibrillator (AED) delivers electrical shocks to a client after it identifies VT or VFib. The device is attached to the client with adhesive sternal-apex pads on flexible cables, which allows "hands-free" defibrillation, a feature available with conventional defibrillation as well. AEDs also have an internal microprocessor-based detection system that analyzes the rhythm for the characteristics of VFib or VT. When VFib or VT is present, the AED "advises" the operator to deliver a shock.

AEDs are "automated," in the sense that the device—not the operator—analyzes the rhythm and determines the presence of VFib or VT.[1, 5] The most common cause of unconsciousness in an adult is VFib. Defibrillation is the only effective treatment. AEDs are thus common in emergency response units.

AUTOMATIC IMPLANTABLE CARDIOVERTER-DEFIBRILLATOR. The AICD consists of a pulse generator and a sensor that continuously monitors heart rhythm. When the device detects a dysrhythmia, it automatically delivers a countershock. For VFib, the AICD gives an electrical countershock within 15 to 20 seconds. It can also detect and treat VT with cardioversion. Compared with external defibrillation, this implanted system does not require as much energy because less energy is lost when the impulse is applied directly to the heart. In addition, a back-up pacemaker helps to control the rhythm.

The AICD is implanted surgically into a pouch into the abdominal wall through a thoracotomy incision or transvenously for two types of conditions[1, 5, 32]:

- Survival of one or more episodes of sudden cardiac death resulting from VT or VFib
- Recurrent, refractory, life-threatening ventricular dysrhythmias that can develop into VT or VFib, or both, despite antidysrhythmic therapy

Clients who require AICDs have a great deal of anxiety. Anxiety can develop from past episodes of near death as well as from feelings of not ever being able to die. Other clients may fear that the AICD will not be able to reverse the dysrhythmia. Be sensitive to these thoughts, and facilitate their discussion.[1, 5, 7, 10, 13, 18]

CARDIOVERSION
Cardioversion, most often an elective procedure, involves the use of a synchronized direct current (DC) electrical countershock that depolarizes all the cells simultaneously, allowing the SA node to resume the pacemaker role. The electrical discharge is synchronized with or triggered by the client's QRS complex for avoidance of accidental discharge during the repolarization phase when the ventricle is vulnerable to the development of VFib. A QRS complex must be present for successful conversion of the dysrhythmia.

Low voltages (50 to 100 J) are tried initially. If the attempt is unsuccessful, cardioversion using larger voltages can be repeated. Only specially trained physicians can perform this procedure.[1, 23, 32]

Cardioversion is used to treat SVT, AFib, and atrial flutter that is resistant to medication, and VT in an unstable patient. The unstable client may be hypotensive or dyspneic, may be experiencing chest pain, or may have evidence of heart failure, MI, or ischemia. Analgesia or sedation may be provided before the electrical shock.

CARE BEFORE CARDIOVERSION. The physician evaluates the ECG to identify the type of dysrhythmia present. The client must sign an informed consent, after which the intervention is scheduled. The client and family must receive a full explanation of cardioversion.

Cardioversion is typically performed at the client's bedside in the critical care unit. If a life-threatening dysrhythmia develops after cardioversion, emergency equipment and trained clinicians must be in the room.

If the client has been taking a digitalis preparation, a therapeutic drug level must be present. Digitalis toxicity may predispose the client to ventricular dysrhythmias during cardioversion. In addition, a low serum potassium level also increases the risk of lethal dysrhythmias. Premedicate the client with prescribed antidysrhythmics to ensure maintenance of postconversion rhythms. Administer oxygen before cardioversion, and discontinue if oxygenation saturation is within normal limits. Keep the client on NPO (fasting) status for several hours before cardioversion. Start an IV line for medication delivery. To reduce fear and to promote amnesia, administer an antianxiety medication IV as prescribed.

CARE DURING CARDIOVERSION. The physician performs the following steps:

1. Sets the machine within a range of 50 to 200 J (more or less, depending on the underlying impedances).

2. Turns the synchronizer switch to "on" to deliver the shock during the QRS complex, not on the downslope of the T wave.

3. Lubricates the paddles and places them exactly as described for defibrillation.

4. Calls for all health care personnel to stand back from the bed.

5. While standing back from the bed, depresses and holds the buttons on the paddles until the shock is delivered.

Newer equipment for cardioversion includes adhesive skin paddles attached to the client's chest and back.

CARE AFTER CARDIOVERSION. Clinicians immediately assess the ECG and pulse after the procedure. In some cases, VFib or VT occurs, an event demanding emergency action. Monitor the client's ECG rhythm and vital signs continuously for at least 2 hours, and carefully assess for rhythm changes and complications. A successful response to cardioversion resolves the dysrhythmia and restores normal sinus rhythm. With a good response and no complications, the client may be discharged later that day when fully awake and able to eat.

SUPPRESSING IRRITABLE FOCI
Improving Myocardial Oxygen

Oxygen is an essential component of dysrhythmia management, especially for dysrhythmias that result from irritable foci in an ischemic myocardium. These include PVCs and other ventricular dysrhythmias. Oxygen should be given to all clients at risk of ventricular dysrhythmias, such as those with chest pain or hypoxemia or during cardiac arrest.

Antidysrhythmic Therapy

Do not attempt to memorize Table 57–2; rather, commit a few drugs to memory (atropine, lidocaine, epinephrine, verapamil, and procainamide). These medications may be administered orally or by continuous IV infusion. You must be diligent in monitoring for the intended effect and side effects of the medication.

ABLATING CONDUCTION PATHWAYS

A variety of procedures can be used to treat dysrhythmias when use of medications are unsuccessful in bringing about conversion of the abnormal rhythm to a normal rhythm. Interventions include (1) chemical and mechanical ablation and (2) radiofrequency of the abnormal pathway. These procedures involve risk to normal conduction tissue, and a pacemaker may be needed either temporarily or permanently.[5, 21, 32]

CHEMICAL ABLATION. Alcohol or phenol is inserted into involved areas of the myocardium through an angioplasty catheter. Test injections with saline or lidocaine are given to determine whether the dysrhythmia ceases before the final injection. Postprocedural care is the same as that for angioplasty.

MECHANICAL ABLATION. The abnormal pathway is surgically removed or treated with a cryoprobe to interrupt its effect on heart rhythms. SVT, AFib, atrial flutter, and WPW syndrome may be treated with this method when the client does not respond to medication. Before the procedure, the myocardium is mapped to determine whether other forms of surgery (e.g., coronary bypass

grafting, valve replacement) may correct the dysrhythmia. Mapping also isolates the area to be treated. The procedure may be performed through open-heart or closed-heart methods.

Postprocedure care and recovery are similar to those following cardiac catheterization.

RADIOFREQUENCY ABLATION. Radiofrequency catheter ablation (RFA) is used primarily for SVT associated with WPW or AV nodal reentry, although it has also been used successfully to treat refractory VT. A steerable pacing catheter directs low-power, high-frequency current to a localized accessory pathway and necroses a small portion of the heart. When this current is applied, the temperature of the contact tissue rises, water is driven out, and coagulation necrosis results. The amount of tissue injury depends on the amount of energy delivered (5 to 50 watts), the length of time it is delivered (10 to 90 seconds), and the resistance at the end of the catheter. RFA produces lesions that are smaller and more controllable than DC catheter ablation lesions.

The major advantage of RFA is the high rate of success (99% at some centers) and low morbidity. RFA is more successful than conventional medical therapies or DC ablation but equal in success to surgical treatment.

Although RFA is a relatively safe procedure, some complications can occur:

- Cardiac tamponade (1%)
- Deep vein thrombosis (1%)
- Trauma to vessel (1%)
- Transient ischemic attack or stroke (0.5%)
- Perforation of AV leaflet (extremely rare)
- Hematoma at introducer site (common)
- Unintentional AV block requiring pacemaker implantation (up to 10%)

Postprocedure nursing care and recovery are similar to those following cardiac catheterization. Specific nursing responsibilities include (1) preprocedure education of client and family, (2) interventions to reduce anxiety before and during the RFA procedure, (3) monitoring of vital signs and lower extremity perfusion during and after the procedure, and (4) discharge instructions. Clients are usually discharged within 24 hours after RFA and are instructed to gradually resume normal activities but to avoid strenuous activities for 7 to 10 days. ECGs are obtained routinely at 1, 3, 6, and 9 months after RFA. Aspirin, 325 mg, is prescribed for 14 days after RFA to prevent clot formation and platelet aggregation at the ablation site.[5, 32]

▉ Surgical Management

RESTORING IMPULSE GENERATION

Pacemakers

Pacemakers provide an artificial SA node or Purkinje system. Pacemakers can be *permanent* or *temporary*.

An artificial pacemaker is indicated if the conduction system fails to transmit impulses from the sinus node to the ventricles, to generate an impulse spontaneously, or to maintain primary control of the pacing function of the heart. Many conditions may affect the ability of the heart's conduction system to function normally, creating

BOX 57–2	Conditions That May Necessitate a Pacemaker

- Ablation
- Acute myocardial infarction
- Autonomic nervous system failure
- Cardiac surgery
- Drug toxicity (antidysrhythmics)
- Electrolyte imbalance
- Myocardial ischemia

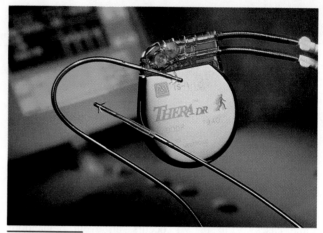

FIGURE 57–9 A permanent pacemaker (pulse generator). (Courtesy of Medtronic, Inc., Minneapolis, MN.)

circumstances that warrant pacing (Box 57–2). Pacemakers can be used temporarily or prophylactically until the condition underlying the disturbance resolves. Pacemakers also can be used on a permanent basis if the client's condition persists despite adequate therapy.

An artificial pacemaker is intended to provide a physiologic back-up for the heart during failure of the conduction system to depolarize the myocardium and maintain adequate cardiac output. When cardiac output is diminished because of lack of depolarization of the ventricles, artificial pacing can provide the necessary stimulus directly to the atria or ventricles, or both, to bring about contraction. If cardiac output is compromised because an ectopic pacemaker is causing the ventricles to depolarize and contract at a rate that does not promote adequate ventricular filling, artificial pacing competes with the ectopic pacemaker to assume the primary pacing function of the heart.

Pacemaker Design

An artificial pacemaker provides an external source of energy for impulse formation and delivery, and stimulation of myocardial tissue. Whereas numerous pacemaker models are available, each with unique capabilities, every pacemaker consists of a pulse generator with circuitry, the lead, and the electrode system.

The pulse generator is essentially the pacemaker's power source. It houses the electronic circuitry responsible for sending out appropriately timed signals and for sensing cardiac activity. The output circuit controls the current pulse delivery rate, pulse duration, and refractory period. The sensing circuit is responsible for identifying and analyzing any spontaneous intrinsic electrical activity and responding appropriately.

The pulse generator can be external or internal. The external unit is designed for temporary pacing, primarily for support of transient dysrhythmias that impair cardiac output.

The unit is the size of a small transistor radio and operates by dry-cell batteries (Fig. 57–9). There are dials for adjustment of power, rate of discharge, and mode. The pulse generator can also be permanently implanted. The surgeon places the permanent pulse generator into a small tunnel burrowed within the subcutaneous tissue below the right (Fig. 57–10) or left clavicle or in the abdominal cavity. The pulse generator is a small—about the size of a stethoscope head—hermetically sealed (to prevent exposure to body fluids) lithium battery. Most of the new generators can be reprogrammed after insertion, as needed.

The lead delivers the electrical impulse from the pulse generator to the myocardium. The leads consist of flexible conductive wires enclosed by insulating material. The electrode is the end of the lead that delivers the impulse directly to the myocardial wall. It is usually made of platinum-iridium, a highly conductive material that also deters the adherence of platelets. This system not only delivers electrical impulses but also relays information about spontaneous intracardiac signals back to the sensing circuit within the pulse generator.

Electrodes can be *unipolar* or *bipolar*. Unipolar designs incorporate the cardiac electrode as the negative

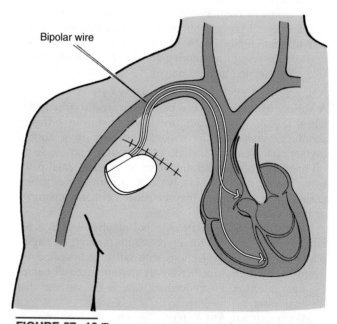

FIGURE 57–10 Transvenous temporary endocardial pacing is routine for most cardiac surgical procedures. This can be established by insertion of electrode wires through a vein (subclavian or internal jugular) and into the right atrium or right ventricle. Temporary pacing wires can also be advanced through pulmonary artery catheters. (From Thelan, L. A., et al. [1998]. *Critical care nursing* [3rd ed.]. St. Louis: Mosby–Year Book.)

terminal of the electrical circuit with the metallic shell or second wire of the impulse generator as the positive electrode. Bipolar systems use two wires, each ending in an electrode a short distance apart.

Single-chamber pacemakers pace either the ventricles or atria; *dual-chamber* pacemakers pace both the ventricles and atria.

Pacemaker Methods

Impulses can be delivered to myocardial tissue by three major modes of artificial pacing: external, epicardial, and endocardial.

EXTERNAL (TRANSCUTANEOUS) PACING. The heart is stimulated through large gelled electrode pads placed anteriorly and posteriorly and connected to an external transcutaneous pacemaker. Transcutaneous pacing is the treatment of choice in emergency cardiac care because it can be started quickly while a temporary transvenous pacemaker is being inserted or as prophylaxis against dysrhythmias. It is also the least invasive pacing technique. Because no vascular puncture is needed for electrode placement, transcutaneous pacing is preferred in clients who are receiving anticoagulation therapy or who may require thrombolytic therapy.

Because the anterior electrode is placed to the left of the sternum and centered close to the point of maximal impulse (PMI), excessive chest hair must be clipped or

TABLE 57-3	PACEMAKER MALFUNCTIONS AND NURSING INTERVENTIONS	
Problem	**Possible Cause**	**Nursing Interventions***
FAILURE TO PACE PROPERLY		
Intermittent or complete absence of pacing artifact Rapid, inappropriate firing of pacemaker (pacemaker-mediated tachycardia)	Battery failure A break or loose connection anywhere along the system Pulse generator failure Circuitry failure "Oversensing" or "undersensing" by the pacemaker	Replace pulse generator Replace battery unit Check and tighten all connections between pulse generator and leads Reduce or increase sensitivity threshold of pacemaker unit Assess client's tolerance of pacemaker failure; have emergency drugs on hand; perform CPR as indicated
FAILURE TO CAPTURE		
Pacing artifact present but is not followed by a QRS complex or P wave	Increased pacing threshold. Can be related to electrolyte imbalance, ischemia, drug toxicity, perforation, or excessive fibrosis of tissue at electrode site Lead displacement due to migration, or idle manipulation of pulse generator ("twiddler's syndrome")	Increase voltage by 1–2 mA (temporary pacemaker) Increase amplitude of pacemaker output/pulse width Reposition client to either side in attempt to improve contact of electrode with endocardium; in temporary pacemaker, try moving arm if lead wire is inserted in antecubital area Obtain chest film to determine pacemaker position Have emergency drugs on hand; initiate CPR if necessary
FAILURE TO SENSE		
Pacing artifact present despite the presence of QRS complexes and P waves A competitive rhythm may develop	Sensitivity threshold set too low Intrinsic beats are of too-low voltage and go undetected by pacemaker's sensing mechanism Dislodged or fractured lead Circuitry failure Electromagnetic interference	Increase sensitivity threshold on pulse generator Reposition client If client's intrinsic rhythm or rate is adequate, turn off pacemaker Increase pacing rate to overdrive client's intrinsic heart rate Give antidysrhythmics to decrease ectopy Notify physician Obtain chest x-ray to determine electrode placement
OVERSENSING		
Results from the inappropriate sensing of extraneous electrical signals or myopotentials (which should be ignored)	Sensitivity threshold set too high T wave sensing myopotentials Electromagnetic interference Two leads touching	Decrease sensitivity threshold Correct conditions that produce large T waves

*For all problems, document malfunction by an electrocardiogram. If pacemaker is programmable, have reprogramming machine available. Monitor client's tolerance to pacemaker malfunction (vital signs, chest pain).

CPR, cardiopulmonary resuscitation.

Modified from Huang, S. H., et al. (1989). *Coronary care nursing* (2nd ed.). Philadelphia: W. B. Saunders; and Thelan, L. A. et al. *Critical care nursing* (3rd ed.). St. Louis: Mosby–Year Book.

shaved to ensure good contact, or alternative pacing electrode positions must be used. The pacing device is usually activated at a rate of 80 BPM. Electrical capture is characterized by widening of the QRS complex and broadening of the T wave. Many clients feel extreme discomfort with each paced beat; this is a significant limitation to transcutaneous pacing.

Narcotic analgesia and sedation may be given to clients who are conscious or who regain consciousness to reduce discomfort and anxiety. Additional complications of external transcutaneous pacing can include skin burns, muscle twitching, psychological reactions, failure to "capture" (inability of the impulse to initiate a contraction), and failure to "sense" (inability of the pacemaker to sense intrinsic electrical activity) (Table 57–3).

EPICARDIAL (TRANSTHORACIC) PACING. With this method of artificial pacing, the electrical energy travels from an external pulse generator through the thoracic musculature directly to the epicardial surface of the heart via lead wires. Epicardial pacing is most commonly used during and immediately after open-heart surgery because there is direct access to the epicardium at this time. Some occasional complications may include lead dislodgment, microshock, cardiac tamponade, infection, psychological reactions, failure to capture, and failure to sense.

ENDOCARDIAL (TRANSVENOUS) PACING. Endocardial pacing is the most common mode of pacing the heart in emergency situations. The surgeon inserts the pacing electrode via the transvenous route (via the antecubital, femoral, jugular, or subclavian vein) and then threads the electrode into the right atrium or right ventricle so that it comes into direct contact with the endocardium. This procedure can be done at the bedside under fluoroscopic control or in a cardiovascular laboratory.

Major drawbacks include thrombophlebitis, infection at the insertion site, sepsis from unsterile technique, increased chance of lead displacement as the client changes position, and the discomfort of having the extremity nearest the insertion site immobilized (Fig. 57–11). Other additional complications occasionally seen are pacer-induced dysrhythmias, hiccups, abdominal twitching, myocardial irritability, perforation of chamber or septum, failure to capture, and failure to sense.

Temporary Pacing

Temporary pacing may be used in emergent or elective situations that require limited, short-term pacing (<2 weeks). The pulse generator is external. Temporary pacemakers can be applied transcutaneously and can be inserted transthoracically or, more commonly, transvenously.

Although the principles of cardiac pacing are the same for temporary and permanent pacemakers, each type presents distinct issues for nurses to assess and to teach to the client and family. Clients with a temporary pacemaker need the following:

- An explanation about the pacemaker
- Monitoring for response to the pacemaker
- Maintenance of electrical safety
- Monitoring for pacing parameters (sensing, capturing, threshold)
- Protection against injury and infection

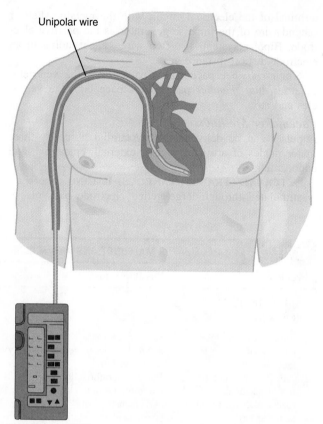

FIGURE 57–11 A temporary endocardial pacemaker.

Before the procedure, explain the purpose of the temporary pacemaker to the client and family. Ensure that a permit for the procedure has been signed and that all questions have been answered. Necessary equipment is gathered, and the external generator is checked (battery and sense and pace modes). Assess the client's vital signs, and obtain a rhythm strip.

During the procedure, monitor the client's ECG and vital signs continuously. Large P waves are seen as the catheter passes through the atrium, and larger QRS complexes are seen in the ventricles. Set and maintain the stimulus and sensitivity settings according to the physician's orders. Tape or suture the electrode at the insertion site.

After the procedure, assess vital signs routinely along with heart rhythm and emotional reactions to the procedure and pacing. Secure and check all connections. Monitor battery and control settings. Clean and dress the incision site according to protocols. Keep the generator dry and protect the controls from mishandling. The client must be protected from electrical microshocks and electromagnetic interference. Wear rubber gloves when exposed wires are handled. Check electrical equipment for adequate grounding. Limit motion of the extremity at the insertion site. Stabilize arm, catheter, and pacemaker to an arm board and avoid movement of the arm above shoulder level. Do not lift the client from under the arm. If the leg is the insertion site, limit its motion, especially hip flexion and outward rotation.

In addition to protecting the client from injury, monitor pacemaker function. Document the location and

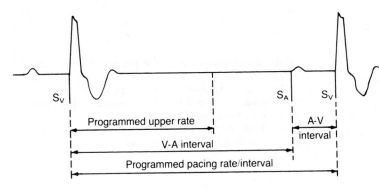

FIGURE 57–12 Pacing intervals. The atrioventricular (A-V, delay) interval can be thought of as an artificial P-R interval. The programmed pacing rate, or interval, is also called the ventriculoventricular (V-V) interval. Ventricular pacing occurs if intrinsic ventricular activity does not occur within the V-V interval. (From *Symbiotics series: Selecting the DDD patient* [1984]. Minneapolis: Medtronic.)

type of pacing lead. Note the pacing mode, stimulus threshold, sensitivity setting, pacing rate and intervals, and intrinsic rhythm. Pacing intervals are shown in Figure 57–12.

Permanent Pacing

Permanent pacing is indicated for chronic or recurrent dysrhythmias that are severe, unresponsive to antiarrhythmic medication, and caused by AV block or sinus node malfunction. The need for permanent pacemakers is confirmed through ECGs, electrophysiology studies, and Holter monitoring. Indications for permanent pacemakers have been grouped into three classes. Class I criteria are identified in Box 57–3.[31, 32]

Clinical manifestations that are directly attributable to the slow heart rate include transient dizziness, lightheadedness, near syncope or frank syncope as manifestations of transient cerebral ischemia, and more generalized manifestations such as marked exercise intolerance or frank heart failure.[12, 31, 32]

BOX 57–3   Clinical Conditions That Warrant Permanent Pacemakers (Class I Criteria)

A. Complete heart block (permanent or intermittent), associated with the following complications:
  1. Symptomatic bradycardia
  2. Left ventricular heart failure
  3. Ectopic rhythms that suppress the automaticity of escape pacemakers and result in symptomatic bradycardia
  4. Documented periods of asystole greater than 3 seconds or any escape rate less than 40 beats per minute in a symptom-free client
  5. Confusional states that clear with temporary pacing
  6. Post-AV (atrioventricular) junctional ablation
B. Second-degree AV block, permanent or intermittent, with symptomatic bradycardia
C. Atrial fibrillation, atrial flutter, supraventricular tachycardia with complete heart block or advanced AV block, bradycardia (the bradycardia must be unrelated to digitalis or drugs known to impair AV conduction)

From Zaim, B, Zaim, S., & Kutalek, S. (1994). Indications for use of permanent cardiac pacemakers. *Heart Disease and Stroke, 3,* 71–76.

Pacemaker Modes

There are two basic kinds of pacemakers:

1. *Fixed-rate* (non-demand or asynchronous). Fixed-rate pacemakers are designed to fire constantly as a preset rate without regard to the electrical activity of the client's heart. This mode of pacing is appropriate in the absence of any electrical activity (asystole) but is dangerous in the presence of an intrinsic rhythm because of the potential of the pacemaker to fire during the vulnerable period of repolarization and initiate lethal ventricular dysrhythmias.

2. *Demand* pacemakers contain a device that senses the heart's electrical activity and fires at a present rate only when the heart's electrical activity drops below a predetermined rate level (Fig. 57–13).

In addition to a variety of capabilities, permanent pacemakers now have special programmable and antitachyarrhythmic functions that are quite complex. In order to communicate all the functions of the individual pacemakers, international codes were developed. Pacemakers are identified with a five-digit letter code. Although the last two letters contain pertinent information, commonly a pacemaker is referred to only by its first three letters (Box 57–4).

Pacemaker Function

Because there are many types of pacemakers with more than 250 programs, the general functions are discussed first. A simple demand pacing system works in the following manner. The cardiac cycle normally begins with the client's own beat. The pacemaker's sensor senses

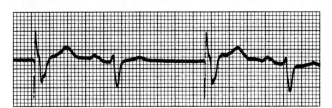

FIGURE 57–13 Demand pacing. The pacemaker initiates an electrical impulse when the sinus node fails to pace the heart. (From Phillips, R. E., & Feeney, M. K. [1990]. *The cardiac rhythms: A systematic approach to interpretation* [3rd ed.]. Philadelphia: W. B. Saunders.)

BOX 57-4   Classification System for Pacemakers

First Letter: Chamber-Paced

Indicates which chamber(s) of the heart will be stimulated.

V = Ventricle
A = Atrium
D = Dual-chamber (both atria and ventricles stimulated)

Second Letter: Chamber-Sensed

Indicates the chamber(s) of the heart in which the lead is capable of recognizing intrinsic electrical activity.

V = Ventricle
A = Atrium
D = Dual-chamber (sensing capabilities in atria and ventricles)
O = No sensing capability

Third Letter: Mode of Response

Indicates how the pacemaker will act based on the information it senses.

T = Triggered (may have energy output triggered)
I = Inhibited (pacing output inhibited by intrinsic activity)
D = Dual-chamber (may be either inhibiting or triggering of both chambers)

Fourth Letter: Programmable Functions

Indicates ability to change function once the pacemaker has been implanted.

P = Programmable for one or two functions
M = Multiprogrammable ability to change functions other than the rate or output

Fifth Letter: Tachyarrhythmic Functions

Indicates specific methods of interrupting tachyarrhythmias.

B = Bursts of pacing
N = Normal rate competition
S = Scanning

Examples

Pacing Modes Within Single-Chamber Pacemakers

Atrial demand pacemaker (AAI). A pacemaker that senses spontaneously occurring P waves and paces the atria when they do not appear.

Atrial fixed-rate pacemaker (AOO). A pacemaker that paces the atria and does not sense.
Ventricular demand pacemaker (VVI). A pacemaker that senses spontaneously occurring QRS complexes and paces the ventricles when they do not appear.
Ventricular fixed-rate pacemaker (VOO). A pacemaker that paces the ventricles and does not sense.

Pacing Modes Within Dual-Chamber Pacemakers

Atrial synchronous ventricular pacemaker (VDD). A pacemaker that senses spontaneously occurring P waves and QRS complexes and paces the ventricles when QRS complexes fail to appear after spontaneously occurring P waves, as in complete atrioventricular (AV) block. In this type of pacemaker, the pacing of ventricles is synchronized with the P waves, so that the ventricular contractions follow the atrial contractions in a normal sequence. A major benefit is that it permits the heart rate to vary, and AV synchrony occurs, depending on the physiologic demands of the body. A built-in safety mechanism causes ventricular depolarizations to occur at a fixed rate should atrial rates become too fast.
AV synchronous pacemaker (VAT). A pacemaker that has ventricular pacing, atrial sensing, and triggered response to sensing. The ventricular pacing stimulus will fire at a set time after sensing of a spontaneous atrial depolarization.
AV sequential pacemaker (DVI). A pacemaker that senses spontaneously occurring QRS complexes and paces both the atria and ventricles (the atria first, followed by the ventricles after a short delay) when QRS complexes do not appear.
AV sequential fixed-rate pacemaker (DOO). A pacemaker that paces both the atria and ventricles, but does not sense.
Optimal sequential pacemaker (DDD). A pacemaker that senses spontaneously occurring P waves and QRS complexes and (1) paces the atria when P waves fail to appear, as in sick sinus syndrome, and (2) paces the ventricles when QRS complexes fail to appear after spontaneously occurring or paced P waves. In this type of pacemaker, like the VDD pacemaker, the pacing of ventricles is synchronized with the P waves, so that the ventricular contractions follow the atrial contractions in a normal sequence.

---

whether the intrinsic beat has occurred; if not, the pacer sends out an impulse to begin myocardial depolarization through a pulse generator. The impulse generator is said to "capture" the myocardium and thereby maintain heart rhythm.

For a predetermined amount of time after the pacemaker impulse, the pacemaker cannot sense incoming signals. This feature prevents the pacer from sensing its own generated electrical current and from acting again. The *refractory period* is followed by the *noise-sampling period*. If any electromagnetic interference is sensed during this phase, the pacemaker goes into a fixed-rate mode of operation, where it remains until the source of interference is removed. At the end of the noise-sampling period, the *alert period* begins and the cycle starts over again. If a PVC or PAC occurs during the alert period, the pacemaker can sense it and start its cycle over again without emitting any impulse.

Electrocardiography of Paced Beats

The ECG appearance of a paced rhythm differs from that of a normal sinus rhythm. A pacing artifact is seen. With atrial pacing, a P wave follows the artifact but may be hidden in some leads. Examination of leads II and V_1 is best for deciding whether a P wave follows a pacer spike. The QRS complex appears normal with atrial pacing; the impulse travels through usual conduction systems.

The ECG with ventricular pacing shows an abnormal QRS complex because the impulse begins in the ventricle. With right ventricular endocardial pacing, a pseudo-LBBB ECG wave is created. If the left ventricle is paced, a pseudo-RBBB is created.

Assess the ECG strip for pacer spikes followed by the expected appearance of a P wave or QRS complex. Spikes not followed by depolarization waves or paced beats that appear too early or too late may signal pacemaker failure.

Pacemaker Failure

Malfunctions can occur in the pacemaker's sensor or pulse generator. Complications associated with the components of the pacemaker system itself (see Table 57–3) may include:

1. *Failure to sense*—an inability of the sensor to detect the client's intrinsic beats; as a result, the pacemaker sends out impulses too early (Fig. 57–14A). The failure may be due to improper position of the catheter, tip or lead dislodgment, battery failure, the sensitivity set too low, or a fractured wire in the catheter.

2. *Failure to pace*—a malfunction of the pulse generator. The ECG shows an absence of any impulse (Fig. 57–14B). Component failure to discharge (pace) can be due to battery failure, lead dislodgment, fracture of the lead wire inside the catheter, disconnections between catheter and generator, or a sensing malfunction.

3. *Failure to capture*—a disorder in the pacemaker electrodes; the impulse does not generate depolarization (Fig. 57–14C). This complication can result from low voltage, battery failure, faulty connections between the pulse generator and catheter, improper position of the catheter, catheter wire fracture, fibrosis at the catheter tip, or a catheter fracture.

Clinical manifestations associated with pacemaker malfunctioning include syncope, bradycardia or tachycardia, and palpitations. When these manifestations occur, the malfunctioning leads or pacemaker must be replaced.

Teach the client and family how to care for the pacemaker and the precautions to follow (see Client Education Guide).[11, 32, 34]

■ Nursing Management of Clients with Pacemakers

ASSESSMENT

Assess the client for *subjective* clinical manifestations of dysrhythmias and alterations in cardiac output. These include palpitations, syncope, fatigue, shortness of breath, chest pain, or skipped beats felt in the chest. The client may also feel anxiety about the heart disorder and may manifest nervousness, fear, sleeplessness, uncertainty, or hopelessness. *Objective* clinical manifestations may include diaphoresis, pallor or cyanosis, variations in radial and apical pulses such as bradycardia or tachycardia, rhythm changes, hypotension, crackles, and decreased mental acuity. The client may be fearful of being left alone. Monitoring is begun, and the heart rhythm is observed continuously by a nurse, a computer, and an ECG technician. Rhythm strips are examined at least every shift.

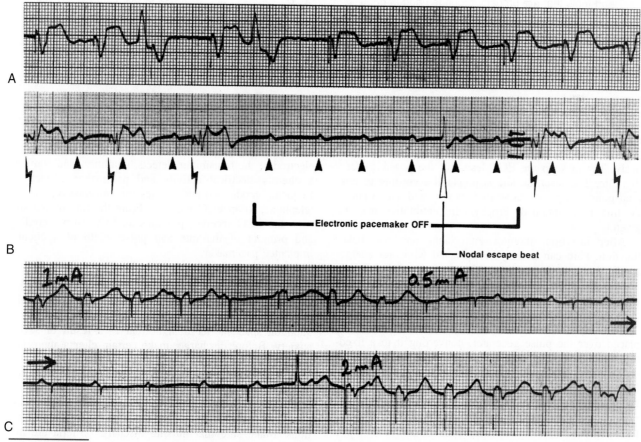

FIGURE 57–14 Pacemaker failures. *A,* Failure to sense. *B,* Failure to pace. *C,* Failure to capture. (From Phillips, R. E., & Feeney, M. K. [1990]. *The cardiac rhythms: A systematic approach to interpretation* [3rd ed.]. Philadelphia: W. B. Saunders.)

CLIENT EDUCATION GUIDE

The Client with a Permanent Pacemaker

Wound Care

1. Assess your wound daily.
2. Report any signs of inflammation (fever, redness, tenderness, discharge, or warmth) to the physician.
3. Avoid constrictive clothing (e.g., tight brassiere straps), which puts excessive pressure on the wound and the pulse generator.
4. Avoid extensive "toying" with the pulse generator, because this may cause pacemaker malfunction and local skin inflammation.

Pacemaker Management

1. Take your pulse daily in your wrist or on your neck. You will be taught how to do this before leaving the hospital.
2. Notify the physician if your pulse is slower than the set rate; also report sensations of feeling your heart "racing," beating irregularly, or of dizziness.
3. Avoid being near areas with high voltage, magnetic force fields, or radiation; this can cause pacemaker problems.
4. Avoid being near large running motors (gas or electric) and standing near high-tension wires, power plants, radio transmitters, large industrial magnets, and arc welding machines. Riding in a car is safe, but do not bring the pacemaker to within 6 to 12 inches of the distributor coil of a running engine.
5. You can continue to safely operate most appliances and tools that are properly grounded and in good repair, including microwave ovens, televisions, video recorders, AM and FM radios, electric blankets, lawn mowers, leaf blowers, and cars.
6. You can safely operate the following office and light industrial equipment that is properly grounded and in

good repair, such as electric typewriters, copying machines, and personal computers.
7. An airport's metal detector may be triggered by the pacemaker's metal casing and the programming magnet. Mention your pacemaker to security guards. The metal detector itself does not harm the pacemaker.
8. At all times, carry a pacemaker identity card (including programming information—pacemaker manufacturer, emergency phone numbers). Wear a medical alert bracelet.
9. Avoid activity that might damage the pulse generator, such as playing football and firing a rifle with the butt end against the affected shoulder.
10. Some stores sell antitheft devices that may affect pacemaker function. If you suddenly become dizzy, move away from the area and notify the store clerk about the pacemaker.
11. If radiation therapy has been prescribed to the area in which the pulse generator was implanted, the pulse generator must be relocated.
12. Do not lift more than 5 to 10 pounds (equivalent to a full grocery sack or a gallon of milk) for the first 6 weeks after surgery. Do not move your arms and shoulders vigorously for the first 6 weeks. Normal activities (including sexual activity) can be resumed in 6 weeks.
13. Discuss with the nurse the purpose, dose, schedule, and possible side effects of prescribed medications. Consult your written information sheets to reinforce learning.
14. Plan to see your physician to test your pacemaker. Your cardiologist will periodically reevaluate pacemaker function and can reprogram it if needed. You may also be able to check your pacemaker by telephone. If this is possible, you will receive instructions.

Explain the purpose of the pacemaker and the experience of having a pacemaker inserted to the client and family. Most permanent pacemakers are inserted transvenously. Try to keep the ECG leads off the possible insertion site. The insertion site is prepared according to hospital policy. A preoperative ECG is obtained, and a patent IV line is maintained. Prophylactic antibiotics may be given.

After insertion, monitor vital signs and pacemaker function. Pain can usually be managed with oral analgesics if the transvenous approach has been used. Initially, instruct the client to avoid excessive extension or abduction of the arm on the operative side. Perform passive range-of-motion exercises on the arm.

Obtain paced and nonpaced ECGs. A magnet may be placed over the pulse generator, converting it to a fixed-rate pacing mode, so that the client's intrinsic rhythm can be determined. The location of the pacemaker electrodes is determined by x-ray. The model and serial numbers of the pulse generator and leads along with the date of implantation and programmed functions of the initial implant are recorded.

Transtelephonic Pacemaker Monitoring

Special telephone monitoring of the client's ECG may be done from time to time on an outpatient basis. Telephone ECG systems are designed for follow-up monitoring of clients with pacemakers. Via finger tip, wrist, or ankle electrodes, the transmitter detects, amplifies, and converts a client's electrical activity and pacemaker artifacts to frequency-modulated audio tones for transmission, via the telephone, to an ECG receiver. From the transmitted signals, the ECG receiver provides an ECG strip recording and printout of the rate and pulse width of a client's implanted pacemaker.

■ Self-Care

It may be necessary to teach about the nature of the disorder several times, because the client may have an attention span shorter than normal as a result of severe anxiety. Before discharge, make certain clients appreciate the importance of taking antidysrhythmic agents as prescribed. Include details concerning medication administration, dosage, and side effects in the discharge plan. If discharged too early and in an unstable condition, many clients risk further exacerbations or additional complications. Make sure that nursing discharge criteria are met and documented.

Clients who have experienced cardiac dysrhythmias

while at a health care facility may be apprehensive about leaving the facility. Those who have experienced innocuous dysrhythmias may need only calm reassurance and an explanation of the cause of their disorder. Clients with recurring life-threatening dysrhythmias, such as VT, require comprehensive and specialized attention. These clients may have experienced many frightening events in the course of their hospitalization.

When a client is at risk for development of a life-threatening dysrhythmia, ascertain whether the client's housemates and significant others know how to perform CPR. Refer them to community agencies that provide CPR training (e.g., the American Heart Association, the American Red Cross, local fire department, local hospital).

Sometimes clients with serious, chronic, or potential dysrhythmias use portable telemetry units for self-monitoring at home after discharge. This allows resumption of daily activities while providing continuous 24-hour surveillance of cardiac rhythm. Nurses are often responsible for instructing clients in the use of these units. Ask the client to keep a diary of daily activities so that clinicians can correlate factors in the client's life that may be contributing to the development of dysrhythmias.

Finally, instruct clients concerning the importance of regular medical follow-up. Advise them to keep regular appointments with their physician after discharge. Explain to the client and significant others how to obtain emergency medical attention if necessary.

Living under the constant threat of sudden death provokes anxiety, depression, and, occasionally, dependent behavior. In some cases, psychological counseling may bolster coping resources. Recommend community and private counseling services for the client and significant others.

CONCLUSIONS

Common dysrhythmias usually do not interfere with everyday activities. In fact, most people with dysrhythmias lead a productive and relatively normal life. Clients need to follow a prescribed medical regimen, to take medications as directed, to report any manifestations and side effects, and to become aware of the importance of continued medical care.

THINKING CRITICALLY

1. **You are walking with a client in the hospital. He is recovering from an MI. A dysrhythmia develops. What assessments should you perform? What care does the client need?**

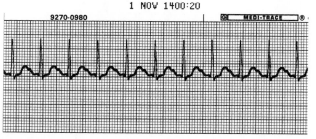

ECG Strip.

Factors to Consider. What is the usual heart rhythm response to activity? How can you assess if your client is tolerating this rhythm? How should the client be returned to his room?

2. **An 82-year-old woman is brought to the emergency department by her son after losing consciousness and hitting her head upon falling. She is now awake and states that she has been having periods of dizziness and blackouts for the past few weeks. During your physical examination, you notice what appears to be a pacemaker device implanted under her left clavicle. What additional assessments should you make? What information should you obtain about the pacemaker?**

Factors to Consider. What might have happened to the pacemaker during the fall? Could a faulty pacemaker be responsible for the loss of consciousness?

BIBLIOGRAPHY

1. American Heart Association. (1996). *Handbook of emergency cardiac care for health care providers 1996.* Dallas: Author.
2. American Heart Association. (1999). *Heart and stroke facts.* Dallas: Author.
3. Aronow, W. S. (1995). Treatment of ventricular arrhythmias in older adults. *Journal of the American Geriatrics Society 43*(6), 688–695.
4. Brown, D. L. (1998). *Cardiac intensive care.* Philadelphia: W. B. Saunders.
5. Bubien, R., et al. (1993). What you need to know about radiofrequency ablation. *American Journal of Nursing, 93*(7), 30–36.
6. Bush, D. E. (1994). Permanent cardiac pacemakers in the elderly. *Journal of the American Geriatrics Society, 42*(3), 326–334.
7. Conover, M. B. (1996). *Understanding electrocardiography* (7th ed.). St. Louis: Mosby–Year Book.
8. Collins, M. A. (1994). When your patient has an implantable cardioverter defibrillator. *American Journal of Nursing, 94*(3), 34–39.
9. Diem, S., Lantos, J., & Tukley, J. (1996). Cardiopulmonary resuscitation on television: Miracles or misinformation. *New England Journal of Medicine 334*(12), 1578–1582.
10. Dunn, F. G. (1990). Prevention of sudden cardiac death. *Cardiovascular Clinics, 20*(3), 95–109.
11. Frye, R. L., et al. (1984). Guidelines for permanent cardiac pacemaker implantation: A report of the Joint American College of Cardiology/American Heart Association Task Force of the Assessment of Cardiovascular Procedures. *Circulation, 70,* 331A–337A.
12. Hasemeier, C. S. (1996). Permanent pacemaker. *American Journal of Nursing, 96*(2), 30–31.
13. Hayes, D. L. (1992). The next 5 years in cardiac pacemakers: A preview. *Mayo Clinic Proceedings, 67*(4), 379–384.
14. Higgins, C. A. (1990). The AICD: A teaching plan for patients and families. *Critical Care Nurse, 10*(6), 69–74.
15. Kater, K. M., et al. (1992). Corralling atrial fibrillation with "maze" surgery. *American Journal of Nursing, 92*(7), 34–38.
16. Karnes, N. (1995). Adenosine: A quick fix for PSVT—paroxysmal supraventricular tachycardia. *Nursing 25*(7), 55–56.
17. King, K. B. (1994). Preparing families for health care procedures. *Heart Disease and Stroke, 3*(2), 95–97.
18. Massie, B. M., & Amidon T. A. (1997). Disturbances in rate and rhythm. In L. M. Tierney, et al. (Eds.), *Current medical diagnosis and treatment* (36th ed.). Stamford, CT: Appleton and Lange.
19. Massie, B. M., & Amidon, T. A. (1997). Conduction disturbances. In L. M. Tierney, et al. (Eds.), *Current medical diagnosis and treatment* (36th ed.). Stamford, CT: Appleton and Lange.
20. Nattel, S. (1995). Newer developments in the management of atrial fibrillation. *American Heart Journal 130*(5), 1094–1106.
21. Moser, S. A., Crawford, D., & Thomas, A. (1993). Updated care guidelines for patients with automatic implantable cardioverter defibrillators. *Critical Care Nurse, 13*(4), 62–71.

22. Ophie, L. H, & Marcus, F. I. (1997). Antiarrhythmic drugs. In L. H. Ophie (Ed.)., *Drugs for the heart* (4th ed.). Philadelphia: W. B. Saunders.

23. Petrosky-Pacini, A. J. (1996). The automatic implantable cardioverter defibrillator in home care. *Home Healthcare Nurse 14*(4), 238–243.

24. Porter, L. A. (1995). Drug profiles: Maximizing therapeutic effectiveness. *Journal of Cardiovascular Nursing, 10*(1), 64–72.

25. Porterfield, L. M., Porterfield, J. G., & Collins, S. W. (1993). The cutting edge in arrhythmias. *Critical Care Nurse, 13*(suppl. 6), 8–9.

26. Rakel, R. E. (1992). *Conn's current therapy.* Philadelphia: W. B. Saunders.

27. Saver, C. L. (1994). Decoding the ACLS algorithms. *American Journal of Nursing, 94*(1), 26–36.

28. Schron, E. B., et al. (1996). Relation of sociodemographic, clinical, and quality of life variables to adherence in the cardiac arrhythmia suppression trial. *Cardiovascular Nursing, 32*(2), 1–5.

29. Simons, L. H., Cunningham, S., & Catanzaro, M. (1992). Emotional responses and experiences of wives of men who survive a sudden cardiac death event. *Cardiovascular Nursing, 28*(2), 17–21.

30. Sims, J. M., & Miracle, V. (1997). Ventricular tachycardia. *Nursing 97, 21*(11), 47.

31. Sirles, A. T., & Selleck, C. S. (1989). Cardiac disease and the family: Impact, assessment, and implications. *Journal of Cardiovascular Nursing, 3*(2), 23–32.

32. Sommers, M. S. (1992). Preventing complications of CPR. *Medical-Surgical Nursing Quarterly, 1*(1), 44–54.

33. Sommers, M. S. (1992). The near-death experience after cardiopulmonary arrest. *Medical-Surgical Nursing Quarterly, 1*(1), 55–62.

34. Stuart, J. V., & Sheehan, A. M. (1991). Permanent pacemakers: The nurse's role in patient education and follow-up care. *Journal of Cardiovascular Nursing, 5*(3), 32–43.

35. Thelan, L. A., et al. (1998). Temporary pacemakers. In L. A. Thelan, et al. (Eds.), *Critical care nursing: Diagnosis and management* (3rd ed.). St. Louis: Mosby–Year Book.

36. Thelan, L. A., et al. (1998). Implantable cardioverter defibrillator. In L. A. Thelan, et al. (Eds.), *Critical care nursing: Diagnosis and management* (3rd ed.). St. Louis: Mosby–Year Book.

37. Whalley, D. W., Wendt, D. J. & Grant, A. O. (1995). Basic concepts in cellular cardiac electrophysiology: II. Block of ion channels by antiarrhythmic drugs. *Pacing and Clinical Electrophysiology, 18,* 1686–1703.

38. Zaim, B., Zaim, S., & Kutalek, S. P. (1994). Indications for use of permanent cardiac pacemakers. *Heart Disease and Stroke, 3*(2), 71–76.

39. Zipes, D. P. (1997). Management of cardiac arrhythmias: Pharmacological, electrical, and surgical techniques. In E. Braunwald (Ed.), *Heart disease* (5th ed.). Philadelphia: W. B. Saunders.

40. Zipes, D. P. (1997). Specific arrhythmias: Diagnosis and treatment. In E. Braunwald (Ed.), *Heart disease* (5th ed.). Philadelphia: W. B. Saunders.

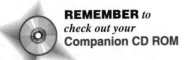

REMEMBER *to*
check out your
Companion CD ROM

CHAPTER

58

Management of Clients with Myocardial Infarction

Janice Tazbir
Peggy Gerard

NURSING OUTCOMES CLASSIFICATION (NOC)
for Nursing Diagnoses—Clients with Myocardial Infarction

Altered Health Maintenance	Vital Signs Status	Health Beliefs: Perceived Control
Health Promoting Behavior	**Fluid Volume Excess**	Health Beliefs: Perceived Resources
Health Seeking Behavior	Electrolyte and Acid-Base Balance	**Risk for Activity Intolerance**
Knowledge: Health Behaviors	Fluid Balance	Cardiac Pump Effectiveness
Participation: Health Care Decisions	Hydration	Circulation Status
Psychosocial Adjustment: Life Change	**Impaired Gas Exchange**	Energy Conservation
Self-Direction of Care	Electrolyte and Acid-Base Balance	Knowledge: Prescribed Activity
Altered Tissue Perfusion	Respiratory Status: Ventilation	**Risk for Constipation**
(Cardiopulmonary)	**Pain**	Bowel Elimination
Pain Level	Comfort Level	Mobility Level
Tissue Perfusion: Cardiac	Pain Control	Nutritional Status: Food and Fluid Intake
Anxiety and Fear	Pain: Disruptive Effects	**Risk for Impaired Skin Integrity**
Anxiety Control	Pain Level	Immobility Consequences: Physiologic
Coping	**Powerlessness**	Tissue Integrity: Skin and Mucous
Fear Control	Depression Control	Membranes
Decreased Cardiac Output	Depression Level	Tissue Perfusion: Peripheral
Cardiac Pump Effectiveness	Health Beliefs: Perceived Ability to	**Risk for Injury**
Circulation Status	Perform	Risk Control

The heart requires a balance between oxygen supply and oxygen demand in order to function properly. The integrity of the coronary arteries is an important determinant of oxygen supply to the heart muscle. Any disorder that reduces the lumen of an artery may cause a decrease in blood flow and oxygen delivery to heart muscle and may result in the acute coronary syndromes of angina, myocardial infarction (MI), and sudden cardiac death. Coronary heart disease (CHD) is the primary underlying cause of these syndromes and is the single largest killer of American men and women.[2]

The clinical syndromes associated with CHD are familiar to most Americans. Almost every day, the news media covers a story on a celebrity who has suffered from or was treated for chest pain, heart attack, or cardiac arrest. Turn on any television hospital drama and you will see someone seeking treatment for an episode of chest pain. Many of us also have had personal experience with CHD through the illness of a relative or close friend.

Acute coronary syndromes are responsible for more than 250,000 deaths annually and result from a progressive atherosclerotic process that culminates in rupture of atherosclerotic plaques and thrombus formation.[2] This chapter reviews the risk factors, pathophysiology, clinical manifestations, and medical and nursing interventions for the acute coronary syndromes of angina pectoris (a type of chest pain) and MI.

ANGINA PECTORIS

As vessels become lined with atherosclerotic plaques, plaques may be disrupted and thrombi may form, leading to clinical manifestations of inadequate blood supply in the tissues supplied by these vessels. Problems such as stroke, claudication, and angina develop. Stroke is described in Chapter 70 and claudication is discussed in Chapter 53.

Angina pectoris is chest pain resulting from myocardial ischemia (inadequate blood supply to the myocardium).[29] It is a common manifestation of CHD and affects about 6,200,000 Americans — 2,300,000 men and 3,900,000 women. According to the Framingham Heart Study, approximately 350,000 new cases of angina occur each year.[2] Angina can also occur in clients with normal coronary arteries, but it is less common. Clients with aortic stenosis, hypertension, and hypertrophic cardiomyopathy can have angina pectoris.

Etiology and Risk Factors

Angina pectoris is associated with atherosclerotic lesions and is a manifestation of CHD (see Chapter 56). Angina can be caused either by chronic or acute blockage of a coronary artery or by coronary artery spasm. Chronic blockages are associated with fixed calcified (type Vb) or fibrotic (type Vc) atherosclerotic lesions that occlude more than 75% of the vessel lumen.[8]

When fixed blockages are present in the coronary arteries, conditions that increase myocardial oxygen demand (e.g., physical exertion, emotion, exposure to cold) may precipitate episodes of angina. Because the severely stenosed arteries cannot deliver enough oxygen to meet the increased demand, ischemia results.[31, 36] In contrast, acute blockage of a coronary artery results from rupture or disruption of vulnerable atherosclerotic plaques that cause platelet aggregation and thrombus formation (see etiology of MI).[2] Acute blockages are associated with unstable angina and MI.

Primary prevention is through the lifelong commitment to reducing the risk factors of CHD (see Chapter 56). Secondary prevention is through recognition and early treatment of anginal attacks. Tertiary prevention is resolution of angina before myocardial damage occurs.

Pathophysiology

The coronary arteries normally supply the myocardium with blood to meet its metabolic needs during varying workloads. The coronary vessels are usually efficient and perfuse the myocardium during diastole. When the heart needs more blood, the vessels dilate. As the vessels become lined and eventually occluded with atherosclerotic plaques and thrombi, the vessels can no longer dilate properly.

Myocardial ischemia develops if the blood supply through the coronary vessels or oxygen content of the blood is not adequate to meet metabolic demands. Disorders of the coronary vessels, the circulation, or the blood may lead to deficits in supply.

Disorders of the coronary vessels include atherosclerosis, arterial spasm, and coronary arteritis. Atherosclerosis increases resistance to flow. Arterial spasm also increases resistance. Coronary *arteritis* is inflammation of the coronary arteries caused by infection or autoimmune disease.

Disorders of circulation include hypotension and aortic stenosis and insufficiency. Hypotension may be a result of spinal anesthesia, potent antihypertensive drugs, blood loss, or other factors that result in decreased blood return to the heart. Aortic valve stenosis or insufficiency results in decreased filling pressure of the coronary arteries.

Blood disorders include anemia, hypoxemia, and polycythemia. Anemia and hypoxemia result in decreased oxygen flow to the myocardium. Polycythemia increases blood viscosity, which slows blood flow through the coronary arteries.

The opposite of supply is demand, and increased demands can be placed on the heart. Conditions that increase demands on the myocardium are those that increase cardiac output or increase myocardial need for oxygen (see Box 58–1).

Myocardial ischemia occurs when either supply or demand is altered. In some people, the coronary arteries can supply adequate blood when the person is at rest; when the person attempts activity or is taxed in some other manner, however, angina develops. Myocardial cells become ischemic within 10 seconds of coronary artery occlusion. After several minutes of ischemia, the pumping function of the heart is reduced. The reduction in pump-

---

BOX 58–1 Factors Influencing Myocardial Supply and Demand

Factors That Decrease Supply

Coronary Vessel Disorders

Atherosclerosis
Arterial spasm
Coronary arteritis

Circulation Disorders

Hypotension
Aortic stenosis
Aortic insufficiency

Blood Disorders

Anemia
Hypoxemia
Polycythemia

Factors That Increase Demand

Increased Cardiac Output

Exercise
Emotion
Digestion of a large meal
Anemia
Hyperthyroidism

Increased Myocardial Need for Oxygen

Damaged myocardium
Myocardial hypertrophy
Aortic stenosis
Aortic insufficiency
Diastolic hypertension
Thyrotoxicosis
Strong emotions
Heavy exertion

ing deprives the ischemic cells of needed oxygen and glucose. The cells convert to anaerobic metabolism, which leaves lactic acid as a waste product. As lactic acid accumulates, pain develops. Angina pectoris is transient, lasting for only 3 to 5 minutes. If blood flow is restored, no permanent myocardial damage occurs.

Clinical Manifestations

CHARACTERISTICS OF ANGINA

Angina pectoris produces transient paroxysmal attacks of substernal or precordial pain with the following characteristics:

Onset. Angina can develop quickly or slowly. Some clients ignore the chest pain, thinking that it will go away or that it is indigestion. Ask what the client was doing when the pain began.

Location. Nearly 90% of clients experience the pain as retrosternal or slightly to the left of the sternum.

Radiation. The pain usually radiates to the left shoulder and upper arm and may then travel down the inner aspect of the left arm to the elbow, wrist, and fourth and fifth fingers. The pain may also radiate to the right shoulder, neck, jaw, or epigastric region. On occasion, the pain may be felt only in the area of radiation and not in the chest. Rarely is the pain localized to any one single small area over the precordium.

Duration. Angina usually lasts less than 5 minutes. However, attacks precipitated by a heavy meal or extreme anger may last 15 to 20 minutes.

Sensation. Clients describe the pain of angina as squeezing, burning, pressing, choking, aching, or bursting pressure. The client often says the pain feels like gas, heartburn, or indigestion. Clients do not describe anginal pain as sharp or knife-like.

Severity. The pain of angina is usually mild or moderate in severity. Rarely is the pain described as severe.

Associated characteristics. Other manifestations that may accompany the pain include dyspnea, pallor, sweating, faintness, palpitations, dizziness, and digestive disturbances.

Atypical presentation. Women and older adults may have atypical presentations of CHD that are equivalent to angina. In women, CHD may be manifested as epigastric pain, dyspnea, or back pain, whereas the elderly frequently experience dyspnea, fatique, or syncope.[3]

Relieving/aggravating factors. Angina is aggravated by continued activity, and most anginal attacks quickly subside with the administration of nitroglycerin and rest. The typical "exertion–pain, rest–relief" pattern is the major clue to the diagnosis of angina pectoris.

Treatment. Has the client treated the pain with nitroglycerin? Did it work? Angina should subside after nitroglycerin use.

PATTERNS OF ANGINA

Classic angina pectoris can be subdivided into the following basic patterns:

Stable angina. Stable angina is paroxysmal chest pain or discomfort triggered by a predictable degree of exertion (e.g., walking 20 feet) or emotion. Characteristi-

cally a stable pattern of onset, duration, severity, and relieving factors is present.[10, 13]

Unstable angina. Unstable angina (preinfarction angina, crescendo angina, or intermittent coronary syndrome) is paroxysmal chest pain triggered by an unpredictable degree of exertion or emotion, which may occur at night. Unstable angina attacks characteristically increase in number, duration, and severity over time. Once unstable angina is diagnosed, the client must receive immediate medical attention.[10, 34]

Variant angina. Variant angina (*Prinzmetal's angina*) is chest discomfort similar to classic angina but of longer duration; it may occur while the client is at rest. These attacks tend to happen in the early hours of the day. Variant angina may result from coronary artery spasm and may be associated with elevation of the ST segment on the electrocardiogram (ECG).

Nocturnal angina. Nocturnal angina is possibly associated with rapid eye movement (REM) sleep during dreaming.

Angina decubitus. Angina decubitus is paroxysmal chest pain that occurs when the client reclines and lessens when the client sits or stands up.

Intractable angina. Intractable angina is chronic incapacitating angina that is unresponsive to intervention.

Post-infarction angina. Pain occurs occurs after MI, when residual ischemia may cause episodes of angina.

DIAGNOSTIC TESTS

The following modalities are described in Chapter 54.

ELECTROCARDIOGRAPHY. The ECG tracings remain normal in 25% to 30% of clients with angina pectoris. An ECG taken in the presence of pain may document transient ischemic attacks with ST-segment elevation or depression. An ECG taken during an episode of pain also suggests coronary artery involvement and the extent of cardiac muscle affected by the ischemic event.[34]

EXERCISE ELECTROCARDIOGRAPHY. During a *stress test,* the client exercises on a treadmill or stationary bicycle until reaching 85% of maximal heart rate. ECG or vital sign changes may indicate ischemia.[34]

RADIOISOTOPE IMAGING. Various nuclear imaging techniques are used to evaluate myocardial muscle. Regions of poor perfusion or ischemia appear as areas of diminished or absent activity (cold spots).

ELECTRON-BEAM (ULTRAFAST) COMPUTED TOMOGRAPHY. This promising noninvasive method enables detection of the amount of calcium in coronary arteries. Because calcification occurs with atherosclerotic plaque formation, measurement of coronary calcium may reflect the extent of coronary atherosclerosis. High coronary calcium values have been associated with obstructive coronary disease.

CORONARY ANGIOGRAPHY. Angiography provides the most accurate information about the patency of the coronary arteries and allows visualization of the artery and any partial or complete blockages.

Outcome Management

The aims of therapy in the treatment of angina are to alleviate manifestations and to prevent the progression of

CHD. The ultimate goal is to reduce the risk of MI and death. This goal is accomplished through (1) pharmacologic intervention, (2) education and counseling regarding the most effective way to control or eliminate known cardiovascular risk factors, and, (3) in some instances, revascularization through interventional cardiology or coronary artery bypass graft (CABG) surgery. Smoking cessation reduces the risk of coronary heart disease by 37%; a 10% reduction in cholesterol lowers the risk of CHD by 20%; and a 6-mm reduction in diastolic blood pressure lowers the risk of CHD by 10%.[2] The American Heart Association (AHA) recommends that people with angina control their modifiable risk factors and seek prompt treatment for episodes of chest pain.

Clients with chronic stable angina (CSA) are usually managed effectively with risk factor reduction and pharmacologic therapy. Revascularization through interventional cardiology procedures or CABG surgery is reserved for these clients with triple-vessel or left main coronary artery disease, with left ventricular dysfunction, or whose manifestations are not adequately controlled by pharmacologic therapy. Revascularization is used most often for clients with unstable angina or MI. Interventional cardiology procedures and CABG are discussed in Chapters 55 and 56.

■ Medical Management

Medical management of clients with angina pectoris focuses on two goals: (1) relief of the acute attack and (2) prevention of further attacks to reduce the risk of MI.

The diagnosis of angina pectoris is confirmed by history and various tests. Obtain a complete history of the pain and its pattern. Encourage clients to describe the pain in their own words. Record a complete analysis of manifestations. This description provides a baseline that can be used in ongoing care.

Most physical findings are transient. The client exhibits pallor or has cold, clammy skin. Tachycardia and hypertension may be recorded. Pulsus alternans (the force of each beat varies) may be present at the onset of ischemic attacks. On auscultation, an S_3 or S_4 gallop or a paradoxical split of S_2 may be noted. If mitral regurgitation is present because of ischemia of the papillary muscle, a murmur can be heard.

RELIEVE ACUTE ATTACK

The primary goal of pharmacologic treatment of angina is to balance myocardial oxygen supply and demand by altering the various components of the process, thereby increasing oxygen supply to the myocardium or reducing myocardial oxygen demand. The components of myocardial oxygen consumption that can be pharmacologically treated are (1) blood pressure, (2) heart rate, (3) contractility, and (4) left ventricular volume. Drugs used in the treatment of angina and associated nursing implications are listed in Table 58–1.

The major types of medications used to treat the acute attack in angina pectoris are as follows:

1. *Opiate analgesics* are used to relieve acute pain.
2. *Vasodilators* help reduce acute pain and prevent further attacks by widening the diameter of coronary arteries and increasing the supply of oxygen to the myocardium. *Nitroglycerin,* a *short-acting* nitrate, has been the treatment of choice against anginal attacks since 1867. Administered sublingually, per tablet, or via translingual spray, nitroglycerin helps relieve anginal pain within 1 to 2 minutes. *Long-acting* nitrates help maintain coronary artery vasodilation, thereby promoting greater flow of blood and oxygen to the heart muscle.
3. *Beta-adrenergic blockers* help reduce the workload of the heart, decrease myocardial oxygen demand, and may decrease the number of anginal attacks.
4. *Calcium-channel blockers* are used to dilate coronary arteries, thereby increasing oxygen supply to the myocardium.
5. *Antiplatelet* agents inhibit platelet aggregation and reduce coagulability, thus preventing clot formation.

PREVENT FURTHER ATTACKS

Education and counseling regarding modification of risk factors are necessary to reduce the progression of CHD and to prevent further attacks. Recommendations should follow the guidelines established by the AHA for primary and secondary prevention of CHD. Specific recommendations for risk factor modification are described in Chapter 56.

■ Nursing Management of the Medical Client

RELIEVE ACUTE ATTACK

In addition to documenting the clinical manifestations of angina, ascertain how long the client has had angina, whether risk factors for CHD are present, and the client's emotional reaction to chest pain. Start cardiac monitoring, obtain a 12-lead ECG, and control ongoing angina. Until the angina is controlled and coronary blood flow is reestablished, the client is at risk for myocardial damage from myocardial ischemia. If the client reports angina, assess the pain and ask the client whether the pain is the same as experienced in the past. Note new characteristics or increased pain.

Give sublingual nitroglycerin tablets or spray as prescribed. Because nitroglycerin causes vasodilation and hypotension, monitor blood pressure. If the pain is not relieved after three nitroglycerin tablets, each taken 5 minutes apart, or after morphine, notify the physician. In addition, an environment that provides rest and security as well as allays fear and anxiety helps reduce pain.

PREVENT FURTHER ATTACKS THROUGH SELF-CARE

The client must be knowledgeable about the care of episodes of angina and how to reduce the risk factors that exacerbate the process. Use the following information as needed to help clients control risk factors for angina pectoris.

1. Educate the client to avoid activities or habits that precipitate angina (eating large meals, drinking coffee, smoking, exercising too strenuously, going out in cold weather, being exposed to excessive stress). If an attack begins, the client should stop the activity and sit down. An antianginal medication (e.g., nitroglycerin) should be taken. One pill can be

Class	Example	Assessment of Therapeutic Responses	Assessment of Adverse Responses	Nursing Implications
Vasodilators	Nitroglycerin	Dilates coronary arteries, improves collateral blood flow, and decreases cardiac oxygen demands. Clinically, a decrease in chest pain, resolving ST segments, is observed.	The client may experience flushing, weakness, headache, postural hypotension, dizziness, and reflex tachycardia.	Monitor client for chest pain and hypotension. IV nitroglycerin should be in non-PVC sets, and blood pressure and heart rate should be continuously monitored. Titrate IV 5 μg/min every 3–5 minutes until pain subsides. Because tablets are inactivated by light, heat, air, and moisture, store in tight-fitting amber glass containers. Nitroglycerin tablets may be taken 5 minutes apart. If pain is not resolved after three tablets, contact physician immediately.
Beta-adrenergic blocking agents	Atenolol	The effects of blockade of beta-adrenergic receptors and the neurohormonal response that inhibits the sympathetic nervous system are seen clinically by a decreased heart rate, and the vasodilatation decreases blood pressure. It also decreases the automaticity, decreasing heart rate and the incidence of dysrhythmias. Over the long term, the client experiences less mortality and less incidence of heart failure.*	The client may experience bronchoconstriction, severe bradycardia, or hypotension. The client may also experience A-V conduction abnormalities, dizziness, confusion, constipation or diarrhea, and vomiting. Male clients may experience impotence.	Do not give to clients with a history of bronchospastic pulmonary disease. If the client has diabetes, it may potentiate hypoglycemia. Monitor the heart rate and blood pressure frequently. Assess pulmonary status for bronchoconstriction.
ACE inhibitor	Captopril	The decrease in afterload increases cardiac output by enhancing contractility. The neurohormonal effects may cause vasodilatation and a decrease in systemic blood pressure. Long-term effects include a decrease in mortality and decrease in the incidence of heart failure.*	The client may experience hypotension, oliguria, palpitations, insomnia, dizziness, fatigue, nausea, vomiting, maculopapular rash, and cough.	Monitor blood pressure closely. Full therapeutic effect may take weeks to achieve. May increase BUN, creatinine, liver enzymes, and potassium levels.

Table continued on following page

TABLE 58-1 NURSING IMPLICATIONS FOR MEDICATIONS USED TO TREAT ANGINA PECTORIS *Continued*

Class	Example	Assessment of Therapeutic Responses	Assessment of Adverse Responses	Nursing Implications
Opiate analgesics	Morphine	Binds with opiate receptors in the CNS causing inhibition of ascending pain pathways altering the perception of pain. Decreases afterload by vasodilatation and may decrease blood pressure.	The client may experience respiratory depression, hypotension, bradycardia, drowsiness, constipation, pruritus, and weakness.	Monitor heart rate, blood pressure, and respiratory status frequently. Naloxone is the antidote for overdose and should be available when giving morphine IV.
Antiplatelet aggregating agent	Acetylsalicylic acid (ASA)	ASA blocks prostaglandin synthesis action, which prevents formation of the platelet aggregating substance thromboxane A_2. Clinically, this limits the formation or progression of a thrombus and decreases mortality.†	The client may experience heartburn, stomach pains, nausea and vomiting, rash, weakness, hemolytic anemia, and gastrointestinal ulceration. Overdose symptoms include tinnitus, headache, dizziness, confusion, and metabolic acidosis.	Avoid use in clients with severe renal or liver disease. Monitor serum concentrations, renal function, hearing changes, skin inflammation, and for abnormal bleeding. Administer with food or large quantities of water to decrease gastrointestinal upset. Instruct the client to avoid concurrent use of over-the-counter products that contain ASA.
Calcium-channel blockers	Diltiazem	Inhibits influx of calcium ion through the cell membrane, resulting in a relaxation of coronary vasculature smooth muscle and coronary vasodilation, decreasing anginal pains.	Clients may experience hypotension, dysrhythmias, syncope, Stevens-Johnson syndrome, and weakness.	Monitor heart rate for dysrhythmias and blood pressure for hypotension. May increase liver enzymes. Use in MI is investigational for non–Q wave MIs.

ACE, angiotensin-converting enzymes; A-V, atrioventricular; BUN, blood urea nitrogen; IV, intravenous; MI, myocardine infarction; CNS, central nervous system; PVC, premature ventricular contraction.
*See Moser D., et al. (1999, October). The role of the critical care nurse in preventing heart failure after acute myocardial infarction. *Critical Care Nurse Supplement*, 11–15.
†See Feldman, M., & Cryer, B. (1999). Aspirin absorption rates and platelet inhibition times with 325-mg buffered aspirin tablets (chewed or swallowed intact) and with buffered aspirin solution. *American Journal of Cardiology, 84,* 404–409.

taken sublingually three times in 5-minute intervals. If the pain does not subside, worsens, or radiates, the client should be taken or driven to an emergency department. Stress this point, because if the client is experiencing an MI, the sooner the treatment is initiated, the lower the mortality rate.[18]

2. Explain the importance of daily management of hypertension. Advise the client to take daily medication even if no clinical manifestations are evident (see also Chapter 53).

3. Encourage and help plan a regular program of daily exercise to promote improved coronary circulation and weight management.

4. Instruct clients who smoke to quit smoking at once. Smoking cigarettes raises carboxyhemoglobin levels in the blood, which reduces the amount of oxygen available to the myocardium. Clients with angina pectoris exposed for 2 hours to cigarette smoke demonstrate elevations in carboxyhemoglobin concentration, decreased exercise time, increased heart rate, and elevated blood pressure. Advise clients to avoid "passive smoking" (i.e., being with a smoker or in a smoke-filled room).

5. Urge overweight clients to lose excess weight. Encourage them to eat small meals, avoid high-calorie and high-cholesterol diets, abstain from gas-forming foods, and rest for short periods after meals. In addition, recommend a high-fiber diet, which not only may prevent constipation and other intestinal tract ailments but also may decrease the number and severity of anginal attacks. Diets high in fiber may also help lower serum cholesterol and triglyceride levels. CHD is less common among clients with a high intake of dietary fiber than in those with a low intake. High-fiber diets can also decrease hypertension.

6. Help the client who leads an active, hectic life to adjust activities to a level below that which precipitates anginal attacks. Encourage brief rest periods throughout the working day, an early bedtime, and longer or more frequent vacations. Advise clients who are anxious and nervous to consider counseling. Relaxation techniques may also be used.

ACUTE MYOCARDIAL INFARCTION

Acute MI, also known as a heart attack, coronary occlusion, or simply a "coronary," is a life-threatening condition characterized by the formation of localized necrotic areas within the myocardium. MI usually follows the sudden occlusion of a coronary artery and the abrupt cessation of blood and oxygen flow to the heart muscle. Because the heart muscle must function continuously, blockage of blood to the muscle and the development of necrotic areas can be lethal.

Every year about 1.1 million Americans have MIs. Indeed, MI is the leading cause of death in America and is responsible for an estimated 500,000 deaths each year. During an MI, men are more likely than women to die before they reach the hospital, whereas women have higher in-hospital mortality than men.[2, 7, 25] This differ-

ence may result from differences in treatment for men and women. In one study, women with MI received aspirin, beta-blocking drugs, coronary thrombolysis, and acute cardiac catherization, percutaneous transluminal coronary angioplasty (PTCA), or CABG surgery less often than did men with MI.[40] About 250,000 people a year die before they reach the hospital. Studies indicate that half of all MI victims wait more than 2 hours before getting help.[45] On the basis of data from the Framingham study, about 45% of all MIs occur in people under age 65 years and 5% occur in those under age 40. Four out of five people who die of MI are 65 years of age or older.[2]

Etiology and Risk Factors

The most common cause of MI is complete or nearly complete occlusion of a coronary artery, usually precipitated by rupture of a vulnerable atherosclerotic plaque and subsequent thrombus formation. Plaque rupture can be precipitated by both internal and external factors.

Internal factors include plaque characteristics, such as the size and consistency of the lipid core and the thickness of the fibrous cap as well as conditions to which it is exposed, such as coagulation status and degree of arterial vasoconstriction. Vulnerable plaques most frequently occur in areas with less than 70% stenosis and are characterized by an eccentric shape with an irregular border; a large, thin lipid core; and a thin, fibrous cap.[8, 28]

External factors result from actions of the client or from external conditions that affect the client. Strenuous physical activity and severe emotional stress, such as anger, increase sympathetic activity that in turn increases hemodynamic stress that may lead to plaque rupture. At the same time, sympathetic activity increases myocardial oxygen demand. Scientists have reported that external factors, such as exposure to cold and time of day, also affect plaque rupture. Acute coronary events occur more frequently with exposure to cold and during the morning hours. Researchers hypothesize that the sudden increases in sympathetic activity associated with these factors may contribute to plaque rupture.[8, 27]

Regardless of the cause, rupture of the atherosclerotic plaque results in (1) exposure of the plaque's lipid-rich core to flowing blood, (2) seepage of blood into the plaque, causing it to expand, (3) triggering of thrombus formation, and (4) partial or complete occlusion of the coronary artery. *Unstable angina* is associated with short-term partial occlusion of a coronary artery, whereas MI results from significant or complete occlusion of a coronary artery that lasts more than 1 hour.[8, 35] When blood flow ceases abruptly, the myocardial tissue supplied by that artery dies. Coronary artery spasm can also cause acute occlusion. The risk factors that predispose a client to a heart attack are the same as for all forms of CHD (see Chapter 56).

Pathophysiology

MI can be considered the end-point of CHD. Unlike the temporary ischemia that occurs with angina, prolonged unrelieved ischemia causes irreversible damage to the

Understanding Myocardial Infarction and Its Treatment

Change in the condition of plaque in the coronary artery

Activation of platelets

Aspirin
Antiplatelet aggregates

Formation of a thrombus

Thrombolytic therapy
Glycoprotein IIB/IIIA receptor antagonists

Nitrates

Ischemia of tissue in the region supplied by the artery

Altered repolarization of the myocardium

Elevated ST segment Q wave appears

Coronary blood supply less than demand

Release of lysosomal enzymes

Elevated CPK-MB
Elevated myoglobin
Troponin T
Troponin I

Beta-blockers

Myocardial cell death

Anaerobic glycolysis

Lactic acid production

Nitroglycerin

Myocardial irritability

Angina

Decreased contractility

Dysrhythmias

Stimulation of the sympathetic nervous system

Antidysrhythmics

Increased heart rate

Increased O₂ needs

Decreased left ventricular function

Angiotensin-converting enzyme inhibitors

Increased afterload

Nitrates

Increased preload

Fluid restriction

Decreased cardiac output

Vasoconstriction

Increased CVP
Increased PCWP

Decreased LV ejection fraction

☐ pathophysiology   ◯ treatment   ◇ clinical manifestations

myocardium. Cardiac cells can withstand ischemia for about 20 minutes before they die. Because the myocardium is metabolically active, signs of ischemia can be seen within 8 to 10 seconds of decreased blood flow. When the heart does not receive blood and oxygen, it converts to *anaerobic metabolism,* creating less adenosine triphosphate (ATP) and more lactic acid as a by-product. Myocardial cells are very sensitive to changes in pH and become less functional. Acidosis causes the myocardium to become more vulnerable to the effects of the lysosomal enzymes within the cell. Acidosis leads to conduction system disorders, and dysrhythmias develop. Contractility is also reduced, decreasing the heart's ability to pump. As the myocardial cells necrose, intracellular enzymes are introduced into the bloodstream, where they can be detected by laboratory tests.

Figure 58–1 illustrates the depth of various types of infarctions in the wall of the ventricle. Cellular necrosis occurs in one layer of myocardial tissue in subendocardial, intramural, and subepicardial infarctions. In a transmural infarction, cellular necrosis is present in all three layers of myocardial tissue. The infarct site is called the *zone of infarction and necrosis.* Around it is a zone of hypoxic injury. This zone can return to normal but may also become necrotic if blood flow is not restored. The outermost zone is called the *zone of ischemia;* damage to this area is reversible.

Transmural infarctions cause changes in the architecture of the left ventricle, called "remodeling," which can result in acute or chronic heart failure. Within the first few hours of an MI, the necrotic area stretches in a process called "infarct expansion." This expansion may continue for up to 6 weeks after an MI and is accompanied by progressive thinning and lengthening of infarcted and noninfarcted areas. This remodeling results in left ventricular dysfunction and produces increases in ventricular volumes and pressures. Remodeling may continue for years after an MI and may result in chronic heart failure (see Chapter 56).[8]

The most common site of MI is the *anterior wall* of the left ventricle near the apex, resulting from thrombosis of the descending branch of the left coronary artery (Fig. 58–2). Other common sites are (1) the *posterior wall* of

the left ventricle near the base and behind the posterior cusp of the mitral valve and (2) the *inferior (diaphragmatic) surface* of the heart. Infarction of the posterior left ventricle results from occlusion of the right coronary artery or circumflex branch of the left coronary artery. An inferior infarction occurs when the right coronary artery is occluded. In nearly 25% of inferior wall MIs, the right ventricle is the site of infarction. Atrial infarctions develop less than 5% of the time. See Understanding Myocardial Infarction and Its Treatment.

Clinical Manifestations

The clinical manifestations associated with MI result from ischemia of the heart muscle and the decrease in function and acidosis associated with it. The major clinical manifestation of MI is chest pain (Fig. 58–3), which is similar to angina pectoris but more severe and unrelieved by nitroglycerin. The pain may radiate to the neck, jaw, shoulder, back, or left arm. The pain also may present near the epigastrium, simulating indigestion. MI may also be associated with less common clinical manifestations, including:

- Atypical chest, stomach, back, or abdominal pain
- Nausea or dizziness
- Shortness of breath and difficulty breathing
- Unexplained anxiety, weakness, or fatigue
- Palpitations, cold sweat, or paleness

Women experiencing MI frequently present with one or more of the less common clinical manifestations.[17]

ELECTROCARDIOGRAPHY

When blood flow to the heart is decreased, ischemia and necrosis of the heart muscle occur. These conditions are reflected in altered Q wave, ST segment, and T wave on the ECG. The Q-wave change is significant; normally, the Q wave is very small or absent. Ischemic tissue produces an elevation in the ST segment and a peaked T wave or inversion of the T wave. Through the course of an MI, changes occur first in the ST segment, then the T wave, and finally the Q wave. As the myocardium heals, the ST segment and T waves return to normal but the Q-wave changes persist (Fig. 58–4).[34]

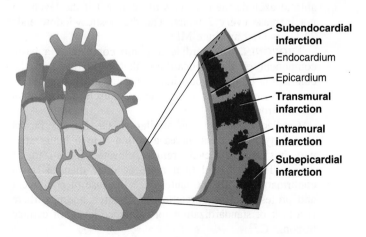

Subendocardial infarction
Endocardium
Epicardium
Transmural infarction
Intramural infarction
Subepicardial infarction

FIGURE 58–1 Depth of infarction in the wall of the ventricle. Subendocardial, intramural, and subepicardial injuries are only in one layer. Transmural infarction extends through all three layers.

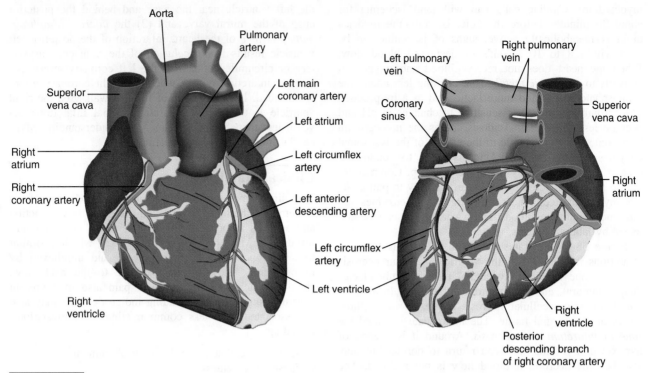

FIGURE 58–2 Areas of the myocardium affected by arterial insufficiency of specific coronary arteries.

LABORATORY TESTS

Laboratory findings include elevated levels of serum creatine kinase (CK)–MB isoenzyme, myoglobin, cardiac troponin T, and cardiac troponin I. Historically, elevations in lactate dehydrogenase (LDH) M1 isoenzyme, serum aspartate transaminase (AST), and leukocytosis (increased leukocytes), and erythrocyte sedimentation rate (ESR) have aided in the diagnosis of acute MI.

CK-MB. Serum levels of CK-MB (an isoenzyme of CK found primarily in cardiac muscle) increase 3 to 6 hours after the onset of chest pain, peak in 12 to 18 hours, and return to normal levels in 3 to 4 days.

MYOGLOBIN. Myoglobin is a heme protein found in striated muscle fibers. Myoglobin is rapidly released when myocardial muscle tissue is damaged. Because of the rapid release, it can be detected within 2 hours after an acute MI. Although many other factors can raise the serum myoglobin level, (strenuous exercise, heavy ethanol use), myoglobin is a highly sensitive indicator of acute MI if serum levels double when a second sample is drawn within 2 hours of the first. Conversely, it is reliable to exclude the diagnosis of acute MI if the levels do not increase every 2 hours. The diagnostic window ends 24 hours after an acute MI.[22]

TROPONIN. The cardiac troponin complex is a basic component of the myocardium that is involved in the contraction of the myocardial muscle. Cardiac troponin T and I are more sensitive to cardiac muscle damage than cardiac troponin C.

Cardiac *troponin T* is similar to CK-MB as far as sensitivity, and levels increase within 3 to 6 hours after pain has started. Levels remain elevated for 14 to 21 days.[16] This is useful (and more accurate than LDH) in confirmation of distant acute MI.[16] Because of equipment and professional interpretation of research findings, there is a lack of standardization for reference levels of cardiac troponin C.[22]

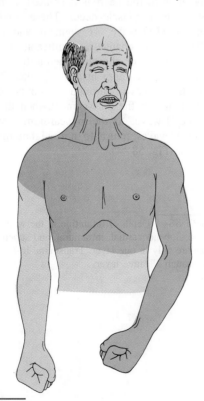

FIGURE 58–3 Possible extent of pain resulting from a myocardial infarction.

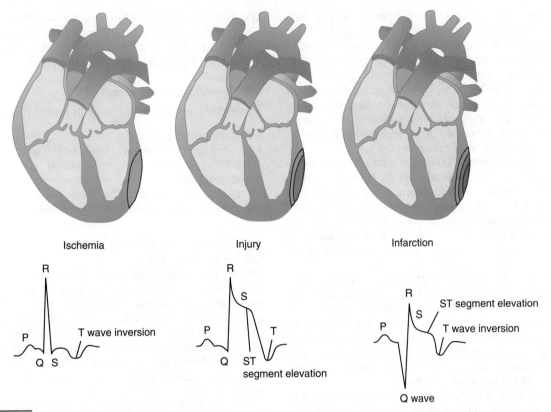

FIGURE 58–4 Zones of hypoxic injury, zone of infarction, and zone of necrosis and the electrocardiographic patterns accompanying these changes during myocardial infarction.

Cardiac *troponin I* levels rise 7 to 14 hours after an acute MI. It is a very specific and sensitive indicator of acute MI and is not affected by any other disease or injury except cardiac muscle.[22] Like cardiac troponin C, it lacks a standardization for reference. Elevation persists for 5 to 7 days.

LDH. The LDH_1 subunit is plentiful in heart muscle and is released into the serum when myocardial damage occurs. Serum levels of LDH elevate 14 to 24 hours after onset of myocardial damage, peak within 48 to 72 hours, and slowly return to normal over the next 7 to 14 days. Figure 58–5 illustrates the pattern of enzyme changes after MI.

AST. Serum levels of AST rise within several hours after the onset of chest pain, peak within 12 to 18 hours, and return to normal within 3 to 4 days.

LEUKOCYTOSIS. Leukocytosis (10,000 to 20,000 mm^3) appears on the second day after an MI and disappears in 1 week.

IMAGING STUDIES

Radionuclide imaging studies provide information on the presence of coronary artery disease as well as the location of ischemic and infarcted tissue. Cardiac imaging studies have been used to provide information for triage decisions and the management of clients who present to the emergency department with acute chest pain.[33]

When a client experiences acute chest pain, perfusion imaging with agents such as thallium, sestamibi, and teboroxime can be used to identify ischemic and infarcted tissue. Perfusion imaging is sometimes called "cold spot" imaging because the radioisotope in the bloodstream is not taken up by ischemic or infarcted tissue.

Infarct, or "hot spot" imaging, is useful in confirming

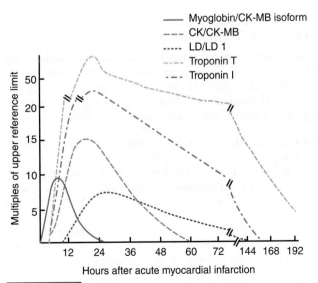

FIGURE 58–5 Isoenzyme alterations in acute myocardial infarction. (From Wong, S. S. [1996.] Strategic ultilization of cardiac markers for the diagnosis of acute myocardial infarction. *Annals of Clinical Laboratory Science, 26,* 301–312. Copyright 1996 by the Institute for Clinical Science, Inc.)

MI in clients who present to the hospital several days after MI. Technetium 99m–tagged pyrophosphate binds with calcium in areas of myocardial necrosis. Areas of uptake (hot spots) seen on nuclear imaging indicate areas of infarction. Because this test does not give positive results for 24 hours however, it cannot be used to identify an acute, early-stage MI. Radiolabeled antimyosin is also used for hot spot imaging, but its diagnostic value is limited because it cannot differentiate between a new infarct and a scar from an earlier infarct.[15]

POSITRON EMISSION TOMOGRAPHY. Positron emission tomography (PET) is used to evaluate cardiac metabolism and to assess tissue perfusion. It can also be used to detect CHD, assess coronary artery flow reserve, measure absolute myocardial blood flow, detect MI, and differentiate ischemic from non-ischemic cardiomyopathy. It may also be used to assess myocardial viability to determine which clients can benefit from CABG.

MAGNETIC RESONANCE IMAGING. Magnetic resonance imaging (MRI) helps to identify the site and extent of an MI, to assess the effects of reperfusion therapy, and to differentiate reversible and irreversible tissue injury. Its use as a diagnostic tool for coronary artery disease is increasing, although MRI cannot be used in clients with implanted metallic devices, such as pacemakers or defibrillators.[37] MRI is discussed in Chapter 11.

ECHOCARDIOGRAPHY. Echocardiography is useful in assessing the ability of the heart walls to contract and relax. The transducer is placed on the chest, and images are relayed to a monitor screen. Wall motion is abnormal in ischemic or infarcted areas.[5]

TRANSESOPHAGEAL ECHOCARDIOGRAPHY. Transesophageal echocardiography (TEE) is an imaging technique in which the transducer is placed against the wall of the esophagus. The image of the myocardium is clearer when the esophageal site is used because no air is between the transducer and the heart. This technique is particularly useful for viewing the posterior wall of the heart.[5]

Outcome Management

Since the advent of coronary care units and devices that aid in promptly recognizing and treating life-threatening dysrhythmias, 70% to 80% of people experiencing an acute MI survive the initial attack. Chances for survival greatly diminish with the presence of the following:

- Old age (clients 80 years or older have a 60% mortality rate)
- Evidence of other cardiovascular disease, respiratory disease, or uncontrolled diabetes mellitus (concomitant angina or previous MI carries a mortality rate above 30%)
- Anterior location of MI (about a 30% mortality rate)
- Hypotension (systolic blood pressure of <55 mm Hg on admission betokens a 60% mortality rate)

Deaths generally result from severe dysrhythmias, cardiogenic shock, heart failure, rupture of the heart, and recurrent MI.

Clients fortunate enough to avoid complications after MI still require 6 to 12 weeks for complete recovery. Unfortunately, however, 50% of those who completely recover from their first coronary die within 5 years; 75% die within 10 years from massive infarctions.

▆ Medical Management

Major goals of care for clients with acute MI are:

- Initiating prompt care
- Delivering successful treatment for the acute attack and prompt reperfusion of the myocardium
- Reducing pain
- Preventing complications and heart failure
- Rehabilitating and educating the client and significant others

TREAT THE ACUTE ATTACK
Give Immediate Care

Clients with manifestations of MI must receive immediate treatment. Delay may increase damage to the heart and reduce the chance of survival. Most communities have an emergency medical system (EMS) that responds quickly (call 9-1-1). Until EMS personnel arrive, keep the client quiet and calm. It is recommended that, if conscious, a client chew an aspirin with the onset of manifestations, because mortality is reduced 23% with this action alone.[11]

Elevate the head and loosen any tight clothing around the neck. Once EMS workers arrive, the client is assessed and transported quickly to an emergency department. The client is given oxygen; an intravenous (IV) line is inserted, and the client is connected to a heart monitor. Clients who become unconscious before reaching the emergency department may require cardiopulmonary resuscitation (CPR).

Many people who experience manifestations of MI delay calling for help because they misinterpret what they are sensing. Their expectations of what an acute MI should "feel like" and their experience are not the same.[44] Many studies have documented an average client delay time that exceeded 7 hours.[44] In women, this delay may even be longer.[40] Community education to "call first, call fast" is important.

The client experiencing an acute MI needs immediate admission to a hospital with a coronary care unit if possible. The first 24 hours after an MI is the time of highest risk for sudden death. There is a significant benefit if treatment is administered within the first 12 hours of onset of manifestations.[18] The first 6 hours after the onset of pain is the crucial time frame for salvage of the myocardium. Because of this, efforts have been made to decrease the time for initial treatment. In 1994, the National Heart Attack Alert Program recommended that all emergency departments treat acute MI clients within 30 minutes of presenting to the hospital. The mnemonic *4D*'s (*d*oor, *d*ata, *d*ecision, and *d*rug), along with treatment algorithms, has been adopted by many emergency departments to treat those with acute MI.

Reduce Pain

Upon admission, the client who complains of chest pain is admitted to the emergency department, given oxygen therapy, and placed on ECG monitoring. An IV line is placed, serum cardiac markers are drawn, and a 12-lead ECG is undertaken. Pain control is a priority, usually with IV morphine. Continued pain is a manifestation of myocardial ischemia. Pain also stimulates the autonomic nervous system and increases preload, which in turn increases myocardial oxygen demand. Oxygen is used to treat tissue hypoxia. Because dysrhythmias are common, ECG monitoring is essential and antidysrhythmic medications should be at hand. A two-dimensional echocardiogram and full exercise stress test may be performed in the emergency department to aid in ruling in or ruling out an acute MI.

Improve Perfusion

The general principles of pharmacologic treatment of acute MI consist of anti-ischemic and antithrombotic therapies.[39] The actions, side effects, and nursing implications of drugs used to treat acute MI are described in Table 58-2. Anti-ischemic therapy usually consists of beta blockade and IV nitroglycerin.

Antithrombotic therapy and the combination of different antithrombotic agents are being studied widely. Antithrombotic therapy is usually initiated with the administration of an aspirin if the client has not taken one before reaching the emergency department. Heparin therapy is the next step.

Clinicians treat acute MI with medications that lyse (dissolve) the clot that forms part of the blockage of the coronary artery. Thrombolytic therapy includes streptokinase, urokinase, tissue-type plasminogen activator (t-PA), anisoylated plasminogen-streptokinase activator complex (anistreplase, APSAC), alteplase, urokinase plasminogen activator, and the newest, reteplase. For best efficacy, thrombolytic agents must be given within 6 hours, (preferably 3 hours) after the onset of chest pain. The choice of thrombolytic agent is not as important as the speed with which it is given.[18] After the thrombolytic agent is administered, IV heparin or a glycoprotein IIB/IIIA is usually continued. All of these thrombolytic agents can be given intravenously. See Understanding Myocardial Infarction and Its Treatment (p. 1586).

Not all clients with MI are suitable candidates for thrombolytic therapy. History of recent cerebral vascular accident, surgery, pregnancy or use of anticoagulants would contraindicate thrombolytic therapy. Complications of thrombolytics include bleeding, allergic reactions, and stroke. Successful reperfusion of the coronary arteries is evidenced by (1) return of ECG changes to normal; (2) relief of chest pain; (3) presence of reperfusion dysrhythmias, usually sudden onset of frequent premature ventricular contractions (PVCs) or short runs of PVCs; and (4) a rapid, early peak of the CK-MB isoenzyme ("washout"). If reperfusion is not attained or if the client is not a candidate for thrombolytic therapy, then primary angioplasty, stenting, or CABG may be performed. Interventional cardiology procedures and bypass surgery are discussed in Chapter 56.

Antidysrhythmic agents are initiated. Some clinicians begin angiotensin-converting enzyme (ACE) inhibitors within 72 hours of onset because ventricular remodeling starts at that time.[21] Stool softeners are used to relieve constipation and to lower the risk of bradycardia from straining that stimulates the vagus nerve.

Monitor for Complications

The possibility of death from complications always accompanies an acute MI. Thus, prime collaborative goals include the prevention of life-threatening complications or at least recognition of them.

DYSRHYTHMIAS. Dysrhythmias are the major cause of death after an MI (40% to 50% of deaths). Ectopic rhythms arise in or near the borders of intensely ischemic and damaged myocardial tissues. Damaged myocardium may also interfere with the conduction system, causing dissociation of the atria and ventricles (*heart block*). Supraventricular tachycardia (SVT) sometimes occurs as a result of heart failure. Spontaneous or pharmacologic reperfusion of a previously ischemic area may also precipitate ventricular dysrhythmias.

Provide continuous cardiac monitoring and frequent counts of PVCs (many monitoring systems count continuously). Notify the physician if more than six PVCs occur per minute and the client is symptomatic (e.g., hypotension, chest pain). For *dysrhythmias*, provide prompt intervention per protocol or orders. For new-onset, symptomatic *ventricular ectopy* (runs, couplets, salvos), administer lidocaine per order. For *ventricular tachycardia,* administer lidocaine, procainamide, or bretylium or provide elective cardioversion. For *ventricular fibrillation,* provide immediate defibrillation. For *SVT,* administer a vagal maneuver, adenosine, verapamil, or lidocaine, and provide elective cardioversion. For *heart block,* administer atropine or isoproterenol (with caution) and use a temporary pacemaker.[26] Dysrhythmias are discussed in Chapter 57.

CARDIOGENIC SHOCK. Cardiogenic shock accounts for only 9% of deaths from MI, but an estimated 80% of clients who develop shock die from it. Causes include decreased (1) myocardial contraction with diminished cardiac output, (2) undetected dysrhythmias, and (3) sepsis.

Clinical manifestations include systolic blood pressure significantly below the client's normal range; diaphoresis; rapid pulse; restlessness; cold, clammy skin; and grayish skin color.

Shock can be prevented with rapid relief of pain and sufficient IV fluids to prevent circulatory collapse. It is also vital to identify dysrhythmias rapidly.

Administer vasopressors (norepinephrine, dopamine, dobutamine, metaraminol [Aramine]) as prescribed, to raise blood pressure by increasing peripheral resistance. In other cases, vasodilators (nitroprusside) promote better blood flow in the microcirculation. Positive inotropic agents (dobutamine, epinephrine, isoproterenol) increase cardiac contractility and cardiac output and improve tissue perfusion. Administer oxygen therapy and antidysrhythmic agents as prescribed, and continuously monitor arterial and pulmonary artery pressures.[26] Chapter 81 explains shock in detail.

HEART FAILURE AND PULMONARY EDEMA. The most common cause of in-hospital death in clients with cardiac disorders is heart failure. Heart failure disables

Class	Example	Assessment of Therapeutic Responses	Assessment of Adverse Responses	Nursing Implications
Antiplatelet aggregating agent	Acetylsalicylic acid (ASA)	ASA blocks prostaglandin synthesis action, which prevents formation of the platelet aggregating substance thromboxane A_2. Clinically, this limits formation or progression of a thrombus and decreases mortality.*	The client may experience heartburn, stomach pains, nausea and vomiting, rash, weakness, hemolytic anemia, and GI ulceration. Overdose manifestations include tinnitus, headache, dizziness, confusion, and metabolic acidosis.	Avoid use in clients with severe renal or liver disease. Monitor serum concentrations, renal function, hearing changes, skin inflammation, and for abnormal bleeding. Administer with food or large quantities of water to decrease GI upset. Instruct client to avoid concurrent use of over-the-counter products containing ASA.
Indirect thrombin inhibitor	Heparin	Heparin increases ability of antithrombin to inactivate circulating thrombin, limiting formation or progression of a thrombus. Clinically, this is seen as a more patent coronary vessel, with resolving ST segments, decreased angina, and lower mortality.†	The client is at risk for bleeding. Monitor for manifestations of occult and overt bleeding. The client may also experience rash or urticaria. Once medication is discontinued, the client is at risk for "rebound" ischemia.	Assess client for manifestations of bleeding or bruising. Monitor ST segments. Monitor aPTT levels during therapy. Protamine sulfate is the antidote for heparin. Many drugs can increase the risk of bleeding if used concurrently with heparin.
Glycoprotein IIB/IIIA receptor antagonists	Abciximab	After atherosclerotic plaque ruptures, platelets attach. Glycoprotein receptor agonists do not allow platelet to become activated, which does not allow fibrinogen to attach to platelet. These actions do not allow further platelet aggregation. Clinically, this is depicted as a more patent coronary vessel, with a decrease in chest pain, resolving ST segments, and a lower mortality.†‡§	Severe bleeding may occur, which rapid transfusion of platelets reverses. Ventricular dysrhythmias, pulmonary emboli, hypotension, and bradycardia may occur.	Assess the client for manifestations of occult and overt bleeding. Monitor platelets while the client is on therapy. Monitor ST segments and chest pain.
Thrombolytic agents	Reteplase	By converting plasminogen to plasmin, the fibrin strands that hold thrombus together are broken down, hence destroying the thrombus. Clinically, this is seen as a decrease in angina, resolving ST segments, and decreased mortality. Long-term effects include preserved ventricular function and reduced incidence of heart failure.†	Clients may experience bleeding, ventricular fibrillation, reperfusion dysrhythmias, and cardiac arrest.	Client must be on cardiac monitor during infusion. Anticipate dysrhythmias, and have appropriate medications on hand. Observe for bleeding. Assess for reduction of chest pain and resolving ST segment elevation. Clients are not candidates for therapy if they have had recent surgery, CVA, or GI bleeding or are currently receiving warfarin or are pregnant. Start treatment as soon as possible for best results.¶

aPTT, activated partial thromboplastin time; CVA, cerebrovascular accident; GI, gastrointestinal.
*See Feldman, M., & Cryer, B. (1999). Aspirin absorption rates and platelet inhibition times with 325-mg buffered aspirin tablets (chewed or swallowed intact) and with buffered aspirin solution. *American Journal of Cardiology*, 84, 404–409.
†See Dracup, K., & Cannon, C. (1999). Combination treatment strategies for management of acute myocardial infarction. *Critical Care Nurse Supplement*, 1–17.
‡See Gensini, G., Comeglio, M., & Falai, M. (1999). Advances in antithrombotic therapy of acute myocardial infarction. *American Heart Journal*, 138(2), S171–S176.
§See Verheugt, F. (1999). What an interventional cardiologist should know about the pharmacological treatment of acute myocardial infarction. *Seminars in Interventional Cardiology*, 4, 17–20.
¶See Kosnik, L. (1999, October). Treatment protocols and pathways: Improving the process of care. *Critical Care Nurse Supplement*, 3–7.

CASE MANAGEMENT

Acute Myocardial Infarction

Clients who have had an acute myocardial infarction (MI) have experienced a serious, life-threatening event. Case management involves prevention of complications, education regarding current treatment plans and rehabilitation, and lifestyle modification. Ideally, modifiable risk factors for coronary artery disease (smoking, hypertension, high cholesterol levels, sedentary lifestyle) should be reduced before MI occurs. The client with an uncomplicated MI usually has a 4-day length of stay with interventions such as angioplasty or stenting during the same admission. The needs of each client vary according to the type, extent, and prognosis as well as age, comorbidities, and plans for intervention.

Assess

- What type of MI has been sustained?
- What should you expect based on the pathophysiology involved (e.g., dysrhythmia, conduction disturbances)?
- Has this client had a previous MI; was there a particular precipitating cause?
- Is unstable angina (pain) part of the clinical picture?
- What other diagnoses might worsen or make it difficult to control this condition (hypertension, heart failure, anemia, diabetes, hyperthyroidism, cardiomyopathy, emotional distress)?
- What were the presenting manifestations, and how long did the client wait before seeking assistance?
- What is the client's pain level? Has pain been relieved?

Advocate

Even if the client has had angina in the past, having a heart attack is an unexpected event that causes anxiety and fear. Being connected to various monitoring devices with warning alarms, being in a special unit with unknown schedules or procedures, and having to make decisions about unfamiliar tests or treatments all contribute to feelings of powerlessness and anxiety. What is routine for the nurse is not routine for the client.

Try to explain tests and procedures thoroughly to the client and family members. Many hospitals have developed educational materials or clinical pathways that may assist. Address difficult questions, such as advanced directives and wishes for resuscitation.

If an emergency occurs, try to remain calm and focused on the situation. Be honest with family members and clients. As recovery progresses, clients may have questions about resuming work or sexual activity. Work with the client and physician to obtain answers and alleviate fear.

Prevent Readmission

As you administer medication, start teaching the name, purpose, and side effects of each medication. If nitroglycerin is prescribed, explain correct use (including prophylactic administration) and storage.

Discuss the factors that caused the need for hospital admission and how the client might prevent future problems by modifying lifestyle or diet; be aware of ethnic or cultural preferences.

Consider appropriate referrals for home care, cardiac rehabilitation or exercise programs, smoking cessation, nutritional counseling, and emergency response systems.

Make sure the client knows how to obtain emergency help, when to call the physician, and the time and date of the first follow-up appointment.

Encourage family members to learn cardiopulmonary resuscitation and to become aware of their own cardiovascular risks.

Investigate support groups and other community resources available through specific institutions, insurers, or the American Heart Association.

Cheryl Noetscher, RN, MS, Director of Case Management, Crouse Hospital and Community–General Hospital, Syracuse, New York

---

20% of clients who experience an MI and is responsible for one third of deaths after an MI.

Heart failure may develop at the onset of the infarction or may occur weeks later. Clinical manifestations include dyspnea, orthopnea, weight gain, edema, enlarged tender liver, distended neck veins, and crackles. It is managed by correcting the underlying cause, relieving clinical manifestations, and enhancing cardiac pump performance.[23, 24, 30] Heart failure is discussed in Chapter 56. The Case Study presents a scenario involving cardiogenic shock, tachycardia, and heart failure.

PULMONARY EMBOLISM. Pulmonary embolism (PE) may develop secondary to phlebitis of the leg or pelvic veins (venous thrombosis) or from atrial flutter or fibrillation. PE occurs in 10% to 20% of clients at some point, during either the acute attack or convalescence. PE is discussed in Chapter 62.

RECURRENT MYOCARDIAL INFARCTION. Within 6 years after an initial MI, 21% of men and 33% of women may experience recurrent MI.[2] Possible causes include overexertion, embolization, and further thrombotic occlusion of a coronary artery by an atheroma. The clinical manifestation is the return of angina. Management is the same as for acute MI.

COMPLICATIONS CAUSED BY MYOCARDIAL NECROSIS. Complications that are due to necrosis of the myocardium include ventricular aneurysm, rupture of the heart (*myocardial rupture*), ventricular septal defect (VSD), and ruptured papillary muscle. These complications are infrequent but serious, usually occurring about 5 to 7 days after MI.[19] Weak, friable necrotic myocardial tissue increases vulnerability to these complications (Fig. 58–6).

Text continued on page 1596

Cardiogenic Shock, Tachycardia, and Heart Failure

Mr. Borg is a 70-year-old retired African American man who was admitted to the ED after arriving by rescue squad. According to his wife, he had been vomiting and experiencing progressive weakness earlier in the day. When the rescue squad arrived at his home, he was in supraventricular tachycardia with a rate over 180 BPM. The squad administered adenosine (Adenocard) 6 mg IV, followed by an additional 12 mg 3 minutes later.

Mr. Borg denied the presence of chest pain or shortness of breath upon admission to the ED. He was cyanotic with no palpable blood pressure and a regular heart rate of 160 BPM. A bolus of diltiazem (Cardizem) 10 mg was administered IV push and normal sinus rhythm was briefly restored. When supraventricular tachycardia returned, a diltiazem drip was initiated. Blood gases drawn in the ED showed a pH of 7.3 and a $PaCO_2$ of 55 mm Hg. Mr. Borg was transferred to the ICU with the diltiazem drip and oxygen at 4 L per nasal cannula.

In the ICU, Mr. Borg's hypotension and tachycardia persisted and a low-dose dopamine drip was initiated at 2 μg/kg/min. Mr. Borg became more hypotensive, tachycardic, and hypoxic. He was then intubated and placed on a ventilator with 100% oxygen. A Swan-Ganz catheter was placed, and his initial PAWP was 30 mm Hg. Furosemide (Lasix) 80 mg and procainamide (Pronestyl) 500 mg IV bolus were administered. A 2 mg/min IV drip of procainamide was continued, and the diltiazem drip was discontinued.

The next morning, Mr. Borg was no longer acidotic, with a pH of 7.36. His heart rate was 140 BPM, and systolic BP was around 100 mm Hg while he was receiving 9 μg/kg/min of dopamine. The ECG revealed that the distal two thirds of the left ventricle was akinetic. Admission and follow-up CPK levels were within normal limits, which indicates that Mr. Borg had an extensive anterior myocardial infarction at an earlier date. Mr. Borg is scheduled to have a right and left heart catheterization at 1:00 PM today. Given his condition, he is not considered a candidate for percutaneous transluminal coronary angiography at this time.

Selected Laboratory Values	
RBC	4.08 million/mm³
Hb	14.2 g/dl
Hct	41.7%
WBC	20,500/mm³
Sodium	135 mEq/L
Potassium	3.3 mEq/L
Chloride	94 mEq/L
Cholesterol	264 mg/dl
Triglycerides	334 mg/dl

Nursing Admission Assessment

Mr. Borg is a former mail carrier who retired 10 years ago. He and his wife recently celebrated their 50th wedding anniversary. Their two sons live in cities 1500 miles away, and they will be flying in to visit their father as soon as possible. His wife reports that he stopped smoking 20 years ago and continues to drink two to four alcoholic beverages per day. He has gained 40 pounds during the past 10 years. His wife is concerned that he eats and drinks too much and that he spends most of the day sitting in front of the television. Mr. Borg's wife also reports that he has been taking benazepril (Lotensin) 10 mg/day.

Nursing Physical Examination

Height: 5'11" Weight: 210 pounds (95.45 kg)
Vital signs: BP = 90/40; TPR = 101, 135, 20

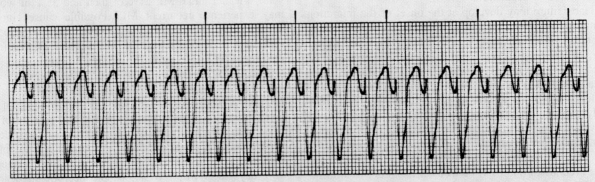

● When the rescue squad arrived at Mr. Borg's home, he was in supraventricular tachycardia, with a rate of more than 180 BPM.

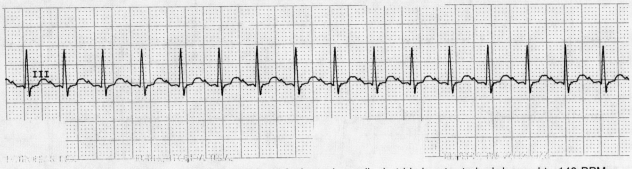

● After initial treatment, Mr. Borg was still in supraventricular tachycardia, but his heart rate had dropped to 140 BPM.

LOC: Sedated and intubated

EENT: Within normal limits

Cardiac: S$_1$, S$_2$ audible without murmur, questionable S$_3$ regular rate, unable to assess neck vein distention

Pulmonary: Rhonchi present throughout lungs with fine basilar rales bilaterally

Abdominal: Within normal limits

Genitourinary: Foley catheter in place draining clear yellow urine.

Peripheral pulses: 1/1 with 1+ pitting edema which extends to midcalf

Current Treatment Plan

Meds: Dopamine 1600 mg in 500 ml D$_5$W; titrate to keep systolic BP >90 mm Hg

Furosemide 40 mg IV tid

Potassium 40 mEq in 100 ml D$_5$W over 4 hr bid

Thiamine 100 mg IM qd

MVI 1 ampule IV qd

Methylprednisolone (Solu-Medrol) 100 mg IV q 8 hr

Ceftriaxone (Rocephin) 1 g q 12 hr IV

Saline lock as needed for medications, flush bid, prn

Diet: NPO

Activity: Bed rest

Respiratory treatments: 70% FIO$_2$, IMV = 10, tidal volume = 750 ml with 5 cm PEEP

Diagnostic tests: Repeat chest x-ray, ECG, CBC, metabolic profile, cardiac enzymes this AM

The results of the cardiac catheterization reveal 100% occlusion of the left coronary artery and severe diffuse disease of the left anterior descending coronary artery. The physicians have determined that the client is a poor surgical risk and plan to treat him medically. Mr. Borg has interpreted this as an indication that his problem is temporary and states, "You can't keep a good man down."

Over the next several days, Mr. Borg's BP stabilizes and he is weaned from the dopamine. Furosemide is changed to an oral dose, and potassium dosage is reduced to 10 mEq PO tid. IV procainamide is discontinued after

oral procainamide (Procan SR) is initiated at 250 mg bid. Mr. Borg is given digitalis and will be maintained on digoxin 0.25 mg qd. His resting heart rate has been approximately 70 BPM. A nitroglycerin (Nitro-Dur) patch is ordered daily to be applied in the morning and removed at bedtime. Mr. Borg is also extubated and placed on a no-added-salt, low-fat diet. He is to begin a cardiac rehabilitation program. The physician is planning to discharge him tomorrow after a recovery treadmill test.

Discharge Criteria

Average length of stay: 5.4 days

Cardiac rehabilitation initiated and follow-up appointments scheduled (includes diet, exercise, stress management, and medication teaching)

Questions to Be Considered

1. Compare and contrast left versus right ventricular, backward versus forward, and high-output versus low-output heart failure. Given the information provided, how would you categorize Mr. Borg's heart failure?

2. Compare and contrast the effects of Mr. Borg's cardiac medications: dopamine, diltiazem, adenosine, procainamide, digoxin, nitroglycerin. Why are the furosemide and potassium ordered?

3. What ramifications does Mr. Borg's lifestyle have on the success of his cardiac rehabilitation program? How might a home health nurse facilitate Mrs. Borg's participation in his rehabilitation program?

4. Eight weeks after discharge, Mr. Borg asks the cardiac rehabilitation nurse if new lights have been installed because "they all have a yellow ring round them and the edges are fuzzy." Upon further investigation the nurse determines that Mr. Borg has also had a decreased appetite, intermittent nausea and vomiting, and decreased ability to complete his entire exercise protocol. What should the nurse suspect? What recommendations should she make?

5. Six months after discharge, the physician resumes Mr. Borg's medication orders for benazepril 10 mg PO qd. Describe the pharmacodynamics of this drug and how it compares with furosemide.

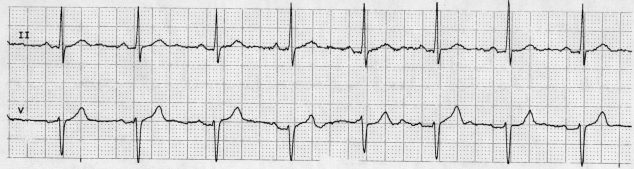

● After several days of treatment, Mr. Borg is in normal sinus rhythm, with a resting heart rate of approximately 70 BPM.

ABG, arterial blood gas; BP, blood pressure; BPM, beats per minute; CBC, complete blood count; CPK, creatine phosphokinase; D_5W, 5% dextrose in water; ECG, electrocardiogram; ED, emergency department; EENT, eyes-ears-nose-throat; Hb, hemoglobin; Hct, hematocrit; ICU, intensive care unit; IMV, intermittent mechanical ventilation; IV, intravenous; LOC, loss of consciousness; PEEP, positive end-expiratory pressure; PAWP, pulmonary artery wedge pressure; PO, by mouth; RBC, red blood cell; TPR, temperature, pulse, respirations; WBC, white blood cell.

Manifestations of heart failure develop with ventricular aneurysm, rupture of the ventricular septum, and rupture of the papillary muscle. Manifestations of severe mitral insufficiency often develop when the papillary muscle of the left ventricle ruptures. Ventricular dysrhythmias (e.g., frequent PVCs and ventricular tachycardia) occur often in the presence of a ventricular aneurysm (the necrotic tissue is very irritable). Manifestations of cardiac tamponade develop with rupture of the heart.

The goal of treatment is to decrease the workload of the heart and increase the oxygen supply to keep the area of infarction and necrotic tissue as small as possible.

Surgery is performed to (1) excise the ventricular aneurysm, (2) replace the mitral valve if the papillary muscle is ruptured, or (3) repair the VSD. Pericardiocentesis and immediate surgery help relieve cardiac tamponade that occurs after rupture of the heart.

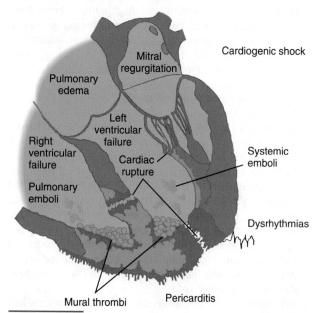

FIGURE 58–6 Major complications of acute myocardial infarction. (From O'Rourke, R. A. [1982]. The bedside diagnosis of the complications of myocardial infarction. In R. S. Eliot [Ed.], *Cardiac emergencies*. Mount Kisco, NY: Futura Publishing.)

PERICARDITIS. Up to 28% of clients with an acute transmural MI develop early pericarditis (within 2 to 4 days). The inflamed area of the infarction rubs against the pericardial surface and causes it to lose its lubricating fluid. A pericardial friction rub can be auscultated across the precordium. The client complains that chest pain is worse with movement, deep inspiration, and cough. The pain of pericarditis is relieved by sitting up and leaning forward.

Frequent assessment may lead to early identification and intervention. Relieve pain with analgesics, such as acetaminophen, nonsteroidal anti-inflammatory drugs (NSAIDs), or other anti-inflammatory agents. Reduce the client's anxiety by differentiating the pain of pericarditis from the pain of MI.

DRESSLER'S SYNDROME (LATE PERICARDITIS). Dressler's syndrome, a form of pericarditis, can occur as late as 6 weeks to months after an MI. Although the etiologic agent is unknown, an autoimmune cause is suggested. The client usually presents with a fever lasting 1 week or longer, pericardial chest pain, pericardial friction rub, and occasionally pleuritis with pleural effusions. This is a self-limiting phenomenon, and no prevention is known. Treatment includes aspirin, prednisone, and narcotic analgesics for pain. Anticoagulation therapy may precipitate cardiac tamponade and should be avoided in these clients.

REHABILITATION AND EDUCATION
Strengthen the Myocardium

A successful rehabilitation program begins the moment the client enters the coronary care unit for emergency care and continues for months and even years after discharge from the health care facility.[1] The overall goal of rehabilitation is to help the client live as full, vital, and productive a life as possible while remaining within the limits of the heart's ability to respond to increases in activity and stress. Six important subgoals of the rehabilitation process are as follows:

- Developing a program of progressive physical activity
- Educating the client and significant others about the cause, prevention, and treatment of CHD
- Helping the client accept the limitations imposed by illness

- Aiding the client in adjusting to changes in occupational goals
- Lessening the exposure to risk factors
- Changing the psychosocial factors adversely affecting recovery from CHD.[42, 43]

Cardiac rehabilitation is a comprehensive, long-term program that involves periodic medical evaluation, prescribed exercises, and education and counseling about cardiac risk factor modification.[42] Cardiac rehabilitation is a multifactorial program that begins when the client is still hospitalized and continues throughout recovery. Cardiac rehabilitation consists of four phases[1]:

- Phase 1 (inpatient)
- Phase II (immediate outpatient)
- Phase III (intermediate outpatient)
- Phase IV (maintenance outpatient)

Phase I (Inpatient)

Phase I begins with admission to the coronary care unit. After an MI, clients usually remain on bed rest for less than 24 hours unless complications such as heart failure or dysrhythmias develop. Although the myocardium must rest, bed rest puts the client at risk for hypovolemia, hypoxemia, muscle atrophy, and pulmonary embolus. Thus, the client must avoid both invalidism and reckless overexertion.

Provide complete bed rest for the first day or so with use of a bedside commode for bowel movements. Most clients receive a 2-g sodium diet. If the client is nauseated, provide a clear liquid diet until nausea subsides. A coronary care nurse or physiotherapist should start passive exercises. As the client regains strength, have the client sit for brief periods on the side of the bed and dangle the feet. Allow the client to ambulate to a bedside chair for 15 to 20 minutes after the first day if dangling has been tolerated. When the client is transferred from the coronary care unit to an intermediate or regular unit, bathroom privileges and self-care activities are encouraged. Wireless heart monitoring (telemetry) may continue. Allow brief walks in the hall with supervision. The length and duration of these walks are increased progressively, working up to 5 to 10 minutes according to the client's endurance.[6]

The client loses 10% to 15% of skeletal muscle and contractile strength within the first week of bed rest and 20% to 25% after 3 weeks of bed rest. The client must increase activities gradually to avoid overtaxing the heart as it pumps oxygenated blood to the muscles. The metabolic equivalent test (MET) provides one way of measuring the amount of oxygen needed to perform an activity:

$$1 \text{ MET} = 3.5 \text{ ml O}_2/\text{kg/min}$$

One MET is about equivalent to the oxygen uptake a client requires when resting. Early mobilization activities after an acute MI should not exceed 1 to 2 METs, as from shaving, washing, and self-feeding. (Later activities can increase to 10 or 11 METs, such as cycling or running.)

With each activity level increase, monitor the heart rate, blood pressure, and fatigue level, adjusting the client's activity level accordingly. During early activities, the heart rate should not rise more than 25% above resting level. Blood pressure must not rise more than 25 mm Hg above normal.[1]

Help the client avoid fatigue. Dyspnea, chest pain, tachycardia, and a sense of exhaustion warn that the client is attempting to do too much. Instruct the client regarding these warning signs of overexertion.

During phase I, client education should include cardiac anatomy and physiology risk factors and management of CHD, behavioral counseling, and home activities.

Phase II (Immediate Outpatient)

If no complications arise, the physician discharges the client to the home by the end of the second week. Nearly 50% of clients after an acute MI have an uncomplicated hospital course without evidence of angina, heart failure, or major dysrhythmias. There is a growing trend toward early discharge of clients with uncomplicated MI. A team at one health care facility discharges post-MI clients at the end of the 4th day but allows clients to go home early only if the household has adequate help and is conducive to rest. Such clients are followed up carefully by trained nurse-clinicians who visit the home and supervise physiologic status, exercise, and diet every other day. Researchers hope that earlier discharge after MI reduces depression as well as hospital expenses. The Bridge to Home Health Care provides suggestions for helping the client to adjust to convalescence at home.

Resuming sexual activity may be one of the most difficult aspects of returning to normal life after an MI. One study reports that more than 50% of a group of women had fear of resuming sexual activity after MI (44% of their partners reported similar concerns). Sexual intercourse may resume 4 to 8 weeks after MI if the physician agrees. The client should be able to climb two flights of stairs before resuming sexual activity. Caution clients not to eat or drink alcoholic beverages immediately before intercourse. Taking nitroglycerin before intercourse may help prevent exertional angina.[20, 32]

Advise the client to stop smoking. Encourage frequent walks, but warn against strenuous activities, such as shoveling snow. The walking program aims for a goal of 2 miles in less than 60 minutes.

A monitored group program may help the client achieve the best possible physical conditioning. These programs typically last from 10 to 12 weeks and are implemented in a supervised setting. They offer various training devices, such as treadmills, stationary bicycles, and rowing machines, to facilitate fitness. During phase II, the client performs large-muscle exercises for at least 20 to 30 minutes three or four times a week. In addition, clients are trained in warm-up and stretching exercises.[1, 6, 42] During the sessions, cardiac rehabilitation staff monitor cardiac rhythm, heart rate, and blood pressure before exercise, at peak exercise, and during recovery. Clients also report their level of perceived exertion several times during the exercise session.

Some clients may be able to return to work at the end of 8 or 9 weeks if they remain asymptomatic. Clients with less physically strenuous jobs can sometimes resume a full-time schedule, but manual laborers may have to work part time or find less taxing work. Occupational evaluations can be done to assess cardiac impairment in relation to job requirements and client skills.[41]

Between the 8th and 10th weeks, the client requires a complete physical examination, including ECG, exercise stress tests, lipid analysis, and chest x-ray study. Clini-

BRIDGE TO HOME HEALTH CARE

Heart-Healthy Living After a Myocardial Infarction

The role of the home health nurse is to help clients who had a myocardial infarction (MI) adjust to their lifestyle by teaching healthy heart living. Focus your teaching on areas that will help clients become responsible for self-care. Assume that you need to repeat health education that was provided in the hospital during the acute MI episode. When stress is high, clients usually recall little of what was taught.

Instruct the client and significant other or family member to monitor for clinical manifestations that may indicate extensions and recurrences of the MI. Clients need to report indigestion, shortness of breath, increased edema, and palpitations. Learning when to call the physician or nurse for these physical problems is very important.

Determine what your clients know about their medications. Knowing what the medication is called, its function, the schedule for taking it, and its side effects is required for client safety. Generally, multiple medications are prescribed, and you need to give the client written instructions and information about each medication. Many pharmacists provide a computer printout of medications and interactions for the client to keep. Medication planners that have compartments for various times of day allow the client to prefill medications for a week at a time and may prevent errors.

The convalescence period for the client and family creates anxiety about daily activities. Instruct the client to avoid prolonged baths or showers to prevent vasodilation. Use tepid water and a stool or bath chair in the shower. Encourage the use of energy-conservation techniques, such as keeping the arms at waist level and getting enough rest to prevent fatigue. Routine household activities and mild recreational activities, such as playing golf, are usually permitted.

Climbing more than two flights of stairs and lifting more than 20 pounds are restricted. If clients do not ask about resuming sexual relations, consider introducing the topic. They may be too timid to consult their physicians about this subject.

An appropriate unsupervised exercise is a prescribed indoor walking program. Exercising after a heavy meal or during mild illness is contraindicated. Instruct the client to begin each exercise session with a warm-up period that may last as long as 15 minutes and to end the session with a cool-down period. Walking should be constant and should last long enough to increase blood flow to the muscles.

The client or caregiver should have an emergency plan that includes having someone available to drive if a ride is needed and someone in the home who knows basic cardiopulmonary resuscitation (CPR). A personal emergency response system may be appropriate for clients who live alone. Some emergency response systems are worn around the neck, and the push of a button summons medical assistance. Caregiver stress, communication problems, and fear of the unknown are valid concerns. Community resources and additional information can be obtained by calling the American Heart Association's toll-free number, 800-242-8721.

Pamela Singh, RN-CS, MSN, FNP, *Family Nurse Practitioner, San Diego, California*

cians must correct pre-existing health problems that might have contributed to the development of CHD (e.g., hypertension, anemia, hyperthyroidism).

Recovery after an MI may be lengthy and difficult. The client may have undergone surgery or may have been managed medically. In either case, a serious threat to integrity has occurred. Initially after an MI, clients attempt to prove that they are not seriously ill. Coping strategies include denial and minimization. Some clients conceal the recurrence of chest pain. As recovery continues, clients begin to comprehend that a heart attack has really occurred, to understand why it happened, and to consider its impact on the future. Clients begin the process of life adjustment to find a lifestyle that can be tolerated and maintained while preserving a sense of self-worth. Several strategies are used to regain self-control, such as gauging progress, seeking reassurance, learning about health, and being cautious. Eventually, clients come to terms with the fact that they will not be living life to the fullest. Clients learn to accept limitations and to refocus on other aspects of life. Some clients are unable to adjust. Sometimes clients find that they have had too many setbacks and are powerless to make changes or gain control. The education and counseling that accompany a structured cardiac rehabilitation program can help to improve psychological well-being, social adjustment, and functioning.[41]

Phase III (Intermediate Outpatient)

The extended outpatient phase of cardiac rehabilitation lasts from 4 to 6 months. Exercise sessions continue to be supervised, and clients are taught how to monitor their exercise intensity by taking their pulse or, if in a walking program, by counting the number of steps they take in a 15-second interval. Clients with dysrhythmias are monitored more closely, and intermittent rhythm strips may be taken. For clients who prefer to exercise at home, clinicians trained in cardiac rehabilitation can provide detailed, written instructions for a long-term exercise program. Various methods are used to determine the appropriate exercise routines. Periodic evaluation is necessary to assess the client's endurance and tolerance to the prescribed exercise program.

Phase IV (Maintenance Outpatient)

Phase IV, the final phase of cardiac rehabilitation, usually takes place in the home or community and is unsupervised. The client maintains a program of regular exercise and other lifestyle modifications to modify cardiac risk. Clients should undergo an exercise testing and risk factor assessment annually.[6]

■ Nursing Management of the Medical Client

The goals of nursing management after an MI are as follows:

Text continued on page 1605

■ THE CLIENT WITH A MYOCARDIAL INFARCTION

Nursing Diagnosis. Pain related to myocardial ischemia resulting from coronary artery occlusion with loss or restriction of blood flow to an area of the myocardium and necrosis of the myocardium.

Outcomes. The client will experience improved comfort in the chest, as evidenced by a decrease in the rating of the chest pain, the ability to rest and sleep comfortably, less need for analgesia or nitroglycerin, and reduced tension.

Interventions

1. Assess the characteristics of chest pain, including location, duration, quality, intensity, presence of radiation, precipitating and alleviating factors, and associated manifestations. Have the client rate pain on a scale of 0 to 10, and document findings in nurses' notes.
2. Assess respirations, blood pressure, and heart rate with each episode of chest pain.

3. Obtain a 12-lead electrocardiogram (ECG) on admission, then each time chest pain recurs for evidence of further infarction.
4. Monitor the response to drug therapy. Notify the physician if pain does not abate within 15 to 20 minutes.
5. Provide care in a calm, efficient manner that will reassure the client and minimize anxiety. Stay with the client until discomfort is relieved.
6. Limit visitors as the client requests.
7. Administer morphine as ordered.

8. Administer nitrates as ordered.

Rationales

1. Pain is an indication of myocardial ischemia. Assisting the client in quantifying pain may differentiate pre-existing and current pain patterns as well as identify complications. Usually a scale of 0 to 10 is used, 10 being the worst pain and 0 being none.
2. Respirations may be increased as a result of pain and associated anxiety. Release of stress-induced catecholamines increases heart rate and blood pressure.
3. Serial ECGs and stat ECGs record changes that can give evidence of further cardiac damage and location of myocardial ischemia.
4. Pain control is a priority because it indicates ischemia.

5. External stimuli may worsen anxiety and cardiac strain and limit coping abilities.

6. Limiting visitors prevents overstimulation and promotes rest.
7. Morphine is an opiate analgesic and alters the client's perception of pain and reduces preload time vasoconstriction.
8. Nitrates relax the smooth muscles of coronary blood vessels, decreasing ischemia and hence decreasing pain.

Evaluation. The client should be pain-free within 15 to 20 minutes after administration of drug therapy. The client will verbalize relief of pain and will not exhibit associated manifestations of pain.

Nursing Diagnosis. Altered Tissue Perfusion (cardiopulmonary) related to thrombus in coronary artery, resulting in altered blood flow to myocardial tissue.

Outcomes. The client will demonstrate improved cardiac tissue perfusion, as evidenced by a decrease in the rating of pain and resolving ST segments.

Interventions

1. Keep the client on bed rest with a quiet environment.

2. Administer oxygen as ordered.
3. Administer thrombolytics as ordered.

4. Monitor ST segments.

Rationales

1. Stress activates the sympathetic nervous system and increases myocardial oxygen needs.
2. Oxygen increases myocardial supply of oxygen.
3. Thrombolytic therapy can break apart the thrombus and increase myocardial tissue perfusion.
4. ST segment elevation indicates myocardial tissue injury; ST segment depression indicates decreased myocardial perfusion.

Evaluation. The client will have a decrease in pain and a normal ST segment.

Collaborative Problem. Dysrhythmias related to electrical instability or irritability secondary to ischemia or infarcted tissue, as evidenced by an increase or decrease in heart rate, change in rhythm, and dysrhythmias.

Outcomes. The client will have no dysrhythmias, as evidenced by normal sinus rhythm or return to the client's own baseline rhythm.

Interventions

1. Teach the client and family about the need for continuous monitoring. Keep alarms on and limits set at all times.
2. Assess the apical heart rate. Auscultate for change in heart sounds (murmurs, rub, S_3, and S_4).
3. Document the rhythm strip every shift and prn (as needed) if dysrhythmias occur. Measure the pulse rate, QRS, PR, and QT segments with each strip. Note and report any deviations from the client's baseline values.

Rationales

1. Continued monitoring keeps staff aware of myocardial changes. Family anxiety is decreased.
2. The apical heart rate suggests early cardiac decompensation and potential loss of cardiac output.
3. Dysrhythmias are the most common complication after a myocardial infarction (MI).

4. Report six or more multifocal premature ventricular contractions (PVCs) per minute to the physician.

5. Give antidysrhythmic agents as ordered.
6. Monitor the effects of antidysrhythmic agents.

7. Monitor serum potassium levels.
8. Maintain a patent intravenous (IV) line or heparin lock at all times.
9. Monitor ST segments, and document changes.

4. Multifocal PVCs indicate ventricular irritability, which decreases cardiac output and may lead to life-threatening dysrhythmias.
5. Antidysrhythmic drugs reduce myocardial irritability.
6. The desired results are increased diastolic threshold potential and decreased action potential duration.
7. Altered potassium levels can affect cardiac rhythms.
8. This measure is for emergency administration of IV cardiac medications.
9. ST depression indicates myocardial ischemia, and ST elevation indicates injury; either may precipitate dysrhythmias.

Evaluation. Within 24 hours of admission, the client's cardiac rhythm will remain stable and the client will exhibit no manifestations of rhythm disturbance.

Nursing Diagnosis. Decreased Cardiac Output related to negative inotropic changes in the heart secondary to myocardial ischemia, injury, or infarction, as evidenced by change in the level of consciousness, weakness, dizziness, loss of peripheral pulses, abnormal heart sounds, hemodynamic compromise, and cardiopulmonary arrest.

Outcomes. The client will have improved cardiac output, as evidenced by normal cardiac rate, rhythm, and hemodynamic parameters, dysrhythmias controlled or absent; and absence of angina.

Interventions

Assess for and document the following as evidence of myocardial dysfunction with decreasing cardiac output:
1. Mental status—be alert to restlessness and decreased responsiveness.

2. Lung sounds—monitor for crackles and rhonchi.

3. Blood pressure—monitor for hypertension or hypotension.

4. Heart sounds—note the presence of gallop, murmur, and increased or decreased heart rate.

5. Urinary output—be alert to output less than 30 ml/hr.

6. Peripheral perfusion—monitor for pallor, mottling, cyanosis, coolness, diaphoresis, and peripheral pulses.
7. Monitor arterial blood gas (ABG) levels.

8. If a pulmonary artery catheter is used, record hemodynamic parameters every 2 to 4 hours and as required (prn). Be alert to pulmonary capillary wedge pressure (PCWP) >18 mm Hg, cardiac output <4 L/min, and cardiac index <2.5 L/min.

9. Maintain hemodynamic stability by monitoring the effects of beta-blockers and inotropic agents.
10. Monitor and assess angina for type severity and duration.

Rationales

1. Cerebral perfusion is directly related to cardiac output and aortic perfusion pressure and is influenced by hypoxia and electrolyte and acid-base variations.
2. Crackles may develop, reflecting pulmonary congestion related to alterations in myocardial function.
3. Hypotension related to hypoperfusion, vagal stimulation, dysrhythmias, or ventricular dysfunction may occur; it may be related to pain, anxiety, catecholamine release, or pre-existing vascular problems.
4. Bradycardia may be present because of vagal stimulation or conduction disturbances related to the area of myocardial injury. Tachycardia may be a compensatory mechanism related to decreased cardiac output. A gallop may be related to fluid volume overload or heart failure, and a murmur may be present if a ruptured chordae tendineae occurred.
5. Urinary output less than 30 ml/hr may reflect reduced renal perfusion and glomerular filtration as a result of reduced cardiac output.
6. Decreased peripheral pulses may indicate a decrease in cardiac output.
7. Acidosis may cause dysrhythmias and depressed cardiac function.
8. A PCWP above 18 may indicate fluid volume overload or heart failure. A cardiac output below 4 and a cardiac index of below 2.5 indicate heart failure or decrease in cardiac output. Use hemodynamic monitoring to assess drug therapy and for prevention or early detection of complications of MI (i.e., extension, heart failure, cardiogenic shock).
9. Assess the effect of drug therapy on myocardial contractility and function.
10. Angina indicates myocardial ischemia, which may decrease cardiac output.

Evaluation. Within 2 to 3 days of admission, the client will have normal hemodynamic pressures, normal vital signs, clear breath sounds, no shortness of breath, normal ABG values. Normal sinus rhythm with rate between 60 to 100 beats/min (BPM).

Nursing Diagnosis. Impaired Gas Exchange related to decreased cardiac output, as evidenced by cyanosis, impaired capillary refill, reduced arterial oxygen tension (PaO_2), and dyspnea.

Outcomes. The client will demonstrate improved gas exchange, as evidenced by absence of cyanosis, brisk cap refill, absence of dyspnea, and ABG levels within normal limits.

■

Interventions

1. Administer oxygen as ordered; maintain continuous oximetry.

2. Monitor ABGs as ordered.

3. Continue to assess the client's skin, capillary refill, and level of consciousness every 2 to 4 hours and prn.

4. Assess respiratory status for dyspnea and crackles.

5. Prepare for intubation and mechanical ventilation if hypoxia increases.

Rationales

1. Increases amount of oxygen available for myocardial uptake; oximetry measures peripheral oxygen saturation.

2. The presence of hypoxia indicates a need for supplemental oxygen. Monitoring provides data on the adequacy of tissue perfusion and oxygenation.

3. Cyanosis (circumoral or at extremities) indicates hypoxia. Capillary refill >3 seconds indicates poor perfusion and possibly hypoxia.

4. Dyspnea may indicate inadequate oxygenation, and the presence of crackles may impair gas exchange because of decreased exchange of oxygen and carbon dioxide through fluid in alveoli.

5. With increasing hypoxia, mechanical ventilation may be necessary to oxygenate the client adequately.

Evaluation. Within 2 to 3 days of admission, client's breath sounds will be clear, and ABG values will be within normal limits.

Nursing Diagnosis. Risk for Injury related to coagulopathies associated with thrombolytic therapy.

Outcomes. The client will maintain hemostasis; if bleeding does occur, it will be recognized and treated at once.

Interventions

1. Obtain coagulation studies as ordered.

2. Monitor invasive line sites for active bleeding.

3. Inspect all body fluids for presence of blood.

4. Hold pressure on any discontinued lines 15 minutes; if arterial, hold for 30 minutes.
5. Observe neurologic status.

6. Avoid intramuscular (IM) injections.
7. Assess for back or flank pain.
8. Keep an IV line patent.

9. Maintain an active type and crossmatch on the client.

Rationales

1. Coagulation studies can help determine the tendency to bleed.

2. Thrombolytic therapy disrupts the normal coagulation process, and bleeding may occur at any invasive site.

3. Internal bleeding may be manifested through body fluids.

4. It takes longer to achieve hemostasis at catheter sites.

5. A change in neurologic status may indicate intracranial bleeding.

6. IM injections may cause bleeding.
7. Flank or back pain may suggest retroperitoneal bleeding.
8. In case of active bleeding, a patent line must be maintained to transfuse blood products.

9. If the client requires blood or blood products, an active type and crossmatch help eliminate any delay in treatment.

Evaluation. The client will be free from overt or occult bleeding.

Nursing Diagnosis. Powerlessness related to the hospital environment and anticipated lifestyle changes, as evidenced by verbalized "feelings of doom," crying, and anger.

Outcomes. The client will regain a sense of "control," as evidenced by feeling able to express feelings of powerlessness over the present situation and future outcomes.

Interventions

1. Provide opportunities for the client to express feelings about oneself and the illness.
2. Explore reality perceptions, and clarify if necessary.

3. Eliminate the unpredictability of events by allowing adequate preparation for tests and procedures.
4. Reinforce the client's right to ask questions.

5. Allow choices when possible.
6. Provide positive reinforcement for increased involvement in self-care.

7. Help the client identify strengths and areas of control.

Rationales

1. These opportunities create a supportive climate and send the message that caregivers are willing to help.
2. Listening to the client's feelings and words can help the client acquire a more hopeful outlook.
3. Information helps the client and family feel more hopeful and be more willing to participate in care.
4. Maintain a supportive climate to let the client feel free to ask questions or have information repeated.
5. Self-care allows the client to feel independent.
6. When clients participate in planning for care, they are more likely to feel a sense of control and to follow through with actions.
7. Self-confidence and security come with a sense of control; foster full client participation.

Evaluation. Within 24 hours of admission, client will verbalize a feeling of control over the situation and will actively participate in decisions regarding care.

Nursing Diagnosis. Anxiety and Fear related to hospital admission and fear of death, as evidenced by client and family appearing restless, hostile, or withdrawn; client and family verbalize fatalism or act extremely emotional as if in the grieving process.

Outcomes. The client will have reduced feelings of anxiety and fear, as evidenced by demonstrating appropriate range of feelings and initial signs of effective coping (participating in the treatment regimen) being able to rest, and asking fewer questions.

Interventions

1. Limit nursing personnel; provide continuity of care.

2. Allow and encourage the client and family to ask questions; do not avoid questions. Bring up common concerns.

3. Allow the client and family to verbalize fears.

4. Stress that frequent assessments are routine and do not necessarily imply a deteriorating condition.

5. Repeat information as necessary because of the reduced attention span of the client and family.
6. Provide a comfortable, quiet environment for the client and family.

Rationales

1. Continuity of care promotes security and development of rapport with and trust of health care providers.
2. Accurate information about the situation reduces fear, strengthens the client-nurse relationship, and assists the client and family to face the situation realistically.
3. Sharing information elicits support and comfort and can relieve tension and unexpressed worries.
4. The client may feel reassured after learning that frequent assessments may prevent development of more serious complications.
5. The client's attention span is short, and time perception may be altered. Anxiety decreases learning and attention.
6. A comfortable environment enhances coping mechanisms and reduces myocardial workload and oxygen consumption.

Evaluation. Within 2 days of admission, client will exhibit signs of effective coping and progression through stages of recovery.

Nursing Diagnosis. Risk for Constipation related to bed rest, pain medications, and NPO (nothing by mouth) or soft diet, as evidenced by subjective feeling of fullness, abdominal cramping, painful defecation, and palpable impaction.

Outcomes. The client will have improved bowel elimination, as evidenced by eliminating a stool without straining or having a vasovagal response (bradycardia).

Interventions

1. Ensure that the client has adequate bulk in diet and adequate fluid intake (without violating fluid restrictions).
2. Monitor the effectiveness of softeners or laxatives. Instruct the client on prevention of straining and avoiding the Valsalva (vasovagal) maneuver.
3. Encourage the client to use a bedside commode rather than a bedpan.

Rationales

1. Bulk and fluid within the colon prevent straining.

2. Stool softeners decrease the myocardial workload of straining. The Valsalva maneuver causes bradycardia, decreasing cardiac output.
3. Use of bedpans necessitates more straining and increases the vasovagal response.

Evaluation. Within 2 to 3 days of admission, client will have normal bowel function.

Nursing Diagnosis. Altered Health Maintenance related to MI and implications for lifestyle changes.

Outcomes. The client and family will learn about the medical regimen and lifestyle changes, as evidenced by verbalizing an understanding of a heart attack and the necessary lifestyle changes regarding diet, medications, stress reduction, quitting smoking, and cholesterol, weight, and blood pressure reduction.

Interventions

1. Explain the following, providing both oral and written instructions: anatomy and functions of heart muscle, coronary arteries, and atherosclerotic process; definition of a "heart attack"; healing process of the heart; and role of collateral circulation.
2. Assist the client with identifying personal risk factors.

3. Assist the client in devising a plan for risk factor modification (e.g., diet; smoking cessation; cholesterol, stress, and blood pressure reduction).
4. Provide guidelines for a diet low in cholesterol and saturated fat. Arrange for dietary consultation before hospital discharge.

Rationales

1. Use of multiple learning methods enhances retention of material; information helps the client understand the underlying problems of overall heart functions.

2. Risk factor identification is the first step before changes can be implemented.
3. This information is helpful in providing opportunity for the client to identify risk factors, assume control, and participate in a treatment regimen.
4. Consultation with other health professionals enhances client learning from others. Guidelines developed with the client and family before discharge help once they are home.

5. Teach the client and family about medications that will be taken after hospital discharge (name, purpose, dosage, schedule, precautions, potential side effects).
6. Discuss post-MI activity progression; arrange for a cardiac rehabilitation consultation.

7. Utilize other professionals to collaborate in the care of the client.

5. The more clients understand the medical regimen and potential side effects, the more adept they will be in monitoring for them.
6. Continued follow-up will let clients know how they are doing; outpatient cardiac rehabilitation supports and assists clients in the lifestyle changes necessary for a healthy recovery and life.
7. Dietitians can assist in diet education; social services can identify assistance in the area; cardiac rehabilitation personnel can assist in exercise regimens; clergy can assist in coping strategies; and support groups can assist in social support.

Evaluation. Within 2 days of admission, the client and family will be able to verbalize understanding of heart attack and identify personal risk factors and necessary lifestyle changes.

Nursing Diagnosis. Risk for Activity Intolerance related to an imbalance between oxygen supply and demand, as evidenced by weakness, fatigue, change in vital signs, dysrhythmias, dyspnea, pallor, and diaphoresis.

Outcomes. The client will have improved activity tolerance, as evidenced by participating in desired activities, meeting activities of daily living (ADL), reduced fatigue and weakness, vital signs within normal limits during activity, absence of cyanosis, diaphoresis, and pain.

Interventions

1. Monitor vital signs before and immediately after activity and 3 minutes later.

2. Monitor for tachycardia, dysrhythmias, dyspnea, diaphoresis, weakness, fatigue, or pallor after activity.

3. Encourage verbalization of feelings or concerns regarding fatigue or limitations.
4. Provide assistance with self-care activities, and provide frequent rest periods, especially after meals.

5. Increase activity per cardiac rehabilitation nurse and physician orders.

Rationales

1. Data are provided about the client's response to increased activity. Vital signs should return to baseline levels in 3 minutes. If blood pressure decreases and heart rate increases, cardiac decompensation is suggested and activity should be decreased. The development of chest pain or dyspnea may indicate a need for an alteration in exercise regimen or medication.
2. These indicators of myocardial oxygen deprivation may call for decreased activity, changes in medications, or use of supplemental oxygen.
3. Knowing limitations prevents exertion and increasing myocardial workload.
4. Large meals may increase myocardial workload and cause vagal stimulation, with resultant bradycardia or ectopic beats; caffeine, a cardiac stimulant, increases heart rate.
5. Gradual increase in activity increases strength and prevents overexertion, enhances collateral circulation, and restores a normal lifestyle as far as possible.

Evaluation. Within 3 to 4 days of admission, the client will progress normally through steps of phase I cardiac rehabilitation without manifestations of exercise intolerance.

Collaborative Problem. Risk for Heart Failure related to disease process, as evidenced by tachycardia, hypotension or hypertension, S_3 or S_4 heart sounds, dysrhythmias, ECG changes, decreased urine output, decreased peripheral pulses, cool ashen skin, diaphoresis, crackles, jugular vein distention, edema, and chest pain.

Outcomes. The nurse will monitor for clinical manifestations of heart failure by assessing cardiac rate, rhythm, hemodynamic parameters, skin perfusion, renal perfusion, and CNS perfusion.

Interventions

1. Auscultate the apical pulse.

2. Assess heart rate and rhythm.

3. Document dysrhythmias, if present, as necessary.

4. Note lung sounds every 2 to 4 hours and as needed.

5. Palpate peripheral pulses every 2 to 4 hours and as necessary.

Rationales

1. Atrial (S_3) or ventricular (S_4) gallop rhythms are common and reflect tissue noncompliance or distention of chambers.
2. Sinus tachycardia, paroxysmal atrial contractions, paroxysmal atrial tachycardia, multifocal atrial tachycardia, and PVCs are commonly seen with heart failure.
3. Dysrhythmias reduce ventricular filling time, decrease myocardial contractility, and increase myocardial oxygen demands, which further compromises cardiac output.
4. Crackles may develop; ineffective cardiac output causes an increase in venous congestion that transcends to the pulmonary vasculature and leaks into the alveolar tissue, resulting in congestion.
5. Pulses may be weak, thready, or difficult to obtain when cardiac output is decreased.

6. Monitor blood pressure every 2 to 4 hours and as needed.

6. Hypotension related to hypoperfusion, vagal stimulation, or ventricular dysfunction may occur. Hypertension may be related to pain, anxiety, catecholamine release, or pre-existing vascular problems.

7. Inspect skin for pallor, cyanosis, and diaphoresis every 2 to 4 hours and as needed.

7. Pallor is associated with vasoconstriction, reduced cardiac output, and anemia. Cyanosis may develop during severe episodes of pulmonary edema. Dependent areas are often blue or mottled with increased venous congestion.

8. Monitor urine output, noting changes or decreasing output and dark or concentrated urine, every 2 to 4 hours and as needed.

8. Urinary output below 20 ml/hr may reflect reduced renal perfusion and glomerular filtration as a result of reduced cardiac output.

9. Assess for chest pain.

9. Chest pain may indicate inadequate cardiac perfusion related to the hypertrophied myocardium.

10. Assess for peripheral edema.

10. In heart failure, especially right-sided, the inability to pump venous blood back to the heart results in venous pooling, increased pressure in the vascular space that leaks in the interstitium and presents as peripheral edema.

11. Assess changes in sensorium.

11. Cerebral perfusion is directly related to cardiac output, and mentation may be a sensitive indicator of deterioration.

12. Provide frequent rest periods.

12. Physical rest decreases the production of catecholamines, which raises heart rate, myocardial oxygen demand, and blood pressure.

13. Instruct the client on avoidance of activities that increase cardiac workload.

13. Avoidance of activities provides an opportunity for myocardial recovery and decreases workload and myocardial oxygen consumption.

14. Provide a bedside commode. Avoid the Valsalva maneuver.

14. The Valsalva maneuver causes bradycardia and temporarily decreases cardiac output.

15. Elevate the client's legs and avoid pressure under the knees. Permit increase in activity as tolerated.

15. This position enhances venous return, reduces dependent swelling, decreases venous stasis, and may reduce the incidence of thrombus and embolus formation.

16. Administer medications as ordered.

16. ACE inhibitors and beta blockade help reduce the incidence of heart failure after MI in clinical trials.[38]

Evaluation. The client will not manifest heart failure after an MI.

Nursing Diagnosis. Fluid Volume Excess related to reduced glomerular filtration rate (GFR), decreased cardiac output, increased antidiuretic hormone (ADH) production, and sodium and water retention, as evidenced by orthopnea, S_3 heart sound, oliguria, edema, jugular neck vein distention, increased weight, increased blood presssure, respiratory distress, and abnormal breath sounds.

Outcomes. The client's fluid volume balance will be adequate, as evidenced by balanced intake and output (I&O), clear or clearing breath sounds, vital signs within normal limits, stable weight, and absence of edema.

Interventions

1. Monitor I&O (especially note color, specific gravity, and amount) every 2 to 4 hours, and as needed, and 24-hour totals.
2. Maintain chair or bed rest in the semi-Fowler position.

3. Involve the client and family in fluid schedules, especially if there are restrictions, and provide frequent oral care.
4. Weigh the client daily.

5. Assess for jugular neck vein distention, edema, peripheral pulses, and presence of anasarca.

6. Auscultate breath sounds. Note adventitious sounds, and monitor for dyspnea or tachypnea.

7. Monitor for sudden extreme shortness of breath and feelings of panic.
8. Palpate for hepatomegaly. Note complaints of right upper quadrant pain or tenderness.

9. Note increased lethargy, hypotension, and muscle cramping.

Rationales

1. Intake greater than output may indicate fluid volume excess. If client receives diuretic therapy, an increase in output is expected.
2. This position promotes diuresis by recumbency-induced increased GFR and reduced ADH hormone production.
3. Involving the client in the therapy regimen may enhance a sense of control and fosters cooperation with restrictions.
4. Daily weights can show the increase or decrease in congestion and edema in response to therapy. A gain of 5 pounds represents about 2 L of fluid.
5. Excessive fluid retention may be demonstrated by venous engorgement and edema formation. Peripheral edema often begins in the feet and ascends upward as heart failure worsens.
6. These manifestations of pulmonary congestion reflect increased vascular volume and pulmonary hypertension or worsening of heart failure.
7. These are manifestations of extreme pulmonary capillary hypertension (pulmonary edema).
8. Advancing heart failure leads to venous congestion, which results in liver engorgement and altered liver function (i.e., impaired drug metabolism, prolonged drug half-life).
9. These are manifestations of hypokalemia and hyponatremia that may occur because of fluid shifts and diuretic therapy.

10. Evaluate the effectiveness of diuretics and potassium supplements.

10. Fluid shifts and use of diuretics can alter electrolytes, especially potassium and chloride, which affects cardiac rhythm and contractility.

11. Assess the need for dietary consultation as needed.

11. Restrictions of foods high in sodium may be necessary. The client may need to eat foods enriched with potassium when taking loop diuretics.

Evaluation. Within 3 days of admission, the client's fluid volume will be normal. I&O will be balanced, breath sounds will be clear, vital signs will be normal, and weight will be stable, with no signs of peripheral or central edema.

Nursing Diagnosis. Risk for Impaired Skin Integrity related to bed rest, edema, and decreased tissue perfusion, as evidenced by reddened areas and the presence of areas of breakdown.

Outcomes. The client will have intact skin integrity, as evidenced by an absence of reddened areas and no areas of breakdown.

Interventions

1. Inspect the client's skin; note bone prominences, edema, altered circulation, pigmentation, obesity, and emaciation.
2. Assist with active or passive range-of-motion (ROM) exercises.

3. Reposition the client every 2 hours in a bed or chair.

4. Provide pressure-reducing devices, sheepskin, or elbow and heel protectors if needed.
5. Assess and provide special air or flotation beds for clients at high risk for pressure ulcers.

Rationales

1. Altered skin color in isolated areas suggests damage caused by pressure or decreased circulation.
2. ROM exercises enhance venous return. Isometric exercises may adversely affect cardiac output by increasing myocardial work and oxygen consumption.
3. Repositioning increases circulation and reduces the time that weight deprives any one area of blood flow.
4. These devices reduce pressure to bone prominences and improve skin integrity.
5. These beds reduce pressure to skin and may improve circulation.

Evaluation. Within 2 to 3 days of admission, the client will have intact skin integrity and will have no reddened areas or skin breakdown.

- Recognize and treat cardiac ischemia
- Administer thrombolytic therapy as ordered, and observe for complications
- Recognize and treat potentially life-threatening dysrhythmias
- Monitor for complications of reduced cardiac output
- Maintain a therapeutic critical care environment
- Identify the psychosocial impact of MI on the client and family
- Educate the client in lifestyle changes and rehabilitation

Nursing diagnoses or collaborative problems that may apply to the client after acute MI are discussed in the Care Plan. Case managers are assigned to these clients to coordinate their care (see Case Management feature).

CONCLUSIONS

CHD is a progressive occlusive disorder that commonly results in reduced coronary blood flow. This reduction is manifested clinically by angina and MI. MI, permanent damage to the myocardium, may be the first indicator of how serious the heart disease is. Your responsibilities in the care of these clients are to educate them about the warning signs of MI, to monitor their response to therapy, to prevent complications, and to promote rehabilitation.

THINKING CRITICALLY

1. **Mrs. Polk, a 62-year-old housewife who cares for her two grandchildren, is admitted to the emergency department with complaints of chest pain. She is diaphoretic and pale and reports pain "under my left breast that pushes to my back." She rates the pain an 8 on a scale of 1 to 10. Her ECG shows a depressed ST segment. She is placed on oxygen therapy, and an IV line is inserted. Cardiac serum markers are drawn and sent to the laboratory. Her vital signs are temperature 36.9° C, apical pulse 110, and blood pressure 108/68.**

Factors to Consider. What additional testing is necessary to rule in or role out an acute MI? What other information from Mrs. Polk's history might aid in the diagnosis?

2. **The physician immediately orders reteplase, a thrombolytic agent, for Mrs. Polk.**

Factors to Consider. What information must be obtained from Mrs. Polk to safely initiate thrombolytic therapy?

3. **You administer the thrombolytic therapy as ordered. Mrs. Polk states her pain is now a 1 on a scale of 1 to 10. ST segments are resolving, and she is no longer diaphoretic.**

Factors to Consider. What effects from the thrombolytic therapy appear to be occurring? Which side effects of the therapy should you be anticipating?

4. **A client with long-standing coronary artery disease experiences severe chest pain unrelieved by**

nitroglycerin. He is admitted with an acute MI to the coronary care unit. What are the priorities on admission? What medical treatment may be instituted in the first hours following the infarction?

Factors to Consider. What time frame is considered most crucial to the salvage of myocardial muscle? What care is given to the newly admitted client?

BIBLIOGRAPHY

1. American Association of Cardiovascular and Pulmonary Rehabilitation. (1995). *Guidelines for cardiac rehabilitation programs.* Champaign, IL: Human Kinetics.
2. American Heart Association. (1998). *1999 Heart and stroke statistical update.* Dallas: Author.
3. Beattie, S. (1999). Management of chronic stable angina. *Nurse Practitioner, 24*(5), 44, 49, 53, 56, 59–61.
4. Braunwald, E., et al. (1994). *Unstable angina: Diagnosis and management. Clinical practice guideline No. 10* (AHCPR Pub. No. 94-0602). Rockville, MD: Agency for Health Care Policy and Research and the National Heart, Lung, and Blood Institute, Public Health Service, U.S. Department of Health and Human Services.
5. Colon, P., et al. (1998). Utility of stress echocardiography in the triage of patients with atypical chest pain from the emergency department. *American Journal of Cardiology, 82,* 1282–1284.
6. Cox, M. H. (1997). Exercise for coronary artery disease. *Physician and Sports Medicine, 25*(12), 27–32.
7. Dempsey, S. J., Dracup, K., & Moser, D. K. (1995). Women's decision to seek care for symptoms of acute myocardial infarction. *Heart and Lung, 24,* 444.
8. Doering, L. V. (1999). Pathophysiology of acute coronary syndromes leading to acute myocardial infarction. *Journal of Cardiovascular Nursing, 13*(3), 1–20.
9. Dracup, K., & Cannon, C. (1999, April). Combination treatment strategies for management of acute myocardial infarction. *Critical Care Nurse Supplement,* 1–17.
10. Fallon, E. M., & Roques, J. (1997). Acute chest pain. *AACN Clinical Issues, 8,* 382–397.
11. Feldman, M., & Cryer, B. (1999). Aspirin absorption rates and platelet inhibition times with 325-mg buffered aspirin tablets (chewed or swallowed intact) and with buffered aspirin solution. *American Journal of Cardiology, 84,* 404–409.
12. Gensini, G., Comeglio, M., & Falai, M. (1999). Advances in antithrombotic therapy of acute myocardial infarction. *American Heart Journal, 138*(2), S171–S176.
13. Gersh, B. J., Braunwald, E., & Rutherford, J. D. (1997). Chronic coronary artery disease. In E. Brunwald (Ed.), *Heart disease: A textbook of cardiovascular medicine.* Philadelphia: W. B. Saunders.
14. Goodwin, M., et al. (1999). Early extubation and early activity after open heart surgery. *Critical Care Nurse 19*(5), 18–26.
15. Hudak, C. M., Gallo, B. M., & Lohr, P. G. (1998). *Critical care nursing* (7th ed.). Philadelphia: Lippincott-Raven.
16. Hudson, M., et al. (1999). Cardiac markers: Point of care testing. *Clinica Chimica Acta, 28*(4), 223–237.
17. Jensen, L., & King, K. M. (1997). Women and heart disease: The issues. *Critical Care Nurse, 17*(2), 45–52.
18. Kosnik, L. (1999, October). Treatment protocols and pathways: Improving the process of care. *Critical Care Nurse Supplement,* 3–7.
19. Kuhn, F. E., & Gersch, B. J. (1996). Mechanical complications of acute myocardial infarction. In V. Fuster, R. Ross, & E. J. Topol (Eds.), *Atherosclerosis and coronary artery disease* (Vol. 2). Philadelphia: Lippincott-Raven.
19a. Lee, T. H., & Goldman, L. (2000). Evaluation of the patient with acute chest pain. *New England Journal of Medicine, 342*(16), 1187–1193.
20. McCauley, K. M. (1995). Assessing social support in patients with cardiac disease. *Journal of Cardiovascular Nursing, 10,* 73–80.
21. Moser, D., et al. (1999, October). The role of the critical care nurse in preventing heart failure after acute myocardial infarction. *Critical Care Nurse Supplement,* 11–15.
22. Murphy, M., & Berding, C. (1999). Use of myoglobins and cardiac troponins in the diagnosis of acute myocardial infarction. *Critical Care Nurse, 19*(1), 58–65.
23. O'Connor, C. M., Gattis, W. A., & Swedberg, K. (1999). Current and novel pharmacologic approaches in advanced heart failure. *Heart and Lung, 28,* 227–239.
24. Rich, M. W. (1999). Heart failure disease management: A critical review. *Journal of Cardiac Failure, 5*(1), 64–75.
25. Riegel, B., & Gocka, I. (1995). Gender differences in adjustment to acute myocardial infarction. *Heart and Lung, 24,* 457.
26. Ryan, T. J., et al. (1996). ACC/AHA guidelines for the management of patients with acute myocardial infarction: A report of the American College of Cardiology/American Heart Association Task Force on practice guidelines (Committee on Management of Acute Myocardial Infarction). *Journal of the American College of Cardiology, 28,* 1328–1428.
27. Sayer, J. W., et al. (1997). Attenuation or absence of circadian and seasonal rhythms of acute myocardial infarction. *Heart, 77,* 325–329.
28. Shah, P. K. (1996). Pathophysiology of plaque rupture and the concept of plaque stabilization. *Cardiology Clinics, 14,* 17–28.
29. Skillings, J. (1998). Atherosclerosis. *Lippincott's Primary Care Practice, 2*(5), 437–451.
30. Soran, O., Schneider, V. M., & Feldman, A. M. (1999). Basic therapy for congestive heart failure: Current practice, new prospects. *Journal of Critical Illness, 14*(2), 78–89.
31. Stary, H. C., et al. (1995). A definition of advanced types of atherosclerotic lesions and a histological classification of atherosclerosis. *Circulation, 92,* 1355–1374.
32. Steinke, E. F., & Patterson, P. (1995). Sexual counseling of MI patients by cardiac nurses. *Journal of Cardiovascular Nursing, 10,* 81–87.
33. Tatum, J., et al. (1997). Comprehensive strategy for the evaluation and triage of the chest pain patient. *Annals of Emergency Medicine, 29,* 116–23.
34. Thelan, L. A., et al. (1998). *Critical care nursing: Diagnosis and management* (3rd ed.). St. Louis: Mosby–Year Book.
35. Theroux, P., & Fuster, V. (1998). Acute coronary syndromes: Unstable angina and non-Q-wave myocardial infarction. *Circulation, 97,* 1195–1206.
36. Tofler, G. H. (1997). Triggering and the pathophysiology of acute coronary syndromes. *American Heart Journal, 134,* S55–S61.
37. van derWall, E. E., et al. (1995). Magnetic resonance imaging in coronary artery disease. *Circulation, 92,* 2723–2739.
38. Vantrimpont, P., et al. (1997). Additive beneficial effects of beta-blockers to angiotensin-converting enzyme inhibitors in the survival and ventricular enlargement (SAVE) study. *Journal of the American College of Cardiology, 29,* 229–236.
39. Verheugt, F. (1999). What an interventional cardiologist should know about the pharmacological treatment of acute myocardial infarction. *Seminars in Interventional Cardiology, 4,* 17–20.
40. Wenger, N. K. (1999). Women, myocardial infarction, and coronary revascularization. *Cardiology in Review, 7,* 117–120.
41. Wenger, N. K. (1997). Cardiac rehabilitation: Implications of the AHCPR guideline. *Hospital Medicine, 33*(4), 31–38.
42. Wenger, N. K., et al. (1995). *Cardiac rehabilitation as secondary prevention. Clinical practice guideline: Quick reference guide for clinicians. No. 17.* Rockville, MD: Agency for Health Care Policy and Research and the National Heart, Lung, and Blood Institute, Public Health Service, U.S. Department of Health and Human Services.
43. Wu, C. Y. (1995). Assessment of postdischarge concerns of coronary artery bypass graft patients. *Journal of Cardiovascular Nursing, 10,* 1–7.
44. Zerwic, J. (1998). Symptoms of acute myocardial infarction: Expectations of a community sample. *Heart and Lung, 27,* 75–81.
45. Zerwic, J. (1999). Patient delay in seeking treatment for acute myocardial infarction symptoms. *Journal of Cardiovascular Nursing, 13,* 21–32.

The Implantable Cardioverter-Defibrillator and Quality of Life

QUESTIONS

How does implantation of a cardioverter-defibrillator affect a recipient's and the family's quality of life (QOL)?
What are their concerns and fears?

CITATION

Gallagher, R. D., McKinley, S., Mangan, B., et al. (1997). The impact of the implantable cardioverter defibrillator on quality of life. *American Journal of Critical Care, 6,* 16–24.

STUDIES

Eighteen studies examined QOL after insertion of an implantable cardioverter defibrillator (ICD). Published between 1993 and 1995, the studies were identified in the critical care, nursing, medical, and technical literature. The method used to identify the studies included in the review was not specified. A total of 489 recipients (average age, 57 years) participated.

Summary of Findings

Overall, recipients felt that the ICD maintained or improved their QOL,[2, 9, 16, 18] and most indicated they had resumed their normal activities.[2, 12, 20] A majority reported having successfully incorporated the device into their body image over time.[13, 18, 20] In one study, QOL initially declined but returned to the pre-implant level by 1 year.[13] Despite overall success, ICDs do cause problems and life changes for clients and their families.

Psychological Issues

Fear

Seventeen per cent to 47% of clients reported pain when a shock was dispensed[2, 16]; in one study, the pain was perceived by most people as being moderate (5 to 7 level on a 10-point Visual Analogue Scale).[2, 6] Descriptions of the shock varied from "like a spark plug" to "a bolt of lightning."[6, 16]

Reported rates of fear vary greatly, from 85% to 12.5%, with most subjects experiencing fear after a shock.[3, 6, 12, 16] Forty-three per cent of recipients reported being afraid that the shocks would not be successful,[12, 16] whereas others feared battery failure.[3, 6] In one study, 88% of recipients reported general nervousness after a shock and felt a need to talk about the experience.[6] The unpredictability of shocks and the possibility of loss of consciousness contribute to their fear.[10, 15]

Many recipients responded to this lack of predictability by attributing the shock to a specific activity (e.g., bending), and then by changing their normal behavior in an effort to prevent further shocks.[6, 19] A small study found that seven of 17 recipients reduced or totally abstained from sexual activity because of fear of shocks.[3] Syncope was unpredictable in these clients; even the absence of earlier syncope did not predict the absence of loss of consciousness during subsequent shocks.[10]

Anxiety

Recipients of ICDs reported higher levels of anxiety than the general population, but the source of the anxiety remains unclear. The anxiety might be due to the presence of the device, but it also might be due to the experience of receiving a shock, the anticipation of being shocked, malfunction of the device,[1, 3, 12, 16] or a residual effect from prior sudden cardiac arrest or ventricular tachycardia experience.[13] Since the ICD is to prevent adverse results of arrest or dysrhythmia, one might argue that recipients should have lower levels of anxiety; indeed, several studies have shown this effect.[16, 20] In one of these studies, 78% of the recipients reported reduced or no anxiety, some even viewed the device as a source of security and a life extender.[16]

It is unclear whether recipients who receive more shocks are more anxious than those who receive fewer shocks.[6, 9, 12] Generally, older people were less anxious than younger people.[12] Body image was a problem for 35% of recipients experiencing shocks[3, 16]; depression, global stress, confusion, and anger were also present.[4, 5, 16, 209]

Psychiatric Disorders

A retrospective study of 20 recipients and their families found that six of the patients had a transient psychiatric disorder (such as adjustment problems or panic attacks), four had major psychiatric disorders, and 9 of the families felt distressed.[14] These incidents are comparable to those found in other groups with chronic medical problems. Like anxiety, these disorders may be related to the presence of cardiac disease with all its implications or to prior experiences of sudden cardiac arrest.

Coping Strategies

Coping strategies of recipients and their families vary widely. Overall, optimism, denial, and confrontation are frequently reported,[4, 5, 11] although evasion is frequently used to cope with physical stresses.[11] Whether coping by recipients and family members improves or declines over the first year is not clear.[4, 13]

Spouses and families tend to be overprotective[18] and to be more concerned about the effects of the ICD and shock experiences on the family than recipients are.[18] Both recipients and families appear to have difficulty seeking and obtaining social support even though they feel a need for it.[4, 11]

Physical Function

Many recipients found that their ability to perform normal physical activities did not return to previous levels.[4, 11, 12, 16, 18] Difficulty sleeping and reduced energy were the most frequently reported limitations.[4, 11, 12, 16, 19] Many of the findings have been contradictory. For example, one study found that only 14% of recipients reported a limited QOL, but 47% of recipients reported an inability to return to an active life.[12] Also, in interpreting the findings regarding physical functioning, remember that many of the recipients have other cardiac conditions; one study reported a 68% incidence of cardiac disease and a 36% incidence of low cardiac output.[17]

Driving has been a controversial issue. About 6% of drivers have received shocks while driving, sometimes with associated syncope, but no accidents resulted.[8]

The Implantable Cardioverter-Defibrillator and Quality of Life *Continued*

Intellectual Function

In a small (n = 15) but comprehensive study of neurocognitive changes, confusion and low global cognitive functioning were often present at the time of implantation, although they returned almost to normal by 1 year.[4] However, memory and construction of thoughts were below normal at implantation and improved only slightly during the recovery year. These findings are limited in credibility by the fact that only 65% of the people contacted participated in the study, and poor coping was given as the main reason for nonparticipation; this suggests that recipients with more severe problems might not have been represented in the data. In another small study, decreased attention span and memory loss were reported.[18]

Work and Social Function

Given the recipients' problems with physical and intellectual activities, it is logical to expect that work and social functioning also would be disrupted after implantation. However, the findings are contradictory; the disparate findings may be the result of the different populations studied, improved technology over the years, or the research methods used.

Of two studies examining social activities after implantation, one noted reduced social interaction (i.e., found more social isolation),[16] whereas the other showed a decrease in social isolation.[19] Several studies have documented a decrease in employment, but estimates range from 38% to 66%.[2, 7, 12, 13, 16] Pre-existing cardiac conditions, voluntary retirement, nearing or reaching retirement age, and a history of sudden cardiac arrest all contributed to the decision to stop working.

Driving is an important issue for recipients. Approximately 92% of recipients have continued to drive even though some of them had been advised not to do so.[8] Several subsequent studies have examined the safety of driving and the advice currently given to ICD recipients (see update).[21–24]

Updated, Annotated Study Reports, 1995–1999

Chevalier, P., et al. (1996). Improved appraisal of the quality of life in patients with automatic implantable cardioverter defibrillator. *Psychotherapy and Psychosomatics, 65,* 49–56.

This French study examined the impact of shock delivery on QOL as well as social, psychological, and physical well-being in ICD recipients. Slightly fewer than half the 32 recipients reported a good or very good physical tolerance of the ICD, whereas 75% reported a good or very good psychological tolerance. Better control of cardiac health was reported by 59%, and 82% felt more secure after receiving an ICD. QOL scores were negatively correlated with anxiety and depression, whereas occurrence of shocks had no influence on psychological well-being. Recipients with a psychiatric diagnosis had less favorable psychosocial and QOL outcomes. The single most important factor leading to negative psychosocial outcomes was low physical tolerance of the device itself, although the current miniaturization of devices might diminish this effect.

Dubin, A. M., Batsford, W. P., Lewis, R. J., and Rosenfeld, L. E. (1996). Quality-of-life in patients receiving implantable cardioverter defibrillators at or before age 40. *Pacing and Clinical Electrophysiology, 19,* 1555–1559.

Sixteen recipients 40 years of age or younger who had an ICD in place for an average of 3 years previously completed a functional health questionnaire; 63% were employed, with most holding the same job before and after ICD placement. Four of the nine women became pregnant after implantation, and all delivered healthy infants. All recipients considered their health good to excellent, with 38% reporting improved health since ICD placement. Moderate physical activities were freely performed by 68% of them. Of the recipients, 75% felt that the ICD interfered with social interactions and 50% were concerned about its effect on sexual relationships.

Jung, W., and Luderitz, B. (1996). Quality of life and driving in recipients of the implantable cardioverter-defibrillator. *American Journal of Cardiology, 78*(suppl 5A), 51–56.

Of the European cardiologists who responded to the survey, 67% recommended temporary abstinence from driving for 3 to 18 months (average 9 ± 4 months) after ICD insertion. Despite medical advice not to drive, most recipients resumed driving within 12 months. However, only two experienced ICD shocks while driving—and no motor vehicle accidents resulted. It was concluded that risk of causing an accident varies considerably, depending on the original reason for the implant as well as the nature of the shock experiences of the recipient during the first 6 months after implantation.

Pinski, S. L., and Fahy, G. J. (1999). Implantable cardioverter-defibrillators. *American Journal of Medicine, 106,* 446–458.

This review article summarizes a broad range of findings from randomized clinical trials. The authors conclude that the studies examining QOL show unchanged or improved QOL after implantation. Most recipients perceive ICD shocks as quite uncomfortable, comparing them with a jolt from an electric socket or a kick in the chest. A small proportion (<15%) lose consciousness as a result of the lag between dysrhythmia and the corrective shock. Serious adjustment difficulties do occur, albeit in a small number of recipients.

A survey of American physicians over a 12-year period revealed that the driving fatality and injury rates for persons with ICDs were significantly lower than in the general population. The American Heart Association has advised that recipients with ICDs inserted for sustained, fast, ventricular dysrhythmias refrain from driving for 6 months after implantation and for 6 months after each subsequent shock.

Rosenqvist, M., Beyer, T., Block, M., den Dulk, K., Minten, J., & Lindemans, F. (1998). Adverse events with transvenous implantable cardioverter-defibrillators: A prospective multicenter study. *Circulation, 98,* 663–670.

The Implantable Cardioverter-Defibrillator and Quality of Life *Continued*

Adverse events associated with one ICD model were classified and their incidences reported; 778 European patients were observed for an average of 4 months after implantation. In total, 356 adverse events were observed in 259 recipients. Of the recipients, 50% experienced an adverse event within the first year after ICD implantation. The most frequently observed severe events included (1) inappropriate detection of dysrhythmia, (2) wound or pocket problems, and (3) lead or ICD dislodgment. The impact of adverse events on QOL was not examined, although clearly there is an association.

Limitations/Reservations. When applying the studies' findings, take into account the caveat that the experiences of older people are represented to a greater extent than the experiences of younger people who are now receiving ICDs. Remember, many of the studies in the review were conducted with 30 or fewer participants.

Research-Based Practice

From the evidence presented, it is clear that ICDs relieve recipients of worries about life-threatening dysrhythmias. Yet they also introduce new concerns, and restraints on how recipients live. The rate of occurrence of an adverse event, be it serious or mild, in the first year after implantation is high enough (50%) to contribute to anxiety at the least and to major adjustment disorders at the worst. These problems and responses highlight the need for educational or supportive interventions that cover the first year. Given the levels of problems and psychological stresses, many recipients might benefit from having access via telephone at all times to a nurse who can advise or reassure them.

Education of recipients and their families must carefully balance the possibility of problems with the benefits to be gained. Counseling in how to deal with problems at both emotional and practical problem-solving levels should be provided. Recipients should be encouraged to discuss problems with the nurse who will be seeing them over the long term. When discussing driving, take into account what driving means to the recipient in terms of practical and self-image ramifications. Counseling regarding driving should follow the guidelines provided by the American Heart Association.

The findings enable us to identify recipients who are at risk for poor adjustment to the ICD, namely those who:

- Had experienced sudden cardiac arrest or symptomatic ventricular tachycardia
- Have experienced loss of consciousness with a dysrhythmia-cardioversion event
- Have other serious cardiac disease (e.g., heart failure)
- Have a history of a psychiatric disorder
- Experience an adverse event

These recipients are in particular need of ongoing support.

Cited References

1. Badger, J., & Morris, P. (1989). Observations of a support group for automatic implantable cardioverter-defibrillator recipients and their spouses. *Heart and Lung, 18,* 238–243.

2. Bainger, E., & Fernsler, J. (1995). Perceived quality of life before and after implantation of an internal cardioverter defibrillator. *American Journal of Critical Care, 4,* 36–43.

3. Cooper, D., et al. (1986). The impact of automatic implantable cardioverter defibrillator on quality of life. *Clinical Progress in Electrophysiologic Pacing, 4,* 306–309.

4. Dougherty, C. (1994). Longitudinal recovery following sudden cardiac arrest and internal cardioverter defibrillator implantation: survivors and their families. *American Journal of Critical Care, 3,* 145–154.

5. Dougherty, C. (1995). Psychological reactions and family adjustment in shock versus nonshock groups after implantation of cardioverter defibrillator. *Heart and Lung, 24,* 281–291.

6. Dunbar, S., Warner, C., & Purcell, J. (1993). Internal cardioverter defibrillator device discharge: Experiences of patients and family members. *Heart and Lung, 22,* 494–501.

7. Kalbfleisch, K., et al. (1989). Reemployment following implantation of the automatic cardioverter defibrillator. *American Journal of Cardiology, 64,* 199–202.

8. Keelan, E., et al. (1995). Driving habits and experiences of patients with implantable cardioverter-defibrillators (Abstract). *Journal of the American College of Cardiology, 25*(pt II, suppl A), 145A.

9. Keren, R., Aaron, D., & Veltri, E. (1991). Anxiety and depression in patients with life-threatening ventricular arrhythmias: Impact of the implantable cardioverter-defibrillator. *PACE Pacing and Clinical Electrophysiology, 14,* 181–186.

10. Kou, W., et al. (1991). Incidence of loss of consciousness during automatic implantable cardioverter-defibrillator shocks. *Annals of Internal Medicine, 115,* 942–945.

11. Kuiper, R., & Nyamathi, A. (1991). Stressors and coping strategies of patients with automatic implantable cardioverter defibrillators. *Journal of Cardiovascular Nursing, 5,* 65–76.

12. Luderitz, B., et al. (1993). Patient acceptance of the implantable cardioverter defibrillator in ventricular tachyarrhythmias. *PACE Pacing and Clinical Electrophysiology, 16,* 1815–1821.

13. May, C., et al. (1995). The impact of the implantable cardioverter defibrillator on quality-of-life. *PACE Pacing and Clinical Electrophysiology 18,* 1411–1418.

14. Morris, P., et al. (1991). Psychiatric morbidity following implantation of the automatic implantable cardioverter defibrillator. *Psychosomatics, 32,* 58–64.

15. Porterfield, J., et al. (1991). A prospective study utilizing a transtelephonic electrocardiographic transmission program to manage patients in the first several months post-ICD implant. *PACE Pacing and Clinical Electrophysiology, 14,* 308–311.

16. Pycha, C., et al. (1990). Patient and spouse acceptance and adaptation to cardioverter-defibrillators. *Cleveland Clinic Journal of Medicine, 57,* 441–444.

17. Saksena, S., et al. (1992). Long-term multicenter experience with a second-generation implantable pacemaker-defibrillator in patients with malignant ventricular arrhythmias. *Journal of the American College of Cardiology, 19,* 490–499.

18. Sneed, N., & Finch, N. (1992). Experiences of patients and significant others with automatic cardioverter defibrillators after discharge from the hospital. *Progress in Cardiovascular Nursing, 7,* 20–24.

19. Vitale, M. B., & Funk, M. (1995). Quality of life in younger persons with an implantable cardioverter defibrillator. *Dimensions of Critical Care Nursing, 14,* 100–111.

20. Vlay, S., et al. (1989). Anxiety and anger in patients with ventricular tachyarrhythmias: Responses after automatic internal cardioverter defibrillator implantation. *PACE Pacing and Clinical Electrophysiology, 12,* 366–372.

The Implantable Cardioverter-Defibrillator and Quality of Life *Continued*

Added References

21. Chevalier, P., et al. (1996). Improved appraisal of the quality of life in patients with automatic implantable cardioverter defibrillator. *Psychotherapy and Psychosomatics, 65,* 49–56.
22. Jung, A., & Luderitz, B. (1996). Quality of life and driving in recipients of the implantable cardioverter-defibrillator. *American Journal of Cardiology, 78*(suppl. 5A), 51–56.
23. Pinski, S. L., & Fahy, G. J. (1999). Implantable cardioverter-defibrillators. *American Journal of Medicine, 106,* 446–458.
24. Rosenqvist, M., et al. (1998). Adverse events with transvenous implantable cardioverter-defibrillators: A prospective multicenter study. *Circulation, 98,* 663–670.

Sarah Jo Brown, PhD, RN, *Principal and Consultant, Practice-Research Integrations, Norwich, Vermont*

Oxygenation Disorders

Anatomy and Physiology Review
The Respiratory System

Robert G. Carroll

Our body needs a constant supply of oxygen to support metabolism. The respiratory system brings oxygen through the airways of the lung into the alveoli, where it diffuses into the blood for transport to the tissues. This process is so vital that difficulty in breathing is experienced as a threat to life itself. Whether death is a real possibility or not, people with respiratory disorders are often very anxious and fearful that they may die, perhaps agonizingly.

The respiratory system also has other essential functions:

1. Expels carbon dioxide (CO_2), a metabolic waste product that is transported from the tissues to the lungs for elimination.
2. Filters and humidifies air that enters the lungs.
3. Traps particulate matter in the mucus of the airways and propels it toward the mouth for elimination by coughing or swallowing.

An active immune system helps prevent the entry of inhaled pathogens.

Respiratory control is tied most closely to arterial blood and brain CO_2 levels as well as to arterial blood oxygen levels. Respiration is also controlled by higher cortical centers. For example, an increase in ventilation accompanies exercise and keeps arterial blood gases within the normal range.

Respiratory problems are widespread. Acute disorders range from minor inconveniences (colds or flu) to more life-threatening problems (asthma, some types of pneumonia, and chest trauma). Chronic disabling conditions include *chronic airflow limitation* (also called chronic obstructive pulmonary disease, or COPD), and certain restrictive lung diseases. Chronic respiratory problems affect many people, often causing them to make radical lifestyle changes, such as retiring from work earlier than they wish.

Respiratory problems are associated with many causes: allergies, occupational factors, genetic factors, smoking and tobacco use, infection, neuromuscular disorders, chest abnormalities, trauma, pleural conditions, and pulmonary vascular abnormalities. The most significant factor in chronic respiratory illness and lung cancer is cigarette smoking.

STRUCTURE OF THE RESPIRATORY SYSTEM

UPPER AIRWAYS

The airways are the regions through which air passes on its way to the exchange areas of the lungs. The upper airways consist of the nasal cavities, pharynx, and larynx.

Nasal Cavity

The nose is formed from both bone and cartilage. The nasal bone forms the bridge, and the remainder of the nose is composed of cartilage and connective tissue (Fig. U13–1). Each opening of the nose on the face (*nostrils* or *nares*) leads to a cavity (*vestibule*). The vestibule is lined anteriorly with skin and hair that filter foreign objects and prevent them from being inhaled. The posterior vestibule is lined with a mucous membrane, composed of columnar epithelial cells, and goblet cells that secrete mucus. The mucous membrane extends throughout the airways, and cilia (hair-like projections) propel mucus to the pharynx for elimination by swallowing or coughing. The portion of mucous membrane that is located at the top of the nasal cavity, just beneath the cribriform plate of the ethmoid bone, is specialized (*olfactory*) epithelium, which provides the sense of smell. Because the olfactory epithelium does not lie along the usual path of air movement, smell is enhanced by sniffing.

Along the sides of the vestibule are *turbinates,* mucous membrane-covered projections that contain a very rich blood supply from the internal and external carotid arteries. They warm and humidify inspired air.

Paranasal sinuses, open areas within the skull, are named for the bones in which they lie—frontal, ethmoid, sphenoid, and maxillary. Passageways from the paranasal sinuses drain into the nasal cavities. The nasolacrimal ducts, which drain tears from the surface of the eyes, also drain into the nasal cavity.

The mouth is considered part of the upper airway but only because it can be used to deliver air to the lungs when the nose is obstructed or when high volumes of air are needed, such as during exercise. The mouth does not perform the nasal functions efficiently, especially those of warming, humidifying, and filtering air.

Pharynx

The pharynx is a funnel-shaped tube that extends from the nose to the larynx. It can be divided into three sections.

The *nasopharynx* is located above the margin of the soft palate and receives air from the nasal cavity. From the ear, the eustachian tubes open into the nasopharynx. The pharyngeal tonsils (called *adenoids* when enlarged) are located on the posterior wall of the nasopharynx.

The *oropharynx* serves both respiration and digestion. It receives air from the nasopharynx and food from the oral cavity. Palatine (faucial) tonsils are located along the sides of the posterior mouth, and the lingual tonsils are located at the base of the tongue.

The *laryngopharynx (hypopharynx),* located below the base of the tongue, is the most inferior portion of the pharynx. It connects to the larynx and serves both respiration and digestion.

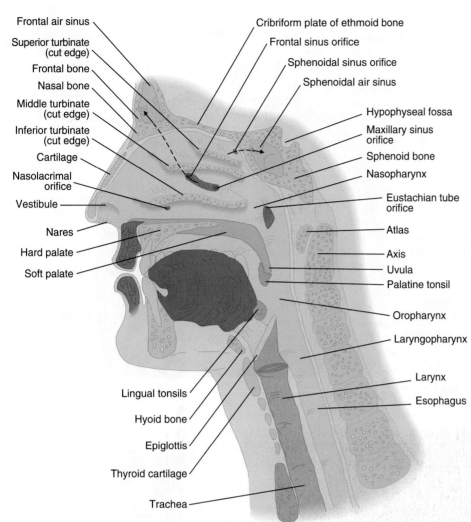

FIGURE U13–1 Structures of the upper airway.

Larynx

The larynx is commonly called the *voice box*. It connects the upper (pharynx) and lower (trachea) airways. The larynx lies just anterior to the upper esophagus. Nine cartilages form the larnyx: three large unpaired cartilages (epiglottis, thyroid, cricoid) and three smaller paired cartilages (arytenoid, corniculate, cuneiform). The cartilages are attached to the hyoid bone above and below the trachea by muscles and ligaments, all of which prevent the larynx from collapse during inspiration and swallowing.

The larynx consists of the endolarynx and a surrounding triangle-shaped bone and cartilage. The endolarynx is formed by two paired folds of tissue, forming the false and the true vocal cords. The slit between the vocal cords forms the *glottis*. The *epiglottis,* a leaf-shaped structure immediately posterior to the base of the tongue, lies above the larynx. When food or liquids are swallowed, the epiglottis closes over the larynx, protecting the lower airways from aspiration.

The thyroid cartilage protrudes in front of the larynx, forming the "Adam's apple." The cricoid cartilage lies just below the thyroid cartilage and is the anatomic site for an artificial opening into the trachea (tracheostomy, or cricothyroidotomy). The internal portion of the larynx is composed of muscles that assist with swallowing, speak-

ing, and respiration and that contribute to the pitch of the voice. The blood supply to the larynx is through the branches of the thyroid arteries. The nerve supply is through the recurrent laryngeal and superior laryngeal nerves.

LOWER AIRWAYS

The lower airway or tracheobronchial tree is composed of the trachea, right and left mainstem bronchi, segmental bronchi, subsegmental bronchi, and terminal bronchioles (Fig. U13–2). Smooth muscle, wound in overlapping clockwise and counterclockwise helical bands, is found in all of these structures. This arrangement allows contraction of the smooth muscle to decrease the diameter of the airways, increasing the resistance to air flow. This muscle is subject to spasm in many airway disorders. The lower airways continue to warm, humidify, and filter inspired air en route to the lungs.

Trachea

The trachea (windpipe) extends from the larynx to the level of the seventh thoracic vertebrae, where it divides into two main *(primary)* bronchi. The point at which the trachea divides is called the *carina.* The trachea is a flexible, muscular, 12-cm long air passage with C-shaped

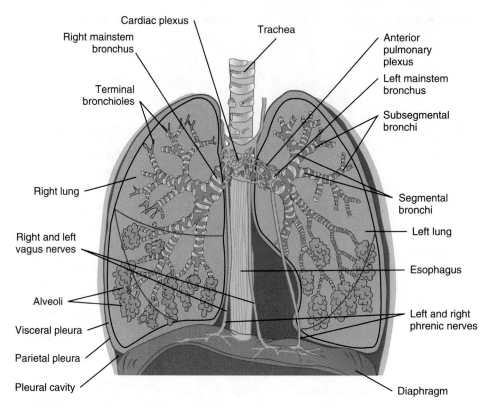

FIGURE U13–2 Structures of the lower airways.

cartilaginous rings. Along with all other regions of the lower airways it is lined with pseudostratified columnar epithelium that contains goblet (mucus-secreting) cells and cilia (Fig. U13–3). Because the cilia beat upward, they tend to carry foreign particles and excessive mucus away from the lungs to the pharynx. (No cilia are present in the alveoli.)

Bronchi and Bronchioles

The right mainstem bronchus is shorter and wider, extending more vertically downward, than the left mainstem bronchus. Thus, foreign bodies are more likely to lodge here than in the left mainstem bronchus. The *segmental* and *subsegmental bronchi* are subdivisions of the main bronchi and spread in an inverted, tree-like formation through each lung. Cartilage surrounds the airway in the bronchi, but the bronchioles (the final pathway to the alveoli) contain no cartilage and thus can collapse and trap air during active exhalation.

The *terminal bronchioles* are the last airways of the conducting system. The area from the nose to the terminal bronchioles does not exchange gas and functions as *anatomic dead space.* The lack of gas exchange means that the first air out of the mouth during exhalation resembles room air, but the last air out (end-tidal air) resembles alveolar air.

LUNGS AND ALVEOLI

Lungs

The lungs lie within the thoracic cavity on either side of the heart (see Fig. U13–2). They are cone-shaped, with

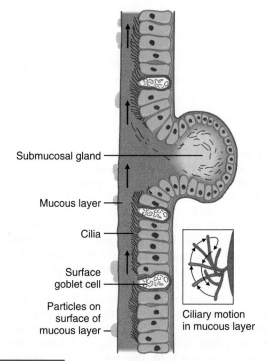

FIGURE U13–3 The mucociliary blanket is an important respiratory defense mechanism. Mucus is secreted by surface goblet cells. About 100 ml of mucus is normally secreted each day by the submucosal glands. Mucus covers the epithelial lining of the tracheobronchial tree in two layers—the watery solution layer close to the mucosal surface and the thicker gel layer. The cilia (hair-like projections) beat in an upward direction toward the upper airway. Particulate matter is trapped on the mucous layer and moved upward by the cilia. Debris-laden mucus is then either swallowed or expectorated as sputum.

the apex above the first rib and the base resting on the diaphragm. Each lung is divided into superior and inferior lobes by an oblique fissure. The right lung is further divided by a horizontal fissure, which bounds a middle lobe. The right lung, therefore, has three lobes; the left lobe has only two. In addition to these five lobes, which are visible externally, each lung can be subdivided into about 10 smaller units *(bronchopulmonary segments).* Each segment represents the portion of the lung that is supplied by a specific tertiary bronchus. These segments are important surgically, because a diseased segment can be resected without the need to remove the entire lobe or lung. The two lungs are separated by a space (the *mediastinum),* where the heart, aorta, vena cava, pulmonary vessels, esophagus, part of the trachea and bronchi, and the thymus gland are located.

The lungs contain gas, blood, thin alveolar walls, and support structures. The alveolar walls contain elastic and collagen fibers; these form a three-dimensional, basket-like structure that allows the lung to inflate in all directions. These fibers are capable of stretching when a pulling force is exerted on them from outside of the body or when they are inflated from within. The elastic recoil helps return the lungs to their resting volume.

Branches of the pulmonary artery provide most of the blood supply to the lungs. The blood is oxygen-poor, but oxygen is supplied by inspired air. The trachea and bronchioles, which are not part of the oxygen exchange surface, receive oxygen-rich blood from branches of the aorta.

Lung Volumes

The lungs of an average 19-year-old man have a total capacity of about 5900 ml. However, a person cannot exhale all the air from the lungs, and about 1200 ml of air always remains, no matter how forceful the expiration. This remaining volume *(residual volume)* prevents the collapse of the lung structures during expiration. The volume of air that moves in and out with each breath is called the *tidal volume.* During quiet breathing, tidal volume is about 500 ml. When we take a deep breath, the

lung is more fully expanded. The amount of extra air inhaled, beyond the tidal volume, is called the *inspiratory reserve volume;* the extra air that can be exhaled after a normal breath is called the *expiratory reserve volume.*

Lung volumes are often combined into capacities:

- *Total lung capacity* (all four volumes)
- *Vital capacity* (all volumes except residual volume), which is the amount we can ventilate
- *Functional reserve capacity* (expiratory reserve plus residual volumes)
- *Inspiratory capacity* (tidal volume plus inspiratory reserve volume)

These volumes and capacities are frequently altered by disease. Lung volumes as measured by spirometry are shown in Figure U13-4. (Pulmonary function tests are described in Chapter 39.)

Alveoli

The lung parenchyma, which consists of millions of alveolar units, is the working area of the lung tissue. At birth, we have about 24 million alveoli; by age 8 years, we have 300 million. The total working alveolar surface area is approximately 750 to 860 square feet. The blood supply flowing toward the alveoli comes from the right ventricle of the heart.

The entire alveolar unit (respiratory zone) is made up of respiratory bronchioles, alveolar ducts, and alveolar sacs (Fig. U13-5). The alveolar walls are extremely thin, with an almost solid network of interconnecting capillaries. Because of the extensiveness of the capillary system, the flow of blood in the alveolar wall has been described as a "sheet" of flowing blood.

Oxygen and CO_2 are exchanged through a respiratory membrane, about 0.2 mm thick (Fig. U13-6). The average diameter of the pulmonary capillary is only about 5 μm, but red blood cells (7 μm in diameter) must squeeze through, actually touching the capillary wall. Thus, the distance across which oxygen and CO_2 must diffuse is greatly reduced. Thickening of the respiratory membrane

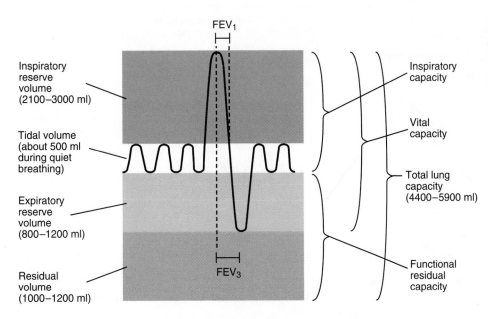

FIGURE U13-4 Lung volumes and capacities as measured by spirometry. The four volumes of the lungs are combined to form four capacities.

FEV$_1$

Inspiratory reserve volume (2100–3000 ml)

Tidal volume (about 500 ml during quiet breathing)

Expiratory reserve volume (800–1200 ml)

Residual volume (1000–1200 ml)

FEV$_3$

Inspiratory capacity

Vital capacity

Total lung capacity (4400–5900 ml)

Functional residual capacity

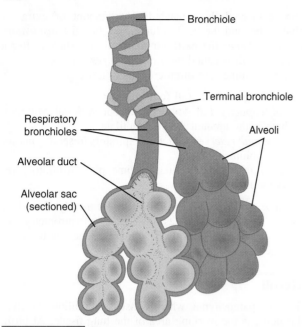

FIGURE U13–5 Gas exchange occurs in the respiratory zone, which consists of the respiratory bronchioles, alveolar ducts, and alveolar sacs.

up of 12 pairs of ribs. The ribs connect posteriorly to the transverse processes of the thoracic vertebrae of the spine. Anteriorly, the first seven pairs of ribs are attached to the sternum by cartilage. The 8th, 9th, and 10th ribs *(false ribs)* are attached to each other by costal cartilage. The 11th and 12th ribs *(floating ribs)* allow full chest expansion because they are not attached in any way to the sternum.

DIAPHRAGM

Breathing is accomplished by skeletal muscle alteration of the thoracic space. The diaphragm is the primary muscle of breathing, and serves as the lower boundary of the thorax (Fig. U13–7). The diaphragm is dome-shaped in the relaxed position, with central muscular attachments to the xiphoid process of the sternum and the lower ribs. Contraction of the diaphragm pulls the muscle downward, increasing the thoracic space and inflating the lungs. The diaphragm's nerve supply (phrenic nerve) comes through

(e.g., with pulmonary edema or fibrosis) may interfere with normal exchange of gases.

The alveolus comprises two cell types: *Type I pneumocytes,* which line the alveolus, are thin and incapable of reproduction but are effective in gas exchange. *Type II pneumocytes* are cuboidal and do not exchange oxygen and CO_2 well. They produce surfactant and are important in lung injury and repair. They differentiate into type I cells; oxygenation is impaired during the transition from type II to type I cells.

THORAX

The bony thorax provides protection for the lungs, heart, and great vessels. The outer shell of the thorax is made

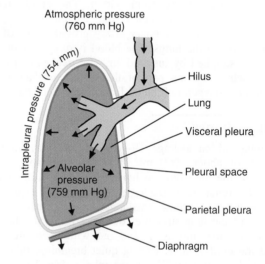

NORMAL INSPIRATION

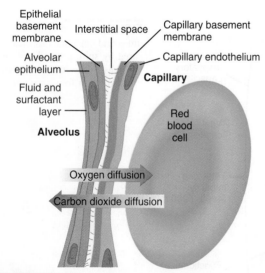

FIGURE U13–6 The ultrastructure of the respiratory membrane, where oxygen is exchanged.

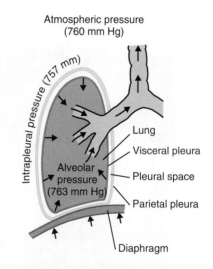

NORMAL EXPIRATION

FIGURE U13–7 Normal inspiration and expiration.

the spinal cord at the level of the third cervical vertebra. Thus, spinal injuries at C3 or above can impair ventilation.

PLEURAE

The pleurae are serous membranes that enclose the lung in a double-walled sac. The *visceral* pleura covers the lung and the fissures between the lobes of the lung. The *parietal* pleura covers the inside of each hemithorax, the mediastinum, and the top of the diaphragm; it joins the visceral pleura at the *hilus* (a notch in the medial surface of the lung, where the mainstem bronchi, pulmonary blood vessels, and nerves enter the lung).

Normally, no space exists between the pleurae; the *pleural space* is a potential space between the two layers of pleura. A thin film (only a few milliliters) of serous fluid acts as a lubricant in the potential space. The fluid also causes the moist pleural membranes to adhere, creating a pulling force that helps to hold the lungs in an expanded position. The action of the pleurae is analogous to coupling two sheets of glass with a thin film of water. It is extremely difficult to separate the sheets of glass at right angles, yet they readily slide along each other. Because of the nature of this coupling, the movement of the lungs closely follows the movement of the thorax. If air or increased amounts of serous fluid, blood, or pus accumulates in the thoracic space, the lungs are compressed and respiratory difficulties follow. These conditions constitute *pneumothorax* (air in the pleural space) or *hemothorax* (blood in the pleural space).

FUNCTION OF THE RESPIRATORY SYSTEM

The respiratory system enhances gas exchange. Inspiration brings oxygen-rich air into the alveoli. The upper and lower airways filter and humidify inspired air. Gas exchange between the air and the blood occurs in the alveolus. Oxygen diffuses into the blood, and CO_2 diffuses from the blood into the alveolar air. The CO_2-enriched air is removed from the body during expiration. The large number and large surface area of alveoli are necessary to meet both resting and exercise gas exchange requirements.

The thorax and diaphragm alter pressures in the thorax to drive air movement. The movement of air depends on pressure gradients between the atmosphere and the air in the lungs, with air flowing from regions of higher pressure to regions of lower pressure. On inspiration, the dome of the diaphragm flattens and the rib cage lifts. As thoracic and lung volumes increase, alveolar pressure decreases and air moves into the lungs.

Airway resistance also affects air movement and is affected primarily by the diameter of the airways. Decreasing the diameter by half results in a 16-fold increase in airway resistance. Thus, a decreased diameter of the airways due to bronchial muscle contraction or to secretions in the airways increases resistance and decreases the rate of air flow. This is a common finding in obstructive airway diseases such as asthma.

During quiet breathing, expiration is usually passive, that is, does not require the use of muscles. The chest wall, in contrast to the lungs, tends to recoil outward. The

opposing forces of lung and chest wall create a subatmospheric (negative) force of about -5 cm of water in the intrapleural space at the end of quiet exhalation. Exhalation is also a result of elastic recoil of the lungs.

VENTILATION

Ventilation, the movement of air in and out of the lungs, involves three forces: (1) compliance properties of the lung and the thorax (chest wall), (2) surface tension, and (3) the muscular efforts of inspiratory muscles.

Compliance

Compliance refers to the ease with which the lung expands and indicates the relationship between the volume and the pressure of the lungs. The lungs are elastic structures that tend to recoil to a volume slightly less than *residual volume* (the volume of gas remaining in the lungs after a full exhalation). The force required to distend the lungs is the difference between the alveolar pressure and the intrapleural pressure. Diseases that cause fibrosis of the lungs result in "stiff" lungs with low compliance; stiff lungs require high inspiratory pressures to achieve a set volume of gas. In contrast, diseases such as emphysema that damage the elastic structure of the alveolar walls result in "floppy" lungs with greater compliance. Relatively low pressures can achieve the same volume of air during inspiration, but passive exhalation is impaired.

Surface Tension

Changes in the surface tension of the liquid film lining the alveoli also affect compliance by changing resistance. *Surface tension,* the result of the air-liquid interface at each alveolus, restricts alveolar expansion on inspiration and aids alveolar collapse on expiration. Surfactant produced by type II cells in the alveolar lining lowers surface tension and thus increases compliance and aids ventilation. A deficiency of surfactant results in stiff lungs. Premature babies lacking surfactant may suffer infant respiratory distress syndrome (IRDS), or hyaline membrane disease.

Muscular Effort

Ventilation also requires muscular effort. For inspiration to occur, the pressure within the lungs (alveolar pressure) must be less than atmospheric pressure. Contraction of the diaphragm and the external intercostal muscles enlarges the size of the thorax. The external intercostal muscles pull the ribs upward and forward, thus increasing the transverse and anteroposterior diameter. Two accessory muscles of inspiration—the scalene and sternocleidomastoid muscles—elevate the first and second ribs during inspiration to enlarge the upper thorax and stabilize the chest wall. The sternocleidomastoid muscle elevates the sternum. The expanding thorax creates a more negative intrapleural pressure, which expands the lungs. When the alveolar pressure becomes lower than the atmospheric pressure, air flows into the lungs.

During exhalation, the inspiratory muscles relax. The elastic recoil of the lung tissue, increases alveolar pressure above atmospheric pressure and causes air to move out of the lungs. Air flow stops when the recoil pressure of the lungs balances the muscular and elastic forces of the chest (see Fig. U13–7).

Although expiration is usually passive, forced expiration and coughing employ accessory muscles to decrease the size of the thoracic space and cause expiration. Contraction of the abdominal muscles forces the diaphragm upward to its dome-shaped position. Contraction of the internal intercostal muscles pulls the ribs inward, thus decreasing the anteroposterior diameter of the chest wall.

Work of Breathing

Respiratory muscle contraction represents a significant metabolic load. Tidal volume and respiratory rate are adjusted to minimize the workload on the body. For example, clients with obstructive lung disease use slower but deeper breaths to maintain appropriate alveolar ventilation. Clients with restrictive lung disease use frequent, shallow breaths to maintain alveolar ventilation.

RESPIRATORY CONTROL

Human metabolism is not one of steady state. The oxygen needs of the tissues change with changing metabolic demands. Respiratory control mechanisms match the elimination of CO_2 and supply of oxygen to the metabolic needs. The lungs have no intrinsic control of themselves; instead, they are controlled by the central nervous system (CNS).

CENTRAL NERVOUS SYSTEM CONTROL. The medulla has several levels of respiratory centers. The dorsal respiratory group primarily provides for inspiration. The ventral respiratory group is normally quiet unless increased ventilation is needed or if active exhalation is performed. The pons has an apneustic center, which contains both expiratory and inspiratory neurons. The upper pons contains the pneumotaxic center, which fine-tunes breathing. For example, the pneumotaxic center allows for talking and breathing.

Output from the respiratory neurons, located in the medulla, descends via the ventral and lateral columns of the spinal cord to phrenic motor neurons of the diaphragm and intercostal motor neurons of the intercostal muscles. The result is rhythmic respiratory movements.

The cortex also allows voluntary control of breathing (holding our breath or altering the rate or depth of breathing).

REFLEX CONTROL. The cough reflex is a neural reflex stimulated by mechanical stimuli (Table U13–1). Inhaled irritants and mucus (mechanical stimuli) excite rapidly adapting pulmonary stretch receptors concentrated in the region of the carina and the large bronchi. The stimulation of the receptors results in high-velocity expiratory gas flow (cough).

PERIPHERAL CONTROL. Peripheral control of respiration is due to the sensing of partial pressure of oxygen (PO_2) and of partial pressure of CO_2 (PCO_2) in the blood. In the blood, CO_2 is an acid. An increase in PCO_2 causes acidosis, or a fall in pH. Receptors that are responsive to changes in oxygen, CO_2, and pH are located in the brain and in structures adjacent to blood vessels. Arterial blood oxygen and CO_2 pressures are sensed by receptors in the

carotid body and the aortic body. The carotid body receptors are located close to the carotid sinus, and the aortic bodies are located near the aortic arch. Chemoreceptors are also located on the brain side of the blood-brain barrier. These receptors respond only to PCO_2 (or pH). An elevated PCO_2 in arterial blood is the normal stimulus to increase ventilation. Low levels of partial pressure of oxygen in arterial blood ($PaCO_2$) can stimulate ventilation, but only when PO_2 drops below 70 mm Hg. There is a powerful synergism between these respiratory stimuli, with the greatest ventilatory drive caused by a simultaneous increase in PCO_2 and decrease in PO_2.

GAS EXCHANGE AND TRANSPORT

The exchange of gases occurs between air and blood in the respiratory membrane. Respiration is the exchange of oxygen and CO_2 at the alveolar-capillary level (*external respiration*) and at the tissue-cellular level (*internal respiration*). During respiration, body tissues are supplied with oxygen for metabolism and CO_2 is released.

In the earth's atmosphere, air contains 20.84% oxygen, 78.62% nitrogen, 0.04% CO_2, and 0.50% water vapor. Each gas exerts a pressure (*partial pressure*) as if it were the only gas present. The sum of the partial pressures is the *barometric pressure*. When a liquid is exposed to a gas, gas enters the liquid in proportion to the individual pressures. PO_2 in the alveoli is about 104 mm Hg, and PCO_2 is about 40 mm Hg. Venous blood has a PO_2 of 40 mm Hg and a PCO_2 of about 45 mm Hg. These differences in concentration result in the movement of oxygen into the pulmonary capillary bloodstream and of CO_2 out of the pulmonary capillary bed into the alveoli (Fig. U13–8).

TABLE U13–1	PHYSIOLOGIC ELEMENTS OF A COUGH
Deep inspiration	Inhaled volume of air must be sufficient to increase lung volume, to increase diameter of bronchi and bronchioles, and to move mucus up and out of airways
Inspiratory pause	Pause (inspiratory pause) allows a buildup and distribution of air and pressure distal to mucus
Closed glottis	Intact muscles and nerves supplying larynx required; allows development of high intrapleural pressures, resulting in a high air flow velocity to propel mucus out of airway
Abdominal muscles	Increase intra-abdominal pressure, which forces diaphragm upward to increase intrapleural pressure against closed glottis
Open glottis	After intrapleural pressures increase, glottis opens suddenly to allow a high velocity of air to leave lungs; flow rates may be as high as 300 L/min
Mucus is expelled	Expulsion due to high velocity of air leaving airway

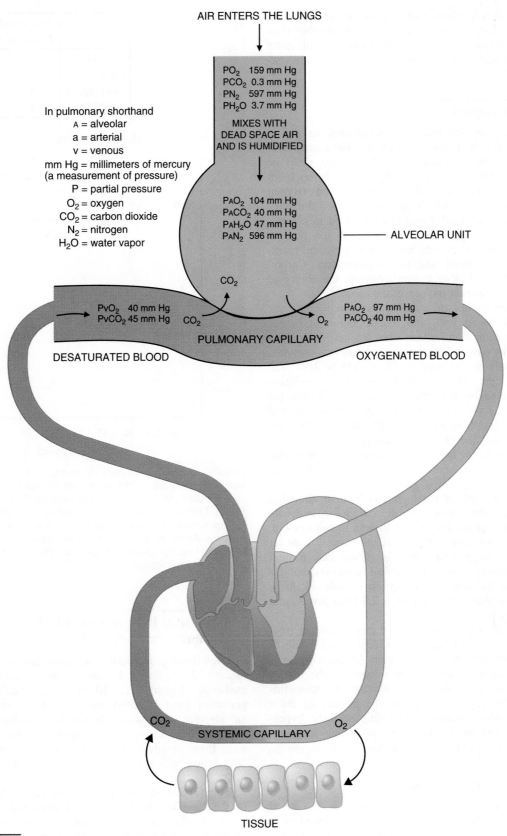

FIGURE U13–8 Partial pressures of gases during normal respiration.

The high PO_2 gradient between the alveolar air and blood is necessary because oxygen is less soluble than CO_2. Diseases that decrease gas diffusion generally alter oxygen exchange before altering carbon dioxide exchange.

Oxygen Transport

After diffusing into the pulmonary capillaries, oxygen is transported throughout the body by the circulatory system. The oxygen is dissolved in the plasma (3%) or bound in the ferrous iron-containing protein hemoglobin (97%). The combination of hemoglobin and oxygen forms *oxyhemoglobin,* which greatly increases the oxygen content of the blood above that dissolved in plasma. Tissues take up oxygen at varying rates; the rate of oxygen consumption creates an oxygen pressure gradient between the blood and the mitochondria. Carbon monoxide (CO) and other chemicals impair the ability of hemoglobin to transport oxygen in the blood.

The *oxyhemoglobin dissociation curve* represents the relationship between PaO_2 and the saturation of hemoglobin. This saturation reflects the amount of oxygen available to the tissues. For a normal curve, it is assumed that the client's temperature is 37° C, pH is 7.40, and PCO_2 is 40 mm Hg. The oxyhemoglobin dissociation curve is affected by a number of factors, including (1) temperature, (2) pH, (3) PCO_2, (4) enzymes in the red blood cell (2,3-diphosphoglycerate [2,3-DPG]), (5) presence of CO, and (6) abnormal hemoglobin. Changes in affinity of oxygen for hemoglobin cause the oxyhemoglobin to move from its normal contour, or to *shift* (Fig. U13–9).

A *shift to the left* of the oxyhemoglobin dissociation curve increases the affinity of the hemoglobin molecule for oxygen. It is easier for oxygen to bind to hemoglobin, but oxygen is not easily released at the tissues. Thus, at any PO_2 level, oxygen saturation is greater than normal but tissue hypoxia is present. Clinical situations that diminish the tissue delivery of oxygen include alkalosis, hypocapnia, hypothermia, decreased 2,3-DPG levels, and CO poisoning.

A *shift to the right* indicates an easier release of oxygen at the tissue level but more difficulty in binding in the lungs. This shift protects the body by allowing oxygen attached to hemoglobin to be released in the tissues to maintain adequate tissue oxygenation. Exercise improves the delivery of oxygen to the tissues, as do a number of clinical situations, including acidosis, hypercapnia, hyperthermia, hyperthyroidism (which increases 2,3-DPG), anemia, and chronic hypoxia.

Carbon Dioxide Transport

CO_2, the waste product of tissue metabolism, is carried by the blood in the following ways: (1) combined with water as carbonic acid (70%), (2) coupled with hemoglobin (23%), or (3) dissolved in plasma (7%). Red blood cells contain the enzyme carbonic anhydrase, which rapidly breaks down CO_2 into hydrogen ions and bicarbonate ions. When venous blood enters the lungs for gas exchange, this reaction reverses, forming CO_2, which is then exhaled.

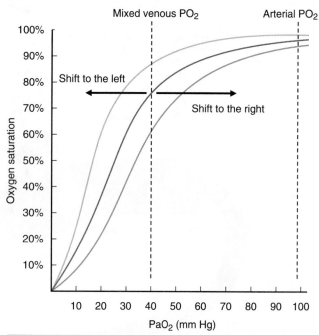

	Factors shifting curve...	
	To the left	To the right
[H⁺], pH	↑	↓
PCO_2	↓	↑
Temperature	↓	↑
2,3 DPG	↓	↑

FIGURE U13–9 The normal oxyhemoglobin wave, showing how changes in the affinity of oxygen for hemoglobin shift the curve to the right or the left. Changes in the PaO_2 at the flattened top portion of the curve result in small changes in oxygen saturation. The opposite is true as the slope of the curve steepens. At the steepest portion of the curve, with the PaO_2 below 60 mm Hg, small changes in the PaO_2 result in large drops in oxygen saturation.

Relationship Between Ventilation and Perfusion

The relationship between *ventilation* (air flow) and *perfusion* (blood flow) determines the efficiency of gas exchange. Figure U13–10 illustrates ventilation with perfusion (unit of dead space), lack of ventilation of an alveolar unit with continued perfusion (a shunt), and total blockage with collapse of alveoli (atelectasis). Low ventilation/perfusion (V/Q) ratios and high V/Q ratios both result in lower oxygen delivery to the body.

The ventilation-perfusion balance differs from the top to the base of the lung. Blood flow and (to a lesser extent) ventilation are greater in the more dependent lung segments at the base of the lung. Consequently, the base of the lung has the lowest V/Q ratio, and the apex of the lung has the highest V/Q ratio.

The V/Q balance is controlled at both the airway and vascular levels. Hypoxia, resulting from underventilation of an alveolar region, causes vasoconstriction, which redirects blood to well-ventilated alveoli. CO_2 in the

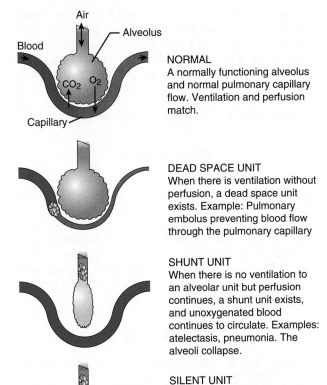

NORMAL
A normally functioning alveolus and normal pulmonary capillary flow. Ventilation and perfusion match.

DEAD SPACE UNIT
When there is ventilation without perfusion, a dead space unit exists. Example: Pulmonary embolus preventing blood flow through the pulmonary capillary

SHUNT UNIT
When there is no ventilation to an alveolar unit but perfusion continues, a shunt unit exists, and unoxygenated blood continues to circulate. Examples: atelectasis, pneumonia. The alveoli collapse.

SILENT UNIT
When there is neither ventilation nor perfusion, a silent unit develops. Example: Pulmonary embolus combined with ARDS (adult respiratory distress syndrome). The alveoli collapse.

FIGURE U13–10 Relationships between ventilation (air flow) and perfusion (blood flow).

airways dilates the airway smooth muscle. Poorly perfused alveoli have low CO_2 levels, and the resultant airway constriction directs ventilation to better-perfused alveoli.

REGULATION OF ACID-BASE BALANCE

The lungs, through gas exchange, have a key role in regulating the acid-base balance of the body. Pulmonary disorders that change the CO_2 level in the blood cause either respiratory acidemia or respiratory alkalemia. Insufficient ventilation causes *hypercapnia,* a respiratory acidemia caused by retention of excessive amounts of CO_2. Hyperventilation, conversely, causes *hypocapnia,* a respiratory alkalemia due to the low amounts of CO_2 in the blood.

The effectiveness of ventilation is best measured by the PCO_2 in the arterial blood ($PaCO_2$). Because the respiratory system is normally set to maintain a $PaCO_2$ between 35 and 45 mm Hg at sea level, a $PaCO_2$ above this range represents *hypoventilation.* Anesthetic agents, sedatives, and narcotics all tend to increase the resting $PaCO_2$. (Acid-base balance is detailed in Chapter 14.)

REACTION TO INJURY

The elaborate defense mechanisms of the lungs involve clearance mechanisms, defense by the respiratory epithelium, and immunologic responses in the lungs. Any injury to the lung affects the barrier between the atmosphere and the bloodstream. This barrier, which lies within the alveolar septum, is made up of epithelial (types I and II pneumocytes) and vascular endothelial cells. Injury resulting from airborne or blood-borne agents may increase vascular permeability and cause pulmonary edema. Inflammatory cells (e.g., neutrophils) arrive soon after acute injury. Then the proportion of lymphocytes, monocytes, and macrophages increases.

The basic lung repair processes include lymphatic drainage of excess fluid and phagocytic removal of protein and debris. This action generally restores lung function and structure. More severe injury requires endothelial and epithelial cell regeneration and proliferation of interstitial cells (fibroblasts). Type II cells that are generated for defense eventually differentiate into thin type I cells, which permit gas exchange. The lung's ability to recreate alveolar septa determines the degree to which normal lung function and structure are restored.

Defense by Clearance Mechanisms

The *upper airways* filter particles. Because the nose has a larger surface-volume ratio and a much more tortuous pathway for airflow than the mouth, particle deposition and conditioning of the air are more efficient when we breathe through the nose. Larger particles (> 10 mm) are generally trapped; smaller particles (< 1 mm) may readily enter the lower airways.

There are four clearance mechanisms of the lower airways and alveoli:

- Cough (first five to eight bronchial generations)
- Mucociliary system (to terminal bronchioles)
- Macrophages (alveoli and respiratory bronchioles)
- Lymphatics (alveoli and interstitium)

The cough, an automatic protective reflex used to clear the trachea, occurs most rapidly in the clearing process (see Table U13–1). If the swallowing reflex is delayed or absent, a cough may be stimulated to avoid aspiration of particles into the lower airways.

Defense by the Respiratory Epithelium

Unlike the upper and lower airways, the alveoli lack a mucous layer to trap foreign particles and cilia to propel them to the pharynx for elimination. The alveolar lining is made up of flat, membranous pneumocytes (type I cells) and rounded granular (type II) cells. The type II cells are resistant to injury and cover most of the alveolar surface after exposure to infectious agents. Alveolar macrophages, derived from blood monocytes that migrate into the lungs, are also found over the surface of the alveoli. Alveolar macrophages are active phagocytes that remove dead cells and protein and that synthesize and secrete substances that regulate the immune system. They leave the lung by the mucociliary system or the lymphatic system.

Defense by Immunologic Mechanisms

The systemic immune system responds to the lung during inflammatory processes by mobilizing blood neutrophils and monocytes. Recruited thymus-dependent (T) and thymus-independent (B) lymphocytes contribute to local cell-mediated immune reactions and the production of specific antibodies within the alveoli. Cell-mediated immunity is a key determinant in resistance to organisms such as *Mycobacterium tuberculosis* and *Pneumocystis carinii*. Immune mechanisms are generally a host defense function. However, hypersensitivity immune reactions lead to tissue injury and are responsible for clinical conditions such as asthma, granuloma formation, and lung transplant rejection. (Chapter 76 describes types I, II, III, and IV hypersensitivity reactions.)

EFFECTS OF AGING

Most of the changes that occur with aging affect the lower airway. Movement of cilia in the upper airway slows and becomes less effective. This change predisposes older clients to a greater number of respiratory infections.

Lung structure also changes with age. The lungs become rounder as a result of increased anteroposterior diameter, circumference, area, and height of the lung. The proportion of the lung formed by alveolar duct air increases, and alveolar air decreases. Loss of alveolar wall tissue and its elastic tissue fibers is seen. The result is a deterioration of lung function.

The air spaces enlarge, although this is not referred to as emphysema because it is not a result of disease. These changes may be due to environmental pollutants rather than to aging alone. An increased incidence of true emphysema and a greater prevalence of chronic cough and sputum production are seen in the elderly population. These findings suggest that environmental or occupational pollutants, in addition to the normal aging process, may be a component in the decline of lung function.

CONCLUSIONS

The primary function of the lungs is gas exchange. The physical structure of the airways allows air to be warmed, filtered, and humidified as it enters the body. In the alveolar sacs, oxygen is exchanged for CO_2. The mechanics of breathing are coordinated by the ribs, diaphragm, pleural space, elastic recoil of the lungs, and the nervous system. The respiratory system also helps regulate acid-base balance. Alterations in structure and function can result in various disorders.

BIBLIOGRAPHY

1. Dickson, S. L. (1995). Understanding the oxyhemoglobin dissociation curve. *Critical Care Nurse, 15*(5), 54–58.
2. Guyton, A. C., and Hall, J. (1996). *Textbook of medical physiology* (9th ed.). Philadelphia: W. B. Saunders.
3. Silverthorn, D. (1998). *Human physiology.* Upper Saddle River, NJ: Prentice-Hall.
4. West, J. (1995). *Respiratory physiology: The essentials* (5th ed.). Baltimore: Williams & Wilkins.
5. West, J. (1997). *Pulmonary pathophysiology: The essentials* (5th ed.). Baltimore: Williams & Wilkins.

CHAPTER 59

Assessment of the Respiratory System

Amy Verst

GENERAL RESPIRATORY ASSESSMENT

Nurses caring for clients experiencing respiratory disorders perform and interpret a variety of assessment procedures. This chapter discusses the physical assessment and diagnostic procedures for clients who have respiratory disorders. The assessment data are used to plan client care.

HISTORY

A respiratory history contains information about a client's present condition and previous respiratory problems. Interview the client and family, and focus on the clinical manifestations of the chief complaint, events leading up to the current condition, past health history, family history, and psychosocial history.

The detail and time taken for a respiratory history depend on the client's condition (e.g., acute, chronic, or emergent). State questions simply using short, easy to understand sentences. When necessary, reword questions to clarify statements the client seems not to understand. Ask questions in the context of the client's daily activities, for instance, Are you able to carry the groceries in from the car? Are you able to make your bed, vacuum the house, bathe yourself, or dress yourself without stopping to rest and catch your breath?

■ BIOGRAPHICAL AND DEMOGRAPHIC DATA

Begin the history by obtaining biographical data. Include the client's name, age, sex, and living situation.

Demographic data are usually recorded on an agency assessment form. Note the client's biologic age and compare it with the client's appearance. Does the client look his or her stated age? Disorders such as lung cancer and chronic lung disorders often make the client appear older. The living situation, whether it be alone, with children, or with significant others, is important in planning for discharge.

■ CURRENT HEALTH

Chief Complaint

The chief complaint helps to establish priorities for intervention and to assess the client's level of understanding of the current condition. Common respiratory complaints include dyspnea (difficulty breathing), cough, sputum production, hemoptysis (blood-stained sputum), wheezing, stridor (a high-pitched respiratory sound), and chest pain. Focus on the manifestations, and prioritize questions to elicit a symptom analysis (see Chapter 9).

In emergency or acute situations, simple questions are all that may be asked until the client is stable and comfortable. Whenever possible, ask significant others for further details.

Take as extensive a respiratory history as the client's condition allows. Detailed questioning provides valuable clues to (1) the client's manifestations, (2) the client's degree of existing respiratory dysfunction, (3) the client's and family's understanding of the condition and its management, and (4) the family's support system and ability to cope with the manifestations and management of the condition on an ongoing basis.

DYSPNEA

Dyspnea (difficulty breathing) is one of the most common manifestations experienced by clients with pulmonary and cardiac disorders. It is a subjective symptom and a reflection of the client's assessment of the degree of work of breathing for a given task or effort. Clients may define dyspnea as shortness of breath, suffocation, tightness, being winded, or being breathless.

The assessment of dyspnea involves several aspects. The subjective nature of dyspnea makes it difficult to quantify objectively. Several methods are used to assess accurately the level of dyspnea experienced by a client. The Visual Analogue Scale (Fig. 59–1) is used to quantify breathlessness in response to particular questions. It is easy to understand, and the amount of dyspnea during various activities can be assessed. The Modified Borg Category Ratio Scale (Table 59–1) is used to rate the intensity of dyspnea. It is simple, and results have been reproduced in several populations.

The Pulmonary Functional Status and Dyspnea Questionnaire (PFSDQ) is used to quantify dyspnea and changes in activity with dyspnea. This instrument was developed and initially tested in a hospital-based pulmonary rehabilitation program.[9]

In addition to subjective assessment, conduct a symptom analysis to document the characteristics of the dysp-

FIGURE 59-1 The Visual Analogue Scale of dyspnea. Although the scale can be in the form of either a vertical or a horizontal line, the most commonly used scale consists of a 100-mm horizontal line, like the one shown here.

How short of breath are you right now?

None   Extremely
                                                                      Severe

nea. Assess all of the characteristics because there are many respiratory and nonrespiratory causes.

COUGH

Detail the many aspects of the client's *cough* by conducting a symptom analysis. Note when and how the cough began (suddenly or gradually) and how long it has been present. Determine the frequency of the cough and the time of day when the cough is better or worse (early morning, late afternoon, nighttime). Use the client's own words to describe the cough. A cough may be described as hacking, dry, hoarse, congested, barking, wheezy, or bubbling.

Determine which medications or treatments the client has used for the cough (e.g., antitussives, codeine, inhalers, nebulizers, rest, sitting up). Find out what precautions are used to prevent the spread of infection (if present). Use the opportunity to remind the person about good hand-washing, proper disposal of soiled tissues, and completion of a full course of antibiotics (if prescribed).

Coughing may lead to stress incontinence; you may want to ask female clients about this embarrassing problem. The incontinence should clear when the coughing subsides; protective padding may be helpful.

SPUTUM PRODUCTION

Sputum is the substance expelled by coughing or clearing the throat. The tracheobronchial tree normally produces about 3 ounces of mucus a day as part of the normal cleaning mechanism; however, sputum production with coughing is not normal. Question the client about sputum color (clear, yellow, green, rusty, bloody), odor, quality (watery, stringy, frothy, thick), and quantity (teaspoon, tablespoon, cup). Document changes in color, odor, qual-

ity, or quantity in the client's medical record. Ascertain whether sputum is produced only after the client is lying in a certain position. The amount of sputum produced is increased in several disorders; for instance, clients with bronchitis may expectorate several cups of sputum daily.

Sputum may be a secretion from the oral or nasopharyngeal area or sinuses rather than from the tracheobronchial tree. For example, draining sinuses may provoke a productive cough.

HEMOPTYSIS

Hemoptysis refers to blood expectorated from the mouth in the form of gross (visible to the naked eye) blood, frankly bloody sputum, or blood-tinged sputum. Attempt to identify the source of the blood—lungs, nosebleed, or stomach. Blood from the lungs is usually bright red because blood in the lungs stimulates an immediate cough reflex. If the blood remains in the lungs for any period of time, it may turn dark red or brown. Ask the client whether the hemoptysis occurred as a result of forceful coughing. Also, obtain an estimate of the amount of blood expectorated (teaspoon, tablespoon, cup).

Pulmonary causes of hemoptysis include chronic bronchitis, bronchiectasis, pulmonary tuberculosis, cystic fibrosis, upper airway necrotizing granulomas, pulmonary embolism, pneumonia, lung cancer, and lung abscesses. Cardiovascular abnormalities, anticoagulants, and immunosuppressive drugs that cause parenchymal (lung tissue) bleeding may also cause hemoptysis.

WHEEZING

Wheezing sounds are produced when air passes through partially obstructed or narrowed airways on inspiration or expiration. *Wheezing* may be audible or may be heard only with a stethoscope. The client may not complain of wheezing but may complain of chest tightness or chest discomfort instead. Ask the client to identify when the wheezing occurs and whether it resolves spontaneously or whether medication (such as inhaled bronchodilators) is required for relief. Not all wheezing is caused by asthma. Wheezing can be caused by mucosal edema, airway secretions, collapsed airways resulting from loss of elastic tissue, and foreign objects or tumors partially obstructing air flow.

STRIDOR

Stridor is the name given to high-pitched sounds produced when air passes through a partially obstructed or narrowed upper airway on inspiration. Stridor is associated with respiratory distress and can be life-threatening because the airway is compromised. Several conditions can lead to stridor: epiglottitis, sleep apnea (cessation of breathing), heart failure, and aspiration. Inquire about changes in voice character, hoarseness, difficulty swallowing, sleep-related disorders such as insomnia, degree of snoring, hypersomnolence (excessive sleepiness) in the morning, early morning headaches, weight gain, fluid retention, apnea, and restlessness.

TABLE 59-1	THE MODIFIED BORG CATEGORY-RATIO SCALE FOR ASSESSMENT OF DYSPNEA
Score	**Intensity**
0	Nothing at all
0.5	Very, very slight
1	Very slight
2	Slight
3	Moderate
4	Somewhat severe
5	Severe
6	
7	Very severe
8	
9	Very, very severe
10	Maximal

Modified from Burden, J., et al. (1982). The perception of breathlessness. *American Review of Respiratory Diseases, 126,* 825–828.

CHEST PAIN

Chest pain may be associated with pulmonary and cardiac problems, and distinguishing between the two is important. Conduct a complete symptom analysis for any chest pain. *Angina pectoris* (from Latin, pain of the chest) may be associated with decreased blood flow to the heart and is a potentially life-threatening problem.

Determine the location, duration, and intensity of the chest pain to provide early clues to the cause. Coughing and pleuritic infections can cause chest pain. Pleuritic chest pain is commonly a sharp, stabbing pain that occurs at one site on the chest wall and increases with chest wall movement or deep breathing. Retrosternal (behind the sternum) pain is usually burning, constant, and aching. Pain can also originate in the bony and cartilaginous parts of the thorax.

The characteristics of angina pectoris and other chest pains differ from each other. Cardiac chest pain is usually described as an aching, heavy, squeezing sensation with pressure or tightness in the substernal area. Angina pectoris can also radiate into the neck or arms (see Chapter 54, Table 54–2, for comparison of types of chest pain). Ask the client what brings on the pain (activity, coughing, movement) and what relieves the pain (nitroglycerin, splinting the chest wall, heat).

Symptom Analysis

To obtain a complete history of the respiratory system, assess the characteristics of any clinical manifestation. Assessment of these characteristics leads to a comprehensive symptom analysis. When the client describes a specific respiratory manifestation, assess the following factors.

SETTING

In what setting does the symptom occur most often? The *setting* refers to the time and place or particular situation—physical setting and psychological environment—in which the client experiences the complaint. For example, the client may cough in the morning after smoking a cigarette or may complain of respiratory distress at work.

TIMING

Timing encompasses both onset (the gradual or sudden appearance of the symptom) and the period (days, weeks, months) during which the problem has occurred. Ask the client whether there is a specific time of day when the problem occurs most frequently, for example, the morning cough or shortness of breath associated with lying flat at night.

CLIENT'S PERCEPTION

Phrase the *client's perception* in the client's own words. Note any unique properties of the complaint. Use a direct quotation to document the client's complaint. For example, client reports a "catch" in the left posterior chest with deep breaths.

QUANTITY AND QUALITY

Describe the *quantity and quality* of the problem in common language. Ask the client to report the amount, size, number, and extent of the chief complaint. Especially with sputum production, ask the client to estimate how much sputum is produced a day—a cup, a tablespoon, or

teaspoon. Avoid using terms such as "a little" or "a lot," which have different meanings among clients and health care providers. Often a scale of 1 to 10, with 1 being the least and 10 the most, is used to describe pain or distress.

In an assessment of a cough, the cough may be described as tight, loose, dry, hacking, or congested. Have clients describe the characteristics of their cough in their own words.

LOCATION

Note the *location* of the manifestation. Ask the client to identify its exact location. Location is especially important when the complaint is chest pain because it is essential to determine whether the pain is cardiac or respiratory in origin.

AGGRAVATING AND RELIEVING FACTORS

The *aggravating* and *relieving factors* precipitate, worsen, or alleviate a symptom. Environmental allergens, such as dog or cat dander, dust mites, mold, and pollen, are often described as aggravating factors. Sitting up or lying down may relieve or exacerbate the symptom. Medication may also worsen or relieve the symptom.

ASSOCIATED MANIFESTATIONS

Associated manifestations occur in conjunction with the chief complaint. Examples include chills, fever, night sweats, anorexia, weight loss, excessive fatigue, anxiety, and hoarseness. You may be able to recognize that chills and fever commonly accompany infectious lung disorders, whereas anorexia and weight loss can occur in clients with disorders that result in dyspnea.

■ PAST HEALTH HISTORY

Examine the past health history of the client and family members for data related to the upper and lower respiratory systems (the upper respiratory history and physical examination are discussed later). These systems are common sources of both acute and chronic health problems. Assess clients with chronic conditions for changes in their ongoing respiratory manifestations (e.g., cough, dyspnea, sputum production, or wheezes) because these changes provide clues to the cause of the new problem. Include questions about the following areas.

Childhood and Infectious Diseases

In addition to obtaining data regarding common childhood diseases and vaccinations, ask the client about the occurrence of tuberculosis, bronchitis, influenza, asthma, and pneumonia and the frequency of lower respiratory infections after upper respiratory infection. Determine the existence of congenital problems, such as cystic fibrosis and premature birth history. These problems are associated with respiratory complications, such as obstructive and restrictive pulmonary disease.

Immunizations

Inquire about vaccination against pneumonia (polyvalent pneumococcal vaccine [Pneumovax]) and influenza. Ask the client to list the dates of these vaccinations. Pneumovax provides lifelong immunity against pneumococcal pneumonia, whereas "flu shots" must be received annually in the fall of the year.

Major Illnesses and Hospitalizations

Ask the client about previous hospitalizations or treatment for respiratory problems. Determine dates of illnesses or hospitalization, the specific respiratory problem, medical treatment (including surgery, use of a ventilator, and inhalation treatments or oxygen therapy), and the present status of the problem.

Has a chest x-ray film been taken? When? Have other pulmonary diagnostic tests been performed? These test results can provide baseline data for the evaluation of the current problem. Inquire about previous injuries to the mouth, nose, throat, or chest (such as blunt trauma, fractured ribs, or pneumothorax).

Medications

Obtain detailed information regarding both prescribed and over-the-counter medications, including herbal remedies, because many products affect the respiratory system. The client may have taken antibiotics for respiratory infections, bronchodilators, or steroids. Specify the route of administration (pill, liquid, or inhalation). Many respiratory medications are inhaled through a metered-dose inhaler (MDI) or mini-nebulizer. If an MDI is used, the client may use a spacer to disperse the medication properly. Ask the client to demonstrate the use of the MDI and spacer.

Herbal medicines for respiratory problems include remedies for nasal discharge and congestion, cough, sore throat, fever and headache, and immunostimulant effects. *Ephedra* (*E. sinica, E. vulgaris*) is a stimulant and is illegal in some areas. Expectorants include anise (*Pimpinella anisum*), coltsfoot (*Tussilago farfara*), and horehound (*Marrubium vulgare*). Coltsfoot and horehound are also believed to have antitussive action.

Sore throat remedies include mint (*Mentha piperita* [peppermint], *Mentha spicata,* [spearmint]) and slippery elm (*Ulmus rubra*). Remedies for the fever and headache that may accompany colds and influenza include boneset (*Eupatorium perfoliatum*), feverfew (*Tanacetum parthenium*), and white willow (*Salix purpurea, Salix fragilis, Salix daphnoides*).

Stimulants of the immune system, believed to help ward off colds and flu, include *Echinacea* (*E. angustifolia, E. pallida, E. purpurea*) and goldenseal (*Hydrastis canadensis*).

Allergies

Question the client about a history of allergies and timing of manifestations to help identify a possible allergic basis for the condition. Ask about precipitating and aggravating factors, such as foods, medications, pollens, smoke, fumes, dust, and animal dander. Sources of molds that may cause allergic manifestations include the water reservoir of a furnace humidifier, air conditioners, and plant soil.

Ask the client to describe the allergic manifestations experienced (e.g., chest tightness, wheezing, cough, rhinitis, watery eyes, scratchy throat) and their severity. Determine the age at which allergies first occurred and whether they have become progressively more severe.

Has the client been tested for allergies? When? Are medications (including allergy shots) taken prophylactically or on an as-needed basis to provide symptomatic relief?

■ FAMILY HEALTH HISTORY

Question the client about the family history of respiratory diseases. Identify blood relatives (in regard to *genetically transmitted* diseases) and family members (in regard to *infectious* conditions) who have had asthma, cystic fibrosis, emphysema or chronic obstructive pulmonary disease (COPD), lung cancer, respiratory infections, tuberculosis, or allergies. List the age and cause of death of each deceased family member.

Do any household members smoke cigarettes, pipes or cigars? Secondary inhalation of smoke often precipitates or worsens respiratory manifestations.

■ PSYCHOSOCIAL HISTORY

Respiratory status is affected by numerous factors that may lead to acute problems or that may affect the client's coping with chronic problems such as COPD. Areas to be assessed are described next.

Occupation

Identify any environmental agents that may contribute to the client's condition. Ask specifically about the work environment and hobbies. Focus on exposure to dust, asbestos, beryllium, silica, and other toxins or pollutants. Farmers are exposed to airborne particles that may be inhaled, such as grain dust, fertilizers, and animal dander. Hobbies may involve chemicals, heat, dust, and airborne particles from grinding, soldering, or welding.

Geographical Location

Ask about recent travel to areas where respiratory diseases are prevalent, such as Asia (tuberculosis), the Ohio River valley (histoplasmosis), or the San Joaquin valley (valley fever). Polluted city air has also been related to increasing incidence and severity of asthma.

Environment

Ask about the client's living conditions. How many people are in the household? Crowded living conditions increase risk of exposure to infectious respiratory diseases such as tuberculosis and cold viruses. Recent exposure to continuous air conditioning in a hotel or motel setting may be related to legionnaires' disease.

Assess for environmental hazards such as stairs or poor air circulation. A client with a chronic respiratory condition may have difficulty climbing stairs or breathing unfiltered air.

Habits

Inquire about any history of smoking tobacco products. Calculate the pack-years, which helps quantify the smoking history, as follows:

years of smoking × packs smoked per day = pack-years

Smoking has been associated with decreased ciliary function of the lungs, increased mucus production, and the development of lung cancer. Ask the client about the use of smokeless tobacco (such as snuff, chewing tobacco) and smoking nontobacco substances (such as marijuana and clove cigarettes).

Ask about alcohol use. Ciliary action is slowed by alcohol, which reduces mucus clearance from the lungs. Heavy alcohol ingestion depresses the cough reflex and increases risk of aspiration. Clients who use and abuse recreational drugs are at risk for drug overdose and respiratory failure. Sharing needles increases the risk of human immunodeficiency virus (HIV) infection and the development of acquired immunodeficiency syndrome (AIDS) and opportunistic infections such as *Pneumocystis carinii.*

Exercise

Clients who are active may describe the onset of coughing and wheezing during exercise. These clients need to be further evaluated for exercise-induced asthma before continuing workouts. Clients with chronic respiratory conditions often do not have the lung capacity to sustain even mild forms of exercise and subsequently become dyspneic. Has tolerance for activity decreased or remained stable? Ask the client to describe typical activities, such as walking, light housekeeping chores, or grocery shopping, that are tolerated or, conversely, that result in shortness of breath.

Nutrition

Maintaining a nutritious diet is important for clients with chronic respiratory disease, which can result in decreased lung capacity and greater workload for the lungs and cardiovascular system. The added workload increases caloric expenditure, and weight loss may occur. Clients may become anorectic because of the effects of medications and fatigue. The client may not have enough energy to consume the needed calories to maintain body weight. Ask the client to recall intake for the last 24 hours. Assess the amount of protein, kilocalories, and sodium intake (see Chapter 28).

■ REVIEW OF SYSTEMS

Ask the client to describe other manifestations associated with the respiratory system. In addition to cough, dyspnea, sputum production, hemoptysis, wheezing, stridor, and chest pain, include breathlessness, fever, hoarseness, night sweats, anorexia, weight loss, and dependent edema. Upper respiratory manifestations include colds, nasal discharge, postnasal drip, sinus pain and swelling, epistaxis (nosebleed), and sinus headaches.

Hypoxia may precipitate subtle neurologic alterations, such as restlessness, fatigue, disorientation, and personality changes. Tachycardia usually accompanies respiratory problems as the body attempts to compensate for decreased oxygen delivery. Stomach upset, nausea, and vomiting can result from accumulation of excess mucus swallowed from draining sinuses. Anorexia and weight loss are seen in many chronic respiratory conditions. Detailed questions for the review of systems may be found in Chapter 9, Box 9–2.

PHYSICAL EXAMINATION

Physical examination follows the health history. Use the techniques of inspection, palpation, percussion, and auscultation. Successful examination requires that you be familiar with the anatomic landmarks of the posterior, lateral, and anterior thorax (Fig. 59–2). Use these landmarks to locate and visualize the underlying structures, particularly the lobes of the lungs, the heart, and major vessels. Compare the findings on one side of the thorax with those on the other side. Palpation, percussion, and auscultation proceed in a back-and-forth or side-to-side manner so that you continually evaluate findings by using the opposite side as the standard for comparison.

Note the condition and color (pale, red, blue) of the client's skin throughout the examination of the thorax, and record abnormalities. Assess respiratory rate, depth, and rhythm, if not assessed previously with the vital signs, during inspection of the thorax (see Chapter 10). Assess the client's level of consciousness and orientation throughout the examination to determine adequate gas exchange. See the Physical Assessment Findings in the Healthy Adult feature for expected respiratory findings.

■ INSPECTION

The physical examination begins during the history-taking stage as you observe the client and the client's response to questions. Note manifestations of respiratory distress at this time: position of comfort, tachypnea (rapid, shallow breathing), gasping, grunting, central cyanosis, open mouth, flared nostrils, dyspnea, color of facial skin and lips, and use of accessory muscles. Note the *inspiratory-to-expiratory (I:E) ratio.* Because the normal length of expiration is twice that of inspiration, the normal ratio is 2:1.

Observe the client's speech pattern. How many words or sentences can be said before another breath is taken? Clients who are short of breath may be able to say only three or four words before taking another breath. During the physical examination, the client should be bare to the waist while privacy and warmth are maintained. Inspection and palpation, often performed together, are discussed separately.

Head and Neck

Begin inspection with observation of the head and neck for any gross abnormalities that would interfere with respiration. Note the odor of the breath and whether sputum is present. Note nasal flaring, breathing with pursed lips, or cyanosis of the mucous membranes. Record the use of accessory muscles, such as flexion of the sternocleidomastoid muscle.

Chest

CHEST WALL CONFIGURATION
Continue inspection by observing the chest wall configuration. Observe chest size and contour, and note the *anteroposterior* (AP) diameter. Calculate the ratio of the AP diameter to the transverse diameter. The transverse diameter is generally twice the AP diameter (Fig. 59–3A).

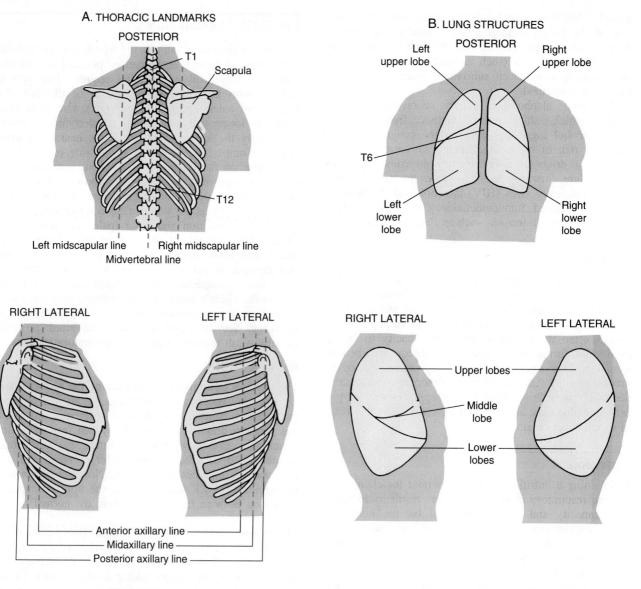

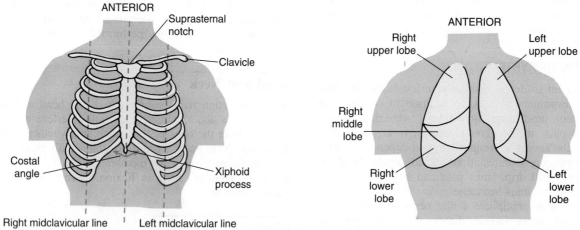

FIGURE 59-2 Thoracic landmarks and underlying lung structures. During chest examination, it is important to document in a universally understood manner the location of unusual or abnormal findings. Use the terminology of thoracic landmarks and lung structure to do so.

PHYSICAL ASSESSMENT FINDINGS IN THE HEALTHY ADULT

Respiratory System

Inspection

Nose. Nose straight, without flaring or discharge; nares patent; mucosa pink and moist; septum midline, without masses or perforation

Sinuses. Transilluminate

Thorax. Even color; regular, even contour; respirations quiet, unlabored, of even depth, and without retractions, bulges, masses, or use of accessory muscles; antero-posterior-transverse diameter ratio 1:2

Digits. Clubbing absent; nail beds pink; immediate capillary refill on blanching

Palpation

Nose. Nontender, without masses or lesions

Sinuses. Nontender, without swelling or bogginess

Trachea. Midline and mobile without crepitus

Thorax. Chest wall symmetrical, smooth, without lumps, masses, tenderness, or crepitus; thoracic excursion symmetrical; tactile fremitus present

Percussion

Sinuses. Nontender

Thorax and Lungs. Resonant throughout peripheral lung fields; cardiac dullness; diaphragmatic excursion ranges from 3 to 6 cm for each hemidiaphragm, with the right side slightly higher than the left

Auscultation

Thorax and Lungs. Vesicular sounds throughout peripheral lung fields; bronchovesicular sounds over the area of tracheal bifurcation, both anteriorly and posteriorly; bronchial sounds over the trachea anteriorly; adventitious sounds absent; vocal resonance absent

BARREL CHEST. Barrel chest is present when the AP diameter is increased and equals the transverse diameter (Fig. 59–3B). It is a characteristic finding in clients with chronic disorders that interfere with ventilation (e.g., emphysema).

PIGEON CHEST. Pigeon chest (pectus carinatum) is the opposite of funnel chest. The sternum juts forward and increases the AP diameter (Fig. 59–3C). Congenital atrial or ventricular septal defects are the most common cause of pigeon chest, but rickets, Marfan's syndrome, and severe primary kyphoscoliosis may contribute to pigeon chest.

FUNNEL CHEST. Funnel chest (pectus excavatum) is a deformity in which the sternum is depressed and the organs that lie below it are compressed (Fig. 59–3D). In severe cases, the sternum may actually touch the spinal column. In most cases, however, pectus excavatum is clinically insignificant. Some causes of funnel chest, including Marfan's syndrome and congenital connective tissue disorders, may be serious.

THORACIC KYPHOSCOLIOSIS. Thoracic kyphoscoliosis is an accentuation of the normal thoracic curve (Fig. 59–3E). The client takes on a hunched-over or hunchback appearance. Causes include congenital defect, osteoporosis secondary to aging, spinal tuberculosis, rheumatoid arthritis, and poor posture over a long period of time. The underlying lungs are distorted, which can make interpretation of lung findings difficult.

CHEST MOVEMENT

Observe chest movement during respiration. Normal respiratory rate is 12 to 22 breaths per minute. Note the amplitude, or depth of expansion, and rhythm. Abdominal breathing is more apparent in men, whereas women use their thoracic muscles. Note the use of accessory muscles, retractions, symmetry, and any paradoxical movements.

Fingers and Toes

Examination of the fingers and toes may reveal *clubbing,* which may be present in clients with pulmonary fibrosis, lung cancer, or bronchiectasis. Clubbing occurs as a compensatory measure in chronic hypoxia. The physiologic cause of clubbing has not yet been identified, although some hypotheses have been proposed. The body develops collateral circulation around an area of impaired circulation to provide more oxygen to that area. With clubbing, the nail bed loses its normal angle of 160 degrees between the nail plate and the finger, and the angle increases to 180 degrees. The base of the nail bed may feel spongy and soft. With advanced clubbing, the finger takes on a bulbous or spoon-like appearance. Assess early clubbing by using the Schamroth technique (Fig. 59–4).

Note the color of the nail beds to assess the status of peripheral tissue oxygenation. Nail beds should be pink, without cyanosis or a dusky blue color. Quickly and gently compress (between thumb and index finger) and release several of the client's nail beds on each extremity. Continuously observe for the *blanch response* and *capillary refill.* With compression, the nail bed becomes pale as capillary blood is squeezed from the tissue. Upon release of the pressure, oxygenated arterial blood fills the capillary bed. Normal capillary refill occurs within 3 seconds; a refill time longer than 3 seconds indicates delayed capillary refill.

■ PALPATION

Palpation is the use of the hands to feel various structures on and below the surface of the body. The technique of palpation is described in Chapter 10.

Trachea

Gently place the thumb of the palpating hand on one side of the trachea and the remaining fingers on the other side. Move the trachea gently from side to side along its length while palpating for masses, *crepitus* (air in the subcutaneous tissues), or deviation from the midline. The trachea is usually slightly movable and quickly returns to the midline position after displacement. A chest mass, goiter, or an acute chest injury may displace the trachea.

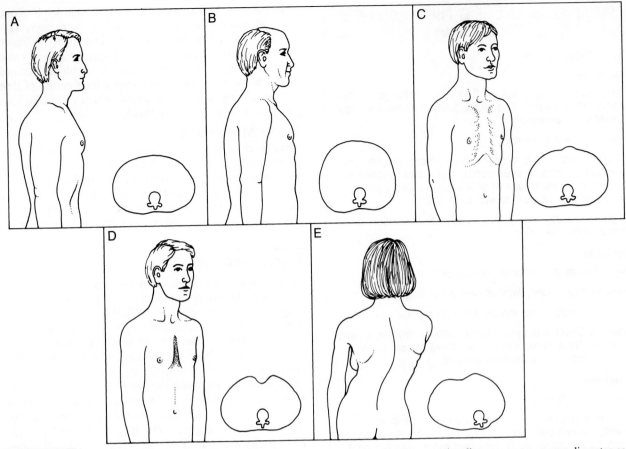

FIGURE 59–3 Chest deformities. *A*, Normal adult, for comparison. The ratio of anteroposterior diameter to transverse diameter can be seen here as 1:2. *B*, Barrel chest. The anteroposterior-transverse diameter ratio is 1:1. *C*, Pigeon chest (pectus carinatum). *D*, Funnel chest (pectus excavatum). *E*, Thoracic kyphoscoliosis.

Chest Wall

Palpate the chest wall, holding the heel or ulnar aspect of your hand against the client's chest. During palpation, continue the investigation of abnormalities found on in-

spection. Palpation combined with inspection is particularly effective in assessing whether the movements, or thoracic excursion of the chest during inspiration and expiration, are symmetrical and equal in amplitude. During palpation, assess for crepitus, defects or tenderness of

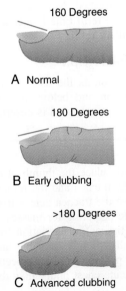

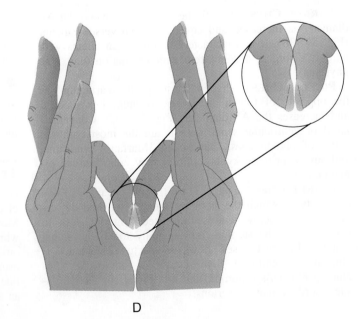

FIGURE 59–4 Clubbing. *A*, A normal digit, with an angle of 160 degrees. *B*, A flattened angle between the nail and the skin, exceeding 180 degrees. *C*, Advanced clubbing, with a rounded nail. *D*, Assess clubbing with the use of the Schamroth technique. Instruct the client to place the nails of the fourth (ring) fingers together while extending the other fingers and to hold the hands up. A diamond-shaped space between the nails is a normal finding and indicates the absence of clubbing.

160 Degrees

A Normal

180 Degrees

B Early clubbing

>180 Degrees

C Advanced clubbing

D

the chest wall, muscle tone, edema, and tactile *fremitus* (the vibration of air movement through the chest wall while the client is speaking).

Thoracic Excursion

For the evaluation of thoracic excursion, the client sits upright. Place your hands on the client's posterior chest wall (Fig. 59–5). The thumbs oppose each other on either side of the spine, and the fingers face upward and out like butterfly wings. As the client inhales, your hands should move up and out symmetrically. Any asymmetry suggests a disease process in that region.

Tactile Fremitus

Palpate the posterior chest wall while the client says words that produce relatively intense vibrations (e.g., "ninety-nine"). The vibrations are transmitted from the larynx via the airways and can be palpated on the chest wall (Fig. 59–6). Compare the intensity of vibrations on both sides for symmetry. Stronger vibrations are felt over areas where there is consolidation of the underlying lung (e.g., pneumonia). Decreased tactile fremitus is usually associated with abnormalities that move the lung farther from the chest wall, such as pleural effusion and pneumothorax.

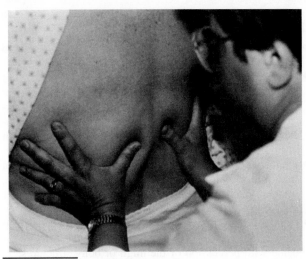

FIGURE 59–5 Assessment of thoracic excursion to determine the degree and symmetry of chest movement.

■ PERCUSSION

Percussion is an assessment technique of producing sounds by tapping on the chest wall with the hand (see Chapter 10). Tapping on the chest wall between the ribs

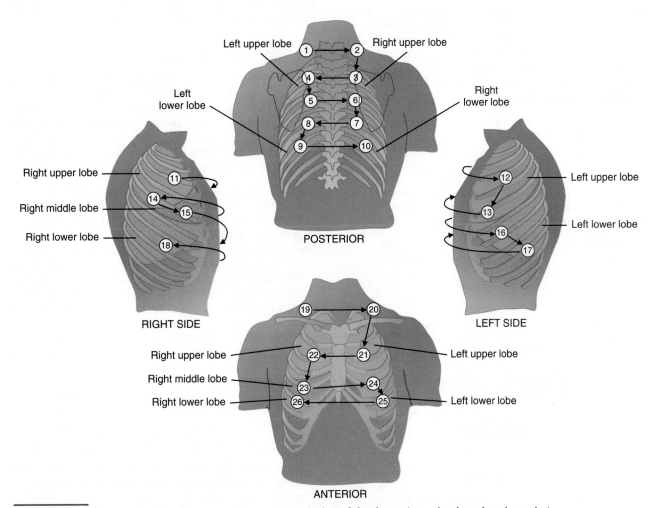

FIGURE 59–6 Sequence of palpation, percussion, and auscultation of the thorax (posterior, lateral, and anterior).

produces various sounds that are described in relation to their acoustic properties:

- *Resonant* sounds are low-pitched, hollow sounds heard over normal lung tissue.
- *Hyperresonant* sounds indicate an increased amount of air in the lungs or pleural space. These sounds are louder and lower-pitched than resonant sounds. Hyperresonant sounds are produced by emphysema and pneumothorax; they are normally heard in children and in very thin adults.
- *Dull* sounds occur over dense lung tissue, such as a tumor or a consolidation. These sounds are thud-like, medium-pitched. They are normally heard over the liver and heart.
- *Flat* notes are soft and high-pitched; they result from percussion over airless tissue. This sound can be replicated with percussion of the thigh or bony structures.
- *Tympanic* notes are high, hollow, drum-like sounds heard with percussion over the stomach, a large tension pneumothorax, or a large air-filled chamber (such as the empty stomach).

Figure 59–7 illustrates the location of percussion sounds of the chest.

Begin percussion at the apices and proceed to the bases, moving from the posterior to the lateral and then to the anterior areas (see Fig. 59–6). The posterior chest is best percussed with the client in an upright position and with arms crossed to separate the scapulae.

Percussion is also used to assess diaphragmatic excursion. Ask the client to take a deep breath and to hold it as you percuss down the posterior lung field and listen for the percussion note to change from resonant to dull. Mark this area with a pen. The process is repeated after the client exhales, and again the area is marked.

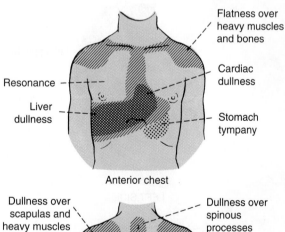

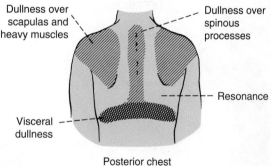

FIGURE 59–7 Location of thoracic percussion sounds and their associated structures.

Assess both right and left sides. The distance between the two marks should be 3 to 6 cm; smaller spans are found in females and larger spans in males. The marks on the right are slightly higher because of the presence of the liver. A client with an elevated diaphragm related to a pathologic process has decreased diaphragmatic excursion.

If the client has lung disease in the lower lobes (e.g., consolidation or pleural fluid), the same dull percussion note is heard. When abnormalities are found, other diagnostic tests should be used to assess the problem fully.

■ AUSCULTATION

Auscultation involves listening to chest sounds with a stethoscope. By listening to the lungs while the client breathes through an open mouth, you can assess:

- The character of the breath sounds
- The presence of adventitious sounds (described later)
- The character of the spoken and whispered voice

Figure 59–6 identifies a sequence for auscultation with comparison of sounds from right to left.

Listen to all areas of the lungs over a bare chest; do not listen to lungs over sheets, gowns, or shirts. The sounds heard may be from the movement of fabric beneath the stethoscope. At each position, listen at the diaphragm for a full respiratory cycle of inspiration and expiration as the client breathes through the mouth.

Normal Breath Sounds

Breath sounds are noises resulting from the transmission of vibrations produced by the movement of air in the respiratory passages. Be familiar with the sounds created by normal air exchange and their location (Table 59–2). Normal breath sounds (vesicular, bronchial, and bronchovesicular) are heard in the locations identified in Figure 59–8. The sounds are described as follows:

Vesicular breath sounds are heard throughout the chest and heard best in the bases of the lungs. They are low-pitched, soft, "swishing" sounds best heard during inspiration with an $I:E$ ratio of $5:2$.

Bronchial breath sounds are heard over the manubrium in the large tracheal airways. Bronchial sounds, heard only anteriorly, are best heard during expiration with an expiratory-to-inspiratory ($E:I$) ratio of $2:1$. These sounds are loud and high-pitched and have a hollow or harsh quality.

Bronchovesicular sounds are heard anteriorly and posteriorly over the central, large airways. They are heard equally during inspiration and expiration and have a tubular or breezy-sounding quality.

Absent or *diminished* breath sounds are confirmed during deep respirations after the client has been instructed to take deep breaths and sounds cannot be heard. "Shallow" breaths may produce diminished sounds in the peripheral lung regions, but "deep" breaths should produce normal vesicular sounds. If absent breath sounds are a new finding, immediate medical attention is required because this finding usually indicates pneumothorax or other respiratory emergency.

	Pitch	Amplitude	Duration	Quality	Normal Location
TABLE 59–2		**CHARACTERISTICS OF NORMAL BREATH SOUNDS**			
Bronchial (tracheal)	High	Loud	Inspiration < expiration	Harsh, hollow, tubular	Trachea and larynx
Bronchovesicular	Moderate	Moderate	Inspiration = expiration	Mixed	Over major bronchi where fewer alveoli are located: posterior, between scapulae, especially on the right; anterior, around the upper sternum in the first and second intercostal spaces
Vesicular	Low	Soft	Inspiration > expiration	Rustling, like the sound of the wind in the trees	Over peripheral lung fields where air flows through smaller bronchioles and alveoli

From Jarvis, C. (1996). *Physical examination and health assessment* (2nd ed.) Philadelphia: W. B. Saunders.

Adventitious Breath Sounds

Adventitious sounds (Table 59–3) are abnormal sounds superimposed on normal breath sounds. The current American Thoracic Society nomenclature for adventitious sounds is used throughout this chapter. Adventitious sounds include (1) crackles, (2) rhonchi, (3) wheezes, and (4) pleural friction rubs.

CRACKLES

Crackles (formerly called *rales*) are audible when there is a sudden opening of small airways that contain fluid. The sound of a crackle can be reproduced by rubbing a lock of hair between the thumb and finger close to the ear. Crackles are usually heard during inspiration and do not clear with a cough. Crackles can be found in clients with pulmonary edema, pulmonary fibrosis, or pneumonia.

RHONCHI

Rhonchi (also called "gurgles") occur as the result of air passing through fluid-filled, narrow passages. Diseases in which there is excess mucus production, such as pneumonia, bronchitis, or bronchiectasis, are associated with rhonchi. Rhonchi are usually heard on expiration and may clear with a cough.

WHEEZES

A wheeze is a continuous musical or hissing noise that results from the passage of air through a narrowed airway. Wheezes are heard during inspiration or expiration or both. Severe wheezes are audible without a stethoscope. Wheezing is commonly associated with asthma and its bronchoconstriction and edema, but foreign bodies can also cause airway narrowing and wheezing.

PLEURAL FRICTION RUBS

Pleural friction rubs are the result of pleural inflammation often associated with pleurisy, pneumonia, or pleural infarct. A rub is described as a creaking, grating noise similar to that made by two pieces of leather rubbing together. A rub is audible on inspiration and expiration over the area of the inflammation. Chest wall splinting can be associated with a pleural friction rub.

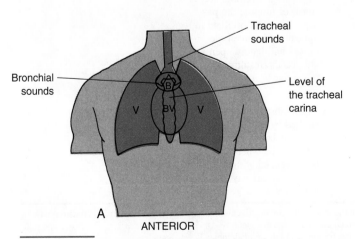
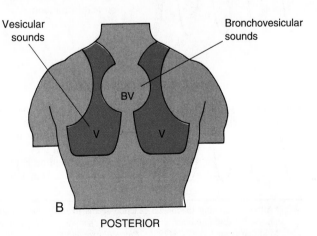

FIGURE 59–8 *A* and *B*, Location of normal breath sounds.

TABLE 59–3   **ADVENTITIOUS BREATH SOUNDS**

Sound*	Description	Mechanism	Clinical Example
DISCONTINUOUS SOUNDS			
Crackles—fine (rales, crepitations) Inspiration Expiration	Discontinuous, high-pitched, short crackling, popping sounds heard during inspiration that are not cleared by coughing; this sound can be simulated by rolling a strand of hair between the fingers near the ear, or by moistening thumb and index finger and separating them near the ear	Inhaled air collides with previously deflated airways; airways suddenly pop open, creating a crackling sound as gas pressures between the two compartments equalize	*Late inspiratory crackles* occur with restrictive disease: pneumonia, heart failure, and interstitial fibrosis *Early inspiratory crackles* occur with obstructive disease: chronic bronchitis, asthma, and emphysema
Crackles—coarse (coarse rales)	Loud, low-pitched, bubbling and gurgling sounds that start in early inspiration and may be present in expiration; may decrease somewhat by suctioning or coughing but will reappear shortly; sound like opening a self-fastening tape (Velcro) fastener	Inhaled air collides with secretions in the trachea and large bronchi	Pulmonary edema, pneumonia, pulmonary fibrosis, and in the terminally ill who have a depressed cough reflex
Atelectatic crackles (atelectatic rales)	Sound like fine crackles, but do not last and are not pathologic; disappear after the first few breaths; heard in axillae and bases (usually dependent) of lungs	When sections of alveoli are not fully aerated, they deflate and accumulate secretions; crackles are heard when these sections reexpand with a few deep breaths	In aging adults, bedridden people, or in people just aroused from sleep
Pleural friction rub	A very superficial sound that is coarse and low-pitched; it has a grating quality as if two pieces of leather are being rubbed together; sounds just like crackles, but *close* to the ear; sounds louder if the stethoscope is pushed harder onto the chest wall; sound is inspiratory and expiratory	Caused when pleurae become inflamed and lose their normal lubricating fluid; their opposing roughened pleural surfaces rub together during respiration; heard best in the anterolateral wall where there is greatest lung mobility	Pleuritis, accompanied by pain with breathing (rub disappears after a few days if pleural fluid accumulates and separates pleurae)
CONTINUOUS SOUNDS			
Wheeze—high-pitched (sibilant rhonchi)	High-pitched, musical squeaking sounds that predominate in expiration but may occur in both expiration and inspiration	Air squeezed or compressed through passageways narrowed almost to closure by collapsing, swelling, secretions, or tumors; the passageway walls oscillate in apposition between the closed and barely open positions; the resulting sound is similar to a vibrating reed	Obstructive lung disease such as asthma or emphysema
Wheeze—low-pitched (sonorous rhonchi)	Low-pitched, musical snoring, moaning sounds; they are heard throughout the cycle, although they are more prominent on expiration; may clear somewhat by coughing	Air flow obstruction as described by the vibrating reed mechanism above; the pitch of the wheeze cannot be correlated with the size of the passageway that generates it	Bronchitis

*Although nothing in clinical practice seems to differ more than the nomenclature of adventitious sounds, most authorities concur on two categories: (1) discontinuous, discrete crackling sounds and (2) continuous, coarse, or musical sounds.

Modified from Jarvis, C. (1996). *Physical examination and health assessment* (2nd ed.). Philadelphia: W. B. Saunders.

Voice Sounds

Assess voice sounds (vocal resonance) by auscultation if tactile fremitus is abnormal. Auscultation while the client speaks normally reveals muffled and indistinct sounds. The sound is louder medially over the larger airways and softens toward the periphery. Consolidation results in *bronchophony* or increased resonance, so that when the client says "ninety-nine," it is heard clearly.

If bronchophony is present, assess for egophony next. *Egophony* involves a change in the sound of the letter *e* to that of the letter *a*, indicating consolidation. The sound also has a nasal or bleating quality.

A third voice test for consolidation is *whispered pectoriloquy.* Ask the client to whisper "one-two-three." If the words are distinct, the abnormal finding of whispered pectoriloquy is present. Consolidation enhances the transmission of sound vibrations and results from lung tumors, pneumonia, or pulmonary fibrosis.

ASSESSMENT OF THE NOSE, PHARYNX, AND SINUSES

HISTORY

Upper respiratory problems can occur alone or progress to lower respiratory complications, such as viral infections.

■ CURRENT HEALTH

Chief Complaint

The client may present with a current complaint of nosebleeds (epistaxis); sinus infection; hay fever; postnasal drip; rhinitis; sneezing; or nasal, facial, or referred ear pain. Obstruction by engorged mucous membranes or nasal polyps may occlude the upper airway. Loss of or a decreased sense of smell may accompany manifestations of the common cold and allergies or may signal a more serious neurologic problem.

Inquire whether the client has experienced these manifestations previously and, if so, when and how often. Ask the client to describe self-treatment measures, such as nasal sprays, decongestants, antihistamines, and other over-the-counter and herbal cold and allergy medications. For example, an herbal remedy for hay fever is nettle (*Urtica dioica*). See the earlier discussion of herbal remedies.

Symptom Analysis

Perform a complete symptom analysis to determine the nature of the problem, including onset, duration, and severity.

AGGRAVATING AND RELIEVING FACTORS

Ask the client about factors that alleviate or worsen the manifestations, such as increased humidity, sitting upright, lying supine, weather and seasonal changes, or allergies. Nasal and sinus problems may be allergy-related and provoked by pollen, fumes, smoke, animal dander, or dust particles. Nosebleeds may increase during the winter months if mucous membranes are dry because of insufficient humidity.

ASSOCIATED MANIFESTATIONS

A foul taste in the mouth, unpleasant breath odor (halitosis), nasal obstruction, and facial pain (particularly over the frontal and maxillary sinuses) may accompany sinusitis. Chronic sinusitis may be accompanied by headache or facial pain present on awakening and diminishing during the day (because the sinuses drain when the client sits or stands).

■ PAST HEALTH HISTORY

Ask about past problems with frequent colds, sinus infections, nasal stuffiness, or trauma (fracture). Explore episodes of epistaxis for cause (e.g., hypertension), frequency, and treatment (e.g., cauterization or nasal packing).

PHYSICAL EXAMINATION

Inspect and palpate the client's nose and sinuses. The structures assessed include the external nose, vestibule, nasal mucosa, septum, turbinates, nasal canals, and sinuses. Function of the first cranial nerve (olfactory) is usually not tested unless a deficit in the sense of smell is reported or suspected.

■ NOSE

External Nose

Inspect and palpate the external nose for deviations from normal alignment, symmetry, color, discharge, nasal flaring, lesions, and tenderness. Normal findings are listed. The skin color over the nose is the same as that of the facial skin. Alignment is straight and symmetrical without deviation from the midline. Discharge from the nares (nostrils) should be absent, and the nares should not flare (spread) with respirations. The client is able to breathe quietly through the nose rather than breathe through the mouth. Masses, lesions, and tenderness are absent.

Check the nasal canals for patency by asking the client to occlude one naris with a finger and to breathe through the open naris while closing the mouth. Repeat this for the opposite naris. The client should be able to breathe without difficulty through both nares. Ask the client to tip the head back, and inspect the outer nares for crusting, bleeding, or dryness, which should be absent.

Internal Nose

Next, inspect the vestibules with a penlight while the client's head is tipped back. Normal findings include coarse hairs, a clear passage without discharge, and a midline septum. Further examination of the internal nose requires use of a nasal speculum and is not conducted unless indicated. If a detailed examination of the internal nose is performed, either attach a nasal speculum tip to the otoscope head or use a metal nasal speculum (Fig. 59–9) and penlight for illumination. While the client tips the head back, gently insert the speculum into one naris, taking care not to scrape the mucosa. Inspect one naris at a time.

Hold the speculum correctly, and insert the blades gently about ½ inch into the nostril. Gain additional control of the speculum by resting the index finger of the dominant hand on the side of the client's nose. Steady the client's head with the nondominant hand. Open the blades gently and vertically, avoiding pressure on the septum and turbinates. Slowly move the head to inspect all areas

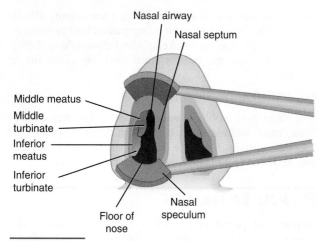

FIGURE 59–9 Internal inspection of the nose with a nasal speculum.

of the nasal chamber. Observe the condition of the mucous membrane (e.g., pallor, redness, swelling). Normally, the mucosa is moist and dark pink without sign of inflammation, pallor, or a blue color. Presence of discharge is abnormal. The septum divides the nasal cavity into halves without deviation, masses, perforation, or exudate. The turbinates are the same color as the mucosa and should be free of exudate, swelling, or inflammation (only the inferior and part of the middle turbinate are visible; the superior is not). Look for polyps and other masses. Observe mucous plugs for color, consistency, amount, and odor.

Inspection may be hampered by nasal congestion. It may be necessary to shrink the nasal mucosa with a topical vasoconstrictor (e.g., phenylephrine hydrochloride) for adequate inspection. When the agent is instilled into the nose, ask the client to say *e* and hold the sound. Use of this technique raises the posterior tongue, occludes the upper airway, and prevents the fluid from running into the pharynx.

■ NASOPHARYNX

The nasopharynx is best examined with a mirror while the tongue is depressed with a tongue blade or pulled forward and grasped with a gauze sponge. Prevent fogging of the mirror by warming it before putting it into the mouth. Hold the mirror to one side of the uvula, and focus light on it. A small part of the nasopharynx can be observed with a nasal speculum. Specialists may use a nasopharyngoscope to examine the nasopharynx.

■ PARANASAL SINUSES

Assess the paranasal sinuses by (1) inspecting and palpating the soft overlying tissues, (2) observing any nasal secretions (it is possible to determine which sinus is infected according to where discharge appears), and (3) transilluminating the maxillary and frontal sinuses. Palpate and percuss the frontal and maxillary sinuses to assess for swelling and tenderness, which are normally absent.

Palpate the frontal sinuses simultaneously by placing the thumbs above the eyes, just under the bony ridge of the orbits, and apply gentle pressure. Palpate the maxillary sinuses by using either the index and third fingers or thumbs to press gently on each side of the nose just under the zygomatic bones. Use direct percussion over the eyebrows for the frontal sinuses and on either side of the nose below the eyes in line with the pupils for the maxillary sinuses.

Transillumination is a technique used to assess the sinuses further if tenderness is present. Either a penlight or the otoscope handle fitted with a transilluminator head (see Chapter 10) is used. Darken the room. Place the light against the orbital bones immediately below the eyebrows and direct upward. Shield the light source with one hand. Normally, a reddish glow appears above the frontal sinus area. Lack of illumination may indicate sinus congestion and purulent fluid accumulation. Assess the maxillary sinuses by placing the light beneath the center of the eyes and the zygomatic bones and directing it down and in toward the roof of the mouth. Ask the client to open the mouth. A glow should appear on the hard palate on the side being illuminated. For a more complete assessment of sinus conditions, radiologic studies may be done. Air, normally present in the sinuses, appears as a dark area on a developed film.

■ SMELL

The senses of taste and smell are closely related. Many conditions affect taste and smell, such as viral infections, normal aging, head injuries, and local obstruction. Some medications can affect smell and taste, such as metronidazole, local anesthetics, clofibrate, some antibiotics, some antineoplastics, allopurinol, phenylbutazone, levodopa, codeine, morphine, carbamazepine, lithium, and trifluoperazine. Smell impairment may be (1) *hyposmia* (decrease in smell sensitivity) or (2) *anosmia* (bilateral and complete absence of smell sensitivity).

Assess smell by having the client identify various odors. Various substances are placed in individual test tubes (covered to eliminate visual cues). Test each nostril separately; have the client sniff the tubes (first with the eyes closed and then with the eyes open). Document whether the client can (1) perceive each odor and (2) identify each odor accurately.

Smell is perceived mainly via the olfactory nerves, although some smell is perceived via the trigeminal nerves. Trigeminal irritants are perceived even by clients with anosmia. (Therefore, a client who claims not to smell trigeminal irritants may be experiencing a conversion hysterical loss of smell rather than hyposmia or anosmia.) A client with a tracheostomy may not be able to smell because of limited upper airway movement. Olfactory stimulants and trigeminal stimulants commonly used to assess smell are listed in Box 59–1. See Chapter 67 for further discussion of smell assessment.

BOX 59–1	**Substances Used in Assessing Smell**
Olfactory stimulants	**Trigeminal stimulants**
Coffee (instant powder)	Ammonia
Phenylethyl alcohol	Acetone
Almond oil	Menthol
Peppermint	Distilled water
Musk	

DIAGNOSTIC TESTS

Diagnostic procedures augment the assessment of clients with respiratory disorders. To clarify which diagnostic test is used when and for what purpose, the tests are discussed here in the framework of what is being evaluated: functional status, anatomy, or specimens. The diagnostic test may be used for any or all of these reasons. This listing is limited to the most commonly used diagnostic tests.

■ TESTS TO EVALUATE RESPIRATORY FUNCTION

The diagnostic tests used to evaluate the functional status of the pulmonary system include:

- Pulmonary function tests
- Pulse oximetry
- Capnography
- Arterial blood gas (ABG) analysis
- Ventilation-perfusion studies

Pulmonary Function Tests

Pulmonary function tests (PFTs) provide information about respiratory function by measuring lung volumes, lung mechanics, and diffusion capabilities of the lungs (Table 59–4). PFTs performed in a pulmonary function laboratory can measure respiratory volumes and capacities. PFTs done outside a laboratory are modified to include ventilation tests of forced expiratory volume, vital capacity, and maximal voluntary ventilation measures. A measure of expiratory flow obtained with a hand-held device is called a *peak flow*. Many clients with asthma use a peak flowmeter (Fig. 59–10) at home to monitor changes in their condition and responses to treatment.

Education about the purpose, procedure, and implications of the test is performed by the nurse and reinforced by the examiner. Explicit instructions for each maneuver are given during the testing. Instruct clients that it is normal to feel short of breath after the test. Clients should not smoke or use a bronchodilator 6 hours before undergoing a PFT.

FORCED SPIROMETRY

The flow and volume capacities of the lungs are measured with forced spirometry. The volume of air inhaled and exhaled is plotted against time during a series of ventilatory maneuvers. Flow volume loops are created as visual patterns. Normal loop spirograms and spirogram patterns with obstructive and restrictive disorders are shown in Figure 59–11. Table 59–4 defines maneuvers used to test lung mechanics.

LUNG VOLUME DETERMINATION

Lung volume is measured by a gas dilution technique or body plethysmography. The two most commonly used gas dilution methods are (1) the *open-circuit* nitrogen method and (2) the *closed-circuit* helium method. These tests are most often used to measure functional residual capacity (FRC).

In the open-circuit method, all exhaled gas is collected while the client breathes pure oxygen. Measurement of the total amount of nitrogen washed out from the lungs permits calculation of the volume of gas present in the lungs at the beginning of the maneuver. The open-circuit method also allows assessment of the uniformity of ventilation in the lungs.

When helium is used to test the lungs in the closed-circuit method, the client inhales a mixture of air with a known concentration of helium. Helium does not significantly diffuse into the pulmonary bed. The helium diffuses throughout the air in the breathing box and lungs. The client exhales and is disconnected from the box. Changes in helium concentration in the box are computed to determine total lung volume.

The body plethysmograph, or *body box* (Fig. 59–12), is a device used to measure lung volumes. The lung volume changes seen with obstructive and restrictive lung disorders are shown in Table 59–5. While sitting in the airtight box, the client is instructed to perform a panting maneuver. Changes in the box pressure reflect changes in thoracic volume. Clients who cannot pant, who cannot tolerate closed spaces, or who have equipment that would interfere with the procedure cannot be tested by this method.

DIFFUSION CAPACITY

Studies of the lung diffusing capacity (DL) or carbon monoxide lung diffusion capacity [DL_{CO}]) measure gas transfer of carbon monoxide (CO) across the alveolar capillary membrane. The DL indicates the ease with which CO diffuses across the alveolar capillary membrane and binds with hemoglobin. (Hemoglobin has 250 times greater affinity for CO than for oxygen.) With normal hemoglobin and normal ventilatory function, the only limiting factor to diffusion of CO is the alveolar capillary membrane. The test involves inhaling room air mixed with 0.3% CO and 10% helium.

In many diseases, such as sarcoidosis, systemic lupus erythematosus, and emphysema, the alveolar membrane is thickened and oxygen transfer and diffusion are impaired, resulting in a decrease in DL. An increased DL is found with exercise, polycythemia, and hypervolemia.

Instruct the client to exhale forcefully, then inhale quickly, and hold the breath for 10 seconds and exhale. A sample of the exhaled air is collected for analysis.

Pulse Oximetry

PROCEDURE

Pulse oximetry is a safe and simple method of assessing oxygenation. It has the advantage that the data are obtained noninvasively and continuously. Previously, oxygenation was most commonly assessed by use of ABG determinations. Pulse oximetry was originally used in surgery but has been extended to most acute care settings. In fact, it is so common that it has been called the "fifth vital sign."

The pulse oximeter (Fig. 59–13) passes a beam of light through the tissue, and a sensor attached to the finger tip, toe, or ear lobe measures the amount of light absorbed by the oxygen-saturated hemoglobin. The oximeter then gives a reading of the percentage of hemoglobin that is saturated with oxygen (SaO_2). SaO_2 is closely correlated with the saturations obtained from the pulse oximeter if it is above 70%. Table 59–6 provides a quick guide for comparison of SaO_2 and partial pressure of arterial oxygen (PaO_2).

TABLE 59–4	PULMONARY FUNCTION TEST (PFT) COMPONENTS

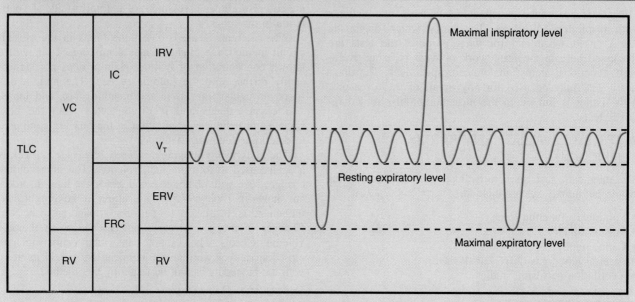

LUNG VOLUMES AND CAPACITIES

VC	*Vital capacity*	Volume of air that is measured during a slow, maximal expiration after a maximal inspiration; normal range varies with age, sex, and body size
IC	*Inspiratory capacity*	Largest volume of air that can be inhaled from resting expiratory volume
ERV	*Expiratory reserve volume*	Largest volume of air exhaled from resting end-expiratory level
FRC	*Functional residual capacity*	Volume of air remaining in lungs at resting end-expiratory level
IRV	*Inspiratory reserve volume*	Volume of air that can be inhaled from a tidal volume level
RV	*Residual volume*	Volume of air remaining in the lungs at the end of maximal expiration
TLC	*Total lung capacity*	Volume of air contained in the lungs after maximal inspiration
V_T	*Tidal volume*	Volume of air inhaled or exhaled during each respiratory cycle; normal range is 400–700 ml

LUNG MECHANICS

FVC	*Forced vital capacity*	Maximal volume of air that can be forcefully expired after a maximal inspiration to total lung capacity
FEV_t	*Forced expiratory volume*	Volume of air expired during a given time interval (t in seconds) from the beginning of an FVC maneuver
$FEF_{25\%-75\%}$	*Forced expiratory flow$_{25\%-75\%}$*	Average of flow during the middle half of an FVC maneuver
PEFR	*Peak expiratory flow rate*	Maximal flow rate attained during an FVC maneuver
MVV	*Maximal voluntary ventilation*	Largest volume that can be breathed during a 10- to 15-second interval with voluntary effort
MIP	*Maximal inspiratory pressure*	Greatest negative or subatmospheric pressure that can be generated during inspiration against an occluded airway
MEP	*Maximal expiratory pressure*	Highest positive pressure that can be generated during a forceful expiratory effort against an occluded airway

Limitations of pulse oximetry are still present despite the advancement of the technology. Motion at the sensor site changes light absorption. The motion mimics the pulsatile motion of blood, and because the detector cannot distinguish between movement of blood and movement of the finger, results can be inaccurate. Hypotension, hypothermia, and vasoconstriction reduce arterial blood flow to the sensor; keeping the finger warm may help with this

problem. There are also sensors for the nose that can be used to improve accuracy. The sensor should not be placed distal to blood pressure cuffs, pressure dressings, arterial lines, or invasive catheters and should not be taped to the client's finger.

Readings for clients with severe right-sided heart failure and those with high levels of positive end-expiratory pressure (PEEP) may be inaccurate because of the creation

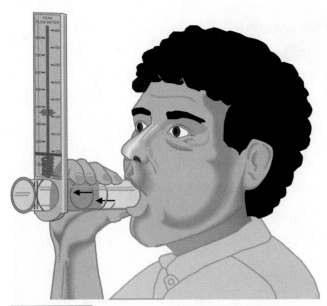

FIGURE 59–10 Use of a peak flowmeter to measure peak expiratory flow volume. The client stands and exhales into the mouthpiece. Normal peak flow values for adults are based on age, sex, height, and underlying lung disorder. Normal values range from 300 to 700 L/min but are best assessed when compared against a client's baseline values.

of pulsatile venous blood. Dark nail polish (especially blue, green, black, and brown-red) may interfere with accuracy. Red nail polish and artificial nails do not affect accuracy. Hyperbilirubinemia can also lead to false results.

Continue to assess the whole client, not just the oxygen saturation monitor. If values fall below preset norms (usually 90%), instruct the client to breathe deeply (if appropriate). Sometimes the amount of inspired oxygen is increased (titrated) to keep oxygen saturation above 90%. If the probe comes off the client's finger, the monitor usually indicates that the probe is off. Seldom is a loose probe the cause for readings of low levels of oxygen saturation.

PREPROCEDURE CARE

Tell the client about the need for the monitor. The test is noninvasive and painless. Explain that an infrared light probe will be attached to a finger, toe, or ear lobe. The client should avoid moving the sensor because movement disrupts the sensor and results in false readings.

Capnography

PROCEDURE

Capnography, another noninvasive procedure, is used to measure exhaled carbon dioxide (CO_2) concentrations of

FIGURE 59–11 A normal flow volume loop pattern and patterns for obstructive and restrictive lung disease. (From Kersten, L. D., et al. [1989]. *Respiratory nursing* [p. 382]. Philadelphia: W. B. Saunders.)

**LOOP SPIROGRAM
PATTERNS AND EXPLANATION**

NORMAL PATTERN

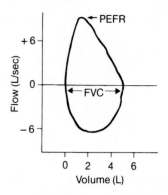

The expiratory curve shows a straight line decrease in flow after peak flow (PEFR). The inspiratory curve has a normal rounded pattern.

OBSTRUCTIVE PATTERN

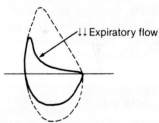

The expiratory curve shows scooping at low lung volumes (minimal to mild obstruction). As obstruction increases, the scooping becomes more marked and is accompanied by a decreased $FEF_{50\%}$ (mild to moderate obstruction).

Severe (e.g., emphysema)

The expiratory curve shows a sudden decrease in PEFR in an "index finger" pattern, followed by a nearly horizontal line.

The inspiratory curve is normal, except for absolute decreases in flow rates.

RESTRICTIVE PATTERN

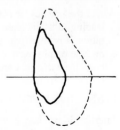

The entire loop resembles a miniature normal flow-volume loop. The FVC is markedly reduced. The expiratory curve shows a straight line decrease in flow with decreasing lung volumes. Peak flow rates may be normal, increased, or decreased, depending on the degree of respiratory impairment.

*The dotted lines represent the boundaries of the normal flow-volume loop.

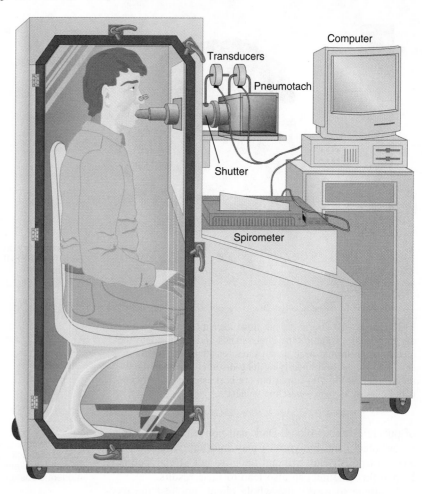

FIGURE 59–12 The volume plethysmograph—the "body box."

clients receiving mechanical ventilation. The amount of CO_2 found in exhaled air, end-tidal carbon dioxide (E_TCO_2), correlates closely with partial pressure of arterial CO_2 ($PaCO_2$) in clients with normal respiratory, cardiovas-

cular, and metabolic function. The normal $PaCO_2$-E_TCO_2 gradient is approximately 5 mm Hg. As the $PaCO_2$ increases with hypoventilation or decreases with hyperventilation, associated changes are noted in E_TCO_2.

TABLE 59–5	CATEGORIZATION OF OBSTRUCTIVE AND RESTRICTIVE PULMONARY DISORDERS AND PULMONARY FUNCTION TEST (PFT) FINDINGS						
		PFT Findings					
		VC	FEV_1	FEV_t/VC	FRC	TLC	RV
OBSTRUCTIVE DISORDERS							
Affect the patency or elasticity of the airways, leading to an increase in airway resistance; expiration is primarily affected. Obstructive disorders include emphysema, chronic bronchitis, asthma, bronchiectasis, and airway inflammation in response to irritants, infections, or allergies.		↓	↓	↓	↑	↑	↑
RESTRICTIVE DISORDERS							
Interfere in or change chest wall or lung parenchyma; inspiration is primarily affected. Restrictive disorders include kyphoscoliosis, pulmonary fibrosis, neuromuscular diseases and disorders, chest wall trauma, congenital chest wall changes, and tumors.		Normal or ↓	Slightly ↓	Normal or ↑	↓	↓	↓

FEV, forced expiratory volume in a unit of time; FRC, functional residual volume; RV, residual volume; TLC, total lung capacity; VC, vital capacity.

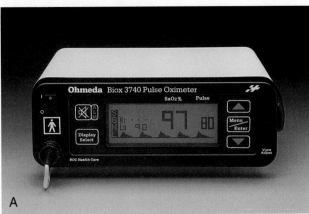

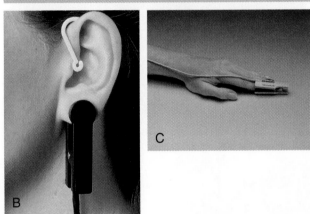

FIGURE 59–13 Oximetry. *A,* Noninvasive monitoring of oxygen saturation (SaO_2) is performed with a pulse oximeter. This unit has an ear probe and a finger probe. The ear probe *(B)* is used during measurements of SaO_2 while the client is exercising. The finger probe *(C)* is most frequently used for stationary measurement. (Courtesy of Ohmeda, Boulder, CO.)

Capnography requires continuous sampling of exhaled air.

PREPROCEDURE CARE

Explain the purpose of this test to the client. The test is noninvasive and painless. Clients who require capnography already have an endotracheal tube or tracheostomy tube in place for mechanical ventilation or airway management. A sensor is attached to the endotracheal tube or tracheostomy tube to measure E_TCO_2.

Arterial Blood Gas Analysis

ABG analysis (see Chapter 14) involves the use of arterial, rather than venous, blood to measure PaO_2, $PaCO_2$,

TABLE 59–6	COMPARING OXYGEN SATURATION TO PARTIAL PRESSURE OF ARTERIAL OXYGEN (PaO_2)	
Oxygen Saturation (%)	PaO_2 (mm Hg)	Client Status
50	25	Life-threatening hypoxemia
75	40	Moderate hypoxemia
90	55	Mild hypoxemia

and pH directly. Other data, such as bicarbonate (HCO_3^-) and SaO_2, are calculated. ABG analysis is an excellent diagnostic tool. PaO_2 reflects the efficiency of gas exchange, whereas $PaCO_2$ reflects the effectiveness of alveolar ventilation. The acid-base status of the body (see Chapter 14) is indicated by the pH of arterial blood. ABG analysis is essential for the assessment of clients who are acutely ill with pulmonary and nonpulmonary disorders, who require an artificial airway, who are dependent on mechanical ventilation, or who are experiencing chronic respiratory disease.

PROCEDURE

A sample of arterial blood is obtained by arterial puncture. A sterile needle (connected to a heparinized syringe) is inserted into one of the superficial arteries (i.e., radial, brachial, or femoral) (Fig. 59–14). Arterial blood is differentiated from venous blood by its bright red color. The radial artery is most commonly used because it is readily accessible, is easily palpated, and is associated with fewer complications. Low complication rates are related to ease of access and presence of collateral circulation via the ulnar artery. Send the sample to the laboratory immediately on ice. For serial ABG analyses or ongoing respiratory monitoring, multiple punctures may be avoided by using an arterial line (i.e., a sterile cannula inserted into one of the arteries).

A systematic approach to ABG interpretation, in conjunction with the client's overall status, can lead to the identification of potentially life-threatening abnormalities. First, assess the client's oxygenation status. Acid-base interpretation then follows to evaluate imbalances. Include the following steps in the ABG analysis: PaO_2, pH, $PaCO_2$, HCO_3^-, the presence and degree of compensation, and identification of the primary disorder.

The physician or other clinician skilled in arterial puncture collects the blood sample. In most hospitals, physicians are the only personnel allowed to draw from the femoral artery; nurses and respiratory therapists with special training can take radial or brachial samples.

PREPROCEDURE CARE

Educate the client about the procedure and the need for the test. Explain that the needle-stick will be painful for a moment and that it is necessary to hold very still during the procedure to avoid inadvertent injury to the nerves, vessels, or tendons. After the test is completed, tell the client that pressure must be held at the puncture site for 5 to 10 minutes and it may be uncomfortable.

An Allen test must be completed before the procedure is initiated (see Fig. 59–14A–C). Before the sample is drawn, treat the site with a disinfectant and allow to dry. Position the area to facilitate the puncture. Help the client remain calm during the test by explaining what is happening. If the client is anxious about the test or other problems and is hyperventilating, the results of the test may be altered. The amount of blood needed for the sample varies from laboratory to laboratory but may be as small as 0.5 ml or as large as 10 ml.

POSTPROCEDURE CARE

After the sample is drawn, apply continuous pressure to the site for 5 minutes for radial and brachial sites and 10 minutes for femoral sites. Pressure bandages are com-

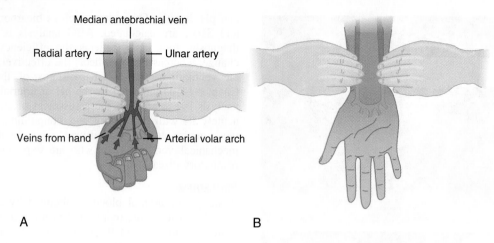

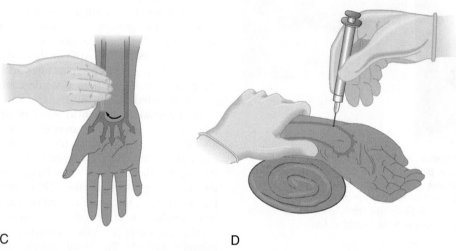

FIGURE 59–14 Obtaining a sample of arterial blood by arterial puncture. First, perform Allen's test, a quick assessment of collateral circulation in the hand. This test is essential before radial artery puncture. *A,* Occlude both the radial and the ulnar arteries with your fingers. Ask the client to close the hand into a fist. *B,* When the client opens the hand with the arteries still occluded, the hand is pale. *C,* When you release either the radial or the ulnar artery, the client's hand should become pink because of collateral circulation. Assess the patency of each of the two arteries in this way, one at a time. *D,* If collateral circulation is adequate, you can draw arterial blood from the radial artery with a heparinized needle and syringe, as shown.

monly used. If the client has a tendency to bleed or is receiving anticoagulant medication, pressure is needed for a longer period.

When interpreting the results, note whether the client is receiving oxygen; record the amount and source of oxygen on the laboratory request form. The results are evaluated in light of the oxygen needed. For example, if the PaO_2 is 85 mm Hg with 50% oxygen, the client has a more significant problem with oxygen transport than a client whose PaO_2 is 85 mm Hg with room air (21% oxygen).

Complications of arterial sampling include bleeding or hematoma formation at the site and injury to the artery and surrounding structures. Report any of these signs to the physician.

Ventilation-Perfusion Lung Scan

Ventilation-perfusion (V/Q) scanning is used to assess lung ventilation and lung perfusion. V/Q scans are valu-

able in identifying pulmonary embolism, pulmonary infarction, emphysema, fibrosis, and bronchiectasis. Quantitative perfusion scans may be helpful in preoperative assessment of clients undergoing surgical resection of thoracic malignancy.

PROCEDURE

The scan consists of two parts, which may be done together or separately: (1) assessment of the distribution of ventilation (ventilation scan) and (2) assessment of the pulmonary vasculature (perfusion scan).

Ventilation Scan. Radioactive gas is inhaled and produces an image of the areas where ventilation is occurring. Assessment of the pattern of deposition of radioactive gas in the alveoli is also possible.

Ventilation images are compared with the pictures taken during the perfusion scan. The same amount of radioactivity should be discernible on both ventilation and perfusion pictures. If there are areas in which there is ventilation but little or no perfusion, a pulmonary embolus is suspected (Fig. 59–15). Further assessment may be needed. If there is doubt about the cause of impaired perfusion, pulmonary angiography may be needed.

Perfusion Scan. Radiologic material (non–iodine-based) is injected intravenously and carried into the pulmonary vasculature. Decreased blood flow to any part of the lungs is revealed as a decrease in the amount of radioactivity shown on either the x-ray film with use of a rectilinear scanner or on Polaroid film with use of a gamma or scintillation camera. Scanning is done in both the anterior and posterior views.

PREPROCEDURE CARE
Explain the procedure to the client. The test is painless except for local discomfort when radiologic material is injected for the perfusion scan. The client will hear clicking noises during the scan, but the noise is not loud. If the client has dyspnea while lying down, reassure the client that sitting up is possible during the procedure. Radiation exposure is minimal. The client may remain dressed with all metal items removed. The procedure takes 30 to 60 minutes to complete.

■ TESTS TO EVALUATE ANATOMIC STRUCTURES

Diagnostic tests used to evaluate anatomic structures include:

- Radiographic imaging
- Radionuclide studies
- Endoscopy
- Alveolar lavage

Chest X-ray Studies

Chest x-ray studies provide information about the chest that may not be available through other assessment means and may be able to graphically illustrate the cause of respiratory dysfunction. Chest films may reveal abnormalities when there are no physical manifestations of pulmonary disease.

Chest films show the bony structures (e.g., ribs, sternum, clavicles, scapulae, and upper portion of the humerus). The vertebral column is visible vertically through the middle of the thorax. The two hemidiaphragms normally appear rounded, smooth, and sharply defined, with

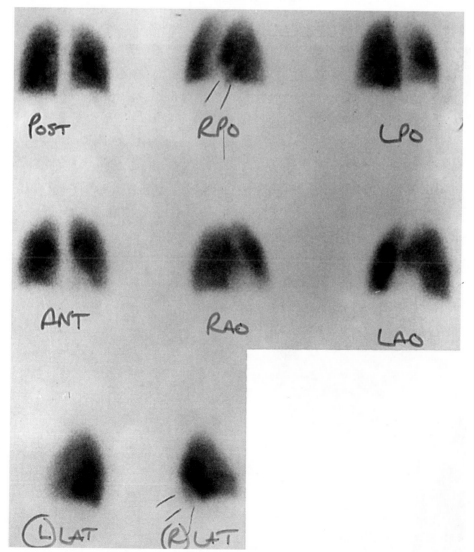

FIGURE 59–15 A ventilation-perfusion scan with technetium 99m. This upright radionuclide pulmonary perfusion study indicates a perfusion deficit of the right posterior basilar segment of the lung, suggesting a pulmonary embolism or pneumonia. This client then underwent a pulmonary venogram (see Chapter 61) that documented the presence of pulmonary embolism.

the right hemidiaphragm slightly higher than the left. The junction of the rib cage and the diaphragm, called the costophrenic angle, is normally clearly visible and angled. Heart tissue is dense and appears white but less intensely white than bone. The heart shadow is normally clearly outlined, extends primarily onto the left side of the thorax, and occupies no more than one third of the chest width. Close observation shows the trachea in the upper middle chest almost superimposed above the cervical and thoracic vertebrae. The trachea bifurcates at the level of the fourth thoracic vertebra into the right and left mainstem bronchi. The pulmonary blood vessels, bronchi, and lymph nodes are located in the hilum on both the right and left sides of the midthorax. Lung tissue appears black on x-ray film. Vascular lung structures are visible as white, thin, wispy strings fanning out from the hilum (Fig. 59–16).

Chest x-ray studies may be performed:

- As part of a routine screening procedure
- When pulmonary disease is suspected
- To monitor the status of respiratory disorders and abnormalities (e.g., pleural effusion, atelectasis, and tubercular lesions)
- To confirm endotracheal or tracheostomy tube placement

- After traumatic chest injury
- In any other situation in which radiographic information helps in the management of a respiratory problem

PROCEDURE

Routine adult chest x-ray studies are performed with the client standing or sitting facing the x-ray film, with the chest and shoulders in direct contact with the film cassette. Several positions are possible.

Posteroanterior View. The client's shoulders are rotated forward to pull the scapulae away from the lung field. The x-ray beam penetrates from the back, for the posteroanterior (PA) position. The radiograph is usually taken on full inspiration, which causes the diaphragm to move downward. Radiographs taken on expiration are sometimes requested in order to demonstrate the degree of diaphragm movement or to assist in the assessment and diagnosis of pneumothorax.

Anteroposterior View. For clients who cannot be transported to the radiology department, portable chest radiography may be performed. These radiographs are usually taken with the film placed behind the client and the x-ray beam entering from the front of the chest—the AP position. Because the x-ray beam enters from the front, the heart appears larger than it really is and larger than on a PA view.

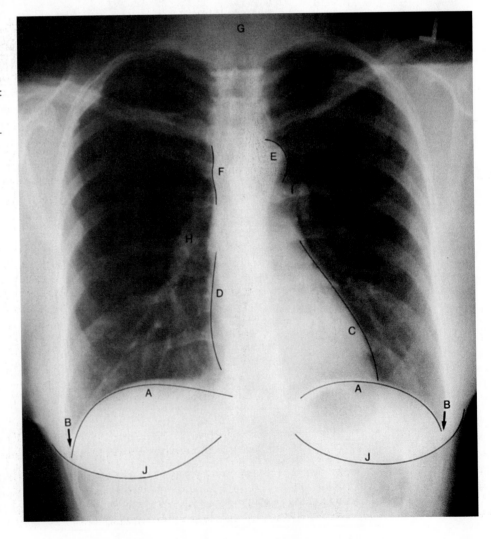

FIGURE 59–16 A normal chest x-ray film taken from the posteroanterior view. The backward "L" in the upper right corner is placed on the film to indicate the left side of the client's chest. A, diaphragm: B, costophrenic angle; C, left ventricle; D, right atrium; E, aortic arch; F, superior vena cava; G, trachea; H, right bronchus; I, left bronchus; J, breast shadows.

Lateral View. The lateral view usually accompanies a standard PA view. It is taken from the right or left side of the chest. The arms are raised above the head, and the side of the chest is placed against the film. The lateral view allows better visualization of the heart and the dome of the diaphragm. In conjunction with a PA film, a lateral radiograph gives a three-dimensional view, allowing more specific identification of the location of an abnormality.

Lateral Decubitus View. The lateral decubitus (from the Latin, lying down) position may be used when it is necessary to determine whether opaque areas on the pleura are due to solid or liquid media. The client lies on the right or left side, depending on which side of the chest is being assessed. In a left lateral decubitus position, the client lies on the left side.

Oblique View. The oblique position is used to visualize behind and around underlying structures. The shoulders are rotated to either the right or left of the film. By turning the client, the examiner can shift the angle at which the x-ray beam passes through the chest. In a right oblique position, the right side is closest to the film. The view may be taken from an anterior or posterior position.

Lordotic View. The lordotic position, consisting of a forward curve of the lumbar spine, is useful if clearer visualization of the upper lung fields is needed. The angle of the cathode x-ray tube is lowered and the beam directed at an upward angle. This angle results in removal of the clavicles and first and second ribs from the field of vision.

PREPROCEDURE CARE

Instruct the client about the need for radiologic testing. The test is painless, and exposure to radiation is minimal. The client must remove all jewelry and underclothes and put on a gown. Assess the client's pregnancy status; pregnant women should not be exposed to radiation. All gonads should be shielded during the study. The test takes 5 to 10 minutes to complete.

Ultrasonography

Ultrasonic waves (sound waves too high in frequency for a human ear to detect) are used diagnostically to assess various body structures. Ultrasonography may be used in conjunction with other pulmonary diagnostic procedures, such as thoracentesis and pleural biopsy, to assess fluid or fibrotic abnormalities. Ultrasonography is especially helpful and accurate in detecting the amount and location of 50 ml or less of pleural fluid. In comparison, positive detection by chest radiography requires at least 500 ml of liquid. If the technique is used in combination with thoracentesis, the ultrasonographer can determine the best location for needle placement as well as the depth of the fluid. This approach facilitates obtaining an adequate amount of fluid for laboratory analysis without unnecessary puncturing and probing.

The client may remain dressed or put on a gown (see Chapter 11 for client preparation needed for ultrasonography). The test takes 15 to 30 minutes to complete.

Fluoroscopy

Fluoroscopy makes it possible for the chest and intrathoracic structures to be observed while they function dy-

namically (see Chapter 11). Fluoroscopy is not used routinely; rather, it is used when continuous observation of the thorax is an advantage (e.g., observing transbronchial passage of biopsy forceps during bronchoscopy). Other uses for fluoroscopy include:

- Observing the diaphragm during inspiration and expiration
- Detecting mediastinal movement during deep breathing
- Assessing the heart, blood vessels, and related structures
- Identifying esophageal abnormalities
- Detecting mediastinal masses

Instruct the client about the need for this test. The test is painless. Sometimes a radiopaque (non–iodine-based) contrast agent is administered intravenously to help distinguish the structures being assessed. The client must remove all jewelry and underclothes and put on a gown. The test takes 30 to 45 minutes to complete. Exposure to radiation is minimal, but pregnant women should not be exposed to fluoroscopy.

Images obtained by fluoroscopy are not as clear and definitive as those obtained on a standard chest film. If abnormalities are discovered, still photographs and cinefluorography may be used to obtain a permanent record. Cinefluorographs are motion pictures that allow more leisurely study and restudy of the area photographed without exposure of radiology personnel or clients to unnecessary radiation.

Computed Tomography

Computed tomography (CT) provides more sophisticated tomography than is possible with conventional x-ray equipment (see Chapter 11).

CT scans are particularly helpful in identifying peripheral (e.g., pleural) or mediastinal disorders. Special techniques can be used to view pulmonary nodules. Thin cuts of CT scans are used in diagnosing interstitial lung disorders such as pulmonary fibrosis and bronchiectasis.

Magnetic Resonance Imaging

Magnetic resonance imaging (MRI) employs magnetic fields rather than radiation to create images of body structures. MRI is used in much the same way as CT. MRI is more definitive than CT because it creates more detailed images of anatomic structures. See Chapter 11 for a detailed discussion of MRI and client preparation.

Gallium Scans

Gallium scanning is usually done 24 to 48 hours after intravenous injection of radioactive gallium citrate. Many organs take up radioactive gallium, as do some tumors and areas of inflammation. A gallium scan might be used to distinguish embolism from pneumonitis as the cause of an infiltrate on a chest radiograph. Gallium has an affinity for areas of inflammation, such as those associated with pneumonia; however, there is little inflammation with a nonseptic pulmonary embolism. Therefore, gallium accumulates around pneumonitis but not around a pulmonary embolism. The usefulness of gallium scanning in clinical pulmonary assessment is limited.

Educate the client about the test. The test is painless except for local pain at the injection site. Gallium is not iodine-based and produces no side effects. The client returns for serial scans at 24, 48, or 72 hours. Scanning is performed with the client supine. The client may remain dressed but must remove all metal objects. The scan takes 45 to 60 minutes to complete.

Bronchoscopy

PROCEDURE

Bronchoscopy involves passage of a lighted bronchoscope into the bronchial tree (Fig. 59–17). It may be performed with rigid steel or flexible fiberoptic instruments. Bronchoscopy may be performed for diagnostic or therapeutic purposes. Diagnostic purposes include:

- Examination of tissue
- Further evaluation of a tumor for potential surgical resection
- Collection of tissue specimens for diagnosis
- Evaluation of bleeding sites

Therapeutic bronchoscopy is used to:

- Remove foreign bodies
- Remove thick, viscous secretions
- Treat postoperative atelectasis
- Destroy and remove lesions

PREPROCEDURE CARE

Explain the procedure to the client and family, and obtain informed consent. Instruct the client not to eat or drink anything 6 hours before the test. Explain that the throat may be sore after bronchoscopy and there will be some initial difficulty in swallowing. Before sedation, the client should remove dentures, contact lenses, and other prostheses. The client undresses and puts on a gown. Local anesthesia and intravenous sedation are used to suppress cough and to relieve anxiety. A topical anesthetic agent is also sprayed into the back of the throat. The test takes 30 to 45 minutes to complete.

During the procedure, the client lies supine with the head hyperextended. Monitor vital signs, talk to and reassure the client, and assist the physician as necessary.

POSTPROCEDURE CARE

After the procedure, monitor vital signs according to agency protocol. Observe the client for signs of respiratory distress, including dyspnea, changes in respiratory rate, use of accessory muscles, and changes in or absent lung sounds. Expectorated secretions are inspected for evidence of hemoptysis. Nothing is given by mouth until the cough and swallow reflexes have returned, usually in 1 to 2 hours. When the client can swallow, feeding may begin with ice chips and small sips of water.

Lung sounds are monitored for 24 hours. Development of asymmetrical or adventitious sounds should be reported to the physician. Pneumothorax has been noted after bronchoscopy.

Alveolar Lavage

Sterile saline can be injected during bronchoscopy to wash tissues. The saline is aspirated and examined for

FIGURE 59–17 Bronchoscopy.

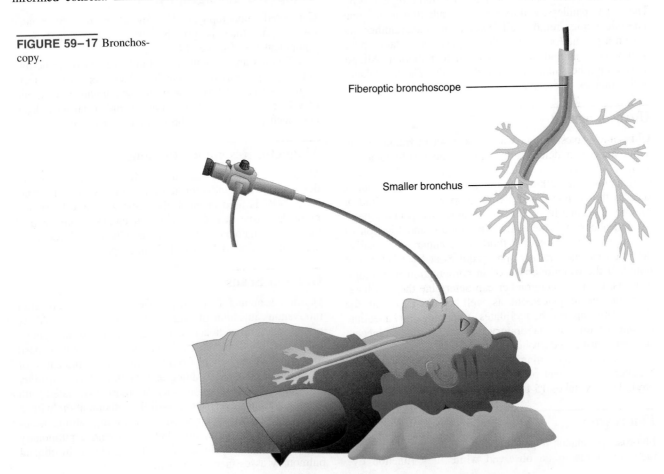

Fiberoptic bronchoscope

Smaller bronchus

atypical cells. Alveolar lavage may be used in the diagnosis of interstitial lung disease, sarcoidosis, hypersensitivity pneumonitis, and *P. carinii* pneumonia. No additional client preparation is needed because this procedure is done during bronchoscopy.

Endoscopic Thoracotomy

Endoscopic thoracotomy is a diagnostic procedure that is an alternative to open-lung biopsy and thoracotomy for pleural surface disorders.

PROCEDURE

Typically, three small incisions are made into the middle chest wall. A scope attached to a camera and video projector is inserted through the first incision to inspect tissue, and tissues are manipulated and biopsy specimens obtained through the other incisions. A chest tube is inserted to promote lung reexpansion. Advantages of the procedure include reduced anesthesia time, less pain, and shortened hospital stay. In addition, biopsy specimens may be obtained from the lower lobes, which is not routinely done during open-lung biopsy procedures.

PREPROCEDURE CARE

Instruct the client about the need for this test, and obtain a signed informed consent form. Endoscopic thoracotomy is a surgical procedure, and general anesthesia is administered (see Chapter 15 for a discussion of the needs of the surgical patient). Explain that a chest tube will be in place and that it will be necessary to perform coughing and deep-breathing exercises.

Pulmonary Angiography

Sometimes the vascular structure of the thorax must be assessed. Angiography and other procedures designed to examine specific vascular structures (i.e., aortography for the aorta) all use similar techniques.

Pulmonary angiography may be done to detect the following:

- Congenital abnormalities of the pulmonary vascular tree
- Abnormalities of the pulmonary venous circulation
- Acquired diseases of the pulmonary arterial and venous circulation (e.g., primary pulmonary arterial hypertension)
- Destructive effects of emphysema
- Potential benefits of resection for bronchogenic carcinoma
- Peripheral pulmonary lesions
- Extent of thromboembolism in the lungs

PROCEDURE

Contrast medium is injected into the vascular system through an indwelling catheter. During pulmonary angiography, the catheter may be inserted either peripherally or directly into the main pulmonary artery or one of its branches. The contrast agent is injected while cinefluorographs or still photographs are taken. (Pulmonary angiography is discussed in Chapter 61.)

Instruct the client about the need for this test, and obtain informed consent. The test is painless and does not involve exposure to radiation. Further preprocedure and postprocedure care of the client is as for angiography (see Chapter 11).

■ SPECIMEN RECOVERY AND ANALYSIS

The following procedures are used for recovery and analysis of pulmonary specimens:

- Sputum collection
- Thoracentesis
- Biopsy

Sputum Collection

Normally, the goblet cells produce 100 ml of mucus a day, but an infectious process can lead to excessive production of mucus (commonly called *sputum*). Assessment of sputum for bacteria, fungus, or cellular elements guides the treatment of an underlying infection.

PROCEDURE

Inspect the sputum for color, quantity, quality, presence of blood, food particles, or other unusual contents. If possible, sputum should be collected before antimicrobial treatment is begun.

Acid-fast smear and culture specimens are collected in the morning, at which time sputum is more plentiful and concentrated because of pooling through the night. Sputum can be collected by (1) the direct method, (2) the indirect method, or (3) gastric lavage.

PREPROCEDURE CARE

Explain the need for and purpose of this test to the client. When a specimen is obtained by the direct method, the client brushes the teeth to reduce contamination and then coughs into a sputum specimen container. Encourage the client to cough, not spit, in order to obtain sputum. Inhaling nebulized saline or water can be used to thin the sputum to facilitate expectoration.

Indirect techniques for obtaining sputum consist of a sterile suction catheter with an attached sputum trap. Sputum can also be obtained by transtracheal aspiration. A puncture is made with a needle through the cricothyroid membrane into the trachea, and sputum is aspirated.

Although gastric lavage is not a common technique for obtaining sputum, it can be used for uncooperative or extremely ill clients. Lavage is based on the assumption that sputum is swallowed during sleep and sometimes after coughing. A nasogastric tube is inserted by appropriate technique. Gastric juice is aspirated with a syringe and sent to the laboratory. The tube is then removed.

The collected sputum is analyzed for Gram's stain, culture, and sensitivity study. Gram's stain is used to classify bacteria as gram-positive or gram-negative and, along with the sputum culture, provides guidelines for appropriate antimicrobial therapy. After the Gram stain, the sputum is incubated for 24 hours or longer on the appropriate culture medium and studied by a microbiologist. Obtaining a specimen for the culture allows further identification of the infecting organism. When the organism is identified, its sensitivity to antibiotic treatment is tested and an appropriate antibiotic is prescribed.

Identification of organisms that cause tuberculosis and similar diseases (acid-fast bacilli) requires tests other than Gram's stain, culture, and sensitivity study.

Regardless of the technique used to obtain the specimen, note the color, consistency, odor, and amount of sputum obtained.

Nose and Throat Cultures

Bacteria in the nose and throat can be identified by culture during assessment of the upper airway. Some bacteria are normally present (e.g., streptococci, staphylococci, pneumococci, *Haemophilus influenzae,* and *Klebsiella pneumoniae*). Other organisms are abnormal (e.g., those causing diphtheria or tuberculosis).

Swab the nose and throat using a sterile cotton swab. Place the swab in a sterile culture tube. Some laboratories require the swab to be suspended in a tube containing 2 ml of fluid to keep air in the tube moist and prevent evaporation and drying of the specimen. Because the fluid is not a culture medium, the swab should not touch the fluid. If Loeffler's medium is used in the tube (i.e., if diphtheria is suspected), the medium should touch the swab. When culture tubes without fluid are used, take the specimen to the laboratory immediately, where the swab is streaked across a culture plate.

Thoracentesis

PROCEDURE

Thoracentesis is performed to drain fluid or air found in the pleural space. Therapeutic thoracentesis removes an accumulation of pleural fluid or air that has caused lung compression and respiratory distress. When the main goal is to determine the cause of an infection or empyema, diagnostic thoracentesis is performed. The fluid collected is sent to the laboratory for assessment of specific gravity, glucose, protein, and pH; culture; sensitivity study; and cytologic evaluation. The color and consistency of the pleural fluid are also documented.

PREPROCEDURE CARE

Obtain informed consent, and instruct the client about the procedure and the need for it. The client must sit upright while leaning over the tray table (Fig. 59–18A). In the upright position, pleural fluid accumulates in the base of the thorax. Alternatively, place the client in a recumbent position with the arm resting under the head. Insertion of the needle is painful. Explain the importance of holding still during the procedure. Sudden movement may force the needle through the pleural space and injure the visceral pleura or lung parenchyma. State that you will help to hold the client, and provide reassurance. The test takes 5 to 15 minutes to complete.

During the procedure, assist the physician; monitor vital signs; and observe for dyspnea, complaints of difficulty breathing, nausea, or pain.

POSTPROCEDURE CARE

After the procedure, the client is usually turned onto the unaffected side for 1 hour to facilitate lung expansion. Assess vital signs according to the facility's policy. Carefully assess the respiratory rate and character and breath sounds. Tachypnea, dyspnea, cyanosis, retractions, or diminished breath sounds, which may indicate pneumothorax, should be reported to the physician.

Record the amount of fluid withdrawn as fluid output. Chest films may be obtained to evaluate the degree of lung reexpansion or pneumothorax. Subcutaneous emphysema may follow this procedure, because air in the pleu-

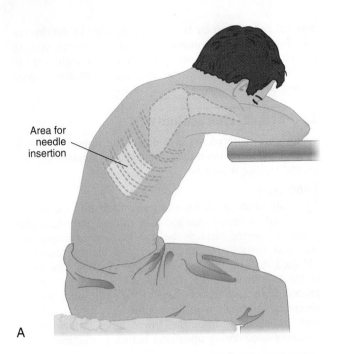

Area for needle insertion

A

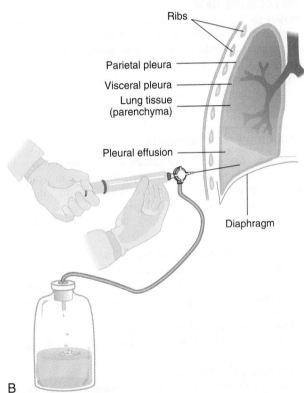

Ribs

Parietal pleura

Visceral pleura

Lung tissue (parenchyma)

Pleural effusion

Diaphragm

B

FIGURE 59–18 Thoracentesis. *A,* Correct position of the client for the procedure. The arms are raised and crossed. The head rests on the folded arms. This position allows the chest wall to be pulled outward in an expanded position. If an institutional overbed table is not available, you may leave the client's arms down, but position them toward the client's hips or cross them in front of the chest. *B,* Usual site for insertion of a thoracentesis needle for a right-sided effusion. The actual site varies, depending on the location and volume of the effusion. The needle is kept as far away from the diaphragm as possible but is inserted close to the base of the effusion so that gravity can help with drainage.

ral cavity leaks into subcutaneous tissues. The tissues feel like lumpy paper and crackle when palpated (crepitus). Usually, subcutaneous emphysema causes no problem unless it is increasing and constricting vital organs (e.g., trachea). Clients often need reassurance about this disorder.

If the client has pleural effusion related to a malignancy, cytotoxic medications may be inserted into the pleural space after thoracentesis. Some of these agents burn; with others, the client must roll about in order to have the medication coat the entire pleural space. Review the interventions used with the various medications.

Biopsy

Biopsy specimens may be taken from various respiratory tissues for examination. As mentioned previously, specimens from tracheobronchial structures may be obtained during bronchoscopy. Biopsy specimens of scalene and mediastinal nodes may be obtained (with local anesthesia) for pathologic study, culture, or cytologic assessment.

PLEURAL BIOPSY

PROCEDURE

Pleural biopsies may be performed surgically through a small thoracotomy incision or during thoracentesis with the use of a Cope needle. Needle biopsy is a relatively safe, simple diagnostic procedure that can help determine the cause of pleural effusions. The needle removes a small fragment of parietal pleura, which is used for microscopic cellular examination and culture. If bacteriologic studies are needed, the biopsy specimen should be obtained before chemotherapy is begun.

PREPROCEDURE CARE

Obtain informed consent, and instruct the client about the need for and purpose of the test. Preparation and positioning of a client for pleural biopsy are similar to those for thoracentesis. The test is painful, and the client must hold still. Assist and reassure the client. The test takes 15 to 30 minutes to complete.

POSTPROCEDURE CARE

Rare complications include temporary pain associated with intercostal nerve injury, pneumothorax, and hemothorax. After the biopsy procedure, observe for indications of complications (e.g., dyspnea, pallor, diaphoresis, excessive pain). A pneumothorax associated with needle biopsy may develop. Chest tubes and chest drainage equipment must be available. Follow-up chest x-ray studies are usually done after the procedure. Development of hemothorax is indicated by a substantial increase in fluid in the pleural space and requires immediate thoracentesis.

LUNG BIOPSY

As with pleural biopsy, lung biopsy may be done by surgical exposure of the lung (open-lung biopsy) with or without endoscopy using a needle designed to remove a core of lung tissue. The tissue is examined for abnormal cellular structure and bacteria. Lung biopsies are most often performed to identify pulmonary tumors or parenchymal changes (e.g., sarcoidosis).

PROCEDURE

Needle puncture (aspiration) biopsy of chest lesions is done with fluoroscopy. After a lesion is identified on a chest film and localized by fluoroscopy, topical anesthesia is administered and the needle is inserted through the chest wall into the lung tissue and lesion. A small sample of cells is aspirated for microscopic study, and the needle is withdrawn. Aspiration biopsy may enable definitive diagnosis of malignant neoplasms, granulomas, or other nonmalignant growths. Possible complications of needle aspiration lung biopsy are hemoptysis, hemothorax, and pneumothorax.

POSTPROCEDURE CARE

After the procedure, examine any sputum closely for evidence of blood. Observe for respiratory distress (may indicate pneumothorax). Monitor the client's vital signs, breath sounds, skin color, and temperature.

CONCLUSIONS

Respiratory assessment begins with obtaining a thorough client history. One of the most essential aspects of history-taking is determining the degree of dyspnea and the impact it has on activities of daily living. Note the client's smoking history and occupational risks because they are common risk factors for respiratory disorders. The chest is inspected for obvious deformity and shape. Percussion, palpation, and auscultation assist in locating areas of possible fluid accumulation or consolidation that interfere with breathing.

Chest x-ray studies, bronchoscopy, pulmonary function tests, and ABG analysis are common diagnostic assessments. Educate the client about the diagnostic modalities, and monitor for potential complications after the study.

BIBLIOGRAPHY

1. Bates, B., et al. (1998). *A guide to physical assessment and history taking* (7th ed.). Philadelphia: J. B. Lippincott.
2. Burton, G., Hodgkin, J., & Ward, J. (1997). *Respiratory care: A guide to clinical practice.* Philadelphia: J. B. Lippincott.
3. Gift, A. G., & Narsavage, G. (1998). Validity of the numeric rating scale as a measure of dyspnea. *American Journal of Critical Care, 7*(3), 200–204.
4. Gift, A. G., & Nield, M. D. (1991). Dyspnea: A case for nursing diagnosis status. *Nursing Diagnosis, 2*(2), 66–71.
5. Govette, L. A. (1994). Back to basics: Interpreting chest x-ray films. *Journal of the American Academy of Physician Assistants, 7*(3), 205–207.
6. Guyton, A. C. (1996). *Textbook of medical physiology* (9th ed.). Philadelphia: W. B. Saunders.
6a. Horne, C., & Derrico, D. (1999). Mastering ABGS: The art of arterial blood gas measurement. *American Journal of Nursing, 99*(8), 26–33.
7. Jarvis, C. (2000). (3rd ed.). *Physical examination and health assessment.* Philadelphia: W. B. Saunders.
8. Kelly-Heidenthal, P., & O'Connor, M. (1994). Nursing assessment of portable AP chest x-rays. *Dimensions of Critical Care Nursing, 13*(3), 127–132.
9. Lareau, S., et al. (1998). Development and testing of the modified version of the Pulmonary Functional Status and Dyspnea Questionnaire (PFSDQ). *Heart and Lung Journal of Critical Care, 27*(3), 159–168.
10. Malley, W. (1990). *Clinical blood gases: Application and noninvasive alternates.* Philadelphia: W. B. Saunders.
11. McCord, M., & Cronin-Stubbs, D. (1992). Operationalizing dyspnea: Focus on measurement. *Heart and Lung, 21*(2), 167.
12. Murray, J. F., & Nadel, J. A. (1994). *The textbook of respiratory medicine* (2nd ed.). Philadelphia: W. B. Saunders.

13. O'Hanlon-Nichols, T. (1998). Basic assessment series: The adult pulmonary system. *American Journal of Nursing, 98*(2), 39–45.

14. Owen, A. (1998). Respiratory assessment revisited. *Nursing, 28*(4), 48–49.

15. Pierson, D., & Kacmarek, R. (1999). *Foundations of respiratory care.* New York: McGraw-Hill.

16. Ripamonti, C., & Bruera, E. (1997). Dyspnea: Pathophysiology and assessment. *Journal of Pain and Symptom Management, 13*(4), 220–232.

17. Ruppel, G. (1994). *Manual of pulmonary function testing* (5th ed.). St. Louis: Mosby–Year Book.

18. Shapiro, B. A., et al. (1991). *Clinical application of respiratory care* (4th ed.). St. Louis: Mosby–Year Book.

19. Shapiro, B. A., et al. (1994). *Clinical application of blood gases* (5th ed.). St. Louis: Mosby–Year Book.

20. Shortall, S. P., & Perkins, L. A. (1999). Interpreting the ins and outs of pulmonary function tests. *Nursing, 29*(12), 41–47.

21. Speck, D., et al. (1993). *Respiratory control: Central peripheral mechanisms.* Lexington, KY: University of Kentucky.

22. Von Rueden, K. T. (1990). Noninvasive assessment of gas exchange in the critically ill. *AACN Clinical Issues in Critical Care Nursing, 1*(2), 239-247.

23. West, J. B. (1995). *Respiratory physiology* (5th ed.). Baltimore: Williams & Wilkins.

24. Wong, F. W. H. (1999). A new approach to ABG interpretation. *American Journal of Nursing, 99*(8), 34–36.

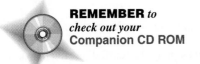

CHAPTER

60

Management of Clients with Upper Airway Disorders

Linda K. Clarke

NURSING OUTCOMES CLASSIFICATION (NOC)
for Nursing Diagnoses—Clients with Upper Airway Disorders

Altered Nutrition: Less Than Body Requirements
Nutritional Status: Food and Fluid Intake
Anxiety and Fear
Anxiety Control
Coping
Fear Control
Social Interaction Skills
Impaired Verbal Communication
Communication Ability
Communication Ability: Expressive Ability
Ineffective Airway Clearance
Aspiration Control
Respiratory Status: Airway Patency

Risk for Aspiration
Respiratory Status: Gas Exchange
Risk Control
Risk Detection
Risk for Constipation
Hydration
Mobility Level
Nutritional Status: Food and Fluid Intake
Risk Control
Risk Detection
Risk for Impaired Gas Exchange
Respiratory Status: Gas Exchange
Vital Signs Status
Risk for Ineffective Management of Therapeutic Regimen (Families)

Family Functioning
Family Participation in Professional Care
Risk for Ineffective Management of Therapeutic Regimen (Individuals)
Compliance Behavior
Knowledge: Treatment Regimen
Risk for Infection
Immobility Consequences: Physiologic
Knowledge: Infection Control
Nutritional Status
Risk Control
Risk Detection
Tissue Integrity: Skin and Mucous Membranes
Wound Healing

The initial complaint for clients with disorders of the upper airway is a problem with breathing. Obstructions to nasal breathing are observed in clients with nasal polyps, deviated nasal septum, or nasal fractures. After surgical interventions, nasal breathing continues to be compromised because of postoperative edema. Laryngeal disorders may also result in breathing problems. Tumors of the larynx create obstruction to air entering the trachea, as well as to air being exhaled. Vocal cord paralysis and laryngospasm may also affect the passage of air through the larynx and vocal cords. Clients with epistaxis and sinusitis exhibit nasal bleeding and drainage, respectively, and may have fever and pain. Inflammation associated with these problems results in obstruction to breathing. Surgical intervention and nasal packing further exacerbate breathing problems.

METHODS OF CONTROLLING THE AIRWAY

Airway obstruction can be prevented or treated with many modalities. Antihistamine treatment is discussed in

Chapter 76. Intubation to support ventilation and oxygenation is discussed in Chapter 63. This chapter begins with tracheostomy because it is a common method of airway management in hospitalized clients.

TRACHEOSTOMY

A *tracheotomy* is a surgical incision into the trachea through overlying skin and muscles for airway management. A *tracheostomy* is the surgical creation of a stoma, or opening, into the trachea through the overlying skin (Fig. 60–1). These terms are often used interchangeably. For simplicity, the term "tracheostomy" is used here.

Tracheostomy can be performed as an emergency procedure or as an elective procedure, depending on the indication. A tracheostomy provides the best route for long-term airway maintenance. Because of the many indications for this procedure, it is discussed at the beginning of this chapter rather than under a particular disorder. Indications for tracheostomy include:

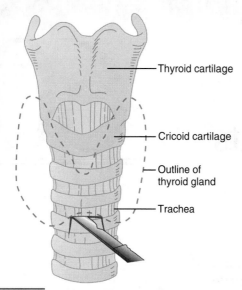

- Thyroid cartilage
- Cricoid cartilage
- Outline of thyroid gland
- Trachea

FIGURE 60–1 Incision for a tracheostomy is made through the fibrous tissue above the third tracheal cartilage. Two small vertical incisions create a flap that can be closed later.

- Relief of acute or chronic upper airway obstruction
- Access for continuous mechanical ventilation
- Prevention of aspiration pneumonia
- Promotion of pulmonary hygiene
- Bilateral vocal cord paralysis
- Prolonged endotracheal tube insertion resulting in erosion or pain

A tracheostomy is by far the most satisfactory artificial airway. It bypasses the upper airway and glottis, making stabilization, suction, and the attachment of respiratory equipment much easier than with other types of artificial airways. The client can eat and, with some adjustments, talk.

■ TRACHEOSTOMY TUBES

The tracheostomy opening is fitted with a tube to maintain airway patency. Tracheostomy tubes vary in their composition, number of separate parts, shape, and size. Tracheostomy tubes are chosen specifically for each client. Incorrectly fitted tubes can precipitate permanent or life-threatening damage.

The diameter of a tracheostomy tube should be smaller than the trachea so that it will lie comfortably within the tracheal lumen. Air should be able to pass between the outer wall of the tracheostomy tube and the tracheal mucosa. Although there is no standard tracheostomy tube sizing system, all packages indicate the inner and outer diameters in millimeters.

The length and curve of a tracheostomy tube are important. Tracheostomy tubes may be long (e.g., Hollinger tube, Shiley single-cannula tube) or short. They may be angled, the angle ranging from 50 to 90 degrees. Short to moderately short tubes with an angle of about 60 degrees are most often used. A tube must be long enough to avoid dislodgment into paratracheal tissue when the client coughs or turns the head. The lower end of a tracheostomy tube should be located above the carina. The tube's curve must allow the tip to be in a straight line with the

trachea, rather than pressing on the anterior or posterior tracheal wall.

Tracheostomy tubes may be cuffed or uncuffed. An inflated cuff permits mechanical ventilation and protects the lower airway by creating a seal between the upper and lower airways (Box 60–1). Tracheostomy cuffs do not hold the tube in place.

Tracheostomy tubes are made of various substances, such as nonreactive plastic, stainless steel, sterling silver, or silicone. Plastic tubes are disposable and used for only one person. Metal tubes may be reused after being sterilized.

UNIVERSAL TRACHEOSTOMY TUBE

The most common tube is a universal, or standard, tracheostomy tube (Fig. 60–2) having three parts: (1) outer cannula with cuff, flange, and pilot tube; (2) inner cannula; and (3) obturator. The parts fit together as one unit and may not be interchanged with other units. Therefore, all three parts of each individual set are kept together.

The outer cannula fits in the tracheostomy stoma to keep it open. The outer cannula has a flange or neckplate that fits flush with the neck and has holes on each side to attach the securing tapes or ties. A tracheostomy tube must be secured in place to prevent accidental extubation, excessive motion, or misalignment. Cloth tape or commercially available self-fastening (Velcro) ties may be used.

The obturator is placed into the outer tube before insertion. Its rounded tip smooths the end of the cannula and facilitates nontraumatic insertion of the tube into the stoma. The obturator is removed immediately after insertion, to open the tube. Place the obturator in a plastic wrapper and tape it to the head of the client's bed in a conspicuous place. If the tracheostomy tube is accidentally displaced, the obturator can be immediately placed into the outer cannula for quick reinsertion.

Once the obturator is removed, the inner cannula is placed into the outer cannula. Lock it into place to prevent accidental removal (e.g., when the client coughs). Frequent removal and cleaning of the inner cannula maintain airway patency. At the distal end, most inner cannulas have a standard 15-mm adapter that fits respiratory therapy and anesthesiology equipment.

SINGLE-CANNULA TRACHEOSTOMY TUBE

A single-cannula tracheostomy tube is slightly longer than a standard, double-cannula tube. Because it does not have an inner cannula that can be cleaned to eliminate secretions, a single-cannula tube should not be used in clients with excessive secretions or difficulty clearing secretions. Clients in whom a single-cannula tube is used must have continuous supplemental humidification to prevent obstruction by accumulated secretions. The longer single-cannula tube is used in the client with a thick neck or with an altered airway in whom a standard tracheostomy tube would be too short.

FENESTRATED TRACHEOSTOMY TUBE

A fenestrated tracheostomy tube has one large opening (Latin, *fenestra*), or several small ones, on the curvature of the posterior wall of the outer cannula. Fenestrated tubes have an inner cannula and may be cuffed or cuffless. When the inner cannula is removed, the fenestration permits air to flow through both the upper airway and the

BOX 60-1   Inflation and Deflation of Tracheostomy Tube Cuff*

Inflation (Minimal Leak Technique)

Objective

Inflate the cuff with the minimum volume of air required to adequately seal the trachea during positive-pressure ventilation and to prevent aspiration of foreign material while exerting the lowest possible cuff–to–tracheal wall pressure.

Intervention

1. Withdraw all residual air from the cuff.
2. Place 6 cc of air in a syringe.
3. Place the diaphragm of a stethoscope over the client's neck in the area of the tracheostomy tube cuff.
4. On inhalation, slowly inject air through the one-way valve into the pilot line in 1-cc increments.
5. Auscultate the neck area over the cuff.
6. Apply positive pressure to the tracheostomy tube with a manual self-inflating bag. An audible air leak can be heard via the stethoscope unless the cuff is inflated.
7. Continue slowly injecting air until the air leak is no longer present during inhalation.
8. When a leak is no longer auscultated, withdraw a small amount of air from the cuff until a very small leak is heard. This is called a *minimal leak.*
9. Note the amount of air necessary to achieve the minimal leak. This is the *minimal occluding volume* (MOV).
10. Once minimal leak is attained, measure the cuff pressure with a manometer.
11. Routinely measure and document cuff pressures.

Deflation

Objective

Allow air to flow around the tracheostomy tube, to permit phonation and to provide an opportunity to blow secretions above the cuff into the oropharynx, where they can be removed by suctioning.

Intervention

Routinely deflating the cuff is not necessary provided that safe cuff inflation and cuff pressure measurements are performed.

1. Remove the ventilator assembly (if present), and attach a self-inflating bag to the 15-mm adapter on the inner cannula.
2. Hyperoxygenate, hyperinflate, and suction the trachea to remove secretions below the cuff. Remove secretions above the cuff by gently applying suction deep into the oropharynx.
3. Insert an empty syringe into the one-way valve, and pull back on the plunger to remove the air in the cuff. At the same time, apply positive pressure with the manual self-inflating bag. This maneuver blows secretions lying directly above the cuff into the mouth, to prevent secretions accumulated above the cuff from draining into the trachea and lower airway.
4. Suction the oropharynx again.
5. If the person is ventilator-dependent, remember that with the cuff "down" or deflated, a portion of ventilation volume will not reach the lungs. Air will escape through the upper airway, which may compromise the person's respiratory status. This volume loss creates an audible leak. Phonation is possible during the exhalation phase of ventilation.

* The same procedure is used for inflation and deflation of endotracheal tube cuffs.

---

tracheostomy opening. This permits speech and more effective coughing. This tube may be used while a client is being weaned from a tracheostomy and for a client in whom use of the tracheostomy is expected to be prolonged. When the inner cannula is in place, the fenestration is closed, and the tube functions as a universal tracheostomy tube. For weaning a mechanically ventilated client, remove the inner cannula and deflate the cuff to allow the client to breathe through the fenestrae and around the tube.

TRACHEOSTOMY SPEAKING VALVES

For a "talking tracheostomy," a one-way valve in a plastic T-piece is attached to the 15-mm end of the inner cannula of a universal tracheostomy tube. This modification permits talking without the need to plug the tracheostomy tube. The one-way valve allows air (and the aerosol of supplemental humidification and oxygen) to flow into the arm of the T-piece during inspiration. On exhalation, the one-way valve closes, directing air from the lungs up through the vocal cords and upper airway. Phonation and effective coughing are facilitated by this normal passage of air.

A talking tracheostomy is *never* used unless there is enough room around the tracheostomy tube to permit sufficient air flow for breathing. *Always deflate* a cuffed tracheostomy tube before the client uses the talking tracheostomy adapter. Cuff inflation prevents exhalation, potentially causing suffocation.

COMMUNITRACH TUBE

The Communitrach tube allows speech by coordination of phonation efforts. Ventilation and phonation are separated because of different air sources. With this device, an air flow tube (that looks like a second pilot tube) runs outside the pilot (main) tube and opens just above the cuff. There is a port at the distal end of the air flow tube. When the port is occluded by a finger and compressed air or oxygen is directed through the air flow tube, a current of air is generated up through the vocal cords. With practice, the client learns to use this air flow for speech, although the "voice" produced in this way does not sound normal. Mucosal irritation may develop from the forced flow of air or oxygen into the upper airway.

TRACHEOSTOMY BUTTON

Use of a tracheostomy button is sometimes indicated during weaning as an intermediate measure between using a standard tracheostomy tube and extubation. A button is a short, straight tracheostomy tube that fits into the stoma of a tracheostomy but is not deep enough to enter the tracheal lumen. It has a removable cap with a one-way flap inside that permits inhalation but not exhalation. Exhalation occurs through the normal upper airway. When the cap is on, the client can talk.

A button cannot be used with a ventilator. It replaces a standard tracheostomy tube for people with retained secretions who do not require ventilatory assistance. A button creates less airway resistance than that produced by a

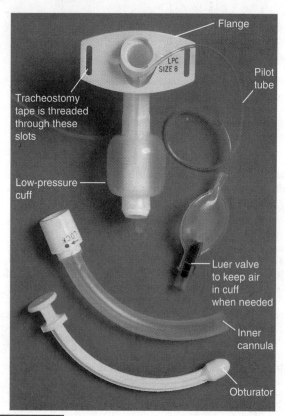

FIGURE 60–2 Parts of a tracheostomy tube. (Courtesy of Shiley, Inc., Irvine, CA.)

plugged standard tracheostomy tube; hence, breathing is easier. Artificial humidification of inspired air is necessary with a button (as with any tracheostomy tube), because the natural airway is bypassed.

PERMANENT TRACHEOSTOMY

Most clients with a permanent tracheostomy use a universal cuffless tracheostomy tube or an Olympic tracheostomy button. For appearance's sake, many people prefer a low-profile inner cannula. This design does not incorporate a 15-mm adapter. Instead, the inner cannula fits into the outer cannula and lies flush with the neck. If the client has had a total laryngectomy, the cut end of the trachea is sutured to the skin, creating a permanent stoma. Once the stoma is healed, most laryngectomy clients do not need a tube.

METAL TRACHEOSTOMY TUBE

Metal tracheostomy tubes are made of sterling silver or stainless steel. The most popular type is the Jackson tracheostomy tube. Metal tubes are cuffless and most often used in clients who have a permanent tracheostomy or laryngectomy. The inner cannula locks together with the outer cannula. Because metal tubes do not have a standard 15-mm adapter, rapid adaptation to respiratory or anesthesia equipment is impossible unless a specific adapter is available. The Hollinger tube is also made of metal and is similar to the Jackson tube.

■ POTENTIAL PROBLEMS ASSOCIATED WITH TRACHEOSTOMY TUBES AND CUFFS

Most tracheostomy tube cuffs are designed to exert a low pressure against the tracheal wall. These cuffs are easily

distensible, so that they accept a high volume of air without generating excessive force (i.e., high-volume, low-pressure cuffs). Low cuff pressure is necessary to prevent damage to the tracheal mucosa. The volume of air in the cuff determines the pressure exerted on the tracheal mucosa. Cuff pressures should not exceed 20 cm H_2O. With pressures above 42 cm H_2O, circulation to the tracheal mucosa is impaired, resulting in ischemia and necrosis. This is because the normal pressure within tracheal arteries is 42 cm H_2O. In the veins and lymphatic vessels the normal pressures are 24 cm H_2O and 7 cm H_2O, respectively.

Tracheal damage from cuff pressure is a frequent complication of intubation. Cuffed tubes can cause tracheal damage in as few as 3 to 5 days.

TRACHEAL WALL NECROSIS

Necrosis of the tracheal wall can lead to the formation of an abnormal opening between the posterior trachea and the esophagus. This problem is called *tracheoesophageal fistula.* The fistula allows air to escape into the stomach, causing distention. It also promotes aspiration of gastric contents. Fistulae most often develop when a cuffed tube is used in conjunction with a standard nasogastric (NG) tube. Use of small-lumen NG tubes can decrease the risk of fistula. Necrosis of the anterior trachea can lead to the rare but life-threatening complication of hemorrhage due to erosion into the innominate artery. This complication is manifested as the bleeding in and around or from the tracheostomy or by pulsation of the tracheostomy tube. Immediate intervention is mandatory because the client can exsanguinate.

When long-term tracheostomy is required, uncuffed tracheostomy tubes are usually used unless the client is at high risk of aspiration. Some clients who require long-term mechanical ventilation can tolerate uncuffed tracheostomy tubes. Tidal volumes and respiratory rates may be adjusted on the ventilator to produce satisfactory ventilation and arterial blood gas (ABG) concentrations while eliminating the risks associated with the use of tracheostomy tube cuffs.

TRACHEAL DILATION

Prolonged intubation can lead to dilation of the trachea from the cuff. This complication should be suspected when increasing amounts of air are needed to seal the cuff, or when bulging of the tracheal wall is seen on x-ray films.

TRACHEAL STENOSIS

Tracheal stenosis is narrowing of the trachea and may be noted 1 week to 2 years after intubation. It results from scar formation in the inflamed trachea. The severity of stenosis can be prevented by choosing the right size of tube, maintaining adequate cuff pressure, keeping intubation time short, preventing infection, and reducing movement of the tube.

AIRWAY OBSTRUCTION

The flow of air through a tracheostomy tube may become occluded for several reasons. The tracheostomy tube may be misaligned so that its opening lies against the tracheal wall, preventing air flow. Cuff overinflation causes the cuff to herniate over the tip of the tube, obstructing air flow. Without adequate airway care, the inner cannula can become occluded with dried secretions or excessive bronchial secretions.

INFECTION

Tracheostomies increase the risk of bronchopulmonary infection because they (1) bypass upper airway protective mechanisms (i.e., filtering, warming, and humidifying) and (2) decrease mucociliary transport and coughing, thus increasing retained secretions. Stoma site infection may occur as well. Nosocomial infection is also a potential problem. The lower airway (below the larynx) is normally sterile. Therefore, all solutions and equipment entering the trachea must be sterile. Organisms (e.g., *Pseudomonas aeruginosa* and other gram-negative bacteria) grow readily in respiratory equipment, which can then contaminate the lower airway. In addition, some bacteria may colonize a tracheostomy without causing infection.

Recommendations for changing tracheostomy tubes vary. Most physicians and health care facilities have established protocols. Some facilities direct that tracheostomy tubes be changed as often as every week, whereas others allow longer periods between tube changes. Ideally, the tube should be changed at least every 6 to 8 weeks, or more frequently if the person is at risk of recurrent tracheobronchial infections. Each client has a unique set of circumstances that dictate the frequency of tracheostomy tube changes.

ACCIDENTAL DECANNULATION

A tracheostomy tube that is not properly secured may be accidentally dislodged from the stoma. Because most new tracheostomy tubes are sutured in place, decannulation is rare, but it is serious nonetheless. Decannulation may occur while the ties are being changed. Manipulation of a tracheostomy tube or suctioning often produces vigorous coughing, which can expel the tube from the stoma unless the tube is held firmly. With accidental extubation, if the stoma is less than 4 days old, it may close, because a tract is not yet formed.

If extubation occurs, call for help immediately. Maintain ventilation and oxygenation by bag and mask. If ventilation is impossible, you must reinsert the tube. To do so, deflate the cuff, remove the tube's inner cannula, insert the obturator in the outer cannula, elevate the person's shoulders with a pillow, and gently hyperextend the neck. You may need to use tracheal dilators (spreaders) to hold the stoma open. Insert the outer cannula with obturator into the client's neck, and immediately remove the obturator. Auscultate for breath sounds. If breath sounds are present, insert the inner cannula and reconnect it to oxygen and ventilation equipment. If the tracheostomy tube cannot be reinserted in 1 minute, (call a code) for respiratory arrest. Unless the client is breathing adequately, an emergency cricothyroidotomy will be necessary (see Chapter 82).

If accidental decannulation occurs once a tract has formed following a tracheostomy, the same procedure is used, but reinsertion of the tube is generally easier. If bleeding occurs or the airway is obstructed, use emergency measures, as indicated earlier.

SUBCUTANEOUS EMPHYSEMA

Subcutaneous emphysema develops when air escapes from the tracheostomy incision into the tissues, dissects fascial planes under the skin, and accumulates around the face, neck, and upper chest. These areas appear puffy, and slight finger pressure produces a crackling sound and sensation. Generally this is not a serious condition; the air is eventually absorbed.

WEANING, REMOVAL, AND RESCUE BREATHING

■ WEANING FROM A TRACHEOSTOMY TUBE

When continuous mechanical ventilation becomes unnecessary, weaning from a tracheostomy tube begins by deflating the cuff to determine the client's ability to manage secretions without aspirating them. A smaller, uncuffed tube may be inserted to ensure adequate ventilation around the tube. The tube is then plugged briefly to assess the client's ability to breathe through the upper airway. The time is gradually lengthened according to the client's respiratory status, general medical condition, and confidence. Eventually, the tracheostomy tube can be removed. The weaning process takes a variable length of time (typically 2 to 5 days) depending on the client's ability to breathe through the upper airway. If the tracheal opening is still needed for some intervention, an uncuffed tube, a fenestrated tube, or a tracheal button may be used.

Plugging a tracheostomy tube is usually done by inserting a tracheostomy plug (decannulation stopper) into the opening of the outer cannula. This closes off the tracheostomy, and air flow and respiration occur normally, through the nose and mouth. *When a cuffed tracheostomy tube is plugged, the cuff must be deflated. If the cuff remains inflated, ventilation cannot occur, and respiratory arrest could result.*

Explain the process to the client and family. Naturally, most clients are anxious about weaning because they fear they may not be able to breathe. Constant, supportive observation during weaning is necessary. Encourage the client to begin to think about breathing through the nose again. This breathing is a strange sensation for people who have used a tracheostomy tube for a long time. Explain ways to facilitate optimal respiration and to maintain control of breathing (e.g., inhale slowly and completely through the nose; avoid holding the breath).

ABG analysis and measurement of spontaneous respiratory mechanics (respiratory rate, tidal volume, vital capacity, inspiratory effort, expiratory effort) are important assessments during weaning. Oximetry and other noninvasive assessment modes may also be used once baseline ABG values are established.

During weaning from tracheostomy, assess for indications of respiratory distress or ventilation impairment. Clinical manifestations of problems may include the following:

- Abnormal respiratory rate and pattern
- Use of accessory muscles to assist breathing
- Abnormal pulse and blood pressure
- Abnormal skin and mucous membrane color
- Abnormal ABG levels or oxygen saturation

Remove the tracheostomy plug immediately if any sign of respiratory distress or ventilation impairment appears. Also assess the client's quality of phonation and ability to deep-breathe and cough effectively. If oxygen has been administered via the tracheostomy, administer it at the prescribed rate of flow using nasal prongs.

■ REMOVING A TRACHEOSTOMY TUBE

A tracheostomy tube is removed after resumption of normal respirations as indicated by the client's ability to breathe comfortably with the tracheostomy plugged, as well as to cough and raise secretions, and normal ABG values or oxygen saturation. Gradually increase the length of plugging sessions until the client is comfortable and confident with the tube plugged continuously for at least 24 hours.

After a tracheostomy tube is removed, place a dry sterile dressing over the stoma. Initially, every 8 hours, clean the skin around the stoma; remove mucus with hydrogen peroxide; rinse the area with normal saline; and apply a fresh, dry dressing over the healing stoma. Document the condition of the stoma and the surrounding skin. If either appears irritated or infected, notify the physician. Topical antibiotic ointment may be prescribed. A tracheostomy stoma closes gradually (over a period of several days). As long as the stoma is open, an air leak is present. Instruct the client to place clean fingers firmly over the dressing to facilitate normal speech and coughing.

After extubation, ongoing assessment of respiratory function is necessary. Some complications of tracheostomy, such as tracheal stenosis, can appear months after tracheostomy tube removal.

■ PERFORMING RESCUE BREATHING

Emergency rescue breathing in the mouth-to-neck mode (i.e., mouth to tracheostomy or mouth to stoma) may be necessary if a client who has a tracheostomy or laryngectomy experiences respiratory depression or respiratory arrest. If a tracheostomy tube is in place, provide ventilation by attaching a manual self-inflating bag to the standard 15-mm adapter on the inner cannula. Some volume is lost from an uncuffed tube. Adequate ventilation can often be compensated for by altering the usual method of manual inflation (e.g., compress the bag more forcefully and quickly). If the tracheostomy tube is cuffed, inflate the cuff and maintain ventilation at the correct rate—that is, 12 to 16 breaths per minute for an adult. If inflation of the cuff impedes ventilation, immediately deflate the cuff, and attempt to compensate for volume loss by compressing the bag more forcefully or quickly. If ventilation continues to be impaired or prevented and you determine the cause is a malfunction in the tube, remove the tube immediately and provide mouth-to-stoma ventilation. Keep the client's nose and mouth closed during mouth-to-stoma rescue breathing to prevent air from escaping through the upper airway.

■ Nursing Management of the Client with a Tracheostomy

PREOPERATIVE CARE

For clients who are to undergo elective tracheostomy, reinforce education provided by the physician. You may delegate some respiratory assistance tasks to other staff members, as discussed in the Management and Delegation feature, Assisting with Respiratory Care. The client's understanding of the tracheostomy tube may be enhanced by looking at anatomic diagrams and by handling a tracheos-

tomy tube. The postoperative changes in ability to speak and eat should be explained. If the tracheostomy is expected to be permanent, information about living a productive life with modifications in clothing can be provided. A visit by a client with a permanent tracheostomy may be desirable.

When an emergency tracheostomy is needed, precious seconds may be all the time available for teaching. The client may be anxious or even unconscious. Education is often provided to the family in lieu of the client.

POSTOPERATIVE CARE
ASSESSMENT

After tracheostomy, frequent assessment is required, including monitoring vital signs; assessing amount, color, and consistency of secretions; and observing for indications of shock, hemorrhage, respiratory insufficiency, or complications related to the client's general condition or the surgical intervention.

DIAGNOSIS, OUTCOMES, INTERVENTIONS

Ineffective Airway Clearance. Numerous factors can lead to ineffective airway clearance in clients with tracheostomy—for example, dehydration, fever, anesthesia, anticholinergic drugs, sedatives, and immobility.

Outcomes. The client will have an effective airway clearance, as evidenced by no retained secretions, clear (or clearing) lung sounds, and no fever.

Interventions. Promote airway clearance and pulmonary aeration by changing the client's position frequently, providing humidification and hydration, using sedatives cautiously, and performing frequent hyperinflation and suctioning to promote lung expansion and reduce the risks of atelectasis, pulmonary infection, and ineffective gas exchange. Hyperinflation creates an "artificial sigh," improving lung aeration and facilitating removal of tracheobronchial secretions by enhancing the cough effort. When the client's condition is stabilized sufficiently, coughing may be enhanced by having the client place a finger over the tracheostomy tube opening while attempting to cough. It is important that the client wash the hands before doing this. Have the person cough into paper tissues and dispose of them carefully.

Perform Suctioning. When a cuffed tracheostomy tube is used, secretions collect above the cuff. It is difficult to remove such secretions by oropharyngeal suctioning. However, the secretions can be "blown" into the mouth by simultaneously deflating the cuff and giving a deep manual inflation. The client may also be instructed to cough during cuff deflation to expel accumulated secretions through the tracheostomy tube. If the client is unable to produce an effective cough, suction the tracheostomy tube during deflation to prevent aspiration of secretions into the lower airway.

Suction the airway as needed. The use of careful technique reduces mucosal trauma, which can lead to tracheal infection. Mucosal trauma is indicated by tracheal irritation, tracheitis, and bloody tracheal secretions. If tracheal secretions are thick and not easily removed, instill 3 to 5 ml of sterile normal saline into the trachea; the saline reduces viscosity of secretions for easier removal and acts to mechanically stimulate the cough reflex. Instill the saline directly into the tracheostomy tube during inha-

MANAGEMENT AND DELEGATION

Assisting with Respiratory Care

Assisting with respiratory care is one of the more controversial areas involving the use of assistive personnel. Opinions differ widely on the role of assistive personnel in caring for clients who need respiratory care. The performance of suctioning in particular is central to this debate. Your clinical facility should provide you with clear guidelines about the role of assistive personnel in this aspect of care.

The following aspects of respiratory care are commonly delegated to unlicensed assistive personnel:

- Setting up of oxygen delivery equipment and suction equipment
- Stocking routine respiratory care supplies at the bedside
- Assisting clients with the use of an incentive spirometer (after client instruction from a nurse or respiratory care clinician)
- Assisting clients with coughing and deep-breathing (after client instruction from a nurse or a respiratory care clinician)
- Performing tracheostomy care
- Measuring peripheral oxygen saturation (SpO$_2$)

Controversial aspects of respiratory care less commonly delegated to unlicensed assistive personnel are as follows:

- Suctioning via an artificial airway
- Performance of chest physiotherapy to promote the loosening of secretions

Before the delegation of any aspect of respiratory care, consider the following:

- What is the client's respiratory status? Complete a thorough respiratory assessment.
- What is the indication for respiratory care? Is the client's condition stable? A client with acute respiratory compromise should receive your full attention and care; the care of such a client should not be delegated.
- Is your client on oxygen therapy? Oxygen is a type of medication for your client. All guidelines that pertain to

medications also apply to oxygen. You may delegate the setup of oxygen delivery equipment to assistive personnel. However, you are responsible to verify that the ordered amount (dose) of oxygen is actually being delivered to the client.

- Has the client been instructed in the use of the incentive spirometer or coughing and deep-breathing exercises? Does the client need reinforcement or reinstruction? Reinforcement can be provided by assistive personnel; education and instruction should always be provided by a registered nurse or a respiratory care clinician.
- Does the client have a *new* artificial airway, such as an oral airway, nasotracheal or endotracheal tube, or tracheostomy? Have you assessed the client during suctioning? How has the client tolerated suctioning previously? Well-tolerated suctioning via an existing artificial airway may be delegated to a skilled assistant, if this is consistent with training and institutional policy.
- Does this client have a new or long-term tracheostomy? A new tracheostomy should always be managed by a registered nurse. The tracheostomy tube that has been placed through a new surgical incision should be evaluated as for any other fresh postoperative site.
- Have the client and family members managed this tracheostomy at home? This is an opportunity to evaluate their sterile technique, to provide reinforcement, and to review instructions with the client and family. After doing so, you may choose to delegate suctioning for this client to assistive personnel.
- Are the assistive personnel aware that suctioning and care of artificial airways are sterile procedures? The sterile technique of assistive personnel should be evaluated intermittently.

Findings that are immediately reportable to you, the Registered Nurse, should be described for the assistive personnel. These include any change or difficulty that the caregiver or the client experiences during the provision of care, changes in the respiratory rate or pattern, and changes in the consistency, color, and quantity of respiratory secretions.

Donna W. Markey, MSN, RN, ACNP-CS, Clinician IV, Surgical Services, University of Virginia Health System, Charlottesville, Virginia

lation. If the client is unable to cough, suction the airway through the tracheostomy tube. Refer to the Management and Delegation feature, Assisting with Respiratory Care, before delegating activities to unlicensed assistive personnel.

Provide Tracheostomy Care. Tracheostomy care is detailed elsewhere in fundamentals textbooks. Reinsertion of the clean inner cannula is shown in Figure 60–3.

Provide Adequate Hydration. The normal hydrating mechanisms of the upper airway are bypassed by a tracheostomy. Hydration can be provided by an oral, parenteral, or inhalation route. Inhalation techniques include increasing the humidity of room air with a room humidifier and administering aerosols with dry gases such as oxygen.

If humidification is insufficient, the body tries to make up the deficit by taking fluid from body water. The result

is inspissated (very thick) mucus, which can compromise airway patency and increases the risk of secretion pooling and subsequent infection. Dried mucus also occludes air passages and leads to atelectasis, pneumonia, and potentially severe gas exchange abnormalities.

Prevent Tube Movement. Secure a tracheostomy tube properly. If the tube tapes for this purpose require knotting, tie a square knot. Avoid placing the knot over the client's carotid artery or spine. Make sure the tapes are not too tight (i.e., allow room for two fingers to slide comfortably under the tape). Inspect the skin under the securing tape for skin irritation. In clients in whom a tracheostomy is required for prolonged periods, the use of fastening devices such as padded straps with self-adhesive fasteners promotes comfort. Secure the tube in midline tracheal alignment. Support ventilator and aerosol tubing to prevent pulling on the tracheostomy tube.

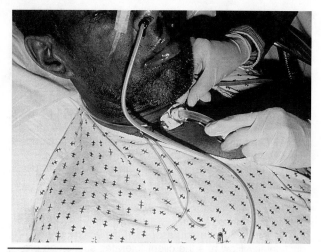

FIGURE 60–3 Reinserting a cleaned inner cannula.

Be careful not to disconnect tubing when turning the client.

Risk for Impaired Gas Exchange. After tracheostomy, impaired gas exchange may occur because of various factors. Factors affecting oxygen delivery include:

- Aspiration of blood, oral secretions, or gastric contents
- Restricted lung expansion from immobility
- Excessive tracheobronchial secretions
- Inability to cough and deep-breathe
- Pre-existing medical conditions (e.g., obesity, fever, inadequate hydration, pneumonia, tracheal injury such as from burns)

Factors affecting the removal of carbon dioxide include (1) the use of sedatives or anesthetic agents, (2) deteriorating level of consciousness, and (3) any other condition potentially affecting ventilatory efficiency and leading to hypoventilation and retention of carbon dioxide.

Outcomes. The client will have adequate gas exchange, as evidenced by maintaining oxygen saturation at greater than 90% (or ABG values within normal limits) and having no manifestations of respiratory distress.

Interventions. Assessment of gas exchange by ABG analysis is important immediately after tracheostomy and whenever there is a change in the client's condition or a change in treatment. Noninvasive monitoring such as pulse oximetry is appropriate once baseline values are established by ABG analysis. Remember, if shock or hypotension exists, or if peripheral vasoconstrictive drugs are used, data obtained by transcutaneous monitoring will be incorrect because of vasoconstriction.

Do not allow smoking in the room of a person who has a tracheostomy. Do not use aerosol spray cans (e.g., room deodorizers) near the person. Do not shake bedding or create dust clouds. Be careful when shaving or tending the person's hair that whiskers or hair does not fall into the trachea. Cover the tracheostomy with a thin cloth towel during shaving.

Risk for Infection. The tracheostomy bypasses normal upper airway protective mechanisms. The client also has an incision. Both areas can become infected.

Outcomes. The client will exhibit no indications of infection, as evidenced by the absence of fever and also a clean and dry tracheostomy site, healing incisions, and clear sputum.

Interventions. Use aseptic technique when working with the tracheostomy. Careful hand-washing, appropriate use of gloves, use of sterile supplies and solutions, and changing and decontaminating respiratory equipment every 24 hours are essential. Create a "loop" in the aerosol or ventilator tubing assembly; that is, let the tube loop down to catch condensate. Drain water and condensate in the tubing away from the tracheostomy into a receptacle.

Clean and inspect the skin around the stoma and the stoma itself. Observe for indications of irritation, inflammation, skin breakdown, and purulent drainage. If skin or stomal infection does occur, a topical antibacterial ointment may be prescribed.

Tracheostomy dressings (Fig. 60–4) are often used, especially in the early postoperative stage. Damp blood- and mucus-soaked dressings constitute a perfect medium for the growth of microorganisms. These conditions promote tissue irritation and breakdown. Change dressings whenever they are soiled or damp. Using hydrogen peroxide and cotton-tipped applicators, carefully clean the skin each time the dressing is changed. Rinse with normal saline and dry the area. Do not use plastic-backed or waterproof dressings. Moisture, secretions, and blood may seep behind the dressings, which hold warmth and moisture in. Skin then becomes irritated and macerated.

Risk for Aspiration. The presence of a tracheostomy increases the risk of aspiration because the tubes tether the larynx, preventing normal upward movement of the larynx and closure by the epiglottis on swallowing.

Outcomes. The client will exhibit no evidence of aspiration—that is, will have clear lung sounds, no fever, and no choking on swallowing.

Interventions. Intravenous fluids are usually given during the first 24 hours after tracheostomy. Then, if the client is alert and swallowing and if gag mechanisms are intact, oral intake of fluid and food may be attempted.

If a cuffed endotracheal tube was used before the tracheostomy, assess for the presence of tracheoesophageal fistula before permitting oral feedings. To assess for fistula, give the client a "test swallow" of water (at room temperature and colored blue with food coloring) before giving fluid or food. Severe coughing or blue fluid suctioned from the tracheostomy tube may indicate aspiration or a fistula. In either case, withhold oral food and fluid, and continue feeding by NG tube or other methods.

A client in whom normal swallowing is not expected to return for some time, or in whom the swallowing mechanism is permanently impaired (e.g., after a cerebrovascular accident), requires gastrostomy feedings or a permanent feeding tube (see Chapter 29). Tube-feedings may cause reflux, and the nutritive substance may be aspirated into the trachea. Before administering tube-feedings, inflate the cuff of the tracheostomy tube. Leave it inflated for at least 1 hour after feeding. Suction above the cuff before deflating it to remove any tube-feeding material.

When feeding a client with a tracheostomy, have the client sit upright. Often, food and fluids with semisolid consistency (e.g., pudding) are easier to swallow than water. Tipping the chin toward the chest narrows the

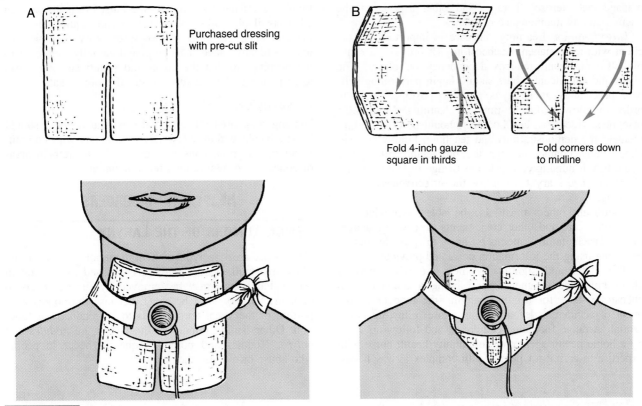

FIGURE 60–4 Tracheostomy dressings. If there is significant bleeding or tracheal secretions, cleaning the skin and changing the dressing frequently may prevent infection and skin breakdown. *A,* Manufactured dressing with a precut slit has no fine threads that could unravel and enter the stoma. Place the dressing around the tracheostomy tube with the slit downward, as shown, or upward. *B,* A 4 × 4 gauze pad is folded and placed under the tracheostomy tube. There should not be any cut edges that might unravel.

airway and helps food enter the esophagus. Overinflation of the cuff causes swallowing difficulty. If oral fluid intake is limited, continue intravenous fluids.

Impaired Verbal Communication. Because the vocal cords are bypassed by the tracheostomy tube, the client cannot talk. The nursing diagnosis of *Impaired Verbal Communication* may need to be combined with the diagnosis of *Fear* or *Anxiety* if the client feels afraid of not being able to summon help.

Outcomes. The client will have a satisfactory method of communicating with the nursing staff, as evidenced by being able to summon help and have needs met.

Interventions. Make sure the client can always reach an emergency call system to summon help. Do not use an intercom system because the client cannot talk. Be sure all staff members know this. Make a written list of common needs, words, and phrases that the client can point to (e.g., "I want to pass urine"; "I am thirsty"; "I have pain") to communicate needs. Provide paper and pencil or a picture communication board to facilitate communication. When possible, assess the client's reading ability preoperatively and select appropriate communication tools to be used postoperatively.

Risk for Constipation. When the glottis and vocal cords are bypassed (as with tracheostomy), the client cannot perform a Valsalva maneuver. This deficit impairs the person's ability to defecate.

Outcomes. The client will have regular bowel movements (according to a usual schedule).

Interventions. Assess for most recent bowel movement. Elimination is a frequently overlooked area of client care. Use prescribed stool softeners, laxatives, and even enemas or suppositories as necessary.

Anxiety and Fear. Anxiety and fear are due to various factors affecting the client with a tracheostomy— for example, inability to talk, fear of suffocating, anxiety about diagnosis, or fear that the tracheostomy tube will come out.

Outcomes. The client will have decreasing manifestations of anxiety and fear, as evidenced by a pulse rate within normal limits, a calm facial expression, the ability to communicate, and no expressed fears.

Interventions. Frequent observation is essential. Your presence and skilled nursing care are reassuring. Be certain to allow the client adequate time to communicate needs and concerns. Assist the family in reassuring the client that nurses are present and that the client is not alone.

Risk for Ineffective Management of Therapeutic Regimen (Individuals) and Risk for Ineffective Management of Therapeutic Regimen (Families). The client and family members need a lot of new information about permanent or long-term tracheostomy care.

Outcomes. Before discharge from the health care facility, the client and significant others will be confident in performing tracheostomy care, suctioning, and preoxygenation and the use of safety measures, emergency airway management, aerosol therapy, and other aspects of the client's airway maintenance regimen.

Interventions. Learning self-care is important for the client with a permanent tracheostomy. It provides a sense of self-control and reduces dependency on others. The client and significant others should begin performing self-care procedures as soon as possible postoperatively in order to allow sufficient time for learning. Multimedia resources, videotape, and booklets should be used to supplement the demonstrations and teaching. Follow-up telephone calls, contact through the physician's office, and home health nursing care (see the Bridge to Home Health Care) are necessary to identify the effectiveness of the teaching.

Significant others must also be able to provide tracheostomy care and other components of airway management. Teach family members how to provide rescue breathing using the information presented previously.

The client and significant others are often anxious about home management. Send home a duplicate tracheostomy tube for use in changing the tube or in the event of accidental decannulation. Close follow-up is essential. Arrange for home equipment and follow-up visits by a home health agency or community health nurse with expertise in caring for people with complex airway needs.

Involve a tracheostomy nurse specialist in client teaching when available. Order home health care equipment from medical suppliers who employ respiratory therapists or nurses. Ideally, have the equipment initially delivered to the hospital, so that the client and significant others can learn its use under the supervision of professionals.

Evaluation

Nursing diagnoses related to airway management should be resolvable within a few days. Problems with communication, infection, constipation, and eating remain areas of concern and require long-term planning.

NEOPLASTIC DISORDERS

BENIGN TUMORS OF THE LARYNX

Papillomas are one type of benign tumor of the larynx. They are small, wartlike growths believed to be viral in origin. Papillomas may be removed by surgical excision or laser. Surgery must be exact, because the nondiseased portion of the vocal cords needs to be retained for function. Other benign tumors of the larynx are *nodules* and *polyps*. Nodules and polyps frequently occur in people who abuse or overuse their voice.

BRIDGE TO HOME HEALTH CARE

Living with a Tracheostomy

Common indications for discharging clients to home health care with tracheostomy tubes include the following:

- Long-term ventilatory support
- Inability to clear secretions
- Presence of a tumor that obstructs breathing
- Swelling from extensive neck surgery
- Vocal cord paralysis

Plastic or metal tracheostomy tubes are appropriate for long-term situations. Metal tubes can be disinfected and reused and are therefore cost-effective for home health care clients. However, metal tubes cannot be used for the client who is dependent on a ventilator because they lack the adapter that attaches to the ventilator tubing.

Daily tracheostomy care at home consists of skin care around the tube, cleaning the inner cannula, and suctioning. The home health nurse needs to teach these procedures to the client, family member, or informal caregiver. Use a clean wash cloth and mild soap and water to cleanse the skin around the tracheostomy tube. Keep the skin clean and dry to avoid skin maceration and potential skin breakdown. Keep a dry, lint-free dressing around the tube. Using a skin barrier after cleansing can help to prevent skin irritation. Remove and clean the inner cannula of the tracheostomy tube once per day or more often, depending upon mucus buildup. Wash inner cannulas in hot soapy water, and then disinfect them by boiling in water or soaking in alcohol or in hydrogen peroxide.

Excess secretions are common in clients with tracheostomy tubes for several reasons: (1) presence of the tube as a foreign body, (2) increased secretions due to respiratory illness, and (3) prevention of the normal process by which mucus is carried to the oropharynx and swallowed. Therefore, it is necessary to teach the process of suctioning. Ideally, family members and informal caregivers should learn to assess the need for suctioning by auscultating the client's lungs for "gurgles" with a stethoscope or by listening for signs of excess mucus. Do not encourage oversuctioning; it can irritate the mucosa. In some cases, clients may be able to cough up secretions on their own, or at least into the tracheostomy tube, which can then be suctioned. The caregiver must never apply suction when the suction catheter is inserted and must never apply suction for more than 10 seconds to avoid deoxygenating the client.

The entire tracheostomy tube is usually changed at least once a month. This procedure may be performed by the home health nurse or taught to a willing and capable client, family member, or informal caregiver. When this procedure is performed for the first time, it must be done in the physician's office or an outpatient setting. There is a risk of bleeding, and the client's response to the procedure is unknown. Once tolerance to the tube change is established, the procedure can be performed regularly in the home. It is best to remove and replace the tracheostomy tube with the client in an upright rather than a supine position, to decrease the sensation of choking and the risk of aspiration. An extra tracheostomy tube in a smaller size should be kept in the home in the event that the home health nurse or the client is unable to replace it with the existing size. It is not uncommon for the tracheostomy stoma to narrow over time.

Lisa A. Gorski, RN, MS, *Clinical Nurse Specialist, Covenant Home Health and Hospice, Milwaukee, Wisconsin*

CANCER OF THE LARYNX

Cancer of the larynx accounts for 2% to 3% of all malignancies. Care of the client with cancer of the larynx presents a unique challenge to the nurse because of the cosmetic and functional deformities commonly resulting from the disorder and its treatment. Benign and early malignant tumors may be treated with limited surgery, and the client recovers with little functional loss. Advanced tumors require extensive treatment, including surgery, radiation treatments, and chemotherapy. When a total laryngectomy is required, postoperatively the client is unable to speak, breathe through the nose or mouth, or eat normally. In addition, the defect left by the operation and its reconstruction may cause a significant deformity, necessitating further surgery to restore appearance.

Laryngeal cancer is classified and treated by its anatomic site. Cancer of the larynx (voice box) may occur on the glottis (true vocal cords), the supraglottic structures (above the vocal cords), or the subglottic structures (below the vocal cords) (Box 60–2).

There are an estimated 10,600 new cases of laryngeal cancer each year, most occurring in men. However, the incidence of cancer of the larynx in women is increasing.[14] If untreated, cancer of the larynx is inevitably fatal; 90% of untreated people die within 3 years. Like other cancers, however, it is potentially curable if discovered early enough.

Etiology and Risk Factors

The primary etiologic agent in laryngeal cancer is cigarette smoking. Three of four clients who develop laryngeal cancer have smoked or currently smoke. Alcohol appears to act synergistically with tobacco to increase the risk of developing a malignant tumor in the upper airway. Additional risk factors include occupational exposure to asbestos, wood dust, mustard gas, and petroleum products and the inhalation of other noxious fumes. Chronic laryngitis and voice abuse may also contribute to the disorder. Research now points to a link between tobacco exposure and mutation of the *p53* gene in squamous cell carcinoma of the head and neck.[28]

Pathophysiology

Squamous cell carcinoma is the most common malignant tumor of the larynx, arising from the membrane lining the respiratory tract. Metastasis from cancer of the glottis is unusual because of the sparse lymphatic drainage from the vocal cords. Cancer elsewhere in the larynx spreads more quickly because there are abundant lymphatic vessels. Metastatic disease often may be palpated as neck masses. Distant metastasis may occur in the lungs. Patterns of spread of head and neck cancer are shown in Figure 60–5.

Clinical Manifestations

The earliest clinical warning signs of laryngeal cancer (Box 60–3) are dependent on the location of the tumor. In general, hoarseness that lasts longer than 2 weeks should be evaluated. Hoarseness occurs when the tumor invades muscle and cartilage surrounding the larynx, causing fixation of the vocal cords. Unfortunately, most clients wait before seeking a diagnosis for chronic hoarseness.

Tumors on the glottis prevent glottic closure during speech, which causes hoarseness or a voice change. Supraglottic tumors may cause pain in the throat (especially with swallowing), aspiration during swallowing, a sensation of a foreign body in the throat, neck masses, or pain radiating to the ear by way of the glossopharyngeal and vagus nerves. Subglottic tumors have no early manifestations; clinical evidence does not appear until the lesion grows to obstruct the airway.[30]

Diagnostic Findings

The diagnosis of laryngeal cancer is made by visual examination of the larynx using direct or indirect laryngoscopy. The nasopharynx and posterior soft palate are inspected indirectly with a small mirror or an instrument resembling a telescope. While the mirror is inserted, slight pressure is applied to the tongue, and the client is instructed to say "a" and then "e," which elevates the soft palate (Fig. 60–6A). The instrument should not touch the tongue, or the client will gag. The nasopharynx is then inspected for drainage, bleeding, ulceration, or masses. Direct visualization of the larynx may be accomplished with use of several different instruments; most devices used are lighted endoscopes. The client is instructed to protrude the tongue, and the examiner *gently* holds the tongue with a gauze sponge and pulls it forward. A laryngeal mirror or telescopic endoscope is inserted into the oropharynx; again, contact with the tongue is avoided. The client is instructed to breathe in and out rapidly through the mouth, or to "pant like a puppy." Panting decreases the gagging sensation caused by the examination. During quiet respiration, the base of the tongue, epiglottis, and vocal cords are examined for signs of infection or tumor (Fig. 60–6B). The client is instructed to vocalize a high-pitched *eee* to approximate (close) the vocal cords. The examiner observes the movement of the cords, the color of the mucous membranes, and the presence of any lesions. If the client is unable to cooperate as described, the examination may be performed with a fiberoptic endoscope inserted through the nose.

Before any definitive treatment for tumor is initiated, a panendoscopy and biopsy should be performed to determine the exact location, size, and extent of the primary tumor. Computed tomography (CT) or magnetic resonance imaging (MRI) is used to assist with this process. Laboratory analysis includes a complete blood count, determination of serum electrolytes including calcium, and kidney and liver function tests. These data help to determine the physiologic readiness of the client for surgery. Because the airway will be altered after surgery, the client requires a thorough pulmonary assessment with ABG analysis for identification of any pre-existing pulmonary disorders that would interfere with breathing. Clients who are to undergo partial laryngectomy must have an adequate pulmonary reserve in order to produce an effective cough postoperatively. The operation is associated with an increased risk of aspiration, and the client must be able to cough to rid the airway of aspirated secretions.

BOX 60–2   **Clinical Manifestations of Laryngeal Cancer**

Area

Glottic Tumor

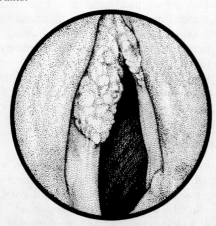

True glottic tumors interfere with normal closure and vibration of the vocal cords

Supraglottic Tumor

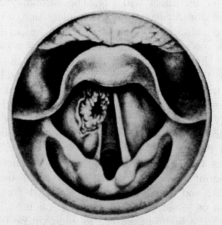

Carcinoma of the false cord partially hiding the true cord

Subglottic Tumor

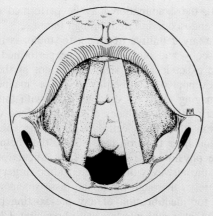

Subglottic polyp; this type of polyp can be single and smooth or lobulated as shown

Manifestations

Early: voice change, hoarseness, hemoptysis
Late: dyspnea, respiratory obstruction, dysphagia, weight loss, pain
Metastasize: through regional lymph nodes (rare except in superior or inferior tumors)

Early: aspiration on swallowing (especially liquids), persistent unilateral sore throat, foreign-body sensation, dysphagia, weight loss, neck mass, hemoptysis (expectoration of blood)
Late: dyspnea, pain in the throat or referred to the ear

Early: None
Late: dyspnea, airway obstruction, dysphagia, weight loss, hemoptysis

Top and bottom figures from DeWeese, D. F., & Saunders, W. H. (1982). *Textbook of otolaryngology* (6th ed.). St. Louis: Mosby–Year Book; middle figure from Del Regato, J. A., et al. (1985). *Ackerman and Del Regato's cancer* (6th ed.). St. Louis: Mosby–Year Book.

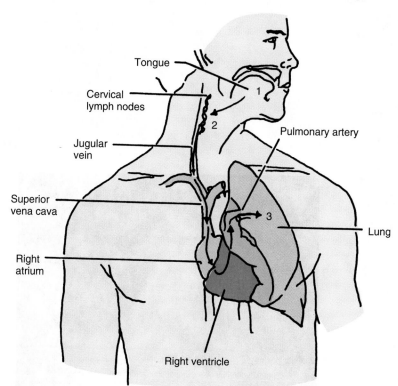

Tongue

Cervical
lymph nodes

Jugular
vein

Pulmonary artery

Superior
vena cava

Lung

Right
atrium

Right ventricle

FIGURE 60–5 Pattern of spread of head and neck cancer. (From Black, J. [1991]. Reconstructive surgery in the elderly. *Plastic Surgical Nursing, 11,* 157.)

Finally, for ascertaining possible tumor spread or other primary tumors, a chest radiography and barium swallow study or esophagography are performed.

Once the tumor has been identified and a biopsy performed, the tumor can be staged. Staging has important implications for treatment choice and outcome. It is essential to determine the extent of the primary tumor in order to select the most appropriate intervention. Staging is accomplished by (1) measuring the size of the primary tumor, (2) determining the presence of enlarged lymphatic nodes, and (3) determining the presence of distant metastasis. This system of staging is called the TNM (tumor-node-metastasis) classification system (see Chapter 19).

Outcome Management

Medical Management

TUMOR ABLATION
The goal of client care is ablation of the tumor, with sparing of undiseased tissue when possible. The choice of treatment for glottic cancer depends on the degree of tumor involvement. If the tumor is limited to the true

BOX 60–3	Clinical Warning Signs of Laryngeal Cancer

- Change in voice quality
- A lump anywhere in the neck or body
- Persistent cough, sore throat, or earache
- Hemoptysis
- Sores within the throat that do not heal
- Difficulty in swallowing or breathing

vocal cord, without causing limitation of the cord's movement, radiation therapy is usually the best treatment, with cure rates of 85% to 95%. The radiation dose depends on the size and location of the tumor; it is usually a minimum dose of 5500 to 6000 cGy (*gray* is a more accurate unit than *rad*) over 5 to 7 weeks. During radiation therapy, the client needs to be assessed for signs of destruction of normal tissue, ability to eat, airway distress, and other side effects. The complications of radiation therapy to the larynx include skin irritation, xerostomia, mucositis, laryngeal edema, and delayed healing. Radiation therapy is discussed fully in Chapter 19.

Supraglottic tumors may be treated with radiation therapy or a partial laryngectomy, with or without lymph node dissection. Subglottic tumors are usually more advanced carcinomas in which the tumor has spread to surrounding tissues. Metastasis is common. Treatment requires a total laryngectomy with or without radical neck dissection on the same or both sides of the tumor. (See later discussion.) The operative site may require reconstruction with pectoralis myocutaneous flaps (see Chapter 49).

Chemotherapy alone is not considered to be curative in treating head and neck cancers. However, it may be administered preoperatively to reduce tumor size, postoperatively to reduce the risk of metastasis, or as palliative treatment. Evidence now exists that larynx preservation may be possible with induction chemotherapy followed by radiation. Chemotherapy is generally not effective in advanced laryngeal cancer, but it may have the ability to control the development of new primary tumors through a process called chemoprevention.

Clients with laryngeal tumors often present in a compromised nutritional state due to dysphagia and weight

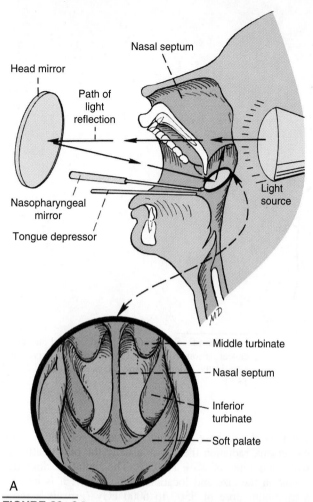

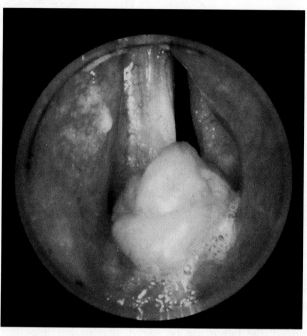

FIGURE 60–6 Laryngoscopy. *A,* Indirect laryngoscopy enables assessment of the pharynx and buccal cavity and some visualization of the larynx. (Laryngeal structure and function are best assessed by direct visualization, such as with flexible or rigid laryngoscopy or flexible fiberoptic bronchoscopy.) A head mirror, tongue depressor, light source, and small examining mirror are used in the indirect method. The mirror is positioned behind the soft palate after the tongue is depressed. To visualize the larynx, gently grasp the tongue with a gauze sponge and pull it forward. Place the mirror against the soft palate in front of the uvula, and move it gently until the cords are visualized. Have the client vocalize the high-pitched sound *eee,* which causes the larynx to move. The larynx is assessed for symmetrical cord motion. *B,* Large granular cell tumor of the true vocal cord, as seen during laryngoscopy. (From Wenig, B. M. [1993]. *Atlas of head and neck pathology.* Philadelphia: W. B. Saunders.)

loss. In addition, surgery, radiation therapy, and chemotherapy can directly affect oropharyngeal structures and impair swallowing. Nutritional intervention should begin before treatment to prevent malnutrition, thereby improving the overall prognosis.

Nursing Management of the Medical Client

The client undergoing radiation therapy for laryngeal cancer should be taught about the procedure and how to assess for and manage any expected problems at home. Written material is usually best, so that the client and family can refer to it as needed. Skin care for the irradiated site should include the use of prescribed creams and sunscreens, which are "patted" onto the skin; avoiding extremes of temperature; avoiding rough or tight garments; and avoiding rubbing or scratching the area.

Surgical Management

The goals of surgical intervention for laryngeal cancer are to (1) remove the cancer, (2) maintain adequate physio-

logic function of the airway, and (3) achieve a personally acceptable physical appearance. Many clients require tracheostomy for airway management (see earlier discussion). Most clients with advanced laryngeal cancer also have malnutrition from obstruction to swallowing by the tumor, as well as from the effects of the cancer. Before surgery, supplemental nutrition may be provided by NG tube-feedings or gastrostomy feedings. If long-term difficulty in swallowing is anticipated, a gastrostomy tube may be inserted at the time of surgery.

LASER SURGERY

Small tumors can often be eradicated with the use of laser. Laser surgery for vocal cord tumors can preserve much of the normal glottis, leaving the client with a usable voice. Sometimes laser surgery is combined with radiation therapy.

PARTIAL LARYNGECTOMY

For cancer involving one true vocal cord, or one cord plus a portion of the other, a partial laryngectomy is

VERTICAL PARTIAL
LARYNGECTOMY
(Hemilaryngectomy)

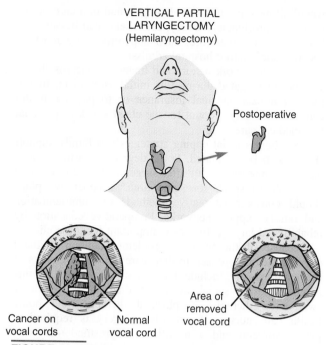

Postoperative

Cancer on
vocal cords

Normal
vocal cord

Area of
removed
vocal cord

FIGURE 60–7 Technique of partial laryngectomy.

feasible. This procedure is also called a vertical partial laryngectomy and involves the removal of half or more of the larynx (Fig. 60–7). A horizontal neck incision is made, and the diseased portion of the vocal cord is removed. Sometimes up to a third of the contralateral cord is also removed. This operation is generally well tolerated, and the client has only mild difficulty swallowing and an altered but adequate voice.

Another form of partial laryngectomy is the supraglottic laryngectomy. This procedure is performed for cancer of the supraglottis. The surgeon removes the superior portion of the larynx from the false vocal cords to the epiglottis and may also remove a portion of the base of the tongue. Lymph node dissection also may be performed. Because the true vocal cords are preserved, voice quality is maintained. The major postoperative problem is risk of aspiration, because the epiglottis, which normally closes over and protects the larynx, has been removed. The airway is managed with a tracheostomy after surgery; when the edema subsides in surrounding tissues, the tracheostomy tube can usually be removed and the stoma allowed to heal. The client then needs to be taught how to swallow to avoid aspiration.

For selected, confined transglottic carcinomas, a supracricoid partial laryngectomy may be indicated. This conservative procedure preserves functional speech and swallowing without a permanent tracheostomy.[34]

TOTAL LARYNGECTOMY

For large glottic tumors with fixation of the vocal cords, a total laryngectomy is required. The larynx is the connection of the pharynx (upper airway) and the trachea (lower airway) (Fig. 60–8A). When the larynx is removed, a permanent opening is made by suturing the trachea to the neck. The esophagus remains attached to the pharynx (Fig. 60–8B). Because no air can enter the nose, the client loses the sense of smell. The biggest problem for the client after laryngectomy is loss of voice. The client should be made aware that without surgery, the voice quality will worsen as the tumor enlarges, but in any case the loss of voice constitutes a serious psychological issue. Because the trachea and esophagus are permanently separated by surgery, there is no risk of aspira-

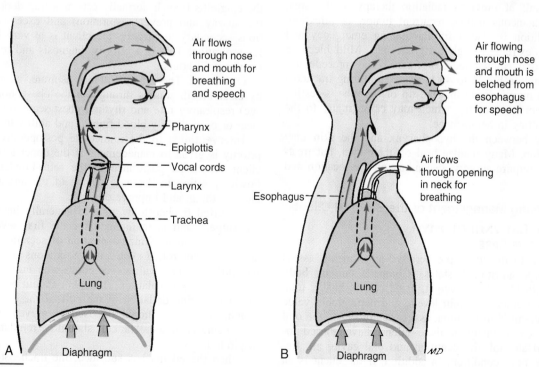

Air flows
through nose
and mouth for
breathing
and speech

Pharynx

Epiglottis

Vocal cords

Larynx

Trachea

Lung

A   Diaphragm

Air flowing
through nose
and mouth is
belched from
esophagus
for speech

Esophagus

Air flows
through opening
in neck for
breathing

Lung

B   Diaphragm

FIGURE 60–8 *A,* Before laryngectomy, air flow is through the nose and mouth. *B,* After surgical removal of the larynx, a new opening must be made for air passage. The trachea and esophagus are separated.

tion unless a fistula forms from the trachea to the esophagus. Besides this, the potential complications of the total laryngectomy are the same as for the partial laryngectomy (see earlier discussion).

CERVICAL LYMPH NODE DISSECTION

Metastasis to the cervical lymph nodes is common with tumors of the upper aerodigestive tract. Surgical management of laryngeal tumors often includes neck dissection. Radical neck dissection (also called en bloc) involves the removal of lymphatic drainage channels and nodes, the sternocleidomastoid muscle, the spinal accessory nerve, the jugular vein, and tissue in the submandibular area. A modified radical neck dissection spares the spinal accessory nerve, and a selective neck dissection removes only the lymph nodes within the area of anticipated spread.[28, 30]

COMPLICATIONS

Possible complications after laryngeal surgery are airway obstruction, hemorrhage, carotid artery rupture, and fistula formation. Airway obstruction is due to edema in the surgical site, bleeding into the airway, or loss of airway from a plugged tracheostomy tube. Airway obstruction constitutes an emergency and requires immediate intervention for restoration of the airway.

Hemorrhage is usually the result of inadequate hemostasis during surgery. Some blood-tinged sputum is expected in the tracheal secretions for the first 48 hours, but frank bleeding from the tracheotomy site or tube is a sign of hemorrhage and must be reported to the physician immediately. Also assess the client for other signs of bleeding such as evident hematoma or unilateral swelling, tachycardia, hypotension, and changes in respiratory patterns.

Carotid artery rupture is usually a late complication and is related to poor condition of the neck tissue. It may be the result of previous radiation therapy to the area, pharyngocutaneous fistula, recurrent tumor, or infection. This condition is also a life-threatening emergency and carries an extremely high mortality rate. Mild bleeding from the oral cavity, neck, or trachea may precede impending rupture by 24 to 48 hours. A pulsating tracheostomy tube may indicate that the tip of the tube is resting on the innominate artery, which may cause injury to the artery resulting in hemorrhage.

Fistulae between the hypopharynx and the skin may also develop. Many fistulae heal on their own, but treatment may require surgery, depending on the location and size.

▎ Nursing Management of the Surgical Client

PARTIAL LARYNGECTOMY
PREOPERATIVE CARE

In addition to the usual preoperative assessments, assess the client's nutritional status. Compare current body weight with ideal body weight, usual caloric intake, total lymphocyte count, albumin levels, and hemoglobin value and hematocrit.[30] In addition, assess dentition and the oral cavity. Because many of these clients have abused tobacco and alcohol, the dentition and oral cavity are frequently in poor condition. In addition, if the client is an active alcoholic, plans should consider support through the period of alcohol withdrawal. The ideal plan of care

would allow some nutritional support and oral care before surgery. Unfortunately, today, few clients can be admitted before surgery; therefore, such supportive care must be accomplished before hospital admission.

The client's work history and financial concerns should also be investigated during this initial assessment. Inability to purchase medical insurance or to pay for health care services may account for the client's lack of personal and medical care.

The client's usual coping strategies and family support should also be evaluated. Some degree of cosmetic (aesthetic) change will result after surgery, and the client will be unable to speak for some time.[6] Preoperative plans should consider alternative methods of communication and family support networks. Preoperative education by rehabilitated laryngectomees is important for these clients.

Because of the multiple problems common in these clients, a team approach to their care is used. Members of the team usually include the primary physician or surgeon, nurses, a social worker, a dietitian, a speech or swallowing therapist, a physical therapist, and home health care nurses. If extensive surgery is required, a plastic surgeon and a maxillofacial prosthodontist may also care for the client during reconstruction.

POSTOPERATIVE CARE
ASSESSMENT

In addition to the routine postoperative assessments, after a partial laryngectomy the client needs to undergo careful assessment of the airway, lung sounds, and position of the tracheostomy tube, as well as checking for potential complications related to the surgical procedure and the tracheostomy tube (see earlier discussion).

DIAGNOSIS, OUTCOMES, INTERVENTIONS

Risk for Aspiration. Because of the removal of the epiglottis (which normally acts as a trap door to close the airway and prevent aspiration) and excessive secretions secondary to surgery, the client is at very high risk for aspiration. This is a priority diagnosis and remains so for about 72 hours.

Outcomes. The client will not aspirate, as evidenced by clear breath sounds throughout the chest, normal (for age) respiratory rate and rhythm, chest secretions that are clear or only slightly blood-tinged, and ability to cough.

Interventions. In the immediate postoperative period, priority is given to management of the upper airway. The client should be positioned in the semi-Fowler to high Fowler position to decrease edema of the airway, facilitate breathing, and improve comfort.

A cuffed tracheostomy tube is generally inserted during surgery and is maintained for the first several days after surgery to minimize aspiration of secretions and for assisted or controlled ventilation. Secretions collect above the cuff. For removal of secretions, the cuff should be deflated during exhalation. The client should be instructed to cough during deflation of the cuff. If the client cannot cough, suctioning should be used to prevent secretions from being aspirated. The cuff should be reinflated during inspiration.

When the edema has subsided, the tracheostomy tube may be removed. The decannulation process is slow and begins with observation of the client for aspiration, as follows. The cuff of the tube is deflated, and the client is observed for the ability to swallow saliva and other secretions without coughing or requiring additional suctioning. If increased secretions are present through and around the tracheostomy tube, aspiration is occurring and the cuff should be reinflated. If no aspiration is occurring, the tracheostomy tube can be replaced with a smaller, uncuffed tube. If the uncuffed tube is tolerated without aspiration, the tube is capped (plugged) to determine the client's ability to breathe through the upper airway. If the client can breathe through the upper airway for 24 hours, the tracheostomy tube is removed, and the stoma is taped closed and covered with an occlusive dressing[2, 29] (Fig. 60–9).

Ineffective Airway Clearance.

The physical alteration in the airway and the presence of a tracheostomy tube interfere with normal movement of mucus up and out of the bronchial tree. In addition, as a result of prior smoking, the cilia have become ineffective. *Ineffective Airway Clearance* is also a priority nursing diagnosis for several days.

Outcomes. The client will have improved airway clearance, as evidenced by effortless, quiet respirations at baseline rate and clear breath sounds.

Interventions. The client may have copious secretions because of the presence of the tracheostomy tube, a history of chronic obstructive lung disease, and aspiration.

There may also be oral secretions that cannot be swallowed. Oral secretions accumulate because of the disruption of normal airflow, and swallowing may be impaired as a result of surgery. In the alert and conscious client, coughing and deep-breathing will mobilize and eliminate many of these secretions. However, in the client who has undergone head and neck surgery and is just emerging from anesthesia, these measures may not be possible. Suctioning of the trachea will be needed for the first 24 to 48 hours after surgery. The frequency of suctioning depends on the client's needs, but suctioning every hour or more often is common for the first 24 hours. Sterile technique must be used to avoid introducing microorganisms into the tracheobronchial tree in a client with impaired immune defenses due to malignancy and surgery. (Suctioning techniques can be found in fundamentals of nursing textbooks.)

The inner cannula of the tracheostomy tube should be cleaned as often as necessary to provide a clear airway. In the immediate postoperative phase, the inner cannula is cleaned after suctioning. Once the client is ambulatory and can handle secretions safely, the cannula can be cleaned three times a day and as necessary.

Chest physiotherapy, ultrasonic nebulization, and aerosol administration of bronchodilators and mucolytics into deeper parts of the respiratory tract for sputum induction are recommended to prevent pulmonary complications.

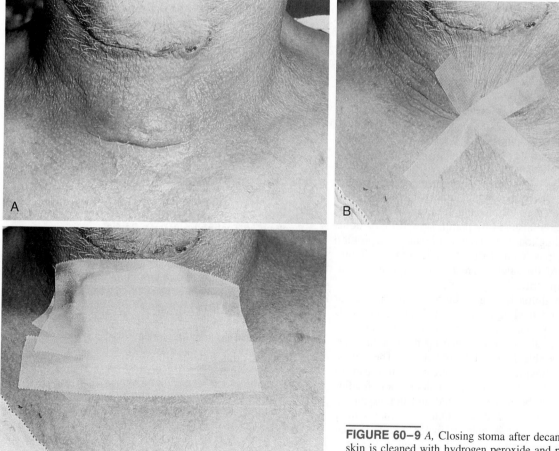

FIGURE 60–9 *A,* Closing stoma after decannulation. The skin is cleaned with hydrogen peroxide and protected with tincture of benzoin. *B,* The skin edges are pulled together and taped in an **X**. *C,* An occlusive dressing is applied.

These treatments are performed every 4 hours for the first few days after surgery and then usually decreased to four times a day once the client can ambulate.[30]

Risk for Impaired Gas Exchange.

Like other postoperative clients, clients with neck surgery have a high risk for atelectasis related to low tidal volume breathing secondary to pain, sedation, and increased mucus production.

Outcomes. The client will have adequate oxygenation, as evidenced by pulse oximetry values above 90%, ABG values within normal limits (that take into consideration any pre-existing lung disorders, such as emphysema), no air hunger, and clear lung sounds.

Interventions. Oxygenation is assessed through ABG analysis or pulse oximetry and the fraction of inspired oxygen (FiO_2) may be adjusted. If the client has pre-existent chronic air flow limitations, oxygen may have to be delivered at lower percentages or not at all. Compressed air with high humidity may be substituted in such cases.

Altered Nutrition: Less Than Body Requirements.

A combination of the pre-existing malignancy and swallowing difficulties sets the stage for malnutrition. In addition, concomitant lung disorders and alcoholism, which are common in this population, increase the tendency for malnutrition.

Outcomes. The client will have an improved nutritional status, as evidenced by maintaining baseline body weight or losing less than 5 pounds; consuming adequate fluid, protein, fat, and carbohydrate each 24 hours; swallowing without aspirating or choking; and hemoglobin, hematocrit, albumin, and total lymphocyte values remaining within normal limits.

Interventions. Immediately after surgery, typically an NG tube is inserted for removal of gastric secretions until postoperative ileus subsides. If long-term difficulty in swallowing is anticipated, a gastrostomy tube may be inserted at the time of surgery. Assess for bowel sounds, passage of flatus, and hunger as signs of returning gastrointestinal function. In some clients, tube-feeding with commercial supplements is indicated. Continually ascertain the correct position of the tube before each feeding. (Techniques for checking feeding tube placement can be found in fundamentals of nursing textbooks.) The tube-feeding can be administered by pump, slow drip, or bolus feeding, depending on the client's tolerance. Aspiration remains a high risk with partial laryngectomy, and precautions to guard the client from this event with its untoward results are critical.

When the epiglottis has been removed, the timing for resumption of oral feeding after a partial laryngectomy is controversial. One approach is to begin oral feedings with the tracheostomy tube in place when edema has subsided and the client is able to swallow secretions. The advantage of this technique is that aspirated liquid can be suctioned. A second technique is to delay oral feeding until the client has been decannulated and the stoma has healed. The advantage of this technique is that with a closed stoma, the client is able to increase intrathoracic pressure and remove any aspirated material through an effective cough.

Whenever the client eats, eating should begin with a nonpourable pureed diet; liquids are reserved until swallowing has been relearned. The accompanying Client Education Guide describes one technique for swallowing after a partial laryngectomy. Once swallowing can be accomplished without aspiration, carbonated beverages may be added. Thin liquids should be withheld until the risk of aspiration is minimal.[2, 29, 30]

Risk for Infection.

The loss of primary defenses of the skin and delayed healing due to pre-existing malignancy and malnutrition make *Risk for Infection* a common nursing diagnosis.

Outcomes. The client will have no clinical manifestations of wound infection, as evidenced by continued approximation of incisional edges; decrease in the amount of wound drainage; absence of purulent drainage; absence of redness, swelling, tenderness, or warmth beyond the suture lines; absence of fever; and a white blood cell count within normal limits.

Interventions. During surgery, a wound drain is placed into the surrounding tissues of the neck and attached to constant suction. A commonly used device for collecting the drainage is a closed wound drainage system (Hemovac) container, which is attached to the client's gown to prevent accidental dislodgment. Using universal precautions, assess the amount and color of the drainage every 4 hours for the first 24 hours. Assess the wound for signs of hematoma or seroma formation by noting whether the amount of drainage is increasing or if there is a change in the color or consistency of the drainage. Also assess the color of the surgical incisions. If the amount of drainage is decreasing, the drain may be removed by the physician. Dressings are placed over the drain puncture sites on the skin. Small to moderate amounts of serosanguineous drainage should be expected for another 48 to 72 hours.

The suture lines should be cleaned at least twice daily with hydrogen peroxide followed by a water or saline rinse. A thin film of antibiotic ointment may be applied to the suture line to prevent crusting of secretions and promote healing.

CLIENT EDUCATION GUIDE

Swallowing Technique After a Partial Laryngectomy

- Begin with soft or semisolid foods.
- Stay with a nurse or swallowing therapist during meals until you master the technique of swallowing without choking.
- Be patient; learning to swallow again is frustrating.

Follow these steps in sequence:

1. Take a deep breath.
2. Bear down to close the vocal cords.
3. Place food into your mouth.
4. Swallow.
5. Cough to rid the closed cord of accumulated food particles.
6. Swallow.
7. Cough.
8. Breathe.

EVALUATION

Expect the problems with airway management to resolve within a few days. Infection, apart from atelectasis, will not arise for about 72 hours. Nutritional problems and problems with healing may require several weeks to resolve.

■ Self-Care

The client who has undergone partial laryngectomy may be discharged from the hospital before completion of wound healing. If upper airway edema has not subsided, the client is discharged with a temporary tracheostomy. The client and significant others should understand and demonstrate proper care of the tube, including inner cannula care, technique for insertion of the entire tube in case of accidental decannulation, suctioning, humidification techniques, and emergency resuscitation measures.

Once decannulation has been performed, the stoma must be cleansed and an occlusive dressing applied at least once a day (see Fig. 60-9). Additional wound care includes cleaning the incision area with hydrogen peroxide and water and applying an antibiotic ointment. All instructions given to the client should be in writing, with additional teaching materials used as available. Ongoing assessment for healing, recurrent tumor, or a new tumor is required.

TOTAL LARYNGECTOMY

The nursing management of the client after a total laryngectomy is the same as the care given to a client with a partial laryngectomy, except for feeding and teaching about permanent stoma care. Clients who have a total laryngectomy will have a permanent tracheostomy and need to learn how to speak using alternative methods.

NUTRITION. Immediately after surgery, the client's nutrition is supplemented with NG tube-feedings. The client remains on tube-feedings until edema has subsided and suture line healing has occurred. When the client can swallow secretions, oral feedings can begin. The diet usually begins with liquid or semisoft foods and progresses as healing occurs.

COMMUNICATION. For the first few days after surgery, the client should communicate by writing. If the client is very fatigued, requests such as "I need something for pain" may be expressed by using a communication board so that the client can just point to the statement. Even though the client cannot speak, conversation should still include the client's input through nodding and pointing and not be directed only to others such as the family. Avoiding conversation with the client because of difficulty in communication is demeaning to the client and leads to frustration.

ARTIFICIAL LARYNX. An artificial larynx may be used as early as 3 to 4 days after surgery. These battery-operated speech devices are held alongside the neck or can be adapted with a plastic tube that is inserted in the mouth. The air inside the mouth is vibrated, and the client articulates as usual (Fig. 60-10). The speech quality is monotone and mechanical-sounding but intelligible.[4, 29]

ESOPHAGEAL SPEECH. Esophageal speech is a technique that requires the client to swallow and hold air in the upper esophagus. By controlling the flow of air, the client can pronounce as many as 6 to 10 words before stopping to reswallow more air. The voice is deep but is loud and effective once the technique is mastered.

TRACHEOESOPHAGEAL PUNCTURE. Tracheoesophageal puncture (TEP) is a surgical technique that also restores speech (Fig. 60-11). A small puncture is made into the upper tracheostoma to the cervical esophagus for creation of a fistula. After the fistula tract has healed, a small one-way valve, or voice prosthesis, is inserted. By occlusion of the prosthesis, air can be shunted into the esophagus and used to produce speech. The TEP may be done concurrently with a total laryngectomy or as a secondary procedure after healing and radiation therapy. These devices require maintenance; therefore, only clients who are highly motivated, are able to perform self-care, and have good manual dexterity are eligible for this procedure. Care of the TEP surgical wound is presented in the accompanying Client Education Guide (see p. 1671).

■ Self-Care

Clients should be discharged with an extra tracheostomy tube to allow daily changes at home (Fig. 60-12). To provide supplemental humidification, normal saline may be instilled into the stoma several times each day to stimulate coughing, moisten the mucosa, and loosen dried secretions and crusts. Use of a bedside humidifier or vaporizer also aids in humidifying the inspired air. A stoma bib or covering should be worn to warm and filter inspired air and to prevent foreign bodies from entering the stoma. These coverings can be purchased, or the client may improvise by using a scarf, necktie, or turtleneck shirt.[4, 30, 31]

The client must be encouraged to continue speech therapy as begun in the hospital. The techniques to restore speech require much time for mastery; the client is seen by a speech therapist after dismissal from the hospital. Community support groups for clients after laryngectomy—the Lost Cord Club and the International Association of Laryngectomees—offer needed reassurance. Much patience is required by the client and family while the client is relearning to speak. The process is time-consuming and frustrating, and progress may sometimes be slow. Encourage the family to give the client enough time to formulate the words and not speak for the client.

Once the incision has completely healed, the tracheostomy tube is no longer required (Fig. 60-13). This process varies but usually takes about 6 to 8 weeks. Occasionally, the tube may be required at night, if the stoma is small or the client does not get adequate air exchange during sleep. Once the tracheostomy tube has been removed, the client can disguise the stoma with clothing and begin to regain a sense of normalcy.

Tub baths or showers are permitted, but the client must use caution to prevent introduction of water into the stoma. Commercial stoma shower covers are available, and the water spray should be aimed at midchest. Water sports are prohibited. If the client fishes, a life preserver must be worn at all times on the boat.

The client should wear a medical alert bracelet or carry an emergency wallet card to identify the fact that resuscitation cannot be performed through the mouth. Information about obtaining these forms of identification is available from the American Cancer Society. The use of mouth-to-stoma rescue breathing is imperative when re-

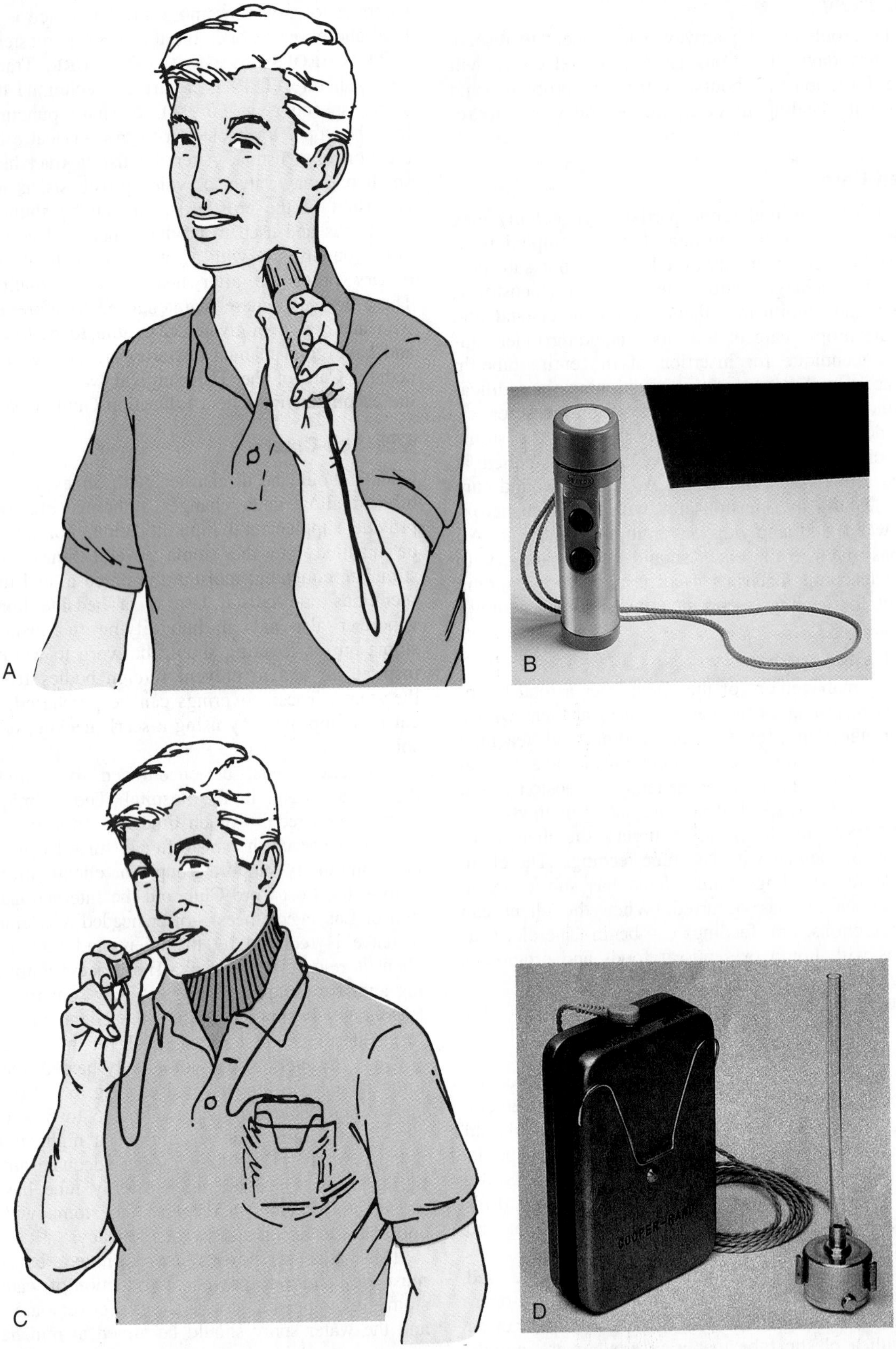

FIGURE 60–10 *A* and *B,* Artificial larynx. This hand-held, battery-powered speech aid is placed against the neck. *A,* When the artificial larynx is activated, it creates a vibration that is transmitted to the neck and into the mouth. Words silently formed by the mouth become sounds from the vibrations emitted by the device. Any type of artificial larynx requires muscle and tongue control and hand strength; usually, such a device is not used until immediate postoperative neck tenderness has subsided. (*B,* Courtesy of Servox Electrolarynx Manufacturing by Siemans Hearing Instruments, Inc., Union, NJ.) *C* and *D,* Electronic speech aid (Cooper Rand) allows the client to adjust tone, pitch, and volume. An oral connector permits speech without the necessity of placing the device against the neck. This is an advantage immediately after surgery, when the neck is too sensitive for a neck-vibrating device. (*D,* Courtesy of Luminaud, Inc., Mentor, OH.)

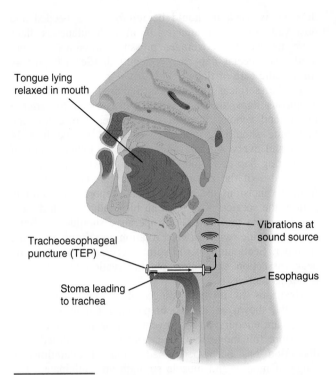

Tongue lying
relaxed in mouth

Vibrations at
sound source

Tracheoesophageal
puncture (TEP)

Esophagus

Stoma leading
to trachea

FIGURE 60–11 Tracheoesophageal puncture for voice rehabilitation after laryngectomy. A prosthesis is inserted into a fistula created in the neck. The prosthesis has a one-way valve that permits air to pass into the esophagus but prevents accidental aspiration. To speak, the client occludes the prosthesis with a finger or attachment. Exhaled air is then shunted through the prosthesis, where it vibrates, and exits the mouth as a spoken word.

suscitation is needed in these clients. Family members should be directed to a community program that teaches mouth-to-stoma resuscitation. For additional security, a wireless "beeper" or automatic response monitoring device can be useful.[8]

The client may require a nutritional plan for the first few weeks at home. The dietitian should work with the client and family to determine the consistency of food easiest to swallow as well as the kinds of foods required to obtain needed protein and calories.

It is essential that the client not smoke so that lung function is preserved and the formation of other aerodigestive tract tumors is prevented. For some clients after laryngectomy, the process of smoking cessation seems pointless. Some clients continue to smoke by inhaling the cigarette smoke through the stoma. The attitude is one of "Why quit now? What else could happen to me?" Use extra support and encouragement with the client, remembering to be an advocate of the client's choice as well as providing assurance that the quality of life after smoking cessation improves.

Follow-up care is important to assess the healing process, to evaluate coping mechanisms, and to examine the client for possible metastasis or new tumors. The client should be taught to report any of the following signs or symptoms to the physician:

- A lump anywhere in the neck or body
- Persistent cough, sore throat, or earache
- Hemoptysis
- Sores around the stoma or within the trachea that do not heal
- Difficulty swallowing or breathing

CLIENT EDUCATION GUIDE

Care of a Tracheoesophageal Puncture Wound

1. A 10 Fr., 12 Fr., or 14 Fr. red rubber catheter is inserted into the puncture site to maintain the opening until a tract has formed (Fig. A).
2. Tie a knot at the end of the catheter to prevent the back-flow of gastric secretions onto your chest.
3. Tape the catheter securely to your chest.
4. If the catheter comes out and cannot be reinserted, contact your physician or speech therapist immediately.
5. Once the voice prosthesis is able to be inserted, clean your neck and stoma. Using the inserter, place the prosthesis into the fistula.
6. Tape the prosthesis to the skin of your neck (Fig. B).
7. To use the prosthesis, take a breath, cover your stoma with your thumb, and speak. The air from your lungs will pass through the prosthesis and vibrate the walls of the throat. The mouth is used for producing the words.
8. If food or fluid leaks around the prosthesis, it may need to be replaced.

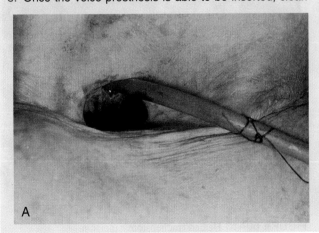

A

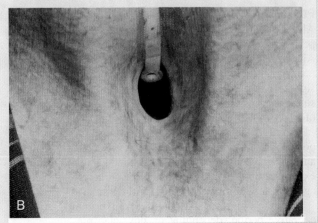

B

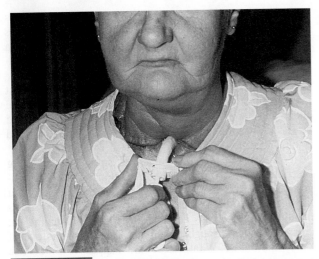

FIGURE 60–12 Insertion of a laryngectomy tube into a permanent tracheostoma. The obturator or guide is inserted into the outer cannula. After the tube is lubricated with water-soluble ointment, the client takes a deep breath and the lubricated tube is inserted. The obturator is removed, and the tube is tied in place.

NECK DISSECTION
PREOPERATIVE CARE

Before surgery, the client's understanding of the plans for surgery should be assessed. Determine what the surgeon has told the client and how much information has been retained or lost because of anxiety. In addition, address the fears the client has about the diagnosis of cancer and fears of deformity after surgery. Assist the client to understand the anatomic and physiologic alterations that will occur as a result of radical surgery. Explain to the client and family what to expect after surgery (e.g., placement in the intensive care unit, tracheostomy, drainage tubes) and review postoperative care (e.g., communication techniques to be used if a tracheostomy is to be placed).

The client's support systems and degree of coping should be assessed. If the client is an alcoholic, the use of alcohol may be the usual coping tool. Because alcohol will not be available, assess the other coping mechanisms available to the client, and encourage the client to use them. Sources may include friends and family. Identify new support systems, if needed, such as interaction with people who have had the same surgery or diagnosis.

POSTOPERATIVE CARE

After surgery, the usual postoperative assessments are performed, with special attention given to the airway. Airway patency can be lost as a result of edema of the neck or bleeding within the area. Assess the client for signs of airway edema or bleeding. Auscultate lung sounds every 2 hours for the first 24 hours. Report signs of airway obstruction immediately.

Place the client in a semi-Fowler position to minimize postoperative edema. Monitor neck drainage for volume and color. Sanguineous or serosanguineous drainage is expected for the first 72 hours after surgery. Once drainage has stopped, the wound drains are removed.

Pressure dressings may be used in the immediate postoperative period, depending on physician preference. If a dressing is used, it should be reinforced as needed and observed for any drainage. If musculocutaneous flaps were needed for coverage, pressure dressings are not used, and special flap care is required. (See Chapter 49 for specific care of flaps.)

If the surgical defect was repaired with musculocutaneous flaps, the flap should be assessed for arterial inflow and venous outflow. Flap temperature, color, and blanching should be noted every hour for the first 24 hours and every 4 hours after that time. Other means of monitoring flap perfusion (Doppler signals) may be used.

Because of the disruption of the sensory nerve fibers from the incisions used, most clients report only minimal pain at the surgical site. If an en bloc radical neck dissection has been performed, postoperative shoulder dysfunction is the rule, with forward rotation and dropping of the shoulder. Sectioning of the spinal accessory nerve during neck dissection also interrupts innervation to the upper trapezius muscle.

Exercises to increase range of motion and muscle strength, shown in the accompanying Client Education Guide, are encouraged to prevent a "frozen shoulder" and to restore full movement. If a selective or modified neck dissection has been performed, minimal alterations in range of motion and muscle strength are anticipated. Encourage use of exercise to prevent permanent disability.[3, 25]

■ Self-Care

After neck dissection, caution clients about the potential for injury to neck tissue due to lack of sensation. The use of a heating pad or exposure to temperature extremes may result in tissue injury (burns, frostbite) in a client who cannot feel these temperatures. Clients who have a tracheostomy need specific instructions for its management. Explain ongoing evaluations and follow-up.

HEMORRHAGIC, INFECTIOUS, AND INFLAMMATORY DISORDERS

EPISTAXIS

Epistaxis (nosebleed) may result from irritation, trauma, infection, foreign bodies, or tumors. In addition, epistaxis

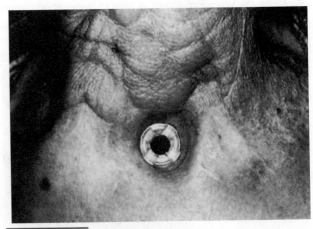

FIGURE 60–13 Healed tracheostomy incision.

CLIENT EDUCATION GUIDE

Exercises After Radical Neck Surgery

Step 1: Begin by gently moving your head from side to side, tipping your ear toward your shoulder on the same side, and moving your chin toward your chest.

Step 2: To exercise your shoulders using the hand on the nonaffected side, lean on or hold onto a low table or chair. Bend your body slightly at the waist and

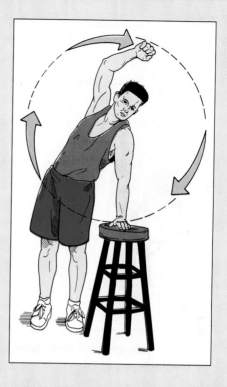

c. Swing your shoulder and arm in a wide circle, gradually bringing your arm all the way over your head.

Step 3: To strengthen your neck muscles, sit on a stool and

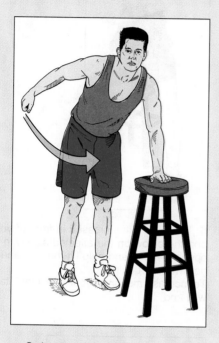

a. Swing your shoulder and arm from left to right

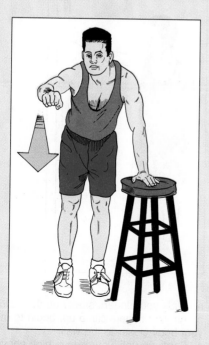

b. Swing your shoulder and arm from front to back.

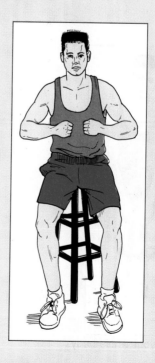

a. Place your hands in front of you with your elbows at right angles, sticking out from your body.

Guide continued on following page

CLIENT EDUCATION GUIDE *Continued*

Exercises After Radical Neck Surgery

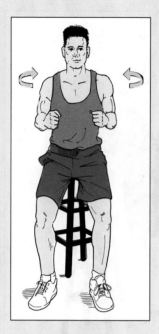

b. Rotate your shoulders back, bringing elbows to your side.

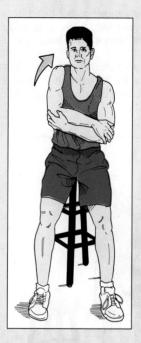

d. With your arms crossed in front of you, support the elbow on the affected side with your opposite hand, and help lift the arm and shoulder while shrugging.

Step 4: To increase motion in your shoulder, stand at a wall and

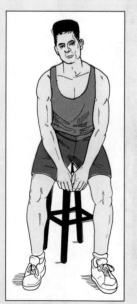

c. Relax your whole body.

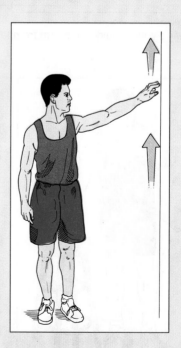

a. Walk your fingers slowly up the wall.
b. As your fingers climb up, begin to move your body closer to the wall.
c. Continue until your arm is high above your head and shoulder.

CLIENT EDUCATION GUIDE *Continued*

Exercises After Radical Neck Surgery

Step 5: To gain shoulder and upper arm strength, attach a hook to a wall or door. Hang a short rope knotted at each end over the hook. Under the hook, place a straight-backed chair or stool. It would be helpful to do this exercise before a mirror.

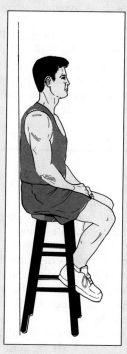

a. Sit straight, with your back against the wall.

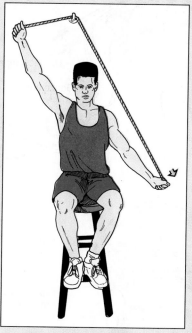

b. Pull one arm and shoulder up with the rope by bringing the other arm and shoulder down. Repeat with the other arm. It is important in this exercise not to bend your body. Keep the motion in the shoulder.

may also be the result of systemic disease (e.g., atherosclerosis, hypertension, blood dyscrasias) or systemic treatment (e.g., chemotherapy or anticoagulants).

Outcome Management

◼ Medical Management

Ninety per cent of nosebleeds are anterior, most occurring in children and young adults. Anterior epistaxis is initially treated by assisting the client to a sitting position. Apply pressure by pinching the anterior portion of the nose for a minimum of 5 to 10 minutes. This maneuver is often successful because the most common source of epistaxis is the anterior part of the septum in an area known as Kisselbach's plexus, a venous plexus vulnerable to trauma. In addition, the application of ice compresses to produce vasoconstriction may also reduce bleeding. If more definitive treatment is necessary, anterior epistaxis can usually be controlled by cauterization of the bleeding vessel with applications of silver nitrate. If these measures do not stop the bleeding, nasal packing may be inserted unilaterally or bilaterally. Antibacterial ointment such as bacitracin or polymyxin B–neomycin (Neosporin) is applied to half-inch gauze, which is then gently but firmly inserted into the anterior nasal cavities to apply

pressure to the bleeding vessels. The use of petrolatum gauze packing should be avoided, because it has no antimicrobial properties, and a malodorous discharge may develop within 1 to 2 days of insertion. Nasal packing should remain in place for a minimum of 48 to 72 hours.[9, 30]

Ten per cent of nosebleeds are posterior, usually occurring in older adults. For clients with posterior epistaxis, a *posterior plug* may be necessary in addition to the anterior nasal packing (Fig. 60–14). Insertion of a posterior plug is very uncomfortable, and a mild analgesic may be required to reduce anxiety and discomfort. A small, red rubber catheter is passed through the nose into the oropharynx and mouth. A gauze pack is tied to the catheter, and the catheter is withdrawn; this moves the pack into proper placement in the nasopharynx and posterior nose to apply pressure. The nasal cavity is packed with half-inch gauze, and the strings from the posterior pack are tied around a rolled gauze or bolus to maintain its position outside the nasal vestibule. The ties from the oral cavity are taped to the client's face to prevent loosening or dislodgment of the plug. A nasal balloon may be substituted for the traditional nasal pack. When the balloon is inflated with normal saline, pressure is applied to the lateral nasal wall.[26]

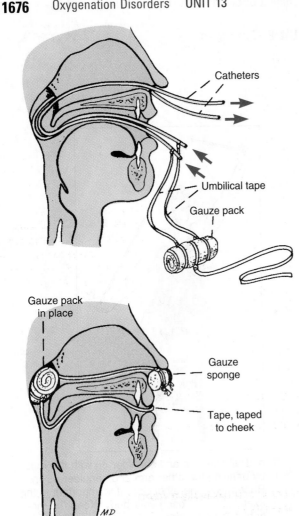

Catheters

Umbilical tape

Gauze pack

Gauze pack in place

Gauze sponge

Tape, taped to cheek

FIGURE 60–14 Instillation of a posterior nasal pack (plug), typically used in an emergency.

Nursing Management of the Medical Client

Clients with a posterior plug and anterior nasal packing are admitted to the hospital and monitored closely for hypoxia. General comfort measures, such as humidification, the use of a drip pad to collect bloody drainage and mucus, and application of water-soluble ointment around the nares to provide lubrication, help to alleviate the discomfort. Monitor the client closely for any signs of airway obstruction and bleeding from the anterior or posterior nares. Inspect the oral cavity for the presence of blood, soft palate necrosis, and proper placement of the posterior plug. If the posterior plug is visible, notify the physician for readjustment of the packing. Posterior nasal packs remain in place for 5 days.[9, 30] Prophylactic antibiotics are used to prevent toxic shock syndrome and sinusitis.

Surgical Management

If anterior and posterior packs fail to control epistaxis, internal maxillary or ethmoidal surgical *artery ligation* may be required. An incision is made in the gum line above the incisor on the affected side, and the maxillary sinus is entered. The artery that supplies the area of bleeding is identified, and a metal clip or suture is used to ligate the artery.

Nursing Management of the Surgical Client

The nasal packing inserted to control epistaxis remains in place for a minimum of 24 hours, during which time the client must be observed for additional bleeding, evidence of hypertension or hypotension, and infection. Upon discharge, the client is instructed to minimize activity for approximately 10 days, such as avoiding strenuous exercise; not blowing the nose; sneezing with the mouth open; and not lifting, stooping, or straining. The use of water-soluble ointment around the nares may provide comfort, and mouth rinses of half-strength hydrogen peroxide mixed with water or saline should be provided for oral hygiene. The use of a humidifier or vaporizer adds supplemental moisture to prevent dryness and crusting of secretions.

SINUSITIS

Sinusitis is a common infection that may occur in any of the paranasal sinuses. *Pansinusitis* is infection of more than one sinus. The term *rhinosinusitis* is thought to more accurately describe respiratory manifestations referable to an inflammatory disease of the nose or sinuses. However, the terms *rhinitis* and *sinusitis* may still be used.

Sinusitis is a common medical condition that affects an estimated 35 million people a year.[12] The sinuses are protected against infection by mucociliary action. The normal mucus produced by the sinuses is removed through small openings in the nose called ostia. When the ciliary action is impaired or the ostia are obstructed, mucus can accumulate in the sinus, which may then become infected. Blockage of the ostia may be due to a deviated nasal septum, bony abnormalities, congenital malformations, infections, or allergy.

A medical diagnosis of sinusitis is suggested by the client's clinical manifestations and confirmed by x-ray findings. Fever and chills along with headaches and facial pain exacerbated with bending, pain or numbness in the upper teeth, and a purulent or discolored nasal discharge may be present. Sinus radiographs or CT scans may show opacification of the sinus, thickened mucous membranes, and an air-fluid level (due to accumulation of secretions in the sinus), all indicative of sinusitis.

Outcome Management

Medical Management

Medical management of sinusitis includes (1) use of the appropriate antibiotic to manage the bacterial infection, (2) decongestants to reduce nasal edema, (3) corticosteroid nasal sprays to reduce mucosal inflammation, and (4) humidification by use of normal saline solution irrigations or a vaporizer or humidifier to prevent nasal crusting and to moisten secretions.

Antral irrigation or sinus lavage may be performed in clients who are not responding to treatment or who have increased purulent exudate in the maxillary sinus. Antral irrigation is performed with the use of a local anesthetic. A trocar (a sharp metal instrument) is inserted through the ostium in the lateral wall of the nose into the sinus. Prepare the client for the procedure with thorough explanations of the anesthetic procedure, the sensation of passage of the trocar through the ostium, and feelings of pressure. Normal saline solution is then injected through the cannula to rinse the sinus of purulent exudate. The client is placed in a sitting position, leaning slightly forward with the mouth open to allow drainage of the irrigating solution through the nose and mouth. A specimen of the exudate may be obtained for culture to determine the causative organism for prescription of an appropriate antibiotic.[30]

Surgical Management

FUNCTIONAL ENDOSCOPIC SINUS SURGERY

If nonoperative measures fail, functional endoscopic sinus surgery (FESS) may be necessary. The major objective of FESS is the reestablishment of sinus ventilation and mucociliary clearance.[13] FEES is usually performed as an outpatient surgical procedure using local anesthesia (with or without conscious sedation) or with the patient under general anesthesia. Small fiberoptic endoscopes are passed through the nasal cavity and into the sinuses to allow direct visualization of the sinuses in order to remove diseased tissue and to enlarge sinus ostia (Fig. 60–15). A more popular method of performing FESS is with the use of small, powered instruments offering precision and safety in the surgical approach.[13]

Possible complications of FESS include nasal bleeding, pain, scar formation, and rarely, cerebrospinal fluid leak and blindness resulting from intraorbital hematoma formation or direct injury to the optic nerve. After FESS, nasal packing may be inserted to minimize nasal bleeding. Packing is removed within a few hours of the surgical procedure.

CALDWELL-LUC PROCEDURE

The Caldwell-Luc procedure is another surgical procedure performed for the management of chronic maxillary sinusitis. An incision is made into the gingival buccal sulcus above the lateral incisor teeth with the patient under general anesthesia, or local anesthesia may be used. Through this opening, the diseased mucous membrane is removed. In addition, an opening between the maxillary sinus and lateral nasal wall (nasal antral window) may be created to increase aeration of the sinus and to permit drainage into the nasal cavity.

After the procedure, the maxillary sinus and anterior nasal cavity are packed with half-inch gauze. Because of the packing, nasal breathing is obstructed. The oral cavity must be frequently evaluated for the presence of blood or packing that may have become dislodged, obstructing the pharynx. If packing is present in the pharynx, the visible portion may be held with a hemostat and cut with scissors. Be certain that the hemostat is holding the trimmed gauze; otherwise, it may be aspirated.[9, 29]

EXTERNAL SPHENOETHMOIDECTOMY

External sphenoethmoidectomy is a surgical procedure performed to remove diseased mucosa from the sphenoidal or ethmoidal sinus. A small incision is made over the ethmoidal sinus on the lateral nasal bridge, and the diseased mucosa is removed. Nasal and ethmoidal packing is then inserted. An eye pressure patch is usually applied to decrease periorbital edema.[30]

Nursing Management of the Surgical Client

After sinus surgery, observe the client for profuse nasal bleeding, respiratory distress, ecchymosis, and orbital and facial edema for the first 24 hours postoperatively. Apply ice compresses to the nose and cheek to minimize edema and control bleeding. Place the client in a semi-Fowler to

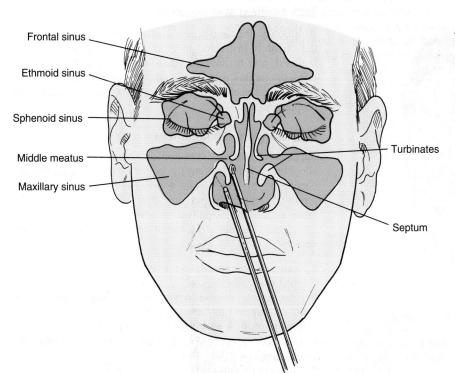

Frontal sinus

Ethmoid sinus

Sphenoid sinus

Middle meatus

Maxillary sinus

Turbinates

Septum

FIGURE 60–15 Functional endoscopic surgery. The middle meatus is the site to which most of the sinuses drain; if it is plugged, drainage is obstructed. With an endoscope, the sinuses can be seen and obstructions removed.

high Fowler position for 24 to 48 hours after surgery to minimize postoperative edema. The nasal packing is generally removed the morning after surgery; however, antral packing may remain in place for 36 to 72 hours. Give mild analgesics to the client to minimize discomfort postoperatively and before removal of the packing.

Instruct clients to increase fluid intake, which maximizes the water content of secretions. Although there may be some pain, a mild analgesic is usually all that is required. Minor nasal bleeding is expected for 24 to 48 hours after surgery. Use of a drip pad under the nose may eliminate the need for constant wiping (Fig. 60–16). Instruct clients to avoid blowing the nose for 7 to 10 days after surgery; tell them to sniff backward or spit, not blow. Teach the client to sneeze only with the mouth open. Nasal saline sprays may be started 3 to 5 days after surgery to moisten the nasal mucosa. Explain that the client is to engage in minimal physical exercise and to avoid strenuous activity, lifting, and straining for approximately 2 weeks. After FESS, the client needs to return to the physician's office for removal of crusts and debris and examination of the nose.

After a Caldwell-Luc procedure, the client may have temporary numbness of the upper teeth caused by interruption of sensory nerves from the mucosal incision. This abnormality may persist for several weeks.[9, 11, 30, 31]

PHARYNGITIS

Pharyngitis is inflammation of the pharynx and may be viral, bacterial, or fungal in origin. Beta-hemolytic streptococci are the most common infecting organisms. A culture of the pharyngeal mucosa is sometimes indicated before treatment is started. Clients may complain of a sore throat, difficulty in swallowing, fever, malaise, and

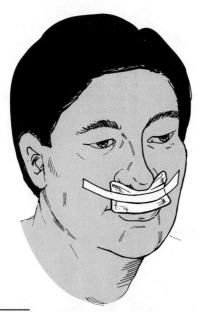

FIGURE 60–16 A nasal drip pad is taped beneath the nares to absorb drainage after nasal or sinus surgery. The usual technique consists of folding 4 × 4 dressings into thirds and taping them in place. These dressings can be changed at the nurse's discretion.

cough and have an elevated white blood cell count. Treatment of pharyngitis depends on the causative agent. Both viral pharyngitis and bacterial pharyngitis are contagious by droplet spread. Good hand-washing technique is essential, and the use of a mask may prevent spread. Antibiotics are used to treat the bacterial pharyngitis; antifungal agents are used to treat fungal infections; and use of comfort measures is required for viral types. Bed rest, fluids, warm saline irrigations or gargles, analgesics, and antipyretics are recommended until the clinical manifestations are alleviated.

Chronic pharyngitis (chronic pharyngeal inflammation) is most common in people who habitually use tobacco and alcohol, have a chronic cough, are employed or live in dusty environments, or use their voices excessively. Clinical manifestations vary according to the degree of irritation and inflammation.

ACUTE TONSILLITIS

Tonsillitis is an infection of the tonsils. *Streptococcus* is the most common infecting organism, although tonsillitis can be caused by *Haemophilus influenzae* and other organisms.

The client with tonsillitis reports throat pain, difficulty in swallowing, otalgia (referred pain to the ear), and generalized malaise. Examination discloses an acutely inflamed mucous membrane around the tonsillar area with or without the presence of purulent exudate. In some clients, lymphadenopathy of the cervical lymph nodes may also be present.

Complications from streptococcal tonsillitis include pneumonia, nephritis, osteomyelitis, and rheumatic fever. Acute tonsillitis may become chronic. Acute otitis media, acute rhinitis, acute sinusitis, and peritonsillar abscess or other deep neck abscesses may also develop.

■ Medical Management

Antibiotics are used to treat acute tonsillitis. In addition, the client is instructed to minimize activity, to maximize bed rest, and to increase fluid intake. Saline throat irrigations or gargles may relieve the discomfort. Mild analgesics such as acetaminophen, with or without codeine, may be prescribed.

■ Surgical Management

Surgical removal of the tonsils (tonsillectomy) and the adenoids (adenoidectomy) is collectively called tonsilloadenectomy, or T&A. The tonsils and adenoids may be removed separately but are most often removed in the same procedure. Removal of chronically diseased tonsil or adenoid tissue is indicated in the following circumstances:

- Recurrent, incapacitating episodes of acute or chronic tonsillitis
- Tonsillar or adenoid hypertrophy causing obstruction of the airway and impaired swallowing
- Resolution of a peritonsillar abscess
- Repeated ear problems related to eustachian tube obstruction
- Sinus complications

T&A is most often done in children. Tonsillectomy may also be indicated for a carrier of diphtheria, because tonsils may "seed" the body with infectious organisms. Adults with recurrent sore throat, ear pain, or hearing dysfunction, or who snore because of hypertrophied adenoid or tonsillar tissue, may also benefit from this procedure. Although T&A is not as routine as in the past, it is indicated in clients who have repeated episodes of infection. T&A is performed as an outpatient procedure or as a same-day surgery procedure. Tonsillectomy may be performed with the use of either general or local anesthesia, although general anesthesia is more commonly used. Surgical intervention is contraindicated during an acute infection, that is, upper respiratory infection. Other contraindications to T&A include hematologic disorders such as hemophilia, aplastic anemia, purpura, and leukemia.

■ Nursing Management of the Surgical Client

After tonsillectomy, place the client in a lateral decubitus position until awake and alert. This position provides for drainage of blood and other secretions through the nose and mouth. Gently inspect the oropharynx and mouth for fresh blood frequently during the first several hours postoperatively. Monitor vital signs closely. Hemorrhage is the most serious complication after tonsillectomy and is most often seen during the first 12 to 24 hours. If postoperative hemorrhage occurs, resuturing or cauterization of the bleeding vessel is mandatory.

The client should begin taking oral feedings once recovery from anesthesia is complete. Encourage cool fluids, and introduce appropriate foods to provide a soft, bland diet, as tolerated. Highly seasoned foods, as well as any food the client finds difficult to swallow, should be avoided.

Pain in the first 7 to 10 postoperative days is common after tonsillectomy. Most clients report generalized throat pain as well as otalgia. Mild analgesics such as acetaminophen with or without codeine may be required to alleviate pain. Increased swallowing of fluids also helps to minimize discomfort. Aspirin is contraindicated because of the risk of bleeding associated with its use.

Encourage clients to seek immediate medical attention if bleeding occurs after hospital discharge. Delayed bleeding may occur once the healing membrane separates from the underlying tissue (7 to 10 days postoperatively). The surgical site is usually well healed in 14 to 21 days, and the client should have little difficulty after this time.[30, 31]

CHRONIC TONSILLITIS

The most frequent manifestation of chronic tonsillitis is recurrent sore throat. Between episodes of acute tonsillitis, the throat remains uncomfortable. The tonsils are often enlarged, and if they are infected, a sharp line may be seen between the color of the buccal mucosa and that of the tonsillar pillar. The most reliable indication of chronic tonsillitis is the expression of purulent material from the tonsillar crypts with a wooden tongue blade. Once chronic tonsillitis is diagnosed, surgical removal is recommended. Surgery is contraindicated during acute tonsillar infection, although tonsillectomy may be performed in a client with acute peritonsillar abscess.

PERITONSILLAR ABSCESS (QUINSY)

Peritonsillar abscess (quinsy) may arise from acute streptococcal or staphylococcal tonsillitis. The tissue between the tonsils and the fascia covering the superior constrictor muscles becomes infected, causing extensive swelling of the soft palate and the pharyngeal wall. The uvula may be pushed to one side, and up to half of the pharyngeal opening may be occluded. Pus formation in the fascial space pushes the tonsil forward toward the midline of the throat.

Peritonsillar abscess is typically manifested several days after the onset of acute tonsillitis. As the tonsillitis-related problems begin to resolve, increasing pain develops on one side of the throat and ear. Inflammation and edema create a partial obstruction to swallowing. Often, the client keeps the mouth partially open to allow drooling, rather than attempting painful swallowing. The voice takes on a characteristic "hot potato" or muffled sound. Thick secretions are raised with difficulty.

A peritonsillar abscess may rupture spontaneously. If spontaneous rupture does not occur, surgical intervention may be necessary. With the client in a sitting position (to allow expectoration of pus and blood), an incision is made and the abscess drained.

Topical anesthetic throat sprays, analgesic agents, hot saline throat irrigations (at temperatures of 40.5° to 43.3° C [105° to 110° F]), saline or alkaline mouthwashes or gargles, and ice collars may be used to make the throat more comfortable. Cool and room-temperature fluids are tolerated best. Ingestion of cool to warm soft foods may also be possible. High-dose antibiotics are often prescribed early to avoid the need for incision and drainage. It takes at least 1 month for the infection of a peritonsillar abscess to subside. Usually, a tonsillectomy is performed following resolution of the abscess and infection, to prevent recurrence. However, a "quinsy tonsillectomy" may be performed during the acute infection.[19, 30, 31]

RHINITIS

Rhinitis, or rhinosinusitis, is inflammation of the nasal mucosa. The classic manifestations of rhinitis are increased nasal drainage, nasal congestion, and paroxysmal sneezing. Normally, nasal drainage is composed of clear mucus. If the infection spreads to the sinuses, however, drainage may become yellow or green. Rhinitis may be classified as acute, allergic, vasomotor, or drug-related (rhinitis medicamentosa).

Acute rhinitis is also known as the common cold, or coryza. Acute rhinitis may be bacterial or viral in origin; it is treated symptomatically. Acute rhinitis usually lasts 5 to 7 days, with or without treatment. Common interventions for acute rhinitis are symptomatic and include supplemental humidification, decongestants to reduce the edema of the nasal mucosa, increased fluids to prevent dehydration, and analgesics to relieve the generalized myalgia. Sometimes antibiotics are given to prevent a secondary infection by bacteria.

Allergic rhinitis occurs most often as a seasonal disorder. In addition to obstruction to nasal breathing, the client may also experience irritation of other mucous membranes (e.g., the conjunctiva, causing tearing and edema of the eyelids). Treatment is symptomatic. A complete allergy evaluation may be required to determine the offending allergen. Most clients are placed on a desensitization program and instructed to avoid the antigen (substance that causes the allergic reaction); treatment is with antihistamines, steroids, or mast cell–stabilizing sprays.[18]

Vasomotor rhinitis causes the same manifestations as those of acute and allergic rhinitis but has no known cause. Clients with vasomotor rhinitis in whom results of culture and allergy evaluation are negative are given symptomatic treatment. If medications have been prescribed for the treatment of rhinitis (especially nasal sprays), the client must be taught the use of medications, including side effects and possible interactions with other medications.

Rhinitis medicamentosa is caused by abuse or overuse of topical nasal decongestant sprays or intranasal cocaine. These substances initially cause vasoconstriction. When used frequently, however, the initial decongestion is followed by severe mucosal edema. The edema is self-treated with more medication, and the rhinitis becomes cyclic. Management of rhinitis medicamentosa consists of avoidance of the causative agent and evaluation and treatment of the original problem.[30, 31]

LARYNGITIS

Laryngitis may be caused by an inflammatory process or vocal abuse. The laryngeal membrane is continuous with the lining of the upper respiratory tract, and infections in other areas of the nose and throat may include the larynx. Edema of the vocal cords caused by the chronic irritation of an upper respiratory tract infection inhibits the normal mobility of the vocal cords, which causes an abnormal sound.

Laryngitis may also be the result of gastroesophageal reflux disorder (GERD). In this syndrome, the cardiac sphincter between the stomach and the esophagus relaxes, and gastric acid is allowed to enter the esophagus. Reflux of gastric secretions, especially during sleep, may result in the aspiration of gastric secretions into the larynx, causing a chemical irritation or burning of the mucous membrane lining the larynx.[18, 25, 30] Clients with gastroesophageal reflux may complain of hoarseness from the chemical irritation of the gastric acid on the vocal cords, increased mucus production from the body's natural tendency to protect the irritated membrane, foreign body sensation, or sore throat. Chronic cough and asthma may also be associated symptoms of GERD.

Hoarseness is a common manifestation of disorders of the larynx and may be caused by inflammation of the vocal cords, abnormal movements of the vocal cords, or a benign or malignant tumor of the vocal cords. All of these problems interfere with normal mobility of the vocal cords, which produces a change in sound. Abnormal voice may also be the result of vocal abuse. Screaming, shouting, and loud speaking over a period of time may produce edema of the vocal cords and the formation of nodules or polyps—outpouchings of inflamed mucous membranes.

The treatment of laryngitis is aimed at the causative factors. If inflammatory laryngitis is suspected, the in-

flammation should be treated. Antibiotics may be used if a bacterial infection is suspected. In severe cases, systemic steroids (e.g., methylprednisolone [Medrol]) may be prescribed to reduce inflammation and edema. Supplemental humidification may add increased moisture to liquify secretions, and mucolytic agents may be prescribed to thin and mobilize mucus. The client with laryngitis may also be placed on voice rest to allow the edema of the vocal cords to subside without added strain. Caution the client to avoid whispering, which also causes excessive vocal cord strain.

Gastroesophageal reflux is initially treated symptomatically. The client is instructed to elevate the head of the bed to minimize reflux; to avoid eating or drinking for 2 to 3 hours before going to sleep; to avoid caffeine, alcohol, and tobacco, which are known to increase gastric secretions; and to use antacids and hydrogen inhibitors (famotidine [Pepcid], ranitidine [Zantac], omeprazole [Prilosec]) to neutralize and decrease acid production.[7, 30, 31]

Chronic laryngitis may stem from repeated infections, allergy, chronic irritant exposure, long-term voice abuse, or reflux esophagitis of acidic gastric contents. Chronic laryngitis is manifested as a tickling sensation in the throat, voice huskiness, and painful or difficult phonation. Management involves correction or removal of the irritation, in addition to measures to increase comfort. Long-term voice retraining may be necessary if improper use or overuse of the voice is the main cause of chronic laryngitis. This retraining includes (1) learning to use the voice without straining and (2) forming and projecting words to use the diaphragm without shouting.[30, 31]

DIPHTHERIA

Diphtheria is an acute, communicable disease caused by *Corynebacterium diphtheriae*. The incidence of diphtheria has declined in the United States as a result of required vaccination. Diphtheria is a highly contagious disease that is spread easily in populations with poor hygiene, crowding, and limited access to medical care.

Humans are the only natural reservoir for *C. diphtheriae*. This organism colonizes the mucosal surface of the nasopharynx and multiplies. The bacteria release a toxin that causes the tissues to necrose, forming a tough pseudomembrane covering the tonsils and pharyngeal walls. This membrane is difficult to dislodge and causes bleeding if removed. Systemic toxins can damage distal sites such as the heart, nerves, and kidneys.

Diphtheria is spread by aerosolization of the pathogen (droplet infection), and when objects used by diphtheria-infected people, such as eating utensils, towels, or handkerchiefs, are used by others. Healthy people, as well as clients recovering from the disease, may harbor the organism in the throat for 2 to 4 weeks.

The clinical manifestations can range from a single, localized lesion without systemic manifestations to those of a rapidly progressive fatal illness.

The two types of diphtheria are tonsillar and pharyngeal. *Tonsillar* diphtheria is seldom life-threatening, although it can progress rapidly to more fatal forms. A low-grade fever, fatigue, headache, and sore throat are common manifestations.

Pharyngeal diphtheria is the more serious form of diphtheria, especially when a membrane covers the larynx or bronchus. The client is gravely ill, with a weak pulse, restlessness, and confusion. Fever may or may not be present. Because of the location of the membrane, the airway is often obstructed, and the client exhibits stridor and cyanosis. The neck may also be swollen and warm.

Diphtheria is diagnosed by culture of the material with the enzyme-linked immunosorbent assay (ELISA) or the Elek test (toxigenicity test). Gram staining or fluorescent antibody staining may also be performed; these tests yield results more quickly. Although cultures are used to identify the organism, treatment begins immediately, before definitive results have been obtained. Treatment consists of antitoxin administration.

To prevent transmission of the disease, the client is placed in strict isolation. Contacts need to be identified, screened, immunized, and treated. Specimens from all contacts should be obtained for culture. People vaccinated 5 or more years previously should receive a booster dose. People who were never immunized should be given vaccine and antibiotics. During antitoxin administration, observe the client for anaphylaxis; epinephrine is kept at the bedside.[23]

Nursing management focuses on management of the airway obstruction. Suction equipment and a tracheotomy tray should be kept at the bedside. Oxygen is administered. Clients experience pain, especially with swallowing. In addition to analgesia, pain can be reduced by limiting the diet to liquids and soft foods. Throat irrigation and fluids may also help control pain.

OBSTRUCTIONS OF THE UPPER AIRWAY

ACUTE LARYNGEAL EDEMA

Acute laryngeal edema may be associated with inflammation, injury, or anaphylaxis. This condition is manifested by hoarseness and dramatic shortness of breath of acute onset. Dyspnea progresses rapidly, and unless a patent airway is established, respiratory arrest occurs. Endotracheal intubation may be very difficult because the larynx is edematous and is likely to bleed. Emergency tracheostomy may be required. If anaphylaxis is the precipitating cause, subcutaneous epinephrine 1:1000 is given. Intravenous corticosteroids are also used.[5]

CHRONIC LARYNGEAL EDEMA

Chronic laryngeal edema may occur when lymph drainage is obstructed, as with infection or tumor or after radiation therapy. If the edema is significant, an artificial airway may be required (either a tracheostomy or an endotracheal tube). The choice of route depends on the severity of the edema.

LARYNGOSPASM

Laryngospasm (spasm of the laryngeal muscles) may occur (1) after administration of some general anesthetic agents, (2) after repeated and traumatic attempts at endotracheal intubation, (3) as a response to some inhaled agents and foreign material, such as industrial fumes, dusts, and chemicals, and (4) from hypocalcemia.

Management is directed at reestablishing the airway as quickly and efficiently as possible. Administer 100% oxygen until the airway is fully reestablished and the larynx relaxes and spasms stop. Titrate FiO$_2$ according to ABG or pulse oximetry values. If the laryngospasm persists, paralysis with neuromuscular blocking agents, such as succinylcholine, may be required to allow intubation until the spasm subsides. Manual or mechanical ventilation is then necessary until the effects of the paralyzing agent have worn off. Occasionally, emergency cricothyroidotomy or tracheotomy may be necessary and should not be delayed.

LARYNGEAL PARALYSIS

Laryngeal paralysis may be the result of neck surgery, peripheral disorders, central nervous system (CNS) disorders, tumor, or viral infections or may be of unknown cause. One of the most common causes of laryngeal paralysis is trauma to the recurrent laryngeal nerve during thyroidectomy. Other causes of laryngeal paralysis are aortic aneurysm; mitral stenosis; thoracic surgery; thyroid gland carcinoma; neck injuries; tuberculosis; tumors of the bronchi, lungs, and mediastinum; metallic poisons (e.g., lead); and infection (e.g., diphtheria). CNS disorders that may lead to laryngeal paralysis include cerebrovascular accident (stroke) and myasthenia gravis. Bilateral laryngeal paralysis is rare, and when it occurs, the client usually exhibits difficulty in breathing or stridor.

With unilateral vocal cord paralysis (in which only one vocal cord is affected), the airway is usually not impaired and the primary manifestation is hoarseness. The client may have a breathy quality of the voice. Aspiration of food or saliva may occur until the normal, moving cord compensates by approximating the paralyzed cord (bringing the cords together). The client must be observed for manifestations of aspiration such as coughing upon swallowing, ineffective cough, decreased breath sounds, and crackles, rhonchi, or wheezes. The client with bilateral vocal cord paralysis can have a near-normal voice if the vocal cords are paralyzed in the adducted position. However, the major concern is airway compromise, especially on exertion. Dyspnea, intercostal muscle retraction, and stridor may occur with activity or upper airway infections.[29, 30]

If the paralyzed cords are bilaterally adducted, an emergency tracheotomy may be required. Surgery, such as arytenoidectomy, in which one or both arytenoid cartilages are removed and the vocal cords are held in an open position, may be used to open the glottis.

Injection of absorbable sponge (Gelfoam), as a temporary measure, or of polytetrafluoroethylene (Teflon), for permanent correction, may be used if the client with unilateral vocal cord paralysis exhibits signs of aspiration or requires strength or projection of the voice. The injected material is placed into the paralyzed cord to add bulk, to allow better approximation with the functioning cord.

Type I thyroplasty is recommended for permanent unilateral vocal cord paralysis. For this procedure, a window is made in the thyroid cartilage through an external incision, and a stent is inserted to move the paralyzed vocal cord into a midline position. The client may show signs of airway edema from both the injection and the thyroplasty and should be observed for respiratory distress.

LARYNGEAL INJURY

Laryngeal injury most often results from trauma during a motor vehicle accident, when the driver's neck strikes the steering wheel. Other causes include inhalation of hot gases and aspiration of caustic liquids. If complete airway obstruction does not occur, carefully assess for post-traumatic edema, which may lead to complete obstruction. Few outward signs may be present. It is often easy to overlook potential problems in the neck structures while focusing on other, possibly more dramatic injuries. Observe for increased dyspnea, intercostal muscle retraction, neck swelling, laryngeal tenderness, dysphagia, stridor, inability to speak, and change in respiration patterns.

The thyroid cartilage may be fractured. This problem leads to soft tissue and laryngeal edema as well as hematoma formation. If airway obstruction occurs, tracheostomy may be necessary. Indications of a fractured thyroid cartilage include (1) a tender, swollen ecchymotic neck; (2) stridor; (3) cyanosis in some cases; and (4) subcutaneous emphysema in some cases.

Damage to the larynx above the cricoid cartilage may lead to tracheal stenosis. The cricoid cartilage forms the only complete circle of cartilage in the upper airway, and it maintains the open lumen of the upper end of the airway.

CHRONIC AIRWAY OBSTRUCTION

NASAL POLYPS

Nasal polyps are outpouchings of mucous membrane lining the nose or paranasal sinuses and may occur as solitary or multiple lesions. Polyps may be exacerbated by allergic symptoms, although they are not caused by allergies.[9] Most people who have symptomatic polyps seek medical attention for obstruction to nasal breathing.

The medical management of clients with nasal polyps is symptomatic. Attempts are made to reduce the size of the polyps by eliminating or treating the causative factor (i.e., allergy). In many clients, surgery is needed to remove nasal polyps in order to restore nasal breathing before allergy treatment. Nasal polypectomy (removal of nasal polyps) can be done in the physician's office or in the operating room. Nasal polypectomy is usually performed with use of a local anesthetic. The anesthetic (commonly lidocaine with epinephrine) eliminates discomfort while also producing vasoconstriction to minimize bleeding during the procedure. A snarelike instrument is used to remove the polyps. The bleeding sites are cauterized, and intranasal packing is inserted. Intranasal splints can be used to prevent formation of adhesions. The nasal packing is maintained for several hours to minimize the possibility of postoperative bleeding and is generally removed before discharge of the client from the health care facility.

Because of the presence of nasal packing and edema, clients need to breathe through the mouth for the first 24

to 48 hours. The use of humidification, frequent mouth care, and increasing oral fluids help to minimize the dryness and oropharyngeal discomfort. Inspect the oral cavity frequently to evaluate the effectiveness of these measures. Clients with polyps frequently also have asthma (when combined with aspirin allergy, this is called "triad disease"). Asthmatic symptoms may be exacerbated after surgery.[9]

The client is placed in a semi-Fowler to high Fowler position after surgery to minimize edema. In addition, continuous use of ice compresses is recommended for the first 48 hours to reduce edema and to control bleeding. With the proper application of nasal packing at the time of surgery and the use of ice compresses in the immediate postoperative period, nasal bleeding should be minimal. However, the client should be assessed for changes in vital signs and the oropharynx inspected for the presence of blood. Because the nasal packing absorbs anterior bleeding, it is essential to observe the client for posterior nasal bleeding. Manifestations of active posterior bleeding include frequent swallowing and the presence of blood in the throat.

Most clients experience only minimal discomfort after a nasal polypectomy. Mild analgesics may be given for any postoperative discomfort. The use of aspirin and aspirin-containing products should be avoided because of their anticoagulant effects. Instruct the client not to blow the nose and to refrain from sneezing if possible. When the stimulus to sneeze cannot be overcome, the client should sneeze through an open mouth.[30, 31]

DEVIATED NASAL SEPTUM AND NASAL FRACTURE

The nasal septum (the dividing structure of the nose) is usually straight and separates the nose into two equal chambers. After trauma, the septum may become deviated, creating asymmetrical breathing passages. For some clients, the deviation may cause an obstruction to nasal breathing, dryness of the nasal mucosa leading to bleeding, and occasionally a cosmetic deformity. A deviated nasal septum changes the velocity of air, altering normal nasal activity resulting in dryness, crusting, nasal bleeding, and changes in the membranes lining the nose.

If a nasal fracture occurs, immediate medical management is advised. Within several hours of nasal injury, severe edema may occur, which causes difficulty in reducing the fracture. Immediately after the injury, ice should be applied. A simple nasal fracture may be reduced in an emergency facility with use of local anesthesia. If immediate reduction of the nasal fracture is not possible, it is advisable to wait several days until edema subsides but before healing begins.

For correction of a deviated nasal septum, reconstruction of a cosmetic deformity of the nose, and reduction of a nasal fracture, the principles of surgical management are similar. All three procedures are usually performed with use of local anesthesia combined with mild sedation. Because of the vasoconstrictor properties of local anesthetics, these agents reduce bleeding during and immediately after surgery. Surgery to correct a deviated nasal septum is known as a nasal septoplasty and consists of making an incision on either side of the septum, elevating the mucous membrane, and straightening or removing the offending portion of the cartilage. If a cosmetic deformity is also of concern or if the deformity interferes with septal reconstruction, a rhinoplasty (reconstruction of the external nose) may be done in conjunction with the nasal septoplasty or as a separate procedure. (See also Chapter 49.)

After these three procedures, intranasal packing and internal splints may be used to maintain the position of the septum, to control bleeding, and to prevent hematoma formation. If the patient has undergone rhinoplasty or reduction of a nasal fracture, an external splint and a small dressing may also be applied. Postoperative care is directed at airway management, control of edema and hemorrhage, and pain relief. Because of the presence of bilateral nasal packing, clients require the same care as discussed for the client who has undergone nasal polypectomy.

CONCLUSIONS

Disorders of the upper airway range from a simple cold to cancer of the larynx. This chapter presents care of clients most commonly hospitalized with upper airway disorders. Nursing management ranges from assessment of life-threatening airway obstruction to teaching techniques that reduce the spread of infection.

THINKING CRITICALLY

1. **The client has a temporary tracheostomy after undergoing a supraglottic laryngectomy. On the second postoperative day, the client indicates to you that he is having trouble breathing. How should you evaluate the client and eliminate the problem?**

Factors to Consider. What principles are used as the basis of tracheostomy care? How does evaluation of pulse oximetry contribute to decision-making for care?

2. **You walk into the room of a client who underwent total laryngectomy 12 hours ago. The client is complaining of severe nausea but has not vomited. What are the client's risks following this type of surgery? How should you respond to the present problem?**

Factors to Consider. What risks are inherent in the occurrence of tracheal interruption? How well can the client communicate with you at this time?

3. **You enter the room of a client in whom a nosebleed has developed. Bright red blood is seeping continuously from the nares, and the client states that it feels like some blood is going down the back of his throat. What is the priority intervention? What are the implications if the bleeding continues?**

Factors to Consider. What are the causes of epistaxis? What are the psychological effects of a nosebleed?

BIBLIOGRAPHY

1. Brennan, J. A., et al. (1995). Association between cigarette smoking and mutation of the *p53* gene in squamous-cell carcinoma of the head and neck. *New England Journal of Medicine, 332,* 712–717.
2. Bryce, J. C. (1995). Aspiration: Causes, consequences and prevention. *ORL—Head and Neck Nursing, 13*(2), 14–20.
3. Byers, R. M., & Roberts, D. B. (1998). The selective neck dissection for upper aerodigestive tract carcinoma: Indications and results. In K. T. Robbins (Ed.), *Advances in head and neck oncology* (pp. 37–45). San Diego: Singular Publishing Group.
4. Clarke, L. C. (1998). Rehabilitation for the head and neck cancer patient. *Oncology, 12*(1), 81–94.
5. Cyr, M. H., Hickey, M. M., & Higgins, T. S. (1998). Tracheal, esophageal conditions and care. In L. L. Harris & M. B. Huntoon (Eds.), *Core curriculum for otorhinolaryngology and head-neck nursing* (pp. 246–271). New Smyrna Beach, FL: Society of Otorhinolaryngology and Head-Neck Nurses.
6. Dropkin, M. J. (1997). Coping with disfigurement/dysfunction and length of hospital stay after head and neck cancer surgery. *ORL—Head and Neck Nursing, 15*(1), 22–26.
7. Goldsmith, C. (1998). Gastroesophageal reflux disease. *American Journal of Nursing, 98*(9), 44–45.
8. Haynes, V. (1996). Caring for the laryngectomy patient. *American Journal of Nursing, 96*(5), 161–164.
9. Higgins, T. S., et al. (1998). Nasal cavity, paranasal sinuses, nasopharynx conditions and care. In L. L. Harris & M. B. Huntoon (Eds.), *Core curriculum for otorhinolaryngology and head-neck nursing* (pp. 169–206). New Smyrna Beach, FL: Society of Otorhinolaryngology and Head-Neck Nurses.
10. Kim, M. J., McFarland, G. K., & McLane, A. M. (1993). *Pocket guide to nursing diagnosis.* St. Louis: Mosby–Year Book.
11. Krouse, H. J., Krouse, J. H., & Christmas, D. A. (1997). Endoscopic sinus surgery in otorhinolaryngology nursing using powered instrumentation. *ORL—Head and Neck Nursing, 15*(2), 22–25.
12. Krouse, J. H. (1999). Introduction to sinus disease: I. Anatomy and physiology. *ORL—Head and Neck Nursing, 17*(2), 7–12.
13. Krouse, J. H., & Krouse, H. J. (1999). Introduction to sinus disease: II. Diagnosis and treatment. *ORL—Head and Neck Nursing, 17*(3), 6–16.
14. Landis, S. H., et al. (1999). Cancer statistics, 1999. *CA: A Cancer Journal for Clinicians, 49*(1), 8–31.
15. Leder, S. B., & Blom, E. D. (1998). Tracheoesophageal voice prosthesis fitting and training. In E. D. Blom, M. I. Singer, & R. C. Hamaker (Eds.), *Tracheoesophageal voice restoration following total laryngectomy* (pp. 57–65). San Diego: Singular Publishing Group.
16. Lockhart, J., & Bryce, J. (1993). Restoring speech with tracheoesophageal puncture. *Nursing 93, 23*(1), 10–13.
17. Lockhart, J., Troff, J., & Artim, L. (1992). Total laryngectomy and radical neck dissection. *AORN Journal, 55*(2), 458–479.
18. Mabry, C. S., & Mabry, R. L. (1996). Making the diagnosis of allergy. *ORL—Head and Neck Nursing, 14*(1), 13–14.
19. McCall, M. (1993). It killed George: Managing the peritonsillar abscess patient effectively. *ORL—Head and Neck Nursing, 11*(1), 10–13.
20. McKenna, M. (1999). Postoperative tonsillectomy/adenoidectomy hemorrhage: A retrospective chart review. *ORL—Head and Neck Nursing, 17*(3), 18–21.
21. Minasian, A., & Dwyer, J. T. (1998). Nutritional implications of dental and swallowing issues in head and neck cancer. *Oncology, 12*(8), 1155–1169.
22. Mood, D. W. (1997). Cancers of the head and neck. In C. Varricchio (Ed.), *A cancer source book for nurses* (7th ed., pp. 271–283). Atlanta: American Cancer Society.
23. Postma, G. N., & Koufman, J. A. (1998). Laryngitis. In B. J. Bailey & K. H. Calhoun (Eds.), *Head and neck surgery—otolaryngology* (2nd ed., Vol. 1, pp. 731–739). Philadelphia: Lippincott-Raven.
24. Repasky, T. M. (1995). Epiglottitis. *American Journal of Nursing, 95*(9), 52.
25. Robbins, K. T. (1998). Targeted cisplatin chemotherapy for advanced head and neck cancer. In K. T. Robbins (Ed.), *Advances in head and neck oncology* (pp. 59–71). San Diego: Singular Publishing Group.
26. Santos, P. M., & Lepore, M. L. (1998). Epistaxis. In B. J. Bailey & K. H. Calhoun (Eds.), *Head and neck surgery—otolaryngology* (2nd ed., Vol. 1, pp. 513–530). Philadelphia: Lippincott-Raven.

27. Seay, S. J., & Gay, S. L. (1997). Problem in tracheostomy patient care: Recognizing the patient with a displaced tracheostomy tube. *ORL—Head and Neck Nursing, 15*(2), 10–11.

28. Sigler, B. A. (1995). Nursing care for head and neck tumor patients. In S. E. Thawley & W. R. Panje (Eds.), *Comprehensive management of head and neck tumors* (pp. 79–100). Philadelphia: W. B. Saunders.

29. Sigler, B. A. (1998). Nursing management of the patient with a tracheostomy. In E. N. Myers, J. T. Johnson, & T. Murray (Eds.), *Tracheotomy—airway management, communication, and swallowing* (pp. 57–65). San Diego: Singular Publishing Group.

30. Sigler, B. A., & Schuring, L. T. (1993). *Ear, nose and throat disorders.* St. Louis: Mosby–Year Book.

31. Society of Otorhinolaryngology and Head and Neck Nurses. (1996). *Guidelines for otorhinolaryngology and head and neck nursing practice.* New Smyrna Beach, FL: Author.

32. Thibodeau, G. A., & Patton, K. T. (1993). *Anatomy and physiology* (2nd ed.). St. Louis: Mosby–Year Book.

33. Weilitz, P. B., & Dettenmeier, P. A. (1994). Back to basics: Testing your knowledge of tracheostomy tubes. *American Journal of Nursing, 94*(2), 46–50.

34. Weinstein, G. S., & Laccoureye, O. (1998). Supracricoid partial laryngectomy. In K. T. Robbins (Ed.), *Advances in head and neck oncology* (pp. 83–98). San Diego: Singular Publishing Group.

CHAPTER

61

Management of Clients with Lower Airway and Pulmonary Vessel Disorders

Sherill Nones Cronin
Kim Miracle

NURSING OUTCOMES CLASSIFICATION (NOC)
for Nursing Diagnoses—Clients with Lower Airway and Pulmonary Vessel Disorders

Activity Intolerance	Respiratory Status: Gas Exchange	**Ineffective Individual Coping**
Activity Tolerance	Respiratory Status: Ventilation	Coping
Altered Nutrition: Less Than Body	**Ineffective Airway Clearance**	Information Processing
Requirements	Respiratory Status: Airway Patency	Role Performance
Nutritional Status	Respiratory Status: Gas Exchange	Social Support
Nutritional Status: Food and Fluid Intake	Respiratory Status: Ventilation	**Knowledge Deficit**
Anxiety	**Ineffective Breathing Pattern**	Knowledge: Disease Process
Anxiety Control	Respiratory Status: Ventilation	Knowledge: Health Behaviors
Coping	Anxiety Control	Knowledge: Medication
Impaired Gas Exchange	Asthma Control	Knowledge: Treatment Regimen

A distinguishing feature of lower airway and pulmonary vessel disorders is the presence of dyspnea. *Dyspnea* (shortness of breath) is a subjective experience that results when air flow, oxygen exchange, or both are impaired. The sensation of uncomfortable breathing can be as distressing as pain and may lead to severe functional disability. The intensity and frequency of dyspnea as well as its association with specific activities must be assessed to develop realistic expectations of treatment outcomes. Because the experience of dyspnea is associated with much anxiety, nursing interventions to relieve this manifestation are essential to the care of clients with conditions of the lower airways and pulmonary vessels.

DISORDERS OF THE LOWER AIRWAYS

ASTHMA

Asthma is a disorder of the bronchial airways characterized by periods of reversible bronchospasm (spasms of prolonged contraction of the airway). Asthma is often called "reactive airway disease." This complex disorder involves biochemical, immunologic, endocrine, infectious, autonomic, and psychological factors. Asthma affects about 5% to 10% of the United States population, making it the most common chronic disease in children and adults. Mortality and morbidity rates from the disease have risen since the mid-1980s, despite a concomitant rise in general knowledge about the disease.[3]

Etiology and Risk Factors

Asthma occurs in families, which suggests that it is an inherited disorder. Apparently, environmental factors (e.g., viral infection, allergens, and pollutants) interact with inherited factors to produce disease. Other inciting factors can include excitatory states (stress, laughing, crying), exercise, changes in temperature, and strong odors. Asthma also is a component of *triad* disease: asthma, nasal polyps, and allergy to aspirin.

Pathophysiology

Asthma involves a chronic inflammatory process that produces mucosal edema, mucus secretion, and airway inflammation. When people with asthma are exposed to extrinsic allergens and irritants (e.g., dust, pollen, smoke, mold, medications, foods, respiratory infections), their airways become inflamed, producing shortness of breath, chest tightness, and wheezing. Initial clinical manifestations, termed *early-phase reaction,* develop immediately and last about an hour.

When a client comes in contact with an allergen, immunoglobulin E (IgE) is produced by B lymphocytes. IgE antibodies attach to mast cells and basophils in the bronchial walls. As shown in the Pathophysiology and Treatment algorithm, the mast cell empties, releasing chemical mediators of inflammation, such as histamine, bradykinin, prostaglandins, and slow-reacting substance of anaphylaxis (SRS-A). The substances induce capillary dilation, leading to edema of the airway in an attempt to dilute the allergen and wash it away. They also induce airway constriction in an attempt to close the airway to prevent inhalation of more allergen.

About half of all asthma clients also experience a *delayed (late-phase) reaction.* Although clinical manifestations are the same as in early phase, they do not begin until 4 to 8 hours after exposure and may last for hours or days.

In both phases, release of chemical mediators produces the airway response. In the late-phase response, however, the mediators attract other inflammatory cells and create a self-sustaining cycle of obstruction and inflammation. This chronic inflammation produces hyperresponsiveness of the airways. This hyperresponsiveness causes subsequent episodes in response not only to specific antigens but also to stimuli, such as physical exertion and breathing cold air. Clinical manifestations may occur with increasing frequency and severity.

Both alpha-adrenergic and beta-adrenergic receptors of the sympathetic nervous system are found in the bronchi. Stimulation of alpha-adrenergic receptors causes bronchoconstriction; conversely, stimulation of beta-adrenergic receptors causes bronchodilation. Cyclic adenosine monophosphate (cAMP) balances the two receptors. Some theories suggest that asthma may be a result of lack of beta-adrenergic stimulation.

Clinical Manifestations

During asthma attacks, clients are dyspneic and have marked respiratory effort. Manifestations of marked respiratory effort include nasal flaring, pursed-lip breathing,

CASE MANAGEMENT

Chronic Obstructive Pulmonary Disease

Chronic obstructive pulmonary disease (COPD) accounts for a high volume of inpatient admissions. Treatment of a COPD exacerbation may be attempted on an outpatient basis, with the administration of nebulized bronchodilators and intravenous steroids in an emergency department or observation unit. Clients who cannot be stabilized or who may have multiple problems are admitted for longer-duration therapy. Case management for these clients involves discovery of underlying risks, education, and health promotion to prevent constant readmission.

Assess

- What manifestations is this client experiencing on admission?
- Are there specific triggers or times when manifestations occur (e.g., stressful situations, environmental factors)?
- What medications does this client take?
- Is the client using the metered-dose inhaler correctly?
- What is the impact of this illness on activities of daily living, family roles, and ability to work or attend school?
- What other co-morbid conditions or practices might worsen this client's respiratory status (e.g., heart failure, cor pulmonale, pneumonia, smoking)?
- Has this client had recent or frequent hospital admissions?

Advocate

Give clients who experience difficulty breathing extra reassurance and attention.

Alleviate their fear and anxiety by anticipating needs and checking frequently to assure them that you are

monitoring their condition and are available to assist them.

Ensure that they understand correct sequencing of medications (e.g., bronchodilator before steroid use); also correct use of metered-dose inhalers, spacers, or other equipment as well as cleaning (to prevent oral thrush).

Discuss home oxygen safety, especially if the client is still smoking. Discourage continued tobacco use and offer resources to assist with smoking cessation.

Help to plan a schedule that includes rest periods and smaller, more frequent meals.

Prevent Readmission

Wean the client from oxygen, if possible, and test oxygen saturation levels during activity as well as at rest. If oxygen will be needed at home, make appropriate referrals. For some clients, especially those with asthma, monitoring peak flow levels is recommended, and a meter should be obtained. Ensure that the client is knowledgeable about medications and how to handle dyspneic episodes correctly.

Discuss prevention of infection, including appropriate flu and pneumonia immunization, disposal of secretions, hand-washing, and care of respiratory equipment. Stress the need for hydration and good nutrition.

Make referrals for nursing care, pulmonary rehabilitation, or smoking cessation programs. The client must also know about planned follow-up, when to call the physician, and how to get emergency assistance.

Encourage participation in community support groups and disease management programs through hospitals, insurer groups, and the American Lung Association.

Cheryl Noetscher, RN, MS, *Director of Case Management, Crouse Hospital and Community–General Hospital, Syracuse, New York*

Understanding Asthma and Its Treatment

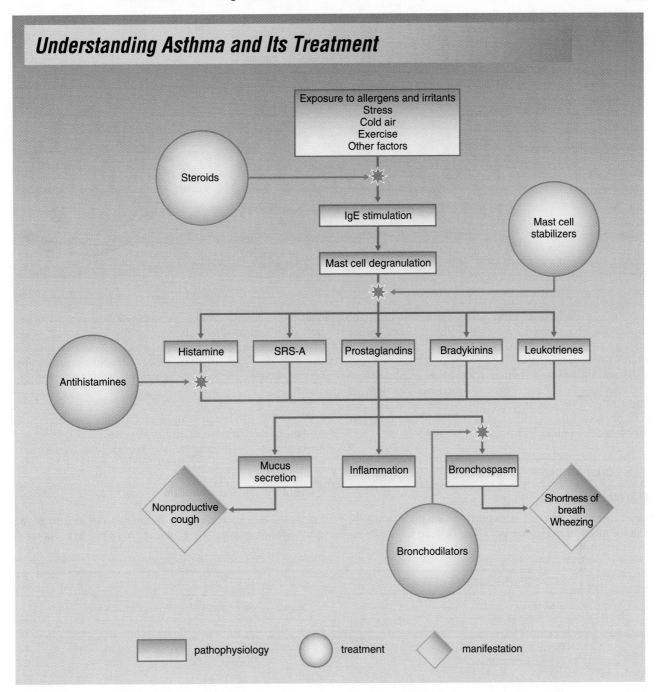

and use of accessory muscles. Cyanosis is a late development.

Auscultation of breath sounds usually reveals wheezing, especially during expiration. The inability to auscultate wheezing in an asthmatic client with acute respiratory distress may be an ominous sign. It may indicate that the small airways are too constricted to allow any air flow. The client may require immediate, aggressive medical intervention. In addition, bronchospasm may lead to almost continuous coughing in an attempt to clear the airway.

The diagnosis of asthma is based on clinical manifestations, spirometry results, and response to treatment. Spirometry reveals decreased peak expiratory flow rate (PEFR), forced expiratory volume timed (FEV_1), and forced vital capacity (FVC). Functional residual capacity

(FRC), total lung capacity (TLC), and residual volume (RV) are increased because air is trapped within the lungs. A 12% improvement in forced expiratory volume in 1 second (FEV_1) after inhaled administration of a beta-agonist bronchodilator implies a reversible air flow obstruction, that is, by definition, asthma. Figure 61–1 shows peak flowmeters for monitoring air flow.

Baseline assessment of pulmonary status also may include pulse oximetry and arterial blood gas (ABG) analysis. Pulse oximetry usually reveals low oxygen saturation. ABGs often show some degree of hypoxemia, with elevated partial pressures of arterial carbon dioxide ($PaCO_2$) in severe cases.

Status asthmaticus is a severe, life-threatening complication of asthma. It is an acute episode of bronchospasm

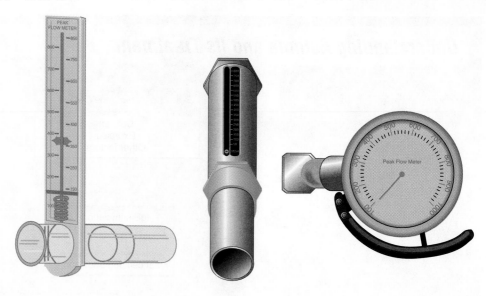

FIGURE 61–1 Peak flowmeters. Several types of portable meters are available for self-monitoring of air flow.

that tends to intensify. With severe bronchospasm, the workload of breathing increases five to 10 times, which can lead to acute cor pulmonale. When air is trapped, a severe paradoxical pulse (i.e., drop in blood pressure >10 mm Hg during inspiration) develops as venous return is obstructed. Pneumothorax commonly develops. If status asthmaticus continues, hypoxemia worsens and acidosis begins. If the condition is untreated or not reversed, respiratory or cardiac arrest ensues.

Outcome Management

Medical Management

Many disorders can cause wheezing, such as sinusitis, gastroesophageal reflux disease (GERD), heart failure, bron-

chitis, and lung tumors. These conditions are ruled out before an asthma diagnosis is given.

Management of asthma is based on the severity of the disease (Table 61–1) and is directed at reversing airway spasm. The general goals of asthma therapy include:

- Prevention of chronic asthma and asthma exacerbations
- Maintenance of normal activity levels
- Maintenance of normal or near-normal lung function
- Minimal or no side effects while receiving optimal medications
- Client satisfaction with asthma care[19]

Emphasis has moved away from episodic treatment of manifestations after they occur to long-term control

TABLE 61–1	CLASSIFYING ASTHMA SEVERITY		
	Symptoms	**Nighttime Symptoms**	**Lung Function**
STEP 4 Severe Persistent	Continual symptoms Limited physical activity Frequent exacerbations	Frequent	FEV_1 or PEF ≤ 60% predicted PEF variability >30%
STEP 3 Moderate Persistent	Daily symptoms Daily use of inhaled short-acting beta$_2$ agonist Exacerbations affect activity Exacerbations ≥2 times a week; may last days	>1 time a week	FEV_1 or PEF > 60% to <80% predicted PEF variability >30%
STEP 2 Mild Persistent	Symptoms >2 times a week but <1 time a day Exacerbations may affect activity	>2 times a month	FEV_1 or PEF ≥ 80% predicted PEF variability 20%–30%
STEP 1 Mild Intermittent	Symptoms ≤2 times a week Asymptomatic and normal PEF between exacerbations Exacerbations brief (from a few hours to a few days); intensity may vary	≤2 times a month	FEV_1 or PEF ≥ 80% predicted PEF variability <20%

FEV_1, forced expiratory volume in 1 second; PEF, peak expiratory flow.
From National Institutes of Health. (1997). *Guidelines for the diagnosis and management of asthma.* NIH Pub. No. 97-4051. Washington, DC: Author.

through inhaled corticosteroids to prevent asthma whenever possible.

Reverse Airway Spasm

A severe asthma episode may constitute a medical emergency. Medical intervention for such episodes is aimed primarily at:

- Maintaining a patent airway by relieving bronchospasm and clearing excess or retained secretions
- Maintaining effective gas exchange
- Preventing complications, such as acute respiratory failure and status asthmaticus

Emergency management of the client begins with inhaled beta$_2$ agonists. Beta$_2$ agonists stimulate the beta-adrenergic receptors and dilate the airways. If the spasm does not abate (i.e., if FEV$_1$ remains < 50% of predicted), nebulized atropine sulfate or intravenous (IV) steroids may be given. Atropine is an anticholinergic that blocks the effect of the parasympathetic system. When the vagus nerve is stimulated, bronchial smooth muscle tone increases. If these treatments do not reverse the clinical manifestations, the client usually is admitted to the hospital for further treatment. If the client has an acute asthma attack and no medications are nearby, the attack sometimes can be lessened by *pursed-lip breathing,* which increases pressure in the airways so that they remain open and so that trapped air can be exhaled more easily.

Supplemental oxygen is indicated if partial pressure of arterial oxygen (PaO$_2$) levels decrease to less than 60 mm Hg. Monitor the client closely for clinical manifestations of increasing anxiety, increased work of breathing, and indications of tiring. Endotracheal intubation and mechanical ventilation may be necessary. Sedation, and in rare cases administration of paralytic agents, may be necessary to blunt the client's respiratory effort and to prevent further air trapping and pressure increases. Status asthmaticus is treated with aggressive use of IV corticosteroids and frequent administration of inhaled beta-adrenergic medications to avoid intubation and mechanical ventilation.

Control Inflammation

Mucosal inflammation is controlled through the use of inhaled corticosteroids. Steroids prevent the mast cell from emptying, reducing the edema and spasm.

Leukotriene inhibitors and mast cell stabilizers are included in special circumstances. Leukotriene inhibitors are thought to be important mediators in the pathogenesis of asthma. Zafirlukast (Accolate) and zileuton (Zyflo) are two such drugs that have been approved for prophylaxis and treatment of mild to moderate asthma. Mast cell stabilizers, such as cromolyn (Nasalcrom, Intal) and nedocromil (Tilade), suppress the release of bronchoconstrictive substances during antigen-antibody reactions.

■ Nursing Management

Assessment

Initially, assess the client for clinical manifestations of airway distress. If present, they constitute an emergency that must be managed before a detailed history of the disease is obtained. The Critical Monitoring feature lists manifestations of acute airway distress.

Asking clients to rate dyspnea on a scale of 0 to 10 is an easy and effective measure of present dyspnea and may help you monitor and evaluate dyspnea in clinic and home care settings: "On a scale of 0 to 10, indicate how much shortness of breath you are having right now, with 0 meaning no shortness of breath and 10 meaning shortness of breath as bad as can be."

Determine known medication allergies so that allergenic medications can be avoided during treatment. Ascertain whether the client has a history of cardiac disease because beta$_2$ agonists can produce tachycardia and stress a diseased heart.

Once the acute episode is controlled, explore the history of the client's asthma. Assist the client to determine whether there is a pattern to the manifestations. These data may help identify a trigger that precipitates the asthmatic manifestations. If an extrinsic trigger can be identified, it may be possible to reduce or eliminate it. For example, if the client is allergic to mold, common sources of mold can be avoided. Ask about current medications. Some clients are inadvertently given medications that may induce bronchospasms. For example, a noncardioselective beta-blocker, such as propranolol (Inderal), prescribed for hypertension may cause bronchospasm.

Within the psychosocial domain, ask about the client's ability to manage the asthma and his or her general adaptation to the illness. Denial of the illness can interfere with early treatment. Determine whether the client feels control over the illness and feels capable of managing it. Clients who have this feeling of control show better compliance with treatments. Determine whether the client is experiencing an increased number of stressors. A stressful lifestyle may exacerbate asthma.

Assess the attitude of the family. The family can be a great source of support and can assist the client in recognizing early manifestations. In contrast, an unsupportive family may contribute to denial or may be an additional source of stress to the client. Involve the Case Manager (see the Case Management feature).

The client with a new diagnosis of asthma may be asked to assess the home and work environment for likely triggers of the clinical manifestations. In addition, skin testing for allergy may be performed. The presence of

---

CRITICAL MONITORING

Asthma

Notify the physician if the client still has the following manifestations after treatment for asthma:

- Increased anxiety
- Increased respiratory rate and effort
- Wheezing, both inspiratory and expiratory
- Almost continuous, nonproductive cough
- Nasal flaring as respiratory distress increases
- Lips pursed while exhaling
- Use of accessory muscles of breathing
- Increasing tachycardia (tachycardia is a normal response to beta-adrenergic drugs)
- Paradoxical pulse as bronchospasm worsens
- Cyanosis and central nervous system depression as late findings

pets that shed hair or dander, cigarette smoke, or occupational exposure to other allergens may require some lifestyle changes. In many cases, the pets can remain in the house but cannot sleep with the asthmatic client. Encourage clients to stop smoking, and teach clients and others about the dangers of second-hand smoke. Elimination of irritants is generally performed in a reasonable fashion, such as removing exposure to one allergen at a time. Potential improvements in a client's manifestations that might result from a major lifestyle change, such as job change or loss of a pet, may be quickly offset by the stress felt from such a change.

DIAGNOSIS, OUTCOMES, INTERVENTIONS

Ineffective Breathing Pattern. Because of airway spasm and edema, the client cannot move air in and out of the lungs as needed to maintain adequate tissue oxygenation. The correct nursing diagnosis would be *Ineffective Breathing Pattern related to impaired exhalation and anxiety.* Anxiety with dyspnea is another cause of breathing pattern problems.

Outcomes. The client will have improved breathing patterns, as evidenced by (1) a decreasing respiratory rate to within normal limits; (2) decreased dyspnea, less nasal flaring, and reduced use of accessory muscles; (3) decreased signs of anxiety; (4) a return of ABG levels to normal limits; (5) oxygen saturation greater than 95%; and (6) vital capacity measurements within normal limits or greater than 40% of those predicted.

Interventions. Assess the client frequently, observing respiratory rate and depth. Assess the breathing pattern for shortness of breath, pursed-lip breathing, nasal flaring, sternal and intercostal retractions, or a prolonged expiratory phase. During an acute asthma attack, these assessments may be conducted continuously.

Place the client in the Fowler position, and give oxygen as ordered. Monitor ABGs and oxygen saturation levels to determine the effectiveness of treatments. Compare pulmonary function test results with normal levels. The degree of dysfunction assists you in planning client activity.

Ineffective Airway Clearance. The excessive production of mucus and spasm in the airway makes it difficult to keep the airway patent. The nursing diagnosis *Ineffective Airway Clearance related to increased production of secretions and bronchospasm* is appropriate.

Outcomes. The client will have effective airway clearance, as evidenced by (1) decreased inspiratory and expiratory wheezing; (2) decreased rhonchi; and (3) decreasing dry, nonproductive cough.

Interventions. If the airway is compromised, the client may require suctioning. Some clients experience asthma episodes as a result of pulmonary infection. Monitor the color and consistency of the sputum, and assist the client to cough effectively. Encourage oral fluids to thin the secretions and to replace fluids lost through rapid respiration. The humidity in the room may be increased slightly. If chest secretions are thick and difficult to expectorate, the client may benefit from postural drainage, lung percussion and vibration, expectorants, and frequent position changes. Give frequent oral care, every 2 to 4 hours, to remove the taste of the secretions.

Impaired Gas Exchange. When air is trapped within alveoli, they are eventually drained of oxygen and the client can become hypoxic. The nursing diagnosis is *Impaired Gas Exchange related to air trapping.*

Outcomes. The client will have adequate gas exchange, as evidenced by (1) decreased inspiratory and expiratory wheezing; (2) decreased rhonchi; (3) PaO_2 greater than 60 mm Hg; (4) $PaCO_2$ equal to or less than 45 mm Hg; (5) pH of 7.35 to 7.45; (6) usual skin color (no cyanosis); and (7) decreasing dry, nonproductive cough.

Interventions. Assess lung sounds every hour during acute episodes to determine the adequacy of gas exchange. Assess skin and mucous membrane color for cyanosis. Cyanosis is a late manifestation of hypoxia and an indication of serious gas exchange problems. Monitor pulse oximetry for oxygen saturation levels. Administer oxygen as ordered.

Refer to the Care Plan for the client with chronic obstructive pulmonary disease (COPD) when working with clients with diagnoses of *Activity Intolerance, Anxiety, Altered Nutrition,* or *Sleep Pattern Disturbance.*

EVALUATION

Generally, asthma episodes can be reversed quickly if there is no underlying problem, such as infection. Expect the client to be hospitalized only briefly; plan a coordinated approach to assessment and follow-up.

■ Self-Care

The approach to pharmacologic therapy often is referred to as *step care,* meaning that the medications ordered and the frequency of administration are adjusted according to the severity of the client's asthma. Asthma medications are categorized into two major classes: (1) *long-term–control* medications, used to achieve and maintain control of persistent asthma, and (2) *quick-relief* medications, used to treat acute air flow obstruction and its accompanying manifestations. The most effective long-term–control medications are those that reduce inflammation, with inhaled steroids being the most potent. Quick-relief medications include short-acting inhaled beta$_2$ agonists and oral steroids (Table 61–2).

For clients who respond poorly to inhaled agents, theophylline and aminophylline are used sometimes. These medications are regarded as weak bronchodilators with wide variations in their rates of metabolism and a high potential for toxicity, however, and their use is declining. Theophylline levels must be monitored to evaluate effectiveness and possible toxicity.

Figure 61–2 depicts a stepwise approach for managing asthma in adults. All clients with asthma require a short-acting inhaled beta$_2$ agonist as needed for acute manifestations. Clients with mild, moderate, or severe persistent asthma require daily long-term–control medications. The preferred treatment strategy is to start with more intensive therapy to achieve rapid control, then "step down" to the minimum therapy needed for maintenance.

Changes in the treatment plan may be needed as asthma severity and control vary over time. Follow-up visits every 1 to 6 months are recommended to monitor the disease and to maintain control. The presence of one or more indicators of poor control (i.e., awakening at night with dyspnea or coughing, increased use of short-

TABLE 61–2	MEDICATIONS USED IN TREATMENT OF CHRONIC OBSTRUCTIVE PULMONARY DISEASE			
Drug Class/ Medication	**Action**	**Expected Outcomes**	**Adverse Effects**	**Dosing**

Steroids
  Beclomethasone (Vanceril) (inhaled)
  Methylprednisolone (Solu-Medrol) (injectable)
  Prednisone (Deltasone) (oral)
	Reduce inflammation and inflammatory response in bronchial walls by suppressing action of WBCs and immune system	Long-term prevention of manifestations; suppression, control, and reversal of inflammation; reduced dyspnea, improved FEV_1	Hypertension, heart failure, peptic ulcer, dysphoria, hyperglycemia, cough, oral thrush, fragile skin, adrenal suppression in high doses	Rinse mouth after inhalation
				Administer oral forms with food
				Taper dose to withdraw

Beta$_2$ agonists Albuterol sulfate (Proventil) (inhaled)	Relax smooth muscles in bronchial tree by acting on beta$_2$ receptors	Prevention of nighttime manifestations and episodes brought on by exercise; increased mucociliary clearance; improved FEV_1	Tachycardia, skeletal muscle tremors, hypokalemia; GI upset, nausea	Monitor blood pressure and pulse rate Monitor potassium levels Shake inhaler well before using; hold breath 10 seconds after inhalation
Leukotriene inhibitors Zafirlukast (Accolate) (oral)	Block leukotriene (a mediater of inflammation)	Long-term control and prevention of manifestations	Inhibits metabolism of warfarin (Coumadin), nausea	Monitor prothrombin times Small frequent meals and good mouth care may reduce any nausea

Methylxanthines
  Theophylline (Theo-Dur) (oral)
  Aminophylline (parenteral)
	Bronchodilator by increasing tissue concentrations of cyclic AMP	Long-term control of manifestations; increased myocardial contractility and mucociliary clearance; improved FEV_1	Gastric upset, tachycardia, nausea and vomiting (possible toxicity), nervousness, diuresis	Monitor blood levels
				Many drug interactions possible
				Charcoal-broiled foods reduce half-life by 50%

Anticholinergics Ipratropium (Atrovent) (inhaled)	Blocks action of acetylcholine at parasympathetic sites in bronchial smooth muscle	Relief of acute symptoms; bronchodilation; decreased mucus secretions; improved FEV_1	Dry mouth, nervousness, dizziness, fatigue, headache	Shake canister well Monitor liquid intake Provide thorough oral care Contraindicated in clients with BPH or glaucoma Assess appropriate use of inhaler or nebulizer Hold breath 10 seconds after inhalation

AMP, adenosine monophosphate; BPH, benign prostatic hypertrophy; FEV_1, forced expiratory volume in 1 second; GI, gastrointestinal.

acting inhaled beta$_2$ agonists, urgent care visits) may suggest a need to "step up" therapy. Before increasing medications, however, consider other possible reasons for poor control (Table 61–3).

Nebulized medications can be difficult to learn how to use. The client must coordinate inhalation with compression of the metered-dose inhaler canister (Fig. 61–3). The Client Education Guide provides directions for using an inhaler. Observe the client's use of the nebulizer to ascertain whether the medication is entering the airway.

Through appropriate use of the peak flowmeter and medications, clients with asthma should be able to anticipate most exacerbations and enhance their quality of life.

Many clients can manage their asthma effectively with a thorough action plan to guide their decisions. An action plan for asthma is presented in Figure 61–4.

CHRONIC OBSTRUCTIVE PULMONARY DISEASE

Also known as *chronic obstructive lung disease*, COPD refers to several disorders that affect the movement of air in and out of the lungs. Although the most important of these—obstructive bronchitis, emphysema, and asthma—may occur in a pure form, they most commonly coexist, with overlapping clinical manifestations. The term *COPD*

Stepwise Approach for Managing Asthma in Adults and Children Over 5 Years Old: Treatment

Long-Term Control

Preferred treatments are in bold print.

Step 4
Severe
Persistent

Daily medications:
- **Anti-inflammatory: inhaled steroid (high dose)** AND
- Long-acting bronchodilator: either **long-acting inhaled beta$_2$-agonist** (adult: 2 puffs q 12 hours; child: 1-2 puffs q 12 hours), sustained-release theophylline, or long-acting beta$_2$-agonist tablets AND
- Steroid tablets or syrup long term; make repeated attempts to reduce systemic steroid and maintain control with high-dose inhaled steroid.

Step 3
Moderate
Persistent

Daily medication:
- Either
  —**Anti-inflammatory: inhaled steroid (medium dose)**
  OR
  —**Inhaled steroid (low-to-medium dose)** and add a long-acting bronchodilator, especially for nighttime symptoms: either **long-acting inhaled beta$_2$-agonist** (adult: 2 puffs q 12 hours; child: 1-2 puffs q 12 hours), sustained-release theophylline, or long-acting beta$_2$-agonist tablets.
- If needed
  —**Anti-inflammatory: inhaled steroids (medium-to-high dose)**
  AND
  —Long-acting bronchodilator, especially for nighttime symptoms; either **long-acting inhaled beta$_2$-agonist**, sustained-release theophylline, or long-acting beta$_2$-agonist tablets.

Step 2
Mild
Persistent

Daily medication:
- **Anti-inflammatory:** either **inhaled steroid (low dose)** or **cromolyn** (adult: 2-4 puffs tid-qid; child: 1-2 puffs tid-qid) **or nedocromil** (adult: 2-4 puffs bid-qid; child: 1-2 puffs bid-qid) (children usually begin with a trial of cromolyn or nedocromil).
- Sustained-release theophylline to serum concentration of 5-15 mcg/mL is an alternative, but not preferred, therapy. Zafirlukast or zileuton may also be considered for those ≥12 years old, although their position in therapy is not fully established.

Step 1
Mild
Intermittent

- No daily medication needed.

Quick-Relief

All Patients

Short-acting bronchodilator: **inhaled beta$_2$-agonist** (2-4 puffs) as needed for symptoms. Intensity of treatment will depend on severity of exacerbation.

NOTES:
- *The stepwise approach presents general guidelines to assist clinical decision-making. Asthma is highly variable; clinicians should tailor medication plans to the needs of individual patients.*
- **Gain control** as quickly as possible. Either start with aggressive therapy (e.g., *add* a course of oral steroids or a higher dose of inhaled steroids to the therapy that corresponds to the patient's initial step of severity); or start at the step that corresponds to the patient's initial severity and step up treatment, if necessary.
- **Step down:** Review treatment every 1 to 6 months. Gradually decrease treatment to the least medication necessary to maintain control.
- **Step up:** If control is not maintained, consider step up. Inadequate control is indicated by increased use of short-acting beta$_2$-agonists and in: step 1 when patient uses a short-acting beta$_2$-agonist more than two times a week; steps 2 and 3 when patient uses short-acting beta$_2$-agonist on a daily basis or more than three to four times in 1 day. But before stepping up: Review patient inhaler technique, compliance, and environmental control (avoidance of allergens or other precipitant factors).
- A course of oral steroids may be needed at any time and at any step.
- Patients with exercise-induced bronchospasm should take two to four puffs of an inhaled beta$_2$-agonist 5 to 60 minutes before exercise.
- Referral to an asthma specialist for consultation or comanagement is *recommended* if there is difficulty maintaining control or if the patient requires step 4 care. Referral may be *considered* for step 3 care.

FIGURE 61–2 Stepwise approach for managing asthma in adults. (From National Institutes of Health. [1997]. *Practical guide for the diagnosis and management of asthma.* NIH Pub. No. 97-4053. Washington, DC: Author.)

commonly is used, but some pulmonologists think that it is not completely accurate and the term *chronic air flow limitation* may be used in its place.

COPD may occur as a result of increased airway resistance secondary to bronchial mucosal edema or smooth muscle contraction. It may also be a result of decreased elastic recoil, as seen in emphysema. Elastic recoil, similar to the recoil of a stretched rubber band, is the force used to passively deflate the lung. Decreased elastic recoil results in a decreased driving force to empty the lung.

COPD is a widespread disorder, affecting more than 14 million Americans. COPD now ranks as the fourth

TABLE 61–3	POSSIBLE REASONS FOR POOR ASTHMA CONTROL—"ICE"
*I*nhaler technique	Check client's technique
*C*ompliance	Ask when and how much medication the client is taking
*E*nvironment	Ask client whether something in the environment has changed
Also consider	
Alternative diagnosis	Assess client for presence of concomitant upper respiratory disease or alternative diagnosis

From National Institutes of Health. (1997). *Practical guide for the diagnosis and management of asthma*. NIH Pub. No. 97-4053. Washington, DC: Author.

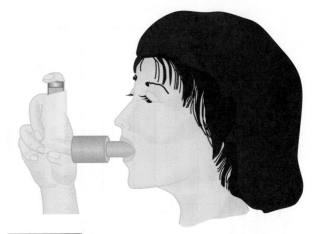

FIGURE 61–3 A client using a metered-dose inhaler with a spacer.

leading cause of death in the United States. The overall cost of caring for clients with COPD has been estimated at $40 billion annually, with $1.6 billion for long-term oxygen therapy alone.[27]

Etiology and Risk Factors

The specific causes of COPD are not clearly understood. The effects of numerous irritants found in cigarette smoke (i.e., stimulation of excess mucus production and coughing, destruction of ciliary function, and inflammation and damage of bronchiolar and alveolar walls), however, make smoking the leading risk factor for COPD development. Chronic respiratory infections, including sinusitis, contribute to development of COPD, as does the aging process. Heredity and genetic predisposition also appear to have a role.

Pathophysiology

COPD is a combination of chronic obstructive bronchitis, emphysema, and asthma. The pathophysiology of bron-

---

CLIENT EDUCATION GUIDE

Asthma

Client Instructions

Asthma may be triggered by pollen, dust, animal dander, molds, smoke, or other allergens. Learn what triggers your asthma and minimize your exposure to it.

Monitor the pollution index and pollen counts. Limit outdoor activities when these indicators are high.

Take all medications as prescribed by your physician. If you are taking both a bronchodilator and a steroid via inhaler, take the bronchodilator first to open the airways.

Use these directions for using an inhaler:

- Remove the cap and shake the inhaler well.
- Hold the canister upright with your index finger on the top and your thumb on the bottom.
- Breathe out through your mouth.
- Place the mouthpiece 1 to 2 inches away from your opened mouth (unless using a spacer).
- Begin with a slow, deep breath. As you breathe in, press the canister down with your finger to give yourself one puff of medication.
- Hold your breath in for at least 5 to 10 seconds.
- Slowly breathe out, holding your lips tight (pursed).
- If your physician has prescribed more than one puff, wait 1 minute between puffs to let the medication open up the upper airway. That way the next puff can reach lower into your lungs.

Pursed-lip breathing, progressive muscle relaxation, and tripod positioning (i.e., leaning on your arms positioned in front of you) may improve your breathing during asthma episodes.

Unless your physician has told you to limit fluids, drink 8 to 10 glasses of water every day. Water helps to thin your sputum so that you can cough it up more easily.

Some forms of asthma may be triggered by exercise. Discuss an exercise plan with your physician before starting.

Keep track of your peak flows. Often they fall about 1 day before an asthma attack.

Follow these directions on how to use a peak flowmeter:

- Attach the mouthpiece and set the pointer to zero (0).
- Stand up and take a deep breath.
- Put the mouthpiece in your mouth, and close your lips tightly around it.
- Blow into the mouthpiece as hard and as fast as you can.
- Record the value and reset the meter.
- Repeat the procedure for a total of three readings.
- Record the highest value on your record sheet.

Call your physician if you experience any of the following manifestations:

- Wheezing and shortness of breath, even though you are taking your medications as prescribed
- Fever, muscle aches, chest pain, or thickening of sputum
- Sputum color changes to yellow, green, gray, or red (bloody)
- Problems that may be related to your medications (e.g., rash, itching, swelling, or trouble breathing)

ASTHMA ACTION PLAN FOR _____

Doctor's Name _____ Date _____

Doctor's Phone Number _____ Hospital/Emergency Room Phone Number _____

GREEN ZONE: Doing Well

- No cough, wheeze, chest tightness, or shortness of breath during the day or night
- Can do usual activities

And, if a peak flow meter is used,
Peak flow: more than _____
(80% or more of my best peak flow)

My best peak flow is: _____

Take These Long-Term-Control Medicines Each Day (include an anti-inflammatory)

Medicine	How much to take	When to take it

Before exercise ☐ _____ ☐ 2 or ☐ 4 puffs 5 to 60 minutes before exercise

YELLOW ZONE: Asthma Is Getting Worse

- Cough, wheeze, chest tightness, or shortness of breath, or
- Waking at night due to asthma, or
- Can do some, but not all, usual activities

-Or-

Peak flow: _____ to _____
(50% - 80% of my best peak flow)

FIRST → **Add: Quick-Relief Medicine – and keep taking your GREEN ZONE medicine**

☐ _____ ☐ 2 or ☐ 4 puffs, every 20 minutes for up to 1 hour
(short-acting beta₂-agonist) ☐ Nebulizer, once

SECOND → **If your symptoms (and peak flow, if used) return to GREEN ZONE after 1 hour of above treatment:**
☐ Take the quick-relief medicine every 4 hours for 1 to 2 days.
☐ Double the dose of your inhaled steroid for _____ (7-10) days.

-Or-

If your symptoms (and peak flow, if used) do not return to GREEN ZONE after 1 hour of above treatment:
☐ Take: _____ ☐ 2 or ☐ 4 puffs or ☐ Nebulizer
(short-acting beta₂-agonist)

☐ Add: _____ _____ mg. per day For _____ (3-10) days
(oral steroid)

☐ Call the doctor ☐ before/ ☐ within _____ hours after taking the oral steroid.

RED ZONE: Medical Alert!

- Very short of breath, or
- Quick-relief medicines have not helped, or
- Cannot do usual activities, or
- Symptoms are same or get worse after 24 hours in Yellow Zone

-Or-

Peak flow: less than _____
(50% of my best peak flow)

Take this medicine:

☐ _____ ☐ 4 or ☐ 6 puffs or ☐ Nebulizer
(short-acting beta₂-agonist)

☐ _____ _____ mg.
(oral steroid)

Then call your doctor NOW. Go to the hospital or call for an ambulance if:
- You are still in the red zone after 15 minutes AND
- You have not reached your doctor.

DANGER SIGNS

- Trouble walking and talking due to shortness of breath
- Lips or fingernails are blue

→ ■ Take ☐ 4 or ☐ 6 puffs of your quick-relief medicine AND
■ Go to the hospital or call for an ambulance (_____) NOW!

FIGURE 61–4 Asthma action plan. (From National Institutes of Health. [1997]. *Practical guide for the diagnosis and management of asthma.* NIH Pub. No. 97-4053. Washington, DC: Author.)

chitis and emphysema is presented here (see pathophysiology of asthma earlier).

CHRONIC OBSTRUCTIVE BRONCHITIS

Inflammation of the bronchi (chronic obstructive bronchitis) causes increased mucus production and chronic cough. In contrast to those of acute bronchitis, the clinical manifestations of chronic bronchitis continue for at least 3 months of the year for 2 consecutive years. Additionally, if the client has a decreased FEV_1/FVC ratio of less than 75% and chronic bronchitis, the client is said to have chronic *obstructive* bronchitis, indicating that the client has obstructive lung disease combined with chronic cough. Chronic bronchitis is characterized by:

- An increase in the size and number of submucous glands in the large bronchi, which increases mucus production
- An increased number of goblet cells, which also secrete mucus
- Impaired ciliary function, which reduces mucus clearance

The lung's mucociliary defenses are impaired, and there is increased susceptibility to infection. When infection occurs, mucus production is greater and the bronchial walls become inflamed and thickened. Chronic bronchitis initially affects only the larger bronchi, but eventually all airways are involved. The thick mucus and inflamed bronchi obstruct airways, especially during expiration. The airways collapse, and air is trapped in the distal portion of the lung. This obstruction leads to reduced alveolar ventilation. An abnormal ventilation-perfusion ($\dot{V}/\dot{Q}$) ratio develops, with a corresponding fall in PaO_2. Impaired ventilation may also result in increased levels of $PaCO_2$. As compensation for the hypoxemia, polycythemia (overproduction of erythrocytes) occurs.

EMPHYSEMA

Emphysema is a disorder in which the alveolar walls are destroyed. This destruction leads to permanent overdistention of the air spaces. Air passages are obstructed as a result of these changes, rather than from mucus production, as in chronic bronchitis. Although the precise cause of emphysema is unknown, research has shown that the enzymes protease and elastase can attack and destroy the connective tissue of the lungs. Emphysema may result from a breakdown in the lung's normal defense mechanisms (alpha$_1$-antitrypsin [AAT]) against these enzymes. Difficult expiration in emphysema is the result of destruction of the walls (septa) between the alveoli, partial airway collapse, and loss of elastic recoil. As the alveoli and septa collapse, pockets of air form between the alveolar spaces (blebs) and within the lung parenchyma (bullae). This process leads to increased ventilatory dead space from areas that do not participate in gas or blood exchange. The work of breathing is increased because there is less functional lung tissue to exchange oxygen and carbon dioxide. Emphysema causes destruction of the pulmonary capillaries, decreasing oxygen perfusion and ventilation further.

There are three types of emphysema (Fig. 61–5): centrilobar, panlobar, and paraseptal.

Centrilobular (or *centriacinar*) *emphysema,* the most common type, produces destruction in the bronchioles, usually in the upper lung regions. Inflammation develops in the bronchioles, but usually the alveolar sac remains intact. *Panlobular emphysema* affects both the bronchioles and the alveoli and most commonly involves the

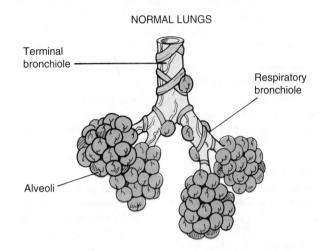

NORMAL LUNGS

Terminal bronchiole

Respiratory bronchiole

Alveoli

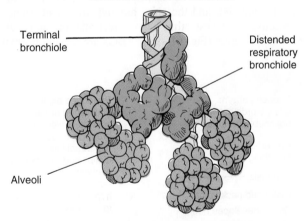

CENTRIACINAR EMPHYSEMA

Terminal bronchiole

Distended respiratory bronchiole

Alveoli

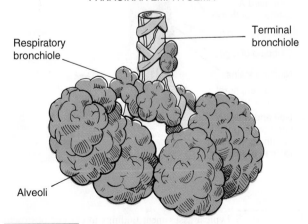

PANACINAR EMPHYSEMA

Respiratory bronchiole

Terminal bronchiole

Alveoli

FIGURE 61–5 Two types of emphysema.

lower lung. These forms of emphysema occur most often in smokers.

Paraseptal (or *panacinar*) *emphysema* destroys the alveoli in the lower lobes of the lungs, resulting in isolated blebs along the lung periphery. It is believed to be the likely cause of spontaneous pneumothorax. Paraseptal emphysema occurs in the elderly and in clients with an inherited deficiency of AAT. Normally, AAT inhibits the action of enzymes that break down proteins. Clients without AAT are at increased risk for COPD because the walls of the lung are at higher risk for destruction. Cigarette smoking is thought to alter the balance of these enzymes and thus to increase destruction of lung tissue.

Clinical Manifestations

All three disorders—asthma, chronic bronchitis, and emphysema—are present to some degree in clients with COPD. Figure 61–6 illustrates the common physical findings in these clients.

Clients with chronic obstructive bronchitis as the major disease have a productive cough, decreased exercise tolerance, wheezing, shortness of breath, and prolonged expiration. As the chronic bronchitis progresses, copious amounts of sputum are produced and pulmonary infection is common. The client suffers from chronic hypoxemia and hypercapnia (Fig. 61–7).

Clients who have primary emphysema have progressive dyspnea on exertion that eventually becomes dyspnea at rest (Fig. 61–8). The anteroposterior diameter of the chest is enlarged, and the chest has hyperresonant sounds to percussion. Chest films show overinflation and flattened diaphragms (Fig. 61–9A). ABGs are usually normal until later stages. Table 61–4 contrasts common findings in chronic bronchitis and emphysema.

Complications

Respiratory infections commonly develop in clients with COPD. This situation is a result of alterations in the normal respiratory defense mechanisms and decreased immune resistance. Because respiratory status already is compromised, infection frequently leads to acute respiratory failure and is a common reason for hospitalization (see Chapter 63).

Spontaneous pneumothorax may develop from rupture of an emphysematous bleb. This rupture results in a closed pneumothorax and requires insertion of a chest tube for reexpansion of the lung (see Chapter 62).

Similar to asthma, chronic obstructive bronchitis and emphysema may worsen at night. Clients often report sleep-onset dyspnea and frequent or early-morning awakenings. During sleep, there is a decrease in the muscle tone and activity of the respiratory muscles. This decreased tone leads to hypoventilation, an increase in resistance of the airways, and $\dot{V}/\dot{Q}$ mismatch. Eventually, the client becomes hypoxemic.

Outcome Management

■ Medical Management

The treatment goals for the client with COPD are to improve ventilation, to facilitate the removal of bronchial secretions, to prevent complications, to slow the progression of clinical manifestations, and to promote health

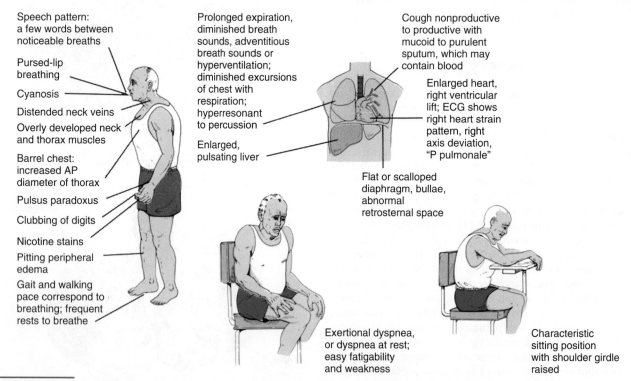

Speech pattern: a few words between noticeable breaths

Pursed-lip breathing

Cyanosis

Distended neck veins

Overly developed neck and thorax muscles

Barrel chest: increased AP diameter of thorax

Pulsus paradoxus

Clubbing of digits

Nicotine stains

Pitting peripheral edema

Gait and walking pace correspond to breathing; frequent rests to breathe

Prolonged expiration, diminished breath sounds, adventitious breath sounds or hyperventilation; diminished excursions of chest with respiration; hyperresonant to percussion

Enlarged, pulsating liver

Cough nonproductive to productive with mucoid to purulent sputum, which may contain blood

Enlarged heart, right ventricular lift; ECG shows right heart strain pattern, right axis deviation, "P pulmonale"

Flat or scalloped diaphragm, bullae, abnormal retrosternal space

Exertional dyspnea, or dyspnea at rest; easy fatigability and weakness

Characteristic sitting position with shoulder girdle raised

FIGURE 61–6 Typical assessment findings in chronic obstructive pulmonary disease (COPD). AP, anterior-posterior; ECG, electrocardiogram.

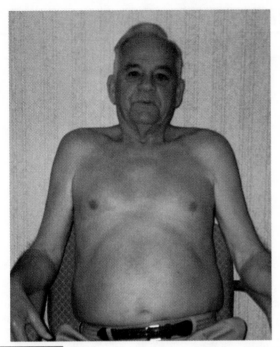

FIGURE 61–7 A client with chronic obstructive bronchitis. Note the stocky build and the presence of pursed-lip breathing and barrel chest. The slight gynecomastia is a side effect of corticosteroid therapy. The client's shoulders are raised because of shortness of breath and increased work of breathing.

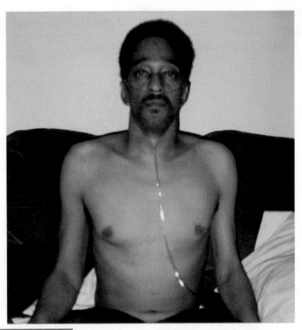

FIGURE 61–8 A client with emphysema. Note the thin appearance and the presence of continuous oxygen therapy. The use of accessory muscles of respiration (neck and shoulder muscles) reflects the client's shortness of breath and increased work of breathing necessary to increase minute ventilation and to maintain adequate arterial blood gas values.

maintenance and client management of the disease. At times, the client may receive continuous mechanical ventilation for adequate oxygenation. Ventilator-dependent clients with COPD may be managed in critical care, although some centers have non–critical care areas for clients on ventilators.

IMPROVE VENTILATION

Bronchodilators and steroids are also used in the treatment of COPD (see Table 61–2). As with asthma, they are used to stop the reversible portion of airway spasm. Narcotics, tranquilizers, and sedatives are used with caution because they depress the respiratory center. The fu-

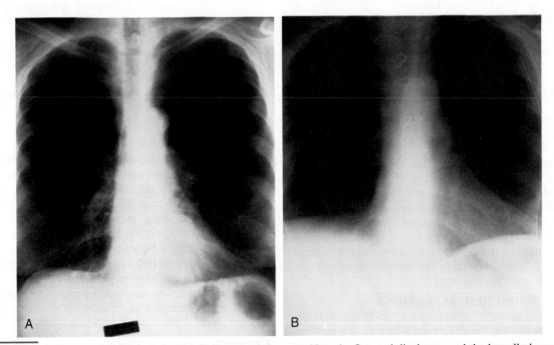

FIGURE 61–9 *A*, Preoperative chest x-ray of a client with emphysema. Note the flattened diaphragm and the laterally hyperexpanded chest walls. *B*, Postoperative chest x-ray after lung volume reduction surgery. The right side of the diaphragm is rounded and no longer flattened by emphysematous lung tissue. (From Allen, G. [1996]. Surgical treatment of emphysema using bovine pericardium strips. *AORN Journal, 63*(2), 373–388.)

TABLE 61-4	PRIMARY CLINICAL MANIFESTATIONS IN CHRONIC BRONCHITIS AND EMPHYSEMA	
Clinical Manifestations	**Chronic Bronchitis**	**Emphysema**
Onset of symptoms	Age 40–50 yr	Age 50–75 yr
Physical appearance	Stocky build with no history of weight loss; use of accessory muscles to breathe in late stages; cyanotic; barrel chest	Cachectic appearance with history of major weight loss; tachypnea and use of accessory muscles to breathe, even in early stages; pink skin color
Chief complaint	Persistent cough and copious sputum production	Persistent shortness of breath with progressive exertional dyspnea
Clinical course	Variable, with exacerbations usually related to respiratory infection	Progressive deterioration
ABGs	Decreased PaO_2, increased $PaCO_2$	PaO_2 normal or slightly decreased; $PaCO_2$ low or normal until end stage
Pulmonary function	Small airways affected early (reduced $FEF_{25\%-75\%}$); FEV_1 reduced later as airway damage progresses; normal to variable diffusion capacity	Reduced $FEF_{25\%-75\%}$ and FEV_1; reduced diffusion capacity because of destruction of alveoli
Associated findings	Frequent episodes of cor pulmonale with dependent edema (especially in late stage); elevated hematocrit	No history of cor pulmonale until very late stage; no edema; on auscultation, diminished breath sounds even with deep breathing

ABGs, arterial blood gases; $FEF_{25\%-75\%}$, forced expiratory flow, midexpiratory phase; FEV_1, forced expiratory volume in 1 second; $PaCO_2$, partial pressure of arterial carbon dioxide; PaO_2, partial pressure of arterial oxygen.

ture looks promising for the treatment of early emphysema with AAT replacement therapy.

Oxygen is used when the client has severe exertional or resting hypoxemia ($PaO_2 < 40$ mm Hg). Oxygen (1 to 3 L) by nasal cannula may be required to raise the PaO_2 to no less than 60 mm Hg. Oxygen is used cautiously in clients with emphysema, however. Because of long-standing hypercapnia, the respiratory drive in emphysematous clients is triggered by low oxygen levels rather than increased carbon dioxide levels. The drive to breathe is the opposite of normal in clients with emphysema. If high levels of oxygen are administered to these clients, their respiratory drive can be obliterated and carbon dioxide retention can occur.

REMOVE BRONCHIAL SECRETIONS

Pulmonary hygiene is needed to rid the lungs of secretions and to reduce the risk of infection. In the hospital, the client may be treated with nebulized bronchodilators and positive-pressure air flow or positive end-expiratory pressure devices to increase the caliber of the airways.

Postural drainage and chest physiotherapy may be prescribed to move the secretions from the small to the large airways, from which they can be expelled.

PROMOTE EXERCISE

Aerobic exercise is used to enhance cardiovascular fitness and to train respiratory muscles to function more effectively. Exercise does not improve lung function. Respiratory muscles can be strengthened even when the lungs are diseased. Progressively increased walking is the most common form of exercise. Before a walking program is begun, ABGs should be assessed and compared with resting levels. Supplemental oxygen should be used during exercise if the client becomes severely hypoxemic.

Breathing exercises may also be prescribed. Encourage diaphragmatic breathing and pursed-lip breathing, and discourage rapid, shallow *panic* breathing.

CONTROL COMPLICATIONS

Edema and cor pulmonale are treated with diuretics and digitalis. Phlebotomy may be used to reduce blood volume in clients with marked elevations in hematocrit (>60%). Phlebotomy also reduces cardiac workload.

IMPROVE GENERAL HEALTH

The most effective way to slow disease progression is for the client to stop smoking. Exposure to known allergens should be minimized. All clients with COPD should avoid high altitudes, and supplemental oxygen may be required for air travel. No specific climate has been shown to alter the course of the disorder.

Adequate nutrition is essential to maintain respiratory muscle strength. Malnutrition is common and contributes to decreased respiratory muscle strength and reduced diaphragmatic mass. Consult a clinical dietitian to assist clients in modifying their diet to meet their caloric needs. Clients with COPD often have difficulty eating because of dyspnea. Offer the client frequent small meals, rather than large meals. When the client must be tube-fed, understand that substrate metabolism also may affect lung function. Macronutrients are metabolized to produce carbon dioxide and water. The ratio of carbon dioxide produced to oxygen consumed is the respiratory quotient (RQ). The RQ of carbohydrate oxidation is 1.0, and the RQ of fat oxidation is 0.7. Excess carbohydrate leads to increased production of carbon dioxide and can lead to respiratory distress. Enteral formulas are designed for pulmonary disease and provide more calories from fat. It is equally important not to overfeed the client with carbohydrates.

Adjust oxygen delivery devices so that the mouth is not obstructed but oxygen is delivered through the nose during eating. Calculate the liter flow of the nasal cannula when converting from a mask style (see formulas in Table 61-5). For example, if a client is using a Venturi oxygen mask at 28%, he or she would receive the same amount of oxygen on 2 L by nasal cannula.

■ Nursing Management of the Medical Client

ASSESSMENT

The nursing history can ascertain whether the client's clinical manifestations are primarily those of chronic bronchitis, emphysema, or asthma. Determine the client's ability to recognize manifestations that require further care. For example, if a client says, "I knew I was developing an infection and went to the doctor," the statement indicates an understanding of the disorder. In contrast, if a client does not fully understand the reasons for hospitalization, educate the client about COPD. A review of past medical history helps determine whether the client has other disorders, such as heart disease, that may affect treatment.

Complete a physical examination with an emphasis on the respiratory and cardiac system. Note the degree of dyspnea, decreased breath sounds, and clinical manifestations of heart failure. Evaluate mental status because confusion and restlessness may be early indicators of increasing hypoxia and hypercapnia.

Consider the impact of stressors that may have led to exacerbations of COPD. Possible factors include the progressive illness itself, marital or other family problems, and financial concerns. Review the client's usual coping strategies. Determine whether these strategies are working

now; if not, why not? Support systems, such as friends and family, also are important components of psychosocial stability. Determine the reliability of the client's support system.

The psychosocial impact of COPD is significant. Clients commonly have feelings of loss of control over their bodies and their social environment. These responses leave the client socially isolated and depressed. A Canadian study found that clients with poor adjustment to COPD used more health care dollars for disease management.[16] Psychosocial intervention is important.

A thorough history may need to be delayed until the client is able to breathe comfortably, or it may be taken over short periods of time or obtained through the family. Likewise, the physical examination should not tire the client.

DIAGNOSIS, OUTCOMES, INTERVENTION

Common nursing diagnoses and interventions for the client with COPD are listed in the Care Plan for the client with COPD. Because COPD is very common, many institutions use care maps to guide care. (See the feature on care maps.)

Evaluation

Dyspnea will be slow to improve. Expect several days for the client to return to baseline levels.

Clients with COPD often continue to deteriorate despite medical care. It is difficult to cope with failing health that limits activity and employment. As much as possible, encourage the client to live an active life with

TABLE 61-5	CONVERTING LOW-FLOW TO HIGH-FLOW OXYGEN SYSTEMS*	
100% Oxygen Flow Rate (L)		**FiO$_2$ (%)**
NASAL CANNULA OR CATHETER		
1		24
2		28
3		32
4		36
5		40
6		44
OXYGEN MASK		
5-6		40
6-7		50
7-8		60
MASK WITH A RESERVOIR BAG		
6		60
7		70
8		80
9		90
10		100

* A normal ventilatory pattern is assumed.
FiO$_2$, fraction of inspired oxygen.

GUIDE TO CLINICAL PATHWAY

Chronic Obstructive Pulmonary Disease

The client hospitalized with acute exacerbation of chronic obstructive pulmonary disease may have increasing dyspnea because of a chest cold or pneumonia. This care map shows a 5-day length of stay with the major focus on the interventions directed at restoring a balance between energy demands for oxygen (activity) and ability to maintain oxygenation (dyspnea).

By day 2 of the care map, the client's underlying problem (such as pneumonia) has been diagnosed and is being treated. It is expected that once the problem is treated, the client can be weaned from the oxygen levels needed while the presenting problem was acute. Carefully assess the degree of dyspnea, pulse oximetry levels, and amount of oxygen needed. Level of activity progresses while you closely monitor the client's ability to tolerate it. If the client is too dyspneic to eat, ask a dietitian to see the client. Foods that are calorie-dense and do not create carbon dioxide are important changes that can be made in the diet.

By day 3, nebulized bronchodilators are changed to metered-dose inhalers. Validate that the client understands and uses these devices correctly. Intravenous corticosteroids (used to decrease the inflammation) are changed to an oral route. Oral steroids are ulcerogenic and given with meals. Shortness of breath is not expected on day 3. Assessment changes to watch for include bronchospasm, which might occur while activity increases.

On day 4, the client's understanding of self-care is validated. Many of these treatments may have been used previously by the client. Record the client's ability to use equipment safely.

The CareMap is reprinted with permission from Baptist Health System. The CareMap shown is an excerpt of one that covers emergency department admission through day of discharge.

Helen Andrews, BSN, RN, *Care Manager, Alegent Health Bergan Mercy Medical Center, Omaha, Nebraska,* and **Linda R. Haddick, MSN, RN,** *Clinical Nurse Specialist, Alegent Health Home Care & Hospice, Omaha, Nebraska*

---

daily exercise. The support of significant others is essential.

■ Surgical Management

Surgery is relatively uncommon in the treatment of COPD. At times, bullectomy (removal of large bullae, which compress the lung and add to dead space) may benefit clients with recurrent spontaneous pneumothorax.

LUNG VOLUME REDUCTION SURGERY

Advances have been made with lung volume reduction surgery (LVRS). Portions of diffusely emphysematous lungs are removed to help restore more normal chest wall configuration and to improve respiratory mechanics and functional capacity (see Fig. 61–9). LVRS also improves quality of life in selected patients. More data are needed regarding the procedure and its long-term effects, however, and multicenter studies are under way.[7]

Candidates for LVRS include people with severely limited pulmonary function (FEV < 30% of normal), maximally flattened diaphragm on radiograph with maximal overdistention of lung volume and evidence of bullae, significant impairment in activities of daily living, and for whom medical management is no longer effective. Before surgery, clients should have stopped smoking for at least 6 months and must complete a 6- to 12-week pulmonary rehabilitation program.[23]

LVRS may be performed via a median sternotomy or thoracotomy. Bovine pericardium strips can be used to reinforce staple lines of resected lung tissue. This technique reduces the problem of air leaks, common in earlier LVRS procedures. Another approach to this intervention is video-assisted thoracoscopy, which avoids a large thoracic incision and may reduce postoperative respiratory complications.[20]

■ Nursing Care of the Surgical Client

After surgery, monitor closely the client's ABG values. Chest assessment and radiograph help determine whether the lungs are expanding. Assess the chest tubes for air leaks and drainage. Intensive pulmonary toilet is essential. Repeated coughing and deep breathing help prevent pulmonary complications. Many clients have chest physiotherapy every 4 hours and nebulized aerosol treatments. Clients usually ambulate soon after surgery, sometimes the same day as the operation. Manage pain aggressively to promote activity and pulmonary hygiene.

After discharge, the client is assessed for adequate ventilation and tissue oxygenation (with pulse oximetry) and progressive wound healing. Pulmonary treatments may continue until lung sounds are clear. The client is weaned from oxygen and placed into a formal pulmonary rehabilitation program.

■ Modifications for Elderly Clients

COPD is the second most significant disorder of people in the middle to late adult years. The elderly client frequently has other problems that influence the treatment of COPD. For example, the client may have decreased exercise tolerance, impaired nutrition, or a long-standing habit of smoking that retards rehabilitation. Also consider the possibility of drug-drug interactions in elderly clients.

The older adult has special requirements when chronic conditions are exacerbated (see the Case Management feature in Chapter 72).

■ Self-Care

Pulmonary rehabilitation is designed to reduce the toll of pulmonary disease for the client and the health care system. The goals of pulmonary rehabilitation are to relieve clinical manifestations, to maximize functional level, and to educate patients to manage their disease process successfully and to maintain an active and independent lifestyle.[27] Clients are taught how to administer medications, what side effects to look for and how to manage them, and the safe and correct use of oxygen. Lower body exercise (walking, cycling) is commonly prescribed. Upper body exercise is also used in some cases.

To facilitate self-care and adherence, the client and significant others need thorough information about the

✝ BAPTIST
HEALTH SYSTEM

COPD CAREMAP

(Addressograph)

	Day 2 Date: _____	INITIAL Met	INITIAL Not Met	Day 3 Date: _____	INITIAL Met	INITIAL Not Met
General Safety:	Bed rails up x 2 Call light within reach Seizure Precautions Fall precautions Bleeding Precautions			Bed rails up x 2 Call light within reach Seizure Precautions Fall precautions Bleeding Precautions		
Activity	Ambulation as tolerated Chair BID			Ambulation as tolerated		
	Goal: Tolerates activity progression without SOB			**Goal:** Tolerates activity progression without bronchospasm		
Dietary: Consult Date/Time Completed _____	Diet type _____			Diet type _____		
	Goal: Tolerates > 50% of diet			**Goal:** Tolerates > 50% of diet		
Respiratory: Consult Date/Time Completed _____	O2 sat per weaning protocol Bronchodilators Virbropercussion/Postural drainage			O2 per protocol Evaluate for home O2 Bronchodilators Switch to MDI if initially on Nebulizer		
	Goal: Respiratory distress improved			**Goal:** SaO2 ≥ 92%		
Rehab: Consult Date/Time Completed _____	Physical Therapy for strengthening and mobilization					
	Goal:			**Goal:**		
Discharge Planning: Consult Date/Time Completed _____	Continue to assess discharge needs Discharge needs identified			TCF unit evaluation for IV steroids or physical therapy indicated. Refer to Home Health Care if applicable. Continue to assess discharge needs. Discharge needs identified		
	Goal: Identify D/C needs prior to day of D/C			**Goal:** Resume pre-hospital services and assure all D/C needs identified and taken care of.		

Nursing:
Consult Date/Time
Completed _____
	D/C telemetry unless
	  a. order continued by MD
	  b. significant arrhythmia
	  c. if heart rate irregular and over 100
	Patient Education continued
				Patient Education continued.
				Assure education and MDI use.
				D/C foley if indicated.		

	Goal:			**Goal:** All medication by mouth		
Tests:						
	Goal:			**Goal:**		
Other:	Change antibiotics to p.o. if appropriate			Steroids IV to po		
	Goal:			**Goal:**		

COPD CAREMAP

G-99-5091-3 PG REV. 6/29/99

disease process. Review the signs of impending respiratory problems (e.g., increased confusion or drowsiness), respiratory infection, and right-sided heart failure (e.g., peripheral edema, distended neck veins) so that prompt intervention can be obtained should these complications develop. The need for routine respiratory follow-up should also be discussed. In your teaching, include a discussion of the hazards of infection and ways to decrease personal risk (i.e., avoid crowds during the flu and colds season, clean respiratory equipment well, obtain pneumococcal and flu vaccines yearly). Review the need for lifestyle modifications.

Text continued on page 1705

■ THE CLIENT WITH CHRONIC OBSTRUCTIVE PULMONARY DISEASE

Nursing Diagnosis. Impaired Gas Exchange related to decreased ventilation and mucous plugs.

Outcomes. The client will maintain adequate gas exchange as evidenced by arterial blood gas (ABG) values (i.e., PaO_2 of at least 60 mm Hg, pH within normal limits, and $PaCO_2$ at baseline).

Interventions	Rationales
1. Regularly monitor the client's respiratory rate and pattern, ABG results, and manifestations of hypoxia or hypercapnia. Report significant changes promptly.	1. Prompt recognition of deteriorating respiratory function can reduce potentially lethal outcomes.
2. Administer low-flow oxygen therapy (1 to 3 L/min on 24% to 31% FiO_2) as needed via nasal prongs or a high-flow Venturi mask.	2. Oxygen corrects existing hypoxemia. Excessive increases in oxygen (55% to 70% FiO_2) may diminish respiratory drive and increase carbon dioxide retention further.
3. Assist the client into the high-Fowler position.	3. The upright position allows full lung excursion and enhances air exchange.
4. Administer bronchodilators if ordered. Monitor for side effects.	4. Bronchodilators relax bronchial smooth muscle, facilitating air flow. Common side effects include tremor, tachycardia, and other cardiac dysrhythmias.
5. Use caution when administering narcotics, sedatives, and tranquilizers.	5. These medications are respiratory depressants and can impair ventilation further.

Evaluation. The client's respirations are regular, unlabored, and between 12 and 20 per minute. ABGs are within normal range.

Nursing Diagnosis. Ineffective Airway Clearance related to excessive secretions and ineffective coughing.

Outcomes. The client will have improved airway clearance, as evidenced by effective coughing techniques and patent airways.

Interventions	Rationales
1. Teach the client to maintain adequate hydration by drinking at least 8 to 10 glasses of fluid per day (if not contraindicated) and increasing the humidity of the ambient air.	1. Hydration helps to thin secretions.
2. Teach and supervise effective coughing techniques.	2. Proper coughing techniques conserve energy, reduce airway collapse, and lessen client frustration.
3. Perform chest physical therapy, if needed, and instruct the client and significant others in these techniques.	3. Chest physical therapy techniques use forces of gravity and motion to facilitate secretion removal.
4. Assess the client's breath sounds before and after coughing episodes.	4. This assessment helps in evaluation of coughing effectiveness.

Evaluation. The client's cough is productive, and breath sounds are clearer.

Nursing Diagnosis. Activity Intolerance related to inadequate oxygenation and dyspnea.

Outcomes. The client will have improved activity tolerance, as evidenced by maintaining a realistic activity level and demonstrating energy conservation techniques.

Interventions	Rationales
1. Advise the client to avoid conditions that increase oxygen demand, such as smoking, temperature extremes, excess weight, and stress.	1. These factors increase peripheral vascular resistance, which increases cardiac workload and oxygen requirements.
2. Instruct the client in energy conservation techniques, such as pacing activities throughout the day, interspersed with adequate rest periods, and alternating high-energy and low-energy tasks.	2. Conservation techniques allow the client to accomplish more tasks with a limited energy supply.
3. Assist the client in scheduling a gradual increase in daily activities and exercise.	3. Gradual increases in physical activity improve respiratory and cardiac conditioning, thus improving activity tolerance.
4. Teach the client to use pursed-lip and diaphragmatic breathing techniques during activities.	4. Breathing retraining ensures maximal use of available respiratory function. Pursed-lip breathing leaves positive end-expiratory pressure in the lungs and helps keep airways open.
5. Schedule active exercise after respiratory therapy or medication (e.g., bronchodilator in metered-dose inhaler).	5. Lung function is maximized during peak periods of treatment and drug effect.
6. Maintain supplemental oxygen therapy as needed.	6. Supplemental oxygen helps alleviate exercise-induced hypoxemia, thus improving activity tolerance.

7. Assess the client for signs of a negative response to activity (e.g., significant change in respiratory rate, failure of pulse to return to near resting rate within 3 minutes of activity, changes in mental status).

7. Significant changes in respiratory, cardiac, or circulatory status signal activity intolerance.

Evaluation. The client performs activities of daily living and other activities with no significant deterioration in respiratory status.

Nursing Diagnosis. Anxiety related to acute breathing difficulties and fear of suffocation.

Outcomes. The client will express an increase in psychological comfort and demonstrate use of effective coping mechanisms.

Interventions

1. Remain with the client during acute episodes of breathing difficulty, and provide care in a calm, reassuring manner.
2. Provide a quiet, calm environment.
3. During acute episodes, open doors and curtains and limit the number of people and unnecessary equipment in the room.
4. Encourage the use of breathing retraining and relaxation techniques.
5. Give sedatives and tranquilizers with extreme caution. Nonpharmaceutical methods of anxiety reduction are more useful.

Rationales

1. Reassures the client that competent help is available if needed. Anxiety can be contagious; remain calm.
2. Reduction of external stimuli helps promote relaxation.
3. Environmental changes may lessen the client's perceptions of suffocation.
4. A feeling of self-control and success in facilitating breathing helps reduce anxiety.
5. Oversedation may cause respiratory depression.

Evaluation. The client's anxiety is decreased; the client demonstrates use of relaxation techniques and appears rested.

Nursing Diagnosis. Altered Nutrition: Less Than Body Requirements related to reduced appetite, decreased energy level, and dyspnea.

Outcomes. The client will maintain body weight within normal limits for gender and body build, and hemoglobin and albumin levels will be within normal ranges.

Interventions

1. Assist the client with mouth care before meals and as needed.
2. Advise the client to eat small, frequent meals (e.g., six meals a day) that are high in protein and calories.

3. Advise the client to avoid gas-producing foods, such as beans and cabbage.
4. Instruct the client in the use of high-calorie liquid supplements if indicated.
5. Advise hypoxemic clients to use oxygen via nasal cannula during meals.
6. Suggest methods to make meal preparation more convenient (e.g., Meals on Wheels program).
7. Monitor the client's food intake, weight, and serum hemoglobin and albumin levels.

Rationales

1. Coughing and sputum production may impair appetite. Mouth-breathing dries mucous membranes.
2. Large meals may create an excessive feeling of fullness that may make breathing uncomfortable and difficult. High protein and calorie levels are needed to maintain nutritional status in light of the increased work of breathing.
3. Gas-forming foods may cause abdominal bloating and distention and thus impair ventilation.
4. Liquid supplements provide high-calorie concentrations in a relatively small volume.
5. Adequate oxygenation increases the energy available for eating.
6. Reducing the energy expenditure of preparation maximizes the energy available for eating.
7. Changes in body weight reflect the degree of nutrition or malnutrition. Hemoglobin and albumin levels reflect protein intake.

Evaluation. The client maintains normal body weight and blood protein levels.

Nursing Diagnosis. Sleep Pattern Disturbance related to dyspnea and external stimuli.

Outcomes. The client will report feeling adequately rested.

Interventions

1. Promote relaxation by providing a darkened, quiet environment; ensuring adequate room ventilation; and following bedtime routines.
2. Schedule care activities to allow periods of uninterrupted sleep.

Rationales

1. The hospital environment can interfere with relaxation and sleep. Using established bedtime rituals increases relaxation.
2. For most people, completing four to five complete sleep cycles (60 to 90 minutes) per night promotes a feeling of being rested.

Care Plan continued on following page

3. Instruct the client in measures to promote sleep;
   a. Plan physical exercise during the day and passive, non-stimulating activities in the evening.
   b. Avoid stimulants, such as caffeine.

   c. Maintain a consistent bedtime and a regular bedtime routine.
   d. Eat a high-protein snack before bedtime.

   e. Use relaxation techniques (e.g., meditation, massage, warm bath, warm beverage).
   f. If the client awakens during the night, suggest a quiet, diverting activity, such as reading, in another room.

   g. If dyspnea is severe, a recliner chair or hospital bed may be more comfortable than a regular bed.

   a. Activity increases the need for sleep and contributes to a feeling of tiredness.
   b. Stimulants increase metabolism and inhibit relaxation.
   c. Consistency promotes relaxation and prevents disruptions of the biologic clock.
   d. Protein digestion produces tryptophan, an amino acid that has a sedative effect.
   e. Sleep is difficult unless the client is relaxed.
   f. Frustration over being awake deters sleep efforts further. The bedroom should be associated mentally with sleep to enhance future sleep promotion.
   g. The upright position facilitates ventilation.

Evaluation. The client gets at least 4 to 5 hours of uninterrupted sleep per night and reports feeling rested.

Nursing Diagnosis. Altered Family Processes related to chronic illness of a family member.

Outcomes. The family will verbalize their feelings, participate in the care of the ill family member, and seek external resources as needed.

Interventions

1. Plan interventions considering the client and significant other as the unit of care. Encourage participation in the planning process.
2. Assess family communication patterns, and intervene if they are ineffective. Family counseling may be needed.

3. Encourage as wide a social support network as feasible.

4. Encourage the client and family to seek support from other sources (e.g., self-help groups and support groups, such as the Better Breathers clubs sponsored by the American Lung Association).
5. Provide the family with anticipatory guidance as the client's COPD progresses.

Rationales

1. COPD affects not only the client experiencing the condition but also the client's significant others.

2. Effective communication helps each member to understand his or her own and others' feelings. Counseling may facilitate healthy interaction.
3. The use of a wide support group prevents a few family members from being overloaded with responsibility.
4. Clients may benefit from opportunities to share common experiences and to learn from others in similar situations.

5. Knowing what to expect facilitates family adjustment.

Evaluation. The client's family copes effectively with the stress of the client's illness, communicates openly, and supports the client.

Nursing Diagnosis. Sexual Dysfunction related to dyspnea, reduced energy, and changes in relationships.

Outcomes. The client will report increased satisfaction with sexual function.

Interventions

1. Provide an opportunity for the client to discuss concerns.

2. Suggest measures that may facilitate sexual activity (e.g., alternative positions, use of bronchodilator therapy before beginning sexual activity).
3. Encourage the client and partner to consider alternative forms of sexual expression (e.g., hugging, cuddling, stroking, kissing).
4. Recommend a professional sex therapist if appropriate.

Rationales

1. Many people are embarrassed or reluctant to talk about their sexual concerns.
2. Such measures can reduce physical exertion and maximize available oxygen levels.

3. Alternative methods require less energy expenditure compared with intercourse.

4. Talking with a skilled professional may assist client with constructive problem-solving.

Evaluation. The client discusses concerns and verbalizes more satisfaction with sexual relations.

Clients with end-stage lung disease experience significant, intensely distressing manifestations. Whether care is provided in the home or an extended-care facility, the focus is on minimizing these manifestations and making the client as comfortable as possible (see Bridge to Home Health Care).

TRACHEOBRONCHITIS

Acute tracheobronchitis is an inflammation of the mucous membranes of the trachea and the bronchial tree. This disorder commonly follows viral infections of the upper respiratory tract. It may also result from inhalation of noxious or irritating gases and particulate matter (including cigarette smoke), bacterial pneumonia, overvigorous tracheobronchial suctioning, and harsh paroxysms of coughing.

Manifestations include a raw burning pain over the upper anterior chest wall over the midsternum. Pain is increased with exposure to cold environments, cigarette smoke, cough, and tracheobronchial suctioning. In addition, the client may have a cough that progresses from dry to productive as the irritation increases. Fever, headache, and malaise may be present. Observe for cough-related syncope. Lightheadedness or fainting may occur with forceful coughing spells. Fainting is caused by prolonged elevation of intrapulmonary pressure during the compressive phase of a cough. The increased pressure impairs venous return to the thorax, causing a decrease in cardiac output.

Outcome Management

Treatment is focused on the cause of the cough. Cough suppressants are rarely effective. Antibiotics, bronchodilators, corticosteroids (inhaled and systemic), and anticholinergics are the primary treatments. Sinusitis is a common accompanying finding as well as a cause of tracheobronchitis.

Priority nursing goals include relief of pain and elimination of the tracheal irritation. Strongly advise the client to stop smoking. Whenever possible, eliminate other irritating gases or substances from the environment. Promote airway clearance by encouraging effective coughing, increased fluid intake, changing positions, and increasing inspired humidity. Inspired humidity may be increased through the use of aerosols. Advise clients to avoid cold air and to cover the mouth and nose before going outdoors.

BRONCHIECTASIS

Bronchiectasis, an extreme form of bronchitis, causes permanent, abnormal dilation and distortion of bronchi and bronchioles. It develops when bronchial walls are weak-

---

BRIDGE TO HOME HEALTH CARE

Conserving Oxygen with Chronic Obstructive Pulmonary Disease

Clients with chronic obstructive pulmonary disease (COPD) are challenged to make the most of their lives, given their available oxygen.

Usually, home health nurses are primarily responsible for monitoring manifestations; reviewing and reinforcing previously taught oxygen-conservation techniques; giving further instructions; and determining whether referrals to registered dietitians and occupational, physical, or respiratory therapists are needed. Evaluate what your clients already know, and proceed from there. Be certain that your clients understand the importance of using pursed-lip breathing, abdominal breathing, and metered-dose inhalers consistently and correctly. Have them demonstrate their technique.

Help your clients develop an oxygen-conservation plan that allows them to participate in activities that are most important to them. Ask them to keep a simple diary and to record their usual behavior during a 1- or 2-day period that includes all waking hours. When you analyze the diary, identify your clients' priorities. Help them relate specific activity to feelings of dyspnea during the day. In this way, you can teach specific oxygen-conservation techniques and pacing of activities to meet their priorities. To increase comfort, have your clients schedule the use of inhalers before activities and keep them within easy reach.

Encourage clients who are concerned about adequate oxygen for sexual activity to assume passive positions and to allow their partner to be more active. If winded, clients should use massage and other relaxation techniques as part of foreplay.

Adequate nutrition is essential to clients who have COPD; they may be malnourished because of respiratory muscle wasting. The diet may be high in protein and calories and low in carbohydrates. Answer your clients' questions, and determine whether they are willing or able to purchase, prepare, and eat the foods that were suggested. Encourage easy food preparation to prevent fatigue. Use foods that are prepackaged or can be heated in the microwave. Consider home-delivered meals. Use liquid food supplements to increase protein and calories; many brands are available, including some that are specially formulated for people who have pulmonary problems.

Encourage clients to rest just before eating and to follow these suggestions. Eat in a relaxed and quiet area. Small, frequent meals are best. Schedule meals early in the day if fatigue increases as the day continues. Snack frequently. Schedule inhalers after meals because inhalers can taint the taste of food and make it more difficult to achieve adequate nutrition.

Clients who have COPD often feel isolated because of their decreased ability to leave their homes. Suggest that they and their families join local support groups where they can share their experiences and feelings about the disease and learn new techniques to improve their quality of life. Many hospitals sponsor groups. Another valuable resource is the American Lung Association, which has local offices throughout the United States; call for information about prevention and the latest developments in treatment.

Rebecca M. Dudley, RN, *Staff Nurse, Fairview Lakes HomeCaring and Hospice, Chisago City, Minnesota*

ened by chronic inflammatory changes in the bronchial mucosa and occurs most often after recurrent inflammatory conditions. Any condition producing a narrowing of the lumen of the bronchioles, however, may result in bronchiectasis, including tuberculosis, adenoviral infections, and pneumonia.

Some forms of bronchiectasis are congenital and are associated with cystic fibrosis, sinusitis, dextrocardia (heart located on right side), and alterations in ciliary activity (Kartagener's syndrome). Bronchiectasis is usually localized to a lung lobe or segment rather than generalized throughout the lungs. At times, however, persistent, nonresolving infection may cause the disorder to spread to other parts of the same lung.

Diagnosis may be confirmed by chest radiograph, bronchogram, or computed tomography (CT) scan.

Manifestations vary according to the etiologic agent. The main manifestations are cough and purulent sputum production in large quantities. Fever, hemoptysis, nasal stuffiness, and drainage from sinusitis also are common. The client may complain of fatigue and weakness. Clubbing of the fingers may be found on physical assessment.

Outcome Management

Management of bronchiectasis is the same as for COPD. Most clients are managed medically to prevent progression of the disorder and to control clinical manifestations. Antibiotics, chest physical therapy, hydration, bronchodilators, and oxygen commonly are prescribed. Severe cases may be treated by surgical resection if the pathologic process is well localized in one lobe or two adjacent lobes and when no contraindications to surgery exist.

DISORDERS OF THE PULMONARY VASCULATURE

PULMONARY EMBOLISM

Pulmonary embolism (PE) is an occlusion of a portion of the pulmonary blood vessels by an embolus. An embolus is a clot or other plug (thrombus) that is carried by the bloodstream from its point of origin to a smaller blood vessel, where it obstructs circulation. Depending on its size, an embolus can be lethal. It is estimated that, in the United States, more than 250,000 people are hospitalized annually for venous thromboembolism. For those with a PE, the mortality rate is approximately 15%.[11]

Etiology and Risk Factors

Virtually all PEs develop from thrombi (clots), most of which originate in the deep calf, femoral, popliteal, or iliac veins. Other sources of emboli include tumors, air, fat, bone marrow, amniotic fluid, septic thrombi, and vegetations on heart valves that develop with endocarditis.

Major operations, especially hip, knee, abdominal, and extensive pelvic procedures, predispose the client to thrombus formation because of the reduced flow of blood through the pelvis. Preventive measures, such as early ambulation, frequent leg exercises, sequential compression stockings, and low-dose heparin prophylaxis, are essential.

Pathophysiology

When emboli travel to the lungs, they lodge in the pulmonary vasculature. The size and number of emboli determine the location. Blood flow is obstructed, leading to decreased perfusion of the section of lung supplied by the vessel. The client continues to ventilate the lung portion, but because the tissue is not perfused, a $\dot{V}/\dot{Q}$ mismatch occurs, resulting in hypoxemia.

If an embolus lodges in a large pulmonary vessel, it increases proximal pulmonary vascular resistance, causes atelectasis, and eventually reduces cardiac output. If the embolus is in a smaller vessel, less dramatic clinical manifestations follow but perfusion is still altered.

The arterioles constrict because of platelet degranulation, accompanied by a release of histamine, serotonin, catecholamines, and prostaglandins. The chemical agents result in bronchial and pulmonary artery constriction. This vasoconstriction probably plays a major role in the hemodynamic instability that follows PE.

PE can lead to right-sided heart failure. Once the clot lodges, affected blood vessels in the lung collapse. This collapse increases the pressure in the pulmonary vasculature. The increased pressure increases the workload of the right side of the heart, leading to failure. Massive PE of the pulmonary artery can also result in cardiopulmonary collapse from lack of perfusion and resulting hypoxia and acidosis.

Clinical Manifestations

The clinical manifestations of PE are nonspecific and, in some clients, may not appear until late in the event. The most common manifestations of PE are tachypnea, dyspnea, anxiety, and chest pain. Because these clinical manifestations are similar to those seen with myocardial infarction and other cardiovascular illnesses, overdiagnosis is as likely as underdiagnosis. Extensive differential diagnosis often is required. The pain usually experienced with PE is pleuritic in nature, caused by an inflammatory reaction of the lung parenchyma or by pulmonary infarction or ischemia, caused by obstruction of small pulmonary arterial branches. Typical pleuritic chest pain is sudden in onset and exacerbated by breathing. The client is usually dyspneic, especially if the embolus has occluded major arteries or major portions of lung tissue. Apprehension, cough, diaphoresis, syncope, and hemoptysis may occur. The presence of hemoptysis indicates that the infarction or areas of atelectasis have produced alveolar damage.

Respirations typically increase. Crackles, an accentuated second heart sound, tachycardia, and fever may also develop. Less common findings include heart gallops, edema, heart murmur, and cyanosis.

Diagnostic Findings

When PE is suspected, the optimal strategy for diagnosis is an integrated approach that includes a thorough history and physical examination, supplemented by selective diagnostic tests. ABG analysis indicates arterial hypoxemia (low PaO_2) and hypocapnia (low $PaCO_2$) in massive PE. There may be a severe respiratory alkalosis. Lactate dehydrogenase (LDH) isoenzymes show an increase in LDH_3

if there is lung tissue injury. A chest radiograph may help to rule out other pulmonary diagnoses.

The best noninvasive diagnostic test for PE is the $\dot{V}/\dot{Q}$ lung scan. A radioisotope lung scan is performed by IV injection of particles of human serum albumin that have been labeled with iodine 131 or technetium 99m. These particles are trapped in the pulmonary microvasculature and are distributed according to pulmonary flow. Both lungs are scanned with a scintillation counter, and the amount of radioactivity counted gives an indication of obstruction to flow. A lung scan can be seen in Chapter 59.

An alternative to lung scanning is spiral CT scan of the chest. This approach is particularly effective for identifying PE in the proximal pulmonary vascular tree.

Pulmonary angiography remains the definitive means of diagnosis of PE (Fig. 61–10). A radiopaque contrast agent is injected into the right atrium and pulmonary artery via a catheter threaded through a peripheral vein. Visualization of any filling defects of the heart and right pulmonary artery is achieved by taking sequential radiographs. Because of the invasive nature of the test, pulmonary angiography typically is reserved for cases in which there is a high index of clinical suspicion despite nondiagnostic findings on other tests.

Outcome Management

■ Medical Care

Successful management of PE depends on prompt recognition of the condition and immediate treatment. Goals are to stabilize the cardiopulmonary system and reduce the threat of a further PE with anticoagulation therapy. For some clients, the clot can be lysed.

STABILIZING THE CARDIOPULMONARY SYSTEM

Maintenance of cardiopulmonary stability is the first priority. Cardiopulmonary support varies with the client's manifestations. Sometimes hypoxemia can be reversed with low-flow oxygen by nasal cannula. Other clients may require endotracheal intubation to maintain PaO_2 greater than 60 mm Hg. Hypotension is treated with fluids. If fluids do not raise the preload (right ventricular end-diastolic pressure) enough to raise blood pressure, inotropic agents may be required. Acidosis, which has a powerful vasoconstricting effect, is corrected with bicarbonate.

ANTICOAGULANT THERAPY

Typically, anticoagulation begins with IV standard (unfractionated) heparin sodium to reduce the risk of further clots and to prevent extension of existing clots. Anticoagulants do not break up existing clots. Clinical trials have shown that subcutaneously administered low-molecular-weight heparin is as safe and effective as standard heparin in the treatment of hemodynamically stable clients with PE. Anticoagulants are administered until a therapeutic partial thromboplastin time (PTT) is achieved. In general, the initial target International Normalized Ratio should be 2.5 to 3.0. Administration of sodium warfarin is begun about 3 to 5 days before heparin is stopped to provide a transition to oral anticoagulation. Because the half-life of warfarin is long, about 2 to 3 days is required to achieve adequate anticoagulation. Clients are maintained on warfarin for 3 to 6 months.

FIBRINOLYTIC THERAPY

The effectiveness of fibrinolytic therapy in the management of a massive PE is not clear, but it may be useful in clients who are hemodynamically unstable. Thrombolytic agents lyse the clots and restore right-sided heart function; however, some clinicians have found that although the clot dissolves, the mortality rate is not improved.

■ Nursing Management of the Medical Client

Monitor the client closely for hypoxemia and respiratory compromise, and assess vital signs and lung sounds frequently. Monitor ABG values, and monitor the client for manifestations of right-sided heart failure. Auscultate heart sounds frequently, assessing for murmurs or extra heart sounds. Check for peripheral edema, distended neck veins, and liver engorgement.

To facilitate breathing, elevate the head of the bed and apply oxygen per physician's orders. Because the usual cause of a PE is thrombus from the lower legs, elevate the legs with caution to avoid severe flexure of the hips. Such flexure would slow blood flow and increase the risk of new thrombi.

The client typically experiences fear with the sudden onset of severe chest pain and inability to breathe. Anxiety, restlessness, and apprehension are common. Emotional support can reduce anxiety and lessen dyspnea. Stay with the client and give calm (yet efficient) nursing care.

Analgesics are given as needed to reduce pain and anxiety. Morphine is the most common agent. Anxiety and pain increase oxygen demand and dyspnea. Administer oral care with soft brushes or rinses while oxygen

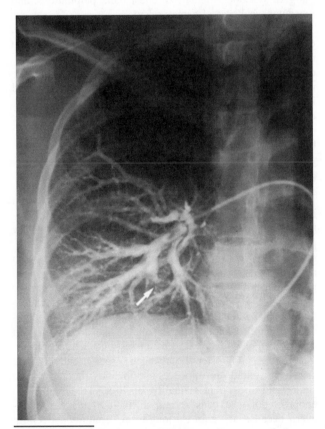

FIGURE 61–10 Angiogram showing a pulmonary embolus (*arrow*).

is in use, especially if the client breathes through the mouth.

Once anticoagulation is achieved, watch for manifestations of excess anticoagulation, such as blood in the urine, in the stool, or along the gums or teeth; subcutaneous bruising; or flank pain. When invasive studies, such as ABGs, are necessary, apply pressure to the puncture site for at least 10 minutes. The client is discharged with oral anticoagulation therapy. Instruct the client about side effects, the importance of follow-up to monitor prothrombin times, and precautions to prevent bleeding. Review methods to reduce thrombophlebitis, if that was the likely cause of the embolus (see Chapter 53).

■ Surgical Management

Surgical interventions that may be used in treatment of PE include (1) vena cava interruption with the insertion of a filter (Fig. 61–11) and (2) pulmonary embolectomy. The Greenfield filter, a basket-like cone of wires bent to look like an umbrella, is the filter most commonly used. The surgeon inserts the filter by threading it up the veins in the leg or neck until it reaches the vena cava at the level of the renal arteries. The filter allows blood flow while trapping emboli.

Embolectomy is used in clients with significant hemodynamic instability caused by the embolus, especially those with unstable circulation and contraindications to thrombolytic therapy. An embolectomy involves surgical removal of emboli from the pulmonary arteries by either a thoracotomy or an embolectomy catheter. Newly developed catheters use high-velocity jets of saline to draw the thrombus toward the catheter tip and pulverize it.[11]

PULMONARY HYPERTENSION

Pulmonary hypertension is defined as a prolonged elevation of the mean pulmonary artery pressure (PAP) above 25 mm Hg at rest (normal, 10 to 20 mm Hg) or above 30

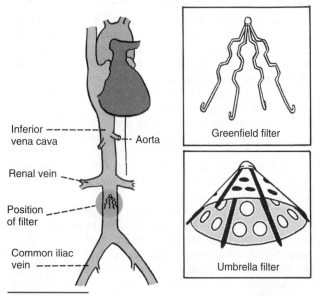

Inferior vena cava

Aorta

Renal vein

Position of filter

Common iliac vein

Greenfield filter

Umbrella filter

FIGURE 61–11 Inferior vena cava filters, such as the Greenfield and umbrella filters, prevent emboli from traveling to the lung.

mm Hg during exercise (normal, 20 to 30 mm Hg). Severe forms of pulmonary hypertension are classified as either *secondary* or *idiopathic (primary)*. Secondary pulmonary hypertension is usually associated with underlying heart or lung disease (e.g., PE, venocclusive disease, COPD). The cause of the idiopathic form is, by definition, unclear. It occurs most often in young adults between the ages of 30 and 40 years. Women are affected more often than men.[29] The condition is progressive, leading to right-sided heart failure and severe dyspnea.

Etiology

The pulmonary circulation is generally a low-pressure, low-resistance system. Increased cardiac output in a healthy person, as with exercise, causes minimal elevations in PAP because of the large pulmonary vascular reserve. When pulmonary vasoconstriction is present, however, pressure elevation occurs because the pulmonary vasculature cannot accommodate increased blood flow.

Mild forms of pulmonary hypertension are normally caused by pulmonary vasoconstriction resulting from chronic hypoxia, acidosis, or both. Administration of oxygen, correction of acid-base imbalance, and use of vasodilating medications in selected cases generally return PAP to normal, either completely or partially.

Clinical Manifestations

Clients with mild pulmonary hypertension may be relatively asymptomatic. In moderate to severe forms, the main (and occasionally only) manifestation is dyspnea. Fatigue, syncope, angina-like chest pain, palpitations, and muscular weakness also may occur.

Chest x-ray study shows right ventricular hypertrophy, enlarged pulmonary arteries, prominent hilar vessels, and normal or reduced intrapulmonary vascular markings. Cardiac catheterization provides the most valuable diagnostic measurements. Typical findings include elevated PAP and increased arteriovenous oxygen differences accompanied by normal systemic blood pressure and normal to low cardiac output. Pulmonary wedge pressures (PWPs) remain normal because left ventricular function is typically unchanged.

Outcome Management

The overall prognosis in severe pulmonary hypertension is poor. There is no known cure for the disorder, although treatment of the underlying cause of secondary pulmonary hypertension may slow its progression. Supportive intervention with supplemental oxygen helps to reduce hypoxemia, whereas anticoagulants may be used to prevent thromboembolic events.

Vasodilator therapy is the cornerstone of pharmacologic management. First-line vasodilators used for treatment are the calcium channel antagonists nifedipine and diltiazem. For clients who do not respond to these drugs, intravenous epoprostenol has been used effectively and has been found to improve significantly hemodynamic status and the client's quality of life.[5] Treatment with epoprostenol is expensive and difficult to manage, however, because it requires long-term, continuous central infusion. Some clients with severe pulmonary hypertension may undergo heart-lung transplantation, although data regarding long-term effectiveness are not yet available. Interventions appropriate for underlying diseases and preparation for diagnostic procedures are incorporated into nursing care.

CONCLUSIONS

Lower airway disorders include asthma, chronic air flow limitations, and inflammations of the airways. Nursing care centers on reversal of any airway spasms and education of the client on how to live with the disorder and to reduce the risk of future problems. PE is a potentially life-threatening disorder that usually can be managed effectively with prompt recognition.

THINKING CRITICALLY

1. **A 52-year-old woman is being treated at the neighborhood health clinic for chronic bronchitis. Her husband of 30 years smoked two to three packs of cigarettes a day. The client never smoked. During this exacerbation, she presents with shortness of breath; wheezing; a deep, throaty, productive cough when she tries to talk; and fatigue. Her blood pressure is 180/90 mm Hg, pulse is 90 beats per minute, respirations are 28 per minute and labored, and temperature is 99.4° F. She tells you that she tried to shovel the driveway on this cold winter day and did not wear a scarf over her mouth as she usually does. She further states that her inhalers did not seem to help her. She is taking a diuretic for hypertension, with blood pressure controlled at about 160/86 mm Hg. What is your priority nursing action? What teaching is appropriate at this time?**

Factors to Consider. What are the clinical manifestations of chronic obstructive emphysema? What nursing assessments are in order?

2. **An elderly client is recovering from pelvic surgery. Because of a previous cerebrovascular accident, she is hemiplegic. She has been on bed rest since the surgery. While the nursing assistant is giving her a bath, she notices the client grimacing as if in pain. The client responds to her question by pointing to her chest and nodding when asked if the pain is severe. The nursing assistant notifies you that the client is in distress. What is the priority assessment?**

Factors to Consider. What complications of surgery and resulting bed rest might pose a risk for this client? How would you compare and contrast the clinical manifestations for pneumonia and pulmonary embolus?

3. **You enter the room of the client from Question 2 and discover that she is apprehensive. She is trying to hold her breath because it hurts to breathe. She is sweating, and there is frothy sputum on her lips. What nursing interventions are appropriate? What treatment might be ordered?**

Factors to Consider. What are the clinical manifestations of a pulmonary embolus? What diagnostic studies may be ordered?

BIBLIOGRAPHY

1. Allen, G. (1996). Surgical treatment of emphysema using bovine pericardium strips. *AORN Journal, 63*(2), 373–388.
2. Bennett, J., & Plum, F. (1996). *Cecil textbook of medicine* (20th ed.). Philadelphia: W. B. Saunders.
3. Bone, R. C. (1996). Goals of asthma management: A step-care approach. *Chest, 109*(4), 1056–1065.
4. Burns, S. M., & Lawson, C. (1999). Pharmacological and ventilatory management of acute asthma exacerbations. *Critical Care Nurse, 19*(4), 39–53.
5. Cheever, K. H., Kitzes, B., & Genthner, D. (1999). Epoprostenol therapy for primary pulmonary hypertension. *Critical Care Nurse, 19*(4), 20–27.
6. Couser, J. I., et al. (1995). Pulmonary rehabilitation improves exercise capacity in older elderly patients with COPD. *Chest, 107*(3), 730–734.
7. Faul, J. L., et al. (1999). Quality of life and lung volume reduction surgery. *American Journal of Critical Care, 8*(6), 359–396.
8. Ferraro, J. (1996). Here's the result of poor treatment for lung infections. *RN, 59*(11), 54–56.
9. Gift, A. G. (1995). Application in research: Issues in asthma self-management. *Perspectives in Respiratory Nursing, 6*(4), 5–6.
10. Gift, A. G., & Narsavage, G. (1998). Validity of the numeric rating scale as a measure of dyspnea. *American Journal of Critical Care, 7*, 200–204.
11. Goldhaber, S. Z. (1998). Medical progress: Pulmonary embolism. *New England Journal of Medicine, 339*(2), 93–104.
12. Graling, P., Hetrick, V., & Kiernan, P. (1996). Bilateral lung volume reduction surgery. *AORN Journal, 63*(2), 389–404.
13. Heslop, A., & Shannon, C. (1995). Assisting patients living with long-term oxygen therapy. *British Journal of Nursing, 4*(19), 1123–1128.
14. Janssen, W. (1996). Treatment for emphysema: An overview of lung volume reduction surgery. *Perspectives in Respiratory Nursing, 7*(1), 1–5.
15. Leidy, N. K. (1995). Functional performance in people with chronic obstructive pulmonary disease. *Image, 27*(1), 23–35.
16. Lewis, D., & Bell, S. K. (1995). Pulmonary rehabilitation, psychological adjustment, and use of healthcare services. *Rehabilitation Nursing, 20*(2), 102–107.
17. Madison, J. M., & Irwin, R. S. (1998). Chronic obstructive pulmonary disease. *Lancet, 352*(9126), 467–473.
18. McKinney, B. (1995). Under new management: Asthma and the elderly. *Journal of Gerontological Nursing, 21*(11), 39–45.
19. National Institutes of Health. (1997). *Guidelines for the diagnosis and management of asthma.* NIH Pub. No. 97-4051. Washington, DC: Author.
20. Newsome, E. A., & Ott, B. B. (1997). Lung volume reduction: Surgical treatment for emphysema. *American Journal of Critical Care, 6*(6), 423–429.
21. Pfister, S. M. (1995). Home oxygen therapy: Indications, administration, recertification, and patient education. *Nurse Practitioner, 20*(7), 44–56.
22. Reid, W. D., & Samrai, B. (1995). Respiratory muscle training for patients with chronic obstructive pulmonary disease. *Physical Therapy, 75*(11), 996–1005.
23. Schedel, E. M., & Connolly, M. A. (1999). Lung volume reduction surgery: New hope for emphysema patients. *Dimensions of Critical Care Nursing, 18*(1), 28–34.
24. Scherer, Y., Schmieder, L., & Shimmel, S. (1995). Outpatient instruction for individuals with COPD. *Perspectives in Respiratory Nursing, 6*(3), 1–8.
25. Shelmerdine, L. (1995). Occupational asthma: Assessing the risk. *Nursing Standard, 10*(4), 25–28.
26. Tarpy, S. P., & Celli, B. R. (1995). Current concepts: Long-term oxygen therapy. *New England Journal of Medicine, 333*(11), 710–714.
27. Tiep, B. L. (1997). Disease management of COPD with pulmonary rehabilitation. *Chest, 112*(6), 1630–1656.
28. Verderber, A., Gallagher, K., & Severino, R. (1995). The effect of nursing interventions on transcutaneous oxygen and carbon dioxide tensions. *Western Journal of Nursing Research, 17*(1), 76–90.
29. Wallace, L. S. (1998). Pulmonary hypertension: A deadly threat. *RN, 61*(10), 48–54.

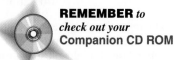

CHAPTER

62

Management of Clients with Parenchymal and Pleural Disorders

Nancy York

NURSING OUTCOMES CLASSIFICATION (NOC)
for Nursing Diagnoses—Clients with Parenchymal and Pleural Disorders

Activity Intolerance
Activity Tolerance
Endurance
Altered Nutrition: Less Than Body
Requirements
Nutritional Status
Nutritional Status: Food and Fluid Intake
Altered Oral Mucous Membrane
Tissue Integrity: Skin and Mucous
   Membrane
Anxiety
Anxiety Control
Coping

Impaired Gas Exchange
Respiratory Status: Gas Exchange
Respiratory Status: Ventilation
Ineffective Airway Clearance
Aspiration Control
Respiratory Status: Airway Patency
Ineffective Breathing Pattern
Respiratory Status: Airway Patency
Respiratory Status: Ventilation
Ineffective Individual Coping
Coping
Information Processing
Role Performance

Social Support
Knowledge Deficit
Knowledge: Disease Process
Knowledge: Health Behaviors
Knowledge: Medication
Knowledge: Treatment Regimen
Pain
Comfort Level
Pain: Disruptive Effects
Sleep Pattern Disturbance
Anxiety Control
Rest
Sleep

The parenchyma of any organ, in this case the lung, is the tissue essential for the function of the organ. This chapter reviews disorders of the lung parenchyma, such as pneumonia, tuberculosis, cystic fibrosis, and cancer.

ATELECTASIS

Atelectasis is the collapse of lung tissue at any structural level (e.g., segmental, basilar, lobar, or microscopic). It develops when there is interference with the natural forces that promote lung expansion. Such interference may result from a reduction in lung distention forces, localized airway obstruction, insufficient pulmonary surfactant, or increased elastic recoil. Examples of each of these causes are given in Box 62–1. Atelectasis is particularly common after surgery, especially upper abdominal or thoracic procedures. Clients who are elderly, obese, or bedridden or have a history of smoking are also susceptible to atelectasis.

Atelectasis may be diagnosed through physical examination, although generally, it is initially detected on chest x-ray. Some clients are asymptomatic. If significant hypoxemia (low level of oxygen in the blood) is present,

however, dyspnea (difficult or labored breathing), tachypnea (rapid breathing), tachycardia (rapid heartbeat), and cyanosis (bluish discoloration of skin and mucous membranes) may occur. Chest auscultation may reveal bronchial or diminished breath sounds and crackles over the involved area. Fever of less than 101° F is common. However, elderly people with atelectasis typically do not exhibit a fever.

If atelectasis is severe, physical assessment findings include the following:

- A tracheal shift toward the side of the atelectasis
- A decrease in tactile fremitus over the affected lung area
- A dull percussion note over the atelectatic region
- Decreased chest movement on the involved side

None of these signs is specific for atelectasis, and the entire clinical picture must always be considered.

One of the primary goals of nursing intervention is to prevent atelectasis in the high-risk client. Frequent position changes and early ambulation help promote drainage of all lung segments. Deep-breathing and effective coughing enhance lung expansion and prevent airway obstruc-

BOX 62–1   Causes of Atelectasis

Reduction in Lung Distention Forces

Pleural space encroachment (e.g., pneumothorax, pleural effusion, pleural tumor)
Chest wall disorders (e.g., scoliosis, flail chest)
Impaired diaphragmatic movement (e.g., ascites, obesity)
Central nervous system dysfunction (e.g., coma, neuromuscular disorders, oversedation)

Localized Airway Obstruction

Mucus plugging
Foreign body aspiration
Bronchiectasis

Insufficient Pulmonary Surfactant

Respiratory distress syndrome
Inhalation anesthesia
High concentrations of oxygen (oxygen toxicity)
Lung contusion
Aspiration of gastric contents
Smoke inhalation

Increased Elastic Recoil

Interstitial fibrosis (e.g., silicosis, radiation pneumonitis)

---

tion. Incentive spirometry is an excellent means of encouraging a client to deep-breathe.

If atelectasis develops, treatment is directed toward the underlying cause. If the client becomes hypoxic, oxygen should be administered as prescribed (e.g., per cannula, 1 to 4 L/min). More aggressive measures to maintain airway patency, such as postural drainage, chest physiotherapy, and tracheal suctioning, may also be ordered. If an airway obstruction is causing atelectasis, bronchoscopy may be used to remove the material.

INFECTIOUS DISORDERS

INFLUENZA

The term "flu" is often used inappropriately to describe many clinical manifestations and disorders. *Influenza* actually refers to an acute viral infection of the respiratory tract.

Influenza usually occurs seasonally in epidemic form. People most at risk are very young children, the elderly, people living in institutional settings, people with chronic diseases, and health care personnel.

The first flu virus was identified in the 1930s. Since then, influenza viruses have been identified as types A, B, and C. Type A is the most prevalent and is associated with the most serious epidemics. Type B outbreaks also can reach epidemic levels, but the disease produced is generally milder than that caused by type A. Type C viruses have never been connected with a large epidemic.

Clinical manifestations of influenza include fever, myalgias (muscular pain), and cough. Influenza predisposes to complications such as viral bronchitis or pneumonia, bacterial pneumonia, and superinfections (infections that occur during the course of antimicrobial therapy).

Influenza differs from a common cold primarily in its sudden onset and widespread occurrence within the population.

Chest findings are usually negative unless pneumonia results. Conversely, colds have a slow onset of manifestations, usually do not cause fever, have malaise as a major manifestation, and commonly cause nasal manifestations.

Outcome Management

Intervention for influenza is based on manifestations as they arise (i.e., supportive measures to relieve fever, myalgia, and cough). In 1999, two new anti-influenza drugs (zanamivir and oseltamivir) were developed that appear to be extremely effective in preventing massive multiplication of the virus. They must be administered within 24 hours of onset. Rimantadine can be used to treat influenza type A in adults, but it has no effect on type B infections. When taken within 48 hours after the onset of illness, rimantadine reduces the duration of fever and other manifestations and allows clients to return to their daily routines more quickly. These drugs do not, however, replace the need for immunization.

Influenza is a communicable disease spread by droplet infection. Prevent the spread of this infection by encouraging clients with influenza to remain at home, practice frequent hand-washing, and cover the nose and mouth when sneezing or coughing.

Encourage clients at risk for influenza to obtain an annual immunization before the start of the "flu season" each winter. Vaccination controls influenza for many high-risk clients. However, clients who are allergic to eggs or have a history of Guillain-Barré syndrome should not receive an influenza immunization.

PNEUMONIA

Pneumonia (pneumonitis) is an inflammatory process in lung parenchyma usually associated with a marked increase in interstitial and alveolar fluid. Advances in antibiotic therapy have led to the widespread perception that pneumonia is no longer a major health problem in the United States. However, pneumonia and influenza are currently the sixth most common cause of death for all ages and one of the most common causes in the elderly. Among all nosocomial infections, pneumonia is the second most common but has the highest mortality.[8, 22]

Etiology and Risk Factors

There are many causes of pneumonia, including bacteria, viruses, mycoplasmas, fungal agents, and protozoa (Table 62–1). Pneumonia may also result from aspiration of food, fluids, or vomitus or from inhalation of toxic or caustic chemicals, smoke, dusts, or gases. Pneumonia may complicate immobility and chronic illnesses. It often follows influenza.

Major risk factors for pneumonia include (1) advanced age, (2) a history of smoking, (3) upper respiratory infection, (4) tracheal intubation, (5) prolonged immobility, (6) immunosuppressive therapy, (7) a nonfunctional immune system, (8) malnutrition, (9) dehydration, and (10) chronic disease states, such as diabetes, heart disease,

TABLE 62-1	ASSESSMENT AND TREATMENT OF PNEUMONIA	
Common Name	**Clinical Manifestations**	**Management**
Pneumococcal pneumonia (caused by *Streptococcus pneumoniae*)	Sudden onset with a single shaking chill, high fever, stabbing-pleuritic chest pain, malaise, weakness, occasional vomiting, tachypnea, dyspnea, and elevated WBC count Single or multiple lobar consolidation on the chest x-ray Cough productive of rusty brown or blood-streaked purulent sputum that turns yellow and mucoid	Primary: penicillinase-resistant penicillin, doxycycline, levofloxacin Alternative: azithromycin or clarithromycin, second- or third-generation cephalosporin Prevention: Vaccine available
Staphylococcal pneumonia (caused by *Staphylococcus aureus*)	Sudden onset with fever, multiple chills, pleuritic pain, dyspnea, rales, decreased breath sounds, elevated WBC count, and exaggerated cough productive of purulent golden-yellow or blood-streaked sputum Chest x-ray may show patchy infiltrates, empyema, abscesses, and pneumothorax Disease may start with headache, cough, and myalgia	Primary: penicillin, cephalosporin; vancomycin for non–penicillinase-producing organism; penicillinase-resistant penicillin if organism produces penicillinase; vancomycin if organism is methicillin resistant
Influenzal pneumonia (caused by *Haemophilus influenzae*)	Similar to those of pneumococcal pneumonia Cough productive of apple- or lime-green purulent sputum, which may be blood-tinged	Primary: cefuroxime, chloramphenicol, ampicillin
Gram-negative bacterial pneumonia (most commonly caused by *Klebsiella pneumoniae*)	Sudden onset with high fever, multiple chills, pleuritic pain, dyspnea, cyanosis, and elevated WBC count Lobar consolidation and cavitation on chest x-ray Cough productive of red sputum resembling currant jelly (mucoid, sticky, and difficult to expectorate)	Primary: aminoglycosides, third-generation cephalosporins, TMP-SMZ, extended-spectrum penicillin, ciprofloxacin
Anaerobic bacterial pneumonia, hypostatic pneumonia (caused by normal oral flora)	Insidious onset with low-grade fever, dyspnea, crackles, cyanosis, hypertension, tachycardia, and elevated WBC count Patchy infiltrates in dependent lung segments on chest x-ray Cough productive of purulent greenish-yellow, foul-smelling sputum	Primary: third-generation cephalosporins (such as cefotaxime) or penicillin G Alternative: cefoxitin, clindamycin, or chloramphenicol
Legionnaires' disease (caused by *Legionella pneumophila*)	Prodrome of 24–48 hours with fever, headache, and malaise followed by high fever with pulse-temperature dissociation, dyspnea, hypoxia, pleuritic pain, nausea, vomiting, diarrhea, confusion, and elevated WBC count Single or multilobar consolidation and small pleural effusions on chest x-ray Dry cough productive of scant mucoid or blood-tinged sputum	Primary: erythromycin Alternative: TMP-SMZ, fluoroquinolone, levofloxacin
Mycoplasma pneumonia (caused by *Mycoplasma* microorganisms)	Insidious onset with slowly rising fever, headache, myalgia, malaise, and normal WBC count Pulmonary infiltrate—sometimes extensive—on chest x-ray Cough productive of scant mucoid sputum Client may show only minimal signs and symptoms	Primary: tetracycline Alternative: erythromycin, ciprofloxacin
Viral pneumonia (caused by influenza A virus)	Prodrome with headache and myalgia followed by high fever, dyspnea, normal breath sounds with occasional wheezing and crackles, and normal or slightly elevated WBC count Diffuse, patchy infiltrates on chest x-ray Dry cough with initial mucoid sputum that later turns purulent Cough may be unproductive	Antiviral agents, symptomatic treatment

TABLE 62-1	ASSESSMENT AND TREATMENT OF PNEUMONIA *Continued*	
Common Name	**Clinical Manifestations**	**Management**
Fungal pneumonia (caused by histoplasmosis, blastomycosis, coccidioidomycosis, aspergillosis, candidiasis)	Usually asymptomatic When manifestations occur, they range from brief periods of malaise to severe, life-threatening illness Typical illness resembles influenza	Amphotericin B and other oral imidazoles (ketoconazole, fluconazole)
Parasitic pneumonia (caused by protozoa, nematodes, platyhelminths); common organism is *Pneumocystis carinii*	Clients who have *P. carinii* pneumonia are invariably immunocompromised (HIV) Cough, dyspnea, pleuritic chest pain, fever and night sweats, crackles	Diamidines, folate antagonists (TMP-SMZ), and other agents (clindamycin)

HIV, human immunodeficiency virus; TMP-SMZ, trimethoprim-sulfamethoxazole; WBC, white blood cell.

chronic lung disease, renal disease, and cancer. Additional risk factors are exposure to air pollution, altered consciousness (from alcoholism, drug overdose, general anesthesia, or a seizure disorder), inhalation of noxious substances, aspiration of foreign or gastric material, and residence in institutional settings where transmission of the disease is more likely.

Pathophysiology

The feature common to all types of pneumonia is an inflammatory pulmonary response to the offending organism or agent. The defense mechanisms of the lungs lose effectiveness and allow organisms to penetrate the sterile lower respiratory tract, where inflammation develops. Disruption of the mechanical defenses of cough and ciliary motility leads to colonization of the lungs and subsequent infection. Inflamed and fluid-filled alveolar sacs cannot exchange oxygen and carbon dioxide effectively. Alveolar exudate tends to consolidate, so it is increasingly difficult to expectorate. Bacterial pneumonia may be associated with significant ventilation-perfusion mismatch as the infection grows.

Clinical Manifestations

The onset of all pneumonias is generally marked by any or all of the following manifestations: fever, chills, sweats, pleuritic chest pain, cough, sputum production, hemoptysis, dyspnea, headache, and fatigue. Elderly clients may present not with fever or respiratory manifestations but with altered mental status and dehydration.

Chest auscultation reveals bronchial breath sounds over areas of *consolidation* (dense white areas on the chest film). Consolidated lung tissue transmits bronchial sound waves to outer lung fields. Crackling sounds (from fluid in interstitial and alveolar areas) and whispered *pectoriloquy* (transmission of the sound of whispered words through the chest wall) may be heard over affected areas. Tactile fremitus is usually increased over areas of pneumonia, whereas percussion sounds are dulled. Unequal chest wall expansion may occur during inspiration if a large area of lung tissue is involved; this is due to decreased distensibility in the affected area. Table 62-1 lists the clinical manifestations of specific types of pneumonia.

Definitive diagnosis is usually determined through sputum culture analysis and sensitivity or serologic testing. At times, fiberoptic bronchoscopy or transcutaneous needle aspiration or biopsy may be necessary for confirmation. Additional diagnostic testing may consist of (1) skin tests, if tuberculosis or coccidioidomycosis is suspected, (2) blood and urine cultures to assess systemic spread, and (3) transcutaneous oxygen level analysis or arterial blood gas (ABG) measurements to assess the need for supplemental oxygen.

Chest x-ray examination provides information about the location and extent of pneumonia. As already mentioned, on a chest film, areas of pneumonia appear as consolidation.

Pneumonia may involve one or more lobe segments of the lungs (*segmental pneumonia*), one or more entire lobes (*lobar pneumonia*) (Fig. 62-1A), or lobes in both lungs (*bilateral pneumonia*). On the basis of location and radiologic appearance, pneumonias may be classified as bronchopneumonia, interstitial pneumonia, alveolar pneumonia, or necrotizing pneumonia. *Bronchopneumonia* (bronchial pneumonia) (Fig. 62-1B) involves the terminal bronchioles and alveoli. *Interstitial (reticular) pneumonia* involves inflammatory responses within lung tissue surrounding the air spaces or vascular structures rather than the air passages themselves. In *alveolar,* or *acinar, pneumonia*, there is fluid accumulation in a lung's distal air spaces. *Necrotizing pneumonia* causes the death of a portion of lung tissue surrounded by viable tissue; x-ray examination may reveal cavity formation at the site of necrosis. Necrotic lung tissue, which does not heal, constitutes a permanent loss of functioning parenchyma.

Outcome Management

Medical Management

Treatment of pneumonia should include specific antibiotic therapy, respiratory support as needed, nutritional support, and fluid and electrolyte management. Initial drug therapy

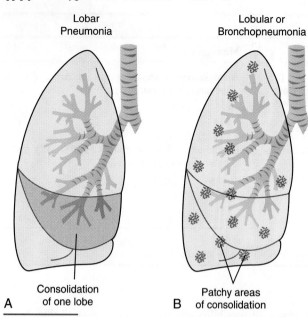

Lobar
Pneumonia

Lobular or
Bronchopneumonia

A Consolidation
of one lobe

B Patchy areas
of consolidation

FIGURE 62-1 Two types of pneumonia. *A*, Lobar pneumonia with consolidation in one lobe of one lung. *B*, Lobular or bronchopneumonia with patchy consolidation throughout lobes of one or both lungs.

should consist of broad-spectrum antibiotics until the specific organism has been identified (see Table 62-1). Oxygen should be administered as ordered, and bronchodilator medications, postural drainage, chest physiotherapy, and tracheal suctioning may be used to maintain airway patency.

■ Nursing Management of the Medical Client

ASSESSMENT

The nursing history should explore the following areas with the client in whom pneumonia is suspected or confirmed:

- Contact with other clients experiencing similar manifestations (suggests viral or mycoplasmal pneumonia)
- Factors suggesting the presence of noninfectious diseases that produce manifestations similar to those of pneumonia (e.g., pulmonary embolism, allergic reaction to drugs or other substances, neoplasm)
- Presence of tuberculosis or contact with others who have active tuberculosis
- Presence and character of any chest pain
- Presence and character of cough and sputum production

Perform respiratory assessment every 4 hours, including determination of the rate and character of respirations, auscultation of breath sounds, and assessment of skin and nail beds to determine the severity of hypoxia. In addition to the physical examination, transcutaneous oxygen level analysis or ABG measurements may be used to evaluate the need for oxygen support.

DIAGNOSIS, PLANNING, INTERVENTIONS

Nursing diagnoses common to pneumonia are described here. Other applicable nursing diagnoses are: *Fluid Volume Deficit related to fever, diaphoresis, and mouth breathing; Altered Nutrition: Less Than Body Requirements related to dyspnea; Pain related to frequent cough-*

ing; and *Altered Oral Mucous Membrane related to mouth breathing and frequent cough.*

Ineffective Airway Clearance. The inflammation and increased secretions seen with pneumonia make it difficult to maintain a patent airway. An appropriate nursing diagnosis is *Ineffective Airway Clearance related to excessive secretions and weak cough.*

Outcomes. The client will maintain effective airway clearance, as evidenced by keeping a patent airway and effectively clearing secretions.

Interventions. Take measures to promote airway patency, such as increasing fluid intake, teaching and encouraging effective coughing and deep-breathing techniques, and frequent turning. Clients with an altered level of consciousness should be turned at least every 2 hours and should be placed in side-lying positions, unless contraindicated, to prevent aspiration. Administer bronchodilating medications, if prescribed. If indicated, more aggressive measures to maintain airway patency may be required (e.g., chest physiotherapy, suctioning, artificial airway).

Ineffective Breathing Pattern. Many clients experience compensatory tachypnea because of an inability to meet metabolic demands. This occurs because affected alveoli cannot effectively exchange oxygen and carbon dioxide. Higher respiratory rates can also develop as a result of chest pain and increased body temperature. An appropriate nursing diagnosis is *Ineffective Breathing Pattern related to tachypnea.*

Outcomes. The client will have improved breathing patterns, as evidenced by (1) a respiratory rate within normal limits, (2) adequate chest expansion, (3) clear breath sounds, and (4) decreased dyspnea.

Intervention. Position the client for comfort and to facilitate breathing (e.g., raise the head of the bed 45 degrees). Teach the client how to splint the chest wall with a pillow for comfort during coughing and about the use of incentive spirometry. Administer prescribed cough suppressants and analgesics; be cautious, however, because narcotics may depress respirations more than desired. Routinely monitor respiratory rate and transcutaneous oxygen levels, auscultate the chest, and document findings. Monitor ABG values, and observe for manifestations of hypoxemia, hypercapnia, and acid-base imbalance.

Activity Intolerance. Depleted energy reserves, due to not eating during periods of dyspnea, and impairment of oxygen and carbon dioxide transport leave little oxygen to meet metabolic demands. An appropriate nursing diagnosis is *Activity Intolerance related to decreased oxygen levels for metabolic demands.*

Outcomes. The client will have improved activity tolerance, as evidenced by an ability to perform activities of daily living and a progressive increase in physical activity without excessive dyspnea and fatigue.

Interventions. Assess the client's baseline activity level and response to activity. Note how well the client tolerates activity by assessing for changes in respiratory and pulse rate, marked dyspnea, fatigue, pallor or cyanosis, and dysrhythmias. Schedule activity after treatments or medications. Use oxygen as needed. Gradually increase activity on the basis of tolerance. Balance activity with adequate rest periods.

Teach the client to avoid conditions that increase oxygen demand, such as smoking, temperature extremes, weight gain, and stress. Pursed-lip and diaphragmatic breathing, as well as techniques to lower energy use, should be reinforced. Activities that are tiring should be interspersed with rest.

Provide psychological support and a quiet environment to reduce anxiety and promote rest. Regulate nursing care and visitors as warranted by the client's condition.

Pneumonia is a very common reason for hospital admission. Many institutions provide care using Care Maps. (See the Case Management feature on pneumonia.)

EVALUATION

The level the client will probably attain is monitored every 2 to 3 days. Pneumonia should resolve quickly once the client is receiving antibiotics, provided there are no immune disorders. Older clients may require additional time to fully recover.

PREVENTION

Prevention is the best defense against the spread of pneumonia. When caring for hospitalized clients, (1) wash hands frequently, (2) use gloves appropriately, (3) encourage fluid intake, (4) turn clients every 2 hours, and (5) control clients' pain so they may breathe deeply and cough adequately. Encourage clients to use their incentive spirometer frequently. For clients who have difficulty swallowing or have nasogastric tubes, raise the head of the bed 45 degrees to decrease the risk of aspiration.

▇ Self-Care

Clients with pneumonia who are ambulatory but have an ongoing health problem may require hospitalization. For clients with intact defense mechanisms and good general health, recuperation can often take place at home with rest and supportive treatment; the term "walking pneumonia" is sometimes used to describe this situation.

Chest physiotherapy may be performed for a pre-

CASE MANAGEMENT

Pneumonia

Community-acquired pneumonia may be treated on an outpatient basis, but this is also a very common inpatient diagnosis. Hospitalization should be considered for (1) clients over 65 years of age (2) clients with other risk factors (underlying chronic obstructive lung disease, heart failure, cardiorespiratory disease), (3) immunocompromised clients, or (4) clients with diabetes or cancer, since infection can pose a serious threat. Many facilities have developed clinical pathways for pneumonia.

Critical issues for case management are as follows:

● Obtaining culture specimens promptly before administration of antibiotics
● Administering the first dose of appropriate antibiotic as soon as possible
● Conversion from intravenous (IV) antibiotics to oral administration on day 2 or 3 (depending on decreased white blood cell count, afebrile status, and ability to take fluids).

Assess

● Has there been outpatient treatment with antibiotics that would void culture results?
● Does your baseline assessment give clues to atypical pneumonia or another condition causing concern (atrial fibrillation, pulmonary embolus)?
● Is this client at risk for aspiration, or are there other conditions that may require special monitoring (e.g., blood glucose level, arterial blood gas values)?
● Is the pneumonia bilateral?
● Has the client been admitted often for pneumonia or related problems?
● Does the client smoke, use oxygen, or receive respiratory therapy at home?

Advocate

Clients, especially older adults, may present in a weakened, debilitated state. Cognitive impairments may be worsened by the lack of oxygen, sometimes resulting in labeling of a client as "confused."

Monitor cognitive functioning as the pneumonia diminishes, and remember that a different environment and sensory impairments can also affect the client's behavior.

Encourage movement and exercise between rest periods to prevent worsening of the pneumonia. Administer antibiotics at prescribed intervals, watching for side effects, especially allergic reaction or gastrointestinal problems. Provide liquids, and monitor any swallowing difficulty. Monitor fluid balance (IV and oral fluids) closely, especially if the client is at risk for heart failure. Frequent, small meals may be better tolerated when breathing is difficult.

Talk with clients about how they are managing at home. What caregiver support is available? Will financial needs prevent the client from obtaining needed medications?

Prevent Readmission

● Teach clients about their condition, and encourage completion of an oral antibiotics course at home.
● Emphasize that antibiotics must never be "saved" or shared with other family members.
● Check the status of influenza and pneumonia immunizations; administer as appropriate.
● Teach avoidance of crowded areas as well as handwashing and secretion disposal.
● Wean the client from oxygen as soon as feasible, and test saturation levels during rest and activity.
● Validate that the client knows how to use any equipment or devices (nebulizer, oxygen, metered dose inhaler) and that the client is familiar with cleaning and safety measures.
● Consider appropriate referrals for home care, pulmonary rehabilitation, and smoking cessation.
● Ensure that the client knows when to follow up with his or her physician any clinical manifestations that require immediate intervention.

Cheryl Noetscher, RN, MS, *Director of Case Management, Crouse Hospital and Community–General Hospital, Syracuse, New York*

scribed period. The client is monitored in a clinic setting until the chest x-ray clears and clinical manifestations abate. Encourage the client to plan for influenza immunization each winter. People who live with the client are also monitored for the onset of pneumonia.

LUNG ABSCESS

Lung abscess is a collection of pus within lung tissue. In its early stages, the abscess resembles a localized pneumonia. If a lung abscess remains unidentified and untreated, tissue necrosis may occur. Lung abscesses are becoming more rare as a result of improved treatment of pneumonia and effective preventive care of clients at high risk for aspiration. Today, abscesses are most often a result of anaerobic bacteria.

Single lung abscesses usually occur distal to a bronchial obstruction. They nearly always create putrid (foul) material. The bronchial obstruction may be due to:

- Aspirated foreign material (e.g., vomitus, mucus, teeth, blood, food, or tissue from upper airway surgery)
- Benign or malignant tumors

Multiple lung abscesses can follow pneumonia caused by necrotizing bacteria (such as *Staphylococcus aureus*, which creates necrotic lung tissue). Bacteria may also arise from septic emboli from infected foci, such as septic phlebitis. Immunosuppressed clients and clients who may aspirate foreign material are at high risk for lung abscesses.

Early assessment findings in a client with a lung abscess are the same as those in a client with bronchopneumonia (i.e., chills, fever, pleuritic pain, cough with abundant sputum). The body attempts to wall off the abscess with fibrous tissue. If the attempt is unsuccessful, the abscess ruptures into a bronchus, causing a cough that produces copious amounts of sputum. The sputum is purulent, foul-smelling, and foul-tasting. After bronchial rupture, hemoptysis often occurs. Chest auscultation reveals decreased breath sounds and dullness to percussion over the affected area. Crackles may be present when the abscess drains.

The diagnosis is commonly confirmed by chest radiography or computed tomography (CT) scan. Sputum cultures assist with identification of the organism.

Outcome Management

Antibiotics are prescribed on the basis of culture results. Although bronchoscopy was once believed to be essential in managing lung abscesses, it is now reserved for clients whose disease fails to improve or who may have malignancy. Surgery is seldom needed because of the success of antibiotic therapy.

Caring for a client with a lung abscess is similar to caring for a client experiencing pneumonia (e.g., promoting hydration, teaching effective cough techniques, and administering postural drainage). Lung abscesses produce copious volumes of sputum. Nursing intervention focuses on removing sputum from the lungs through postural drainage and expectoration. Note the color, quantity, quality, and smell of the expectorated material, including the presence of blood. Use gloves when handling articles contaminated with sputum.

GUIDE TO CLINICAL PATHWAY

Pneumonia

Treatment of the client with pneumonia begins immediately. The care map delineates care beginning 2 hours after admission because immediate treatment has been shown to reduce morbidity. The entire hospital stay is projected as 4 days.

The critical element in early care is to initiate antibiotics. Broad-spectrum intravenous antibiotics are prescribed and must be started within 2 hours of admission, after the drawing of blood for culture analysis, even if no sputum culture specimen has been collected. Then more specific antibiotics are prescribed according to the type of organism being eradicated. Once antibiotics are started, it is expected that the client's dyspnea will improve and that needs for oxygen to maintain oxygen saturation greater than 92% will decrease. Within the first 24 hours, the client is helped to sit in a chair or to walk three times a day. During periods of activity, assess for oxygen desaturation. Use the portable pulse oximetry instrument to continuously monitor oxygen saturation in response to activity.

On day 2 or 3, antibiotics are changed to oral routes if the client has improved clinically, is taking oral foods and fluids, and is afebrile. It is important to instruct the client to complete the entire course of antibiotics after discharge.

The CareMap is reprinted with permission from Baptist Health System.

The CareMap shown is an excerpt of one that covers emergency department to 24 hours.

Helen Andrews, BSN, RN, *Care Manager, Alegent Health Bergan Mercy Medical Center, Omaha, Nebraska,* and **Linda R. Haddick, MSN, RN,** *Clinical Nurse Specialist, Alegent Health Home Care & Hospice, Omaha, Nebraska*

The sputum may have a foul taste. Provide frequent opportunities for the client to use mouthwash, brush the teeth, and floss. Because long-term antibiotic administration is usually necessary, observe oral mucous membranes for indications of *Candida albicans* overgrowth (i.e., white, cheesy patches). Encourage long-term dental care. Oral nystatin (which the client swishes around the mouth and swallows) may be ordered.

Antibiotic therapy for a lung abscess may be needed for 8 weeks or longer. Clients with lung abscesses must understand the importance of compliance with the medication schedule. The entire course of antibiotics must be taken. Teaching about medications should cover (1) the reasons for taking them, (2) specific directions, such as time of day, frequency, and when to take in relation to food, (3) potential side effects, and (4) what to do if side effects occur. Reassessment after the antibiotics course is completed (e.g., with culture of sputum or chest films) is essential to evaluate the effectiveness of treatment.

PULMONARY TUBERCULOSIS

Tuberculosis (TB) is one of the two most prominent mycobacterial diseases known to humankind. Currently, TB

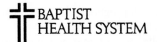
BAPTIST
HEALTH SYSTEM

PNEUMONIA CAREMAP
ER 0-2 HRS. AND ER 2-24 HRS.

(Addressograph)

	ER 0-2 HOURS Date: _____	INITIAL Met	Not Met	ER 2-24 HOURS Date: _____	INITIAL Met	Not Met
General Safety:	Bed rails up x 2, airway precautions, call bell within reach, bed in low position.			Bed rails up x 2, airway precautions, call bell within reach, bed in low position.		
Activity	Up ad lib	___	___	Up ad lib in chair or ambulating at least TID.		
				Goal: Activity Plan established.	___	___
Dietary: Consult Date/Time Completed _____	Diet type _____			Diet type _____		
	Goal: Tolerates > 50% diet.	___	___	**Goal:** Tolerates > 50% diet. 1500-2000cc fluid intake / 24 hr.	___	___
Respiratory: Consult Date/Time Completed _____	SaO2 _____ On (RA) O2 per protocol.			O2 per protocol. Instruct in use of MDI with spacer if indicated.		
	Goal: O2 Sat. > or = 92% Reduced or no respiratory distress.	___	___	**Goal:** O2 Sat. > or = 92%	___	___
Rehab: Consult Date/Time Completed _____						
Discharge Planning: Consult Date/Time Completed _____	Anticipated disposition TCF ___ NH ___ HOME ___ REHAB ___ OTHER ___			Assess discharge needs Refer to Case Management if indicated		
	Goal: Discharge needs identifed	___	___	**Goal:** Discharge needs identified.	___	___
Nursing: Consult Date/Time Completed _____	Elevate head of bed. IV fluids ___ at ___ ml/hr or IV saline lock. **Initial dose of IV ABX within 2 hours. DO NOT hold ABX's awaiting collection of sputum specimen.** Instruct in appropriate method of sputum specimen collection. Notify MD if temp > 101.5 if respiration are > 30, SBP < 100.			I&O q 8 hr (D/C when IV fluids stopped D/C IV fluids if tolerating adequate po fluid intake. Elevate head of bed. IV fluids ___ at ___ ml/hr or IV saline lock. If on Vancomycin or Aminoglycoside refer to protocol. Notify MD of temp >101.5, if resp. > 30, SBP < 100. Instruct to cough/deep breathe q 2 hrs. while awake. Encourage increased oral fluid intake. Provide/review patient/family caremap		
	Goal: Initial ABX administered within 2 hrs of arrival. Able to clear upper airway. Able to collect sputum specimen. Sputum specimen acceptable.	___ ___	___ ___	**Goal:** Able to clear upper airway.	___	___
Tests:	CBC, with differential S7, EKG CXR, PA Lateral view, if not already done Blood cultures from 2 sites (prior to 1st dose of ABX) Sputum C&S and gram stain per protocoll					
	Goal: Blood cultures obtained prior to ABX.	___	___			
Other:	Avoid oral antacids if receiving po Quinolones (Consider H2 Blockers).			Pharmacist to review results of gram stain. Avoid oral antacids if receiving PO Quinolones (Consider H2 blocker)		

PNEUMONIA CAREMAP

G-99-5043-2 PG REV. 5/4/99

kills more people than any other infectious disease in the world.[4] Before the development of anti-TB drugs in the late 1940s, TB was the leading cause of all deaths in the United States. Drug therapy, along with improvements in public health and general living standards, resulted in a marked decline in incidence over the next three decades. However, between 1985 and 1992, the number of reported TB cases increased by 20%. This increase was attributed to the emergence of the human immunodeficiency virus (HIV) epidemic, recent influxes of immigrants from developing Third World countries, and the deterioration of the nation's health care infrastructure. As a result of renewed efforts at prevention and detection, the number of TB cases is currently declining below the 1985 rate.[42]

There are two prevalent public health concerns in the

United States related to TB. First is the rise in cases of TB due to infection by multidrug-resistant organisms (MDR-TB), which are extremely difficult to treat. It is believed that resistance develops because people either stop taking their medication once they begin to feel well or are noncompliant with treatment as a result of other health problems, such as substance abuse.

The second public health concern is that clients with HIV infection are particularly susceptible to TB because *Mycobacterium tuberculosis*, the organism causing TB, is an extremely *opportunistic* pathogen. In some HIV-seropositive populations, the TB infection rate is 1000-fold higher than the annual rate in the United States. Clients with HIV are at greater risk for acquiring a new infection with rapid progression to active disease or for experiencing reinfection from dormant lesions.

Etiology and Risk Factors

TB is a communicable disease caused by *M. tuberculosis*, an aerobic, acid-fast bacillus (AFB). Tuberculosis is an airborne infection. In nearly all instances, tuberculosis infection is acquired by inhalation of a particle small enough (1 to 5 mm in diameter) to reach the alveolus. Droplets are emitted during coughing, talking, laughing, sneezing, or singing. Infected droplet nuclei may then be inhaled by a susceptible person (host). Before pulmonary infection can occur, the inhaled organisms must resist the lung's defense mechanisms and actually penetrate lung tissue.

Brief exposure to TB does not usually cause infection. People most commonly infected are those who have repeated close contact with an infected person whose disease is not yet diagnosed. Such people include anyone who has repeated contacts with medically underserved clients, low-income populations, foreign-born people, or residents of long-term care facilities or institutional settings. Other high-risk populations are intravenous drug users, homeless people, and people who are occupationally exposed to active TB (health care workers).

In countries that do not have public health programs and those in which TB commonly occurs in cattle, humans may experience bovine TB after drinking raw milk from infected cattle. This form of TB can be prevented by pasteurizing milk and maintaining tuberculin skin-testing programs for cattle.

Pathophysiology

PRIMARY (FIRST) INFECTION

The first time a client is infected with TB, the disease is said to be a *primary infection*. Primary TB infections are usually located in the apices of the lungs or near the pleurae of the lower lobes. Although a primary infection may be only microscopic (and hence may not appear on x-ray), the following sequence of events is typically observed.

A small area of bronchopneumonia develops in the lung tissue. Many of the infecting tubercle bacilli are phagocytosed (ingested) by wandering macrophages. However, before the development of hypersensitivity and immunity, many of the bacilli may survive within these blood cells and may be carried into regional bronchopulmonary (hilar) lymph nodes via the lymphatic system.

The bacilli may even spread throughout the body. Thus, the infection, although small, spreads rapidly.

The primary infection site may or may not undergo a process of necrotic degeneration (*caseation*), which produces cavities filled with a cheese-like mass of tubercle bacilli, dead white blood cells (WBCs), and necrotic lung tissue. In time, this material liquifies, may drain into the tracheobronchial tree, and may be coughed up. The air-filled cavities remain and may be detected on an x-ray.

Most primary tubercles heal over a period of months by forming scars and then calcified lesions, also known as Ghon tubercles. These lesions may contain living bacilli that can be reactivated, even after many years, and cause secondary infection.

Primary TB infections cause the body to develop an allergic reaction to tubercle bacilli or their proteins. This cell-mediated immune response appears in the form of sensitized T cells and is detectable as a positive reaction to a tuberculin skin test. The development of this tuberculin sensitivity occurs in all body cells 2 to 6 weeks after the primary infection. It is maintained as long as living bacilli remain in the body. This acquired immunity usually inhibits further growth of the bacilli and the development of active infection.

The reason active TB disease develops in some clients (instead of being controlled by the acquired immune response and thereby remaining dormant) is poorly understood. However, factors that seem to play a role in the progression from a dormant TB infection to active disease are (1) advanced age, (2) HIV infection, (3) immunosuppression, (4) prolonged corticosteroid therapy, (5) malabsorption syndromes, (6) low body weight (10% or more below ideal weight), (7) substance abuse, (8) presence of other diseases (e.g., diabetes mellitus, end-stage renal disease, or malignancy), and (9) genetic predisposition.

SECONDARY INFECTION

In addition to progressive primary disease, reinfection may also lead to a clinical form of active TB, or secondary infection. Primary sites of infection containing TB bacilli may remain latent for years and then may be reactivated if the client's resistance is lowered. Because reinfection is possible and because dormant lesions may be reactivated, it is extremely important for clients who have had a TB infection to be reassessed periodically for new evidence of active disease.

Clinical Manifestations

The detection and diagnosis of TB are achieved through subjective assessment findings and objective test results. The diagnosis can be difficult because TB mimics many other diseases and may occur concurrently with other pulmonary diseases. Nurses and other health care providers should maintain a high index of suspicion for TB in high-risk clients.

The history includes assessing the probability of recent or past exposure to TB as well as the client's occupation, other usual activities, and travel to or residence in countries with a high incidence of TB. A history of exposure to TB is certainly important, but most clients are unaware of exposure. It is advisable to determine whether the client has been previously tested for TB and to obtain the results of that testing.

Figure 62–2 shows the logical progression of the diagnosis and management of TB. Typical findings in pulmonary TB are (1) nonproductive or productive cough, (2) fatigue, (3) anorexia (loss of appetite) and weight loss, (4) low-grade fever, (5) chills and sweats (often at night), (6) dyspnea, (7) hemoptysis, (8) chest pain that may be pleuritic or dull, and (9) chest tightness. Crackles may be present on auscultation.

Primary TB infections may remain unrecognized because they are relatively asymptomatic. Calcified lesions on chest x-ray and a positive skin test reaction are frequently the only indications that a primary TB infection has occurred. Most clients harbor tubercle bacilli for life and never experience active disease because their body defenses are adequate to arrest primary infection. The tubercles heal through fibrosis and calcification. However, infected people face a 10% risk that the primary infection will progress to active disease sometime in their lives. In this situation, the primary complex sites progress and worsen, possibly causing cavitation and the spread of active infection, and the client becomes clinically ill.

Diagnostic Findings

TUBERCULIN SKIN TESTING

Tuberculin skin testing, typically the Mantoux test, is performed on a routine basis in high-risk groups when active TB is suspected. Mantoux testing uses purified protein derivative (PPD) tuberculin to identify TB infection. A small amount of the derivative is administered intradermally to form a wheal in the lower left forearm. The wheal must be examined ("read") in 48 to 72 hours by a trained professional. The presence of induration, not erythema, indicates a positive test result as follows[19]:

- More than 5 mm of induration is considered a positive result for clients with known or suspected HIV infection, intravenous drug users, people in close contact with a known case of TB, and the client with a chest x-ray suggestive of previous TB.
- More than 10 mm of induration is considered positive for clients in all other high-risk groups.
- 15 mm or more of induration is considered positive for clients in low-risk groups.

False-positive reactions to tuberculin skin testing can occur in clients who have other mycobacterial infections or who have received the bacille Calmette-Guérin (BCG) vaccination. False-negative reactions are also possible, especially in people who are immunosuppressed or anergic (impaired ability to react to antigens). For these clients, and for anyone who has a positive skin test reaction, the AFB sputum smear examination and chest x-ray are used to identify active disease. It is critical to initiate respiratory isolation of such clients until AFB sputum results are known.

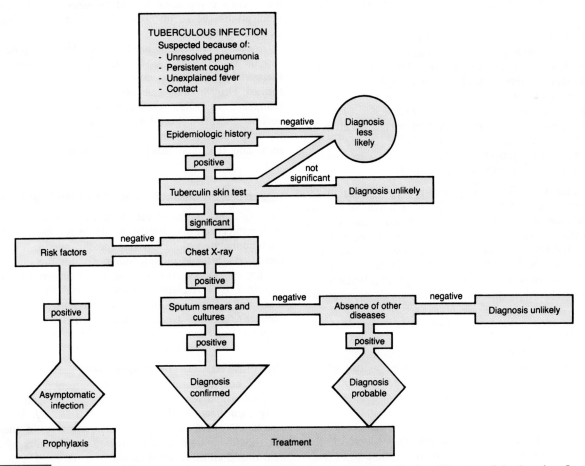

FIGURE 62–2 Algorithm for diagnosis and management of tuberculosis: a logical progression. (Courtesy of the American Lung Association, The Christmas Seal People.)

The term *tuberculin converter* refers to a client who does not show radiologic or bacteriologic evidence of pulmonary TB but whose tuberculin skin test "converts" from a known negative reaction to a known positive reaction. Keep in mind that the absence of a positive (reactive) tuberculin test result does not always mean that TB is absent.

ACID-FAST BACILLUS SMEAR AND CULTURE

A more definitive diagnosis of TB is made from the AFB smear and culture. Three different sputum specimens should be collected on three consecutive mornings. Sputum AFB smears are not extremely sensitive, but the positive result of a sputum AFB smear confirms active disease. A more reliable indicator is a positive culture for *M. tuberculosis*, which does confirm active TB; however, final culture results may not be available for 2 to 12 weeks. Although newer detection tests can generate faster results and show clinical promise, the prevalence of MDR-TB still mandates the use of traditional culture methods for diagnosis.

Outcome Management

■ Medical Management

Most people with newly diagnosed active TB are not hospitalized. If pulmonary TB is diagnosed in the hospitalized client, the client may be kept in the hospital until therapeutic drug levels are established. Some clients with active TB may be hospitalized for the following reasons:

- They are acutely ill.
- Their living situation is considered a high risk.
- They are thought to be noncompliant with therapy.
- They have a history of previous TB and noncompliance, and the disease has been reactivated.
- Concomitant diseases are present and acute.
- Improvement does not occur after treatment.
- The organisms are highly resistant to the usual treatment, requiring second-line or third-line drugs. In this situation, brief hospitalization is necessary to monitor the effects and side effects of the drugs.

Treatment of TB is a long-term process that should be initiated immediately upon suspicion of infection. Clients with a diagnosis of active TB are usually started on a minimum of two or three medications to ensure elimination of the resistant organisms. The dose of some drugs may initially be large because the bacilli are difficult to kill. Treatment continues long enough to eliminate or substantially reduce the number of dormant or semidormant bacilli.

Medications used for TB may include *first-line* and *second-line* agents (Table 62–2). Primary agents are almost always initially prescribed until results of culture and sensitivity tests are available. In clients with a previous history of incomplete TB treatment, resistant organisms may have developed and secondary agents are used.

The U.S. Centers for Disease Control and Prevention (CDC) currently recommends a two-phase approach for treatment, consisting of (1) an *intensive* phase using two or three drugs, aimed at destroying large numbers of rapidly multiplying organisms and (2) a *maintenance* phase, usually using two drugs, directed at eliminating most remaining bacilli.

The recommended basic treatment regimen for previously untreated clients is 2 months of daily doses of isoniazid and rifampin, plus one or two other drugs, depending on type of organism. This treatment is followed with 4 months of isoniazid and rifampin. Ethambutol or streptomycin may also be used initially until culture and sensitivity test results are obtained and the correct medications are identified. The length of time a client remains infectious varies. Sputum cultures and clinical responses (absence of fever and dyspnea, reduction in cough) are used to evaluate the effectiveness of the therapy.

If compliance with daily dosing is a problem, some TB protocols call for administration of medications two or three times a week rather than daily. Additionally, clients may be assigned to receive *directly observed therapy* (DOT). Such a program is administered in a clinic or physician's office to ensure that clients ingest each dose of medication. In some cities, a noncompliant client may be confined to a hospital or other institution for treatment, according to that city's law. Completion of treatment is critical because incomplete treatment leads to reactivation of TB and the development of drug-resistant strains of TB.

If the medication regimen does not seem effective (e.g., worsening manifestations, continued presence of AFB in sputum, increasing infiltrates or cavity formation on x-ray), the treatment program needs reevaluation, and the client's compliance should be assessed. At least two medications (never just one) are added to a failing TB treatment program.

Because medications used to treat TB have potentially serious side effects (see Table 62–2), baseline studies (depending on the specific drugs prescribed) are performed. Drug toxicity can limit the treatment of TB. Drug tolerance, drug effect, and drug toxicity depend on factors such as the medication dosage, the time since last dosage, the medication's chemical formula, and the client's age, renal and intestinal function, and compliance with treatment.

■ Nursing Management of the Medical Client

Nursing management of the client with TB includes many of the interventions already discussed for the client with pneumonia, depending on the specific nursing diagnoses identified. Possible nursing diagnoses for the client with TB are as follows: *Anxiety; Ineffective Airway Clearance; Impaired Gas Exchange; Pain; Altered Nutrition: Less than Body Requirements; Ineffective Individual Coping; Ineffective Family Coping; Altered Health Maintenance; Knowledge Deficit related to treatment or noncompliance;* and *Sleep Pattern Disturbance.*

PREVENTION OF TRANSMISSION

During hospitalization, appropriate infection control and hospital employee health practices are essential. First, early identification of clients with TB is key. High-risk clients and clients with clinical manifestations of pneumonia should be immediately isolated until results of AFB smears and cultures are obtained.

Private respiratory isolation rooms should be available. These rooms should be maintained at negative pressure

TABLE 62-2	NURSING IMPLICATIONS FOR MEDICATIONS USED TO TREAT TUBERCULOSIS			
Medication and Dosage	**Actions**	**Methods to Evaluate Therapeutic Outcomes**	**Methods to Evaluate Adverse Outcomes**	**Nursing Considerations**
FIRST-LINE AGENTS				
Isoniazid (INH) 5 mg/kg/day up to 300 mg PO	Unknown; may cause inhibition of myocolic acid synthesis, resulting in disruption of the bacterial cell wall	Decrease of symptoms (cough, night sweats, fever) Fewer bacilli on sputum smear	Monitor hepatic enzymes during the first 3 months of treatment and in clients who are older than 35 years or are alcohol abusers Perform initial eye examination and repeat if visual problems occur	Can cause fatigue, weakness, anorexia, malaise Must be taken on an empty stomach When administered with phenytoin, may lead to phenytoin toxicity
Rifampin (Rifadin) 10 mg/kg/day up to 600 mg PO	Inhibits bacterial RNA synthesis	Decrease of symptoms (cough, night sweats, fever) Fewer bacilli on sputum smear	Use of alcohol or INH increases risk of hepatotoxicity Periodic monitoring of hepatic enzymes required	Should be taken on empty stomach; however, may be taken with meals if severe GI symptoms occur Reduces levels of many drugs; methadone, theophylline, oral contraceptives, oral antidiabetics, oral anticoagulants, protease inhibitors, non-nucleoside reverse transcriptase inhibitors
Rifapentine (Priftin) 600 mg twice weekly PO	Bactericidal activity against intracellular and extracellular *Mycobacterium tuberculosis*	Decrease of symptoms (cough, night sweats, fever) Fewer bacilli on sputum smear	Increases the metabolism of indinavir sulfate (Crixivan), protease inhibitor used in clients with AIDS Monitor hepatic and serum uric acid levels monthly	May turn body secretions red-orange Must be taken with food, as nausea, vomiting, and GI upset are possible Reduces effects of warfarin, phenytoin, sildenafil, oral antiarrhythmics, oral contraceptives, oral antidiabetic agents
SECOND-LINE AGENTS				
Capreomycin or kanamycin 15–30 mg/kg up to 1 g IM	Polypeptide antibiotic	Decrease of symptoms (cough, night sweats, fever) Fewer bacilli on sputum smear	Observe for ototoxicity by obtaining baseline audiology parameters and nephrotoxicity by obtaining baseline renal function measurements Monitor both periodically	Tell client to report dizziness and hearing loss Encourage adequate hydration
Ethionamide (Trecator-SC) 15–20 mg/kg up to 1 g PO	Inhibits peptide synthesis	Decrease of symptoms (cough, night sweats, fever) Fewer bacilli on sputum smear	Observe for hepatotoxicity by obtaining baseline liver function measurements Transient increase in results may occur	Inform client of potential for distorted sense of smell and metallic taste Instruct client to report signs of hypothyroidism

AIDS, acquired immunodeficiency syndrome; GI, gastrointestinal; IM, intramuscularly; PO, by mouth; RNA, ribonucleic acid.

relative to the hallway; negative pressure keeps room air from flowing out into the hallway when the door is opened, thereby avoiding the spread of infectious particles outside the room. Negative-pressure ventilation sends room air directly to the outside, with at least six air exchanges per hour. Additional equipment, such as ultra-violet lamps (proven to kill mycobacteria) and high-efficiency particulate air (HEPA) filters, may also be used.

Personal protective equipment, called *particulate respirators*, is required for all health care workers entering a TB isolation room. When fitted properly, these respirators filter droplet nuclei; the fit of a particulate respirator should be reassessed if there is a change in the wearer's facial shape.

Monitoring health care workers' TB status is essential. Skin testing should be performed yearly in all health care workers who may be exposed to TB. Semi-annual testing should be completed in high-risk areas or where high rates of TB skin test conversion are occurring.

When a client is determined to have TB, public health officials (often nurses) talk with the client and develop a contact list. Everyone with whom the client has had contact is then assessed with a tuberculin skin test and chest x-ray to check for TB infection.

PREVENTIVE THERAPY

Between 10 and 15 million people in the United States have dormant or asymptomatic TB. Chemoprophylaxis may help many of them avoid active TB and may also prevent initial infection in people recently exposed. Isoniazid preventive therapy (IPT) consists of 300 mg of the drug daily for 6 to 12 months. IPT stops the growth of the bacilli, thus preventing active pulmonary or extrapulmonary TB. IPT is recommended for clients who:

- Are newly infected (have converted tuberculin skin test results but no other indication of active disease)
- Live or closely associate with others who have active TB
- Have significant tuberculin skin test reactions and abnormal chest x-ray findings compatible with those of inactive TB
- Have positive tuberculin skin tests and conditions (e.g., steroid therapy, diabetes mellitus, acquired immunodeficiency syndrome [AIDS]) that place them at increased risk for TB
- Are younger than 35 years of age and have significant tuberculin skin test reactions, even though they may have a normal chest x-ray and no other risk factors

▋ Self-Care

TB treatment is a long process. Nurses in clinics and public health facilities are often responsible for follow-up assessment and monitoring, including (1) determining medication compliance, (2) understanding the pharmacologic actions of medications, (3) monitoring unwanted side effects, (4) collecting follow-up sputum specimens, (5) obtaining serial chest x-rays, and (6) observing for reversal or worsening of initial assessment findings, all of which are part of the ongoing follow-up. It is essential that clients with TB, and their significant others, receive the information summarized in the Client Education Guide for Tuberculosis. Providing complete information and ongoing support helps clients understand the long-

term recovery process. The more information clients have and the more personal control they feel they have, the more likely they are to comply with treatment.

EXTRAPULMONARY TUBERCULOSIS

Extrapulmonary tuberculosis (XPTB) is TB that occurs anywhere outside the lungs. Pulmonary TB is the most common form of the disease, but after initial invasion, tubercle bacilli can spread throughout the body via the blood and lymph. *M. tuberculosis* thrives in oxygen-rich areas. Highly aerobic sites, such as the renal cortex, bone growth plates, and meninges, are where XPTB most commonly grows. It may also occur in the genitourinary tract, lymph nodes, pleurae, pericardium, abdomen, and endocrine glands.

Widespread dissemination throughout the body *(miliary tuberculosis)* involves the lungs and many other organs. It is more common in clients who are HIV-seropositive or are 50 years or older. Miliary TB may develop from delayed or late dissemination after immune system compromise in older people who were infected with TB many years earlier.

Despite the severity of the disease, XPTB is often difficult to detect. Assessment findings are frequently nondistinct. Weight loss, fatigue, malaise, fever, and night sweats may or may not be present. The only physical finding that is specific for disseminated TB is a granuloma in the choroid of the retina. Clinical manifestations may precede changes in the chest x-ray.

CLIENT EDUCATION GUIDE

Tuberculosis

- Tuberculosis (TB) is infectious, but it may be cured or arrested if you take your medication as prescribed.
- TB is transmitted by droplet infection and is not carried on articles such as clothing, books, or eating utensils. You do not need to dispose of any possessions.
- Cover your nose and mouth when coughing, laughing, or sneezing.
- Wash your hands very carefully after any contact with body substances, masks, or soiled tissues. Sputum is highly contaminated. Cough into paper tissues, and dispose of them properly.
- Wear a mask in appropriate situations as advised. Make sure the mask is tight-fitting, and change it frequently.
- Activities are usually not restricted for more than 2 to 4 weeks after medication is begun, and you should not be isolated from others as long as you are compliant with the medication therapy.
- Treatment may be needed for a long time. Take your medication exactly as prescribed, and report all side effects to your physician. Do not stop the medication for any reason without the physician's supervision. Keep an adequate supply of medication available at all times to avoid running out. Compliance with treatment is essential.
- Because TB drugs can cause serious side effects, periodic blood work will be required.

Outcome Management

The diagnosis and treatment of XPTB proceed similarly to those of pulmonary TB. However, the treatment period may be longer, and more medications may be used. Treatment depends on the extent, severity, course, and complications of the disease.

NONTUBERCULOUS MYCOBACTERIAL INFECTION

Pathophysiology

Nontuberculous mycobacteria (NTM), also known as MOTT (mycobacteria other than tubercle [bacilli]), are responsible for growing numbers of mycobacterial infections. Although NTM infection is still relatively uncommon, the following changes in disease patterns have appeared: (1) more cases, (2) wider geographical distribution, and (3) new groups of vulnerable hosts, most notably, clients with HIV infection.

NTM are widely distributed in nature (i.e., in food, standing fresh water, salt water, animal bedding, soil, animals, and birds), and most clients acquire their infections from environmental sources rather than from other diseased clients. Infection is common in the southeastern part of the United States and more prevalent in rural areas.

Etiology

The most commonly occurring NTM diseases are caused by *Mycobacterium avium* complex, *Mycobacterium kansasii*, and *Mycobacterium fortuitum*. The primary site of NTM disease is the lungs, although extrapulmonary sites (e.g., liver, spleen, lymph nodes, skin, joints) may occur. Disseminated disease with multiple organ involvement is also possible, most commonly in immunosuppressed clients.

Clinical Manifestations

Pulmonary NTM disease is very similar to TB, although the clinical manifestations may be less severe. Clinical manifestations of the disease include (1) fever, (2) anorexia, (3) night sweats, (4) diarrhea, (5) abdominal pain, and (6) weight loss. Clients with pre-existing bronchopulmonary disease (e.g., bronchiectasis, chronic obstructive pulmonary disease [COPD], or healed pulmonary TB) are at highest risk of pulmonary involvement.

Diagnosis of NTM disease is often difficult because of the widespread distribution of the organisms in the environment. Definitive diagnosis of disease is possible only if NTM are isolated from specimens collected from normally sterile sites (e.g., blood, cerebrospinal fluid, bone marrow, lymph nodes) or through biopsy. However, NTM disease is strongly suspected when (1) a client presents with a clinical syndrome that is compatible with NTM, (2) no other pathogens can be identified, and (3) repeated sputum cultures reveal large numbers of NTM.

Outcome Management

The same medications used to treat TB are prescribed for NTM disease. However, NTM are considerably more resistant to drugs than *M. tuberculosis*. Consequently, combined drug regimens and longer treatment periods are necessary. Treatment typically consists of three to six different medications and lasts for a minimum of 18 to 24 months, continuing until there are no AFB in the sputum specimens collected consecutively for a period of 1 year. As a result, adherence to medical therapy is critical. Clients are often instructed that chemotherapy will be continued for life.[14]

Unsuccessful treatment may result in further lung damage and general debilitation. Regular, daily medication is essential. The more clients understand about the condition and its management, the more likely they will be to complete the full course of medication.

Other aspects of the nursing management of NTM disease are the same as for pulmonary TB (see preceding discussion). Because these diseases are not believed to be transmitted from person to person, however, isolation and measures to control infection, other than good hygiene, are not necessary.

FUNGAL PULMONARY INFECTIONS

Most fungi that are pathogenic to humans limit their activities to the skin. However, the spores of some fungi become airborne and can be inhaled into the respiratory tract, causing pulmonary diseases that, in their chronic forms, produce granulomatous conditions similar to TB. The most common of these are coccidioidomycosis and histoplasmosis. Each has a specific geographical distribution and occurs in people living or traveling in the regions where these fungi are found. Person-to-person transmission is virtually unknown. Opportunistic fungal infections occur in clients with impaired immunity including those who require long-term high dose immunosuppressant therapy, have hematologic malignancies, or have undiagnosed HIV. In fact, histoplasmosis is often a sentinel infection, the first hint that a client is HIV infected.[16]

Coccidioidomycosis is found in the Western Hemisphere, primarily in the San Joaquin Valley of California, Utah, Nevada, New Mexico, Arizona, western Texas, and northern Mexico. The disease is most likely to develop in people engaging in desert recreational activities or working in construction or other occupations that involve digging (e.g., archaeology). The disease is mild and self-limiting in 60% of those affected. Such clients either are asymptomatic or have only mild upper respiratory assessment findings. The remaining 40% experience a syndrome similar to influenza, with cough, fever, pleuritic chest pain, myalgias, and arthralgias. *Erythema multiforme*, a flat, red rash that erupts with dark red papules, occurs in some people.

Etiology

The causative organism of *histoplasmosis*, the fungus *Histoplasma capsulatum*, is endemic to the central and eastern portions of North America, most notably the Ohio River, Missouri River, and Mississippi River valleys. It is also found in South and Central America, India, and Cyprus. This fungus lives in moist soil of appropriate chemical composition, in mushroom cellars, on the floors of chicken houses and bat caves, and in bird droppings, especially those from starlings and blackbirds.

Clinical Manifestations

As with coccidioidomycosis, *H. capsulatum* infections are usually asymptomatic or mild. Clinical manifestations include fever, fatigue, cough, dyspnea, and weight loss of 1 to 2 months in duration.

The diagnosis of fungal pulmonary diseases is usually based on history and clinical assessment findings. Skin testing is also used for coccidioidomycosis and can indicate exposure but not active infection. Chest x-rays may show hilar adenopathy (lymph gland enlargement), small areas of infiltrates, or manifestations of pneumonia. Sometimes, cavities and calcified nodules may form, usually remaining in the lungs as permanent indicators of previous infection.

A few clients may demonstrate disseminated or chronic forms of pulmonary fungal disease. When disseminated disease occurs, central nervous system, liver, spleen, gastrointestinal tract, or musculoskeletal involvement may be present. Chronic disease may result in progressive changes similar to those seen with TB. Emphysema-like pulmonary structural changes may also occur.

Outcome Management

Mild, primary forms of fungal pulmonary disease usually do not require treatment. Progressive, disseminated, or chronic forms are usually treated with intravenous amphotericin B until the client is asymptomatic for 7 to 10 days. This fungicidal antibiotic is quite toxic, and acute reactions (e.g., chills, fever, vomiting, headache, decreased renal function) may occur during its infusion. Antiemetics, antihistamines, antipyretics, or hydrocortisone may be prescribed as premedications. In order to reduce the common problem of thrombophlebitis at the intravenous site, a small amount of heparin may be added to the infusion. Ketoconazole, a less toxic oral medication, may also be used. If the disorder is not responsive to drug therapy, surgical removal of affected areas (e.g., lung cavities) may be necessary.

Nursing management in relation to fungal pulmonary infection consists of (1) providing preventive education to minimize exposure of clients to infectious fungi (i.e., learning to avoid high-risk situations and to recognize early indications of infection) and (2) appropriate support and education for infected clients and their significant others, along with symptomatic management of the disease. Education involves teaching about not only the disease and intervention measures but also reportable indications of complications.

In addition to the pathogenic fungi, common fungal spores may cause serious, potentially fatal pulmonary disease in immunocompromised people. These fungi include *Aspergillus, Blastomyces dermatitidis, Candida,* and *Cryptococcus neoformans.* These infections are also treated with amphotericin B.

CYSTIC FIBROSIS

Cystic fibrosis is a congenital restrictive lung disorder in which the secretions of the exocrine (mucus-producing) glands are abnormal. This disorder affects the sweat glands, respiratory system, digestive tract (particularly the pancreas), and reproductive tract. Cystic fibrosis is the most common inherited genetic disease in the Caucasian population, affecting approximately 1 in 2000 newborns in the United States.

Previously, this condition was considered a "pediatric problem" because it was fatal in childhood. However, advances in early diagnosis and treatment, including antibiotics, chest physiotherapy, and nutrition programs, have extended the median life expectancy into the late 20s or early 30s, with maximum survival documented as high as the seventh decade of life.[37]

Pathophysiology

The mucus-producing glands of the pancreas and lungs hypertrophy and produce excessive secretions that are thick mucoproteins. Tenacious mucus results from failure of the chloride channels to function. Decreased flow of ions and water results in viscid mucus that causes obstruction of the airway. The thick mucus also decreases action of the cilia, leading to stasis of mucus and a medium for infection.

The thick mucus plugs the glands and ducts of the pancreatic acini, intestinal glands, intrahepatic bile ducts, and the gallbladder, causing dilation and fibrosis. These changes result in decreased production of pancreatic enzymes needed for digestion of carbohydrates, fats, and proteins.

Sweat glands, salivary glands, and lacrimal glands are also affected, leading to high concentrations of sodium and chloride in these secretions.

Clinical Manifestations

Pulmonary involvement is the most common and severe manifestation of cystic fibrosis. More than 90% of clients with cystic fibrosis die of severe pulmonary disease. The disease process causes tracheobronchial secretions to become thick and viscous, leading to (1) interference with normal ciliary action, (2) plugging of airways, and (3) creation of a reservoir for bacterial growth and infection. Bronchiectasis may also develop, compounding the infection risk.

Outcome Management

The goals of therapy for cystic fibrosis are to ensure a reasonable quality of life for as long as possible and to prevent or slow the decline in pulmonary functioning. They are achieved by removing secretions, improving aeration, and administering antibiotic agents. Effective clearing of tracheobronchial secretions is promoted by (1) ensuring adequate hydration, (2) administering prescribed mucolytic aerosols, and (3) teaching and supervising effective coughing techniques, use of positive expiratory pressure devices, postural drainage, and chest vibration and percussion. Auscultate the chest before and after therapy, taking note of the quality of lung sounds and the effectiveness of therapy.

Ensure adequate aeration by following the techniques for maintaining clear airways, administering oxygen if hypoxemia is present, maintaining correct body position to facilitate breathing (i.e., sitting up), and performing exercise to improve pulmonary function. Assess the client for manifestations of hypercapnia and other indications of respiratory failure.

Antibiotic therapy has played an important role in extending the life expectancy of clients with cystic fibrosis. Oral antibiotics are often given prophylactically on a routine basis. Intravenous antibiotics are essential during acute infections. Inhaled antibiotics are also being used with more regularity. The choice of antibiotic should be determined by results of sputum culture and sensitivity testing. Infections are most commonly caused by *Pseudomonas aeruginosa,* followed by *S. aureus.* Sputum should be assessed for color, quality, and quantity. All respiratory equipment should be thoroughly cleaned on a routine basis to prevent reinfection from contaminated equipment.

Persistent pulmonary infection with *Pseudomonas* organisms is common in the end stages of cystic fibrosis. Continuous treatment with large doses of intravenous antibiotics is usually indicated. Moderate to severe hemoptysis can occur if the infection causes erosion of pulmonary blood vessels. Blood replacement and temporary cessation of postural drainage may be required.

New treatments for cystic fibrosis have shown moderate success and are still being studied for long-term effects, including:

- Use of synthetically produced DNase, an enzyme that breaks down the deoxyribonucleic acid (DNA) released from neutrophils and causes the "stickiness" of mucus
- Administration of anti-inflammatory drugs (corticosteroids and nonsteroidal anti-inflammatory drugs [NSAIDs]) to decrease the inflammatory response in the respiratory tract epithelium
- Augmentation of the immune defense with supplemental gamma-globulin
- Use of drugs that alter ion movement and thin secretions

Gene therapy is also being evaluated. Gene transfer is possible, but positive results are transient in duration.[37]

Treatment of end-stage disease is primarily concerned with the management of severe complications. Obstruction of the airways leads to a state of hyperinflation. In time, restrictive lung disease is superimposed on the obstructive disease. Pneumothorax (air in the chest cavity) develops in 20% of all adult clients, requiring lung reinflation with chest tubes.

Over time, pulmonary obstruction leads to chronic hypoxemia, hypercapnia, and acidosis. Pulmonary hypertension and, eventually, cor pulmonale may result. Treatment consists of digitalis, diuretics, and oxygen therapy. Clients with severely reduced lung function (forced expiratory volume in 1 second [FEV_1] less than 30% of predicted) whose disease no longer responds to maximal therapy and who are experiencing a decline in quality of life may be candidates for bilateral lung transplantation.

Attention to psychosocial concerns is a nursing priority throughout the course of the disease. In the adult client with cystic fibrosis, psychosocial concerns center on three major areas:

- Disease management (e.g., treatment compliance, sleep disturbance, hemoptysis, nutrition, and hospitalizations)
- Growth and development (e.g., daily activities, work, and sex and reproduction)
- Family relations (e.g., substance abuse, depression, anxiety, and marital problems)

Nursing intervention involves helping clients cope with these problem areas as well as providing emotional support to both clients and their families.

INTERSTITIAL LUNG DISEASE

Interstitial lung diseases (ILDs) comprise a group of diffuse, inflammatory lower respiratory tract disorders. The term *interstitial* is used to indicate that the interstitium of the alveolar walls is thickened and usually fibrotic. The alveolar walls thicken as a result of the accumulation of inflammatory cells. The thickened alveolus becomes nonfunctional.

Etiology

The cause of ILD is not clearly defined. It most commonly develops from idiopathic pulmonary fibrosis, sarcoidosis, and collagen-vascular disorders. ILD can also result from the inhalation of inorganic dust, such as crystalline silica, asbestos, and coal dust, or of organic dust from organisms encountered in farming, use of air conditioning, and animal husbandry. Other possible causes are radiation damage and infectious agents.

Clinical Manifestations

Manifestations of ILD are insidious and nonspecific, such as fatigue, dyspnea, and nonproductive cough. Because the clinical manifestations are nonspecific, ILD may remain undiagnosed for years. The client's history plays a major part in diagnosis because it is important to determine the agents to which the client has been exposed. Clients report progressive dyspnea and often have dyspnea at rest. Physical examination may reveal reduced chest expansion, reflected as a decrease in total lung capacity (TLC). Inspiratory and expiratory crackles are frequently heard. The crackles have a characteristic sound, like the sound of hook-and-loop tape (Velcro) being pulled apart. Clubbing of the finger tips may be present.

Diagnostic assessment includes gallium ventilation-perfusion scans. These scans usually reveal impaired perfusion in the lower lobes and multiple areas of impaired ventilation. The ventilation-perfusion mismatch results in hypoxemia and carbon dioxide retention. Bronchoscopy and biopsy may also be used to confirm ILD.

Outcome Management

Management of a client with ILD is based on the level of respiratory impairment. Inflammation is controlled with corticosteroids. Explain to the client that corticosteroids reduce further impairment but previously injured alveolar-capillary units are permanently damaged. Clients often show subjective improvement while taking steroids, dosage of which can eventually be tapered and stopped. If the offending agent is known, the initial treatment is to remove the client from exposure to the agent. As the disorder progresses, clients are usually treated with inhaled corticosteroids and bronchodilators to help mobilize secretions and oxygen during periods of exercise.

Nursing management is the same as that for clients with restrictive lung disorders.

SARCOIDOSIS

Sarcoidosis is an inflammatory condition that affects many body systems. The disease is characterized by the formation of widespread granulomatous lesions. In addition to lung involvement, which occurs in more than 90% of cases, clients may present with clinical manifestations involving the peripheral lymphatic system, skin, liver, eyes, spleen, bones, salivary glands, joints, nervous system, and heart.

The onset of sarcoidosis is generally between ages 20 and 40 years. The disorder is approximately 14 times more common in African Americans than in Caucasians. Although the male-to-female ratio is about even in the non–African American population, African American women have sarcoidosis twice as frequently as African American men.

Etiology

The cause of sarcoidosis remains unknown, but the disease itself is becoming more fully understood. It is suggested that a triggering agent, which may be genetic, infectious, immunologic, or toxic, stimulates enhanced cell-mediated immune processes at the site of involvement. A series of interactions between T lymphocytes and monocytes-macrophages leads to the formation of *noncaseating* (i.e., having no cheesy necrotic degeneration) granulomas, which are characteristic of the disease. Granuloma formation may regress with therapy or as a result of the disorder's natural course but may also progress to fibrosis and restrictive lung disease. In chronic cases, approximately 10% of clients die of the disease.

Clinical Manifestations

Of clients with sarcoidosis, 30% to 60% are asymptomatic, and the diagnosis is confirmed by chest x-ray.[23] Clients who have pulmonary manifestations usually present with a dry cough and shortness of breath. Chest pain, hemoptysis, or pneumothorax may also be present. Systemic manifestations include fatigue, weakness, malaise, weight loss, and fever. A definitive diagnosis of sarcoidosis is made from tissue biopsy. When lung involvement is suspected, bronchoscopy, bronchoalveolar lavage, mediastinoscopy, or open lung biopsy may be performed.

Outcome Management

Medical management is primarily determined by the extent to which the client's life is disturbed by the manifestations experienced. If the client with sarcoidosis is asymptomatic, management involves ongoing assessment for further disease progression. Obtaining chest x-rays at 6-month intervals is often indicated. When manifestations are present, medical treatment usually consists of systemic corticosteroids to suppress the immune process and often leads to dramatic improvement.

Nursing intervention in clients with sarcoidosis is the same as that in clients with other restrictive lung diseases and hypoxemia. Assess for drug side effects, especially adverse responses to corticosteroids (such as weight gain, change in mood, development of diabetes mellitus). Also assess for signs of improvement, such as increased exercise tolerance, disappearance of initial assessment findings, improved pulmonary function studies, and better oxygenation. If assessment findings worsen, document them, and notify the physician.

NEOPLASTIC LUNG DISORDERS

MALIGNANT LUNG TUMORS

Lung cancer is malignancy in the epithelium of the respiratory tract. At least a dozen different cell types of tumors are included in the classification of lung cancer. The four major types of lung cancer are

- Small cell carcinoma (oat cell carcinoma)
- Squamous cell carcinoma (epidermoid)
- Adenocarcinoma
- Large cell carcinoma

There is no current effective screening test for lung cancer, and the range of treatment options is limited, resulting in frequent poor prognoses. Lung cancer is the leading cause of cancer deaths both in the United States and worldwide. The term *lung cancer* excludes other disorders, such as sarcoma, lymphoma, blastoma, and mesothelioma.

Etiology and Risk Factors

Cigarette smoking is by far the most important risk factor for lung cancer. Ninety per cent of clients who experience lung cancer are, or have been, smokers. Cigarette smoke contains several organ-specific carcinogens. Other carcinogens are inhaled toxins, such as asbestos, arsenic, and pollutants. Genetic predisposition to the development of lung cancer also plays a role in the etiology, as does age, with lung cancer rarely occurring in people younger than 40 years. Finally, TB and low-level radiation are risks for lung cancer.

Pathophysiology

Lung cancers are divided into two major categories: (1) small cell lung cancers (SCLCs) and (2) non–small cell lung cancers (NSCLCs), which include squamous cell carcinoma, adenocarcinoma, and large cell carcinoma. The characteristics of each of these types are described in Table 62–3. In general, survival rates are best for NSCLC, especially with treatment in the early stages. Despite growing knowledge and improving technology, however, overall survival of lung cancer remains low, especially for clients with small cell carcinomas.

Tumor cells grow and invade surrounding lung tissue. The cancerous lung tissue cannot exchange oxygen and carbon dioxide. Airways are invaded, obstructing the flow of air.

TABLE 62-3	OVERVIEW OF MALIGNANT PULMONARY NEOPLASMS		
Cell Type	Approximate Incidence	Specific Characteristics	Growth Rate
Epidermoid (squamous cell)	30%–35%	Arises from bronchial epithelium As growth occurs, cavitation may develop in lung distal to tumor; Pancoast's tumor arises in apex and upper lung zones Secondary infections distal to obstructive tumor in bronchioles frequently occur	Slow growth with metastasis not common If metastasis occurs, usually to lymph, adrenals, and liver
Adenocarcinoma	35%–40%	Majority arises from bronchial mucous gland Often subpleural; rarely cavitates; often arises in previously scarred lung tissue Incidence strongly linked to cigarette smoking Increasing incidence in women Bronchioloalveolar cell carcinoma is a subtype	Slow growth Can metastasize throughout lung or to other organs of the body
Large cell	15%–20%	More often peripheral mass, either single or multiple masses Cavitation common May be located centrally, midlung, or peripherally Rare hilar involvement Often grows to large tumor mass before diagnosis	Slow Metastasis may occur to kidney, liver, and adrenals
Small cell (oat cell)	20%–25%	65%–75% manifest as hilar or central mass May compress bronchi Involvement of diaphragm through paralysis of phrenic nerve and hoarseness through paralysis of recurrent laryngeal nerve Pleural and pericardial effusions and tamponade often seen Does not form cavities	Rapid growth Metastasis to mediastinum and to thoracic and extrathoracic structures occurs early

Clinical Manifestations

The warning signals of lung cancer are presented in Box 62-2. In many instances, lung cancer may mimic other pulmonary conditions. Extrapulmonary manifestations may occur before pulmonary manifestations. Specific clinical assessment findings vary according to tumor type, location, and extent as well as pre-existing pulmonary health.

Centrally located pulmonary tumors usually obstruct air flow, producing clinical manifestations such as coughing, wheezing, stridor, and dyspnea. As obstruction increases, bronchopulmonary infection often occurs distal to the obstruction. Chest, shoulder, arm, and back pain may develop as the tumor invades the perivascular nerves. Squamous and small cell tumors often cause hemoptysis. Small cell tumors may also extend into the pericardium, causing pericardial effusion and, possibly, tamponade. Cardiac dysrhythmias are also likely.

Diagnostic Findings

Central pulmonary tumors are easiest to locate and identify with fiberoptic bronchoscopy and sputum cytologic study. During bronchoscopy, bronchial washings or

---

BOX 62-2   Warning Signals of Lung Cancer

- Any change in respiratory patterns
- Persistent cough
- Sputum streaked with blood
- Frank hemoptysis
- Rust-colored or purulent sputum
- Unexplained weight loss
- Chest, shoulder, back, or arm pain
- Recurring episodes of pleural effusion, pneumonia, or bronchitis
- Unexplained dyspnea

brushings are performed to obtain tumor cells for cytologic and pathologic study. Positive tissue diagnosis is possible 90% of the time.

Peripheral pulmonary tumors often do not produce early assessment findings. In time, pleural pain develops that increases on inspiration, is sharp and severe, and is usually localized. Pleural effusion (see later) also occurs and, along with the pain, limits lung expansion. Only 30% of peripheral lung tumors are successfully categorized by bronchoscopic and cytologic examination.

Pancoast's tumor occurs in the apices of the lungs in both squamous cell and adenocarcinomatous cancers. The tumor is asymptomatic until it extends into surrounding structures. Clinical manifestations are caused by compression of the brachial plexus in the distribution from the eighth cervical nerve to the first two thoracic nerves. This results in arm and shoulder pain on the affected side along with atrophy of the arm and hand muscles. With continuing tumor growth, the ribs over the tumor (usually the first and second ribs) may be invaded, resulting in bone pain. Later, involvement of the cervical sympathetic nerve ganglia may lead to Horner's syndrome. This syndrome consists of miosis (contraction of the pupil), partial ptosis (drooping upper eyelid), and anhidrosis (absence of sweating) on the affected side of the face.

Numerous diagnostic tests may be used to determine the presence and extent of lung cancer. Sputum cytologic study and chest x-ray are most commonly used. CT scans are used to provide detailed anatomic assessment. Magnetic resonance imaging (MRI) can provide high-quality images of the lung and mediastinum to assess for tumor invasion. New imaging techniques use monoclonal antibodies that have an affinity for cancer cells. The antibodies are tagged with technetium and injected into the client. They concentrate in the area of tumor and can be detected by single photon emission computed tomographic (SPECT) images.

Percutaneous transthoracic needle biopsy, mediastinoscopy, or direct surgical biopsy may be required to confirm the diagnosis of certain lung cancers. Radionuclide scans may be used to detect metastasis to the bone, liver, or brain (see Chapter 11).

The tumor-node-metastasis (TNM) classification scheme is used for lung cancer staging (Boxes 62–3 and 62–4; Fig. 62–3). Staging is performed to provide a guideline for the selection of appropriate therapies and the estimation of prognosis. Staging information is valuable in helping clients and their families make treatment decisions and set appropriate short-term and long-term goals.

BOX 62–3   *Tumor-Node-Metastasis (TNM) Descriptors for Pulmonary Malignancy*

Primary Tumor (T)

Tx

A tumor proven by presence of malignant cells in bronchopulmonary secretions, but not visualized on x-ray or during bronchoscopy, or any tumor that cannot be assessed as in a re-treatment staging

T0

No evidence of primary tumor

Tis

Carcinoma in situ

T1

A tumor that is 3 cm or less in greatest dimension, surrounded by lung or visceral pleura and without evidence of invasion proximal to a lobar bronchus at bronchoscopy

T2

A tumor more than 3 cm in greatest dimension or a tumor of any size that either invades the visceral pleura or has associated atelectasis or obstructive pneumonitis extending to the hilar region; at bronchoscopy, the proximal extent of demonstrable tumor must be within a lobar bronchus or at least 2 cm distal to the carina; any associated atelectasis or obstructive pneumonitis must involve less than an entire lung

T3

A tumor of any size with direct extension into the chest wall (including superior sulcus tumors), the diaphragm, or the mediastinal pleura or pericardium without involving the heart, great vessels, trachea, esophagus, or vertebral body; or a

tumor in the main bronchus within 2 cm of the carina without involving the carina

T4

A tumor of any size with invasion of the mediastinum or involving the heart, great vessels, trachea, esophagus, vertebral body, or carina in the presence of malignant pleural effusion

Lymph Nodes (N)

N0

No demonstrable metastases to regional lymph nodes

N1

Metastasis to lymph nodes in the peribronchial or the ipsilateral hilar region or both, including direct extension

N2

Metastasis to ipsilateral mediastinal lymph nodes and subcarinal lymph nodes

N3

Metastasis to contralateral mediastinal, contralateral hilar, ipsilateral or contralateral scalene, or supraclavicular lymph nodes

Distant Metastasis (M)

M0

No (known) distant metastasis

M1

Distant metastasis present; specify site(s)

Modified from the American Joint Committee on Cancer. In Mountain, C. F. (1997). Revisions in the International System for Staging Lung Cancer. *Chest, 111*(6), 1710.

BOX 62–4	Pulmonary Malignancy Staging by Tumor-Node-Metastasis

Stage	TNM Subset
0	Carcinoma in situ
IA	T1N0M0
IB	T2N0M0
IIA	T1N1M0
IIB	T2N1M0
	T3N0M0
IIIA	T3N1M0
	T1N2M0
	T2N2M0
	T3N2M0
IIIB	T4N0M0
	T4N1M0
	T4N2M0
	T1N3M0
	T2N3M0
	T3N3M0
	T4N3M0
IV	Any T, any N, and M1

Modified from the American Joint Committee on Cancer. In Mountain, C. F. (1997). Revisions in the International System for Staging Lung Cancer. *Chest, 111*(6), 1710.

METASTASIS

If tumors spread, by either direct extension or metastasis, further clinical manifestations may result. Direct extension to the recurrent laryngeal nerve produces hoarseness. Compression of the esophagus may cause dysphagia. Invasion or compression of the superior vena cava produces superior vena cava syndrome, a potentially life-threatening emergency. Obstruction of venous blood flow leads to clinical manifestations, including (1) shortness of breath, (2) facial, arm, and trunk swelling, (3) distended neck veins, (4) chest pain, and (5) venous stasis. Immediate, palliative surgical treatment may be necessary.

Regional lymph node involvement may produce manifestations due to impaired lymph drainage. Involvement of the mediastinal lymph nodes may result in vocal cord paralysis, dysphagia, diaphragmatic paralysis on the affected side (due to phrenic nerve compression), vena cava compression, and malignant pleural effusion (see later). Usually, when mediastinal lymph nodes are involved, surgical excision of the pulmonary tumor is no longer possible.

Outcome Management

▉ Medical Management

EARLY IDENTIFICATION

Early detection is the key to improving survival rates for clients with lung cancer. When premalignant changes begin, dysplastic cells are identifiable with fiberoptic bronchoscopy and sputum cytologic studies. At this stage, lesions are potentially curable. However, a tumor must be at least 1 cm in diameter before it is detectable on a chest x-ray. Unfortunately, invasion and metastasis have usually already occurred once the tumor reaches this size.

Management of the client with lung cancer depends on tumor type and stage as well as the client's underlying health status. Following diagnosis, primary treatment modalities are surgery, radiation therapy, and chemotherapy.

RADIATION THERAPY

Radiation therapy (radiotherapy) may be used as a potentially curative treatment in clients with locally advanced disease (1) for whom surgery poses an unacceptably high risk, (2) who have technically inoperable tumors, or (3) who refuse thoracotomy. Radiation therapy may also be used in combination with surgery or chemotherapy to improve treatment outcomes.

Radiotherapy is administered over a period of 5 to 6 weeks, either consecutively or in split courses. Doses are limited by the presence of other structures in the treatment area and by normal tissue tolerance. Irreversible fibrotic changes and other pulmonary side effects may

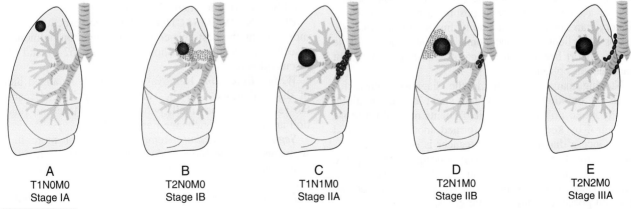

	A	B	C	D	E
	T1N0M0	T2N0M0	T1N1M0	T2N1M0	T2N2M0
	Stage IA	Stage IB	Stage IIA	Stage IIB	Stage IIIA

FIGURE 62–3 Example of various stages of lung cancer by the tumor-node-metastasis (TNM) classification system. *A* and *B*, Stage IA and IB disease includes tumors classified as T1 and T2, respectively, with no node involvement or distant metastasis. *C* and *D*, Stage IIA and IIB disease includes tumors classified as T1 and T2, respectively, with metastasis only to the peribronchial or ipsilateral hilar nodes. *E*, Stage IIIA disease includes tumors classified as T2 with metastasis to ipsilateral mediastinal or subcarinal nodes without distant metastasis.

occur. To delineate precisely the area to be irradiated, CT scanning is often performed before treatment begins. This method also minimizes tissue damage to surrounding areas.

Radiotherapy may also be used for palliation of manifestations such as pain, shortness of breath, hemoptysis, and obstruction or compression of bronchi, blood vessels, or esophagus. Irradiation of metastases to the brain and bone may reduce the distressing manifestations associated with these sequelae as well.

CHEMOTHERAPY

The response of lung cancer to chemotherapy depends on the tumor's cell type. SCLC responds well to chemotherapeutic agents because of its rapid growth rate. Results of clinical trials have demonstrated that long-term survival in clients with SCLC can be improved with intensive combination chemotherapy. As a result, chemotherapy is the cornerstone of management of SCLC.

The effectiveness of chemotherapy in the treatment of NSCLC remains controversial. This modality is commonly used in clients treated with surgery or radiation who experience recurrent disease or distant metastasis. However, large-scale studies have failed to demonstrate significantly improved long-term survival rates for such clients. As a result, the decision to use chemotherapy is usually made on an individual basis, depending on the client's previous history, current condition, and acceptance of the risks and side effects involved.

▓ Nursing Management of the Medical Client

DIAGNOSTIC PHASE

The client who is undergoing diagnostic tests for lung cancer faces an uncertain future. If the diagnosis is confirmed, the client can anticipate a variety of physical difficulties, potentially extensive medical treatment, and many emotional changes. The nursing assessment plays a critical role in developing a plan of care that will provide needed support.

The nursing history should include an exploration of the client's chief complaints, particularly cough (productive or nonproductive), dyspnea, pain, and recurrent infection. Ask the client about the presence of risk factors, such as a smoking history, exposure to occupational respiratory carcinogens, or a family history of the disease. Assess the client's socioeconomic situation and available social support because these factors will affect subsequent management options.

Nursing management during the diagnostic phase focuses on emotional support and client education along with required physical care. Help clients maintain a sense of control by keeping them informed about all scheduled tests. Once a diagnosis of lung cancer is confirmed, nursing care must incorporate measures designed to help the client cope with anxiety and fear, family responses, financial considerations, absence from work and social activities, and possible changes in life goals.

TREATMENT PHASE

Nursing care of the client receiving radiation and chemotherapy is detailed in Chapters 18 and 19.

▓ Surgical Management

Surgical intervention is the treatment of choice in early-stage NSCLC. Cure is possible if the disease is still localized to the thoracic cavity and no distant metastases are present. However, only 20% to 25% of clients with NSCLC meet these criteria at the time of diagnosis. For patients who successfully undergo surgical resection, the 5-year survival rate is approximately 35% to 40%.[33]

The role of surgical resection in the treatment of SCLC is limited. Surgery may be effective for clients with the early stages of SCLC, as a component of combined modality therapy. For clients with more advanced disease, surgery causes unnecessary risk and stress, with no valid benefits.

The primary aim of surgical resection is to remove the tumor completely while preserving as much of the normal surrounding lung tissue as possible. The extent of the operation depends on the location and size of the pulmonary tumor and the severity of the underlying pathologic process. Clients with pre-existing pulmonary disease may not be able to tolerate extensive removal of lung tissue.

PREOPERATIVE MANAGEMENT

Extensive pulmonary function testing may be performed before surgery to determine the client's ability to tolerate the proposed surgical intervention. Clients with impaired pulmonary function may be treated with antibiotics, bronchodilating medications, intermittent positive-pressure breathing procedures, and supervised breathing exercises to improve respiratory efficiency. Clients are encouraged to refrain from smoking during the preoperative period because smoking will increase pulmonary secretions and diminish blood oxygen saturation.

SURGICAL PROCEDURES

LASER SURGERY. One surgical treatment modality is laser therapy. Currently, laser therapy is used as a palliative measure for relief of endobronchial obstructions that are not resectable. Laser procedures do not produce systemic or cumulative toxic effects and are well tolerated. Laser therapy may be given in an outpatient setting. However, in order for the laser to be used, the tumor mass must be accessible by bronchoscopy. Therefore, tumors pressing on bronchial tissue from outside the bronchial lumen are not amenable to laser therapy.

PULMONARY RESECTION. Complete resection of tumor remains the best chance of cure. Common pulmonary resection procedures are shown in Figure 62–4 and are discussed here.

Wedge Resection. Removal of a small, localized area of diseased tissue near the surface of the lung. Because the resected area is small, pulmonary structure and function are relatively unchanged after healing.

Segmental Resection. Removal of one or more lung segments (a bronchiole and its alveoli). The remaining lung tissue overexpands to fill the previously occupied space.

Lobectomy. Removal of an entire lobe of the lung. Postoperatively, the remaining lung overexpands to fill the open portion of the thoracic space.

Pneumonectomy. Removal of an entire lung. Once the lung is removed, the involved side of the thoracic cavity

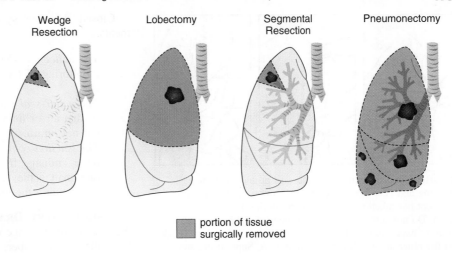

FIGURE 62-4 Pulmonary resections.

portion of tissue surgically removed

is an empty space. In order to reduce the size of the cavity, the surgeon severs the phrenic nerve on the affected side to paralyze the diaphragm in an elevated position. A thoracoplasty, which is the removal of several ribs or portions of ribs to further reduce the thoracic space, may also be performed.

Closed-chest drainage is usually not used after pneumonectomy. The serous fluid that accumulates in the empty thoracic cavity eventually consolidates. The consolidation prevents shifts of the mediastinum, heart, and remaining lung.

CHEST TUBES. Chest surgery causes a pneumothorax on the operated side. During thoracotomy, the parietal pleura is incised, and the pleural space is entered. Atmospheric air rushes into the pleural space. This changes the normally negative pressure in that pleural space to a positive pressure. As a result, the lung recoils to its unexpanded size and remains collapsed. Chest trauma, such as rib fractures, leads to pneumothorax in the same manner. Chest tubes are usually inserted in an operating room during chest surgery. However, in some emergencies, a chest tube may be inserted in a treatment room or at the bedside.

Two catheters are usually placed in the chest following resectional surgery (except pneumonectomy). One catheter (the upper, or anterior, tube) is placed anteriorly through the second intercostal space to permit the escape of air rising in the pleural space. The other catheter (the lower, or posterior, tube) is placed posteriorly through the eighth or ninth intercostal space in the midaxillary line to drain off serosanguineous (consisting of serum and blood) fluid accumulating in the lower portion of the pleural space. The lower tube may have a larger diameter than the upper tube, to enhance fluid drainage. Chest tubes are brought out of the chest wall through stab wounds or through the incisional line. The catheters are secured to the client's skin with sutures.

The two chest tubes may be joined to each other with a plastic Y-junction (and then attached to one closed-chest drainage system). However, it is preferable to leave them separate and to attach them to separate drainage systems. This arrangement makes it possible to monitor air and fluid drainage from each tube and, later, to remove a nondraining tube without disrupting the rest of

the system. Flexible drainage tubing connects the chest tube to the drainage collection apparatus. Usually, chest tubes are connected to a closed-chest drainage apparatus before the client leaves the operating room.

■ **Nursing Management of the Surgical Client**

PREOPERATIVE ASSESSMENT
Preoperative preparation of the client with lung cancer who is to undergo surgery is the same as for any surgical client but with greater emphasis on assessment and preparation of the respiratory system (see Chapter 15 for discussion of preoperative nursing care).

PREOPERATIVE CARE
Nursing interventions during the preoperative period are aimed primarily at reducing the client's anxiety level. Anxiety results from fear of cancer and its prognosis as well as from fear of the surgical procedure and insufficient knowledge of surgical routines and postoperative self-care activities. The client and family are taught about the following issues:

The anticipated surgical procedure: Assess the client's (and family's) understanding, and give further information as needed.

The early postoperative period: Talk specifically about what will be happening to the client and how he or she can participate in recovery activities. Specific explanations should be given about the presence of chest tubes (except with pneumonectomy) and drainage tubes, intubation and mechanical ventilation, oxygen therapy, and available pain relief measures.

Postoperative exercises: They include (1) respiratory exercises, such as the use of incentive spirometry to maintain effective pulmonary function, (2) splinting techniques to promote effective coughing and deep-breathing (Fig. 62-5), and (3) leg exercises to prevent thrombophlebitis. All of these exercises should be demonstrated preoperatively, and opportunity given for practice and return demonstration.

POSTOPERATIVE ASSESSMENT
During the immediate postoperative period, thorough assessment is essential. Make observations as often as the client's condition warrants. Frequency of observations is determined by the following factors:

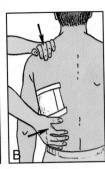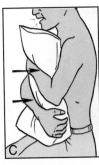

FIGURE 62–5 Splinting techniques to promote effective coughing and deep-breathing. Apply firm, even pressure after the client has taken a deep breath and during forced expiratory cough. Do not squeeze the chest or interfere with chest inspiratory expansion. *A,* Place one hand around the client's back and the other around the incisional area. *B,* Support the area below the incision with one hand while exerting downward pressure on the shoulder on the affected side with the other. *C,* Have the person hug a pillow during forced expiratory cough.

- Amount of anesthesia received and the client's reaction to it
- Amount of intraoperative blood loss
- The client's preoperative condition (e.g., presence of pre-existing medical conditions, such as diabetes and heart disorders)
- The client's response to pain
- Facility protocols

POSTOPERATIVE CARE

Nursing interventions are based on careful assessment and appropriate nursing diagnoses. General postoperative nursing measures are applicable (see Chapter 15). Nursing management specific to thoracic surgery is discussed in the Care Plan.

MAINTAIN CLOSED-CHEST DRAINAGE. Clients have closed-chest drainage after all forms of chest surgery (except pneumonectomy) and some forms of chest trauma.

In closed-chest drainage, the chest drainage system is airtight, or closed, to prevent the effects of atmospheric pressure. Historically, closed-chest drainage was performed with the use of a glass bottle water-seal apparatus (one-, two-, or three-bottle setup) with or without controlled mechanical suction. Most health care facilities have replaced glass bottle water-seal drainage systems with disposable single units, such as the Pleur-evac, Atrium, or Aqua-Seal (Fig. 62–6). However, a knowledge of the basic principles of closed-chest drainage will aid in understanding any specific system.

Closed-chest drainage after thoracotomy or chest trauma is used to:

- Promote evacuation of air and serosanguineous fluid from the pleural space and prevent their reflux
- Help reexpand the remaining lung tissue by reestablishing normal negative pressure in the pleural space
- Prevent mediastinal shift and pneumothorax by equalizing pressures on the two sides of the thoracic cavity

Closed drainage systems have three main compartments:

1. The *collection chamber* collects drainage and allows monitoring of the volume, rate, and nature of drainage.
2. The *water-seal chamber* is used as a one-way valve so that air or fluids can drain from the client's chest but not return.
3. The *suction-control chamber* uses suction to promote drainage from the pleural space (at a greater rate than achieved by gravity alone) and assist in reexpanding the lung.

ASSESS CHEST DRAINAGE. Measure *and* document the amount of drainage coming from the pleural space in the collection chamber. This record helps determine the amount of blood loss and the flow rate of drainage from the pleural space. Disposable plastic systems are manufactured with a marked write-on surface on which to record the amount of drainage. Drainage rates and amounts are used in planning blood replacement therapy and assessing the client's status. As much as 500 to 1000 ml of drainage may occur in the first 24 hours after chest surgery. Between 100 and 300 ml of drainage may accumulate during the first 2 hours; after this time, the drainage should lessen. Excessive drainage or a sudden large increase may require further surgery to determine its cause.

Normally, chest drainage is grossly bloody immediately following surgery, but it should not continue to be so for more than several hours. Assess blood loss by monitoring the rising fluid level in the collection chamber. Suspect hemorrhage if the blood pressure drops and the pulse rate becomes rapid. Check fluid in the drainage collection chamber. If the fluid level has not risen, check the tubes for patency. Notify the surgeon if (1) the drainage remains frankly bloody for longer than the first few postoperative hours, (2) bleeding recurs after it has slowed, or (3) there are any other manifestations of hemorrhage.

ASSESS WATER-SEAL FUNCTION. A water seal provides a one-way valve between atmospheric pressure and subatmospheric (negative) intrapleural pressure. It allows air and fluid to leave the intrapleural space but prevents the back-flow of atmospheric air into the chest.

On expiration, air and fluid in the pleural space travel through the drainage tubing. The air bubbles up through the water seal and enters atmospheric air. On inspiration, the water seal prevents atmospheric air from being sucked back into the pleural space (which would collapse the lung). The fluid in the water-seal compartment is not drawn into the chest cavity because the negative pressures generated during inspiration in the intrapleural space are not high enough to pull the fluid through the drainage tubing. However, fluctuation of the fluid occurs during respiration; this fluctuation is known as "tidaling" (tidal movement) or vacillation.

A closed-chest drainage system must be airtight between the pleural space and the water-seal compartment. Any air leak allows the entry of atmospheric air into the pleural space during inspiration, creating a positive pres-

Text continued on page 1736

■ THE CLIENT UNDERGOING THORACIC SURGERY

Collaborative Problem. Potential complications of thoracic surgery: pulmonary edema; respiratory insufficiency; tension pneumothorax and mediastinal shift; subcutaneous emphysema; pulmonary embolus; cardiac dysrhythmias; hemorrhage, hemothorax, and hypovolemic shock; and thrombophlebitis.

Outcomes. The nurse will monitor for respiratory, cardiac, and vascular complications.

Interventions	Rationales

1. Monitor for manifestations of respiratory failure:
  a. Increased respiratory rate
  b. Dyspnea
  c. Use of accessory muscles or retractions
  d. Cyanosis
  e. Decreased pulse oximetry
  f. Decreased PaO_2 levels and increased $PaCO_2$ levels
  g. Restlessness
  h. Increase in adventitious breath sounds
	1. Postoperatively, respiratory insufficiency may result from an altered level of consciousness due to anesthesia and pain medications, incomplete lung reinflation, decreased respiratory effort due to chest pain, and inadequate airway clearance.

2. Monitor for manifestations of tension pneumothorax:
  a. Severe dyspnea
  b. Tachypnea and tachycardia
  c. Extreme restlessness and agitation
  d. Progressive cyanosis
  e. Laryngeal and tracheal deviation to unaffected side
  f. Laterally or medial PMI shift
	2. Postoperative tension pneumothorax can result from air leaking through pleural incision lines if closed chest drainage fails to function properly.

3. Observe for subcutaneous emphysema around incision and in the chest and neck:
  a. Assess progression by periodically marking the chest with a skin-marking pencil at the outer periphery of emphysematous tissue. If neck involvement occurs, measure neck circumference at least every 2 to 4 hours.
  b. Keep emergency tracheostomy tray at bedside
	3. Subcutaneous emphysema may result from air leakage at pulmonary incision site.
	  a. Rapid progression (i.e., an increase of more than a hand's width in 1 hour) may indicate leakage through the bronchial stump.
	
	  b. Severe subcutaneous emphysema in the neck may compress the trachea and may require tracheostomy.

4. Monitor for manifestations of pulmonary embolus:
  a. Chest pain
  b. Dyspnea and tachypnea
  c. Fever
  d. Hemoptysis
  e. Indications of right-sided heart failure
	4. Pulmonary embolism is a serious potential complication after chest surgery and a significant cause of postoperative hypoxemia.

5. Monitor for signs of acute pulmonary edema:
  a. Dyspnea
  b. Crackles
  c. Persistent cough
  d. Frothy sputum
  e. Cyanosis
  f. Decreased pulse oximetry reading
	5. Circulatory overload may result from the reduced size of the pulmonary vascular bed due to surgical removal of pulmonary tissue and delayed reexpansion of the affected lung. Additionally, hypoxia increases capillary permeability, causing fluid to enter pulmonary tissue.

6. Monitor intravenous flow rates. Consult physician if fluid amounts (maintenance plus intermittent medications [e.g., antibiotics]) exceed 125 ml/hr.	6. After chest surgery, intravenous fluids should not exceed 125 ml/hr because of possible circulatory overload.
7. Assess cardiac monitor for the development of cardiac dysrhythmias, particularly atrial fibrillation, atrial flutter, and paroxysmal atrial tachycardia.	7. Cardiac dysrhythmias are fairly common after chest surgery. Rhythm disturbances result from a combination of factors, including increased vagal tone, hypoxia, mediastinal shift, and abnormal blood pH.
8. Assess dressing and incisional area every 4 hours for evidence of bleeding (increase to every 1 to 2 hours if bleeding develops). Assess drainage in closed chest drainage system for signs of bleeding.	8. Blood loss may be great with major thoracic surgery because blood vessels in the thorax are of large diameter and the incision is often large and produces considerable capillary oozing.

9. Monitor for signs of hypovolemic shock:
  a. Increased pulse
  b. Decreased blood pressure
  c. Restlessness and decreased level of consciousness
  d. Decreased urine output (<30 ml/hr)
  e. Cool, pale, clammy skin
  f. Increased respirations
	9. The body compensates for lost blood volume by increasing blood flow (through increased heart rate) to vital organs and decreasing peripheral circulation.

10. Monitor for thrombophlebitis:
  a. Unilateral leg edema
  b. Calf tenderness, redness, unusual warmth
	10. Anesthesia and immobility reduce vasomotor tone, leading to decreased venous return and peripheral pooling of blood.

Care Plan continued on following page

■

11. Encourage client to perform leg exercises. Discourage placing pillows under knees, crossing the legs, or prolonged sitting. Apply elastic hose or pneumatic compression stockings, if ordered.

11. These measures prevent venous stasis, thus reducing the risk of thrombophlebitis.

Evaluation. The nurse monitors for the development of these complications. Most occur early after surgery, except for pulmonary embolus.

Nursing Diagnosis. Ineffective Airway Clearance related to increased secretions and to decreased coughing effectiveness due to pain.

Outcomes. The client will demonstrate effective airway clearance, as evidenced by clear breath sounds, effective coughing, and adequate air exchange in the lungs.

Interventions

1. Once the vital signs are stable, place the client in semi-Fowler position.
2. Help the client cough and deep-breathe at least every 1 or 2 hours during the first 24 to 48 postoperative hours.
3. Instruct the client to take a deep breath slowly and to hold it for 3–5 seconds, then exhale; to take a second breath and then, while exhaling, to cough forcefully twice.
4. When possible, schedule coughing and deep-breathing sessions at times when pain medication is maximally effective.
5. Assess breath sounds before and after coughing. Provide support and reassurance:
   a. Explain that breathing exercises will not damage the lungs or the suture line.
   b. Manually splint the incision area during coughing and deep-breathing.
   c. Offer sips of warm water.

   d. Maintain adequate level of hydration and adequate humidity of inspired air.
   e. Monitor results of chest x-rays.
   f. Evaluate the need for suctioning.

Rationales

1. The upright position enhances lung expansion and facilitates ventilation with minimal effort.
2. Increasing the volume of air in lungs promotes expulsion of secretions.
3. Coughing helps move tracheobronchial secretions out of the lung. Deep-breathing dilates the airways, stimulates surfactant production, and expands lung tissue.
4. The less postoperative pain a client experiences, the more effective are coughing and deep-breathing.
5. This will help in evaluation of coughing effectiveness.

   a. Client's fear of "splitting open" the incision may hamper coughing efforts.
   b. Physical support of the incision is both comforting and reassuring.
   c. Warm water can aid relaxation and produce more effective coughing.
   d. Fluids and moisture help thin secretions, making them easier to expectorate.
   e. Frequent chest films help detect atelectasis and infection.
   f. If coughing is ineffective, suctioning may be required to remove pulmonary secretions. Suctioning should be performed cautiously so that disruption of pulmonary suture lines is avoided.

Evaluation. Outcomes on effective airway clearance will require days to achieve.

Nursing Diagnosis. Pain related to surgical procedure.

Outcomes. The client will be more comfortable, as evidenced by verbalizing that discomfort is reduced, using less narcotic medication, and moving in bed with less pain.

Interventions

1. Assess pain intensity using a self-report measurement tool.

2. Administer pain medication as ordered.

3. Observe for side effects of medication used.
4. Offer and instruct clients to ask for pain medication before pain becomes severe.
5. Assess medication effectiveness and avoid overmedication.

6. Use nonpharmacologic pain relief measures concurrently.

Rationales

1. Use of a consistent, valid tool promotes communication and evaluation of pain intervention effectiveness.
2. Use of narcotics is a common method of postoperative pain control. Narcotics bind to opiate receptors, decreasing sensations of pain.
3. Side effects are monitored.
4. A preventive approach to pain control provides a more consistent level of relief and reduces client anxiety.
5. Adequate pain relief must be obtained. However, overmedication can depress respirations and the cough reflex.
6. Proper positioning, relaxation techniques, and like measures can augment effects of medications.

Evaluation. Pain will be most acute for 48 to 72 hours postoperatively, requiring narcotics for pain control. Expect pain to subside after that time, and offer less potent narcotics or analgesics.

Nursing Diagnosis. Impaired Physical Mobility related to pain, muscle dissection, restricted positioning, and chest tubes.

Outcomes. The client will maintain physical mobility in the arm and shoulder, as evidenced by regaining of preoperative arm and shoulder function.

■

Interventions

1. Position client as indicated by phase of recovery and surgical procedure:

   a. Nonoperative side–lying position may be used until consciousness is regained.
   b. Semi-Fowler position (head of bed elevated 30 to 45 degrees) is recommended once vital signs are stable.
   c. Avoid positioning client on operative side if a wedge resection or segmentectomy has been performed.

   d. Avoid complete lateral positioning after pneumonectomy.

2. Gently turn the client every 1 to 2 hours, unless contraindicated.

3. Avoid traction on chest tubes while changing client position. Check for kinking or compression of tubing.

4. Encourage regular ambulation, once client's condition is stable. Maintain supplemental oxygen, if ordered.
5. Begin passive ROM exercises of the arm and shoulder on the affected side 4 hours after recovery from anesthesia. Exercises should be performed two times every 4 to 6 hours through the first 24 postoperative hours, with progression to 10 to 20 times every 2 hours.
6. Active ROM exercises are begun once the client's condition permits.
7. Encourage client to use the arm on the affected side in daily activities (e.g., eating, reaching, grooming). Keep bedside stand on the operative side to encourage reaching. Teach the importance of continued use of the arm after discharge.
8. Carefully assess client's response to activity and exercise. Observe for signs of dyspnea and fatigue.

9. Allow adequate rest periods between activities.

Rationales

1. Repositioning maximizes long expansion and drainage of secretions, promotes ventilation and oxygenation, and enhances comfort.
   a. This position prevents aspiration.

   b. The upright position enhances lung expansion and facilitates chest tube drainage.
   c. Lying on the operative side hinders expansion of remaining lung tissue and may accentuate perfusion of poorly ventilated tissue, thus further impeding normal gas exchange.
   d. Because the mediastinum is no longer held in place on both sides by lung tissue, extreme turning may cause mediastinal shift and compression of the remaining lung.
2. Frequent turning promotes mobilization and drainage of air and fluid from the pleural space. Turning also improves circulation, promotes lung aeration, and enhances comfort.
3. Traction may dislodge the chest tubes. Kinking or compression inhibits drainage and reestablishment of negative intrapleural pressure.
4. Early ambulation improves ventilation, circulation, and morale. Oxygen therapy is used to avoid hypoxia.
5. ROM exercises help prevent adhesion formation in the operative area, which can lead to dysfunction syndrome (i.e., "frozen shoulder").

6. Active ROM exercises prevent adhesions of the incised muscle layers.
7. Regular use of the affected arm and shoulder reduces the possibility of contractures.

8. It may take time for the client's activity tolerance to increase, because the body must adjust to reduced respiratory capacity after resectional surgery.
9. Adequate rest will enable the client to cooperate more fully with activities.

Evaluation. Expect the client to be able to turn independently after 24 hours. Improvement in ROM will require a few days, until pain subsides and the chest tube is removed.

Nursing Diagnosis. Risk for Ineffective Individual Coping related to temporary dependence and loss of full respiratory function.

Outcomes. The client will use adaptive coping mechanisms, as evidenced by verbalizing feelings related to emotional state and taking appropriate actions to regain self-care capabilities.

Interventions

1. Provide opportunity for client to express feelings.

2. Encourage use of positive coping strategies that have been successful in the past.
3. Allow client to have as much control over daily activities and decision-making as is possible.
4. Support and praise all independent activities that promote recovery.

Rationales

1. Loss of normal body function and self-care capabilities can lead to feelings of powerlessness, anger, and grief. Open expression of these feelings can help client begin coping.
2. The use of effective coping actions can decrease feelings of hopelessness and helplessness.
3. Active involvement in the plan of care gives the client a sense of control and promotes return to independence.
4. Emotional support and encouragement help motivate client to continue progress toward independence.

Evaluation. The use of effective coping mechanisms depends on prior coping strategies. This outcome may be met quickly if the client is able to cope with a diagnosis of cancer and has hope for recovery and a support system. On the contrary, coping in the face of a dreaded diagnosis, fear of pain, little hope for recovery, and limited support systems will tax coping mechanisms.

Nursing Diagnosis. Altered Health Maintenance related to self-care after discharge.

Outcomes. Client will be able to maintain health, as evidenced by stating or demonstrating discharge plans.

continued

Interventions

1. Provide thorough instruction and preparation for hospital discharge:

   a. Proper wound care

   b. Continuation of exercise program

   c. Precautions regarding activity and environmental irritants

   d. Clinical manifestations to be reported to health care professional

   e. Importance of regular follow-up care

   f. Community agencies that can provide resources, as needed

Rationales

1. Thorough understanding promotes compliance and enhances self-care capabilities.

   a. Wound care will vary according to condition of incision and client.

   b. Continued exercise increases activity tolerance and prevents complications.

   c. Heavy lifting should be avoided. Return to work will depend on client's condition and type of job. However, it is usually possible to return to work within 4 to 6 weeks. Environmental irritants can cause severe coughing episodes.

   d. Evidence of infection, deteriorating respiratory status, or other complications should be reported promptly.

   e. The client should be monitored closely for signs of surgical complications, recurrence of malignancy, and metastasis.

   f. Community resources can facilitate home management.

Evaluation. Client and family must demonstrate understanding of discharge teaching.

$PaCO_2$, partial pressure of arterial carbon dioxide; PaO_2, partial pressure of arterial oxygen; PMI, point of maximal impulse; ROM, range of motion.

---

sure that collapses the lung. All connections within the drainage system must be tight and secure. However, the water-seal chamber itself *must* have an air vent to provide an escape route for air passing through the water seal from the pleural space.

Observe the Water Seal. Fluid in the water-seal compartment should rise with inspiration and fall with expiration (tidaling). When tidaling is occurring, the drainage tubes are patent and the apparatus is functioning properly. Tidaling stops when the lung has reexpanded or if the chest drainage tubes are kinked or obstructed. If tidaling does not occur:

1. Check to make sure the tubing is not kinked or compressed.
2. Change the client's position.
3. Have the client deep-breathe and cough.
4. *If indicated*, milk the tube (see later). If these measures do not restore tidaling, notify the surgeon. (*Note*: Tidaling may not occur or may be minimal in systems using suction.)

Observe for Bubbling in the Water-Seal Compartment. Bubbling in the water-seal compartment is caused by air passing out of the pleural space into the fluid in the chamber. *Intermittent* bubbling is normal and indicates that the system is accomplishing one of its purposes, that is, removing air from the pleural space.

Continuous bubbling during both inspiration and expiration, however, indicates that air is leaking into the drainage system or pleural cavity. Because air entering the system also enters the pleural space, this situation must be corrected:

1. Locate the source of the air leak, and repair it if you can. Begin by inspecting the chest wall where the catheters are inserted.

2. If a chest catheter is loose or has been partially removed, gently squeeze the skin up around the catheter or apply sterile petrolatum gauze around the insertion site. Determine whether this measure stops the continuous bubbling in the chamber.
3. If the air leak continues, check the tubing, inch by inch, and all the connections. A break in the tubing or a loose connection may be found that can be sealed with tape.
4. If the leak still cannot be located, it may be necessary to replace the drainage system.

Rapid bubbling in the absence of an air leak indicates considerable loss of air, as from an incision or tear in the pulmonary pleura. When this occurs, notify the physician *immediately* so that appropriate measures can be taken to prevent collapse of the lung or mediastinal shift, such as (1) application of suction, (2) increase in the amount of suction, or (3) thoracotomy.

When caring for a client with water-seal drainage, find out whether this particular client's water-seal chamber should be bubbling. Having this knowledge facilitates accurate assessment of the drainage pattern (e.g., if intermittent bubbling changes to constant bubbling or if an apparatus that has not been bubbling begins to bubble).

SUCTION. Suction at 10 to 20 cm H_2O may be applied to a chest drainage system if gravity drainage is not adequate or if a client's cough and respirations are too weak to force air and fluid out of the pleural space through the chest catheters. Additionally, suction may be applied to closed-chest drainage (1) if air is leaking into the pleural space faster than it can be removed by a water-seal apparatus or (2) to speed up the removal of air from the pleural space. Suction is regulated by the height of the water column in the suction chamber. The more fluid in the chamber, the more suction (subatmos-

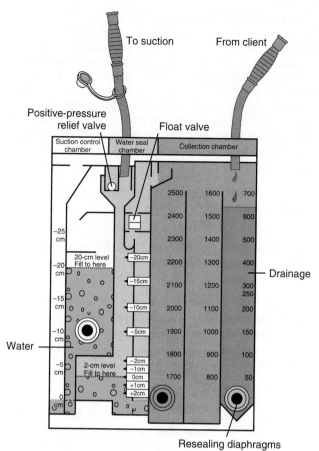

FIGURE 62–6 A commonly used disposable chest drainage system combines the three bottles into a single device. (Courtesy of Deknatel, Fall River, MA.)

pheric pressure) is created. Most clients who require a chest tube postoperatively also need suction for 24 to 72 hours.

If there were no water in the chamber, atmospheric air would go straight from the air vent into the suction source as fast as the suction was applied. Passage of the air through water slows it, and the suction force is controlled. Increasing the source of suction only causes more air to travel through the air vent. The suction applied to the client remains stable. An occluded atmospheric air vent is dangerous because it causes the suction to be applied directly to the pleural cavity. A suction force greater than 50 cm H_2O may cause lung damage.

ASSESS SUCTION APPARATUS FUNCTION. Because most suction regulators can create potentially damaging amounts of suction, the amount of suction in the system must be controlled. Proper functioning of a wet suction control compartment is indicated by continuous bubbling in the suction control chamber. Vigorous bubbling does not increase the amount of suction; rather, it causes the water in the bottle to evaporate more rapidly.

Absence of bubbling in a suction control chamber means that the system is not functioning properly and that the correct level of suction is not being maintained. Possible reasons for malfunction of a mechanical suction

apparatus include (1) large amounts of air leaking into the pleural space or into the drainage apparatus and (2) mechanical problems in the regulator (suction power source). The most serious problem is air leaking into the pleural space.

If bubbling in the suction control chamber stops, check for air leaks by briefly clamping the chest drainage tube close to the client's body and observing the chamber.

If bubbling begins in the suction control chamber, there is nothing wrong with either the drainage apparatus or the regulator. The problem is therefore an air leak into the pleural space around the chest tubes. If the air leak cannot be sealed off (e.g., with petrolatum gauze), notify the surgeon immediately.

If bubbling does not begin in the suction control chamber when the chest catheter is clamped, the problem is in the drainage connections or the regulator. Check the system carefully, looking for loose connections and for air leaks around compartment tops and in the tubing (e.g., split tubing). Make sure that the tubing is not kinked, is correctly positioned, and has no dependent loops. If the suction power source appears to be causing the problem, obtain another suction canister and regulator.

Because the chest catheter remains clamped during this inspection, observe the client closely for indications of tension pneumothorax (e.g., dyspnea, tachycardia, hypotension, trachea shift). As soon as the problem is corrected, the fluid in the suction control chamber will begin to bubble. Immediately remove the clamps on the chest catheter.

Some newer drainage systems feature dry suction, which uses a spring or dial mechanism in place of a water column to control the suction level. The advantages include ease in setup, no noise, and provision of higher, more precise levels of suction. However, because you cannot directly visualize the suction level via bubbling with such a system, it is important to assess the suction indicator frequently.

PROMOTE CHEST DRAINAGE
Closed-chest drainage systems must always be placed lower (preferably 2 to 3 feet) than the client's chest. Drainage by gravity is thus maintained, and fluid is not forced back into the pleural space. Chest drainage systems must be placed upright on the floor or hung from the foot of the bed.

If the drainage apparatus is on the floor, be careful not to lower a high-low bed or side rails onto it. If a client with closed-chest drainage is to be moved, always keep the chest drainage system below the level of the client's chest.

If the apparatus is placed above the level of the client's chest, even for a moment, fluid from the drainage chamber is siphoned back into the pleural cavity. If absolutely necessary, chest tubes may be double-clamped very briefly during momentary movement of the apparatus above the level of the person's chest (e.g., when moving drainage apparatus from one side of the bed to the other if the tubing is not long enough to allow movement around an end of the bed).

Follow positioning orders carefully. If a client can be positioned on the side that has chest tubes, be sure the client is not lying on (compressing or kinking) the catheters or tubing. This may impair drainage, cause retrograde pressure (forcing drainage back into the pleural cavity), and increase the client's discomfort. Coil the drainage tubing (connecting the chest tube to the drainage apparatus) on the client's mattress so that it falls straight to the drainage apparatus, with no dependent loops. Dependent loops of tubing that contain fluid obstruct fluid flow and create back-pressure, thus impairing air or fluid drainage.

Drainage tubing should be neither too short nor too long. Excessive tubing length causes tangling and kinking. However, make sure the tubing is long enough to allow the person to turn and sit up without pulling on the chest tubes. Each time the client is turned or moved, check the chest tubes to make sure they are not being pulled or displaced. Check the drainage tubing to be certain it is properly positioned.

Tube patency is unlikely to be a problem when chest tubes are evacuating only air or when fluid or blood is draining well by gravity. However, if fragments of a blood clot or lung tissue are visible in the tube, use of chest tube clearance techniques *may* be indicated. Traditionally, nurses have manipulated chest tubes by *milking* or *stripping* (Fig. 62–7).

- To strip a chest tube, gently compress it, and slide one hand down the tubing, away from the client's chest and toward the drainage system. Stabilize the tubing with the other hand so that the tube will not be pulled on or displaced during stripping.
- To milk a chest tube, compress the tube intermittently using a twisting or squeezing motion.

Theoretically, these techniques dislodge clot material from the tube lumen and propel it toward the drainage collection chamber. However, studies have demonstrated no difference in tube patency with or without such manipulation. Additionally, stripping a chest tube can cause complications because it creates excessive negative intrapleural pressure (>100 cm H_2O). Therefore, these techniques should be used with extreme caution, if at all.

ENCOURAGE ACTIVITY

Encourage a client with closed-chest drainage to cough and deep-breathe frequently. In addition to clearing the bronchi of secretions, these activities promote lung expansion and the expulsion of air and fluid from the pleural space by increasing intrapulmonary and intrapleural pressures.

A client with a chest drainage system can sit up in bed, get in and out of bed, and ambulate without clamping of the chest tubes as long as the apparatus stays upright. Do not exert traction (pull) on the tubing. Various arrangements are used to hold a chest drainage system below waist level during ambulation. The device may be placed in a wheelchair in front of the client. Many disposable units have handles to allow for carrying. If the client's condition warrants, removal of suction during ambulation may be ordered, allowing gravity drainage.

CLAMP CHEST DRAINAGE TUBING

In most situations, clamping of chest tubes is contraindicated. When the client has a residual air leak or pneumothorax, clamping the chest tube may precipitate a tension pneumothorax because the air has no escape route. If the tube becomes disconnected, it is best to immediately reattach it to the drainage system or to submerge the end in a bottle of sterile water or saline to reestablish a water seal. If fluid is not readily available, it is preferable to leave the tube open because the risk of tension pneumothorax outweighs the consequences of an open tube.

There are occasions, however, when clamping is appropriate, such as:

- Assessing a persistent air leak
- Evaluating the client's readiness for removal of the drainage system
- Changing the drainage system

Except for those occasions in which clamping is clearly indicated, *never* clamp chest drainage tubes without an order to do so. If clamps must be used, the best time to apply them is after an expiration. Remove the clamps as soon as possible.

REMOVE CHEST TUBES

The physician determines when to remove chest tubes and closed-chest drainage. One indication is that the lung has reexpanded, as signified by the cessation of fluctua-

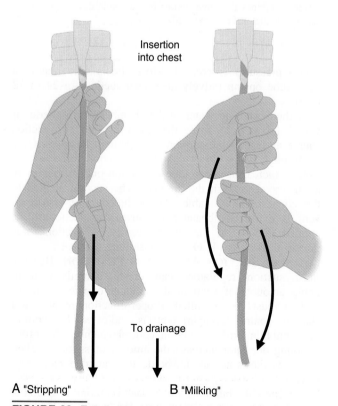

FIGURE 62–7 Stripping *(A)* and milking *(B)* of chest tubes are performed carefully to remove blood clots, but these procedures are not performed routinely.

tion in the water-seal chamber (if suction is not applied). Chest auscultation, chest percussion, and chest x-ray studies confirm lung reexpansion.

Usually, a lung is fully reexpanded after 2 or 3 postoperative days of chest drainage. Chest tubes are generally left in place and connected to drainage systems for an additional 24 hours after all air and significant fluid drainage have stopped. The tubes may be temporarily clamped to see how the client will tolerate their removal. Chest tubes may not be removed if the chest is draining more than 50 to 70 ml of fluid daily. The sooner the chest tubes can be removed, the better. Their presence often contributes to postoperative pain and inactivity. The longer the tubes are in place, the greater the risk of infection. Chest tubes used for treatment of empyema (see later) may be in place longer than tubes placed after chest surgery.

Removal of chest tubes can be moderately painful. The prescribed premedication for pain relief should be administered approximately 30 minutes before the procedure. Assemble equipment as necessary, such as sterile scissors or a suture set to cut sutures securing the tubes, sterile petrolatum gauze, 4×4-inch gauze to cover the wound, and tape.

If chest tubes are accidentally removed, cover the insertion site with sterile petrolatum gauze and notify the surgeon. Observe the client for respiratory distress because tension pneumothorax may develop. If it does, remove the petrolatum gauze to allow air to escape.

BENIGN LUNG TUMORS

Benign pulmonary neoplasms account for fewer than 10% of all primary pulmonary tumors. The term benign may be misleading because although they are not directly harmful to the body, some benign tumors may still have serious physiologic effects. Mechanical interference with lung function (e.g., obstruction of a major bronchus) may occur, depending on the tumor's location. In addition, some such tumors may become malignant over time.

The most common benign lung tumor is the hamartoma, which usually arises in peripheral lung parenchyma. This tumor is more common in older men. Other benign tumor types are fibroma, hemangioma, lipoma, and papilloma.

Benign lung tumors are often difficult to diagnose because clients may be asymptomatic. Unless there is pre-existing lung disease or major airway obstruction, pulmonary function study results and ABG values are usually within normal limits. The tumor may be first detected on chest x-ray. Confirmatory diagnosis usually requires bronchoscopy or, more commonly, thoracotomy.

Until the diagnosis is confirmed, most clients are quite anxious and fearful of the possibility of cancer. Emotional support is an important adjunct to the physical preparation required for diagnostic procedures.

Surgical intervention is the treatment of choice for all benign neoplasms. Tumor removal promptly alleviates any respiratory manifestations that may have resulted from pressure on lung structures. Postoperative management is the same as that after surgical treatment of malignant lung disease.

OCCUPATIONAL LUNG DISEASES

Etiology and Classification

Lung diseases are among the most common occupational health problems. They are caused by the inhalation of various chemicals, dusts, and other particulate matter that are present in certain settings. Not all clients exposed to occupational inhalants experience lung disease. Harmful effects depend on:

1. Nature of the exposure.
2. Duration and intensity of the exposure.
3. Particle size and water solubility of the inhalant; the larger the particle, the lower the probability of its reaching the lower respiratory tract. Highly water-soluble inhalants tend to dissolve and react in the upper respiratory tract; poorly soluble substances may travel as far as the alveoli.
4. The client's smoking history.
5. Presence or absence of underlying pulmonary disease.

The most commonly encountered occupational lung diseases are described in Table 62–4.

Acute respiratory irritation results from the inhalation of chemicals such as ammonia, chlorine, and nitrogen oxides in the form of gases, aerosols, or particulate matter. If such irritants reach the lower airways, alveolar damage and pulmonary edema can result. Although the effects of acute irritants are usually short-lived, some may cause chronic alveolar damage or airway obstruction.

Occupational asthma is defined as variable air flow obstruction caused by a specific agent in the workplace. It is estimated that between 5% and 20% of all adult asthma cases can be attributed to workplace exposure.[36] By far the greatest number of occupational agents causing asthma are those with known or suspected allergenic properties, such as plant and animal proteins (e.g., wheat flour, cotton, flax, and grain mites). In most cases, the asthma resolves after exposure is terminated. However, hyperactivity of the airways may persist for years.

Hypersensitivity pneumonitis, or allergic alveolitis, is most commonly due to the inhalation of organic antigens of fungal, bacterial, or animal origin. The nature of the exposure and the client's immunologic reactivity determine the pulmonary response. Nonatopic people (i.e., those with no history of allergies) demonstrate a pulmonary response to organic dusts more often than atopic people, although atopic people, too, may exhibit pulmonary reactions.

Pneumoconioses, or the "dust diseases," result from inhalation of minerals, notably silica, coal dust, or asbestos. These diseases are most commonly seen in miners, construction workers, sandblasters, potters, and foundry and quarry workers. Pneumoconioses usually develop gradually over a period of years, eventually leading to diffuse pulmonary fibrosis that diminishes lung capacity and produces restrictive lung disease. Early clinical manifestations are cough and dyspnea on exertion. Chest pain, productive cough, and dyspnea at rest develop as the condition progresses.

TABLE 62–4	CHARACTERISTICS OF OCCUPATIONAL LUNG DISEASE			
Disease	**Onset of Symptoms**	**Diagnosis**	**Treatment**	**Clinical Course**
Acute respiratory irritation	Immediate—within minutes of exposure Pulmonary edema may be delayed for hours	Consistent history Physical findings of respiratory tract irritation	Avoidance of exposure Respiratory support as needed	Resolves in hours to days Pulmonary edema may last days to weeks
Occupational asthma	Immediate—within minutes of exposure Can be delayed up to 6 hours	PFTs demonstrate reduced rates of FEV_1 to FVC Chest x-ray usually normal	Avoidance of exposure Asthma medication Steroids	Resolves within hours Permanent loss of physiologic lung function may occur
Hypersensitivity pneumonitis	Within a few hours of exposure	Chest x-ray findings range from normal to fine or diffuse infiltrates PFTs demonstrate a reduction in vital capacity	Avoidance of exposure Steroids	Symptoms typically lessen in 48 hours Chest x-ray and PFT findings may last for weeks to months or may be permanent
Pneumoconiosis	Requires long-term exposure First manifestation often cough progressing to dyspnea	Restrictive pattern on PFTs Chest x-ray with asbestosis shows interstitial markings in lower lobes and with silicosis shows opacities in upper lobes	Avoidance of exposure Cessation of smoking	Gradual worsening with fatigue, loss of appetite, chest pain, respiratory failure, and death

FEV_1, forced expiratory volume in 1 second; FVC, forced vital capacity; PFTs, pulmonary function tests.

Outcome Management

Early detection is one way to prevent progression of occupational lung disease. The respiratory history should consist of a (1) complete occupational history and questions about the actual job performed rather than title or job description, (2) past as well as current occupations, and (3) exposure to organic and inorganic substances in each job. The physical examination should include assessment of respiratory pattern and effort, presence of cough, lung sounds, and other manifestations indicating potential lung disease. Some employers support ongoing assessment programs (e.g., routine pulmonary function studies or chest x-rays) for workers at risk for occupational lung disorders.

Exposure precautions are essential for avoiding permanent pulmonary disability. Safety measures include adequate ventilation, the wearing of masks, and care in the handling of garments worn in dusty environments.

Nursing intervention for clients experiencing occupational lung diseases is similar to that for clients with other restrictive lung disorders (see following discussion). Supportive measures can help clients adjust their lifestyles to their conditions.

If occupational lung disease is significant, the client may qualify for a disability allowance. Refer clients to community resources, such as federal or state departments of labor, if they have questions about their eligibility for such allowances.

RESTRICTIVE LUNG DISORDERS

Restrictive lung disorders constitute a major category of pulmonary problems. The category includes any disorder that limits lung expansion and produces a pattern of abnormal function on pulmonary function tests characterized by a decrease in TLC.

Etiology

There are many causes of restrictive lung diseases. They may result from conditions affecting lung tissues or extrapulmonary causes. Extrapulmonary causes include neurologic and neuromuscular disorders and disorders affecting the thoracic cage, pleura, and movement of the diaphragm. Obesity may also lead to restrictive lung disorders. Box 62–5 lists restrictive lung disorders.

Clinical Manifestations and Diagnostic Findings

Manifestations vary according to the cause of the restrictive disorder. For example, kyphosis, scoliosis, and kyphoscoliosis result in changes in the thoracic cage (Fig. 62–8). Generally, clients with restrictive lung disease exhibit a rapid, shallow respiratory pattern. Chronic hyperventilation occurs in an effort to overcome the effects of reduced lung volume and compliance. Shortness of breath is experienced, at first only with exertion, but later at rest. ABG measurements reveal alveolar hyperventilation (i.e., reduced partial pressure of arterial carbon dioxide [$PaCO_2$]) during the initial and intermediate phases of the disease process. As the disease progresses, respiratory muscle fatigue may occur, leading to inadequate alveolar ventilation and carbon dioxide retention. Hypoxemia is a common finding, especially in the later stages of restrictive lung disease.

Pulmonary function tests demonstrate impairment of the lungs' bellows action. Commonly, the ratio of FEV_1 to forced vital capacity (FVC), or FEV_1/FVC ratio, is normal or increased (i.e., 75% or more of expected values). The FEV_1/FVC ratio by itself is not an absolute indicator of restrictive lung disorders. Reduced TLC is the primary indicator of the disease. TLC is less than 80% of expected values in clients with restrictive lung disease.

Often a specific diagnosis of restrictive lung disease is made only after extensive testing, including chest x-ray, biopsy, immunologic testing, and tests to differentiate neurologic dysfunction, such as electromyography and cerebrospinal fluid analysis.

Outcome Management

Management is based on the severity of impairment and the ability to reverse the condition. Clients with spinal deformities may be helped by corrective spinal surgery. Likewise, obese clients breathe better after weight loss. Selected clients may benefit from the use of transtracheal oxygen administration or nighttime mechanical ventilation with a mask or cuirass respirator (a device that covers the chest and moves the chest wall out and back through changes in pressure), especially clients who have postpoliomyelitis syndrome.

The primary goals of nursing management of the client with restrictive lung disease are (1) promotion of adequate oxygenation, (2) maintenance of a patent airway, and (3) achievement of the highest possible functional level. Interventions to attain these goals are similar to those used in the treatment of COPD (see Chapter 61). ABG analysis is important for monitoring oxygen needs, acid-base balance, and the effects of physical activity. $PaCO_2$ values should be monitored because rising carbon dioxide level is an indicator of impending respiratory failure.

Most restrictive lung disorders are not reversible. End-stage disease is characterized by the development of pulmonary hypertension, cor pulmonale, severe hypoxemia, and eventual respiratory failure. Efforts should be made to maintain the client's functional status and quality of life at as high a level as possible.

LUNG TRANSPLANTATION

Lung transplantation is appropriate for clients who have end-stage lung disease that is unresponsive to medical therapy and who are experiencing progressive deterioration in health status. This procedure involves replacement of one or both of the diseased lungs with a lungs from a cadaver donor. Live donor lobar transplantation has also been performed. The success of lung transplantation has improved significantly since the early 1980s and has become a widely accepted treatment for certain pulmonary diseases, such as COPD, cystic fibrosis, pulmonary fibrosis, and pulmonary hypertension.

PREOPERATIVE CARE

Preoperative assessment consists of both medical and psychosocial evaluation. Once the severity of lung disease is established, the client's physical health is assessed to determine candidacy for transplantation. A battery of tests is performed to rule out active infection and to evaluate cardiac, hepatic, hematopoietic, and renal functions. Psychosocial evaluation focuses on assessing the client's his-

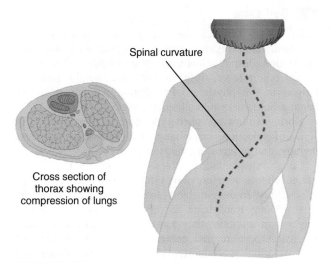

Spinal curvature

Cross section of thorax showing compression of lungs

FIGURE 62–8 Thoracic scoliosis. Note the S shape of the spine. These thoracic deformities alter the chest cage space. Lung tissue may be compressed, producing altered lung function (restrictive lung disease).

tory of compliance with medical therapy and medical recommendations as well as his or her ability to cope with stress.[40]

POSTOPERATIVE CARE

Postoperatively, the client is observed for excessive bleeding. Monitor vital signs, hemodynamic pressures, electrocardiogram (ECG), ABG values, transcutaneous oxygen level analysis, and chest tube drainage. Pulmonary edema may develop in the denervated transplanted lung. Therefore, the client may be started on mechanical ventilation with positive end-expiratory pressure (PEEP) for 24 to 48 hours.

Chest x-rays are obtained at least daily. Fluids are restricted, lung sounds are auscultated, and the severity of peripheral edema is monitored. Pain control is extremely important to allow deep-breathing and coughing in addition to chest physiotherapy. Many clients benefit from epidural analgesia. Following extubation, maintain good pain control, and help the client cough, deep-breathe, and use incentive spirometry to expand the lung.

The client who has received a lung is at high risk for infection and transplant rejection. Isolation is used to decrease inadvertent exposure to pathogens. Laboratory values are monitored, especially the WBC and absolute neutrophil counts. Monitor the client for clinical manifestations of infection, such as (1) changes in vital signs (especially fever), (2) local infections at intravenous access sites and incision lines, and (3) changes in respiratory status (excessive secretions, tachypnea, dyspnea, fatigue). Rejection of the transplanted lung may manifest as dyspnea, development of infiltrates on chest x-ray, need for ventilatory support, and fatigue.

Following the initial procedure, the client may experience alterations in self-concept related to changes in (1) appearance, from the side effects of medications such as steroids and immunosuppressants, (2) lifestyle, or (3) work ability and role performance. Be sensitive to these issues, and encourage the client and family to discuss their feelings and explore options.

■ Self-Care

Before discharge from the facility, teach the client about the medication regimen, and stress the need for daily medication despite a lack of manifestations. The client should report fever, dyspnea, excessive weight gain, and fatigue to the physician. In addition, the client should begin a pulmonary rehabilitation program.

During follow-up visits, the client is monitored for signs of rejection, compliance with immunosuppressive therapy, and progress in functional status.

Lung transplantation offers some hope for extended life to clients with previously fatal conditions. However, it is a very frightening and stressful surgery. Clients receiving lung transplants are always critically ill before surgery. In addition, they must undergo a radical, major surgical procedure and endure prolonged intensive care and isolation procedures. People with transplants also must adapt to an altered self-concept. The client and significant others need constant emotional support for achievement of a successful outcome.

DISORDERS OF THE PLEURA AND PLEURAL SPACE

PLEURAL PAIN

Pleural pain is a common pulmonary manifestation associated with a variety of disorders. It arises from the parietal pleura, which is richly supplied with sensory nerve endings. Pleuritic pain indicates the presence of pleural inflammation (*pleurisy*) due to pneumonia, pulmonary infarction, pleural effusion (see later), or pneumothorax, among others. It is often accompanied by a pleural friction rub that is discovered during chest auscultation.

Pleuritic chest pain often develops abruptly and is usually severe enough that the client seeks medical attention. It commonly occurs on only one side of the chest, usually in the lower lateral portions of the chest wall, and is aggravated by deep-breathing or coughing. Often the client can point directly to the exact location of the pain. However, pleural pain may also be referred to the neck, shoulder, or abdomen. Because other types of chest pain (e.g., cardiac pain, chest wall pain) may be misinterpreted as pleuritic pain, careful assessment is necessary.

Pleuritic pain may restrict normal respiratory efforts, leading to problems with gas exchange and airway clearance. If pain-relieving measures, including administration of prescribed analgesics, do not relieve the pain, the physician may perform an intercostal nerve block (see Chapter 23).

PLEURAL EFFUSION

Pleural effusion is an accumulation of fluid in the pleural space. Pleural fluid normally seeps continually into the pleural space from the capillaries lining the parietal pleura and is reabsorbed by the visceral pleural capillaries and lymphatic system. Any condition that interferes with either secretion or drainage of this fluid leads to pleural effusion.

Causes of pleural effusion can be grouped into four major categories. They are conditions that:

- Increase systemic hydrostatic pressure (e.g., heart failure)
- Reduce capillary oncotic pressure (e.g., liver or renal failure)
- Increase capillary permeability (e.g., infections or trauma)
- Impair lymphatic function (e.g., lymphatic obstruction due to tumor)

Clinical manifestations depend on the amount of fluid present and the severity of lung compression. If the effusion is small (i.e., 250 ml), its presence may be discovered only on a chest x-ray. With large effusions, lung expansion may be restricted, and the client may experience dyspnea, primarily on exertion, and a dry, nonproductive cough caused by bronchial irritation or mediastinal shift. Tactile fremitus may be decreased or absent, and percussion notes may be dull or flat.

■ PRIMARY PLEURAL EFFUSION

Thoracentesis (see Chapter 59) is used to remove excess pleural fluid. The removed fluid is analyzed to determine whether it is transudate or exudate. *Transudates* are substances that have passed through a membrane or tissue surface. They occur primarily in conditions in which there is protein loss and low protein content (e.g., hypoalbuminemia, cirrhosis, nephrosis) or increased hydrostatic pressure (e.g., heart failure). *Exudates* are substances that have escaped from blood vessels. They contain an accumulation of cells, have a high specific gravity and a high lactate dehydrogenase (LDH) level, and occur in response to malignancies, infections, or inflammatory processes. Exudates occur when there is an increase in capillary permeability.

Differentiating between transudates and exudates helps establish a specific diagnosis. Diagnosis may also require analysis of the fluid for white and red blood cells, malignant cells, bacteria, glucose content, pH, and LDH. Large pleural effusions, whether transudates or exudates, should be drained if they are causing severe respiratory manifestations.

Pleural fluid may be (1) hemorrhagic, or bloody (e.g., if tumor is present or after trauma or pulmonary embolus with infarction), (2) chylous, or thick and white (e.g., after lymphatic obstruction or trauma to the thoracic duct), or (3) rich in cholesterol (e.g., chronic, recurrent effusions due to tuberculosis or rheumatoid arthritis).

If there is a high WBC count and the pleural fluid is purulent, the effusion is called an *empyema*. An empyema of any volume requires drainage and treatment of the infection.

If the pus is not drained, it may become thick and almost solidified or loculated (containing cavities), a condition called *fibrothorax*. Fibrothorax may significantly restrict lung expansion and may require surgical intervention. The procedure, known as *decortication*, involves removal of the restrictive mass of fibrin and inflammatory cells. Decortication is usually not performed until the fibrothorax is relatively solid, so it can be easily removed.

After the procedure, closed-chest drainage with suction is used to reexpand the lung rapidly and fill the pleural space. If the fibrous material has restricted the lung for some time, the lung may not reexpand effectively and further intervention (usually thoracoplasty) may be needed.

■ RECURRENT PLEURAL EFFUSION

In some cases, pleural effusions may recur despite repeated thoracenteses (e.g., malignancy-induced effusions), with resultant compromise of lung function or persistent pleural pain. Treatment of recurrent effusions is accomplished through obliteration of the pleural space. Methods of obliterating the pleural space are as follows:

Pleurectomy (pleural stripping): Surgical stripping of the parietal pleura away from the visceral pleura, which produces an intense inflammatory reaction that promotes adhesion formation between the two layers during healing.
Pleurodesis: Instillation of a sclerosing substance (e.g., unbuffered tetracycline, nitrogen mustard, talc) into the pleural space via a chest tube to create an inflammatory response that causes the pleura to adhere and sclerose to each other.

Because pleural space obliteration creates permanent changes, the client's existing and predicted postprocedure respiratory status must be carefully evaluated. If a large area is involved, significant alterations in ventilatory mechanics (e.g., deep-breathing, coughing) may occur, leading to compromised respiratory function.

After the procedure, closely monitor lung function, including respiratory rate and ventilation pattern. Document alleviation or persistence of pleural pain and watch for indications of a return of the pleural effusion. Pulmonary function studies (see Chapter 59) and ABG measurements should also be performed.

BRONCHOPLEURAL FISTULA

A bronchopleural fistula is a communication between the pleural space and a bronchus. It may occur when an undrained empyema erodes into a bronchus or when the pleural space does not heal spontaneously after removal of a chest tube. A bronchopleural fistula raises the risk of pleural infection and may compromise ventilation and oxygenation.

The management of a client with a bronchopleural fistula is often complex. Bronchopleural fistulae may be slow to heal. The client may be discharged home with a chest tube still in place and connected to a collection system. Teach the client and family how to care for the chest tube and collection system and to recognize both manifestations of irritation at the chest puncture site and changes in chest drainage (e.g., blood) that require the physician to be notified.

METASTATIC PLEURAL TUMORS

Primary tumors in the lungs and other organs often metastasize to the pleura. The primary tumor is usually in a lung but may occur in the breast, ovaries, liver, kidneys, uterus, testicles, or larynx or may result from leukemia or lymphoma. Metastatic pleural disease frequently causes pleural effusions.

Assessment findings in malignant pleural effusion are the same as those in pleural effusion from other causes. Diagnosis of pleural effusion is by chest x-ray examination. The source of the effusion is determined from cytologic examination of pleural fluid obtained by thoracentesis.

Intervention is the same as for any pleural effusion, along with treatment of the primary malignancy.

DISORDERS OF THE DIAPHRAGM

SUBDIAPHRAGMATIC ABSCESS

A subdiaphragmatic abscess may develop as a result of (1) gastrointestinal perforation, (2) surgery of the upper gastrointestinal system, liver, or biliary tract, (3) abdominal trauma, or (4) other intra-abdominal surgery. A subdiaphragmatic abscess produces abdominal and thoracic clinical manifestations that potentially compromise respiratory status.

Thoracic assessment findings consist of pleuritic pain

or pain referred to the shoulder on the affected side. Dyspnea and poor or no diaphragmatic movement are common. Abdominal assessment findings include flank pain or tenderness and a palpable abdominal mass in the region of the abscess. Generalized assessment findings are fever, anorexia, weight loss, and vomiting.

The diagnosis of a subdiaphragmatic abscess is confirmed by chest x-ray. The diaphragm is generally elevated on the affected side. Fluoroscopic studies of diaphragmatic movement reveal limitation or absence of diaphragmatic movement on the affected side. Pleural effusion also commonly occurs. Thoracentesis and analysis of the pleural fluid reveal an exudate. Subdiaphragmatic abscesses may erode and perforate the diaphragm.

Intervention for subdiaphragmatic abscess comprises antibiotic administration, drainage of the abscess, and supportive measures to maintain ventilation and respiratory status. An untreated subdiaphragmatic abscess is nearly always fatal. With treatment, the mortality rate is still high but drops to approximately 25%.

DIAPHRAGMATIC PARALYSIS

Many conditions may affect diaphragm function and result in paralysis, either unilateral or bilateral. The unilateral type of paralysis is more common than the bilateral type.

Etiology

Causes of unilateral diaphragmatic paralysis are as follows:

- Severing of the phrenic nerve during surgery
- Bronchogenic or metastatic tumors
- Neurologic disorders, such as poliomyelitis, encephalitis, herpes zoster, and diphtheria
- Accidental or birth trauma
- Mechanical obstruction (e.g., from aortic aneurysm)
- Infectious processes, such as tuberculosis, pneumonia, pleuritic disorders, and subdiaphragmatic abscess
- Other disorders (e.g., pulmonary infarction, congenital abnormalities)

Causes of bilateral diaphragmatic paralysis include:

- Many neuromuscular disorders, such as amyotrophic lateral sclerosis, muscular dystrophy, and Guillain-Barré syndrome
- Alcohol and lead neuropathies
- Closed-chest trauma
- Anatomic defects, such as congenital absence of the phrenic nerve, traumatic diaphragmatic rupture, and spinal injuries

Clinical Manifestations

Although the diaphragm is the primary muscle of respiration, its role can be assumed in part by the accessory and abdominal muscles. As a result, diaphragmatic paralysis is often difficult to detect.

The diagnosis of unilateral diaphragmatic paralysis is confirmed by fluoroscopy. During the fluoroscopic procedure, the client is asked to "sniff." If paralysis is present, the nonparalyzed side of the diaphragm descends during inspiration (the sniff), and the paralyzed side paradoxically rises. Clients with unilateral diaphragmatic paralysis usually experience dyspnea when lying on the affected side. Dyspnea on exertion is not usual unless there is underlying lung disease. Both TLC and vital capacity (VC) are reduced by about 20%. There is also less ventilation to the affected side, and mild hypoxemia occurs because of shifts of ventilation and blood flow. Pre-existing lung disease combined with unilateral diaphragmatic paralysis may be disabling, depending on the extent of the lung disease.

The effects of bilateral diaphragmatic paralysis are potentially much more severe than those of unilateral paralysis. However, the problem is often subtle and overlooked, especially if the client has a neuromuscular disorder.

Fatigue, disturbed sleep, and morning headache are frequently the only manifestations. A classic manifestation of bilateral paralysis of the diaphragm is increased dyspnea when the client is lying flat on the back (supine). Paradoxical inward abdominal movement during inspiration in the supine position and active use of the accessory muscles of inspiration also occur. The pulmonary effects of bilateral paralysis are pronounced when the client is supine. Functional residual capacity (FRC) is also decreased, as is lung compliance. In the side-lying position, ventilation is preferentially distributed to the uppermost lung tissue and away from blood flow, leading to a significant mismatch of ventilation and perfusion. Severe hypoxemia results. Reduced tidal volume leads to retention of carbon dioxide and respiratory acidosis. Respiratory muscle function decreases during rest and sleep, further compromising respiratory status.

Outcome Management

Little can be done to treat diaphragmatic paralysis. Management is aimed at supporting ventilatory function as needed. If the phrenic nerve is intact, a phrenic nerve pacer may be surgically inserted. However, this measure is possible only if the phrenic nerve can be stimulated (its status is tested first during a fluoroscopic procedure). Use of a phrenic nerve pacer is useful primarily for clients with spinal cord injuries.

Assess the client for subjective indications of hypoxemia or hypercapnia. Monitor ventilatory mechanics (e.g., inspiratory effort, spontaneous VC) and ABGs, observing for trends that indicate deterioration.

Nursing management focuses on maintenance of a patent airway and detection of deteriorating gas exchange. Because inspiration is impaired, the client may need assistance to cough and deep-breathe effectively. Position the client on the unaffected side in the semi-sitting or sitting position. Suction as necessary. Increase hydration to liquify secretions. Administer oxygen as prescribed. If respiratory function declines significantly, the physician and client (or possibly significant others) must decide whether a permanent tracheostomy should be placed and whether mechanical ventilation or other assistance devices (e.g., rocking bed, cuirass respirator) should be used.

CONCLUSIONS

Clients with lung disorders are a challenge to the nurse providing care. In addition to common nursing diagnoses centering on *Impaired Gas Exchange* and *Ineffective Airway Clearance,* the client is often anxious because of the feelings of dyspnea and air hunger. Management of lung disorders consists of methods to open the airway (bronchodilators), clear infection (antibiotics), and improve oxygenation (position, coughing and deep-breathing, oxygen).

THINKING CRITICALLY

1. **Your client, who has undergone thoracotomy, has a pleural chest tube connected to water-seal drainage. While your client is being positioned for a bedside chest x-ray, the drainage tubing is inadvertently disconnected from the chest drainage apparatus. What actions should you take?**

Factors to Consider. What happens to the normally negative pressure in the pleural space when it is exposed to room air? Is this a dangerous problem?

2. **A client with exertional dyspnea is admitted to the unit with a diagnosis of pleural effusion. He has difficulty breathing during the transfer from the cart to bed. You are asked to prepare the client for a thoracentesis. How would you prioritize care? What preparations are necessary for a thoracentesis?**

Factors to Consider. What is the purpose of a thoracentesis? How are complications avoided? What clients are at risk for pleural effusion?

BIBLIOGRAPHY

1. Bates, D. V., et al. (1992). Prevention of occupational lung disease. *Chest, 102*(3), 257S.
2. Blumenthal, N. P., Miller, W. T., & Kotloff, R. M. (1997). Radiographic pulmonary infiltrates. *AACN Clinical Issues, 8*(3), 411.
3. Bongard, F. S., Stamos, M. J., & Passaro E. (Eds.). (1997). *Surgery: A clinical approach.* New York: Churchill Livingstone.
4. Boutotte, J. M. (1999). Keeping TB in check. *Nursing 99, 29*(3), 34.
5. Breeding, D. C. (1998). Controlling silica exposures. *Occupational Health and Safety, 67*(10), 178.
6. Brewer, T. F., Heymann, S. J., & Ettling, M. (1998). An effectiveness and cost analysis of presumptive treatment for *Mycobacterium tuberculosis. American Journal of Infection Control, 26*(3), 232.
7. Brogdon, C. F. (1998). Women and cancer. *Journal of Intravenous Nursing, 21*(6), 344.
8. Calianno, C. (1996). Nosocomial pneumonia: Repelling a deadly invader. *Nursing 96, 26*(5), 34.
9. Carpenito, L. J. (2000). *Nursing diagnosis: Application to clinical practice* (8th ed.). Philadelphia: J. B. Lippincott.
10. Clarkson, E. F. (1999). Tuberculosis: An overview. *Journal of Intravenous Nursing, 22*(4), 216.
11. Colice, G. L., & Rubins, J. B. (1999). Practical management of pleural effusions. *Postgraduate Medicine, 105*(7), 67.
12. Corris, P. A. (1997). Prophylaxis post-transplant. *Clinics in Chest Medicine, 18*(2), 311.
13. Donohoe-Dennison, R. (1997). Nurse's guide to common postoperative complications. *Nursing 97, 27*(11), 56.
14. French, A. L., Benator, D. A., & Gordin, F. M. (1997). Nontuberculous mycobacterial infections. *Medical Clinics of North America, 81*(2), 361.
15. Gonzalez-Rothi, R. J. (1997). Resurgent TB: Stopping the spread. *Patient Care, 31*(9), 97.
16. Graybill, J. R., Kaufmann, C. A., & Patel, R. (1999). Treatment of systemic fungal infections. *Patient Care, 33*(19), 50.
17. Hiley, G. J. (1998). Managing the patient with a chest drain: A review. *Nursing Standard, 12*(32), 35.
18. Kemp, C. (1999). Metastatic spread and common symptoms. Part four: Lung cancer, malignant melanoma, multiple myeloma. *American Journal of Hospice and Palliative Care, 16*(3), 545.
19. King, A. B. (1999). Accurately interpreting ppd skin test results. *Nurse Practitioner, 24*(5), 144.
20. King, M. A., & Tomasic, D. M. (1999). Treating TB today. *RN, 99, 62*(6), 26.
21. Konstan, M. W. (1998). Therapies aimed at airway inflammation in cystic fibrosis. *Clinics in Chest Medicine, 19*(3), 505.
22. Long, C. O., Ismeurt, R., & Wilson, L. W. (1995). The elderly and pneumonia: Prevention and management. *Home Healthcare Nurse, 13*(5), 43.
23. Lynch, J. P., Kazerooni, E. A., & Gay, S. E. (1997). Pulmonary sarcoidosis. *Clinics in Chest Medicine, 18*(4), 755.
24. Mandel, J. H., & Baker, B. A. (1989). Recognizing occupational lung disease. *Hospital Practice, 24*(1), 21.
25. Marelich, G. P., & Cross, C. E. (1996). Cystic fibrosis in adults. *Western Journal of Medicine, 164*(4), 321.
26. Markowitz, N., et al. (1997). Incidence of tuberculosis in the united states among HIV-infected persons. *Annals of Internal Medicine, 126*(2), 123.
27. Marshall, B. C., & Samuelson, W. M. (1998). Basic therapies in cystic fibrosis: Does standard therapy work? *Clinics in Chest Medicine, 19*(3), 457.
28. Maurer, J. R., et al. (1998). International guidelines for the selection of lung transplant candidates. *Heart and Lung, 27*(4), 223.
29. Mays, M., & Leiner, S. (1997). Pharmacologic management of common lower respiratory tract disorders in women. *Journal of Nurse-Midwifery, 42*(3), 163.
30. Mountain, C. F. (1997). Revisions in the International System for Staging Lung Cancer. *Chest, 111*(6), 1710.
31. O'Hanlon-Nichols, T. (1996). Commonly asked questions about chest tubes. *American Journal of Nursing, 96*(5), 60.
32. Patterson, G. A. (1997). Indications for unilateral, bilateral, heart-lung, and lobar transplant procedures. *Clinics in Chest Medicine, 18*(2), 225.
33. Quinn, S. (1999). Lung cancer: The role of the nurse in treatment and prevention. *Nursing Standard, 13*(41), 49.
34. Rakel, R. E. (Ed.). (1998). *Conn's current therapy 1998.* Philadelphia: W. B. Saunders.
35. Ramsey, B. W. (1996). Management of pulmonary disease in patients with cystic fibrosis. *New England Journal of Medicine, 335*(13), 179.
36. Redlich, C. A., & Anwar, M. S. (1998). Occupational asthma: Keys to diagnosis and management. *Journal of Respiratory Diseases, 19*(6), 508.
37. Rosenstein, B. J., & Zeitlin, P. L. (1998). Cystic fibrosis. *Lancet, 351*(9098), 277.
38. Ruppert, S. D., Kernicki, J. G., & Dolan, J. T. (1996). *Critical care nursing* (2nd ed.). Philadelphia: F. A. Davis.
39. Sheffield, E. A. (1997). Pathology of sarcoidosis. *Clinics in Chest Medicine, 18*(4), 741.
40. Smith, C. M. (1997). Patient selection, evaluation, and preoperative management for lung transplant candidates. *Clinics in Chest Medicine, 18*(2), 183.
41. Smith, E. L. (1998). Pulmonary metastasis. *Seminars in Oncology Nursing, 14*(3), 178.
42. Sotir, M. J., et al. (1999). Tuberculosis in the inner city: Impact of a continuing epidemic in the 1990s. *Clinical Infectious Diseases, 29*(5), 1138.
43. Stalam, M., & Kaye, D. (2000). Antibiotic agents in the elderly. *Infectious Disease Clinics of North America, 14*(2), 357.
44. Stenton, C. (1998). Managing allergic alveolitis. *The Practitioner, 242*(1584), 200.
45. Vaz, A., et al. (1998). Coccidioidomycosis: An update. *Hospital Practice, 33*(9), 113.
46. Von Nessen, S. (1995). Exercise for patients with cystic fibrosis. *Perspectives in Respiratory Nursing, 6*(2), 5.
47. Yagan, M. B. (1997). Hospital-acquired pneumonia and its management. *Critical Care Nursing Quarterly, 20*(3), 36.
48. Yankaskas, J. R., & Knowles, M. R. (1999). *Cystic fibrosis in adults.* Philadelphia: Lippincott–Williams & Wilkins.

CHAPTER

Management of Clients with Acute Pulmonary Disorders

Joyce M. Black

NURSING OUTCOMES CLASSIFICATION (NOC)
for Nursing Diagnoses—Clients with Acute Pulmonary Disorders

Impaired Gas Exchange
Respiratory Status: Gas Exchange
Respiratory Status: Ventilation
Vital Signs Status
Fluid Volume Excess
Electrolyte and Acid-Base Balance
Hydration
Respiratory Status: Ventilation
Inability to Sustain Spontaneous Ventilation
Vital Signs Status
Respiratory Status: Gas Exchange
Respiratory Status: Ventilation

Ineffective Airway Clearance
Aspiration Control
Respiratory Status
Respiratory Status: Gas Exchange
Respiratory Status: Ventilation
Anxiety
Anxiety Control
Symptom Control
Risk for Infection
Immune Status
Risk Control
Tissue Integrity: Skin and Mucous
   Membranes

Altered Nutrition: Less Than Body Requirements
Nutritional Status
Nutritional Status: Food and Fluid Intake
Nutritional Status: Nutrient Intake
Nutritional Status: Biochemical Measures
Impaired Verbal Communication
Communication Ability
Communication: Expressive Ability
Communication: Receptive Ability
Altered Oral Mucous Membrane
Tissue Integrity: Skin and Mucous
   Membranes

RESPIRATORY FAILURE

Respiratory failure is a broad, nonspecific clinical diagnosis indicating that the respiratory system is unable to supply the oxygen necessary to maintain metabolism or cannot eliminate sufficient carbon dioxide (CO_2). *Acute respiratory failure* is defined as a partial pressure of arterial oxygen (PaO_2) of 50 mm Hg or less or a partial pressure of arterial CO_2 ($PaCO_2$) of 50 mm Hg or more. In clients with chronic hypercapnia, $PaCO_2$ elevations of 5 mm Hg or more from their previously stable levels indicate acute respiratory failure superimposed on chronic respiratory failure.

There are two general types of respiratory failure: (1) hypoxemic and (2) ventilatory. Clients with severe arterial hypoxemia who are minimally responsive to supplemental oxygen despite adequate ventilation have acute *hypoxemic respiratory failure*. Hypoxemic respiratory failure may be caused by diffuse problems such as pulmonary edema, near drowning or adult respiratory distress syndrome (ARDS), or localized problems such as pneumonia, bleeding into the chest, or lung tumors.

Ventilatory failure can result from central nervous sys-

tem (CNS) depression, inadequate neuromuscular ability to sustain breathing, or excessive respiratory system load. Conditions such as acute deterioration of chronic obstructive pulmonary disease (COPD, sometimes called chronic airflow limitation) and status asthmaticus are other causes of ventilatory failure.

Classically, a client in acute respiratory failure has an elevated $PaCO_2$ directly related to alveolar hypoventilation from either (1) decreased minute ventilation with normal dead space ventilation or (2) normal or increased minute ventilation with increased dead space ventilation. In the first category are clients with normal lungs whose respiratory status is impaired by drugs or diseases affecting respiration (e.g., neuromuscular disorders). In the second category are clients with intrinsic lung diseases such as COPD or severe pneumonia. Lung damage in these clients increases the amount of nonfunctional lung tissue, thus increasing dead space (or wasted) ventilation. Even with normal or increased minute ventilation, they cannot "blow off" (exhale) a sufficient amount of CO_2.

The following material addresses both types of respiratory failure, the conditions that commonly lead to the problem, and the usual management options.

HYPOXEMIC RESPIRATORY FAILURE

■ PULMONARY EDEMA

Pulmonary edema is the abnormal accumulation of fluid in the interstitial spaces surrounding the alveoli with advancement of fluid accumulation in the alveolar sacs. Pulmonary edema is classified by its underlying causes: *Cardiogenic* causes include left ventricular failure, mitral valve stenosis, cardiogenic shock, hypertension, and cardiomyopathy. *Noncardiogenic* causes are shown in Box 63–1. Pulmonary edema can also develop after catastrophic injury to the CNS, such as head injury; this form of pulmonary edema is called *neurogenic* pulmonary edema.

Etiology

Recall the processes guiding fluid movement (see Chapter 12). Normally, fluid moves into the interstitial space at the arterial end of the capillary as a result of hydrostatic pressure in the vessel and returns to the venous end of the capillary due to oncotic pressure and increases in interstitial hydrostatic pressure. Fluid in the interstitial spaces of the lungs is not uncommon. It normally escapes from the microcirculation and enters the interstitium, providing nutrients for the cells. The residual fluid is returned via the lymphatic system. Increased volume of fluid in the pulmonary arteries due to obstruction of forward flow is the most common cause of pulmonary edema. Heart failure is the most common example. Lung

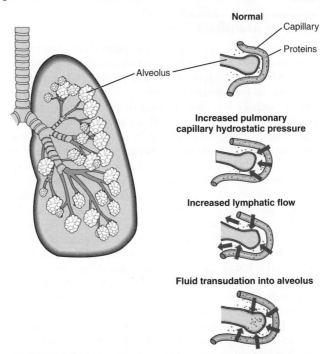

FIGURE 63–1 Progression of pulmonary edema. Pulmonary edema occurs when capillary hydrostatic pressure is increased, promoting movement of fluid into the interstitial space of the alveolar-capillary membrane. Initially, increased lymphatic flow removes the excess fluids but continued leakage eventually overwhelms this mechanism. Gas exchange becomes impaired by the thick membrane. Increasing interstitial fluid pressure ultimately causes leaks into the alveolar sacs, impairing ventilation and gas exchange. (From Hansen, M. [1998]. *Pathophysiology.* Philadelphia: W. B. Saunders.)

tumors can obstruct lymphatic flow and can also lead to pulmonary edema.

Pathophysiology

Increased hydrostatic pressure in the pulmonary vessels creates an imbalance in the Starling forces, leading to an increase in the fluid filtration into the interstitial spaces of the lung that exceeds the lymphatic capacity to drain the fluid away. Increasing volumes of fluid leak into the alveolar spaces (Fig. 63–1). The lymphatic system drains excess interstitial fluid volume. Additional fluid in the pleura drains into the hilar lymph nodes. If this pathway becomes overwhelmed, however, fluid moves from the interstitium into the alveolar walls. If the alveolar epithelium is damaged, the fluid accumulates in the alveoli. Alveolar edema is a serious late sign in the progression of fluid imbalance.

Hypoxemia develops when the alveolar membrane is thickened by fluid that impairs exchange of oxygen and CO_2. As fluid fills the interstitium and alveolar spaces, lung compliance decreases and oxygen diffusion is impaired. If pulmonary edema has developed because of left ventricular failure, right ventricular failure may occur because the pulmonary artery pressure is elevated. This elevation increases afterload for the right ventricle, resulting in manifestations of right ventricular failure.

BOX 63–1 Causes of Noncardiogenic Pulmonary Edema

Aspiration of gastric contents, especially if a large amount of HCl is present
Barotrauma (e.g., with PEEP with mechanical ventilation)
Drugs (e.g., after administration of narcotics)
Fluid overload from IV fluids or renal failure
Hypoalbuminemia (e.g., nephrotic syndrome, hepatic disease, malnutrition)
Sepsis
Inhalation of toxic chemicals (e.g., sulfur dioxide, paraquat, phosgene, chlorine, nitrogen oxides)
High altitudes (>8000 ft)
Neurogenic stimulus (e.g., increased intracranial pressure, epileptic seizures, head trauma)
Near-drowning syndrome
Mechanical ventilation, oxygen toxicity, ARDS
Malignancies blocking outflow of lymph within the lungs
Pancreatitis
Pneumonia
Smoke inhalation (e.g., trapped in a burning building)
Unilaterally, after reexpansion of collapsed lung (pneumothorax)

ARDS, adult respiratory distress syndrome; HCl, hydrochloric acid; IV, intravenous; PEEP, positive end-expiratory pressure.

Clinical Manifestations

The manifestations of pulmonary edema are due to an impairment in the regulatory factors guiding fluid movement. Most manifestations are seen in the respiratory system and include marked dyspnea, tachypnea, weak and thready tachycardia, hypertension (if cardiogenic), orthopnea at less than 90 degrees, and use of accessory muscles. The client's frequent coughing is an attempt to rid the chest of fluid. The sputum is thin and frothy because it is combined with water. If the hydrostatic pressure is very high, small capillaries break and sputum becomes pink-tinged. The client may be anxious from dyspnea and restless from hypoxemia. Chest auscultation reveals crackles, rhonchi, wheezes, and the presence of an S_3 heart sound. Heart murmur may be noted if the cause is mitral valve disease. Pulse oximetry is commonly less than 85% and arterial blood gas (ABG) determinations may reveal an arterial PaO_2 of 30 to 50 mm Hg. Respiratory alkalosis is common because of the tachypnea. Pressure in the pulmonary artery and pulmonary artery wedge pressure (PAWP) are elevated. The chest x-ray shows areas of "white-out" where fluid has replaced air-filled lung tissue, which normally appears black. Right ventricular failure may also be noted, with manifestations of hepatomegaly, jugular venous distention, and peripheral edema.

Outcome Management

■ Medical Management

Medical management addresses four areas: (1) correction of hypoxemia, (2) reduction in preload, (3) reduction of afterload, and (4) support of perfusion.

CORRECTING HYPOXEMIA

It is imperative to maintain adequate oxygenation, and clients with severe pulmonary edema commonly require oxygen therapy at high FiO_2 levels and may require mechanical ventilation or continuous positive airway pressure (CPAP) if they cannot meet the work of breathing.

REDUCING PRELOAD

The client is placed in an upright position. Usually, the client does not lie down because of orthopnea and a feeling of choking when supine. Diuretics are prescribed to promote fluid excretion. Nitrates, such as nitroglycerin, are used for their vasodilative properties. Phlebotomy can be used to remove excessive volumes of blood, although this practice is fairly rare. Older methods of preload reduction included the use of rotating tourniquets; this practice is also rare today. Other management strategies consist of treating the underlying condition.

REDUCING AFTERLOAD

Afterload is reduced to diminish workload on the left ventricle. Antihypertensive agents, including potent agents such as nitroprusside, are prescribed. Morphine is prescribed to reduce the sympathetic nervous system response and to reduce anxiety from the dyspnea.

SUPPORTING PERFUSION

Left ventricular failure is supported by using inotropic medications such as dobutamine. Urine output is monitored closely to determine whether renal perfusion is adequate. An intra-aortic balloon pump (IABP) may be needed (see Chapter 55).

■ Nursing Management

ASSESSMENT

The client with pulmonary edema is assessed quickly upon admission. Anxiety is often marked, and control of dyspnea is imperative. A complete assessment is carried out over the following hours, when the client can breathe more comfortably and answer questions. A baseline weight is recorded, and baseline lung assessment is noted.

DIAGNOSIS, OUTCOMES, INTERVENTIONS

Impaired Gas Exchange. The fluid-filled alveoli retard the exchange of gases. Use the nursing diagnosis *Impaired Gas Exchange related to capillary membrane obstruction from fluid* to plan care.

Outcomes. The client will demonstrate improved gas exchange, as evidenced by rising PaO_2 to 55 or 60 mm Hg, oxygen saturation above 90%, normalizing pH, decreasing anxiety and dyspnea, and fewer crackles and rhonchi within 12 hours.

Interventions. Monitor vital signs every 15 minutes initially, until the client is stable, and the electrocardiogram (ECG). Administer oxygen as ordered using a high-flow rebreather bag to maintain oxygenation. Titrate the actual liter flow of oxygen to maintain saturation above 90%. Continuous assessment is needed because the client may not be able to tolerate the work of breathing and may require intubation and mechanical ventilation. Mechanical ventilation and intubation equipment should be nearby. To reduce preload, position the client with the legs in a dependent position. Raising edematous legs increases venous return and will stress the overtaxed left ventricle. Preload is reduced with morphine and nitroglycerin. Morphine can be used to reduce anxiety. Because perfusion to the skin is often compromised, repositioning is important.

Air hunger can lead to panic and feelings of suffocation. Feelings of anxiety in the client can lead to the nurse's empathetic reaction of being out of breath also. Be aware of the "contagiousness" of anxiety and its effect on decision-making. Administer opioids and anxiolytics to control both dyspnea and anxiety. Stay with the client and give breathing using 1:1 techniques, such as "Breathe with me, in and out, slowly."[13a]

Fluid Volume Excess. Accumulation of fluid from several causes leads to fluid overload. Use the nursing diagnosis *Fluid Volume Excess related to excess preload.*

Outcomes. The client will demonstrate fluid balance, as evidenced by diuresis (input < ouput), decreased number of crackles and rhonchi, eupnea, weight loss, resolving peripheral edema, and decreased anxiety.

Interventions. Administer furosemide as prescribed to promote diuresis. Place an indwelling catheter to monitor response to diuretics. Monitor urine output, weight, and potassium levels (potassium loss is a side effect of furosemide). Monitor blood pressure to determine whether the client can maintain perfusion without inotropic support. Because oral fluids are restricted, oral care is completed every 2 hours.

TABLE 63–1	RISK FACTORS FOR ACUTE VENTILATORY FAILURE

Imbalances in Load	Imbalances in Neuromuscular Competence
Increased resistance	*Depressed drive*
Bronchospasm	Drug overdose
Airway edema	Brain stem lesions
Retained secretions	Hypothyroidism
Airway obstruction	
Obstructive sleep	*Impaired neuromuscular trans-*
apnea	*mission*
	Phrenic nerve injury
Elastic recoil in lung	Spinal cord lesion
Alveolar edema	Neuromuscular blocking agents
Infection	Aminoglycosides
Atelectasis	Guillain-Barré syndrome
	Myasthenia gravis
Elastic recoil in chest	Amyotrophic lateral sclerosis
wall	Botulism
Pleural effusion	
Pneumothorax	*Muscle weakness*
Rib fractures	Fatigue
Tumors	Electrolyte imbalance
Obesity	Malnutrition
Ascites	Hypoperfusion
Abdominal disten-	Hypoxemia
tion	Myopathy
Minute ventilation	
Sepsis	

From Schmidt, G., Hall, J., & Wood, L. (1994). Ventilatory failure. In J. Murray & J. Nadel (Eds.), *Textbook of respiratory medicine* (2nd ed.). Philadelphia: W. B. Saunders.

EVALUATION

Expect a fairly rapid response to diuresis and oxygen therapy.

Self-Care

Consider the reasons for development of pulmonary edema when developing a plan for self-care. Clients may need further education on daily weights, dietary choices, and scheduling of medications. Teach the early manifestations of fluid overload so that early intervention is possible.

ACUTE VENTILATORY FAILURE

Ventilatory failure is the inability of the CNS to sustain respiratory drive or inability of the chest wall and muscles to mechanically move air in and out of the lungs.

Etiology and Risk Factors

Two broad categories of problems can lead to acute ventilatory failure: (1) increased load for ventilation and (2) decreased ability or competence of the chest wall and lung to meet oxygen need. The respiratory load placed on the lung to exchange oxygen and CO_2 is impaired by (1) problems of resistance to moving air in and out of the lung, (2) ability of the lung to expand and contract (elastic recoil), and (3) conditions that increase the production of CO_2 or decrease the surface available for exchange of gases. The competence of the nerves and muscles coordinating the movement of the chest can also be impaired by loss of drive to breathe, impaired transmission of signals to the chest and diaphragm, and muscle fatigue. Conditions that can lead to acute ventilatory failure are listed in Table 63–1.

Pathophysiology

Alveolar ventilation is maintained by the CNS acting through nerves and the muscles of respiration to drive breathing. Failure of alveolar ventilation leads to hypercapnia (rising CO_2 levels). When CO_2 levels rise, acidosis develops. Untreated, ventilatory failure leads to death.

In obstructive forms of ventilatory failure, the residual pressure in the chest impairs inhalation and increases the workload of breathing. Functional residual capacity (FRC) is the volume of air remaining in the lung after normal expiration. When end-expiratory alveolar volumes remain above their critical closing point, the alveoli remain open and functioning, allowing oxygen to diffuse into the bloodstream. If alveolar volumes fall below the closing point, the alveoli tend to collapse. When alveoli collapse, no oxygenation of blood flow to the alveoli occurs (Fig. 63–2). The residual volume and FRC are decreased, resulting in a true intrapulmonary shunt (perfusion without oxygenation). Lung compliance is also affected.

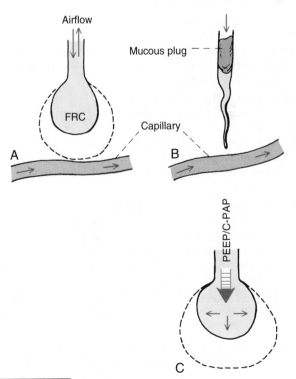

FIGURE 63–2 Effects of positive airway pressure on alveolus. *A,* Normal alveolus. *Dotted line* represents expansion during inspiration. *B,* Collapsed alveolus. Perfusion (continued). *C,* The alveolus is opened by positive pressure. *Dotted line* indicates alveolus during inspiration, and *solid line* indicates end-expiratory alveolar volume. FRC, functional reserve capacity; PEEP, peak end-expiratory pressure; C-PAP, continuous positive airway pressure.

Once alveolar collapse occurs, reinflation necessitates very high opening pressures, the generation of which significantly increases the work of breathing. The hypoxemia resulting from alveolar collapse and the increased oxygen consumption caused by the increased work of breathing may severely compromise the client.

Clinical Manifestations

To avoid frank apnea, recognizing impending ventilatory failure is crucial. Continuous monitoring of high-risk clients indicates changes in respiratory rate, mental status, and patterns of breathing. The client may also verbalize that dyspnea is increasing despite treatment. Altered respiratory patterns can herald impending ventilatory failure. The client's respiratory rate can rise to 50 to 60 breaths per minute, but the breaths are shallow and impaired by spasm of the airway. The rate can also fall to four to six per minute. Clients become confused, less conversant, and less arousable. If the cause is obstruction of the airway, during inspiration the systolic pressure falls as a result of intrathoracic resistance. This change, called *pulsus paradoxus,* is present when systolic blood pressure falls more than 10 mm Hg during inspiration. Pulse oximetry indicates steadily decreasing values, and ABG analysis shows falling PaO_2 and rising $PaCO_2$.

Outcome Management

◼ Medical Management

Medical management is directed at reversing bronchospasm, maintaining oxygenation, treating the underlying problem, and providing ventilatory assistance. Mechanical ventilation is not used until other methods of maintaining ventilation have been tried.

REVERSING BRONCHOSPASM

Several forms of bronchodilators are used to treat obstructions to airflow in clients with COPD and asthma. These agents include inhaled beta$_2$-selective agonists (albuterol), ipratropium, theophylline, and corticosteroids. If infection is the underlying cause, broad-spectrum antibiotics are given.

MAINTAINING OXYGENATION

Oxygen by mask may be adequate to support oxygenation. Using forms of CPAP, such as a mask, reduces the workload of breathing by decreasing the force needed to overcome the pressure in the chest. Outcomes after ventilation with lower tidal volumes may be better than the traditional formula (10 to 15 ml of body weight per kilogram), which sometimes led to stretch-induced lung injury.

MANAGING THE UNDERLYING PROBLEM

Table 63–1 demonstrates the many causes of ventilatory failure. Some of these causes can be quickly managed, such as drug overdose with naloxone, but others require more aggressive treatment. Supportive therapies are used to reverse or control the underlying problem.

MAINTAINING VENTILATION

Mechanical ventilation helps to minimize the work of breathing while effectively promoting gas exchange (oxygenation and ventilation). The client requires an artificial airway (usually by endotracheal tube [ET] intubation initially) and the use of positive-pressure ventilation (PPV). If prolonged intubation is required, the ET tube is replaced with a tracheostomy.

Intubation

The ET tube, a long, slender, hollow tube usually made of polyvinyl chloride, is inserted into the trachea via the mouth or nose. It passes through the vocal cords, and the distal tip is positioned just above the bifurcation of the mainstem of the bronchus (carina). Oral intubation is usually used for short-term airway management. Nasal intubation, a more secure method, is believed to be more comfortable because the tube does not move as much in the airway. However, nasal intubation is not being used in many hospitals because of the risk of sinusitis. The client is supine with all dental bridgework and plates and loose teeth removed because these items can be jarred loose and aspirated during intubation. The client's head is hyperextended, the lower aspect of the neck flexed, and the mouth opened (Fig. 63–3). This position brings the mouth, pharynx, and larynx into a straight line. A laryngoscope is used to hold the airway open, expose the vocal cords, and serve as a guide for the tube into the trachea. ET tubes are inserted only by fully trained health care team members.

Intubation should not cause or exacerbate hypoxia. If the client's neck and mandible are mobile, the procedure usually takes about 30 seconds. Certain pre-existing conditions, such as rheumatoid arthritis of the neck, can make intubation difficult. For clients with expected difficulty of intubation, an oxygen mask can be used to provide oxygen through the mouth. An oxygen saturation monitor may also be used to warn of hypoxemia.

A good practice to remember during difficult intubation is to hold your breath while intubation is attempted. If you must stop to breathe before the client is intubated, the intubation is taking too long. Stop the intubation, reoxygenate the client by mask, and reattempt intubation.

Immediately after ET tube insertion, tube placement is verified by auscultation and chest x-ray to ensure aeration of both sides of the chest. Record in the nurses' notes and on the respiratory flow sheet the point at which the tube meets the lips or nostrils by using the numbers listed on the side of the ET tube. If the tube slips, its correct position can be reestablished quickly.

Secure the ET tube immediately after intubation with adhesive tape, twill tape, or specially designed ET tube holders (Fig. 63–4). Secure a nasotracheal tube in the same way, but place the second of the small strips across the bridge of the nose instead of on the upper lip. Retaping is required only if the tape becomes loose or soiled.

Cuff Inflation

The cuff of an ET tube seals the tube against the tracheal wall to facilitate PPV and protects the respiratory tract from aspiration of foreign material.

The amount of air required to seal an ET tube cuff is reflected by the cuff pressure, which is usually maintained at less than 20 mm Hg. Most ET tubes are designed with soft plastic cuffs for use of high volumes at low pressures. Cuffs are inflated with a volume of air high enough to seal the trachea while exerting the lowest possible pressure on the tracheal wall. Low cuff pressure is neces-

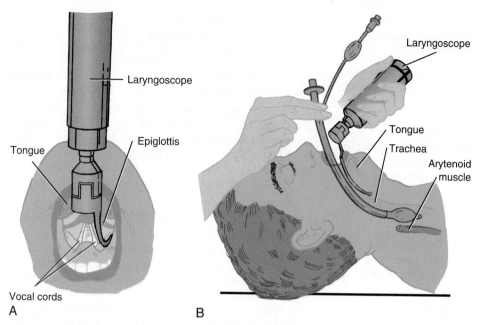

FIGURE 63-3 *A,* A laryngoscope is used to visualize the vocal cords. *B,* The endotracheal tube is inserted with the client's head extended to align the airway.

sary to prevent damage to the tracheal mucosa. Arterial pressures in the tracheal wall are approximately 20 to 25 mm Hg; venous pressures are 18 to 20 mm Hg. Therefore, cuff pressures greater than 18 to 20 mm Hg impair circulation to the tracheal mucosa and necrosis may develop. Assess cuff pressures every 8 hours.

The most common method of cuff inflation (*minimal*

occlusion volume technique) aims to provide an adequate seal in the trachea at the lowest possible cuff pressure. Slowly inject air into the cuff while auscultating with a stethoscope placed over the larynx (over the cuff) during a positive-pressure breath. At the point when sounds (from air movement) cease, inflation is stopped, indicating that the cuff is sealed against the tracheal wall.

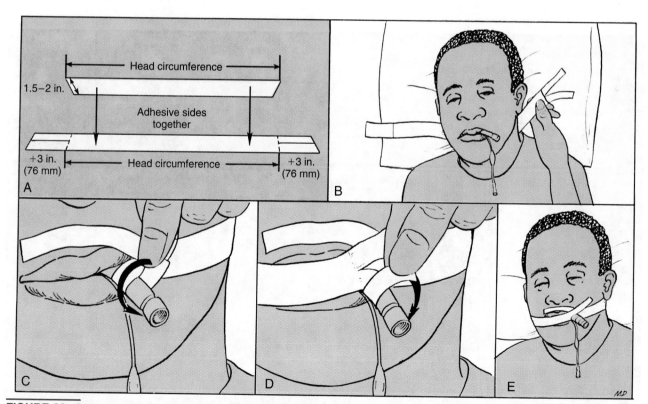

FIGURE 63-4 Securing a cuffed endotracheal tube with tape. *A,* Two strips of tape are torn; one is used to measure head circumference, and the other is 6 inches longer. The tape is placed with the adhesive sides together to form a strip. *B,* Place the strip behind the head and tear one end of the strip in half. *C,* Secure the tube to the upper lip with the untorn end. *D,* Wrap the torn segments around the tube to secure it (*E*).

Cuff Deflation

Generally, ET cuffs should remain inflated at all times. If cuff deflation is required for any reason:

1. Suction the trachea (with the client being hyperventilated and hyperoxygenated before and during this procedure).
2. Clean the area above the cuff of secretions by gently suctioning deep into the oropharynx.
3. Advance the suction catheter to the end of the ET tube. Deflate the cuff while applying suction to the suction catheter so that any secretions lying above the cuff can be removed.
4. Repeat pharyngeal suctioning.

Cuff Leaks

Cuff leaks can be a major problem. They may be caused by a rupture or tear in the cuff or pilot system or by a change in ET tube position in the trachea. There are several signs of a leak in or around the ET tube cuff:

- The pilot balloon is not filling when air is injected.
- The client can talk when the cuff is inflated.
- Air is heard leaking during positive pressure breathing.

If the system is not functional, the ET tube is replaced. Before replacement, increasing tidal volume may help maintain ventilation by compensating for the escaping gas. The client is at high risk for aspiration while the cuff is leaking.

CONTINUOUS MECHANICAL VENTILATION

The goals of continuous mechanical ventilation (CMV) are to:

- Maintain adequate ventilation
- Deliver precise concentrations of FiO_2
- Deliver adequate tidal volumes to obtain an adequate minute ventilation and oxygenation
- Lessen the work of breathing in those clients who cannot sustain adequate ventilation on their own.

Normal respiration begins with the contraction of the diaphragm and respiratory muscles to create negative pressure in the chest: A vacuum is created and air flows in. When a ventilator is used, positive pressure forces air into the lungs. The positive pressure can damage the alveoli and may retard venous return and cardiac output.

Types of Ventilators

Several types of mechanical ventilators are available. A control panel is shown in Figure 63–5.

Pressure-cycled ventilators deliver a volume of gas to the airway using positive pressure during inspiration. This positive pressure is delivered until the preselected pressure has been reached. When the preset pressure is reached, the machine cycles into exhalation. Pressure-cycled ventilators are used in only a small portion of clients who require CMV.

Volume-cycled (*volume-controlled* or *volume-limited*) ventilators deliver a preset tidal volume of inspired gas. The tidal volume that has been preselected is delivered to the client regardless of the pressure required to deliver this volume. A pressure limit can be set to prevent the occurrence of dangerously high airway pressures.

Time-cycled ventilators terminate when a preset inspiratory time has elapsed. In most of these devices, a pressure limit is also incorporated.

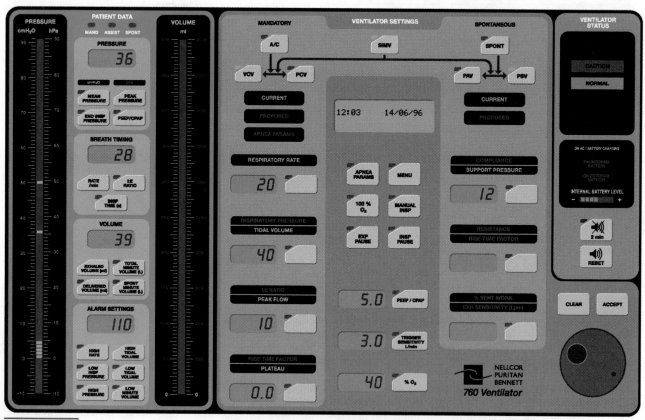

FIGURE 63–5 Nellcor Puritan Bennett 760 Ventilator. (Courtesy of Mallinckrodt, Inc., Nellcor Puritan Bennett Ventilator Division.)

BRIDGE TO CRITICAL CARE

Example of a Ventilator Control Panel

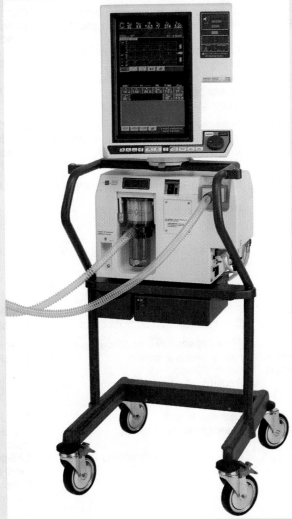

Puritan Bennett 840 Ventilator.

Troubleshooting Alarms

Display Message	Possible Cause	Remedy
HIGH CONTINUOUS PRESSURE	Airway pressure higher than set PEEP plus 15 cm H_2O for more than 15 sec	Check client Check circuit Check ventilator settings and alarm limits
CHECK TUBINGS	Disconnected pressure transducer (expiratory) Blocked pressure transducer (expiratory) Water in expiratory limb of ventilator Wet bacterial filter Clogged bacterial filter	Check ventilator internals on expiratory side Refer to service Replace filter Remove water from tubing and check humidifier settings, i.e., relative humidity Check heater wires in humidifier (if present)
AIRWAY PRESSURE TOO HIGH *Note:* If airway pressure rises 6 cm H_2O above set upper pressure limit, the safety valve opens. Safety valve also opens if system pressure exceeds 120 cm H_2O.	Kinked or blocked client tubing Mucus or secretion plug in endotracheal tube or in airways Client coughing or fighting ventilator Inspiratory flow rate too high Improper alarm setting	Check client Check ventilator settings and alarm limits

Bridge continued on following page

BRIDGE TO CRITICAL CARE *Continued*

Display Message	Possible Cause	Remedy
LIMITED PRESSURE *Note:* Alarm is active only in PRVC and VS modes	Kinked or blocked client tubing Mucus or secretion plug in endotracheal tube or in airways Client coughing or fighting ventilator Improper alarm setting Client's lung/thorax compliance decreasing Client's airway resistance increasing	Check client Check ventilator settings and alarm limits
EXPIRED MINUTE VOLUME TOO HIGH	Increased client activity Ventilator selftriggering (autocycling) Improper alarm limit setting Wet flow transducer	Check client Check trigger sensitivity setting Check alarm limit settings Dry the flow transducer
EXPIRED MINUTE VOLUME TOO LOW	Low spontaneous client breathing activity Leakage in cuff Leakage in client circuit Improper alarm limit setting	Check client Check cuff pressure Check client circuit (perform leakage test if necessary) Check pause time and graphics to verify Consider more ventilatory support for client
EXPIRED MINUTE VOLUME DISPLAY READS 0	Flow transducer faulty Circuit disconnected from client	Replace flow transducer Connect Y-piece to client
APNEA ALARM *Note:* If in VS, ventilator will revert to PRVC. Back-up rate and time must be set.	Time between two consecutive inspiratory efforts exceeds: Adult: 20 sec. Pediatric: 15 sec. Neonate: 10 sec.	Check client Check ventilator settings
PEEP/CPAP AND/OR PLATEAU PRESSURE FAILS TO BE MAINTAINED	Leakage in cuff Leakage in client circuit Improper alarm limit setting	Check cuff pressure Check client circuit (perform leakage test if necessary) Check pause time and graphics to verify Consider more ventilatory support for client

CPAP, continuous positive airway pressure; PEEP, positive end-expiratory pressure; PRVC, pressure-regulated volume control; VS, volume support.

Modified from *Servo Ventilator 300 operating manual 8.0* (1996). Solna, Sweden: Siemens-Elema AB.

Flow-cycled ventilators are triggered to stop when a preset flow rate has been achieved.

Modes of Ventilation

The ventilation mode refers to the way the client receives breaths from the ventilator. There are several conventional modes of CMV (Table 63–2).

Triggering Mechanisms

All breaths given to the client must be initiated or triggered. Triggering mechanisms can be based on (1) time, (2) negative pressure, (3) flow, or (4) volume.

Time-triggered inhalation is used to manage clients who cannot breathe on their own. The ventilator will trigger a breath after a preset time, serving as a back-up in case a client's own breathing rate falls below a preset value.

Negative pressure inhalation is triggered by the initial negative pressure that begins inspiration. As soon as the client initiates a breath, the ventilator is triggered to produce inhalation. The sensitivity of the system is set to reduce the workload of breathing. Pressure fluctuations (e.g., hiccoughs, leaks) can cause premature triggering.

Flow-triggered inhalation occurs when the client can initiate a breath. The ventilator completes the breath by sensing the flow of air into the chest. This system works well in combination with positive end-expiratory pressure (PEEP).

Volume-triggered ventilation occurs when the ventilator completes the breath to maximize inhaled gas volumes.

Alarms

Ventilators have several alarms to assist with their safe use (see Bridge to Critical Care).

Positive End-Expiratory Pressure and Continuous Positive Airway Pressure

PEEP and CPAP are techniques applied during expiration whereby intrathoracic pressures are not allowed to return to ambient atmospheric pressure. The PEEP and CPAP

TABLE 63–2	MODES OF MECHANICAL VENTILATION
Mode	**Description**
STANDARD MODES	
Continuous mechanical ventilation (CMV)	Ventilator delivers preset tidal volume and respiratory rate. No allowance for spontaneous breaths. Since ventilator is not responsive to client, this can lead to agitation and asynchrony.
Assist/control ventilation (A/C)	Spontaneous inspiratory effort of client triggers ventilator to deliver preset tidal volume. If client does not trigger an assisted breath, ventilator delivers breaths at preset respiratory rate.
Intermittent mandatory ventilation (IMV)	Ventilator delivers preset tidal volume and respiratory rate. Client can take unassisted spontaneous breaths between preset breaths. "Stacking" can occur when voluntary preset breaths occur simultaneously.
Synchronized intermittent mandatory ventilation (SIMV)	Similar to IMV except that preset ventilator breaths are synchronized with client's spontaneous breaths to avoid "stacking" of breaths. Can develop "stacking" of breaths and asynchrony.
Positive end-expiratory pressure (PEEP)	Preset amount of pressure stays in the lungs at the end of exhalation, keeping alveoli open. Used in conjunction with CMV, A/C, IMV, or SIMV
High-frequency ventilation (HFV)	Ventilator delivers breaths at a rate of greater than 60/min and at tidal volumes considerably lower than normal
Inverse ventilation ratio	Inspiration time is lengthened to over half of respiratory cycle. Reduces tendency to collapse alveoli, since they do not empty
Differential lung ventilation	Each lung is ventilated separately; special intubation needed with bifurcated endotracheal tube or two endotracheal tubes
WEANING MODES	
Continuous positive airway pressure (CPAP)	Similar to PEEP, but for the client who is breathing entirely on own (i.e., no ventilator-generated breaths)
Pressure support ventilation (PSV)	Client breathes spontaneously, but ventilator provides a preset level of pressure assistance with each spontaneous breath (inspiration only)
Volume support	Same as pressure support; tidal volume guaranteed
USE OF UNCONVENTIONAL GASES	
Nitric oxide	Relaxes smooth muscle of airway and arterioles. Used in ARDS
Helium	Carries oxygen at a lower density. Used to treat obstruction of large airways
GAS EXCHANGE DEVICES	
Extracorporeal membrane oxygenator (ECMO)	External oxygenation of blood. Blood is removed, oxygenated, and returned to the body without use of heart or lungs
Intravascular oxygenator	An oxygen/carbon dioxide exchange device is implanted in the inferior vena cava

Adapted from Boggs, R. L., & Wooldridge-King, M. (1993). *AACN procedure manual for critical care.* Philadelphia: W. B. Saunders.

are used to apply positive airway pressure that keeps the alveoli open and reduces the amount of shunting, allowing the use of lower levels of FiO$_2$ (Fig. 63–2C). This increased pressure also increases FRC and enhances oxygenation as a result of the enlarged surface area that is available for diffusion. CPAP is applied to a client with spontaneous respiration; PEEP is applied during mechanical ventilation. Positive pressures of 5 to 20 cm H$_2$O are typically used in adults. Pressures may be adjusted until the level is found that produces the best PaO$_2$ without producing adverse effects. This level is called "best PEEP."

Risks of PEEP include overdistention of the alveoli, ventilation-perfusion ($\dot{V}/\dot{Q}$) mismatch, subcutaneous emphysema, and decreased cardiac output from increased intrathoracic pressure.

PHYSIOLOGIC CHANGES AFTER MECHANICAL VENTILATION

Many physiologic changes occur when a client is placed on mechanical ventilation. Decreased cardiac output is the most common of these. Normal unassisted respiration begins with subatmospheric pressure. Negative pressure increases during inhalation and decreases during exhalation. Positive pressure applied to the airway has the opposite effect. As positive pressure inflates the lungs, pressure in the thorax builds, decreasing the flow of blood to the vena cava and reducing blood flow to the right atrium of the heart. Exhalation is passive, and pressures return to their normal, resting, subatmospheric level. Positive pressure also briefly affects the left side of the heart by increasing filling and output. This increase is due to the displacement of blood from the pulmonary system into the left ventricle. However, this effect is noted only immediately after institution of PPV.

If PPV is continued for more than a few minutes, blood flow to and from the right ventricle is decreased. This, in turn, decreases the filling of the left ventricle, leading to a lowered cardiac output. The lowered cardiac output is reflected in the hypotension that clients commonly exhibit immediately after receiving mechanical ventilation. It is imperative that blood pressures be monitored closely.

Stretch injury may develop in the alveoli and release inflammatory mediators. The lowest possible tidal volume and PEEP are used.

Other body systems are also affected by PPV. As the diaphragm descends into the abdomen during the inspiratory phase, blood flow to the splanchnic area decreases, sometimes leading to ischemia of the gastric mucosa. Ischemia of the gastric mucosa may be one of the reasons that clients receiving PPV for an extended period have a high incidence of gastrointestinal (GI) bleeding and stress ulcerations. Decreasing blood flow to the splanchnic region also results in decreased blood flow to the kidneys. Decreased blood flow signals the posterior pituitary gland to increase secretion of vasopressin (antidiuretic hormone [ADH]). Elevated vasopressin levels lead to reabsorption of free water in the renal tubular cells, thereby increasing water retention. Lymphatic flow also decreases.

PPV can also cause neurophysiologic changes. When ABG values improve in acute, uncompensated respiratory failure, improved cerebral oxygenation results. A client with compensated *respiratory acidosis* (chronic CO_2 retention) may be adversely affected by positive-pressure breathing owing to "blowing off" (exhalation) of CO_2. Acute alkalosis may occur, producing faintness, dizziness, lightheadedness, and anxiety. If severe alkalosis persists, convulsions, cardiac dysrhythmias, and cerebral edema may occur. Cerebral edema may contribute to intensive care unit (ICU) psychosis.

Oxygen toxicity can develop in clients who receive oxygen at concentrations greater than 70% for as little as 16 to 24 hours. Oxygen free radicals are produced in excess of their normal consumption by antioxidants; oxygen free radicals damage cell membranes, which increases the risk of pulmonary fibrosis. Manifestations of oxygen toxicity include fatigue, lethargy, weakness, restlessness, and nausea and vomiting. Later manifestations include severe dyspnea, coughing, tachycardia, tachypnea, crackles, and cyanosis. Because these manifestations are vague, oxygen concentration is limited to the minimal amount needed to maintain oxygenation.

■ Nursing Management

The nurse coordinates efforts of the health care team, teaches and supports the client and family, monitors the client's response to ventilation, intervenes to maintain oxygenation and ventilation, and ensures that the client's complex needs are met. See the Care Plan for the Mechanically Ventilated Client.

NEUROMUSCULAR BLOCKING AGENTS

Sedation is often necessary to maintain ventilation by creating a synchronous respiratory pattern and reduce oxygen demand. In some clients, paralysis with neuromuscular blocking agents is also needed. The most common agents given are vecuronium (Norcuron) and pancuronium (Pavulon). Because neuromuscular blocking agents do not inhibit pain or awareness, they are combined with a sedative or an anxiolytic agent. Pain medication may also be required if the client has pain. If the client is awake, be aware of anxiety or fear related to inability to breathe independently. The story of a nurse on a ventilator is an excellent reminder of a client's perceptions.[13]

Several nursing precautions are needed while these medications are administered. Reorient the client often, and explain all procedures because the client can still hear but cannot move or see. Eye care with lubricating ointment is important.

Long-term use of neuromuscular blocking agents has been associated with prolonged neuromuscular weakness. To avoid these complications, carefully monitor the client's level of paralysis using a peripheral nerve simulator (PNS) (Fig. 63–6). The PNS delivers an electrical stimulus (single, tetanic, or train-of-four) to a nerve. The train of four is the most common stimulus used. The facial, ulnar, posterior tibial, or peroneal nerve can be used; most commonly, the ulnar nerve is used for ongoing evaluation.

Problems with the PNS can give false readings. Poor skin contact, improper electrode placement, or edema of the arm can lead to false-negative readings, suggesting that the client has too high of a blockade. Direct stimulation of the muscle can lead to finger-twitching and may give an erroneous reading. This direct stimulus would provide a false-positive twitch and may lead to administration of more medication than needed. Correlate the PNS response to your clinical observation of the client.

WEANING FROM A VENTILATOR

The physician decides when to begin gradually removing, or "weaning," the client from CMV. The modes of the ventilator that depend on the client's initiating a breath can be used as modes for weaning. The decision is usually based on assessments made by nurses and respiratory therapists. The length of time required for successful weaning generally relates to the underlying disease process and to the client's state of health before the ventilator was used. For example, a young client who is recovering from an overdose of drugs can usually be weaned rapidly, but a client with COPD who develops acute respiratory failure and has little or no pulmonary reserve often takes longer and requires much professional patience and skill. Criteria for weaning are shown in Box 63–2.

Techniques for Weaning

Weaning from mechanical ventilation can be accomplished in two ways.

"RAPID" WEANING. The rapid, or T-piece weaning, technique is often used when mechanical ventilation has been instituted only briefly. Start in the morning after the client has had a good night's rest. Place the client in the semi-Fowler position. The ventilator's respiratory rate may be reduced to half the original rate; in some cases, this step may be eliminated. Obtain ABG values in 30 minutes.

Text continued on page 1760

■ THE MECHANICALLY VENTILATED CLIENT

Nursing Diagnosis. Inability to Sustain Spontaneous Ventilation related to imbalance between ventilatory capacity and ventilatory demand

Outcomes. The client will have a normal respiratory rate and pattern, return of arterial blood gases (ABGs) and pulse oximetry to normal, decreased dyspnea, absence of air trapping, and no complications after continuous mechanical ventilation (CMV).

Interventions	Rationales
1. Check ventilator settings, FiO$_2$, alarms, and connections and endotracheal (ET) tube placement (use cm markings) at beginning of each shift, hourly thereafter, and after any changes.	1. Determine baseline values, and validate that settings are accurate. Ensure that alarms are functional.
2. Assess lung sounds.	2. Lung sounds should be present bilaterally (unless a previous change in lung sounds is known).
3. Check placement of the ET tube, and secure the tube.	3. The visible portion of the ET tube should not change. Check previous records for a mark that is visible (in cm). Securing prevents dislodgment.
4. Use a bite block.	4. A bite block prevents the client from chewing on the tube and ET tube compression.
5. Move the ET tube daily from one side of mouth to the other. Assess for signs of skin or mucous membrane irritation.	5. ET tubes can place pressure on the lips and oral mucosa.
6. Assess for agitation, distress, and "fighting" the ventilator.	6. An incorrect ventilator setup may be providing less air than the client requires.
7. Assess for an obstructed airway. If it is obstructed, manually inflate lungs with a resuscitation bag and 100% oxygen and suction the airway.	7. Airway obstruction with mucus may prevent oxygenation. Providing air to the client is imperative. A common cause of obstruction is retained secretions.
8. Sedate and paralyze the client if ventilator settings and oxygenation are adequate.	8. Sedation and paralysis may be required to prevent mismatch.
9. Medicate the client if pain is indicated.	9. Pain can lead to agitation.
10. Perform passive range-of-motion (ROM) or assisted ROM exercises; transfer the client to a chair when feasible.	10. Immobility leads to decreased respiratory muscle strength.

Evaluation. The timing of goal attainment will vary greatly because of underlying co-morbid conditions. Expect postoperative clients to require CMV for 24 hours or less. Clients with end-stage pulmonary disease may require prolonged ventilatory support.

Nursing Diagnosis. Impaired Gas Exchange and Ineffective Breathing Pattern related to underlying disease process and artificial airway and ventilator system

Outcomes. The client will have improved gas exchange and breathing pattern, ventilation of both lungs, no signs of hypoxemia (O$_2$ saturation > 92%, respiratory rate < 24/min, no restlessness); ABGs and acid-base balance will return to preintubation level or normal values.

Interventions	Rationales
1. Auscultate lung sounds and respiratory rate and pattern every 1 to 2 hours as needed.	1. Auscultation reveals the amount of fluid and secretion in the lungs; validates that the ET tube is placed correctly so that both lungs can be ventilated; determines ventilatory effectiveness.
2. Provide adequate humidity via the ventilator or nebulizer.	2. This step replaces the function of the upper airway to warm and humidify the inspired air; thins secretions to facilitate their removal.
3. Turn and reposition the client every 2 hours (see Fig. 63–8).	3. Both lungs can be fully ventilated; secretions can be mobilized.
4. Monitor ABG values and pulse oximetry.	4. Degree of oxygenation can be indicated; lack of improvement in ABGs may require a change in interventions.

Evaluation. If the client's underlying problem has been corrected by mechanical ventilation, these outcomes will be met quickly. If the client has a pre-existing pulmonary disease or is acutely ill, it may take several days for attainment of outcomes.

Nursing Diagnosis. Ineffective Airway Clearance related to inability to cough and stimulation of increased secretion formation in the lower tracheobronchial tree from the ET tube.

Outcomes. The client will have improved airway clearance, as evidenced by fewer crackles, fewer rhonchi, and an absence of fever.

Care Plan continued on following page

Interventions

1. Assess the need for suctioning: noisy, wet respirations; restlessness; increased pulse and respirations; visible mucus bubbling into the ET tube; rhonchi; and an increase in peak airway pressure.
2. Thoroughly explain the procedure before starting, and provide reassurance to the client throughout.
3. Airway suctioning is performed on an "as-needed" basis, not at regularly scheduled intervals.
4. Select a catheter of appropriate size. The most common sizes for adults are 12F and 14F.
5. Avoid excessive vacuum pressures that may traumatize the airway.
6. Maintain sterility throughout the procedure. Use closed system for suctioning. Clean gloves can be used for closed suctioning; sterile gloves are needed for open suctioning.
7. Hyperoxygenate before and after each suctioning attempt and after the procedure. Increase the FiO_2 on the ventilator or manually ventilate the client.

Rationales

1. Detecting the need for suctioning early can prevent desaturation.
2. Suctioning can be an uncomfortable and frightening experience.
3. Suctioning can traumatize the airway and mucosa.
4. The suction catheter should never exceed half the diameter of an artificial airway or the natural airway it is to enter.
5. The safe range of pressure for adults is 80 to 120 mm Hg.
6. Usual cilia clearance and cough are suppressed. Closed systems avoid opening the ET tube and exposing the airway to the environment.
7. Providing extra oxygen prevents desaturation from suctioning.

Evaluation. The ability to maintain a clear airway will require several days until the underlying problem (e.g., pneumonia) is stabilized and the client's strength returns.

Nursing Diagnosis. Anxiety related to dependence on CMV for breathing

Outcomes. The client will exhibit decreased anxiety as evidenced by reduction in the level of stress or anxiety and decreased feelings of powerlessness.

Interventions

1. Develop a means of communication.
2. Place a nurse call device within the client's reach.
3. Be available and visible.
4. Provide distractions (e.g., television, radio).

5. Explain all procedures.
6. Medicate as necessary for anxiety.

7. Provide privacy.
8. Respect the client's rights and opinions.

9. Provide a calm environment.

10. Explain to the client and family that the client's vocal cords have been bypassed, which prevents talking; encourage them to use other modes of communication.

Rationales

1. Communication allows the client to have needs met.
2. Anxiety is increased when fear of being alone is present.
3. The client's anxiety is alleviated when not alone.
4. Anxiety is reduced because the client does not focus on the ventilator and noises.
5. The client feels respected and fears are alleviated.
6. Antianxiety medications and narcotics may be needed, but use them with caution during weaning because these drugs suppress respiratory drive.
7. Providing privacy demonstrates respect for the client.
8. The client feels respected and maintains dignity when included in discussion.
9. A frenzied environment engenders anxiety; if the client becomes anxious, ventilation is more difficult and oxygen needs increase.
10. Clients can hear and respond even though they cannot talk.

Evaluation. Expect the client to remain moderately anxious while receiving CMV.

Collaborative Problem. High Risk for Complications of CMV and Positive-Pressure Ventilation (PPV)

Outcomes. The nurse will monitor the client for pulmonary barotrauma, cardiovascular depression, inadvertent extubation, and malposition of the ET tube.

Interventions

1. Assess for acute, increasing, or severe dyspnea; agitation; panic; decreased or absent breath sounds; localized hyperresonance; increased breathing effort; tracheal deviation away from the side with abnormal findings; subcutaneous emphysema; and decreasing PaO_2 levels.
2. Assess for an acute or gradual fall in blood pressure, tachycardia (early sign), bradycardia (late sign), dysrhythmias, weak peripheral pulses, acute or gradual increase in pulmonary capillary wedge pressure (PCWP), and respiratory "swing" (depression) in arterial or pulmonary artery wave forms during inspiration.

Rationales

1. Barotrauma can lead to pneumothorax or tension pneumothorax.

2. Cardiovascular depression can occur after an increase in tidal volume, positive end-expiratory pressure (PEEP), continuous positive airway pressure (CPAP), or with hyperinflation; positive pressure decreases venous return and cardiac output because of an increase in intrathoracic pressure.

3. Monitor for signs of inadvertent extubation: vocalization, low-pressure alarm, bilateral decrease in upper lobe airway sounds, gastric distention, clinical manifestations of inadequate ventilation; change in length of portion of ET tube that extends beyond the lip. If inadvertent extubation occurs, notify the physician, because reintubation is necessary; manage ventilation and oxygenation with a self-inflating resuscitation bag.
4. Keep an intubation tray readily available.

3. Inadvertent extubation can be obvious, as when the tube is found in the client's hand; it can also be obscure, as when the tube slips into the hypopharynx or esophagus.

4. Intubation supplies may be needed quickly.

Evaluation. Most complications of PPV occur within 48 hours after intubation. Inadvertent extubation can occur at any time.

Nursing Diagnosis. Risk for Infection related to impaired primary defenses in respiratory tract

Outcomes. The client will remain free of infection, as evidenced by clear sputum, no fever, clear lung sounds, no increased difficulty with ventilation (e.g., increased peak inspiratory pressure), white blood cell (WBC) count within normal limits, and respiratory rate less than 24 breaths/min.

Interventions

1. Wash your hands thoroughly.
2. Use sterile technique for suctioning.
3. Monitor the client for increased breathing effort, localized changes on auscultation, and changes in PaO_2.
4. Provide oral care every 2 hours.

5. Drain water from ventilator tubing; do not drain water back into the humidifier.
6. Monitor laboratory values, WBC count, and differential.
7. Monitor sputum for changes in color, consistency, amount, and odor.

Rationales

1. Hand-washing reduces spread of infection.
2. The respiratory tract is considered sterile.
3. Infected lung segments transmit sound differently (more solid) and do not permit gas exchange.
4. The client's mouth becomes dry, and stomatitis may develop from lack of oral secretions.
5. Water may become a source of contamination, especially with *Pseudomonas*.
6. WBC count increases may indicate pulmonary infection.
7. Infection may cause sputum to increase, darken, thicken, and become malodorous.

Evaluation. Infection usually develops after 72 hours of intubation unless the client is immunosuppressed.

Nursing Diagnosis. Altered Nutrition: Less Than Body Requirements related to lack of ability to eat while on a ventilator and to increased metabolic needs

Outcomes. The client will exhibit adequate nutritional intake, as evidenced by (1) stable weight or weight appropriate to height, (2) intake of adequate calorie levels, (3) no signs of catabolism, (4) wound healing, (5) absence of infection, (6) laboratory value within normal limits (prealbumin, total protein, transferrin), and adequate muscle strength to breathe spontaneously.

Interventions

1. Provide adequate nutrition (high calorie intake, protein, vitamins, and minerals); provide a nutrition consult, as needed.

2. Begin tube-feeding as soon as it is evident that the client will remain on CMV for a length of time (usually 2–3 days).
3. Avoid excessive carbohydrate loads.

4. Weigh the client daily.

5. Monitor intake and output.
6. Assess for complications of tube-feeding: aspiration, diarrhea, constipation.

7. If the client cannot tolerate enteral feeding, consider total parenteral feeding (TPN).
8. Monitor bowel sounds.

9. Before tube-feeding or between bolus feedings, obtain pH and guaiac test every 8 hours.

Rationales

1. Intake of about 1200 kcal is adequate to maintain weight; inadequate nutrition decreases diaphragmatic muscle mass, decreases pulmonary function, and increases mechanical ventilation requirements.
2. The client should not be allowed to go into a catabolic state.

3. Carbohydrate loads may increase carbon dioxide production to the point of producing hypercapnia.
4. Changes in body weight are a reliable indicator of nutritional balance.
5. Fluids are still required, and output should match intake.
6. Feed the client while he or she is sitting upright, with the cuff inflated. Check for residual tube feeding every 4 hours (continuous feeding) or before beginning another feeding (intermittent feeding). Diarrhea is often caused by osmotic changes from an excessive concentration of tube feeding or the use of sorbitol-based elixirs; consider reducing the concentration or changing to crushed pills. Constipation is caused by a lack of free water within the feeding; add 100 ml of water every 4 to 6 hours if allowable.
7. Clients with decreased gastrointestinal (GI) function may require parenteral nutrition to meet metabolic needs.
8. Bowel obstruction and ileus present as changes in bowel sounds.
9. A change in pH may indicate an increased risk of gastric stress ulcer. A positive guaiac test indicates bleeding.

Care Plan continued on following page

■

Evaluation. Malnutrition is preventable. Expect the client's weight to stabilize (unless there is fluid imbalance).

Nursing Diagnosis. Impaired Verbal Communication related to mute state when the ET tube is in place

Outcomes. The client will be able to communicate with health care providers in order to have basic needs met.

Interventions	Rationales
1. Help the client develop a means of communication. Keep a pencil and paper pad or a picture board readily available. 2. Be patient and willing to spend time communicating.	1. With an ET tube passing through the vocal cords, the client cannot cough effectively or speak. 2. Prevents feelings of frustration, and reduces anxiety.

Evaluation. Depending on preexisting problems (language), disease-related problems (confusion), or treatment-related problems (restraints) affecting communication, the timing to develop effective communication may be long or short.

Nursing Diagnosis. Altered Oral Mucous Membranes related to nothing by mouth (NPO) status

Outcomes. The client's gums and mouth will remain moist and ulcer-free.

Interventions	Rationales
1. Provide oral hygiene every 2 hours. 2. Moisten the mouth with solutions that do not contain alcohol or lemon. 3. Moisten lips with lubricant. 4. Brush the client's teeth twice daily. 5. Suction oral secretions from mouth. 6. Assess for pressure areas at the corner of the mouth from the ET tube.	1. Oral mucous membranes dry in 2 hours. 2. Alcohol and lemon solutions dry mucous membranes. 3. Lubricants prevent drying, cracking, and excoriation. 4. Dental caries are prevented by saliva. 5. Secretions pool in the oropharynx because of the inflated tracheal cuff. 6. ET tube repositioning may be required.

Evaluation. Oral mucous membranes can be restored to pink and moist within 24 hours. Oral care, however, is an ongoing need.

If these values are at or near baseline level, place the client on a T-piece at the same FiO₂. Obtain ABG values in 30 minutes. If the ABGs are again at or near baseline level and the respiratory rate is below 25 to 30 breaths/min, extubate. Apply a face tent for high humidity.

Some nurse researchers are questioning the practice of beginning a weaning program in the morning. You may see changes in practice in the next few years based on the correlation of circadian rhythms with ideal time frames for weaning.

"GRADUAL" (SLOW) WEANING. This technique is used after prolonged mechanical ventilation or if a neuromuscular disorder is present. The first step is to ascertain whether spontaneous breathing is present. Once spontaneous breathing has been established, slowly reduce the amount of ventilatory support. Continue to reduce ventilatory support until the client can accept full responsibility for his or her own ventilatory requirements. This process may be accomplished through increasingly longer periods of time on a T-piece (followed by periods of CMV support) or by decreasing the rate of intermittent mandatory ventilation (IMV) or synchronized IMV (SIMV) breaths. This technique may take weeks or even months. Patience is crucial.

Difficulties in Weaning

A first weaning attempt may not be successful for several reasons:

- Decreased muscular strength caused by protein-carbohydrate malnutrition or certain disease processes or caused by incoordination of respiratory muscles from disuse after prolonged CMV

- Increased work of breathing due to increased airway resistance, abdominal distention, a small-diameter artificial airway, upper airway obstruction, or unresolved acute lung diseases
- Increased ventilation requirements
- Difficulty managing secretions
- Psychological factors, such as fear

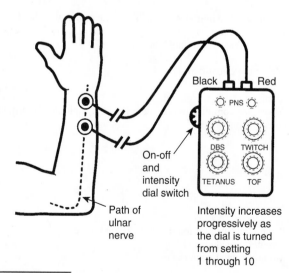

FIGURE 63–6 Peripheral nerve function is assessed with a nerve stimulator. (From Thelan, L. A., et al. [1998]. *Critical care nursing: Diagnosis and management* [3rd ed.]. St. Louis: Mosby–Year Book.)

Respiratory Criteria

Minute ventilation ≤ 15/L min
Respiratory rate ≤ 38 breaths/min
Tidal volume ≥ 325 ml
Maximum inspiratory pressure ≤ −15 cm H_2O
FiO_2 ≤ 50%

Other Criteria

Improvement, correction, or stabilization of the active disease process
Nutritional and fluid status sufficient to maintain the increased metabolic needs and demands of spontaneous respiration
Adequate physical strength and mental alertness
Afebrile status (any infections controlled)
Stable cardiovascular, renal, and cerebral status
Optimal levels of arterial blood gases, electrolytes, hemoglobin, and other laboratory tests

If the first attempt at weaning is not successful, determine the reasons and try to eliminate them in subsequent attempts. Clients who require prolonged ventilatory support and extended periods of weaning often do best in a setting that promotes rehabilitation concepts. These clients can usually be transferred to subacute or extended care facilities.

Extubation

Once the client has been weaned successfully and has demonstrated adequate ventilatory effort and an acceptable level of consciousness to sustain spontaneous respiration, the ET tube may be removed. ET tubes are removed on physician's orders and only by health care team members qualified to reintubate if necessary. The occurrence of laryngospasm and tracheal edema after extubation may occlude the airway, requiring reintubation.

The ET tube is suctioned, the cuff deflated, and the tube removed. Immediately after extubation, the client is usually given oxygen. Assess the client for signs of respiratory distress and hypoxemia, as evidenced by restlessness, irritability, tachycardia, tachypnea, and decreased PaO_2 or increased $PaCO_2$. If these signs are noted, notify the physician and prepare for reintubation.

Some clients are restless and extubate themselves. Because the cuff is not deflated, the tracheal wall can be damaged and bleeding can ensue. In most cases, the client requires reintubation, which must be done swiftly to prevent hypoxemia and to avoid needing to insert the ET tube through swollen tissues. Sometimes, however, the client can be monitored and not reintubated, especially if the time for extubation was approaching.

Dysfunctional Ventilatory Weaning Response

Some clients cannot adjust to lowered levels of mechanical ventilation, and the process of weaning them from the ventilator is delayed. The nursing diagnosis *Dysfunctional Ventilatory Weaning Response related to respiratory muscle fatigue or anxiety* may be used. Manifestations of respiratory muscle fatigue include a respiratory rate more than 30 breaths/min, increased $PaCO_2$, abnormal patterns

of breathing, hemodynamic changes such as dysrhythmias, diaphoresis, anxiety, and dyspnea.

An unsuccessful attempt to wean the client may have taken place, resulting in reventilation. When the client can not sustain ventilation independently, the ventilator is set at full ventilation; the client has no spontaneous breaths and, therefore, can rest.

Once the client has rested, attempts at weaning should begin again. Some clients can never be weaned from mechanical ventilation. Those clients can be managed in less acute care units or at home for many years.

Home Care of Ventilater-Dependent Clients

Some clients become stable and can be discharged from acute care and return home. The Bridge to Home Health Care feature provides ways to assist the ventilator-dependent client.

ADULT RESPIRATORY DISTRESS SYNDROME

ARDS is a sudden, progressive form of respiratory failure characterized by severe dyspnea, hypoxemia, and diffuse bilateral infiltrates. It follows acute and massive lung injury that results from a variety of clinical states, often occurring in previously healthy persons. The syndrome was first described in 1967 and has been alternatively referred to by several terms, including shock lung, wet lung, Da Nang lung (from the Vietnam War era), posttraumatic lung, congestive atelectasis, capillary leak syndrome, and adult hyaline membrane disease. Tremendous advances in the treatment of this condition have occurred over the last two decades.

Etiology and Risk Factors

ARDS develops as a result of ischemia during shock, oxygen toxicity, inhalation of noxious fumes or fluids (e.g, gastric acid), or inflammation from pneumonia or sepsis that traumatizes the alveolar capillary membrane. The insult may be directly to lung tissue or indirect, occurring in other body areas. Conditions leading to ARDS are listed in Box 63-3. Early recognition and treatment of these conditions may reduce the risk of ARDS.

Pathophysiology

The hallmark of ARDS is increased permeability of the alveolar membrane, with resultant movement of fluid into the interstitial and alveolar spaces. This leads to the development of noncardiogenic pulmonary edema, which decreases lung compliance and impairs oxygen transport.

Four phases of ARDS have been described:

Phase 1 consists of damage to the capillary endothelium with adhesion of neutrophils and initiation of protease enzymes. Inflammatory responses accompany the pulmonary parenchymal damage, leading to the release of toxic mediators, the activation of complement, the mobilization of macrophages, and the release of vasoactive substances from mast cells.

Phase 2 is further damage to the basement membrane, interstitial space, and alveolar epithelium. Fibrin, blood, fluid, and protein exude into the interstitial

BRIDGE TO HOME HEALTH CARE

Living with a Ventilator

It is essential that the ventilator-dependent child or adult client, family members, and informal caregivers have good communication with the home health nurse, the physician, and community resources. As soon as you obtain physician's orders and establish a plan of care, call the durable medical equipment (DME) supplier to review all of the equipment that will be required in the home setting. You may want to plan a shared visit with the DME supplier to evaluate and coordinate all of the client's equipment needs.

Next, check with the local electric company to ensure that your client will be placed on a list of people to receive priority attention and whose power service will be restored immediately in the event of an electrical failure. The client should have a portable battery-operated ventilator in the home in case of a power failure.

Plan to spend several hours with the family and informal caregivers during your initial home visit. Instruct them about the equipment, ventilator alarms, suctioning devices, dressing changes, and other care requirements. Be certain that they give satisfactory return demonstrations to you. The equipment may be very intimidating to the family. Write as much information as possible; provide the telephone numbers of the home health agency, the equipment supplier, the physician, other pertinent agencies, and yourself to use in case of emergency.

Write instructions about the use of the equipment in terms that the caregivers and family understand. Using large print, use a large piece of paper to make it easy to read and easy to find. It is not unusual to have families or caregivers forget most of the information you have presented after you leave. Remember, the client is probably happy to be back in the home environment, but the family may be very anxious and frightened. Address the availability of respite care or other community resources to provide the family with periods of rest and relaxation.

Equipment noise may be a nuisance. Suggest a radio, television, or cassette player with earphones. If clients can communicate through writing, make sure they have a computer, small chalkboard, or dry erase board. The family and client may want to hire a tutor to teach sign language, but most people learn to read lips.

Keep the room light and open; a bed by a window offers extrasensory stimuli. Caution the family to avoid irritants or pollutants (smoke, animal fur or dander, bird feathers, heavy dust).

Your creativity and imagination can help provide a safe and secure home setting when a ventilator is needed.

Terri Sellin Brown, RN, BSN, *School Nurse, Omaha Public Schools, Omaha, Nebraska*

---

spaces around the alveoli and increase the distance across the capillary membrane.

Phase 3 occurs when the source of injury persists and more mediators of inflammation are released.

Phase 4 is the irreversible deposition of fibrin into the lung, further decreasing compliance and oxygenation.

Throughout the process, the type II alveolar cells, which produce pulmonary surfactant, are also damaged, which leads to atelectasis and further impairment in lung distensibility and gas exchange. The end result is a significant $\dot{V}/\dot{Q}$ imbalance and profound arterial hypoxemia (see Understanding ARDS and Its Treatment).

Clinical Manifestations

The initial insult of ARDS is followed by a period of apparently normal lung function that may last from 1 to 96 hours. Then hypoxemia rapidly develops and progresses along with decreasing lung compliance and development of diffuse lung infiltrates.

The earliest clinical manifestation of ARDS is usually an increased respiratory rate. Breathing becomes increasingly labored; the client may exhibit air hunger, retractions, and cyanosis. Chest auscultation may or may not reveal the presence of adventitious sounds. If present, abnormal sounds may range from fine inspiratory crackles to widespread coarse crackles. ABG analysis reveals increasing hypoxemia ($PaO_2 < 60$ mm Hg) that does not respond to increased fraction of inspired oxygen levels ($FiO_2 < 40\%$) and compensatory hypocapnia. In the early stages, respiratory alkalosis is present because of hyperventilation. Later, metabolic acidosis develops from increased work of breathing and hypoxemia. The chest x-ray usually demonstrates diffuse, bilateral, and rapidly progressing interstitial or alveolar infiltrates (Fig. 63–7). Bronchial washing and biopsy may be used to determine whether infection is present.

Outcome Management

The keys to successful management of ARDS are early detection and initiation of treatment. The goals of medical management are (1) respiratory support, (2) maintenance of hemodynamic stability, (3) treatment of the underlying cause, when possible, and (4) prevention of complications.

■ Medical Management

Support Respiration and Ventilation

ET intubation, mechanical ventilation, and PEEP are usually required to maintain adequate blood oxygen levels. Smaller tidal volumes may be used to reduce the risk of lung injury. Other alternative modes of ventilation (e.g., extracorporeal membrane oxygenation [ECMO], intravascular oxygenation) may be employed in some situations. Inverse ratio ventilation (IRV) is one method of increasing mean airway pressure without creating further peak pressures in the alveolus from PEEP. IRV increases the inspiratory portion of each breath to more than half the respiratory cycle.

Nitric oxide (NO) is now being used more often in the treatment of ARDS. NO prevents calcium influx into cells and thereby causes vasodilation. Inhaled NO dilates the capillary bed of the lungs, which in turn reduces the

*Understanding ARDS and Its Treatment**

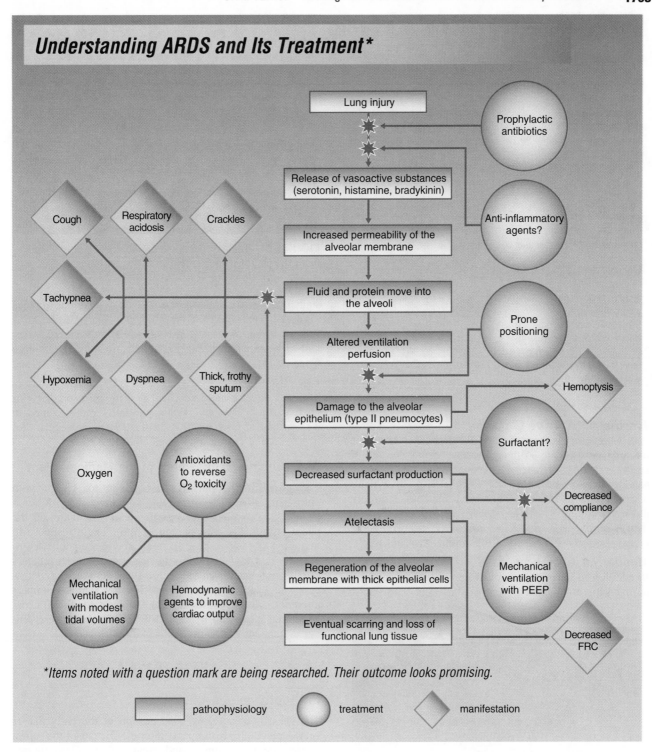

Items noted with a question mark are being researched. Their outcome looks promising.

pathophysiology   treatment   manifestation

pressure in the pulmonary arteries without lowering systemic blood pressure.

Scavengers of oxygen free radicals are being used. Alpha$_1$-antitrypsin has also been effective in reducing the degradative effect of the proteases. Pharmacologic efforts to inhibit the substances released by the endotoxins, neutrophils, and macrophages are also being explored.[42] To date, no effective method of administering surfactant has been developed.

The prone position has been used to improve oxygenation by changing the distribution of perfusion, sometimes by 50%.[12] Side effects include hypotension, desaturation, and dysrhythmias, although these appear to be short term. The prone position is shown in Figure 63–8.

Maintain Hemodynamic Stability

Hemodynamic monitoring is used to observe the effect of fluids and degree of pulmonary edema. The use of pharmacologic agents in the treatment of ARDS varies according to the client's underlying disease process. Inotropic agents (e.g., dobutamine) may be indicated to improve cardiac output and to increase systemic blood pressure. Fluids are restricted, and diuresis is produced.

Risk Factors for Adult Respiratory Distress Syndrome

Direct Pulmonary Trauma

Viral, bacterial, or fungal pneumonias
Lung contusion
Fat embolus
Aspiration (e.g., foreign material, drowning, vomitus)
Massive smoke inhalation
Inhaled toxins
Prolonged exposure to high concentrations of oxygen

Indirect Pulmonary Trauma

Sepsis
Shock
Multisystem trauma
Disseminated intravascular coagulation
Pancreatitis
Uremia
Drug overdose
Anaphylaxis
Idiopathic
Prolonged heart bypass surgery
Massive blood transfusions
Pregnancy-induced hypertension
Increased intracranial pressure
Radiation therapy

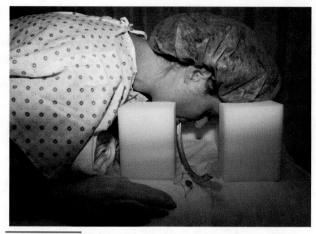

FIGURE 63-8 Use of the prone position to improve ventilation-perfusion. (Courtesy of H.E.A.D. Prone, Inc.)

such as cardiac dysrhythmias due to hypoxemia, oxygen toxicity, renal failure, thrombocytopenia, GI bleeding secondary to stress ulcers, sepsis from invasive lines, and disseminated intravascular coagulation (DIC) (see Chapter 75).

PROGNOSIS

The outcome for any one client is difficult to predict. For most of the 1970s and 1980s, mortality rates seemed to be constant at 60% to 70%. In the 1990s, however, rates improved and current rates are about 40%.[13]

Nursing Management of the Medical Client

The principles of nursing management of clients with pulmonary edema and care of the client requiring mechanical ventilation are appropriate in the care of the client with ARDS. Evaluation of the client's response to treatment as well as careful monitoring for potential complications is essential. Emotional support for the client's family and significant others is also important. The disease can progress very rapidly, leaving family members unprepared for the severity of the client's condition. Clear communications and frequent condition updates are essential to keeping the family adequately informed.

Treating Underlying Condition

Antibiotics are administered if suspected or confirmed infection is present. Although controversial, the use of large doses of corticosteroids is also common. The rationale for steroid administration is to reduce inflammatory response and to promote pulmonary membrane stability; however, controlled clinical trials have not demonstrated their effectiveness in ARDS, and their use is avoided unless the client is in shock from adrenal insufficiency.

Monitor for Complications

In addition to lung fibrosis, other complications may arise during supportive management of the client with ARDS,

CHEST TRAUMA

Pathophysiology

The chest is a large, exposed portion of the body that is very vulnerable to impact injuries. Because the chest houses the heart, lungs, and great vessels, chest trauma frequently produces life-threatening disruptions. Injury to the thoracic cage and its contents can restrict the heart's ability to pump blood or the lungs' ability to exchange air and oxygenate blood. Major dangers associated with chest injuries are internal bleeding and punctured organs.

Chest injuries can range from relatively minor bumps and scrapes to severe crushing or penetrating trauma. Chest injuries may be *penetrating* or *nonpenetrating (blunt)*. Penetrating chest injuries may cause an open chest wound, permitting atmospheric air into the pleural space and disrupting the normal ventilation mechanism.

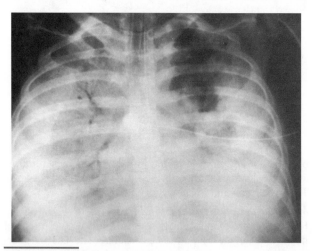

FIGURE 63-7 Adult respiratory distress syndrome (ARDS). This chest x-ray study shows massive consolidation from pulmonary edema following multisystem trauma. (From Fraser, R. G., et al. [1990]. *Diagnosis of diseases of the chest* [3rd ed., p. 493]. Philadelphia: W. B. Saunders.)

Penetrating chest injuries may seriously damage the lungs, heart, and other thoracic structures.

Blunt injuries are most commonly deceleration injuries associated with motor vehicle crashes. Blunt chest trauma may also result from falls or blows to the chest.

Initial assessment is directed toward identifying and treating immediate life-threatening conditions. Any client with chest trauma should be considered to have a serious injury until it is proved otherwise. Airway patency, adequacy of breathing, and circulatory sufficiency (i.e., presence of shock), or ABCs, are always of primary concern.

Once initial emergencies have been addressed, assess the client more thoroughly (Box 63–4). A medical history helps identify any pre-existing conditions that may further complicate the injury. A thorough physical examination should be performed, with care being taken not to focus only on obvious injuries. Information about the accident (obtained from the injured client or witnesses) assists in the diagnosis of regional as well as anatomic injuries. A chest film and ECG are obtained for detection of possible pulmonary or cardiac impairment.

Outcome Management

Ventilation-perfusion imbalances may result from atelectasis, hemopneumothorax, flail chest, aspiration, or pulmonary contusion. Oxygen or mechanical ventilation may be required. General respiratory status (e.g., rate and depth of respirations, chest movement, spontaneous vital volumes) and ABG values should be monitored closely. Deterioration may indicate previously undetected injury or late-developing complications.

Therapeutic measures such as thoracentesis, chest tube insertion, bronchoscopic aspiration, and thoracotomy (see Chapters 59 and 62) may be indicated. Maintain effective functioning of any equipment used (e.g., chest drainage system). Help the client and significant others understand these procedures and the rationale for their use. Clients with chest injuries may experience significant hypovolemia. Fluid replacement is with blood and blood products, if indicated, or with crystalloid IV solutions (e.g., lactated Ringer's solution, normal saline).

Monitor continually for clinical manifestations of shock. Shock often results from hypovolemia, but in the chest-injured client it may also be caused by cardiac tamponade, cardiac contusion, flail chest, or tension pneumothorax. Central vascular pressure readings (central venous pressure [CVP] or pulmonary artery pressure [PAP]) require careful interpretation. Once the cause of shock is determined, rapid treatment is crucial (see Chapter 81).

Excessive blood loss may further compromise oxygenation. Assess external bleeding carefully, and estimate blood loss. Internal bleeding may result from injuries to the thoracic or abdominal viscera, torn muscles, or fractures. Considerable bleeding (2 L or more) into the pleural space may occur. This is usually detected quickly. Bleeding into areas such as the chest wall (e.g., from torn intercostal muscles) is more difficult to assess. A liter of blood can accumulate between the chest wall muscles without producing much swelling.

A chest-injured person may require large quantities of blood replacement. Until the results of typing and cross-matching are available, the client is given O-negative blood. The volume of blood replacement is determined through assessment of clinical findings, hemodynamic measurements, and laboratory results (e.g., hemoglobin and hematocrit). When possible, surgery is delayed until blood volume is restored.

Pain associated with chest injuries may cause the client to breathe rapidly and shallowly, which leads to atelectasis and pooling of tracheobronchial secretions. Analgesics minimize pain, permit periods of rest and relaxation, and allow the client to cough and to take deeper breaths. Narcotics are most effective if given via the IV route. Intercostal nerve blocks or epidural analgesia may be used in clients with underlying health problems. Splinting the chest may also be helpful.

PNEUMOTHORAX

Pathophysiology

Pneumothorax is the presence of air in the pleural space that prohibits complete lung expansion. Air may escape into the pleural space from a puncture or tear in an internal respiratory structure (e.g., bronchus, bronchioles, alveoli). This form of pneumothorax is called *closed* (*spontaneous*) *pneumothorax* (Fig. 63–9A). Fractured ribs commonly lead to closed pneumothorax. Air may enter

---

BOX 63–4	Chest Trauma: Assessment and Interventions

1. Assess "ABCs":
   a. Maintain *a*irway, *b*reathing, and *c*irculation.
   b. Ensure adequate air movement.
2. Obtain a quick history:
   a. What happened?
   b. What was the mechanism of injury?
   c. How long ago did it happen?
   d. Where is the pain? Does it radiate?
   e. Is there anything that makes the pain better or worse?
   f. What does the pain feel like?
   g. How severe is the pain on a scale of 1 to 10?
   h. Is there a significant medical history?
3. Perform a quick (1-minute) assessment for:
   a. Shortness of breath and cyanosis
   b. Vital signs
   c. Skin color and temperature
   d. Wound size and location
   e. Paradoxical chest movement
   f. Distended neck veins
   g. Tracheal deviation
   h. Respiratory stridor
   i. Bilateral breath sounds
   j. Use of accessory muscles
   k. Estimated tidal volume
   l. Subcutaneous emphysema
   m. Sucking chest wounds
   n. Heart sounds
   o. Dysrhythmias
4. Quickly intervene:
   a. Administer oxygen.
   b. Cover any open chest wound.
   c. Control flail segment.
   d. Prepare to insert a chest tube.
   e. Initiate a large-bore intravenous line.

the pleural space directly through a hole in the chest wall (*open pneumothorax*) or diaphragm.

Clinical Manifestations

Clinical manifestations of *moderate* pneumothorax include tachypnea; dyspnea; sudden sharp pain on the affected side with chest movement, breathing, or coughing; asymmetrical chest expansion; diminished or absent breath sounds on the affected side; hyperresonance (tympany) to percussion on the affected side; restlessness; anxiety; and tachycardia.

Clinical manifestations of *severe* pneumothorax include all the preceding and distended neck veins; point of maximal impulse (PMI) of heart beat, or PMI shift; subcutaneous emphysema; decreased tactile and vocal fremitus; tracheal deviation toward the unaffected side; and progressive cyanosis.

Chest x-ray may reveal a slight tracheal shift away from the affected side and retraction of the lung back

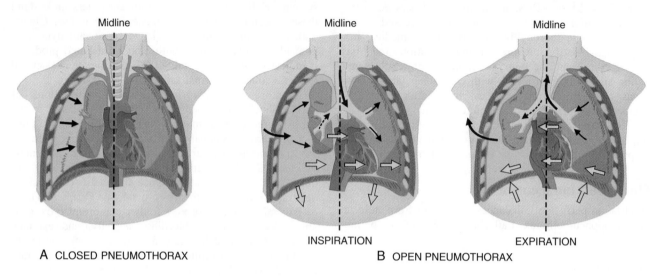

A CLOSED PNEUMOTHORAX

INSPIRATION   EXPIRATION
B OPEN PNEUMOTHORAX

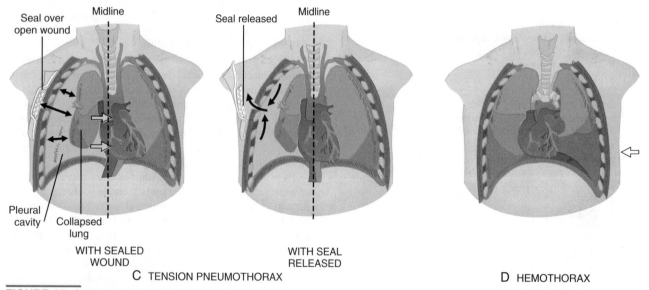

WITH SEALED WOUND   WITH SEAL RELEASED
C TENSION PNEUMOTHORAX

D HEMOTHORAX

FIGURE 63–9 Pneumothorax.

A, Closed pneumothorax. The lung collapses as air gathers in the pleural space.

B, Open pneumothorax (sucking chest wound). *Solid and dashed arrows* indicate air movement; *open arrows* indicate structural movement. A chest wall wound connects the pleural space with atmospheric air. During inspiration, atmospheric air is sucked into the pleural space through the chest wall wound. Positive pressure in the pleural space collapses the lung on the affected side and pushes the mediastinal contents toward the unaffected side. This reduces the volume of air in the unaffected side considerably. During expiration, air escapes through the chest wall wound, lessening positive pressure in the affected side and allowing the mediastinal contents to swing back toward the affected side. Movement of mediastinal structures from side to side is called mediastinal flutter.

C, Tension pneumothorax. *Left,* If an open pneumothorax is covered (e.g., with a dressing), it forms a seal, resulting in tension pneumothorax with a mediastinal shift. A tear in lung structure continues to allow air into the pleural space. As positive pressure builds in the pleural space, the affected lung collapses, and the mediastinal contents shift to the unaffected side. *Right,* Tension pneumothorax is corrected by removing the seal (e.g., dressing), allowing air trapped in the pleural space to escape.

D, Massive hemothorax (*arrow*) below the left lung, causing collapse of lung tissue.

from the parietal pleura. (In pneumothorax, the collection of air is between the visceral and parietal pleura.) On chest x-ray, pneumothorax is expressed as a percentage. For example, a client may have a complete 100% to a partial 10% pneumothorax. The use of percentages allows for evaluation of progress on subsequent x-rays. If pneumothorax is suspected (but respiratory distress is too severe to permit x-ray confirmation), the physician may insert an 18-gauge needle (emergency thoracentesis) into the second or third intercostal space in the midclavicular line. Aspiration demonstrates whether free air is present in the pleural space.

Outcome Management

Most physicians prefer to insert a chest tube immediately into the pleural space via the fourth intercostal space at the midaxillary or anterior axillary line. The chest catheter is connected to closed chest drainage (see Chapter 62). The catheter permits the continuous escape of air and blood from the pleural space, thus helping the lung expand by reestablishing subatmospheric (negative) pressure in the pleural space (necessary for normal ventilation). Sometimes thoracotomy is done to explore the chest surgically and to repair the site of origin of the pneumothorax or hemothorax.

■ OPEN PNEUMOTHORAX AND MEDIASTINAL FLUTTER

Pathophysiology

An open pneumothorax occurs with sucking chest wounds. With this type of wound, a traumatic opening in the chest wall is large enough for air to move freely in and out of the chest cavity during ventilation (Fig. 63–9B). This abnormal movement of air through the chest wound produces a slurping or sucking noise that is audible in a quiet environment.

Etiology

Open sucking chest wounds may result from accidental injuries or surgical trauma. For example, if a chest drainage catheter is accidentally pulled out of a chest, the remaining puncture incision in the chest wall may become a sucking wound.

Outcome Management

When an open sucking chest wound is detected, emergency intervention includes immediately covering the wound securely with anything available. An airtight covering usually prevents tension pneumothorax and preserves ventilation of the opposite lung. Do not waste time looking for a sterile gauze petrolatum dressing (the ideal covering for such a wound) if it is not immediately available. Cover the wound with whatever is at hand (e.g., a towel) right away until someone can bring a sterile petrolatum dressing. When possible, fix the temporary dressing firmly in place with several strips of wide tape.

If the client is conscious and cooperative, ask him or her to take a very deep breath and to try to blow it out while keeping the mouth and nose closed. This pushing effort against a closed glottis helps push air out through the chest wound and reexpand the lung. When the client does this, apply the dressing before the client inhales again.

Stay with the chest-injured client after a dressing has been applied to a sucking wound. Carefully assess for indications of tension pneumothorax and *mediastinal shift* (contents of mediastinum are pushed to the unaffected side of the chest). These complications may develop if the air leak is in the lung or a bronchus; such a situation allows air to escape into the pleural space. In such instances, closing the chest wall wound with an airtight dressing prevents the outflow of escaping air. Thus, an open pneumothorax has been accidentally converted into a tension pneumothorax. If tension pneumothorax appears to be developing after the wound is sealed, immediately unplug the seal to allow the air to escape. Closed chest drainage is necessary to (1) remove the air from the pleural space and (2) allow the lung to reexpand if it is collapsed.

In addition to experiencing dyspnea and collapse of the lung on the affected side, the client with an open pneumothorax may experience *mediastinal flutter*. This complication results from air rushing in and out of the thoracic cavity on the affected side. With inspiration, the mediastinal structures (heart, trachea, esophagus) and collapsed lung are pushed toward the unaffected side. With expiration, these structures then move back toward the affected side. Fluttering, back-and-forth movements of these vital mediastinal structures produce severe cardiopulmonary embarrassment, which is fatal if not treated promptly.

Chest tubes are inserted on the affected side away from the open wound. Surgical closure of the wound may follow. Supplemental high-flow oxygen should be administered.

■ TENSION PNEUMOTHORAX AND MEDIASTINAL SHIFT

Although it is dangerous to have air moving in and out of the pleural space with each respiration (open pneumothorax), the client is at even greater risk when air moves only into the pleural space and cannot move back out (tension pneumothorax). Tension pneumothorax (Fig. 63–9C) is a true emergency. Air enters the pleural space with each inspiration, becomes trapped there, and is not expelled during expiration (i.e., one-way valve effect). Pressure builds in the chest as the accumulation of air in the pleural space increases. Tension pneumothorax most commonly occurs with blunt traumatic injuries and is frequently associated with flail chest injuries.

If untreated, tension pneumothorax collapses the lung on the affected side as intrapleural pressure or tension increases, causing a mediastinal shift (mediastinal contents—heart, trachea, esophagus, great vessels—pushed or "shifted" toward the chest's unaffected side). Mediastinal shift may cause (1) compression of the lung in the direction of the shift (i.e., the lung opposite the pneumothorax) and (2) compression, traction, torsion, or kinking of the great vessels; thus, blood return to the heart is dangerously impaired. The latter situation causes a subsequent decrease in cardiac output and blood pressure. Tension pneumothorax produces serious circulatory and pulmonary impairment that can be rapidly fatal. This is a high-priority emergency requiring prompt assessment and intervention.

Clinical Manifestations

Clinical manifestations of tension pneumothorax include (1) marked, severe dyspnea; (2) tachypnea; (3) subcutaneous emphysema in the neck and upper chest; (4) progressive cyanosis; (5) acute chest pain on the affected side; (6) hyperresonance (tympany) to percussion on the affected side; (7) tachycardia; (8) asymmetrical chest wall movement; (9) diminished or absent breath sounds on the affected side; and (10) extreme restlessness and agitation. Other manifestations include (1) neck vein distention; (2) laryngeal and tracheal deviation or shift to the unaffected side; (3) a feeling of tightness or pressure within the chest; (4) a PMI shift laterally or medially; (5) severe hypotension leading to shock; and (6) muffled heart sounds.

A suspected mediastinal shift may be confirmed by x-ray study. Laryngeal and tracheal deviation toward the unaffected side can be detected by gentle palpation and with x-ray study. ABG analysis demonstrates hypoxia and respiratory alkalosis. When mediastinal shift is severe and not immediately corrected, respiratory acidosis may ensue.

Outcome Management

The immediate intervention is to convert *tension* pneumothorax into *open* pneumothorax (a less serious disorder). Large-bore chest tubes (36 to 40 Fr.) are inserted on the affected side at the fifth intercostal space anterior to the midaxillary line. Once tubes are inserted, suction drainage should be established. If a delay is anticipated, a 14- to 18-gauge needle is inserted into the pleural space of the affected side at the level of the second intercostal space at the midclavicular line. Prompt thoracentesis to remove air may be life-saving. As trapped air rushes from a tension pneumothorax, the tension is relieved, the lung should reexpand, and if mediastinal shift is present, it corrects itself. Supplemental oxygen is administered.

HEMOTHORAX

Hemothorax may be present in clients with chest injuries. A small amount of blood (<300 ml) in the pleural space may cause no clinical manifestations and may require no intervention (blood is reabsorbed spontaneously). Severe hemothorax (1400 to 2500 ml) may be life-threatening because of resultant hypovolemia and tension (Fig. 63–9D). Massive hemothorax is associated with 50% to 75% mortality.

Clinical manifestations include respiratory distress, shock, and mediastinal shift. There is dullness to percussion on the affected side.

A chest film confirms a diagnosis of hemothorax. If the client is in severe distress, the physician may aspirate blood from the pleural space by inserting a 16-gauge needle into the fifth or sixth intercostal space at the midaxillary line. To drain intrathoracic accumulations of blood, the physician inserts a large-caliber (36F or larger)

chest catheter, which is then connected to a drainage system. An initial drainage of 500 to 1000 ml is considered moderate, and additional treatment may not be required. An initial drainage of 1500 ml or more or continued large amounts of drainage (200 ml/hr) warrants immediate exploratory thoracotomy. Fluid replacement with O-negative blood or autotransfusion of blood should be used.

Surgical repair of active bleeding may be needed.

CHEST FRACTURES

■ FLAIL CHEST

Severe chest injuries that compress the rib cage often produce a "crushed" chest in which the ribs are pushed in on lung tissue. By definition, a flail chest consists of fractures of two or more adjacent ribs on the same side and, possibly, the sternum, with each bone fractured into two or more segments (Fig. 63–10). The flail segment most commonly involves the lateral side of the chest. It is common for a fractured rib end to tear the pleura and lung surface (thereby producing *hemopneumothorax*) and for a crushed chest to have a flail segment. Pulmonary edema, pneumonitis, and atelectasis often develop rapidly when the chest is crushed because fluids tend to increase and collect at the injured site.

The "flail" segment no longer has bony or cartilaginous connections with the rest of the rib cage. Lacking attachment to the thoracic skeleton, the flail section "floats," moving independently of the chest wall during ventilation. This abnormality disrupts the normal bellows action of the thorax by causing *paradoxical motion,* during which the flail portion of the chest and its underlying lung tissue are (1) "sucked in" with inspiration (instead of expanding outward as normal) and (2) "blown out" with expiration, instead of collapsing normally inward. This alteration in normal chest wall mechanics diminishes the client's ability to achieve an adequate tidal volume and to produce an adequate cough. Hypoventilation and hypoxia may result, leading to respiratory failure. Furthermore, mediastinal structures tend to swing back and forth (mediastinal flutter) with significant paradoxical motion. These swings may seriously affect circulatory dynamics, producing elevated venous pressure, impaired filling of the right side of the heart, and decreased arterial pressure.

In addition, pulmonary contusion occurs, resulting in an accumulation of fluid in the affected alveoli, which leads to intrapulmonary shunting and further hypoxia. The full effects of pulmonary contusion may not be manifested until the height of the body's inflammatory response in 24 to 48 hours.

The client with a flail chest commonly experiences emotional and physical distress while trying to breathe in spite of excruciating pain. The client is typically cyanotic and severely dyspneic. Respirations are usually rapid, shallow, and grunting. Paradoxical movement of the chest wall is usually obvious. Hypercapnia and hypoxia worsen as the effort necessary to breathe further depletes the already diminished oxygen supply. Frequent assessment of ABGs is needed to monitor respiratory effectiveness and to detect acidosis. Various factors produce metabolic and respiratory acidosis in chest-injured clients.

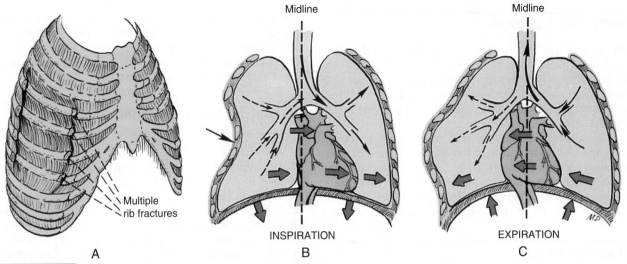

FIGURE 63–10 Flail chest. *Solid and dashed arrows* indicate air movement; *open arrows* indicate structural movement. *A,* A flail chest consists of fractured rib segments that are unattached (free-floating) to the rest of the chest wall. *B,* On inspiration, the flail segment of ribs is sucked inward. The affected lung and mediastinal structures shift to the unaffected side. This compromises the amount of inspired air in the unaffected lung. *C,* On expiration, the flail segment of ribs bellows outward. The affected lung and mediastinal structures shift to the affected side. Some air within the lungs is shunted back and forth between the lungs instead of passing through the upper airway.

Outcome Management

Treatment is usually with intubation and mechanical ventilation, which can accomplish the following:

- Restore adequate ventilation, thus reducing hypoxia and hypercapnia.
- Decrease paradoxical motion by using positive pressure to stabilize the chest wall internally.
- Relieve pain by decreasing movement of the fractured ribs.
- Provide an avenue for removal of secretions.

Internal stabilization with continuous ventilation may require 21 days or more. Muscle relaxants or musculoskeletal paralyzing agents may be administered to reduce the risk of separation of the healing costochondral junctions.

FRACTURED RIBS

Etiology

Rib fractures are common chest injuries, particularly in older adults. Such fractures are usually associated with a blunt injury, such as a fall, a blow to the chest, coughing or sneezing or (more frequently) the impact of the chest against a steering wheel during rapid deceleration. The fifth through the ninth ribs are most commonly affected.

Clinical Manifestations

Clinical manifestations include (1) localized pain and tenderness over the fracture area on inspiration and palpation, (2) shallow respirations, (3) the client's tendency to hold the chest protectively or to breathe shallowly in order to minimize chest movements, (4) bruising or surface markings (sometimes present) at the site of injury,

(5) protruding bone splinters if the fracture is compound, and (6) a clicking sensation during inspiration when costochondral separation or dislocation is present.

Fractured ribs predispose to atelectasis and pneumonia because the pain causes shallow breathing and prevents effective coughing. Thus, secretions accumulate, which obstruct the bronchi and become a site of infection. Shallow breathing also reduces lung compliance.

Bone splinters from fractured ribs may cause pneumothorax or hemothorax by puncturing the lung and pleura. Chest films are carefully reviewed for 24 to 48 hours after injury for indications of these complications. Bright-red sputum may be coughed up if the lung has been penetrated. Assess the client for signs of pneumothorax or hemothorax, and report such findings promptly.

Outcome Management

Fractured ribs are generally treated conservatively with rest, local heat, and analgesics. Strapping the ribs is no longer recommended because it restricts deep breathing and can increase the incidence of atelectasis and pneumonia. The pain from fractured ribs usually lasts 5 to 7 days. Complete healing occurs in approximately 6 to 8 weeks.

If pain is severe enough to impair ventilation significantly, a local anesthetic solution may be injected at the fracture site itself. Intercostal nerve blocks may also be used. A client with an underlying chest or heart disease (e.g., COPD, heart failure) may benefit particularly from this type of pain management. A chest film should be taken after this procedure to ensure that pneumothorax has not occurred. Adequate pain control and splinting of the chest during coughing and deep breathing help the client with rib fractures to carry out these painful but vital activities more comfortably. Hospitalization may be required, especially in the elderly, whose vital capacity may be significantly compromised.

FRACTURED STERNUM

Sternal fractures usually result from blunt deceleration injuries, such as impact from a steering wheel. They are usually accompanied by other major injuries, such as flail chest; pulmonary and myocardial contusions; ruptured aorta, trachea, bronchus, or esophagus; and hemothorax or pneumothorax.

Clinical manifestations include sharp, stabbing pain; swelling and discoloration over the fracture site; and crepitus. The main priority is to control associated injuries. A client with a nondisplaced fracture may need analgesics or intercostal nerve blocks for pain relief. Surgical fixation may be required for severe sternal fractures.

NEAR-DROWNING

Clients who initially survive suffocation after submersion in a water or fluid medium are said to have experienced a near-drowning or *immersion syndrome.* Freshwater drowning (i.e., in a swimming pool) is more common than saltwater drowning. Alcohol or drug ingestion, over-estimation of swimming skills, hypothermia, hyperventilation, and hypoglycemia are risk factors.

Both freshwater and saltwater wash out alveolar surfactant. Freshwater also changes the surface tension of surfactant. The loss of surfactant leads to alveolar collapse, intrapulmonary shunting, and hypoxemia. Poor perfusion and hypoxemia result in acidosis and eventual pulmonary edema. Near-drowning also compromises the respiratory system and leads to hypoxia, hypercapnia, cardiac arrest, and severe alterations in fluid-electrolyte balance. Bronchospasm, from aspirating water into the lungs, causes most drowning deaths. Cerebral edema from metabolic derangement is a major cause of death.

Outcome Management

Begin assessment and interventions with the ABCs. Obtain a history of the submersion. Include the length of submersion, temperature of the water, any associated injuries, and type of water. Note any respiratory efforts and adventitious sounds. Open the airway while maintaining spinal immobility. Assess the level of consciousness. Look for signs of hypoxia, such as confusion, irritability, lethargy, or unconsciousness. Obtain a complete set of vital signs. Additional injuries may be present, including associated trauma, spinal cord injury from diving, air embolism from scuba diving, and seizures.

For respiratory insufficiency, intubate and ventilate with 100% oxygen and 5 to 10 cm of PEEP to prevent the alveoli from collapsing. If the client is breathing, provide respiratory support with a non-rebreather mask.

Remove the client's wet clothing, and wrap the client in a warm blanket. Core rewarming may be indicated if the client is hypothermic. Rewarm the client slowly to avoid a rapid influx of metabolites (lactic acid) that may be trapped in the cold extremities.

Once the vital functions are stabilized, correct any acid-base or electrolyte abnormalities. Diagnostic studies include ABG analysis, complete blood count, electrolytes, appropriate toxicology studies if alcohol or drug ingestion

is suspected, and a chest film. Clients are at high risk for pulmonary edema even several hours after a near-drowning incident. Monitor neurologic status carefully. A deteriorating level of consciousness may indicate cerebral edema, severe acidosis, or increased hypoxia.

CARBON MONOXIDE POISONING

Etiology and Risk Factors

Carbon monoxide (CO) is a colorless, odorless, tasteless gas that is formed by the incomplete combustion of any carbon fuel. Intoxication by CO is the leading cause of death by poisoning. CO preferentially binds to hemoglobin, with an affinity for hemoglobin 200 to 230 times greater than that of oxygen. CO displaces oxygen, leading to reduced supplies of oxygen in the arterial blood and development of tissue hypoxia.

Generally, the client gives a history of exposure to CO after being found in an enclosed space in the presence of gases or fire. Faulty furnaces are also associated with CO poisoning. If CO poisoning is due to smoke inhalation, hoarseness, stridor, burns, or soot on the mouth or nose is present. Sputum may be black because of inhalation of soot. In a small number of clients, the skin will appear "cherry red" from high levels of oxygen in arterial blood.

Clinical Manifestations

Clinical manifestations are vague until levels of CO bound to hemoglobin (carboxyhemoglobin, or COHb) are around 40%. Manifestations include headache, vertigo, dizziness, nausea, and dyspnea on exertion when levels are below 20%. Above 20%, the client may have impaired concentration, clumsiness, and throbbing headache. Only when levels exceed 30% are manifestations more evident: irritability, visual changes, impaired thought, and vomiting. At 40% vital signs change and eventually coma ensues when levels are over 50%. The diagnosis is confirmed by measurement of carboxyhemoglobin levels in the blood.

Outcome Management

CO poisoning is treated by inhalation of 100% oxygen to shorten the half-life of CO to around an hour. Hyperbaric oxygen may be required to reduce the half-life of CO to minutes by forcing it off of the hemoglobin molecule. Reasons for CO poisoning must be explored and interventions directed at correcting those problems begun before hospital discharge. If the client's home furnace is faulty, it must be repaired. If the CO poisoning was a suicide attempt, crisis counselors should be used. Long-term neurologic and psychiatric consequences may develop, and the clients should be observed and followed up by their usual health care provider.

CONCLUSIONS

Two forms of respiratory failure exist: hypoxemic and ventilatory. Hypoxemic failure includes problems that lead to failure to transport oxygen and CO_2 across the capillary. Ventilatory failure includes disorders that impair neurologic triggers to breath and neuromuscular movement with respiration. Mechanical ventilation is a common method of treatment for both problems. Chest trauma involves life-threatening problems that demand prompt recognition and treatment.

THINKING CRITICALLY

1. **You are caring for a client who is receiving mechanical ventilation. You have just suctioned the client's airway and begin to leave the room when the high-pressure alarm sounds. What should you do?**

Factors to Consider. What changes in the client can trigger the high-pressure alarm? What changes in the ventilator can cause high pressure?

2. **You are going to position the client prone to improve ventilation and perfusion. What considerations should be made before, during, and after the prone position is used?**

Factors to Consider. How can the tubes be moved safely with the client? What complications might occur in a prone position? What procedures cannot be done while the client is prone?

BIBLIOGRAPHY

1. Burns, S. M., et al. (1995). Weaning from long-term mechanical ventilation. *American Journal of Critical Care, 4,* 4.
2. Butler, K. (1995). Psychological care of the ventilated patient. *Journal of Clinical Nursing, 4,* 398.
3. Carroll, P. (1995). A med/surg nurse's guide to mechanical ventilation. *RN, 58*(2), 26.
4. Connelly, B., et. al. (2000). A pilot study exploring mood state and dyspnea in mechanically ventilated patients. *Heart and Lung, 29*(3), 173–179.
5. Jones, C. (1998). Inhaled nitric oxide: Are the safety issues being addressed? *International Critical Care Nursing, 14*(6), 271–275.
6. Kacmarek, R. (1999). Ventilator-associated lung injury. *International Anesthesiology Clinics, 37*(3), 47–64.
7. Klein, D. (1999). Prone positioning in patients with acute respiratory distress syndrome: The Vollman Prone Positioner. *Critical Care Nurse, 19*(4), 66–71.
8. Kosmos, C. (1995). Multype trauma. In S. Kitt (Ed.), *Emergency nursing.* Philadelphia: W. B. Saunders.
9. Lenart, S., & Garrity, J. (2000). Eye care for patients receiving neuromuscular blocking agents or propofol during mechanical ventilation. *American Journal of Critical Care, 9*(3), 188–191.
10. Rice, R. (1995). Home mechanical ventilator management. *Home Healthcare Nurse, 13,* 73.
11. Ruppert, S. D., Kernicki, J. G., & Dolan, J. T. (1996). *Critical Care Nursing* (2nd ed.). Philadelphia: F. A. Davis.
12. Schuster, D., & Kollef, M. (1998). Acute respiratory distress syndrome. In D. Dantzker & S. Scharf (Eds.), *Cardiopulmonary critical care* (3rd ed., pp 415–433). Philadelphia: W. B. Saunders.
13. Spencer, K. (1998). Near breathing: Nurse on a vent. *Plastic Surgical Nursing, 18*(3), 139–140.
13a. Tarizan, A. J. (2000). Caring for dying patients who have air hunger. *Journal of Nursing Scholarship, 32*(2), 137–143.
14. The acute respiratory distress syndrome network. (2000). Ventilation with lower tidal volumes as compared to traditional tidal volumes for acute lung injury and the acute respiratory distress syndrome. *New England Journal of Medicine, 342*(18), 1301–1308.
15. Valta, P., et al. (1999). Acute respiratory distress syndrome: Frequency, clinical course and cost of care. *Critical Care Medicine, 27*(11), 2367–2374.
16. Voggenreiter, G., et al. (1999). Intermittent prone positioning in the treatment of severe and moderate posttraumatic lung injury. *Critical Care Medicine, 27*(11), 2375–2382.
17. Woodruff, D. (1999). How to ward off complication of mechanical ventilation. *Nursing99, 29*(11), 35–39.
18. Wright, J., Doyle, P., & Yoshihara, G. (1996). Mechanical ventilation: Current uses and advances. In J. Clochesy, et al. (Eds.), *Critical care nursing.* Philadelphia: W. B. Saunders.

Arterial Oxygen Saturation Monitoring by Pulse Oximetry

QUESTIONS

How accurately do measures of oxygenation using pulse oximetry agree with measures by standard arterial blood gas (ABG) analysis?

What factors affect the accuracy of pulse oximetry?

CITATION

Jensen, L. A., Onyskiw, J. E., & Prasad, N. G. N. (1998). Meta-analysis of arterial oxygen saturation monitoring by pulse oximetry in adults. *Heart and Lung, 27*, 387–408.

STUDIES

Published studies of pulse oximetry in adult clients were located by searching four health science indexes. Because this review used a statistical technique called *meta-analysis* to summarize and compare findings, only studies that supplied the necessary statistics were included. Seventy-four studies published between 1976 and 1994 met the inclusion criteria; approximately 30% were published in the early 1990s.

Many studies compared the percentage of oxygen saturation of hemoglobin (SaO_2) using pulse oximetry with that obtained at the same time using standard ABG analysis (an approach called *repeated measures design*). A variety of participants were represented in the studies, including healthy volunteers, hospitalized clients, cardiac surgical clients, and critically ill clients. Forty-one models of pulse oximeters from 25 manufacturers were studied.

Summary of Findings

Accuracy

The percentage of SaO_2 in arterial blood is widely used as a clinically significant index of oxygenation, and ABG analysis has been the "gold standard" for measuring it. However, the disadvantages of ABG analysis include:

- The need to perform multiple arterial punctures
- The intermittent nature of the information it provides
- Delay between time of sampling and availability of results
- Cost

Pulse oximetry using a finger or ear probe and an oximeter unit is noninvasive, provides immediate and continuous measures, and is relatively inexpensive. Clearly, if pulse oximetry can be established as accurate and precise, it should be widely used.

Pulse oximeters are most accurate when the SaO_2 is in the range of 70% to 100%; in this range, most models were found to be accurate within 2% of the standard ABG analysis value. Overall, few pulse oximeters performed well at an SaO_2 level below 70%.

In 39 studies that provided the essential data for the statistical analysis, the oximetry value and the ABG value had a weighted, average correlation coefficient of .895. (The value is weighted because it has taken into account the number of subjects in each study.) A correlation coefficient (r) of 1.0 would indicate perfect correlation between the values from the two methods. In the studies conducted during the 1990s, the weighted mean correlation coefficient was .899. The highest correlation was in healthy adult volunteers and the lowest in critically ill patients ($r = .760$).

Four studies compared pulse oximetry accuracy with ear and finger probes. Finger probes were found to have a statistically higher correlation with ABG SaO_2 (weighted $r = .967$) than ear probes (weighted $r = .938$).

Factors Affecting Pulse Oximetry Accuracy

Most difficulties in using pulse oximeters produce a blank screen or an error message, indicating problems; however, some circumstances may result in false readings. As mentioned, pulse oximetry readings become less accurate when clients are extremely hypoxic (SaO_2 level <70%).[2, 9, 11, 13, 17] Readings are also inaccurate when abnormalities of the hemoglobin's oxygen-carrying ability (as in carbon monoxide poisoning)[5, 14, 16] or severe anemia is present.[17]

In the three studies on which data were available, the accuracy of pulse oximetry decreased when the blood pressure was low; the weighted average r between pulse oximetry values and ABG values was .582. In one study, the oximeter alarm sounded for systolic blood pressure below 100 mm Hg and accuracy was decreased.[6] In contrast, another study using a different manufacturer's model obtained reliable data when mean arterial pressure was less than 60 mm Hg.[11]

Five studies examined the effect of hypothermia on pulse oximetry. The weighted r from the three studies with the necessary statistics was .665, indicating a relatively low level of accuracy when the client is hypothermic. However, findings are quite variable. In one study, the oximeter did not work properly[17]; in another study the oximeter overestimated the SaO_2[7]; and in another study, high correlations existed whether or not the client was hypothermic.[12]

Whether skin pigmentation affects the accuracy of pulse oximetry is even more uncertain. In the one study in which essential data were provided, the weighted r was .800. In a study that involved testing of two manufacturers' models, there was greater inaccuracy in the subset of African Americans than in the total sample.[3] In clients with high serum bilirubin levels, there was a low correlation between pulse oximetry and ABG—the SaO_2 value was underestimated by the oximeter.[4]

Limitations/Reservations. This soundly conducted statistical analysis of findings from many studies details the extent to which SaO_2 values determined by pulse oximetry correspond with ABG values under a variety of clinical conditions. The report provides much information about the accuracy of specific models of pulse oximeters.

Research-Based Practice

Most pulse oximeters are adequately accurate under various clinical circumstances, but in some clinical situations they may not produce accurate readings. Be aware that pulse oximetry may not record accurate SaO_2 values if the client has any of the following conditions.*

---

* The direction of error for each of these conditions is provided in the review report.

Arterial Oxygen Saturation Monitoring by Pulse Oximetry Continued

- Severe hypoxia (e.g., respiratory arrest)
- Severe anemia
- Sepsis
- Shock
- Hypotension, severe hypertension
- Hypothermia
- Cardiac arrest
- Poor peripheral blood flow (e.g., hypovolemia, peripheral edema, cardiogenic shock)
- Carbon monoxide poisoning (e.g., smoke inhalation, inhalation of fumes from a heating system or motor vehicle)
- High bilirubin levels (liver dysfunction)
- Dark skin pigmentation
- Diseases in which the hemoglobin's oxygen-carrying ability is abnormal
- After receiving intravenous methylene blue dye for a diagnostic procedure

When these conditions exist, pulse oximetry should not be used or it should be used only as a trend detector and the true value of the patient's SaO_2 determined by ABG analysis.

Unfortunately, one or several of these conditions may be present in most critically ill clients. Nevertheless, pulse oximetry is valuable in early detection of a decrease in SaO_2 by providing opportunity to notice deviations from baseline status. The evidence favors the use of finger probes rather than ear probes.

The authors of this meta-analysis caution that pulse oximetry does not present a complete picture of how well body tissues are being oxygenated. Information is not provided about the adequacy of the hemoglobin level, cardiac output, delivery of oxygen to the tissues, or oxygen consumption. Also, carbon dioxide levels and acid-base balance can be obtained only by ABG analysis.

Cited References

1. Barker, S. J., et al. (1993). The effect of sensor malpositioning on pulse oximeter accuracy during hypoxemia. *Anesthesiology, 79,* 248–254.
2. Brodsky, J. B., et al. (1985). Pulse oximetry during one-lung ventilation. *Anesthesiology, 63,* 212–214.
3. Cecil, W. T., et al. (1988). A clinical evaluation of the accuracy of the Nellcor N-100 and the Ohmeda 3700 pulse oximeters. *Journal of Clinical Monitoring, 4,* 31–36.
4. Chaudhary, B. A., & Burki, N. K. (1978). Ear oximetry in clinical practice. *American Review of Respiratory Disease, 117,* 173–175.
5. Douglas, N. J., et al. (1979). Accuracy, sensitivity to carboxyhemoglobin, and speed of response of the Hewlett-Packard 47201A ear oximeter. *American Review of Respiratory Disease, 119,* 311–313.
6. Fahey, P. J., et al. (1983). Clinical evaluation of a new ear oximeter (Abstract). *American Review of Respiratory Disease, 127*(4part2), 129.
7. Gabrielczyk, M. R., & Buist, R. J. (1988). Pulse oximetry and postoperative hypothermia: An evaluation of the Nellcor N-100 in a cardiac surgical intensive care unit. *Anaesthesia, 43,* 402–404.
8. Huffman, L. M. (1989). Pulse oximetry: Accuracy and clinical performance in different practice settings. *Journal of American Association of Nurse Anesthetists, 57,* 475–476.
9. Kagle, D. M., et al. (1987). Evaluation of the Ohmeda 3700 pulse oximeter: Steady state and transient response characteristics. *Anesthesiology, 66,* 376–380.
10. Kissinger, D. P., Hamilton, I. N., & Rozycki, G. S. (1991). The current practice of pulse oximetry and capnometry/capnography in the prehospital setting. *Emergency Care Quarterly, 7,* 44–50.
11. Mihm, F. G., & Halperin, B. D. (1985). Noninvasive detection of profound arterial desaturation using a pulse oximetry device. *Anesthesiology, 62,* 85–87.
12. Peters, K., et al. (1990). Increasing clinical use of pulse oximetry. *Dimensions of Critical Care Nursing, 9,* 107–111.
13. Severinghaus, J. W., Naifeh, K. H., & Koh, S. O. (1989). Errors in 14 pulse oximeters during profound hypoxia. *Journal of Clinical Monitoring, 5,* 72–81.
14. Shippy, M. B., et al. (1984). A clinical evaluation of the BTI BIOX II ear oximeter. *Respiratory Care, 29,* 730–735.
15. Strohl, K. P., et al. (1986). Comparison of three transmittance oximeters. *Medical Instrumentation, 20,* 143–149.
16. Tashiro, C., et al. (1988). Effects of carboxyhemoglobin on pulse oximetry in humans. *Journal of Anesthesia, 2,* 36–40.
17. Tremper, K. K., et al. (1985). Accuracy of pulse oximetry in the critically ill adult: Effect of temperature and hemodynamics (Abstract). *Anesthesiology, 63,* A175.
18. Webb, R. K., Ralston, A. C., & Runciman, W. B. (1991). Potential errors in pulse oximetry: II: Effects of changes in saturation and signal quality. *Anaesthesia, 46,* 207–212.

Sarah Jo Brown, PhD, RN, *Principal and Consultant, Practice-Research Integrations, Norwich, Vermont*

Respiratory Care of Older Adults After Cardiac Surgery

QUESTION

What nursing interventions prevent and decrease the incidence of adverse respiratory-related outcomes in older adults after cardiac surgery?

CITATION

Bezanson, J. (1997). Respiratory care of older adults after cardiac surgery. *Journal of Cardiovascular Nursing, 12*, 71–83.

STUDIES

Although many studies were cited in this review of research-based interventions, the method of identifying the studies cited was not described. Studies from nursing, medical, and interdisciplinary research were included.

A conceptual framework of ventilatory support was used to group the variables that influence respiratory outcomes. The major grouping concepts are (1) pre-episode patient characteristics, (2) processes of patient management, and (3) respiratory-related clinical outcomes. Pre-episode characteristics are depicted as having direct influences on clinical outcomes as well as having indirect influences through their effect on processes of client management. Processes of client management directly influence clinical outcomes.

Summary of Findings

Pre-episode Characteristics of Older Adults (p. 73)

Many respiratory system alterations involving the chest wall and lungs occur as a consequence of aging. Among these changes are diminished respiratory muscle strength,[38] decreased elasticity and recoil of the alveoli,[22, 23, 36] increased chest wall stiffness,[22, 36] and reduced ventilatory responsiveness to hypoxia and hypercapnia.[17] Collectively, these alterations contribute to a decrease in respiratory reserve, which is clinically manifested by reduced coughing efficiency and reduced arterial oxygenation. A study of age and gender differences in clients requiring mechanical ventilation found that men older than 70 years of age had a statistically significant increased incidence of respiratory insufficiency compared with younger men (<70 years). Differences in incidence of respiratory insufficiency were not statistically significant between older and younger women or between older men and women (p. 74).[14]

The presence of disease in adults undergoing cardiac surgery has been associated with development of postoperative pulmonary complications and prolonged mechanical ventilation; these co-morbidities include impaired left ventricular function, angina (pain), diabetes mellitus, and heart failure.[12, 30] Other risk factors include an emergent operation, very low weight, chronic obstructive pulmonary disease (COPD), previous stroke, smoking, and left coronary artery disease.[12] Interestingly, receiving intravenous (IV) antibiotics prior to mechanical ventilation has been associated with ventilator-associated pneumonia.[15] In a study examining the association between psychosocial characteristics and duration of mechanical ventilation,[13] depression, anxiety, and hostility were not associated with either earlier or later extubation. However, a higher positive effect was associated with earlier extubation.

Processes of Patient Management (p. 75)

Anticipated physiologic responses after cardiac surgery include lung injury related to having the heart-lung bypass machine,[25] atelectasis,[6, 19] and increased oxygen consumption related to hypermetabolism.[35] These physiologic responses together with the age-related alterations may contribute to pulmonary complications and prolonged duration of mechanical ventilation in older adults (p. 75). Additionally, decreased level of consciousness following administration of anesthesia and narcotics increases the risk of aspiration and hinders productive coughing effort (p. 75).

Older adults also may have increased vulnerability for aspiration when lying supine, and avoidance of that position may reduce the risk of aspiration.[34] In a study of clients in an intensive care unit (ICU), being over 60 years of age and being supine during the first 24 hours of mechanical ventilation were independently related with development of ventilator-associated pneumonia.[15] Several studies have demonstrated the benefits of right lateral positioning on arterial oxygenation[1, 2]; however, a decrease in pulmonary complications did not occur in a sample of postoperative cardiac surgical clients.[7]

Research findings show that hyperoxygenation prior to endotracheal suctioning with a closed suction system promotes arterial oxygenation.[10] This result is best accomplished using the mechanism of the ventilator rather than the manual resuscitation bag.[24] However, in postoperative cardiac surgery clients hyperinflation of the lungs during hyperoxygenation prior to endotracheal suctioning appears to increase the arterial pressure, which can cause problems in clients with postoperative hypertension.[31, 32] The optimal frequency of endotracheal suctioning remains controversial.[27]

The author of a review of the literature on normal saline instillation before suctioning concluded that this practice may decrease oxygen saturation values[26]; the article was published in 1995. Since then, several studies have demonstrated that saline instillation prior to endotracheal suction adversely affects oxygenation during and after suctioning.[40, 41] The study of 35 clients after coronary artery bypass grafting showed that the group receiving 5 ml of normal saline at the start of suctioning took 3.78 minutes longer to return to baseline mixed venous oxygenation saturation values compared with those not receiving saline.[41]

Predictors of readiness for weaning from mechanical ventilation have been studied in critically ill clients. One study of postoperative cardiac surgery patients identified vital capacity, arterial pH, and mean arterial blood pressure as interdependent predictors of weaning readiness.[9] However, different factors and strategies should probably be used for older adults.[16] Early extubation, defined as less than 8 hours of mechanical ventilation, has been successful in cardiac surgery clients,[4, 8] but its appropriateness in older adults is not certain. In one study, it was considered appropriate in people older than 70 years of age in the absence of co-morbidities and impaired left ventricular functioning (ejection fraction <45%).[8]

The presence of an endotracheal tube after cardiac surgery is stressful to clients,[29] and makes communication with them diffi-

Respiratory Care of Older Adults After Cardiac Surgery *Continued*

cult. Two studies have examined the effects of preoperative arrangements for postoperative communication.[5, 33] In one of the studies,[33] introducing the use of a communication board preoperatively resulted in increased patient satisfaction with communication after discharge from the ICU.

A few studies have examined the role of psychosocial support in promoting comfort and early discontinuation of mechanical ventilation. In a study of men (average age 58 years), a high frequency of spousal visitation was contributory to reduced length of stays in the cardiac surgical ICU.[18] When surgical ICU clients were interviewed 3 days after surgery, closeness and affirming behaviors of visiting family members were often remembered and a majority reported that family visitation provided feelings of comfort and relaxation.[28]

Although effective pain management clearly affects client comfort and ventilation, studies have found inconsistent assessment, administration, and documentation practices in postoperative cardiac surgery clients.[20, 21, 37] In a study of 80 patients, women received smaller doses of IV morphine than men, and older adults were less likely than younger adults to receive prescriptions of acetaminophen with oxycodone.[20] When pain management was documented using a standardized pain flowsheet, clients experienced reduced pain intensity.[37]

Limitations/Reservations. Although this review used research findings as the basis for its recommendations, it is not clear whether *all* studies regarding each recommendation were considered when a recommendation was made. This area of practice is changing rapidly; as a result, much research has been conducted on the various issues related to respiratory care of the postoperative cardiac surgical client since this review was published.

Research-Based Practice

Preoperative assessment of physiologic status, chronic conditions, and pychosocial characteristics helps identify older patients at risk for prolonged ventilatory assistance and pulmonary complications. A cardiac severity scoring system has been developed to assess these risks but has not been validated among older adults.[12] Preoperative assessment can also help identify those clients who are candidates for early extubation. Special arrangements for systematic assessment and client teaching need to be made when clients are admitted on the day of surgery.

Teaching clients slow deep-breathing maneuvers preoperatively can help to improve oxygenation postoperatively. Establishing a simple method for communicating before surgery is important for some people. A picture or word board depicting a few common problems may be useful. Clients also benefit emotionally, and perhaps physiologically, from being allowed frequent, short visits of one or two people who are close to them while they are in the ICU.

The four processes of care that affect respiratory outcomes are (1) suctioning practices, (2) positioning practices, (3) assessing weaning readiness, and (4) pain management. Hyperoxygenation using the mechanical ventilator mechanism prior to endotracheal suctioning has proven benefit. However, the use of normal saline instillation prior to endotracheal suctioning is discouraged, as it has not shown benefit and may adversely affect oxygenation. Elevation of the head of the bed, especially early after intubation, and right lateral positioning, reduce the risk of pneumonia.

Early extubation can be considered for older adults who do not have other conditions precluding it. Algorithms and perioperative clinical pathways have been developed to guide all members of the cardiac surgery team through the processes of care that must be optimized and the decision points involved in providing a safe and timely early extubation. Finally, well-planned pain assessment and management approaches and standardized documentation can improve clients' pain experiences and probably improve their respiratory outcomes.

Cited References

1. Banasik, J. L., et al. (1987). Effect of position on arterial oxygenation in postoperative coronary revascularization patients. *Heart and Lung, 16,* 652–657.
2. Banasik, J. L., & Emerson, R. J. (1996). Effect of lateral position on arterial and venous blood gases in postoperative cardiac surgery patients. *American Journal of Critical Care, 5,* 121–126.
3. Bostick, J., & Wendelgass, S. T. (1987). Normal saline instillation as part of the suctioning procedure: Effects on PaO_2 and amount of secretions. *Heart and Lung, 16,* 532–537.
4. Cheng, DCH. (1995). Pro: Early extubation after cardiac surgery decreases intensive care unit stay and cost. *Journal of Cardiothoracic Vascular Anesthesia, 9,* 460–464.
5. Cronin, L., & Carrizosa, A. (1984). The computer as a communication device for ventilator and tracheostomy patients in the intensive care unit. *Critical Care Nurse, 4,* 72–76.
6. Gamsu, G., et al. (1976). Postoperative impairment of mucous transport in the lung. *American Review of Respiratory Diseases, 114,* 673–679.
7. Gavigan, M., Kline-O'Sullivant, C., & Klumpp-Lybrand, B. (1990). The effect of regular turning on CABG patients. *Critical Care Nursing Quarterly, 12,* 69–76.
8. Gross, S. B. (1995). Early extubation: Preliminary experience in the cardiothoracic patient population. *American Journal of Critical Care, 4,* 262–266.
9. Hanneman, S. K. G. (1994). Multidimensional predictors of success or failure with early weaning from mechanical ventilation after cardiac surgery. *Nursing Research, 43,* 4–10.
10. Harshbarger, S. A., Hoffman, L. A., Zullo, T. G., & Pinsky, M. R. (1992). Effects of a closed tracheal suction system on ventilatory and cardiovascular parameters. *American Journal of Critical Care, 3,* 57–61.
11. Higgins, T. L., et al. (1991). Risk factors for respiratory complications after cardiac surgery (Abstract). *Anesthesia, 75,* A258.
12. Higgins, T. L., et al. (1992). Stratification of morbidity and mortality outcome by preoperative risk factors in coronary artery bypass patients. *Journal of the American Medical Association, 267,* 2344–2348.
13. Ingersoll, G. L., & Grippi, M. A. (1991). Preoperative pulmonary status and postoperative extubation outcome of patients undergoing elective cardiac surgery. *Heart and Lung, 20,* 137–143.
14. King, K. B., et al. (1992). Coronary artery bypass graft surgery in older women and men. *American Journal of Critical Care, 1,* 28–35.
15. Kollef, M. H. (1993). Ventilator-associated pneumonia. *Journal of the American Medical Association, 270,* 1965–1970.
16. Krieger, B. P., et al. (1989). Evaluation of conventional criteria for predicting successful weaning from mechanical ventilatory support in elderly patients. *Critical Care Medicine, 17,* 858–861.
17. Kronenberg, R. S., & Drage, C. W. (1973). Attenuation of the ventilatory and heart rate responses to hypoxia and hypercapnia with aging in normal men. *Journal of Clinical Investigation, 52,* 1812–1819.
18. Kulik, J. A., & Mahler, H. I. M. (1989). Social support and recovery from surgery. *Health Psychology, 8,* 221–238.

Bridge continues on following page

Respiratory Care of Older Adults After Cardiac Surgery *Continued*

19. Matthay, M. A., & Wiener-Kronish, J. P. (1989). Respiratory management after cardiac surgery. *Respiratory Management of Cardiac Surgery, 95,* 424–434.

20. Maxam-Moore, V. A., Wilkie, D. J., & Woods, S. L. (1994). Analgesics for cardiac surgery patients in critical care: Describing current practice. *American Journal of Critical Care, 3,* 31–39.

21. Meehan, D. A., et al. (1995). Analgesic administration, pain intensity, and patient satisfaction in cardiac surgical patients. *American Journal of Critical Care, 4,* 435–442.

22. Mittman, C., et al. (1965). Relationship between chest wall and pulmonary compliance with age. *Journal of Applied Physiology, 20,* 1211–1216.

23. Pierce, J. A., & Ebert, R. V. (1965). Fibrous network of the lung and its changes with age. *Thorax, 20,* 469–476.

24. Preusser, B. A., et al. (1988). Effects of two methods of preoxygenation on mean arterial pressure, cardiac output, peak airway pressure, and post suctioning hypoxemia. *Heart and Lung, 17,* 290–299.

25. Ratliff, N. B., et al. (1973). Pulmonary injury secondary to extracorporeal circulation. *Journal of Thoracic and Cardiovascular Surgery, 65,* 425–432.

26. Raymond, S. J. (1995). Normal saline instillation before suctioning: Helpful or harmful? A review of the literature. *American Journal of Critical Care, 4,* 267–271.

27. Simmons, C. L. (1997). How frequently should endotracheal suctioning be undertaken? *American Journal of Critical Care, 6,* 4–6.

28. Simpson, T. (1991). The family as a source of support for the critically ill adult. *AACN Clinical Issues, 2,* 229–235.

29. Soehren, P. (1995). Stressors perceived by cardiac surgical patients in the intensive care unit. *American Journal of Critical Care, 4,* 71–76.

30. Spivak, S. D., et al. (1996). Preoperative prediction of postoperative respiratory outcome. *Chest, 109,* 1222–1230.

31. Stone, K. S., et al. (1989). Effects of lung hyperinflation on mean arterial pressure and post suctioning hypoxemia, *Heart and Lung, 18,* 377–385.

32. Stone, K. S., et al. (1988). Effect of lung hyperinflation on cardiopulmonary hemodynamics and post suctioning hypoxemia (Abstract). *Heart and Lung, 17,* 309.

33. Stovsky, B., Rudy, E., & Dragonette, P. (1988). Comparison of two types of communication methods used after cardiac surgery with patients with endotracheal tubes. *Heart and Lung, 17,* 281–289.

34. Torres, A., et al. (1992). Pulmonary aspiration of gastric contents in patients receiving mechanical ventilation: The effect of body position. *Annals of Internal Medicine, 116,* 540–543.

35. Tulla, H., et al. (1991). Hypermetabolism after coronary artery bypass. *Journal of Thoracic and Cardiovascular Surgery, 101,* 598–600.

36. Turner, J. M., Mead, J., & Wohl, M. E. (1968). Elasticity of human lungs in relation to age. *Journal of Applied Physiology, 25,* 644–671.

37. Voigt, L., Paice, J. A., & Pouliot, J. (1995). Standardized pain flowsheet: Impact on patient-reported pain experiences after cardiovascular surgery. *American Journal of Critical Care, 4,* 308–313.

38. Wahba, W. M. (1983). Influence of aging on lung function: Clinical significance of changes from age twenty. *Anesthesia and Analgesia, 62,* 764–776.

39. Zuckerman, M., Lubin, B., & Rinck, C. M. (1983). Construction of new scales for the multiple affect adjective check list. *Journal of Behavioral Assessment, 5,* 119–129.

Added References

40. Ackerman, M. H., & Mick, D. J. (1998). Instillation of normal saline before suctioning in patients with pulmonary infections: A prospective randomized controlled trial. *American Journal of Critical Care, 7,* 261–266.

41. Kinloch, D. (1999). Instillation of normal saline during endotracheal suctioning: Effects on mixed venous oxygen saturation. *American Journal of Critical Care, 8,* 231–240.

Sarah Jo Brown, PhD, RN, *Principal and Consultant, Practice-Research Integrations, Norwich, Vermont*

UNIT 14

Sensory Disorders

Anatomy and Physiology Review
The Eyes and Ears
Robert G. Carroll

OVERVIEW

The visual, auditory, and olfactory systems are "distance" senses, bringing information about our environment to our perception. Each system detects the intensity and quality of stimuli, encodes and processes this information, and transmits it to the cerebral cortex. Together these senses provide much of the available information about our environment. This review covers vision and hearing, smell is described in Unit 6.

The *visual apparatus* is specialized to detect light. Light passes through the cornea, aqueous humor, lens, and vitreous humor before striking the retina. The visual receptors —rods and cones—encode data about the intensity and wavelength of light. This information is processed and transmitted through nerve cells of the retina, the optic nerve, and the thalamus before arriving at the visual cortex. The information is constructed in the primary and associated visual cortex into a conscious perception.

The *auditory apparatus* is specialized to detect sound. Sound waves pass through the pinna to the ear drum (tympanic membrane), through the bones of the middle ear, and then to the receptors in the cochlea. The auditory hair cells are arranged on the organ of Corti (the end organ for hearing) and are coded to detect the intensity and frequency of sound. This information passes through the auditory nerve through the lateral lemniscus and, finally, to the auditory cortex. Within the primary and secondary auditory cortex, auditory discrimination occurs.

VISUAL SYSTEM

STRUCTURE OF THE VISUAL SYSTEM

■ EXTERNAL STRUCTURES

The visual system is a complex group of structures that includes the eyeballs, muscles, nerves, fat, and bones. The *ocular adnexa* (Fig. U14–1A) are the acessory structures of the eye (muscles, fat, and bone) that support and protect it. The bony orbit (eye socket) surrounds and protects most of the eye so that only a small portion is visible. The orbit is formed from portions of the frontal, lacrimal, ethmoid, maxillary, zygomatous, sphenoid, and palatine bones. These bones are thin and fragile and break easily when pressure is applied to the eye (as in a fistfight). In addition to bone, the orbit also contains fat, various connective tissues, blood vessels, and nerves.

The *eyeball* is moved by six ocular muscles, which are attached to the surface of the globe (Fig. U14–2) and which move the eye through six cardinal gazes. The four rectus muscles (the medial, lateral, superior, and inferior) move the eyes horizontally and vertically. The two oblique muscles (superior and inferior) rotate the eye in circular movements to allow vision at all angles.

The upper and lower *eyelids* are elastic folds of skin that close to protect the anterior eyeball. When the eyelids close, they distribute tear film, which prevents evaporation and drying of the surface epithelium. The elliptic space between the two open lids is the *palpebral fissure*. The corners of the fissure are called the *canthi*. The medial, or inner, canthus is next to the nose; the lateral, or outer, canthus is the outside corner. Oil-secreting *meibomian glands* are embedded in both upper and lower lids (Fig. U14–1B).

The *lacrimal gland,* in the upper lid over the outer canthus, produces tears that reach the eyeball through secretory ducts. Tiny openings *(puncti)* in both the upper and lower lids at the inner canthus direct tears to the lacrimal sac. The *nasolacrimal duct* directs the flow of tears into the nose. The tear film is composed of lipids secreted by the meibomian glands and dissolved salts, glucose, urea, protein, and lysozyme secreted by the lacrimal glands. The tear film lubricates, cleans, and protects the ocular surface. Mucus, secreted by goblet cells located in the lids, assists these processes.

■ INNER EYE

The *conjunctiva* is a thin transparent layer of mucous membrane that lines the eyelids and covers the eyeball (Fig. U14–1C). The *cornea* is a transparent avascular structure with a brilliant, shiny surface. It is convex in shape, about 0.5 mm thick, and acts as a powerful lens to bend and direct (refract) rays of light to the retina. The cornea is composed of five layers. It derives oxygen from the atmosphere. A rich network of nerve fibers in the outer layer (epithelium) produces a sensation of pain whenever the fibers are exposed or stimulated.

The *sclera* is the fibrous protective coating of the eye. It is white, dense, and continuous with the cornea. In children, the sclera is thin and appears bluish because of the underlying pigmented structures. In old age, it may become yellowish from degeneration.

The *uveal tract,* the middle vascular layer of the eye that furnishes the blood supply to the retina, consists of three structures:

1. The *iris* is a thin, pigmented diaphragm with a central aperture, the pupil. Iris color is determined by the degree of pigmentation in the stromal melanocytes. The interaction of the two iris muscles (sphincter and dilator) determines pupil diameter. Expansion and contraction of the iris regulate the amount of light entering the eye.
2. The *ciliary body* produces and secretes *aqueous humor,* a clear alkaline fluid composed mainly of water, which occupies the space between the iris and the cornea (the anterior chamber of the eye). The ciliary body is in direct continuity with the iris and

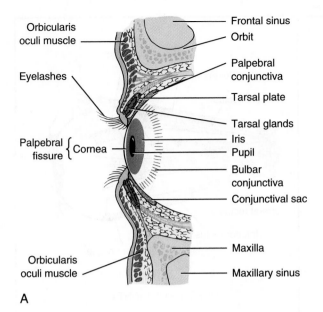

A

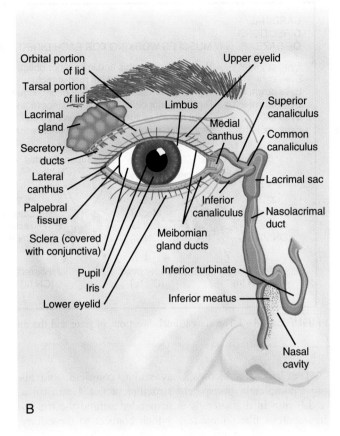

B

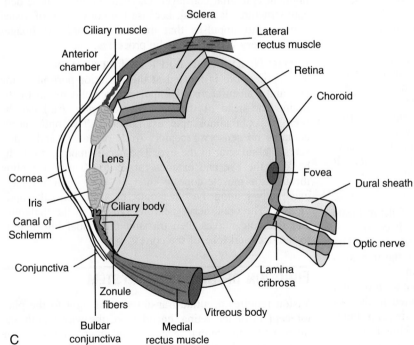

C

FIGURE U14–1 Surface anatomy of the eye. *A,* Ocular adnexa. *B,* Frontal view of the lacrimal drainage system. *C,* Horizontal section of the eye.

is circular, surrounding the lens. Aqueous humor circulates from the posterior chamber through the pupil into the anterior chamber. The flow continues into the anterior chamber angle and is filtered out through the trabecular meshwork into Schlemm's canal. From there, the aqueous humor is channeled into a capillary network and into episcleral veins.

Normal intraocular pressure is maintained as long as there is a balance between the aqueous production and the aqueous humor outflow.

3. The *choroid* is the posterior segment of the uveal tract between the retina and the sclera. It is composed of three layers of vessels and is attached to both the ciliary body and the optic nerve.

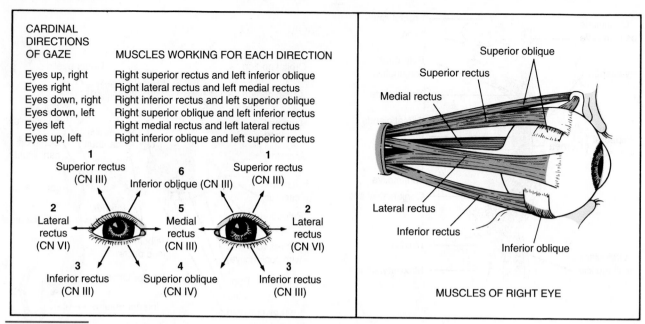

CARDINAL DIRECTIONS OF GAZE	MUSCLES WORKING FOR EACH DIRECTION
Eyes up, right	Right superior rectus and left inferior oblique
Eyes right	Right lateral rectus and left medial rectus
Eyes down, right	Right inferior rectus and left superior oblique
Eyes down, left	Right superior oblique and left inferior rectus
Eyes left	Right medial rectus and left lateral rectus
Eyes up, left	Right inferior oblique and left superior rectus

1 Superior rectus (CN III)
6 Inferior oblique (CN III)
1 Superior rectus (CN III)
2 Lateral rectus (CN VI)
5 Medial rectus (CN III)
2 Lateral rectus (CN VI)
3 Inferior rectus (CN III)
4 Superior oblique (CN IV)
3 Inferior rectus (CN III)

MUSCLES OF RIGHT EYE

Superior oblique
Superior rectus
Medial rectus
Lateral rectus
Inferior rectus
Inferior oblique

FIGURE U14–2 The six cardinal directions of gaze and the muscles responsible for each.

The *lens* is a biconvex, avascular, colorless, and almost completely transparent structure, about 4 mm thick and 9 mm in diameter. It is suspended behind the iris by ligamentous fibers *(zonules),* which connect to the ciliary body. The sole purpose of the lens is to focus light on the retina. The physiologic interplay of the zonular fibers and elasticity of the lens allows for focusing on nearby or distant objects. The change of focus from distant to near is called *accommodation.* There are no pain fibers or blood vessels in the lens. The lens is surrounded by a transparent envelope (the capsule). The lens of the eye consists of about 65% water and 35% protein.

The *vitreous body* is a clear, avascular, jelly-like structure. Vitreous fluid is thick and viscous, and occupies a space called the *vitreous chamber.* It fills the largest cavity of the eye, accounting for two thirds of its volume. It helps maintain the shape and transparency of the eye.

RETINA

The retina is a thin, semitransparent layer of nerve tissue that forms the innermost lining of the eye. It consists of 10 distinct layers of highly organized, delicate tissue. The retina contains all the sensory receptors for the transmission of light and is actually part of the brain.

There are two types of retinal receptors: rods and cones. About 125 million *rods* are distributed in the periphery of the retina; they function best in dim light. Damage to these structures results in night blindness. The *cones,* numbering about 6 million and concentrated in the center of the retina, provide resolution of small visual angles, resulting in perception of fine details. They are also responsible for color vision.

The center of the retina *(macula)* is an area about 5 mm in diameter. In an ophthalmoscopic examination, it appears as a yellowish spot with a depressed center, the *fovea.* An area 1.5 mm in diameter where only cones are present, the fovea is the point of finest vision. Damage to the fovea can severely reduce central vision.

The retina is composed of many fine layers of neural tissue attached to a single layer of pigmented epithelial cells. The photoreceptor cells in the retina are nourished by the capillaries of the choroid layer just beneath the pigment epithelial cell layer. Oxygen supply to these delicate structures is crucial, because the conversion of visual stimuli into impulses that the brain records as images requires very active metabolic processes.

OPTIC NERVE AND NEURAL PATHWAYS

The optic nerve is located at the posterior portion of the eye and transmits visual impulses from the retina to the brain. The head of the optic nerve *(optic disc)* can be seen by ophthalmoscopic examination. The optic nerve contains no sensory receptors (rods or cones) and represents a blind spot in the eye. The nerve emerges from the back of the eye and extends for 25 to 30 mm, traveling through the muscle cone to enter the bony optic foramen, eventually joining the other optic nerve to form the optic chiasm. The optic nerve neurons synapse in the thalamus, and thalamic nerves then transmit the visual information to the occipital lobe of the cortex.

FUNCTION OF THE VISUAL SYSTEM

Vision requires accurate transmission of light to the photoreceptors of the retina, encoding of the wavelength and intensity by the retinal receptors and interpretation of the coded signals by the visual cortex.

■ TRANSMISSION OF LIGHT

Light passes through the cornea, aqueous humor, lens, and vitreous humor before striking the retina. Blood vessels are opaque, and the cornea, lens, and fovea are sparsely vascularized, which enhances light transmission. The cornea and lens refract light, allowing it to converge to a focal point on the fovea of the retina. Refraction at the lens is regulated by contraction of the ciliary muscles.

Near vision is accomplished by contraction of the ciliary muscles, which increases curvature of the lens and brings near objects into focus on the retina. *Far vision* is accomplished by relaxing the ciliary muscles and flattening the lens. With age, lens elasticity decreases, reducing the ability to accommodate for near vision. Visual abnormalities are corrected by placing an appropriate refractor (eye glasses or contact lens) in the light pathway.

■ VISUAL RECEPTORS OF THE RETINA; CONES AND RODS

Three types of cones are sensitive to specific wavelengths of light, with peak sensitivities in the red, green, and blue wavelengths. Density of the cone receptors is highest in the fovea (the area of highest visual acuity). Bright light causes contraction of the iris, limiting the light entering the eye and focusing the light on the fovea. Exposure to light bleaches retinal photopigments, reducing the receptor responsiveness to subsequent exposure (light adaptation). However, prolonged exposure to dark allows the receptors to recover; cones recover completely in about 5 minutes.

Rods are sensitive to light in the green and yellow wavelengths and impart night *(scotopic)* vision. Rods are distributed throughout the retina, but few rods are in the fovea. In the dark, the iris dilates, admitting light to large portions of the retina. Consequently, night vision is enhanced by looking just to the side of the object of inter-

est. After light exposure, rods recover slowly, taking about 20 minutes to return to peak sensitivity (dark adaptation). Because the rod photopigments are not sensitive to red light, exposure to red light does not interfere with dark adaptation.

■ IMAGE PROCESSING AND THE VISUAL CORTEX

Interneurons in the retina process the receptor output and transmit information via the optic nerve to the thalamus. The thalamus processes information about the wavelength and intensity of the light and relays the information to the visual cortex. Visual space in the cortex is completely crossed; objects appearing on the left side of the body are represented on the right visual cortex and vice versa (Fig. U14–3). The two eyes work as though they were one, focusing on the same point in space and fusing their images so that a single mental impression is obtained. The ability of the eyes to fuse two images into a single image is called *binocular vision,* accounting for one aspect of depth perception.

EFFECTS OF AGING ON VISION

STRUCTURAL CHANGES

Several age-related changes occur in the structures of the eye and surrounding tissue. Eyebrows and eyelashes turn

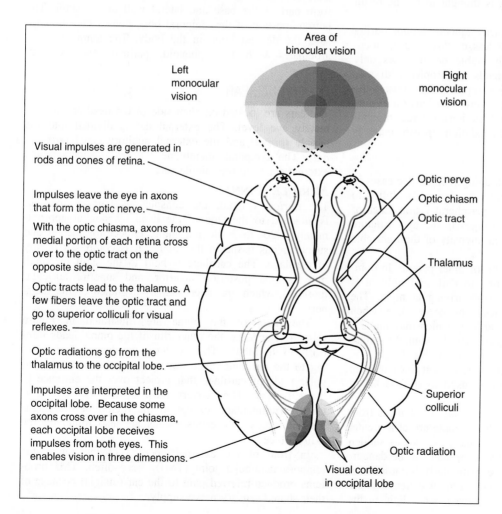

Visual impulses are generated in rods and cones of retina.

Impulses leave the eye in axons that form the optic nerve.

With the optic chiasma, axons from medial portion of each retina cross over to the optic tract on the opposite side.

Optic tracts lead to the thalamus. A few fibers leave the optic tract and go to superior colliculi for visual reflexes.

Optic radiations go from the thalamus to the occipital lobe.

Impulses are interpreted in the occipital lobe. Because some axons cross over in the chiasma, each occipital lobe receives impulses from both eyes. This enables vision in three dimensions.

Area of binocular vision

Left monocular vision

Right monocular vision

Optic nerve
Optic chiasm
Optic tract
Thalamus
Superior colliculi
Optic radiation
Visual cortex in occipital lobe

FIGURE U14–3 Visual pathways from the retina to the occipital lobe. The pathway is partially crossed, so that objects in the visual space of one side are interpreted in the contralateral visual cortex.

gray, and skin around the eyelids becomes wrinkled and loose because of loss of muscle tone and elasticity. Loss of orbital fat causes the eyes to sink deeper into the orbit and sometimes limits the upward gaze. Tear secretions may also diminish, resulting in the condition of dry eyes.

The most frequent and significant age-related change in the eye is the formation of a *cataract.* With age, the thickness and density of the lens increase and the lens becomes progressively yellowed and opaque. Throughout the life span, the lens continues to grow by forming new fiber cells. Although the rate of growth gradually diminishes, the accumulation of cells over time contributes to lens density. Loss of transparency also results from molecular deterioration from absorption of ultraviolet radiation. The yellow material is associated with the development of abnormal fluorescent substances in the aging lens. Although the cloudiness of the lens that occurs with aging decreases visual acuity, it does provide a natural protection for the retina against ultraviolet light. The lens accommodation diminishes because of ciliary muscle atrophy.

The cells of the inner layer of the cornea (endothelium) decrease in number with age. Because this layer does not reproduce lost cells, the ability of this layer to heal after injury or surgery may be compromised. The corneal reflex also may be diminished or absent. Another phenomenon characteristic of aging is the *arcus senilis,* a grayish yellow ring found on the periphery of the cornea surrounding the iris. This ring is thought to be the result of the accumulation of lipids.

The ciliary body produces less aqueous humor during the aging process, but there is less outflow and intraocular pressure remains relatively stable or increases only slightly. The ciliary muscle tends to atrophy with age, and sometimes connective tissue replaces lost muscle tissue. The loss in muscle action along with lens thickening decreases the focusing ability of the lens. Decreasing ability to focus at near accommodation *(presbyopia)* is common.

VISUAL CHANGES

The major visual changes with aging include decreases in (1) visual acuity, (2) tolerance of glare, (3) ability to adapt to dark and light, and (4) peripheral vision. Each of these decreases is related to changes in the eye structure and each affects the quality and intensity of the light able to reach the retina.

Glare is a particular problem for older people. In combination with difficulty adjusting to dark and light, it is often the reason older adults stop driving at night. The lights from oncoming vehicles produce a glare when passing through both cornea and lens, which may make it very difficult to discern objects. Bright sunlight, either indoors or outdoors, causes an equally blinding glare. Indoor rooms should be lighted with soft incandescent lights, and sheer curtains can be used to diffuse bright sunlight.

Because the eye takes longer to adapt to changes from dark to light and vice versa, older people are at a greater risk for falls and injuries. Any place subject to sudden changes in lighting (e.g., inside a theater) can be dangerous. Getting up at night can be particularly hazardous for older adults. However, because red wavelengths are longer and are perceived by the cones, a red light in the bathroom at night allows enough vision to function without interfering with dark vision.

Peripheral vision decreases with age and may interfere with social interactions and physical activities. Older adults suffering from loss of peripheral vision may not notice someone sitting next to them. They may also have difficulty finding objects out of their range of vision.

The iris loses pigment with age, and older people may thus appear to have grayish or light blue eyes. The pupil becomes gradually smaller with age. A decrease in pupil size results in a smaller amount of light reaching the retina, meaning that the light must pass through the densest, most opaque area of the lens.

In the posterior chamber, the vitreous body begins to liquefy and collapse. Small pieces of debris from separation and shrinkage of the vitreous body may become visible as "floaters." Although floaters may not obstruct vision, they are an annoyance. Vitreal shrinkage may result in retinal detachment. Additionally, the retina may degenerate as a result of local ischemia and loss of neural function.

AUDITORY SYSTEM

STRUCTURE OF THE AUDITORY SYSTEM

The ear is housed in the *temporal bone* of the skull. The temporal bones are two of the eight cranial bones that form part of the base and lateral wall of the skull. The petrous portion of the temporal bone houses the otic capsule, the densest bone in the body. The temporal bone articulates with the sphenoid, parietal, and occipital bones.

■ EXTERNAL EAR

The ears are located on each side of the head at approximately eye level. The external ear is divided into the auricle *(pinna)* and the external auditory canal *(ear canal).* The tympanic membrane *(eardrum)* separates the external ear from the middle ear.

AURICLE (PINNA)

The *auricle* (pinna), the conspicuous part of the ear, is attached to the side of the head by skin at approximately a 20- to 30-degree angle. Except for the fat and subcutaneous tissue in the lobule, it is composed mostly of cartilage. The cartilage is held to the skull by small muscles (the posterior, anterior, and superior auricular muscles), which are innervated by a branch of the facial nerve.

The parts of the pinna are illustrated in Figure U14-4. The *helix,* the outer rim of the pinna, leads inferiorly to the lobule. The *concha* is the deepest part, leading to the ear canal. The tragus and antitragus are triangular folds of cartilage that project over the entrance to the ear canal. Hair covers most of the ear, but it is usually rudimentary, except in the region of the tragus and antitragus. Sebaceous glands are also found on the skin surface.

In front of the external opening of the ear is the temporomandibular joint (TMJ). Very often, TMJ problems produce referred pain to the ear (otalgia) because of their shared sensory nerve supply.

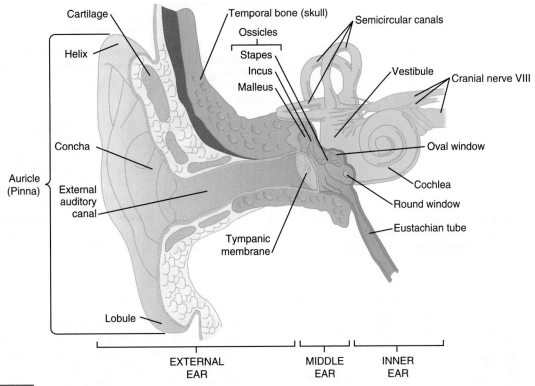

FIGURE U14–4 Anatomy of the ear.

EXTERNAL AUDITORY CANAL (EAR CANAL)

The ear canal extends from the concha of the pinna to the tympanic membrane (see Fig. U14–4). This slightly S-shaped canal is approximately 2.5 cm (1 inch) in length and follows an inward, forward, and downward path. The skeleton of cartilage in the outer third is continuous with the cartilage of the pinna. The inner two thirds is a bony canal entering the skull. The lumen of the ear canal is irregularly shaped and is narrowest where the transition from cartilage to bone occurs. The skin covering the cartilage portion is thick, containing sebaceous and ceruminous glands and hair follicles. The sebaceous and ceruminous glands secrete a golden to black substance called *cerumen* (wax). The skin covering the bony portion is very thin.

TYMPANIC MEMBRANE

The tympanic membrane (eardrum) is an oval disc (~1 cm in diameter); it covers the end of the auditory canal and separates the canal from the middle ear (Fig. U14–4). The eardrum is a thin, translucent, pearly gray membrane obliquely directed downward and inward, so that the posterior part is more accessible than the anterior part. The eardrum consists of three tissue layers:

- An outer epithelial layer continuous with the skin of the ear canal
- A fibrous supporting middle layer
- An inner mucosal layer continuous with the mucosal lining of the middle ear cavity

■ MIDDLE EAR

The middle ear consists of the middle ear cleft and contents: ossicles, oval and round windows, eustachian tube,

and facial nerve (see Fig. U14–4). The middle ear lies between the ear canal and the *labyrinth* (inner ear). The middle ear cavity has a mucosal lining.

OSSICLES

The middle ear contains the three smallest bones (*ossicles*) of the body, named according to their appearance. The outermost and largest ossicle is the *malleus* (hammer), which is firmly attached to the tympanic membrane. The innermost and smallest ossicle is the *stapes* (stirrup); its footplate occupies the oval window, in direct contact with the perilymph of the inner ear. The *incus* (anvil) lies between the other two and is shaped like a tooth with two roots (see Fig. U14–4).

WINDOWS

The middle ear contains two windows, whose names reflect their shape. The *round window* is an opening in the inner ear from which sound vibrations exit. The *oval window* is an opening in the inner ear into which sound vibrations enter. The oval window is not a true window because the footplate of the stapes bone covers it.

EUSTACHIAN TUBE

The eustachian tube is a narrow channel approximately 35 mm (1½ inches) long and only 1 mm wide at its narrowest end. This tube connects the middle ear to the nasopharynx (see Fig. U14–4). The structure consists mostly of fibrous tissue, cartilage, and bone; it extends downward, forward, and inward from each middle ear. The eustachian tube is lined with a mucous membrane that is continuous with the lining of the middle ear at one end and with the nasopharynx at the other end. A small section of this tube, originating in the middle ear, remains permanently open. Otherwise, the walls of the tube lightly

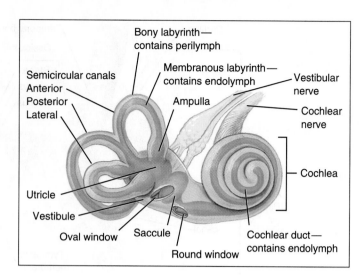

FIGURE U14–5 The labyrinths of the inner ear. (From Applegate, E. J. [2000]. *The anatomy and physiology learning system* [2nd ed.]. Philadelphia: W. B. Saunders.)

oppose or touch each other, closing the tube to both the throat and ear and preventing the sound of normal nasal respiration and of one's own voice from passing up the eustachian tube.

MASTOID BONE

The mastoid section of the temporal bone includes the cone-shaped *mastoid process;* the *mastoid antrum,* a large cavity posteriorly continuous with the middle ear; and the *mastoid air cells,* which extend from the antrum and fill the temporal bone with air pockets.

The mastoid bone is a bony protuberance behind the lower portion of the pinna. The mastoid cavity is close to several important cranial structures: the dura of the temporal lobe, the cerebellar dura, the sigmoid sinus, and the jugular bulb. The middle ear is also bounded by the internal carotid artery. Therefore, infection of the middle ear and mastoid cavities can also involve these structures.

■ INNER EAR (LABYRINTH)

The inner ear or labyrinth is located deep within the petrous section of the temporal bone; it contains the sense organs for hearing and balance, which form the eighth cranial nerve (Fig. U14–5). The inner ear is a complicated system of intercommunicating chambers and connecting tubes composed of two structures:

1. The *bony labyrinth* is the rigid capsule (otic capsule) that surrounds and protects the delicate membranous labyrinth. The *vestibule* connects the cochlea (for hearing) to the three semicircular canals (for balance). The *cochlea,* which looks like a snail shell with 2½ turns, is approximately 7 mm in diameter at the widest part and is structurally divided into three compartments (Fig. U14–6). The upper compartment *(scala vestibuli)* leads from the oval window to the apex of the cochlear spiral. The

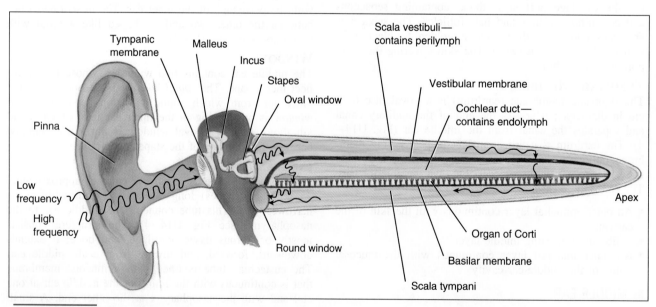

FIGURE U14–6 The uncoiled cochlea, showing the pathway of pressure waves. (From Applegate, E. J. [2000]. *The anatomy and physiology learning system* [2nd ed.]. Philadelphia: W. B. Saunders.)

lower compartment *(scala tympani)* leads from the apex of the cochlear spiral to the round window. The *scala media,* which contains the organ of Corti, lies between the scala vestibuli and scala tympani.

2. The *membranous labyrinth,* lying within but not completely filling the bony labyrinth, is bathed in a fluid called *perilymph,* which communicates with the cerebrospinal fluid (CSF) via the cochlear duct. The membranous labyrinth consists of the utricle, the saccule, the semicircular canals, the cochlear duct, and the *organ of Corti* (the end organ for hearing). The membranous labyrinth contains a different fluid *(endolymph).* This fluid also protects the end organ because it acts as a cushion against abrupt movements of the head.

The three *semicircular canals* are at right angles to each other and are named the anterior (superior), the posterior, and the lateral (horizontal) canal. The horizontal canal lies closest to the middle ear. This arrangement allows detection of movement in all three dimensions.

FUNCTION OF THE AUDITORY SYSTEM

■ EXTERNAL EAR

The ears are a pair of complex sensory organs for both hearing and balance. Their location on either side of the head produces binaural hearing, allows the detection of sound direction, and aids in maintaining equilibrium. The temporal bone provides protection for the organs of hearing and balance. It houses (1) the external and internal auditory canals; (2) the mastoid air cells, which provide an air reservoir for the middle ear; (3) the blood vessels; (4) the facial, vestibular, and auditory nerves; (5) the labyrinth; and (6) the cochlea.

SOUND WAVE CONDUCTION

The head, pinna, and ear canal act as an integrated system to transmit sound vibrations to the eardrum. The external ear actually amplifies certain frequencies. Sound is transmitted from the external ear through the middle ear (which amplifies the sound) to the inner ear (see Fig. U14–6). The funnel shape of the pinna collects and directs sound to the eardrum.

The tympanic membrane, a common membrane between the external ear canal and the middle ear space, protects the middle ear and conducts sound vibrations from the external ear to the ossicles. The sound pressure applied to the stapes (the smallest ossicle) in the oval window is 22 times greater than the sound pressure exerted on the eardrum. The pressure of the sound vibrations is increased as a result of transmission from a larger area to a smaller area, and the lever effect of the ossicular chain. The sound energy, after transformation, is carried by neural elements to the brain for decoding and, thus, hearing.

WAX PRODUCTION

Cerumen (wax) protects the ear. Wax is to the ear what tears are to the eyes. The sticky consistency of the wax and the fine hairs of the ear canal help clean the ear canal of foreign matter and protect it from water damage. Impacted cerumen can cause hearing losses in clients of all ages. At times, wax must be mechanically removed.

■ MIDDLE EAR

SOUND WAVE CONDUCTION

The ossicles transmit sound vibrations mechanically (see Fig. U14–6). The ossicles are held in place by joints, muscles, and ligaments, which also offer some protection from loud sounds. The light weight and the configuration of the ossicles provide an efficient means of transmitting sound vibrations from the air molecules of the external ear to the fluid molecules of the inner ear. Fluids offer more resistance than air and need more force to transmit movement. The ossicular chain produces and magnifies this force in order to move the inner ear fluids.

VENTILATION AND PRESSURE REGULATION

The eustachian tube provides an air passage from the nasopharynx to the middle ear to equalize pressure on both sides of the eardrum. This tube regulates ventilation and pressure, both of which are necessary for normal hearing. During yawning, swallowing, and sneezing, the eustachian tube is opened by the *tensor veli palatini* muscle. The natural opening and closing of the eustachian tube also allows drainage of exudate from the middle ear mucosa. The tube can be forcibly opened by increasing nasopharyngeal pressure. This act (the Valsalva maneuver) is accomplished by attempting to blow air through the nose while holding the nose closed.

The cavity of the mastoid bone and the interconnected arrangement of the air-filled spaces aid the middle ear in adjusting to changes in pressure. The mastoid system acts as a buffer for the middle ear. The system of cavities and air cells also lightens the skull.

■ INNER EAR

HEARING

Sound waves are transmitted by the ossicles to the delicate membrane of the oval window (see Fig. U14–6). These vibrations move the perilymph in the scala vestibuli. The perilymph of the scala vestibuli is continuous with that of the scala tympani at the extreme tip of the "snail shell," called the *helicotrema.* The sound energy vibrations enter through the oval window and exit through the round window.

Vibrations in the perilymph of the scala vestibuli are transmitted through the vestibular membrane *(Reissner's membrane)* to the endolymph that fills the cochlear duct. The cochlear duct is located between the scala vestibuli and the scala tympani. The *organ of Corti,* which is bathed in the endolymph, lies on the basilar membrane in a spiral strip from the basal turn near the round window to the apex at the helicotrema. This organ transforms mechanical sound vibrations into neural activity and separates sound into different frequencies. The electrochemical impulse travels via the acoustic nerve to the brain stem. Auditory nerve input from both ears joins at the lateral lemniscus, reducing the possibility of unilateral deafness from CNS damage. The auditory nerves ascend to the cortex by a variety of pathways, reaching both the primary and secondary auditory regions of the temporal cortex of the brain. Efferent innervation via the acoustic nerve (eighth cranial nerve) reaches the cochlea and vestibule via the internal auditory canal, which also carries the facial nerve (seventh cranial nerve).

Sound is filtered by the ear components. Human auditory sensitivity ranges from 15 to 20,000 Hz. The auditory canal diminishes the passage of sounds with frequencies above 3500 Hz, the higher end of the human voice frequency. The middle ear diminishes passage of sounds with frequencies below 1000 Hz, the lower end of human voice frequency. The muscles of the middle ear decrease sound transmission by uncoupling the ossicles. For example, contraction of the tensor tympani allows reflex adaptation to a noisy environment. Contraction of the stapedius decreases sound transmission while speaking.

BALANCE

The *utricle* and *saccule* are vestibular receptors that position the head as it relates to the pull of gravity. The *semicircular canals* are arranged to sense rotational movements, such as movements or changes in position. Each of the semicircular canals connects with the utricle. Where the canals connect with the utricle is an enlarged portion *(ampulla).* The ampulla contains a cluster of hair cells *(crista),* concerned with dynamic balance. For example, when head position is changed, movement of the endolymph stimulates the hair cells, initiating increased impulses that travel over the vestibular division of the acoustic nerve to the brain. Balance functions in the vestibular system, along with visual cues and musculoskeletal cues, combine to maintain balance. Hearing and balance are partially maintained with the loss of function of one ear.

EFFECTS OF AGING ON HEARING

Many physiologic changes lead to changes in hearing in older people. The hairs become coarser during the aging process; thus, retention of wax is more of a problem.

Presbycusis, a gradual sensorineural loss caused by nerve degeneration in the inner ear or auditory nerve, is a type of hearing loss that occurs with aging, even in people living in a quiet environment. Loss of auditory neurons in the organ of Corti and cochlear hair cell degeneration create an inability to hear high-frequency sounds. There may also be degeneration of the cochlear conductive membrane and decreased blood supply to the cochlea, leading to inability to hear at all (but especially higher) frequencies. Finally, a loss of cortical auditory neurons leads to diminished hearing and speech comprehension.

CONCLUSIONS

Vision and hearing are two senses that allow distance perception of the environment. Because we rely on these senses for communication with those around us, alterations in either sense can have a profound social and emotional impact. Some reductions in the ability to see or to hear are a normal part of age-related changes.

BIBLIOGRAPHY

1. Applegate, E. J. (2000). *The anatomy and physiology learning system* (2nd ed.). Philadelphia: W. B. Saunders.
2. Guyton, A. C., & Hall, J. (1996). *Textbook of medical physiology* (9th ed.). Philadelphia: W. B. Saunders.
3. Kandel, E. R., Schwartz, J. H., & Jessell, T. M. (1999). *Principles of neural science* (4th ed.). Norwalk, CT: Appleton & Lange.
4. McPhee, S. J., et al. (1999). *Pathophysiology of disease.* New York, McGraw-Hill.
5. Nolte, J. (1999). *The human brain* (4th ed.). St. Louis: Mosby.
6. Silverthorn, D. (1998). *Human physiology.* Upper Saddle River, NJ: Prentice Hall.

64

Assessment of the Eyes and Ears

Linda A. Vader
Helene J. Krouse

ASSESSMENT OF THE EYE

One of the most important considerations in an ocular assessment is that many ophthalmic disorders are asymptomatic. The four most common preventable causes of permanent vision loss in developed nations are (1) *amblyopia* (reduced visual acuity that is uncorrectable with glasses in the absence of anatomic defects in the eye or visual pathways), (2) diabetic retinopathy, (3) age-related maculopathy, and (4) glaucoma. Routine eye examinations are therefore imperative.

The eye is a unique organ because its external anatomy may be easily assessed. Even the internal eye is visible through the cornea, where blood vessels and central nervous system (CNS) tissue (the retina and optic nerve) may be visualized without the use of x-rays or invasive procedures. The effects of many systemic problems, such as infections, cancer, and vascular and autoimmune disorders, can be detected with an internal eye examination. Clients may voice misconceptions about vision and the eyes (Box 64–1). If you encounter such misconceptions while conducting a physical examination, be prepared to address them.

HISTORY

An ophthalmic history includes (1) demographic data, (2) exploration of current manifestations, (3) past health history, (4) family health history, (5) psychosocial history and lifestyle, and (6) review of systems.

■ BIOGRAPHICAL AND DEMOGRAPHIC DATA

Demographic data relevant to ocular assessment include age and sex. The incidence of cataracts, dry eye, retinal detachment, glaucoma, entropion (eyes turning inward), and ectropion (eyes turning outward) increases with age. Hereditary color vision deficits are more common in men than in women.

■ CURRENT HEALTH

Ocular manifestations may be divided into three basic categories: (1) vision, (2) appearance, and (3) sensations of pain and discomfort.

Chief Complaint

The most common chief complaint is a change or loss of vision, but the complaint may also be less specific, such as headache or eyestrain. Commonly, the client is unable to verbalize a specific complaint. The chief complaint may be as vague as "something is wrong with my eyes."

Symptom Analysis

Whenever possible, characterize clinical manifestations according to rapidity of onset, location, duration, and characteristics (such as frequency and severity). The circumstances surrounding onset as well as the client's response to treatment are important. Record current eye and systemic medications being used and all other current and past ocular disorders.

ABNORMAL VISION

Visual changes or loss of vision may be caused by abnormalities in the eye or anywhere along the visual pathway. Considerations include (1) a refractive (focusing) error; (2) interference from lid *ptosis* (drooping eyelid); (3) clouding or interference in the cornea, lens, aqueous or vitreous space; and (4) malfunction of the retina, optic nerve, or intracranial visual pathway.

Glare or halos may result from uncorrected refractive error, scratches on glasses, dilated pupils, corneal edema, or cataract. Flashing or flickering lights may indicate retinal traction or migraine. Floating spots may represent normal vitreous body strands or the pathologic presence of blood, pigment, or inflammatory cells in the vitreous body. *Diplopia* (double vision) may occur in one eye or both and may be caused by refractive correction, muscle imbalance, or neurologic disorders.

ABNORMAL APPEARANCE

The most common abnormal appearance is a *red eye*. Causes include minor irritation, vascular congestion, subconjunctival hemorrhage, inflammatory disorders, infection, allergy, and trauma (Box 64–2). Other external changes in appearance include growths or lesions, edema, and abnormal position.

The following statements are often passed along as "advice." They are all false.

1. Reading in the dark is harmful to the eyes.
2. Children will outgrow crossed eyes.
3. A cataract is a film growing over the surface of the eye.
4. Cataracts must "ripen" before they are removed.
5. The surgeon takes out the eye to operate on it.
6. A person with failing eyesight should avoid reading to save the eyes.
7. Children must be cautioned not to sit too close to the television.
8. Wearing someone else's glasses may damage your eyes.
9. Misuse of the eyes in childhood results in the need for glasses later in life.
10. Cataracts can be removed by a laser.
11. Emotional stress increases intraocular pressure.

ABNORMAL SENSATION

Eye pain is often poorly localized. Nonspecific complaints include eyestrain, pulling, pressure, fullness, or generalized headache. The pain may be periocular, ocular, or retrobulbar (behind the globe). Foreign-body sensation produces a sharp superficial pain that can be relieved by topical anesthesia. Deeper internal aching may indicate glaucoma, inflammation, muscle spasm, or infection. Reflex spasm of the ciliary muscle and iris sphincter that occurs with inflammation may produce brow ache and *photophobia* (sensitivity to light) or a constricted pupil (*miosis*). Itching is usually a sign of an allergic response. Dryness, burning, grittiness, and mild foreign-body sensation can occur with dry eyes or mild corneal irritation.

Tearing may be due to irritation or an abnormality of the lacrimal system. Increased ocular secretions usually indicate viral or bacterial infections and may also be present in allergic and noninfectious irritations.

■ PAST HEALTH HISTORY

The past health history focuses on systemic disorders commonly associated with ocular manifestations, such as diabetes mellitus, arthritis, hypertension, and thyroid disease.

Childhood and Infectious Diseases

Diseases occurring in childhood with possible ocular sequelae include diabetes mellitus, retinoblastoma, thyroid disorders, rheumatoid arthritis, exposure to sexually transmitted diseases (STDs) such as syphilis and acquired immunodeficiency syndrome (AIDS), and muscular dystrophy. Inquire about vaccinations, particularly for measles (rubella).

Major Illnesses and Hospitalizations

In addition to the just-mentioned systemic diseases, ask about hypertension, multiple sclerosis, myasthenia gravis, and adult onset of thyroid disorders, rheumatoid arthritis, and diabetes mellitus. Ocular diseases and structural problems include refractive errors (and corrective lenses used), strabismus, amblyopia, cataracts, glaucoma, and retinal detachment. If the client wears eyeglasses or contact lenses, ask when the last eye examination took place and when the prescription was last changed. Has the client has been hospitalized or undergone surgery related to the eyes or brain? Is there a history of head trauma or eye trauma related to motor vehicle accidents, sports injury, or other unintentional events?

Medications

Many medications affect the eyes. Prescription drugs include insulin, corticosteroids, oral hypoglycemics, and thyroid replacement hormones. Ask whether the client uses eye drops, and note the name, dose, and frequency taken. Specifically ask about use of over-the-counter eye drops such as natural tears. Over-the-counter preparations that may dry the eyes include antihistamines and decongestants.

Inquire about the use of herbal remedies, dietary supplements such as vitamins, and the consumption of specific foods. Some clients may consume large doses of vitamins A and C and certain foods, believing that these substances will prevent the development of vision problems such as cataracts and macular degeneration.

Nurses often encounter a client whose chief complaint is a "red eye." The condition causing the eye to be red (engorgement of the conjunctival vessels) may be a subconjunctival hemorrhage that requires no treatment, or it may be a sign of a serious eye disorder requiring immediate attention. Disorders involving red eye include:

Conjunctivitis—Bacterial, viral, allergic, and irritative
Herpes simplex keratitis—inflammation of the cornea
Scleritis—inflammation of the sclera
Angle-closure glaucoma—sudden occlusion of the anterior chamber angle by iris tissue
Adnexal disease—stye, dacryocystitis, blepharitis, lid lesions (carcinoma), thyroid disease, and vascular lesions
Subconjunctival hemorrhage—accumulation of blood in the potential space between the conjunctiva and the sclera
Pterygium—abnormal growth of tissue that progresses over the cornea
Keratoconjunctivitis sicca—inflammation associated with lacrimal deficiency
Abrasions and foreign bodies—hyperemic response
Abnormal lid function—Bell's palsy, thyroid ophthalmopathy, or lesions that cause ocular exposure

To evaluate a red eye:

1. Check the client's visual acuity with a Snellen chart.
2. Inspect for a pattern of redness.
3. Observe for the presence of discharge.
4. Using a penlight or slit lamp, observe for corneal opacities.
5. Using fluorescein stain, observe corneal defects.
6. Examine the anterior chamber for depth, blood cells, or pus.
7. Examine the pupils for irregularity.
8. Check intraocular pressure.
9. Observe for the pressure of proptosis or a lid disorder.

Allergies

Note allergies to medications and other substances. Has the client ever had an allergic reaction to eye drops or other medications that have affected the eyes? Allergic manifestations include eye redness, tearing, and itching. Determine past allergic reactions not only to medications but also to inhalants (dust, chemicals, or pollens) and contactants (cosmetics or pollens).

■ FAMILY HEALTH HISTORY

Because many ocular disorders tend to be familial, ask specifically about strabismus, glaucoma, *myopia* (near-sightedness), and *hyperopia* (farsightedness). Other common familial disorders include migraine, retinoblastoma, macular degeneration, retinitis pigmentosa, sickle cell anemia, keratoconus, and diabetes mellitus. Lack of a family health history does not necessarily rule out the possibility of a genetic disorder. Some clients do not know the ocular history of family members, and some may be embarrassed or hesitant to share the information.

■ PSYCHOSOCIAL HISTORY

Psychosocial history and lifestyle data significant to the ocular health history include occupational hazards, leisure activities and hobbies, and health management behaviors. A driving history can reveal a vision problem. Ask about the nature of the client's work and hobbies. Is the client exposed to irritating fumes, smoke, or airborne particles? Are safety goggles worn in situations in which eye injury may occur from fragments of metal or sand? Is there insufficient lighting, leading to eyestrain or harsh, glaring light? Leisure and sports activities associated with increased incidence of eye injury include baseball, racquetball, and contact sports; football is associated with a potential for head trauma. Participation in active outdoor activities, such as gardening, hiking, and cross-country skiing, increases the risk of foreign-body injury, abrasion, or penetrating injury. Does the client wear sunglasses or other protective eye gear when outdoors?

Explore health management behaviors related to the eyes. If the client has a systemic disease that affects the eyes, ask whether the client practices self-care measures. For example, does the diabetic client aggressively manage the disease by attempting to regulate blood glucose levels with diet and medication? If the client wears contact lenses, are the lenses cleaned and stored as recommended? Is the client capable of safely taking care of the lenses?

Visual ability is one of several capabilities necessary for a person to operate a motor vehicle. Use tact when assessing a client who may have impaired vision. Clients may not answer truthfully if they feel that driving privileges will be lost.

Briefly review the client's driving history for information that can indicate a vision deficit. Ask if driving at night is difficult because of the need to adjust to the glare from oncoming headlights. Does the client have trouble seeing the dashboard instrument panel at night because of dim lighting? Are traffic or street signs difficult to read while driving? Is the client able to drive in conditions of reduced visibility, such as in rain or fog? Do other vehicles, pedestrians, bicyclists, or objects appear unexpectedly in the peripheral vision while the client is looking straight ahead? Has the client had a motor vehicle accident or "close call" within the past year?

The social stigma of blindness underlies the anxiety that clients experience with actual or potential vision loss. Total loss of vision isolates a person within a different reality. Although most clients are successfully rehabilitated, some losses are permanent. Some people, for a variety of reasons, remain socially isolated. The image of a blind person who is pitied and must accept the charity of others is disturbing.

Not all work environments can be adapted for someone who is visually impaired. Clients with actual or potential vision loss may be faced with barriers in their vocations that force an unwanted change. Age may be a major factor in the client's ability to meet this challenge. Self-esteem is closely related to one's roles in a particular lifestyle. Loss of control in personal, family, and work situations can be devastating. The issue of dependence versus independence may also be a factor in the client's ability to cope with the stressors of vision loss.

■ REVIEW OF SYSTEMS

The review of systems (ROS) relevant to the eyes includes asking about manifestations such as headaches and problems with sinusitis. Determine whether manifestations occur in association with pain or discomfort, visual changes, swelling, redness, or drainage from the eye. Ask about the time of day and the season of year during which manifestations occur as well as about sensitivity to light. Detailed questions are presented in Box 9–2.

PHYSICAL EXAMINATION

Your role and scope of practice in ophthalmic assessment and examination vary according to state nurse practice acts, institutions, and employer guidelines. Regardless of the level of responsibility in any practice situation, you must be knowledgeable about ophthalmic clinical manifestations and diagnoses as they relate to the holistic approach to client care.

Examination of the eyes includes assessment of external structures, using inspection and palpation, extraocular movements (EOMs), visual acuity, and visual fields (peripheral vision). If you have advanced clinical assessment skills, you may perform tonometry and examine the internal eye structures with an ophthalmoscope. For an example of an assessment recording, see Physical Assessment Findings in the Healthy Adult: The Eye.

Observe the client's body structure and features for obvious deformities and apparent age. For example, the hand deformities or abnormal gait of a client with arthritis may be a clue to the diagnosis of an associated eye disorder of keratoconjunctivitis sicca (*dry eye syndrome*) in a client who reports itching and burning eyes.

■ EXTERNAL EYE

External eye structures include the eyebrows, eyelashes, eyelids, the lacrimal apparatus, anterior portion of the eyeballs, conjunctivae, sclerae, corneas, anterior chambers, pupils, and irises. Inspect and palpate these structures while the client sits at eye level.

PHYSICAL ASSESSMENT FINDINGS IN THE HEALTHY ADULT

The Eye

Inspection

Visual acuity 20/20. Eyebrows full, mobile. Eyelashes curve out and away from eyelids. Ptosis absent. Eyelids without lesions or inflammation. Eyes moist. Palpebral conjunctivae pink; bulbar conjunctivae clear. Scleral color even, without redness. Corneal light reflection symmetrical. PERRLA, directly and consensually. Cornea smooth; lens and anterior chamber clear. Irises evenly colored. EOMs full, without nystagmus. Conjugate movement. No strabismus. Visual fields full to confrontation.

Palpation

Eyeballs firm. Orbits without edema. No regurgitation from puncta. Tenderness absent over lacrimal apparatus.

Funduscopic Examination

Red reflexes visualized. AV ratio approximately 2:3. Vessels without tortuosity, narrowing, pulsation, or nicking. Disc margins clear, no cupping, cup-to-disc ratio 1:3. No evidence of retinal hemorrhage, patches, spots.

AV, artery-to-vein; EOM, extraocular movement; PERRLA, pupils equal, round, reactive to light and accommodation.

Eye Position

Assess eye position for symmetry and alignment. Sunken or protruding eyes, such as protrusion of one eye or both eyes (*exophthalmos*) are an abnormal finding.

Eyebrows

Inspect the eyebrows for symmetry, hair distribution, skin conditions, and movement. The eyebrows normally move up and down smoothly under control of the facial nerves. Hair loss of the lateral aspects occurs with aging. The skin may be dry and flaking (i.e., dandruff), which is abnormal.

Eyelids and Eyelashes

Examine the eyelids and eyelashes for placement and symmetry. When open, the upper lids rest at the top of the irises and the lower lids at the bottom so that the sclerae are not visible above or below the irises. Sagging of the upper lids that covers part of the pupil (ptosis) is abnormal. Ptosis may occur with aging but also results from edema, third cranial nerve disorders, and neuromuscular disorders. Check for effective closure by asking the client to close the eyes. Eyelids that turn inward (*entropion*) or outward (*ectropion*) can result in corneal irritation. Lid eversion and inversion are often related to aging tissues but may result from facial nerve paresis, scarring, or allergies. Elevate the eyebrows to inspect the upper lids for lesions. Inspect the lower lids by asking the client to open the eyes. Examine the skin of the eyelids and orbit by palpating for texture, firmness, mobility, and integrity of the underlying tissues.

Blink Response

Blinking is an involuntary reflex that occurs bilaterally up to 20 times a minute. Rapid, infrequent, or asymmetrical blinking is abnormal.

Eyeballs

Palpate the eyeballs for symmetry and firmness. Instruct the client to close the eyes and look down. Place the tip of the index fingers on the upper eyelids, over the sclerae, and palpate gently. Normally, the eyeballs feel firm and symmetrical, not asymmetrical, hard, or soft. If you have advanced clinical skills, you may perform tonometry to measure ocular pressure (see Internal Eye Examination).

Lacrimal Apparatus

Examine the lacrimal apparatus by retracting the upper lid and having the client look down so that part of the lacrimal gland may be visualized. Observe this area for swelling or tenderness. The eye surface should be moist, without excess tearing. Inspect the area between the lower lid and the nose, which should be free of edema. Gently palpate the area over the lower orbit rim near the inner canthus (over the lacrimal sac). There should be no regurgitation of fluid from the sac or puncta.

Conjunctivae and Sclerae

Inspect the conjunctivae and sclerae for color changes, texture, vascularity, lesions, thickness, secretions, and foreign bodies. The bulbar conjunctivae are colorless and transparent, allowing the sclerae to be seen. Small blood vessels may be visible. In white people, the sclerae are white; in people with dark skin, they may appear light yellow. Wear gloves to inspect the palpebral conjunctivae, and wash your hands both before and after this portion of the examination.

Retract the lower eyelids to expose the conjunctivae without applying pressure to the eyeballs. You (or the client) should gently push the lower lids down against the bony orbit while the client looks up. Healthy conjunctivae are pink to light red; paleness or a bright red color is abnormal. If the lower palpebral conjunctivae are normal, the upper palpebral conjunctivae usually are not inspected. If examination is necessary, evert the upper eyelids by gently grasping the eyelashes of the upper lid and pulling down while the client looks down. Place a cotton-tipped applicator just above the lid margin, and turn the upper lid inside out over the applicator. After the inspection, return the eyelid to its normal position by gently pulling the eyelashes forward while the client looks up.

Corneal Reflex

The corneal reflex test is performed to assess the function of the fifth (trigeminal) cranial nerve. Instruct the client to keep the eyes open and look straight ahead. Bring a sterile cotton wisp from behind the client and touch it lightly to the cornea. Blinking and tearing indicate that the nerves are intact. Use a separate wisp for each eye. An alternative method is to use a syringe or the bulb from an otoscope to gently puff air across the cornea, eliciting the blink-and-tear response. A client wearing contact lenses may not respond to the same degree as someone who does not wear them because of insensitivity to the stimulus.

Cornea

Inspect the cornea from an oblique angle while shining a penlight on the corneal surface. The irises are easily visible. In older adults, a thin, grayish white ring around the edge of the cornea (arcus senilis) may be seen. Abnormalities include surface irregularity and cloudiness (opacity).

Anterior Chamber

Using the same oblique angle and penlight, inspect the anterior chamber while observing the cornea. The chambers should appear clear and transparent with no cloudiness or shadows cast upon the irises. The depth of the chamber between the cornea and iris normally is about 3 mm. Shallower or deeper chambers are abnormal; refer the client to an ophthalmologist.

Iris and Pupil

Inspect the iris and pupil. The iris should light up with oblique lighting from the penlight and should have a consistent color. Bulging or uneven coloring is abnormal. When light shines into the eyes, the iris constricts as the optic nerves are stimulated, causing the pupil to become smaller. Dim lighting causes the pupil to dilate. Inspect the pupils for size, equality, shape, and ability to react to light and accommodation. Pupils are normally black, round, with smooth borders, and the same size. The actual size depends on the level of lighting, effect of medications that alter iris contractility, changes in intracranial pressure, or lesions impinging on the optic nerve.

Dim the light to test pupil reactions to light and accommodation. Instruct the client to look straight ahead. To test direct response to light, bring the penlight in from the side to shine directly over the center of the pupil. The illuminated pupil should constrict briskly and evenly. Repeat this maneuver on the other eye. Both eyes should react to the same degree. Test consensual response by observing one pupil while the penlight is shone on the opposite pupil. Both pupils should constrict to the same degree, although the consensual response is slightly slower.

Test accommodation by holding the penlight 4 to 6 inches (10 to 15 cm) away from the client's nose. Instruct the client to look first at the penlight, then at the distant wall straight ahead, and then back at the penlight. While the client gazes from near to far and back again, observe the pupils' response to changes in distance. The pupils should dilate when the client looks at the far point and should constrict when the client looks at the near object. Then move the penlight toward the bridge of the client's nose, observing the pupils for convergence and constriction.

Results of the pupil assessment that are normal are recorded as PERRLA (pupils equal, round, and reactive to light, and accommodation). Abnormal results include light intolerance (photophobia), irregular or unequal pupils, or pupils that do not react to light or accommodation. Pupil abnormalities may be caused by neurologic disease, intraocular inflammation, iris adhesions, systemic or ocular medication side effects, or surgical alteration, or they may be benign variations of normal findings.

Ocular Motility

Evaluation of ocular motility provides information about the extraocular muscles; the orbit; the oculomotor, trochlear, and abducent nerves; their brain stem connections; and the cerebral cortex. Ask the client to track a target with both eyes as it is moved in each of the six cardinal directions of gaze (see Fig. 64–1). Note the speed, smoothness, range, and symmetry of movements and observe for unsteadiness of fixation (nystagmus).

The eyes normally move in parallel to each other, smoothly and in unison. Test the function of the oculomotor, trochlear, and abducent nerves by asking the client to look straight ahead while you stand directly in front. Hold a penlight approximately 12 inches (30 cm) from the client's eyes. Instruct the client to keep the head still and to follow the penlight's movements with the eyes only. Move the penlight slowly and smoothly through the six cardinal positions of gaze, being careful not to go beyond the client's field of vision. Move the penlight in an orderly manner from the center outward along each of the six directions; pause briefly to observe for nystagmus, then return to the center. Nystagmus is an involuntary rapid, oscillating movement of the eyeball and is considered an abnormal finding except for slight nystagmus in the extreme lateral gazes (e.g., end-point nystagmus). If the eyes do not move in parallel or if the upper eyelid covers more than a tiny portion of the iris, note the conditions as abnormal findings.

CORNEAL LIGHT REFLEX TEST

The corneal light reflex test (Hirschberg's test) determines eye alignment. Shine a penlight at the bridge of the client's nose from a distance of 12 to 15 inches (30 to 38 cm) while the client stares straight ahead. Observe where the light reflects from both corneas; the reflection should be symmetrical. Asymmetrical reflection is abnormal and may indicate strabismus, a disorder in which the eye axes cannot be directed to the same object. A constant deviation of ocular alignment is termed tropia. Deviation toward the nose is called esoptropia, a deviation away from the nose is called exotropia, and a vertical (up or down) deviation is called hypertropia. Latent deviations are seen only when one eye is covered and are called phorias (e.g., esophoria and exophoria).

COVER-UNCOVER TEST

This test assesses eye muscle function and alignment for tropia and phoria. Ask the client to stare straight ahead at a fixed point approximately 20 inches (51 cm) away. Cover one of the client's eyes with an opaque card while you observe the uncovered eye for lateral or medial movement as it focuses on the fixed point. There should be no movement. Remove the eye cover, and observe that

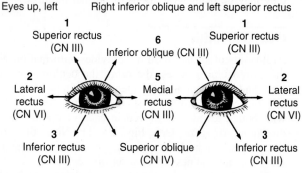

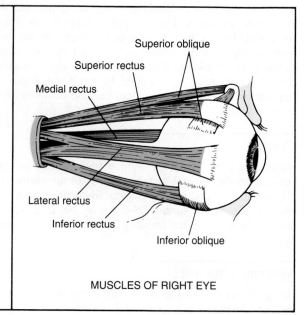

CARDINAL DIRECTIONS OF GAZE

	MUSCLES WORKING FOR EACH DIRECTION
Eyes up, right	Right superior rectus and left inferior oblique
Eyes right	Right lateral rectus and left medial rectus
Eyes down, right	Right inferior rectus and left superior oblique
Eyes down, left	Right superior oblique and left inferior rectus
Eyes left	Right medial rectus and left lateral rectus
Eyes up, left	Right inferior oblique and left superior rectus

1 Superior rectus (CN III)
6 Inferior oblique (CN III)
1 Superior rectus (CN III)
2 Lateral rectus (CN VI)
5 Medial rectus (CN III)
2 Lateral rectus (CN VI)
3 Inferior rectus (CN III)
4 Superior oblique (CN IV)
3 Inferior rectus (CN III)

MUSCLES OF RIGHT EYE

Superior oblique
Superior rectus
Medial rectus
Lateral rectus
Inferior rectus
Inferior oblique

FIGURE 64–1 The six cardinal directions of gaze and the muscles responsible for each: (1) right, (2) left, (3) up and right, (4) up and left, (5) down and right, and (6) down and left. CN, cranial nerve.

eye for movement as it focuses on the fixed point; again, there should be no movement. Repeat the maneuvers for the opposite eye. The test may need to be repeated several times to confirm abnormal findings of strabismus.

Vision

VISUAL ACUITY

Testing visual acuity is the standard and routine method used to determine the clarity of the ocular media (cornea, lens, and vitreous) and the function of the visual pathway from the retina to the brain. Although abnormal acuity implies an uncorrected refractive error or pathologic process, normal acuity does not exclude disease of the visual system. Visual acuity is assessed in one eye at a time, then in both eyes together, with the client comfortably seated. Begin with the right eye while covering the left eye with an occluder or opaque card. Test visual acuity with and without corrective lenses. Visual acuity is traditionally measured with the Snellen chart (Fig. 64–2A) at a distance of 20 feet; at this distance, rays of light from an object are practically parallel and little effort of accommodation is required. In rooms that are shorter than 20 feet, mirrors or projection may be used to achieve the required distance. Charts may also be reduced proportionately to compensate for distance. Adaptations may be needed for the client who is illiterate or who does not speak English; variations of the Snellen chart are available for these clients. The numbers and symbols can be used in lieu of letters. There must be adequate lighting for the client to see.

Begin by asking the client to read the smallest line of symbols or letters that is seen. Credit the client for the smallest line of print that is read with more than 50% accuracy. Record the results according to the standardized numbers printed next to the lines on the chart. The sizes of the symbols are identified according to the distances at which they are normally visible. For example, the largest symbols can be read 200 feet away by people with unimpaired vision. The results of visual acuity testing are expressed as a fraction. The numerator denotes the distance the client is from the chart letters, and the denominator denotes the distance from the chart at which a client with normal vision can see the chart letters. Examples of results are as follows:

- Vision that is 20/20 is normal; that is, the client is able to read at 20 feet what a person with normal vision can read at 20 feet.
- A client with a visual acuity of 20/60 can read at a distance of 20 feet only what a client with normal vision can read at 60 feet.
- The client with *myopia* (nearsightedness) has results of 20/30 or greater, signifying that the client can read at 20 feet only what a person with normal vision can read at 30 feet (or greater).
- *Hyperopia* (farsightedness) results are 20/15 or less; that is, the client can read at 20 feet what a person with normal vision can read at 15 feet (or less).
- A result of 20/15 indicates better-than-average visual acuity.
- *Legal blindness* is defined as 20/200 or less with corrected vision (glasses or contact lenses) or less than 20 degrees of visual field in the better eye.

When the client cannot distinguish the largest letter on the chart, ask the client to read the number of fingers held up in front of him or her at a distance of 3 feet (CF = count fingers). If the client cannot distinguish fingers, ask whether the client perceives hand movements (HM = hand motion). Finally, determine whether the client can perceive light (LP = light perception). NLP indicates no light perception.

Test near vision with a card or newsprint held 12 to 14 inches (30 to 36 cm) from the client's eyes (Fig. 64–

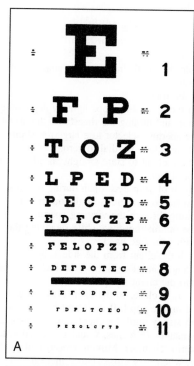

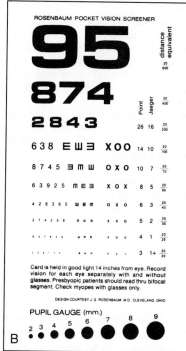

FIGURE 64–2 *A,* Snellen's chart, for assessment of visual acuity. *B,* A Rosenbaum pocket vision screener. The charts are not pictured to scale with respect to one another. (*B,* Courtesy of SMP Division, Cooper Laboratories [P.R.], Inc., San German, Puerto Rico.)

2*B*). Corrective lenses are worn if needed. The client with normal vision can read the material at that distance. Complaints of blurring or attempts by the client to move the card either closer or farther away signal abnormal near vision.

If the client becomes familiar with the letters through repeated examination, have the client read the letters

backward. If the client can read most of the letters in a particular line but misses one or two, document the visual acuity as 20/40–2.

VISUAL FIELDS

Visual field testing is used to evaluate peripheral vision. It may be accomplished by the *confrontational method* (Fig. 64–3) or with a computerized instrument. The confrontational method assumes that the examiner has normal peripheral vision.

The client sits facing you approximately 2 feet (60 cm) away. The client's eyes and yours should be at the same level. Both you and the client cover the eyes directly opposite to one another with an opaque cover (e.g., your right eye and the client's left eye) and stare at each other's uncovered eye. Hold a small object, such as a penlight, in your free hand, holding it equidistant between yourself and the client, just out of view at the periphery of the visual field. Starting with the superior field, slowly bring the penlight down between the client and yourself until the client states that he or she can see it. (You should be able to see the penlight at the same time.)

Repeat this maneuver at 45-degree angles, progressing through the superior, temporal, inferior, and nasal fields until all are tested. You may need to position the penlight slightly behind the client to adequately test the temporal fields. Repeat the test for the other eye. Normal visual fields extend approximately 50 degrees superiorly, 90 degrees laterally, 70 degrees inferiorly, and 60 degrees medially. Gross visual field defects can be detected and, if found, refer the client for further examination.

A variety of manual and computerized visual field testing equipment may be used to permit more accurate, reproducible detection and quantification of *scotoma* (an area of decreased visual function). CNS disorders, such as a brain lesion or syphilis, and ocular disorders, such as glaucoma or retinal detachment, can alter visual fields.

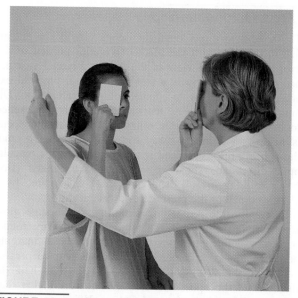

FIGURE 64–3 Confrontational method of assessment of visual fields. (From Jarvis, C. [1996]. *Physical examination and health assessment* [2nd ed.]. Philadelphia: W. B. Saunders.)

Special Testing of Vision

COLOR VISION

Color vision problems are genetic and acquired in both men and women. Men are more often affected with inherited losses in color vision (7%), and women are affected to a lesser degree (0.5%). Nutritional problems, optic nerve disorders, and problems with the fovea centralis can also alter color perception.

Color vision testing is not always part of a routine eye examination. It is used most often in screening people seeking a license to operate a motor vehicle or for employment in which color discrimination is important. A common test involves the use of color plates on which numbers are outlined in primary colors and surrounded by "confusion" colors. The person with color vision problems is unable to recognize the figure. One such test consists of 84 chips of color that are matched in terms of increasing hues.

Central Area Blindness Assessment

The Amsler grid is a 20-cm square that is divided into 5-mm squares with a dot in the center. The grid is used to detect and follow the development of central area blindness (scotoma), such as occurs in macular degeneration. The client wears glasses, closes one eye, and holds the grid 12 inches from the face (the usual reading distance). The client fixes vision on the central dot and describes any areas of distortion or absences in the grid.

■ INTERNAL EYE

Internal eye structures are visible only with illumination such as that provided by an ophthalmoscope. This instrument is used to inspect the structures posterior to the iris, including the lens and fundus (which includes the retina, retinal vessels, choroid, optic disc, macula, and fovea). Using the ophthalmoscope requires considerable skill and practice.

Direct Ophthalmoscopy

The hand-held direct ophthalmoscope provides a magnified ($\times 15$) image of the fundus (posterior portion of the eye) and a detailed view of the disc and retinal vascular bed. Ophthalmoscopy is a part of a general physical examination as well as an ophthalmologic examination. Dilating the eye enhances the view, although a darkened room may cause adequate dilation. The ophthalmoscope is held 1 to 2 inches away from the client's eye and, through a light source and reflective mirrors, the macula, optic disc, and retinal vessels can be examined (Box 64–3 and Fig. 64–4). The view may be impaired by a cloudy cornea or the presence of a cataract.

Normally, the red reflex is a bright red-orange glow seen through the pupil. The optic disc appears round, with well-defined margins (except in the nasal margin), and a creamy pink color. The physiologic cup (depressed center of the disc) should be no larger than half the diameter of the optic disc. Retinal veins are darker than arteries and radiate from the disc. Veins are slightly thicker than arteries and should be free of pulsation. Tor-

---

BOX 64–3   Guidelines for Using an Ophthalmoscope

1. Assemble the ophthalmoscope by attaching the head to the handle.
2. Darken the room.
3. Turn on the ophthalmoscope light by depressing the rheostat button and turning the rheostat to the brightest light.
4. Turn the aperture selector to a large round circle of light.
5. Turn the lens selector dial to zero.
6. Instruct the client to stare straight ahead and to focus on a distant object.
7. Leave both of your eyes open during the examination. Learn to suppress visual stimulation from the eye that is not looking through the viewing aperture.
8. Hold the ophthalmoscope while steadying the client's head with your free hand.
9. Approach the client from the side at approximately a 45-degree angle and a distance of 15 inches. Direct the light into the client's pupil.
10. Move slowly closer to the client's eye, keeping the light directed on the pupil. If the client blinks, hold your position steady until the client's eye opens again. At approximately 15 inches, visualize the red reflex, then the anterior chamber. Moving closer, look at the lens. Finally, when very close (1 to 2 inches), vessels of the fundus may be seen.
11. Adjust the lens selector with your index finger to focus on a blood vessel and follow it into the optic disc.
12. Focus on the disc, adjusting the lens selector as needed to correct for visual deficits of both you and the client. Once the focus is adjusted, examine the optic disc (for color, margins, shape, and presence of physiologic cup; see Fig. 64–6).
13. Follow the major blood vessels from the disc and look for evidence of tortuosity, pulsation, diameter, ratio of arteries to veins (normally 2:3), and areas where arteries and veins cross for signs of nicking.
14. Note the retinal background color. Look for the presence of exudate or hemorrhage.
15. Last, ask the client to look into the light so that you can examine the fovea centralis. The fovea may be seen as a tiny bright light in the center of the macula. Only a very brief glimpse is possible because the light is too bright for the client to look at for long.
16. Repeat the examination for the opposite eye.

---

tuous vessels or straightened arteries are abnormal, as is nicking (i.e., the disappearance of a vessel where an artery and vein cross each other so that one vessel looks discontinuous). The retinal background is pink in whites, and dark and heavily pigmented in people with a dark complexion. Choroidal vessels may appear as linear orange streaks. A normal retina is shown in Figure 64–4.

The fundus is the only site in the body where the vascular bed may be observed directly. Thus, funduscopic examination yields information about many systemic diseases. Abnormal findings include an altered arteriovenous ratio, narrowed arteries, widened veins, pinched-off vessels, abnormal arterial light reflex, excessive tortuosity, numerous arteriovenous nickings, exudates, white patches, and focal hemorrhage.

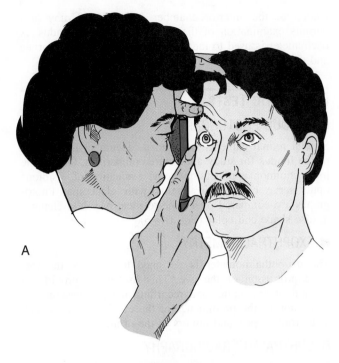

A

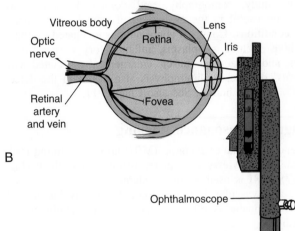

Vitreous body

Optic nerve

Retinal artery and vein

Retina

Lens

Iris

Fovea

B

Ophthalmoscope

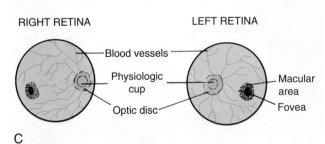

RIGHT RETINA   LEFT RETINA

Blood vessels

Physiologic cup

Optic disc

Macular area

Fovea

C

FIGURE 64–4 *A,* The examiner uses the right hand to hold the ophthalmoscope to the right eye to examine the client's right eye. The examiner uses the left hand and left eye when examining the client's left eye. Note the positioning of the examiner's free hand, which is placed to steady the client's head and to slightly retract the eyebrow. *B,* The examiner sees what appears in the angle of light through the viewing aperture. *C,* The actual area of retina visualized depends on the dilation of the pupil. Note the structures that may be examined.

Indirect Ophthalmoscopy

Indirect ophthalmoscopy provides a stereoscopic picture over a large area of the retina. The light source comes from a head-mounted light. The examiner holds a convex lens in front of the client's eye and, through a viewing device attached to the headband, sees an inverted reversed image. The indirect ophthalmoscope provides for binocular visual inspection with depth perception and permits a wider field of view compared with the direct method.

Tonometry

Tonometry is a method of measuring intraocular fluid pressure with the use of calibrated instruments that indent or flatten the corneal apex. The eye can be thought of as an enclosed compartment through which there is a constant circulation of *aqueous humor,* which maintains the shape of the eye with a relatively uniform pressure within the globe. As the pressure increases, the eye becomes firmer and a greater force is required to cause the same amount of indentation. Pressures between 8 and 21 mm Hg are considered within the normal range.

The two most common types of tonometers are the hand-held tonometer and applanation tonometer (Fig. 64–5). The portable hand-held instrument may be used in an office, clinic, emergency department, or operating room or at the bedside. It measures the amount of tension on the cornea. First the cornea is anesthetized with a topical anesthetic eye drop. While the client sits and looks straight forward, the tonopen is held perpendicular to the cornea and tapped several times directly on the

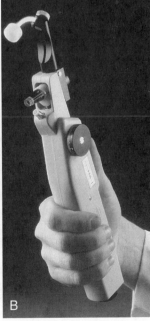
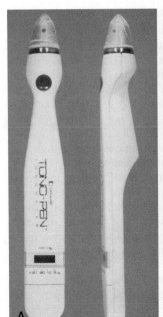

A

B

FIGURE 64–5 *A, Left and right,* Tonometer, seen from two viewpoints (Courtesy of Ophthalmic Photography at the University of Michigan W. K. Kellogg Eye Center, Ann Arbor.) *B,* Hand-held applanation tonometer. (Courtesy of Kowa Optimed, Torrance, CA.)

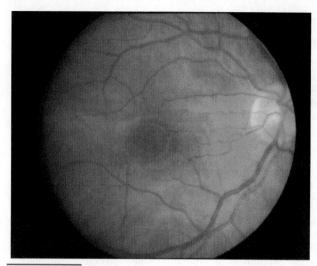

FIGURE 64–6 A normal fundus. (Courtesy of Ophthalmic Photography at the University of Michigan W. K. Kellogg Eye Center, Ann Arbor.)

cornea. A computer chip in the instrument averages the readings and notes the standard deviation.

An applanation tonometer, which may either be hand-held or attached to a slit-lamp microscope, measures the amount of force required to flatten the corneal apex by a standard amount. Anesthetic eye drops are also used beforehand.

Intraocular pressure is noted in the client record with a large T. The top number indicates the pressure in the right eye and the bottom number, the left eye.

Slit-Lamp Examination

The slit-lamp microscope is used to illuminate and examine the anterior segment of the eye under magnification. A linear slit beam of incandescent light is projected onto the globe, illuminating an optical cross-section of the anterior chamber. The angle of illumination, length, width, and intensity of the light may be adjusted. The client sits, and the head is stabilized by an adjustable chin rest and forehead strap. Details of the lid margins, lashes, conjunctiva, tear film, cornea, iris, lens, and aqueous humor can be studied. At the highest magnification setting, the abnormal presence of red or white blood cells in the aqueous humor may be visualized. The presence of protein (flare), called an *anterior chamber reaction,* that accompanies intraocular inflammation may also be detected. Normal aqueous humor is optically clear, without cells or flare. The presence of cells and flare is documented as 1 to 4+.

Fluorescein dye is often used in a slit-lamp examination to highlight corneal irregularities. Sterile paper strips containing fluorescein dye are wetted and touched against the inner surface of the lower lid, instilling the yellow dye into the tear film and onto the corneal surface. A blue filter is attached to the light beam, causing the dye to fluoresce. The dye highlights defects in the cornea.

In addition to the applanation tonometer, several other devices may be attached to the slit lamp to expand the scope of the examination. A gonioscope provides visual-

ization of the anterior chamber angle. The Hruby lens permits examination of the vitreous body and fundus. A pachymeter is used to measure the thickness of the cornea and the anterior chamber.

DIAGNOSTIC TESTS

■ FUNDUS PHOTOGRAPHY

Special retinal cameras are used to document fine details of the fundus for study and future comparison. One of the most common applications is the evaluation of insidious optic nerve changes in clients with glaucoma. Photographs are compared over time to identify subtle changes in disc shape and color (Fig. 64–6).

■ EXOPHTHALMOMETRY

The exophthalmometer is designed to measure the forward protrusion of the eye. This instrument provides a method of evaluating and recording the progression and regression of the prominence of the eye in disorders such as thyroid disease and tumors of the orbit.

■ OPHTHALMIC RADIOGRAPHY

X-ray study, tomography, and computed tomography (CT) are useful in the evaluation of orbital and intracranial conditions. Common abnormalities evaluated by these methods include neoplasms, inflammatory masses, fractures, and extraocular muscle enlargement associated with Graves' disease. Radiography is also useful in the detection of foreign bodies. See also Chapter 11.

Magnetic Resonance Imaging

Magnetic resonance imaging (MRI) allows obtaining multidimensional views without repositioning the client (Fig. 64–7). MRI is used to image edema, areas of demyelination, and vascular lesions. However, the availability of MRI equipment is often limited and the examination is lengthy.

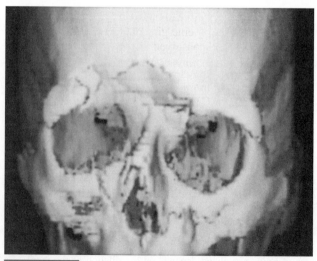

FIGURE 64–7 A magnetic resonance imaging (MRI) scan showing massive facial fractures. Note the three-dimensional appearance obtained with MRI.

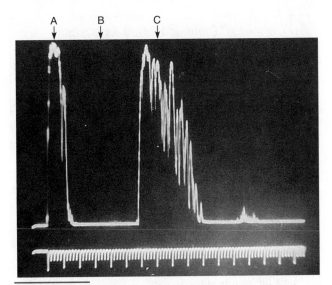

FIGURE 64–8 A normal A-scan ultrasound study of the eye. The sound beam is aimed in a straight line, and echoes are displayed as spikes. The amplitude depends on the density of the reflecting tissue and perpendicularity of the probe. *A,* Cornea and lens. *B,* Clear vitreous. *C,* Retina and choroid.

Ultrasonography

Ultrasonography uses high-frequency sound waves transmitted through a probe placed directly on the eyeball. As the sound waves bounce back off the various tissue components, they are collected by a receiver and amplified on an oscilloscope screen. Sound waves derived from the most distal structures arrive last, having traveled the farthest (Fig. 64–8). A-scan ultrasonography is used to measure axial length, the distance from the cornea to the retina, to determine the refractive power of an intraocular lens in cataract surgery. B-scan ultrasonography may be used to evaluate the characteristics of a lesion, as well as its size and growth over time, or the presence of a foreign body.

■ OPHTHALMODYNAMOMETRY

Ophthalmodynamometry is a test that consists of exerting pressure on the sclera with a spring plunger while the central retinal vessels emerging from the disc through an ophthalmoscope are observed. This instrument gives an approximate measurement of the relative pressures in the central retinal arteries and indirectly assesses carotid arterial flow on either side. Ophthalmodynamometry is indicated in the neurologic evaluation of clients who complain of "blacking out" of vision in one eye (*amaurosis*), spells of weakness on one side of the body, or other manifestations of cerebral ischemia. A difference of more than 20% in the diastolic pressures between the two eyes suggests insufficiency of the carotid arterial system on the side with the lower pressure.

■ ELECTRORETINOGRAPHY

An electrical potential exists between the cornea and retina of the eye. Because the retina is neurologic tissue, the retina exhibits certain electrical responses when stimulated by light. Electroretinography (ERG) measures the change in electrical potential of the eye caused by a diffuse flash of light. For this test, electrodes incorporated into a contact lens are placed directly on the anesthetized eye. Because eye movements disrupt the values of the test, the client must be able to fixate on a target while keeping the eyes still. Normal ERG findings signify functional integrity of the retina. Retinal diseases that may be evaluated with ERG include retinitis pigmentosa (progressive degeneration of photoreceptor cells), massive ischemia, disseminated infection, or toxic effects from drugs or chemicals.

■ VISUAL EVOKED RESPONSE

Visual evoked response (VER) is similar to ERG, in that it also measures the electrical potential resulting from a visual stimulus. The entire visual pathway from the retina to the cortex may be evaluated through the placement of electrodes on the scalp. Reduced speed of neuronal conduction, as with demyelination in optic neuritis, results in an abnormal response. Retinal or optic nerve disease may be diagnosed by stimulation of each eye separately.

■ FLUORESCEIN ANGIOGRAPHY

Fundus photography is enhanced by the use of fluorescein dye whose molecules emit green light when stimulated by blue light. The client sits in front of a retina camera after the pupils are dilated. A small amount of fluorescein dye is injected into an antecubital vein. The dye circulates throughout the body before eventual excretion by the kidneys. As the dye passes through the retinal and choroidal circulation, it can be visualized and photographed because of its ability to fluoresce (Fig. 64–9). A rapid sequence of pictures captures the initial rapid perfusion of the retinal and choroidal vessels. Later photos may demonstrate the gradual leakage of dye from abnormal vessels. Changes in blood flow, ischemia, and hemorrhage may be detected. Because it can so precisely delineate areas of

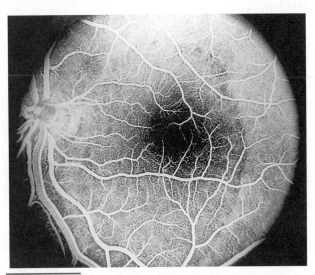

FIGURE 64–9 A normal fluorescein angiogram. The normal pattern of fluorescein angiography can be divided into three phases: (1) The *filling phase* (pictured) takes 8 to 20 seconds. (2) The *recirculation phase* starts 0.5 second after the filling phase and lasts 3 to 5 minutes. (3) The *late phase* lasts 30 to 60 minutes. Photographs are taken before injection, at half-second intervals for 20 seconds, then at intervals of 5 minutes.

abnormality, it is an essential guide for planning laser treatment of retinal vascular disease.

You may administer the intravenous (IV) fluorescein dye injection under an ophthalmologist's direction. First assess the client's general health status and identify any allergies. Allergic reactions to other dye injections, such as for an IV pyelogram [IVP] or cholangiogram, should be considered before the fluorescein injection. Diphenhydramine may be prescribed prophylactically. Although anaphylactic shock is a rare occurrence, emergency equipment should be located nearby. Occasionally, a client's vasovagal response to the dye may include vertigo, nausea, and momentary loss of consciousness. Obtain a consent for the procedure. Explain that during the injection the client may experience a warm sensation. The client will also hear the mechanics of the camera taking rapid-sequence photographs and experience bright flashes of light.

After the examination, encourage the client to increase intake of fluids because the dye is excreted through the kidneys. During the next 24 hours, the urine will be yellowish, and light-complexioned clients may experience a temporary yellow tint to the skin that will fade within a few hours as the dye is excreted. Because the pupils are dilated before the examination, it may be necessary to wear dark glasses for several hours until the pupils can constrict again in the presence of light.

ASSESSMENT OF THE EAR

The otologic history can be an important assessment tool and should be obtained before audiometric testing. Certain behavioral cues can indicate hearing impairment (Box 64–4). Collect significant data by conducting a thorough interview. Include the specific items in the otologic history (Box 64–5).

HISTORY

An otologic history includes demographic data, current clinical manifestations, past health history, family health

---

BOX 64–4   Clues Suggesting Hearing Impairment

Any adult who exhibits one or more of the following traits may be experiencing hearing impairment:

- Is irritable, hostile, hypersensitive in intercliental relations
- Has difficulty hearing upper frequency consonants (Sl, Sh)
- Complains about people mumbling
- Turns up volume on television
- Asks for frequent repetition and answers questions inappropriately
- Loses sense of humor, becomes grim
- Leans forward to hear better or turns head to preferred side
- Shuns large-group and small-group audience situations
- Shuns areas with increased background noise
- Might appear aloof and "stuck up"
- Complains of ringing in the ears
- Has an unusually soft or loud voice

BOX 64–5   Otologic History Assessment Guide

Current Problem

What changes are you having in your hearing?
Do you have any of the following manifestations?

Distortion of hearing	Yes No
Differences in the pitch of sound	Yes No
Noise in your ear	Yes No
Fullness or pressure in your ear	Yes No
Pain in your ear	Yes No
Drainage from your ear	Yes No
Have you ever had a hearing examination?	Yes No

If yes, why?
What were the results?

Use of Hearing Aids

Are you wearing hearing aids now?	Yes No
Are your hearing aids effective?	Yes No
How old are your hearing aids?	L ___ yr R ___ yr

Associated Problems

Do you have any of the following manifestations?

Head noise or ringing	Yes No
Feeling dizzy or unsteady	Yes No
Blurred vision	Yes No
Double vision	Yes No
Numbness in the hands or feet	Yes No
Weakness in the arms or legs	Yes No
Tingling around the mouth or face	Yes No
Loss of consciousness or blackouts	Yes No
Fainting	Yes No
Convulsions or seizures	Yes No

Risk Factors

Have you ever worked around loud noises?	Yes No
How long? _____ yr	
Do you still work around loud noise?	Yes No
Do you wear ear protection?	Yes No

Past Health History

Did you have hearing problems as a child?	Yes No
Did you have frequent ear infections as a child?	Yes No
Did you ever have a perforation in your eardrum?	Yes No
Did you ever get hit in the ear?	Yes No
Have you had ear surgery?	Yes No

If yes,

	Date	Operation	Surgeon
Right ear			
Left ear			

Do you have any food or medication allergies?
Please list and describe your reaction.

Family History

Do you have family members who were hard of hearing before 50 years old?
If yes, explain.

Have any members of your family ever had ear surgery?
If yes, explain.

history, psychosocial history, and review of systems. Ear problems often result from childhood illnesses or abnormalities associated with adjacent structures. The history interview is essential for determining current problems related to the ear.

■ BIOGRAPHICAL AND DEMOGRAPHIC DATA

Demographic data relevant to otologic assessment include the client's age. Hearing impairment may occur as a consequence of the aging process (Table 64–1).

■ CURRENT HEALTH

Chief Complaint

The most common chief complaints include the following:

- Hearing loss
- Pain
- Tinnitus
- Ear drainage
- Loss of balance
- Vertigo
- Dizziness

The client may also complain of associated nausea or vomiting. Complete a symptom analysis to determine onset, duration, frequency, and precipitating and relieving factors. Explore the client's past health history to determine the chronicity of the problem and the probable cause (see Box 64–5).

Symptom Analysis

Hearing loss may occur suddenly or gradually and can accompany the normal aging processes. The loss may be conductive, sensorineural, or related to a CNS disorder. The client may report inability to hear certain words or sounds or that sounds are muffled.

Pain may be perceived as a feeling of fullness in the ear. It may be intensified by movement and relieved by holding the head still or by applying heat. Ear pain may occur as a result of related problems of the nose, sinuses, oral cavity, or pharynx.

Ear drainage can be bloody (sanguineous), clear (se-

rous), mixed (serosanguineous), or contain pus (purulent). Drainage may also be accompanied by an odor.

Tinnitus (ringing in the ears) may be reported as high-pitched or low-pitched, roaring, humming, hissing, or loud and persistent. Tinnitus may occur more commonly at certain times of the day and may involve one or both ears.

Loss of balance may be accompanied by vertigo or dizziness. *Vertigo* is a sensation of motion while the person is not moving. A client may feel that either he or she or the room is moving. *Dizziness* is a sensation of unsteadiness and a feeling of movement within the head or lightheadedness.

■ PAST HEALTH HISTORY

Childhood and Infectious Diseases

Common childhood diseases involving the ears include the following:

- Acute middle ear infections (otitis media)
- Eardrum perforations resulting from otitis media
- Complications of ear infections such as chronic otitis media, frequent upper respiratory tract infection, and acute and chronic sinus infections

Infectious diseases with ear sequelae include mumps, measles, and meningitis. Specifically inquire whether the client has been immunized for mumps, measles, and *Haemophilus influenzae* type b (Hib). In utero exposure to maternal influenza or rubella may result in congenital hearing loss in the child. Premature birth is also associated with hearing problems.

Major Illnesses and Hospitalizations

Inquire about a history of upper respiratory tract infections. Has the client had a tonsillectomy or adenoidectomy? Does the history include ear surgery? Has the client had trauma to the head or ear, such as a severe blow or sustained loud noise exposure or concussion from sudden changes in air pressure (such as may occur in an explosion)? Does the history include chronic eardrum perforation?

Medications

Certain medications can damage the vestibulocochlear nerve (eighth cranial nerve), with resultant hearing loss, tinnitus, or disturbances in equilibrium. Aspirin is a common cause of tinnitus. Other drugs include aminoglycosides, analgesics, salicylates, quinine, chemotherapeutic agents, and antiprotozoal agents (Box 64–6). Obtain a complete medication history for prescription and over-the-counter drugs and herbal remedies.

Review the use of herbal remedies. Ginger (*Zingiber officinale*) is known for its anti-nausea effect and may be used for the relief of motion sickness. Ginkgo biloba (*Ginkgo biloba*) has been used for tinnitus and vertigo.

Allergies

In addition to asking about allergies to medications and other substances, inquire about allergies resulting in nasal

TABLE 64–1	CHANGES IN AUDITORY ACUITY CAUSED BY AGING
Anatomic Changes	**Physiologic Changes**
Degeneration of basilar conductive membrane of cochlea	Decreased ability to hear at all frequencies but greater at higher frequencies
Degeneration of cochlear hair cells	Decreased ability to hear high-frequency sounds
Decreased vascularity of cochlea	Loss of hearing equal at all frequencies
Loss of auditory neurons in spiral ganglia of organ of Corti	Loss of ability to hear high-frequency sounds
Loss of cortical auditory neurons	Diminished hearing and speech comprehension

---

BOX 64–6 Selected Ototoxic* Drugs

Aminoglycoside Antibiotics

Streptomycin
Neomycin
Gentamicin
Tobramycin
Amikacin
Kanamycin
Minocycline
Netilmicin

Other Antibiotics

Vancomycin
Viomycin
Polymyxin B
Polymyxin E
Erythromycin
Capreomycin
Chloramphenicol

Other Drugs

Chemotherapeutic agents (bleomycin, cisplatin, nitrogen
  mustard)
Salicylates
Quinine drugs
Quinidine
Chloroquine

Diuretics

Furosemide
Ethacrynic acid
Acetazolamide
Bumetanide
Mannitol

Chemicals

Metals (lead, mercury, gold, arsenic)
Alcohol
Aniline dyes
Caffeine
Carbon monoxide
Nicotine
Potassium bromate
Povidone-iodine

---

* Substances toxic to the ear.

---

stuffiness and congestion. Close proximity of the eustachian tubes to the nasal mucosa may also result in edema, which obstructs the flow of air between the middle ear and nose so that air pressure cannot be equalized.

■ FAMILY HEALTH HISTORY

Ask about a history of hearing loss or ear surgery among family members. Determine the age at onset for hearing loss or changes in hearing acuity.

■ PSYCHOSOCIAL HISTORY

Psychosocial and lifestyle factors that influence the incidence of hearing impairment include occupational hazards, environmental exposure, and leisure activities and

hobbies. Ask about exposure to loud noises (Table 64–2), including type, frequency, and duration. Is protective ear gear worn? Sound intensity is measured in units known as *decibels*. Ordinary speech level measures about 50 decibels (dB); heavy traffic is about 70 dB; at above 80 dB, noise becomes uncomfortable to the human ear. Exposure to levels greater than 85 to 90 dB for months or years causes cochlear damage.

Does the client swim, especially in water that may be contaminated? Has the client had problems with "swimmer's ear"? Does the client use earplugs to prevent water from entering the ear canal? Contaminated water can provoke an external ear infection and, if the tympanic membrane is perforated, may lead to infection in the middle ear.

Explore the client's ear hygiene habits. Does the client put objects into the ear, such as pencils, hairpins, or cotton-tipped applicators? Inserting objects such as these can traumatize the ear canal and damage or perforate the tympanic membrane.

■ REVIEW OF SYSTEMS

The review of systems related to the ear includes asking about problems with the nose, sinuses, mouth, pharynx, and throat. Has the client experienced head trauma, loss of balance, dizziness, or vertigo. Detailed questions for the review of systems are found in Box 9–2.

PHYSICAL EXAMINATION

Physical examination of the ear includes assessment of hearing acuity, balance, and equilibrium. Because the external ear is completely visible, it is easy to identify anatomic landmarks and to assess abnormalities. The eardrum reveals important information regarding the middle ear. However, because much of the middle ear and inner ear is inaccessible to direct examination, you must make inferences indirectly by testing auditory and vestibular function. See Physical Assessment Findings in the Healthy Adult: The Ear.

■ INSPECTION AND PALPATION

External Ear

Gross examination of both ears should precede individual examination of either ear. Use inspection and palpation to assess the external ear. Note size, configuration, and angle of attachment to the head. Observe the configuration of the pinna for gross deformity. Note whether the ears protrude and the degree of protrusion, the color of the skin of the ears, and whether additional skin tags are present. The skin of the ear should be smooth and without breaks or inflammation, especially in the crevice behind the ear. Note any lumps, skin lesions, or cysts, and record approximate size and location.

Perform palpation and manipulation of the pinna to detect tenderness, nodules, or *tophi* (small, hard nodules in the helix that are deposits of uric acid crystals characteristic of gout). During palpation, move the pinna, feel the mastoid area, and press on the tragus, noting any pain or discomfort, which may indicate inflammation or infection.

TABLE 64–2	DECIBEL (dB) RATINGS AND HAZARDOUS TIME EXPOSURE OF COMMON NOISES	
Typical Level* (dB)	**Example**	**Dangerous Time Exposure**
0	Lowest sound audible to human ear	
30	Quiet library, soft whisper	
40	Quiet office, living room, bedroom away from traffic	
50	Light traffic at a distance, refrigerator, gentle breeze	
60	Air conditioner at 20 ft, conversation, sewing machine	
70	Busy traffic, noisy restaurant (constant exposure)	Critical level begins
80	Subway, heavy city traffic, alarm clock at 2 ft, factory noise	More than 8 hr
90	Truck traffic, noisy home appliances, shop tools, lawnmower	Less than 8 hr
100	Chain saw, boiler shop, pneumatic drill	2 hr
120	Rock concert in front of speakers, sandblasting, thunderclap	Immediate danger
140	Gunshot blast, jet plane	Any length of exposure time is dangerous
180	Rocket launching pad	Hearing loss is inevitable

*Sound levels refer to intensity experienced at typical working distances. Intensity drops 6 dB with every doubling of distance from noise source. (Courtesy of American Academy of Otolaryngology–Head and Neck Surgery, Washington, DC.)

Ear Canal

DIRECT OBSERVATION

Inspection of the ear canal is carried out by direct observation, otoscopy, or microscopic examination. For direct observation, ask the adult to tip his or her head slightly to the opposite side while you pull the pinna up, back, and out. Use a penlight to inspect the ear canal for any abnormalities such as extreme narrowing, excessive wax, redness, scaliness, swelling, drainage, cysts, or foreign objects. None of these signs should be present. Visualization of the eardrum with this method would be unlikely.

OTOSCOPY

The eardrum is located at the end of the only skin-lined canal in the body. Proper visualization requires illumina-tion and magnification for accurate assessment. An otoscope is portable, and otoscopic examination is the most common method used. An otoscope is a device (Fig. 64–10) consisting of a handle, a light source, a magnifying lens, and an attachment for visualizing the ear canal and eardrum. A pneumatic device attached to the otoscope is used for injecting air into the ear canal to test the mobility and integrity of the eardrum.

Specula for the otoscope come in various sizes. Since

PHYSICAL ASSESSMENT FINDINGS IN THE HEALTHY ADULT

The Ear

Inspection

Auricles symmetrical, superior portion level with outer canthus of eye. Outer canals clear. Preauricular and postauricular areas without swelling, masses, or lesions. AC > BC, bilaterally. No lateralization. Whisper heard at 3 feet.

Palpation

Tenderness over tragus and mastoid absent. No masses.

Otoscopic Examination

Soft cerumen present in canals. No discharge. TMs intact, gray. Cone of light at 4:00 in right ear and at 7:00 in left ear. Landmarks visualized. No retraction or bulging. TM freely movable with pneumatic pressure.

AC, air conduction; BC, bone conduction; TM, tympanic membrane.

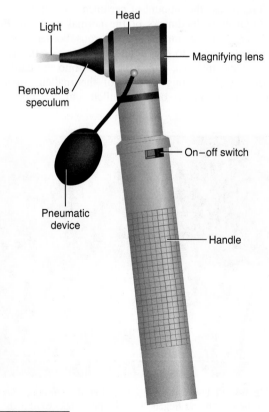

FIGURE 64–10 An otoscope.

the diameter of the meatus and the length of the ear canal vary, select the speculum with the largest diameter that fits comfortably into the ear canal. Check the light source for brightness. If the light appears yellowish or dim (like a flashlight with weak batteries), recharge or replace the batteries.

Hold the otoscope with the dominant hand, positioning it so that your hand rests against the client's head (Fig. 64–11). If the client moves suddenly, the otoscope will also move, thereby reducing the likelihood of damaging the external canal during examination. With your non-dominant hand, pull the pinna up, back, and out (in the adult), thus straightening the ear canal. While this is done, gently tilt the client's head away from you and insert the speculum slowly and carefully into the ear canal. Bring your eye close to the magnifying lens to visualize the ear canal and eardrum. When a pneumatic bulb is present, advance the otoscope far enough to make a secure seal.

Observe the ear canal while the speculum is entering and leaving. Move the otoscope in a circular fashion to visualize the entire ear canal. Note abnormalities such as extreme narrowing of the ear canal, nodules, redness, scaliness, swelling, drainage, cysts, foreign objects, and excessive wax. Visualization of the eardrum is impaired by most of these abnormalities. Sometimes the ear canal must be cleaned of wax, dead skin, and other debris. Wax and debris can be removed with a cerumen spoon (wax curet), suction aspirator, or irrigation.

Cerumen should not interfere with the examination when the amount is small. Cerumen is normally present in the external ear and varies in color from light yellow to black. Cerumen that is impacted in the ear canal is a common cause of hearing loss, especially in the elderly. Therefore, assess the amount of cerumen present.

Distinguishing landmarks of the normal eardrum (Fig. 64–12) are (1) the annulus, the fibrous border that attaches the eardrum to the temporal bone; (2) the short process of the malleus, which protrudes into the eardrum superiorly; (3) the long process of the malleus (manubrium); (4) the umbo of the malleus, at the point of

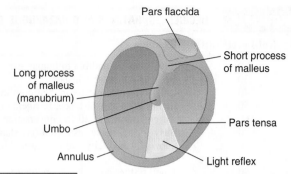

FIGURE 64–12 Normal right eardrum (tympanic membrane).

maximal concavity and attaches to the center of the eardrum; (5) the pars flaccida, a small triangular area above the short process of the malleus; and (6) the pars tensa, the remaining and largest portion of the eardrum.

The normal eardrum is slightly conical, translucent, shiny and smooth, and pearly gray in color. The position of the drumhead is oblique with respect to the ear canal. In the presence of disease, not only does the color of the eardrum change; other abnormalities are also manifested, such as retraction, bulging, or perforation of the eardrum and a white plaque (*tympanosclerosis*) on the eardrum.

Carefully inspect the entire eardrum, including the border (annulus), rotating the otoscope as needed. A cone of light reflex should be present on the eardrum in the lower anterior quadrant. The umbo and the long and short process of the malleus should be easily visible through the eardrum.

Test the mobility of the eardrum by using the pneumatic device of the otoscope to inject a small puff of air into the ear canal. Observe the eardrum for normal movement. An adequate seal is important to perform this maneuver accurately.

■ TESTS FOR AUDITORY ACUITY

Assessment of the middle and inner ear for hearing is accomplished by sophisticated methods of indirect testing (e.g., audiometry and vestibular testing). However, a gross assessment of hearing can be made simply through conversation, by evaluating the logical sequence of replies and the appropriateness of the responses. Gross assessments can be made at the bedside or in the office.

Test each ear separately to estimate hearing ability. Begin by occluding one of the client's ears with a finger. Then, while standing a foot away, whisper two-syllable numbers softly toward the unoccluded ear and ask the client to repeat the numbers. Increase the intensity of your voice from a soft, medium, or loud whisper to a soft, medium, or loud voice. If you suspect that the client is lip-reading, turn the client's face to one side. Ask the client whether hearing is better in one ear than in the other ear. If auditory acuity between the two ears is different, test the ear that hears better first. Next, produce noise in the better-hearing ear by rapidly but gently moving the finger in the client's ear canal while the other ear is tested.

Although the ticking of a watch tick can also be used to test hearing, it produces a higher-pitched sound, which is less relevant to functional hearing compared with the voice test.

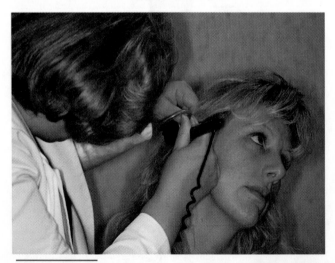

FIGURE 64–11 Use of the otoscope. Hold the otoscope handle between the thumb and fingers. Pull the pinna backward and upward in the adult to straighten the auditory canal.

The tuning fork also provides a general estimate of hearing loss. A frequency of 512 Hz is recommended. The two major tuning fork tests date from the 19th century and are named after their originators: Weber and Rinne.

Weber Test

The Weber test is used to assess conduction of sound through bone. Set the tuning fork into vibration by striking the tines on your hand. Place the rounded tip of the handle on the center of the client's forehead or nasal bone (Fig. 64–13A). Placement on the teeth (even false teeth) is a reliable option. Does the client hear the tone in the center of the head, the right ear, or the left ear? Normally, the sound is heard equally in both ears by bone conduction. If there is a sensorineural (nerve) hear-

ing loss in one ear, the sound is heard in the unaffected ear. With a conductive (air conduction) hearing loss, the sound is heard better in the affected ear.

Rinne Test

The Rinne test compares air conduction to bone conduction and helps to differentiate conductive from sensorineural hearing loss. Shift the vibrating tuning fork between two positions: first against the mastoid bone for bone conduction (Fig. 64–13B) and then 2 inches from the opening of the ear canal for air conduction (Fig. 64–13C). Move the tuning fork when the client no longer hears the sound by bone conduction, and ask the client to indicate whether the tone is louder in front of or behind the ear. Ask the client to state when the tone is no longer heard by air conduction.

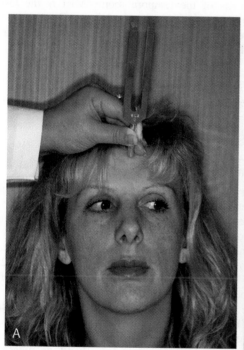
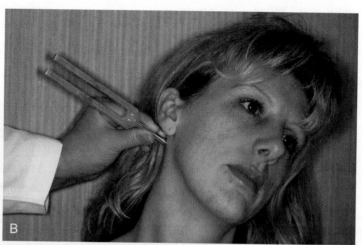
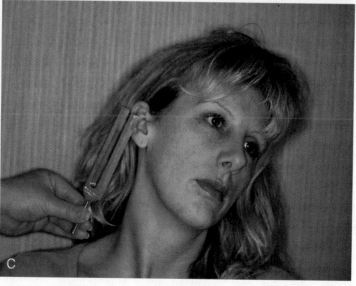

FIGURE 64–13 Weber and Rinne tests for hearing impairment. The Weber test is used to detect lateralization of hearing; the Rinne test distinguishes conductive hearing loss from sensorineural hearing loss. The two tests should be performed consecutively. *A,* For the Weber test, use a vibrating tuning fork, placed on the client's head to produce a centrally located stimulus. The client should hear the sound equally in both ears. The tone is louder in an ear with unilateral conductive loss and quieter in an ear with unilateral sensorineural loss. *B,* Perform the Rinne test to characterize the unilateral hearing loss as either conductive or sensorineural. Hold a vibrating tuning fork on the mastoid bone. *C,* When the client no longer hears the sound, place the tuning fork about 2 inches from the external ear. When the tone is louder through air than through bone, the Rinne test finding is positive, which indicates either normal hearing or a sensorineural hearing loss. A negative Rinne test finding, or louder bone conduction than air conduction, indicates a conductive loss.

Normally, sound is heard twice as long or as loud by air conduction than it is by bone conduction. Results are as follows:

- In *normal* hearing, air conduction is greater than bone conduction (a positive Rinne test finding).
- With a *conductive* hearing loss, bone conduction sounds louder or longer than air conduction sounds (a negative Rinne test finding).
- With a *sensorineural* hearing loss, the client hears better by air conduction (a positive Rinne test finding).

Conductive hearing loss results when the pathways of normal sound conduction are blocked. Because vibrations against the mastoid bone can bypass the obstruction, bone conduction lasts longer or sounds louder than air conduction. In *sensorineural* hearing loss, the acoustic nerve is less able to perceive vibrations from either bone or air; therefore, normal patterns are reported by the client.

■ TESTS FOR VESTIBULAR ACUITY

Romberg Test

Assess the inner ear for balance by performing a Romberg test. The client stands with feet together, arms by the sides, and eyes closed. Note the ability to maintain an upright posture with only a minimal amount of sway. Stand close to the client to offer balance support if needed. If the client loses balance, this is a positive Romberg sign, suggesting a vestibular ear problem or cerebellar ataxia.

A *tandem* Romberg test should also be performed. Instruct the client to walk forward and backward, heel-to-toe. A peripheral vestibular lesion may cause marked swaying or falling. A client without pathologic vestibular change can usually maintain balance, depending on age.

A *past-pointing test* can also indicate a labyrinthine disorder. While the client is seated, facing you with eyes open, hold out your index finger at the client's shoulder level. Instruct the client to touch your finger with the right index finger. Ask the client to lower the arm, close the eyes, and touch your finger again. Repeat the procedure, testing the client's left index finger. Observe and record the presence or absence, as well as the degree and direction, of past-pointing. A labyrinthine disorder can lead to past-pointing when the eyes are closed. Cerebral lesions are indicated when past-pointing occurs whether the eyes are open or closed.

Test for Nystagmus

Nystagmus is involuntary, rhythmic oscillation of the eyes associated with vestibular dysfunction. Nystagmus occurs normally when a client watches a rapidly moving object or looks beyond 30 degrees laterally (*end-point nystagmus*). To assess for *gaze nystagmus,* place your finger directly in front of the client at eye level. Ask the client to follow (track) the finger without moving the head. Starting at the midline, slowly move your finger toward the client's right ear and then the left ear, but not more than 30 degrees laterally, superiorly, or inferiorly. Observe the client's eyes for any jerking movements. For example, if the eyes jerk quickly to the left, and drift slowly back to the right, the client has left spontaneous (*horizontal*) nystagmus. Nystagmus is named for the direction of the fast phase. Nystagmus can be horizontal, vertical, or rotary.

DIAGNOSTIC TESTS

■ TESTS FOR AURAL STRUCTURE

The temporal bone and its structures are easily examined by radiography (x-ray study). The oldest, but not necessarily most useful, study is x-ray examination of the mastoid bone. More recent radiographic techniques have largely been replaced by imaging studies (see Chapter 11).

Computed Tomography

CT without contrast medium is the most commonly ordered CT scan for imaging of the temporal bone. Contrast is not generally needed because most bony structures are well seen. Contrast may be used to delineate vascular or soft tissue structures.

Magnetic Resonance Imaging

MRI reveals membranous organs as well as nerves and blood vessels of the temporal bone. MRI is the test of choice for tumors of the temporal bone. Contrast can be used for enhancement. For certain diagnostic assessments, both MRI and CT scans are obtained.

Arteriography

Arteriography is used to assess vascular abnormalities in the temporal bone.

■ TESTS FOR AUDITORY FUNCTION

Audiometric Tests

Audiology may be broadly called the science of hearing. Audiometric tests are performed to measure hearing and comprehension. A hearing test is performed in a sound-proof booth by an audiologist. An audiometer is an electronic instrument used to test hearing by producing sounds of varying pure-tone frequencies between 250–8000 Hz and loudness. The unit of measure of hearing, the decibel (dB), is a logarithmic function of sound intensity. The average normal adult has a hearing threshold of 0 to 20 dB hearing loss. The greater the threshold level, the poorer the hearing sensivity. The client is asked to signal the audiologist by raising a hand or pressing a button when a tone is heard; the responses are plotted on a graph called an *audiogram* (Fig. 64–14). Earphones are used for the audiogram.

Normal hearing is a range established nationally by testing the hearing levels of people of all ages. A client with normal hearing ability has 80% or more hearing, depending on age.

Some audiometric tests are performed by computer-assisted instruments. The objective of these special tests is to reveal whether a disorder is in the cochlea, acoustic nerve, or brain stem.

AUDIOGRAPHY

The components of hearing are tested through assessment of air conduction, bone conduction, and speech. Air con-

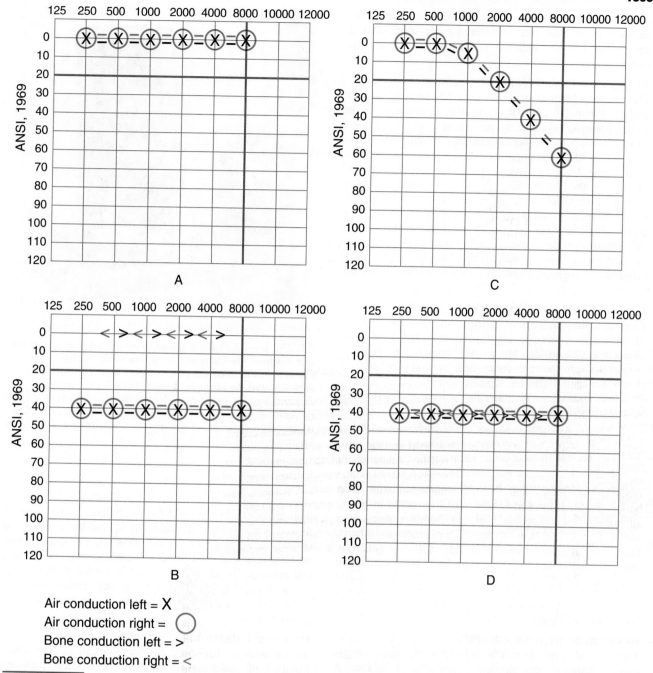

Air conduction left = X

Air conduction right = ◯

Bone conduction left = >

Bone conduction right = <

FIGURE 64-14 Audiograms showing types of hearing. *A,* Normal hearing. *B,* Conductive hearing loss. *C,* High-frequency hearing loss. *D,* Sensorineural hearing loss. (Courtesy of Arnold G. Schuring, M.D.)

duction is assessed by presenting tones through the earphones. When the examiner varies the loudness and frequency of tones, a hearing level is established. Bone conduction is assessed by presenting tones through a bone conduction oscillator placed behind the ear on the mastoid bone. The bone conduction level is the level at which the cochlea can hear, bypassing the middle ear structures, and is referred to as the *nerve hearing level.* A difference between air and bone conduction signifies a conductive hearing loss. When air and bone conduction are the same, either normal hearing or a *sensorineural* (nerve) hearing loss exists. Speech evaluation includes (1) *speech reception threshold* (the level of speech hearing),

which serves as a check on the reliability of the air conduction test, and *speech discrimination* (the ability to understand the spoken word).

TYMPANOMETRY

A popular test used for differentiating problems in the middle ear is tympanometry, or impedance audiometry. This test measures compliance (mobility) and impedance (opposition to movement) of the tympanic membrane and ossicles of the middle ear. The examiner applies positive, normal, and negative air pressure into the external meatus and measures the resultant sound energy flow, which is traced on a graph called a *tympanogram.* Abnormalities on the tympanogram reveal dysfunction of the middle ear, eustachian tube, and ossicles. Tympanometry can also be used to measure the stapedial muscle reflex and its decay. This test also indicates the function of the acoustic nerve.

TESTS FOR BRAIN STEM RESPONSE
The auditory brain stem response test is currently one of the most popular approaches to the assessment of the auditory nervous system. By presenting a sound to the ear and measuring the response (computer averaging) in the brain stem, the examiner can obtain specific diagnostic information. Imaging tests of the head are usually ordered to confirm the abnormality. Brain stem auditory evoked responses (BAERs) can be recorded from scalp electrodes. The early potentials reflect activity in the cochlea, eighth cranial nerve, and brain stem. Later evoked potentials reflect cortical activity. Early evoked responses may be used to estimate the magnitude of the hearing loss and differentiate cochlea, eighth cranial nerve, and brain stem lesions.

ELECTROCOCHLEOGRAPHY
Electrocochleography is designed to measure the response of the cochlea and the eighth cranial nerve to acoustic stimulation. Electrodes are placed through the tympanic membrane onto the promontary near the round window or in the ear canal, and an acoustic stimulation is applied. This test is used to evaluate the presence of Ménière's disease or perilymphatic fistula.

OTOACOUSTIC EMISSIONS
Otoacoustic emissions (OAEs) are low-level sounds, produced by the cochlea, that are involved in modulation of the hearing mechanism. OAEs can be recorded spontaneously or can be evoked through stimulation with short bursts of sound. Evoked OAEs can be observed in nearly all normal-hearing people, and can therefore serve as a useful screen for hearing acuity, especially in infants. Since they can be measured quickly, they are generally easier to obtain than BAERs, especially in uncooperative and crying infants.

Vestibular Tests

ELECTRONYSTAGMOGRAPHY
The vestibular system can be tested by electrophysiologic means. Although the physical assessment of balance is important, the most common objective measurement of balance is accomplished by electronystagmography (ENG). The ENG instrument was developed to measure nystagmus (involuntary, rapid eye movement) in response to stimulation of the vestibular system. This stimulation includes testing the client at rest in different positions for both the eyes and the head, and with different temperatures of air or water in the ear canals, thus stimulating the semicircular canals. The different test results give a recording (electronystagmogram) that reflects the status of each labyrinth and can indicate CNS system disorders.

PLATFORM POSTUROGRAPHY
Platform posturography, performed while the client is standing, is another balance test that helps to identify, quantify, and localize the source of balance disorders

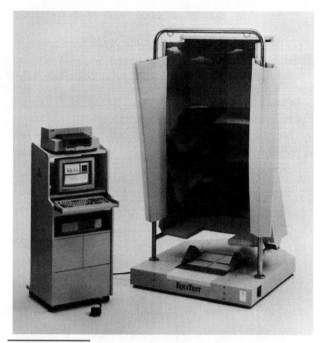

FIGURE 64–15 Platform posturography, used to assess vestibular function. The client stands on a movable platform, and vision is restricted by the panels with clouds. The platform is moved so that the client must compensate for the postural changes. Without visual cues, the vestibular system is tested for its ability to compensate. Because of the risk of falls, the client is strapped to the sides of the apparatus. (Courtesy of Neurocom International, Inc.)

(Fig. 64–15). The client stands in a tall box-like device that provides no visual cues for balance. The floor is moved while the client stands on it, and the response to correcting balance is recorded. Most people correct posture changes with adjustments in muscles (e.g., of the feet and ankles). The client is strapped in for safety in case he or she loses balance. This test can help isolate the etiologic basis of balance disorders as vestibular, visual, or proprioceptive.

ROTARY CHAIR ASSESSMENT
Rotary chair or harmonic acceleration can also be used. Rotation of the client in a chair in darkness provides information about vestibular dysfunction and the level of central compensation.

■ LABORATORY TESTS

Blood Tests

Blood tests that are diagnostic for systemic abnormalities are only secondarily significant for ear disease. For example, an elevated white blood cell (WBC) count suggests an infection but is not diagnostic of ear disease. In the presence of clinical signs of ear infection, and in the absence of other signs of infection, however, an elevated WBC count does suggest acute ear infection. Other blood tests are useful for diagnosis of autoimmune diseases and other systemic illnesses that can affect hearing and balance.

Cultures

Drainage samples from the ear canal are sometimes obtained for culture to identify an infecting organism. This is rarely necessary in choosing an antibiotic for acute infections. When long-term drainage is present, such as in chronic otitis media, cultures are more helpful because multiple pathogenic organisms can be present.

Tests for the Presence of Cerebrospinal Fluid

When clear drainage is found in the ear, a dilemma is presented. Is this cerebrospinal fluid (CSF) or serous drainage? A fistula from the inner ear to the middle ear can drain CSF. This pathway can also lead to meningitis by retrograde contamination. Therefore, an analysis of clear fluid drainage from the ear or nose is often helpful in the diagnosis.

Tissue Specimens

Biopsy specimens of abnormal tissue from the ear canal or from other tissue harvested during surgery are necessary to rule out a malignancy and to identify unusual problems. In an infected ear, abnormal tissue is readily identified with visual assessment. If the surgeon is in doubt about the findings, a tissue sample is taken for pathologic examination.

CONCLUSIONS

Understanding the complexity of ocular structures and the physiology of vision is essential to providing comprehensive nursing care for clients with ocular disorders. Ophthalmic Registered Nurses perform the roles of educator, technician, counselor, and coordinator in the diagnostic setting.

Hearing and balance are vital to a person's safety and independence. Understanding the physiology of hearing and balance is essential to providing comprehensive nursing care for clients with ear disorders.

BIBLIOGRAPHY

1. Eagle, R. (1999). *Eye pathology: An atlas and basic text.* Philadelphia: W. B. Saunders.
2. Goldblum, K. (Ed.). (1997). *Ophthalmic nursing core curriculum.* Dubuque, IA: Kendall.
3. Jarvis, C. (2000). *Physical examination and health assessment* (3rd ed.). Philadelphia: W. B. Saunders.
4. Kanski, J. (1999). *Clinical ophthalmology* (4th ed.). Oxford: Butterworth Heinemann.
5. Sigler, B., & Schuring, L. T. (1993). *Ear, nose and throat disorders.* St. Louis: Mosby–Year Book.
6. Silverman, C. A. (1998). Audiologic assessment and amplification. *Primary Care, 25* (3), 545–581.
7. Thompson, J. M., & Wilson, S. F. (1996). *Health assessment for nursing practice.* St. Louis: Mosby–Year Book.
8. Vaughan, D, Asbury, T., & Riordan-Eva, P. (1995). *General ophthalmology* (14th ed.). Norwalk, CT: Appleton & Lange.

CHAPTER 65

Management of Clients with Visual Disorders

Linda A. Vader

NURSING OUTCOMES CLASSIFICATION (NOC)
for Nursing Diagnoses—Clients with Visual Disorders

Anticipatory Grieving	Compliance Behavior	Knowledge Deficit: Regimen
Coping	Knowledge: Treatment Regimen	**Sensory/Perceptual Alterations (Visual)**
Grief Resolution	Participation: Health Care Regimen	Anxiety Control
Psychosocial Adjustment: Life Change	Treatment Behavior: Illness or Injury	Body Image
Ineffective Management of Therapeutic	**Knowledge Deficit**	Vision Compensation Behavior
Regimen	Knowledge Deficit: Treatment Procedure	

The role that vision plays in our lives is difficult to define because it is so deeply personal and intimate. It is the connection between the mind and the body and the rest of the world. The visual pathway is a multidimensional system with many structures and processes subject to trauma or disorders. When there is a failure of any part along the visual pathway, the result is loss of vision.

Loss of vision is closely associated with the loss of independence. Even simple tasks become difficult to perform without assistance. Seeing what food is being served at the table, selecting clothes for color and design, avoiding objects while walking, and reading books, magazines, or personal mail are no longer possible. The visually impaired person must adapt to this loss in order to maintain control in the daily affairs of life.

The nursing diagnosis *Sensory/Perceptual Alterations* is commonly identified for clients with visual problems or impairment. Nursing interventions focus on providing a safe environment and education for self-care. The most important assessment you can make, however, should address your client's grieving process. Visual impairment is more than a physiologic deficit. It is a loss that has physical, emotional, and spiritual effects on the person afflicted. Even minor changes in vision can provoke feelings of anger and frustration in people who must rely on clear and sharp vision in their work (e.g., airline pilots, artists, photographers, architects). Permanent and profound loss of vision can result in morbid grieving, in which an individual is unable to cope with or adapt to life changes.

Surveys have shown that most people are more afraid of going blind than dying of cancer. Although we have made some improvements in the way our society views and provides for people who are physically challenged, blind people are frequently regarded with pity. Loss of vision is a threat to a person's independence, self-esteem, and self-control.

GLAUCOMA

Glaucoma comprises a group of ocular disorders characterized by increased intraocular pressure, optic nerve atrophy, and visual field loss. It is estimated that more than 80,000 people in the United States are blind as a result of glaucoma. The incidence of glaucoma is about 1.5%, and in blacks between ages 45 and 65 years, the prevalence is at least five times that of whites in the same age group. In most cases, blindness can be prevented if treatment is begun early.

Classification

Many terms are used to describe the various types of glaucoma:

Primary and *secondary glaucoma* refer to whether the cause is the disease alone or another condition.

Acute and *chronic* refer to the onset and duration of the disorder.

Open (wide) and *closed* (narrow) describe the width of the angle between the cornea and the iris (Fig. 65–1A). Anatomically narrow anterior chamber angles predispose people to an acute onset of *angle-closure glaucoma.*

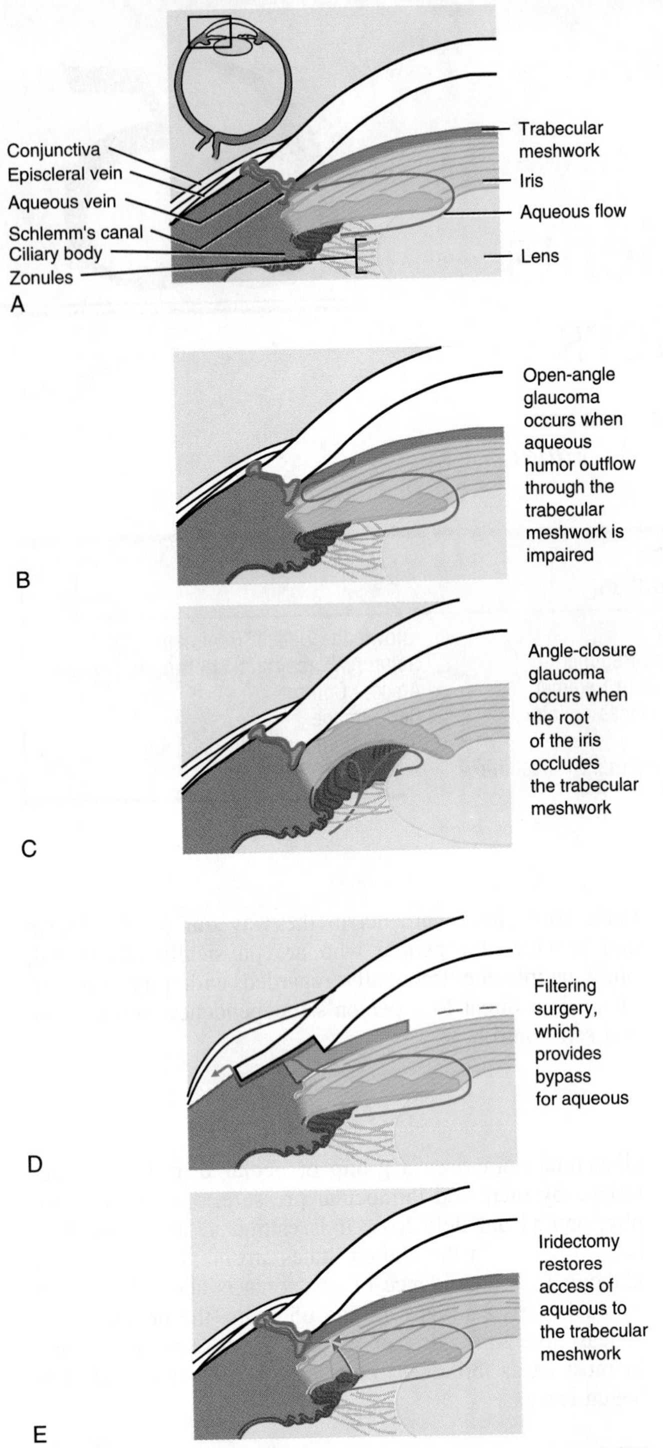

Conjunctiva
Episcleral vein
Aqueous vein
Schlemm's canal
Ciliary body
Zonules

A

Trabecular meshwork
Iris
Aqueous flow
Lens

B

Open-angle glaucoma occurs when aqueous humor outflow through the trabecular meshwork is impaired

C

Angle-closure glaucoma occurs when the root of the iris occludes the trabecular meshwork

D

Filtering surgery, which provides bypass for aqueous

E

Iridectomy restores access of aqueous to the trabecular meshwork

FIGURE 65–1 *A,* Normal flow of aqueous humor. *B,* Open-angle glaucoma occurs when aqueous humor outflow is impaired by the trabecular meshwork. *C,* Angle-closure glaucoma occurs when the root of the iris occludes the trabecular meshwork. Filtering surgery (*D*) and iridectomy (*E*) restore flow of aqueous humor through the trabecular meshwork.

PRIMARY OPEN-ANGLE GLAUCOMA

Primary open-angle glaucoma, the most common form, is a multifactorial disorder that is often genetically determined, bilateral, insidious in onset, and slow to progress. This type of glaucoma is often referred to as the "thief in

the night" because no early clinical manifestations are present to alert the client that vision is being lost. Aqueous humor flow is slowed or stopped because of obstruction by the trabecular meshwork (Fig. 65–1*B*).

ANGLE-CLOSURE GLAUCOMA

An acute attack of angle-closure glaucoma can develop only in an eye in which the anterior chamber angle is anatomically narrow. The attack occurs because of a sudden blockage of the anterior angle by the base of the iris (Fig. 65–1*C*).

OTHER FORMS OF GLAUCOMA

Low-tension glaucoma resembles primary open-angle glaucoma. The angle is normal, the optic nerves are cupped, and the visual fields show characteristic glaucomatous effects (peripheral vision deficits). These changes, however, develop in the presence of statistically normal intraocular pressures. Although the pressure readings are in the normal range, treatment is indicated to lower the pressure even further to avoid progressive optic nerve damage and visual field loss.

Secondary glaucoma is a result of increased intraocular pressure that has developed for other problems, such as postoperative edema. Edematous tissue may inhibit the outflow of aqueous humor through the trabecular meshwork. Delayed healing of corneal wound edges may result in epithelial cell growth into the anterior chamber.

Congenital glaucoma is rare, the result of developmental abnormalities in anterior chamber angle structures, the cornea, and the iris.

Etiology and Risk Factors

Approximately 90% of primary glaucoma occurs in people with open angles. Because there are no early warning clinical manifestations, it is imperative that regular ophthalmic examinations include tonometry and assessment of the optic nerve head (disc). The most common cause of chronic open-angle glaucoma is degenerative change in the trabecular meshwork, resulting in decreased outflow of aqueous humor. Hypertension, cardiovascular disease, diabetes, and obesity are associated with the development of glaucoma. Increased intraocular pressure also results from inflammation of filtering structures in uveitis. Encroachment by a rapidly growing tumor and chronic use of topical corticosteroids may also produce manifestations of open-angle glaucoma. The cause of *low-tension glaucoma* is not known.

Secondary glaucoma may occur as a result of trauma. Lens displacement, hemorrhage into the anterior chamber, lacerations, and contusions can disrupt the flow pattern of aqueous humor. Smoking, ingestion of caffeine or large amounts of fluids, alcohol, illicit drugs, corticosteroids, altered hormone levels, posture, and eye movements may cause varying transient increases in intraocular pressure.

Congenital glaucoma is caused by an arrest of development of the anterior chamber angle structures at about the 7th month of fetal life.

Pathophysiology

Intraocular pressure is determined by the rate of aqueous humor production in the ciliary body and the resistance to outflow of aqueous humor from the eye. Intraocular pressure varies with diurnal cycles (the highest pressure is usually on awakening) and body position (increased when lying down). Normal variations do not usually exceed 2 to 3 mm Hg. Intraocular pressure and blood pressure are independent of each other, but variations in systemic blood pressure may be associated with corresponding variations in intraocular pressure. Increased intraocular pressure may result from hyperproduction of aqueous humor or obstruction of outflow. As aqueous fluid builds up in the eye, the increased pressure inhibits blood supply to the optic nerve and the retina. These delicate tissues become ischemic and gradually lose function.

Clinical Manifestations

Clinical manifestations of glaucoma include increased intraocular pressure, cupping or indentation of the optic nerve head (disc), and visual field defects. As intraocular pressure increases, the head of the optic nerve is pressed inward. Visual field defects are the result of the loss of blood supply to areas in the retina. The individual response to intraocular pressure varies; some clients sustain damage from relatively low pressures, whereas others sustain no damage from high pressure. The degree of increased pressure that causes ocular damage is not the same in every eye, and some clients may tolerate a pressure for long periods that would rapidly blind another.

In clients with *acute angle-closure glaucoma*, the aqueous flow is obstructed and intraocular pressure becomes markedly elevated, causing severe pain and blurred vision or vision loss. Some clients see rainbow halos around lights, and some experience nausea and vomiting.

Depending on the primary factor, *secondary glaucoma* may be acute or chronic. The ocular manifestations, however, are the same as in angle-closure glaucoma.

An ophthalmoscopic examination shows atrophy (pale color) and cupping (indentation) of the optic nerve head. The visual field examination is used to determine the extent of peripheral vision loss (see visual fields earlier). In *chronic open-angle glaucoma*, a small crescent-shaped *scotoma* (blind spot) appears early in the disease. In *acute angle-closure glaucoma*, the fields demonstrate larger areas of significant loss of vision.

In clients with *angle-closure glaucoma*, a slit-lamp examination may demonstrate an erythematous conjunctiva and corneal cloudiness. The anterior chamber aqueous humor may also appear turbid (hazy), and the pupil may be nonreactive. Slit-lamp examination is used in *open-angle glaucoma* to look for secondary causes and associated findings. Intraocular pressure is measured at the slit lamp with the applanation tonometer. Increased intraocular pressure (>23 mm Hg) indicates the need for further evaluation. Gonioscopy is performed to determine the depth of the anterior chamber angle and to examine the entire circumference of the angle for any abnormal changes in the filtering meshwork.

Outcome Management

The goal of management is to facilitate the outflow of aqueous humor through remaining channels and to maintain intraocular pressure within a range that prevents further damage to the optic nerve. If intraocular pressure is very high, it must be reduced to retain vision. If vision is lost, the goals are to restore independence for the client.

■ Medical Management

REDUCE INTRAOCULAR PRESSURE (PROMOTE AQUEOUS FLOW)

Several medications are used to promote aqueous flow in *narrow-angle glaucoma:* (1) topical miotics, which act by constricting the pupil, (2) topical epinephrine, which increases outflow, (3) topical beta-blockers or alpha-adrenergics, which suppress the secretion of aqueous humor, and (4) oral carbonic anhydrase inhibitors, which also reduce the production of aqueous humor. Figure 65–2 shows the sites of action for various drugs.

Also shown in the figure are sites of action for drugs used to treat *open-angle glaucoma.* Mydriatic agents dilate the pupil by inhibiting the parasympathetic nervous system and blocking acetylcholine. Cycloplegic agents paralyze the ciliary muscle and the dilator muscle of the iris, causing both pupillary dilation and paralysis of accommodation. These dilating agents are contraindicated in narrow-angle glaucoma, because further dilation of the pupil restricts outflow of aqueous humor.

REDUCE INTRAOCULAR PRESSURE

In emergent situations in which intraocular pressure must be brought under control, an oral osmotic agent may be administered in the form of glycerin (Osmoglyn). The agent is supplied in a variety of strengths, and the percentage of the solution ordered is closely checked against what is supplied. The diuretic action of glycerin lowers intraocular pressure. Diabetic clients often receive a synthetic glycerin such as isosorbide (Ismotic) to reduce the effect on blood glucose levels. The average dose for an adult is 1.5 g/kg oral solution of 100 g/220 ml (45%), which may be repeated several times until the intraocular

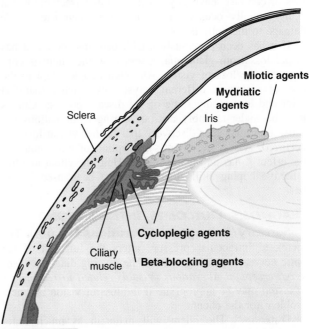

FIGURE 65–2 Sites of action of mydriatic, beta-blocking, cycloplegic, and miotic agents.

pressure is reduced to a tolerable level. If the glycerin is not already flavored, the extreme sweetness and viscosity may be made more palatable by mixing it with equal parts of a tart juice such as lemon. Serving the solution over cracked ice also makes it more palatable. After 3 hours, encourage the intake of water and other liquids to prevent mild to moderate dehydration and make sure the client can get to the bathroom during the diuretic phase.

Intravenous (IV) mannitol, a potent osmotic diuretic, may be used to arrest extremely high intraocular pressure. It should be used only for management of a glaucoma crisis under close nursing and medical supervision. Carefully evaluate the client's cardiovascular and renal status before treatment is begun. Document baseline vital signs before treatment and frequently during the infusion. Because mannitol tends to crystallize, the bottle may need to be warmed before it is administered. Do not use the vial while crystals are present. An in-line micropore filter should also be used to prevent infusion of any crystal particles.

▆ Nursing Management of the Medical Client

ASSESSMENT

Nursing assessment includes establishing demographic data of age and race because open-angle glaucoma occurs most often in clients over 40 years of age and in blacks. Determine whether there is a family history of glaucoma or other eye problems and whether the client has had ocular surgery, infections, or trauma. An accurate list of current medications is imperative because over-the-counter medications (such as antihistamines) may dilate the pupil, increasing the risk for angle-closure glaucoma. Always note a history of allergic reactions, particularly to medications or dyes.

Ask the client to describe any changes in vision. Although the manifestations of primary open-angle glaucoma are insidious, the client may describe blind spots in the periphery or an overall decreased visual acuity with loss of contrast sensitivity. Decreased uncorrectable visual acuity usually occurs when there has been irreversible damage to the optic nerve.

If it has been previously established that the client has visual loss from glaucoma, assess how the client is coping with the loss of vision. Although people adapt to the loss of vision in different ways, they usually manifest grief and loss at any stage of the disease process. Clients may be understandably anxious during examinations because they may fear discovery that further vision loss has occurred. Assess the client's perception of glaucoma and the effect it has on quality of life. Help the client identify effective coping skills that may have been used in the past.

DIAGNOSIS, OUTCOMES, INTERVENTIONS

Sensory/Perceptual Alterations (Visual). The increased intraocular pressure alters the function of the optic nerve, decreasing vision. The nursing diagnosis *Sensory/Perceptual Alterations (Visual) related to recent loss of vision* may be appropriate if the loss of vision is a new problem for the client.

Outcomes. The client will maintain as much functional vision as possible, report no further loss of vision, adapt to any visual loss, be able to perform activities of

daily living (ADL), and recognize clinical manifestations of complications.

Interventions. Reassure the client that although some vision has been lost and cannot be restored, further loss may be prevented by adhering to the treatment plan.

Anticipatory Grieving. Vision lost to glaucoma is irreparable. Even with the most aggressive medical and surgical management, vision loss may progress. A typical nursing diagnosis would therefore be *Anticipatory Grieving related to loss of vision.* Significant loss of vision represents the need for compromise and adaptation for both client and family.

Outcomes. The client will express grief, describe the meaning of the loss, and share the grief with significant others.

Interventions. Assess the causative and contributing factors that may delay the work of grieving and promote family cohesiveness. The social stigma of blindness underlies the anxiety that clients experience with actual or potential loss of vision. Total loss of vision isolates a person within a different reality. Although most clients are successfully rehabilitated, some losses are permanent. Also, some people, for a variety of reasons, remain socially isolated. The image of a blind person who is pitied and must accept the charity of others is disturbing.

Use therapeutic communication to express empathy as the client relates expected and actual losses that are due to loss of vision. People with actual or potential loss of vision may be faced with barriers in their vocations that force an unwanted change. Not all jobs and work environments are adaptable for a person who is visually impaired. Age may be a major factor in the person's ability to meet this challenge.

Self-esteem is closely related to the roles of people in their particular lifestyle. Loss of control in personal, family, and work situations can be devastating. The issue of dependence versus independence may also be a factor in the person's ability to cope with the stressors of vision loss.

Risk for Ineffective Management of Therapeutic Regimen (Individuals). The regimen for eye drops and oral medications to control glaucoma ranges from simple to complex. This diagnosis should be stated as *Risk for Ineffective Management of Therapeutic Regimen (Individuals) related to complex medication schedule.*

Outcomes. The client will describe the disease process and the regimen for disease control, and will relate how the medication routine will be incorporated into ADL.

Interventions. The client may need to instill as many as three or four different eye drops from one to six times a day. Constricting eye drops are usually prescribed four times a day, and beta-blockers are usually prescribed every 12 hours; however, the eye drops may be needed every 4 to 6 hours. The schedule is designed to provide the best possible control of intraocular pressure around the clock.

Medications are an integral part of the treatment and care of a client with glaucoma, and nursing interventions must thus be directed at the client's ability to understand and comply with prescribed therapy.

First, determine the client's current level of knowledge. Provide necessary information about glaucoma and its treatment in understandable terms. Diagrams may be helpful to the client and significant others. Because treatment for glaucoma is often complex, involving both oral and topical ophthalmic medications, review a written plan of care in large print with the client and family. To maximize compliance, ensure that the plan of care fits into the client's lifestyle.

The administration of eye drops is a critical component of self-care for the client with glaucoma. After instructing the client and family on the technique of instillation, validate the client's or family's ability to properly instill eye drops by asking for a demonstration. Be sure to include discussion of medications and their side effects. Table 65–1 lists additional guidelines for teaching the client about eye drops.

EVALUATION

Independent self-care is the area for evaluation in the medically managed client. Evaluate the client's ability for self-care (a short-term outcome) and compliance with the medical regimen (a long-term outcome).

Modifications for Elderly Clients

Older clients with arthritic or shaking hands have difficulty instilling their own eye drops. Instruct the client to lie down on a bed or sofa. Tilting the head back can lead to loss of balance. The eye drop regimen for glaucoma requires accurate timing. Older clients may need visual reminders, such as a check-off list, and may also need to use a timer or an alarm clock to help them remember.

TABLE 65–1	TEACHING THE CLIENT ABOUT EYE DROPS FOR GLAUCOMA
Medication	**Teaching Aspects**
Pilocarpine HCl	Usually given three to four times a day A miotic, causing pupillary constriction to open Schlemm's canal Space out administration, beginning on awakening and ending at bedtime. May cause blurred vision after instillation Brow ache has been reported Consider use of thin gel strips (a timed-release form) to improve compliance
Timolol maleate and other beta-blockers (e.g., levobunolol)	Usually given every 12 hours Decreases production of aqueous humor Space out administration Contraindicated in clients with asthma and chronic obstructive pulmonary disease Assess for bradycardia before administration
Carbonic anhydrase inhibitors (e.g., acetazolamide)	Inhibits production of aqueous humor Available as tablets and in sustained-release capsules Side effects include anorexia and tingling in the hands and feet

Surgical Management

When maximal medical therapy fails to halt the progression of visual field loss and optic nerve damage, surgical intervention is recommended. Many procedures are used to improve aqueous humor outflow; however, no operation has been uniformly successful.

LASER TRABECULOPLASTY. The use of the laser to create an opening in the trabecular meshwork is often indicated before filtering surgery is considered. The laser produces scars in the trabecular meshwork, causing tightening of meshwork fibers. The tightened fibers allow increased outflow of aqueous humor. Intraocular pressure is reduced through improved outflow in about 80% of cases. The effect of the laser treatment decreases with time, and the procedure may need to be repeated. Medical treatment is usually continued.

TRABECULECTOMY. Trabeculectomy is the creation of an opening through which the aqueous fluid escapes. A half-thickness scleral flap is loosely sutured over the created opening through which the fluid escapes, again resulting in subconjunctival absorption of aqueous humor (Fig. 65–1C).

FILTERING PROCEDURES. Operations such as trephination, thermal sclerostomy, and sclerectomy create an outflow channel from the anterior chamber into the subconjunctival space (Fig. 65–1D). Aqueous humor is absorbed through the conjunctival vessels. In about 25% of cases, the opening closes because of scar tissue formation and reoperation is necessary. Such filtering procedures are less successful in young and black clients, who tend to have an increased ability to produce thicker scar tissue. Topical corticosteroids are used postoperatively because their anti-inflammatory action inhibits proliferation of fibroblasts at the surgical site.

IRIDECTOMY. Iridectomy is the creation of a new route for the flow of aqueous humor to the trabecular meshwork. The laser is used to create the new opening in the iris (Fig. 65–1E).

OTHER TECHNIQUES. 5-Fluorouracil (5-FU), mitomycin, and other antimetabolites are sometimes injected subconjunctivally because they also inhibit fibroblast proliferation and thereby reduce postoperative scarring. Ocular implantation devices (e.g., Molteno implant, Baerveldt seton) are sometimes used to control the flow of aqueous humor in clients with complicated types of glaucoma. A device is sutured to the outer surface of the eyeball on the sclera between the ocular muscles. A tiny probe is inserted under the scleral flap directly into the anterior chamber that directs the flow of aqueous humor more posteriorly than in the more common filtering procedures.

CYCLODESTRUCTIVE PROCEDURES. When other surgical procedures have failed, cyclocryotherapy (application of a freezing tip) or cyclophotocoagulation may be used to damage the ciliary body and decrease production of aqueous humor.

Nursing Management of the Surgical Client

PREOPERATIVE CARE

Preoperative nursing care includes preparing the client for a surgical procedure that may be performed in either an outpatient or inpatient setting (see Chapter 15).

Laser therapy is most commonly performed in a clinic or office, including use of a topical anesthetic. Explain both the expected outcome of the procedure and the "popping" sounds and flashing lights that the client will experience. Explain that there will be a waiting period (usually 1 to 2 hours) after the procedure to evaluate a possible rise in intraocular pressure. Because of the instability of the intraocular pressure, the client should arrange for a friend or family member to accompany him or her and to provide transportation.

POSTOPERATIVE CARE

When the client returns from the operating room, the eye is covered with a patch and a metal or plastic shield for protection. Instruct the client not to lie on the operative side to avoid pressure on the surgical site. When the effects of perioperative sedation have diminished, the client may walk about and eat as desired.

Frequent monitoring of intraocular pressure is necessary because the surgical site is microscopic. Assess the client for unrelieved pain, nausea, and decreased vision. When healing is delayed, the anterior chamber may not re-form. Intraocular pressure readings may be 2 to 5 mm Hg, or the anterior chamber may even be flat. If the anterior chamber does not re-form, another surgical procedure may be required. The wound also may seal tightly, causing intraocular pressure to rise above normal levels; such a case also warrants reoperation.

■ Self-Care

The postoperative plan must include client education and evaluation of the home environment and available care. Because the level of independence varies with each client, use information supplied by the client and family or friends to assess how much support may be needed. Although many clients with glaucoma undergo repeated surgical procedures, carefully review the information each time. Client and family education includes the following steps:

1. Manifestations of infection (redness, swelling, drainage, blurred vision, pain).
2. Manifestations of increased intraocular pressure (unrelieved pain, nausea, decrease in vision).
3. The rationale for eye protection (shield or eyeglasses at all times) to protect from light and trauma.
4. Medications and eye drop instillation technique.
5. Scheduled return visit date and time.
6. Treatment of the surgical site:
   a. Carefully clean the area around the eye with warm tap water and a clean washcloth.
   b. Do not rub or apply pressure over the closed eye, which may damage healing tissue.

CATARACTS

A *cataract* is an opacity of the lens. Although cataract formation is usually associated with aging, there are several other causes. Some degree of cataract formation is to be expected in most people over 70 years of age. More than a million cataract operations are now being performed annually in the United States. A person with a normal life span is likely to undergo a cataract operation more than any other major surgical procedure.

The most common cataract is the *age-related* or *senile* type. Worldwide, cataract is the primary cause of reduced vision and blindness. Senile cataracts usually begin around the age of 50 years and consist of cortical, nuclear, or posterior subcapsular opacities, which may coexist in various combinations. In *cortical* cataracts, spoke-like opacifications are found in the periphery of the lens. They progress slowly, infrequently involve the visual axis, and often do not cause severe loss of vision. Nuclear sclerotic cataracts are a result of a progressive yellowing and hardening of the central lens (nucleus). Most people over age 70 years have some degree of nuclear sclerosis. Posterior subcapsular opacities occur centrally on the posterior lens capsule and cause visual loss early in their development because they lie directly on the visual axis.

Etiology and Risk Factors

The cumulative exposure to ultraviolet light over a person's life span is the single most important risk factor in cataract development. People who live at high altitudes or who work in bright sunlight, such as commercial fishermen, appear to experience cataract formation earlier in life. Glass blowers and welders without eye protection are also at higher risk.

Cataracts may develop as a result of many other systemic, ocular, and congenital disorders.

Systemic disorders include diabetes, tetany, myotonic dystrophy, neurodermatitis, galactosemia, Lowe's syndrome, Werner's syndrome, and Down syndrome.
Intraocular disorders include iridocyclitis, retinitis, retinal detachment, and onchocerciasis.
Infections (German measles, mumps, hepatitis, poliomyelitis, chickenpox, infectious mononucleosis) during the first trimester of pregnancy may cause *congenital* cataracts.

Blunt trauma, lacerations, foreign bodies, radiation, exposure to infrared light, and chronic use of corticosteroids may also result in cataracts.

Pathophysiology

Cataract formation is characterized chemically by a reduction in oxygen uptake and an initial increase in water content followed by dehydration of the lens. Sodium and calcium contents are increased; potassium, ascorbic acid, and protein contents are decreased. The protein in the lens undergoes numerous age-related changes, including yellowing from formation of fluorescent compounds and molecular changes. These changes, along with the photoabsorption of ultraviolet radiation throughout life, suggest that cataracts may be caused by a photochemical process.

Cataracts progress through the following clinical stages of development:

Immature cataracts are not completely opaque, and some light is transmitted through them, allowing useful vision.
Mature cataracts are completely opaque. The former term for this stage was *ripe*. Vision is significantly reduced.
Intumescent cataracts are those in which the lens absorbs water and increases in size. The lens may be mature or immature. The increase in size may result in glaucoma.

Hypermature cataracts are those in which the lens proteins break down into short-chain polypeptides that leak out through the lens capsule. The pieces of protein are engulfed by macrophages, which may obstruct the trabecular meshwork, causing phacolytic glaucoma.

Clinical Manifestations

Clients experience blurred vision, sometimes monocular diplopia (double vision), photophobia (light sensitivity), and glare because the opacity of the lens obstructs the reception of light and images by the retina. Clients usually see better in low light when the pupil is dilated, which allows for vision around a central opacity. There is no complaint of pain. A cloudy lens can be observed (Fig. 65–3).

A cataract should be suspected when the red reflex seen with the direct ophthalmoscope is distorted or absent. Although cataracts can usually be easily identified with the direct ophthalmoscope, an accurate determination of the type and extent of the lens change requires a slit-lamp examination.

Outcome Management

■ Surgical Management

There is no known treatment other than surgery that prevents or reduces cataract formation. The goal of cataract surgery is to remove the opacified lens. Since the 1980s, cataract surgery has improved dramatically as a result of the operating microscope, new instrumentation, improved suture material, smaller incisions, and refinement of the intraocular lens implant. The lens is surgically removed by an intracapsular or extracapsular procedure (Fig. 65–4).

Intracapsular cataract extraction (ICCE) consists of removing the lens, including the lens capsule. *Extracapsular* cataract extraction (ECCE) consists of removing the lens and the anterior portion of the lens capsule. The posterior lens capsule is left intact. Although ICCE is

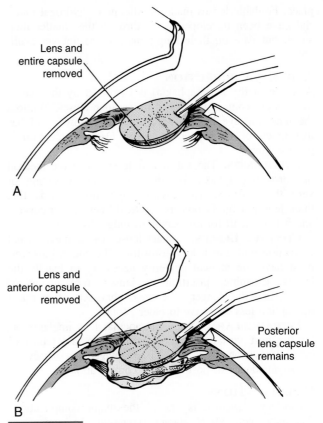

FIGURE 65–4 Surgical approaches to lens removal for cataracts. *A,* Intracapsular cataract extraction. *B,* Extracapsular cataract extraction.

highly successful and still performed, ECCE is by far the most common procedure in the United States. The primary reason for performing ECCE is to allow insertion of a posterior chamber intraocular lens inside the remaining capsule, which results in fewer postoperative complications.

Phacoemulsification is an extracapsular technique that uses ultrasound vibrations to break up the lens material. Pieces of the anterior lens capsule and the lens are removed by suction through the phacoemulsifier tip. With this "small incision" technique, a much smaller incision in the eye is necessary. Only one to three sutures are needed, and in some cases none at all is required. Wound healing in small-incision surgery occurs at the same rate as in larger-incision techniques.

Cataract surgery is often performed while the client is under IV conscious sedation. An IV injection of methohexital sodium (Brevital) or thiopental (Pentothal) induces a few minutes of light anesthesia while the retrobulbar injection of local anesthetic solution is given. Cataract surgery is also successfully performed with a topical anesthetic.

INTRAOCULAR LENS IMPLANTATION

After extraction of the cataract, a new lens is inserted in the posterior chamber, or the client is left without a lens. Although there are many styles of intraocular lenses, they all consist of two basic parts: (1) a clear spherical optic lens usually made of polymethyl methacrylate (Plexiglas) and (2) footplates or haptic lenses to hold the lens in

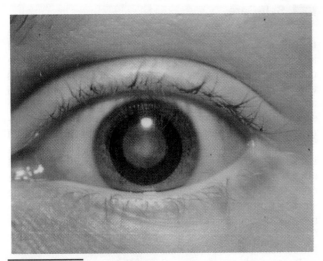

FIGURE 65–3 The cloudy appearance of a lens affected by cataract. (Courtesy of Ophthalmic Photography at the University of Michigan W. K. Kellogg Eye Center, Ann Arbor.)

place. Foldable lenses made of silicone or hydrogel material have been developed to fit through the smaller incisions, but data on their long-term use are not yet available.

APHAKIA CORRECTION

Absence of the lens (aphakia) is corrected by the use of eyeglasses, contact lenses, or intraocular lenses. Without the lens, the eye has no accommodative power and has lost much of its refractive power. Depth perception is greatly altered.

EYEGLASSES. The safest and least expensive method of correcting aphakia is with eyeglasses consisting of very thick lenses. The disadvantage, however, is that thick lenses magnify objects. Vertical lines appear curved, and it is difficult for the person to judge distances.

CONTACT LENSES. Contact lenses can achieve visual correction with much less distortion. The client, however, must have the manual dexterity necessary to handle the lenses. Cleaning, insertion of lenses, replacement of lenses, and the danger of corneal abrasions often make this option less attractive to older people.

INTRAOCULAR LENSES. Intraocular lens implants offer the best visual correction, with immediate return of binocular vision. The main disadvantage is a somewhat higher incidence of postoperative complications.

COMPLICATIONS

Secondary glaucoma is one of the major complications that may occur after cataract extraction. As a result of postoperative edema in the ocular tissues, a certain rise in intraocular pressure is anticipated and expected. This elevation most often resolves within 24 to 72 hours. If prolonged intraocular pressure persists, medical therapy may be necessary.

Postoperative infection, bleeding, macular edema, and wound leaks are also possible. The incidence of retinal detachment is higher in the first 12 months after cataract surgery.

Following ECCE, the posterior capsule may become opacified, which is called an *after-cataract* or *secondary membrane*. Subcapsular lens epithelial cells may regenerate lens fibers, which can obstruct vision. This postoperative complication occurs fairly frequently and used to require a second operation to remove the opacified tissue. The neodymium:yttrium-aluminum-garnet (Nd:YAG) laser is being used to create an opening in the capsule through pulses of laser energy that cause tiny "explosions" in the target tissue. Complications of this technique include a transient rise in intraocular pressure and possible damage to the intraocular lens.

■ Nursing Management of the Surgical Client

ASSESSMENT

During the history and physical examination, ask the client about any predisposing factors (trauma, systemic diseases, medications such as corticosteroids, and other ocular problems). Visual acuity (both distant and near) in each eye is documented. Ask the client to describe visual disturbances. The client's visual acuity may be relatively close to normal ranges, yet the client may experience difficulty in performing ADL. The client's individual perception of the quality of vision is an important factor in determining the need for surgery.

DIAGNOSIS, OUTCOMES, INTERVENTIONS

Sensory/Perceptual Alterations (Visual). Removal of the clouded lens reduces glare and cloudy vision. Improvement in visual acuity is related to the type of correction. Intraocular lens implantation provides the best visual correction. Contact lenses provide a good correction, and eyeglasses provide functional correction. None of these corrections provide the same visual acuity as the natural lens of the eye. Although vision may be greatly improved, there may still be varying degrees of change in depth perception. Write the nursing diagnosis as *Sensory/Perceptual Alterations (Visual) related to lens extraction and replacement.*

Outcomes. The client will gain improved vision and will adapt to changes in visual correction.

Interventions. Adaptation is the key issue in caring for the client having cataract surgery. Nursing interventions are based on assisting the client to gain or maintain as much independence as possible. Evaluate the client's lifestyle, abilities, and home environment. A 55-year-old client who is an architect and otherwise healthy may have an early cataract removed because it interferes with his work in areas where bright light is used. A 75-year-old diabetic client who is retired and mainly watches television has entirely different needs.

Unless there are other ocular complications or health factors, cataract surgery is performed on an outpatient basis. When clients are admitted to the hospital or surgical facility, determine their current level of knowledge and understanding of the perioperative events. Preoperative eye drops may include a dilating agent such as tropicamide (Mydriacyl) to facilitate the surgery. A cycloplegic cyclopentolate (Cyclogyl) may also be administered to paralyze the ciliary muscles.

EVALUATION

Adaptation to restored normal vision is usually rapid. Adaptation to limited vision requires more time based on individual variations.

■ Self-Care

After cataract surgery, clients are expected to return for a follow-up visit the next morning and again at 1 week and at 1 month. Postoperative care includes observation of the ocular dressing, if present, and assessment of the client's ability to perform ADL at the preoperative level. Nausea and vomiting are no longer an expected outcome of the surgical procedure but, if present, should be reported immediately. Prolonged vomiting may result in increased intraocular pressure and wound dehiscence. The eye patch is usually removed the next morning but may be removed after a few hours if the client has limited vision in the other eye. Instruct the client to wear a metal or plastic shield to protect the eye from accidental injury and not to rub the eye. Glasses may be worn during the day. The Client Education Guide provides instructions to be followed after cataract removal.

Restrictions on postoperative activity vary according to the practice of the ophthalmologist. Generally, the client

CLIENT EDUCATION GUIDE

Care After Cataract Removal

Leave the eye patch in place.

For 24 hours, limit your activity to sitting in a chair, resting in bed, and walking to the bathroom.

Do not rub your eye.

You can wear your glasses.

Do not lift more than 5 pounds (the weight of a gallon of milk).

Do not strain (or bear down).

Do not sleep on the side of your body that was operated on.

Take your eye drops.

Take acetaminophen (e.g., Tylenol) as needed for pain or itching.

DO NOT take aspirin or drugs containing aspirin.

Report any pain that is unrelieved, redness around the eye, nausea, or vomiting.

Wear eye shield to protect your eye.

should avoid heavy lifting (>5 pounds) or straining in the early postoperative period.

Eye care for the client after cataract surgery is the same as that for glaucoma clients (see Glaucoma). Postoperative eye medications may include antibiotics, corticosteroids, or both. Assess the client's or family's ability to instill eye drops appropriately. Review the rationale and schedule for the medications with the client and family. Postoperative discomfort should be minimal to moderate and is usually relieved by acetaminophen. Clients commonly experience an itching sensation after cataract surgery. Instruct the client to report any pain that is unrelieved. Review the clinical manifestations of infection and increased intraocular pressure with the client and family.

Depending on the client's age, ability, and availability of assistance, make a referral for home health care if indicated. Adjustment to changes in vision also varies with the individual client.

RETINAL DISORDERS

RETINAL DETACHMENT

Rhegmatogenous retinal detachment (secondary to a tear in the retina) is characterized by a retinal hole, liquid in the vitreous body with access to the hole, and subsequent fluid accumulation between the retina and the retinal pigment epithelium. The liquid seeps through the hole and separates the retina from its blood supply. Without intervention, the detachment continues to spread and the detached retina loses the ability to function. It may become increasingly detached over a period of hours to years.

Etiology and Risk Factors

Retinal detachment occurs mainly in the adult eye. The overall incidence is 1 in 15,000 people per year, but the risk of detachment increases after age 40 and most often occurs between the ages of 50 and 70.

Predisposing factors to retinal detachment include aging, cataract extraction, degeneration of the retina, trauma, severe myopia, previous retinal detachment in the other eye, and a family history of retinal detachment. Retinal holes and tears usually occur from spontaneous vitreous traction, but there may be abnormal adhesions between the retina and vitreous body secondary to diabetic retinopathy, injury, or other ocular disorders. Atrophy of the vitreous body may also result in a retinal tear.

Pathophysiology

If the retina is separated from its choroidal blood supply, it will die. The retinal tissues are at a high risk for avascular necrosis because they are delicate structures and have a high metabolic rate.

Clinical Manifestations

Characteristic clinical manifestations of retinal detachment are described by clients as a shadow or curtain falling across the field of vision. Shadows or black areas in the field of vision are the result of separation of visual receptors from the neural pathway (Fig. 65–5). No pain is associated with a detached retina. The onset is usually sudden and may be accompanied by a burst of black spots or floaters indicating that bleeding has occurred as a result of the detachment. The person may also see flashes of light caused by separation of the retina.

Examination with a direct and indirect ophthalmoscope reveals the portion of the retina involved and the extent of the detachment (Fig. 65–6). A scleral depressor also may be used externally on the lid or conjunctiva to assist in rotating the eyeball and to indent the retina for increased viewing ability. Areas of detachment appear bluish gray, as opposed to the normal red-pink color. Retinal tears are most often horseshoe-shaped but may be round.

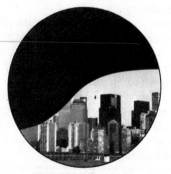

Detached Retina

FIGURE 65–5 Vision of a client with retinal detachment. (Courtesy of National Industries of the Blind, Wayne, NJ.)

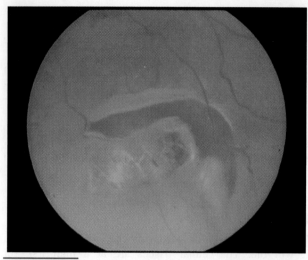

FIGURE 65–6 Bluish-gray appearance of areas of retinal detachment. (Courtesy of Ophthalmic Photography at the University of Michigan W. K. Kellogg Eye Center, Ann Arbor.)

■ Surgical Management

There is no known medical treatment for a detached retina. The goal of surgical repair of retinal detachment is to place the retina back in contact with the choroid and to seal the accompanying holes and breaks. Often *cryopexy* (use of a freezing probe) or laser photocoagulation is used to seal the hole if it has not progressed to detachment. Both methods create inflammation around the area, which scars and seals the hole. If not treated promptly, a retinal detachment may progress to involve the macula, which greatly compromises visual acuity. A retinal detachment requires urgent intervention.

The surgical procedure to place the retina back in contact with the choroid is called *scleral buckling* (Fig. 65–7). The sclera is actually depressed from the outside by rubber-like silicone (Silastic) sponges or bands that are sutured in place permanently. In addition to the buckling procedure, an intraocular injection of air or sulfahexafluoride (SF6) gas bubble, or both, may be used to apply pressure on the retina from the inside of the eye. This holds the retina in place by gravitational force during the healing phase. Postoperative positioning of the client maximizes the tamponade effect of the air or gas bubble. The bubble is slowly absorbed.

Postoperative swelling of tissues and cells in the anterior chamber caused by the inflammatory process or compromise of the venous drainage system may result in increased intraocular pressure. Because of the fragility of the tissues involved in the repair, re-detachment of the retina may occur at any time. At times, the retina has been separated from its blood supply long enough so that, even when reattached, it no longer has useful function and the client's vision does not improve significantly. Postoperative infection is also a risk.

The client should not expect immediate return of vision. Postoperative inflammation and the dilating drops interfere with vision. As healing takes place over weeks and months, vision may improve gradually.

■ Nursing Management of the Preoperative Client

ASSESSMENT

When the history has been obtained and the physical examination is being performed, assess the client's visual changes in both eyes. Visual field loss occurs in the opposite quadrant of the actual detachment. For example, a tear in the temporal region, which is affected more frequently, creates a visual defect in the nasal area. The pupil must be widely dilated for a retinal examination. Tell clients that they will experience an extremely bright light and will be asked to change their gaze frequently to facilitate the examination.

DIAGNOSIS, OUTCOMES, INTERVENTION

Sensory/Perceptual Alterations (Visual). The extent of loss of vision is related to the portion of the retina involved. Giant retinal tears involving the entire retina may result in temporary blindness, whereas peripheral tears may not interfere with central vision at all.

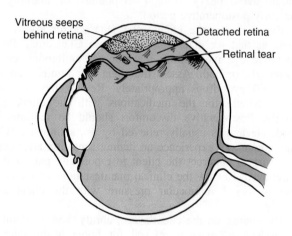

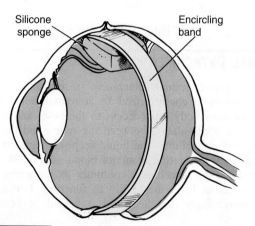

FIGURE 65–7 Scleral buckling to repair a detached retina. A silicone sponge implant is placed over the tear and held in place with an encircling band. When the buckle is tightened, the implant indents the sclera, holding the choroid and retina together.

Healing involves delicate neurologic tissue, and visual improvement may be gradual over several months. Write the nursing diagnosis as *Sensory/Perceptual Alterations (Visual) related to decreased retinal function.*

Outcomes. The client will maintain as much functional vision as possible, as evidenced by reporting no further loss of vision; adapting to any visual loss; and demonstrating an ability to perform ADL, to instill eye medications, and to recognize clinical manifestations of complications.

Interventions. The focus of the care plan is to help the client cope with the fears and reality of loss of vision and adapt to changes in vision. The client must be aware of the clinical manifestations of further loss of vision. See the Bridge to Home Health Care feature for suggestions on how to assist clients.

Knowledge Deficit. Assess the client's current level of knowledge and understanding of the implications of retinal detachment and the expectations for the surgical procedure The most common nursing diagnosis used before surgery is *Knowledge Deficit related to impending surgery, unknown outcomes, and expectations.*

Outcomes. The client will express understanding of the planned operation, expected outcomes for restoration of vision, and role in his or her own care after surgery.

Interventions. Provide preoperative teaching. Preoperative nursing care involves preparing the client for outpatient surgery or an overnight stay in the hospital. Because retinal detachment repair may take several hours, general anesthesia is used commonly. The pupil must be widely dilated before the operation, and the client may be given a sedative.

EVALUATION

Determine whether the client has adapted to imposed changes in vision. You may need to find help at home for independent living until sight returns or the client adapts to changes in vision.

■ Nursing Management of the Postoperative Client

Observe the eye patch for any drainage. Blood loss in retinal detachment surgery is minimal, and only serous drainage is expected on the postoperative dressing. Assess level of pain and presence of nausea.

Activity restrictions may be necessary if an air or gas bubble has been injected. The client needs to be positioned so that the bubble can apply maximal pressure on the retina by the force of gravity. This position, usually head down and to one side, is maintained for several days. Provide suggestions for comfort and support with the positioning (pillows under stomach, elbows, or ankles).

Posterior segment surgery, such as scleral buckling procedures, causes considerably more discomfort than anterior segment procedures do. Ocular muscles are separated, and the globe is manipulated to reach the posterior portions of the eyeball. Narcotics may be needed during the first 24 hours after surgery. Nausea and vomiting may also require management.

BRIDGE TO HOME HEALTH CARE

Coping with Failing Vision

Providing a safe home environment for the client with failing vision is essential. Promoting an autonomous lifestyle is desirable. Assessing the client's ability to remain safely at home is an important responsibility of home health care nurses.

Basic emergency procedures can be implemented by the use of nationwide services such as Lifeline. This service provides a portable electronic device usually worn around the client's neck or wrist. By simply pushing the button, immediate contact is made with emergency personnel. The toll-free phone number is 1-800-852-5433.

Local telephone companies can provide special adaptive equipment for 9-1-1 access. Telephones that can be programmed and have lighted or large numbers are available in most retail stores.

Home safety precautions can be simple. Burns can be prevented by color-coding water faucets. Use red for hot water and blue for cold water. Marking the "Off" dials on stoves and microwave ovens with colored tape or paint reduces the chance of injury.

Adequate lighting is essential. During the day, natural light is preferable. Open drapes or shades to provide ample light. Replace light bulbs with the highest wattage recommended.

Removal of hazards, such as throw rugs, clutter, and unnecessary furniture, can promote unrestricted ambulation. Handrails can be installed in hallways, in bathrooms, and on steps to prevent falls. Equipment such as canes, walkers, raised toilet seats, and bathtub rails promote safety. These items are available at medical supply stores.

Many commercial products are now marketed that can be of great assistance in the home. Pill organizers are clearly marked boxes with the day of the week and the times pills are to be taken. These can be filled by family members for a week at a time. Electronic lamp timers and voice-activated switches will allow the client to function more independently.

Access to a television and a radio is important. Large-print newspapers and reading materials help keep the client in touch with current events. The local library and the American Association for the Blind can provide assistance in obtaining needed items.

Creativity and planning can allow the client to remain at home in a safe environment for as long as possible.

Bernadette Mruz, RN, *Clinical Manager, Visiting Nurse Association of Omaha, Omaha, Nebraska*

IV acetazolamide (Diamox) may be used to reduce increased intraocular pressure. The intraocular pressure is monitored closely during the first 24 hours. Encourage the client to resume a regular diet and fluids as tolerated. The eye patch and shield are removed the next morning. Redness and swelling of the lids and conjunctiva should be expected from the surgical manipulation. After several days, the swelling and ecchymosis of the lids subside, but the conjunctiva may remain red or pink for a few weeks.

Postoperative eye medications generally include an antibiotic-steroid combination eye drop to prevent infection and reduce inflammation. Cycloplegic agents are prescribed to dilate the pupil and relax the ciliary muscles, which decreases discomfort and helps prevent the formation of iris adhesions to the corneal endothelium (synechiae). Either warm or cold compresses may be applied for comfort several times a day.

■ Self-Care

Because retinal detachment surgery is often performed on an urgent basis, the client rarely has an opportunity to plan for the surgery. Evaluate the home environment, and assist the client and family in preparing for any necessary support. Although the eye patch is usually removed early in the postoperative period, clients commonly have decreased functional vision in the eye.

Instruct the client to clean the eye with warm tap water using a clean washcloth. Warm compresses may be continued at home. Either an eye shield or glasses should be worn during the day, and the shield should be worn during naps and at night. Advise the client to avoid vigorous activities and heavy lifting during the immediate postoperative period. If an air or gas bubble has been injected, it may take several weeks to be totally absorbed. Clients are advised to avoid air travel during this time because the gas and air expand at high altitudes.

DIABETIC RETINOPATHY

Diabetic retinopathy is a progressive disorder of the retina characterized by microscopic damage to the retinal vessels, resulting in occlusion of the vessels. As a result of inadequate blood supply, sections of the retina deteriorate and vision is permanently lost.

Etiology and Risk Factors

Diabetic retinopathy is one of the leading causes of blindness worldwide. All diabetic people are at risk for retinopathy, although there appears to be a strong correlation between incidence and severity of retinopathy and duration of the disease and blood glucose control. Approximately 30% to 40% of the diabetic population has some degree of retinopathy. Clients who have had diabetes for 15 to 20 years have an 80% to 90% risk for development of retinopathy.

Pathophysiology

There are two types of diabetic retinopathy: (1) background *(nonproliferative)* and (2) *proliferative*. In background retinopathy, early pathologic changes demonstrate the hyperpermeability and weakening of the retinal vessels. The capillaries develop tiny dot-like outpouchings (microaneurysms), and the retinal veins become dilated and tortuous. Multiple hemorrhages occur from these defective vessels. Retinal edema is caused by leaking capillaries, and after the serous fluid is absorbed, a yellowish precipitate ("hard exudate") remains. Hemor-

rhages, exudates, and ischemia contribute to impaired vision, particularly if these occur on or around the macula. Progressive retinal ischemia stimulates the growth of new but ineffective blood vessels. These new and fragile blood vessels proliferate and grow into the vitreous body. These vessels leak, hemorrhage, and undergo fibrous changes that may form bands that pull on the retina, causing detachment. This process is called *proliferative retinopathy* (Fig. 65–8). With increasing ischemia, microinfarcts of the nerve fiber layer, called "cotton-wool spots," appear.

Clinical Manifestations

Clients experience a wide range of visual disturbances and fluctuations. Retinal vessel hemorrhage into the vitreous space obstructs vision with black spots or floaters or may result in complete loss of vision. Areas of retinal ischemia become blind spots. Macular edema causes decreased central vision.

Outcome Management

To reduce the occurrence of hemorrhage and retinal detachment in progressive retinopathy, the argon laser is used to photocoagulate the blood vessels. Hundreds and even thousands of microscopic photocoagulation applications (burns) are systematically placed around the peripheral retina, avoiding the central area that includes the macula and the optic disc. When a hemorrhage does not clear spontaneously over time, a vitrectomy (removal of a portion of the vitreous humor) may be performed. A vitrectomy may also be needed to release the traction of membranes on the retina.

Nursing interventions for the client with diabetic retinopathy are focused on assessment and management of diabetes. Elevations in blood glucose levels cause a temporary decrease in visual acuity. Because retinopathy is generally progressive, the client will need to cope with increasing visual deficits. Community referrals for rehabilitation and aids for low vision often provide useful assistance. Visiting nurses often prepare insulin injections for the upcoming week, because clients cannot see well enough to do this accurately.

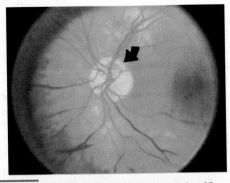

FIGURE 65–8 Proliferative diabetic retinopathy. Neovascularization covers one fourth to one third of the optic disc (*arrow*). (Standard photograph No. 10A of the Modified Airlee House Classification of Diabetic Retinopathy. Courtesy of the Early Treatment Diabetic Retinopathy Study Research Group.)

RETINITIS PIGMENTOSA

Retinitis pigmentosa is a genetic disorder that initially destroys the rods of the eye. Because the rods perceive black and white vision, the earliest manifestation is noticed during childhood as night blindness. Over the next several years, manifestations progress until a total loss of peripheral vision occurs. In time, central vision is also lost. No treatment is available to slow or stop this disorder. Genetic counseling is advised.

Retinal infections in clients with acquired immunodeficiency syndrome (AIDS) are discussed at the end of this chapter.

AGE-RELATED MACULAR DEGENERATION

Previously known as *senile macular degeneration,* age-related macular degeneration is an atrophic degenerative process that affects the macula and surrounding tissues, resulting in central visual deficits. Age-related macular degeneration is found to some degree in most adults over age 65 years. It is one of the most common causes of visual loss in older people. The exact cause is unknown, but the incidence increases with each decade in people over 50 years of age. It may be hereditary.

Age-related macular degeneration falls into two groups: (1) nonexudative *(dry)* and (2) exudative *(wet).* Both types are usually bilateral and progressive.

DRY MACULAR DEGENERATION
Nonexudative age-related macular degeneration is characterized by atrophy and degeneration of the outer retina and underlying structures. Yellowish round spots *(drusen)* may be seen on the retina and macula with an ophthalmoscope. Drusen are deposits of amorphous material from the pigment epithelial cells of the retina. Over time, these spots increase, enlarge, and may calcify.

WET MACULAR DEGENERATION
At the exudative stage of age-related macular degeneration, Bruch's membrane, which lies just beneath the pigment epithelial cell layer of the retina, becomes compromised. This results in serous fluid leaks from the choroid, with accompanying proliferation of choroidal blood vessels. A dome-shaped retinal pigment epithelium may be seen when examining the fundus. These leaks produce a visual effect called *metamorphopsia,* which is the blurred, wavy distortion of vision. The client may also notice a blurred scotoma or decreased central visual acuity (Fig. 65–9). Fundus photography and angiography may be performed on a regular basis to document and evaluate changes.

Outcome Management

There is no known means of medical treatment or prevention of age-related macular degeneration. Further damage from exudative macular degeneration sometimes may be arrested by the use of argon photocoagulation, even though laser damage to the retina in this area results in a blind spot. When the fovea is involved, central vision is lost and the only helpful measures are low-vision aids.

The client with age-related macular degeneration is threatened with the loss of central vision (see Bridge to Home Health Care). To evaluate changes in vision, teach

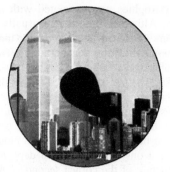

Macular Degeneration

FIGURE 65–9 Vision of a client with macular degeneration. (Courtesy of National Industries for the Blind, Wayne, NJ.)

the client to use the Amsler chart at home. You may assist the client to maximize remaining vision with low-vision aids and community referral to a low-vision specialist and low-vision support groups.

RETINAL ARTERY OCCLUSION

Occlusion of the retinal artery or vein can cause loss of vision. The most common causes of occlusion are emboli from atherosclerosis, valvular heart disease, and increases in blood viscosity. The retinal artery can also be occluded from embolized plaque in the carotid artery or from spasm. Retinal artery occlusion causes a sudden, unilateral, painless loss of vision. The severity of the visual loss ranges from total loss, when the central artery is occluded, to a loss of a visual field, when a branch of the artery is blocked. Retinal vein occlusion is due to systemic vascular disorders, venous stasis, hypertension, or increased blood viscosity.

Outcome Management

Retinal artery occlusion is an emergency. Management includes intermittent massage of the eyeball by a physician to move an embolus from the central artery into a branch and increased oxygenation (95% oxygen for 10 minutes). Surgery can include anterior chamber paracentesis to reduce intraocular pressure and to move the embolus. Anticoagulants are used in the early phases of occlusion.

CORNEAL DISORDERS

CORNEAL DYSTROPHIES

Corneal dystrophies comprise a group of hereditary and acquired disorders of unknown cause, characterized by deposits in the layers of the cornea and alteration of the corneal structure. Specific corneal dystrophies characteristically appear at different ages. They may be stationary or slowly progressive throughout life. The most common form, Fuchs' dystrophy, usually begins in a person's 20s or 30s, affects more women than men, and is slowly progressive.

Corneal dystrophies are associated with all five layers of the cornea. Although the disease usually originates in the inner layers (Descemet's membrane, the stroma, and Bowman's membrane), the degeneration, erosion, and deposits affect all layers.

Fuchs' dystrophy is characterized by deposits in Descemet's membrane that look like warts. Descemet's membrane becomes thickened, and defects appear in the endothelial layer. Because the integrity of the cornea is compromised, it becomes edematous and cloudy. Vision is compromised not only by the corneal deposits but also by the altered structure of the cornea secondary to the edema.

The cornea is evaluated by slit-lamp examination. Fluorescein staining is used to enhance visualization of surface corneal defects. Corneal scrapings may be taken with a sterile spatula for further staining and microscopic evaluation. Specular micrography (see Diagnostic Tests in Chapter 64) may be used to evaluate the corneal endothelium.

■ Surgical Management

CORNEAL TRANSPLANTATION

The goal of corneal transplantation *(keratoplasty)* is to improve the clarity of vision. This operation may be indicated for serious corneal conditions, including corneal dystrophy. *Penetrating* keratoplasty denotes full-thickness corneal replacement; *lamellar* keratoplasty denotes a partial-thickness procedure.

Because there is a direct relationship between age and health of the endothelial layer of the cornea, young donor tissue is preferred. Donor eyes are obtained from cadavers, must be enucleated soon after death because of rapid endothelial cell death, and must be stored in a preserving solution. Storage, handling, and coordination of donor tissue with surgeons are provide by a network of state eye bank associations around the country.

Corneal transplantation surgery is usually performed with the client under local anesthesia (Fig. 65–10). The surgeon prepares a donor cornea first by using a trephine

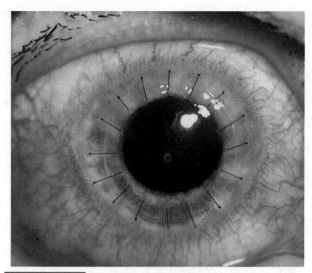

FIGURE 65–11 Clinical appearance of the eye after keratoplasty. (Courtesy of Ophthalmic Photography at the University of Michigan W. K. Kellogg Eye Center, Ann Arbor.)

to cut a corneal button with a radius of usually 7.0 to 8.5 mm. The recipient cornea is prepared in the same manner; however, it is usually cut 0.5 mm smaller so that there is an overlap by the donor cornea, which is then sutured into place. Figure 65–11 shows the eye after keratoplasty.

Graft rejection or failure may occur at any time after transplantation. It can result from unsuitable storage of donor tissue, dystrophy of the donor's endothelium, surgical trauma, or immunologic rejection. Wound leakage, bleeding into the anterior chamber, glaucoma, cataract, and infection are other complications that may occur. At the first sign of graft rejection, when the cornea becomes cloudy and edematous and when there is an anterior chamber reaction (presence of white blood cells or protein) (Fig. 65–12), topical steroids are prescribed in fre-

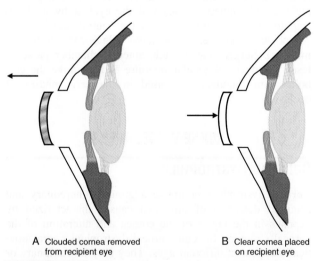

A Clouded cornea removed from recipient eye   B Clear cornea placed on recipient eye

FIGURE 65–10 Steps for corneal transplantation (penetrating keratoplasty). *A,* The diseased cornea is removed with a trephine. *B,* The donor cornea is placed on the eye and stitched in place with extremely fine suture material.

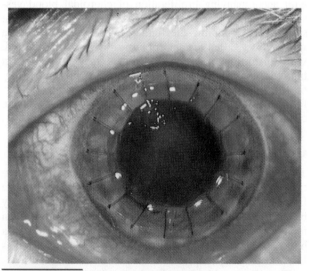

FIGURE 65–12 Acute graft rejection. (Courtesy of Ophthalmic Photography at the University of Michigan W. K. Kellogg Eye Center, Ann Arbor.)

quent doses to control the inflammatory response and to reverse the rejection reaction. In severe cases, a second transplantation may be necessary.

Nursing Management of the Postoperative Client

Corneal transplant surgery is usually performed as outpatient surgery. Postoperatively, the client returns from the operating room with an eye patch and protective shield in place. Observe the patch for signs of drainage. There is no blood loss associated with this procedure. The client should experience only mild to moderate discomfort, which should be relieved by acetaminophen. Unrelieved pain may indicate a rise in intraocular pressure and should be reported to the surgeon. Because the eye patch is to be in place until the following morning, assess the client's ability for self-care and advise the client and family about the hazards of monocular vision (see postoperative care for retinal detachment).

The eye is examined the next morning with the slit lamp. Depending on the extent of preoperative visual limitations, most clients experience improved vision immediately. Instruct clients, however, not to raise their expectations for full vision too high. Vision continues to improve gradually because the healing process may take up to a year or more. Glasses or contact lenses are usually needed to obtain the best result. Many months may be required for restoration of vision, and revisions in the care plan may be needed.

Self-Care

Postoperative eye drops usually include an antibiotic and a corticosteroid. Topical corticosteroid therapy may be needed indefinitely. Discharge instructions include the rationale for the medications and proper instillation technique. It is important for the client to wear eye protection in the form of regular glasses, sunglasses, or a protective shield to prevent injury to the eye. Advise the client never to rub the eye. The area around the eye may be cleaned with warm tap water using a clean washcloth.

Teach the client and family to recognize the clinical manifestations of graft rejection. A mnemonic tool may be useful in teaching the client to remember the signs of graft rejection (RSVP):

R, redness
S, swelling
V, decreased vision
P, pain

Teach the client and family to recognize the signs of increased intraocular pressure and infection.

Advise the client to evaluate vision in the eye each day. A picture on the wall or some object in a well-lighted room should be selected as a point of reference. If a change in vision from the day before is noted, the client should reevaluate his or her vision in a few hours. If no improvement is noted or if vision is worse, the client should notify the physician. Because graft rejection may occur at any time (even years) after the surgery, advise the client to make the vision check a routine part of ADL for the rest of his or her life.

CORNEAL INFECTION: KERATITIS

The corneal epithelium is normally an effective barrier against microorganisms. Once it is compromised from disease or trauma, the underlying stromal layer becomes an excellent culture medium for a variety of organisms. Dry eyes or ineffective eyelid closure predisposes the eye to keratitis. Clients who have a systemic collagen disorder, such as rheumatoid arthritis, are particularly susceptible to corneal infections and ulceration.

The client's eyes tear more than usual because the cornea produces tears to reduce the irritation. Sensitivity to light is due to the irritated nerve endings in the cornea, and blurred vision results from the inability of the cornea to provide the proper refractive surface. Clients with a corneal defect from an infection experience a great deal of discomfort, which is worsened by eyelid movement. The eye appears infected and indurated. Fluorescein staining of the cornea outlines the affected area, which can be viewed through the slit lamp or with a hand-held flashlight.

Corneal infections may develop into ulcerations that severely compromise the integrity of the eye (Fig. 65–13). Sources of infection include bacteria (e.g., *Staphylococcus aureus, Pseudomonas aeruginosa, Streptococcus pneumoniae*), fungi *(Candida, Aspergillus)*, viruses (adenovirus, herpes simplex, herpes zoster), and protozoa *(Acanthamoeba)*. Clinical findings under slit-lamp examination are specific to particular organisms. Hypopyon (a layer of white cells in the anterior chamber) may accompany corneal ulceration.

Outcome Management

The goal of treatment is to eradicate the infection, prevent further injury to the cornea, and promote comfort and healing.

Medical Management

Topical antibiotic, antifungal, and antiviral therapy is prescribed, with the frequency of instillation based on the

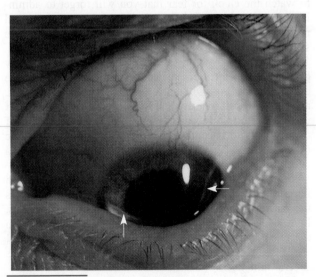

FIGURE 65–13 A corneal ulcer (*arrows*). (Courtesy of Ophthalmic Photography at the University of Michigan W. K. Kellogg Eye Center, Ann Arbor.)

severity of the infection to prevent progression to perforation and to promote healing. Maximal therapy includes the alternating instillation of two broad-spectrum eye drops every 15 minutes around the clock. As the infection begins to respond to the medication, frequency of administration is gradually decreased. Systemic IV medication may be prescribed as well.

To aid the healing process, surgical intervention may be necessary. *Tarsorrhaphy* (suturing the eyelid closed) promotes healing by decreasing eyelid blinking and by decreasing evaporation of the corneal tear film. For corneal perforation, a conjunctival flap may be performed to cover the defect. Tissue adhesive, a kind of "superglue," may also be used to seal the perforation. A soft contact lens may be used as a bandage to maintain the seal. Large perforations may require either lamellar (partial-thickness) or penetrating (full-thickness) keratoplasty.

When medical and surgical interventions fail, *enucleation* (removal of the entire eyeball) may be necessary (see nursing care of ocular melanoma). In some cases, *evisceration* (removal of orbital contents only) may be indicated. The scleral shell is left intact along with the ocular muscles, which allows for improved ocular prosthetic fit and function.

■ Nursing Management

Although the early stages of corneal infection are often managed at home, the client may need to be hospitalized for the management of a severe corneal ulcer. If the client and family have been instilling frequent eye drops at home, the client may be fatigued from lack of sleep as well as anxious about possible loss of vision. Assess the client's level of discomfort and methods of coping with the stress of pain and lack of sleep. Often at this stage, the client is not coping well at all. When eye drops are given every 15 minutes around the clock, the schedule is a challenge not only for the client but for you as well. Hand-washing is particularly important in this situation and is carried out even if gloves are worn to instill the drops. The threat of losing eyesight compels many clients to watch the clock for fear that you will forget to administer the eye drops. You can build the client's trust and reduce anxiety by scrupulous adherence to the time schedule.

The client's eye may need to be cleaned frequently because the medications and excessive tears will become dried and the lids will stick together. Warm tap water, applied with soft gauze pads, is used. The combination of tearing, medications, and cleaning may cause the skin of older clients to become excoriated. Antibiotic ophthalmic ointment may be applied to the lower lid margin and cheek to reduce irritation.

Effective sleep and rest are nearly impossible, with interruptions every 15 minutes. The client rarely reaches the deeper stages of sleep, and most experience restless, light sleep in stages 1 and 2. In addition to the eye pain the client may already be experiencing, some eye drops, such as fortified bacitracin, may cause stinging that lasts several minutes.

You can institute several measures to comfort the client. Outline a daily routine of care, based as much as possible on the client's normal routine at home. Because there are many interruptions to the client's personal time and space, identify at least two periods of time during the day when the client may rest or nap, with the only interruption being the nurse who comes in to administer the eye drops. Post a sign on the door to the client's room for privacy during these rest times. You and the client may also agree that you will not open topics of conversation during this time but will quietly instill the eye drops. Adopt this same routine during the client's normal nighttime. Some clients are actually able to sleep during instillation of eye drops at night; however, establish this routine with the client in advance. Older clients, who are accustomed to more stage 2 sleep than younger clients, are able to rest more effectively. Because younger clients tend to become confused and irritable more often, speak to the client before touching him or her. Oral analgesics are given at regular intervals, and mild sleeping medications may be helpful at bedtime.

Clients usually become adapted to this regimen of interruptions after the first 48 hours. As the cornea begins to show improvement, the eye drops may be reduced in frequency to every 30 minutes and then to every hour. Most clients do not notice a great deal of difference in the every-30-minute routine, but when the routine is reduced to every hour, they begin to sleep more heavily as the body attempts to compensate for lost sleep. At the end of an hour, the client may complain to you that it has seemed like only a few minutes since the last interruption. Intense dreaming may also be experienced during this time.

■ Self-Care

At discharge from the facility, the client should be able to demonstrate how to properly instill eye drops. The client will also understand the importance of complying with the medication regimen. Instruct the client and family about the clinical manifestations of increasing infections. The eye may continue to be cleaned with warm tap water at home. Assess the home environment if the client's vision is greatly reduced. Referrals for rehabilitation also may be necessary.

UVEAL TRACT DISORDERS: UVEITIS

Uveitis is an inflammation of the uveal tract that can affect one or more parts (iris, ciliary body, choroid). Uveitis commonly occurs in its acute form from a hypersensitivity reaction or in its chronic form following microbial infection. Clients complain of pain, blurred vision, and photophobia. There is marked redness of the eye, and the pupil is usually constricted. Cells (white blood cells) and flare (protein), called an "anterior chamber reaction," are seen in the anterior chamber fluid with the slit lamp.

The primary cause of discomfort in clients with uveitis is ciliary body muscle spasm. A cycloplegic medication such as atropine effectively relieves the spasm, and the dilation of the pupil prevents the inflamed iris from adhering to the lens and the corneal endothelium from forming synechiae. Topical steroid drops are prescribed to reduce the inflammation.

MALIGNANT OCULAR TUMORS

OCULAR MELANOMA

Although fewer than 1% of the people in the United States are affected by malignant ocular tumors, treatment of these tumors can be a challenge for both client and nurse. Choroidal melanomas are often detected during a routine ocular examination because there is no pain associated with the development of the tumor. By the time the tumor has grown large enough to obstruct vision, there may be involvement of the macula and metastasis.

Outcome Management

The goal of treatment is to care for the malignancy while preserving the eye.

■ Medical Management

When ocular melanoma is discovered early, radiation therapy alone may be the treatment of choice. Radiation therapy to the eye is accomplished through insertion of a tiny plate or plaque about the size of a dime that holds tiny seeds of radioactive iodine 125. The plaque is sutured to the sclera directly over the site of the tumor. It is left in place for several days, depending on the required dose, and then removed. Both insertion and removal are performed in the operating room.

During treatment, a lead shield is placed over the eye. Radiation exposure to the nurse who cares for the client is minimal—a small fraction of a chest x-ray study. Despite this extremely low exposure, the routine restrictions for hospital personnel and visitors are implemented for the sake of consistency. Hospitalization for treatment with radioactive iodine is required, depending on regulations.

During the client's hospitalization for this treatment, provide support and encouragement for the client. The plaque is only mildly to moderately uncomfortable, and discomfort should be relieved with acetaminophen. The difficult challenge for clients is confinement to their room with limitations on visitors at a time when support is essential. Eye medications include a cycloplegic agent and an antibiotic-steroid eye drop.

■ Surgical Management

ENUCLEATION

The goal of surgical removal is to preserve life by removing the tumor. Removal of the entire eyeball (enucleation) has been the traditional method of treatment and may be combined with radiation treatments. Exenteration (removal of the eyeball and surrounding tissues and bone) may also be necessary. The goal for clients following enucleation is adaptation to monocular vision and return to their former level of independence.

Enucleation surgery is usually performed with the client under general anesthesia, but IV conscious sedation may also be used. The ocular muscles are dissected from the eyeball, which is removed by severing the optic nerve and vessels at the back. An acrylic sphere covered by donor scleral tissue is usually placed within the capsule of tissue that formerly held the eyeball. Scleral tissue encourages fibrovascular ingrowth, which prevents migra-

tion and extrusion of the implant. A soft plastic scleral shell is placed in the visible outer portion of the socket as a support until a permanent prosthesis can be made. A newer type of implant, hydroxyapatite, which is made of the same inorganic material present in human bone, is now being used.

Several weeks later, a central hole is drilled into the sphere and covering tissues. A peg (which later fits into a depression on the posterior surface of the artificial eye) is then inserted into the hole. The movement of the implant by the muscle cone is transferred directly to the prosthesis. With the artificial eye being primarily supported by the peg instead of the lids and socket tissues, there are fewer cosmetic and structural complications.

■ Nursing Management

The client undergoing enucleation for a malignant tumor is stressed not only by the threat of cancer but also by disfigurement of the face. Assess the client's response, home, and family for support mechanisms. Nursing interventions are focused on assisting the client to grieve for the lost body part and lost vision and to identify coping mechanisms that will facilitate rehabilitation.

PREOPERATIVE CARE

Assist the client in preparing for the surgical procedure. Most often, the client is made aware of the tumor at a routine office visit. Surgery is usually scheduled within a few days. Recognizing that the client is most appropriately in a state of shock and denial, carefully explain the perioperative events. Although it is possible to have an enucleation as an outpatient procedure, the client may stay overnight in the hospital.

POSTOPERATIVE CARE

Provide routine postoperative care. The client returns from the operating room with a pressure dressing over the eye. Assess the dressing for bleeding using standard postoperative routines. Clients are understandably anxious about the removal of the dressing the next morning. Prepare the client by explaining how the eye and conformer will appear. The socket and lids will be swollen, and the white plastic conformer is visible. Determine the client's or family's ability to care for the wound postoperatively.

Some clients fear that their appearance will frighten others, especially children. In this case, an eye patch may be worn during the 4 to 6 weeks before the prosthesis is fitted but should not be worn continuously. Eventually, the eye prosthesis can be worn and looks pleasingly normal (Fig. 65–14). Refer to a fundamentals of nursing textbook for insertion and removal of the prosthesis.

The area around the lids may be cleaned with warm tap water with a clean washcloth. Soap and water should be kept away from the socket. If the plastic conformer accidentally comes out, it should be washed and replaced. Antibiotic ophthalmic ointment is usually ordered to be instilled in the socket once or twice a day.

■ Self-Care

Adjustment to monocular vision is a challenge the client begins to face immediately. Depth perception is altered, and the client needs to exercise caution in walking,

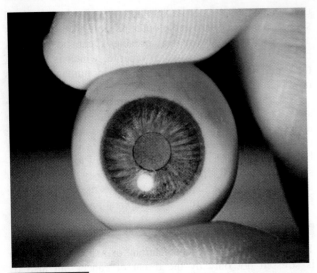

FIGURE 65-14 An ocular prosthesis. (Courtesy of Ophthalmic Photography at the University of Michigan W. K. Kellogg Eye Center, Ann Arbor.)

crossing streets, and driving. Advise the client to practice ADLs until visual and body adjustments are made.

Emphasize the need for extra precaution with the remaining eye. Eye protection should be worn when engaging in any activity that might even remotely result in an injury. Many clients are advised to wear glasses even if no correction is needed.

RETINOBLASTOMA

Retinoblastoma is a highly malignant intraocular tumor. The tumor occurs in two forms: sporadic (60%) and inherited (40%). The neoplasm arises from mutations in the primitive neuroectodermal tissue of the retina. It is a relatively rare form of cancer, occurring most often in children.

Clinical manifestations are difficult to detect early because they are not obvious. In children, parents usually notice a whitish appearance of the pupil (*cat's eye reflex*) and strabismus. Decreased vision, *proptosis* (protruding eye), and pain are late signs. Retinoblastomas grow rapidly along the optic nerve and invade the brain.

Treatment of mild or moderate forms of retinoblastoma includes radiation, photocoagulation, and cryotherapy to save vision. Eyes with extensive retinal destruction or glaucoma are enucleated (see later). Adults who have survived retinoblastoma are at increased risk for other malignancies, especially osteogenic sarcoma.

EYELID TUMORS

Basal cell and squamous cell carcinomas of the lids are the most common malignant tumors of the eyelids. These tumors appear more frequently in people with fair complexions who have had chronic exposure to the sun. Malignant lid tumors are most often (90% to 95%) of the basal cell type and frequently appear on the lower lid as nodules that gradually enlarge, becoming scaly and ulcerated. Benign tumors of the lids are very common and

often increase in frequency as people age. Melanocytic nevi (moles) and verrucae (warts) commonly appear on the lids and lid margins. Xanthelasma appears as yellow, wrinkled patches, which are actually lipid deposits under the skin of the eyelids. These benign lesions may be removed for cosmetic reasons.

Malignant tumors may be removed and treated by various methods, such as electrodesiccation, cryotherapy, and surgery. When the tumor is large, reconstruction may be required.

EYELID, LACRIMAL, AND CONJUNCTIVAL DISORDERS

DRY EYE SYNDROME

Dry eye syndrome is a condition in which tear production is inadequate. It most commonly occurs in women between 50 and 60 years of age. Three primary causes are lacrimal gland malfunction, mucin deficiency, and mechanical abnormalities that prevent the spread of tears across the surface of the eye. The lacrimal gland can be genetically malformed or malformed because of injury or infection. Tear production is also decreased in Sjögren's syndrome, an autoimmune disorder that commonly accompanies rheumatoid arthritis. Facial nerve (seventh cranial nerve) palsy disrupts tear production. Conjunctivitis and mumps can obstruct the gland. Some medications, such as antihistamines, atropine, and beta-adrenergic blocking agents, decrease tear production.

Mucin, a substance produced by the goblet cells in the eyelid, maintains an even layer of tears across the surface of the eye. The absence of mucin allows the tear film to break up, leaving "dry spots" on the cornea. Mucin deficiency is seen in clients with vitamin A deficiency and those taking medications such as antihistamines and beta-adrenergic blocking agents.

Mechanical abnormalities include problems with eyelid structure, eyeball extrusion, and misuse of contact lenses.

Manifestations include burning, itching eyes and a sensation of "something" in the eye. The term *keratoconjunctivitis sicca* is used to describe the problem.

Management includes determining the degree of injury to the cornea. Artificial tears (eye drops and lubricants) can be used. In addition, some clients benefit from using airtight goggles at night to prevent tear evaporation. Postmenopausal women have found some relief from estrogen replacement. Surgery can be used to open the lacrimal duct or to repair lid problems.

Other eyelid, lacrimal, and conjunctival disorders are discussed in Table 65-2.

REFRACTIVE DISORDERS

Light is bent (refracted) as it passes through the cornea and lens of the eye. Refractive errors exist when light rays are not focused appropriately on the retina of the eye.

Three basic abnormalities of refraction occur in the eye: (1) myopia, (2) hyperopia, and (3) astigmatism. Optical correction is important to distinguish between visual loss caused by disease and visual loss caused by refractive error. *Refractometry* is the measurement of refractive error and should not be confused with *refraction*, the

TABLE 65–2	EYELID, LACRIMAL, AND CONJUNCTIVAL DISORDERS		
Disorder	**Definition**	**Appearance**	**Management**
Dacryocystitis	Inflammation of lacrimal gland		Antibiotics, daily massage of the lacrimal system
Hordeolum (stye)	Infection of glands of eyelids	Redness and swelling of a localized area of the eyelid	Warm compresses and antibiotics; may need to be incised and drained
Chalazion	Chronic granuloma of meibomian gland	Painless, localized swelling of the lid margin	If cosmetically distracting, may be surgically removed
Blepharitis	Chronic, bilateral inflammation of eyelids	Itching and burning of the eyes, eyes appear red, scales noted on the lashes	Wash eyelids with baby shampoo, water, and cotton-tipped applicators; antibiotic ointments may be prescribed
Conjunctivitis	Inflammation of conjunctiva from various microorganisms	Redness, tearing, and exudation of eyelid; may progress to eyelid drooping, abnormal tissue growth	Antibiotic eye drops
Entropion	Turning in eyelid margin	Inversion of lower eyelid; dry and irritated eyes	Surgical resection
Ptosis	Drooping of eyelid from several causes	Irritation of eye caused by drying, loss of tears	Artificial tears; surgical correction needed; sometimes glasses used to life redundant skin
Lagophthalmos	Inadequate closure of eyelids	Irritation of eye caused by drying	Artificial tears, eye shields at night; surgical correction
Absence of blinking	Lack of blinking seen with Parkinson's disease and hyperthyroidism	Blinking less than 20 times a minute	Artificial tears; eye shields at night

method used to determine which lens or lenses (if any) will most benefit the client.

MYOPIA

Myopia, or *nearsightedness,* is a condition in which the light rays come into focus in front of the retina (Fig. 65–15A). In this case, the refractive power of the eye is too strong and a concave, or minus, lens is used to focus light rays on the eye. In most cases, myopia is caused by an eyeball that is longer than normal, which may be a familial trait. Transient myopia may occur with the administration of a variety of medications (sulfonamides, acetazolamide, salicylates, and steroids) and has been associated with other disorders, such as influenza, typhoid fever, severe dehydration, and large intakes of antacids (for stomach ulcers).

Correction is accomplished with eyeglasses or contact lenses.

HYPEROPIA

The hyperopic, or *farsighted,* eye is deficient in its ability to focus light rays. The focal point falls behind the eye, and, consequently, the image that falls on the retina is blurred (see Fig. 65–15B). Vision may be brought into focus by placing a convex, or plus, lens in front of the eye. The lens supplies the magnifying power that the eye is lacking. Hyperopia may be caused by an eyeball that is shorter than normal or a cornea that has less curvature than normal. Because children have a greater ability to

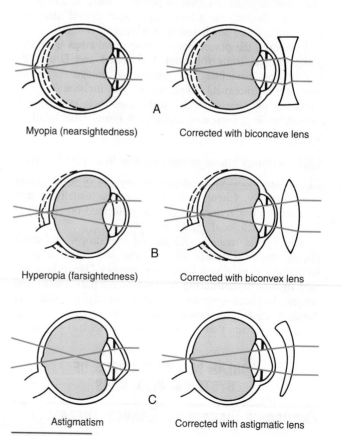

Myopia (nearsightedness)   Corrected with biconcave lens

A

Hyperopia (farsightedness)   Corrected with biconvex lens

B

Astigmatism   Corrected with astigmatic lens

C

FIGURE 65–15 *A–C,* Common refractive disorders and their correction. *Dashed lines* in *A* and *B* indicate normal eye contour.

accommodate, they are less often affected than adults. Demands for close work and reading usually bring on manifestations of headache or eyestrain.

Correction is based on a person's age and individual needs and complaints.

ASTIGMATISM

Astigmatism is a refractive condition in which rays of light are not bent equally by the cornea in all directions, so that a point of focus is not attained (see Fig. 65-15*C*). In most instances, astigmatism is caused because the curvature of the cornea is not perfectly spherical. This is the cause of poor vision for both distant and near objects.

Astigmatism is corrected with cylindrical lenses.

■ Surgical Management

Several techniques and methods of surgical correction for myopia and hyperopia were developed in the 1990s. Short-wavelength, high-energy ultraviolet radiation lasers are being used to reshape the corneal surface. In photorefractive keratectomy (PRK) for myopia, the central cornea is flattened with the excimer laser. The same laser may be used to reshape the cornea by steepening the central curvature to correct hyperopia.

Laser in situ keratomileusis (LASIK) is a procedure in which an extremely thin layer of the cornea is peeled back for the laser reshaping on the middle layer of the cornea and then put back in place. Although the LASIK procedure is more difficult to perform, there is less postoperative discomfort, a more rapid recovery of clear vision, and quicker stabilization of refractive change.

Currently, the placement of intracorneal rings is undergoing clinical trials following U.S. Food and Drug Administration guidelines. Theoretical advantages of using synthetic intracorneal implants versus incisional, excisional, or ablative refractive techniques include improved wound healing, increased rapidity of visual rehabilitation, and reversibility.

■ Nursing Management of the Surgical Client

Clients are assessed for degree of myopia or astigmatism preoperatively. Clients with a severe case usually cannot achieve full correction. Surgery is performed on an outpatient basis with local anesthesia.

The eye is treated with steroid eye drops, and most clients report watering of the eyes and minimal pain. Refraction slowly stabilizes after surgery. There is a period of adjustment during which visual acuity waxes and wanes. Reduced contrast sensitivity in night vision and daytime glare is common. Some clients require re-treatment for scarring that is unresponsive to topical steroids.

OCULAR MANIFESTATIONS OF SYSTEMIC DISORDERS

ENDOCRINE DISORDERS: GRAVES' DISEASE

Graves' disease may exist with or without any clinical evidence of thyroid dysfunction. Ocular manifestations include retraction of both upper and lower lids, resulting in

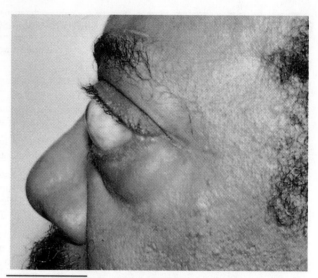

FIGURE 65-16 Graves' exophthalmos. (Courtesy of Ophthalmic Photography at the University of Michigan W. K. Kellogg Eye Center, Ann Arbor.)

a staring or frightened expression (Stellwag's sign), and lid lag (Graefe's sign), the retarded lowering of the upper lid when looking down (Fig. 65-16). When the gaze is changed from down to up, the globe then lags behind the upper lid. Other signs are infrequent blinking, marked fine tremor with lid closure, and jerky movements on lid opening.

The globes enlarge because of the increased size of extraocular muscles, edema of tissues, and excess orbital fat. The eye develops proptosis (forward protrusion of the eyeballs), which is called exophthalmos. Subsequent degeneration of muscle tissue leads to fibrosis, which restricts muscle movement, resulting in double vision.

Outcome Management

As a primary measure, adequate control of thyroid abnormalities is essential. Diuretics as well as steroid therapy and radiotherapy may be indicated.

Surgical interventions include corrective lid surgery and tarsorrhaphy for lid retraction to protect the cornea. Decompression of the orbit, which usually involves removal of the inferior and medial walls of the orbit, may be necessary to accommodate proliferative orbital fat and enlarged ocular muscles. Ocular muscle surgery may also be indicated.

The extent of the surgical procedure is likely to determine whether the client undergoing an orbital decompression requires a hospital stay. If the surgery is extensive, suction drains may be placed at the operative sites. Drainage is usually serosanguineous. It is important that the client sleep with the head elevated to reduce postoperative swelling.

Advise the client to expect redness, swelling, and ecchymoses around the eyes and lids. In the immediate postoperative period, check the client's visual acuity with a near vision card every hour to monitor the possibility of pressure on the optic nerve (see Thinking Critically). Caution the client to modify normal activities for the first 2 weeks after surgery.

RHEUMATOID AND CONNECTIVE TISSUE DISORDERS

Sjögren's syndrome includes keratoconjunctivitis sicca, a common condition in which tear secretion is reduced, in association with a systemic disorder such as rheumatoid arthritis, psoriatic arthritis, connective tissue disorders, sarcoidosis, or Crohn's disease. Manifestations include ocular irritation and foreign-body sensation. Frequent instillation of lubricating eye drops or ointment is effective in most cases.

Several ocular problems may be associated with systemic lupus erythematosus (SLE), a connective tissue disorder. The eyelids may be involved, with the discoid lesions characteristic of the disease. Punctate epithelial keratopathy and secondary Sjögren's syndrome may also occur. Retinopathy of SLE produces cotton-wool spots and increased retinal vessel fragility, as in diabetes. Optic neuropathy can also occur.

NEUROLOGIC DISORDERS

Approximately 90% of clients with myasthenia gravis have ocular involvement. In most cases, it is the presenting manifestation. *Ptosis* (drooping of the eyelid) is bilateral but may be asymmetrical. Diplopia is frequently in the vertical plane. Nystagmus is also present. Ocular myopathy and cranial nerve palsy may develop later, as may *ophthalmoplegia* (paralysis of all extraocular muscles). Medical treatment is supportive and includes systemic steroids.

There is also a close association between optic neuritis and multiple sclerosis. Approximately three fourths of women and one third of men with optic neuritis have multiple sclerosis at 15-year follow-up. Typically, an attack of optic neuritis starts with acute onset of loss of vision in one eye, with periocular discomfort made worse by movement of the eye. Visual impairment is progressive over 2 weeks and usually resolves after 4 to 6 weeks. Recovery may take longer and may be incomplete. Medical treatment consists of oral, IV, and retrobulbar steroids.

CIRCULATORY DISORDERS

The primary response of retinal arterioles to hypertension is a narrowing. In clients with chronic hypertension, the blood-retina barrier is disrupted in small areas, resulting in increased vascular permeability. Funduscopic examination reveals vasoconstriction, leakage, and arteriosclerosis. Hypertensive retinopathy is graded for severity on a scale of 1 to 4, with 4 the most severe. Systemic hypertension is also associated with an increased risk of retinal vein occlusion. There is no known treatment for retinal vein occlusion.

IMMUNOLOGIC DISORDERS

Ocular complications affect approximately 75% of clients with acquired immunodeficiency syndrome (AIDS). In many cases, it is the presenting ocular manifestations that may lead to diagnosis of human immunodeficiency virus (HIV) infection. Cytomegalovirus (CMV) *retinitis* is the most common opportunistic ocular infection. This sight-threatening condition occurs in 30% of clients with AIDS. It is often asymptomatic until it is well established, when the client begins to notice visual field loss, "floaters," or other vague vision problems. A unilateral lesion with the appearance of a cotton-wool spot often develops with white irregular borders associated with hemorrhages. Small lesions may be seen beyond the edges. The retina in the center of the lesion becomes thin and tears easily. Loss of vision is involved and central vision is greatly diminished.

Clients with CMV retinitis require IV therapy, usually through placement of a long-term indwelling catheter. Ganciclovir or foscarnet sodium is administered over several weeks in the hospital or through home care. Because progression is rapid, early treatment is essential and may prevent involvement of the other eye. Careful monitoring of side effects and response to the medication is imperative.

Other infectious ocular conditions that may occur in people with HIV disease are bacterial corneal ulcers (syphilis, staphylococcosis), fungal corneal ulcers (candidiasis, cryptococcosis, histoplasmosis, sporotrichosis), and protozoan (toxoplasmosis, pneumocystosis) and viral infections (herpes simplex).

Noninfectious ocular manifestations in people with HIV infection include HIV retinopathy and neoplastic processes such as Kaposi's sarcoma and non-Hodgkin's lymphoma, which appear around the ocular adnexa. AIDS retinopathy is seen in more than 50% of clients with HIV infection. Direct ophthalmoscopy reveals the presence of cotton-wool spots, retinal hemorrhages, and other microvascular anomalies. The lesions of AIDS retinopathy are indistinguishable from the retinopathy of diabetes or hypertension. They usually occur in the superficial retina and resolve over a period of a few weeks, whereas CMV retinitis lesions will expand. Kaposi's sarcoma and non-Hodgkin's lymphoma present around the eyelids and orbit with diplopia, ptosis, conjunctival edema, or hemorrhage. Diagnosis is confirmed with imaging, needle biopsy, and systemic work-up. Treatment of Kaposi's sarcoma is usually conservative and may include radiotherapy.

Evaluation of extraocular muscle function is important because lymphoma may increase intracranial pressure, which may lead to cranial nerve palsies and altered eye position. Surgical correction of extraocular muscle positioning may be necessary for resolving diplopia or for cosmetic reasons.

LYME DISEASE

Lyme disease (*Borrelia burgdorferi),* transmitted by the bite of a tick, consists of three stages. The initial stage involves a lesion and erythema around the bite, accompanied by regional lymphadenopathy, malaise, fever, headache, myalgia, arthralgia, and frequently conjunctivitis. Several weeks to months later, the second phase is associated with neurologic and cardiac problems. Along with these problems, there may be cranial nerve palsies, uveitis, optic neuropathy, keratitis, choroiditis, and exudative retinal detachments. Rheumatologic complications may develop in the third stage, which may occur over several years. Tetracycline and penicillin are effective in treating the initial infection and in preventing late complications.

CONCLUSIONS

To provide comprehensive nursing care for clients, it is essential to understand the complexity of ocular structures and the physiology of vision. The specialty practice of ophthalmic nursing is devoted to caring for clients with eye disorders. Ophthalmic Registered Nurses perform the roles of caregiver, advocate, educator, counselor, technician, coordinator, and researcher. Ophthalmic nursing care not only is directed at those biologic systems that are affected by an actual or potential deficit but also is an integration of how actual or potential visual deficits affect the individual as an entire being.

THINKING CRITICALLY

1. **Your client is a 72-year-old retired carpenter who has undergone outpatient cataract surgery. He and his wife live an hour away from the surgery center, where they received instructions to call the emergency number if any unusual pain or nausea. They have an appointment to return for a follow-up evaluation the next morning. After supper, the client's wife calls to report that her husband has a headache. She says that her husband also has an upset stomach, but she thinks he feels queasy because he ate some spicy food. The client does not want his wife to drive him back at night and thinks she should not have bothered to call because they have an appointment in the morning. How would you proceed? What further assessment data are needed? What are the likely complications following cataract surgery, and what are their clinical manifestations?**

Factors to Consider. Might the headache and upset stomach be related to the cataract surgery, or are they likely to be unrelated?

2. **Your client, a 55-year-old woman with Graves' ophthalmopathy, has undergone surgery in the late afternoon today for a right orbital decompression. An incisional drain is in place at the right temple with a bulb attached for suction. The surgeon has ordered postoperative vision checks with a near vision card every hour throughout the night. The surgery lasted more than 3 hours; general anesthesia was used, and the client is still sedated. Her right eye is extremely swollen; she is unable to open it to read the vision card. She winces and cries when her operative eye is touched, and she is so sleepy that she cannot respond by reading the vision card. What should you do to carry out the surgeon's postoperative orders?**

Factors to Consider. Are such severe eye pain and swelling normal postoperative findings? How would you assess the eye? How would you rouse the client to perform these crucial eye assessments?

BIBLIOGRAPHY

1. Allen, P., & Shepherd, J. (1998). The ophthalmic registered nurse's responsibility to the adult patient with low vision. *Insight, 23*(2), 53.
2. Benson, W., & Lanier, J. (1998). Current diagnosis and treatment of corneal ulcers. *Current Opinion in Ophthalmology, 9*(4), 45.
3. Burris, T. (1998). Intrastomal corneal ring technology: Results and indications. *Current Opinion in Ophthalmology, 9*(4), 9.
4. D'Ambrosio, F. (1999). Assessing disability in the patient with cataracts. *Current Opinion in Ophthalmology, 10*(1), 42.
5. Dolphin, K. (1998). Complications of postenucleation/evisceration implants. *Current Opinion in Ophthalmology, 9*(5), 75.
6. Eagle, R. (1999). *Eye pathology: An atlas and basic text.* Philadelphia: W. B. Saunders.
7. Emery, J. (1999). Capsular opacification after cataract surgery. *Current Opinion in Ophthalmology, 10*(1), 42.
8. Fishbaugh, J. (1995). Look who's driving now? Visual standards for driver's licensing in the United States. *Insight, 20*(4), 11–20
9. Gills, J., Loyd, T., & Cherchio, M. (1995). Anesthesia, preoperative, and postoperative medications. *Current Opinion in Ophthalmology, 6,* 31–35.
10. Gimbel, H., & Levy, S. (1998). Indications, results, and complications of LASIK. *Current Opinion in Ophthalmology, 9*(4), 3.
11. Goldblum, K. (Ed.). (1997). *Ophthalmic nursing core curriculum.* Dubuque, IA: Kendall Publishing.
12. Gramer, E., & Tausch, M. (1995). The risk profile of the glaucomatous patient. *Current Opinion in Ophthalmology, 6,* 78–88.
13. Grehn, F. (1995). The value of trabeculotomy in glaucoma surgery. *Current Opinion in Ophthalmology, 6,* 52–60.
14. Harding, J. (1995). Epidemiology, pathophysiology, and world blindness. *Current Opinion in Ophthalmology, 6,* 27–30.
15. Haller, J. (1998). Retinal detachment. *Focal Points, 16*(5), 1–14.
16. Kanski, J. (1999). *Clinical ophthalmology* (4th ed.). Oxford: Butterworth Heinemann.
17. L'Esperance, F. (1998). Choosing the appropriate photorefractive keratoplasty patient. *Focal Points, 16*(9), 1–14.
18. Miller, N., & Newman, N. (1999). *Clinical neuro-ophthalmology: The essentials* (5th ed.). Baltimore: Williams & Wilkins.
19. O'Brart, D. (1999). The status of hyperopic LASIK. *Current Opinion in Ophthalmology, 10*(4), 247.
20. O'Day, B. (1999). Employment barriers for people with visual impairments. *Journal of Visual Impairment and Blindness, 93*(10), 627–642.
21. Pieramici, D., & Bressler, S. (1998). Age-related macular degeneration and risk factors for the development of choroidal neovascularization in the fellow eye. *Current Opinion in Ophthalmology, 38.*
22. Recchia, F., Conolly, B., & Benson, W. (1998). Ocular manifestations of diabetes. *Current Opinion of Ophthalmology, 9*(6), 64.
23. Rowen, S. (1999). Preoperative and postoperative medications used for cataract surgery. *Current Opinion in Ophthalmology, 10*(1), 29.
24. Schubert, H. (1998). Ocular manifestations of systemic hypertension. *Current Opinion in Ophthalmology, 9*(6), 93.
25. Shields, J., & Shields, C. (1999). *Atlas of eyelid and conjunctival tumors.* Philadelphia: Lippincott–Williams & Wilkins.
26. Smith, S. (1999). Non-proliferative diabetic retinopathy and macular edema. *Insight, 24*(2), 59–64.
27. Sperber, L., & Dodick, J. (1995). Laser therapy in cataract surgery. *Current Opinion in Ophthalmology, 6,* 22–26.
28. Stewart, W. (1995). The effect of lifestyle on the relative risk to develop open-angle glaucoma. *Current Opinion in Ophthalmology, 6,* 3–9.
29. Stewart, W. (1999). Perspectives in the medical treatment of glaucoma. *Current Opinion in Ophthalmology, 10*(2), 99.
30. Trobe, J. (1993). *The physician's guide to eye care.* San Francisco: American Academy of Ophthalmology.
31. Vader, L. (1996). The significance of cultural values in vision loss. *ABNF Journal, 1*(3), 69–71.
32. Vader, L. (2000). Ophthalmic nursing. In N. Burden (Ed.), *Ambulatory surgery nursing.* Philadelphia: W. B. Saunders.
33. Vaughan, D., Asbury, T., & Riordan-Eva, P. (1995). *General ophthalmology* (14th ed.). Norwalk, CT: Appleton & Lange.
34. Wason, B., & McMillan, J. (1998). *Macular degeneration.* Berkeley, CA: Hunter House Publishers.
35. Whitaker, R., & Whitaker, V. (1999). Glaucoma: What the ophthalmic nurse should know. *Insight, 24*(3), 86.

REMEMBER *to*
check out your
Companion CD ROM

CHAPTER 66

Management of Clients with Hearing and Balance Disorders

Helene J. Krouse

HEARING IMPAIRMENT

Hearing impairment ranges from minor difficulty in understanding words or hearing certain sounds to total deafness. Hearing impairment is the nation's primary disability: one in 15 Americans is affected. By the year 2050, approximately one in five clients in the United States will be 55 years or older; of these estimated 58 million people, 26 million are expected to have hearing impairment. Of the 10 million people in the United States with a hearing loss who are now 65 years or older, more than 90% have a sensorineural hearing loss. Because of fear, misinformation, lack of information, and vanity, many clients do not admit that they have a hearing problem. Up to 80% of all hearing impairments are caused by hearing nerve disorders, for which no cure is currently available. Hearing impairments diminish the quality of life for a third of adults between 65 and 75 years of age.

Etiology and Risk Factors

Many factors influence the type and amount of hearing loss. Hearing loss is not an actual disorder but is a clinical manifestation of many possible problems. Both common and uncommon causes of hearing impairment are examined in this chapter. Hearing loss can be classified into three main areas:

- Conductive hearing loss (i.e., otosclerosis, trauma)
- Sensorineural hearing loss (i.e., presbycusis, noise-induced, and sudden hearing loss)
- Mixed hearing loss

Conductive hearing loss results from interference of sound transmission through the external ear and middle ear. It may be caused by (1) anything that blocks the external ear, such as wax, infection, or a foreign body, (2) thickening, retraction, scarring, or perforation of the tympanic membrane, or (3) any pathophysiologic changes in the middle ear that affect or freeze one or more of the ossicles.

Sensorineural hearing loss is caused by impairment of the function of the inner ear, the eighth cranial nerve, or the brain. Causes are congenital and hereditary factors, noise injury, aging and degenerative processes, Ménière's disease, and ototoxicity. Systemic disorders, such as autoimmune disease, syphilis, certain collagen disorders, and diabetes, may cause sensorineural hearing losses. Most recently, cigarette smoking and exposure to environmental tobacco smoke have been associated with age-related hearing loss.

In a *mixed hearing loss*, both conductive and sensorineural hearing components are present simultaneously. A client with a perforated eardrum and presbycusis has both conductive and sensorineural hearing losses.

CONDUCTIVE HEARING LOSS
Ear Obstructions

Obstruction of the ear is most commonly caused by impacted cerumen. Although the ear canal is self-cleaning, cerumen may become impacted from a disorder or from improper cleaning. The elderly are more susceptible to cerumen impaction because hair in the ear becomes coarser with age and traps the wax. Some people produce more cerumen in the ear canal and require a regular routine for eliminating excessive buildup of wax in the ear canal. Insertion of cotton-tipped swabs into the ear canal can create further impaction of ear wax or can even traumatize the ear canal or perforate the eardrum.

Ear obstruction can also be caused by a wide array of foreign bodies that fit into the ear canal and impede conduction of sound waves. The most common foreign bodies found in the adult ear are pieces of cotton and insects. Foreign bodies commonly seen in children consist of small toys, beads, insects, and food, such as kernels of corn. Teach clients to avoid inserting hard instruments into the ear and to avoid obstructing the ear canal with objects.

Infection

Many infections can lead to hearing loss. An infection of the inner ear, called *labyrinthitis,* can be either viral or bacterial in origin. Viral labyrinthitis can be associated with recent respiratory tract infections, measles, mumps, or rubella. Bacterial labyrinthitis, which is rare, is associated with otitis media or meningitis. Otitis media is a common disorder of the middle ear. Repeated infections or allergic inflammation can lead to fluid accumulation behind the eardrum, causing dampening of the sound being conducted to the inner ear. In addition, drainage, perforation, or scarring of the tympanic membrane can result in a conductive hearing loss. Otitis media and other infectious ear processes are discussed later in the chapter, under the heading Otalgia.

Otosclerosis

Otosclerosis, or hardening of the inner ear, is a genetic disorder in which repeated resorption and redeposition of abnormal bone gradually leads to fixation of the footplate of the stapes in the oval window (Fig. 66–1A). The immobility of the footplate prevents transmission of sound vibration into the inner ear, leading to conductive hearing loss. This disorder occurs twice as often in women and is ten times more prevalent in whites. The disorder is autosomally dominant with variable penetrance and, therefore, can be transmitted to offspring if only one parent has the disorder.

Tympanosclerosis

Tympanosclerosis is the result of repeated infection and trauma to the tympanic membrane. It consists of a deposit of collagen and calcium within the middle ear that can harden around the ossicles, causing a conductive hearing loss. Tympanosclerotic deposits can also be found mounded in the middle ear or as plaque on the tympanic membrane.

Trauma to the Tympanic Membrane

The tympanic membrane can be damaged by trauma. Increased pressure from a hand slap, falling in water, sports injuries, cleaning the ear with a sharp instrument, and industrial accidents involving welding sparks can rupture the thin membrane. Trauma to the tympanic membrane from a blast or blunt injury can involve the middle ear, causing a fracture or dislocation of the ossicles and tearing of the tympanic membrane. Also, the facial nerve is vulnerable to trauma. A basilar skull fracture involves the temporal bone and, depending on the fracture site, causes ossicular damage as well as facial nerve paralysis and sensorineural hearing loss. Care of clients with facial fracture is discussed in Chapter 49. When the tympanic membrane is perforated, infection is a concern.

SENSORINEURAL HEARING LOSS
Presbycusis

Presbycusis is a progressive hearing loss found predominantly in the elderly. This degenerative process involves changes in the labyrinthine structures over time. The client initially experiences a decrease in high-frequency sound. At times, *tinnitus,* or the perception of noise in the ear, accompanies this decline in hearing.

Sudden Hearing Loss

Sudden (idiopathic) hearing loss (SHL) is a fairly common condition in which the client loses hearing in an ear

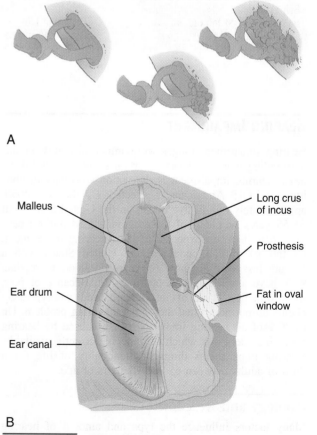

A

Malleus

Long crus of incus

Prosthesis

Ear drum

Fat in oval window

Ear canal

B

FIGURE 66–1 *A,* Stapedial otosclerosis. The immovable footplate prevents sound transmission. *B,* Stapedectomy.

within minutes or hours. This condition is almost exclusively unilateral. Although the exact cause of sudden sensorineural hearing loss has not been determined, postmortem examinations of temporal bones suggest that the disease involves a viral infection of the inner ear. Prompt early intervention with oral corticosteroids has been shown to at least partially restore the lost hearing in many patients with sudden hearing loss. In the United States alone, approximately 4000 new cases of sudden hearing loss are reported annually.

Sensorineural hearing loss of abrupt onset can sometimes occur from discrete causes. Some of these specific causes are (1) rapid infectious processes, such as meningitis or mumps, (2) ototoxic agents, (3) trauma, (4) metabolic disturbances, and (5) immunologic disorders. In most cases of SHL, however, no specific cause is found.

Congenital Hearing Loss
Congenital episodes of sensorineural hearing loss are not uncommon. These losses can be severe and present at the time of birth or can develop during childhood or early adulthood and gradually worsen with time. Congenital hearing loss often results in total deafness. It can occur either in a genetic pattern within families or spontaneously. Both autosomal recessive and autosomal dominant methods of transmission have been documented. In milder cases of congenital hearing loss, the individual may not be aware of a loss until hearing is screened for work or school. In families with a history of congenital hearing loss, infant screening is essential to allow early detection of the problem and rehabilitation of congenitally deaf infants.

Noise-Induced Hearing Loss
Noise-induced hearing loss is a specific type of sensorineural hearing loss that most often occurs over time from repeated acoustic trauma from loud noise. The major causes are industrial noise, use of firearms, and listening to loud music. Traumatic injury associated with a sudden loud noise, such as a blast, can also result in noise-induced hearing loss.

Benign and Malignant Tumors
Both benign and malignant tumors of the temporal bone can involve the inner ear and lead to sensorineural hearing loss. The most common benign tumor is an acoustic neuroma or schwannoma of the eighth cranial nerve. The tumor usually develops in the internal auditory canal, the bony channel through which the vestibular nerve passes as it leaves the inner ear. The tumor presses on the nerve, which then sends false signals to the brain. If the vestibular portion of the nerve is compressed, the client is unable to interpret stimuli about position and movement. If the cochlear branch is compressed, the client experiences tinnitus. The first clinical manifestation is often partial or complete sensorineural hearing loss followed by tinnitus. The client may also report dizziness.

Other tumors in the cerebellopontine angle likewise involve the seventh and eighth cranial nerves as they enter the internal acoustic meatus. Malignant tumors invade the entire inner ear, usually spreading from the middle ear and mastoid system.

Meniérè's Disease
Méniére's disease is a disorder that affects both vestibular and auditory function. It is caused by excess endolymph (clear intracellular fluid in the membranous labyrinth of the inner ear) in the vestibular and semicircular canals. Hearing loss is fluctuant, and usually subtle and reversible in the early stages. Later, the hearing loss becomes permanent. Although Ménière's disease is associated with sensorineural hearing loss, the most prominent clinical manifestation is vertigo (feeling that the surroundings or one's own body is revolving). Therefore, it is fully discussed in the section Balance Disorders.

Central Auditory Dysfunction
Central auditory dysfunction is a phenomenon whereby the central nervous system (CNS) cannot interpret normal auditory signals. Central auditory dysfunction, also known as central deafness, is a rare form of sensorineural hearing loss. Diseases that alter the CNS, such as cerebrovascular accidents and tumors, can cause central deafness.

MIXED HEARING LOSS
Some causes of hearing impairment can result in both sensorineural and conductive hearing losses. These types of losses are referred to as *mixed hearing loss*. Clients with mixed hearing loss present with clinical manifestations associated with both sensorineural and conductive hearing losses.

Prevention and Screening

A major nursing responsibility is the identification of hearing impairment in clients in both hospital and community settings. The different types of hearing loss are listed in Box 66-1. Identification of clients at risk for hearing loss and adequate protection of the ears are important to maintain normal function. The American

---

BOX 66-1   Types of Hearing Loss

Air conduction hearing loss: Loss of hearing through the external and middle ear.

Bone conduction hearing loss: Loss of hearing through the inner ear.

Central hearing loss: Loss of hearing from damage to the brain's auditory pathways or auditory center.

Conductive hearing loss: Loss of hearing in which air conduction is worse than bone conduction and involves the external and middle ear.

Fluctuating hearing loss: A sensorineural hearing loss that varies with time.

Functional hearing loss: Loss of hearing for which no organic lesion can be found.

Mixed hearing loss: Both sensorineural and conductive hearing loss.

Neural hearing loss: A sensorineural hearing loss originating in the eighth cranial nerve or brain stem.

Sensorineural hearing loss: Loss of hearing involving the cochlea and hearing nerve; bone and air conduction equal but diminished.

Sensory hearing loss: A sensorineural hearing loss in the cochlea and involving the hair cells and nerve endings.

Sudden hearing loss: A sensorineural hearing loss with a sudden onset.

Conductive hearing loss results from interference with conduction in the external and middle ear; sensorineural hearing loss in the inner ear; and mixed hearing loss in all three areas.

Speech-Language-Hearing Association (ASHA) has recommended specific guidelines for annual hearing screenings for children 3 to 10 years old who are at risk for hearing impairment.

Primary prevention is aimed at minimizing the risks from trauma, noise exposure, use of ototoxic drugs, and infectious diseases, such as meningitis, mumps, and measles. To reduce the risk of head trauma, young clients should be instructed to wear protective headgear or helmets when participating in sports. People should avoid insertion of hard instruments or objects into the ear canal to prevent obstruction, trauma, or perforation. Individuals in occupations with high noise exposure should be instructed to wear earplugs and to avoid prolonged exposure. Exposure to noise levels in excess of 80 decibels (dB) throughout an 8-hour day is considered excessive and should be avoided. In addition, teenagers need to be aware that listening to extremely loud music in enclosed spaces, such as cars, can contribute to hearing loss.

Secondary prevention involves early detection of hearing impairment through screening and referral of any ear problems. Hearing screenings are important to detect hearing impairment in children that can be related to congenital, infectious, or allergic processes. Hearing tests and ear examinations should be performed in clients 65 years and older and in people experiencing hearing difficulties. When administering drugs with ototoxic side effects, monitor clients for vertigo, lessened hearing acuity, and tinnitus. If any of these manifestations occurs, the client or nurse must stop the ototoxic medication and promptly notify the physician.

Tertiary prevention focuses on maintenance of optimal function through hearing rehabilitation programs, proper use and care of hearing aids, and implementation of coping and communication strategies.

Pathophysiology

Conductive hearing loss is the result of interference of sound transmission into and through the external ear and middle ear. The inner ear is not affected in a pure conductive loss; therefore, sound transmission from the inner ear to the brain is normal. Normal movement of sound vibrations through the ear canal, tympanic membrane, or ossicles is impeded because of the nature of the disease process involved in the conductive loss. Sound is perceived as faint or distant, but it remains relatively clear. Most conductive hearing losses are correctable by medical or surgical treatment.

Sensorineural hearing loss, however, results from disease or trauma to the organ of Corti or auditory nerve pathways of the inner ear leading to the brain stem. Normal reception and transmission of sound waves is disrupted. Sound is distorted and faint. Sensorineural hearing losses are usually permanent and are generally not correctable by medical or surgical treatment.

Clinical Manifestations

Most hearing loss is gradual and goes unnoticed by the client until several incidents of communication problems have occurred. Significant others and co-workers are usually aware of the client's hearing problem long before the

client realizes or admits to the problem. However, a small loss of hearing goes unnoticed and does not cause manifestations. Health care providers should be alert for the following manifestations of hearing loss in a client:

- Failure to respond to oral communication
- Inappropriate response to oral communication
- Excessively loud speech
- Abnormal awareness of sounds
- Strained facial expressions
- Tilting of head when listening
- Constant need for clarification of conversation
- Faulty speech articulation
- Listening to radio and television at increased volume

The hearing impaired, or "hard-of-hearing" client may repeat the information, even incorrectly, or may ask for clarification. Clients with a hearing loss can also experience distorted or abnormal sounds. Sometimes a sound is heard at different pitches for each ear; this is called *diplacusis*. A sound may cause a rapid increase in loudness; this is called *recruitment*. These abnormal sounds can cause discomfort.

The onset of a conductive hearing loss can be sudden or progressive. In cases of fluid in the middle ear, hearing loss is often bilateral but is usually restored with medical or surgical treatment. In other conductive processes, such as otosclerosis, clinical manifestations consist of slow progressive hearing loss with changes noted even in adolescence. Hearing loss is usually bilateral but may be asymmetrical. Other manifestations are mild tinnitus, recurrent vertigo, and postural imbalance. It is common for the client to speak in a very soft voice.

If damage to the tympanic membrane is suspected, such as perforation, examination of the client may reveal a conductive hearing loss and serous drainage in the ear canal. The hearing loss found with a total perforation of the eardrum is approximately 35 dB (one third of the hearing range). With small perforations, no loss may be present. If a perforation is present, damage to the ossicles should be suspected. Diagnostic findings of conductive hearing loss include greater bone conduction than air conduction on Rinne's test. If hearing loss is greater in one ear, Weber's test shows lateralization to the more affected ear. Pure tone audiometry confirms hearing loss. *Speech discrimination* (understanding of words) is usually maintained.

Noise-induced hearing loss is characterized by a greater loss in the higher frequencies. Sudden or fluctuating hearing losses are recognized as separate disorders from routine sensorineural hearing loss. Although fluctuating losses usually suggest syphilis or Ménière's disease, sudden sensorineural hearing losses are believed to be viral in origin. Recognition of these patterns is important because medical treatment of such disorders can result in significant improvements in hearing.

A characteristic of a severe hearing loss is the loss of discrimination. To some clients, a hearing loss feels like a blockage or fullness in the ear or an inability to distinguish the direction of sounds.

Tinnitus accompanies most sensorineural hearing losses and is very annoying. Tinnitus literally means "ringing" but can actually sound like roaring, the chirping of crickets, or, occasionally, music. Tinnitus is not a disease but a very distressing manifestation, and it is sometimes a warning sign of hearing loss or other, more serious problems. Ear noise that cannot be heard by an observer is classified as *subjective tinnitus*, which is the most common kind. Any ear noise that can be heard by someone other than the client is called *objective tinnitus*. In some clients, the tinnitus becomes the problem, and the underlying cause may be forgotten.

The major nursing responsibility in a client with tinnitus is to perform a thorough history and assessment of the onset, frequency, constancy, and level of intensity of the tinnitus. Unilateral tinnitus merits a complete neuro-otologic evaluation with the goal of ruling out the possibility of a tumor, most likely an acoustic neuroma. The nurse must keep in mind that tinnitus is a manifestation of an underlying pathologic process that warrants further referral.

Table 66–1 presents clinical manifestations of conductive and sensorineural hearing losses. Diagnostic measures include (1) testing for hearing of pure tones on audiometry, (2) speech reception and discrimination, (3) tympanometry, and, (4) sometimes, brain stem auditory evoked responses. Tones are presented using earphones (air conduction) and vibrators (bone conduction). The minimal level at which the client can hear is determined. The *speech reception threshold* is the lowest intensity at which the client can correctly repeat 50% of the words presented. The speech discrimination test is a measure of the client's ability to understand speech when it is presented at a volume that is easily heard.

Outcome Management

Medical Management

The goals for medical management of the client with hearing impairment are (1) to restore hearing loss, (2) to assist hearing, (3) to manage tinnitus, and (4) to implement aural rehabilitation.

RESTORE HEARING LOSS
Hearing loss that results from blockage or fullness in the ear associated with an infectious process may be restored to normal with administration of antibiotics for bacterial infections or acyclovir and oral corticosteroids for herpesvirus infections. In the case of sudden hearing loss, prompt administration of oral corticosteroids is used in an attempt to lessen the progressive hearing loss or to reverse a sudden loss. If ototoxicity is suspected, the administration of all ototoxic medications is discontinued. Most sensorineural hearing loss cannot be reversed with

medical or surgical intervention. Conductive hearing loss, in contrast, is often amenable to surgical correction.

ASSIST HEARING
Unfortunately, most hearing losses are permanent, and hearing cannot be restored. The use of hearing aids and assistive listening devices can greatly improve the client's ability to communicate and interact with others.

Hearing aids amplify sound in a controlled manner. They are used by both *hearing-impaired* clients (those with slight or moderate hearing loss) and *deaf* clients (those with severe or profound hearing loss). Hearing aids make sound louder but do not improve the quality of sound. Therefore, clients with decreased discrimination benefit less from a hearing aid. The hearing aid amplifies all background noises, such as hospital machinery, background conversation in restaurants, footsteps, and department store noises, as well as speech. These noises may mask conversation or confuse the hearing-impaired client, especially one who is elderly.

A client should undergo a trial period before purchasing a hearing aid to see whether he or she can adapt to its use. In fact, in most states, such a trial period is mandatory. Bilateral (binaural) aids may be desirable.

Several types of hearing aids are available, and they vary according to size and location. Hearing aids can be worn in the following locations:

• In the ear
• In the ear canal
• Behind the ear (postauricular)
• In eyeglasses
• In the middle of the chest (body-worn aid)

Regardless of type, the hearing aid consists of four parts:

1. Microphone to receive sound waves from the air and change sounds into electrical signals.
2. Amplifier to increase the strength of electrical signals.
3. Receiver (loudspeaker) to change the electrical signals into sound waves.
4. Battery to provide the electrical energy needed to operate the hearing aid.

On all types of hearing aids but the body-worn type, all four components are housed in one small case. The louder sounds are then directed into the ear through a custom-molded earpiece (Fig. 66–2).

The evolution in hearing aid design has led to smaller and more effective aids. Small hearing aids are available

TABLE 66–1	CLINICAL MANIFESTATIONS OF CONDUCTIVE AND SENSORINEURAL HEARING LOSSES	
	Conductive Hearing Loss	**Sensorineural Hearing Loss**
Voice quality	Soft voice	Loud voice
Effect of environmental noise on hearing	Hearing improved	Hearing made worse
Speech discrimination	Good	Poor
Ability to hear on telephone	Good	Poor
Lateralization on Weber's test	To diseased ear	To normal ear
Result of Rinne's test	Negative, AC<BC	Positive, AC>BC

AC, air conduction; BC, bone conduction.

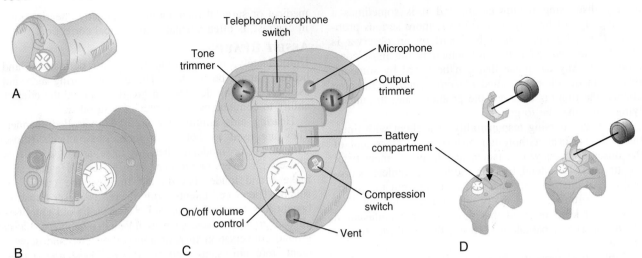

FIGURE 66-2 Types of hearing aids and components. *A*, In-the-canal aid. *B*, In-the-ear aid. *C*, Hearing aid components. *D*, Battery compartment. (Courtesy of Arnold G. Schuring, M.D.)

that fit into the ear canal. The latest advancement in hearing aids is digital processing. Another advancement is directional microphones, which enhance the voice of a speaker in front of the client and suppress background noise. Programmable hearing aids allow the selection of various amplification patterns by the user, and may have some added benefit for clients. Hearing aid technology will continue to advance.

Assistive listening devices help the hearing-impaired client hear the television or radio as well as use the telephone. Stationary devices called teletypewriters and a portable instrument called a Telecommunication Device for the Deaf (TDD) are used for telephone communication by the profoundly deaf. A flashing light signals the presence of a dial tone, a busy signal, or a ring. When another teletypewriter or TDD is reached, messages are typed and displayed on a screen or printed. Other devices, such as flashing lights that alert a deaf person to a ringing doorbell, alarm clock, or smoke alarm, are available. Hearing dogs are trained to be sensitive to certain noises, such as the telephone, doorbells, and crying children. On hearing the sound, a hearing dog moves back and forth between the client and the sound to alert the client.

MANAGE TINNITUS

Tinnitus can be a very distressing disorder associated with the sensorineural hearing loss. Many approaches have been tried to alleviate this problem, including biofeedback, electrostimulation, hypnosis, medication, hearing aids, and tinnitus maskers. They have all met with minimal success. Tinnitus maskers appear quite similar to hearing aids except that they generate noise. The tinnitus masker is of benefit only while it is being used. However, every approach for the relief from tinnitus is only moderately successful, at best. Clients should be counseled to avoid unproven treatments for tinnitus. The nurse and family must be alert to manifestations of depression if the tinnitus is chronic. The quality of the spouse's support of the client with tinnitus has been shown to be strongly correlated with role function. In addition, the nurse

should be alert to spousal interaction and should facilitate problem-solving as needed.

IMPLEMENT AURAL REHABILITATION

Aural rehabilitation may improve communication if (1) hearing loss is irreversible or is not amenable to surgical intervention or (2) the client elects not to have surgery. The purpose of aural rehabilitation is to maximize the hearing-impaired client's communication skills.

Hearing is one of our primary modes of communication. Rehabilitation is directed toward teaching the client to more effectively use the other senses, those of vision, touch, and vibration, and to maximize the use of any remaining hearing ability. The outcome of rehabilitation is affected by all demographic variables and the severity of impairment. As with other forms of rehabilitation, success depends partly on the client's level of motivation.

Speech reading, the current term used for lip reading, is an important means of communication. Speech reading is the process of understanding vocal communication by the integration of lip movements with facial expressions, gestures, environmental clues, and conversation contexts. Speech reading is difficult without auditory cues, for several reasons. Many movements for speech are rapid, many sounds are similar (*b, m, p*), and the production of certain sounds in any language is not visible. The hearing-impaired client must guess at a high percentage of words. Knowledge of this fact alone helps the nurse be more understanding of the client who is using this communication approach.

Because of reduced auditory feedback (the inability of hearing-impaired clients to monitor their own speech), the clearness, pitch quality, or rate of the client's speech may deteriorate. These changes may alter the efficiency of communication and reduce the intelligibility of speech. The goal of speech training is to conserve, develop, or prevent deterioration of speech skills.

Last, but still important, is sign language. Sign language allows communication by hand signals that represent different letters of the alphabet, words, and phrases.

■ Nursing Management of the Medical Client

ASSESSMENT

The client's ability to communicate may be informally assessed during the history. The nurse should assess the client's ability to follow conversation. During the interview, the nurse should look for answers to the following questions:

1. Does the client admit to having a hearing loss and difficulty communicating or blame other people for not speaking clearly?
2. In what settings does the client have more problems with hearing or communicating?
3. Are family members, co-workers, and friends aware of the hearing problem? Are they supportive of the client, making communication easier and including him or her in conversation? Do others feel frustrated or angry when the client cannot hear correctly or does not respond? Does the client feel left out? Embarrassed?
4. Does the client try to understand spoken words? Or does he or she withdraw or refuse to participate, letting others do the talking?
5. Does the client wear a hearing aid? Does it appear to work?

Occasionally, laboratory, radiologic, and vestibular examinations are used for assessment. In an otology office, the nurse may have the responsibility of performing the history, otologic examination, and screening audiometry. The history is often the most important part of the clinical assessment, as previously described (see questionnaire in Chapter 64). The extent of assessment of the sensorineural hearing loss depends on the setting and the nurse's educational preparation and experience. Nurses should be able to inspect the outer ear and grossly assess auditory acuity.

Visualization of the ear canal and tympanic membrane is accomplished with the otoscope. Cerumen in the canal or on the eardrum can interfere with the examination and may need to be removed. The blind removal of ear wax with an ear syringe should be performed only if the ear is free of other abnormalities, such as an infection or perforation of the eardrum.

Impacted accumulations of ear wax may be softened and loosened for removal by alternating instillations of glycerin and hydrogen peroxide eardrops. The eardrops are warmed to body temperature and used daily as directed for 1 to 2 weeks. The ear is then irrigated gently with warm water for removal of the softened wax or cleaned under magnification with a cerumen spoon. Wax on the tympanic membrane should be removed by a otolaryngologist or an advanced-practice nurse in otaryngology. However, the removal of cerumen can lead to irritation from mildly caustic commercial products.

DIAGNOSIS, OUTCOMES, INTERVENTIONS

Impaired Verbal Communication. Clients who have lost their ability to hear are best managed with the nursing diagnosis *Impaired Verbal Communication related to effects of hearing loss.*

Outcomes. The client will develop effective methods to communicate needs and will be included in conversation.

Interventions. When normal conversation is impossible, writing may be used successfully by clients who have good comprehension of English (or their primary language). Writing may cause frustration when the client's primary language is American Sign Language because it is grammatically different from standard English. Visual aids, such as pictures, diagrams, and models, may also improve the nurse's ability to explain medical terminology or procedures. An expert interpreter should be used when other attempts to communicate have failed or when speed and accuracy are critical. The National Registry of Interpreters for the Deaf (NRID) has local chapters and offers certification for qualified individuals. Box 66–2 lists common nursing interventions to improve communication with hearing-impaired clients. They can apply to all clients, regardless of the type or severity of hearing loss.

Many hearing-impaired clients live in the community. Nurses may see these clients for their hearing problems or for many other problems. The Bridge to Home Health Care addresses approaches to home care of hearing-impaired clients.

BOX 66–2   Common Nursing Interventions for Hearing-Impaired Clients

- Get the client's attention by raising your arm or hand.
- Stand with a light on your face; this helps the client to speech-read.
- Talk directly to the client while facing him or her.
- Speak clearly, but do not overaccentuate words.
- Speak in a normal tone; do not shout. Shouting overuses normal speaking movements so may cause distortion, and may be too loud for the client with sensorineural damage. If the client has conductive loss only, it is sometimes helpful to make the voice louder without shouting.
- If the client does not seem to understand what is said, express it differently. Some words are difficult to "see" in speech reading, such as "white" and "red."
- Move closer to the client and toward the better-hearing ear.
- Write out proper names or any statement that you are not sure was understood.
- Do not smile, chew gum, or cover the mouth when talking.
- Remember that a client's inattention may indicate tiredness or lack of understanding.
- Use phrases to convey meaning rather than one-word answers. State the major topic of the discussion first, and then give details.
- Do not show annoyance by careless facial expressions. Clients who are hard of hearing depend more on visual clues for understanding.
- Encourage the use of a hearing aid if it is available; allow the client to adjust it before speaking.
- In a group, repeat important statements, and avoid making asides to others in the group.
- Avoid the use of the intercommunication system, because this may distort sound and cause poor communication.
- Do not avoid conversation with a client who has hearing loss. It has been said that to live in a silent world is much more devastating than to live in darkness, and clients with hearing loss appear to have more emotional difficulties than do those who are blind.

BRIDGE TO HOME HEALTH CARE

Living with a Severe Hearing Loss

People are often reluctant to admit that they have a hearing impairment. This reluctance results in difficulty with verbal communication, inability to follow instructions, and social isolation. To maximize communication, reduce background noise (turn off the television or radio), face the person, and speak clearly without shouting. Sometimes, the only way to communicate is by writing. Develop written materials for repeated use. Include introduction materials (e.g., your name, your agency's name, the purpose of your visit), reportable problems, and treatment regimens.

In many cases, hearing loss is due to accumulation of cerumen. Use an otoscope to visualize the ear canal. If cerumen is present, a physician may need to remove it. If you are responsible for removing the cerumen, contact the physician to discuss a prescription for an ear irrigation solution, instill the solution, and evaluate the amount and color of drainage.

When people experience a hearing loss, they need a medical evaluation and a hearing aid evaluation. Many older adults are reluctant to wear a hearing aid for various reasons. It is a visual sign of an impairment, it is expensive, and it necessitates leaving home for evaluation, fitting, and follow-up appointments. If a client's reluctance is due to cosmetic reasons, show pictures of hearing aids and discuss individuals who wear hearing aids, such as former President George Bush.

If cost is a problem, consider a referral to a social worker to identify local resources. Currently, Medicare pays for the cost of a hearing evaluation and little for the hearing aid; Medicaid usually pays for the hearing aid. Consider other financial resources, such as the American Association of Retired Persons and local hearing aid vendors. When leaving home is a problem, check whether a vendor will make a home visit. If this is not a possible, suggest that the client use a head-set amplifier that can be purchased from a local electronics store.

Teaching is an important nursing intervention related to hearing impairment. It involves cleaning the devices and changing the batteries. Also, evaluate the client's ability to use the telephone and answer the door. Local telephone companies can equip the telephone with an adjustable volume control, hearing aid adapters, loud ringing signals, and a Telecommunication Device for the Deaf (TDD). A TDD allows the hearing-impaired individual to communicate by typing information into a specially designed device. To receive information, the receiver must have a specific TDD telephone number. Teach the client with a TDD about TDD telephone numbers for an emergency response, and provide information about the home health agency and community resources.

It is important to involve informal caregivers, significant others, and family members in the management of a hearing impairment. Teach these people to maximize communication with a variety of techniques and adaptive equipment.

Gail F. Wilkerson, RN, MSN, CS, *Disease Management Specialist, Heart Failure, Group Health Plan, St. Louis, Missouri*

Ineffective Individual Coping. The individual with a loss of hearing goes through the same stages of grieving as others experiencing a loss. Rehabilitation cannot begin until some acceptance of the hearing loss has taken place, leading to the nursing diagnosis *Ineffective Individual Coping related to recent loss of hearing.*

Outcomes. The client will discuss or will demonstrate problem-solving–based coping strategies, as evidenced by the following:

1. Taking the initiative to inform others of the hearing impairment and requesting that they assist with communication by using techniques that promote comprehension.
2. Not experiencing feelings of embarrassment, frustration, or withdrawal.
3. Not blaming others for failure to communicate effectively.
4. Avoiding situations and environments, such as noisy areas, that impair hearing.

Interventions. Work with the client and family on methods to enhance communication and thereby enhance coping. Encourage the client to role-play how he or she might tell people about the hearing impairment and indicate what techniques should be used to help hearing. Self-help groups, such as Self-Help for Hard of Hearing People (SHHH), located in Bethesda, Md., can assist with resources, information, and support for clients and their families.

Impaired Social Interaction. Clients with hearing losses can experience fears of inadequacy, feelings of inferiority, depression, and varying degrees of stress and isolation. The nursing diagnosis *Impaired Social Interaction related to perceived inability to interact with others secondary to hearing loss* can be used to guide interventions.

Outcomes. The client will exhibit a willingness to be involved in social situations, as evidenced by (1) attempting to become a part of social events, (2) conversing with others, (3) indicating lessened feelings of inadequacy, and (4) responding appropriately to questions asked (not fabricating answers to cover hearing loss).

Interventions. The ASHA urges that all clients with hearing impairments *not* be grouped into one category. Each client is unique and has an individual hearing problem. The nurse functions as a role model in accepting the client as an individual and demonstrating effective communication techniques.

Work with the client to enhance coping, encourage continued social involvement, and advocate the use of various organizations to their fullest extent. Many agencies and associations exist for the hearing-impaired client. Services are offered by audiology clinics and sponsored by universities, hospitals, community programs, state or local departments of health, the Department of Veterans Affairs (VA), and national organizations.

Knowledge Deficit. Clients with new hearing aids need information about their care and proper use. Therefore, *Knowledge Deficit related to lack of previous exposure to a hearing aid* is an important nursing diagnosis.

Outcomes. The client will have greater knowledge about the hearing aid, as evidenced by proper use and care of the aid.

Interventions. The hearing aid user should know how to care for the aid (Box 66–3) and what to do if the device does not work. Gain a basic knowledge of the hearing aid to help with insertion for clients who are ill. Encourage the client to use the hearing aid and to store it safely when not using it. Turn the device off before removal to prevent squealing feedback. The maintenance of a hearing aid is becoming less of a problem today. Usually, the aid is returned to the dealer for factory repair while the client uses a "loaner" hearing aid. Unlicensed assistive personnel often care for clients with hearing aids. Delegation of care of the hearing aid and the hearing-impaired client is shown in the Management and Delegation feature.

Cost has been cited as a major factor in the non-use of hearing aids. Clients needing financial assistance should be referred to the state department of vocational rehabilitation, the local Lions Club, and, in some states, Medicaid.

EVALUATION

A client with a new hearing loss or disorder needs frequent evaluation to determine the severity of hearing loss, coping strategies, and ability to adequately communicate. Because many forms of hearing loss are permanent or progressive, long-term evaluation should also be performed to be certain the client is adapting positively. Also determine whether the client has questions about the equipment used for hearing rehabilitation and the need for further education.

BOX 66–3 Care of a Hearing Aid

- Turn the hearing aid off when it is not in use.
- Open the battery compartment at night to avoid accidental drainage of battery power.
- Keep an extra battery available at all times.
- Wash the ear mold frequently (daily if necessary) with mild soap and warm water, and use a pipe cleaner to cleanse the cannula.
- Dry the ear mold completely before reconnecting it to the hearing aid.
- Do not wear the hearing aid when you have an ear infection.

What to Do if the Hearing Aid Fails to Work

- Check the on-off switch.
- Inspect the ear mold for cleanliness.
- Examine the battery for correct insertion.
- Examine the cord plug for correct insertion.
- Examine the cord for breaks.
- Replace the battery, cord, or both, if necessary. The life of batteries varies according to the amount of use and power requirements of the aid. Batteries last 2 to 14 days.
- Check the position of the ear mold in the ear. If the hearing aid "whistles," the ear mold is probably not inserted properly into the ear canal, or you need to have a new ear mold made.

MANAGEMENT AND DELEGATION

Hearing Aids

Caring for hearing aids and helping clients with maintenance of these devices may be delegated to unlicensed assistive personnel. Clients with new hearing aids need individualized teaching provided by you, the Registered Nurse. You are to evaluate the client's understanding of the instruction. Before delegating hearing aid care, consider the following issues:

- The client's learning needs. Are these new hearing aids? Does the client have a new hearing loss disorder? If so, you should instruct the client to care for these devices and provide consistent teaching.
- The competency level of the unlicensed assistive personnel who will potentially perform hearing aid care. Unlicensed assistive personnel may not provide the initial instruction but may reinforce the instructions that you have provided.

Instruct unlicensed assistive personnel caring for the client with hearing aids to:

- Encourage the use of hearing aids and independent care by clients without cognitive impairment.
- Provide safe storage of the hearing aids when not in use (in the client's personal case or another small storage device). If the client is hospitalized, ensure that the case is labeled with the client's name and location.
- Turn the device off when it is not in use. If the aid is to be off for a prolonged duration (such as during the night or sleeping hours), open the battery compartment to avoid additional drainage of battery power.
- Cleanse the ear mold with mild soap and water each day or as needed.
- Completely dry the ear mold prior to reconnecting it to the hearing aid.
- Help the client insert the ear mold into the ear. If the hearing aid makes a whistling noise, the device is not inserted properly into the ear. At this point, it may be necessary for you to further assess placement in the ear canal.
- Allow the client to adjust the volume prior to speaking.
- Speak clearly in a normal tone to the client. Do not shout.
- Turn off the device before removing it to prevent squealing "feedback."

Findings that are immediately reportable to you are (1) difficulty with placement in the ear, (2) redness or drainage in the ear, (3) mechanical failure of the device, and (4) other issues of concern to the client.

Kimberly Elgin, BSN, RN, *Clinician III, Clinical Manager, Surgical Services, University of Virginia Health System, Charlottesville, Virginia*

Surgical Management

Surgery is usually not warranted for sensorineural hearing loss. However, because mixed, conductive, and sensorineural hearing loss exists, surgery may be performed (1) to restore the conductive hearing loss, (2) to remove tumor, and (3) to assist hearing in profoundly deaf people.

RESTORE CONDUCTIVE HEARING

The most common cause of conductive hearing loss is serous otitis media (see later). Although most commonly seen in children, this disorder can occur at any age. In cases of serous otitis media and persistent conductive hearing loss that do not resolve after 2 to 3 months of medical management, an incision into the tympanic membrane and an evacuation of fluid can be performed with the client under local or general anesthesia. This procedure, known as *myringotomy*, will restore hearing. It is discussed later in this chapter.

Another type of conductive hearing loss that can be treated medically or corrected surgically results from otosclerosis. Because speech discrimination is usually unimpaired, simple amplification of sound is quite effective. People who are at high risk of otosclerosis or who are not candidates for surgery can be given medications in an attempt to reduce the severity of the bony fusion. Sodium fluoride has been given to replace the hydroxyl ion in bone and decrease resorption. In addition, calcium gluconate and vitamin D have been used to retard bone resorption. If hearing is stable, these minerals and vitamins are given for only 2 years. The clinical efficacy of these medications remains unsubstantiated.

STAPEDECTOMY. Surgical intervention for otosclerosis has been very successful. *Stapedectomy* is a surgical procedure whereby the damaged stapes is removed and replaced with a stainless steel, polytetrafluoroethylene (Teflon), or plastic prosthesis (Fig. 66–1*B*). The oval window is grafted with absorbable gelatin sponge (Gelfoam) or tissue grafts. Stapedectomy was once a common middle ear procedure. However, the pool of clients with otosclerosis is dwindling, and today, stapedectomy is performed less and less often.

The client must be free of otitis externa and otitis media before surgery. To reduce the risk of bleeding, the client should use no aspirin or products with aspirin for 1 week before surgery. Preoperative and postoperative audiograms and tympanograms are performed to test hearing acuity levels.

After surgery, the client is often instructed to lie on the nonoperative ear with the head of the bed elevated. This position helps reduce edema and prevent dislodgment of the prosthesis. Antibiotics are prescribed. The packing in the ear canal should not be disturbed. Upon discharge from the hospital, the client is told to report the acute onset of vertigo. To reduce the risk of development of a perilymph fistula (rupture of the oval window, which permits leakage of perilymph fluid), the client should avoid excessive exercise, straining, and activities that may lead to head trauma. If the client needs to blow the nose, it should be done gently, one nostril at a time. The client should sneeze with the mouth open. No airplane travel is allowed for a month.

Hearing aids may still be required after stapedectomy, and the client's hearing will need to be reevaluated. Complications of the operation include granuloma formation and perilymph fistula. Either complication may result in profound deafness and persistent vertigo. Hearing loss may also develop after surgery from middle ear adhesions or shifting of the prosthesis.

TUMOR EXCISION

Surgery is usually recommended for treatment of acoustic neuroma. Current microsurgical techniques often allow preservation of hearing and usually enable resection of the tumor without injury to the facial nerve. In older clients, especially those with total deafness in the affected ear, a more conservative, nonsurgical approach is sometimes taken, because acoustic neuroma is benign and very slow growing.

ASSIST HEARING IN PROFOUND DEAFNESS

Use of implantable hearing devices (IHDs) may be appropriate in various clients. There are three types of implantable hearing devices: cochlear implants, temporal bone stimulators, and middle ear implants.

COCHLEAR IMPLANTS. Cochlear implants provide auditory sensation to clients with severe to profound sensorineural hearing loss who cannot benefit from a hearing aid (Fig. 66–3). Preoperative vestibular testing is highly recommended for all clients in whom a cochlear implant is being considered.

The cochlear implant contains a small computer that changes the spoken word to electrical impulses. The impulses are transmitted across the skin to an implanted coil that carries the impulse to the hearing nerve endings in the cochlea by means of an electrode introduced through the round window. The most effective cochlear implants use multiple-frequency channels. In multichannel cochlear implants, up to 22 electrodes are inserted along the cochlear partition. The surgery for insertion of a cochlear implant is similar to mastoid surgery. The success of a cochlear implant varies widely, ranging from minimal improvement in auditory awareness to the ability to understand speech on the telephone.

TEMPORAL BONE STIMULATORS (BONE HEARING DEVICES). In some cases of hearing loss, sound can be transmitted by applying a stimulation directly to the temporal bone, thereby transmitting sound through the skull to the inner ear. For clients with a conductive hearing loss, a device is available in which the receiver is implanted under the skin into the skull. The external device transmits the sound through the skin. This device is worn above the ear rather than in the ear canal. Because some conductive hearing losses cannot be surgically repaired, the temporal bone stimulator may provide an alternative rehabilitative method to conventional hearing aids. It is not widely used at the present time.

MIDDLE EAR IMPLANTS (SEMI-IMPLANTABLE DEVICE). A variety of implantable devices are being evaluated for sound amplification. However, many challenges have to be met before a workable device is available. This method of hearing aid technology is still in the research stage.

OTALGIA

Otalgia is defined as pain in the ear, or earache. Otalgia can be primary in origin (i.e., coming from a disorder in

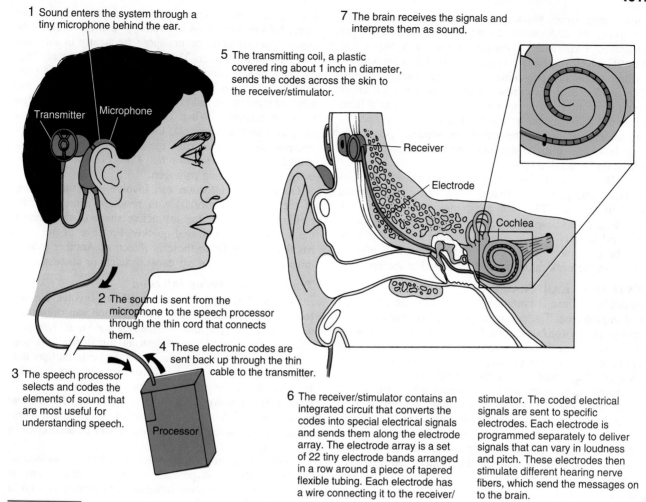

1 Sound enters the system through a tiny microphone behind the ear.

7 The brain receives the signals and interprets them as sound.

5 The transmitting coil, a plastic covered ring about 1 inch in diameter, sends the codes across the skin to the receiver/stimulator.

Transmitter   Microphone

Receiver

Electrode

Cochlea

2 The sound is sent from the microphone to the speech processor through the thin cord that connects them.

4 These electronic codes are sent back up through the thin cable to the transmitter.

3 The speech processor selects and codes the elements of sound that are most useful for understanding speech.

Processor

6 The receiver/stimulator contains an integrated circuit that converts the codes into special electrical signals and sends them along the electrode array. The electrode array is a set of 22 tiny electrode bands arranged in a row around a piece of tapered flexible tubing. Each electrode has a wire connecting it to the receiver/ stimulator. The coded electrical signals are sent to specific electrodes. Each electrode is programmed separately to deliver signals that can vary in loudness and pitch. These electrodes then stimulate different hearing nerve fibers, which send the messages on to the brain.

FIGURE 66–3 Cochlear implant to restore hearing.

the ear) infectious, or referred (i.e., coming from a disorder outside the ear). Otalgia from ear pain can be the result of infection in the external or middle ear or of trauma to the ear and head. Referred otalgia can be caused by disorders in the temporomandibular joint (TMJ), cranial nerves, face, scalp, pharynx, tonsils, thyroid, trachea, teeth, or cervical muscles.

Etiology and Risk Factors

Otalgia can be related to infectious processes in the external ear and middle ear. Bacterial contaminants can enter the ear through insertion of unclean articles, such as fingers or toys. Insertion of any sharp objects into the ear canal can traumatize the skin and provide an open medium for infection. Instillation of contaminated solutions into the ear or swimming in polluted water raises the risk for development of ear infection and inflammation. Clients with recent upper respiratory infections, eustachian tube dysfunction, and allergies are also at increased risk for ear infections.

Infectious and neoplastic processes of the pharynx can also cause referred otalgia. It is not uncommon for patients with acute tonsillitis to complain of significant ear pain, even though the ears may be normal on examina-

tion. Otalgia following tonsillectomy is universal and is not a manifestation of infection. In clients with unilateral otalgia and a history of smoking, consideration must be given to a neoplastic process of the lateral pharynx, especially if there are concurrent manifestations, such as hoarseness or dysphagia. Examination of the lower pharynx by means of a fiberoptic endoscope is necessary in the smoker with persistent hoarseness, and referral to an otolaryngologist is indicated.

Trauma to the head, temporal bone, and ear can also result in ear pain. Engaging in contact sports without protective headgear can result in severe trauma to the head, injuring the hearing apparatus. A blow to the ear by an object such as a ball or hand can cause local or diffuse pain in the area. Noise trauma from a blast or loud noise may create a ringing sensation that is perceived as painful and uncomfortable. Nerve damage may be accompanied by an intolerance to even soft sounds, resulting in severe pain. Exposure to extremely hot or cold temperatures can lead to burns or severe frostbite, respectively, of the external ear.

Blockage of the eustachian tube and otalgia can be the result of enlarged adenoid tissue and tonsils in children, middle ear infections often associated with upper respiratory infections, and *barotrauma* (pressure injury to the middle ear). Acute blockage from altitude changes caused by flying or underwater diving will cause middle ear problems. Hyperbaric oxygen treatments can also cause barotrauma. Hyperbaric oxygen treatment is common for carbon monoxide poisoning as well as other disorders. The incidence of barotrauma is increased when an upper respiratory infection is present. *Aerotitis media* is a form of serous otitis media in which fluid or air is trapped in the middle ear during descent in an airplane. Any long-term blockage of the eustachian tube leads to serous otitis media and a hearing loss.

TMJ pain, mouth and gum pain, cervical muscle tenderness, and pain from dental work can cause referred pain to the ear. TMJ arthralgia may result from teeth grinding, gum chewing, excessive talking, or biting down on hard objects. The resultant inflammation to this joint can be perceived by the client as an earache. Similarly, stress on the neck muscles can be referred to the ear.

EXTERNAL EAR TRAUMA

Auricular trauma is common because ears are prominent and unprotected. The pinna is subject to lacerations, blunt injury, abrasions, burns, and frostbite. A special concern with ear trauma is that a hematoma can quickly develop between the skin and cartilage (called *perichondrial hematoma*). The hematoma exerts pressure on the cartilage, impairing its healing. Such hematomas are common after blunt injuries such as occur in wrestling, fighting, or boxing and are responsible for so-called cauliflower ear.

People can often avoid ear trauma by wearing headgear for contact sports, wide-brimmed hats in the summer, and earmuffs or hats in the winter; heavy pierced earrings should not be worn because they can lacerate the lobule.

FOREIGN BODIES

Surprisingly, a wide array of foreign bodies fit into the ear canal. The most common foreign body found in the adult ear is either a piece of cotton or, most annoying, an insect.

Ear pain from obstruction usually results from the buildup of matter in the ear canal, which leads to pressure and pain. Clients may also report decreased hearing, a sense of fullness, a throbbing sensation, and itching. The onset, duration, frequency, and intensity of manifestations should be noted.

EUSTACHIAN TUBE DISORDERS

Because the eustachian tube connects the middle ear to the nasopharynx, pharyngeal disorders also cause eustachian tube dysfunction and, thus, secondary middle ear problems. For example, a common disorder is blockage of the eustachian tube by enlarged adenoid tissue in children. In adults, swelling of the mucosa in the eustachian tube during an upper respiratory infection can lead to serous otitis media (see later). For persistent unilateral blocked eustachian tube, a malignant tumor must be ruled out as the cause.

EAR INFECTIONS

Otitis Externa

The most common problems found in the external ear are infections, primarily bacterial or fungal. The most frequent infection, called *external otitis,* involves the external ear canal. Infection begins when the protective waxy coating has been damaged by dryness, moisture, or treatment. Infection can lead to edema, which can occlude the canal. External otitis occurs more frequently in the summer than in the winter. The most common form of external otitis is also called *swimmer's ear,* because it is prevalent in clients in whom water remains in the ear canal after swimming. In addition, opportunistic fungal infections are common. When a debilitating systemic disease such as diabetes is present, the external otitis can spread aggressively through cartilage and bone and is then named *malignant external otitis; Pseudomonas aeruginosa* is the usual offending pathogen.

Occasionally, infection can involve only the cartilage of the pinna (chondritis), with resultant necrosis of the cartilage and loss of the distinctive shape of the pinna if the infection is not treated quickly. Frostbite of the pinna has findings similar to those of infection. Another form of infection is seen as an ear canal furuncle or abscess.

Tympanic Membrane Infection

Infections of the external ear canal can involve the surface of the tympanic membrane. Infection can cause hard deposits in the tympanic membrane, known as *tympanosclerosis* (see discussion of hearing impairment). A specific infection of the tympanic membrane is bullous myringitis. This inflammatory disease forms blisters or bullae between the layers of the eardrum, which are extremely painful. It is usually caused by the bacterium *Mycoplasma pneumoniae.* Holes or perforations of the tympanic membrane can be caused by infection and can be accompanied by drainage.

Tympanic membrane disorders can lead to perforation of the membrane. A perforation may be either acute, as seen in trauma and acute infection, or chronic, as seen in repeated infection. An acute perforation has a better chance of healing spontaneously than does a chronic perforation.

Otitis Media

Otitis media is the most prevalent disorder of the middle ear. It is most common in children, but it does occur in adults. When an infection is sudden in onset and short in duration, the diagnosis is acute suppurative otitis media. When the infection is repeated, usually causing drainage and perforation, the problem is chronic otitis media. Chronic otitis media is often due to gram-negative organisms, such as *Pseudomonas, Staphylococcus,* and *Klebsiella.* Anaerobes such as *Bacteroides* have also been identified in culture analysis of specimens from the ear. Infection can cause swelling of the mucosa throughout the middle ear and eustachian tube. At times, *serous otitis media* is found in conjunction with upper respiratory infections or allergies.

Chronic otitis media can lead to tympanic membrane retraction, adhesive otitis media, or necrosis of the tympanic membrane (perforations) or of the ossicles. Both problems create a conductive hearing loss. Necrosis of the bone covering of the facial nerve may cause facial paralysis. Because of the anatomy of the temporal bone, middle ear infection can also lead to brain abscesses that are life-threatening if not treated properly. Cholesteatoma, another complication, is discussed later.

Subsequent to infectious otitis media or allergic disease, fluid may form in the middle ear, known as serous otitis media. This fluid is formed when a vacuum develops in the middle ear, caused by a blocked eustachian tube. When the swelling subsides, the fluid may be too thick to drain. Tympanometry is a useful diagnostic assessment to distinguish a normal ear from one with a middle ear effusion.

Mastoiditis

The mastoid system is a series of air cells contained within the temporal bone that communicate with the middle ear. Before the discovery of antibiotics, a mastoid infection was a life-threatening event. Now, acute mastoiditis is very rare, although chronic mastoiditis does sometimes occur. With repeated middle ear infections, the mastoid cavity becomes a significant part of the problem, increasing the amount of drainage. A chronic infection also leads to the development of cholesteatoma (see later).

Drainage from the mastoid cavity via the ear canal is the most likely sign to appear. The drainage courses through the middle ear and out the tympanic membrane through a perforation. Tenderness over the mastoid cavity behind the ear points to an infection but usually is caused by an acute exacerbation of chronic mastoiditis rather than an acute mastoiditis. The protrusion of the pinna as a result of swelling over the mastoid may be part of this process.

Cholesteatoma

Cholesteatoma is a cyst in the middle ear or mastoid system that is lined with squamous epithelium and filled with keratin debris. Often, infection is present in the mass of the cholesteatoma. Although cholesterol granules can be present in the specimen, yielding the term cholesteatoma, they are not the primary pathologic process.

Cholesteatoma most often results from chronic otitis media or marginal perforation of the tympanic membrane. Clients have conductive hearing loss and foul-smelling discharge from the ears. Although it is a benign growth, the cholesteatoma causes erosion of the surrounding structures, leading to other problems, such as brain abscesses, vertigo, and facial paralysis. Fortunately, these complications are uncommon.

OTHER MASSES

Benign masses of the external ear canal are usually cysts that arise from a sebaceous gland or, more rarely, from the cerumen glands. Cysts can also be congenital in nature. Bony protrusions seen in the bony portion of the ear canal are called *exostoses*. The skin covering an exostosis is normal. If the skin is red, the mass is usually an abscess. Infectious polyps found in the ear canal arise from either the tympanic membrane or, more commonly, the middle ear, through a hole in the tympanic membrane.

Malignant tumors are also found in the external ear. The cutaneous carcinomas are most often basal cell carcinoma on the pinna and squamous cell carcinoma in the ear canal. If not treated, the carcinomas can invade underlying structures; squamous cell carcinoma may spread throughout the temporal bone. Rare tumors of the cerumen glands are of the adenoma cell type. Masses of the external ear are diagnosed through physical examination and biopsy to rule out malignancy. Surgical excision may be required.

Both benign and malignant tumors can involve the tympanic membrane, but they seldom arise from it. However, an infectious glandular polyp can be isolated to the tympanic membrane. Tumors in the middle ear can be seen through or may protrude through the tympanic membrane.

The most common benign growth in the middle ear is an infectious polyp. A facial nerve neuroma is found along the course of the facial nerve. Malignant tumors involving the middle ear can be primary or secondary.

The same tumors that arise in the middle ear can be found in the mastoid cavity. Because the mastoid cavity is connected to other air cells throughout the temporal bone and is close to the brain, malignant tumors at this location carry a poor prognosis.

Pathophysiology

Otalgia related to a problem in the ear is usually the result of an inflammatory process that can be caused by trauma or infection. Inflammation causes chemical mediators to be released into the tissue and the chemotaxis of leukocytes to the damaged area, resulting in tissue edema, pain, heat, and redness. This inflammatory process results in swelling of tissue that impinges on nerve endings and surrounding areas, causing the otalgia. Masses such as tumors grow and press on nearby tissue and nerves, causing pain. Sometimes, the infection or mass erodes into tissue and bone as in cholesteatoma and causes further inflammation and pain.

Otalgia can also be caused by referred pain to the ear. In conditions such as TMJ or cervical adenopathy, the pain does not originate in the ear. However, the neuronal pain pathways for these processes cross over and are perceived in the ear. Although the perception of pain in the ear is real, the cause of the pain is not related to a pathologic process in that area.

Clinical Manifestations

In the case of head trauma and damage to the tympanic membrane, clients often report an episode of brief but intense otalgia. Blunt injury to the auricle can result in a blue or reddish purple, tense swelling over the pinna. Perichondrial hematomas can develop and, left untreated, form a hypertrophic scar known as a cauliflower ear, which is an occupational hazard for boxers. However, if the tympanic membrane is ruptured from barotrauma or otitis media, the client often notes a sudden *relief of pressure and pain*. Pain is not usually elicited on palpation of the external ear; this phenomenon usually provides a differential diagnosis between problems of the external ear and middle ear. Disorders involving the tympanic membrane are painful, perhaps the most painful of all middle ear disorders. Hearing loss may be noted but is often reversible.

Ear pain from obstruction usually results from the buildup of matter in the ear canal, which leads to pressure and pain. Clients may also report decreased hearing, a sense of fullness, a throbbing sensation, and itching. The onset, duration, frequency, and intensity of manifestations should be noted.

Pain in the external ear is the most common clinical

manifestation of infection. Pain ranges from mild to severe and is generally unilateral. Pain is more intense when the ear canal is swollen. Painful sites are tender because of the close proximity of bone (a hard surface) when the ear is palpated. A clue to early external otitis is tenderness when the pinna is gently pulled on, in contrast to otitis media, in which touching the ear does not cause pain. A forerunner of pain in external otitis is itching in the ear canal. Inflammation (redness) is easily identified with an otoscope. At different stages of infection, drainage will be found from the ear canal. In early infectious disorders, the drainage may be clear rather than discolored by pus.

Manifestations of otitis media include ear pain and an immobile tympanic membrane. Because the tympanic membrane is a semitransparent membrane, what lies beneath it is visible. It can also become discolored or displaced. Therefore, both fluid and infection can be seen in the middle ear. The tympanic membrane may be dull or red instead of the normal pearly gray. The eardrum may be normal, perforated, infected, retracted, or bulging, according to the disease process involved.

In addition, the client may report bubbling, crackling, or popping sensations in the ear, especially during swallowing. There is a sense of fullness in the ear and conductive hearing loss that fluctuates.

Suppurative otitis media is invasion of the middle ear by virulent organisms and formation of pus, often accompanied by purulent *otorrhea* (drainage). Clinical manifestations include intense ear pain, fever, mild to moderate conductive hearing loss, thickened and bulging tympanic membrane, and occasional dizziness.

Outcome Management

■ Medical Management

The goals of medical management are to (1) promote healing, (2) alleviate pain, and (3) restore normal function of the ears.

PROMOTE HEALING

EAR IRRIGATION. The ear is commonly irrigated to cleanse the external auditory canal or to remove impacted wax, debris, or foreign bodies in order to promote healing. Irrigation is not used in clients with a history or clinical suspicion of perforated eardrum. Ear irrigation is performed as follows.

Warm the irrigating solution (usually water) to body temperature, and place it in the irrigating syringe. Protect the client's clothes with a plastic drape, and place a kidney-shaped basin below the ear to catch the irrigating solution. Have the client sit with the ear to be irrigated toward you and the head tilted toward the other ear. In the adult, pull the external ear upward and backward (or in children pull external ear directly back) and direct the tip of the syringe along the upper wall of the ear canal (Fig. 66–4). The canal should not be completely obstructed by the syringe to allow the back-flow of solution.

Sometimes the client is instructed to use a medicinal ear irrigation solution. The most common solution for ear irrigation is boric acid and alcohol, which is obtained by prescription. This solution cleanses the ear of debris and infection and provides a drying agent. A 2- or 3-oz ear

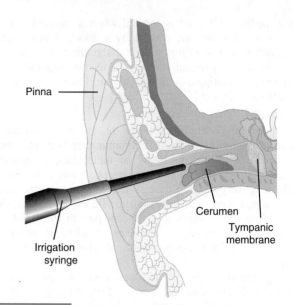

FIGURE 66–4 Ear irrigation. The tip of the syringe is directed along the upper wall of the ear canal.

syringe is needed for irrigation. A family member performs the irrigation for the client. Usually, the ear irrigation is followed by the use of eardrops.

When charting the ear irrigation, include the type of irrigation solution used and the nature of returned solution, regarding amount, texture, color of cerumen, and type of debris. In addition, instruct the client to report pain, vertigo, or nausea during the procedure.

ANTIBIOTICS. Local and systemic antibiotics are the cornerstone of preventing and managing infectious processes. However, the first rule of treating infection is meticulous cleaning of the site so that the local antibiotic can reach the infected area. Suction, irrigation, or manual removal of matter with a cotton-tipped swab can be used. Regular application of antibiotic-steroid eardrops for a week is required.

If the ear canal is swollen shut, a wick must be inserted to allow the drops to penetrate the canal. Eardrops are placed directly on the wick. Commercially prepared wicks or single pieces of ¼-inch gauze can be used. The wick serves not only as a bandage but also as an excellent vehicle to medicate the ear canal. The wick is gently inserted into the ear canal by means of forceps while the external ear is gently pulled upward and backward. The wick is usually slightly less than 1 inch in length (Fig. 66–5). The client should lie on the unaffected side for 3 to 5 minutes to allow gravity to promote movement of the medication into the ear canal. If the infection is generalized or severe, systemic antibiotics are used. An infection that involves cartilage has to be treated aggressively and quickly with systemic antibiotics to avoid complications.

With any form of otitis media, appropriate antibiotic therapy may be necessary. If drainage is present, a specimen may be collected for culture analysis and sensitivity testing. However, most episodes of acute otitis media do not produce drainage, and the specific bacterial cause need not be identified. Otitis media is generally a very easily managed disease, but if it is not treated properly, it

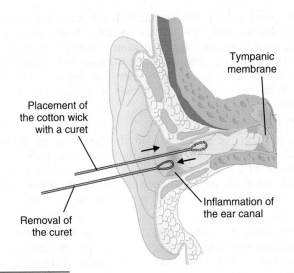

FIGURE 66–5 Administration of antibiotics for otitis externa. A curet with a cotton wick around it is placed into the ear canal. The wick is gently placed into the canal, and an antibiotic or treatment solution is added to the wick.

can lead to sinusitis, meningitis, and brain abscess because of the proximity of the ear to other tissues.

Suppurative otitis media is managed with systemic antibiotics, topical antibiotic drops, and analgesics. If otitis media becomes chronic, myringotomy may be required to ventilate the middle ear and equalize pressure between the middle ear and external ear. Because infection starts in the middle ear, the problems in the mastoid cavity are avoided by early use of antibiotics with otitis media.

ALLEVIATE PAIN

Because external otitis is one of the most painful disorders of the ear, appropriate analgesics are required. Pain persists for 24 to 48 hours after treatment is initiated. Once the swelling and drainage are reduced by treatment, in about 48 hours, the pain subsides.

RESTORE NORMAL FUNCTION AND REMOVE FOREIGN BODIES

Removal of foreign bodies from the ear canal can be quite difficult. The external auditory canal is an exquisitely sensitive, elliptical, cylinder-like structure. In adults, it is about 24 mm long and has two anatomic points of narrowing. Objects caught behind these narrow points create the greatest problems for removal. If perforation of the tympanic membrane is deemed unlikely and the object is not tightly wedged, you can irrigate the external canal with warm water. Direct the stream of water superiorly and anteriorly into the ear canal and around the object (see Fig. 66–4). Water pressure builds up and forces the object outward. It often takes about 200 to 300 ml of water to remove an object. Do not irrigate vegetable foreign proteins, such as beans, because they would swell and become even more difficult to remove.

For removal of a live insect, the ear canal is filled with mineral oil, lidocaine, or an ether-soaked cotton ball, *not water,* to kill or stupefy the insect. Water would cause the insect to swell and become more difficult to remove.

The least traumatic method of removing a foreign body is with the aid of an operating microscope. The

nurse should not spend a long time attempting to remove an object from the ear without asking for help. After removing the object, inspect the tympanic membrane and ear canal for manifestations of trauma. If trauma is noted, the client should be treated for external otitis and seen again in 4 to 5 days.

◼ Nursing Management of the Medical Client

ASSESSMENT

When obtaining the history of the pain, ask the client about what events have triggered the ear pain, paying special attention to a recent history of:

- Upper respiratory tract infection
- Travel by airplane
- Exposure to very loud noises
- Trauma to the head
- Stressors that lead to teeth grinding or dental work

The nurse first observes the external ear for redness, swelling, lumps, scaling, crusting, or drainage, either serous or purulent. During assessment of the external ear, manipulation of the ear is important. If the client complains of pain when any part of the ear is palpated, an abscess, a lesion, or some kind of inflammatory process of the ear canal is suspected. If an otoscopic examination is performed, care must be taken not to cause the client unnecessary pain. An abscess may be close to the opening of the canal, where the pressure of the speculum may cause greater pain.

During physical examination, determine the presence of pain with swallowing, neck rotation, palpation of the face and head (over the sinuses), palpation of the mastoid process, and manipulation of the pinna. Assess the TMJ by inserting your index fingers into the external auditory canals and applying pressure anteriorly while the client opens and closes the mouth. TMJ syndrome may cause pain, clicking, or crepitation of the joint during movement.

DIAGNOSIS, OUTCOMES, INTERVENTIONS

Altered Protection. Because of tissue damage from trauma, foreign body, or pathogen, the nursing diagnosis *Altered Protection related to tissue destruction* may be appropriate in the client with otalgia.

Outcomes. The client will not develop an infectious process or will experience resolution of infection without complications.

Interventions. Monitor for clinical manifestations of infection, and administer antibiotics as prescribed. Other medications, such as antihistamines, decongestants, and steroid nasal sprays, may be ordered to reduce inflammation that can damage tissue. Teach the client to complete the entire prescription of the antibiotic even though manifestations may have cleared (see the Client Education Guide).

During an infectious process, instruct the client to avoid getting water in the ear while bathing or showering by using earplugs or placing cotton balls coated with petroleum jelly in the ear canal.

Eardrops may also be prescribed for bacterial or fungal infections, which are often seen in otitis externa. Various irrigations of the mastoid system and middle ear are used for chronic infections along with antibiotic eardrops or powders. In chronic otitis media with discharge, both broad-spectrum oral antibiotics and topical antibiotic drops are used.

Pain. Otalgia may be caused by a process in the ear or may be referred from a source outside the ear, resulting in the nursing diagnosis *Pain related to inflammation in the external or middle ear or from referred pain in the head and neck area.*

Outcomes. The client will be able to relieve pain and achieve an acceptable comfort level.

Interventions. Otalgia is managed by treating the primary problem. Comfort can be promoted by using anesthetic ear solutions or systemic analgesics. After the physician has prescribed the analgesic therapy, instruct the client as to the amount, frequency, and duration. Other measures are application of heat by warm compress, a soft diet, a quiet environment, and positioning of the client with the affected ear down.

The client with TMJ syndrome should avoid chewing and hyperextension of the jaw (e.g., for dental examination and care). He or she should also try to stop grinding the teeth. A specially fitted mouth guard to be worn while sleeping can be helpful in preventing teeth grinding at night.

In the case of eustachian tube dysfunction or barotrauma, teach the client how to facilitate opening of the eustachian tube. Chewing gum, sucking hard candy and swallowing often, yawning, and blowing air out against closed nostrils (Valsalva maneuver) help open the tube.

EVALUATION

The positive outcome for the client with otalgia depends on (1) the thoroughness of the instructions provided by the nurse and (2) the client's compliance with the prescribed treatment regimen. Ongoing assessment of the client to achieve resolution of infectious and inflammatory processes contributing to the otalgia are key to effective management.

Surgical Management

The surgical treatment of infections involves incision and drainage in the acute phase for abscesses and, at times,

for perichondritis. Perichondrial hematomas are incised and drained and then dressed in large bulky dressings. The most common surgical treatment is excision of cysts and cutaneous carcinomas. For conditions that occlude the ear canal, more extensive surgery that involves removal of bone and skin grafting, known as a *canaloplasty,* is performed.

MYRINGOPLASTY

Surgery can be performed on the tympanic membrane with use of an operating microscope for magnification. Closure of a simple perforation is called a *myringoplasty.* If the tympanic membrane needs to be reconstructed, temporalis fascia or other connective tissue can be used.

TYMPANOPLASTY

Tympanoplasty is the surgical correction of a perforated tympanic membrane. There are four types of corrections based on medial position of the placement of the graft, as follows:

Type I: Graft rests on malleus
Type II: Graft rests on incus
Type III: Graft attaches to head of stapes
Type IV: Graft attaches to footplate of stapes

When the eustachian tube is stable, postoperative hearing results worsen as one proceeds from type I to type IV tympanoplasty. Under favorable conditions, type I tympanoplasty should result in normal or near-normal restoration of conductive hearing loss, whereas type IV should result in approximately a 30-db air-bone gap. In tympanoplasty, a graft is placed to restore the damaged tympanic membrane. The location of the graft depends on the original defect. Sometimes tympanostomy (ventilation) tubes are inserted.

OSSICULOPLASTY

The surgical procedure of ossicular reconstruction is called *ossiculoplasty.* Various methods of repositioning these tiny ear bones are now in use. In addition, various synthetic prostheses have been used to reconnect the ossicles to carry sound. In an attempt to prevent extrusion of the prostheses, tissue is combined with the prostheses to rebuild the ossicles. This semibiologic method is used in different forms by most otologic surgeons (Fig. 66–6).

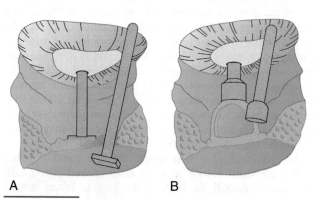

A   **B**

FIGURE 66–6 Middle ear prostheses used for reconstruction. *A,* Ossicle columella prosthesis (total ossicular replacement). *B,* Ossicle cup prosthesis (partial ossicular replacement). (Courtesy of Arnold G. Shuring, M.D.)

Laser surgery can be performed in chronic ear disease for a cholesteatoma associated with the stapes.

MYRINGOTOMY

An incision into the tympanic membrane through which fluid is removed by suction is called *myringotomy*. To keep the incision open and to prevent a recurrence of fluid, various types of transtympanic tubes can be inserted into the incision. These tubes extrude by themselves in 3 to 12 months and rarely have to be removed. More permanent tubes (T tubes) with larger flanges may be used for clients who require repeated myringotomies.

MASTOIDECTOMY

Radical mastoidectomy removes the contents of the mastoid bone for control of infection and cholesteatoma. However, because the radical mastoidectomy sacrificed hearing, a modified radical mastoidectomy was developed to save the remaining middle ear structures. With the advent of antibiotics, simple mastoidectomy became possible, which maintained a normal-appearing ear canal. Because radical and modified mastoidectomies exteriorize the mastoid cavity to the external ear canal, they are known as *open* or *canal wall–down mastoidectomies*. *Closed* or *canal wall–up mastoidectomies* are simple mastoidectomies with modifications that are performed in conjunction with tympanoplasty and ossiculoplasty to retain or regain hearing. Today, even the open mastoidectomy is performed with various tympanoplasties.

■ Nursing Management of the Surgical Client

PREOPERATIVE CARE

The scope of nursing activities for the client undergoing surgery for otalgia can be as broad as a preoperative assessment performed in an office or clinic or as limited as an assessment performed in the holding area of the surgical suite. Before surgery, an audiogram and tympanogram are obtained to assess preoperative hearing acuity. The client's level of knowledge about the procedure, expectations, and mental readiness for surgery are evaluated along with the physiologic status.

The client undergoing ear surgery should be told what to expect during the procedure, because local anesthesia with sedation is often used. Instructions should be given about the duration of the procedure, the estimated length of hospital stay, and immediate postoperative instructions. Very often, fear of the unknown can be decreased by an understanding of the events that will occur.

POSTOPERATIVE CARE

Pain is not usually a major problem, but mild analgesia may be required. Vertigo or lightheadedness may occur when the client ambulates for the first time. Clients should be supervised when ambulating on the day of surgery to protect them from falling. Some clients who are quite vertiginous exhibit nystagmus (see Chapter 64) from stimulation of the inner ear. The vertigo usually passes very quickly and seldom requires medication.

The ear rarely bleeds after surgery. A small amount of serosanguineous drainage on a cotton ball is expected. After most ear procedures, only a cotton ball is needed in the ear, although a dressing over the ear may be necessary after tympanomastoidectomy. The Client Education

Guide lists precautions that the client should be aware of after ear surgery.

Immediate postoperative instructions may include the following:

1. Positioning should be specified, such as the client lying with operated ear up for several hours after surgery.
2. If necessary, the client should blow the nose gently one side at a time.
3. The client should sneeze or cough with the mouth open.
4. Participation in water sports or activities is prohibited.

Normal occurrences in the initial period after ear surgery may include the following:

- Decreased hearing in operated ear from surgical packing (people may sound like they are talking in a barrel)
- Noises in the ear, such as cracking or popping
- Minor earache and discomfort in cheek and jaw
- Ear swelling

BALANCE DISORDERS

As already described, *vertigo* is the perception that either oneself or one's surroundings are moving. The person with vertigo usually remains seated or supine to prevent falling. Vertigo is often described as "dizziness." However, dizziness, which can involve feelings of disorientation in space or lightheadedness, is different. Vertigo results from imbalance of neural signals from the vestibular system in the ears. The imbalance of signals is interpreted by the brain as constant motion in space.

Disorders of balance and coordination result from problems of the vestibular system and "righting" reflexes. Balance can also be affected by problems outside the

---

CLIENT EDUCATION GUIDE

Precautions After Ear Surgery

To prevent injury and promote healing:

- Continue to blow your nose gently one side at a time and to sneeze or cough with your mouth open for 1 week after surgery.
- Avoid physical activity for 1 week and exercises or sports for 3 weeks after surgery.
- Return to work as recommended, usually 3 to 7 days after surgery (3 weeks if work is strenuous).
- Avoid heavy lifting, especially after stapedectomy.
- Change the cotton ball in your ear daily as prescribed.
- Keep your ear dry for 4 to 6 weeks after surgery.
- Do not shampoo for 1 week after surgery.
- Protect your ear when necessary with two pieces of cotton (outer piece saturated with petroleum jelly).
- Avoid airplane flights for the first week after surgery. For sensation of ear pressure, hold your nose, close your mouth, and swallow to equalize pressure.
- Wear noise defenders in loud environments.
- Report any drainage other than a slight amount of bleeding to the physician.

vestibular system. Very few problems are more private than those involving one's sense of balance. Balance problems may be debilitating and may also cause embarrassing gait problems, which can jeopardize safety. More than 90 million Americans aged 17 years or older have experienced vertigo or a balance problem. Vertigo is second only to chronic pain as the most common symptom reported in America today.

Etiology and Risk Factors

Although vertigo and dizziness are not synonymous, they both relate to a sense of balance and equilibrium. Dizziness, vertigo, and syncope (fainting) are all manifestations of one of the following types of problems:

- Peripheral vestibular disorders (i.e., labyrinthine or inner ear)
- Central disorders (i.e., medullary, cerebellar, or cortical)
- Systemic disorders (i.e., cardiovascular or metabolic)

Peripheral vestibular disorders involve a disorder in the labyrinth or internal ear. Central disorders result from a problem in the brain or nerves, such as a tumor of the eighth cranial nerve (acoustic neuroma) or stroke. Systemic disorders begin in a nerve or organ outside the cranium (e.g., orthostatic hypotension, hypoglycemia). Examples of common causes of vertigo and dizziness, grouped by etiology, are presented in Box 66–4.

Little can be done to reduce the risk of balance disorders. Clients should be treated early for manifestations of ear problems. Clients at high risk for falling as a result of vertigo should stand up slowly to prevent injury and should keep a light on at all times to enable visual cues to lessen the disequilibrium. Finally, situations that lead to vertigo should be avoided. Motion sickness occurs normally if the provocative stimulus is present. Humans are not evolutionarily adapted to special environmental situations, such as deep-sea diving, high-speed flying, and space travel. Vertigo or dizziness may occur in these environments.

PERIPHERAL VESTIBULAR DISORDERS
Benign Paroxysmal Positional Vertigo

Benign paroxysmal positional vertigo (BPPV) is a common cause of vertigo. It tends to follow head injury and viral infections of the inner ear. BPPV is due to *cupulolithiasis,* the presence of calcium crystals in the semicircular canals. These crystals are normally deposited on small hair-like structures in the ear called otoliths, and they slow responses to head movement. When they are dislodged, head movement creates a hypersensitive response. BPPV is provoked when the head is placed in certain positions, usually hyperextended and to one side. Clinical manifestations usually consist of brief attacks of rotational vertigo, a rapid head tilt to the affected ear, and a lag time of 3 to 6 seconds between change of position and vertigo with nystagmus. It is usually self-limited and resolves spontaneously over weeks to months.

Labyrinthitis (Vestibular Neuronitis)

Labyrinthitis is infection or inflammation of the cochlear or vestibular portion of the inner ear or both. Causes are not fully understood, but the syndrome tends to occur in spring and early summer and to be preceded by an upper respiratory infection. A virus has therefore been implicated but has never been isolated. Three classic manifestations are reported: vertigo, nausea, and vomiting. There are no hearing changes. Vertigo is usually sudden in onset; it peaks in 24 to 48 hours and then gradually subsides over 1 to 2 weeks. Supportive treatment is usually given during the wait for the underlying problems to clear.

Ménière's Disease

As mentioned previously, Ménière's disease is caused by excess endolymph in the vestibular and semicircular canals. Normal vestibular activity depends on stability of fluid pressure. Ménière's disease causes hearing changes and vertigo. It is discussed under balance disorders because the vertigo is often the most troublesome manifestation in the early stages.

Ménière's disease is an episodic illness that waxes and wanes, often remaining quiescent for many years and then reappearing. A cluster of manifestations develops, consisting of (1) paroxysmal whirling vertigo, (2) fluctuating hearing loss, (3) tinnitus, and (4) aural fullness. Only one or two manifestations may be present initially. Vertigo is characterized by remission and relapses without apparent cause, although the manifestations become less severe in time. The initial attacks consist of approximately 30 minutes of intense vertigo, which commonly provokes nausea and vomiting. Remaining stationary reduces vertigo.

A sensorineural hearing loss (see hearing impairment) that may be reversible in the early stages is a serious consequence of Ménière's disease. Control of episodes of the disease is usually possible, although a cure is not yet available. Clients are treated with low-sodium diets, diuretics, and balance exercises. Surgery, which is another option, is discussed later.

BOX 66–4   **Disorders Associated with Vertigo and Dizziness**

Peripheral Labyrinthine (Inner Ear) Disorders

Benign paroxysmal positional vertigo (BPPV)
Labyrinthitis
Ménière's disease
Cholesteatoma

Central Nervous System Disorders

Cerebellar lesions
Temporal lobe lesions
Tumors of cranial nerve VIII (e.g., acoustic neuroma)
Stroke

Systemic Disorders

Diabetes
Postural hypotension
Arthritis
Hypoglycemia
Multiple sclerosis
Parkinson's disease
Allergies

CENTRAL DISORDERS OF BALANCE

Dizziness may be a manifestation of a transient ischemic attack (TIA) ("small stroke"). A temporary loss of blood flow to the brain leads to several manifestations, depending on the brain area that is not being perfused. Clients can experience momentary losses of consciousness, transient numbness, tingling, weakness, and changes in speech. TIAs should be reported and treated aggressively to prevent true ischemic changes.

SYSTEMIC DISORDERS LEADING TO VERTIGO

Physiologic Vertigo

Physiologic vertigo is involved in common disorders such as motion sickness. In these conditions, vertigo is minimal or absent, but autonomic manifestations are present. Motion sickness leads to perspiration, nausea, vomiting, increased salivation, yawning, and malaise. Physiologic vertigo can usually be suppressed by supplying sensory cues that come from other stimuli. For example, motion sickness from reading in a car can be reduced by looking out the window at the moving environment.

Presbystasis

A disorder that is recognized more and more is presbystasis, or disequilibrium of aging. Because of the generalized degenerative changes that occur in aging, balance and stability are affected. In addition to the labyrinth, balance also depends on the visual system and the proprioceptive changes in the muscles. Because all three systems are involved in aging, the elderly have difficulty with stability, which results in falls and subsequent trauma.

Orthostatic Hypotension

Orthostatic hypotension is a sudden drop in blood pressure and dizziness upon sitting or standing. The manifestations noted are lightheadedness and faintness, not vertigo, which is due to inadequate cerebral blood flow. The elderly are at high risk of orthostatic hypotension because of atherosclerosis and the use of medications that lead to diuresis or hypotension (e.g., furosemide, calcium-channel blockers). Orthostasis is diagnosed through assessment of positional blood pressure changes. Clients should be taught to change position slowly, and medications may require adjustment if blood pressure is too low.

Pathophysiology

The body maintains balance and equilibrium by responding to an intricate network of information. The ability to maintain balance depends on the intactness of four systems:

- Vestibular system (the labyrinth or inner ear)
- Visual system (the eyes)
- Proprioceptive system (the somatosensory nerves of joints and muscles)
- Cerebellar system (the coordinator)

The sensations transmitted from the ears, the eyes, and the somatosensory nerves are integrated in the brain stem and cerebellum and perceived in the cerebral cortex. Gradual interference of vestibular input causes compensatory changes that allow the brain to adjust slowly. Quick changes demand more adjustments than can be made. Infections can destroy the nerve and alter transmission of messages. Overproduction of endolymph can slow transmission of messages and lead to the perception that the body is in constant motion. Head trauma can shake free calcium carbonate crystals on the utricular macule and alter endolymph movement.

Clinical Manifestations

Vertigo is the most common clinical manifestation in a client with a balance problem. The clinical manifestations of balance disorders vary widely depending on (1) the cause, (2) the location (one or both ears), (3) the client's age at onset, (4) the extent of the loss of vestibular function, and (5) the rapidity with which damage occurs. Disease in the external ear, middle ear, and inner ear usually leads to vertigo that is sudden, transient, and accompanied by vagal manifestations (e.g., nausea, vomiting, sweating, and pallor). The vertigo that is associated with cerebrovascular lesions does not follow a pattern; however, tinnitus and hearing loss are usually not present.

An important differentiation is whether the vertigo is associated with hearing loss. The close anatomic relationship between the balance and hearing systems sometimes causes the sensation of vertigo in conjunction with a hearing loss. However, in most instances, vertigo is present without a hearing loss. It is also important to distinguish between vertigo from vestibular problems and other forms of vertigo. Table 66-2 differentiates the two forms of vertigo.

Dizziness is described by clients in such varied terms that it is almost impossible to define. Not all the terms listed here suggest true vertigo. The nurse should record

TABLE 66-2	VESTIBULAR AND NONVESTIBULAR VERTIGO	
	Vestibular	**Nonvestibular**
Common descriptions	Spinning (environment moves), on a merry-go-round	Lightheadedness, feeling of being dissociated from body, swimming, giddiness, spinning inside (environment stationary)
Clinical manifestations	Drunkenness, tilting, motion sickness, off-balance	
Course of illness	Episodic	Constant
Precipitating factors	Head movement, position change	Stress, hyperventilation, cardiac dysrhythmia, orthostatic hypotension
Associated manifestations	Nausea, vomiting, tinnitus, hearing loss, impaired vision, unsteadiness	Perspiration, pallor, paresthesias, palpitations, syncope, difficulty concentrating, tension headache; anxiety

the terms or description the client uses to help find the actual cause. Clinical manifestations include, but are not limited to:

- Staggering
- Giddiness
- Lightheadedness
- Disorientation
- Visual blurring
- Veering in one direction while walking
- Unsteadiness
- Reeling
- Faintness
- Wooziness
- Shakiness
- Instability
- Wobbliness
- Bewilderment
- Confusion
- Being dazed
- Clumsiness
- Sense of floating
- Sense of falling
- Weakness
- Vague feeling of uncertainty

Even after the vertigo has abated, anxiety tends to persist. Clients are very worried about having another "attack."

For the client with vertigo, the differential diagnosis may be accomplished by means of a thorough medical assessment, including audiometry, vestibular tests, imaging evaluation, and, sometimes, laboratory studies. Clients who have had vertigo may become quite anxious when they think about experiencing it again. Because vertigo is only a clinical manifestation, the diagnosis and treatment of the underlying disease are important. Unlike with vision or hearing problems, no single organ is responsible for balance problems. Therefore, the diagnosis, treatment, and rehabilitation of the client with a balance problem can be difficult as well as frustrating.

Outcome Management

▨ Medical Management

Two main treatment goals guide the medical management of the client with vertigo. They are (1) suppression of the CNS and the vestibular system and (2) vestibular rehabilitation.

SUPPRESS THE CENTRAL NERVOUS SYSTEM AND VESTIBULAR SYSTEM
Treatment of acute vertigo involves several medicines, which are called antivertigo agents. These medicines tend to suppress the balance system or the CNS, allowing recovery over time. They should be used judiciously in clients with BPPV because they slow recovery of function. Other medicines used for specific disorders are antibiotics, steroids, diuretics, tranquilizers, and vitamins.

PROMOTE VESTIBULAR REHABILITATION
Vestibular rehabilitation is a recognized form of control for vertigo. Because the balance system can compensate,

head and total body exercises are performed by the client to hasten compensation. Usually, physical therapists are involved in structuring this treatment. Vestibular rehabilitation uses all three organ systems that provide balance.

The exercises included in vestibular rehabilitation are performed as follows:

1. While lying in bed, slowly then quickly turn the eyes up, down, and from side to side, and the head forward, backward, and from side to side.
2. Perform the same exercises while sitting; in addition, bend forward and pick up objects from the ground.
3. While standing, perform the previously mentioned exercises; in addition, change from sitting to standing position with the eyes open and then closed, and turn around in between (i.e., change direction as well as position with eyes open and closed).
4. While moving about, walk up and down steps with the eyes open and then closed, or play games involving stooping and stretching, such as basketball.

It is believed that when vertigo is induced by these exercises, a tolerance for it is acquired. Clients should perform these exercises from the time of the acute attack and continue until they are free of manifestations for two consecutive days. Driving a car safely needs to be addressed with clients who have vertigo.

A specific intervention strategy that is currently being utilized involves a series of manipulative interventions known as the *Epley maneuvers*. These maneuvers, which are used specifically for BPPV, are designed to facilitate return of dislodged otoliths to their more normal position within the labyrinth. The Epley maneuvers are essentially a more direct, rapid method to restore normal function and are of variable efficacy.

▨ Nursing Management of the Medical Client
ASSESSMENT
Nursing assessment of the client with a balance problem should consist of the following areas:

1. A client interview to obtain a health history and specific information about the onset and characteristics of the balance problem and associated hearing problems. Attempt to distinguish the type of vertigo reported, and note aggravating conditions (e.g., head movement).
2. An interview with a family member to determine the effects of the client's balance problem on others.
3. Assessment of the effect of the vertigo on the client's performance of the activities of daily living.

The importance of the history and interview cannot be overemphasized. An adequate description of vertigo should include information about the onset, exacerbating and alleviating factors, associated clinical manifestations, and predisposing factors in the medical history, as previously described. All clients bring some degree of anxiety regarding this illness to the examina-

A. When you are dizzy, do you experience any of the following sensations? Please read the entire list first. Then circle the numbers of those sensations that describe what you experience most accurately.
  1. Lightheadedness
  2. Tendency to lose balance or to fall
  3. Objects spinning or turning around you
  4. Sensation that you are turning
  5. Headache
  6. Nausea or vomiting
  7. Pressure in the head
B. Please fill in the blank spaces.
  1. When did the dizziness first occur? _____
  2. Is your vertigo constant? _____
  3. Does it come in attacks? _____
  4. How often do attacks occur? _____
  5. How long are the attacks? _____
  6. Does vertigo occur only in certain positions? _____

     When upright? _____
     When lying flat? _____
     Turning to the right? _____
     Turning to the left? _____
  7. Have you ever stumbled or fallen because of vertigo? _____
  8. Do you know of anything that will stop the vertigo or make it better? _____

     Make your vertigo worse? _____

     Bring on an attack? _____

  9. Did you ever injure your head? _____
  10. Do you take any medications regularly (e.g., tranquilizers; oral contraceptives; barbiturates; a course of antibiotics, such as streptomycin, neomycin)?
     _____
  11. Do you use tobacco in any form? _____
     Alcohol? _____
  12. Have you worked for long in a noisy environment?
     _____
  13. Do you suffer easily from motion sickness? _____
     _____

tion. Balance problems can have devastating effects on a client's behavior. The disruption of the client's routine, the severity of the "attacks," and the fear of the unknown can make the client agitated, anxious, or depressed. The nurse must be aware of these feelings and must demonstrate self-confidence, patience, courtesy, and gentleness.

A structured questionnaire such as the one shown in Box 66-5 should be completed by the client. These questions can also be used to facilitate the interview. However, the interview should be guided by client cues. A gross assessment of the client's balance can be made by watching the client's gait. Evidence of instability may be noted if the client touches the wall or walks with a wide-based, waddling gait.

The same inspection, palpation, and otoscopic examination should be performed for the client with a balance problem as was performed for the client with hearing loss (see earlier discussion). The client must be questioned for the loss of hearing and tinnitus, which can accompany a balance problem.

DIAGNOSIS, OUTCOMES, INTERVENTIONS

Nursing care of the client with vertigo is detailed in the Care Plan.

Surgical Management

Approximately 5% or less of all clients with vertigo undergo surgical intervention.

ENDOLYMPHATIC SAC SURGERY

The endolymphatic sac procedures include decompression and various forms of shunts to the CNS or mastoid cavity. The intent of these procedures is to lessen the fluid pressure within the labyrinth and control the vertigo of Ménière's disease. Forty-four studies have been conducted over the past decade to determine the efficacy of endolymphatic sac procedures. A collective review of the results of 1800 cases of various surgical approaches to the endolymphatic sac found that 22% of clients had improved hearing, 53% had no change in hearing acuity, and 25% had worsened hearing as determined by the established guidelines. Refinement of surgical approaches and outcomes research on these techniques continues to be important.

LABYRINTHECTOMY

Labyrinthectomy is a form of surgery designed to destroy the labyrinth and eliminate its abnormal input. It is performed through the oval or round window (membranous limits of cochlear and inner ear). This is a destructive procedure that removes the membranous labyrinth, either subtotally through the oval window or totally through the mastoid bone. Any remaining hearing is sacrificed.

In a nonsurgical approach to labyrinthectomy, an ototoxic drug can be injected through the tympanic membrane into the middle ear in order to destroy the hair cells of the vestibular system. This procedure is carried out over a series of visits and is designed to decrease the abnormal vestibular signal in the affected ear. A secondary and sometimes unavoidable effect is concurrent cochlear toxicity. Clients are treated until their vestibular manifestations improve significantly, with the goal of preserving as much hearing as possible.

VESTIBULAR NERVE RESECTION

Vestibular nerve resection is a highly effective procedure performed to alleviate vertigo. Vestibular nerve resection can be performed through the labyrinth (sacrificing hearing) or around the labyrinth (saving hearing). The retrolabyrinthine surgical approach is the most common form of surgical control for vertigo today. This method preserves the inner ear structures and approaches the vestibular nerve from behind the semicircular canal. Alleviation of the client's vertigo is usually immediate. Because of the compensation by all of the other structures related to maintaining balance, a client can function with only one labyrinth.

■ THE CLIENT WITH VERTIGO

Nursing Diagnosis. Risk for Injury related to tendency to lose balance.

Outcomes. The client will reduce the risk of injury by moving slowly, remaining immobile when dizzy, and using aids for ambulation if gait and balance are unstable.

Interventions	Rationales

1. While the client is at bed rest:
  a. Encourage the client to move in bed slowly.
 	
  b. Minimize the client's head movement during acute attacks.
  c. Darken the room.
  d. Avoid startling the client to reduce reflexic head movement.
  e. Help the client with hygiene as needed while encouraging independence.
  f. Keep the side rails up and the bed in low position when the client is in bed. Place call light, phone, and personal articles within the client's reach.
 	
  g. Help with ambulation as needed.
	1. Basis for intervention:
	  a. Slow movement allows the vestibular system time to regain balance and integrate messages.
	  b. Eye and head movements often aggravate vertigo.
	  c. Darkness may help reduce acute vertigo.
	  d. The risk of vertigo caused by sudden movement is reduced.
	  e. Assistance protects the client from slipping. Complete care may be needed.
	  f. Side rails remind the client to call for help. A low bed position limits distance to the floor in case of falls from bed. Placing articles within reach decreases the client's risk of falling when reaching for articles.
	  g. Reduces risk of falls.

Evaluation. Expect this outcome to be met over several days. Look for small improvements, and encourage the client.

Nursing Diagnosis. Risk for Impaired Adjustment related to a required change in lifestyle secondary to unpredictability of vertigo.

Outcomes. The client will adjust to or modify his or her lifestyle to decrease disability and exert maximal control and independence within limits imposed by vertigo and balance disorder.

Interventions	Rationales
1. Encourage the client to identify personal strengths and roles that can still be fulfilled.	1. Encouragement fosters positive self-esteem.
2. Encourage the client to talk about feelings, personal perception of danger, and perception of his or her own coping skills and limitations.	2. Allows nurse to provide individualized support.
3. Encourage the client to make decisions and assume responsibility for self-care.	3. Personal responsibility helps the client to maintain a sense of control.
4. Provide information about vertigo and how to prepare for attacks.	4. Education promotes a problem-solving approach to managing the disorder.
5. Encourage the client to perform balance exercises.	5. Balance exercises reduce the severity of attacks by training the central nervous system to adjust to changes in position.
6. Include the client's family and significant others in discussions.	6. Family involvement promotes awareness and, hopefully fosters support.

Evaluation. Achievement of this outcome rests almost entirely on the client's willingness to modify a previous lifestyle and his or her ability to overcome limits that can be felt from vertigo.

Nursing Diagnosis. Impaired Verbal Communication related to decreased hearing and tinnitus.

Outcomes. The client will report satisfaction with ability to communicate.

Interventions	Rationales
1. Assess the client's hearing acuity and audiogram results.	1. Assessment results provide factual information on the severity of hearing loss.
2. Speak distinctly and enunciate words without shouting.	2. Clear speech facilitates hearing and comprehension.
3. Use picture boards or write to communicate.	3. These are alternate methods of communication.
4. Assess the client for hearing aid candidacy, and make needed referrals.	4. Hearing aids augment sound.

■ **Evaluation.** This outcome may require several days to achieve. Hearing loss is reversible in early stages but may become permanent if prolonged.

Nursing Diagnosis. Risk for Fluid Volume Deficit related to decreased oral intake and loss of fluids through emesis.

Outcomes. The client will maintain adequate fluid volume, as evidenced by normal blood pressure, normal pulse rate, quick skin turgor, moist oral mucous membranes, and adequate urine output.

Interventions

1. Assess the client's pulse, respiration, and blood pressure every 4 hours (if stable).
2. Assess the client's skin turgor, oral mucous membranes, oral intake, and urine output every 8 hours (if stable).
3. Compare intake with output, and consider intravenous fluids if the output is greater than intake for several hours.
4. Encourage the client to drink fluids.
5. Teach the client to avoid caffeinated beverages.
6. Administer antiemetics as ordered, and observe for side effects of medications given.
7. Encourage the client to try resting on the unaffected ear.

Rationales

1. Hypotension and tachycardia are indicators of dehydration.
2. Decreased skin turgor, dry mucous membranes, and oliguria are indicators of dehydration.
3. Intake should equal output over 24 hours. Urine output should be 20–30ml/hr. Intravenous fluids are another access for fluids.
4. Lost fluids should be replaced.
5. Caffeine is a vestibular stimulant.
6. Antiemetics reduce the risk of emesis and allow for increased oral intake.
7. Gravity facilitates drainage from the affected ear.

Evaluation. If the client's nausea can be controlled, fluid balance should be achievable within 24 to 48 hours.

Nursing Diagnosis. Powerlessness related to feelings of loss of control secondary to unpredictability of vertigo.

Outcomes. The client will verbalize ways to maintain control and respond to vertigo.

Interventions

1. Assess the client's cognitive appraisal of illness.

2. Assess the client's previous coping strategies.

3. Help the client develop coping strategies based on past coping skills and situational support available to the client.
4. Stress the importance of maintaining or resuming normal activities or developing diversionary activities.
5. Provide needed information about vertigo:

   a. Information about prescribed medications
   b. Manifestations requiring medical attention (e.g., a sudden loss of hearing, a change in the current level of hearing, visual disturbances, weakness or numbness in the extremities, seizures, loss of consciousness, or progressive worsening of vertigo)

6. Refer the client to support groups in the community.

Rationales

1. Cognitive appraisal of the illness provides information about the client's perception of the illness and how much control the client feels he or she has over vertigo.
2. The client will use previous coping strategies during this new stress.
3. Reuse effective past coping strategies. Situation support can help bridge the client's return to society.
4. Reduces the risk that client will become disabled by vertigo. Activity also reduces depression.
5. Encourages the use of problem-solving and coping.

6. The client may benefit from interaction with others and may learn effective methods to cope with the disorder.

Evaluation. Feelings of powerlessness may require weeks to months to resolve, especially if vertigo is chronic.

CONCLUSIONS

Nurses caring for clients with hearing and balance problems need to focus on safety and on promoting independence. Many hearing-impaired clients live a normal life with hearing augmentation and aural rehabilitation. Clients who have diminished hearing or balance disorders are at increased risk for injury because of lack of awareness of the risks or from losing balance. Infections of the ears remain common, but excellent antibiotics have reduced the incidence of chronic problems caused by infections. Tumors of the ear are rare, but when they occur, they are quite destructive.

THINKING CRITICALLY

1. **A middle-aged man comes to the health clinic with ear pain and difficulty hearing. He had some serous drainage 1 day ago but does not recall any recent infection (throat or ear). The problem has persisted intermittently over the past 6 months and is getting progressively more painful and occurring more frequently. If surgery were deemed necessary for this client, how would you prepare him? What discharge teaching might need to be completed for this client after ear surgery?**

Factors to Consider. What preoperative assessments are needed? How should equal pressures be maintained on the tympanic membrane? What normal occurrences might the client expect in the initial period following surgery?

2. **An elderly woman reveals a 10-year history of ear infection. She is experiencing sensorineural hearing loss associated with presbycusis, which affects older people. During her clinic appointment, she tells the nurse that her right ear is painful and is keeping her awake at night. She explains that she can hear most sounds, although sounds on the right side seem to be coming through a filter. She has been using her eardrops as directed but has stopped taking her oral antibiotic because she felt better 2 days ago. She requests information about daily medication or a surgical procedure that might alleviate the problem. How should you respond to this client's request? How do age-related changes contribute to her problem?**

Factors to Consider. What is the assessment focus for this client? What is the prognosis for the client with presbycusis? What type of teaching does the client require?

BIBLIOGRAPHY

1. Balkany, T., Hodges, A. V., & Luntz, M. (1996). Update on cochlear implantation. *Otolaryngologic Clinics of North America, 29*(2), 277–289.
2. Clendaniel, R. A., & Tucci, D. L. (1997). Vestibular rehabilitation strategies in Ménière's disease. *Otolaryngologic Clinics of North America, 30*(6), 1145–1158.
3. Cruickshanks, K. J., et al. (1998). Cigarette smoking and hearing loss: The epidemiology of hearing loss study. *Journal of the American Medical Association, 279*, 1715–1719.
4. Cummings, C. W., et al. (1998). *Otolaryngology-head and neck surgery* (3rd ed.). St. Louis: Mosby–Year Book.
5. Fairbanks, D. N. F. (1999). *Antimicrobial therapy in otolaryngology–head and neck surgery* (9th ed.). Alexandria, VA: American Academy of Otolaryngology–Head and Neck Surgery.
6. Gershman, K., & Nielsen, C. (1995). Prevention and screening in the nursing home. *Clinics in Primary Care, 22*(4), 731–753.
7. Girardi, M., & Konrad, H. R. (1998). Vestibular rehabilitation therapy for the patient with dizziness and balance disorders. *ORL–Head and Neck Nursing, 16*(4), 13–21.
8. Glasscock, M. E., & Stambaugh, G. E. (1990). *Surgery of the ear.* Philadelphia: W. B. Saunders.
9. Grant, I. L. & Welling, D. B. (1997). The treatment of hearing loss in Ménière's disease. *Otolaryngologic Clinics of North America, 30*(6), 1123–1144.
10. Hughes, G. B., et al. (1996). Sudden sensorineural hearing loss. *Otolaryngologic Clinics of North America, 29*(3), 393–405.
11. Jamieson, D. G., Brennan, R. L., & Cornelisse, L. E. (1995). Evaluation of speech enhancement strategy with normal-hearing and hearing-impaired listeners. *Ear and Hearing, 16*(3), 274–286.
12. Jerger, J., et al. (1995). Hearing impairment in older adults: New concepts. *Journal of the American Geriatric Society, 43*(8), 928–935.
13. Karver, S. B. (1998). Otitis media. *Primary Care, 25*(3), 619–632.
14. La Rosa, S. (1998). Primary care management of otitis externa. *The Nurse Practitioner, 23*(6), 125–128, 131–133.
15. Linstrom, C. J. (1998). Cochlear implantation: Practical information for the generalist. *Primary Care, 25*(3), 583–612.
16. Maniglia, A. J. (1996). State of the art on the development of the implantable hearing device for partial hearing loss. *Otolaryngologic Clinics of North America, 29*(2), 225–243.
17. Monsell, E. M., & Harley, R. E. (1996). Eustachian tube dysfunction. *Otolaryngologic Clinics of North America, 29*(3), 466–444.
18. Nobel, W., Ter-Horst, K., & Byrne, D. (1995). Disabilities and handicaps associated with impaired auditory localization. *Journal of the American Academy of Audiology, 6*(2), 129–140.
19. Pollock, K. J. (1995). Ménière's disease: A review of the problem. *ORL–Head and Neck Nursing, 13*(2), 10–13.
20. Seidman, M. D., & Jacobson, G. P. (1996). Update on tinnitus. *Otolaryngologic Clinics of North America, 29*(3), 455–465.
21. Sigler, B., & Schuring, L. T. (1993). *Ear, nose and throat disorders.* St. Louis: Mosby–Year Book.
22. Silverman, C. A. (1998). Audiologic assessment and amplification. *Primary Care, 25*(3), 545–581.
23. Slattery, W. H., & Fayad, J. N. (1997). Medical treatment of Ménière's disease. *Otolaryngologic Clinics of North America, 30*(6), 1027–1066.
24. Society of Otorhinolaryngology–Head and Neck Nurses. (1994). *Guidelines for otorhinolaryngology head and neck nursing practice.* New Smyrna Beach, FL: Author.
25. Telian, S. A., & Shepard, N. T. (1996). Update on vestibular rehabilitation therapy. *Otolaryngologic Clinics of North America, 29*(2), 359–661.
26. Weber, P. C., & Adkins, W. Y., Jr. (1997). The differential diagnosis of Ménière's disease. *Otolaryngologic Clinics of North America, 30*(6), 977–986.

Cognitive and Perceptual Disorders

Anatomy and Physiology Review
The Neurologic System
Joyce M. Black

The nervous system is the body's most organized and complex structural and functional system. It profoundly affects both psychological and physiologic function. This unit discusses the importance of the nervous system to human function and the major consequences of neurologic disorders.

CENTRAL NERVOUS SYSTEM

The brain and spinal cord are known collectively as the *central nervous system* (CNS). The CNS is divided into three major functional divisions:

1. Higher-level brain or cerebral cortex
2. Lower brain level (basal ganglia, thalamus, hypothalamus, midbrain, pons, medulla, cerebellum)
3. Spinal cord

These structures are protected by a rigid bony encasement, three layers of membranes, a fluid cushion, and a blood-brain or blood–spinal cord barrier.

BRAIN

The brain is the largest and most complex part of the nervous system. It is composed of more than 100 billion neurons and associated fibers. The brain tissues have a gelatin-like consistency. This semi-solid organ weighs about 1400 g (~3 pounds) in the adult.

■ CEREBRUM

The cerebrum is divided by a deep groove (longitudinal fissure) into two sections called *cerebral hemispheres.* A transverse fissure separates the cerebrum from the cerebellum. The outermost layer of the cerebrum, the *cerebral cortex,* is only 2 to 5 mm thick. Directly beneath the cerebral cortex are varying thicknesses of association tracts above the commisural tracts, known as the *corpus callosum* (Fig. U15–1).

The cerebral cortex is composed of gray matter (predominantly nerve cell bodies and dendrites) formed into raised convolutions, or gyri. Approximately 75% of the neuronal cell bodies in the brain are found in the cortex. The shallow grooves between the gyri *(sulci)* divide the cerebral cortex into five lobes: frontal, parietal, occipital, temporal, and central (insula) (Fig. U15–2).

The term *neocortex* is often used to refer to the cerebral cortex. The neocortex includes all of the cerebral cortex except the olfactory portions and the hippocampal regions.

Both the left cortex and the right cortex interpret sensory data, store memories, learn, and form concepts. However, each hemisphere dominates the other in many functions. In most people, for example, the *left* cortex has dominance for systematic analysis, language and speech,

mathematics, abstraction, and reasoning. The *right* cortex has dominance for assimilation of sensory experiences, such as visual-spatial information, and activities such as dancing, gymnastics, music, and art appreciation.

In the frontal lobes, the precentral gyrus (motor cortex) controls voluntary motor activity. Most of these fibers cross to the opposite side of the brain at the medulla and descend via the spinal cord as the lateral corticospinal tracts. The area anterior to the precentral gyrus (the premotor area) is also associated with voluntary motor activities. *Broca's area,* lying anterior to the primary motor cortex and superior to the lateral sulcus, coordinates the complex muscular activity of the mouth, tongue, and larynx, which makes expressive (motor) speech possible. Damage to this area leaves the client unable to speak clearly, a disorder called *Broca's aphasia.*

The *prefrontal areas* control (1) attention over time (concentration); (2) motivation, (3) ability to formulate or select goals; (4) ability to plan; (5) ability to initiate, maintain, or terminate actions; (6) ability to self-monitor, and (7) ability to use feedback (called "executive functions"). These same areas are thought to contribute to reasoning, problem-solving activities, and emotional stability by inhibiting the limbic areas of the cerebrum (see later).

Each *parietal lobe,* located posterior to the central sulcus of Rolando, contains a primary somatic (tactile) receptive area and the somatic (tactile) association areas. The post-central gyrus and the posterior portion of the paracentral lobule are the primary receptive (interpretation) areas for tactile sensations (e.g., temperature, touch, pressure). The association areas occupy the remainder of the parietal lobe. Concept formation and abstraction are carried out by the parietal association areas. The right parietal areas are also dominant for spatial orientation and awareness of size and shapes (stereognosis) and body position (proprioception). The left parietal areas assist with right-left orientation and mathematics.

Each *occipital lobe* contains a primary visual receptive (interpretation) area and visual association areas. The primary visual cortex is on either side of the calcarine sulcus. The other areas of the occipital cortices are visual association areas. Visual memories are stored in these areas, which contribute to our ability to visually recognize and understand our environment.

Each *temporal lobe* is located under (caudal to) the lateral sulcus. The temporal lobe contains a primary auditory receptive area and secondary auditory association areas. Spoken language memories are stored in the left temporal auditory association areas. All other sound memories that are not language (e.g., music, various animal sounds, other noises) are stored in the right temporal lobe auditory areas. Damage to these areas would leave us unable to understand spoken or written language or

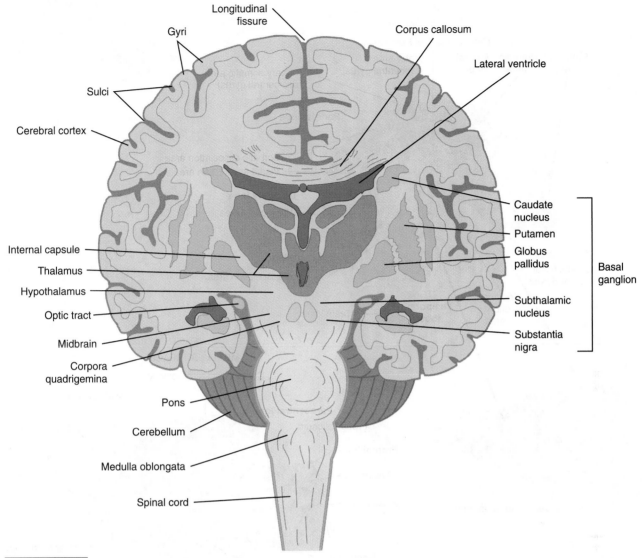

FIGURE U15-1 Structures of the brain (coronal section).

to recognize music or other environmental sounds. Cells that facilitate understanding language reside in Wernicke's area.

The *central (insula) lobe* is located deep within the lateral sulcus and is surrounded by the frontal, parietal, and temporal lobes. Nerve fibers for taste pass through the parietal lobe to the insular lobe. Many association fibers leading to other parts of the cerebral cortex pass through this lobe.

■ HIPPOCAMPUS

The hippocampus, a part of the medial section of the temporal lobe, plays an essential role in the process of *memory,* a very complex phenomenon. Three levels of memory have been identified:

1. *Short-term (recent) memory* is lost after seconds or minutes.
2. *Intermediate memory* lasts days to weeks and eventually is lost.
3. *Long-term (remote) memory* is stored and lasts a lifetime.

Theories about the physiologic basis of memory suggest that reverberating neuronal messages cause short-term memory and that actual neuronal structural changes lead to long-term memory. The hippocampus assists in the conversion of short-term memory into intermediate and long-term memory in the thalamus. The association fibers of the frontal, parietal, temporal, and occipital lobes as well as the diencephalon is important in long-term memory.[2]

■ BASAL GANGLIA

The basal ganglia consist of several structures of subcortical gray matter buried deep in the cerebral hemispheres. These structures include the caudate nucleus, putamen, globus pallidus, substantia nigra, and subthalamic nucleus. The basal ganglia serve as processing stations linking the cerebral cortex to thalamic nuclei. Almost all the motor and sensory fibers connecting the cerebral cortex and the spinal cord travel through the white matter pathways near the caudate nucleus and putamen ganglia. These pathways are known as the *in-*

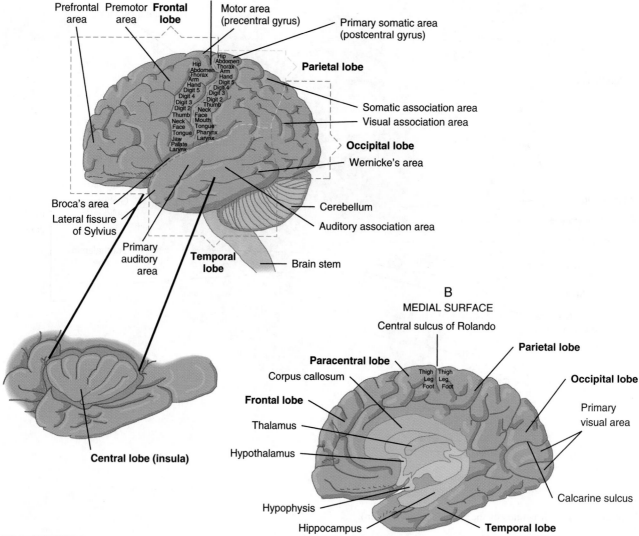

A
LATERAL SURFACE

Central sulcus of Rolando

Prefrontal   Premotor   **Frontal**   Motor area
area   area   **lobe**   (precentral gyrus)

Primary somatic area
(postcentral gyrus)

Hip
Abdomen
Thorax
Arm
Hand
Digit 5
Digit 4
Digit 3
Digit 2
Thumb
Neck
Face
Tongue
Jaw
Palate
Larynx

Hip
Abdomen
Thorax
Arm
Hand
Digit 5
Digit 4
Digit 3
Digit 2
Thumb
Neck
Face
Mouth
Tongue
Pharynx
Larynx

Parietal lobe

Somatic association area
Visual association area

Occipital lobe

Wernicke's area

Broca's area

Lateral fissure
of Sylvius

Cerebellum

Auditory association area

Primary
auditory
area

**Temporal
lobe**

Brain stem

Central lobe (insula)

B
MEDIAL SURFACE

Central sulcus of Rolando

Parietal lobe

Paracentral lobe

Corpus callosum

Thigh
Leg
Foot

Thigh
Leg
Foot

Occipital lobe

Frontal lobe

Thalamus

Primary
visual area

Hypothalamus

Calcarine sulcus

Hypophysis

Hippocampus

Temporal lobe

FIGURE U15–2 The lateral *(A)* and medial *(B)* surfaces of the cerebral cortex. The central lobe is the fifth lobe.

ternal capsule. The basal ganglia, along with the cortico-spinal tract, is important in controlling complex motor activity.

■ DIENCEPHALON

The diencephalon is composed of the thalamus and the hypothalamus. The *thalamus* lies between the cerebral hemispheres and superior to the brain stem. Its gray matter surrounds the lateral edges of the third ventricle. The *hypothalamus* forms the floor of the third ventricle. Other important structures found in and near the diencephalon include (1) the optic tracts and optic chiasm, (2) the pituitary gland on the floor of the diencephalon, and (3) the pineal gland on the roof of the diencephalon.

The thalamus channels all ascending (sensory) information, except smell, to the appropriate cortical cells. The hypothalamus regulates autonomic nervous system (ANS) functions such as heart rate, blood pressure, water and electrolyte balance, stomach and intestinal motility, glan-

dular activity, body temperature, hunger, body weight, and sleep-wakefulness. It also serves as the master over the pituitary gland by releasing factors that stimulate or inhibit pituitary gland output.

■ LIMBIC SYSTEM

The limbic system is made up of many nuclei, including parts of the medial portion of the frontal and temporal lobes (hippocampus), thalamus, hypothalamus, and the basal ganglia. It is considered the center for feelings and control of emotional expression (fear, anger, pleasure, sorrow). The limbic system (the temporal lobe component) also receives nerve fibers from the olfactory bulbs and thus plays an essential role in the interpretation of smells.

■ BRAIN STEM

The brain stem is composed of the midbrain, pons, and medulla oblongata (Table U15–1). These structures are

TABLE U15–1	BRAIN STEM STRUCTURES AND THEIR FUNCTIONS

Structures	Functions
MIDBRAIN	
Corpora quadrigemina	
Superior colliculi	Visual reflexes
Inferior colliculi	Auditory reflexes
Cerebral aqueduct	
Origin of CN III and IV	
Ascending sensory pathways	
Reticular formation	
Red nuclei	Motor pathways to spinal cord, cerebellum
Paired crura cerebri	Afferent/efferent cerebellar pathways
Substantia nigra	Part of basal ganglia
Descending motor pathways	
PONS	
Fourth ventricle	
Nuclei of inferior colliculus	Auditory processing
Nuclei of CN V, VI, VII	
Locus ceruleus	Secretes norepinephrine
Raphe nuclei	Secretes serotonin
Ascending sensory pathways	
Medial lemniscus, auditory pathway	Proprioceptive pathways
Descending motor pathways	
Medial longitudinal fasciculi	Efferent pathway to spinal cord
Pyramids (corticospinal, corticobulbar, corticopontine)	Voluntary motor
Reticular formation	
Respiratory centers	
Pontine nuclei; pontocerebellar fibers	
MEDULLA OBLONGATA	
Fourth ventricle	
Central canal	
Raphe nuclei	Secretes serotonin
Ascending sensory pathways	
Medial lemniscal pathways	Proprioceptive pathways
Spinothalamic tracts	Pain pathways
Trigeminothalamic tracts	Tactile, temperature
Lateral lemnisci	Auditory pathways
Nuclei of CN VIII, IX, X, XI, XII	
Olive and vestibular-cerebellar systems	
Reflex centers: respiratory, vasomotor, cardiac, coughing, swallowing, sneezing, vomiting	
Reticular formation	
Descending motor pathways (pyramids)	Voluntary motor

CN, cranial nerve.

continuous segments of the diencephalon nuclei. They are composed of ascending pathways, the reticular formation, cranial nerves and their nuclei, and descending autonomic and motor pathways.

■ RETICULAR FORMATION

The reticular formation is composed of a complex network of gray matter (nuclei), ascending reticular pathways, and descending reticular pathways. Its nuclei extend from the superior part of the spinal cord to the diencephalon and communicate with the basal ganglia, cerebrum, and cerebellum.

The reticular formation assists in regulation of skeletal motor movement and spinal reflexes. It also filters incoming sensory information to the cerebral cortex. Approximately 99% of sensory information is disregarded as unessential. One component of the reticular formation, the reticular activating system, controls the sleep-wake cycle (see Chapter 22) and consciousness.

■ CEREBELLUM

The cerebellum is composed of gray and white matter. The cortex of the cerebellum is a thin layer of gray matter arranged in parallel long and deep gyri, called *folia,* and separated by cerebellar sulci (Fig. U15–3). Deep fissures divide the cerebellum into three lobes, but the functional division of the cerebellum consists of a right and left hemisphere separated by a narrow band of white matter called the *vermis.* An extension of dura mater, the falx cerebelli, partially separates the hemispheres.

The cerebellum integrates sensory information related to position of body parts, coordinates skeletal muscle movement, and regulates muscle tension, which is necessary for balance and posture. Three pairs of nerve tracts (cerebellar peduncles) provide the communication pathways. The inferior peduncles are sensory (afferent) pathways from the spinal cord and medulla, which carry information related to the position of body parts to the cerebellum. The middle peduncles carry information from the cerebral cortex to effector cells that control voluntary (purposeful) motor activities. The cerebellum also receives sensory input from the receptors in the muscles, tendons, joints, eyes, and inner ear. After this information is integrated and analyzed, the cerebellum sends impulses via the superior peduncles (efferent pathways) to the brain stem and spinal cord and then to the appropriate body parts (effectors) to make connections.

Most of the tracts in the cerebellum travel through various nuclei without crossing. Therefore, the right cerebellar hemisphere predominantly affects the right (ipsilateral) side of the body and vice versa.

SPINAL CORD

The spinal cord, that portion of the CNS surrounded and protected by the vertebral column, is continuous with the medulla and lies within the upper two thirds of the vertebral canal (the cavity within the vertebral column). The lower spinal cord terminates caudally in a cone-shaped structure known as the *conus medullaris* at the level of the first (L1) and second (L2) lumbar vertebrae. The spinal cord is subdivided into four areas: (1) cervical cord, (2) thoracic cord, (3) lumbar area, and (4) sacral cord (conus medullaris) (Fig. U15–4).

Within the spinal cord, butterfly-shaped gray matter (mostly unmyelinated) is surrounded by mostly myelinated white matter. The white matter consists of *ascend-*

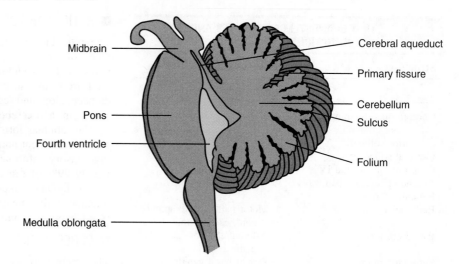

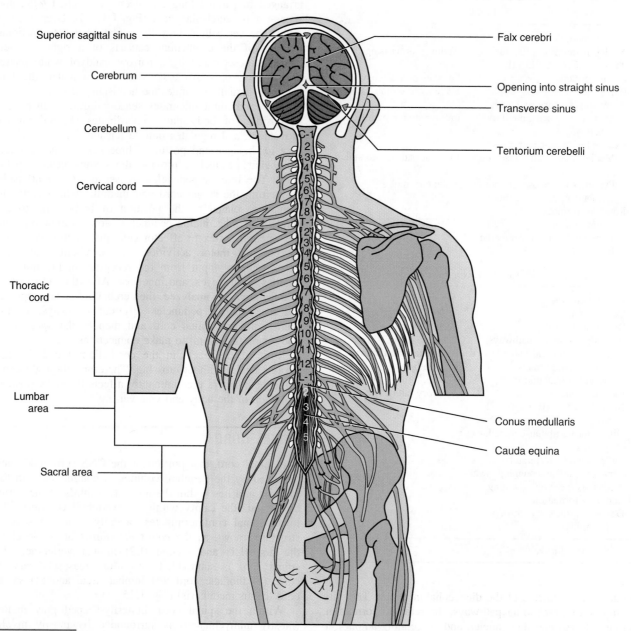

FIGURE U15-3 Sagittal view of the brain stem, fourth ventricle, and cerebellum.

FIGURE U15-4 Cranial vault, vertebral column, and peripheral nerves.

ing tracts and *descending tracts* that conduct nerve impulses between the brain and the cells outside the CNS. The cell bodies in the gray matter are grouped into clusters of nuclei and laminae (a defined group or column of cells). The tracts in the white matter are arranged into three paired columns: posterior, lateral, and anterior (Fig. U15–5, *inset*).

■ ASCENDING AND DESCENDING PATHWAYS

The *ascending (sensory) pathways* in the spinal cord eventually terminate in the cerebral and cerebellar cortex. Motor impulses from the brain, which travel through the *descending pathways,* terminate in the muscles and glands. For example, a spinothalamic tract, which is a sensory tract, begins in the spinal cord and ends in the parietal lobe. The corticospinal tract is a descending tract that originates in the frontal lobe of the cerebral cortex, travels through the spinal cord, and terminates in the muscle cells. These motor neurons, which originate in the frontal lobe and continue through the corticospinal tract, are also referred to as *upper motor neurons. Lower motor neurons* are cells that begin in the anterior horn of the spinal cord and pass into the spinal nerves.

Table U15–2 summarizes the specific functions of the major brain and spinal cord tracts.

Many of the tracts communicating with the cerebral cortex cross (decussate), but not all cross at the same place. The term *contralateral* refers to tracts that cross at the medulla and ascend or descend to the opposite side of the body; *ipsilateral* (same-sided) tracts do not cross. For example, sensory tracts (including the anterior spinothalamic, posterior, and anterior spinocerebellar tracts) cross in the medulla as they ascend to the cerebral cortex. Therefore, the sensory neurons in the cerebral cortex interpret sensory stimuli from the contralateral side of the body.

The lateral corticospinal spinal tract (the pyramidal tract) crosses at the medulla as it descends from the frontal lobe of the cerebral cortex to the spinal cord. The posterior spinocerebellar tracts are ipsilateral tracts and thus coordinate muscular function on the same side of the body. The crossing of the lateral spinothalamic tract is unique.

PROTECTIVE AND NUTRITIONAL STRUCTURES

■ CRANIUM AND VERTEBRAL COLUMN

Eight bones that fuse early in childhood compose the cranium. The fused junctions are called *sutures.* The cranium encloses the brain structures and serves as a source of protection.

The floor, or basilar plate, of the cranial vault has three depressions, called *fossae.* The frontal lobes lie in the anterior fossa. The temporal lobes and the base of the diencephalon lie in the middle fossa. The cerebellum rests in the posterior fossa.

The vertebral column, a flexible series of vertebrae, surrounds and protects the spinal cord. The vertebral column consists of seven cervical vertebrae, 12 thoracic vertebrae, five lumbar vertebrae, five sacral vertebrae fused into a sacrum, and four coccygeal vertebrae fused into a coccyx. Ligaments hold the vertebrae together, and discs between the vertebrae prevent the bones from rubbing together.

■ MENINGES

The meninges, three membranes enveloping the brain and spinal cord, are predominantly for protection (Fig.

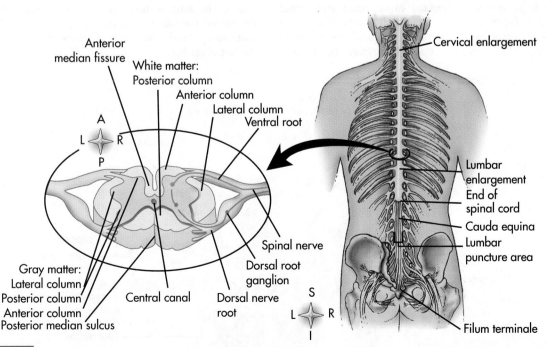

FIGURE U15–5 The spinal cord ends at L-2. *Inset,* Transverse section *(left)* of the spinal cord. (From Thibodeau, G., & Patton, K. [1999]. *Anatomy and physiology* [4th ed., p. 381]. St. Louis: Mosby.)

TABLE U15–2	MAJOR NERVE TRACTS OF THE SPINAL CORD	
Tract	**Location**	**Function**
ASCENDING TRACTS		
Fasciculus gracilis	Posterior column	Touch, pressure, body movement, position
Fasciculus cuneatus	Posterior column	
Spinothalamic		
Lateral	Lateral column	Pain, temperature
Anterior	Anterior column	Light (crude) touch
Spinocerebellar		
Posterior	Lateral column	Coordination of muscle movements
Anterior	Lateral column	
DESCENDING TRACTS		
Corticospinal		
Lateral	Lateral column	Voluntary motor
Ventral	Anterior column	Voluntary motor
Reticulospinal		
Lateral	Lateral column	Autonomic nervous system fibers, muscle tone, sweat glands
Anterior	Anterior column	
Medial	Anterior column	
Rubrospinal	Lateral column	Coordination of muscle movements

The pia mater and astrocytes together form the membrane part of the blood-brain barrier (see Blood-Brain Barrier).

The *arachnoid,* a thin layer of connective tissue, extends from the top of each gyrus to the top of the adjacent gyrus; it does not extend into the sulci and fissures. The space between this layer and the pia mater is known as the *subarachnoid space.* Cerebrospinal fluid (CSF) flows through this space.

The cranial *dura mater* is a tough, nonstretchable vascular membrane with two layers. The *outer* dura mater is actually the membrane (periosteum) of the cranial bones. The *inner* dura mater forms the plates that separate the two cerebral hemispheres (falx cerebri), the cerebrum and the brain stem and cerebellum (tentorium cerebelli), and the cerebellar hemispheres (faly cerebelli). The tentorium cerebelli is a landmark term that is often used by clinicians to separate parts of the brain; it is often referred to as "tentorium." *Supratentorial* refers to the cerebrum and all the structures superior to the tentorium cerebelli; *infratentorial* refers to structures inferior to the tentorium cerebelli—the brain stem and the cerebellum.

Brain spaces that often fill with blood after head trauma include the potential space (the *subdural space*) between the inner dura mater and the arachnoid and the *epidural space* between the dura mater and the periosteum.

The meninges anchor the spinal cord. The pia mater, which closely surrounds the spinal cord, continues from the tip of the conus as a thread-like structure (the *filum terminale*) to the end of the vertebral column, where it is anchored into the ligament on the posterior side of the coccyx. The denticulate ligaments extend laterally from the pia mater to the dura mater to suspend the spinal cord from the dura mater.

Two common spaces that are commonly accessed by physicians are the subarachnoid space (for diagnostic studies) and the epidural space (for delivery of medications). The subarachnoid space extends below the level of the spinal cord to the second sacral (S2) vertebral level, and the epidural space lies between the dural sheath and the vertebral bones.

U15–6). Each layer, the pia mater, arachnoid, and dura mater, is a separate membrane.

The *pia mater* is a vascular layer of connective tissue and is so closely connected to the brain and spinal cord that it follows every sulcus and fissure. This layer serves as a supporting structure for blood vessels passing through to the tissues of the brain and spinal cord.

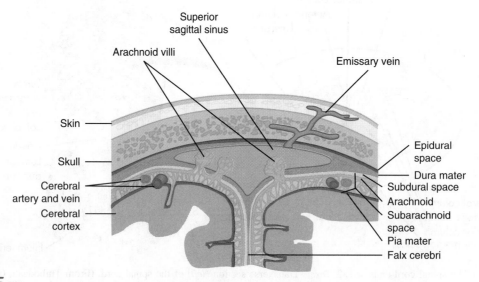

FIGURE U15–6 The meninges (coronal section through the superior sagittal sinus).

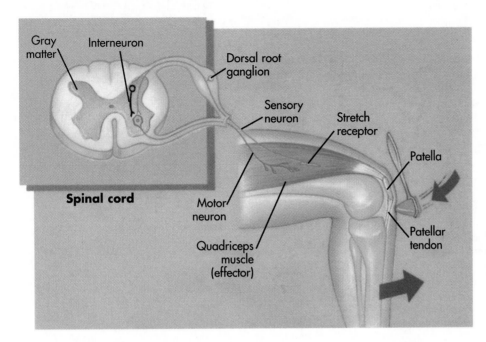

Gray matter
Interneuron
Dorsal root ganglion
Sensory neuron
Stretch receptor
Patella
Spinal cord
Motor neuron
Quadriceps muscle (effector)
Patellar tendon

FIGURE U15–7 Patellar reflex and neural pathway involved in the reflex response. (From Thibodeau, G., & Patton, K. [1999]. *Anatomy and physiology* [4th ed., p. 428]. St. Louis: Mosby.)

■ REFLEX MECHANISMS

Our unconscious automatic responses to internal and external stimuli, known as *reflex responses,* provide many homeostatic functions. Although the spinal cord is often thought of as the reflex center, it is not the only site for reflex regulation. Many of the complex reflexes controlling heart rate, breathing, blood pressure, swallowing, sneezing, coughing, and vomiting are found in the brain stem.

Some intrinsic reflex circuits in the spinal cord create patterns of movement (flexion and extension) that are the basis for posture and forward progression. Other reflex circuits are the bases for spinal cord reflexes, which include the myotatic (deep tendon, stretch) reflex, the flexor withdrawal reflex, the crossed extension reflex, and the extensor thrust reflex. Visceral-somatic reflexes can also excite or inhibit the motor neurons, producing changes in muscle tone and even movement.

Neuromuscular spindles monitor muscle stretch. As a muscle stretches, increased firing of spindles leads to contraction of the same muscle, commonly seen as the *knee-jerk reflex.* The Golgi tendon organs are sensory nerve endings that protect against excessive contraction.

Simple reflexes require only two or three neurons; for example, the knee-jerk reflex requires only a sensory and a motor neuron. The *withdrawal reflex* helps prevent or decrease tissue injury when a body part touches a potentially harmful object. The harmful stimuli are sent via the sensory neuron to the interneuron in the spinal cord for interpretation and the response message is sent via the motor neuron, resulting in the withdrawal response (Fig. U15–7).

■ CEREBROSPINAL FLUID AND THE VENTRICULAR SYSTEM

CSF is a clear, colorless fluid. Approximately 100 to 160 ml of CSF circulates through the ventricles and within the subarachnoid space. When a person is lying in a horizontal position, the average CSF pressure is 100 to 180 mm Hg.

About two thirds of the CSF is made in the choroid plexus of the four ventricles, primarily in the lateral ven-tricles. Small amounts are produced by ependymal, arachnoid, and other brain cells. The choroid plexus is a network of blood vessels within the pia mater that is in direct contact with the lining of the ventricles. The choroid plexuses together produce approximately 500 ml of CSF per day. If CSF were allowed to accumulate, it would exert enough pressure to damage the brain. Normally, however, it is absorbed into the blood at the same rate at which it is formed.

The ventricular system is a series of cavities within the brain. CSF flows from each of the lateral ventricles via the foramen of Monro into the third ventricle (Fig. U15–8). The third ventricle is midline just beneath the fornix. CSF drains from the third ventricle through the aqueduct of Sylvius into the fourth ventricle. The fourth ventricle is located in the brain stem just anterior to the cerebellum. From the fourth ventricle, CSF passes via one of three foramina (two foramina of Luschka and one foramen of Magendie) into a large subarachnoid space that lies behind the medulla and below the cerebellum, called the *cisterna magna.* The cisterna magna is continuous with the subarachnoid space, which surrounds the brain and spinal cord.

Eventually, the CSF circulates upward into the region of the superior sagittal sinus where it is absorbed across the arachnoid villi. The arachnoid granulations are extensive tufts of pia-arachnoid that along with the inner dura extend into the superior sagittal sinus and permit one-way flow of CSF into the sinus.

■ BLOOD-BRAIN BARRIER

Three brain barriers (blood-brain, blood–CSF, and brain-CSF) primarily regulate and maintain an optimal and stable chemical environment for neurons. Brain barriers are either physical barriers or physiologic processes (transport systems) that slow movement of certain substances from one CNS compartment to another by regulating ion movement between the compartments. Physical barriers include tight junctions of the endothelial cells lining the capillaries, pores of the capillaries of the choroid plexuses, the

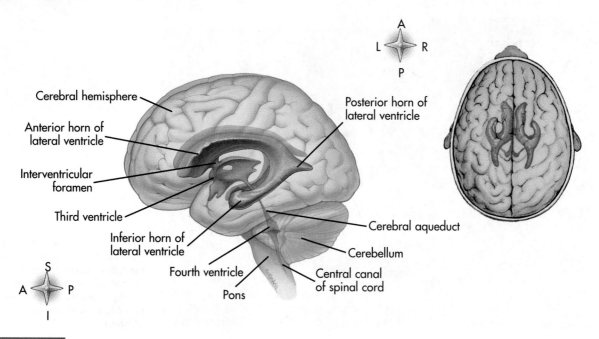

FIGURE U15–8 The ventricles of the brain produce and circulate cerebrospinal fluid. (From Thibodeau, G., & Patton, K. [1999]. *Anatomy and physiology* [4th ed., p. 378]. St. Louis: Mosby.)

basement membrane (ependymal cells) next to the choroid plexuses, and the pial-glial membrane.

An intact blood-brain barrier may prevent some drugs from crossing into the brain, a fact that must be considered when medications are prescribed for nervous system disorders. Certain events, including dilutional hyponatremia, acute hypertension, high doses of some anesthetics, vasodilation, and hypercarbia, can increase the permeability of the blood-brain barrier.

BLOOD SUPPLY

The brain requires one third of the cardiac output and uses 20% of the body's oxygen. Glucose is catabolized or burned for its energy. Gray matter has higher metabolic needs than white matter. The brain receives 750 to 900 ml of blood flow per minute. Blood flow is regulated by

levels of carbon dioxide. When carbon dioxide levels rise, a negative feedback mechanism causes vasodilation.

The vertebral arteries and the internal carotid arteries (Fig. U15–9) provide the arterial supply to the brain.

■ ARTERIAL SUPPLY

The *vertebral arteries* branch from the subclavian arteries, travel through the transverse foramina in the cervical vertebrae, and enter the cranial vault through the foramen magnum. The vertebral arteries are located on the anterolateral surface of the medulla. At the junction of the medulla and pons, the vertebral arteries join to form the basilar artery. The basilar artery bifurcates at the midbrain level to form two posterior cerebral arteries. The vertebral artery system supplies the brain stem, the cerebellum, the lower portion of the diencephalon, and the medial and inferior regions of the temporal and occipital lobes.

FIGURE U15–9 Inferior view of the cerebral circulation.

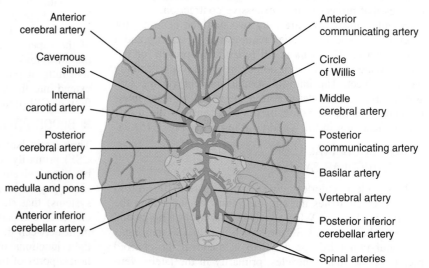

The *internal carotid arteries* branch from the common carotid arteries and enter through the carotid canals at the base of the skull. The internal carotid arteries bifurcate into the anterior and middle cerebral arteries. Near this bifurcation, the circle of Willis (a ring of blood vessels at the base of the brain) is formed by the posterior cerebral arteries, posterior communicating arteries, internal carotid arteries, anterior cerebral arteries, and anterior communicating branches. The internal carotid arteries supply the upper diencephalon, basal ganglia, lateral temporal and occipital lobes, and parietal and frontal lobes. The middle cerebral arteries supply large portions of the frontal, parietal, temporal, occipital, and insular lobes and the basal ganglia, internal capsule, and thalamus. The anterior cerebral arteries supply the medial portions of the frontal and parietal lobes and the upper basal ganglia and internal capsule (see Fig. U15–9).

The spinal cord derives its arterial blood supply from small spinal arteries that branch off larger arteries, including the vertebral, ascending cervical, deep cervical, intercostal, lumbar, and sacral arteries. These arteries and their branches form the three main arteries of the spinal cord, the anterior spinal artery and a pair of posterior spinal arteries, which extend the length of the cord.

■ VENOUS SUPPLY

Most of the venous blood from the head returns to the heart through the internal jugular veins, the external jugular veins, and the vertebral veins.

Venous distribution is similar to arterial distribution of the spinal cord. The venous system drains into the venous sinuses located between the dura mater and the periosteum of the vertebral column.

Cells of the Nervous System

■ STRUCTURE

Nervous tissue consists mainly of *neuroglia* and *neurons* (as well as vascular and some connective tissues). Neurons are responsible for communication, and neurological cells provide support for the activity of neurons. The brain and spinal cord constitute the CNS.

■ NEUROGLIA

Glial cells, collectively called neuroglia, provide structure and support for neurons. They are plentiful, with a ratio of glial cells to neurons high as 50:1! They also control ion concentrations within the extracellular space and contribute to the transport of nutrients, gases, and waste products between neurons and the vascular system and the CSF. Clinically, these cells are responsible for the development of many intracranial tumors. Four types of neuroglial cells exist (Fig. U15–10).

In addition to these functions, each type of glial cell has specific functions.

Astrocytes supply nutrients to the neurons. They have specialized contacts with blood vessels in the pial-glial

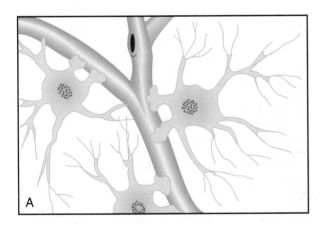
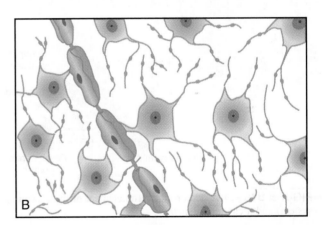
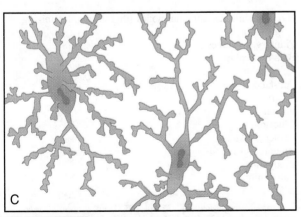
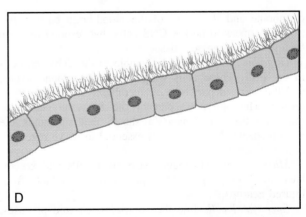

FIGURE U15–10 Neuroglial cells. *A,* Astrocytes along the capillary. *B,* Oligodendrocytes along the nerves. *C,* Microglia (phagocytes). *D,* Ependymal cells form a sheet that lines fluid cavities in the brain.

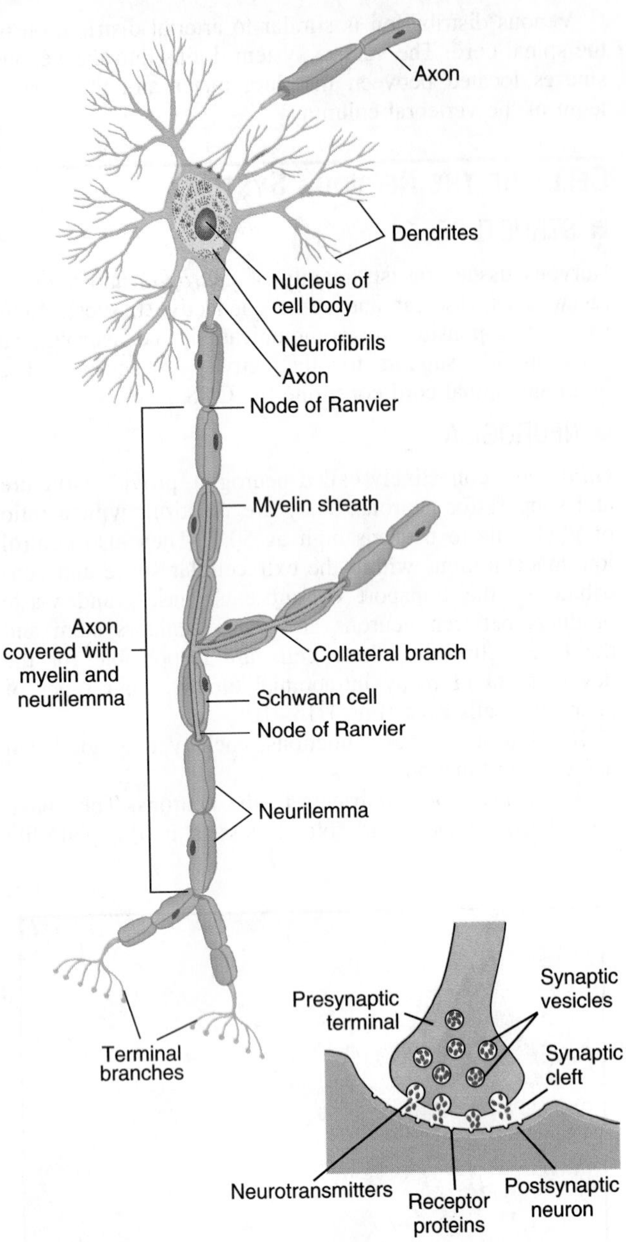

FIGURE U15–11 A neuron (the basic element of the nervous system) and a chemical synapse.

They create a one-cell-layered membrane that allows regulated diffusion of substances between the interstitial fluid and the CSF.

■ NEURONS

A neuronal cell body *(soma)* is like other cells, in that it contains most of the organelles seen in other cells. Unique structures in the neuron include *neurofibrils,* which are networks of thread-like structures supporting other structures. *Nissl bodies* are dark-staining sections of rough endoplasmic reticulum and are unique to the neuron.

Tree-like *dendrites* carry messages to the neuronal cell body; *axons* carry messages away from the cell body (Fig. U15–11).

Three types of neurons exist:

1. *Unipolar* neurons have only one nerve fiber leaving the cell body, but they branch to form a dendrite and axon. Unipolar neurons often send general sensory signals.
2. *Multipolar* neurons send motor signals.
3. *Bipolar* neurons are often utilized in the pathways of special sensory systems (eyes, nose, and ears).

Synapses, very important in nerve function, are small spaces between neurons and their muscular or glandular target organs. As a message travels down the neuron, it reaches a synapse that it must cross in order to "jump" to

---

membrane and form part of the blood-brain barrier. Astrocytes appear to be the CNS cells that respond to brain trauma by forming scar tissue.

Oligodendrocytes are comparable to the Schwann cells in the PNS. These cells wrap themselves around axons, and the spiraled part of their membrane is referred to as *myelin.* The outermost part of the Schwann cells also make up the *neurilemma,* a sheath that surrounds the myelin sheath. Neurilemma is essential to nerve regeneration (see later).

Microglia are phagocytic scavenger cells and are related to macrophages. They phagocytose products from injured neurons.

Ependymal cells line the ventricles, choroid plexuses, and the central canal that extends through the spinal cord.

BOX U15–1   Common Neurotransmitters and Neuropeptides

Small-Molecule Transmitters

Acetylcholine
Dopamine
Norepinephrine
Epinephrine
Histamine
Serotonin
Gamma-aminobutyric acid (GABA)
Glycine
Glutamate
Aspartate
Nitric oxide

Neuropeptides

Hypothalamic-releasing hormones (thyrotropin, luteinizing, growth)
Pituitary hormones
Beta-endorphin
Enkephalin
Substance P
Gastrin
Insulin
Glucagon
Cholecystokinin
Angiotensin II
Bradykinin
Calcitonin

Adapted from Guyton, A. C., & Hall, J. E. (1996). *Textbook of medical science* (9th ed., pp. 572–573). Philadelphia: W. B. Saunders.

the next neuron. There are two types of synapses; *chemical* synapses dominate. In an *electrical synapse,* the electrical nerve impulses of two cells cross directly through a very small separation (called *gap junctions* or a *nexus*) from the presynaptic to the postsynaptic cell; this type of synapse is found in smooth and cardiac muscle cells.

Chemical substances called *neurotransmitters* are discharged into the space *(cleft)* between two neurons and propel the message onto the next neuron. Transmitters are manufactured in the cell body, and transported anterograde to the terminals *(knobs),* stored, and secreted from the vesicles in the first neuron *(presynaptic neuron)* into the synaptic cleft (see Fig. U15–11). The neurotransmitter excites, inhibits, or modifies signals to the second neuron (postsynaptic neuron) by interacting with the receptors on its membrane. More than 100 neurotransmitters have been identified. Box U15–1 lists the more common transmitters.

IMPULSE CONDUCTION

■ RESTING POTENTIAL

A neuron not conducting a nerve impulse is said to be "resting." Although it is resting, it remains charged and potentially ready to fire. The potential to fire is produced by a difference in electrical charge between the interstitial fluid outside the neuron and the intracellular fluid within (Fig. U15–12). The inside of the nerve cell is electrically negative, the interstitial fluid electrically positive. A resulting membrane potential, measured in millivolts (mV) results from this difference in electrical potential between the two compartments. The *resting membrane potential* (RMP) of neurons is between −45 and −75 mV. The RMP in a neuron is −70 mV; in cardiac and skeletal cells it is −90 mV.

The cell is *depolarized* when an influx of sodium makes the membrane potential more positive (i.e., rising to zero). In most cells, this is due to an electrical stimulus transmitted by an adjacent cell.

As the membrane potential rises during depolarization, it reaches a specified level *(threshold).* When threshold is reached, the excited cell is committed to full action

potential because the cell follows an all-or-none phenomenon.

Repolarization is the restoration of the membrane polarity, and sodium and potassium are returned to their usual places via the sodium-potassium pump.

After an action potential is generated, no segment of the nerve fiber can conduct another action potential for a brief period of time (<1 ms). This interval is called the *absolute refractory period.* Sodium and potassium are returning to their original locations during this period, and sodium cannot enter the nerve cell. During the next period, called the *relative refractory period,* only a stimulus stronger than ordinary can produce an action potential. On average, a return to a resting potential takes approximately 10 to 30 ms.

■ NERVE IMPULSES

Because neurons are arranged in chain-like pathways, impulses must travel from one cell to another quickly. In nerve cells, the impulse begins at the axon. When the action potential reaches the presynaptic knob at the dendrite, the membrane's permeability to calcium increases, allowing increased calcium influx. Calcium promotes fusing of the vesicles with the membrane and release of the neurotransmitters inside. Some neurotransmitters are transported back into the vesicles *(reuptake).* Others are decomposed by an enzyme process. For example, acetylcholinesterase decomposes acetylcholine at the postsynaptic membrane.

■ MYELIN

Myelin surrounds most large nerve fibers and is separated by nodes of Ranvier. Action potentials are generated only at the nodes and thus they skip between them rather than depolarize the entire membrane. This jumping characteristic is known as "saltatory conduction." Conduction using this process is very rapid. Neurons with their axons covered by myelin are called *myelinated nerve fibers;* neurons with little or no myelin are called *unmyelinated nerve fibers.* Myelinated fibers in the CNS compose the *white matter* in the brain and spinal cord. *Gray matter* consists of cell bodies which are unmyelinated. The speed of the nerve impulse conduction is also related to the

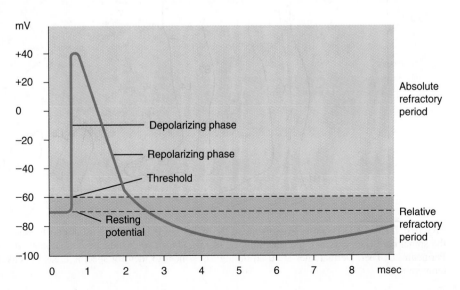

FIGURE U15–12 Generation of nerve impulses. The resting membrane potential is shown at −70 mV.

diameter of the fiber; the greater the diameter, the faster the impulse.

■ RECEPTORS

Receptors are biologic transducers, using the stimulus of one form of energy—mechanical, electrical, chemical, thermal or light—to initiate the "electrical" energy of the nerve impulse. Although sensory receptors may be stimulated by more than one form of energy, each receptor is especially sensitive to a particular form of energy.

Receptors exhibit a phenomenon known as *adaptation,* a decreased receptor sensitivity in response to steady continuous stimuli. Slow-adapting receptors can maintain the lower rate of discharge for minutes to even hours. Fast-adapting receptor bursts of impulses terminate less than 1 second after initiation of the stimulus. The mechanism of adaptation is not known.

Receptors respond more effectively to change than to continuous stimulation. This characteristic of nerve "fatigue" is protective.

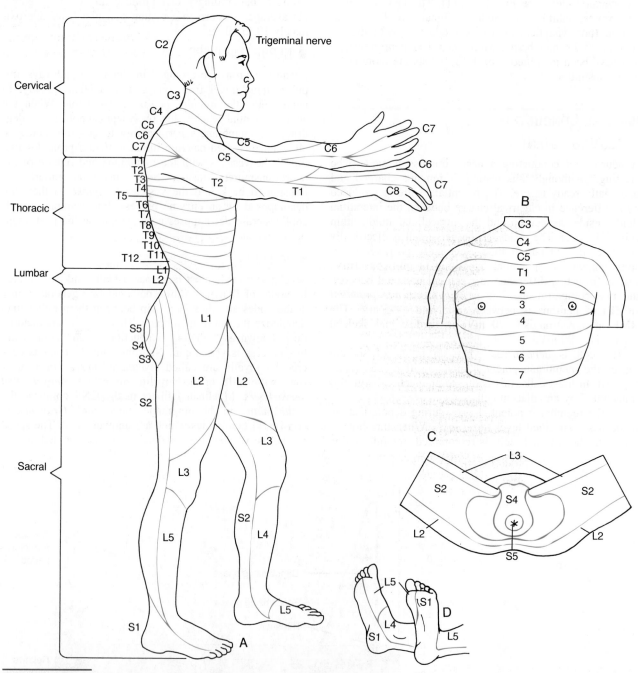

FIGURE U15–13 Dermatomes (segments of the spinal cord) indicate distribution of spinal nerves. *Solid lines* divide the regions of the spinal cord (i.e., cervical, thoracic, lumbar, sacral). *Dotted lines* indicate dermatomes. *A,* Torso and limbs. *B,* Anterior chest. *C,* Perineum. *D,* Feet. Dermatomes are used during assessment to identify specific areas of sensory impairment (e.g., touch, pain, temperature).

PERIPHERAL NERVOUS SYSTEM

The PNS includes all neurons other than those in the brain and spinal cord. It consists of pathways of nerve fibers between the CNS and all outlying structures in the body. Included in the PNS are 12 pairs of cranial nerves and 31 pairs of spinal nerves.

Nerves that conduct impulses to the brain and spinal cord are called *sensory (afferent) neurons*. Nerves that conduct impulses away from the brain and spinal cord are called *motor (efferent) neurons*. Most nerves are mixed, having both sensory and motor components.

SPINAL NERVES

The spinal nerves develop from a series of nerve rootlets that collect laterally as spinal roots. Each spinal nerve consists of a *dorsal (sensory) root* and a *ventral (motor) root* which unite to form a spinal nerve. The dorsal root emerges from the posterolateral cord. The ventral root emerges from the anterolateral spinal cord. There are 31 pairs of spinal nerves: eight pairs of cervical nerves, 12 pairs of thoracic nerves, five pairs of lumbar nerves, five pairs of sacral nerves, and usually one pair of coccygeal nerves (see Fig. U15–4). The specific area of sensory reception for each dorsal root is called a *sensory dermatome* (Fig. U15–13).

The peripheral nerves that are formed into plexuses have specific names. There are three major plexuses:

1. The *cervical plexus* supplies the muscles and skin of the neck and branches to form the phrenic nerve, which innervates the diaphragm.
2. The *brachial plexus* supplies the muscles and skin of the shoulder, axilla, arm, forearm, and hand. It branches to form the ulnar, median, and radial nerves.
3. The *lumbosacral plexus* supplies sensory and motor impulses to the muscles and skin of the perineum, gluteal region, thighs, legs, and feet. Its many branches include the pudendal, gluteal, femoral, sciatic, tibial, and common fibular nerves.

CRANIAL NERVES

Twelve pairs of cranial nerves arise from the brain. Most of the cranial nerves are composed of both motor and sensory neurons, although a few cranial nerves carry only sensory impulses (Fig. U15–14). Except for the olfactory and optic nerves, whose nuclei lie just below the cere-

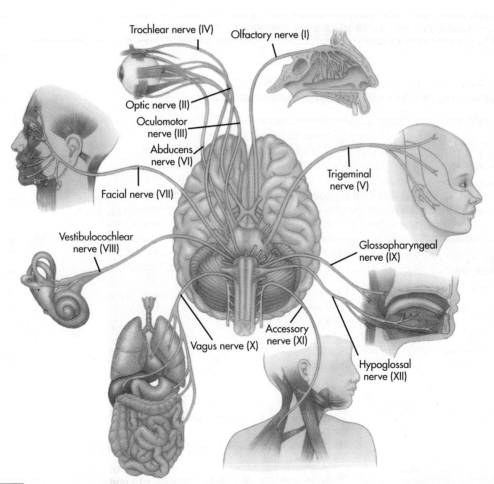

FIGURE U15–14 Ventral surface of the brain showing the attachment of the cranial nerves. (From Thibodeau, G., & Patton, K. [1999]. *Anatomy and physiology* [4th ed., p. 420]. St. Louis: Mosby.)

brum, all the other cranial nerve nuclei lie within the brain stem. Table U15–3 presents the 12 pairs of cranial nerves.

AUTONOMIC NERVOUS SYSTEM

The autonomic nervous system (ANS) is the part of the PNS that coordinates involuntary activities, such as visceral functions, smooth and cardiac muscle changes, and glandular responses. Although it can function independently, its primary control is from the brain and spinal cord. The ANS has two divisions: the *sympathetic* and *parasympathetic nervous systems.* The efferent ANS fibers travel within some cranial and spinal nerves. These two systems are highly integrated and interact with each other to maintain a stable internal environment.

Unlike the *somatic* neurons, which usually are single neurons linking the CNS to a muscle or gland, the ANS has a *two-neuron chain* prior to the effector organ. The terminal of the first neuron is located in the CNS and synapses with nerve fibers whose cell bodies are within an autonomic ganglion. The axon of the second neuron (postganglionic fiber) carries impulses to the target viscera. An exception is the adrenal medulla, which is innervated directly by preganglionic fibers. The medulla is actually composed of postganglionic neurons that secrete adrenaline into the bloodstream during an "adrenaline rush."

The *sympathetic nervous system* coordinates activities used to handle stress and is geared for action as a whole for short periods of time. The preganglionic neurons of the sympathetic nervous system emerge from the spinal cord via the motor (ventral) roots of the thoracic and upper two lumbar spinal nerves (T1-L2) (see Fig. U15–14). Preganglionic axons are short; postganglionic axons are long.

The *parasympathetic nervous system* is associated with conservation and restoration of energy stores and is geared to act locally and discretely for a longer duration. The preganglionic fibers emerge from the brain stem via the cranial nerves and from the spinal cord via the sacral spinal nerves at S2-4. These preganglionic fibers have long axons that synapse with the postganglionic neurons in ganglia close to or located within the organs to be innervated. Each postganglionic neuron has a relatively short axon. Most organ systems, but not all, have both parasympathetic and sympathetic innervation. Approximately 75% of the parasympathetic fibers are in the vagus nerve.

Table U15–4 lists the effects of both the sympa-

TABLE U15–3	FUNCTIONS AND TYPES OF CRANIAL NERVES		
	Name	**Function**	**Type**
I	Olfactory	Olfaction (smell)	Sensory
II	Optic	Vision	Sensory
III	Oculomotor	Extraocular eye movement	Motor
		Elevation of eyelid	
		Pupil constriction	Parasympathetic
IV	Trochlear	Extraocular eye movement	Motor
V	Trigeminal		
	Ophthalmic division	Somatic sensations of cornea, nasal mucous membranes, face	Sensory
	Maxillary division	Somatic sensations of face, oral cavity, anterior two thirds of tongue, teeth	Sensory
	Mandibular division	Somatic sensation of lower face	Sensory
		Mastication (chewing)	Motor
VI	Abducens	Lateral eye movement	Motor
VII	Facial	Facial expression	Motor
		Taste, anterior two thirds of tongue	Sensory
		Salivation	Parasympathetic
VIII	Vestibulocochlear		
	Vestibular	Equilibrium	Sensory
	Cochlear	Hearing	Sensory
IX	Glossopharyngeal	Taste, posterior third of tongue; pharyngeal sensation	Sensory
		Swallowing	Motor
X	Vagus	Sensation in pharynx, larynx, external ear	Sensory
		Swallowing	Motor
		Thoracic and abdominal visceral parasympathetic nervous system activities	Parasympathetic
XI	Spinal accessory	Neck and shoulder movement	Motor
XII	Hypoglossal	Tongue movement	Motor

TABLE U15–4	EFFECTS OF THE SYMPATHETIC AND PARASYMPATHETIC NERVOUS SYSTEMS ON ORGANS	
Organ	**Effect of Sympathetic Stimulation**	**Effect of Parasympathetic Stimulation**
Eye		
Pupil	Dilation (alpha)*	Constriction
Ciliary muscle	Slight relaxation (far vision)	Constriction (near vision)
Glands	Vasoconstriction and slight secretion	Stimulation of copious secretion (containing many
Nasal		enzymes for enzyme-secreting glands)
Lacrimal		
Parotid		
Submandibular		
Gastric		
Pancreatic		
Sweat glands	Copious sweating (cholinergic)	Sweating on palms of hands
Apocrine glands	Thick, odoriferous secretion	None
Heart		
Muscle	Increased rate ($beta_1$)	Slowed rate
	Increased force of contraction ($beta_1$)	Decreased force of contraction (especially of atria)
Coronaries	Dilated ($beta_2$); constricted (alpha)	Dilation
Lungs		
Bronchi	Dilation ($beta_2$)	Constriction
Blood vessels	Mild constriction	? Dilation
Gut		
Lumen	Decreased peristalsis and tone ($beta_2$)	Increased peristalsis and tone
Sphincter	Increased tone (alpha)	Relaxation (most times)
Liver	Gluconeogenesis, glycogenolysis ($beta_2$)	Slight glycogen synthesis
Gallbladder and bile ducts	Relaxation	Contraction
Kidney	Decreased output and renin secretion	None
Bladder		
Detrusor	Relaxation (slight) ($beta_2$)	Contraction
Trigone	Contraction (alpha)	Relaxation
Penis	Ejaculation	Erection
Systemic arterioles		
Abdominal viscera	Constriction (alpha)	None
Muscle	Constriction (alpha)	None
	Dilation ($beta_2$)	
	Dilation (cholinergic)	
Skin	Constriction	None
Blood		
Coagulation	Increase	None
Glucose	Increase	None
Lipids	Increase	None
Basal metabolism	Increase up to 100%	None
Adrenal medullary secretion	Increase	None
Mental activity	Increase	None
Piloerector muscles	Contraction (alpha)	None
Skeletal muscle	Increased glycogenolysis ($beta_2$)	None
	Increased strength	
Fat cells	Lipolysis ($beta_1$)	None

*Sympathetic nervous system composed of alpha, $beta_1$, and $beta_2$ receptors.
Adapted from Guyton, A. C., & Hall, J. E. (1996). *Textbook of medical science* (9th ed., pp. 774–775). Philadelphia: W. B. Saunders.

thetic and parasympathetic nervous systems on different organs. These functions and responses are related to the type of neurotransmitter released. The preganglionic fibers of the sympathetic and parasympathetic nerves and the postganglionic fibers of the parasympathetic nerves release acetycholine. The postganglionic fibers of the sympathetic nerves release norepinephrine. Fibers secreting acetylcholine are called *cholinergic fibers;*

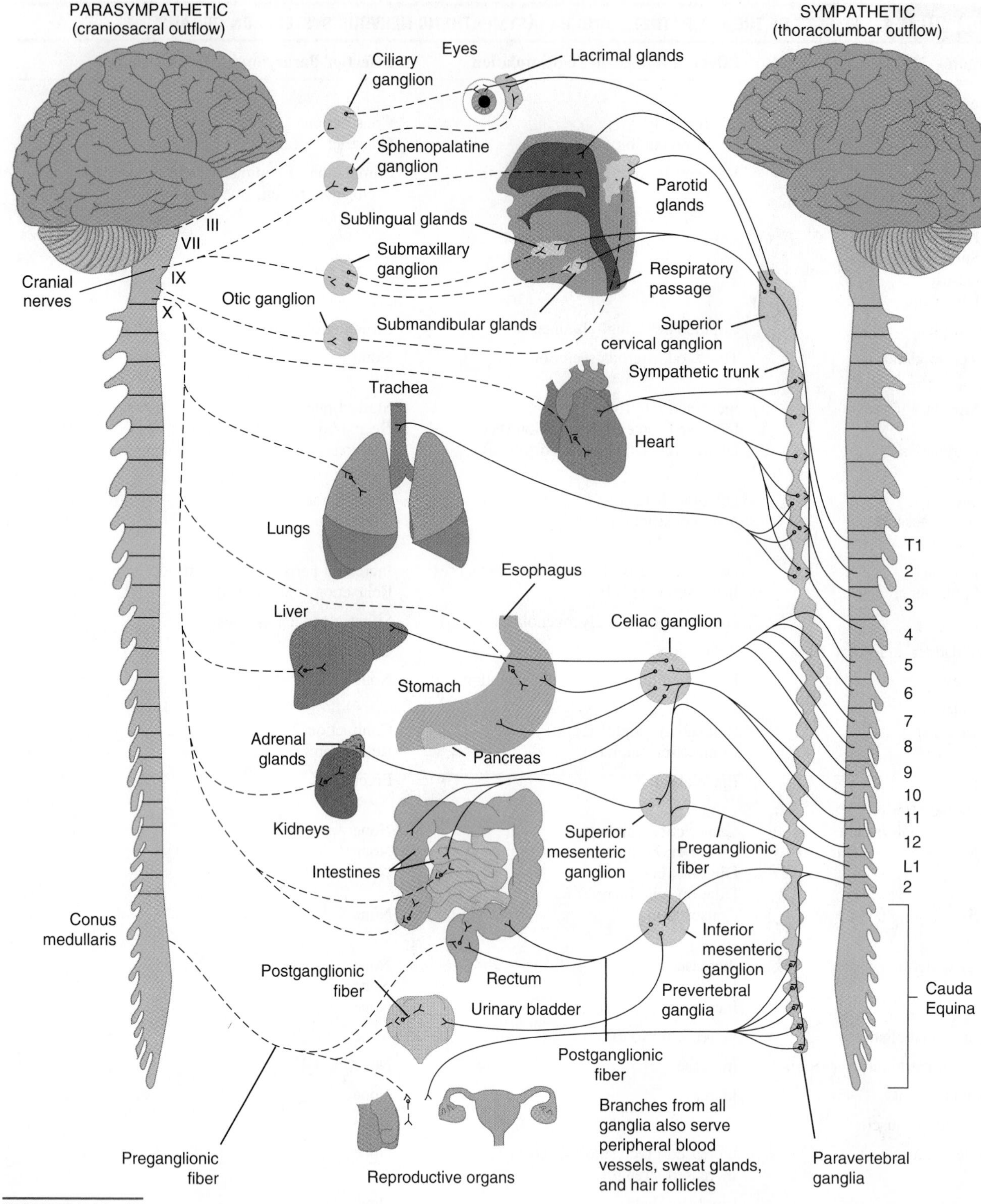

FIGURE U15-15 Autonomic nervous system.

fibers secreting norepinephrine are called *adrenergic fibers.*

The complexity of the sympathetic and parasympathetic response also depends on the type of receptor that combines with the neurotransmitter. The sympathetic nervous system has four types of receptors: alpha$_1$, alpha$_2$, beta$_1$, and beta$_2$. The parasympathetic nervous system has muscarinic and nicotinic receptors.

EFFECTS OF INJURY ON THE NERVOUS SYSTEM

■ REGENERATION

For many years, it was thought that nerve cell bodies were not able to regenerate; however, it appears that CNS cortical neurons do attempt to regenerate. PNS regeneration can occur if only the axon in the PNS is injured. Initially, there is breakdown of the myelin sheath and axon. The axon swells and fragments while the myelin sheath disintegrates distal to the injury. The cell body takes up water. Macrophages phagocytose the breakdown products. Neurilemma cells migrate into the emerging space (Fig. U15–16).

The injured axon tip forms a new plasma membrane. A few days after injury, sprouts emerge from the tip. Peripheral nerve sprouts enter the distal stump and often come in contact with a neurilemma cord, which serves as a guide. The regenerating axon grows along the cord at a rate of 4 mm/day. Later, the neurilemma cells encapsulate the regenerating nerve fibers. With time, the axon and myelin sheath both thicken. Axons within the CNS sprout and form growing tips but appear unable to sustain the metabolic responses necessary for extensive regeneration. It is believed that the axon tip is not able to penetrate the glial scar formed at the injury site, such as after spinal cord injury.

An uninjured axon may sprout a collateral branch at a node of Ranvier that may enter into an adjacent denervated neurilemma cord. Collateral nerve regeneration occurs in both the PNS and the CNS, for example, after peripheral nerve trauma or inflammation of a peripheral nerve, as in Bell's palsy.

EFFECTS OF AGING ON THE NERVOUS SYSTEM

Neurons undergo senescence. Intracellular, cellular, and biochemical changes occur. Lipofuscin accumulates in the cell. Neurofibrillary tangles and senile plaques develop. After we reach 30 years of age, neurons decrease in number and neuroglial cells increase in size and number. The number of dendrites decreases, but the intrinsic dendritic changes are quite variable in hippocampal areas of the brain on postmortem examination in the normal aging population. Variations in dendrite length, stability, and growth have been attributed to compensatory response to death of dendrites.

Aging has little effect on sensory and primary memory but causes a decrease in working memory, including longer retrieval times for short-term memory, categorization, and episodic memory. Dendritic changes are quite pronounced in pathologic conditions such as Alzheimer's disease (see Chapter 72). The axons also change in normal aging; their diameters thin, and the receptors decrease in number.

CONCLUSIONS

The nervous system has three major divisions:

1. The CNS regulates higher-level process, such as thought and vital functions.
2. The PNS provides pathways to the CNS.

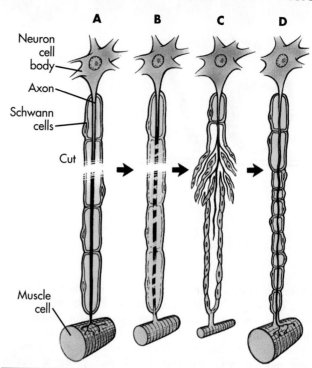

FIGURE U15–16 Regeneration of peripheral nerve tissue. *A*, An injury results in a cut nerve. *B*, Immediately after the injury, the distal portion of the axon degenerates, as does its myelin sheath. *C*, The remaining neurilemma cells tunnel from the point of injury to the effector. New Schwann cells grow within this tunnel, maintaining a path for regrowth of the axon. Meanwhile, several growing fibers reach the tunnel. *D*, The neuron's attachment is reestablished. (From Thibodeau, G., & Patton, K. [1999]. *Anatomy and physiology* [4th ed., p. 353]. St. Louis: Mosby.)

3. The ANS coordinates involuntary activities such as digestion.

The neuron is the structural and functional unit of the nervous system. The typical neuron is composed of a cell body, one axon, and several dendrites. The impulses along the nerve are carried through the action of several electrolytes. Neurotransmitters carry the impulse from neuron to neuron.

BIBLIOGRAPHY

1. Guyton, A. C., & Hall, J. E. (1996). *Textbook of medical science* (9th ed.). Philadelphia: W. B. Saunders.
2. Hanson, M. (1998). *Pathophysiology.* Philadelphia: W. B. Saunders.
3. Lewis, B. (1992). *AANA Journal* Course: Update for nurse anesthetists: Blood-brain barrier function alteration during anesthesia. *Journal of the American Association of Nurse Anesthetists, 60*(6), 573–577.
4. Sur, M., & Cowey, A. (1995). Cerebral cortex: Function and development. *Neuron, 15,* 497–505.
5. Tower, D. B. (1992). A century of neuronal and neuroglial interactions, and their pathological implications: An overview. In A. C. H. Yu, et al. (Eds.), *Progress in brain research* (Vol. 94, pp. 3–17). New York: Elsevier Science.

CHAPTER

67

Assessment of the Neurologic System

Mary Vorder Bruegge

Assessment of a client experiencing a neurologic disorder is a challenge. Neurologic disorders range from simple to complex and have profound consequences for activities of daily living (ADL) and survival. Neurologic assessment establishes baseline data that are used to compare ongoing assessments, diagnose actual and potential health problems, manage client care, and evaluate the outcome. Because of the complexity of the nervous system, neurologic assessment is both multifaceted and lengthy. The three main components of a neurologic assessment are

- A comprehensive history
- A neurologic physical examination
- General and specific neurodiagnostic studies

Assessment is both anatomic and functional. Continuous observations of the client are made and compared with baseline data. Astute observations are essential because many neurologic changes occur subtly. Nurses collect data on the client's ability to function physically (e.g., self-care deficit) and mentally (e.g., confusion and altered problem solving). Finally, because many neurologic disorders are serious, the nurse provides skillful, crisis-oriented support for the client and significant others.

This chapter presents basic neurologic assessment procedures. Additional assessment techniques for specific neurologic disorders are discussed throughout Unit 15. Novice practitioners may follow the assessment sequence described in this chapter to avoid missing parts of a complex examination. Advanced clinicians may develop a preferred sequence based on experience. The sequence suggested in Table 67–1 integrates cranial nerve and reflex testing into motor and sensory examinations.

HISTORY

The history consists of biographical data, the chief complaint and symptom analysis, past health history, family health history, psychosocial history, and review of systems.

■ BIOGRAPHICAL AND DEMOGRAPHIC DATA

Biographical data comprise demographic, administrative, and insurance information. Often included are (1) a per-

sonal profile or brief description of the client, (2) the source of the history (e.g., client or a significant other), and (3) the client's mental status (indicating the reliability of the data). Neurologic problems often affect mental status, sometimes making it difficult to obtain an accurate history directly from the client.

■ CURRENT HEALTH

Chief Complaint

Obtain a detailed description of the events that have led the client to seek care. Avoid suggesting manifestations to the client, and use open-ended questions.

Symptom Analysis

Determine the onset and sequence of manifestations and their progress. Describe neurologic disease processes accurately to facilitate the diagnostic process. Ask the client to describe manifestations using his or her own words. Use a symptom analysis to elicit manifestation characteristics and their progression (see Chapter 9).

The health history guides the physical examination. For example, a complaint of dizziness cues a focus on examination of the eyes, ears (vestibular nerve), and cerebellar function instead of motor and sensory functions. Detailed neurologic examination is indicated when the client reports behavioral changes, altered level of consciousness (LOC), growth and development problems, pain, changes in motor or sensory function, infection, or trauma. Assess for neurologic problems that may be related to other problems, such as alcohol and recreational drug use, metabolic imbalances, and metastatic lesions.

■ PAST HEALTH HISTORY

Childhood and Infectious Diseases and Immunizations

Collect data regarding common childhood diseases and immunizations. Diseases associated with neurologic sequelae include rubella, rubeola, cytomegalovirus infection, herpes simplex, influenza, and meningitis. Ask whether the client has completed the recommended immunization schedule. Public health resources provide schedules for

Text continued on page 1879

TABLE 67–1   NEUROLOGIC ASSESSMENT GUIDELINES

Functional Category	Specific Category	Area of Nervous System Involved	Assessment Technique	Examples of Disorders
1. Consciousness (awareness of self and environment)	Arousal response to verbal, tactile, and visual stimuli	Reticular activating system (mesencephalon, diencephalon) Both hemispheres	Is client alert? What is attention span? Is there normal response to visual and auditory stimuli? Reaction to loud noises, shaking, deep pressure over eye orbits or sternum? Are vital signs, pupils, and reflexes normal?	Elevation: insomnia, agitation, mania, delirium Depression: somnolence, lethargy, semicoma, coma
2. Mentation	Thinking	Cerebral hemispheres plus specific regional functions	Is client oriented (time, place, person)?	Disorientation
	Insight, judgment, planning	Frontal lobe, with association fibers to other areas of cerebrum	Does client recognize implication of illness? Are goals congruent with abilities? How would client respond to given situation (e.g., house on fire)?	Lack of judgment, inattention to grooming, appearance, and personal habits
	Fund of information	Basic biologic intellect (frontal lobe) integrated into other areas	Calculation ability, knowledge of current events consistent with educational level. Who is U.S. president?	Impairment—functioning not congruent with level of education
	Memory	Temporal lobe and association to most other areas of cortex		
	Recent	Hippocampus	What did client eat for breakfast? What happened yesterday?	Organic brain disease
	Past	Frontal lobe	Recall past events during taking of history	Lapses of memory for past events may coincide with past CNS problems (e.g., trauma, infection, psychic trauma)
	Feeling (affect) (congruence of response to stimulus)	Limbic system (usually involves both hemispheres)	Compare observed with expected reactions. Are emotions labile? Appropriate?	Blunted affect: hysteria, schizophrenia, bilateral frontal lobe lesions
	Perceptual distortions (illusions, hallucinations)	General and specific cortical areas in hallucinations	Observations for behavior indicating perceptual problems. Ask client	Irritative lesions of cortex may → hallucinations (occipital cortex → visual, postcentral gyrus → somatic sensation, uncus → smell)
3. Language and speech	Dysarthria (defects in articulation, enunciation), and rhythm in speech	Impairment of muscles of tongue, palate, pharynx, or lips (may be due to ↓ impulses or incoordination) Brain stem, cerebellum, or extraneural causes; CN V, VII, IX, X, XII	Have client repeat a difficult phrase (e.g., "Susie sells seashells by the seashore")	Slurring, slowness, indistinctness, nasality, break in normal speech rhythm (i.e., speech of intoxication); amyotrophic lateral sclerosis; pseudobulbar palsy; myasthenia gravis

Table continued on following page

TABLE 67–1   NEUROLOGIC ASSESSMENT GUIDELINES *Continued*

Functional Category	Specific Category	Area of Nervous System Involved	Assessment Technique	Examples of Disorders
	Dysphonia (abnormal production of sounds from larynx)	Many extraneural causes Recurrent laryngeal nerve problems (part of vagus); CN X Medulla (area of nucleus of CN X)	Is client hoarse? Whispered voice is intact Use indirect laryngoscopy findings	Compression of recurrent laryngeal nerve by bronchogenic carcinoma of left mainstem bronchus Left atrial hypertrophy Brain stem tumors, occlusion of posterior inferior cerebellar or vertebral artery
	Aphasia (inability to use and understand written and spoken words)	Fluent (receptive) left temporal and parietal lobes (Wernicke's area) Nonfluent (expressive) Broca's area (lateral) inferior portion of frontal lobe of dominant side Global (combined)	Observe vocal expression, written expression, comprehension of spoken and written language, and gesture communication	Cerebrovascular disease of middle cerebral artery Trauma, tumor, abscess, etc., in left temporal and parietal lobe areas Damage to Broca's area or association fibers (stroke, tumor, etc.)
	Agnosia (inability to recognize objects or symbols by means of senses)	Primarily in parietal temporal and occipital areas	Sense organs intact? Can the client recognize objects by sight, touch, hearing, etc.?	Cerebrovascular disease
4. Motor function	Expression (facial)	CN VII	Symmetry of smile, frown, raising of eyebrows	Central facial weakness (upper motor neuron dysfunction); weakness of lower half of face Causes: cerebral vascular accident, corticobulbar tract Peripheral facial weakness (lower motor dysfunction); weakness of entire half of face Causes: Bell's palsy, brain stem tumor, fracture of temporal bone
	Eating (chewing, swallowing)	CN V, VII, IX, X, XII	Strength of masticator muscles, gag reflexes, ability to swallow	Tetanus, peripheral spasm of muscle; amyotrophic lateral sclerosis, medullary tumor; pseudobulbar palsy may be associated with dysarthria
	Eye movements	CN III, IV, VI	Extraocular movement, pupil size, reactivity, pupils react equally to accommodation, diplopia, nystagmus	Cerebral peduncle pressure → CN III dysfunction, cavernous sinus thrombus → CN III, IV, VI problem Muscular problems (e.g., myasthenia gravis, hyperthyroid) Horner's syndrome (ptosis, constricted pupil), anisocoria

TABLE 67–1	NEUROLOGIC ASSESSMENT GUIDELINES *Continued*

Functional Category	Specific Category	Area of Nervous System Involved	Assessment Technique	Examples of Disorders
	Moving	Motor precentral gyrus (pyramidal) and cerebellar systems, basal ganglia, CN XI, spinal cord, upper motor neuron, (brain → spinal cord via corticospinal tract)	Gait, heel-to-toe walking, presence or absence of involuntary movements, coordination, muscle tone, mass, strength, Romberg's test, ability to shrug shoulders and to rise from chair	*Upper motor neuron:* Brain and cord-sparing anterior horn cell Tone ↑ ↑ (spastic) Bulk ↓ due to atrophy of disuse Reflexes ↑ ↑ due to loss of central inhibition No fasciculations Frequent clonus
		Lower motor neuron (motor cells of cranial and spinal nerves and anterior horn cells → peripheral muscles)		*Lower motor neuron:* Segment anterior horn cell peripheral nerve Tone ↓ ↓ (flaccid) Bulk ↓ due to tone loss Reflexes ↓ or absent due to loss of anterior horn cell Fasciculations No clonus
	Involves cerebellum			*Cerebellar problem →* loss of coordination and balance
5. Sensory function	Seeing	CN II: optic, occipital lobe	Acuity, visual fields, funduscopy	Field test: loss in retina or optic nerve → loss in eye involved, optic chiasm → bitemporal hemianopsia Optic tract → homonymous hemianopsia, parietal lobe → quadrant problems (inferior), temporal lobe → superior quadrant problems ↑ Intracranial pressure → papilledema (raised disc → hemorrhage)
	Smelling	CN I: temporal lobe (uncus)	Ability to detect familiar odors	Usually ↓ smell due to extraneural causes (e.g., upper respiratory infection, allergy, smoking), olfactory groove; meningioma, olfactory hallucinations

Table continued on following page

TABLE 67-1	NEUROLOGIC ASSESSMENT GUIDELINES *Continued*

Functional Category	Specific Category	Area of Nervous System Involved	Assessment Technique	Examples of Disorders
	Hearing	CN VIII: cochlear division, temporal lobe	Acuity of hearing, presence or absence of unusual sounds, Weber's and Rinne tests	May have conductive (nerve OK) or neural hearing loss; Ménière's syndrome (tinnitus, hearing loss, vertigo, and nystagmus), basilar skull fracture → otorrhea. Brain stem vascular dysfunction or tumors → ↓ hearing
	Taste	CN VII, IX: insula lobe	Ability to differentiate sweet, salt, sour, and bitter	Brain stem or insula lesions → ↓ taste; extraneural causes, smoking, poor oral hygiene
	Feeling (sensory)	Peripheral nerves → Dermatomes → Spinal cord → Tracts (leading to) Pain-temperature–tactile, anterolateral system, proprioception, stereognosis, dorsal roots → thalamus leading to somasthetic area (postcentral gyrus, parietal lobe)	Pain: pinprick. Touch: cotton touched to skin. Proprioception: check where digit is in space. Vibration: place vibrating tuning fork on bony prominence. Temperature: test tubes of cold and warm water laid against skin; person identifies whether hot or cold	Polyneuropathy (e.g., diabetes, anemia). Spinal cord lesions → dermatome alterations. Upper pons → thalamus, contralateral loss. Thalamus → contralateral loss + paresthesia. Thalamus → cortex → cortical sensory loss
6. Bowel and bladder function	Bowel function	Afferent Spinal nerve S3–5 External sphincter (voluntary control) Internal sphincter Spinal nerve S3–5 Autonomic nervous system Cerebral cortex	Check for fecal impaction or incontinence. Check muscle tone	Fecal incontinence with lesions S3–5. Anal anesthesia—conus medullaris and tabes dorsalis. May be extraneural causes. Loss of inhibitory control (e.g., stroke)
	Bladder function	Autonomic nervous system Afferent Spinal nerve T9–L2, S2–4 Pudendal nerve Efferent Spinal nerve T11–L2 External sphincter (voluntary) Spinal nerve S2–4 Cerebral cortex	Feels when bladder is full, complete emptying. Does client have urgency, frequency?	Urinary incontinence. Flaccid bladder. Spastic bladder. Loss of inhibitory control (e.g., stroke). May be extraneural causes

C, cervical; CN, cranial nerve; CNS, central nervous system; L, lumbar; S, sacral; T, thoracic.
↑, increase; ↑ ↑, significantly increased; ↓, decreased; ↓ ↓, significantly decreased; →, may affect or lead to.

childhood immunizations as well as recommendations for travelers to foreign countries.

Major Illnesses and Hospitalizations

A number of major illnesses are associated with neurologic changes, such as diabetes mellitus, pernicious anemia, cancer, infections, and hypertension. Advanced liver disease and renal disease result in metabolic disturbances, fluid and electrolyte imbalances, and acid-base changes that affect mental function. Inquire about hospitalization, injury, or surgery for neurologic system problems, such as head trauma, seizures, stroke, and crushing tissue injury. Has the client undergone a neurologic diagnostic study, such as electroencephalography (EEG), electromyography (EMG), or computed tomography (CT)? Results of such diagnostic studies provide valuable data for future comparison.

Medications

The medication history covers all medicines that the client is taking or has taken, both prescription and over-the-counter, including herbal preparations. Specifically, ask about aspirin, anticonvulsants, stimulants and depressants, sedatives, anticoagulants, narcotics, tranquilizers, and antihypertensive medications. Many preparations for allergies and colds contain ingredients that cause drowsiness. Inquire about the current or past use of recreational drugs, the type of drug, and the duration of use.

Common herbal preparations used for neurologic problems are as follows:

- CNS stimulants: betel nut (*Areca catechu*); ephedra (*Ephedra sinica, E. vulgaris, E. nevadensis*), also known as Ma huang, and illegal in some areas; nutmeg (*Myristica fragrans*).
- Sedatives/hypnotics: chamomile (*Matricaria recutita, Chamaemelum nobile*); gotu kola (*Centella asiatica*); hops (*Humulus lupulus*); kava kava (*Piper mythysticum*); St. John's wort (*Hypericum perforatum*); valerian (*Valeriana officinalis*).
- Antidepressives: *Ginkgo biloba*; sage (*Salvia officinalis*); St. John's wort. Sage can be used as an aid for dizziness, as can *G. biloba*. *G. biloba* has also been indicated for treating tinnitus, short-term memory loss, and headache.
- Analgesics: cayenne (*Capsicum*), taken internally for headache and toothache or applied externally for neuralgia; feverfew (*Tanacetum parthenium*), used in the treatment and prophylaxis of migraine headaches; white willow (*Salix purpurea, S. fragilis, S. daphnoides*), used as an analgesic and antipyretic.
- Antihypertensive or anti-stroke effects: garlic (*Allium sativum*); *G. biloba*; onion (*Allium cepa*); reishi mushroom (*Ganoderma lucidum*).

Growth and Development

The growth and development history may help determine whether neurologic dysfunction was present at an early age. The perinatal history may contain data about in utero exposure to viruses (rubella), maternal consumption of alcohol, tobacco, or other drugs, and radiation. Ask whether the client's mother carried to full term during her pregnancy. Premature birth increases the risk of neurologic damage from inadequate oxygenation and intracranial bleeding if ventilator support was used. A difficult or prolonged labor and delivery can result in hypoxia or use of forceps for delivery, with consequent central and peripheral neurologic damage.

At what age did the client accomplish major developmental tasks, such as walking and talking? Was the client able to participate in games, sports, and other childhood activities with peers? Did the client have any problems with coordination, balance, or agility?

■ FAMILY HEALTH HISTORY

Ask about a family history of neurologic disorders to determine the presence of genetic risk factors. Inquire about epilepsy, Huntington's disease, amyotrophic lateral sclerosis, muscular dystrophy, hypertension, stroke, mental retardation, and psychiatric disorders.

■ PSYCHOSOCIAL HISTORY

An understanding of personal psychosocial factors (e.g., educational background, level of performance, and personality changes) enhances assessment. Inquire about changes that have occurred in daily routines. Ask about changes in sleep patterns, exercise routines, hobbies and recreation, occupation, perceived stressors, and sexual interest and performance. Is there risk of exposure to neurotoxic fumes or chemicals, such as pesticides, paints, or bonding agents (glue), or does the client spend time in an inadequately ventilated living area or workspace?

■ REVIEW OF SYSTEMS

Neurologic disorders often subtly affect the ability to function in an integrated fashion. Ask the client to describe any neurologic manifestations, such as behavior changes, mood swings, loss of consciousness, seizures, headaches, dizziness, vertigo, memory deficits, speech or motor function problems (e.g., unstable balance or posture, gait changes, tics, tremors), and sensory function problems (e.g., vision changes, pain, paresthesia or tingling, paralysis). Significant neurologic assessment data include those given in Box 67-1. Detailed questions for the review of systems can be found in Chapter 9, Box 9-2.

The client who has a neurologic problem may be unaware of its presence. Attempt to supplement and corroborate the history and review of systems by speaking with a family member or significant other who knows the client well. Ask specifically about mental or physical changes that have been noticed.

PHYSICAL EXAMINATION

The physical examination is intended to detect abnormalities in neurologic functioning. Variations in client age, physical condition, and LOC determine how detailed an examination can be. A comprehensive neurologic examination is described here. Adapt the examination to the client's level of neurologic function. Box 67-2 is a guide for adapting the assessment in various situations. A suggested sequence for the physical examination is as follows:

BOX 67-1   Manifestations Related to Neurologic Assessment

Eye

Visual loss
Diplopia
Ptosis
Proptosis

Ear, Nose, and Throat

Infections
Hearing loss
Tinnitus
Dizziness
Vertigo
Voice change
Dysphagia
Changes in taste or smell
Experiences of unusual smells

Cardiovascular

Syncope
Palpitations
Hypotension
Hypertension
Vertigo
Transient ischemic attacks
Stroke

Neurologic

Weakness
Numbness

Paresthesias
Headache
Pain
Altered thinking
Speech difficulty
Vomiting
Vertigo
Ataxia
Fainting
Seizures
Any loss of consciousness
Distortions of reality
Use of consciousness-altering drugs
Disorientation
Altered sleep patterns
Changes in ability to speak, read, or understand language
Changes in memory of recent or remote events
Changes in ability to concentrate

Skin

Hair and nail changes

Musculoskeletal

Tremor
Weakness
Altered coordination
Staggering
Difficulty climbing stairs

---

1. Vital signs.
2. Mental status (including language and communication).
3. Head, neck, and back.
4. Cranial nerves (including pupils).
5. Motor system.
6. Sensory function.
7. Reflexes.
8. Autonomic nervous system.

Neurologic findings are summarized in the accompanying feature called Physical Assessment Findings in the Healthy Adult: Neurologic System.

■ VITAL SIGNS

Although cortical changes occur first (e.g., LOC), vital signs are assessed first because neurologic disorders can cause life-threatening changes in vital signs. Clients who have cervical spinal cord injuries exhibit a classic triad of hypotension, bradycardia, and hypothermia related to the loss of sympathetic nervous system function. Inadequate perfusion of vital organs may result from hypotension if the blood pressure is not sustained.

Changes in vital signs can also accompany the late stages of increased intracranial pressure (ICP). The body attempts to provide an adequate supply of oxygen and glucose to the brain by increasing the blood flow to the brain to compensate for the elevated ICP. *Cushing's response* consists of elevated systolic blood pressure, widened pulse pressure, and bradycardia. Respiratory rate and rhythm can be altered by increased ICP on the brain stem.

■ MENTAL STATUS

Document general data about the client's mental status (e.g., LOC, orientation, memory, mood and affect, intellectual performance, judgment and insight, and language and communication). The mental status examination is discussed in Chapter 9.

Level of Consciousness

The *LOC* is the most sensitive indicator of changes in neurologic status. Consciousness is maintained by the cerebral hemispheres and reticular activating system. Test LOC by using stimuli to determine arousal. Stimuli include verbal, visual, tactile, and noxious agents, such as painful pressure.

When assessing LOC, begin by observing spontaneous behavior before using stimuli; then provide stimuli, and make observations regarding the response. Start with a visual cue, such as walking in front of the client or waving hello. If a response is not elicited, provide verbal stimulation. Use touch and painful (noxious) stimuli only if the client does not respond to the milder forms of stimulation.

If a painful stimulus is needed to elicit a response, it should be a central stimulus, such as sternal pressure, supraorbital ridge pressure, or sternocleidomastoid muscle pinch. Although nail bed pressure may be used, it is a

---

BOX 67-2   The Initial Neurologic Examination in the Clinical Setting

The sequence in which the neurologic examination is performed and the amount of time devoted to each step are dictated by the client's situation. For example, assessment of the head-injured client in the emergency department requires evaluation of vital signs, pupil reactivity, level of consciousness, and motor response. These clients may not be stable or cooperative enough to allow completion of the cranial nerve and sensory response assessment. Spinal cord–injured clients, however, are usually coherent and able to participate in the sensory examination. The sensory assessment information is essential for documenting changes in the status of spinal cord–injured clients.

As clients become more stable and cooperative, the examination can be performed in more depth and with less frequency. Remember that neurologically impaired clients frequently experience fluctuations in status. Alter the assessment schedule and technique to detect and report these fluctuations.

Following are suggested modifications in the screening neurologic examination that may be made on the basis of the client's initial presentation:

- *Initial examination for diagnosis and triage*:

  - Client history based on chief complaint
  - Physical examination including vital signs
  - Level of consciousness
  - Pupillary response
  - Brain stem function (corneal reflex)
  - Motor and sensory functions in all four extremities

- *If the client is conscious and stable*:

  - Complete baseline neurologic examination
  - Focused examinations at prescribed levels

- *If the client is conscious and unstable*:

  - Quick baseline physical assessment
  - Frequent focused examinations until client is stable

- Vital signs
- Level of consciousness
- Pupillary response
- Brain stem function
- Motor and sensory functions in extremities
- Spinal cord function

- *If the patient is unconscious but stable*:

  - Vital signs
  - Level of consciousness and ability to arouse
  - Cranial nerve function
  - Motor and sensory functions
  - Pathologic reflexes

- *If the patient is unconscious and unstable*:

  - Vital signs
  - Level of consciousness
  - Cranial nerve function
  - Motor and sensory functions relative to the ability to test for them
  - Pathologic reflexes
  - Frequent focused examinations on ongoing basis (hourly or more often)

- *If spinal cord involvement is suspected*:

  - Motor functions in detail with testing of specific muscle groups
  - Sensory function
  - Reflexes
  - Bowel and bladder functions
  - Vital signs

---

peripheral stimulation and may elicit a spinal reflex response rather than a central, or brain, response. Noxious stimuli are also discussed in Chapter 68.

Document the location and type of stimuli applied along with the client's response so that the results can be accurately compared with those of future examinations. Terms such as "alert," "lethargic," "stuporous," "semicomatose," and "comatose" are vague. Avoid these terms unless your agency has explicit definitions for them to maintain consistency.

The *Glasgow Coma Scale* is an assessment tool designed to note trends in a client's response to stimuli (see Chapter 73). The original Glasgow Coma Scale was developed for use with head-injured clients. Many variations of this scale now exist for use with other client populations.

Orientation

Establish *orientation* to time, place, person, and event (or situation); for instance, ask What is your name? What year is this? What kind of place is this? Where are you? What brought you to the hospital today?

Memory

Identify gross deficits in long-term and short-term memory with simple tests. Test *long-term memory* when the client relates the past health history. (Of course, another source must be able to validate the data.) Test *short-term memory* by (1) stating three words for the client to remember (e.g., red, Broadway, three), (2) asking the client to say the words immediately, and (3) then asking the client to repeat them after a few minutes.

Mood and Affect

Assess mood by asking the client to describe how he or she feels. Assess affect (1) by the way the client appears (e.g., euphoric, depressed) and (2) from the reports of significant others. Is the client's affect appropriate to the situation?

Intellectual Performance

Intellectual performance consists of the fund of knowledge and calculation ability. Ask the client to identify com-

PHYSICAL ASSESSMENT FINDINGS IN THE HEALTHY ADULT

Neurologic System

Inspection

Mental Status. Oriented to person, place, time, and situation. No difficulty recalling recent and past events. Serial 7s deferred. Mood and affect congruent; cooperative, and pleasant. Thought process clear and logical. Demonstrates effective problem solving. Speech articulate, clear, and fluent.

Head, Neck, and Back. Normocephalic without obvious lesions. Maintains head position. Spine in straight alignment with normal cervical, thoracic, and lumbar curves. Neck and back have full range of motion.

Cranial Nerves.

CN I. Discerns smell of coffee, cinnamon, alcohol.

CN II. Visual acuity per Snellen's chart is OU = 20/20. Visual fields full to confrontation. Optic disc margins sharp, no cupping; cup-to-disc ratio is 1:3. Retina: Arteriovenous ratio is 2:3, without nicking. Fovea visualized.

CN III, CN IV, CN VI. PERRLA, direct and consensual. Accommodation present. EOMs intact without nystagmus or strabismus. Cover-uncover test negative. Corneal light reflections symmetrical.

CN V. Opens and closes mouth; chews, clenches teeth, and moves jaw side to side voluntarily. Sensation intact to forehead, cheeks, and chin. Corneal reflexes present.

CN VII. Face movements symmetrical with smiling, frowning, eyebrow raising, lip pursing, and cheek puffing. Discerns sweet, salty, sour, and bitter tastes (also CN IX).

CN VIII. Gross hearing intact. Whisper heard at 3 ft. Air conduction greater than bone conduction bilaterally.

CN IX and CN X. Tongue and uvula midline. Uvula and soft palate rise in midline with phonation. Gag reflex present bilaterally. Swallows, coughs, and speaks without difficulty.

CN XI. Performs shoulder shrugs. Turns head against resistance. Maintains head position against resistance.

CN XII. Tongue protrudes midline without deviation; pushes side to side with equal strength.

Motor Function. Muscle groups symmetrical. Gross and fine motor coordination intact. Moves all extremities through range of motion. Romberg's test negative. Pronator drift absent. Gait smooth, steady. Maintains balance walking on toes and heels. Rapid alternating movements and point-to-point maneuvers performed without difficulty.

Sensory Function. Sensation to light touch, pain, and vibration intact distally and over trunk, neck, and face. Position sense of fingers and toes intact. Stereognosis and graphism present bilaterally. Two-point discrimination: 2 mm on index fingers. Discerns two-point simultaneous stimulation.

Palpation

Head, Neck, and Back. Skull without lesions or tenderness; smooth and firm. Neck and paravertebral muscles firm, relaxed, and nontender. No pain or tenderness over spinous processes.

Motor Function. Muscle groups firm and elastic; strength rated as 5/5.

Percussion

Reflexes. Deep tendon reflexes rated 2+ (on a scale of 0–4+) in triceps, biceps, wrists, knees, and ankles. Plantar reflexes present. Abdominal reflexes present in all four quadrants.

Auscultation

Vascular Flow. Absence of bruit over carotid arteries bilaterally.

---

monly known people, places, events, and the like. Assess calculation ability by asking the client to count by 7s (*serial 7s*) or 3s. If the client is unable to perform reversed serial 7s, have the client perform simple addition or subtraction (e.g., 3 + 4 = ?, 13 − 5 = ?).

Judgment and Insight

Judgment and insight include reasoning, abstract thinking, problem solving, and the client's perception of the situation. Assess reasoning, abstract thinking, and problem-solving for indications of major problems with thought content (see Chapter 9).

Listen to how the client answers questions. Are the answers logical? Do they relate to the question? Can the client concentrate and remain focused, or is the client easily distracted? Assess abstract thinking by asking the client to explain a proverb such as "A rolling stone gathers no moss." Evaluate reasoning and problem-solving by

describing a situation and asking the client to give a solution. For example, "What would you do if you lost your house keys?" Assess insight and perception by asking the client to give an opinion about what might be the cause of the chief complaint.

Language and Communication

Language and communication assessment tests the ability to express and comprehend one's environment. Grossly evaluate *expression* and *comprehension* during the initial interview. Does the client initiate speech? Is speech fluent and appropriate?

Assess speech quality. Is speech clear and intelligible, or garbled because of facial droop or poor dentition? Note the content of speech (orientation, intellect, logic). Assess speech for articulation problems (usually motor disorders) or comprehension or expression problems (aphasic disorders).

Does the client follow verbal commands? Evaluate the client's ability to communicate and understand verbally, in writing, mathematically, and nonverbally.

COMPREHENSION AND EXPRESSION. Comprehension and expression are then assessed in more depth. Test the *ability to comprehend spoken language* by asking the client to follow basic commands ("Show me your right thumb," "Stick out your tongue"). To determine comprehension of written language, ask the client to read several words or sentences and explain them. Write a simple command ("Stick out your tongue"), and have the client read and then perform the command.

Evaluate *expression* as the client responds to questions that require more than a nod or a *yes* or *no* answer. Evaluate speech for flow, choice of words, and completion of phrases or sentences. If the client is expressively aphasic), test comprehension by asking *yes* or *no* questions or by having the client follow simple verbal commands. Assess written expression by having the client write answers to simple questions on paper (e.g., "Write your name and address").

INTEGRATED SENSORY FUNCTIONS. *Integrated sensory functions* involving language are often tested with this portion of the neurologic examination. Have the client perform simple addition or subtraction without writing. Ask the client to orally identify common objects, such as a pen, a key, and a watch. These skills require integration of cortical functioning (calculation) and visual recognition with expressive speech.

■ HEAD, NECK, AND BACK

Examine the head, neck, and spine using inspection, palpation, percussion, and auscultation. Tumors, vascular disorders, traumatic disorders, and problems involving the vertebrae and surrounding muscles may be detected through examination.

Inspection

Inspect the head for size, shape, contour, and symmetry. Note any ecchymosis (bruising) around the eyes or behind the ears. Anterior basilar skull fractures often result in "raccoon eyes," with periorbital ecchymosis and, occasionally, drainage of cerebrospinal fluid (CSF) from the nares. Middle fossa basilar skull fractures often result in ecchymosis over the mastoid process behind the ears (Battle's sign) and drainage of blood, CSF, or both from the ears.

Palpation

Palpate the skull lightly for nodules or masses and to supplement inspection findings. Wear gloves if there are open or draining areas. The skull normally feels smooth and firm. Areas of bogginess or depressions are abnormal. Palpation of neck muscles may identify masses or tender areas. Ask the client to flex the neck with the chin touching the chest; look for nuchal (back of the neck) rigidity, which is a sign of meningeal irritation.

Inspect and palpate spine alignment. Note any deviation from the normal curvatures. Palpate the paravertebral muscles for masses, tenderness, and spasm (also see Chapter 25).

Percussion

Gentle percussion over the spinous processes may produce pain or tenderness, which are abnormal findings.

Auscultation

Auscultation of major neck and other vessels may reveal bruits or other abnormal sounds suggesting an abnormality. Use the bell of the stethoscope to auscultate the carotid arteries. Bruits result from turbulent flow, usually a sign of atherosclerotic disease.

■ CRANIAL NERVES

The cranial nerves are referred to by specific name or Roman numeral. Cranial nerve (CN) examination is important for two reasons. First, CN III through CN XII arise in the brain stem. Testing their function provides information about the brain stem and related pathways. Second, three reflexes involving cranial nerves are called *protective reflexes* (corneal, gag, and cough reflexes). The presence or absence of protective reflexes indicates the ability to protect the eye surfaces and airway. This is especially important in unconscious patients.

Normal cranial nerve reflexes require an appropriately received stimulus (input) that produces an appropriate response (output). During testing of cranial nerves, the absence of a normal response may indicate (1) failure to receive stimuli (input failure), (2) failure to respond appropriately (output failure), or (3) a combination of input and output failure. Determining which problems exist is often a challenge. For example, vision is a function of CN II, and pupillary light response is a function of both CN II and CN III (Fig. 67–1; see Table 67–1). The structure and function of the cranial nerves are discussed in the Anatomy and Physiology review for Unit 15.

Olfactory Nerve (CN I): Smell

The function of CN I is purely sensory. Ask the client to smell and then identify an aromatic, nonirritating odor (e.g., coffee, isopropyl alcohol, toothpaste) with each nostril separately and with the eyes closed. Test with several different odors. If the client can perceive any one smell, consider the nerve functional.

Although inability to smell (*anosmia*) may develop in older people, problems such as basal skull fracture or olfactory groove tumor also may be responsible. Other possible causes of anosmia are cribriform plate fracture, an olfactory bulb or a tract tumor, and previous sinus disorders or surgery.

Optic Nerve (CN II): Vision

CN II has a purely sensory function. Assessment of the optic nerve involves the following steps:

1. Inspecting the globe for foreign bodies, cataracts, inflammation, or other obvious abnormalities. Details of eye assessment are given in Chapter 64.
2. Testing *visual acuity*. Have the client read a newspaper, a sign (from a distance), or a Snellen's chart. Eyeglasses should be worn during the test if the

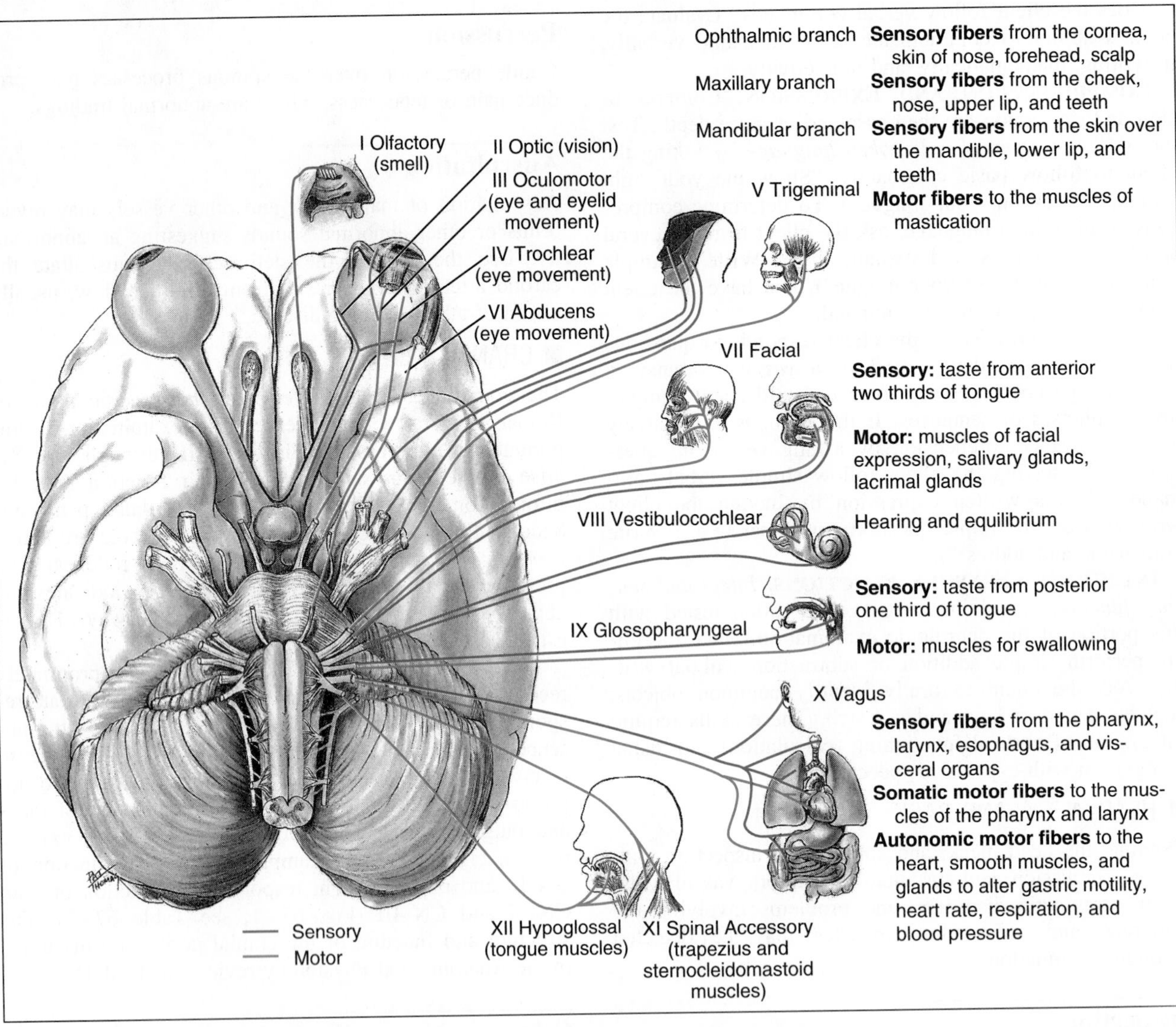

Ophthalmic branch **Sensory fibers** from the cornea, skin of nose, forehead, scalp

Maxillary branch **Sensory fibers** from the cheek, nose, upper lip, and teeth

Mandibular branch **Sensory fibers** from the skin over the mandible, lower lip, and teeth

V Trigeminal **Motor fibers** to the muscles of mastication

I Olfactory (smell)

II Optic (vision)

III Oculomotor (eye and eyelid movement)

IV Trochlear (eye movement)

VI Abducens (eye movement)

VII Facial

Sensory: taste from anterior two thirds of tongue

Motor: muscles of facial expression, salivary glands, lacrimal glands

VIII Vestibulocochlear — Hearing and equilibrium

IX Glossopharyngeal

Sensory: taste from posterior one third of tongue

Motor: muscles for swallowing

X Vagus

Sensory fibers from the pharynx, larynx, esophagus, and visceral organs

Somatic motor fibers to the muscles of the pharynx and larynx

Autonomic motor fibers to the heart, smooth muscles, and glands to alter gastric motility, heart rate, respiration, and blood pressure

— Sensory
— Motor

XII Hypoglossal (tongue muscles)

XI Spinal Accessory (trapezius and sternocleidomastoid muscles)

FIGURE 67–1 Distribution of the cranial nerves. Study this figure along with Table 67–1.

client usually wears them. Refraction errors are not significant in neurologic assessment.

3. Testing *visual fields* to determine whether vision is absent in one or more directions or in a portion of the visual field, such as half of the visual field, the middle portion, or both sides. Such losses may indicate various problems and may correlate with the area of the brain involved.

4. Examining the eye fundus with an ophthalmoscope. Gross inspection of the eyes and examination of the fundus can provide information about neurologic disease. Possible causes of abnormal findings include trauma to orbit or eyeball; fracture of optic foramen; diabetic retinopathy; laceration or blood clot in the brain's temporal, parietal, or occipital lobes; and increased ICP (e.g., papilledema).

Oculomotor (CN III), Trochlear (CN IV), and Abducens (CN VI) Nerves: Eyes and Eye Movement

CN III, CN IV, and CN VI have only motor components. CN III controls pupil constriction and elevation of the

upper lid. Pupils should be equal in size and round. In approximately 20% of the population, *anisocoria* (unequal pupils) is a normal finding. Older clients who have undergone cataract surgery with lens implants may have irregular, nonreactive pupils. This finding does not indicate neurologic damage. Note pupil size before shining a light into the client's eyes. Document each pupil's size and shape.

Approach the pupil from the temporal side while the client looks straight ahead. Test each pupil for both direct and consensual responses (pupillary constriction) to a light. A *direct response* occurs in the eye being tested. A *consensual response* occurs in the other eye. A direct response indicates an intact connection in the midbrain between CN II and the ipsilateral CN III. An intact consensual response indicates a connection between CN II and the contralateral CN III via a connection in the midbrain.

Test *accommodation* (eyes able to focus on both near and far objects) by having the client look across the room (away from the light source) and then at your fingers held about 6 inches from the client's nose. Normally, the lens shape changes and the pupils constrict. The notation

PERRLA (pupils *e*qual, *r*ound, *r*eactive to *l*ight and *ac*commodation) indicates that these functions are normal. When testing *pupillary light reflex* only (not accommodation), the abbreviation *PERL* (pupils *e*qual, *r*eactive to *l*ight) is used.

CN III lies over the edge of the uncal portion of the temporal lobe. Increased ICP or edema causes that area of the brain to shift, and CN III is stretched. This disruption of the CN III pathway causes either a sluggish response or absence of response to light. This response can be unilateral or bilateral, depending on the site and severity of edema. *Hippus*, the rhythmic constriction and dilation of a pupil, is caused by early compromise of CN III with increased ICP; it is not seen in all clients. Destruction of part of CN III can cause *ptosis* (drooping of the eyelid). Disorders or pressure on a specific side of CN III can cause the ipsilateral pupil to dilate, the eyelid to droop, and the eye to deviate outward.

CN III, CN IV, and CN VI coordinate to control eye movements in all six cardinal directions of gaze (see Chapter 64). Test the function of these nerves by having the client hold the head still and follow your finger or another object as it is moved in all directions of gaze. *Conjugate gaze* allows for the eyes to move in a coordinated effort for binocular vision (two images "merged" into one). *Disconjugate gaze* often occurs due to weakness of one or more extraocular muscles. *Diplopia* (double vision) occurs with disconjugate gaze because the two images are not "merged." If a client has diplopia but no muscle weakness can be demonstrated, shine a light so it reflects on both eyes. The area of reflection is normally symmetrical, meaning that the client has a conjugate gaze. In disconjugate gaze, the light's reflection is asymmetrical (i.e., not the same in both eyes).

If *extraocular movements* are intact, document as "EOMs intact." Also observe for *nystagmus* (involuntary eye movements), seen as fine, rhythmic eye movements that can be vertical or horizontal. Possible causes of abnormal findings include (1) pressure on CN III, CN IV, or CN VI at the brain stem due to fracture of the orbit; (2) increased ICP; and (3) tumor at or trauma to the base of the brain. An inability to look down or to walk down steps because of a visual disturbance might be related to CN IV dysfunction. Inability of an eye to move laterally outward is associated with compression of or damage to CN VI.

Trigeminal Nerve (CN V)

CN V has a motor division and a sensory division. The motor division innervates the muscles of mastication. Test CN V function by asking the client to clamp the jaws shut, open the mouth against resistance, open the mouth widely, move the jaw from side to side, and make chewing movements. A normal CN V allows all these activities. Document any asymmetry in the temporal muscles.

The sensory division mediates all sensations for the entire face, scalp, cornea, and nasal and oral cavities. With the client's eyes closed, test sensations such as pain (e.g., pinprick), touch (e.g., wisp of cotton), and temperature (e.g., hot and cold test tubes of water) on both sides of the face from the top of the head (vertex) to the chin.

Test the *corneal reflexes* by gently touching the cornea with a sterile wisp of cotton or gently stroking the eyelash. (Omit this test during the screening examination.) The normal response is brisk eyelid blinking. The corneal reflex involves CN V and CN VII. CN V is the afferent (sensory) arc, and CN VII controls closure of the eye (motor). Possible causes of abnormal findings include a tumor at or trauma to the base of the brain, a fracture of the orbit, and trigeminal neuralgia.

Facial Nerve (CN VII)

CN VII has both a motor division and a sensory division. The motor division innervates muscles controlling facial expression. Observe the face for symmetry and the ability to use facial muscles. Ask the client to smile, frown, raise the forehead and eyebrows, tightly close the eyes and resist attempts to open them, whistle, show the teeth, and puff out the cheeks. Test the anterior part of the tongue for taste by asking the client to close the eyes and protrude (stick out) the tongue. Then place a taste substance on one side of the anterior tongue. Have the client keep the tongue protruded while identifying the taste. Ask the client to rinse the mouth or drink a small amount of water before testing the other side. Test taste on each side with sweet, salty, acidic or sour (e.g., vinegar or lemon), and bitter (e.g., coffee) substances.

Common abnormalities noted with CN VII dysfunction include (1) loss of the nasolabial fold, (2) inability to close the eye and blink reflexively, (3) facial asymmetry, (4) drooling, (5) difficulty swallowing secretions, (6) loss of tearing, and (7) loss of taste on the anterior two thirds of the tongue. Possible causes of abnormal findings are Bell's palsy, temporal bone fracture, and peripheral laceration or contusion of the parotid region.

The lower half of the facial muscles, especially around the mouth, also receive innervation from the voluntary motor area of the frontal lobes. Deficits of lower facial muscles can be related to a lesion in the contralateral frontal lobe (i.e., client who has had a stroke and has a flattened nasolabial fold and facial droop on the opposite side retains the ability to close the eyelid on the same side of the face). Deficits on the lower half of the face only are called *central deficits* because the lesion is in the CNS. A deficit involving both the upper face and lower face is called a *peripheral deficit* because the lesion involves CN VII, which is a peripheral nerve.

Vestibulocochlear or Acoustic Nerve (CN VIII)

CN VIII is a sensory nerve with two divisions: cochlear and vestibular. The cochlear nerve permits hearing. Test *auditory acuity* by having the client listen to and report on a whispered voice, rustling fingers, or a tuning fork at various distances from the ear. Test *bone and air conduction* with a tuning fork. Audiometry may be used for a precise assessment.

The vestibular nerve helps maintain equilibrium by coordinating the muscles of the eye, neck, trunk, and extremities. *Equilibrium tests* include Romberg's and caloric tests (oculovestibular reflex) and electronystagmography. (Hearing and equilibrium assessment is described in Chapter 64.) Possible causes of abnormal findings include Ménière's syndrome and acoustic neuroma.

Glossopharyngeal (CN IX) and Vagus (CN X) Nerves

CN IX and CN X have both motor and sensory components. Because of overlapping innervation of the pharynx, assess these nerves together. Ask the client to open the mouth widely and say "Ah." Observe the position and movement of the uvula and palate. The palate should rise symmetrically, and the uvula should at the midline. Test the *gag reflex* by gently touching each side of the pharynx with a tongue depressor, which normally elicits a brisk response. Use a small amount of water to assess the ability to swallow. Test the posterior third of the tongue for taste, as with CN VII (perform when testing CN VII). Dysfunction of CN IX includes loss of taste and sensation of the glossopharyngeal nerve.

To test the function of CN X, ask the client to cough and to speak. Damage to CN X causes an ineffective cough and a weak, hoarse voice. To differentiate areas of weakness, ask the client to vocalize different sounds: "kuh-kuh" (soft palate), "mi-mi" (lips), "la-la" (tongue). Possible causes of abnormal findings include brain stem trauma or tumors, neck trauma, and stroke.

Spinal Accessory Nerve (CN XI)

CN XI has only a motor component. It innervates the sternocleidomastoid muscle and the upper portion of the trapezius muscle. Ask the client to (1) elevate the shoulders (with and without resistance), (2) turn (not tilt) the head to one side and then the other, (3) resist attempts to pull the chin back toward the midline, and (4) push the head forward against resistance. Disorders may produce drooping of a shoulder, muscle atrophy, weak shoulder shrug, or weak turn of the head. Possible causes of abnormal findings include neck trauma, radical neck surgery, and torticollis.

Hypoglossal Nerve (CN XII)

CN XII has only a motor component. This nerve innervates the tongue. Ask the client to open the mouth widely, stick out the tongue, and rapidly move the tongue from side to side and in and out. Document any deviation from midline. Assess strength by having the client push the tongue against the inside of the cheek while applying external pressure. Possible causes of abnormal findings include neck trauma associated with major blood vessel damage.

■ MOTOR SYSTEM

Assessing the motor system thoroughly involves numerous procedures. The following discussion focuses on the screening examinations and common abnormalities.

Muscle Size

Inspect all major muscle groups bilaterally for symmetry, hypertrophy, and atrophy.

Muscle Strength

Assess the power in major muscle groups against resistance (see Chapter 25). Assess and rate muscle strength on a 5-point scale in all four extremities, comparing one side with the other, as follows:

5/5 = Normal full strength. Muscle is able to move actively through the full range of motion against the effects of gravity and applied resistance.

4/5 = Muscle is able to move actively through the full range of motion against the effect of gravity with weakness to applied resistance.

3/5 = Muscle is able to move actively against the effect of gravity alone.

2/5 = Muscle is able to move across a surface but cannot overcome gravity.

1/5 = Muscle contraction is palpable and visible; trace or flicker movement occurs.

0/5 = Muscle contraction or movement is undetectable.

Next, test for subtle weakness in upper and lower extremities. For upper extremities, have the client hold the arms straight out in front with the palms up ("like holding a tray"). Ask the client to close the eyes and to maintain the position. A *pronator drift* is said to be present if one arm pronates and falls lower than the other. For the lower extremities, have the client walk on the heels, then on the toes. This tests dorsiflexion, plantiflexion, and balance.

Assessment of specific muscle groups evaluates deficits in certain areas, such as spinal cord disorders. Disorders of muscle strength may be exhibited as weakness on one side of the body, in both lower extremities, or in both upper and lower extremities.

If asymmetry is detected, ask the client or family whether it is long-standing or recent. Consider the client's age and physical condition when interpreting the results of muscle strength testing. One would not expect the same strength from a physically fit young client as from an elderly or debilitated client. If abnormalities are found in muscle power, more detailed assessment may be conducted with procedures such as EMG (see later in this chapter).

Muscle Tone

Assess muscle tone while moving each extremity through its range of passive motion. When tone is decreased *(hypotonicity),* the muscles are soft, flabby, or flaccid; when tone is increased *(hypertonicity),* the muscles are resistant to movement, rigid, or spastic. Note the presence of abnormal flexion or extension posture.

Muscle Coordination

Muscle coordination assessment consists of testing rapid alternating movements, point-to-point maneuvers, and maintenance of truncal balance and head position. Test *rapid alternating movements* by asking the client to touch (approximate) each finger to the thumb quickly in succession. Alternatively, ask the client to pat the thighs first with the palms, then with the back of the hands, and to repeat the patting quickly.

For *point-to-point testing*, hold up an index finger approximately 18 inches from the client. Ask the client to first touch his or her nose with a finger, then touch your index finger, and then touch the nose again. Repeat this several times while you move your index finger to different locations. Perform the test for the client's right and left hands. Test lower extremity coordination by asking the client to place the heel of the foot below the other knee and then to slide the heel down the shin toward the great toe. Repeat for the other leg.

Assess *truncal balance* with the client sitting. Can the client remain upright without support? Gently push the client to a leaning position. Can the client return to an upright position? Note *head position* by observing the ability to move the head while following your movements.

Disorders related to coordination indicate cerebellar or posterior column lesions. The defining characteristics of cerebellar dysfunction are (1) ataxia, (2) intention tremor (tremor upon nearing the object), (3) nystagmus, (4) ocular dysmetria (inability to gaze on an object), and (5) dysdiadochokinesia (arresting one motor impulse and substituting an opposite one).

Gait and Station

Assess gait and station by having the client stand still, walk, and walk in tandem (i.e., one foot in front of the other in a straight line). Walking involves the functions of motor power, sensation, and coordination. The ability to stand quietly with the feet together requires coordination and intact *proprioception* (sense of body position). If the client has difficulty standing, assess further to determine whether the client is weak or unsteady. If the client is weak, you need to protect the client from falling. Box 67–3 includes terms used to describe gait disorders.

Movement

Examine the muscles for fine and gross abnormal movements. Examples of fine movements are *fasciculations* (involuntary ripples or twitches that occur while the client

---

BOX 67–4	**Abnormal Movements Associated with Extrapyramidal Disease**

Akinesia: reduced body movement in the absence of weakness or paralysis; habitual movements (e.g., swinging arms) limited or absent
Athetosis: gross, writhing, worm-like movements of body, face, or extremities
Ballismus: a form of chorea; involuntary dramatic movements of arms and legs (*hemiballismus* involves only one side)
Bradykinesia: slow movement
Chorea: discrete, jerky, purposeless movements in distal extremities and face
Dystonia: prolonged twisting movements
Myoclonus: sudden muscle contractions of varying intensity that may involve a small part of one extremity or the entire body; may violently fling a client to the floor
Tic: involuntary movement of groups of muscles in stereotypic patterns; may be physical or psychogenic in origin; pathologic causes of tics include Tourette's syndrome and tic douloureux
Tremors: involuntary trembling or quivering; may vary in direction, amplitude, rhythmicity, parts involved, speed, and timing in relation to rest or activity; types include parkinsonian, familial, and senile

---

is relaxed), which may indicate lower motor neuron disease. Examples of more grossly abnormal movements, often representing extrapyramidal disease, are described in Box 67–4.

Move all joints through a full range of passive motion. Abnormal findings include pain, contractures, and muscle resistance.

Test for *apraxia* (inability to carry out a learned movement on command in the absence of weakness or paralysis). Ask the client to perform a common activity, such as tying shoes or combing hair. Apraxia is present if a client can follow other commands (indicating intact comprehension), has the motor strength to move the extremity involved, but cannot carry out the command.

Motor Testing of Unconscious Patients

In this chapter, the term "patient" is used to describe the client who is unconscious and who cannot be an active participant in care. The family is considered the client in these situations.

An unresponsive patient can be tested only for response to painful stimuli (e.g., reflex withdrawal of limbs, wincing, grimacing). Although a pain stimulus is used, the response is usually recorded as a motor system response. These responses are often incorporated into the motor scale of the Glasgow Coma Scale.

Use deep pain to elicit a sensory response when an unconscious patient is unresponsive to superficial stimuli. Use minimal stimulation to assess cerebral response to pain with techniques such as rubbing the sternum, applying pressure to the orbital rim, or squeezing the sternocleidomastoid muscle. Nail bed pressure may be used; however, the stimulus is a peripheral source of pain and may produce a spinal segment reflex response even in the absence of cerebral function. Document the site and type of stimulus used so that the examination can be ade-

---

BOX 67–3	**Terms Associated with Gait Disorders**

Ataxic: staggering and unsteady
Double step: alternate steps differing in length or rate
Dystonic: irregular and nondirective
Dystrophic or broad-based: legs far apart; weight shifting from side to side (waddling)
Equine: high steps
Festinating: walking on toes at an accelerating pace
Helicopod: feet (or foot) making a half-circle with each step
Hemiplegic: paralyzed on one side; paralyzed limb swings outward; foot drags; arm on affected side does not swing freely
Parkinsonian: short, accelerating steps; shuffling; forward-leaning posture; head, hips, and knees flexed; difficulty starting and stopping
Scissors: legs crossed while walking with short, slow steps
Spastic: stiff, short steps; toes catch and drag; legs held together; hips and knees flexed
Steppage: foot and toes lifted high; heel comes down heavily
Tabetic: high steps; foot slaps down

quately reproduced at a later time. Note the patient's response to the noxious stimuli. Following are the most common responses to painful stimuli:

- *Localization:* Patient reaches for the source of the stimulus and attempts to push the examiner away.
- *Flexion withdrawal:* Patient moves without purpose and may exhibit minimal movement, grimacing, or wincing.
- *Abnormal flexion (decorticate posturing):* Patient flexes, adducts, and internally rotates the wrists and arms to the chest and rigidly extends the legs. This posture indicates damage in the corticospinal tracts near the cerebral hemispheres that has left the rubrospinal tract intact.
- *Abnormal extension (decerebrate posturing):* Patient extends and pronates the arms while rigidly extending the legs. This posture indicates damage in the upper brain stem.
- *No response:* There is no visible reaction to painful stimuli.

■ SENSORY FUNCTION

The sensory function examination incorporates assessment of responses to superficial and mechanical sensations as well as cortical discrimination. Sensory assessment involves testing for touch, pain, vibration, position (proprioception), and discrimination. Assessment of hearing, vision, smell, and taste is also sensory assessment. Sensory assessment may identify dermatomes as having normal, absent, reduced, exaggerated, or delayed sensation. Dermatomes are discussed in the Anatomy and Physiology review for Unit 15.

A complete sensory examination is possible only on a conscious client because the client's cooperation is required. Always test sensation with the client's eyes closed. Help the client relax.

Conduct sensory assessment systematically. Test a particular area of the body, then test the corresponding area on the other side. Begin testing a selection of dermatomes that represent cervical, thoracic, lumbar, and sacral segments of the spinal cord. If you note a sensory loss, you can perform a more detailed testing of surrounding dermatomes. Document asymmetrical findings (those varying from one side to the other). If the client has a sensory loss, document the area of loss and where normal sensation begins. Sensation assessment may be documented on a body chart of dermatomes.

Superficial Sensation

Test superficial sensations by stimulating the skin in symmetrical areas on each side of the body according to dermatome distribution. Test *superficial pain* by alternating the sharp and dull ends of a broken cotton applicator. The wooden broken end is pointed enough for testing sharp sensation, yet dull enough not to break the skin. The cotton swab end serves as the dull stimulus. Use a new swab for each client to eliminate concern about cross-contamination from one client to another.

TOUCH AND PAIN

Ask the client to close the eyes. Explain that the client will feel a sharp or a dull stimulus. Demonstrate how sharp and dull feel. Touch the client with the dull end of the swab. Then apply a painful stimulus with the pointed end. Move from the fingers to the shoulders. Alternate the

two stimuli inconsistently (so that the client cannot predict which is being used), and ask the client to distinguish sharp from dull. Then test from the toes to the thighs. Finally, test the anterior and posterior trunk and the buttocks.

Keep the dermatomal pattern in mind while testing. Where there is a loss of the sense of pain, test for awareness of temperature. Otherwise, it is not necessary to test for temperature because pain and temperature sensations travel on related pathways.

OTHER MODALITIES

Other modalities for testing superficial sensation in the conscious client include using a cotton wisp to assess *light touch.* Follow the same guidelines as for testing superficial pain sensation, stimulating symmetrical areas of the dermatomes.

Temperature sensation is not assessed routinely. Perform the test only when pain and light touch responses are abnormal. Use two test tubes, one filled with warm water and one with cold water. Check first to ensure that the warm water is not too hot. Assess each major dermatome symmetrically. Alternatively, use the side of the tuning fork, which is usually cold, to test for awareness of temperature.

Mechanical Sensation

Mechanical sensations are assessed with vibration and proprioception.

VIBRATION

Use a tuning fork to test for vibration. Place the end of a vibrating tuning fork on a distal bony prominence, such as a finger or great toe joint. Ask the client to indicate when the vibration is felt and when it is no longer felt. Once the client indicates that the sensation has stopped, test your own joint to see whether you can feel vibration. You serve as the control. If the client reports that the sensation has stopped but you can still sense a clear vibration, the client has reduced vibratory sense. If the client does not feel vibration at all, move the tuning fork proximally to test the wrist, elbow, or ankle.

PROPRIOCEPTION

Test proprioception by holding the side of the client's fingertips, then the great toes, between thumb and index finger. As each of the client's fingers and toes are gently flexed and extended, ask the client to state when movement is felt and in what direction. If impairment is detected, test more proximal joints.

Discrimination

Cortical discrimination depends on the ability to integrate and interpret sensory stimuli in the parietal lobe. Included are tests for stereognosis, graphism, extinction phenomenon, and simultaneous two-point stimulation.

To test *stereognosis* (i.e., discernment of the form and configuration of objects felt, or three-dimensional discrimination), place three small, familiar objects, such as a coin, a key, and a paper clip, one at a time in the client's hands. Ask the client to identify each with the eyes closed.

To test *graphism* (recognition of the form and configuration of written symbols), trace different separate letters and numbers on the client's palm with the blunt end of a pen. Ask the client to identify each with the eyes closed. Orient the figures so that they are right-side-up for the client.

To test for the *extinction phenomenon* (simultaneous stimulation), prick the client's skin at the same point on the two sides of the body at the same time. Ask the client to state whether one or two pricks are felt.

To perform *two-point stimulation* (two-point discrimination), simultaneously prick the skin with two pins at varying distances apart to identify the smallest distance at which the client can perceive two pricks. Normal distances at which two-point discrimination is lost are: upper arms, 75 mm; thighs, 75 mm; back, 40 to 70 mm; chest, 40 mm; forearms, 40 mm; palms, 8 to 12 mm; toes, 3 to 8 mm; fingertips, 2.8 mm; and tongue, 1 mm.

Abnormalities of sensation include:

- *Dysesthesias:* well-localized irritating sensations, such as warmth, cold, itching, tickling, crawling, prickling, and tingling
- *Paresthesias:* distortions of sensory stimuli (e.g., light touch may be experienced as burning or painful sensation)
- *Anesthesia:* absence of the sense of touch
- *Hypoesthesia:* reduced sense of touch
- *Hyperesthesia:* pathologic (abnormal) overperception of touch
- *Analgesia:* absence of the sense of pain
- *Hypalgesia:* reduced sense of pain
- *Hyperalgesia:* increased sense of pain
- *Agraphesthesia:* inability to identify symbols traced on the palm when the eyes are closed
- *Astereognosis:* loss of sense of three-dimensional discrimination

Figure 67–2 summarizes patterns of sensory loss. Sensory changes are part of the normal aging process. Careful assessment of such changes is the basis of nursing intervention for elderly clients. Table 67–1 contains guidelines for assessment.

■ REFLEX ACTIVITY

Reflex testing evaluates the integrity of specific sensory and motor pathways. Reflex arcs consist of:

- Receptor (sensory) organ
- Afferent (sensory) nerve
- Connection in the central nervous system (brain or spinal cord)
- Efferent (motor) nerve
- Effector (motor) organ

Reflex activity assessment, always a part of neurologic assessment, provides information about the nature, location, and progression of neurologic disorders.

Normal Reflexes

Two types of reflexes are normally present: (1) superficial, or cutaneous, reflexes and (2) deep tendon, or muscle-stretch, reflexes (Table 67–2).

SUPERFICIAL (CUTANEOUS) REFLEXES

Superficial (cutaneous) reflexes are elicited by stimulation of the skin or mucous membranes. The stimulus is produced by stroking a sensory zone with an object that will not cause damage. Superficial reflexes (i.e., abdominal, plantar, corneal, pharyngeal [gag], cremasteric, and anal) are absent in pyramidal tract disorders. For example, they are absent on the affected side after a cerebrovascular accident (stroke).

ABDOMINAL REFLEX. Lightly stroking the skin on an abdominal quadrant normally contracts the abdominal muscle, moving the umbilicus toward the stimulated side.

PLANTAR REFLEX. Scratching the foot's outer aspect of the plantar surface (outer sole) from the heel toward the toes normally contracts or flexes the toes in clients older than 2 years of age.

CORNEAL REFLEX. Gently touching the cornea with a wisp of cotton causes reflex blinking. For example, to test the left eye, have the client look up and to the right, and bring the cotton wisp in from the side so the client cannot see your hand; then very gently touch the outer edge of the cornea.

In an unconscious patient, you can test the corneal reflex by holding the eyelids open and placing a drop of sterile saline on the cornea. This technique prevents inadvertent corneal abrasions.

PHARYNGEAL (GAG) REFLEX. Gentle stimulation with a tongue blade at the back of the throat and pharynx normally produces gagging. The corneal and pharyngeal reflexes are usually assessed with the cranial nerves, discussed earlier.

CREMASTERIC REFLEX. Stroking the inner thigh of a man normally elevates the ipsilateral testicle.

ANAL REFLEX. Stimulate the perianal skin or gently insert a gloved finger into the rectum. Normal response is contraction of the rectal sphincter.

DEEP TENDON (MUSCLE-STRETCH) REFLEXES

Deep tendon reflexes are also called muscle-stretch, or myotactic, reflexes because reflex muscle contraction normally results from rapid stretching of the muscle. This is produced by sharply striking a muscle tendon's point of insertion with a sudden, brief blow of a reflex hammer (Fig. 67–3 and Box 67–5).

Reflexes commonly assessed include the Achilles tendon, patella, biceps, and triceps as follows:

- An *ankle jerk* (plantiflexion of the foot) is produced by tapping the Achilles tendon.
- A *knee jerk, quadriceps jerk,* or *patellar reflex* (leg extension) is produced by tapping the quadriceps femoris tendon just below the patella.
- A *biceps jerk* (forearm flexion) is produced by tapping the biceps brachii tendon.
- A *triceps jerk* (forearm extension) is produced by tapping the triceps brachii tendon at the elbow.

OTHER NORMAL REFLEXES

Some normal reflexes involve structures other than skeletal muscles. For example, reflex mechanisms help maintain respiration and keep blood pressure within normal limits. Reflex salivation may follow the taste (or smell) of food. Flashing a light in an eye causes the pupils of both eyes to constrict (*light reflex* or *pupillary reflex*; see also the discussion of cranial nerve assessment).

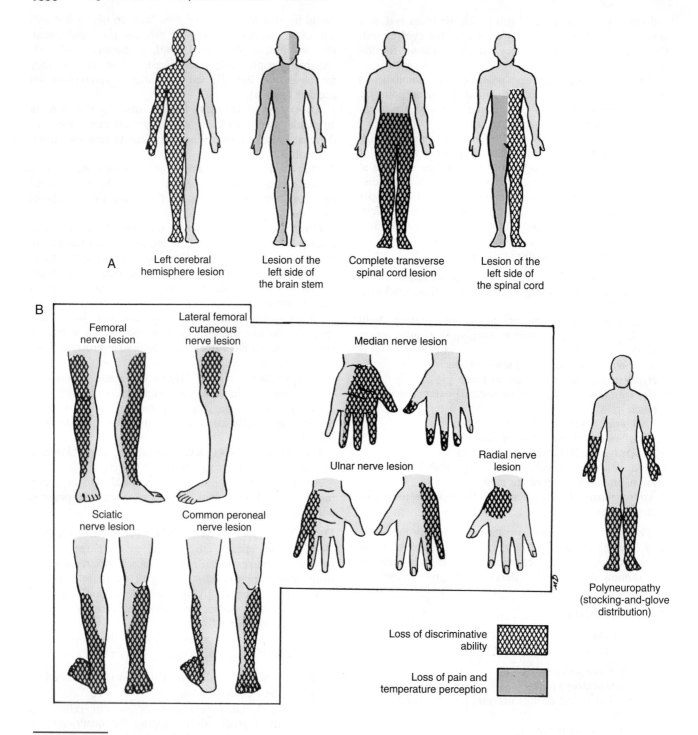

A Left cerebral hemisphere lesion

Lesion of the left side of the brain stem

Complete transverse spinal cord lesion

Lesion of the left side of the spinal cord

B

Femoral nerve lesion

Lateral femoral cutaneous nerve lesion

Median nerve lesion

Sciatic nerve lesion

Common peroneal nerve lesion

Ulnar nerve lesion

Radial nerve lesion

Polyneuropathy (stocking-and-glove distribution)

Loss of discriminative ability

Loss of pain and temperature perception

FIGURE 67–2 Patterns of sensory loss with brain and spinal cord disorders *(A)* and peripheral nerve lesions *(B).*

Abnormal Reflexes

Pathologic reflexes indicate neurologic disorders, often related to the spinal cord or higher centers. These responses include Babinski's, jaw, palm-chin (palmomental), clonus, snout, rooting, sucking, glabella, grasp, and chewing reflexes.

BABINSKI'S REFLEX. Test Babinski's reflex by gently scraping the sole of the foot with a blunt object. To elicit the reflex, start the stimulus at the midpoint of the heel,

and move upward and laterally along the outer border of the sole to the ball of the foot. Continue the stimulus across the ball of the foot (without touching the toes) toward the medial side and off the foot. Alternatively, start the stimulus at the midlateral sole and carry it down toward the heel. A normal response is plantiflexion of the toes. An abnormal response (presence of Babinski's reflex) is dorsiflexion of the great toe and, often, fanning of the other toes (Fig. 67–4). In extreme circumstances, a Babinski reflex may be accompanied by dorsiflexion of

TABLE 67-2	IMPORTANT REFLEXES		
Reflex	**Assessment Technique**	**Expected Response**	**Pathway Involved**
TENDON REFLEXES			
Biceps reflex	A blow on the examiner's thumb placed over the biceps tendon	Flexion of elbow	C5-6
Brachioradialis reflex (supinator)	Styloid process of radius is tapped while forearm is in semiflexion and semipronation	Flexion of elbow, fingers, and hand with supination of forearm	C5-6
Triceps reflex	Strike on triceps tendon just above the olecranon	Extension of elbow	C6-8 (C7 primarily)
Patellar reflex (knee jerk)	Tap on patellar tendon	Leg extends	L2-4
Achilles reflex (ankle jerk)	Tap on Achilles tendon	Plantar flexion of foot	S1-2
SUPERFICIAL REFLEXES			
Corneal reflex	Light touch at the corneoscleral junction	Closure of eyelids	CN V, VII
Palatal and pharyngeal reflexes	Light touch to soft palate and pharynx	Elevation of palate; gagging	CN IX, X
Abdominal reflexes	Stroke skin of upper, middle, and lower abdomen toward umbilicus	Contraction of abdominal wall toward stimulus	Upper: T7-9 Middle: T9-11 Lower: T11-12
Cremasteric reflex	Stroke medial surface of upper thigh	Elevation of ipsilateral scrotum and testicle	T12-L2
Anal reflex	Stroke perianal region	Contraction of external anal sphincter	S3-5
Plantar reflex (normal)	Stroke sole of foot	Flexion of toes	L4-S2
Plantar reflex (pathologic; Babinski's sign)	Stroke sole of foot	Dorsiflexion of great toe and fanning of other toes	L4-S2

C, cervical; CN, cranial nerve; L, lumbar; S, sacral; T, thoracic.
Adapted from Mitchell, P. A., et al. (1988). *AANN's neuroscience nursing: Phenomena and practice.* Norwalk, CT: Appleton & Lange.

the foot at the ankle and flexion at the knee and hip (called triple flexion).

When exaggerated deep reflexes are present, superficial reflexes are usually diminished or absent and pathologic reflexes (e.g., Babinski's reflex) are observed.

JAW REFLEX. The jaw reflex is also called mandibular reflex or "jaw jerk." Have the client relax the mouth, leaving it open slightly. Then tap gently on the lower jaw below the mouth. The jaw normally contracts and closes the mouth as a result of downward tapping. This reflex is absent in most clients but may be present in clients who have lesions in the corticobulbar tract above the midpons.

PALM-CHIN (PALMOMENTAL) REFLEX. The palm-chin reflex is produced by vigorous, rapid irritation on the mound of the palm at the thumb's base with a blunt instrument, which causes the chin muscles to pull up on the same side.

CLONUS. Clonus consists of rapidly alternating joint flexions and extensions resulting from continuous rhythmic contractions of a stretched muscle. This is not like a normal stretch reflex, which typically produces one reflex action. With clonus, the action continues. Support the leg at the knee, and help the client relax the leg. Rapidly flex the foot, and hold it in a flexed position. The flexion stretches the calf muscles and causes repeated "beats" of clonus if this reflex is present.

SNOUT REFLEX. A brisk midline tap above or below the mouth results in pursing of the lips. This reflex is normal in infants but is abnormal in adults.

ROOTING REFLEX. Stroking the side of the face causes the mouth to open and the head to turn to the stimulated side. This reflex is normal in infants but is abnormal in adults.

SUCKING REFLEX. Touching the lips with a blunt object results in movement of the tongue, lips, and jaws. This reflex is normal in infants but is abnormal in adults.

GLABELLA REFLEX. Tapping the forehead between the eyebrows results in sustained closure of the eyelids.

GRASP REFLEX. Placing an object in the palm of the hand causes the fingers to curl around it.

CHEWING REFLEX. A tongue blade placed between the teeth results in the tight closing of the jaws.

Grading Reflex Activity

Figure 67–5 shows the grading and documentation of superficial reflexes. Although 1+ or 3+ responses are not

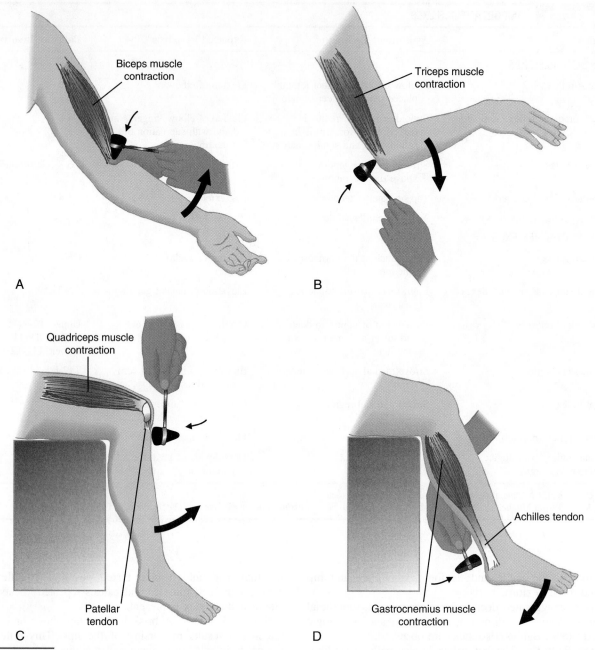

FIGURE 67-3 Deep tendon (muscle-stretch) reflexes. *A*, Biceps jerk (C5-6). *B*, Triceps jerk (C7-8). *C*, Patellar reflexes (L2-4). *D*, Ankle jerk (S1-2).

considered normal, they may not be significant findings. Asymmetrical responses are more significant. Abnormal reflexes may be present in both neurologic and metabolic disorders. Table 67-2 summarizes important reflexes.

■ AUTONOMIC NERVOUS SYSTEM

The autonomic nervous system cannot be examined directly. The system consists of sympathetic and parasympathetic innervation of many body organs. The functioning of the system is evaluated by a full body systems assessment. Clinical manifestations of autonomic nervous system disorders occur in many body systems. Unit 15 focuses on neurologic disorders (e.g., heatstroke, autonomic dysreflexia). Disorders of other portions of the autonomic system are discussed in the cardiac, urinary, digestive, reproductive, and endocrine chapters of this book.

Examples of activity under autonomic nervous system influence are:

- Increased or decreased heart rate
- Peripheral vasoconstriction or vasodilation
- Bronchoconstriction or bronchodilation
- Increased or decreased peristalsis
- Constriction or dilation of the pupil

Review any medications the client is taking. Many medications have side effects involving the parasympathetic or sympathetic nervous system.

BOX 67–5   Guidelines for Assessment of Deep Tendon Reflexes

Use the following guidelines when assessing deep tendon reflexes:

1. Test deep tendon reflexes with the client either sitting or supine.
2. Support the joint where the tendon is being tested so that the attached muscle is relaxed.
3. Use the pointed end of a triangular reflex hammer to strike over small areas while you place your thumb over the biceps tendon. Use the flat end of the hammer to strike over larger areas, such as the Achilles tendon.
4. Hold the reflex hammer loosely between thumb and fingers so it can swing in an arc.
5. Swing the reflex hammer using only wrist motion, not the arm or elbow.
6. Tap the tendon briskly.
7. Note the speed, force, and amplitude of reflex responses.
8. Compare reflex responses on the two sides of the body.
9. Grade reflexes on a 0 to 4+ scale. Consider the strength of the reflex in relation to the bulk of the muscle mass.

Repeat testing of reflexes graded 0 or 1+ by using the technique of reinforcement (see next phase). Note in the record that *reinforcement* was used. Reinforcement is a maneuver used to enhance deep tendon reflex responses when they are graded 0 or 1+. Reinforcement maneuvers for various deep tendon reflexes are as follows:

1. Ask the client to perform isometric contraction of other muscles, which may increase the generalized reflex response.
2. For the upper extremities, have the client either clench the teeth together or contract the quadriceps muscles (i.e., push the thighs against the table).
3. For the lower extremities, have the client lock the fingers together and try to pull them apart at the same time you test the tendon.

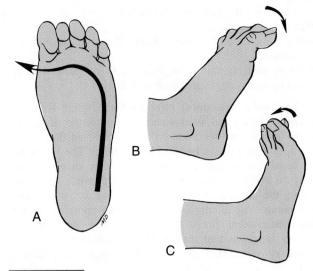

FIGURE 67–4 Babinski's reflex. *A,* Test maneuver: Using a blunt point, scratch the sole of foot as shown. *B,* Normal response (absence of Babinski's response) is plantiflexion of the toes. *C,* Abnormal response (presence of Babinski's response) is dorsiflexion of the big toe and often a fanning of the other toes.

- *Right gaze preference:* The client overcomes gaze preference and moves the eyes past the midline to the left when asked. The client turns the head to the left to see visitors enter a room.

■ CLINICAL APPLICATIONS

Initial assessment for diagnosis and triage of the client with a possible neurologic deficit consists of a history, a *brief* physical examination, and a neurologic examination. The *initial* neurologic examination usually includes assessments of the following (see Box 67–2):

■ FUNCTIONAL ASSESSMENT

A client who has a neurologic disorder may experience problems that disrupt basic function either permanently or temporarily. Ability to cope effectively with ADL (ability to meet basic needs) is often altered. For example, a client may have problems seeing, hearing, breathing, walking, talking, or eating. Remember, a client with a neurologic disorder may be frustrated just trying to do the things most people take for granted.

Functional assessment can be incorporated into the neurologic examination as well as into the daily care of the client. During the examination, note any deficits the client experiences and how the client manages them. Ask the client or family what changes have been made in daily routines to accommodate deficits. Document not only the deficit but also the functional response. Examples include:

- *Motor strength of right arm 4/5:* The client reports independence in ADL but notices difficulty in carrying books or groceries with the right arm.
- *Diplopia:* The client uses an eye patch, alternating the side covered every few hours to reduce the headache and nausea caused by diplopia.

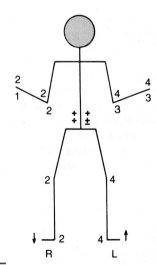

FIGURE 67–5 Documentation of muscle-stretch and superficial reflexes in left hemiparesis. Muscle-stretch reflex grades: 0, absent; 1, diminished; 2, normal; 3, brisker than normal; 4, hyperactive (clonus). Superficial reflex grades: 0, absent, ±, equivocal or barely present; +, normally active.

- LOC using the Glasgow Coma Scale
- Pupillary response
- Focal motor and sensory abnormalities in all four extremities
- Brain stem function via assessment of protective reflexes (gag, cough, and corneal reflexes)

The initial assessment provides the baseline for comparison when serial assessments are completed. If assessment findings are recorded on a time-oriented flow sheet, changes in status can be quickly identified. The frequency of serial assessments is determined by the diagnosis and may be every 15 minutes. You are responsible for monitoring the client's progress and reporting any unexpected deviations. All clients initially undergo complete neurologic assessment. Serial examinations may focus on deficits or functions that may indicate potential danger (e.g., pupillary responses and LOC for suspected increased ICP).

Thorough assessment and reporting of changes in a client serve a major role in determining the plan of care. Often the client's current condition (e.g., a decreased level of responsiveness and a change in pupillary reaction) is compared with initial data.

Because nurses are with clients consistently, it is the nurse's responsibility to develop sound assessment skills and to recognize trends in the client's condition that warrant further care. In no other area of practice are subtle changes as important to detect and act on than in the care of the client with a neurologic disorder.

DIAGNOSTIC TESTS

The complexity of the CNS combined with the relative inaccessibility of the brain requires study by indirect techniques. Early techniques, such as lumbar puncture, plain x-ray study, EEG, and pneumoencephalography, have provided the foundation for new techniques that allow more detailed examination of the brain structure, blood supply, and metabolism.

Air contrast studies, such as pneumoencephalography and ventriculography, were performed for assessment before the development of CT and magnetic resonance imaging (MRI). Results of such early tests may be found recorded in the history of a client who has had neurologic disorders for many years. As their name implied, the tests used air to provide contrast so that various portions of the brain could be viewed on an x-ray film. Air contrast studies were painful and had potentially serious side effects. Today's neurodiagnostic studies are much safer. This description of tests begins with the least invasive and moves to the more invasive tests of structure and then of function.

The focus of nursing care for the client who is to undergo diagnostic studies centers on physical and psychological preparation for the tests. You must plan for the specific assessments that must be made after the study is completed, such as continued neurologic assessment. Determine which components of the neurologic examination you will use in serial assessments before and after the test. These findings will be compared with results of the baseline neurologic examination. Before a diagnostic study, educate the client and family about the purpose of the study, the preparation needed, and the client's role during the test.

After the diagnostic procedures have been performed, assess the client for possible side effects and neurologic changes, and help the client understand the results of the studies, as needed. More information on diagnostic testing can be found in Chapter 11.

■ NONINVASIVE TESTS OF STRUCTURE

Skull and Spinal X-ray Studies

Skull x-ray studies reveal the size and shape of the skull bones, suture separation in infants, fractures or bony defects, erosion, calcification, sella turcica erosion, and pineal gland shift (>12 years of age). Spinal x-ray studies show fractures, dislocation, compressions, curvature, erosion, narrowed spinal cord, and degenerative processes.

The nurse may accompany clients who are confused, combative, or ventilator dependent to the radiology department to assist with client positioning and cooperation during the examination. If a spinal fracture is suspected, the neck is immobilized before the client is moved for the x-ray films. A lateral view of the cervical spine is taken first because the x-ray study can usually be conducted with minimal movement to determine whether fractures have occurred. Multiple views of the cervical spine are needed to rule out fracture. Until the results are known, maintain preprocedure precautions, such as spinal immobilization.

Computed Tomography

PROCEDURE

The primary purpose of CT scanning is to detect intracranial bleeding, space-occupying lesions, cerebral edema, and shifts of brain structures. Infarctions, hydrocephalus, and cerebral atrophy can also be identified. Advances in technology have expanded the uses of CT. Spiral CT utilizes injection of contrast material followed by rapid image sequencing to study movement of the contrast material through the cerebral blood vessels. Xenon CT uses inhaled xenon gas, which is absorbed into the blood stream, to enhance views that depict regional cerebral blood flow.

Aneurysms and arteriovenous malformations (AVMs) are best detected by angiography. The basilar cisterns and posterior fossa are not as well visualized on CT scans because these areas reveal high-density contrast between bone and air-filled sinuses (Fig. 67–6).

CT scans can be used for stereotactic procedures. Before the scan, a frame is applied to the client's head with pins inserted into the skull. The scan is performed with the frame in place. The computer marks reference measurements on the scan to guide the location of treatment.

PREPROCEDURE CARE

Answer any questions the client and family have about the CT scan. Explain that fasting usually is not required for CT of the head. If you think that the client might become nauseated, adjust the intake of food and fluids accordingly. For example, some clients prefer a light meal to reduce nausea, with others preferring an empty stomach before the test.

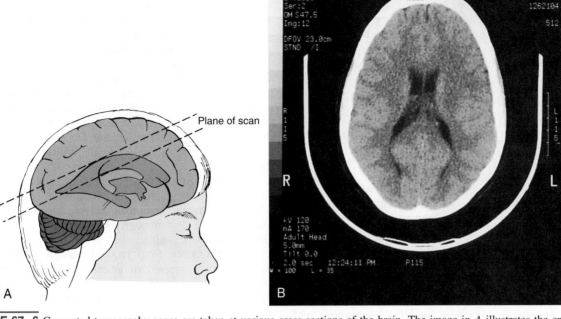

FIGURE 67–6 Computed tomography scans are taken at various cross-sections of the brain. The image in *A* illustrates the cross-section used for the scan shown in *B*.

Explain that a contrast agent may be used. Because some agents are iodine-based, ask whether the client has allergies to iodine or contrast material (see Chapter 11). If the client does not have an intravenous (IV) infusion, such an infusion will be established before the study begins. Before the test in which contrast material is to be used, check that informed consent has been obtained.

POSTPROCEDURE CARE

After the test, assess the client for reactions to contrast media and check other specific observations, such as presence of hematoma at the injection site and manifestations of IV infiltration of contrast material or fluids. Report infiltration of contrast medium to the radiologist. The client can resume normal activities unless other diagnostic tests are planned.

If a stereotactic frame was used during CT, it is to be left in place until the stereotactic procedure is completed. The frame may be a source of anxiety, and light sedation may be ordered to help keep the client relaxed.

Serial neurologic examinations are necessary after any testing to evaluate the potential effects on the client's neurologic function from contrast media, transportation to a new environment, or sedation. Assess the client before and after the CT scan.

Magnetic Resonance Imaging

PROCEDURE

MRI provides more anatomically detailed pictures than are available with CT (Fig. 67–7). MRI has several advantages over CT. MRI can detect disorders in white matter pathways caused by loss of myelin, as in multiple sclerosis, better than CT. MRI can evaluate cerebral infarction within hours of the event; CT would not demonstrate the stroke for several days. Contrast material

can be used with MRI to delineate blood flow through cerebral blood vessels in more detail than is possible with CT.

PREPROCEDURE CARE

Teach the client and family about the purpose of the test, what the client will hear and feel during the examination, and the client's role during the test. Before the test, the client should remove all metal-containing objects. IV fluid pumps must be removed immediately before the test. Spe-

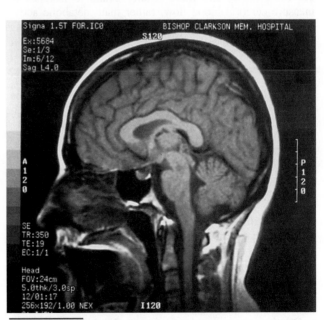

FIGURE 67–7 A normal magnetic resonance image. This sagittal section shows the cerebrum, ventricles, cerebellum, and medulla.

cial MRI-compatible monitoring devices, such as pulse oximeters and ECG leads, can be left in place.

Usually, the client may eat and may take prescribed medications before the examination. If contrast material is to be used, ask whether the client tends to become nauseated easily and adjust the intake of food and fluids accordingly. Chapter 11 details the MRI procedure and client care.

POSTPROCEDURE CARE
After the test, the client can resume previous activities.

Positron Emission Tomography

PROCEDURE
Positron emission tomography (PET) enables visualization of physiologic function in body areas. Often, the function of diseased tissue is different from that of normal tissues. PET has three primary uses:

- Determining the amount of blood flow to specific body tissues
- Revealing how adequately tissues use blood or nutrients, such as oxygen
- Mapping specific receptors, such as medications and neurotransmitters

PET can be used to measure cerebral blood flow, cerebral glucose metabolism, and oxygen extraction. PET is used in the diagnosis of stroke, brain tumors, and epilepsy, and to chart the progress of Alzheimer's disease, Parkinson's disease, head injury, schizophrenia, and manic-depressive illness.

A major disadvantage of PET is its high cost. The procedure requires its own positron to manufacture high-energy radioactive tracers; a PET system can cost $5 million initially. As a result, a modification of the procedure, called single-photon emission computed tomography (SPECT), has been developed. SPECT uses less precise but more stable and more readily available isotopes to measure cerebral blood flow, rather than metabolic activity as measured with PET. SPECT appears to be an effective diagnostic tool. A PET scan is shown in Chapter 11, Figure 11–6.

PREPROCEDURE CARE
Educate the client and family about the purpose of the test, what the client will hear and feel during the examination, and the client's role during the test. In contrast to CT and MRI equipment, the PET scanner is absolutely quiet. Clients must fast for 4 hours before the scan. If the client is diabetic, it is preferred that the blood glucose level be below 150 g/dl. Clients who are agitated may require sedation before the scan.

POSTPROCEDURE CARE
After the test, the client can resume usual activities.

Tests for Vascular Abnormalities

The noninvasive tests described here are useful in assessing cerebrovascular disorders.

OPHTHALMODYNAMOMETRY. Ophthalmodynamometry is used to compare the retinal artery pressures in the eyes. It may help in the diagnosis of extracranial vascular disease. While the retina is observed through an ophthalmoscope, pressure (or suction) is applied to the eyeball with a dynamometer and readings are obtained. A reduction in retinal artery pressure suggests insufficient carotid flow on the ipsilateral side.

DOPPLER ULTRASONOGRAPHY. Doppler ultrasonography may be used to measure blood flow (including direction and velocity) in the supraorbital region. In clients with occlusion or stenosis of the internal carotid artery, the direction of blood flow is altered (reversed) in the supraorbital artery, a change that may be detected by ultrasonography. Transcranial Doppler studies evaluate arterial flow in the circle of Willis and its major branches.

DOPPLER SCANNING. Doppler scanning combines Doppler ultrasonography with pulsed wave echocardiography. Visual representation of moving blood is obtained. Assessment of flow through carotid arteries is a common use of Doppler scanning.

QUANTITATIVE SPECTRAL PHONOANGIOGRAPHY. A noninvasive method of assessing the extent of carotid stenosis, quantitative spectral phonoangiography is spectral analysis of bruits arising from the carotid bifurcation.

■ INVASIVE TESTS OF STRUCTURE

Lumbar Puncture

PROCEDURE
In a client undergoing a lumbar puncture (LP), also known as a *spinal tap*, a needle is inserted into the subarachnoid space in the lumbar region of the spine below the level of the spinal cord. CSF can be withdrawn from or substances can be injected into this space.

LP is performed for assessment and therapeutic purposes. LP enables assessment of CSF pressure and collection of CSF for evaluation. When meningitis or subarachnoid hemorrhage is suspected, the CSF is examined for white blood cells and blood. A *myelogram* is a x-ray study in which contrast material is injected into the subarachnoid space after CSF is removed in order to examine the spinal canal. Therapeutically, LP is used to administer spinal medications and anesthetics.

Even though LP is generally a safe procedure, it is associated with potential hazards. The procedure can be uncomfortable. The client feels pressure in the lower back and may experience pain if a nerve root is touched with the needle during insertion. The potential complications of LP are CSF leakage, infection, intervertebral disc damage, and brain herniation.

A space-occupying lesion within the cranium, such as a tumor or bleeding, increases ICP. Therefore, LP is not performed in clients with papilledema (a sign of increased ICP), suspected intracranial lesions, increased ICP, or infection of the skin at the puncture site. CT scans are used in these clients to rule out masses before an LP is performed. If an LP were performed in a client with increased ICP, there would be a rapid decrease in CSF pressure around the spinal cord. This change in pressure might allow the structures within the brain to drop (herniate) into the spinal canal. The process of herniation creates pressure on the vital centers in the medulla (cardiac and respiratory centers) and may cause sudden death.

PREPROCEDURE CARE

Educate the client and the family about the purpose of LP, what the client will feel, and the client's role during the examination. Obtain an informed consent. If possible, the client should empty the bladder and bowels before the procedure. The client lies on one side with the legs pulled onto the abdomen and the head tucked into the chest in order to open the spaces between the vertebrae. The client must lie still during the test. Sedation may be ordered before the procedure.

Assemble the necessary equipment in the client's room. Lumbar puncture trays containing all the needed equipment are available. In addition, have laboratory request forms available and a marking pencil to label the samples of spinal fluid.

INTRAPROCEDURE CARE

LP to remove a sample of CSF is described here; however, the same general principles apply to any LP procedure.

1. Position the client on the side (lateral recumbency) with the back close to the edge of the bed. Place a pillow under the flank so that the spinous processes are horizontal. Use additional pillows between the knees and under the head to keep the spine horizontal.
2. Ask the client to draw the knees up to the abdomen and the chin onto the chest (Fig. 67–8). Help the client maintain this curved position to separate and increase space between the vertebrae so that the needle can be inserted more easily.
3. Stand in front of the client, and place one hand behind the client's knees and the other around the neck. Keep the client's upper shoulder from falling forward, thus preventing rotation of the spine. (An alternative position is to have the client sitting up with the head and chest bent toward the knees.)
4. After a local anesthetic is given, the physician places a small needle into the space between the vertebrae in the lower back. In adults, the needle is inserted about level with the top of the iliac crests (hip bones) or at the next lower vertebral level (usually between the third and fourth or fourth and fifth lumbar vertebrae). In adults, the spinal cord normally ends at the lower border of the first lumbar vertebra. Thus, the puncture site is low enough to avoid spinal cord injury.
5. The needle bevel is usually held parallel to the longitudinal fibers of the dura. This position limits the size of the dural tear and reduces the risk of CSF leak.
6. Local pain may occur as the needle passes the dura mater. Ask the client to mention additional discomfort, which may indicate misplacement of the needle.

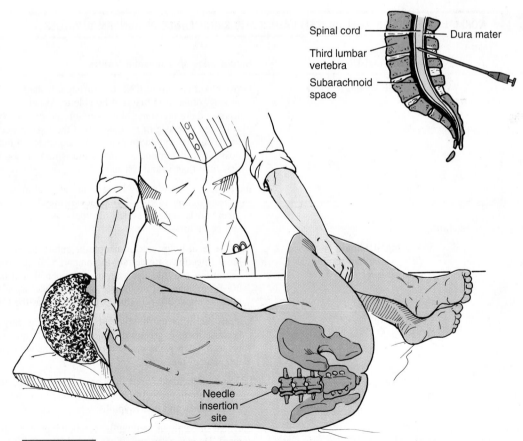

FIGURE 67–8 Lumbar puncture. Position the client laterally, with the knees drawn up to the abdomen and the chin brought down to the chest. This position increases the spaces between the vertebrae. The sterile lumbar puncture needle is inserted as shown, between the third and fourth (or fourth and fifth) vertebrae and enters the subarachnoid space.

7. When the needle has entered the subarachnoid space, the physician removes the stylus and attaches a stopcock and manometer to measure CSF pressure. The first stabilized CSF pressure is the opening pressure. Normal opening CSF pressure with the client in a horizontal position is 6 to 13 mm Hg (80 to 180 mm H_2O). Pressures exceeding 15 mm Hg (200 mm H_2O) are abnormal. Normally, CSF pressure oscillates (fluctuates) in the manometer, readily responding to coughing, straining, and changes in the person's breathing. If there is a blockage in the spinal canal, the CSF pressure may not oscillate.

8. CSF specimens are collected in a series of small sterile test tubes, numbered in sequence of collection (e.g., No. 1, No. 2). Two to 3 ml of CSF is collected in each tube; 8 to 10 ml may be removed.

9. The needle is withdrawn, and the physician places a dry sterile dressing over the puncture site.

In adults, CSF is assessed for cells, chloride, glucose, protein, and lactate dehydrogenase (LDH) as well as pressure. Table 67–3 lists common abnormalities of CSF. In the analysis of CSF, the first vial obtained is not assessed for blood because it may contain blood from the puncture.

POSTPROCEDURE CARE

Record vital signs after the LP. Sometimes, lying flat for several hours is prescribed. The client can eat and drink as before the test. Drinking extra fluids will help restore CSF volume. If the CSF pressure measurement indicated a high ICP, assess the client for decreasing LOC, which would indicate rising ICP.

Post-LP headache (spinal puncture headache, spinal headache) is typically throbbing, bifrontal, and suboccipital, developing a few hours to several days after an LP. The headache is probably due to continuing CSF leakage through the opening in the dura made by the needle. As a result of the leak, the CSF circulating around the cranium is depleted. The fluid loss allows abnormal movement of the brain in the skull. When the brain moves, tension is placed on the meninges and venous sinuses, causing pain. The headache is usually relieved when the client lies down and is made worse with sitting up or with a sudden jolt of the head. Such headaches usually disappear within 24 hours but may last for several days.

To reduce the risk of post-LP headache, have the client remain in bed after the examination. Although physician's orders may differ, an average time in bed is 3 hours. Encourage fluids to replace the CSF withdrawn during the test. Once a headache begins, treatment may be bed rest in a dark, quiet room and the administration of analgesics and fluids.

If the headache continues, an epidural blood patch may be required. Blood is withdrawn from the client's vein and injected into the epidural space, usually at the LP site. The blood acts as a fibrin patch to seal the hole in

TABLE 67–3	NORMAL CEREBROSPINAL FLUID (CSF) VALUES AND SIGNIFICANCE OF ABNORMAL VALUES	
Substance	**Normal Value (Conventional Units)**	**Significance of Abnormal Values**
Blood	None; CSF should be clear	Gross blood is seen in CNS hemorrhage. If the CSF is grossly bloody, other tests may not be able to be performed. Rarely, there are some blood cells in the first tube of CSF collected, because of trauma during the tap. The collection of specimens should be marked in sequence, so that it is possible to determine whether there is more blood in the first tube than in the last tube.
Cells	0–5 mononuclear	Increased neutrophils may be seen in bacterial infections such as bacterial meningitis. Lymphocytes may be increased in tuberculosis and some viral disorders. Aerobic pathogens can be cultured.
Glucose	50–75 mg/dl, should be 20 mg less than serum glucose level	Glucose level is lowered in neoplasm, inflammation, and bacterial infections. Be certain to compare CSF glucose with serum glucose. Ideally, a serum specimen should be drawn 30–60 minutes before lumbar puncture, because it takes glucose about 30–60 minutes to diffuse into the CSF.
Protein Albumin	15–45 mg/dl 10–30 mg/dl	Lesions that interrupt the blood-brain barrier increase proteins because there is greater diffusion. Decreased proteins can be seen when water reabsorption occurs, as with elevated intracranial pressure.
IgG Oligoclonal bands	1–4 mg/dl Absent	IgG and oligoclonal bands (an abnormal type of protein band seen on immunoelectrophoresis) are often present in multiple sclerosis and neurosyphilis.
Pressure	70–180 mm H_2O	Elevated in bacterial meningitis, cerebral bleeding, and tumors. Decreased in conditions that obstruct CSF flow, such as tumors of the spinal canal.

CNS, central nervous system; CSF, cerebrospinal fluid; IgG, immunoglobulin G.

the dura and prevent further CSF leakage. Blood patches cannot be performed in a client who has bleeding tendencies or infection at the puncture site.

Myelography

Myelography is an x-ray examination of the spinal cord and vertebral canal following introduction of contrast material into the spinal subarachnoid space (Fig. 67–9). It is used to study the spinal canal and subarachnoid space. This study is a valuable assessment tool when the spinal cord is thought to be compressed (e.g., by a herniated intervertebral disc or an encroaching tumor). Myelography is used to identify spinal cord disorders, such as intramedullary tumors, AVMs, and syringomyelia.

In the radiology department, an LP is performed, a small amount of CSF is withdrawn, and contrast material is injected. With the needle in place, the client is turned onto the abdomen and secured to the table. While the radiologist observes with fluoroscopy, the table is slowly tilted. Tilting causes the column of contrast material to move up or down within the subarachnoid space, permitting visualization of the desired areas. Standard films are taken. If the contrast material used is water-soluble, it is not removed from the spinal column. In some cases, the myelogram is followed by a CT scan of the spine to evaluate the contrast-enhanced structures.

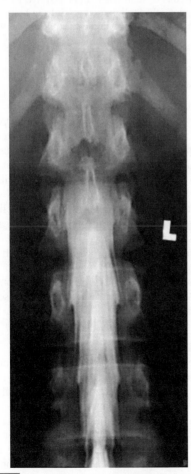

FIGURE 67–9 A myelogram of the lumbar spine shows contrast dye flowing throughout the subarachnoid space without obstruction.

Preparation for a myelogram requires hydration for at least 12 hours before the procedure. After the myelogram, the client remains flat in bed if oil-based contrast material was used; the head of the bed is elevated 15 to 30 degrees if water-based contrast material was used. Usually, the client remains in bed 6 to 8 hours and then resumes normal activity. Encourage the client to drink extra fluids. Assess neurologic status frequently.

Back pain (ranging from mild discomfort to severe pain) in the area of the needle insertion may develop and may last a few days. Also, the client may experience a stiff neck and headache for a few days, particularly if the contrast medium was allowed to rise to high cervical levels. The discomfort is usually relieved by having the client lie flat and by administration of fluids and analgesics (see LP discussion).

Cisternal Puncture

Cisternal puncture involves puncture of the cisterna magna (a small reservoir of CSF between the cerebellum and medulla). This procedure is performed either to drain CSF or to obtain a specimen if there is a block in the spinal subarachnoid space or if LP is contraindicated. CT and MRI have largely replaced this procedure.

A short-beveled needle is inserted below the occipital bone, between the first cervical lamina and the rim of the foramen magnum. Fluoroscopy is used to guide exact placement of the needle. If the client has a lesion on the spinal cord, the upper edge of the lesion can be determined by contrast material injected via the cisternal puncture. If there is any concern about the client's ability to cooperate and hold still, sedation or general anesthesia may be used. Positioning the client and subsequent assessments and interventions are essentially the same as those for LP.

Cerebral Angiography

A *cerebral angiogram* consists of injection of contrast material into an artery to visualize intracranial circulation (Fig. 67–10). Angiography is the procedure used most often to visualize aneurysms, AVMs, major vessel displacement, vascular occlusion, and thrombi. Cerebral angiography is not only invasive; it is also a procedure in which small errors can result in permanent disability or death. Meticulous attention must be given to the client before, during, and after angiography.

PROCEDURE

A catheter is inserted into the femoral artery and guided with a fluoroscope into the carotid or vertebral arteries. This approach has replaced previous approaches in which the carotid, vertebral, or brachial vessel was punctured directly. A femoral artery puncture is less traumatic, and local complications, such as infection and bleeding at the puncture site, occur away from the neck. Once the vessels are reached, the contrast agent is injected and a series of x-ray films is taken from lateral, anteroposterior, and oblique approaches. Sequential views show the movement of the contrast material in the vessels.

After the catheter is removed, a sterile dressing is placed over the puncture site and firm pressure is applied to the site for 10 minutes to prevent hematoma formation.

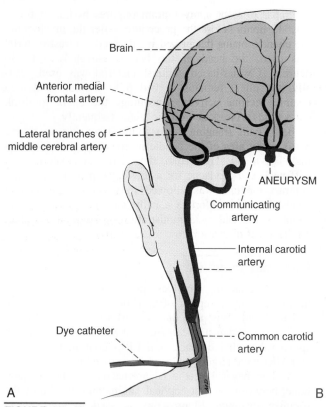

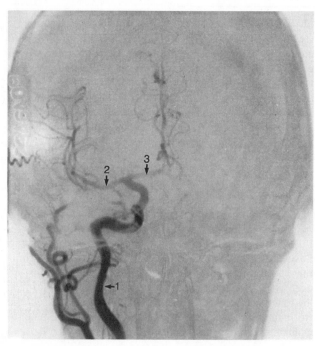

FIGURE 67–10 Cerebral angiography allows x-ray visualization of the brain's vascular system when a contrast dye is injected arterially. *A*, Insertion of dye through a catheter in the common carotid artery, subsequently outlining vessels of the brain. *B*, An angiogram using the subtraction technique. 1, Internal carotid artery. 2, Middle cerebral artery. 3, Middle meningeal artery.

Sandbags and a pressure dressing may be used to provide firm pressure after the first 10 minutes. The injection site may be tender.

INTERVENTIONAL ANGIOGRAPHY. A polymer glue or small balloons are used to occlude feeding vessels in tumors or AVMs. Blocking the feeding vessels reduces the size and vascularity of the tumor or AVM, thus diminishing the need for, and the complications of, its surgical removal. Interventional angiography also enables balloon angioplasty to be performed in order to expand atherosclerotically narrowed cerebral vessels.

DIGITAL VENOUS ANGIOGRAPHY. Computerized digital video subtraction systems allow visualization of vascular structures. Much less contrast medium is required compared with that needed for cerebral angiography. A central venous line is necessary to inject the contrast medium. Raw data are stored in digital form and can be retrieved at any time. Images with the best vascular visualization are selected and subjected to electronic manipulation to improve image detail.

Indications for digital venous angiography include:

- Assessment for transient ischemic attacks
- Serial follow-up evaluations for known carotid stenoses
- Assessment of intracranial tumors
- Postoperative assessment of aneurysms
- Follow-up evaluations after extracranial-intracranial bypass procedures
- Assessment of dural venous sinuses

Three to four venous injections of contrast material are usually required for a complete diagnostic craniocerebral study. The only potential complication is a reaction to the contrast material.

PREPROCEDURE CARE

Educate the client and family about the purpose of the test, what the client will experience, and the client's role during the procedure. Before the test, the client may not take anything by mouth for 4 to 6 hours but should be kept well hydrated. IV fluids may be prescribed. Document the neurologic status of the client to serve as a baseline measure after the examination. The client should remove any metal items from the head, such as barrettes and earrings. Report allergies to iodine.

During the test, the client is given an injection of local anesthetic before placement of the catheter. The client may have a warm flushed feeling when the contrast material is injected. The client is continually assessed for neurologic deterioration while the angiogram is being performed.

POSTPROCEDURE CARE

After the test, assess for complications, which are rare. They include (1) local and systemic allergic reactions to the contrast medium, (2) spasm or occlusion of the vessel by a clot, (3) hemorrhage, and (4) obstructive clot formation above a femoral injection site. Assess for reactions to the contrast material. Spasm or occlusion of the target vessels causes symptoms similar to those of a stroke (see Chapter 70.) Clot formation at the injection site also causes ischemic reactions in the affected area. These adverse reactions are usually reversible and rarely cause permanent damage.

Complications vary according to their cause. For example, indications of centrally located reactions include changes in LOC, aphasia, hemiplegia (paralysis of one side of the body), hemiparesis (muscular weakness or partial paralysis of one side of the body), convulsive seizures, and increased focal symptoms. A hematoma in the neck may cause difficulty in breathing or swallowing. If the hematoma is large, it may compress the trachea and esophagus, requiring emergency tracheostomy. Nausea, vomiting, extremity numbness or weakness, speech disturbances, profuse sweating, and alterations in LOC may indicate a delayed reaction to the contrast material.

After angiography, position the client safely and comfortably and maintain the prescribed bed rest. Clients undergoing diagnostic angiograms may need to stay in bed only 4 hours. If interventional treatment was performed, the client may have to remain in bed longer.

Check the injection site frequently for bleeding and hematoma formation. Keep the affected extremity (arm or leg) or neck straight to prevent vessel kinking and clot formation. Assess vital signs (every 15 minutes for 1 hour, then every 30 minutes for 1 hour, then every hour for 4 hours), pulses distal to the puncture site, color and temperature of the extremity, and the ability to move the distal extremity. The client can usually resume a regular diet.

Cerebral Perfusion Studies

When brain death is suspected, cerebral perfusion can be assessed. The patient is injected with technetium 99m (^{99m}Tc), a radioisotope. The ability of ^{99m}Tc to perfuse from blood vessels into brain tissue is assessed with a scanner. In patients who are clinically brain-dead, there is no uptake of the substance by the cerebrum or cerebellum. The radioisotope is injected, and the scanner can be brought to the bedside to evaluate perfusion. Although

brain death can be determined by clinical examination, the perfusion study is used when the clinical findings are clouded by the previous use of long-acting sedative medications.

■ NONINVASIVE TESTS OF FUNCTION

Electroencephalogram

An electroencephalogram is a measurement of the electrical activity of the superficial layers of the cerebral cortex. It records the electrical potentials from neuron activity within the brain in the form of wave patterns. The intensity and pattern of electrical activity are influenced by the reticular activating system. The wave characteristics depend on the extent of cortical activity. Waveform patterns can be affected by (1) structural lesions, such as tumors, subdural hematomas, and areas of infarction, (2) infections, (3) degenerative processes, and (4) metabolic disorders.

Several distinct wave patterns are found in recordings of clients without brain disorders. Wave patterns are called delta, theta, alpha, or beta, depending on their appearance (amplitude and frequency). EEG waves are shown in Figure 67–11. EEG wave patterns change with aging and disease; for example, beta activity increases with age.

PROCEDURE

Electrodes are attached to the client's scalp (Fig. 67–12). The waveforms are amplified and recorded on a moving paper strip, much as for an electrocardiogram. The recordings are interpreted according to the characteristics, frequency, and amplitude of brain waves.

If the patient is comatose or is unable to be moved, a bedside study can be performed. For routine diagnostic examination, the client is taken to an EEG laboratory, a more controlled environment. The scalp is cleaned, and

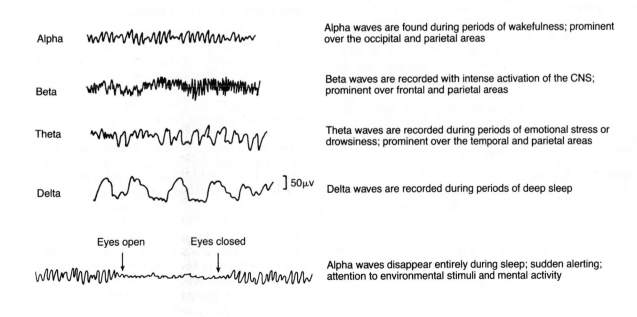

Alpha — Alpha waves are found during periods of wakefulness; prominent over the occipital and parietal areas

Beta — Beta waves are recorded with intense activation of the CNS; prominent over frontal and parietal areas

Theta — Theta waves are recorded during periods of emotional stress or drowsiness; prominent over the temporal and parietal areas

Delta — 50μv — Delta waves are recorded during periods of deep sleep

Eyes open   Eyes closed — Alpha waves disappear entirely during sleep; sudden alerting; attention to environmental stimuli and mental activity

1 sec

FIGURE 67–11 Electroencephalographic waves. (Modified from Guyton, A. C., & Hall, J. [Eds.]. [1996]. *Textbook of medical physiology* [9th ed.]. Philadelphia: W. B. Saunders.)

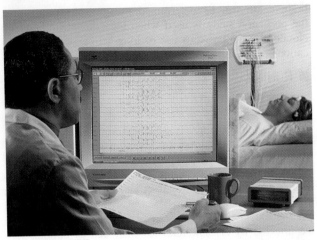

FIGURE 67–12 Client undergoing an electroencephalogram.

electrodes are applied to the scalp and ear lobe (for reference) with special conductive gel. Leads can also be placed in the nasopharynx to assess waveforms from the temporal lobe.

The first portion of the test is performed with the client as relaxed as possible to obtain a baseline recording. Further readings are taken while the client is hyperventilating, sleeping, or viewing flickering lights. Hyperventilation alters acid-base balance (respiratory alkalosis) and decreases cerebral blood flow. Flickering lights may trigger seizures. Sleep may evoke abnormal EEG patterns not present while the client is awake. The client may be kept awake the night preceding the test or may be sedated to induce sleep.

The electroencephalogram is used to assess seizure disorders. The results are diffusely abnormal in various metabolic disturbances, toxic conditions (e.g., drug overdose), coma, organic brain syndrome, and infections such as meningitis and encephalitis. The device may be used in the operating room to monitor cerebral activity during surgery on the blood vessels in the head or neck. Sleep patterns in depressed clients may also be assessed. Some clients are assessed for temporal lobe epilepsy with the use of a 24-hour recording. The device also facilitates diagnosis of narcolepsy and insomnia.

Absence of waves on the recording ("flat lines") may be one of the criteria for defining brain death. EEG studies of comatose patients show a high correlation of flat EEGs with death of the client in a coma.

PREPROCEDURE CARE
Explain the purpose of the test and the procedure to the client and family. Reassure them that electricity does not enter the brain (shock is not given) and that the machine cannot read minds.

Before EEG is performed, the client's hair must be shampooed. Stimulants (e.g., coffee, alcohol, tea, cola, and cigarettes), antidepressants, tranquilizers, and anticonvulsants should be avoided for 24 to 48 hours before the test. Sometimes sleep is withheld. If the client will be asked to sleep for a portion of the test, sleep should be minimized the night before the test. The client will be asked to relax during the test because anxiety can block alpha rhythms and produce artifacts from increased muscle

tone in the head and neck. Send adequate supplies (i.e., IV fluids or oxygen) to the laboratory with the client.

If EEG is being performed to evaluate the possibility of brain death, artifacts must be kept to a minimum. Electrode manipulation, electrical interference, respirator cycling, and someone walking in the room can cause artifacts. Follow agency guidelines when EEG is performed at the bedside.

POSTPROCEDURE CARE
After EEG, the client can resume previous activity, medications, and diet. If seizure activity is possible, follow precautions to avoid seizures. The hair can be washed, and acetone may be used to remove the electrode paste or gel from the scalp and hair.

Evoked Potential Studies

Evoked potential (EP) studies are a form of EEG in which brain waves are monitored as various stimuli are given. The test is used to assess the function of the cerebral hemispheres and the brain stem. A variety of types of stimuli are used, such as auditory, somatosensory, and visual. Typical stimuli are flashing lights, buzzing tones, and peripheral nerve stimulation. EP studies can be used to assess blindness, deafness, and brain stem injury. Specific brain signals can be accentuated and others filtered out, allowing assessment of brain waves from other areas.

EP studies are carried out in the same fashion as EEG studies. EP studies can detect abnormalities even if the client is sedated or paralyzed with neuromuscular blocking agents. Some clinicians believe that EP studies are more reliable than clinical assessments in predicting neurologic recovery in comatose, head-injured patients. Nursing interventions are the same as for the client undergoing an EEG study except in the explanation of the variations between the tests.

Neuropsychological Testing

Neuropsychological testing involves a series of tests to evaluate cortical function by localizing the area and extent of impairment and determining the rate of progression or recovery. The tests gauge many types of abilities, such as motor, perceptual, language, visuospatial, and cognitive. Test results can provide information regarding the extent of cognitive impairment and the effect it may have on functional ability. Clinical manifestations as well as results of neuropsychological evaluations, neurologic examinations, and neurodiagnostic studies are correlated and used to plan rehabilitation. Serial testing is valuable for monitoring rehabilitative progress and recovery in clients with problems such as head injury and epilepsy.

A client may be referred for neuropsychological assessment either in the acute phase of or months after an injury. For example, after a head injury in which the physical neurologic assessment is normal and the EEG reveals only mild generalized abnormalities, the client may complain of being unable to work because of persistent headaches. Test results may be used to make recommendations about treatment, including educational and vocational rehabilitation.

Neuropsychological tests measure deficits in coping skills by assessing the skills directly. They may be helpful when deficits in adaptive abilities are suspected. An individual test may be performed in the case of a disorder with only one specific manifestation, or a complete series of tests with extended evaluation may require several hours or days of testing. The client's level of performance is compared with scores representing normal performance levels. General measures of intelligence (e.g., Wechsler Adult Intelligence Scale) as well as tests of emotional and personal adjustment (e.g., the Minnesota Multiphasic Personality Inventory) are used.

Testing may be nonspecific in implicating the presence of brain damage or very narrow in scope with sensitivity for certain areas of the brain. Results may indicate that something is wrong but may be unable to identify the specific problem.

Memory loss is common after head injury and in neurologic disorders. Skills such as reading, which have been stored in the brain over the years, may be retained, in contrast to new learning or short-term memory, which may be impaired. An impaired memory may interfere with the effectiveness of client teaching and the client's ability to learn. A brain-injured client with damage to the limbic system, especially the hippocampus, amygdala, or areas of the temporal and prefrontal lobes, is a candidate for neuropsychological testing to determine memory loss.

Testing can identify problems in cognitive, psychomotor, and affective domains. Left hemisphere lesions impair factual information functions, like problem-solving, decision-making, and judgment. Client and family teaching must be modified to address these deficits.

Both the right and left hemispheres are involved with psychomotor learning. The right hemisphere controls visuospatial abilities, and the left controls verbal instructions and sequencing of activities. Repetition and time are needed for the individual to perform activities automatically. Memory loss that is identified from damage to the right or left hemisphere and is causing affective learning deficits can be improved with role modeling and one-to-one and group therapy. Documentation of client behavior and functional abilities assists the neuropsychologist in following the client's progress and recovery.

■ INVASIVE TESTS OF FUNCTION

Caloric Testing

The oculovestibular reflex, or *caloric test,* provides information about the function of the vestibular portion of CN VIII and pathways in the pons and midbrain. It aids in the differential diagnosis of brain stem lesions (see also Chapter 68).

The test is performed only in an unconscious patient to determine the presence of brain stem function. Check that the ear canal is patent and that the tympanic membrane is intact. Ice-cold water is introduced into the auditory canal. If brain stem function is intact, the eyes move in a conjugate fashion slowly toward the irrigated side and then quickly move back to midline. With brain stem death, this nystagmus pattern does not occur. Oculovestibular tests are contraindicated for patients with perforated eardrums or with acute labyrinthine disease. As with pupil signs, abnormalities in eye movements help to localize the area of a disorder. They also help differentiate between structural and metabolic causes of coma.

Peripheral Nerve Studies

ELECTROMYOGRAPHY. EMG is used to measure and document electrical currents produced by skeletal muscles, called *muscle action potentials.* Small needle electrodes are inserted into muscles. The electrical potentials of each muscle are amplified, transmitted to an oscilloscope, and displayed on a screen. The recording can be made audible and documented on paper (Fig. 67–13).

EMG provides objective diagnostic information for various neuromuscular disorders. EMG can differentiate between primary muscle disease and disease secondary to denervation. It helps identify specific primary muscle diseases. The results may indicate a transmission defect at the neuromuscular junction, such as myasthenia gravis. The procedure can be used to help differentiate diseases of the anterior horn cells from those primarily of peripheral nerves. Peripheral nerve degeneration and regeneration can be monitored with EMG before clinical manifestations appear.

NERVE CONDUCTION VELOCITY STUDY. A nerve conduction velocity study, often performed in conjunction with EMG, is used to evaluate the excitability and conduction velocities of motor and sensory nerves. It is helpful in identifying peripheral nerve disorders. A stimulating electrode and a recording electrode are placed to test specific nerves (usually on a limb). The time required for the passage of a nerve impulse from the point of stimulation to the point of recording is measured precisely. Conduction velocity is calculated. Both motor and sensory modalities are altered in peripheral nervous system disorders (e.g., carpal tunnel syndrome), whereas only motor

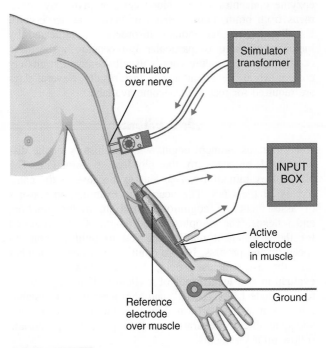

FIGURE 67–13 Electromyography measures and documents electrical currents produced by skeletal muscles. A stimulator is placed over the peripheral nerve being tested. A small pin is inserted into the muscle being assessed for nerve innervation, and a ground wire is placed on the client's skin.

fibers are affected in chronic disease of the anterior horn cell or motor nerve roots.

Explain the procedure. The client should avoid all stimulants, depressants, and sedatives for 24 hours before the test. There may be discomfort when the electrodes are inserted. If many muscles are tested, there may be residual discomfort. There may be a mild electrical shock during the procedure. The client lies flat and may be asked to move various muscles at specific times during the test. Clients with neuritis may have residual pain after testing. Mild analgesic medications may be needed.

Muscle Biopsy

Muscle biopsy is used in the diagnosis of neuropathies and myopathies. It is useful in distinguishing neurogenic from myopathic processes. However, muscle histologic findings are nonspecific for any neurogenic atrophy. An EMG is helpful in locating those muscle areas that are most abnormal. It is important that areas that have been traumatized by needle electrodes be avoided when tissue is taken for biopsy. Care of the biopsy site is needed.

Cellular Assessment

Chromosome analysis assists diagnosis of some abnormal neurologic conditions and provides the basis for genetic counseling in families with evidence of congenital neurologic malformations. Chromosomes can be prepared for microscopic examination from tissue culture of cells obtained from peripheral blood, bone marrow, or skin.

Mental retardation and convulsive seizures may result from neurologic dysfunction associated with inborn errors of metabolism. Diagnosis of carbohydrate and lipid metabolism disorders may require measurements of specific enzyme concentrations in blood cells or in biopsy specimens from brain, muscle, liver, or peripheral nerve cells. Usually, protein metabolism disorders are indicated by increased amounts of particular amino acids in the urine or blood. Postprocedure care is usually directed at anxiety control while the client awaits test results. Several days are required for results to become available.

CONCLUSIONS

Neurologic assessment begins with the history of the disorder and proceeds to the physical examination. The physical examination can be lengthy because of the complexity of the CNS. The neurologic examination consists of assessments of cognition, sensation, motor function, and reflexes. The complexity and length of time required for the assessment may tempt you to omit portions to speed up the process. Before omitting portions, remember that the assessments provide baseline data for further evaluation and legal proof of a client's status. Diagnostic tests include LP, CT, MRI, and angiography. Understanding how a test is performed enables the nurse to provide adequate client preparation and to perform appropriate follow-up assessments.

BIBLIOGRAPHY

1. ———. (1996). Adult screening for cognitive and functional impairment. *Nurse Practitioner, 21*(4), 112–115.

2. The American Association for Neuroscience Nurses. (1996). *Core curriculum for neuroscience nursing.* Chicago: Author.

3. Baker, D. (1993). Assessment and management of impairments in swallowing. *Nursing Clinics of North America, 28*(4), 793–805.

4. Barker, E. (1994). *Neuroscience nursing.* St. Louis: Mosby–Year Book.

5. Barker, E., & Moore, K. (1992). Neurological assessment. *RN, 55*(4), 28–35.

6. Bell, T. A., et al. (1992). Transcranial Doppler: Correlation of blood velocity measurement with clinical status in subarachnoid hemorrhage. *Journal of Neuroscience Nursing, 24*(4), 215–219.

7. Biller, J. (1997). *Practical neurology.* Philadelphia: Lippincott-Raven.

8. Bondy, K. (1994). Assessing cognitive function: A guide to neuropsychological testing. *Rehabilitation Nursing, 19*(1), 24–30.

9. Brocklehurst, R., Tallis, J., & Fillit, H. (1992). *Textbook of geriatric medicine and gerontology* (4th ed.). New York: Churchill Livingstone.

10. Buzea, C. E. (1995). Understanding computerized EEG monitoring in the ICU. *Journal of Neuroscience Nursing, 27*(5), 292–297.

11. Cason, C. L., & Sample, J. C. (1995). Preparatory information for myelogram. *Journal of Neuroscience Nursing, 27*(3), 182–187.

12. Chernecky, C., & Berger, B. (1997). *Laboratory tests and diagnostic procedures* (2nd ed.). Philadelphia: W. B. Saunders.

13. DiDonato, O., & Schaffer, V. (1994). The importance of outcome data in brain injury. *Rehabilitation Nursing, 19*(4), 219–228.

14. Gilman, S. (1992). Advances in neurology: Part 2. *New England Journal of Medicine, 326*(25), 1671–1676.

15. Gilman, S. (1998). Imaging the brain: Part I. *New England Journal of Medicine, 338*(12), 812–820.

16. Gilman, S. (1998). Imaging the brain: Part II. *New England Journal of Medicine, 338*(13), 889–896.

17. Gilroy, J. (1990). *Basic neurology* (2nd ed.). New York: Pergamon Press.

18. Guyton, A., & Hall, J. (1996). *Textbook of medical physiology* (9th ed.). Philadelphia: W. B. Saunders.

19. Hickey, J. V. (1997). *Clinical practice of neurological and neuroscience nursing.* Philadelphia: Lippincott-Raven.

20. Hudak, C. M., & Gallo, B. M. (1997). Quick review of neurodiagnostic testing. *American Journal of Nursing, 97*(7), 16CC–16FF.

21. Jarvis, C. (2000). *Physical examination and health assessment* (3rd ed.). Philadelphia: W. B. Saunders.

22. Lauren, N., et al. (1989). Cerebral perfusion imaging with technetium-99m HM-PAO in brain death and severe central nervous system injury. *Journal of Nuclear Medicine, 30*(10), 1627–1635.

23. Lederman, R. (1996). Lumbar puncture: Essential steps to a safe and valid procedure. *Geriatrics, 51*(6), 51–58.

24. Lewis, A. M. (1999). Neurologic emergency! *Nursing, 29*(10), 54–56.

25. Lower, J. (1992). Rapid neuroassessment. *American Journal of Nursing, 92*(6), 38–48.

26. Lucke, K. T., Kerr, M. E., & Chovanes, G. (1995). Continuous bedside cerebral blood flow monitoring. *Journal of Neuroscience Nursing, 27*(3), 164–173.

27. McDonagh, A. (1991). Getting your patient ready for a nuclear medicine scan. *Nursing 91, 21*(2), 53–57.

28. McGruder, J., et al. (1988). Headache after lumbar puncture: Review of the epidural blood patch. *Southern Medical Journal, 81*(10), 1249–1252.

29. Monti, E., Kerr, M., & Bender, C. (1995). Monitoring neuromuscular function. *Journal of Neuroscience Nursing, 27*(4), 252–256.

30. O'Hanlon-Nichols, T. (1999). Neurologic assessment. *American Journal of Nursing, 99*(6), 44–50.

31. Pressman, E., Zeidman, S., & Summers, L. (1995). Primary care for women: Comprehensive assessment of the neurological system. *Journal of Nurse-Midwifery, 40*(2), 163–71.

32. Reid, R., et al. (1989). Clinical use of technetium-99m HM-PAO for determination of brain death. *Journal of Nuclear Medicine, 30*(10), 1621–1626.

33. Shier, D., et al. (1996). *Hole's human anatomy and physiology* (7th ed.). Dubuque, IA: Wm. C. Brown.

34. Solomon, E. P. (1992). *An introduction to human anatomy and physiology* (2nd ed.). Philadelphia: W. B. Saunders.

35. Sur, M., & Cowey, A. (1995). Cerebral cortex: Functional development. *Neuron, 15,* 497–505.

36. Swartz, M. H. (1997). *Textbook of physical diagnosis* (3rd ed.). Philadelphia: W. B. Saunders.

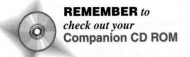

68

Management of Comatose or Confused Clients

Chris Stewart Amidei

NURSING OUTCOMES CLASSIFICATION (NOC)
for Nursing Diagnoses—Comatose or Confused Clients

Altered Family Processes	**Caregiver Role Strain**	Hydration
Family Coping	Caregiver Emotional Health	Nutritional Status: Food and Fluid Intake
Family Normalization	Caregiver Lifestyle Disruption	Thermoregulation
Family Participation in Professional Care	Caregiver Performance: Direct Care	Urinary Elimination
Grief Resolution	Caregiver Physical Health	**Risk for Impaired Skin Integrity**
Social Support	Caregiver Stressors	Immobility Consequences: Physiologic
Altered Nutrition: Less Than Body	Caregiver Home Care Readiness	Tissue Integrity: Skin and Mucous
Requirements	Caregiver Patient Relationship	Membranes
Nutritional Status: Nutrient Intake	Knowledge: Health Resources	Tissue Perfusion: Peripheral
Nutritional Status: Biochemical Measures	Social Support	**Risk for Injury**
Nutritional Status: Body Mass	**Risk for Aspiration**	Neurologic Status
Altered Oral Mucous Membranes	Neurologic Status	Risk Control
Oral Health	Respiratory Status: Gas Exchange	Safety Status: Falls
Tissue Integrity: Skin and Mucous	Respiratory Status: Ventilation	Safety Status: Physical Injury
Membranes	**Risk for Disuse Syndrome**	**Risk for Suffocation**
Altered Thought Processes	**(Contractures)**	Aspiration Control
Cognitive Orientation	Immobility Consequences: Physiologic	Neurological Status: Consciousness
Distorted Thought Control	Joint Movement: Passive	Respiratory Status: Gas Exchange
Communication Ability	Mobility Level	**Sleep Pattern Disturbance**
Bowel Incontinence	Muscle Function	Rest
Bowel Elimination	**Risk for Fluid Volume Deficit**	Sleep
Bowel Continence	Electrolyte and Acid-Base Balance	

Perhaps more than any other clients we encounter, clients who are comatose or confused need to be cared for in a holistic manner. All aspects of physiologic and psychological function need to be addressed. Even if clients cannot interact with the environment, the nurse must care for them in a respectful and dignified manner. It is important for family members to see that their loved ones are spoken to and cared for in a professional and caring way.

The brain serves many functions in the body. In contrast to other body systems that monitor and regulate a group of functions, such as the gastrointestinal (GI) tract regulating digestion, the nervous system monitors and regulates all other body systems. Some of these functions are self-protective, including the ability to think, be awake, respond appropriately to the environment, and

move about. Other functions are automatic, such as the regulation of body temperature and protective reflex responses. When these protective functions are lost, the clinical manifestations reflect the complexity of the nervous system.

The term *patient* is used in this chapter to describe the client who is comatose. It is assumed that such a client cannot be an active participant in care and that the *family* serves as the *client* in these circumstances.

DISORDERS OF CONSCIOUSNESS

Consciousness is a state of being that has two important aspects: (1) wakefulness and (2) awareness of self, environment, and time. *Awareness of self* means that the client can identify himself or herself. *Awareness of environment* indicates that the client can identify his or her present location and reason for being there. *Awareness of time* indicates that a client knows the date, month, and year and can identify common current facts, such as the name of the President of the United States.

Unconsciousness can be brief, lasting for a few seconds to an hour or so, or sustained, lasting for a few hours or longer. To produce unconsciousness, a disorder must (1) disrupt the ascending reticular activating system, which extends the length of the brain stem and up into the thalamus, (2) significantly disrupt the function of both cerebral hemispheres, or (3) metabolically depress overall brain function, as in a drug overdose.

Coma is a state of sustained unconsciousness in which the patient (1) does not respond to verbal stimuli, (2) may have varying responses to painful stimuli, (3) does not move voluntarily, (4) may have altered respiratory patterns, (5) may have altered pupillary responses to light, and (6) does not blink. In general, the longer the coma lasts, the more likely that it is irreversible and due to a permanent disorder in the brain structure. Duration of coma is also associated with mortality and outcome; the longer the coma, the higher the mortality rates, and the poorer the neurologic outcome.[4]

Etiology and Risk Factors

Two kinds of disorders produce sustained coma (Fig. 68–1):

1. Structural lesions in the brain that place pressure on the brain stem or the structures within the posterior

cranial fossa, including the cerebellum, midbrain, pons, and medulla. These types of lesions affect the reticular activating system (RAS).

2. Metabolic disorders and diffuse lesions, which impair wakefulness and awareness by reducing the supply of oxygen and glucose, which are necessary energy substrates, or by allowing waste products to accumulate in the brain.

Structural causes of coma include brain tumors, head trauma, and cerebral hemorrhage. The brain can be a site for tumors to metastasize from many organs, such as breast and lung, or tumors may arise from the brain itself. Automobile and motorcycle accidents, physical assaults, gunshot wounds, and falls are common causes of head injury. The impact of the initial injury causes damage. A cascade of events also occurs in response to the initial injury, characterized by edema and ischemia. Clients with head injury (see Chapter 73) may also have sustained injury to the chest or airway, which increases the risk of hypoxia. Cerebral hemorrhage can occur as a consequence of hypertension or from rupture of a vascular anomaly. Hemorrhage causes coma by placing pressure on brain tissue.

There are many metabolic causes of coma. The term *metabolic* is used to describe any problem that alters brain metabolism. Most metabolic comas originate in organ systems outside the brain. *Hypoxia* is a common cause of metabolic coma. Blood loss, high altitudes, or carbon monoxide poisoning may deprive the brain of oxygen. *Ischemia,* inadequate tissue levels of oxygen, may occur with cardiac disorders in which cardiac output is decreased, such as cardiac arrest or even

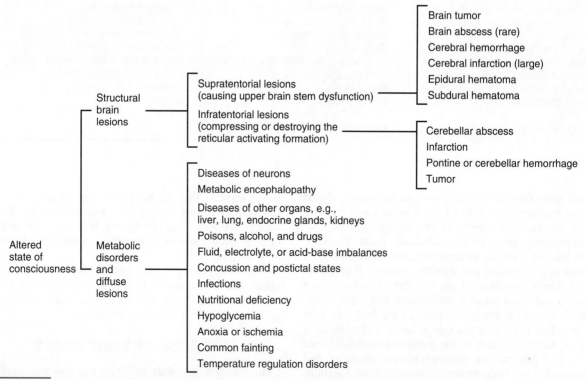

FIGURE 68–1 Some causes of altered states of consciousness. *Supratentorial* lesions are located *above* the dura roofing in the cerebellum, which separates the cerebellum from the cerebrum. *Infratentorial* lesions lie *beneath* the dura roofing in the cerebellum.

fainting. Disorders of the liver, lungs, and kidney may produce coma through the accumulation of metabolic waste products. Many other factors affect brain metabolism, including toxins, hypoglycemia, fever, infections such as encephalitis, and fluid, electrolyte, or acid-base imbalances.

Pathophysiology

Consciousness is a complex function controlled by the RAS and its integrated components. The RAS begins in the medulla as the reticular formation (RF) (Fig. 68–2). The reticular formation connects to the RAS, which is located in the midbrain, which then connects to the hypothalamus and thalamus. Integrated pathways connect to the cortex via the thalamus and to the limbic system via the hypothalamus. Feedback systems also connect at the brain stem level. The reticular formation produces wakefulness, whereas the RAS and higher connections are responsible for awareness of self and the environment. Diffuse cortical connections allow maximum integration of all conscious-related activities.

Disorders that affect any part of the RAS can produce coma. To produce coma, a disorder must affect both cerebral hemispheres or the brain stem itself. Disorders affect these areas in one of three ways:

1. Direct compression or destruction of structures responsible for consciousness. A tumor or hemorrhage in the brain stem or swelling in the cerebral hemispheres can cause coma in this manner.
2. Decrease in availability of oxygen or glucose, both of which are needed for cerebral metabolism. Hypoxia and ischemia are the most common

TABLE 68–1	DIFFERENTIAL MANIFESTATIONS OF STRUCTURALLY INDUCED AND METABOLIC COMA
Mechanism	**Manifestations**
Supratentorial mass lesions compressing or displacing the diencephalon or brain stem	Initiating sign is usually focal cerebral dysfunction Signs of dysfunction progress cephalocaudad Neurologic signs at any given time point to one anatomic area (e.g., frontal lobes, thalamus) Motor signs are often asymmetrical
Infratentorial mass of destruction causing coma	History of sudden onset of coma Localizing brain stem signs precede or accompany onset of coma and always include oculovestibular abnormality Cranial nerve palsies "Bizarre" respiratory patterns that appear at coma onset
Metabolic coma	Confusion and stupor commonly precede motor signs Motor signs usually are symmetrical Pupillary reactions usually are preserved Asterixis, myoclonus, tremor, and seizures are common Acid-base imbalance with hyperventilation or hypoventilation is common

causes; without oxygen and glucose, the brain cannot form the chemicals necessary to carry out its functions.
3. Toxic effects of substances on structures of the RAS. Toxic wastes from liver or kidney disease, bacterial invasion from meningitis, and metabolites from drug overdose are examples of such substances.

The causes may overlap. The exact location of involvement as well as the extent of the problem and the time frame of its occurrence determine the depth of coma.

Clinical Manifestations

Masses located in the supratentorial area (above the dura roofing the cerebellum) of the brain cause a fairly predictable set of clinical manifestations (Table 68–1). Supratentorial lesions can involve the entire cortical or subcortical level of the brain tissue, as with ischemia. The disorder may also be located in one hemisphere, as with tumor. These masses first produce manifestations such as headache, localized sensorimotor deficits, aphasia, visual loss, and seizures. The manifestations are related to the specific area of the brain affected.

For example, if the client has a mass in the frontal lobe, early clinical manifestations may consist of headaches, memory deficits, or partial seizures. *Partial seizures* are seizures occurring in one area of the body, such

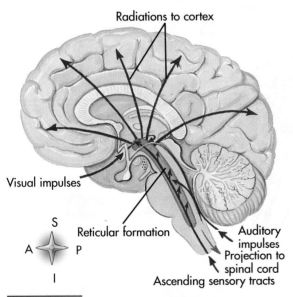

FIGURE 68–2 The reticular activating system (RAS) consists of centers in the brain stem reticular formation along with fibers conducting to the centers from below and fibers conducting from the centers to widespread areas of the cerebral cortex. A functioning RAS is essential for consciousness. (From Thibodeau, G., & Patton, K. [1999]. *Anatomy and physiology* [4th ed., p. 395]. St. Louis: Mosby.)

as the hand. As the mass expands, manifestations worsen because the mass places pressure on nearby areas. This pressure may cause a unilateral sensorimotor deficit (e.g., client cannot raise the right leg or has numbness in the right leg), aphasia, or a deficit in the visual field (blind in one half of the visual field). The client usually has intact pupillary and oculocephalic reflexes (see later). If the mass is not detected or cannot be treated and so progresses, coma eventually develops. Coma indicates that the mass has grown and now compresses structures deep in the brain stem.

Disorders of the infratentorial area (located beneath the dura roofing the cerebellum) cause the client to suddenly lose consciousness either (1) by directly affecting the RAS or its pathways or (2) by invading the brain stem or reducing its blood supply. Infratentorial lesions may produce unusual respiratory patterns (Fig. 68–3). The medulla houses the center for rhythmic breathing. This center's function is lost as consciousness decreases, and the lower brain stem begins to regulate breathing by responding to changes primarily in the carbon dioxide levels as well as in acid-base balance and oxygen levels. The result is a very irregular breathing depth and pattern. The mass or edema in the brain commonly compresses the cranial nerves, and various cranial nerve palsies can be seen, in particular, abnormal eye movements and loss of pupillary reactivity to light. Specific patterns of pupil size and reactivity to light occur when pressure is exerted at various levels (see Fig. 68–3).

Coma caused by a metabolic disorder more often is manifested as the presence of bilateral or symmetrical findings, because the disorder affects the entire brain rather than just one section. The patient usually demonstrates confusion and stupor before any physical signs are noticed. Physical signs of coma due to a metabolic disorder include tremor, asterixis (flapping tremors of the hands), myoclonus (a single, sudden jerking movement), and seizures. Pupillary response is usually normal unless the condition is related to drug overdose. Depending on the underlying cause, acid-base imbalances may be noted. For example, metabolic acidosis would be present in a patient with diabetic coma.

Level of consciousness is the single most important indicator of neurologic function. In the comatose patient, this indicator is lost and other indicators of neurologic function must be evaluated. Information about motor response, pupil size and reactivity to light, presence or absence of oculocephalic and oculovestibular responses, and breathing pattern can localize the level of involvement and determine the depth of coma. For discussion on these indicators, see Chapter 73.

Some patients in coma awaken slowly and begin to respond normally. They often require physical, occupational, and speech therapy in order to return to maximal levels of function. Irreversible coma is caused by damage to any area of the brain that destroys the patient's ability to respond to the environment. The brain stem and cerebellum remain intact, however, so that vital functions, such as heart, lung, and gastrointestinal functions, continue. Patients can remain in irreversible coma for years. Significant ethical and legal debates have arisen regarding the maintenance of nutritional intake for such a patient, particularly when a patient's family questions the rationale for artificial feeding.

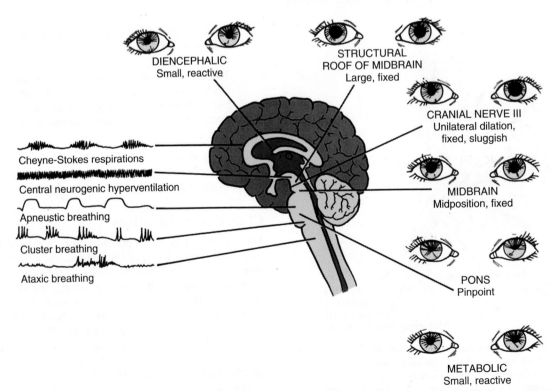

FIGURE 68–3 Respiratory patterns and appearances of the pupil associated with lesions of various neurologic structures. Cheyne-Stokes respiration may occur because of altered cerebral perfusion deep within the cerebral hemisphere or from within the diencephalon.

Diagnostic Findings

The neurologic examination is supplemented by diagnostic testing. Tests identify structural or physiologic abnormalities that affect brain function.

COMPUTED TOMOGRAPHY AND MAGNETIC RESONANCE IMAGING. A computed tomography (CT) or magnetic resonance imaging (MRI) scan usually provides data that indicate whether the cause of the coma is structural. In coma, a CT scan is usually performed first because it is quicker. Tumors or areas of bleeding are evident on the scan. Sometimes the patient requires emergency surgery to remove the mass or drain the fluid and thereby relieve pressure. In metabolic coma, the structures may appear unremarkable, or edema or diffuse nonspecific changes may be seen.

LUMBAR PUNCTURE. A lumbar puncture can be performed when it is known, from data provided by the CT or MRI scans, that the patient does not have an expanding intracranial mass. Obtaining this information prior to lumbar puncture avoids the risk of herniation due to sudden changes in cerebrospinal fluid (CSF) pressures (low in the spinal column and high in the ventricles). A lumbar puncture can assist in the diagnosis of infection or bleeding as a cause of coma. CSF may be cloudy or bloody when the patient has an infection or bleeding into the ventricles or the subarachnoid space.

ELECTROENCEPHALOGRAPHY. Electroencephalography (EEG) can be used to determine whether the patient is comatose because of continuous seizures. EEG results are abnormal in many patients with structural and metabolic coma and do not serve as a clear diagnostic tool. A portion of the general population may have abnormal EEG results as well.

LABORATORY TESTS. Liver and kidney function as well as glucose level may be evaluated through blood tests. A urine or blood toxicology screen may be useful in distinguishing drug-induced coma. Blood oxygenation tests may be used to evaluate for hypoxia. Other laboratory tests may be ordered specific to the patient's situation. Chapter 67 covers specific neurologic diagnostic tests.

TESTS FOR ABNORMAL REFLEXES

OCULOCEPHALIC REFLEX RESPONSE. The *doll's eye reflex* is movement of the eyes in the direction opposite to that in which the head is moved; for example, doll's eye reflex is considered present if the eyes move to the right when the head is rotated to the left, and vice versa (Fig. 68–4). This test can be performed only in unconscious patients, because conscious patients have voluntary control over eye movements. The presence of the doll's eye reflex indicates that brain stem function is preserved. The reflex is absent or impaired in patients with brain stem problems. The doll's eye test should never be performed in comatose patients with suspected or known cervical spine injury because the head movement required may produce permanent spinal cord damage.

Patients in metabolic coma, except for that caused by barbiturate or phenytoin (Dilantin) poisoning, retain ocular reflexes. The brain stem in a comatose patient may be functioning even in the absence of the doll's eye reflex. Other agents and disorders can block the eye's response.

Neuromuscular drugs, such as succinylcholine, and Ménière's disease, which destroys the labyrinth in the ear, cause absence of the oculocephalic response. In the patient without Ménière's disease or evidence of neuromuscular drugs, however, absence of the oculocephalogyric response supports the diagnosis of brain death.[4, 6]

OCULOVESTIBULAR REFLEX RESPONSE. If oculocephalic responses are absent, an oculovestibular (caloric) test can be performed to test cranial nerves III, IV, VI, and VIII (see Chapter 67). A normal response to instillation of iced water into one ear canal is seen as smooth movement of both eyes with nystagmus toward the irrigated ear (see Fig. 68–4C). Instillation of warm water results in eye movement away from the irrigated ear. *Nystagmus* is the involuntary oscillation of the eyeballs; it may be horizontal, vertical, oblique, rotary, or mixed, with various rates of movement.

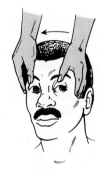
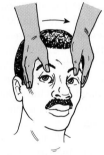

A. NORMAL REACTION:
Eyes move in direction opposite to head movement when head is turned

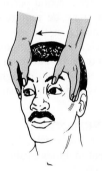
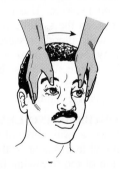

B. ABNORMAL REACTION:
Eyes remain in fixed position in skull when head is turned

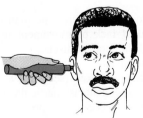
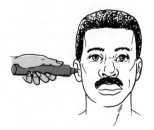

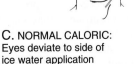

C. NORMAL CALORIC:
Eyes deviate to side of ice water application

D. ABNORMAL CALORIC:
Eyes do not deviate

FIGURE 68–4 *A* and *B,* Normal and abnormal doll's eye reflexes (oculocephalic response). *C* and *D,* Normal and abnormal caloric test results (oculovestibular response).

Failure to produce eye movement and nystagmus with the instillation of warm or cold water into the ear canal indicates an altered brain stem, with a few exceptions. The use of ototoxic drugs, barbiturates, sedatives, phenytoin, or tricyclic antidepressants or the presence of Ménière's disease may produce a false-negative caloric test result. In a patient without these conditions, the absence of an oculovestibular reflex supports the diagnosis of brain death.

A caloric test is contraindicated in a patient with a ruptured tympanic membrane (eardrum) or otorrhea (ear discharge). This test is usually performed only in comatose patients because awake patients may vomit in response to the stimulation of CN VIII.

Outcome Management

The goals of medical management are to preserve brain function and to prevent additional brain injury. The primary focus is on maintaining the supply of oxygen and glucose to the brain.

The patient's airway, breathing, and circulation ("ABCs") must be maintained. A nasal or oral airway may be inserted for a short time. If the patient is breathing spontaneously, closely monitor the airway and respirations because the airway may become obstructed and aspiration may occur as consciousness decreases. If the patient is completely unresponsive or respiratory patterns become ineffective, an endotracheal tube is inserted, with care taken to avoid injury to the cervical spine (see also Chapter 63). Ventilation and supplemental oxygen are given.

Normal cerebral perfusion is promoted through monitoring of blood pressure and maintenance of the systolic pressure between 100 and 160 mm Hg. Blood pressures lower or higher than these levels may alter cerebral perfusion pressure. Use of vasoactive agents may be required to keep the systolic pressure at 100 mm Hg or the *mean* systolic blood pressure above 80 mm Hg, or medications may be needed to lower the blood pressure. However, blood pressure must be cautiously lowered because high blood pressure may represent a compensatory mechanism to perfuse the brain.

DETERMINING LEVEL OF INVOLVEMENT

Once airway, breathing, and circulation are established, initial assessment of the comatose patient includes evaluation of the following factors:[11]

1. Level of consciousness, through observation of response to stimuli.
2. Presence or absence of localizing neurologic manifestations, such as unilateral lack of movement or posturing, indicating focal intracranial disease.
3. Pupil size and reactivity to light.
4. Deep tendon and superficial reflexes (see Chapter 67). Superficial reflex assessment is particularly valuable in comatose patients because it provides objective information about brain stem function in the absence of consciousness. Assess the corneal reflex carefully to avoid corneal abrasion.
5. Response to noxious stimuli. First, loud verbal stimuli and then shaking are performed to produce a response. If none is noted, the examiner applies a painful stimulus, such as pressure to the sternum, nail beds, or supraorbital notch. Care must be taken not to damage skin underlying the areas where pressure is applied. Other aspects of sensory assessment are not possible or are unreliable in comatose patients.
6. Evidence of trauma. Trauma may be the result of coma rather than the cause of it (e.g., a tongue bite may result from a seizure). Examine the ears for ruptured eardrums and otorrhea.
7. Determination of serum oxygenation, blood alcohol, blood urea nitrogen, ammonia, and glucose levels if manifestations suggest a metabolic disorder.
8. History from significant others (or observers of what has happened), if possible.

REVERSING COMMON CAUSES OF COMA

Immediate interventions for the patient in a coma include treatment of common causes of coma while assessment of neurologic status and diagnostic testing continue. For example, after a blood specimen is drawn for testing, intravenous (IV) glucose is given to reverse potential insulin reactions. Many comatose patients are malnourished and subject to Wernicke's encephalopathy related to alcohol abuse. These patients are commonly given thiamine, especially if they are given glucose.

If the patient is having repetitive seizures, coma and brain damage can follow. The patient is given IV diazepam or lorazepam to stop the seizures. If the patient is not intubated, closely monitor the airway because of the respiratory depressant effects of these medications.

Many metabolic causes of coma lead to acid-base, fluid, and electrolyte imbalances. The patient's acid-base balance should be restored quickly. Fluid imbalances should be restored slowly to prevent rebound fluid shifts into the brain (see Chapter 12). Isotonic saline is usually given if the patient is dehydrated, and fluids are withheld if the patient is fluid-overloaded. If cerebral edema is present, osmotic diuretics may be used to promote shifting of extracellular brain fluid back into the plasma. Other medications, such as steroids, barbiturate therapy, and neuromuscular blocking agents, decrease intracranial pressure (ICP) through more indirect means. (Electrolyte imbalances are covered in Chapter 13.)

If infection is suspected, specimens for culture are obtained from the blood, nose, throat, and wounds (if present). Once such specimens have been collected, antibiotics are given if infection is suspected. Body temperature should be normalized as much as possible by means of antipyretics, air circulation, and cooling mattresses. Care must be taken to ensure that the patient does not shiver, because shivering increases ICP.

Coma from drug overdose may be reversed by specific antidotes if the ingested drug can be identified. Often, however, the specific drug ingested is not known. A blood specimen should be collected for a toxicity screen. Narcotic overdose may be reversed with naloxone. Because the duration of action of naloxone is 2 to 3 hours shorter than that of most narcotics, naloxone may need to be readministered. Seizures resulting from cocaine overdose can be treated with diazepam. Patients with cocaine overdose often have cardiac dysrhythmias and irregular respirations. Gastric lavage may be used to remove ingested agents, followed by instillation of activated charcoal.

Structural causes of coma may require surgery to decompress the cranial vault. Burr holes may be created to drain a subdural hematoma. A craniotomy may be performed to remove a tumor or intracerebral hematoma. A ventricular catheter or shunt may be placed to relieve hydrocephalus.

To stimulate your thought process, see Thinking Critically at the end of this chapter for the description of a scenario involving a client with coma from a hypertensive hemorrhage.

PREVENTING COMPLICATIONS

If the coma is prolonged, initiate enteral feeding to promote nutrition and prevent muscle wasting. Parenteral nutrition may be used if paralytic ileus is present. Take care to avoid hyperglycemia, which can exacerbate brain injury in the presence of ischemia. However, brain cells have a high glucose need compared with other cells; supplying the cell need without causing brain damage requires a delicate balance.

Prevent the complications of immobility, such as pneumonia and pressure ulcers, with frequent turning or the use of an oscillating bed. Continue to reposition the patient to relieve skin pressure unless the bed provides more than 40 degrees of rotation. The eyes may need to be taped closed to avoid corneal abrasion. Suctioning may be needed to keep the airway clear and prevent pneumonia. Passive range-of-motion exercises keep joints mobile and minimize muscle wasting. Position the extremities in correct alignment to prevent contractures. Use sequential compression stockings to prevent deep venous thrombosis (DVT); low-dose heparin may also be ordered. All of these complications are continually assessed for and are treated promptly if they occur.

OUTCOMES

In the past, little information was available on which to base a prediction about the outcome for a patient in coma. Most of the time, a "wait-and-see" approach was taken. Today, the family and the health care team should have some idea of the probable eventual outcome for the patient. It is discouraging and inappropriate to vigorously treat a patient who has no chance of recovery, but it is even more inappropriate to deny treatment to a patient with a reasonable chance of recovery.

Coma after head injury has a statistically better outcome than coma associated with medical illness.[9] About 50% of patients in coma from head injury die, many instantly. Immediate treatment may somewhat improve the outcome for those who reach the hospital. Recovery in traumatic cases is closely linked to age; the younger the patient, the better the recovery. Severely abnormal neuro-ophthalmologic signs reflecting brain stem dysfunction imply a poor prognosis; approximately 90% of patients with such signs either die or remain in near-vegetative states.[4]

The absence of pupillary, corneal, or oculovestibular responses during the early stages of coma is highly predictive of mortality or significant morbidity (e.g., persistent vegetative state). The recovery of these responses and a return to purposeful movement correlate with a better prognosis. Patients who lapse into coma as a result of metabolic disorders have an extremely poor prognosis if the coma lasts more than 1 week.

Coma stimulation, application of planned meaningful, multimodality sensory stimulation, has been suggested as a measure to enhance outcome from coma. Clinical validity of coma stimulation has not been clearly established. The type of stimulation, timing of application, and outcomes measures used vary among studies, making it difficult to determine whether coma stimulation is of benefit.[5] Nonetheless, the nurse is encouraged to interact with comatose patients through all their sensory systems.

■ Nursing Management of the Medical Client
ASSESSMENT

Frequent, systematic, and objective nursing assessment of the comatose patient, including neurologic status, is essential. Serial observations are important for comparison and to facilitate prompt reporting of even subtle changes in status. Even if assessment findings seem insignificant for long periods, documentation provides an objective pattern and an important baseline for future observations. Assessment of consciousness is most effective when the assessments are performed by a consistent nurse. The neurologic assessment is performed as often as every 15 minutes during the first few hours of coma. Depending on the patient's condition, assessments may need to be continued hourly for several days.

The Critical Monitoring feature lists the neurologic manifestations of a person who is unconscious. Presenting manifestations are ordered according to the degree of seriousness. Remembering these subtle changes in assessment helps in early identification of a patient's improvement or worsening. A decrease in the patient's Glasgow Coma Scale (GCS) score also indicates worsening. The GCS is the most common neurologic assessment tool used in clinical practice (see Chapter 73).

Although neurologic assessment is the priority evaluation, the entire body of a comatose patient must be periodically observed because the patient is unable to offer any specific complaints. Complications either of the initial condition causing coma or of immobility can arise at any time during the course of care. If surgery has been performed, postoperative assessments must be performed as well.

DIAGNOSIS, OUTCOMES, INTERVENTIONS

This section describes interventions appropriate for all comatose patients regardless of the cause of the coma. Interventions specific to particular etiologic factors are described elsewhere (e.g., hepatic coma in Chapter 47, and uremic coma in Chapter 34).

Comatose patients are completely dependent on others because their protective reflexes are impaired. Nursing intervention provides the safety normally afforded by protective reflexes. Coma is often life-threatening and requires aggressive medical intervention. Physicians are concerned with establishing a medical diagnosis and prescribing appropriate treatment; nurses are responsible for meeting basic human needs and preventing the complications associated with coma. Nurses are also responsible for assessing and intervening to reduce ICP.

Altered cerebral tissue perfusion is one of the highest risks for a patient with an altered level of consciousness. This outcome is often seen as a direct consequence of

CRITICAL MONITORING

Manifestations of Changes in Neurologic Status

"Change" is the key word. Notify the physician whenever there is a change in the client's neurologic status. The following manifestations are listed in the order that indicates a *worsening* in the client's condition. Remember, a client may display a "transient" deterioration in neurologic responses that does not warrant calling a physician. For example, after you have just performed suctioning of the client's airway or have turned the client, you would anticipate a possible change in neurologic status. If you hyperoxygenate the client and ensure proper positioning for venous return from the jugular veins and airway maintenance, however, any signs of increased deficit should last only a few seconds or no more than 4 or 5 minutes. Signs of increased deficit that last longer than this increase the risk for irreversible brain injury.

Normal

Alert, oriented to person, place, time
Responds appropriately to verbal commands
Eyes open spontaneously with any stimulus, unless in a deep sleep

Abnormal; Changes Due to Altered Perfusion of the Cerebral Cortex

Altered level of consciousness
Altered perception of time, then place, and lastly person
Motor deficits (e.g., hemiparesis, hemiplegia)
Speech deficits (e.g., expressive or receptive speech or both)
Memory deficits (e.g., recent, intermediate, remote)
Hyperreflexia
Babinski's sign
Seizures
Decorticate rigidity
Emotional lability
Altered sensory interpretation
Cheyne-Stokes respiration
Headache, nausea, vomiting, papilledema

Abnormal; Changes Due to Altered Perfusion Just Inferior to the Cortex

Pupillary changes: asymmetry of size, shape, or time-responsiveness
Loss of reaction to direct light
Visual field changes (e.g., homonymous hemianopsia; see Chapter 69)

Abnormal; Changes Due to Altered Perfusion of the Diencephalon

Altered temperature; first high fevers, then hypothermia
Cheyne-Stokes respiration

—————
CN, cranial nerve.

Abnormal; Changes Due to Altered Perfusion of the Posterior Pituitary Gland

Diabetes insipidus (decreased antidiuretic hormone)

Abnormal; Changes Due to Altered Perfusion of the Midbrain

Dysfunction of CN III (loss of reaction to indirect or consensual light, dysconjugate eye movement)
Dysfunction of CN IV (dysconjugate eye movement)
Central neurogenic hyperventilation

Abnormal; Changes Due to Altered Perfusion of the Upper Pons

Dysfunction of CN V (altered sensory function to cornea, nasal membranes, face, oral cavity, tongue, teeth, or altered mastication)
Dysfunction of CN VI (altered lateral eye movement)
Dysfunction of CN VII (altered facial expression, taste, and salivation)
Central neurogenic hyperventilation
Abnormal extension posture
Pinpoint pupils

Abnormal; Changes Due to Altered Perfusion of the Lower Pons

Apneustic breathing
Flaccidity

Abnormal; Changes Due to Altered Perfusion of the Medulla

Dysfunction of CN VIII (altered equilibrium and hearing)
Dysfunction of CN IX (altered taste, pharyngeal sensations, and cough and swallowing)
Dysfunction of CN X (altered sensations in pharynx, larynx, external ear, and altered cough and swallowing; altered parasympathetic nervous system functions in thoracic and abdominal viscera)
Dysfunction of CN XI (altered neck and shoulder movement)
Dysfunction of CN XII (altered tongue movement)
Projectile vomiting
Cushing's triad (increased systolic blood pressure, wide pulse pressure, bradycardia)
Ataxic (Biot's respiration)

increasing ICP. Nursing management of this problem is described in Chapter 73.

Risk for Suffocation. Clients who are unconscious cannot swallow because of loss or suppression of the gag or coughing reflex and thus are at risk for suffocation. Airway obstruction is the most common source of harm to patients with decreased consciousness. Write the diagnosis as *Risk for Suffocation related to loss of gag reflex.*

Outcomes. The client will exhibit no signs of accidental suffocation or airway obstruction as evidenced by (1) clear lung sounds, (2) equal lung expansion, and (3) absence of stridor, cyanosis, and pallor.

Interventions. For initial airway management, an oral airway can be inserted in an unconscious patient. Endotracheal intubation, with the use of a ventilator, may be required to maintain airway patency or improve ventilation.

For extended airway management, a tracheostomy may be required to (1) allow long-term continuous mechanical ventilation, (2) facilitate removal of tracheobronchial secretions, and (3) separate the upper and lower airways (see Chapter 60).

Risk for Aspiration. The lack of effective airway clearance and gag reflex puts the comatose patient at very high risk for aspiration. Write the diagnosis as *Risk for Aspiration related to lack of effective airway clearance and loss of gag reflex.*

Outcomes. The patient will exhibit no signs of aspiration, as evidenced by (1) clear lung sounds, (2) no stridor, (3) absence of fever, (4) minimal amounts of clear mucus upon suctioning, and (5) clear lungs as demonstrated by chest x-ray.

Interventions. Monitor results of arterial blood gas (ABG) analysis and pulse oximetry to determine the level of oxygenation provided by ventilators or oxygen. Assess breath sounds every 1 to 2 hours in acutely ill patients. Keep suctioning equipment available.

Perform tracheobronchial suctioning as needed, not routinely, to prevent or decrease the accumulation of secretions from immobility, the lack of a cough and sigh reflex, or pneumonia. Not suctioning a person who cannot expectorate his or her own secretions can cause hypoxia and result in neurologic damage. Suctioning should be gentle, and the catheter should not remain in the airway for longer than 10 seconds. While suctioning, observe the cardiac monitor for dysrhythmias (e.g., premature ventricular contractions) secondary to hypoxia. Hyperoxygenating the patient before, during, and after suctioning decreases the risk of dysrhythmias. Hyperoxygenation and limiting the suctioning time to 10 seconds also minimizes increased ICP associated with suctioning. Never suction the nasal passages in the patient with a basilar skull fracture because the suction catheter can enter the cranial cavity.

A comatose patient may lack pharyngeal reflexes and be unable to swallow. Pneumonia secondary to aspiration is a common cause of death in unconscious patients. To reduce the risk of aspiration, never give a comatose patient fluids to swallow. Secretions also accumulate in the posterior pharynx and may be aspirated. If the patient is intubated, make sure the cuff is inflated. Suction the upper trachea and posterior pharynx as often as necessary to remove secretions. After tracheal suctioning, the same suction catheter can be used for oral or pharyngeal suctioning, but not vice versa. Also, turn the patient from side to side every 2 hours to facilitate drainage of secretions and prevent pneumonia.

While performing mouth care, place a comatose patient in a lateral position to prevent aspiration. If facial paralysis is present, keep the affected side uppermost. Keep the patient's mouth open by placing an oral airway or bite block between the teeth. Pay close attention to the roof of the mouth in patients who breathe through the mouth for long periods. Crusts of dried sputum may form, break off, and be aspirated. Use of artificial moisturizers may help prevent crust formation; however, frequent oral care is the best prevention.

As consciousness returns and the client begins to respond to verbal stimuli and has a gag reflex, test the client's ability to suck and to swallow liquids. Before the test, position the client in high Fowler's position, and have suction equipment nearby in case it is needed. Use a thick juice, nectar, or ice chips rather than water; liquid of a thick consistency is easier to swallow. Place about 1 teaspoon of liquid into the back of the mouth. Observe for swallowing. Suction as needed to prevent aspiration. If a client cannot suck through a straw or drink from a glass because of facial paralysis, place fluids into the unaffected side of the mouth with an aseptic (Asepto) syringe. Watch for difficulty in swallowing. Suction as needed.

If there is any question about a client's ability to swallow, a formal swallowing evaluation should be performed by a speech therapist. Clients who cannot swallow for long periods may require placement of a gastrostomy tube. Many rehabilitation and extended-care facilities require the use of gastrostomy tubes rather than nasogastric (NG) tubes because there is less risk of aspiration with gastrostomy tube-feedings.

Clients with impaired swallowing require special instruction. Swallowing can be stimulated by having the client lean the head forward and, after taking fluid, quickly tip the head backward. Stroking the anterior neck may also promote swallowing.

Once a client can safely swallow, begin oral nutrition with small liquid feedings, progressing to a soft diet. Discontinue tube-feedings only when the client can take adequate nutrition orally. Many clients are fed orally during the daytime and tube-fed at night to maintain adequate nutrition.

When changing from tube-feeding to oral feeding, turn off the tube-feeding several hours before the meal. This will stimulate the appetite. When a client begins to eat independently, be reassuring and encouraging. Remind the client to eat slowly and to swallow after each bite. Position the client sitting up as tolerated.

Altered Oral Mucous Membranes. Several factors can lead to altered oral mucous membranes. The comatose patient usually has an NPO (nothing by mouth) order, is unable to swallow, and breathes through the mouth. A possible nursing diagnosis might be *Altered Oral Mucous Membranes related to mouth breathing.*

Outcomes. The patient will maintain intact oral mucous membranes, as evidenced by oral and nasal mucous membranes that are pink, moist, and without lesions, crusts, or bloody drainage.

Interventions. Using a flashlight and tongue depressor, inspect the patient's mouth every 8 hours. Keep the patient's lips coated with a water-soluble lubricant to prevent encrustation, drying, and cracking. Carefully inspect a paralyzed cheek for crusts or other conditions requiring intervention. Provide oral hygiene to prevent excessive drying of oral mucous membranes and complications such as parotitis, aspiration, and respiratory tract infections.

At least twice a day, brush the patient's teeth with a small toothbrush, and rinse the mouth. Clean the oral mucous membranes (especially the roof of the mouth), tongue, and gums with sponge toothbrushes. Avoid using agents containing lemon or alcohol, because they dry the membranes. While performing mouth care in an unconscious patient, suction excess secretions to prevent aspiration. Toothbrushes with suction attachments are now available in many health care agencies.

Nasal passages may become occluded because an unconscious patient is unable to sniff, blow, sneeze, or otherwise clear the nose. To clear the nasal passages of mucus and crust formations, gently swab the nose with an applicator moistened with water or normal saline. Then apply a thin coat of water-soluble lubricant with a cotton-tipped applicator.

Do *not* clean the nasal passages or ears of a patient with a basilar skull fracture. If bleeding occurs from the ears or nose, or if CSF (a watery discharge) appears to be draining from these areas, notify the physician.

Risk for Impaired Skin Integrity. Normal reflexes reduce the risk of skin ischemia by signaling conscious (even sleeping) persons to shift their body weight. Comatose patients have lost these protective reflexes and are completely immobile. Sometimes patients are agitated and can shear the skin with frequent nonpurposeful movements; this diagnosis also applies to these patients. Write the diagnosis as *Risk for Impaired Skin Integrity related to immobility.*

Outcomes. The patient will have intact skin, as evidenced by no reddened areas over bony prominences and no areas or signs of skin irritation or dryness.

Interventions. Provide nursing intervention for all self-care needs, including bathing and care of the hair, skin, and nails. Patients often scratch themselves as the depth of unconsciousness lessens; therefore, keep the nails trimmed. Patients who are comatose for long periods may be lifted occasionally into a bathtub half-filled with warm water. It may be helpful to apply solutions high in fatty acids (e.g., Castile soap, baby oil, or cold cream) daily and to bathe the patient weekly to prevent loss of cutaneous oils as well as skin irritation and dryness.

Perineal care should be performed at least every 8 hours and after every episode of incontinence. If perineal care is not effective for a woman with vaginal discharge or odor, consult the physician about the use of cleansing douches.

When the patient cannot respond to local tissue hypoxia from being in one position for an extended time, the risk of pressure ulcers increases. Patients should be repositioned at least every 2 hours. If repositioning is impossible because of the patient's medical condition, place the patient on a special mattress or bed (Fig. 68–5). However, the use of a special bed does not eliminate the need to pad bony prominences and assess the skin every 4 hours. In addition, meet the nutritional needs of the patient to reduce the risk of pressure ulcers.

Risk for Contractures. Normal movement and stretch are needed to prevent tightening of one group of muscles. When muscle groups are not used during periods of immobility, contractures of joints can develop. Footdrop is of special concern. Write the diagnosis as *Risk for Contractures related to disuse.*

Outcomes. The patient will maintain full range of motion in any joint, as evidenced by an absence of contractures. Another outcome could be that the client will have a reduced risk of contractures, as evidenced by (1) a

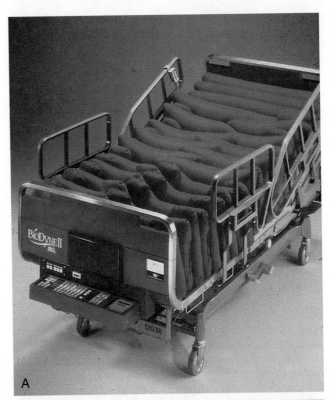

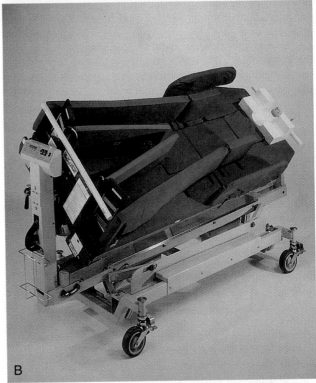

FIGURE 68–5 *A,* BioDyne, an oscillating air support surface. *B,* Roto Rest, an oscillating bed. Both devices are used to treat hypoxemia and to reduce the incidence of nosocomial pneumonia. Roto Rest is also used for clients with spinal cord injury and skeletal traction. (Courtesy of Kinetic Concepts, Inc., San Antonio, TX.)

normal range of motion, (2) an absence of flexed arms and legs, and (3) no manifestations of footdrop.

Interventions. Prevent contractures by maintaining the patient's extremities in functional positions with proper support. Hand and forearm splints prevent flexion contracture of the fingers and wrists. Orthotic devices or high-top athletic shoes are used to support the feet. Remove the support devices every 4 hours to perform skin care and passive exercises. Assess the heel closely.

Altered Nutrition: Less Than Body Requirements.
Comatose patients cannot eat and yet have normal or even increased metabolic needs, so they can quickly become malnourished. Write the diagnosis as *Altered Nutrition: Less Than Body Requirements related to inability to eat and swallow.*

Outcomes. The patient will demonstrate the following signs of adequate nutrition: (1) stable weight, (2) adequate calories for age, height, and weight, (3) intake equaling output, (4) healing of incisions and wounds within 12 to 14 days, and (5) hemoglobin, blood urea nitrogen, total lymphocyte count, total protein, and serum albumin values within normal limits for age and sex.

Interventions. IV fluids are begun on admission for comatose patients. Initially the IV site provides access to the circulatory system for the administration of medications. Because fluid intake is restricted and only limited amounts of glucose and few electrolytes are given by the IV route, an IV infusion cannot be considered nutritional support. Consider that a 1-L solution of 5% dextrose provides only 200 kilocalories!

Just because a patient is comatose, never assume that hunger is not present and that caloric needs are reduced. In fact, the opposite is true; such a patient's caloric needs are usually increased. Nutritional and fluid needs of comatose patients are usually met through enteral feedings because of the risk of aspiration with the oral route. If the patient does not have paralytic ileus or delayed gastric emptying and if bowel sounds are audible, start enteral feedings (see Management and Delegation feature on enteral nutrition).

The nutritional requirements of a patient in coma are complex; a complete nutritional assessment with comparison of height and weight charts, laboratory tests, and clinical examination is essential. There is a marked increase in metabolic needs. Malnutrition increases the morbidity and mortality of neurologically ill patients. Diarrhea and delayed gastric emptying may result from malabsorption. Healing cannot take place in the presence of a negative nitrogen state. Immunodeficiency, with increased risk of infection, sepsis, stress ulcers, weight loss, skeletal muscle protein wasting, and lung tissue catabolism leading to diaphragmatic weakness with respiratory reduction, results from prolonged calorie and protein deprivation. Starvation can lead to death.

Nursing responsibilities in tube-feeding of comatose patients are critical because these patients cannot communicate and may have lost protective cough and gag reflexes. The possible complications from enteral feeding, and their prevention, are described here:

1. Vomiting and aspiration if the stomach is overfilled or the head of the patient is below the level of the

---

MANAGEMENT AND DELEGATION

Preparing Enteral Nutrition

Enteral nutrition may be delivered via oral, nasal, gastrostomy, or jejunostomy tubes. Gastrostomy or jejunostomy tubes are most commonly used because they pose a lower risk of aspiration. The delivery of enteral nutrition, including the verification of tube placement, is your responsibility. You may choose to delegate the reconstitution or preparation of enteral feedings to assistive personnel. Before delegating the preparation of tube feeding or refilling the nutrition reservoir bag, consider the following:

- Your abdominal assessment does not reveal abdominal distention, pain, discomfort, or complaints of nausea. Your examination includes verification of tube placement, and the residual volume is less than 50% of the previous hour's intake. The presence of any of these findings would prompt you to delay the tube feeding and notify the physician of your examination findings.
- You have checked the physician's order for the type and rate of tube feeding to be delivered.
- Instruct assistive personnel in the proper dilution and handling of enteral feeding. (*Hint:* When mixing powdered enteral feedings, always place the powder in the mixing container before the water; this will ensure that the powder dissolves fully.)
- Instruct assistive personnel to place a 4-hour supply of feeding in the reservoir bag and to store the remaining mixture in a refrigerator for future use. Label the storage container with the client's name, date on which mixture was prepared, and description of mixture.
- Although assistive personnel may prime the pump, you must set the pump and ensure that the flow rate matches the ordered flow rate.
- You are responsible for performing any irrigation of the tube.
- You may delegate care of gastrostomy and jejunostomy tube site to assistive personnel.
- You are responsible for monitoring fluid and nutritional balance via input and output and changes in weight.

Describe findings that are immediately reportable to you for assistive personnel. They include any difficulty in preparing the enteral feeding and client complaints of fullness, nausea, or vomiting.

Verify the competence of assistive personnel in performing these tasks during orientation and annually thereafter.

Donna W. Markey, MSN, RN, ACNP-CS, *Clinician IV, Surgical Services, University of Virginia Health System, Charlottesville, Virginia*

---

stomach, such as during chest physiotherapy. When tube-feeding a patient, elevate the head of the bed at least 30 degrees to minimize possible aspiration.

2. Tube dislocation into trachea or lungs, causing aspiration. Some facilities use blue food coloring to tint the formula; then, if suctioned secretions are blue, aspiration is suspected. Comatose patients are often

restless. Tape the tube securely to prevent dislodgment. Aspiration may occur if a feeding tube is pulled out during a feeding session or whenever it is unclamped. During feeding sessions, cloth wristlets or wrist restraints may be needed.

Verify NG tube placement by aspirating for gastric contents. Some agency policies and some manufacturers of small-bore tubes require checking tube placement by listening with a stethoscope for "whooshing" while instilling air through the tube. Never tube-feed a patient in the supine position unless all other positions are impossible. Leave the head of the bed elevated 30 degrees for at least 30 minutes after bolus feedings.

3. Ulcerated or crusted nares due to local pressure from the feeding tube.
4. Tracheoesophageal fistula, that is, breakdown of the anterior esophageal wall from prolonged contact between the NG tube and a tracheostomy tube. This complication is manifested by gastric contents in tracheal secretions. Notify the physician immediately.
5. Trauma to the gastric mucosa if the tube's distal end hardens, as may happen over time.
6. Delayed gastric emptying. Check residual volumes every 4 hours. If the residual volume is more than 100 ml, delay the feeding for 1 hour, then reassess. Assess bowel sounds, and check for gastric distention; if this complication persists after several hours, notify the physician. If there is a high suspicion that the patient has a bowel obstruction, do not return the gastric residue to the stomach.
7. Fluid volume deficit if hypertonic tube-feedings are given. To prevent this problem, ensure that the patient receives approximately 1 ml of fluid for every kilocalorie of feeding. Depending on the agency's policy, this intervention may require consultation with the dietitian or the physician.
8. Constipation or diarrhea, which may develop from the osmolarity of the feeding, the use of liquid medications with a sorbitol base, or a too rapid infusion.
9. Sacral pressure ulcers from continued positioning in the semi-Fowler position. Turn the patient 30 degrees lateral (to the side) with the head of the bed elevated to reduce pressure on the sacrum.

Risk for Fluid Volume Deficit. The comatose patient cannot drink fluids or respond to normal thirst mechanisms. Such a patient is therefore at *Risk for Fluid Volume Deficit.* Recall that hypertonic tube-feedings also increase this risk.

Outcomes. The patient will demonstrate these indications of fluid balance: (1) intake and output being equal for 24, 48, and 72 hours, (2) stable body weight, (3) no signs of excessive perspiration, diarrhea, or vomiting, (4) serum glucose, hematocrit, and blood urea nitrogen, creatinine, sodium, potassium, and chloride values within normal limits, and (5) moist oral mucous membranes with absence of tongue furrows.

Interventions. Important aspects in maintaining fluid and electrolyte balance in unconscious patients are (1) accurate documentation of intake and output, (2) daily weighing with comparison of trends, and (3) assessment and documentation of conditions that may increase fluid volume deficit (e.g., diaphoresis, polyuria, diarrhea, vomiting, hypertonic tube-feedings).

Before fluid and electrolyte intervention is planned for a comatose patient, carefully assess the fluid-electrolyte status. The coma itself may have a fluid or electrolyte cause. Blood tests such as blood glucose, hematocrit, blood urea nitrogen, or creatinine, serum sodium, potassium, chloride, and carbon dioxide measurements help determine fluid and electrolyte status (see Chapters 12 and 13). Dehydration and water intoxication (true hyponatremia) are common causes of electrolyte imbalance associated with coma.

Always avoid overhydration in a patient receiving IV fluids because of the risk of cerebral edema. Diuretics may be prescribed to correct fluid overload and reduce edema. Monitor the response to these medications. When evaluating the response to any diuretic, empty the indwelling catheter before administering the diuretic. Evaluation of the response should consider the diuretic given, the dose, and the patient's renal status.

Risk for Injury. It may not be apparent that the comatose patient is at *Risk for Injury* because he or she does not move. If the coma starts to lighten, however, the patient can move and, without protection, could fall or be injured. In addition, use caution when moving the patient, who cannot voice pain. Although the loss of the corneal blink reflex, which increases the risk of corneal abrasions, is also a type of injury, it is addressed as a collaborative problem. Nursing interventions for a loss of the corneal blink reflex are discussed in Chapter 73.

Outcomes. The patient will not sustain injury, as evidenced by an absence of abrasions or bruises and experiencing no falls from bed.

Interventions. Keep the side rails up on the bed and the bed in the lowest position whenever the patient is not receiving direct care or is unattended. Observe seizure precautions for anyone who has a history of seizure or is at risk of seizure. Protect the patient from injury during seizures or periods of agitation (e.g., use padded side rails, keep the patient's nails short and filed). It is of utmost importance to protect the patient's head. Give the prescribed seizure medication on time to maintain a high seizure threshold. If a dose of the medication is missed for any reason (e.g., vomiting), notify the physician. Anti-epileptic medication should not be withheld without a physician order.

Give adequate support to the limbs and head when moving or turning an unconscious patient. Limbs without tone may dislocate if they are allowed to fall unsupported. Always turn an unconscious patient toward you or someone else to prevent falls. Protect an unconscious patient from external sources of heat (e.g., heating pads).

Do not restrain the patient unless it is absolutely necessary because restraint is likely to worsen confused and combative behavior. If restraints are used, they must be released at least every 2 hours for range-of-motion exercises and skin checks. Do not leave unstable patients unattended. Attempt to manage the patient's behaviors without restraints first. "Sitters," hospital volunteers, or family members or friends may be able to provide attendant services. Avoid oversedation because it may alter respirations, which increases ICP and masks changes in a patient's level of consciousness.

Fecal Incontinence. Once a paralytic ileus is corrected, the patient will produce feces. Most patients are incontinent because voluntary control is required for the function of the external anal sphincter. Write the diagnosis as *Fecal Incontinence related to inability to respond to normal cues about evacuation;* also consider *High Risk for Impaired Skin Integrity related to fecal incontinence.*

Outcomes. The patient will have reduced fecal incontinence, as evidenced by (1) a bowel movement every 2 to 3 days and (2) no signs of fecal impaction.

Interventions. Plan interventions to (1) control bowel movements, (2) maintain the patient's normal elimination schedule, and (3) prevent fecal impaction or constipation. As soon as the patient is able, begin a program of bowel retraining. Maintain a regular schedule, administering stool softeners and suppositories, and performing digital removal of stool at approximately the same times each day. Examine the abdomen frequently for distention. Constipation and fecal impaction may occur. Small, frequent liquid stools may indicate impaction. If diarrhea or constipation persists, assess for possible causes, such as medications, enteral feedings, and intestinal bacterial infections.

Caution: Consult with the physician prior to performing digital removal of stool in a patient with an altered level of consciousness. This intervention has been known to induce seizures and may increase ICP. Rectal application of an anesthetic jelly prior to the stimulus decreases this risk.

Altered Family Processes. Having a family member in a coma is a significant stressor for the family. A possible diagnosis is *Altered Family Processes related to uncertain future or impending death of a family member.* Individualize the etiology portion of the diagnosis to fit the specific patient and family.

Outcomes. Family members will exhibit positive coping behaviors, as evidenced by (1) showing an ability to solve problems, (2) meeting the needs of other family members, and (3) asking questions about the patient that indicate understanding of previous teaching.

Interventions. The significant others of a comatose patient are often very stressed. It is difficult for the family when they cannot communicate with the patient. The uncertainty of not knowing whether the patient will recover is a major stressor. Include family members in the patient's care to the extent that they can and want to be involved. Family members need information and realistic hope.

It is important for the family to see the patient receiving high-quality, professional, and caring nursing care. For example, talk to the patient as if he or she can understand. Initially, this behavior will seem awkward, but in time, it will feel appropriate. Tell the patient that he or she will be turned to the side, bathed, and so on, before performing the task. Depending on the depth of the coma, the patient's sense of hearing may still be intact. Therefore, speak to the patient as if he or she can hear, and tell the family to do the same. Comatose patients have awakened and reported that they remember hearing specific voices.

The family is often in a state of shock, needing someone to recognize their needs and help them through this difficult situation. They may experience various conflicting feelings, such as guilt and anger. The Client Education Guide suggests ways for the patient's family members to cope with these feelings.

Allow significant others to stay with the patient when and where possible. At times, family members may become zealous about attending and may stay at the patient's bedside continuously. Encourage family members to care for themselves also by eating regular meals and obtaining adequate sleep. Have them consider using external support systems (e.g., neighbors and church groups). Tell them that they will be telephoned if any significant changes occur in their loved one's status, and ask them to leave a phone number where they can be reached. Encourage family members to phone if they have questions or concerns.

Social workers may be contacted to provide additional support. Some hospitals, especially tertiary care centers, have "family homes," where family members who must travel a long distance to the hospital may stay to be close to the hospital and the patient.

EVALUATION

The patient may remain comatose for a few hours or even months. Some comatose patients (e.g., patients with diabetic coma) awaken and make a complete recovery while in the hospital. Therefore, some expected outcomes have brief time frames (e.g., airway obstruction), whereas others are prolonged, requiring frequent reevaluation (e.g.,

---

CLIENT EDUCATION GUIDE

When a Loved One Is in an Altered State of Consciousness

Family Instructions

Seeing a loved one in this state causes a roller coaster of feelings (e.g., denial, anger, depression, guilt, bargaining). There is no "correct" order for these feelings; they may recur even after one thinks they have been worked through. These and other feelings are normal. It is important to "give yourself permission" to feel, so that you can work through the grieving process.

Talk to and touch your loved one. Research supports the positive benefit of talking to and touching the person.

Become involved in the care of your loved one, including decisions about how he or she will be cared for.

Learn about the devices and equipment used to monitor and treat your loved one.

Stay informed of your loved one's condition. Ask a nurse to repeat or explain information provided by the physician and to clarify any medical jargon that you do not understand.

If the physician has indicated that there is no chance for your loved one's recovery, refocus your energies into hoping for a peaceful death. Consider organ donation; this has helped other families with their healing.

Join a support group, whether your loved one is expected to die or to stay at this level of altered consciousness for an indeterminate time. Through reaching out, you may be able to find strength and meaning in this tragedy.

family coping). Your evaluation may identify a need for revision of the care plan.

■ Modifications for Elderly Clients

The older patient in a coma requires the same quality of care as patients in other age groups. However, the older patient is at higher risk for all complications of immobility, especially pressure ulcers and pneumonia. Urinary retention is common in elderly men because of prostatic enlargement. Finally, fully assess the patient for the common disorders of aging (e.g., diabetes) that might be the cause of the coma.

■ Self-Care

The site to which a patient with coma is discharged from an acute care setting depends totally on (1) the condition of the patient, (2) the cause of the coma, and (3) the level of family support available. If the patient is recovering from coma, plan for placement in a rehabilitation center. Patients remaining in coma but showing slow recovery may be placed in an extended-care facility until they can participate in rehabilitation.[3, 12] Coma stimulation programs, although not readily available, provide an alternative for the patient who is slow to recover.[3-5]

If the patient is in a coma and is not expected to awaken but may live for a time with nutritional support, placement in a skilled nursing center is common.[4] In these centers, supportive care is given. Family members usually specify how aggressively they wish the patient to be treated in the event of a deterioration in status. Your role in discharge of the comatose patient centers on communication with the receiving nurses and the family. If the patient is ventilator-dependent or combative, special consideration is required for transport to the new facility. Provide a complete plan of care.

CONFUSIONAL STATES

Confusion is a mental state marked by alterations in thought and attention deficit, followed by problems in comprehension. It is accompanied by a loss of short-term memory and, often, irritability alternating with drowsiness. Confusion is a common clinical manifestation in many neurologic and metabolic disorders.

Sundowning is defined as agitation, confusion, and restlessness that occurs after the sun sets.[12] However, diurnal variations may be responsible for these changes as well.[1]

Confusion has been shown to increase both morbidity and length of hospital stay. This relationship has major implications in terms of cost containment, especially because people older than 85 years are the fastest-growing age group in the United States.

Etiology and Risk Factors

There are many causes of confusion. Common causes of acute confusion are alcohol withdrawal and drug ingestion. Confusion can also follow fever, heart failure, head injury, and use of anesthetics. Other causes of confusion are hypoxia, hypoglycemia, severe fluid and electrolyte disorders, sepsis, liver or renal failure, poisons, and drug overdose.

Delirium and dementia are classifications of types of confusion. Three features are common to all types of *delirium:*

- A disturbance of consciousness with a reduced ability to focus, sustain, or shift attention
- A change in cognition (memory, language, disorientation) or development of a perceptual disturbance that is not better accounted for by a pre-existing, established, or evolving dementia
- A change that develops over a short time (hours to days) and may fluctuate during the course of the day

Several classifications of delirium have each of the three common features but specific causes. They are (1) delirium related to a general medical condition, (2) delirium due to substance intoxication (prescribed drugs, over-the-counter medications, or street drugs), (3) delirium due to substance withdrawal, (4) delirium with multiple causes, and (5) delirium "not otherwise specified."[7, 10]

Dementia is the chronic form of confusion. As with delirium, there are common features in the many types of dementia. They are as follows:

- The development of multiple memory impairments
- One or more of the following cognitive disturbances: *aphasia* (problems with expressing speech or understanding sounds), *apraxia* (inability to convert a thought to action), *agnosia,* (inability to recognize objects), impaired executive functioning
- Significant impairment and decline in social or occupational functioning
- A gradual onset and continuing cognitive decline

The classifications of dementia include the four common features with variable causes and characteristics. There are many subtypes of dementia of the Alzheimer's type. Essentially, all other causes, such as central nervous system (CNS) disorders, systemic conditions, substance-induced conditions, depression, and schizophrenia, must be ruled out. The other types of dementia are (1) vascular dementia (multi-infarct), (2) dementia secondary to other general medical conditions, (3) substance-induced persisting dementia, (4) dementia with multiple causes, and (5) dementia "not otherwise specified."[6, 9]

An in-depth discussion of the care related to specific types of delirium and dementia, as well as the memory changes that occur in clients with amnesic disorders and other cognitive disorders not meeting the criteria for any of the preceding classifications, is beyond the scope of this book. The reader should refer to a psychiatric textbook for this information. This discussion focuses on the general care of a client with confusion. However, because dementia of the Alzheimer's type is a growing problem, Chapter 72 details the pathologic processes and care related to this type of degenerative disease.

Risk factors leading to confusion vary with the specific etiologic factors. In general, the proper management of various diseases, such as diabetes mellitus, would reduce the incidence of confusion. Disorders such as Alzheimer's disease have no known prevention at this time, although new drugs may slow disease progression. Avoid the use of any medications that contribute to confusion in people who are at risk for confusion.

Pathophysiology

Three mechanisms account for the development of *acute confusion:* (1) damage to the brain with swelling or loss of oxygen, blood, or both (functional disorder), (2) impairment of the action of the nervous system by chemicals or other substances (metabolic disorder), and (3) the rebound overactivity of a previously depressed center in the brain. Chemicals that cross the blood-brain barrier, such as alcohol, impair the metabolism of neuronal cells. When the drug action wears off or the drug is withdrawn from the client, the lower centers in the brain are overactive. This overactivity accounts for the development of acute confusion, combativeness, and other abnormal behaviors.

Chronic confusional states are due to disorders that cause brain tissue destruction, biochemical imbalances, or compression of the brain. For example, people with Alzheimer's disease lack acetylcholine, a neurotransmitter that is necessary for short-term memory. Other disorders causing chronic confusion may be inherited; may be secondary to a transmissible agent, as with Creutzfeldt-Jakob disease; or may follow diseases such as encephalitis.

Clinical Manifestations

The earliest sign of a brain disorder is a *disorder of attention.* The client may report the loss of concentration or may appear preoccupied. At the same time, restlessness, emotional lability, insomnia or drowsiness, and vivid nightmares may begin. Clients may appear anxious and may fear that they are "going crazy." As the disorder progresses, stupor and coma develop. Behaviors seen in the client are reflective not of personality but of the cause of the disorder. For example, barbiturate or alcohol abuse and withdrawal and liver disorders cause agitated delirium. In contrast, anoxia and kidney and lung disorders are associated with a quieter response. Disorders that develop rapidly are more likely to cause an agitated response than those that develop slowly.

Fluctuations in cognition (the ability to think and reason) are common in clients with metabolic brain disorders. Clients may be totally irrational one moment and lucid the next. Some of the fluctuations are caused by the environment. Delirious clients become more disoriented at night, in unfamiliar surroundings, when they hear unfamiliar noises or see unfamiliar people, or when restraints are used. The lack of a window in the room has caused many clients to become disoriented.

Loss of memory for recent events is a hallmark of metabolic brain disorders. The client commonly has difficulty with both immediate recall and abstract thought. Clients who are delirious quickly lose orientation to time. Normal people can readily recall six or seven digits forward and five or six backward and identify the commonalities between an orange and an apple or a tree and a bush; delirious clients cannot do these things. However, the client's general intelligence level can affect the behaviors observed. If possible, the client's level of education should be known before the assessment.

Perceptual errors (e.g., mistaking the nurse for a daughter) as well as hallucinations, illusions, and delusions are common accompaniments of delirium.

Hallucinations are sensations occurring in the absence of external stimuli. A client may hear, see, feel, smell, or taste something that is not present. The client may or may not realize that the experience is "not real." Unfortunately, the most common hallucinations involve rodents and unfriendly animals (e.g., snakes, spiders). These visions are very frightening.

Illusions differ from hallucinations, in that illusions are the misinterpretation of something actually in the environment. For example, if a client sees a shadow on the drape and mistakes it for a real person, the client is experiencing an illusion.

Delusions are thoughts or beliefs that have no basis in fact. For example, a client may think that he or she has been robbed or poisoned, when there is no basis for this belief.

There are no specific diagnostic tests for confusion. The client may undergo CT or MRI scanning to determine whether there is a structural cause for the confusion, such as a tumor or stroke. In addition, a series of laboratory studies may be performed to look for a metabolic cause. Common studies include a complete blood count, electrolyte measurements, determination of vitamin B_{12} and folate levels, thyroid and liver function studies, drug toxicity screening tests, and an EEG. A lumbar puncture may be performed for the analysis of CSF.

Outcome Management

■ Medical Management

In all care settings, the medical management of the confused client begins by determining the cause of the confusion and correcting it, if possible.[7] When no specific cause is found, the medical management focuses on controlling manifestations. Sometimes medications can be given to calm agitation. Nutritional needs also must be monitored.

■ Nursing Management of the Medical Client
ASSESSMENT

A thorough history is required for assessment of the confused client. The history should include the onset of the confusion, past medical illnesses, work and occupational history, and past injuries. Disorders such as diabetes or liver failure may be out of control and responsible for the confusion. The client may have been exposed to heavy metals or toxic wastes at work. Record past injuries, especially head injury. Depending on the level of confusion, the client may not be able to answer each question, and you may need to rely on the family or others who have been with the client. Review medications, including over-the-counter drugs and nutritional supplements.

Specific questions about the client's ability to handle routine financial transactions or home safety with tasks such as cooking, dressing, and driving will help determine whether the client can be safely returned home or is in need of an alternative arrangement. At times, the family may report a change in personality, such as apathy, social isolation, disinterest in current events, and irritability. Record these observations because they may be clinical manifestations of Alzheimer's disease or frontal lobe lesions.

The confused client requires ongoing assessment with the Mini-Mental State Examination (see Chapter 67). This examination is much more sensitive than other tools for serial evaluations of confused clients.[13] Analyze the data collected to determine whether the confusion is improving, worsening, or unchanged.

The confused client is often combative and argumentative. Observe for factors in the client's environment that may affect confusion. Assess whether the client is able to refrain from self-injury or injury to others. If not bedridden, the client may wander about and become lost or injured if harmful items are not secured (e.g., knives).

Confusion can occur in clients of any age or culture and from variable causes. The nurse's role as a client advocate supersedes personal bias related to any of these variables.

DIAGNOSIS, OUTCOMES, INTERVENTIONS

This section describes interventions appropriate to the confused client, regardless of the cause, with an emphasis on the issue of safety.

Altered Thought Processes. Use the nursing diagnosis *Altered Thought Processes related to failure in memory and lack of self-protective behavior to address needs for safety.*

Outcomes. The client will have improved thought processes, as evidenced by (1) higher scores on the Mini-Mental State Examination and (2) decreased frequency of hallucinations, illusions, and delusions.

Interventions. The confused client will benefit from consistency in the environment and care routine. Keep objects, such as the tray table and bedside chair, in the same place. If possible, the same staff member should care for the client. Give the client short explanations as events occur, such as "You need an x-ray" and "Please sit in the wheelchair." Saying to a confused client, "In 2 hours, an x-ray tech will be coming to take you for a CT scan," is useless, because such a client will neither understand nor remember it. Response time may be slowed in confusion; allow the client time to respond.

Reorient the client as often as necessary, but use caution about the specific communication used. Clients with chronic untreatable confusion do not benefit from reorientation and may become more agitated when you attempt to reorient them. For example, in one study in which a 92-year-old client was told repeatedly that her mother or father could not possibly be alive, the client reacted each time as if it was the first time she had been told and grieved deeply.[13] For these selected clients, avoid reorienting, and "go along" with the confusion. Of course, when the client is at risk of injury, safety precautions are foremost. Clocks and calendars in the room also help with reorientation. The use of familiar objects is helpful when a client's remote memory is intact. For example, the use of a quilt from home on the bed may help the confused client recognize the bed as his or her own.

Promote reduction of unfamiliar noise because it adds to confusion. The client's room should be quiet and softly lighted without producing shadows.

Consistency in care of a client with confusion requires communication among caregivers. This communication occurs not only through the oral reporting method but also in the care plan and documentation records.

Risk for Injury. Confusion greatly increases risk of harm. The client cannot interpret, or may not be able to

respond to, environmental stimuli that precede danger. Write the nursing diagnosis as *Risk for Injury related to the unpredictable behavior and inability to interpret environmental stimuli.*

Outcomes. The client will not sustain injury and will not injure others.

Interventions. The client must be protected from self-injury. The client should be in a room near the nursing station so that assessments can be performed every 30 to 60 minutes. In addition, the bed should be in the low position. Structure the client's environment to minimize injury; remove any extraneous equipment.

The routine use of physical restraints (e.g., side rails, cloth restraints) or chemical restraints (e.g., medication) is discouraged.[8] The use of side rails and restraints does not guarantee that clients will not fall and often either makes them more agitated or leads to more severe injury when they do fall. Alternatives to restraints include the use of sitters for ongoing observation and placement of the patient in an area permitting constant observation, such as the nursing station. If all other alternatives have been unsuccessful and restraints are used, make frequent assessments and record the data. Cloth restraints must be removed every 2 hours to assess the skin beneath them and perform range-of-motion exercises. Chemical restraint (e.g., tranquilizers) can result in greater confusion and tremors (extrapyramidal symptoms).

The client with brain alteration is not in control of his or her behavior. Behaviors may be unpredictable, irrational, or impulsive, or the client may be frightened and suspicious. Never "punish" a confused client for inappropriate behavior or remarks. Instead, remember that these personality changes are a result of brain lesions, and adjust the care plan accordingly. If a client is agitated, provide reassurance and a calm environment. Redirect or distract the client. Monitoring systems may be used for clients who wander.

Confused elderly clients are at increased risk for falls. A formal fall risk assessment should be completed. Some institutions have programs for clients who are at risk for falling or who have fallen. These programs include frequent assessments, routine toileting, bed and wandering monitors, and environmental changes (mattress on the floor, use of a lap buddy). Trying to ambulate to the bathroom is a common time for falls, and toileting should be offered routinely (every 2 hours).

Sleep Pattern Disturbance. A common problem seen in confused clients consists of daytime napping and nighttime hallucinations. This problem is stated as *Sleep Pattern Disturbance related to alterations in usual sleep habits.*

Outcomes. The client will have improved sleep patterns, as evidenced by (1) sleeping 4 to 6 hours continuously at night and (2) not sleeping as often during the day.

Interventions. Plan nighttime interventions to allow 4 to 6 hours of uninterrupted sleep. Recall that a sleep cycle requires 1½ to 2 hours, and the loss of REM (rapid eye movement) sleep can increase confusion. When you enter the room at night, assess the client for REM. If REM is present, the client should be allowed to complete the REM portion of the sleep cycle. You should return later to care for the client.

Keep the client active during the day so that there is

some fatigue by nighttime. Daytime sleeping is a difficult pattern to break, and the client may have to be kept awake for this pattern to be reversed. Bedtime routines should be developed. Avoid the use of caffeinated beverages and alcohol, which may prevent sleep. For the elderly client, the normal changes in sleep with aging need to be considered, such as the greater use of short naps and less sleep during the night. Sleeping medications are seldom given to the confused client because they often alter sleep cycles and rob the client of REM sleep. See Chapter 21 for further information about sleep disorders.

Risk for Caregiver Role Strain. The unfamiliar behavior of the confused client or the stress of providing continual care for the client at home may increase stress in the family and alter their ability to cope. This diagnosis is stated as *Risk for Caregiver Role Strain related to long-term, stressful, and complex care required by family member.*

Outcomes. The client's family members will maintain their own physical and psychological health, as evidenced by (1) improved use of support systems, (2) obtaining of adequate equipment to provide care, (3) limited use of addictive drugs for coping, (4) interaction with friends and extended family (as desired), and (5) appropriate analysis of the client's condition.

Interventions. Teach the family to monitor for the effects of confusion. When confusion is a new problem for the client, the family will be distressed by the behavior. Explain to the family that the client is not able to control behavior or speech at this time. Assess whether the client becomes calm or agitated when the family is present, and advise visitations accordingly. If possible, the need for and use of restraints should be explained to the family before they see a client in restraints. The family may become very upset when they see their loved one "tied" to a bed. Advance explanations can avert some of this reaction. There have been instances in which a client suffered an injury because the family did not understand the purpose for the restraints and untied them.

See Management and Delegation: Physical Restraints.

MANAGEMENT AND DELEGATION

Physical Restraints

The use of physical restraints to protect a client from self-harm or injury, or to manage a client at risk for disruption of medical therapies, is a decision made collaboratively between you and the physician and may include consultation with other members of the interdisciplinary team. The serious decision to use physical restraints is made after your comprehensive assessment and evaluation of previous interventions and alternatives.

A clear goal is the use of the least restrictive device for the shortest interval possible. Regulatory agencies consider the use of restraints to be a high-risk intervention. Death and injury have been associated with restraint use in hospital environments. Your clinical site should provide you with clear guidelines regarding the use of restraints and the role of unlicensed assistive personnel in caring for restrained clients.

Before delegating care of the client in physical restraints, consider the following:

- Have the client and family been informed and educated regarding the need for restraints to protect the client? Your education of the client and family should include standards of care and discussion of what factors lead to discontinuation of restraints.
- Have you assessed the client to determine the most appropriate type of restraint? The restraint must be the right size. Follow the manufacturer's recommendations for sizing. Never use anything other than a manufactured device that has been approved by the Food and Drug Administration.
- Have you obtained a physician's order for the use of restraints? In addition to the initiation order for restraints, there should be ongoing discussion of the need to continue restraint use with the interdisciplinary team and physician order updates every 24 hours.

Your assessment of the client's safety and comfort needs must occur at regular intervals as defined by your institution. You are accountable for assessing and documenting the client's condition, the client's response to restraints, and the safety and comfort interventions provided.

Consider the following points when delegating components of care to assistive personnel:

- Be very clear about the type of restraint being used. In addition to applying restraints according to the manufacturer's instructions, restraints are to be secured only to the bed frame or chair with slip knots.
- Explain that restraints are never used as a punishment.
- Clients with altered mental status experiencing unmet elimination needs may become agitated. Instruct assistive personnel to offer assistance with elimination at regular intervals.
- Provide specific expectations and a time schedule for observation of the client.
- Instruct on how to remove restraints one at a time in agitated clients.
- How to respond to clients who ask for the restraints to "be cut-off" by re-explaining the need for them.

You may delegate these components of care to assistive personnel:

- Assistance with activities of daily living, such as bathing, grooming, and feeding
- Active or passive range of motion
- Turning and repositioning the client. They should be instructed to re-secure restraints after position changes.

Describe for the assistive personnel the findings that are immediately reportable to you. Such findings may include skin redness or irritation noted at points of contact with the restraint device, changes in color or movement of areas distal to the restraint, the client's unplanned removal of a restraint, disruption of a medical therapy, and the client's complaints of discomfort or distress. Verify the competency of assistive personnel in caring for restrained patients during orientation and in an ongoing manner thereafter.

Kathleen Rea, BSN, RN, *Clinician III, Clinical Manager, Surgical Services, University of Virginia Health System, Charlottesville, Virginia*

Choosing the placement site for a confused client being discharged from the hospital varies with the cause of confusion. If the confusion is acute and full recovery is expected, the patient may be able to go home under the care of family members. If the confusion is chronic, the patient needs either care or supervision at home or placement in an extended-care facility. Some communities offer adult day care and respite services that give family members relief from the constant care of the confused person. See Chapter 72 for care of the client with Alzheimer's disease at home.

Advise the family to have legal counsel determine the client's competence and the need for guardianship or durable power of attorney. The family may also need to grieve the loss of the client's previous functional role, personality, companionship, and so on. Assess for evidence of violence in the caregiver and the client. Caregiver violence is possible, especially if the client was violent toward the caregiver in the past.

Help the caregiver find respite care and personal time to meet his or her own needs and to learn stress management techniques. Female caregivers are especially vulnerable to social isolation.

EVALUATION

Most of the time, confusion will require many months to abate. The diagnosis of a chronic, progressive condition such as Alzheimer's disease or dementia of the Alzheimer type may require an entire change in care plan prioritization. These conditions are discussed in Chapter 72.

▇ Modifications for Elderly Clients

It is common, but incorrect, to believe that elderly people naturally undergo a marked deterioration in mental function. In general, elderly people have difficulty recalling new information but their remote memory is intact. In addition, depression occurs in 20% to 30% of the elderly. Depression may follow the loss of friends, spouse, health, and independence and may lead to manifestations such as memory loss and confusion.

Older adults are particularly at risk for confusion during hospitalization.[10] They are dealing not only with the stress of being ill but also with the stress of an unfamiliar environment. Elderly clients may rely heavily on familiar landmarks and routines to help them maintain an independent lifestyle. These cues are often lost in the hospital or extended-care setting. A large percentage of the population in hospital and extended-care settings are elderly, who typically have other conditions that contribute to confusion. Confusion is best managed by using a team approach and teaching unlicensed personnel to (1) introduce themselves at the beginning of a work shift, (2) use the same time for the client's sleep, naps, and meals, (3) routinely place the client on the toilet or commode, (4) talk to the client about the past, (5) gently redirect lost or wandering clients, and (6) encourage self-care (eating, dressing, and so on).

CONCLUSIONS

Clients who are confused or comatose are vulnerable to many complications, including injury, aspiration, malnu-trition, and skin breakdown. Nurses provide a lifeline for these clients, giving protection and promoting normal body functions. The families of these clients require therapeutic management because they face many difficult decisions.

THINKING CRITICALLY

1. **A 48-year-old man is brought to the emergency department by ambulance. His wife states that he had been shaving in the bathroom when she heard a thud. She found him unresponsive on the floor. How do you intervene?**

Factors to Consider. What was the client's neurologic baseline when he was received in the emergency department? What other clinical manifestations did the client display? Were there any physical signs of injury to his head or other parts of his body? Does he have any other significant medical history or allergies?

2. **You are caring for a 72-year-old woman who recently underwent repair of a hip fracture. Her husband indicates that she had recently been confused, which led to her falling and fracturing her hip. How do you intervene?**

Factors to Consider. What do you include in your assessment? What kinds of interventions do you need to consider? How do you involve her family?

BIBLIOGRAPHY

1. Davis, A. E., & White, J. J. (1995). Innovative sensory input for the comatose brain-injured patient. *Critical Care Nursing Clinics of North America, 7*(2):351–361.
2. Foreman, M. D., et al. (1999). Standard of practice protocol: Acute confusion/delirium. *Geriatric Nursing 20*(3), 147–152.
3. Giacino, J. T., et al. (1997). Development of practice guidelines for assessment and management of the vegetative and minimally conscious states. *Journal of Head Trauma Rehabilitation, 12*(4), 36–51.
4. Hamel, M. B., et al. (1995). Identification of comatose patients at high risk for death or severe disability. *Journal of the American Medical Association, 273*(23), 1842–1848.
5. Helwick, L. D. (1994). Stimulation programs for coma patients. *Critical Care Nurse, 8,* 47–51.
6. Hickey, J. V. (1997). Management of the unconscious patient. In *The clinical practice of neurological and neurosurgical nursing* (4th ed.). Philadelphia: J. B. Lippincott. 275–294.
7. Mentes, J., et al. (1999). Acute confusion indicators: Risk factors and prevalence using MDS data. *Research in Nursing and Health, 22*(2), 95–105.
8. Rogers, P. D., & Bocchino, N. L. (1999). Restraint-free care: Is it possible? *American Journal of Nursing, 99*(10), 26–34.
9 Rosenwasser, R. H., & Schneck, M. J. (1996). Initial evaluation and management of acute coma. *Hospital Medicine, 32*(12), 39–44.
10. Shedd, P. P., Kobokovich, L. J., & Slattery, M. J. (1995). Confused patients in the acute care setting: Prevalence, intervention, and outcomes. *Journal of Gerontological Nursing, 21*(4), 5–12.
11. Stewart-Amidei, C. (1991). Assessing the comatose patient in the intensive care unit. *AACN Clinical Issues in Critical Care Nursing, 2*(4), 613–622.
12. Talbot, L. R., & Joanette, Y. (1998). Postcomatose unawareness in a brain-injured populaton. *Journal of Neuroscience Nursing, 30*(2), 129–134.
13. Wallace, M. (1994). The sundown syndrome. *Geriatric Nursing, 15*(3), 164–166.

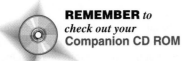

CHAPTER

69

Management of Clients with Cerebral Disorders

Melanie Minton

NURSING OUTCOMES CLASSIFICATION (NOC)
for Nursing Diagnoses—Clients with Cerebral Disorders

Altered Health Maintenance	Grief Resolution	Decision-Making
Knowledge: Health Behaviors	Psychosocial Adjustment: Life Change	Impulse Control
Knowledge: Treatment Regimen	**Anxiety**	Role Performance
Treatment Behavior: Illness	Aggression Control	**Risk of Injury**
Altered Thought Processes	Anxiety Control	Safety Status: Falls Occurrence
Cognitive Ability	Coping	Safety Status: Physical Injury
Cognitive Orientation	**Decreased Adaptive Capacity:**	Symptom Control
Decision-Making	**Intracranial**	**Risk for Spiritual Distress**
Altered Tissue Perfusion: Cerebral	Electrolyte and Acid-Base Balance	Anxiety Control
Cognitive Ability	Fluid Balance	Coping
Neurologic Status	Neurologic Status: Autonomic	Grief Resolution
Neurologic Status: Central Motor Control	Neurologic Status: Cranial Sensory/Motor	Hope
Neurologic Status: Consciousness	Function	Quality of Life
Tissue Perfusion: Cerebral	Neurologic Status: Spinal Sensory/Motor	Spiritual Well-Being
Anticipatory Grieving	Function	
Aggression Control	**Ineffective Individual Coping**	
Coping	Aggression Control	
Family Coping	Coping	

SEIZURE DISORDERS

In this chapter, an important distinction is made between seizures and epilepsy. A *seizure* is a sudden, abnormal electrical discharge from the brain that results in changes in sensation, behavior, movements, perception, or consciousness. A seizure may occur in isolation or with some acute problem within the central nervous system (CNS), such as a low blood glucose level, drug or alcohol withdrawal, or traumatic brain injury. *Epilepsy* is a chronic disorder of recurrent seizures. An isolated, single seizure does not constitute epilepsy.[20, 24, 46, 48]

EPILEPSY

Epilepsy is derived from the Greek *epilepsia,* meaning "seizure." In early times, epilepsy was viewed as being of divine origin and was called the "sacred disease" because someone with epilepsy was thought to be "seized" or struck down by the gods. An epileptic syndrome is composed of paroxysmal neurologic dysfunction causing recurrent episodes of one or more of the following manifestations: loss of consciousness, convulsive movements or other motor activity, sensory phenomena, and behavioral abnormalities. About 2.3 million Americans are known to have seizures or epilepsy. About 181,000 new cases of seizures and epilepsy are documented annually.[20, 24, 45, 47]

The last two decades have brought significant advances in the understanding, diagnosis, and treatment of epilepsy. Despite improvements in electroencephalographic monitoring, neuroimaging, and surgery, however, a cure has not been found.

Etiology and Risk Factors

Epilepsy can be caused by any process that disrupts the stability of the neuronal cell membrane. A variety of conditions are associated with an extremely high likelihood of onset of a chronic seizure disorder. One of the best examples of such conditions is severe, penetrating head trauma, which is associated with up to a 50% risk of the development of epilepsy. This association suggests that the injury results in a long-lasting pathologic change in the CNS that transforms a presumably normal neural network into one that is abnormally hyperexcitable.

The identified mechanism responsible for such malfunction is unknown. Possible theories include neuronal structural impairment, abnormalities involving the sodium-potassium pump, and changes in various neurochemicals.[20, 48] Hypersensitive neurons can be found throughout the brain and spinal cord. The neuronal cell membrane appears to be more permeable and more sensitive to various offending factors. An epileptogenic focus may develop at the location of increased cell membrane permeability. The epileptogenic focus may be limited to a specific area or encompass the entire cortical surface.

Seizures are classified as *genetic, acquired,* or *idiopathic.*[39] What is not well understood is how these three factors may cause the seizure threshold to be lowered, thereby increasing the possibility of seizures. For example, with idiopathic seizures, what is the offending agent? Is it structural, neurochemical, or a combination of several factors?

Idiopathic epilepsy most often begins before the age of 20 years and rarely begins after age 30. Seizures beginning in newborns and infants are often caused by congenital brain defects, birth injuries, or metabolic problems such as anoxia, hypoglycemia, or hypocalcemia. Although the underlying cause may be perinatal, seizures may not begin for many years, often with onset during puberty. Other than in children under age 5 years, the highest incidence of new-onset epilepsy is in people older than 65. The increased risk in this age group is attributed to the increase in conditions that cause neurologic changes in this group. These include cerebrovascular disease, tumor, delirium, Alzheimer's disease, infection, accumulated trauma, and chronic alcoholism, as well as the aging process itself.[20, 24, 26, 46, 48]

When the cause of seizures is known, the disorder is called *secondary epilepsy.* After age 20, generalized seizures usually have an identifiable cause. These causes include traumatic brain injury, brain tumor, and infection. Approximately two thirds of cases of epilepsy are idiopathic; the remainder are from secondary causes.

Pathophysiology

When the integrity of the neuronal cell membrane is altered, the cell begins firing with increased frequency and amplitude.[20, 46, 48] When the intensity of the discharges reaches a threshold, the neuronal firing spreads to adjacent normal neurons. Discharges in the brain stem cause muscle contraction and possibly loss of consciousness. The excitation of the cells can spread to the spinal cord.

Normally, excitatory messages from a single hypersensitive neuron in the cerebral cortex are modulated by deeper structures (e.g., thalamus and brain stem) (Fig. 69-1). In epilepsy, these bursts of electrical activity from the cortex are not controlled or modulated. These discharges block normal inhibition and perpetuate a feedback loop. Eventually, inhibitory neurons in the cortex,

anterior thalamus, and basal ganglia slow the neuronal firing. This inhibition interrupts the seizure and produces an intermittent contraction-relaxation phase. Once the epileptogenic neurons are exhausted and inhibitory processes build, the seizure stops. These later events depress CNS action and impair consciousness. This period of impaired consciousness after a seizure, called a *postictal state,* may be manifested as sleep, confusion, or fatigue.

Seizure activity increases the need for adenosine triphosphate (ATP) and also cerebral oxygen consumption. Supplies of oxygen and glucose are rapidly consumed. To meet these demands, the cerebral blood flow increases by during a seizure. If the seizure is ongoing (as in status epilepticus), severe hypoxia and lactic acidosis occur and may result in brain tissue destruction.[20, 34, 45]

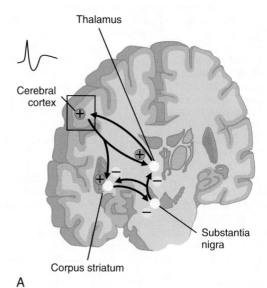

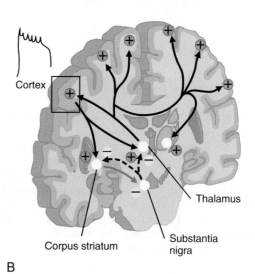

FIGURE 69-1 *A,* Normally, excitatory messages from the cerebral cortex are modulated by deeper structures. *B,* In clients with epilepsy, bursts of activity from the cortex are not modulated and these bursts spread. (From Devinsky, O. [1994]. Seizure disorders. *Clinical Symposia, 46*(1), 1–54. Adapted from an original illustration in *Clinical Symposia,* illustrated by John Craig, M.D., copyright by Ciba-Geigy Corporation.)

Clinical Manifestations

Epilepsy has been classified according to the age at onset, cause, area of origin, abnormalities on the electroencephalogram (EEG), and clinical type of seizure. The International Classification of Epileptic Seizures, used here, is based on the clinical seizure type and on EEG findings during seizures (the ictal period) and between seizures (the interictal period). According to this classification of epilepsy, the neurologic abnormality may be limited to a specific part or focus of the brain—hence the term "partial seizures"—may involve the entire cortical surface, to produce a generalized seizure. Using these two major categories, epileptologists can classify the major forms of epilepsy.[41]

PARTIAL (FOCAL, LOCAL) SEIZURES WITH NO LOSS OF CONSCIOUSNESS

Partial seizures are the most common type of epilepsy. The first clinical and electroencephalographic changes indicate initial activation of neurons in one part of the cerebral hemisphere. They are further classified according to whether or not consciousness is impaired. There are four types of simple partial seizures that do not impair consciousness. These include seizures with motor signs, those with somatosensory or "special senses" signs, those with autonomic manifestations, and psychic manifestations.[41]

MOTOR SIGNS. Partial seizures with motor signs arise from a focus in the region of the brain's motor cortex. The resulting motor activity (seizure) occurs in the part of the body innervated by motor neurons originating in the affected region of the cortex. Because the hand and fingers have the largest cortical representation, many focal motor seizures begin with convulsive movement in an upper extremity. Involuntary movements may spread centrally and involve the entire limb, and even the same side of the face and lower extremity. This progression or spread is known as the jacksonian march. The client also may exhibit changes in posture or spoken utterances.[41]

SOMATOSENSORY OR "SPECIAL SENSES" MANIFESTATIONS. If the epileptogenic focus is in the parietal region, the client experiences sensory phenomena such as numbness and tingling in the affected area. If the focus is in the occipital region, the client may experience bright, flashing lights in the field of vision opposite the side of the focus. Likewise, the client can have changes in speech or taste. Involvement of the posterior temporal area of the dominant hemisphere (usually the left) causes difficulty with speaking, or aphasia.[41]

AUTONOMIC MANIFESTATIONS. Stimulation of the autonomic system produces epigastric sensations, pallor, sweating, flushing, piloerection (goose flesh), pupillary dilation, tachycardia, and tachypnea.[41]

PSYCHIC MANIFESTATIONS. Seizures arising in the anterior temporal lobe can begin with psychic manifestations. These seizures frequently begin with an aura, a subjective sensation that helps localize the focus. An aura may be a strange smell, noise, or sensation preceding a seizure, or a sense of "rising" or "welling up" in the epigastric region. Visual distortions and feelings such as déjà vu are common.[41]

COMPLEX PARTIAL SEIZURES

There are two types of complex partial seizures: complex partial seizures with automatisms and partial seizures evolving into generalized seizures.

COMPLEX PARTIAL SEIZURES WITH AUTOMATISMS. The most characteristic features of a complex partial seizure are the accompanying *automatisms*. These automatic behaviors include purposeless repetitive activities such as lip-smacking, chewing, patting a part of the body, or picking at clothes while in a dreamy state. Inappropriate or antisocial behavior may also automatically occur during the seizure. This unusual behavior may cause the client to be viewed as psychotic or otherwise mentally disturbed. However, some abnormalities are very subtle and may not be detected by an untrained observer.

Temporal lobe seizures usually last 2 to 3 minutes but may last up to 15 minutes. The client is usually unaware of any activity during the seizure and may be confused or drowsy postictally. Attempts to restrain the client during a seizure may induce combative and uncooperative behavior.[41]

PARTIAL SEIZURES EVOLVING TO SECONDARY GENERALIZED SEIZURES. These seizures start from a particular focus, and then the electrical discharges spread throughout the brain. Clinically, the client first shows focal signs; for example, one side of the face moves, and then the whole body becomes involved. Consciousness is lost if the discharges spread throughout the brain.[41]

GENERALIZED SEIZURES

Generalized seizures lead to a loss of consciousness. They can be convulsive or nonconvulsive. Generalized seizures begin with manifestations involving both hemispheres. Consciousness may be impaired, which may be the first clinical manifestation. About one third of seizures are generalized. Types of generalized seizures are absence, myoclonic, clonic, tonic, tonic-clonic, and atonic.[41]

ABSENCE SEIZURES. Absence seizures occur in childhood and early adolescence. "Grand mal" or partial seizures may develop at any time in patients who have had absence seizures.[41]

MYOCLONIC SEIZURES. Myoclonic seizures involve sudden uncontrollable jerking movements of either a single muscle group or multiple groups, sometimes causing the client to fall. The client loses consciousness for a moment and then is confused postictally. These seizures often occur in the morning, and clients often report that they spill their coffee with their fall.[41]

CLONIC SEIZURES. The clinical manifestations of clonic seizures include rhythmic muscular contraction and relaxation lasting several minutes. Distinct phases of clonic seizures are not easily observed.[41]

TONIC SEIZURES. Tonic seizures include an abrupt increase in muscular tone and muscular contraction. In addition, with tonic seizures there is a loss of consciousness and the presence of autonomic signs. Tonic seizures may last from 30 seconds to several minutes.[41]

TONIC-CLONIC SEIZURES. Formerly known as "grand mal" seizures, tonic-clonic seizures are the type of seizures most closely associated with epilepsy. Actually, however, this type of generalized seizure comprises only 10% of all seizures. A tonic-clonic seizure typically proceeds as follows:

1. Aura may or may not be present.
2. Sudden loss of consciousness may occur.
3. In the tonic phase, the entire body becomes rigid (Fig. 69–2A). If standing or sitting, the client falls stiffly to the floor. A cry may be uttered. Respirations are interrupted temporarily, and the client may become cyanotic. The jaw is fixed and the hands are clenched. The eyes may be opened wide; the pupils are dilated and fixed. The tonic phase lasts 30 to 60 seconds. At the end of this phase the client breathes deeply.
4. The clonic phase begins next, with rhythmic, jerky contraction and relaxation of all body muscles, especially those of the extremities (Fig. 69–2B). The client is usually incontinent and may bite the lips, tongue, or inside of the mouth. Excessive saliva is blown from the mouth, which creates frothing at the lips.
5. An entire tonic-clonic seizure may last from 2 to 5 minutes, after which the client enters the postictal phase, during which he or she relaxes and remains totally unresponsive for a time. The client may rouse briefly and then go into a postictal sleep lasting 30 minutes to several hours. This sleep may be followed by general fatigue, depression, confusion, or headache, all of which gradually resolve. The client has complete amnesia for the seizure episode and may feel nauseated, stiff, and sore. Bruising may occur as the result of falls. Petechial hemorrhages may develop on the face and chest due to the vasovagal responses. Falling during the seizure may cause other injury.

Tonic-clonic seizures vary in frequency from many times daily to once or twice a year. Tonic-only and clonic-only seizures may also occur.[20, 41, 45]

ATONIC SEIZURES. Atonic seizures are associated with a total loss of muscle tone. They may be mild, with the client briefly nodding the head, or the client may fall to the floor. Consciousness is impaired only briefly.[41]

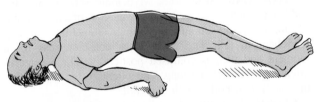

A Tonic phase

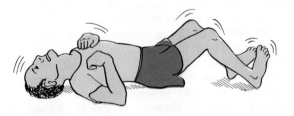

B Clonic phase

FIGURE 69–2 *A,* The tonic phase of a seizure is marked by loss of consciousness, falling, crying, and generalized stiffness. There may be incontinence. *B,* During the clonic phase, there is jerking of the limbs and salivary frothing.

DIAGNOSTIC TESTS

The major diagnostic tool for assessment of clients suspected of having epilepsy is the EEG (see Chapter 68). This test assists in (1) locating the focus of abnormal electrical discharges, if present; (2) establishing a diagnosis of epilepsy; and (3) identifying the specific type of seizures. The EEG records only the electrical activity of the cerebral cortex. With this limitation, a normal EEG tracing does not always exclude a diagnosis of epilepsy, and EEG abnormalities do not always confirm the diagnosis. During a seizure, EEG abnormalities involve all parts of the cortex. Between seizures, clients with epilepsy may show EEG abnormalities not characteristic of seizure disorders. An ambulatory EEG study can be used to clarify suspected seizures that are occurring frequently. The monitor used is similar to a Holter monitor. Long-term video EEG monitoring may also be used to rule out pseudoseizures.

Occasionally, diagnostic tests such as skull radiography, computed tomography (CT), and magnetic resonance imaging (MRI) are used to rule out brain lesions that can trigger seizures. Positron emission tomography (PET) and single photon emission computed tomography (SPECT) may be helpful to measure cerebral blood flow in clients undergoing surgery for epilepsy. As important as the EEG and other diagnostic studies are, a complete seizure profile and history must be established. The seizure profile includes a baseline neurologic examination and description of the seizure activity, as well as laboratory studies.[20, 47]

Outcome Management

■ Medical Management

The goals of management of clients with seizures and epilepsy are to prevent injury during seizures, to eliminate factors that precipitate seizures, to diagnose and treat the cause of the seizure, and to control seizures to allow a desired lifestyle.

PREVENTION OF INJURY DURING A SEIZURE

During a seizure, the major goals are to maintain the airway, to prevent injury to the client, to observe the seizure activity, and to administer appropriate anticonvulsant medications. Today, "seizure precautions" as identified in a hospital setting refers to the availability of an oral airway and suction equipment. In the home or the community, turning the person to his or her side displaces the tongue and usually results in an open airway once the tonic phase has ceased. Any tight clothing around the person's neck is loosened.

The person experiencing a seizure usually requires protection from the environment. For example, objects should be moved out of the way so that he or she does not strike the head or extremities. Put a pillow or folded blanket under the affected person's head, but do not flex the neck sharply or close the airway.

Observers' descriptions of a seizure can be very helpful in making a diagnosis, especially if the descriptions include details such as the sequence in which phenomena occurred. Instruct the family and unlicensed assistive personnel to make the following observations:

- How long did the seizure last?
- Where in the body did the seizure begin and how did it progress?
- Did the client's eyes and/or head deviate?
- Were the respirations labored or frothy?
- Was the client incontinent?
- Did the client lose consciousness?
- What were the types of movements and what body parts moved?
- Eliminating factors that precipitate seizures

For decades the main antiepileptic drugs (AEDs) were phenytoin (Dilantin), phenobarbital, carbamazepine (Tegretol), and valproate sodium (Depakote). Since the 1990s, other AEDs have been approved and show promising effectiveness. Currently available antiepileptic drugs appear to act primarily by blocking the initiation or spread of seizures.

Phenytoin, carbamazepine, valproic acid, and lamotrigine inhibit sodium-dependent action potentials, blocking the burst and firing neurons in a seizure focus. Phenytoin also appears to suppress seizure spread through inhibition of specific voltage-gated calcium channels.

Benzodiazepines and barbiturates augment inhibition by distinct interactions with gamma-aminobutyric acid (GABA) receptors (see Anatomy and Physiology review). Valproic acid elevates the concentration of GABA in the brain, perhaps through interaction with enzymes involved in the synthesis (glutamic acid decarboxylase) and catabolism (GABA transaminase) of GABA. Gabapentin, which is a structural analog of GABA, appears to increase GABA levels by enhancing GABA synthesis and release and may also cause a decrease in glutamate synthesis. The two most effective drugs for absence seizures, ethosuximide and valproic acid, probably acts by reducing calcium conduction in thalamic neurons.

In contrast to the relatively large number of antiepileptic drugs that can attenuate seizure activity, there are no drugs known to prevent the formation of a seizure focus after CNS injury in humans. The eventual development of such "antiepileptogenic" drugs will provide an important means of preventing the emergence of epilepsy after injuries such as head trauma, stroke, and CNS infection.

The use of AEDs is not without adverse effects. Although myriad adverse effects can occur, for the most part they can be grouped into three categories; idiosyncratic, dose-related, and allergic reactions. It is the responsibility of the nurse, as well as of other health care team members, to instruct the client about the action, dosing, and possible side effects of the various AEDs.

Medical intervention focuses on prescribing AEDs to arrest or prevent seizures. Table 69–1 lists and describes the most common anticonvulsants. Developing a program of correctly prescribed anticonvulsants requires weeks of medication adjustment by trial and error. The desired outcome pharmacologic management is monotherapy (use of

TABLE 69–1	MEDICATIONS USED TO TREAT EPILEPSY			
Proposed Mechanism/ Drug	Action	Therapeutic Outcome	Adverse Outcomes	Dosing
Phenytoin	Stabilizes the neuronal membrane	Reduces partial and generalized tonic-clonic seizures	Unsteady gait, slurred speech, confusion, nausea, hypothermia, coma	Narrow window of therapeutic effectiveness; requires frequent monitoring of blood levels to prevent overdosage Associated with many drug-drug interactions Can be given IV for seizures; however, can suppress respirations and heart rate
Phenobarbital	Prolongs postsynaptic potential; prolongs chloride channel opening and GABA activity	Reduces partial and generalized tonic-clonic seizures	Hypotension, cardiac dysrhythmias, dizziness, lethargy, CNS excitement	Parenteral solutions are highly alkaline; dilute and monitor closely Controlled substance Long half-life; use cautiously in clients with impaired renal or hepatic function Abrupt withdrawal may precipitate seizures in clients with epilepsy
Ethosuximide (Zarotin)	Reduces calcium conductance in thalamus	Drug of choice for simple absence seizures	Ataxia, drowsiness, sedation, behavioral changes	Use cautiously in clients with hepatic disease

CNS, central nervous system; GABA, gamma-aminobutyric acid.

one anticonvulsant medication).[20, 46] Large doses of a single anticonvulsant are often more helpful than smaller doses of several drugs.

Ideally, initial treatment begins with a single drug (primary anticonvulsant) until either seizure control is attained or unacceptable side effects appear. If side effects become intolerable before seizures are controlled, another drug is added. Combining medications does carry the potential risk of drug-drug interactions, which decrease effectiveness.

▇ Nursing Management of the Medical Client

The management of epilepsy does not usually involve hospitalization. However, a client may initially be hospitalized for assessment, diagnosis, and education immediately after a first seizure (i.e., in a person with previously undiagnosed epilepsy). Hospitalization may also be required if seizures become uncontrolled or if status epilepticus develops. Nurses have a role in assessing for altered health maintenance related to knowledge deficit or other barriers, anticipating risk of injury, and providing support for clients and their families who experience life changes related to seizure disorders.

ASSESSMENT

Assessment of clients not actively experiencing seizures includes the following:

*   History, including prenatal, birth, and developmental history; family history; age at seizure onset; history of all illnesses and trauma; previous brain surgery or stroke; complete description of seizures, including precipitating factors; and presence of an aura
*   Medication use and postictal symptoms
*   Psychosocial assessment, including mental status examination
*   Complete physical examination, focusing on neurologic signs (usually, physical findings between seizures are normal)

DIAGNOSIS, OUTCOMES, INTERVENTIONS

Altered Health Maintenance. This nursing diagnosis is appropriate for clients who are having difficulty adjusting their life to their epileptic condition. Knowledge deficit of the significance of managing the AED regimen is a common problem. State the diagnosis as *Altered Health Maintenance related to chronic disorder (epilepsy) management.*

Outcomes. The client will have improved health maintenance related to knowledge deficit, as evidenced by maintaining routine dosing, consulting a physician whenever there is a problem, and wearing a medical alert identification tag or bracelet.

Intervention. Provide the client with verbal information and written reinforcement about (1) how anticonvulsants prevent seizures, (2) the importance of taking prescribed medication regularly, and (3) care during seizures. Consult with the client to plan ways to make taking medication part of daily activities (e.g., keeping medication by the toothbrush). Also, help the client to identify factors that precipitate seizures and ways of avoiding these factors. Such factors include increased stress, lack of sleep, emotional upset, and alcohol use. See the Client

Education Guide on Epilepsy for other important teaching information.

EVALUATION

The short-term outcomes for the client who is experiencing a seizure are usually met within hours. An example is that the seizure stops and the client returns to the previous level of functioning. Nursing care of clients with confirmed epilepsy should focus on the long-term outcomes with self-care.

▇ Modifications for Elderly Clients

With the increasing frequency of epilepsy in the elderly population, nurses need to be more aware of the changes in pharmacokinetics in this age group. Concurrent disease, foods, and drug-drug interactions affect absorption of anticonvulsant medication. A decrease in albumin, as is commonly seen in the older adult, can increase the free plasma level of these drugs. Decreased metabolism can increase the half-life of these drugs, and decreased elimination can result in higher plasma levels.

Enteral feedings inhibit the absorption of phenytoin (Dilantin). Therefore, the feeding should be turned off 2 hours before and after administration of phenytoin, or the dose should be altered on the basis of plasma levels. Altered vitamin D metabolism with phenytoin increases the risk of osteoporosis. Carbamazepine (Tegretol) carries an increased risk of slowed cardiac conduction and heart failure; hyponatremia secondary to increased secretion of antidiuretic hormone, especially if the client is on a low-sodium diet; and altered cholesterol metabolism in the elderly population. Valproate (Depakene) carries an increased risk of causing hyperammonemia in older clients, leading to hepatic dysfunction, decrease in platelets, and toxicity related to its longer half-life in this population.[20, 24, 46-48]

▇ Surgical Management

For approximately 75% of clients with seizures, medical management with AEDs and follow-up evaluation suf-

---

CLIENT EDUCATION GUIDE

Epilepsy

Client Instructions

*   Take prescribed dosages of medications to maintain your blood levels.
*   Consult your physician if you are unable to take medication because of illness.
*   Observe for side effects of anticonvulsant drugs. Do not stop taking medications because of annoying side effects; this is very dangerous. Consult your physician first.
*   Notify the physician if seizure activity is not being controlled. Provide specific descriptions of the seizure activity.
*   Do not take any over-the-counter medications without consulting with your physician.
*   Obtain a medical alert identification card (or bracelet or tag) with the name of the drug, dosage, and frequency, and your physician's name and phone number. Carry this identification with you at all times.

fices. The remaining 25% continue to have seizures. For about 5% of people with epilepsy, surgery is recommended to control the disease.

The safest and most effective surgical treatment is cortical resection of the anterior temporal lobe for complex partial seizures.[10, 13] Criteria for resection include (1) failure of the medical approach and (2) localization and identification of a focus of abnormal discharge that is easily accessible surgically and is located in the "dispensable" areas of the cerebral cortex. Dispensable areas are those for which there is a duplicative area in the cortex.

Thorough assessment is necessary before surgery. This is usually done in three phases:

Phase 1 involves using video EEG to locate the epileptogenic focus. This stage can also include SPECT and PET studies.[41] Intelligence quotient (IQ) testing and psychological assessments are usually performed.[45, 63]

Phase 2 is used when surface EEG electrodes are not sensitive enough to locate the seizure focus exactly. Depth electrodes are placed in the temporal and frontal lobes of the brain or in the subdural space. These techniques allow detailed maps of the brain for surgery.[17]

Phase 3 involves cerebral angiography with *Wada's test* to determine hemispheric dominance and location of the speech center. The functional supremacy of one cerebral hemisphere is crucial to language function.

Wada's test is a method of determining which side of the brain is dominant for speech production. An injection of amobarbital sodium (Amytal Sodium) is introduced into the left internal carotid artery. If the left hemisphere is dominant, speech is arrested for 1 or 2 minutes, followed by misnaming and misreading for 8 to 9 minutes altogether. After 30 minutes, the process is repeated in the right internal carotid artery. The physician looks for changes in sensation, abstract thought, and coordination. Postprocedural care is the same as for cerebral angiography (see Chapter 68).[49]

CORTICAL RESECTION/CORPUS CALLOSOTOMY. Corpus callosal resection is considered palliative surgery designed to make the seizures more tolerable. It involves the excision of one section of cortex to reduce the spread of epileptic discharges (Fig. 69–3A). One complication, called *disconnection syndrome,* results when the pathways responsible for communication from one hemisphere to another are severed. Clinical manifestations range from motor apraxias and mutism to minimal losses detected only on neuropsychological testing. Staged resections are now performed to reduce the risk of disconnection syndrome.[44, 62]

TEMPORAL LOBECTOMY. This form of curative surgery for epilepsy is performed to remove the area in which the seizures begin without causing neurologic or cognitive deficits (Fig. 69–3B). If the dominant hemisphere is removed, the client experiences some language defects for a few weeks. Visual defects from loss of visual projection fibers are compensated for quickly.[44, 62]

HEMISPHERECTOMY. Removal of most of the cortex of one hemisphere is done in children with intractable seizures to control those that are injurious, not to stop all seizures (Fig. 69–3C).[44, 62]

VAGAL NERVE STIMULATOR IMPLANTATION. The implantation of a vagal nerve stimulator (VNS) offers clients another treatment modality. Although the underlying mechanism is not fully understood, the VNS is believed to provide a stimulus that desynchronizes the abnormal uncontrolled electrical discharge of the brain activity during a seizure. One study has reported that the benefit from VNS increases over time. For example, 40%

Corpus callosotomy

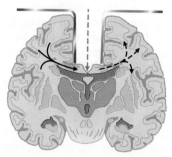

Division of the corpus callosum disrupts the interhemispheric pathway for secondary generalization of partial A seizures (unilateral seizure focus)

Temporal lobectomy

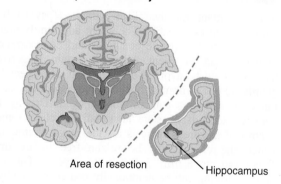

B   Area of resection   Hippocampus

Hemispherectomy

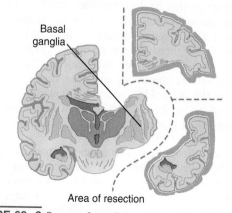

Basal ganglia

C   Area of resection

FIGURE 69–3 Surgery for epilepsy can consist of corpus callosotomy *(A)*, temporal lobectomy *(B)*, or hemispherectomy *(C)*. (From Devinsky, O. [1994]. Seizure disorders. *Clinical Symposia, 46*(1), 1–54. Adapted from an original illustration in *Clinical Symposia,* illustrated by John Craig, M.D., copyright by Ciba-Geigy Corporation.)

to 45% of clients continue to experience a decrease in the frequency of seizures at 18 months after implantation of the VNS.[36, 45, 52, 59]

■ Nursing Management of the Surgical Client

PREOPERATIVE CARE

The role of the nurse during the evaluation phase before surgery is to provide support and education. Clients who have epilepsy have been trying to control their seizures for most of their lives. Now, as part of the preoperative assessment, the health care team needs to observe the client during seizure activity. Therefore, AEDs are tapered and discontinued. This withdrawal of effective medication is often confusing and frightening. In addition, some clients are far from family and may be rethinking their decision to undergo surgery. Memory impairments are common because of both the side effects of medications and postictal states. Be certain to provide written material and reinforce education often.[26, 33, 45]

POSTOPERATIVE CARE

Postoperative nursing care is the same as for any client undergoing a craniotomy (see later). The client is often placed in an intensive care unit (ICU) to facilitate frequent assessment. Anticonvulsant medications are resumed immediately after surgery as well as after leaving the hospital.[33, 43]

■ Self-Care

It is important for the client with epilepsy to live as normal a life as possible. The client and family members must learn to accept the condition and not exaggerate it or overprotect the client. Although certain dangerous activities should be avoided or performed with special safeguards (e.g,. swimming or horseback riding), a wide range of activities can still be enjoyed. Driving motor vehicles depends on state laws and the client's medical control of seizures. There is a wide range of time during which the client must be seizure-free before driving. Times can range from 3 months to 2 years. This restriction on driving can be emotionally and economically devastating for clients of all ages and socioeconomic backgrounds.

A regular pattern of adequate diet, fluid intake, sleep, and moderate recreation and exercise is helpful. Many clients find that skipping meals or not getting enough sleep lowers the threshold for seizures. Alcoholic beverages are contraindicated for two reasons. First, alcohol lowers the seizure threshold, and second, alcohol is detoxified by the liver. Most anticonvulsant drugs are also metabolized by the liver. Consuming alcohol while taking an anticonvulsant places an increased strain on the metabolizing functions of the liver.

For some clients, the psychosocial impact of epilepsy is overwhelming. Because most seizures occur without warning, many clients spend their lives anticipating inappropriate behavior, embarrassment, and self-injury. Clients with epilepsy often have a poor self-image, feelings of inferiority, self-consciousness, guilt, anger, depression, and other emotional problems. Education and support groups can help clients deal with the emotional impact of epilepsy.

The client and family members should be taught that epilepsy is a chronic disorder that requires long-term management. Even though the client may have been seizure-free for some time, it is important to take medication as prescribed. Phenytoin, a common anticonvulsant, leads to excessive gingival (gum tissue) growth. Brushing two to three times daily helps retard gingival growth. Some clients have excess gingival tissue excised every 6 to 12 months. Medications may also cause diplopia, ataxia, sedation, and bone marrow depression. Most anticonvulsant drugs require periodic monitoring of serum drug levels, liver function, and complete blood counts. Clients with epilepsy should always wear or carry identification stating that they have epilepsy and providing the name and telephone number of their physician.

If the client is able to recognize that certain activities trigger the seizure, the activities can be avoided, or the client can be desensitized in some cases. For example, flickering lights can trigger seizures. Fluorescent lights and flickering shadows from trees on the road while driving during the late afternoon are common precipitants of seizures. If the client experiences an aura, precautions should be taken immediately to prevent self-injury from the impending seizure—for example, lying down on the ground or floor or, if driving a vehicle, pulling over to the side of the road and lying on the seat. Instruct clients to carry a large pillow in the vehicle or to use the arms to protect the head.

Some clients with epilepsy cannot find employment if they admit to having seizures. However, falsifying job applications can result in dismissal from employment. These factors contribute to a higher incidence of depression among clients with epilepsy. Nurses can educate the public regarding epilepsy and help to dissipate prejudices. When discussing the long-term impact of epilepsy with the client, be empathetic but realistic. It is hoped the client can accept the lifestyle limitations of the disorder and not be overwhelmed by them.[5]

The client's family needs to know what to do in the event of a seizure. The affected person should be protected from self-injury. Clothing should be loosened, the head protected from impact, and sharp objects in the environment removed. The person should not be forcibly restrained during a seizure but protected from self-injury. Hard objects or fingers should not be inserted into the mouth. People experiencing a seizure do not swallow the tongue—a common misconception. However, the tongue can occlude the airway, and positioning the head is important to protect the airway. After the head is protected from injury, the person should be placed in a side-lying position to displace the tongue and allow oral secretions to drain from the airway. Someone should stay with the person until full consciousness has returned. An ambulance should be called if the seizure lasts for longer than 10 minutes, if another seizure occurs before consciousness returns, if there is respiratory difficulty on evidence of injury, or if the person is pregnant.

Various organizations are working at public education, introduction of appropriate legislation, and assisting people with epilepsy. In the United States, these include the Epilepsy Foundation of America and Epilepsy Services. Similar organizations exist in other countries.

SEIZURES

Not all seizures are epilepsy. Not only do clients differ in their susceptibility to experiencing a seizure; there are also variations in seizure thresholds. For example, seizures may be induced by high fevers in children who are otherwise normal and who never develop other neurologic problems, including epilepsy.

The cause of seizures varies widely in adults. Brain tumors are the most common cause. Seizures are often the first manifestation of an intracranial mass. Traumatic brain injury is another common cause of seizures in young adults. With severe closed head injuries, seizures occur in a small percentage of clients. However, with open head injuries in which the skull and dura are penetrated, the incidence of seizures rises markedly.

Cerebrovascular disease is the most common cause of seizures in clients over age 50. These seizures usually accompany a stroke. In other vascular lesions, such as arteriovenous malformations (AVMs), seizures may be the first manifestation.

CNS infections frequently produce seizures, either in the acute phase of infection or chronically thereafter. Seizures can be a sequela of viral infections, brain abscesses, and meningitis. Postinfectious encephalitis can cause persistent seizures.

Toxic substances that interfere with brain metabolism or with the supply of oxygen or glucose to the brain can cause seizures. Alcohol is one of the most frequently ingested toxins and can cause seizures either during ingestion or during withdrawal. Chronic substance abuse, especially of barbiturates, can lead to seizures when the drug is withdrawn (see Chapter 24).

Simulated convulsive episodes may occur in clients with psychiatric disorders. These are called "pseudoseizures." One key to differentiating between pseudoseizures and actual seizures is to look for stereotypical movements and a paroxysmal nature of the episodes. Clients with recurrent seizures exhibit the same stereotypic movements with each seizure. Clients exhibiting pseudoseizure make different movements with each seizure.[33, 47]

Management of the client who is experiencing a single seizure focuses on protecting the client during the seizure and then identifying and correcting the underlying problem. Care of clients during a seizure is as discussed earlier.

Controversy exists over the best pharmacologic approach to seizure management. Many authorities recommend a single antiepileptic drug therapy approach, which decreases the risk of drug interactions and adverse effects, makes monitoring easier, and increases client compliance.

STATUS EPILEPTICUS

Etiology

Status epilepticus, a medical emergency, is a state in which a client has continuous seizures or seizures in rapid succession, without regaining consciousness, lasting at least 30 minutes. The most common cause of status epilepticus is the sudden withdrawal of anticonvulsant medication. During a seizure, the brain's metabolic needs increase dramatically. If these heightened requirements continue without opportunity for the body to recover, the supply of glucose and oxygen to the brain becomes inadequate, and permanent brain damage may occur.

Outcome Management

The major goals in managing a client with status epilepticus are to establish and protect the airway, to control the seizure, and to monitor for cessation or other outcomes.

The airway is maintained and aspiration prevented by placing the client in a side-lying position, suctioning the airway, and providing oxygen. Recall that oxygen offers nothing to a client who is apneic; therefore, intubation may be necessary to ventilate and oxygenate the client.

Anticonvulsant medications are given to terminate seizures and to prevent exhaustion. Intravenous (IV) infusion is begun immediately and maintained during treatment. Status epilepticus is treated with diazepam in doses of 5 to 10 mg (0.2 mg/kg) given every 10 to 20 minutes, for a total dose of up to 30 mg in an 8-hour period. Lorazepam (0.1 mg/kg) can also be given in 4-mg doses given over 2 to 5 minutes, repeated every 10 to 15 minutes to a maximum of 8 mg (0.2 mg/kg). In addition, phenytoin can be given to a total dose of 15 to 18 mg/kg by slow IV push (no more than 50 mg/min). Assess the client for bradycardia and heart block while phenytoin is given. If this agent is not effective, diazepam or lorazepam can be used. Because all of these medications can depress respiration, emergency ventilation equipment should be readily available.

If diazepam or lorazepam is not effective, pentobarbital can be used to bring on a barbiturate coma and suppress brain activity. Inducing coma is used only after the anticonvulsant treatments have been tried and have not been unsuccessful. The client in barbiturate coma is ventilator-dependent and requires nursing care in an ICU.

A last resort involves the use of general anesthesia. If a general anesthetic agent or a neuromuscular blocking agent such as vecuronium bromide (Norcuron) is required, the client requires mechanical ventilation, continuous EEG monitoring, and hemodynamic monitoring.

The client's neurologic status is assessed frequently. Even when the status epilepticus has been controlled, the client may be unresponsive for a period of time. Absence of signs of seizure does not mean the seizure has stopped. The manifestations may not be evident. Semiconscious clients thought to be in a postictal state have been found to be still experiencing seizure. After the seizures have been controlled, maintenance anticonvulsants are prescribed.

Clients experiencing status epilepticus are especially difficult for significant others to watch. They need support and assessment. Always explain to family members the treatment being given.[20, 24, 33, 45–47]

BRAIN TUMORS

Brain tumors are identified as primary or secondary lesions. Tumors arising from the brain or its supporting structures are called *primary* brain tumors; those metastasizing from other areas in the body are *secondary* tumors. Brain tumors may also be referred to as *intra-axial* or *extra-axial*. Intra-axial tumors are those originating from the glial cells (cells supporting the neurons) and arise from within the cerebrum, cerebellum, or the brain stem. Extra-axial tumors have their origin in the skull, meninges, cranial nerves, or pituitary gland.

The Central Brain Tumor Registry for the United States (CBTRUS) estimates that the overall incidence for primary brain and CNS tumors is 11.5 cases per 100,000 person-years. This registry estimates that 35,000 new primary brain tumors are diagnosed yearly. The incidence of brain tumors appears to be increasing but may reflect improved and earlier diagnosis.[2, 12, 50, 51]

Etiology

A clear etiologic factor has not been established for any of the primary brain tumors. Although the type of cell that gives rise to the tumor can often be identified, the mechanism causing the cells to act abnormally remains unknown. Most primary brain tumors do not metastasize out of the brain to other areas. Neuroscience researchers are searching for the answers. Familial tendencies, immunosuppression, and environmental factors are being considered.[2, 12, 14, 50, 51]

Pathophysiology

SPACE-OCCUPYING LESIONS

Brain tumors are described as "space-occupying lesions." This phrase explains that the tumor displaces normal tissue or occupies normal tissue spaces. When normal brain tissue is compressed, normal brain tissue cannot function and may become necrotic.

INCREASED INTRACRANIAL PRESSURE

Not only are the tumors space-occupying lesions; they often produce considerable cerebral edema. The skull is a rigid, box-like structure, containing little room for expansion of any of the intracranial contents. Brain tumors cause progressively increased intracranial pressure (ICP) which leads to displacement of brain structures with herniation of the brain (see Chapter 72).

INTRACRANIAL TUMORS

Intracranial tumors may arise from neurons (neuromas) or from the support cells, the neuroglial cells (gliomas). Brain tumors can be encapsulated, nonencapsulated, and/or invasive. Much confusion exists with regard to the pathologic and histologic nomenclature. Historically, staging or grading scales identified tumors as grade I (benign) through grade IV or V (malignant). A more recent, three-tiered system from the World Health Organization (WHO) labels tumors according to the maturity of the tumor cells—for example, "mature cells, benign," or "immature cells, malignant"[32, 44, 62] (see Box 69-1).

GLIAL TUMORS. Gliomas are tumors of the neuroglia (supporting brain tissue). Astrocytomas are the most common type of glial cell tumor and can be found throughout the brain and/or spinal cord. These tumors occur in adults and children. Depending upon the exact location, clinical manifestations may result in increased ICP or focal compression.[44, 62]

OLIGODENDROGLIOMAS. Oligodendroglial cells are found in the CNS and produce myelin. Oligodendrogliomas are tumors of the white matter of the brain. They tend to develop in the cortex of the frontal and parietal lobes. This tumor is fairly slow-growing and calcifies, which makes it recognizable on x-ray studies. The calcification may contribute to the development of seizures as a presenting clinical manifestation. Oligodendrogliomas peak in clients between the ages of 30 and 50 years. Clinical manifestations in addition to seizures are headache, personality changes, and papilledema.[44, 62]

EPENDYMOMAS. The ependymal cells line the ventricles and form the inner lining of the spinal cord. Ependymomas may be found anywhere within the CNS; however, there is an increased incidence in the fourth ventricle and intramedullary (within the spinal cord tissue). This tumor affects all age groups. Manifestations are caused by ventricular obstruction and include headache, vomiting, diplopia, dizziness, ataxia, vision changes, and motor and sensory abnormalities.[44, 62]

PITUITARY TUMORS. Pituitary tumors are usually slow-growing tumors that involve only the anterior lobe of the pituitary gland or extend into the floor of the third ventricle. Most of these are benign, small, and encapsulated. Manifestations can be related to hypofunctioning of the gland and include visual field defects, irregular or absent menstrual cycles, infertility, decreased libido, impotence, decreased body hair, and decreased production of pituitary-stimulating hormones; this decrease results in decreased thyroid and adrenal function. Hypersecretion can also occur and is related to the hormones that are in excess. Combinations of hyposecretion and hypersecretion can also be seen. Manifestations of pituitary tumors are often overlooked for months because they are so diverse. Clients are usually diagnosed by testing blood for the presence of pituitary-stimulating hormones.[44, 62]

TUMORS OF SUPPORTING STRUCTURES. These tumors include meningiomas and acoustic neuromas.

Meningiomas. Meningiomas are common benign tumors that may involve all meningeal layers; however,

BOX 69-1	Schema for Classifying Brain Tumors*
Astrocytoma	Increased number of astrocytes; mature astrocytes; normally developed astrocytes
Anaplastic astrocytoma	Increased number of less mature astrocytes; possibility of mitotic figures (mitotic figures represent increased cellular division and malignant changes)
Glioblastoma multiforme	Increased number of astrocyte cells; immature astrocytes; presence of mitotic figures; hemorrhage, necrosis, swelling, and obscure tumor margins

* This schema of astrocytoma, anaplastic tumor, and glioblastoma multiforme is also used for the astrocytoma, ependymoma, and oligodendroglioma.

these tumors are believed to originate in the arachnoid cells (Fig. 69–4). Most meningiomas are benign, but some tumors may become malignant.[13] Meningiomas may be found in the brain or spinal cord. They are slow-growing and occur at any age, most commonly at midlife and in women. Manifestations depend on location of the tumor and can be quite diverse. Outcomes are related to the site of the tumor. Recurrence is a concern.[33, 44, 62]

Acoustic Neuromas. Acoustic neuromas are tumors of the Schwann cells of the eighth cranial nerve, the acoustic nerve. Manifestations are tinnitus, dizziness, and unilateral hearing loss. If the tumor is allowed to grow, it can displace the other cranial nerves—especially cranial nerves IV to X—and the brain stem. An excellent outcome can be expected with surgical resection and preservation of the remaining cranial nerves. However, most clients experience at least temporary tinnitus, balance problems, and facial weakness after surgery.[23, 44, 62]

METASTATIC BRAIN TUMORS. Metastatic brain tumors are those with primary sites outside of the brain. Cancers of the lung, breast, and kidney and malignant melanoma are the major sources of metastatic brain cancers. The tumor location may also be within the brain or on the arachnoid. The common locations of brain tumors are shown in Figure 69–4.

Clinical Manifestations

General clinical manifestations are caused by changes in cerebral function resulting from edema and increased ICP. The classic triad of clinical manifestations is headache, nausea, and vomiting. Papilledema, which for diagnostic purposes is often substituted for one component of the triad, is not a manifestation; however, it is a hallmark of increased ICP.

MENTAL STATUS CHANGES

As in any neurologic or neurosurgical disorder, a change in the level of consciousness (LOC) or sensorium is often

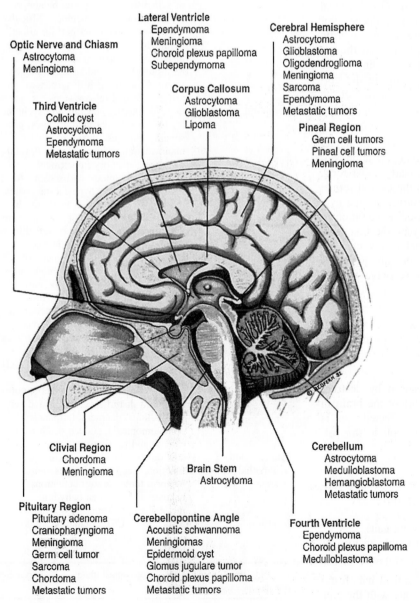

Optic Nerve and Chiasm
Astrocytoma
Meningioma

Third Ventricle
Colloid cyst
Astrocycloma
Ependymoma
Metastatic tumors

Lateral Ventricle
Ependymoma
Meningioma
Choroid plexus papilloma
Subependymoma

Corpus Callosum
Astrocytoma
Glioblastoma
Lipoma

Cerebral Hemisphere
Astrocytoma
Glioblastoma
Oligodendroglioma
Meningioma
Sarcoma
Ependymoma
Metastatic tumors

Pineal Region
Germ cell tumors
Pineal cell tumors
Meningioma

Clivial Region
Chordoma
Meningioma

Brain Stem
Astrocytoma

Cerebellum
Astrocytoma
Medulloblastoma
Hemangioblastoma
Metastatic tumors

Pituitary Region
Pituitary adenoma
Craniopharyngioma
Meningioma
Germ cell tumor
Sarcoma
Chordoma
Metastatic tumors

Cerebellopontine Angle
Acoustic schwannoma
Meningiomas
Epidermoid cyst
Glomus jugulare tumor
Choroid plexus papilloma
Metastatic tumors

Fourth Ventricle
Ependymoma
Choroid plexus papilloma
Medulloblastoma

FIGURE 69–4 Common intracranial tumors and their usual locations. (From Murphy, G. P., Lawrence, W., & Lenhard, R. E. [1995]. American Cancer Society *Textbook of clinical oncology* [2nd ed., p. 381]. Atlanta: American Cancer Society.)

noted. Mental and emotional status changes such as lethargy and drowsiness, confusion, disorientation, and personality changes may be found.

HEADACHES

Headaches may be localized or generalized and are most severe in the frontal or occipital region. They are usually intermittent, are of increasing duration, and may be intensified by a change in posture or straining. Recurrent, severe headaches in a client who was previously free of headaches, or recurrent headaches in the morning, increasing in frequency and severity, may indicate an intracranial tumor and indicate the need for further assessment.

NAUSEA AND VOMITING

Classically, the clinical manifestations of nausea and vomiting are believed to occur because of pressure on the medulla, where the vomiting center is found. The occurrence of these manifestations may be related to generalized swelling, cerebral edema, increasing headache, and/or stimulation of the chemoemetic trigger zone (CETZ). The CETZ has numerous neural connections from areas within the cerebral hemispheres that transmit or synapse with the vomiting center in the medulla. In a frequent clinical scenario, the client complains of a severe headache after lying flat in bed. As the headache increases in severity, the client may also experience nausea related to the involvement of the CETZ. With increasing signaling to the vomiting center, the client then vomits. During the episode of emesis the client may hyperventilate and after the episode may note that the headache is less severe.

PAPILLEDEMA

Compression of the second cranial nerve, the optic nerve, may result in papilledema. The underlying pathophysiologic mechanism of papilledema is not clearly understood. The cause may be increased pressure in the central retinal vein as a result of obstructed venous return from the eye. Papilledema, also known as "choked disc," is common in clients with intracranial tumors and may be the first sign. Early papilledema does not cause visual acuity changes and can be detected only through an ophthalmologic examination. Prolonged papilledema causes optic atrophy and severely diminished visual acuity.

SEIZURES

Seizures, focal or generalized, are common in clients with intracranial tumors, especially cerebral hemisphere tumors. See previous discussion in this chapter.

LOCALIZED MANIFESTATIONS

Localized clinical manifestations are caused by destruction, irritation, or compression of the part of the brain in or near the tumor. Blood supply to the affected area is also impaired. Localized manifestations include the following:

* Focal weaknesses (e.g., hemiparesis)
* Sensory disturbances, including absence of feeling (anesthesia) or abnormal sensation (paresthesia)
* Language disturbances
* Coordination disturbances (e.g., staggering gait)
* Visual disturbance such as diplopia (double vision) or visual field deficit (monopia)

As with other cranial disorders, the clinical manifestations associated with a brain tumor correlate with the area of the brain involved. Table 69–2 lists specific clinical manifestations based on tumor location. As an intracranial tumor enlarges, it shifts intracranial structures, which may lead to herniation.

Despite the availability of extremely sensitive and sophisticated equipment, brain tumor diagnosis is often delayed because of difficulty recognizing early manifestations. No two adults with the diagnosis of brain tumor present with the same clinical manifestations. Older clients, especially, fail to report such problems during regular examinations because they forget or think that the manifestations are "just part of growing old."

TABLE 69–2	CLINICAL MANIFESTATIONS OF BRAIN TUMORS BY LOCATION
Location	**Clinical Manifestations**
Frontal lobe	Disturbed mental state, apathy, inappropriate behavior, dementia, depression, emotional lability, inattentiveness, inability to concentrate, indifference, loss of self-restraint and social behavior, impaired long-term memory, difficulty with abstraction, quiet but flat affect, dominant hemisphere expressive speech disturbance, impaired sphincter control with bowel and bladder incontinence, motor disorders, gait disturbances, paralysis, "frontal release signs," seizures
Temporal lobe	Receptive aphasia, generalized psychomotor seizures, visual field changes, personality changes, ataxia, headache, manifestations of increased ICP, tinnitus, recent memory impairment
Parietal lobe	Sensory deficits, motor and sensory focal seizures, agnosias, hypesthesias, paresthesias, dyslexia, visual field cut, diminished appreciation of side opposite the tumor, headache, apraxia, tactile inattention, right/left disorientation
Occipital lobe	Headache, manifestations of increased ICP, visual impairment (homonymous hemianopsia), visual agnosia, cortical blindness, hallucinations, seizures
Cerebellar	Unsteady gait, falling, ataxia, incoordination, tremors, head tilt, nystagmus, CSF obstruction/hydrocephalus, truncal ataxia if vermis is tumor site
Brain stem	Vertigo, dizziness, vomiting, CN III–XII palsies/dysfunction, nystagmus, decreased corneal reflex, headache, vomiting, gait disturbance, motor and sensory deficits, deafness, intranuclear ophthalmoplegia, sudden death from cardiac and respiratory failure
Pituitary and hypothalamus	Visual deficits, headache, hormonal dysfunction, sleep disturbances, water imbalance, temperature fluctuations, imbalance in fat and carbohydrate metabolism, Cushing's syndrome
Ventricle	Obstruction of CSF circulation, hydrocephalus, rapid rise in ICP, postural headache

CN, cranial nerve; CSF, cerebrospinal fluid; ICP, intracranial pressure.

Diagnostic Findings

If an intracranial tumor is suspected, noninvasive studies such as CT, MRI, and x-ray examination are performed (Fig. 69–5). Other disorders may be ruled out with EEG, radionuclide scans, angiogram, or a lumbar puncture. A stereotactic biopsy may confirm the diagnosis of a brain tumor and help in planning chemotherapy and radiation therapy. Three-dimensional thresholding techniques help visualize the tumor's location in the brain and can assist with plans for resection. PET scans can also be used to study the biochemical and physiologic effects of the tumor.

Outcome Management

▇ Medical Management

For the adult client with a brain tumor, there are many options for treatment. Regardless of which treatment modality is selected, there are several goals. First and foremost, the initial goal is to remove and/or reduce as much of the tumor burden as possible. Additional goals include managing increased ICP, controlling and/or preventing of seizures, and monitoring for motor or sensory deficits and cranial nerve deficits.

Intervention depends on the type and location of the intracranial tumor and the client's medical condition. Management is always interdisciplinary, with several members forming a clinical team to support the client through care.

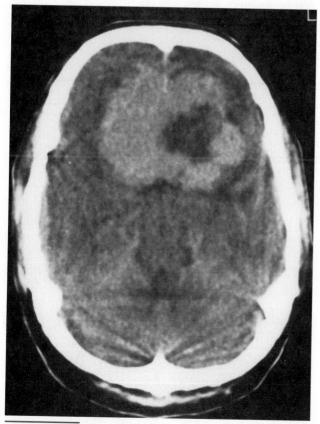

FIGURE 69–5 Magnetic resonance image revealing a midline frontal meningioma.

Surgical intervention may range from biopsy to total removal of the brain tumor. The primary goal of surgery, whether biopsy or resection, is to arrive at the histologic/pathologic diagnosis. Surgical resection decreases the tumor bulk or burden, making other treatments and adjunctive therapeutic treatments more effective. With only a few exceptions, all clients with brain tumors require surgical intervention.

▇ Surgical Management

CRANIOTOMY

The term *craniotomy* means to surgically create an opening into the skull. A craniectomy (removal of a portion of the cranium) may be performed for decompression. Regardless of the type of tumor and the extent of tumor removed, today the neurosurgeon has many methods to remove tumor (see Table 69–3).

Intraoperatively the client may be positioned in various ways to facilitate exposure and visualization. Such positions and/or head-supporting frames have the potential to cause skin pressure on the head, edema of the face, and muscle soreness, especially in the neck. Preoperatively and/or postoperatively, a ventriculostomy—in which a catheter is inserted through a burr hole into the ventricle—may be needed to drain cerebrospinal fluid (CSF) or blood. Drains may be used if a large area of dead space remains after the removal of the tumor.

TRANSSPHENOIDAL HYPOPHYSECTOMY

Transsphenoidal hypophysectomy may be used for clients with pituitary tumors, if the tumor is small and housed within the sella turcica (bony structure housing the pituitary gland). The initial incision for this procedure is made horizontally at the junction of the inner aspect of the upper lip and gingiva, extending bilaterally to the canine teeth. From this incision a surgical area is created beneath the nasal cartilage, extending superiorly through and up to the floor of the sella turcica. At this location, the area of the floor of the sella turcica is accessed, and the tumor is removed (Fig. 69–6). Fat and/or muscle grafts, using tissue from the abdomen or upper thigh, are implanted at the surgical site to assist in healing of the hypophysectomy operative wound. Nasal packing may or may not be used.

After any brain surgery the client is closely assessed for injury to and edema of the brain. Specific complications from intracranial surgery depend on the area of surgery and the procedure being performed. Examples include increased ICP, motor or sensory deficits and cranial deficits, seizures, CSF leak, wound infection, and CNS infections. If there is loss of significant functions, these problems can be psychosocially and physically devastating. Some postoperative complications gradually resolve, but others are permanent.

General postoperative complications after intracranial surgery do not differ from those after other forms of surgery. Complications may occur as the result of anesthesia, narcotics, or immobility. Ecchymosis and periorbital edema may be present after intracranial surgery but are transient. These changes affecting the appearance of the eyes and the face overall can be very frightening to the client as well as to the family members.

TABLE 69–3	SURGICAL OPTIONS FOR BRAIN TUMOR DIAGNOSIS AND EXCISION
Procedure	**Description**
Cortical mapping	Intraoperative cortical EEG recording and monitoring, facilitating areas for greater resection without loss of eloquent motor and/or sensory functions
Stereotactic surgery	Localization of a specific target within a three-dimensional space: with the client stabilized in a head frame, the tumor is imaged using either CT or MRI; data from the scans are analyzed by a computer and a trajectory location is identified; stereotactic procedures may be used for biopsy or craniotomy
Frameless stereotactic localization systems	External devices are placed preoperatively and the client's body is scanned using CT or MRI; scanning data are transferred to the operating room, allowing determination of the boundaries of the lesion by means of a surgical "wand"
Brain-mapping technique	Utilizes viewing wand to precisely identify location of specific anatomical functions—i.e., motor, sensory, and/or speech; methods developed include localizing tumors not only with ultrasound techniques but with various wandlike structures
Intraoperative ultrasonography	Utilizes a hand-held device to differentiate tumors with a cystic component; ultrasound techniques allow identification of tumor margins
Laser surgery	Destroys tumor tissue without causing adjacent edema or damage
Neuro-endoscopic techniques	For treatment of third and/or lateral ventricle lesions; this approach provides access to lesions in areas otherwise difficult to locate
Intraoperative imaging techniques	Real-time CT or MRI imaging in the operating room is evolving and holds great promise; such imaging affords safer and better resections as a result of improved visualization
Ultrasonic aspirator	Suction-like device used in removing solid tumors
Direct cortical stimulation	Electrical current is directed to a specific area in the brain, causing a visible movement of the corresponding body part
Somatosensory evoked potentials (SSEPs)	Measurement of electrical response of specific areas (e.g., visual, auditory, brain stem); after the function of such critical areas has been determined, these areas can be avoided during surgical manipulation
Embolization	Decreases blood supply to the tumor; may be used in conjunction with surgical procedures
Photodynamic therapy	Combination of a sensitizing agent and laser surgery; goal is for the "sensitizing" agent to make the tumor more visible or "fluorescent" when the laser is used
Polymer wafer implants	Chemotherapeutic wafers are placed in the tumor bed; currently, carmustine is available, and other agents are being tested

CT, computed tomography; EEG, electroencephalography; MRI, magnetic resonance imaging.

Nursing Management of the Surgical Client

PREOPERATIVE CARE

Today more than at any other time, the role of the nurse caring for the client with the diagnosis of a brain tumor is diverse. The nurse in the neurosurgeon's office begins preoperative teaching. The nurse is usually the first person the client sees when being admitted for diagnostic procedures. During the perioperative and the postoperative periods, the nurse prepares the client for various transitions in the continuum of care.

Preoperative assessment includes the routine assessment data (see Chapter 15). In addition, obtain a detailed history and physical examination to provide a baseline for comparison of neurologic data. Obtain and record data on the following:

- Vital signs; LOC, orientation to person, place and time; ability to follow instructions; pupil equality, size, reactivity, accommodation, and reaction to light; extraocular eye movements; and cranial nerve function
- Limb strength and movement—note limited or exaggerated movements, pronator drift, hand grip, dorsiflex-

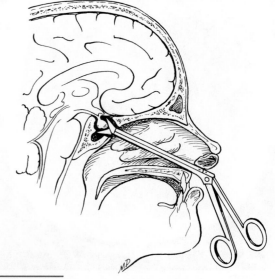

FIGURE 69–6 Transsphenoidal hypophysectomy for the excision of pituitary tumors.

ion/plantiflexion, any paresis or paralysis, or sensory abnormalities

- Manifestations of increased ICP, such as changes in Glasgow Coma Scale score, difficulties in problem-solving, limited memory, changes in pupil response, or loss of limb strength or movement

Preoperative interventions are similar to those for the care of other clients before surgery (see Chapter 15). In addition, the client undergoing a craniotomy requires hair removal at the surgical site. If the operation is for treatment of cancer, the client and family members may have considerable anxiety over the potential outcome. Offer explanations and clarification as needed. Be certain not to offer empty promises about recovery.

POSTOPERATIVE CARE

The postoperative care of the client after craniotomy is shown in the accompanying Care Plan. See also the information on care of clients with increased ICP in Chapter 74.

Postoperative care after pituitary surgery using a transsphenoidal approach includes prohibition of the use of straws for drinking any fluid, to prevent trauma to oral/gingival incision site. Frequent oral hygiene is provided, and a cool vaporizer mist may be used to keep oral mucous membranes moist. The nasal drip pad ("moustache" dressing pad) is assessed frequently for bloody and/or clear fluid (CSF). The donor site and dressings are also assessed, and dressings are changed as needed.

A fairly common effect of pituitary surgery is the development of transient diabetes insipidus (DI) as a result of decreased secretion of antidiuretic hormone (ADH). The main clinical manifestations of DI are polyuria (large urine volumes) and polydipsia (increased thirst). Clients with DI produce large volumes (2 to 15 L/day) of dilute urine with a specific gravity of 1.005 or less. These clients require laboratory assessment of serum and urine levels of sodium and osmolality. Aside from the inconvenience of polyuria, the client often suffers no serious side effects from DI unless deprived of oral or IV fluids. When this happens, circulatory collapse (hypovolemic shock) and hypertonic encephalopathy occur as a result of fluid shifts in the brain. Usual treatment is with IV vasopressin (Pitressin) or inhalation desmopressin (DDAVP). Long-acting forms of these agents can be used for the treatment of chronic DI.

◼ Medical Management

Surgical excision is completed initially to reduce the bulk of the brain tumor, or to excise it completely, in most clients. After surgery when an exact histological diagnosis has been obtained, the client is given adjuvant therapy including radiation therapy and chemotherapy. A complete discussion of these modes of cancer treatment can be found in Chapters 18 and 19; this material is also applicable to the care of clients with brain cancer.

RADIATION THERAPY

Conventional radiotherapy utilizes two different machines to deliver the radiation: the linear accelerator and the cobalt machine. Both of these machine are used in treating brain tumors. With conventional radiotherapy, the standard dose for primary brain tumors is approximately 6000 Gy given four to five times a week for a 4- to 6-week period. For clients with metastatic tumors, a standard dose of radiation is approximately 3000 Gy. The exact dose depends on tumor characteristics, volume of tissue to be irradiated, and the goals of radiation therapy. Radiation treatments are usually given over shorter periods of time to allow for protection of normal surrounding tissues. The cancer cells in CNS tumors tend to be more slowly dividing; therefore, the tumor response often takes longer. This concept is important for clients to understand, as they may be disappointed when they do not see effects during or immediately following irradiation.

As in many areas of medicine, new methods of treatment and improved delivery devices are helping clients daily. This is also the case with radiation therapy. Newer methods of delivery and more sophisticated machines are available. Table 69–4 offers examples of advances made in the area of radiotherapy for clients with brain tumors.[2] Additional forms of radiation therapy, although not considered conventional and, more important, not readily available are heavy particle radiation therapy, fast neutron radiotherapy, photodynamic therapy, and boron neutron capture therapy.[2] In spite of its wide use, radiation therapy is not without consequences. Effects may be acute, early, delayed, or late delayed; see Chapter 19.

CHEMOTHERAPY

In addition to surgery and radiotherapy, chemotherapy is used in the management of brain tumors. As part of a multimodality approach, chemotherapy may be given before, during, or after other therapies. The goal of chemotherapy is to match the appropriate agent with the appropriate cell cycle phase and then attack the rapidly dividing cells. However, there are several challenges in the use of chemotherapy in the treatment of brain tumors: the blood-brain barrier blocks transportation, there are few data to guide specific dose schedules, and the mitotic cycle of brain tumor cells is very long. Today, there does not appear to be one chemotherapy agent that can overcome all of the challenges.

The nitrosoureas are the most frequently used and effective chemotherapy agent for brain tumors. Examples of these drugs are carmustine (BCNU) and lomustine (CCNU). For the client with a brain tumor, the chemotherapy regimen may involve oral medication; IV solutions; intra-arterial routes; or intraventricular, intra-tumor, or epidural administration; or the use of other implanted devices, such as the Ommaya reservoir[8] (see Chapter 19, Fig. 19–3).

Some progress has been made in delivery of chemotherapy across the blood-brain barrier. Of recent interest is the use of substances to open up the blood-brain barrier. In opening or unlocking the blood-brain barrier, certain agents may enter and directly bind with the CSF and/or have a direct effect on the tumor. The osmotic diuretic mannitol may be used to disrupt the blood-brain barrier, allowing for greater drug concentration. There are also newer chemotherapeutic agents that cross the blood-brain barrier.[2, 5, 16, 18] As with the treatment of any cancer invading the body and especially the brain, the hope lies in future research. Biologic response modifiers and modula-

■ THE CLIENT WHO HAS UNDERGONE CRANIOTOMY

Nursing Diagnosis. Risk for Altered Tissue Perfusion: Cerebral related to edema or bleeding after craniotomy.

Outcomes. The client will have intracranial pressure (ICP) less than 15 mm Hg, mean arterial pressure (MAP) greater than 70 mm Hg, cerebral perfusion pressure (CPP) greater than 50 mm Hg, neurologic assessments and vital signs at baseline values or improved, no clinical manifestations of increased ICP and/or herniation, and body temperature less than 38.5° C.

Interventions

1. Assess neurologic status and vital signs frequently and compare with baseline values.
2. Elevated head of bed to 30 degrees.
3. Maintain head and neck in neutral alignment.
4. Change position slowly.

5. Avoid a Valsalva maneuver.

6. Monitor intake and output frequently.

7. Monitor pulse oximetry and arterial blood gases.

8. Suction airway as needed.

Rationales

1. A change in level of consciousness is the first sign of increasing intracranial pressure (ICP).
2. Elevation facilitates venous drainage and reduces edema.
3. This facilitates venous drainage and reduces edema.
4. Rapid changes in position increase cerebral blood flow and pressure.
5. Straining during coughing, movement in bed, or moving bowels increases ICP.
6. Excess fluids can promote edema; dehydration can decrease cerebral arterial flow.
7. The cerebrum is sensitive to lack of oxygen, and damage can occur within minutes after onset of hypoxia.
8. Routine suctioning not advised because it stimulates cough and increases ICP; however, sputum plugs cause retention of carbon dioxide and need to be removed because carbon dioxide increases cerebral blood flow and pressure.

Evaluation. Depending on the etiology of edema or amount of bleeding, it may require hours to days to control ICP.

Nursing Diagnosis. Ineffective Individual Coping related to fear of changes in body image, role performance, or life expectancy.

Outcomes. The client will have improved individual coping, as evidenced by statements indicating feelings of self-worth, behaviors demonstrating self-worth, and less use of dependent behaviors.

Interventions

1. Encourage family members/significant others to assist in meeting need for close contact.
2. Anticipate needs.
3. Offer praise and encouragement during ongoing assessment of client's readiness to move toward more competent coping.
4. Reduce environmental stress by minimizing interruptions and stimuli.
5. Provide opportunities for expression and ventilation of feelings.
6. Utilize consistent personnel.
7. Establish trust relationship; follow through on promises.

Rationales

1. Family members may also fear that they will injure the client.
2. Anxiety increases feelings of loneliness.
3. Positive reinforcement helps to guide future steps toward independence.
4. Noise and frequent interruptions may decrease needed sleep and alter ability to cope.
5. Problem-solving coping styles are initiated by talking about feelings and issues.
6. A therapeutic relationship is easier to maintain than to build.
7. Feelings of fear and anxiety are reduced.

Evaluation. Coping skills will wax and wane over time. Expect periods of coping and periods of failure to cope with changes in prognosis.

Nursing Diagnosis. Anxiety related to uncertain future and prognosis.

Outcomes. The client will have decreased anxiety and express fears and concerns openly.

Interventions

1. Repeat information; provide information in different forms; encourage the client and/or significant other to write down questions and/or concerns.

2. Encourage open communication between the client, significant others, and members of the health care team.

3. Involve the client's clergy or hospital chaplain if desired.

Rationales

1. Depending on the type of tumor, the location of the tumor, and/or motor or sensory deficits, the client may be faced with the loss of specific functions and the possibility of having a malignancy. Appropriate interventions may help the client better understand the prescribed plan of care.
2. Having a diagnosis of brain cancer may immobilize all of the normal coping mechanisms of the client and significant others.
3. Spiritual support is crucial at times of serious illness for the client, family members, and significant others. The client need not be "religious" to gain support from clergy.

Evaluation. Anxiety should be controllable in a short time. However, changes in response to therapy or other outcomes will increase anxiety.

Nursing Diagnosis. Risk for Altered Thought Processes related to neurologic changes from edema or surgical excision of sections of brain or tumor.

Outcomes. The client will make decisions and process information at expected levels, express and identify anger, exercise control over own behavior, and make appropriate choices, and/or cease hostile behavior.

Interventions	Rationales
1. Allow client to verbalize concerns, and channel these concerns to the appropriate person.	1. Problem-solving coping begins with verbalization of concerns.
2. Offer reasonable choices to client.	2. Feelings of control can be reestablished by offering choices to client. All options must be safe and implementable for the client.
3. Assist client to recognize alternatives and the implications of choices.	3. This measure helps client with problem-solving abilities.
4. Report client's status to client, and allow for opportunity to make decisions about treatment or no treatment.	4. Do not keep facts from the client. The client has the right to know his or her diagnosis and to be a part of decisions about care.
5. Inform family about physiologic reasons for behavior, and teach them how to respond to client.	5. The family needs to be informed about any abnormal behavior and how best to respond to it.
6. Use a consistent approach to inappropriate behavior; establish contracts if needed.	6. Consistent approaches help the client relearn acceptable ways of personal expression.
7. Maintain nonjudgmental behavior.	7. The nurse realizes that the client's outbursts are not personal attacks but due to the disease or feelings of loss of control.

Evaluation. Expect restoration of thought and behavior control to take weeks or months. Long-term coping by the family is important.

Nursing Diagnosis. Anticipatory Grief related to potential loss of function, previous abilities, or life from brain cancer or surgery.

Outcomes. The client will have resolution of grief or progression through stages of grief, as evidenced by expression of feelings, maintaining hope, identifying problems with changes in body function, seeking help with anticipated problems, or developing realistic plans for the future.

Interventions	Rationales
1. Acknowledge reality, but do not force its acceptance.	1. Denial is a powerful defense mechanism; clients will examine reality when they are ready.
2. Establish regular time to spend with client, family members, and/or significant others for the exclusive purpose of discussing feelings and concerns.	2. Discussions about feelings can be difficult; giving the client time to plan and prepare facilitates the discussion.
3. If denial is beneficial, respond by listening with and reflecting statements by client.	3. It is important to understand that not all clients reach acceptance of their disease; some remain in complete denial.
4. Accept emotions and assist client, family members, and/or significant others to clarify them.	4. This measure reinforces the ideas that emotional response is normal and that family members should be accepting of the client at all stages of grief.
5. Assess perceptions about realistic goals and the future.	5. Inaccurate perceptions about the future can prevent or stall planning.
6. Have the client list those activities he or she wants to perform/resume.	6. Plans for the future can be uplifting.

Evaluation. Expect each client and family to cope differently with grief over losses or impending death. Clients may go through the "typical" stages in order or go back and forth between them.

tion of the immune system are two of the keys that scientists hope may hold the answers.

The care of the client with a brain tumor is a challenging task for all involved. The client should not feel abandoned or uninformed during any portion of the care or treatment. To assist the client, family members, significant others, and the health care team, the American Cancer Society as well as the American Brain Tumor Association provides valuable information.

HEMORRHAGIC CEREBROVASCULAR DISORDERS

There are two types of hemorrhagic cerebrovascular disorders (CVDs): (1) intracerebral hemorrhage (ICH) (see Chapter 70) and (2) subarachnoid hemorrhage (SAH). The following section discusses SAH resulting from bleeding due to intracranial aneurysms and AVMs.

TABLE 69-4	RADIATION THERAPY MODALITIES FOR TREATMENT OF BRAIN TUMORS
Procedure	**Description**
Interstitial radiation Also called brachytherapy, tumor implants, tumor seeding, and/or radioactive pellets	Temporary or permanent placement of radioactive substances in the tumor bed Advantages include minimal effects to the surrounding tissue Generally not advised in large tumors because of secondary swelling and edema Disadvantages: implantation does require a surgical procedure; because of the radioactive substances, the client must be protected and isolated to prevent exposure to family members and health care personnel
Stereotactic radiosurgery, stereotactic radiotherapy	Allows for a high dose of radiation beams to be directed precisely to a small brain tumor in a single session If multiple sessions are required, technique is called stereotactic radiotherapy Gamma knife, linear accelerator, or cyclotron is used to deliver the radiation Best used on small, round, well-defined tumors The Peacock technique incorporates stereotaxis, radiosurgery, and computers to deliver radiation exactly to the tumor, skipping over vital areas that may be embedded in the tumor such as nerves or blood vessels
Hyperthermia	Application of heat into the tumor; electrodes with small catheters/antennae are placed through burr holes in the skull into the tumor bed; using computer-assisted stereotactic methods, the heat is delivered into the tumor Several features of brain tumors make tumor cells more susceptible to the increased temperature: poor blood supply, hypoxic areas, and increased acidity; these factors alone allow the increased temperature to kill the tumor cells Nerve cells in the brain can tolerate temperatures up to 40° C before cellular death occurs Hyperthermia uses heat from radiofrequency or microwave sources
Radiation sensitizing therapy	Use of various pharmacologic agents as "sensitizers" to make the tumor more responsive to radiation therapy and other therapies
Intraoperative radiation	Direct irradiation of the tumor while exposed in surgery; bypasses normal tissues
Conformal radiation	High or higher dose of external radiation "conformed" to match tumor's shape; the goal is to deliver a uniform amount of radiation to the entire tumor
Radioactive monoclonal antibodies	Antibodies that are cloned or mated to kill tumor cells

SUBARACHNOID HEMORRHAGE

SAH is the occurrence of bleeding into the subarachnoid space. SAH most often develops from traumatic brain injury (TBI) (see Chapter 73), intracranial aneurysms, and AVMs. Other potential causes of SAH include brain tumors (see earlier discussion), blood dyscrasias, and anticoagulant therapy.

Etiology

An SAH can occur when any of the aforementioned conditions weakens the artery, causing either a leaking or rupturing of the artery. Trauma is the leading cause of SAH, and intracranial aneurysms are the second leading cause of SAH. The majority of intracranial aneurysms are congenital or developmental.

ANEURYSMS

An intracranial aneurysm is from a weakness in the tunica media, the middle layer of the blood vessel. The most common type of intracranial aneurysm is the saccular or berry aneurysm. These congenital aneurysms are present from birth and begin to weaken over time. The muscular walls of the artery weaken and lead to formation of a sac-like or berry-like structure.

Conditions that hasten the development of this type of aneurysm are hypertension, atherosclerosis, the aging process, and stress.[44, 62] Greater than 25% of all clients with intracranial aneurysms present with multiple intracranial aneurysms. Statistically, SAH is more common in females than in males.[44, 62]

Intracranial aneurysms are found more often in the anterior cerebral circulation (internal carotid artery and its branches—the anterior cerebral artery [ACA], the middle cerebral artery [MCA], and the posterior cerebral artery [PCA])—than in the posterior cerebral circulation, including the vertebral and basilar arteries. Intracranial aneurysms are found in locations where normal anatomic weaknesses occur—that is, in bifurcations and trifurcations.

Pathophysiology

Saccular aneurysms occur at the bifurcations of the large arteries at the base of the brain and rupture into the subarachnoid space in the basal cisterns. Approximately 85% of aneurysms occur in the anterior circulation, mostly in the circle of Willis. The common sites include the junction of the anterior communicating artery with the ACA, the junction of the PCA with the internal carotid artery, and the bifurcation of the MCA. The top of the basilar artery, the junction of the basilar artery and the superior cerebellar artery or the anterior inferior cerebellar artery, and the junction of the vertebral artery and the posterior inferior cerebellar artery comprise most of the remainder (see Fig. 69–7).

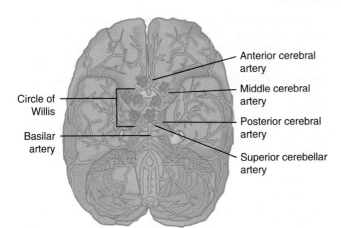

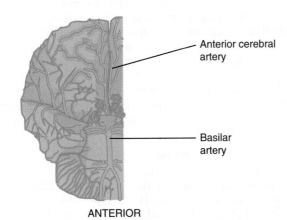

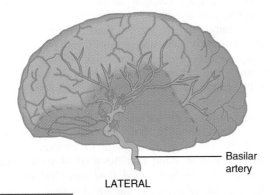

FIGURE 69–7 Common locations of cerebral aneurysms.

As an aneurysm develops, it often forms a neck with a dome. The arterial internal elastic lamina disappears at the base of the neck. The media thins, and connective tissue replaces smooth muscle cells. At the site of rupture (most often the dome), the wall thins, and the tear that allows bleeding is often no more than 0.5 mm long. It is not possible to predict which aneurysms are likely to rupture, but limited data suggest that most ruptured aneurysms are large, averaging 7 mm in diameter.

Vasospasm is defined as the constriction or narrowing of the cerebral vessels. Narrowing of the arteries at the base of the brain regularly occurs after SAH. This vasospasm causes ischemia and infarction. Vasospasm is a very serious consequence and is the major cause of de-

layed morbidity or death. Although the precise mechanism of delayed vasospasm is uncertain, it seems related to direct effects of clotted blood and its breakdown products on the artery. In general, the more blood there is surrounding the arteries, the more likely that there will be symptomatic vasospasm.

Clinical Manifestations

Aneurysms are found during incidental assessment, such as a work-up for headache, or may be detected because of a mass effect, when the accumulated blood pushes on other structures. Occasionally, mild premonitory manifestations are present, such as mild headache, confusion, fainting, or vertigo. However, the onset of the hemorrhage is usually sudden. The client experiences a sudden, severe headache, often accompanied by vomiting, often describing the headache as "the worst headache I have ever had."

The client may lose consciousness immediately or may become confused and lethargic and gradually become comatose within hours, or may remain conscious and coherent. Generalized seizures may occur. Manifestations of meningeal irritation (e.g., nuchal rigidity, photophobia, back pain) are often present, caused by blood in the subarachnoid space. Depending on the location and size of the aneurysm and the SAH, focal clinical manifestations may be noted (e.g., motor or sensory deficits, speech and cranial nerve deficits). Retinal hemorrhages may be present. Various grading scales have been developed. Table 69–5 presents criteria for the Hunt-Hess scale and the Fisher scale.

Manifestations of vasospasm vary according to the specific arterial territories involved. However, collateral

TABLE 69–5	GRADING SCALES FOR SUBARACHNOID HEMORRHAGE

HUNT-HESS CLINICAL GRADING SCALE FOR CLIENTS WITH ANEURYSMAL SAH

Grade	Clinical Criteria
I	Alert, minimal headache
II	Alert, moderate to severe headache (cranial nerve palsy allowed)
III	Lethargic or confused or mild focal deficit
IV	Stuporous, moderate to severe hemiparesis, possibly early decerebrate rigidity
V	Deep coma, decerebrate rigidity, moribund appearance

FISHER SCALE FOR CT GRADING OF CLIENTS WITH SUSPECTED ANEURYSMAL SAH

Grade	CT Criteria
1	No SAH on CT scan
2	Thin SAH (<1 mm)
3	Thick SAH (>1 mm)
4	Intracerebral or intraventricular hemorrhage, with no or thin SAH (<1 mm)

CT, computed tomography; SAH, subarachnoid hemorrhage.

blood flow may prevent the appearance of some expected manifestations. Spasm of the MCA typically causes contralateral hemiparesis and dysphasia (dominant hemisphere). Proximal ACA vasospasm causes abulia (faulty problem-solving) and incontinence, whereas severe vasospasm of the PCA causes hemianopia. Severe spasm of the basilar or vertebral arteries occasionally produces focal brain stem ischemia. All of these focal neurologic manifestations may develop over a few days, fluctuate, or present abruptly.

Manifestations of ischemia appear 4 to 14 days after the hemorrhage, most frequently at about 7 days. The severity and distribution of vasospasm determine whether infarction occurs subsequently.

Diagnosis of SAH is usually based on history and physical examination. The hallmark of aneurysmal rupture is presence of blood in the CSF. In about 80% of affected clients, enough blood is present to be visualized on a non-contrast CT scan obtained within 72 hours. A small hemorrhage may not be seen on CT scan. If the scan neither establishes the diagnosis of SAH nor demonstrates a mass lesion or obstructive hydrocephalus, a lumbar puncture is performed to establish the presence of subarachnoid blood. Lumbar puncture is contraindicated when pressure is high in the cerebrum.

CT scan may identify blood in the subarachnoid space, intracerebral clots, and large clots surrounding an aneurysm. However, cerebral angiography is the definitive diagnostic test. A four-vessel study provides adequate visualization of the carotid and vertebrobasilar circulation. An angiogram usually provides information about the aneurysm location and type, vessels supplying the aneurysm, presence of an intracerebral blood clot, and presence of cerebral vasospasm.[44, 62] Depending on the client's condition, angiography may be performed immediately or when the client's condition stabilizes. (See Chapter 11 regarding angiography.)

Outcome Management

Medical Management

The client with an SAH resulting from an intracranial aneurysm presents a challenge to all members of the interdisciplinary health care team. Until the 1980s it was not unusual to place a client on bedrest, imposing severe physical and environmental limitations (complete bedrest for 10 to 14 days, dimming lights, feeding the client, keeping the room quiet, and minimizing visitors). This management approach was believed to lessen the effects of the SAH, allowing for better visualization during surgery and decreasing swelling and cerebral edema. Many innovations have developed over the intervening years to cause a paradigm shift not only in the treatment interventions but also in the medical and nursing management.[44, 62] Today, treatment is often instituted within 24 hours of onset of the headache, and the client typically makes a full recovery.

The goals for the management of a client with SAH include maintaining cerebral perfusion pressure, controlled ICP, minimizing effects of vasospasm, managing hydrocephalus, managing cardiac dysrhythmias, and preventing bleeding (or rebleeding).

Ongoing neurologic assessment is essential regardless of the setting in which care is provided. For the first 24 to 72 hours, the nurse examines the serial data to note trends in the neurologic assessments that suggest changes and/or deterioration. The client with an intracranial aneurysm is at great risk for the development of increased ICP. The LOC is the most sensitive and early indicator of neurologic change, usually evident before pupillary changes, new hemiparesis, or changes in respiratory patterns are noted. The onset of lethargy or restlessness may be the first clinical manifestation of increased ICP, hydrocephalus, or vasospasm.

Cardiac and respiratory function is also closely monitored, particularly because of the direct role in providing adequate cerebral perfusion pressure (CPP) and oxygen supply to the brain. Because cardiovascular disease is common in people with aneurysms, continuous electrocardiographic monitoring is necessary to identify life-threatening dysrhythmias. Pulse oximetry is imperative to monitor peripheral oxygen saturation. In the ICU setting, most clients have a central IV line and/or a pulmonary artery catheter in place to monitor hemodynamic status for prescription of fluids and vasoactive medications. The pulmonary capillary wedge pressure is often used for targeted therapy to manage fluid administration.[11, 21, 44, 54, 55, 63]

REDUCE VASOSPASM
In order to reduce the damaging effects of vasospasm, hypervolemic therapy is the treatment of choice (often referred to as the "triple-H" therapy—for hypertension, hypervolemia, and hemodilution). Various therapies are utilized. For example, calcium channel blockers, vasopressor agents, and hyperosmotic diuretics may be indicated. It is important to realize that the treatment of vasospasm in these clients necessitates consideration of a delicate balance between benefit and risk. With the major goal of improving and increasing cerebral blood flow, as well as CPP, many measures utilized have the potential to precipitate a cardiopulmonary crisis. Simply stated, if the client cannot tolerate an increase in fluid status or an increase in blood pressure, how can the vasospasm be relieved? Table 69–6 gives a guide to various clinical interventions. Keep in mind that the goal of such therapies is to increase cerebral blood flow and CPP without producing cerebral infarction or cardiopulmonary compromise.[11, 54, 60]

MAINTAIN CEREBRAL PERFUSION PRESSURE
Medical and nursing management focuses on maintaining blood pressure to facilitate CPP. The blood pressure must be maintained to keep the systemic pressure at a level high enough to provide adequate CPP, yet not so high to cause rebleeding. Various medications and or infusions are used to maintain the blood pressure approximately 10% above the patient's normal pressure. In addition to medications supporting the blood pressure, blood products, and albumin are used when indicated. When the blood pressure exceeds the acceptable range, antihypertensive and diuretic agents are used to decrease the blood pressure slowly. Any sudden decrease in blood pressure will have a dramatic effect on the cerebral blood flow, as well as on the CPP, and may increase the risk of cerebral infarction.[60]

TABLE 69–6	EXAMPLE TREATMENT PROTOCOL FOR VASOSPASM
Intervention	**Rationale**
1. Continuous observation and assessment of neurologic status.	Alterations provide information concerning increasing vasospasm.
2. Maintain patent airway with PO_2 values greater than 85 mm Hg and PCO_2 between 25 and 30 mm Hg.	Prevent cerebral hypoxia; hypercapnia increases cerebral blood flow.
3. Hemodynamic monitoring used with assessment parameters to be determined. For example, check PA pressures q 1 to 2 hr, PCWP q 2 to 4 hr, and cardiac outputs q 8 hr.	Desired wedge pressures 14–16 mm Hg. Hemodynamic readings give indications of effects of "triple-H" therapy (see text) not only on cardiopulmonary system but on intracranial vessels as well.
4. If PCWP <10 mm Hg, notify physician; may order fluid challenge. If PCWP >20 mm Hg, notify physician; may order diuretic.	Desired state of fluid balance to maintain an increase in cerebral blood flow.
5. Maintain infusion rate at 100–150 ml/hr to 225–250 ml/hr; albumin or plasma if needed; IV mannitol 1–2 ampules q 4–6 hr.	Maintain perfusion via "triple-H" therapy. Mannitol produces some vasodilation, which can increase cerebral blood flow.
6. Packed RBCs or whole blood if hematocrit less than 30%.	For volume replacement if hemodilution becomes excessive in client.
7. Dopamine 400 mg in 250 D_5W to maintain systolic BP and/or MAP between specified values.	Increases cardiac output and increases cerebral blood flow.
8. Nimodipine (Nimotop) 60 mg q 4 hr for at least 3 wk.	Calcium channel blocker; promotes relaxation of blood vessels, decreasing vasospasm.
9. Morphine as required.	Sedative effect; allows for continuous monitoring.
10. Accurate I&O q 1 hr.	Fluid balance is crucial to maintaining CPP.

BP, blood pressure; CPP, cerebral perfusion pressure; D_5W, 5% dextrose in water; I&O, (fluid) input and output; MAP, mean arterial pressure; PA, pulmonary artery; PCO_2, partial pressure of carbon dioxide; PCWP, pulmonary capillary wedge pressure; PO_2, partial pressure of oxygen; RBCs, red blood cells.

■ Surgical Management

To successfully treat the aneurysm requires either a surgical procedure or endovascular intervention. If surgery is the chosen treatment, many different procedures may be used; however, the one most commonly used is clipping of the intracranial aneurysm. Aneurysms not anatomically suited to clipping can be wrapped in a surgical gauze material and/or coated with an acrylic material.[44, 60, 62]

ENDOVASCULAR THERAPY AND EMBOLIZATION

An embolization procedure involves clotting of the aneurysm by means of platinum coils, wires, or embolic substances. An interventional radiologist performs the procedure in an angiography suite. An cerebral angiogram is first performed to facilitate advancing a catheter to the selected vessel(s) in the brain. Once the neck of the aneurysm is visualized, a small platinum wire is guided carefully into the aneurysm. Each coil is advanced until it curls into a ball shape inside the aneurysm, not allowing arterial blood to flow into the aneurysmal sac. As each coil is fitted into the sac, a small current of electricity is deployed that breaks the solder and leaves the coils in the aneurysm. When the aneurysm becomes embolized, thrombosing begins. To complete the procedure, an angiogram is performed.

After embolization, the client is admitted to the ICU. The client may receive heparin for 12 to 24 hours after the procedure. The catheter sheath (from the angiogram site) remains in the femoral/groin area with a saline infusion to maintain patency of the artery. Care of the femoral/groin site includes assessing the puncture site for bleeding and hematoma formation, as well as frequent checking of peripheral pulses of the legs. The client is instructed to remain flat in bed and to avoid bending the leg at the groin. Nursing measures to maintain comfort are provided as indicated. Ongoing and frequent assessment of neurologic status is required.

COMPLICATIONS. Minimal complications result from the embolization procedure. If the aneurysm has not bled, there is a risk of bleeding at the time of embolization. Other problems may be related to the cerebral angiogram (see Chapter 67). Regardless of the treatment utilized, one factor of importance not only in selection of the treatment protocol but also in the clinical course is whether or not the aneurysm has ruptured or bled.[37, 54, 57, 60] If the SAH aneurysm ruptures, the client experiences a hemorrhagic stroke (see Chapter 70).

ANEURYSM CLIPPING

Surgical obliteration of the aneurysm with a metal clip eliminates the risk of rebleeding. A craniotomy incision is used, and the aneurysm is isolated. A metal clip is placed over the neck of the aneurysm. The timing of surgery is based on the clinical status and the grade of the aneurysm. Clients with grade I or II aneurysms are operated on within 3 days of the SAH event. Clients with lesions of grades III to V undergo clipping later on, between 10 and 14 days. Surgery is delayed while vasospasm is present. Operating on vessels in spasm increases mortality and morbidity. For clients with high-grade aneurysms, the risk of rebleeding is less than that for morbidity and mortality of early surgery. Unfortunately, medical instability, delay in transfer from one hospital to another, or client or family reluctance to consent to surgery may also delay prompt intervention.

Postoperatively, the client's neurologic status is carefully monitored. The usual postoperative care is given, including cardiac monitoring. As with any neurologic disorder, the physician must be promptly notified about any neurologic changes.

ARTERIOVENOUS MALFORMATIONS

Etiology and Pathophysiology

AVMs are vascular lesions composed of a tangled array of arteries and veins. AVMs have abnormal communication between artery and vein, wherein the blood is shunted directly from artery to vein, skipping the capillary bed. One major artery (a common example is the MCA) and an adjacent vein form the origin of the AVM, called the *nidus* of the malformation. Going to and from the nidus are multiple feeding vessels. Most AVMs are congenital, resulting from failure of capillary formation in utero. Some AVMs have been associated with traumatic brain injuries, wherein the blood is shunted around a hematoma.[45, 61, 63] AVMs range in size from small to those encompassing an entire hemisphere.

AVMs may be found in the brain or spinal cord. Intracranially, the majority of AVMs are found in the cerebral hemispheres. In the spinal cord, AVMs predominantly occur on the posterior aspect of the cord. Depending on the size of the malformation, the number of feeders, and the magnitude of circulatory steal, the AVM can bleed or undergo thrombosis, resulting in transient to permanent spinal cord damage.

Clinical Manifestations

The onset of clinical manifestations may be seen at any age; however, increased incidence is noted in clients under 40 years of age. Manifestations are related to the anatomy of the malformation and the vessels involved and occur as the result of the vessels' weakening and shunting of blood in the tortuous mass. Manifestations may also be due to increasing size of the AVM. As the AVM expands, the anomalous vessels dilate and require more blood. The process of acquiring more blood flow is referred to as circulatory "steal." In this phenomenon, blood is diverted (stolen) from normal areas to maintain flow through the anomalous vessels. Consequently, localized hypoperfusion and hypoxia occur in the tissue adjacent to the AVM.

When the AVM bleeds, the client may present with any of the following: complaints of headache, seizures, SAH, or infracerebral hemorrhage. Once an AVM has bled, there is a 25% chance of rebleeding.

Outcome Management

The management of AVMs is similar to that of intracranial aneurysm. Nursing goals are comparable to those for aneurysm management, with limitation of activity, seizure control, and blood pressure management. The goals of AVM treatment are complete and permanent obliteration of the lesion. This goal may be accomplished with surgery, endovascular embolizations, or radiosurgery. The client's condition and the characteristics of the AVM determine the course of treatment. For example, in a client who has had a large SAH, vasospasm may develop. In this case, treatment is delayed until the vasospasm is decreased or resolved. With an improvement in the clinical status of the client, a treatment plan can then be developed.[44, 60, 62]

Clients commonly require a combination of treatments. Surgical resection may be the preferred treatment. Depending upon the size and location of the aneurysm, the client may undergo serial embolizations, and surgery is the final form of treatment. For the serial embolizations, a thrombosing agent, histoacryl glue may be used. The goal of the embolization is to place the glue as close to the nidus of the AVM as possible.

Another treatment option for cerebral AVMs is radiosurgery. This approach may constitute the main treatment or may be used in combination with other therapies. Radiosurgery consists of direction of a focused beam of radiation toward the nidus of the AVM. The dose delivered is determined by the size of the AVM. The use of radiotherapy is recommended with small AVMs.

For example, research is ongoing with "liquid coils" (coils that take the shape within the vascular lesion) and new coatings on currently used coils. The future holds the answers to the treatment and management of hemorrhagic cerebral disorders.[44, 60, 62]

INFECTIONS

BACTERIAL MENINGITIS

Bacterial meningitis is characterized by inflammation of all the meninges; however, the organisms predominantly involve the arachnoid and subarachnoid spaces. The infection spreads throughout the subarachnoid space via the CSF around the brain and spinal cord and usually involves the ventricles.

Etiology

Almost any bacteria entering the body can cause meningitis. The most common are meningococci (*Neisseria meningitidis*), pneumococci (*Streptococcus pneumoniae*), and *Haemophilus influenzae*. These organisms are often present in the nasopharynx. It is not known how they enter the bloodstream and the subarachnoid space. *S. pneumoniae* and *N. meningitidis* are found most often in adults. Factors predisposing to bacterial meningitis include traumatic brain injury, systemic infection, postsurgical infection, meningeal infection, anatomic defects, and other systemic illnesses. Toxins such as intrathecal drugs or tumor cytokines may directly trigger meningeal irritation.

Pathophysiology

The route of entry into the intact CNS is uncertain. Invasion may occur through the choroid plexus (across the blood-brain barrier) or within monocytes as a component of normal cellular movement. Little change occurs in brain structure in the early stages of meningitis. Later in bacterial meningitis, inflammation leads to formation of exudate. The arachnoid and pia tissues become thickened, and adhesions form, especially in areas where there normally is an increased amount of CSF. The arteries supplying the subarachnoid space, may be engorged with blood, leading to rupture or thrombosis of these vessels.

Clinical Manifestations

The classic manifestations of meningitis are nuchal rigidity (rigidity of the neck), Brudzinski's sign and Kernig's sign, and photophobia. To assess for *Kernig's sign,* begin with the client recumbent and the thigh flexed at a right angle to the abdomen, and with the knee flexed at a 90-degree angle to the thigh. Then extend the client's lower leg. In meningeal irritation, extending the leg upward causes pain, spasm of the hamstring muscles, and resistance to further leg extension at the knee (Fig. 69–8A). To assess for *Brudzinski's sign,* with the client supine lift the head rapidly up from the bed. If meningeal irritation is present, forward neck flexion produces flexion of both thighs at the hips and flexure movements of the ankles and knees (Fig. 69–8B).

Other general manifestations related to infection are also present, such as fever, tachycardia, headache, prostration, chills, fever, nausea, and vomiting. The client may be irritable at first but, as the infection progresses, appears acutely ill and confused, stuporous, or semicomatose. Seizures may occur. A petechial or hemorrhagic rash may develop. CSF is cloudy. Gram stain of the CSF reveals organisms in 70% to 80% of cases.[39] When the organism cannot be identified, bacterial antigens can be determined. *Haemophilus influenzae* is frequently detected with this technique. Clients with bacterial pneumomeningitis demonstrate the following:

- Moderately elevated CSF pressures
- Elevated CSF protein (normal, 15 to 45 mg/dl)
- Decreased CSF glucose (normal 60 to 80 mg/dl, or two-thirds of the serum glucose value)
- Elevated white blood cell count, usually increased (100 to 10,000/cm³), with predominantly polymorphonuclear leukocytes

Outcome Management

Bacterial meningitis constitutes a medical emergency. If untreated, it can be fatal within hours to days. Medical diagnosis is made by assessment of clinical manifestations and is confirmed by isolating the causative organism from the CSF. The use of antibiotics has reduced the mortality rate for all types of bacterial meningitis. Prognosis varies according to the causative organism. The mortality rate is less than 5%.[40] Deaths most often occur in newborn infants and in older adults. Complications are rare but may include septic shock, vasomotor collapse, seizures, and increased ICP due to hydrocephalus, brain swelling, and fluid overload. Residual neurologic deficits are rare in adults.[31]

Intervention depends on the causative microorganism and the source of the infection. Empiric therapy in bacterial meningitis includes cephalosporins, rifampin, and vancomycin. The empirical use of penicillin or ampicillin in the treatment of CNS infections is avoided because of the beta-lactamase–producing *H. influenzae* and *N. meningitidis.* It is believed that the cephalosporins are more potent against the beta-lactamase organisms. Chloramphenicol and trimethoprim-sulfamethoxazole are recommended for clients allergic to penicillin. Once the organism is known, antibiotics with greater sensitivity may be used. High doses of the appropriate antibiotic are usually prescribed for at least 10 days. If the primary focus of infection is located in the frontal area, such as the parasinuses, or if cranial osteomyelitis is present, surgery may be indicated after the acute phases of meningitis have subsided.

A unique problem in treating CNS infection is that an intact blood-brain barrier prevents complete penetration of the antibiotic. However, inflammation inhibits the blood-brain barrier, so for a short time, antibiotics penetrate the CNS. Antibiotics are given intravenously; the blood-brain barrier recovers as inflammation subsides, and high doses are required in order to reach the CSF.

Adequate fluid and electrolyte balance must be maintained. Frequent assessment of the neurologic status is indicated to detect early signs of increasing ICP and seizures. Anticonvulsants may be prescribed for seizure prevention.

Outbreaks of meningitis can be a major health problem in the community, especially when they occur in schools. Refer to your facility's isolation protocols.

BACTERIAL TOXINS

Toxins produced by several pathogenic bacteria have a special affinity for the nervous system. They cause conditions such as tetanus, diphtheria, and botulism. Tetanus, a preventable disease, is caused by the anaerobic spore-forming rod *Clostridium tetani.* Tetanus may be found in

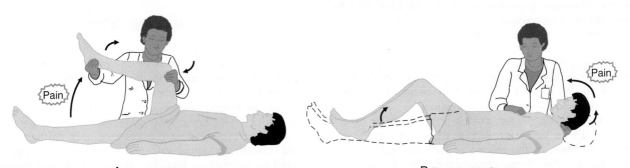

A Kernig's Sign   B Brudzinski's Sign

FIGURE 69–8 Assessment of meningeal irritation. *A,* Kernig's sign. *B,* Brudzinski's sign.

people with some form of trauma and no history of tetanus immunization. Bacteria enter the CNS from a wound in which the spores were introduced and produced a toxin. The toxin enters the blood stream from the wound and travels to the central and peripheral nervous systems. It is important to note that with wounds that are closer to the head, the neurotoxin causes tetanus more quickly.

Clinical Manifestations

Clinical manifestations may be limited to painful muscular spasms and contractions in the affected extremity. However, generalized tetanus is more common, with painful, involuntary muscular contractions involving the neck and facial muscles, especially cheek muscles, the jaw becomes locked closed (trismus), resulting in a grotesque grinning expression (risus sardonicus). The involuntary muscular contractions may further involve the pharyngeal and respiratory muscles, neck, trunk, and limbs. The affected muscles become rigid, with occurrence of painful paroxysms of tonic contractions in response to even the slightest external stimuli. The client may also exhibit seizures as a result of airway problems and/or hypoxia.

Outcome Management

Interventions for the acute care of the client with tetanus include the respiratory support with possible mechanical ventilation, use of neuromuscular blocking agents, surgery to debride any associated wounds, a single dose of tetanus immune globulin (Hyper-Tet), a 10-day course of penicillin G (tetracycline, erythromycin, and chloramphenicol are alternative agents), enteral feedings, and prophylactic anticoagulation to prevent thrombus. The overall mortality rate for tetanus is 25% to 50%, even in modern facilities with extensive resources. Tetanus is best prevented by immunization and regular booster doses of the toxoid.

BRAIN ABSCESS

A brain abscess is a collection of either encapsulated or free pus within brain tissue arising from a primary focus elsewhere (e.g., ear, mastoid sinuses, nasal sinuses, heart, distal bones, lungs, or primary bacteremia). The frontal lobe is the most common site of a brain abscess. They vary in size. A large abscess may involve most of one cerebral hemisphere. Other abscesses are microscopic. Brain abscesses are relatively rare and when they occur, it is most common in persons under age 30. Morbidity and mortality increase greatly with multiple brain abscesses.

A brain abscess may occur after penetrating traumatic brain injuries or intracranial surgery. Staphylococci are the most common organisms in trauma-related cases; however, many organisms may be implicated. *Toxoplasma* is the usual agent found in clients with human immunodeficiency virus (HIV) infection.

In its early stages, the abscess produces inflammation, necrotic tissue, and surrounding edema. Within several days, the center of the abscess is purulent, and a wall of granulation tissue forms, encapsulating the abscess. Infection may spread through thin places in the wall of the capsule, resulting in development of additional abscesses.

Clinical Manifestations

Clinical manifestations of a brain abscess are essentially the same as those seen with any space-occupying brain lesion. Headache and lethargy are the most common manifestations. Manifestations of infection (e.g., fever, chills) are present about half the time. The client may experience drowsiness, confusion, and a depressed mental status as a result of the cerebral edema, increasing ICP, and the intracranial effects of the brain abscess. Transient focal neurologic disorders (e.g., weakness on one side, loss of speech) occur when the abscess is located in a specific area such as the motor or speech area. Early manifestations may subside, and then within a few days or weeks, indications of increasing ICP may develop (e.g., recurrent headaches, changes in LOC focal or generalized seizures).

Medical diagnosis of brain abscess is made by CT and MRI.

Outcome Management

Pyogenic brain abscess may be treated with antibiotic therapy alone or antibiotics combined with surgical aspiration or excision. Needle aspiration may be performed stereotactically (guided by CT imaging) with the use of local anesthesia. Corticosteroids may also be given to reduce cerebral edema. Penicillin is the antibiotic of choice for this type of infection. When antibiotics are used to treat the abscess, follow-up CT scans are used to monitor progress.[6, 31]

VIRAL INFECTIONS

Neurologic viral infections are usually associated with systemic viral infections and can be devastating. Viruses may enter the body via the respiratory system, mouth, or genitalia or from an insect or animal bite. The organism invades the CNS via the cerebral capillaries and choroid plexus or along peripheral nerves. Viruses multiply in the body and cause viremia (blood infected with viruses). Some viruses appear to have an affinity for specific cell types within the CNS.

There is no adequate treatment for most CNS viral infections. Immunizations are available for a few viral conditions (e.g., poliomyelitis, rabies). However, they are not available for most viral encephalitides. At present, mass immunization is practical only for acute anterior poliomyelitis. The best control of other viral disorders is to identify and eliminate vectors responsible for their transmission.[29, 31]

VIRAL MENINGITIS

Acute viral meningitis ("aseptic meningitis") is most often caused by the mumps virus or one of the picornaviruses. Aseptic meningitis infecting the subarachnoid space usually resolves within 2 weeks.

Clinical manifestations are mild. The client may be drowsy or photophobic, may have headache and pain on moving the eyes, and may experience neck stiffness (nuchal rigidity) and spine stiffness on flexion. Other generalized manifestations include weakness, rash, and painful extremities. Fever and signs of meningeal irritation may be present. Physical examination reveals the presence of nuchal rigidity and Brudzinski's and Kernig's signs. Acute and convalescent serologic testing and appropriate viral cultures may identify the specific virus.

Interventions for clients with aseptic meningitis are related to symptom management. Keep the client at bed rest during the acute phase. Plan interventions to relieve headache, control fever, and increase comfort. If seizures occur, anticonvulsants are prescribed.[29, 31]

VIRAL ENCEPHALITIS

Encephalitis is an inflammation of the brain parenchyma from viral invasion. The two most common viral infections are arthropod-borne virus (arbovirus) encephalitis and herpes simplex type 1 virus encephalitis. Also, the viruses that cause viral meningitis may cause severe viral encephalitis.

The course of the illness is unpredictable. Of the clients who recover, a significant percentage have some disability, including mental deterioration, personality changes, and hemiparesis. Residual disability is even higher with eastern equine encephalitis.

Viral encephalitis begins like any acute febrile illness with headache, fever, malaise, and sore throat. Later the client experiences alterations in level of consciousness and sensorium (confusion progressing to disorientation and lethargy progressing to coma). In addition, motor or sensory deficits, seizures, hyperirritability, cranial nerve involvement, and increased ICP may be present.

Arbovirus Encephalitis

Arbovirus encephalitis is caused by arboviruses that multiply in a blood-sucking vector (e.g., mosquito, tick) and are transmitted to humans by the insect's bite. The incidence of diseases caused by arboviruses is characteristically seasonal and geographic. Become familiar with those in your area. In the United States, they occur in late summer and early fall. The most common types of encephalitides are the St. Louis and eastern and western equine forms of encephalitis.

The infection sites are usually microscopic and scattered throughout the cerebral gray and white matter except in eastern equine encephalitis, in which major parts of a lobe or hemisphere may be destroyed. Two thirds of people who acquire eastern equine encephalitis either die or develop severe residual disabilities including mental retardation, seizures, blindness, deafness, speech disorders, and hemiplegia.

Clinical manifestations with all arbovirus encephalitides are similar. The onset is gradual in adults and older children, with headache, nausea, vomiting, listlessness, and fever. After a few days, seizures, nuchal rigidity, stupor, and coma develop. Photophobia, hemiparesis, and asymmetrical reflexes may be present. Fever and neurologic manifestations subside within 2 weeks if the client does not develop irreversible CNS changes or die.[29, 31]

Herpes Simplex Virus Encephalitis

Herpes simplex virus encephalitis occurs at any time of year and throughout the world. It affects particularly middle-aged people.

The gradually evolving initial clinical manifestations are similar to those of other acute encephalitides. However, this virus has an affinity for the inferomedial portions of the frontal and temporal lobes. The client soon becomes acutely ill with headache, fever, vomiting, and, often, seizures. If the infection is not aggressively treated, temporal lobe swelling leads to transtentorial herniation, coma, and brain death.

A biopsy may be done in an attempt to identify the herpes virus. Although biopsy is definitive for the disease, there are risks. MRI is an effective and safe diagnostic tool.

Intervention for herpes simplex encephalitis is a 10-day course of IV acyclovir, an antiviral agent. To be effective, it must be given early in the course of the disease. Despite treatment, the course of the disease may be unrelenting. The prognosis is grave but not hopeless, however, there is significant mortality with this infection. Of people who survive, many are left with severe neurologic and mental disabilities such as global dementia, seizures, and aphasia.

Nursing intervention is a challenge. An acutely ill client is often restless and combative and exhibits bizarre behavior. Extensive rehabilitation is often needed. The client needs careful protection from injury, and the family requires supportive care. If residual behavior changes and mental deterioration develop, assist the family to adjust to changes in the client. Refer the family to agency or community support groups.[29, 31]

FUNGAL INFECTIONS

Fungi may cause meningitis, meningoencephalitis, intracranial thrombophlebitis, or brain abscess. CNS fungal infections are rare. When they do occur, these infections are usually complications of another condition. Conditions that increase the risk of fungal infections include those that interfere with the body's normal flora or suppress the immune response, such as acquired immunodeficiency syndrome (AIDS), leukemia, organ transplantation, diabetes, and collagen-vascular disease.

Cryptococcosis is the most frequent CNS fungal infection. The cryptococcus, a common soil fungus, can cause granulomatous meningitis. Small granulomas and cysts are found within the cortex, and large granulomas and cystic nodules are found deep within the brain. This organism is an opportunist, and the incidence of cryptococcosis has risen since the onset of the AIDS epidemic. Clinical manifestations vary, and diagnosis is confirmed by finding *Cryptococcus neoformans* in the CSF. If untreated, this infection is fatal within a few weeks.

Mucormycosis, a malignant infection of cerebral vessels, is a rare complication of diabetic acidosis. It begins in the nose and paranasal sinuses and spreads to the brain. It may be associated with fungal meningitis.

CNS fungal infections produce clinical manifestations similar to those of bacterial infections. The main intervention for these infections is administration of IV amphotericin B, flucytosine, or fluconazole. With this treatment, recovery is almost certain, except for clients with advanced infection or other, overwhelming, fatal diseases. Cryptococcal meningitis in clients with AIDS is highly refractory and is associated with a 50% to 60% relapse rate.

PARASITIC INFESTATIONS

In South America and Mexico, the parasite most commonly affecting the CNS is *Cysticercus*. The tapeworm, in larval form, causes a systemic infestation. Raw or undercooked pork may contain tapeworms, which are passed into the gastrointestinal tract, where they grow. The worm enters the bloodstream and establishes a cyst, commonly within the muscles and brain tissue. The cyst, which may be 3 to 15 mm in diameter, contains the larvae of the tapeworm. These larvae die approximately 18 months after infestation. Calcification of the cyst and inflammation follow. Clients may have more than one cyst.

CT or MRI studies identify the cysts. Cysticercosis titers may be identified in the blood and CSF; however, surgical biopsy is often performed to confirm the diagnosis.

The drug praziquantel is used to treat cysticercosis. The mechanism of action is to eliminate the tapeworm from the gastrointestinal system. If pharmacologic treatment is ineffective, surgical excision of the cyst may be recommended.[29, 31]

TOXOPLASMOSIS

The most common opportunistic infection of the CNS in clients who have AIDS is toxoplasmosis. It is usually manifested as single or multiple brain abscesses. Initial clinical manifestations are headache, confusion, lethargy, and low-grade fever. More than 65% of clients develop such focal signs as weakness, ataxia, speech disturbances, apraxia, seizures, and sensory disturbances.[34]

Treatment consists of administration of pyrimethamine (Daraprim), sulfadiazine or clindamycin (Cleocin), and leucovorin (folinic acid or Wellcovorin). If a therapeutic response is seen, the client is kept on maintenance dosages.

HEADACHE

Headache, the most common of pains, may occur either in the absence of organic disease or as a manifestation of serious disease. Most headaches are transient and of only moderate or slight severity. However, a few types are chronic, intense, and recurrent over a period of months or years. Headache is a manifestation of an underlying disorder, rather than a disease itself. The cause of headache must be identified so that appropriate treatment can be given.

Clients often self-treat headaches with over-the-counter medications. Most headaches do not indicate serious disease. However, encourage clients with persistent or recurrent headaches to seek neurologic assessment. Serious disorders that typically produce headache include intracranial tumors and hemorrhage, CNS infections, acute systemic infections, TBI, cerebral hypoxia, severe hypertension, and acute or chronic diseases of the eye, ear, nose, or throat.

Assessment of headaches includes detailed history, psychosocial assessment, and physical examination. Neurologic assessment is particularly important. Possible neurologic diagnostic tests include skull x-ray studies, CT, EEG, and lumbar puncture with CSF examination.

History should determine (1) location of the pain, intensity, and paths of radiation; (2) character of the headache (e.g., sharp, dull, throbbing); (3) mode of headache onset, duration, and frequency; (4) methods used to treat the headache; (5) presence of localized tenderness; (6) associated phenomena or precipitating factors; and (7) familial incidence.

Classification and Etiology

TENSION HEADACHE

Tension headaches result from muscle contraction (Fig. 69–9A). This type of headache is described as a tight bandlike discomfort that is unrelenting, with few headache-free intervals. The pain typically builds slowly, fluctuates in severity, and may persist more or less continuously for many days. Triggers include fatigue and stress. The diagnosis of tension headache is confirmed when the headaches occur more often than 15 days a month. Clients may report that the head feels as if it is in a vise or that the posterior neck muscles are tight. In some patients, anxiety or depression coexists with tension headache.

CLUSTER HEADACHES

Cluster headaches are sometimes classified as a form of migraine (Fig. 69–9B). These headaches have a cyclical pattern of one to three short-lived attacks of periorbital pain lasting from 4 to 8 weeks, with an increased incidence in spring and fall. These headaches also have quiescent periods lasting months to years. Cluster headaches occur more often in men.

The headache lasts between 15 minutes and 3 hours. It may occur one to four times each day and may awaken the client from sleep. The pain is described as deep, boring, intense pain of such severity that the client has difficulty remaining still. The client may also develop Horner's syndrome with constricted pupils, injected conjunctiva, unilateral lacrimation, and rhinorrhea during the headaches. Cluster headaches are triggered by consumption of alcohol.

Propranolol and amitriptyline are largely ineffective. Lithium is beneficial for cluster headache and ineffective in migraine. The most satisfactory treatment is the administration of drugs to prevent cluster attacks until the bout is over. Effective prophylactic drugs are prednisone, lithium, methysergide, ergotamine, and verapamil. Lithium appears to be particularly useful for the chronic form of the disorder. A 10-day course of prednisone, followed by a rapid taper, may interrupt the pain bout for many clients.

For the attacks themselves, oxygen inhalation (9 L/min via a loose mask) is the most effective modality; inhalation of 100% oxygen for 15 minutes is often necessary. The self-administration of intranasal lidocaine, either 4% topical or 2% viscous, to the most caudal aspect of the inferior nasal turbinate can produce a ganglionic block that is usually remarkably effective in terminating an attack.

MIGRAINE HEADACHES

Migraine headache is often considered to be a "vascular" headache, vasospasm and ischemia of intracranial vessels being the cause of the pain (Fig. 69–9C). These head-

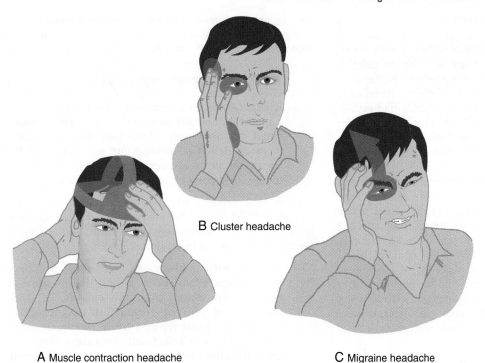

B Cluster headache

A Muscle contraction headache

C Migraine headache

FIGURE 69-9 Types of headaches. The red areas show the regions of greatest pain. *A*, Muscle contraction headache. *B*, Cluster headache. *C*, Migraine headache.

aches usually begin in puberty and are more common in women, often associated with hormonal changes following the menstrual cycle. About 66% of cases of migraine are familial.

Migraine headaches last between 4 and 72 hours, with headache-free intervals between attacks. The headache is most often unilateral, but pain may occur on alternate sides with different attacks. Pain is described as throbbing and pulsatile. Photophobia, phonophobia, anorexia, nausea, vomiting, and focal neurologic signs are often present. Some clients have a visual aura that precedes the headache by 10 to 60 minutes (usually 20 minutes). The client sees a jagged edge of light in the visual fields. Other premonitory manifestations occur 12 to 24 hours before an attack and may include euphoria, fatigue, yawning, and craving for sweets. Migraine headache can be triggered by relief of intense stress, missing meals, or tyramine-rich foods. See the accompanying Client Education Guide.

Typically, the client finds pain relief in a quiet, dark environment. When aspirin and acetaminophen alone fail, the addition of butalbital, caffeine, ibuprofen (600 to 800 mg), and naproxen (375 to 750 mg) is often useful. Isometheptene compound, 1 to 2 capsules, is effective for mild to moderate "common migraine." When these measures fail, more aggressive therapy should be considered. Drug absorption is impaired during migrainous attacks because of reduced gastrointestinal motility. Delayed absorption occurs in the absence of nausea and is related to the severity of the attack and not its duration. Therefore, when oral agents fail to cure, alternative therapies, including rectal ergotamine, subcutaneous sumatriptan, parenteral dihydroergotamine, and IV chlorpromazine and prochlorperazine, should be tried.

Today a number of drugs are available with the capacity to stabilize migraine. They must be taken daily. The decision of whether to use this approach depends on the frequency of attacks and on how well acute treatment is working. The occurrence of at least two or three attacks per month may be an indication for this approach. There is usually a lag of 2 weeks before an effect is seen. The major drugs are propranolol, amitriptyline, valproate, verapamil, phenelzine, and methysergide.

CLIENT EDUCATION GUIDE

Migraine Headache

Client Instructions

- Many things can trigger a migraine headache. Find out what things trigger your headaches and avoid those triggers. If this is not possible, consult your physician about adjusting the dosage of your medication.
- If menstruation and ovulation are triggers, consult your physician for adjustments to your medication dosage.
- Alcohol temporarily increases the diameter of your blood vessels (a process called vasodilation), which may trigger migraines.
- Some foods, such as chocolate, cheese, citrus fruits, coffee, pork, and dairy products, contain substances that may trigger migraines.
- Low food intake may lead to a low blood glucose (sugar) level (hypoglycemia), which can trigger migraines. Eat small, frequent meals to decrease this risk.
- Stress management is essential. Adjust your lifestyle to reduce fatigue and exposure to bright sunlight, heat, or humidity. Get enough sleep. If you are having trouble managing the stresses in your life, seek expert guidance.

LUMBAR PUNCTURE HEADACHE

Loss of CSF volume with lumbar puncture decreases the brain's supportive cushion. Headache after lumbar puncture usually begins within 48 hours but may be delayed for up to 12 days. Head pain is dramatically positional; it begins when the client sits or stands upright, and relief is obtained upon reclining or with abdominal compression. The longer the client is upright, the longer the latency before head pain subsides. It is worsened by head shaking and jugular vein compression. The pain is usually a dull ache but may be throbbing; its location is occipitofrontal. Nausea and stiff neck often accompany headache, and occasionally blurred vision, photophobia, tinnitus, and vertigo are reported. The pain usually resolves over a few days but may on occasion persist for weeks to months.

Treatment with IV caffeine sodium benzoate promptly terminates headache in most clients. An epidural blood patch accomplished by injection of 15 ml of autologous whole blood rarely fails for those who do not respond to caffeine. The mechanism for these treatment effects is not certain. The blood patch has an immediate effect, making it unlikely that sealing off a dural hole with blood clot is its mechanism of action.

POSTCONCUSSION HEADACHE AND SYNDROME

After seemingly trivial head injuries and particularly after rear-end motor vehicle collisions, many clients report varying combinations of headache, dizziness, vertigo, and impaired memory. Anxiety, irritability, and difficulty with concentration are other hallmarks of *postconcussion syndrome*. Manifestations may remit after several weeks or persist for months and even years after the injury.

Postconcussion headaches may occur whether or not a client was rendered unconscious by head trauma. Typically, findings on neurologic examination are normal, with the exception of the behavioral abnormalities. Chronic subdural hematoma may on occasion mimic this disorder. Although the cause of postconcussive headache disorder is not known, it should not in general be viewed as a primary psychological disturbance. It often persists long after the settlement of pending lawsuits.

Treatment is symptomatic support. Repeated encouragement that the syndrome eventually remits is important.

OTHER CAUSES OF HEADACHE

Head pain may also develop from disorders of the eyes, ears, teeth, and paranasal structures. Headaches may result from errors of refraction, glaucoma (with increased intraocular pressure), inflammation, and ocular muscle disturbances (see Chapter 65). Pain associated with sinus infection is usually caused by irritation and inflammation of sinus openings. Sinus walls are less sensitive. The pain of a sinus headache may be relieved or eliminated by decongestants and analgesics. Sometimes antibiotics are needed. Surgery to drain the sinuses may also be required (see Chapter 60).

CONCLUSIONS

Because of the complexity of brain disorders and the emotional reactions of the client and family members to these problems, neurologic nursing is one of the most challenging areas of nursing practice. Common nursing problems center on cerebral perfusion and cognition as well as on those related to functional rehabilitation. Prevention and early intervention are key to optimal client outcome.

THINKING CRITICALLY

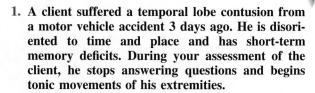

1. **A client suffered a temporal lobe contusion from a motor vehicle accident 3 days ago. He is disoriented to time and place and has short-term memory deficits. During your assessment of the client, he stops answering questions and begins tonic movements of his extremities.**

Factors to Consider. What are the highest priorities for this client? What are the interventions related to these priorities? What interventions come next? What significance does the site of injury have?

2. **A client with a history of headaches, dizziness, and vertigo experienced a first-time seizure at age 27. Immediately after this episode, he noted the onset of blurred vision. Subsequent studies revealed the presence of a brain tumor, and cranial surgery was scheduled. Two days after surgery, the client is transferred to the regular unit. What are your responsibilities regarding monitoring for an increase in intracranial pressure? What are the general interventions for the client after craniotomy?**

Factors to Consider. What is the major complication following intracranial surgery? How do the general interventions prevent complications associated with this type of surgery?

3. **A client is seen in the emergency department at 9 AM on Monday morning. His chief complaint is a severe headache. He states: "I am having the worst headache of my life. The pain awakened me around 5 AM and has gotten worse and worse." On examination the patient is found to have a score of 15 on the Glasgow Coma Scale, complains of nausea, and has a stiff neck. The left-hand grip is slightly weaker than the right-hand grip, and there is a slight pronator drift of the left arm. In addition, there is flattening of the left nasolabial fold. A computed tomography scan of the brain reveals moderate hemorrhage on the right side with increased blood present in the right sylvian fissure. What tests would you expect to be ordered? What complications are important to assess for in this client?**

Factors to Consider. What problem is probably in progress? Is the client a surgical candidate, either at present or later on?

4. **You are caring for a client who had a malignant brain tumor resected 72 hours ago. During previous assessments, she was alert and oriented; her pupils were equal, round, reactive to light, and accommodative (PERRLA), her eyes opened spontaneously; and she was moving all four extremities equally and on command. Her Glasgow Coma Scale (GCS) score was 15. Now, however, she is slow to respond, although still oriented to**

person, place, and time. Her right pupil is equal in size to the left but exhibits a sluggish reaction to direct light. Her left pupil responds normally. She still responds to verbal commands appropriately, has equal motor strength, and opens her eyes spontaneously. Thus, her score on the GCS is still 15. You decide to notify the physician. Why?

Factors to Consider. How sensitive is the Glasgow Coma Scale? What abnormality may be indicated by the decreased response time and the change in pupil reaction?

BIBLIOGRAPHY

1. American Association of Neuroscience Nursing. (1978). *Core Curriculum for Neurosurgical Nurses.* Chicago.
2. American Brain Tumor Association. (2000). *A Primer of Brain Tumors* (7th ed.). Chicago.
3. American Council for Headache Education. (1996). Available: *http://www.achnet.org/whatcause.html,* 1–9.
4. Anderson, S. I., et al. (1999). Mood disorders in patients after treatment for primary intracranial tumors. *British Journal of Neurosurgery, 13*(5), 480–485.
5. Barad, M. B. (1999). Functional assessment for transitions in patient acuity. In *Nursing Clinics of North America, 34*(3), 607–620.
6. Bauman, C. K. (1997). Multiple bilateral cerebral abscesses with hemorrhage. *Journal of Neuroscience Nursing, 29*(1), 4–14.
7. Bauman, G. S., et al. (1998). Bihemispheric malignant glioma: One size does not fit all. *Journal of Neuro-oncology, 28,* 83–89.
8. Berweiler, U., et al. (1998). Reservoir systems for intraventricular chemotherapy. *Journal of Neuro-Oncology, 38,* 141–143.
9. Billings, C. V. (1980). Emotional first aid. *American Journal of Nursing, 80*(11), 2006–2009.
10. Breslau, N., et al. (2000). Headache and major depression. *Neurology, 54*(2), 308–313.
11. Brisman, M. H., & Bederson, J. B. (1997). Surgical management of subarachnoid hemorrhage. *New Horizons, 5*(4), 376–386.
12. (2000). *CA: A Cancer Journal for Clinicans, 50*(1), 12–13.
13. Coke, C. B., et al. (1998). Atypical and malignant meningiomas: An outcome report of 17 cases. *Journal of Neuro-oncology, 39,* 65–70.
14. Davis, F., & Preston-Martin, S. (1998). The epidemiology of brain tumors. In D. Bigner, et al. (Eds.), *Russell and Rubinstein's pathology of tumors of the nervous system* (6th ed.). London: Edward Arnold.
15. Davis, M., & Lucatorto, M. (1994). Mannitol revisited. *Journal of Neuroscience Nursing, 26*(3), 170–174.
16. Dawson, H., & Segal, M. B. (1996). *Physiology of the CSF and blood-brain barriers.* New York: CRC Press.
17. Dewar, S., et al. (1996). Intracranial electrode monitoring for seizure location: Indications, methods and the prevention of complications. *Journal of Neuroscience Nursing, 28*(5), 280–292.
18. Doolittle, N., et al. (1998). Blood-brain barrier disruption for the treatment of malignant brain tumors: The national program. *Journal of Neuroscience Nursing, 30*(2), 81–90.
19. Engle, G. (1964). Grief and grieving. *American Journal of Nursing, 64*(9), 93–98.
20. Engle, J., & Pedley, T. A. (Eds.). (1998). *Epilepsy—a comprehensive textbook* (Vols. I, II, and III). Philadelphia: Lippincott-Raven.
21. Faylor, C. R. (1999). Using transcranial Doppler to augment the neurological examination after aneurysmal subarachnoid hemorrhage. *Journal of Neuroscience Nursing, 31*(5), 285–293.
22. Fisher, C. M., et al. (1980). Relation of cerebrovasospasm to subarachnoid hemorrhage visualized by computerized tomographic scanning. *Neurosurgery, 6*(1), 1–9.
23. Gormely, W. B., et al. (1997). Acoustic neuromas: Results of current surgical management. *Neurosurgery, 41*(1), 50–60.
24. Gumnit, R. (1997). *Living well with epilepsy* (2nd ed.). Minneapolis: Demos Vermande.
25. Gurney, J., et al. (1999). The contribution of nonmalignant tumors to CNS tumor incidence rates among children in the United States. *Cancer Causes and Control, 10*(2), 101–105.
26. Hickey, J. V. (1997). *The clinical practice of neurological and neurosurgical nursing.* Philadelphia: Lippincott-Raven.
27. Huether, S. E., & McCance, K. L. (1996). *Understanding pathophysiology.* St. Louis: Mosby–Year Book.
28. Hunt, W. E., & Hess, R. M. (1968). Surgical risks as related to time of intervention in the repair of intracranial aneurysms. *Journal of Neurosurgery, 28,* 14–20.
29. Johnson, R. T. (1996). Emerging viral infections. *Archives of Neurology, 53,* 18–22.
30. Kajs-Wylie, M. (1999). Antihypertensive therapy for the neurological patient: A nursing challenge. *Journal of Neuroscience Nursing, 31*(3), 142–151.
31. King, D. (1999). Central nervous system infection. *Nursing Clinics of North America, 34*(3), 761–771.
32. Kleihues, P., et al. (1993). The new WHO classification of brain tumors. *Brain Pathology, 3,* 225–268.
33. Long, L., & Reeves, A. (1997). The practical aspects of epilepsy: Critical components of comprehensive patient care. *Journal of Neuroscience Nursing, 29*(4), 249–254.
34. McCarthy, B., et al. (1998). Factors associated with survival in patients with meningioma. *Journal of Neurosurgery, 88,* 831–839.
35. Moloney, M. F., et al. (2000). Caring for the woman with migraine headaches. *Nurse Practitioner,* 2000 Feb.; *25*(2), 17–41.
36. Morris, G. L., et al. (1999). Long-term treatment with vagus nerve stimulation in patients with refractory epilepsy. *Neurology, 53*(7), 1731–1735.
37. Morrison, S. R. (1997). Guglielmi detachable coils: An alternative therapy for surgically high-risk aneurysms. *Journal of Neuroscience Nursing, 29*(4), 232–237.
38. Noebels, J. (1998). Genetics and epilepsy. In Ozuna, J., et al. (Eds.), *Clinical nursing practice in epilepsy* (Vol. 2, pp. 4–7). Secaucus: Churchill Communications.
39. *Radiation therapy and you: A guide to self-help during treatment.* Bethesda, MD: National Institutes of Health, National Cancer Institute. NIH Publ. No. 97–2227, Revised October 1993; reprinted January 1997.
40. Raskin, N. H. (1996). Approach to the patient with migraine. *Hospital Practice, 31*(2), 93–106.
41. Santillli, N., & Sierzant, T. (1987). Advances in the treatment of epilepsy. *Journal of Neuroscience Nursing, 19,* 143–144.
42. Sargent, J., et al. (1995). Oral sumatriptan is effective and well tolerated for the acute treatment of migraine. *Neurology, 45*(suppl. 7), S10–S14.
43. Schiller, Y., et al. (2000). Discontinuation of antiepileptic drugs after successful epilepsy surgery. *Neurology, 54*(2), 346–349.
44. Schmidek, H. H., & Sweet, W. H. (1995). *Operative neurosurgical techniques* (3rd ed., Vols. I and II). Philadelphia: W. B. Saunders.
45. Shafer, P. O. (1999). Epilepsy and seizures—advances in seizure assessment, treatment and self-management. *Nursing Clinics of North America, 34*(3), 743–759.
46. Shafer, P. O. (1999). New therapies in the management of acute or cluster seizures and seizure emergencies. *Journal of Neuroscience Nursing, 31*(4), 224–230.
47. Shah, S. M., & Kelly, K. M. (1999). *Emergency, neurology—principles and practices.* Cambridge: Cambridge University Press.
48. Spencer, D. C., et al. (2000). The role of intracarotid amobarbital procedure in evaluation of patients for epilepsy. *Surgery, 42*(3), 302–325.
49. Surawiez, T. S., et al. (1998) Brain tumor survival: Results from the National Cancer Data Base. *Journal of Neuro-Oncology, 40,* 151–160.
50. Surawiez, T. S., et al. (1999). Results from the Central Brain Tumor Registry of the United States, 1990–1994. *Neuro-oncology* [On-line]. Available: Doc No. 98–13.
51. Surveillance, Epidemiology, and End Results (SEER). (1998). Cancer statistics review, 1973–1995 U.S. populations. Bethesda, MD: National Cancer Institute.
52. Snively, C., et al. (1998). Vagal nerve stimulator as a treatment for intractable epilepsy. *Journal of Neuroscience Nursing, 30*(5), 286–289.
53. Solomon, G. (1997). Update on therapeutics of headache—diagnosis and treatment of headache in the primary care setting. Available: *http://www.sgim.org/meetings/am20/ws/headache.html,* 1–13.
54. Tamargo, R. J., et al. (1997). Aneurysmal subarachnoid hemorrhage: prognostic features and outcomes. *New Horizons, 5*(4), 364–374.

55. Vale, F. L., et al. (1997). The relationship of subarachnoid hemorrhage and the need for postoperative shunting. *Journal of Neurosurgery, 86,* 462–466.

56. Vannemreddy, P. S. S. V., et al. (2000). Glioblastoma multiforme in a case of acquired immunodeficiency syndrome: Investigating a possible oncogenic influence of human immunodeficiency virus on glial cells. *Journal of Neurosurgery, 92,* 161–164.

57. Vinuela, F., et al. (1997) Guglielmi detachable coil embolization of acute intracranial aneurysm: Perioperative anatomical and clinical outcome in 403 patients. *Journal of Neurosurgery, 86,* 475–482.

58. Vitners, H. V. (1998). *Diagnostic neuropathology.* New York: Marcel Dekker.

59. Vonck, K., et al. (1999). Long-term results of vagus nerve stimulation in refractory epilepsy. *Seizure, 8,* 328–334.

60. Walters, K. (2000). Personal communication.

61. Walters, P. 1990). Chemo: A nurse's guide to action, administration, and side effects. *RN, 53*(2), 52–67.

62. Youmans, J. R. (Ed). (1996). *Neurological surgery: A comprehensive reference guide to the diagnosis and management of neurosurgical problems.* Philadelphia: W. B. Saunders.

63. Yundt, K. D., et al.(1996). Hospital resource utilization in the treatment of cerebral aneurysms. *Journal of Neurosurgery, 85,* 403–409.

REMEMBER *to*
check out your
Companion CD ROM

Management of Clients with Stroke

Catherine A. Kernich

NURSING OUTCOMES CLASSIFICATION (NOC)
for Nursing Diagnoses—Clients with Stroke

Altered Cerebral Tissue Perfusion	**Self-Care Deficit**	Communication: Receptive Ability
Neurologic Status: Consciousness	Self-Care: Activities of Daily Living	Muscle Function
Tissue Perfusion: Cerebral	Self-Care: Eating	**Altered Thought Processes**
Altered Tissue Perfusion	Self-Care: Dressing	Cognitive Ability
Risk for Aspiration	Self-Care: Bathing	Cognitive Orientation
Neurologic Status	Self-Care: Hygiene	Information Processing
Swallowing Status	**Risk for Injury**	Memory
Impaired Physical Mobility	Neurologic Status	**Visual Sensory/Perceptual Alteration**
Ambulation: Walking	Safety Behavior: Fall Prevention	Vision Compensation Behavior
Ambulation: Wheelchair	Safety Behavior: Home Physical	Risk Control: Visual Impairment
Body Positioning: Self-Initiated	Environment	**Unilateral Neglect**
Joint Movement: Active	Safety Status: Falls Occurrence	Self-Care: Activities of Daily Living
Mobility Level	Safety Status: Physical Injury	**Ineffective Individual Coping**
Transfer Performance	**Altered Nutrition: Less Than Body**	Coping
Hyperthermia	**Requirements**	Role Performance
Thermoregulation	Nutritional Status: Food and Fluid Intake	Social Support
Risk for Impaired Skin Integrity	Nutritional Status: Biochemical Measures	Caregiver-Patient Relationship
Immobility Consequences: Physiologic	Nutritional Status: Body Mass	
Tissue Integrity: Skin and Mucous	**Impaired Verbal Communication**	
Membranes	Communication: Expressive Ability	

STROKE—SCOPE OF THE PROBLEM

Stroke is a term used to describe neurologic changes caused by an interruption in the blood supply to a part of the brain. The two major types of stroke are *ischemic* and *hemorrhagic*. Ischemic stroke is caused by a thrombotic or embolic blockage of blood flow to the brain. Bleeding into the brain tissue or the subarachnoid space causes a hemorrhagic stroke. Ischemic strokes account for approximately 83% of all strokes. The remaining 17% of strokes are hemorrhagic.

Cerebrovascular disorders are the third leading cause of death in the United States and account for approximately 150,000 mortalities annually. An estimated 550,000 people experience a stroke each year.[42] When second strokes are considered in the estimates, the incidence increases to 700,000 per year in the United States alone.[6] Stroke is both the leading cause of adult disability and the primary diagnosis for long-term care.[14] There are

3 million stroke survivors living with varying degrees of disability in the United States. Along with a high mortality rate, strokes produce significant morbidity in people who survive them. Of the stroke survivors, 31% require assistance with self-care, 20% require assistance with ambulation, 71% have some impairment in vocational ability up to 7 years following the stroke, and 16% are institutionalized.[31]

The advent of thrombolytic therapy for the treatment of acute ischemic stroke has revolutionized the care of the client following a stroke. Before 1995, health care professionals could offer only supportive measures and rehabilitation to stroke survivors.[12] New therapies can now prevent or limit the extent of brain tissue damage caused by acute ischemic stroke. Thrombolytic therapy must be administered as soon as possible after the onset of the stroke; a treatment window of 3 hours from the onset of manifestations has been established. To convey this sense of urgency regarding the evaluation and treatment of stroke, health care professionals now refer to stroke as brain attack. Public education is focused on prevention, recognition of manifestations, and early treatment of brain attack.[42, 49]

Etiology and Risk Factors

ISCHEMIA

Ischemia occurs when the blood supply to a part of the brain is interrupted or totally occluded. Ultimate survival of ischemic brain tissue depends on the length of time it is deprived plus the degree of altered brain metabolism. Ischemia is commonly due to thrombosis or embolism (Fig. 70–1). Thrombotic strokes are more common than embolic strokes.

Strokes can also be "large vessel" and "small vessel." Large vessel strokes are caused by blockage of a major cerebral artery, such as the internal carotid, anterior cerebral, middle cerebral, posterior cerebral, vertebral, and basilar arteries. Small vessel strokes affect smaller vessels that branch off the larger vessels to penetrate deep into the brain.

Thrombosis

A thrombus starts with damage to the endothelial lining of the vessel. Atherosclerosis is the primary culprit. Atherosclerosis causes fatty material to deposit and form plaques on vessel walls. These plaques continue to enlarge and cause stenosis of the artery. Stenosis alters the usual smooth flow of blood through the artery. Blood swirls around the irregular surface of the plaques, causing platelets to adhere to the plaque. Eventually, the vessel lumen becomes obstructed. Rarely, occlusion is due to inflammation of the arteries, called *arteritis* or *vasculitis.*

A thrombus may develop anywhere along a carotid artery or its branches. A common site is at the bifurcation of the common carotid into the internal and external carotid arteries. Thrombotic stroke is the most common type of stroke in people with diabetes.

Lacunar strokes are small vessel strokes. The endothelium of smaller vessels is primarily affected by hypertension, which causes a thickening of the vessel wall and stenosis. Lacunar infarctions are also common in people with diabetes mellitus.

Embolism

The occlusion of a cerebral artery by an embolus causes an embolic stroke. An embolus forms outside the brain, detaches, and travels through the cerebral circulation until it lodges in and occludes a cerebral artery. A common embolus is plaque. A thrombus can detach from the internal carotid artery at the site of an ulcerated plaque and travel into the cerebral circulation. Chronic atrial fibrillation is associated with a high incidence of embolic stroke. Blood pools in the poorly emptying atria. Tiny clots form in the left atrium and move through the heart and into the cerebral circulation. Mechanical prosthetic heart valves have a rougher surface than the normal endocardium and can cause an increased risk of clots. Both bacterial and nonbacterial endocarditis can be sources of emboli. Other sources of emboli include tumor, fat, bacteria, and air. Any cerebrovascular territory may be affected. The incidence of cerebral embolism increases with age.

HEMORRHAGE

Intracerebral hemorrhage results from rupture of a cerebral vessel, which causes bleeding into brain tissue. Intracerebral hemorrhage is most often secondary to hypertension and is most common after age 50 years. These hemorrhages usually produce extensive residual functional

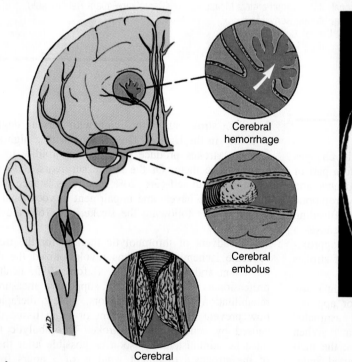

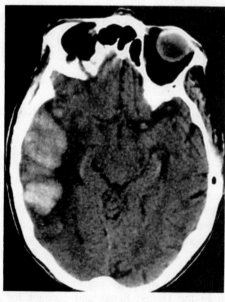

A

B

FIGURE 70–1 *A,* Events causing stroke. *B,* Magnetic resonance image showing a hemorrhagic stroke in the left cerebrum.

loss and have the slowest recovery of all types of stroke. The overall mortality of intracerebral hemorrhage varies between 25% and 60%.[22] The volume of the hemorrhage is the single most important predictor of client outcome.[20, 22] Bleeding may also occur from rupture of an aneurysm or a vascular malformation. The effects of these hemorrhages depend on the site and the extent of the bleeding.

OTHER CAUSES

Cerebral arterial spasm, caused by irritation, reduces blood flow to the area of the brain supplied by the constricted vessel. Spasm of short duration does not necessarily cause permanent brain damage.

Hypercoagulable states, including protein C and protein S deficiencies and disorders of the clotting cascade, can cause thrombosis and ischemic stroke. Compression of cerebral vessels may result from a tumor, large blood clot, swollen brain tissue, brain abscess, or other disorders. These causes are fairly rare.

RISK FACTORS

There has been a gradual decline in the incidence of stroke and stroke mortalities in many industrialized countries in recent years. This is due to stroke prevention through the increased recognition and treatment of risk factors. Modifiable risk factors can be reduced or eliminated through lifestyle changes. Hypertension is the most important modifiable risk factor for both ischemic and hemorrhagic stroke. Adequate blood pressure control is associated with a 38% reduction in stroke incidence.[4]

Cardiovascular disease and atrial fibrillation are also associated with an increased risk of stroke. Diabetes mellitus increases the risk of stroke and morbidity and mortality after stroke. The mechanism is related to macrovascular changes in people with diabetes mellitus. Prior stroke, carotid stenosis, and a history of transient ischemic attacks (TIAs) are considered modifiable risk factors for stroke. Reduction in the risk factors for initial stroke may prevent stroke recurrence.[41] Early recognition and treatment of carotid stenosis and treatment of TIAs with antiplatelet agents reduce the risk of stroke.

Other modifiable risk factors for stroke include hyperlipidemia, cigarette smoking, excessive alcohol consumption, cocaine use, and obesity. Stroke is uncommon in women of childbearing age. However, high-dose estrogen oral contraceptives combined with hypertension, cigarette smoking, migraine headaches, and increasing age increase the risk of stroke in women.[17] Conversely, hormone replacement therapy in postmenopausal women may decrease their risk of stroke.

Client education is aimed at stroke prevention. *Primary* prevention of stroke includes:

- Maintaining an ideal body weight
- Maintaining safe cholesterol levels
- Smoking cessation
- Using low-dose estrogen contraceptives only in the absence of other risk factors
- Reducing alcohol consumption
- Eliminating illicit drug use

Secondary prevention includes:

- Adequate blood pressure control
- Care of diabetes mellitus

- Treatment of cardiovascular disease, TIA, and atrial fibrillation

Nonmodifiable risk factors cannot be prevented or treated. Advancing age is one of the most significant risk factors for stroke. The incidence of stroke in men is slightly higher than that in women. Stroke is more prevalent in African Americans than in whites or Hispanics.[25] This is probably related to the increased incidence of hypertension and diabetes mellitus in this group.[6] Family history of stroke increases one's risk for stroke.

Pathophysiology

The brain is very sensitive to a loss of blood supply. Unlike other body tissues, such as muscle, the brain cannot resort to anaerobic metabolism in the absence of oxygen and glucose. The brain is perfused at the expense of other less vital organs to preserve cerebral metabolism. Hypoxia can cause cerebral ischemia. Short-term ischemia leads to temporary neurologic deficits or a TIA. If blood flow is not restored, brain tissue sustains irreversible damage or infarction within minutes. The extent of infarction depends on the location and size of the occluded artery and the adequacy of collateral circulation to the area it supplies.

Ischemia quickly alters cerebral metabolism. Cell death and permanent changes can occur within 3 to 10 minutes. The client's baseline oxygen level and ability to compensate determine how quickly irreversible changes occur. Blood flow can be altered by localized perfusion problems, such as stroke, or generalized perfusion problems, such as hypotension or cardiac arrest. Cerebral perfusion pressure must fall to two thirds of normal (a mean arterial pressure of 50 mm Hg or below) before the brain does not receive adequate blood flow. These numbers assume a normal baseline of blood flow. A client who has lost compensatory autoregulation experiences manifestations of neurologic deficit sooner.

Decreased cerebral perfusion is usually caused by occlusion of a cerebral artery or intracerebral hemorrhage. Occlusion produces ischemia in the brain tissue supplied by the affected artery and edema in the surrounding tissue. Cells in the center of the stroke area, or the core, die almost immediately following stroke onset. This is referred to as *primary neuronal injury*. A zone of hypoperfusion also exists around the infarcted core. This zone is called the *penumbra*.[19] The size of this zone depends on the amount of collateral circulation present. Collateral circulation describes the vessels that augment the major circulatory vessels of the brain. Differences in the size and number of collateral vessels help explain variations in the severity of manifestations experienced by clients with strokes in the same anatomic area.

A cascade of biochemical processes occurs within minutes of cerebral ischemia. Neurotoxins including oxygen free radicals, nitric oxide, and glutamate are released. Local acidosis develops. Membrane depolarization occurs. This results in an influx of calcium and sodium. Cytotoxic edema and cell death are a result. This is secondary neuronal injury. Penumbral neurons are highly susceptible to the effects of the ischemic cascade. The area of edema after ischemia may lead to temporary neurologic deficits.

Edema may subside in a few hours or sometimes in several days, and the client may regain some function.

Most intracerebral hemorrhages are caused by the rupture of arteriosclerotic and hypertensive vessels. Most intracerebral hemorrhages are very large. Therefore, it is not surprising that hemorrhage into the brain causes the most fatalities of all strokes. Aneurysms are weakened outpouchings in a vessel wall. Although cerebral aneurysms are usually small (2 to 6 mm in diameter), they can rupture. An estimated 6% of all strokes are caused by aneurysm rupture. A stroke secondary to bleeding often produces spasm of cerebral vessels and cerebral ischemia because the blood outside of the vessels acts as an irritant to the tissues.

Clinical Manifestations

General findings of stroke unrelated to specific vessel sites include headache, vomiting, seizures, changes in mental status, fever, and changes on the electrocardiogram (ECG). ECG changes include T-wave changes, shortened PR interval, prolonged QT interval, premature ventricular contractions, sinus bradycardia, and ventricular and supraventricular tachycardias.[7]

EARLY WARNINGS
Manifestations of impending ischemic stroke include transient hemiparesis, loss of speech, and hemisensory loss. Manifestations of a thrombotic stroke develop over minutes to hours to days. The slow onset is related to the increasing size of the thrombus, with partial and then complete occlusion of the affected vessel. In contrast, manifestations of embolic strokes occur suddenly and without warning.

Hemorrhagic stroke occurs rapidly, with manifestations developing over minutes to hours. Common manifestations include severe occipital or nuchal headaches, vertigo or syncope, paresthesias, transient paralysis, epistaxis, and retinal hemorrhages.

Manifestations of deficit must persist longer than 24 hours to be diagnostic of stroke. TIAs are focal neurologic deficits lasting less than 24 hours.

SPECIFIC DEFICITS AFTER STROKE
Stroke manifestations can be correlated with the cause (Table 70–1) and with the area of the brain in which perfusion is impaired (Table 70–2). The middle cerebral artery is the most common site of ischemic stroke. The client's deficit also varies according to whether the dominant or the nondominant side of the brain is affected. The degree of deficit can also vary from little impairment to serious functional loss.

Hemiparesis and Hemiplegia
Hemiparesis (weakness) or hemiplegia (paralysis) of one side of the body may occur after a stroke. These deficits are usually caused by a stroke in the anterior or middle cerebral artery, leading to an infarction in the motor strip of the frontal cortex. Complete hemiplegia involves half of the face and tongue as well as the arm and leg of the ipsilateral side of the body. Infarction in the right side of the brain causes left-sided hemiplegia, and vice versa, because nerve fibers cross over in the pyramidal tract as they pass from the brain to the spinal cord. Strokes causing hemiparesis or hemiplegia usually affect other cortical

areas in addition to the motor strip. As a result, hemiparesis and hemiplegia are often accompanied by other manifestations of stroke, including hemisensory loss, hemianopia, apraxia, agnosia, and aphasia. Muscles of the thorax and abdomen are usually not affected because they are innervated from both cerebral hemispheres.

When voluntary muscle control is lost, strong flexor muscles overbalance the extensors. This imbalance can cause serious contractures. For example, a hemiplegic client's affected arm tends to rotate internally and to adduct, because adductor muscles are stronger than abductors. The elbow, wrist, and fingers also tend to flex. The affected leg tends to rotate externally at the hip joint, flex at the knee, and plantar flex and supinate at the ankle joint (Fig. 70–2).

Aphasia
Aphasia is a deficit in the ability to communicate. Aphasia may involve any or all aspects of communication, including speaking, reading, writing, and understanding spoken language. The primary language center is usually located in the left cerebral hemisphere and is affected by stroke in the left middle cerebral artery. There are several different types of aphasia. The most common are described here.

Wernicke's (sensory or *receptive) aphasia* affects speech comprehension as a result of an infarction in the temporal lobe of the brain. *Broca's (expressive* or *motor) aphasia* affects speech production as a result of an infarction in the frontal lobe of the brain. Branches of the

TABLE 70–1	CLINICAL MANIFESTATIONS OF THE VARIOUS CAUSES OF CEREBROVASCULAR ACCIDENT
Cause	**Clinical Manifestations**
Thrombosis	Tends to develop during sleep or within 1 hour of arising Ischemia is produced gradually; therefore, the clinical manifestations develop more slowly than those caused by hemorrhage or emboli Relative preservation of consciousness Hypertension
Embolism	No discernible time pattern, unrelated to activity Clinical manifestations occur rapidly, within 10–30 seconds, and often without warning May have rapid improvement Relative preservation of consciousness Normotension
Hemorrhage	Typically occurs during active, waking hours Severe headache and nuchal rigidity occur (if client is able to report manifestations) Rapid onset of complete hemiplegia, occurs over minutes to 1 hour Usually results in extensive, permanent loss of function with slower, less complete recovery Rapid progression into coma

TABLE 70-2

CLINICAL MANIFESTATIONS OF CEREBROVASCULAR ACCIDENTS ASSOCIATED WITH AREA OF BRAIN AFFECTED

Location	Middle Cerebral Artery	Anterior Cerebral Artery	Posterior Cerebral Artery	Internal Carotid Artery	Vertebrobasilar System	Anteroinferior Cerebellar (Lateral Pontine)	Posteroinferior Cerebellar
Motor changes	Contralateral hemiparesis or hemiplegia, face and arm deficits greater than leg	Contralateral hemiparesis, foot and leg deficits greater than arm, footdrop, gait disturbances	Mild contralateral hemiparesis (with thalamic or subthalamic involvement) Intention tremor	Contralateral hemiparesis with facial asymmetry	Alternating motor weaknesses Ataxic gait, dysmetria (uncoordinated actions)	Ipsilateral ataxia Facial paralysis	Ataxia Paralysis of larynx and soft palate
Sensory changes	Contralateral hemisensory alterations Neglect of involved extremities	Contralateral hemisensory alterations	Diffuse sensory loss (thalamic)	Contralateral sensory alterations	Contralateral hemisensory impairments	Ipsilateral loss of sensation in face, sensation changes on trunk and limbs	Ipsilateral loss of sensation in face, contralateral on body
Visual or ocular changes	Homonymous hemianopia Inability to turn eyes toward affected side	Deviation of eyes toward affected side	Pupillary dysfunction (brain stem) Loss of conjugate gaze, nystagmus Loss of depth perception Cortical blindness Homonymous hemianopia	Homonymous hemianopia Ipsilateral periods of blindness (amaurosis fugax)	Double vision Homonymous hemianopia Nystagmus, conjugate gaze paralysis	Nystagmus	Nystagmus
Speech changes	Dyslexia, dysgraphia, aphasia	Expressive aphasia	Perseveration Dyslexia	Aphasia if dominant hemisphere is involved	Dysarthria		Dysarthria
Mental changes	Memory deficits	Confusion, amnesia Flat affect, apathy Shortened attention span Loss of mental acuity	Memory deficits		Memory loss Disorientation		
Other changes	Vomiting may occur	Apraxia (inability to carry out purposeful movements in nonaffected areas) Incontinence	Visual hallucinations	Mild Horner's syndrome Carotid bruits	Drop attacks Tinnitus, hearing loss Vertigo Dysphagia Coma or locked-in syndrome	Horner's syndrome Tinnitus, hearing loss	Horner's syndrome Hiccups and coughing Vertigo Nausea, vomiting

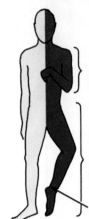

"Frozen" shoulder
Subluxation of the shoulder
Painful shoulder-hand dystrophy

Adduction of arm with internal rotation. Flexion of elbow wrist and fingers.
External rotation of leg at hip joint; flexion at knee; and plantar flexion and supination at ankle.

Shortened heel cord

FIGURE 70–2 Hemiplegic contractures. The elbow is bent, the wrist is flexed, and the fingers are curled into palmar flexion; the knee is bent and the heel cord is shortened.

middle cerebral artery supply both areas. *Global aphasia* affects both speech comprehension and speech production.

Other methods of classifying aphasia are by fluency or by the degree of difficulty in articulation. Clients with fluent aphasia (Wernicke's) have speech that is well articulated and grammatically correct but lacks content. Clients with nonfluent aphasia (Broca's) have varying degrees of difficulty in producing speech, and what words are spoken are uttered slowly, with great effort and poor articulation. Clients with global aphasia typically repeat the same sounds they hear and have poor comprehension.

Sensory or fluent aphasias involve loss of the ability to comprehend written, printed, or spoken words. A client with acoustic aphasia can hear the sounds of speech, but the parts of the brain that give meaning to these sounds are damaged. Clients have difficulty understanding what is being said. They hear sound but cannot make sense of it, because they cannot understand the symbolic communication associated with the sound. Visual aphasia is similar. Affected clients cannot read words but can see them. They cannot understand the symbolic content of printed or written symbols.

Motor or nonfluent aphasias include aphasias in which the ability to write, make signs, or speak is lost. For example, with motor aphasia, words may be recalled but the client cannot combine speech sounds into words and syllables. Pure motor or pure sensory aphasias are rare. Most aphasias are mixed, affecting both expressive and receptive elements.

Most aphasias are partial rather than complete. The severity of aphasia varies with the area involved and the extent of cerebral damage. Severe damage may deprive the client of any meaningful relationship with the environment and family. Global aphasia can be so extensive that neither expressive nor receptive language abilities are retained. Early determination of the client's yes-no reliability facilitates communication. Verbal skills are often the best. Reading and writing are usually more impaired. The use of gestures can aid in communication.

Aphasia is frequently associated with hemiplegia involving the dominant hemisphere. The speech center for a right-handed client is usually located in the left cerebral hemisphere; the speech center for a left-handed client may be in the brain's right or left side. Thus, a right-handed client with right-sided hemiplegia usually has aphasia because the speech center is in the damaged left hemisphere. Most people have left-sided speech dominance.

Dysarthria

Dysarthria is imperfect articulation that causes difficulty in speaking. It is important to differentiate between dysarthria and aphasia. With dysarthria, the client understands language but has difficulty pronouncing words and may slur them, enunciating poorly. No disturbance is evident in grammar or in sentence construction. A dysarthric client can understand verbal speech and can read and write (unless the dominant hand is paralyzed, absent, or injured).

Dysarthria is caused by cranial nerve dysfunction from a stroke in the vertebrobasilar artery or its branches. It may result from weakness or paralysis of the muscles of the lips, tongue, and larynx or from a loss of sensation. In addition to speaking problems, clients with dysarthria often have difficulty chewing and swallowing because of poor muscle control.

Dysphagia

Swallowing is a complex process requiring the function of several cranial nerves. The mouth must open (cranial nerve V), the lips must close (cranial nerve VII), and the tongue must move (cranial nerve XII). The mouth must sense the quantity and quality of the food bolus (cranial nerves V and VII) and must send messages to the swallowing center (cranial nerves V and IX). During swallowing, the tongue moves the food bolus toward the oropharynx. The pharynx elevates and the glottis closes. Contraction of the pharyngeal muscles transports food from the pharynx to the esophagus. Peristalsis moves food to the stomach. A stroke in the territory of the vertebrobasilar system causes dysphagia.

Apraxia

Apraxia is a condition affecting complex motor integration and therefore can result from a stroke in several areas in the brain. In apraxia, the client cannot carry out a skilled act such as dressing in the absence of paralysis. A client with apraxia may be able to conceive or conceptualize the content of messages to send to muscles. However, the motor patterns or schema necessary to convey the impulse message cannot be reconstructed. Thus, accurate "instructions" do not reach the limb from the brain, and the desired action or movement does not happen. Apraxia ranges from relatively simple to highly complex disorders. For example, a client may have less difficulty writing than speaking or vice versa.

Visual Changes

Vision is a complex process controlled by several areas in the brain. Parietal and temporal lobe strokes may interrupt visual fibers of the optic tract en route to the occipital cortex and impair visual acuity. Depth perception and visual perception of horizontal and vertical planes may also be impaired. In clients with hemiplegia, this causes motor performance problems in gait and posture (Fig. 70–3). Clients may or may not be aware of a perceptual difficulty, but it may cause them to be accident-prone and

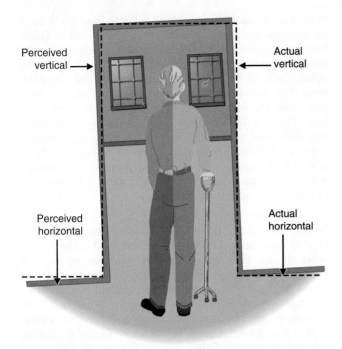

Perceived vertical →

← Actual vertical

Perceived horizontal →

← Actual horizontal

FIGURE 70–3 Perceptual disturbances in hemiplegia. Such disturbances can be both unpleasant and unsafe.

their behavior to appear bizarre. Visual disorders may interfere with a client's ability to relearn motor skills. Infarcts affecting the function of cranial nerves III, IV, and VI may produce cranial nerve palsies and result in diplopia.

HOMONYMOUS HEMIANOPIA. Homonymous hemianopia (Fig. 70–4) is a visual loss in the same half of the visual field of each eye, so the client has only half of normal vision. For example, the client may see clearly on one side of the midline but see nothing on the other side. Clients with homonymous hemianopia cannot see past the midline without turning the head toward that side.

HORNER'S SYNDROME. Horner's syndrome is the paralysis of sympathetic nerves to the eye, causing sinking of the eyeball, ptosis of the upper eyelid, slight elevation of the lower lid, constriction of the pupil, and lack of tearing in the eye.

Agnosia

Agnosia is a disturbance in the ability to recognize familiar objects through the senses. The most common types are visual and auditory. Agnosia may result from an occlusion of the middle or posterior cerebral arteries supplying the temporal or occipital lobes.

A client with visual agnosia sees objects but is unable to recognize or attach meaning to them. Disorientation occurs because of an inability to recognize environmental cues, familiar faces, or symbols. Such a client may examine objects curiously but be unable to determine their function. This can cause considerable self-care deficit when common, necessary objects, such as silverware, clothing, or toilet articles, are unfamiliar. Visual agnosia greatly increases the risk for injury because the client cannot recognize danger or symbols that warn of danger. Extensive visual agnosia can produce such extreme be-

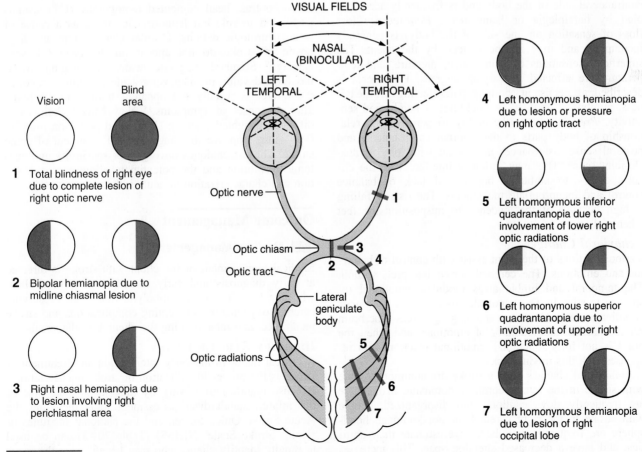

FIGURE 70–4 Visual field defects associated with optic nerve lesions.

havioral effects that the client's condition may be inaccurately diagnosed as diffuse dementia.

A client with auditory agnosia cannot attach meaning to sounds in the absence of hearing loss or decreased level of consciousness. Some degree of aphasia is almost always present. Often, these people are initially considered hysterical or psychotic.

Unilateral Neglect

Unilateral neglect is the inability of a person to respond to stimulus on the contralateral side of a cerebral infarction. Clients with injury to the temporoparietal lobe, inferior parietal lobe, lateral frontal lobe, cingulate gyrus, thalamus, and striatum as a result of a middle cerebral artery occlusion most commonly develop neglect. Because of the dominance of the right hemisphere in directing attention, neglect is most commonly seen in clients with right hemisphere damage.

Clinical manifestations of unilateral neglect include failure to (1) attend to one side of the body, (2) report or respond to stimuli on one side of the body, (3) use one extremity, and (4) orient the head and eyes to one side. Unilateral neglect may be accompanied by inaccurate beliefs about the position of a limb in space or its existence or ownership. For example, a man with unilateral neglect may not believe that his arm is part of his body, he may be unaware of his arm's position, or he may deny that a limb is paralyzed when it is.

Sensory Deficits

Several types of sensory changes can result from a stroke in the sensory strip of the parietal lobe supplied by the anterior or middle cerebral artery. The deficit is on the contralateral side of the body and is frequently accompanied by hemiplegia or hemiparesis. *Hemisensory* loss (loss of sensation on one side of the body) is generally incomplete and may not be noticed by the client. The superficial sensations of pain, touch, pressure, and temperature are affected in varying degrees. Paresthesia is described as persistent, burning pain; feelings of heaviness, numbness, tingling, or prickling; or heightened sensitivity. *Proprioception* (the ability to perceive the relationship of body parts to the external environment) and postural sense disturbances may occur with loss of muscle-joint sense. This may seriously interfere with the client's ability to ambulate because of lack of balance control and inappropriate movements. The risk of falling is high because of the tendency to misposition the feet when walking.

Behavioral Changes

Various portions of the brain assist with control of behavior and emotions. The cerebral cortex interprets stimuli. The temporal and limbic areas modulate emotional responses to stimuli. The hypothalamus and pituitary glands coordinate the motor cortex and language areas. The brain can be seen as a modulator of emotions, and when the brain is not fully functional, emotional reactions and responses lack this modulation.

Behavioral changes after a stroke are common. People with stroke in the left cerebral, or dominant, hemisphere are frequently slow, cautious, and disorganized. People with stroke in the right cerebral, or nondominant, hemisphere are frequently impulsive, overestimate their abilities, and have a decreased attention span. This increases

their risk of injury. Frontal lobe infarcts from a stroke in the anterior or middle cerebral arteries may lead to disturbances in memory, judgment, abstract thinking, insight, inhibition, and emotion.[49] The client may exhibit a flat affect, lack of spontaneity, distractibility, and forgetfulness. The client may have emotional lability and burst into tears or, less commonly, laughter without provocation. There is little or no relationship between the emotion and what is occurring in the person's environment. Significant clinical depression occurs in 25% to 60% of clients with strokes.[18, 23] Because depression can interfere with rehabilitation and functional recovery, it is important to identify it and initiate treatment.[35]

Incontinence

Stroke may cause bowel and bladder dysfunction. One type of neurogenic bladder, an uninhibited bladder, sometimes occurs after stroke. Nerves send the message of bladder filling to the brain, but the brain does not correctly interpret the message and does not transmit the message not to urinate to the bladder. This results in frequency, urgency, and incontinence. Sometimes clients with a type of neurogenic bowel seem fixated on having a bowel movement. Other causes of incontinence may be memory lapses, inattention, emotional factors, inability to communicate, impaired physical mobility, and infection. The duration and severity of the dysfunction depend on the extent and location of the infarct.[9]

DIAGNOSTIC FINDINGS

With the advent of thrombolytic therapy in the treatment of acute ischemic stroke, accurate brain imaging plays an important role in the diagnosis and treatment of stroke.[15] A noncontrast head computed tomography (CT) scan is performed to rule out hemorrhagic stroke as a cause of acute neurologic deficits. Cellular changes that are diagnostic of stroke do not appear on the head CT scan acutely.[39] Standard magnetic resonance imaging (MRI) has limited value in diagnosing acute ischemic stroke, as the infarct is usually not apparent until 8 to 12 hours after the onset of symptoms.[15] New MRI techniques—diffusion-weighted imaging (DWI) and perfusion imaging (PI)—may improve the diagnosis and treatment of acute stroke. These techniques have greater sensitivity and anatomic resolution and the potential to allow earlier detection and characterization of acute ischemic stroke.[37]

Outcome Management

■ Medical Management

Medical management of the client with stroke is directed at early diagnosis and early identification of the client who can benefit from thrombolytic treatment. Preserving cerebral oxygenation, preventing complications and stroke recurrence, and rehabilitating the client are other goals.

IDENTIFY STROKE EARLY

A critical factor in the early intervention and treatment of stroke is the proper identification of stroke manifestations. Because manifestations vary by the location and size of the infarct, standardized assessment tools including the Acute Stroke Quick Screen and the National Institutes of Health Stroke Scale (NIHSS) (Table 70–3) can be used to rapidly identify clients who may benefit from thrombo-

Text continued on page 1963

TABLE 70-3	NATIONAL INSTITUTES OF HEALTH (NIH) STROKE SCALE

Administer stroke scale items in the order listed. Scores should reflect what the patient does, not what the clinician thinks the patient can do. Except where indicated, the patient should not be coached (i.e., repeated requests to patient to make a special effort).

Instruction	Scale Definition
1a. Level of Consciousness The investigator must choose a response, even if a full evaluation is prevented by such obstacles as an endotracheal tube, language barrier, or orotracheal trauma or bandages. A **3** is scored only if the patient makes no movement (other than reflexive posturing) in response to noxious stimulation.	0 = Alert, keenly responsive 1 = Not alert, but arousable by minor stimulation to obey, answer, or respond 2 = Not alert, requires repeated stimulation or painful stimulation to make movements (not stereotyped) 3 = Responds only with reflex motor or autonomic effects, or totally unresponsive, flaccid, areflexic
1b. LOC Questions The patient is asked the month and his or her age. The answer must be correct—there is no partial credit for being close. Aphasic and stuporous patients who do not comprehend the questions will score **2**. Patients unable to speak because of endotracheal intubation, orotracheal trauma, severe dysarthria from any cause, language barrier, or any other problem not secondary to aphasia are given a **1**. It is important that only the initial answer be graded and that the examiner not "help" the patient with verbal or nonverbal cues.	0 = Answers both questions correctly 1 = Answers one question correctly 2 = Answers neither question correctly
1c. LOC Commands The patient is asked to open and close the eyes and then to grip and release the nonparetic hand. Substitute another one-step command if the hands cannot be used. Credit is given if an unequivocal attempt is made but not completed due to weakness. If patients do not respond to command, the task should be demonstrated to them (pantomime) and score the result (i.e., follows none, one, or two commands). Patients with trauma, amputation, or other physical impediments should be given suitable one-step commands. Only the first attempt is scored.	0 = Performs both tasks correctly 1 = Performs one task correctly 2 = Performs neither task correctly
2. Best Gaze Only horizontal eye movements will be tested. Voluntary or reflexive (oculocephalic) eye movements will be scored, but caloric testing is not done. If the patient has a conjugate deviation of the eyes that can be overcome by voluntary or reflexive activity, the score will be **1**. If a patient has an isolated peripheral nerve paresis (CN III, IV, or VI), score a **1**. Gaze is testable in all aphasic patients. Patients with ocular trauma, bandages, pre-existing blindness, or other disorder of visual acuity or fields should be tested with reflexive movements, and a choice made by the investigator. Establishing eye contact and then moving about the patient from side to side will occasionally clarify the presence of a gaze palsy.	0 = Normal 1 = Partial gaze palsy; this score is given when gaze is abnormal in one or both eyes, but where forced deviation or total gaze paresis is not present 2 = Forced deviation or total gaze paresis not overcome by the oculocephalic maneuver
3. Visual Visual fields (upper and lower quadrants) are tested by confrontation, using finger counting or visual threat as appropriate. Patient must be encouraged, but if he or she looks at the side of the moving fingers appropriately, this can be scored as normal. If there is unilateral blindness or enucleation, visual fields in the remaining eye are scored. Score **1** only if a clear-cut asymmetry, including quadrantanopia, is found. If patient is blind from any cause, score **3**. Double simultaneous stimulation is performed at this point. If there is extinction, patient receives a **1** and the results are used to answer question 11.	0 = No visual loss 1 = Partial hemianopia 2 = Complete hemianopia 3 = Bilateral hemianopia (blind including cortical blindness)

Table continued on following page

TABLE 70–3	NATIONAL INSTITUTES OF HEALTH (NIH) STROKE SCALE *Continued*

Instruction	Scale Definition
4. Facial Palsy Ask or use pantomime to encourage the patient to show teeth or smile and close eyes. Score symmetry of grimace in response to noxious stimuli in the poorly responsive or noncomprehending patient. If facial trauma or bandages, orotracheal tube, tape, or other physical barrier obscures the face, these should be removed to the extent possible.	0 = Normal symmetrical movement 1 = Minor paralysis (flattened nasolabial fold, asymmetry on smiling) 2 = Partial paralysis (total or near total paralysis of lower face) 3 = Complete paralysis (absence of facial movement in the upper and lower face)
5 and 6. Motor Arm and Leg The limb is placed in the appropriate position: extend the arms 90 degrees (if sitting) or 45 degrees (if supine) and the leg 30 degrees (always tested supine). Drift is scored if the arm falls before 10 seconds or the leg before 5 seconds. The aphasic patient is encouraged using urgency in the voice and pantomime but not noxious stimulation. Each limb is tested in turn, beginning with the nonparetic arm. Only in the case of amputation or joint fusion at the shoulder or hip may the score be **9**, and the examiner must clearly write the explanation for scoring as a **9**.	0 = No drift; limb holds 90 degrees (or 45 degrees) for full 10 seconds 1 = Drift; limb holds 90 degrees (or 45 degrees) but drifts down before full 10 seconds; does not hit bed or other support 2 = Some effort against gravity; limb cannot get to or maintain (if cued) 90 degrees (or 45 degrees), drifts down to bed but has some effort against gravity 3 = No effort against gravity; limb falls 4 = No movement 9 = Amputation, joint fusion; explain: 5a = Left arm 5b = Right arm 0 = No drift; leg holds 30 degrees for full 5 seconds 1 = Drift; leg falls by the end of the 5-second period but does not hit bed 2 = Some effort against gravity; leg falls to bed by 5 seconds but has some effort against gravity 3 = No effort against gravity; leg falls to bed immediately 4 = No movement 9 = Amputation, joint fusion; explain: 6a = Left leg 6b = Right leg

7. Limb Ataxia
This item is aimed at finding evidence of a unilateral cerebellar lesion. Test with eyes open. In case of visual defect, ensure testing is done in intact visual field. The finger-nose-finger and heel-shin tests are performed on both sides, and ataxia is scored only if present out of proportion to weakness. Ataxia is absent in the patient who cannot understand or is hemiplegic. Only in the case of amputation or joint fusion may the item be scored **9**, and the examiner must clearly write the explanation for not scoring. In case of blindness, test by touching nose from extended arm position.
	0 = Absent
	1 = Present in one limb
	2 = Present in two limbs
	If present, is ataxia in
	  Right arm: 1 = Yes 2 = No
	    9 = Amputation or joint fusion;
	    explain:
	  Left arm: 1 = Yes 2 = No
	    9 = Amputation or joint fusion;
	    explain:
	  Right leg: 1 = Yes 2 = No
	    9 = Amputation or joint fusion;
	    explain:
	  Left leg: 1 = Yes 2 = No
	    9 = Amputation or joint fusion;
	    explain:

8. Sensory Sensation or grimace to pinprick when tested or withdrawal from noxious stimulus in the obtunded or aphasic patient. Only sensory loss attributed to stroke is scored as abnormal, and the examiner should test as many body areas (arms [not hands], legs, trunk, face) as needed to accurately check for hemisensory loss. A score of **2**, "severe or total," should only be given when a severe or total loss of sensation can be clearly demonstrated. Stuporous and aphasic patients will therefore probably score **1** or **0**. The patient with brain stem stroke who has bilateral loss of sensation is scored **2**. If the patient does not respond and is quadriplegic, score **2**. Patients in coma (question 1a = 3) are arbitrarily given a **2** on this item.	0 = Normal; no sensory loss 1 = Mild to moderate sensory loss; patient feels pinprick is less sharp or is dull on the affected side, or there is a loss of superficial pain with pinprick but patient is aware he or she is being touched 2 = Severe to total sensory loss; patient is not aware of being touched

TABLE 70–3	NATIONAL INSTITUTES OF HEALTH (NIH) STROKE SCALE *Continued*

Instruction	Scale Definition
9. Best Language A great deal of information about comprehension will be obtained during the preceding sections of the examination. The patient is asked to describe what is happening in the attached picture, to name the items on the attached naming sheet, and to read from the attached list of sentences. Comprehension is judged from responses here as well as to all of the commands in the preceding general neurologic examination. If visual loss interferes with the tests, ask the patient to identify objects placed in the hand, repeat, and produce speech. The intubated patient should be asked to write a sentence. The patient in coma (question 1a = 3) will arbitrarily score **3** on this item. The examiner must choose a score in the patient with stupor or limited cooperation, but a score of **3** should be used only if the patient is mute and follows no one-step commands.	0 = No aphasia; normal 1 = Mild to moderate aphasia; some obvious loss of fluency or facility of comprehension, without significant limitation on ideas expressed or form of expression. Reduction of speech and/or comprehension, however, makes conversation about provided material difficult or impossible. For example, in conversation about provided materials examiner can identify picture or naming card from patient's response. 2 = Severe aphasia; all communication is through fragmentary expression; great need for inference, questioning, and guessing by the listener. Range of information that can be exchanged is limited; listener carries burden of communication. Examiner cannot identify materials provided from patient response. 3 = Mute, global aphasia; no usable speech or auditory comprehension
10. Dysarthria If the patient is thought to be normal, an adequate sample of speech must be obtained by asking patient to read or repeat words from the attached list. If the patient has severe aphasia, the clarity of articulation of spontaneous speech can be rated. Only if the patient is intubated or has other physical barriers to producing speech may the item be scored **9**, and the examiner must clearly write an explanation for not scoring. Do not tell the patient why he or she is being tested.	0 = Normal 1 = Mild to moderate; patient slurs at least some words and, at worst, can be understood with some difficulty 2 = Severe; patient's speech is so slurred as to be unintelligible in the absence of or out of proportion to any dysphasia, or is mute/anarthric 9 = Intubated or other physical barrier; explain:
11. Extinction and Inattention (formerly Neglect) Sufficient information to identify neglect may be obtained during the prior testing. If the patient has severe visual loss preventing visual double simultaneous stimulation, and the cutaneous stimuli are normal, the score is normal. If the patient has aphasia but does appear to attend to both sides, the score is normal. The presence of visual spatial neglect or anosognosia may also be taken as evidence of neglect. Because neglect is scored only if present, the item is never untestable.	0 = No abnormality 1 = Visual, tactile, auditory, spatial, or personal inattention or extinction to bilateral simultaneous stimulation in one of the sensory modalities 2 = Profound hemi-inattention or hemi-inattention to more than one modality; does not recognize own hand or orients to only one side of space

Additional item, not part of the NIH Stroke Scale score.
 	
12. Distal Motor Function
The patient's hand is held up at the forearm by the examiner, and patient is asked to extend his or her fingers as much as possible. If the patient cannot or does not extend the fingers, the examiner places the fingers in full extension and observes for any flexion movement for 5 seconds. The patient's first attempts only are scored. Repetition of the instructions or of the testing is prohibited.
	0 = Normal (no flexion after 5 seconds)
	1 = At least some extension after 5 seconds but not fully extended; any movement of the fingers that is not a command is not scored
	2 = No voluntary extension after 5 seconds; movement of the fingers at another time is not scored
	    a. Left arm
	    b. Right arm

CN, cranial nerve; LOC, level of consciousness.
Modified from National Institutes of Health, Bethesda, MD.

lytic therapy.[39, 46] The assessment must be complete and accurate to provide a baseline for ongoing assessments.

The initial assessment of the client who is thought to have had a stroke includes level of consciousness, pupillary response to light, visual fields, movement of extremities, speech, sensation, reflexes, ataxia, and vital signs. These data are often recorded and scored on the Glasgow Coma Scale (GCS). In addition, if intracranial pressure monitors are in place, baseline pressure values and waveforms should be noted.

A complete history of the presenting problem as well as past medical and social history provides data about the cause of the stroke. This information also guides stroke treatment. The time of onset of manifestations must be determined, as thrombolytic therapy must be administered within 3 hours of the onset of manifestations. A history of hypertension or cardiac valve disorders is commonly associated with stroke.

MAINTAIN CEREBRAL OXYGENATION

Emergency care of the client with stroke includes maintaining a patent airway. The client should be turned on the affected side if he or she is unconscious, to promote drainage of saliva from the airway. The collar of the shirt should be loosened to facilitate venous return. The head should be elevated, but the neck should not be flexed. The person should be kept quiet, and emergency help should be contacted.

Once the client is in the emergency department (ED), a patent airway is maintained and oxygen is supplied. If the client demonstrates poor ventilatory effort, intubation and mechanical ventilation may be required to prevent hypoxia and increased cerebral ischemia. An ECG is performed to assess for cardiac disorders, such as atrial fibrillation, that increase the risk for embolic stroke. Blood pressure is also evaluated, and hypertension may be reduced with vasodilators. Caution is exercised when treating blood pressure, as lowering the blood pressure too far may lower cerebral perfusion pressure and increase cerebral ischemia.[19, 39] Laboratory tests for hematology, chemistry, and coagulation are obtained to rule out stroke-mimicking conditions and to detect bleeding disorders that would increase the risk of bleeding during thrombolytic therapy.

RESTORE CEREBRAL BLOOD FLOW

The client is evaluated as a candidate for thrombolytic therapy once an intracerebral hemorrhage is ruled out. The goal of thrombolytic therapy is recanalization of the occluded vessel and reperfusion of ischemic brain tissue.[13, 26] Thrombolytic agents are exogenous plasminogen activators, which dissolve the thrombus or embolus blocking the cerebral blood flow.[27] Clients who receive recombinant tissue plasminogen activator (rt-PA) within 3 hours of the onset of stroke are 30% more likely to have minimal or no disability from acute ischemic stroke without an increase in mortality.[31, 38]

There are several contraindications to thrombolytic therapy:

• More than 3 hours from onset
• Intracranial hemorrhage on CT scan
• Rapidly improving stroke manifestations or TIA
• Recent stroke, intracranial surgery, or head trauma
• Uncontrolled hypertension
• Conditions that may increase the risk for systemic bleeding, such as active internal bleeding within 21 days, a major surgery within 14 days, or current use of oral anticoagulants, are also contraindications for thrombolytic therapy.

Treatment should begin immediately after the client is deemed to be a candidate for rt-PA. The dose of rt-PA for acute ischemic stroke is 0.9 mg/kg administered intravenously over 1 hour. Ten per cent of the total dose is given as a bolus over 1 minute prior to the initiation of the intravenous dose.[32, 38, 39] The pharmacologic half-life of rt-PA is approximately 5 to 7 minutes. After thrombolytic therapy, the client is sent to the intensive care unit (ICU) for careful monitoring of blood pressure, neurologic status, and bleeding.

The risk-benefit ratio for the use of thrombolytic therapy must be considered in certain client populations. The choice of whether to pursue aggressive treatment focuses on several factors, such as the client's age, his or her preference (if known), the presence and severity of other disorders, the size of the infarction, how much time has elapsed since the infarction, and the rehabilitation potential. The risk of intracerebral hemorrhage after rt-PA is greater in clients with early signs of a major infarct on CT scan.[47, 50] People with severe neurologic deficits at presentation (NIHSS > 22) are at increased risk for intracerebral hemorrhage and poor outcome.[39, 50]

At present, the treatment for most clients with large areas of infarction or large intracerebral hemorrhage is supportive care. It is hoped that future research can improve the treatment outcomes for these clients.

PREVENT COMPLICATIONS

Bleeding

Following the administration of rt-PA, the client is monitored for potential complications of rt-PA, which may include intracranial hemorrhage and systemic bleeding.[1] In the initial studies of rt-PA in acute ischemic stroke, symptomatic intracranial hemorrhage occurred in 6.4% of clients within the first 36 hours after treatment.[31] Intracranial hemorrhage carries a mortality rate of greater than 50%.[26] All fatal intracranial hemorrhages occurred within the first 24 hours of treatment.[1] The expanding clot of an intracranial hemorrhage destroys brain tissue. The pressure of the clot also disrupts blood flow and causes additional ischemia. Increased intracranial pressure (ICP) results from the space-occupying clot and surrounding edema of ischemic tissue. This can lead to midline shift of intracranial contents, possible brain stem herniation, and death. To decrease the risk of intracranial or systemic bleeding, anticoagulants and antiplatelet medications are not recommended until 24 hours after administration of rt-PA.[5]

Stringent blood pressure management is the single most important measure to prevent intracranial hemorrhage after thrombolysis.[1] Frequent vital signs and neurologic checks are necessary to prevent hypertension and detect signs of intracranial hemorrhage. Hypertension frequently accompanies acute ischemic stroke. Therefore, blood pressure is usually not treated unless it increases to 185 mm Hg systolic or 105 mm Hg diastolic.[1] In addition, the mean arterial pressure should be lowered no more than 10% and in gradual increments.[43] This is less likely to lead to hypoperfusion and worsening cerebral ischemia.

An intracranial hemorrhage should be suspected if the client has new complaints of headache, nausea and vomiting, or sudden change in level of consciousness. An intracranial hemorrhage should be assumed with any acute worsening of neurologic function until it can be ruled out by CT scan. If the rt-PA is still infusing, the infusion should be stopped. A complete blood count, coagulation studies, and type and cross are done. If a head CT scan reveals intracranial hemorrhage, fresh frozen plasma with fibrinogen or cryoprecipitate is administered to correct coagulopathies.

Systemic bleeding may also occur as a complication of rt-PA. Clinical manifestations include change in level of consciousness (LOC), tachycardia, hypotension, and cool, clammy, and pale skin. Thrombolytic therapy may be stopped depending on the site and severity of the bleeding.[19]

Cerebral Edema

Increased ICP is a potential complication of large ischemic strokes.[29] Increased ICP is also a potential complication of intracerebral hemorrhage, either primary or secondary to thrombolytic therapy. Manifestations of increased ICP include change in LOC, reflex hypertension, and worsening neurologic status. Invasive monitoring of ICP is done for those clients with decreased LOC who are at high risk for increased ICP. All clients are placed on bed rest with the head of the bed elevated to 30 degrees to decrease ICP and to facilitate venous drainage. Ideally, the degree of head elevation is based on the response of the client's ICP for those clients on ICP monitoring.[30, 44]

External *ventriculostomy* drainage is sometimes used to reduce pressure from cerebrospinal fluid (CSF) accumulation. A burr hole is placed through the skull, and a catheter is passed into the lateral ventricle to allow for controlled drainage of CSF. Blood pressure is closely monitored. The goal is to maintain blood pressure low enough to prevent another stroke or hemorrhage without decreasing cerebral perfusion. The client may require continuous mechanical ventilation and hyperventilation to decrease ICP. Mannitol, an osmotic diuretic, helps in lowering increased ICP. Surgical evacuation of the intracerebral hematoma may be performed. Increasing ICP, central herniation, and brain stem hemorrhage lead to death from depression of the vital centers in the medulla, that is, brain stem failure.

Stroke Recurrence

The incidence of stroke recurrence in the first 4 weeks after acute ischemic stroke ranges from 0.6% to 2.2% per week.[48] The risks of anticoagulation include intracranial hemorrhage, systemic bleeding, and death. Therefore, the general use of heparin in all clients with acute ischemic stroke is no longer recommended. Heparin is indicated to prevent stroke recurrence in clients at risk for cardiogenic emboli. Initially, unfractionated heparin is administered intravenously, and then warfarin is administered orally. Intravenous (IV) heparin is delivered with an infusion pump for accurate and safe delivery. Monitoring of clotting times is important to detect overanticoagulation, which increases the risk of bleeding. Activated partial thromboplastin time (aPTT) should be at 1.5 to 2.5 times control for anticoagulation to be effective.

After a therapeutic anticoagulant level has been achieved with heparin therapy, warfarin is begun. Because warfarin has a long half-life, the physician initiates the warfarin therapy while the client is still receiving IV heparin. Once the client has a therapeutic response to warfarin, in about 24 to 48 hours, the physician discontinues the heparin and continues the warfarin therapy. The therapeutic International Normalized Ratio (INR) for prophylaxis against cardiogenic embolization is 2.0 to 3.0.[43] Clients receiving anticoagulation therapy should be assessed for bruising, hematuria, blood in feces, bleeding from mucous membranes, and new-onset or worsening headaches.

The long-term risk for stroke recurrence is 4% to 14%

per year.[1] Antiplatelet agents, including aspirin, ticlopidine, and clopidogrel, decrease the risk for secondary stroke by 20% to 25%.[7, 40] Antiplatelet agents inhibit platelet function to decrease the risk of thrombus formation. The selection of the specific antiplatelet agent is individualized according to the client's medical history.

Aspiration

Clients with stroke are at high risk for aspiration pneumonia, which is the direct cause of death in 6% of strokes.[3] Aspiration is most common in the early period and is related to loss of pharyngeal sensation, loss of oropharyngeal motor control, and decreased LOC. Oral food and fluids are generally withheld for 24 to 48 hours. If the client cannot eat or drink after 48 hours, alternate feeding routes are used, such as tube-feeding or hyperalimentation. When the swallowing mechanism has returned, the client can be fed orally. Progressive feeding programs for dysphagia are based on the degree of swallowing ability.

Other Potential Complications

Other complications of stroke depend primarily on the location of the lesion or infarcted tissue. If the brain stem is affected, blood pressure fluctuations, altered respiratory patterns, and cardiac dysrhythmias are all possible. Physical injury related to the client's inability to realize his or her limitations can occur. Complications of immobility can also occur.

Coma can follow strokes of various causes. The blood supply to the brain stem or reticular activating system, which controls consciousness, may have been directly occluded. Similarly, the deep structures of the thalamus that relay information to the cerebral cortex may be involved. Vascular occlusion of the internal carotid artery or one of its major branches may also decrease LOC. Sometimes the cerebral edema that follows stroke may produce midline shifts, resulting in coma.

Hyperthermia is treated immediately with antipyretics. Temperature elevations lead to increased cerebral metabolic needs, which in turn cause cerebral edema and increased risk for cerebral ischemia. In addition, a hypothermia blanket or ice packs may be required to reduce body temperature. Causing the client to shiver should be avoided, however, because shivering increases oxygen consumption and ICP. If seizures develop, phenytoin (Dilantin) or phenobarbital may be used.

Strokes caused by occlusive disease (e.g., thrombus, embolus) rarely cause sudden death. When stroke is fatal, death may occur within 3 to 12 hours, but it more often occurs between 1 and 14 days after the original episode. Typically, with any type of fatal stroke, a rise in temperature, heart rate, and respiratory rate occurs along with deepening coma several hours or days before death. These are a result of damage to the vasomotor and heat-regulating centers. See the Case Study.

REHABILITATION AFTER STROKE

From the onset of stroke, interventions are aimed at maximizing the client's physical and cognitive recovery.[16] Early premobilization efforts are aimed at preventing the complications of neurologic deficit and immobility. After the first few days of the acute event, cerebral edema has usually subsided and the residual deficits of stroke can be identified. Clients with stroke and their families face diffi-

Meningioma, Fractured Hip, and Possible Cerebrovascular Accident

Mrs. Olsen is a 72-year-old white woman who resides at Shady Oaks Care Center. She fell today and could not get up again because of the pain. An x-ray obtained at the nursing home showed a proximal femoral fracture near the right hip joint. She has been transferred to your hospital for a preoperative medical evaluation in preparation for possible surgical repair of her right hip fracture later today.

Mrs. Olsen has a history of a meningioma, which has been resected three times. Two days ago, the client had an episode of apparent dysfunction of the left upper and

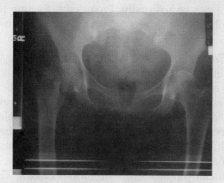

■ Radiograph of Mrs. Olsen's fracture of the proximal femur, near the right hip joint.

lower extremities associated with a period of hypertension and agitation, all of which resolved within 24 hours. Mrs. Olsen also has a history of deep vein thrombosis (DVT) following one of her surgical procedures, but is not receiving long-term anticoagulation therapy. What ramifications will this have for her current treatment?

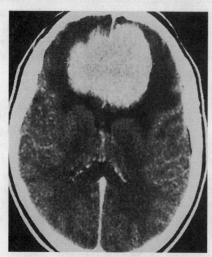

■ This contrast CT scan shows Mrs. Olsen's meningioma before resection.

Nursing Admission Assessment

Mrs. Olsen has lived at Shady Oaks since her last craniotomy, after which she developed seizures and was given

a regimen of phenytoin. The daughter states that her mother has had several falls during the past several days and seems imbalanced at times when she changes position.

Mrs. Olsen is a World War II immigrant from Denmark, where her siblings continue to live. Since her last craniotomy, she has been lapsing into intervals during which she uses her native language and believes that her daughter is her sister Ingrid. Consider the implications of this in your preoperative preparations. Mrs. Olsen denies discomfort at this time.

Mrs. Olsen taught high school mathematics until the time of her first craniotomy 10 years ago. Her husband died of a myocardial infarction last year.

Selected Admission Laboratory Values	
RBC	3.76 million/mm³
Hb	11.7 g/dl
Hct	34%
WBC	10,200/mm³
Sodium	141 mEq/L
Potassium	4.3 mEq/L
Chloride	101 mEq/L
CO_2	22 mEq/L
Glucose	157 mg/dl
ABO/Rh type	O⁺
Phenytoin level	7.6 μg/ml

Nursing Physical Examination

Height: 5'6"
Weight: 135 lb (61.4 kg)
Vital signs: BP = 170/90;
    TPR = 99.6, 102, 22
LOC: Awake, alert, slightly confused; daughter states that she is asking in Danish where she is and what happened
EENT: PERRLA, evidence of cranial surgical scars on right frontal region, slight left facial droop, hand grasps equal
Cardiac: Regular rate and rhythm without gallop or murmur
Pulmonary: Clear bilaterally
Abdominal: Soft, nontender, active bowel sounds
Genitourinary: Foley catheter inserted in ER draining clear yellow urine
Peripheral pulses: 3/4 without edema, some shortening of right lower extremity

Initial Treatment Plan

Meds: Phenytoin (Dilantin) 200 mg PO or IV bid
IV: D₅LR TKO
Diet: NPO
Activity: Bed rest with mattress overlay and trapeze

Additional assessments: Vital signs, neurologic checks, and neurovascular assessments checks q 4 h
Treatments: Ice to right hip continuously
Diagnostic tests: CT scan of head

Mrs. Olsen's CT scan revealed no further progression of her meningioma. She successfully underwent surgery for endoprosthetic replacement of the right proximal femur. Postoperatively, the surgeon orders:

- Advance diet as tolerated
- Soft wrist and Posey restraints as needed to protect self
- Physical therapy to initiate progressive ambulation with weight-bearing as tolerated
- Incentive spirometer while awake
- Medical therapy: cefazolin (Ancef) 1 g IV q 8 h × 4, Lovenox 30 mg SC q 12 h, docusate sodium (Colace) 100 mg PO daily, meperidine (Demerol) 75 mg with hydroxyzine (Vistaril) 25 mg IM q 3 h prn; and Vicodin 500 mg q 4 h prn.

Mrs. Olsen pulls out her Foley catheter 36 hours postoperatively. The urine had become cloudy and odorous. Recordings of the time and amount of voiding and trimethoprim-sulfamethoxazole (Bactrim) 1 tablet PO bid are ordered. Consider the factors that precipitated the need for this drug.

Mrs. Olsen continues to speak primarily in Danish. Because she is incontinent, she requires disposable undergarments. She also refuses to eat, and the nurse is unable to determine why. The IV infusion was discontinued after Mrs. Olsen pulled it out during her bath. Attempts at ambulation have been unsuccessful because of communication difficulties. A Danish interpreter is not available, and although Mrs. Olsen's daughter speaks Danish, she has had to return to her job and family responsibilities. The physician is planning to release Mrs. Olsen to Shady Oaks tomorrow.

Discharge Criteria

Average LOS (insurance certification): 8.5 days with transfer to skilled care on day 5.

Complete transfer form.
Initiate social services referral to coordinate transfer.

Questions to Be Considered

1. Mrs. Olsen becomes increasingly agitated while in restraints. What alternative measures might the nurse consider to protect Mrs. Olsen? Discuss the ethical implications surrounding physical and chemical restraints.
2. Consider the implications that Mrs. Olsen's neurologic problems—the meningioma, seizures, and a possible CVA—may have had in relationship to her fall. What other factors may have contributed to the fall? What actions should the nurse take to protect her from future injury?
3. Based on her admission assessment data, calculate Mrs. Olsen's score on the Glasgow Coma Scale. What influence does Mrs. Olsen's use of the Danish language have on your calculation? How is her situation different from someone who is not bilingual?
4. How has Mrs. Olsen's recovery been compromised because of her lack of mobilization? Identify potential complications that may occur as a result of immobility. How may they be prevented? Discuss methods of communication you might use to facilitate Mrs. Olsen's recovery and rehabilitation.
5. Discuss the effects that Mrs. Olsen's refusal to eat will have on the processes of wound healing and immunity.
6. Review the nursing implications and related patient education for administration of phenytoin and trimethoprim-sulfamethoxazole.
7. Compare and contrast brain tumors in terms of treatment and prognosis.

bid, twice daily; CO_2, carbon dioxide; CT, computed tomography; CVA, cerebrovascular accident; D_5LR, 5% dextrose in lactated Ringer's solution; ER, emergency room; EENT, ears, eyes, nose, throat; Hb, hemoglobin; Hct, hematocrit; μg, micrograms; IV, intravenous; LOC, level of consciousness; LOS, length of stay; NPO, nothing by mouth; PERRLA, pupils equal, round, reactive to light and accommodation; PO, orally; prn, as needed; RBC, red blood cell; SC, subcutaneous; TKO, to keep open; TPR, temperature, pulse, respirations; WBC, white blood cell count.

cult adjustments as the acute stages pass and residual disabilities become obvious.

Previously it had been thought that damage to the central nervous system (CNS) was irreversible. Now it has been shown that even in adults with significant brain injury, relearning can take place. It is extremely important that relearning take place as soon as possible after the injury. Early rehabilitation makes this relearning possible. Clients recover most of their function during the first 3 to 6 months after stroke but may continue to demonstrate modest improvement for 6 to 12 months after stroke.[23]

An interdisciplinary rehabilitation team is necessary to assist and support clients and their families during this time. Assessing the functional abilities of the client and setting realistic goals are part of this approach. To optimize recovery, all clinicians should use the Clinical Practice Guidelines developed by the Agency for Health Care Policy and Research (AHCPR) on post-stroke rehabilitation to guide care of a client suffering from a stroke.[35, 36]

Because stroke is a common health care problem, many facilities have developed clinical pathways to guide care. (See CareMap and Guide to Clinical Pathway.)

The recommended plan of care includes using interdisciplinary services to:

- Document the client's condition and course fully, including deficits, status of other diseases, complications, changes in status, and functional status before stroke
- Begin physical activity as soon as the client's medical condition is stable; use caution with early mobilization in clients with progressing neurologic deficit, subarachnoid or intracerebral hemorrhage, severe orthostatic hypotension, acute myocardial infarction, or acute deep vein thrombosis
- Assist in managing general health functions throughout all stages of treatment, such as managing dysphagia, nutrition, hydration, bladder and bowel function, sleep and rest, co-morbid conditions, and acute illnesses

- Prevent complications, including deep vein thrombosis and pulmonary embolism, aspiration, skin breakdown, urinary tract infections, falls, spasticity and contractures, shoulder injury, and seizures
- Prevent recurrent strokes through control of modifiable risk factors, oral anticoagulation, antiplatelet therapy, or surgical intervention
- Assess throughout acute and rehabilitation stages
- Use reliable standardized instruments for evaluation
- Evaluate for formal rehabilitation during acute stage
- Choose individual or interdisciplinary program based on the client's and family's needs; success of the program requires full support and active participation of the client and family; families must be involved at the outset
- Choose the local rehabilitation program that best meets the client's and family's needs

INTERDISCIPLINARY MANAGEMENT

Several other disciplines join to facilitate recovery of the client following a stroke. It is the coordinated effort of the entire team that best serves the client and family.

GUIDE TO CLINICAL PATHWAY

Stroke

The care of a client with a stroke revolves around quick diagnosis and treatment. Some strokes, if detected early, can be treated with fibrinolytic medications. This care map guides the care of a client with a completed stroke. The expected length of stay is 5 days to diagnose and treat the stroke and to begin rehabilitation of the client and family.

By the second day of hospitalization, the client will have undergone computed tomography, carotid Doppler imaging, and echocardiography. On day 2, a key aspect of recovery is to initiate rehabilitation by the physical, occupational, and speech-language therapists. These therapists continue to treat the client following hospital discharge.

Because the stroke can still be evolving at day 2, neurologic status must be accurately assessed; review the techniques for this assessment. Assessment of changes in cognition is the key indicator of changes in intracranial pressure. Continue to teach the client not to get up without assistance. Monitor the client for aspiration, seizures, and bleeding from anticoagulant therapy. Expect to monitor prothrombin time, partial thromboplastin time, and the International Normalized Ratio to regulate the amount of anticoagulation needed. The amount of heparin infused may vary throughout the day.

Monitor blood pressure carefully; elevations in blood pressure can injure the brain and increase the risk of bleeding. Follow precautions closely to maintain blood pressure in desired range.

The CareMap is reprinted with permission from Baptist Health System.

The CareMap shown is an excerpt of one that covers emergency department admission through day 5.

Helen Andrews, BSN, RN, *Care Manager, Alegent Health Bergan Mercy Medical Center, Omaha, Nebraska,* and
Linda R. Haddick, MSN, RN, *Clinical Nurse Specialist, Alegent Health Home Care & Hospice, Omaha, Nebraska*

Physical Therapy

Physical therapists work with the client to build strength and preserve range of motion (ROM) and tone in noninvolved muscles. Physical therapy also builds ROM and tone and retrains muscles affected by the stroke. The client also works on balance and proprioception skills. This may enable the client, with continued improvement, to sit on the edge of the bed and to eventually ambulate. Exercise and bed mobility skills are taught at the client's bedside, as are wheelchair mobility and transfers. Clients who would benefit from the use of an orthosis are identified and instructed on how to apply and remove it. A hemiplegic client is usually able to ambulate using a quad cane following gait training.

Occupational Therapy

Occupational therapists work with the client to relearn activities of daily living (ADL) and to use assistive devices that promote independence. For example, a client with hemiplegia may be able to dress if the clothing can be closed with self-fastening tape (Velcro) fasteners rather than buttons.

Many clients experience severe pain in the affected shoulder and hand after a stroke. This pain can be so severe that it results in lack of balance and loss of ROM, which further restricts mobility and self-care. Overstretching from turns and transfers can aggravate the problem. Some clients have experienced partial dislocation or subluxation of the shoulder both from having the shoulder pulled on and from the weight of the arm pulling it. Chronic subluxation results in shoulder-hand syndrome, characterized by a painful or frozen shoulder and hand edema. Occupational therapists assist in treating this problem and in instructing the client and caregivers in proper transfer and positioning techniques to prevent further injury.

Speech Therapy

Speech pathologists work with the client to foster the maximum amount of speech recovery possible through relearning, accentuation of speech sounds, or use of alternative communication devices. The speech pathologist also assesses the client's swallowing mechanism and makes recommendations for initiation and progression of foods and fluids to decrease the risk of aspiration.

Case Management

Case managers are often assigned to clients following stroke. Their role is to facilitate all care providers and to advocate for the client and family. (See Case Management feature.)

■ Nursing Management of the Medical Client

ASSESSMENT

Ongoing assessments of all body systems are needed. The use of a standardized neurologic assessment tool such as the GCS assists the nurse in documenting changes in the client's status and in monitoring progress. In addition to the neurologic assessment, the client's heart sounds, heart rate and rhythm, respiratory rate and rhythm, temperature, levels of nutrition, ability to swallow, bladder and bowel elimination, communication, and sexuality need to be assessed. The client's and family's psychosocial and learning needs should be assessed daily.

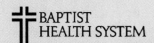

BAPTIST
HEALTH SYSTEM

CVA/TIA CAREMAP
DAY 2 AND DAY 3

	DAY 2 Date: _____	INITIAL Met	INITIAL Not Met	DAY 3 Date: _____	INITIAL Met	INITIAL Not Met
General Safety:	Bed rails up, call light within reach, fall precautions, seizure precautions, bleeding precautions, airway precautions.			Bed rails up, call light within reach, fall precautions, seizure precautions, bleeding precautions, airway precautions.		
Activity	Note PT/OT/ST treatment recommendations &/or activity as tolerated.			Progress as tolerated.		
	Goal: Tolerates activity progression.			**Goal:** Performs ADL's as independently as possible with adaptive equipment.		
Dietary: Consult Date/Time Completed _____	Diet as tolerated. If not tolerating diet, consider calorie counts.			Diet as tolerated. If not tolerating diet, consider calorie counts. Instruct re: food/drug interaction if applicable.		
	Goal: Tolerates > 50% diet.			**Goal:** Tolerates > 50% diet. Food/Drug Interaction Education Initiated.		
Respiratory: Consult Date/Time Completed _____	Wean O2 if indicated.			Wean O2 as indicated		
	Goal: SaO2 ≥ 92% on RA &/or with supplemental O2.			**Goal:** SaO2 ≥ 92% on RA or with supplemental O2.		
Rehab: Consult Date/Time Completed _____	Continue PT/OT/ST as ordered.			Continue PT/OT/ST as ordered.		
	Goal: Tolerates activities/Rehab			**Goal:** Tolerates activities/Rehab progression.		
Discharge Planning: Consult Date/Time Completed _____	Continue to assess discharge disposition Rehab to recommend appropriate disposition/ needs @ D/C.			Continue to assess discharge disposition. Rehab to recommend appropriate disposition/ needs @ D/C. Assess home equipment needs if planned discharged to home. Identify community resources needed.		
	Goal: Discharge plan initiated.			**Goal:** Refer to TCF/Rehab (Easy St)/NH/ Home Health as ordered.		
Nursing: Consult Date/Time Completed _____	VS & neuro checks q 4 h, I & O q 8 h. Notify MD if: Change in neuro status Systolic BP≥220 &/or DBP≥110 HR ≥ 150 or ≤ 50 RR ≥ 30 Temp ≥ 101 IV fluids - NS (Avoid D5W). DVT prophylaxis: Sequential hose for non-ambulating patients. Following swallowing guidelines as indicated. Elevate weak/flaccid upper extremity on pillow. Refer to CVA/TIA Patient Info. Handbook and CVA Patient/Family Caremap.			VS & neuro checks q 8 h, I & O q 8 h. Notify MD if: Change in neuro status Systolic BP≥220 &/or DBP≥110 HR ≥ 150 or ≤ 50 RR ≥ 30 Temp ≥ 101 IV fluids - NS (Avoid D5W). DVT prophylaxis: Sequential hose for non-ambulating patients. Swallowing guidelines as indicated. Elevate weak/flaccid upper extremity on pillow. Refer to CVA/TIA Patient Info. Handbook and CVA Patient/Family Caremap.		
	Goals: Neuro status stable with no deterioration. No evidence of aspiration, swallowing management continues. Vital signs within parameters. Pt./Family education continued.			**Goals:** Neuro status stable with no deterioration. No evidence of aspiration, swallowing management continues. Vital signs within parameters. Pt./Family education continued.		
Tests:	PT monitoring if on heparin protocol. PT/INR if on Coumadin.			PT monitoring if on heparin protocol. PT/INR if on Coumadin.		
Other:	BP/Anticoagulation/DVT prophylaxis option (see orders). Avoid Nifedipine (Procardia).			BP/Anticoagulation/DVT prophylaxis option (see orders). Avoid Nifedipine (Procardia).		

CVA/TIA CAREMAP

G-99-5013A-3 PG REV. 11/8/99

DIAGNOSIS, OUTCOMES, INTERVENTIONS

Altered Cerebral Tissue Perfusion. Perfusion of the cerebrum is critical for survival and long-term outcome. Therefore, it should be the first priority in care of clients with acute stroke. Decreased cerebral blood flow may be secondary to thrombus, embolus, hemorrhage, edema, or spasm. Ongoing assessment and intervention are required beyond the critical stage. Data that indicate that the risk for altered perfusion has become an actual problem are shown in Box 70–1.

Outcomes. The client will have improved cerebral tissue perfusion, as evidenced by ICP less than 15 mm Hg, cerebral perfusion pressure (CPP) greater than 65 mm Hg, no type A waves (when using intracranial monitors), no

CASE MANAGEMENT

Stroke

Because of the prevalence of cardiovascular disease in the United States, stroke (brain attack) is one of the most common conditions seen in acute care. It can also be a high-cost diagnosis-related group (DRG) and can result in a prolonged length of stay. Many hospitals have developed clinical pathways in an attempt to decrease the variability of treatment, to decrease the length of stay, and to control cost. These measures result in positive outcomes for clients, because transfer to rehabilitation occurs earlier, allowing clients to start recovery sooner.

Assess

- Has the client had an ischemic or hemorrhagic stroke?
- What manifestations is the client experiencing?
- Has the client had previous transient ischemic attacks or strokes?
- Is this a life-threatening situation, with the client in critical care, or is the stroke completed, allowing therapy to begin?
- In the case of hemorrhagic stroke, is surgery anticipated?
- What other conditions are present that might make it more difficult to treat the stroke (hypertension, diabetes, atrial fibrillation, polycythemia)?

Assess the client's ability to swallow immediately; take measures to prevent aspiration. In the case of continued swallowing difficulty, assess the need for a feeding tube.

Assess deficits and determine how they will affect the client's care plan (e.g., hemiparesis, hemiplegia, aphasia, visual changes, incontinence). Although it may be difficult, begin exercises and physical therapy evaluation and treatments as soon as possible. Assess the need for referral to other professionals such as social workers or speech therapists.

Advocate

Stroke is an unexpected event causing many life decisions and changes for the client and family. Depending on the severity of the stroke and whether deficits are transitory or permanent, family members may be called on to determine treatment or resuscitation decisions.

Try to determine whether the client has advance directives or has named a health care proxy. Because many clients and family members will be older, they may be overwhelmed and need assistance from pastoral care or social work staff. Depending on the need for rehabilitation or long-term placement, financial assessments or applications for assistance may be necessary.

Be aware of the emotional stress on the client and family as they deal with the impact of change, possibly from a fully independent state to one requiring a great deal of assistance. Carefully explain diagnostic tests and treatments such as computed tomography (CT) scans, magnetic resonance imaging (MRI), Doppler studies, and anticoagulant therapy.

Prevent Readmission

If the stroke has been minor and the client can return home, assess the need for ongoing nursing care and physical or speech therapy. Focus on returning the client to optimal functioning.

Ensure that manifestations of stroke are recognized and that the client understands the urgency of care. Work with the client to reduce risk factors such as hypertension, hypercholesterolemia, obesity, and smoking. Ensure that medication regimens are understood, especially anticoagulant therapy and follow-up blood work. Families must know about and be prepared to deal with depression or emotional lability, which may occur.

Many clients need short-term rehabilitation before returning home. Entrance into a rehabilitation program is advisable as soon as the client is stable and can tolerate the program requirements. Intensive speech, physical, and occupational therapy can assist the client to regain function and to develop living skills despite deficits.

Cheryl Noetscher, RN, MS, *Director of Case Management, Crouse Hospital and Community–General Hospital, Syracuse, New York*

---

reports of headache, no decreases in LOC, and stable or improving GCS score.

Interventions. Serial assessments of these data may be required as often as every 15 minutes for unstable clients to every 2 to 4 hours for stable clients. Analyze data for trends, and if the client is deteriorating neurologically, notify the physician. Manifestations of progressive deterioration include decreasing LOC, changes in motor or sensory function, pupillary changes, respiratory difficulty, and development of visual or perceptual defects or aphasia.

Maintain the client's blood pressure, within the range prescribed by the physician, to maintain perfusion without promoting cerebral edema. Maintain normothermia to reduce cerebral glucose and oxygen consumption. Cluster nursing interventions to reduce unneeded movement and stimulation. Elevate the head of the bed 30 degrees to reduce cerebral edema. Maintain the client's head in neutral position to improve venous drainage.

BOX 70–1   Manifestations Indicating an Actual Change in Cerebral Perfusion

- Intracranial pressure greater than 15 mm Hg sustained for 15 to 30 seconds or longer
- Cerebral perfusion pressure less than 70 mm Hg
- Decrease in Glasgow Coma Scale score of two or more points from baseline
- Decreasing levels of consciousness
- Mean arterial pressure of less than 80 mm Hg or systolic blood pressure less than 100 mm Hg
- Bradycardia
- Altered pattern of breathing
- Loss of response to painful stimuli
- Change in pupil size or response to light
- Headache
- Vomiting
- Abnormal flexion or extension posturing

Administer medications to improve cerebral tissue perfusion as prescribed. The drugs prescribed to decrease risk for further thrombus formation include anticoagulants or antiplatelet agents. Nimodipine, a calcium-channel blocker, is used to treat vasospasm secondary to subarachnoid hemorrhage.[11]

Delirium and restlessness should be controlled, with sedatives if necessary. Be certain, however, that restlessness is not the result of treatable causes, such as hypoxia, full bladder, bowel impaction, or pain. Restraints should be avoided, because they often increase agitation and intracerebral pressure.

Straining at stool or with excessive coughing, vomiting, lifting, or use of the arms to change position should be avoided, because the Valsalva maneuver increases intracerebral pressure. Mild laxatives and stool softeners are often prescribed.

Altered Tissue Perfusion. Because of the increased risk for systemic bleeding secondary to the use of thrombolytic therapy or anticoagulation, altered tissue perfusion is an important nursing diagnosis. Write the nursing diagnosis as *Altered Tissue Perfusion related to prolonged bleeding times secondary to use of thrombolytic agents or anticoagulation.*

Outcomes. Hemorrhage will be prevented, as evidenced by the absence of bleeding and by normal vital signs.

Interventions. For the client who is receiving thrombolytic therapy, certain interventions can prevent systemic bleeding. These include no arterial punctures or insertions of nasogastric tubes for 24 hours after the infusion; monitor all puncture sites and body fluids for signs of bleeding for 24 hours; and maintain bed rest for 24 hours after completion of the infusion. Gingival bleeding and oozing from intravenous sites were associated with intracranial hemorrhage.[1] Pressure may be applied to any compressible bleeding sites.

For the client who is receiving anticoagulation, monitor the aPPT and INR and adjust the client's dosage based on the physician's orders. Report any signs of bleeding to the physician immediately.

Risk of Aspiration. An increased risk for aspiration is listed here because of its importance in maintaining airway and oxygenation. Not all clients are at risk for aspiration after stroke, and their risk depends on the time since injury and area of infarction. When considering this diagnosis, use the following causes of aspiration to guide your problem-solving: impaired swallowing, depressed cough and gag reflexes, and decreased LOC.

Outcomes. The client will remain free of clinical manifestations of aspiration, as evidenced by easily managing saliva, no choking or coughing while eating, no fever, and no crackles or rhonchi.

Interventions. Assess the client for clinical manifestations of aspiration, such as fever, dyspnea, crackles and rhonchi, confusion, and decreased PaO$_2$ in arterial blood gases. Use caution in feeding the client, either orally or enterally. If the client is receiving enteral feedings, add food coloring to the tube-feeding to assist with identifying aspiration via suctioned aspirate. Monitor chest x-ray results, and report findings of pulmonary infiltrate.

Impaired Physical Mobility. Almost all clients have some degree of immobility after a stroke. In the early phases of stroke recovery, the client may be completely immobile and need assistance just to turn over in bed. Later in recovery, mobility may only be hampered in one extremity. Various causes can be used to individualize this diagnosis. These include (1) loss of muscle tone secondary to flaccid paralysis or spasticity and (2) reluctance to move associated with fear of self-injury or prolonged disuse.

Outcomes. The client will achieve maximal physical mobility within the limitations imposed by the stroke, as evidenced by more normal movement of the affected extremity, improved muscle strength, and effective use of adaptive devices.

Interventions. Assess the client's degree of muscle strength to use as a baseline value and for determining and evaluating outcomes. A comprehensive assessment by a physical therapist helps to determine appropriate activity levels.

Encourage Bed Exercises. Encouraging clients with hemiplegia to exercise while they are at bed rest not only prepares them for later activities but also offers hope and a sense of optimism about recovery. A hemiplegic client can learn to move the weak leg by sliding the unaffected leg under it to lift and move the weak leg. The client can also use the unaffected arm to move the affected arm and hand. Keep in mind that clients may have difficulty crossing the midline.

Frequent gluteal and quadriceps muscle setting exercises during the day help prepare the client for later ambulation. Begin with five repetitions, and increase gradually to 20 repetitions each time. Instruct the client as follows:

1. *Gluteal setting:* "Pinch" or contract the buttocks together and count to five. Then relax and count to five. Repeat.
2. *Quadriceps setting:* Contract the quadriceps muscles, on the anterior portion of the thigh, while raising the heel and trying to squash a rolled towel placed under the popliteal fossa against the mattress. While keeping the muscle contracted, count to five. Then relax and count to five. Repeat. Perform on both legs if possible. Start quadriceps setting exercise as soon as the client is conscious. The quadriceps muscle is the most important in giving knee joint stability in walking.

Help the Client Sit Up. Help the client out of bed as soon as the client's condition is medically stable. Remember, however, that hemiplegia can severely affect balance. Assistance is needed to provide security and safety. Raise the head of the bed slowly to reduce orthostatic hypotension.

When the client first sits up, support the affected side, especially the back and the head. Gradually, the client learns to sit alone with the head of the bed elevated and then to sit on the edge of the bed with the feet on a firm surface. Help the client maintain balance by extending the affected arm and placing the palm flat on the bed. Be patient and encouraging as the client regains balance. When the client is sitting in a chair, support the weak side with pillows.

Eventually, the client learns to raise the weak leg with the unaffected leg and to swing both legs laterally over the side of the bed onto the floor. It is safest to have the client pivot on the unaffected leg. Therefore, position the chair at a right angle to the unaffected side.

Teach the Client How to Use a Wheelchair. A hemiplegic client needs to learn safe transfers from the bed to the chair, commode, or wheelchair. The Client Education Guide shows one method. The client with hemiplegia can propel a wheelchair with the unaffected arm and leg; one-arm-drive wheelchairs also are available. Once the client is in a wheelchair, his or her level of independence increases greatly. Deficits in spatial relations, decreased awareness, and unilateral neglect can result in problems such as falling and running into doors. Clients must not be allowed to perform wheelchair self-transfers until they have demonstrated competence.

Promote Walking. A tilt table may be used in physical therapy to help the client assume a standing position if difficulty with balance is a problem. The client can begin standing as soon as the quadriceps muscles on the unaffected side have normal strength. Have the client seated on the edge of the bed. Encourage the client to rise, using the muscle power of the unaffected leg. The client may tend to swing around toward the affected side. Gradually, the client learns to take increasing amounts of weight onto the weaker side.

Despite weakness in the affected limb, a hemiplegic

CLIENT EDUCATION GUIDE

Transfer from Bed to Wheelchair by a Hemiplegic Client

Lock the wheelchair for safety, and keep it beside the bed on your unaffected side.
Use your unaffected arm and leg (*A* and *B*) to move your affected arm and leg.
As your legs drop over the edge of the bed, swing your torso up to a sitting position (*C*).

Push yourself up to a standing position (*D*) by using your unaffected arm and leg.
Reach across the wheelchair (*E*) to grasp the far arm of the chair, and turn to seat yourself.

Shading on the right side of the client indicates the affected side.

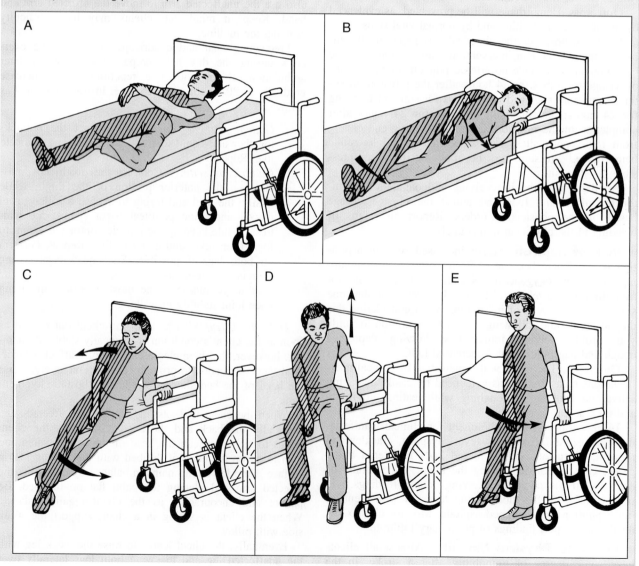

client often develops an extensor reflex, which facilitates standing. Position yourself on the weaker side when helping the client to stand. To avoid pulling on the affected arm and increasing the risk for shoulder injury, provide support with ambulation by using a gait belt. A quad cane should be used on the unaffected side to allow walking with a three-point gait.

Most hemiplegic clients can be taught to walk. Remind them to keep the body weight forward over the feet. Practice is important for learning to walk correctly. Incorrect habits, once developed, may be difficult to overcome later. Supervise clients carefully until they can safely walk alone without fear of falling. When walking, the client should not show circumduction or toe scraping or stoop forward. Heel-toe walking with a reciprocal gait pattern is the goal of ambulation.

Teach Bracing. If bracing is used, teach the client and family how to apply and remove the brace, to observe skin for breakdown, to give proper skin care, and to care for the brace itself.

Hyperthermia. Bleeding or edema of the hypothalamus can lead to ischemia of the thermoregulatory center of the brain.

Outcomes. The client will experience decreasing temperature or will have normal temperature.

Interventions. Treat fever with antipyretics. A hypothermia blanket may be used to bring down a high temperature quickly. When hypothermia blankets are used, assess the skin frequently for pressure points and cold injury. Shivering must be avoided because the muscle activity increases body temperature. Keeping the feet warm with blankets may decrease shivering. Phenothiazines may be used to help stabilize neuronal membranes if fever is related to damaged brain structures.

Risk for Impaired Skin Integrity. The loss of protective sensation and decreased ability to move increases the risk for injury to the skin. In addition, skin damage may develop from friction and shearing or increased skin fragility from inadequate nutritional status or edema.

Outcomes. The client's skin will remain intact, as evidenced by an absence of stage I pressure ulcer development and an absence of manifestations of redness from friction or shearing.

Interventions. Assess the skin every 2 hours. Change the position of a client with hemiplegia or decreased LOC every 2 hours. Develop a written turning schedule for other health care providers and family members to follow. When positioning the client on the affected side, make sure that body weight does not harm affected limbs. Support the affected arm and leg when turning and positioning a hemiplegic client. Complete shoulder and hip dislocation can occur if the flaccid extremity is not supported properly. Place a pillow between the client's legs to provide support. The client may be able to tolerate lying only for 30 minutes on the affected side because of the impaired circulation or pain.

Risk for Contracture. One of the normal activities of the brain is to inhibit spastic muscle contraction. Early in stroke recovery, flaccidity is usually present because of a loss of cerebral connections for afferent sensory and efferent motor nerves. During recovery, affected muscles may be spastic because the injured brain cannot inhibit spastic muscle contraction. Therefore, the diagnosis *Risk for Contracture* is due to flaccid paralysis or spasticity.

Outcomes. The client will have absence of contractures, joint ankylosis, and muscle shortening, as evidenced by maintaining normal ROM.

Interventions. Assess the client's ROM in both the involved and noninvolved joints. These findings can be used as a baseline and as an expected outcome.

Perform passive ROM exercises two times daily after the first 24 hours following a stroke unless otherwise prescribed. Motor impulses usually begin to return between 2 and 14 days after a stroke. The affected part (initially flaccid) becomes spastic as the spinal cord motor systems establish their autonomy and the potential for contractures increases. Passive ROM exercises are more difficult to perform once affected muscles begin to tighten.

Do not force extremities beyond the point of initiating pain or continuous spasm. Always support the joint you are exercising, and move the extremity smoothly, without jerking movements. Frequent passive ROM exercises (1) prevent joint immobility, tendon contractures, and muscle atrophy; (2) stimulate circulation; and (3) help reestablish neuromuscular pathways. By performing these exercises before dressing and undressing the client, you may facilitate self-care.

Teach the client to use the unaffected hand to lift the weak arm and to put it through ROM exercises. Exercise each finger separately. While the client is in bed, teach him or her (1) to exercise the affected arm by grasping it at the wrist with the unaffected hand and raising it above the head and (2) to stretch and rub the fingers of the affected hand several times each day. Active ROM to the unaffected extremities assists in maintaining or increasing muscle strength.

Once some voluntary movement returns, encourage the client with assisted movements. As motor strength increases, resisted movements may strengthen weakened muscles and help restore muscle bulk. Shoulder slings are not recommended because they may increase the risk of contractures.

Several interventions are used to reduce the risk for joint contracture:

1. Allow the client to sit upright for short periods only; sitting can contribute to hip and knee flexion deformities.
2. When the client is on one side, do not flex the hip acutely.
3. Do not place a pillow under the affected knee when the client is supine; this encourages flexion deformity and impedes circulation.
4. If the client's knees tend to hyperextend, place a folded towel under the knee for short periods while the client is lying supine.

If the client can tolerate the prone position, place the client in this position for 15 to 30 minutes several times a day, with a small pillow placed under the pelvis (from the umbilicus to the upper third of the thigh) to hyperextend the hip joints.

Prevent foot drop, heel cord shortening, and plantiflexion by (1) avoiding pressure on the feet, (2) performing frequent passive ROM exercises, and (3) having the client sit in a chair as soon as possible with the feet flat on the floor. While the client is in bed, keep the foot flexed at 90 degrees by using high-top tennis shoes or orthotics.

A trochanter roll, extending from the crest of the ilium to midthigh, prevents external hip rotation by wedging under the projection of the greater trochanter and stopping the femur from rolling. Trochanter rolls increase the risk of skin impairment; assess the skin beneath the roll often.

When the client is in bed, prevent adduction of the affected shoulder by placing a pillow in the axilla, between the upper arm and the chest wall, to keep the arm abducted about 60 degrees. Keep the arm slightly flexed in a neutral position. Place the forearm on another pillow with the elbow above the shoulder and the wrist above the elbow. This position stretches the shoulder's internal rotators. Elevating the arm also helps prevent edema and resultant fibrosis.

Place the affected hand in a position of function (i.e., slightly supinated with fingers slightly flexed and the thumb in opposition). Frequent passive ROM exercises are important. The use of splints to prevent flexion contractures is more effective if the splints are designed individually by occupational therapists and scheduled for on-and-off periods to allow for skin assessment and ROM. Squeezing a rubber ball is not recommended because it promotes flexion when extension is desired.

The weight of an immobile arm may cause pain and movement limitation (frozen shoulder) or subluxation of the shoulder joint. Prevent these by supporting a completely flaccid arm with a pillow when the client is in bed or seated in a chair.

Self-Care Deficit. Self-care deficits may range from not being able to reach with a weak arm to full dependence on others. This diagnosis is applicable if an achievable outcome can be obtained. Clients with complete paralysis and cognitive deficits may not be able to perform self-care. Other diagnoses may be more applicable, such as *Impaired Physical Mobility* and *Impaired Skin Integrity*. Several diagnoses can be used to describe *Self-Care Deficit*, including *Impaired Physical Mobility, Visual Sensory/Perceptual Alterations, Unilateral Neglect,* or *Altered Thought Processes.*

Outcomes. The client will perform as many ADL as possible within limitations, as evidenced by use of adaptive devices and techniques.

Interventions. Initially, a client who has had a stroke may need considerable help with all self-care activities, including washing, eating, and grooming. Encourage clients to perform as many self-care activities as possible and to use the affected arm to avoid the tendency to do everything with the unaffected arm. This activity helps preserve independent self-care, prevents complications of immobility, and enhances self-esteem.

Remember, stroke clients are easily frustrated and may need a lot of encouragement. Self-care activities provide an excellent opportunity for family teaching. Family members find it very difficult to watch a loved one struggle with a task, and they often perform the task for the client. Explain how it benefits the client to be as independent as possible.

In clients with diplopia, an eye patch over one eye removes the second image and promotes better vision. Alternating the patch daily helps to maintain the function and strength of the extraocular muscles in both eyes. Provide mouth care at least three or four times a day, giving special attention to the affected side of the tongue and mouth. Focus rehabilitation plans on self-care deficits and ADL.

Risk for Injury. The *Risk for Injury* and trauma continues throughout recovery from stroke. It may also extend into the home environment, where clients attempt to perform former activities, such as cooking or driving. Factors that increase the risk for injury include decreased LOC, weakness, flaccidity, spasticity, impulsive behavior, altered thought processes, and motor, visual, and spatial-perceptual impairments.

Outcomes. The client will remain free from injury, as evidenced by an absence of abrasions, burns, or falls. The client will also seek needed help to perform tasks that are beyond his or her capabilities.

Interventions. Keep the side rails of the bed raised for clients with recent hemiplegia to protect them from rolling out of bed. As recovery proceeds, the client may pull against side rails when sitting up or turning. Once the client can get out of bed unassisted, half side rails may be more useful. Full side rails hinder ambulation.

A client with impaired sensation is especially prone to injury. Frequent skin inspections for manifestations of injury are essential. Visual disturbances may also increase a hemiplegic client's potential for injury. Weakness on one side makes clients susceptible to falls. Remind clients to walk slowly, rest adequately between intervals of walking, use effective lighting, and look where they are going. Be especially alert during toileting. Make sure that support staff and family members know not to leave these clients alone in the bathroom.

Altered Nutrition. Use the nursing diagnosis *Altered Nutrition: Less Than Body Requirements* if your client has an inability to swallow secondary to stroke. Support the diagnosis with data on intake and output, ability to swallow, caloric intake and weight change over the past 3 days, hemoglobin, hematocrit, albumin, prealbumin, and lymphocyte count over the past 3 days.

Outcomes. The client will demonstrate signs of adequate nutrition, as evidenced by (1) maintenance of stable weight; (2) consumption of adequate calories for age, height, and weight; (3) intake equaling output; (4) hemoglobin and hematocrit levels within normal limits for age and sex; (5) lymphocyte count, prealbumin, and albumin levels within normal limits; and (6) healing of incisions and wounds within 12 to 14 days, as applicable.

Interventions. Carefully assess the client's diet to ensure adequate nutrition. Assess total intake. Feeding clients with partial paralysis of the tongue, mouth, and throat requires patience and care for prevention of choking and aspiration. Clients often fear choking and are embarrassed and frustrated by eating difficulties. Consequently, they may avoid eating and may not obtain adequate nutrition. Give supplemental meals as necessary. If the client cannot swallow at all, tube-feeding may be used. With help and encouragement, hemiplegic clients can usually learn to feed themselves. Many helpful orthotic devices are available through consultation with an occupational therapist. These might include utensils with built-up handles or scoop plates. Make mealtimes pleasant and unhurried. Serve food attractively and at an appropriate temperature.

Feeding can be very frustrating for a dysphagic client, especially if the caregiver is not familiar with the client's specific disabilities. Support personnel and family members need to be taught basic feeding techniques. These people also need to be informed of each client's individual needs and limitations. To facilitate feeding, assess the following and intervene as necessary. The speech pathologist can recommend additional feeding techniques based on the client's specific deficits and needs.

Promote Head Control. If the client has limited or no voluntary head control, placing a hand on the forehead may help. The caregiver approaches the client from the midline rather than from the side so that the client does not have to turn the head to be fed. Remind the client not to throw the head back to propel food, because this can lead to aspiration. The head should be midline and flexed slightly forward.

Assist in Positioning. Have the client in an upright position, as close to 90 degrees as possible, either in bed or in a chair. Support the client's head to counteract hyperextension.

Promote Mouth Opening. If the client does not open the mouth, lightly touch both lips with the tip of a spoon.

If this does not work, apply light pressure with a finger to the chin just below the lower lip. Ask the client to open at the same time. Stroking the muscle under the chin (digastric muscle), without crossing the midline, also stimulates mouth opening.

Stimulate Mouth Closing. If a client does not close the lips, swallowing is more difficult. Stimulate lip closure by stroking the lips with a finger or ice or by applying gentle pressure just above the upper lip with your thumb or forefinger.

Help the Client with Swallowing. A dysphagic client must concentrate on swallowing. A quiet environment, free from distractions, is helpful. Feed the client slowly and offer small amounts. Begin feeding the client with foods that require no chewing and are easy to swallow (Table 70–4). Gradually progress to foods that require more chewing and swallowing effort as tolerated. Alternate liquids with solids whenever possible to prevent food from being left in the mouth. Avoid nonthickened liquids. Place food in the unaffected side of the mouth. Encourage the client to chew each bite thoroughly. After clients have swallowed, teach them to check for food on the paralyzed side by turning the head to the unaffected side and sweeping the mouth with the tongue.

Impaired Verbal Communication. The inability to speak is very frustrating for clients. Early recognition of this problem decreases some of the frustration in meeting everyday needs. Loss of verbal communication is

TABLE 70–4	PROGRESSIVE FEEDING PROGRAM FOR CLIENTS WITH DYSPHAGIA			
	Stage I	**Stage II**	**Stage III**	**Stage IV**
Description	Severe swallowing difficulty	Chewing and swallowing difficulty with various textures	Less difficulty swallowing, beginning to control foods better in mouth, able to tolerate various food textures and consistencies	Able to swallow most foods very well
Meats	Puréed meat with gravy, baby food, egg yolks	Junior baby food meats with gravy; scrambled, soft, or poached eggs; cottage cheese	Ground meat with gravy, soft meats (tuna) in casseroles, macaroni and cheese, fish without bones, chopped meats	Soft diet
Starch	Mashed potatoes with gravy	Muffins (no seeds), pancakes, French toast, cooked cereal (thick)	Toast (no seeds), rice, soft baked potato	Soft foods
Vegetables	Puréed	Junior vegetables	Peas, squash, cooked carrots; avoid stringy foods (celery, spinach)	Soft foods
Fruits	Puréed	Cooked fruit, ripe banana, soft canned fruit	Grapefruit and orange sections; peeled ripe peaches, pears, and nectarines	Soft foods
Dessert	Custard, pudding	Cakes (no seeds, nuts)	Pies, cakes, sherbet, ice cream	Soft foods
Liquids	None	None	Thick liquids, nectars, strained cream soups, eggnog, liquid caloric supplements, milk shakes	May be able to have thickened liquids

usually caused by ischemia of the dominant cerebral hemisphere, leading to loss of the function of muscles that produce speech.

Outcomes. The client will be able to effectively communicate, the client's needs will be understood and met, and the client will indicate understanding of the communication of others.

Interventions. Communication involves the dual processes of sending and receiving language. Although either can be affected, the expressive deficit is usually greater than the receptive deficit after initial recovery. Clients may understand more than they can respond to.

Most aphasic clients regain some speech through spontaneous recovery or speech therapy. Speech therapy should be started early. Occasionally, residual brain function is not adequate for an aphasic client to relearn the complicated processes of communication. A picture board may be helpful.

Assessment of dysarthria usually includes examination of the peripheral muscles of speech, tests for specific speech skills, and assessment of the client's functional ability based on the clarity of speech in conversation. Speech therapy is beneficial for many dysarthric clients.

Reinforce the lessons that a speech therapist has initiated. Remember, the client may have a short attention span. Use every encounter to encourage and support communication, yet be careful not to cause frustration and fatigue. In general, when working with an aphasic client, speak at a slower rate and give the client time to respond. Listen and watch carefully when an aphasic client attempts to communicate. Try hard to understand. This reduces the client's frustration. Anticipate an aphasic client's needs, to reduce feelings of communication helplessness.

When a client *cannot identify objects by name,* give the client practice in receiving word images. For example, point to an object and clearly state its name. Then ask the client to repeat the word.

When a client *cannot understand spoken words or has receptive difficulty,* repeat simple directions until they are understood. Do not shout. The client can hear. Speak slowly and clearly. Talk without pressing for a response. Use nonverbal methods of communication to reinforce your words. Stand within 6 feet, and face the client directly. Gradually shift topics of conversation, and tell the client when you are going to change the topic.

When a client has *difficulty with verbal expression,* give the client practice in repeating words after you. Begin with simple words and then progress to simple sentences.

Help the family to communicate with the aphasic client. Act as a role model for such communication by being calm, patient, and gentle. Explain how damaging it can be to the client's self-image if others appear embarrassed or amused by the client's attempts to communicate. Likewise, the family should not do all of the speaking for the client.

Always try to put aphasic clients at ease. Reduce the feelings of panic that may occur when they first realize that they cannot communicate as before. The fact that others understand the problem is helpful. Offer calm reassurance. Demonstrate use of the call light and allow the client to practice. Use gestures and one-step commands.

Risk for Corneal Abrasion. Following stroke, clients may lose their ability to blink. Without a blink reflex, the cornea will dry and become abraded. The collaborative problem is *Risk for Corneal Abrasion.*

Outcomes. Monitor the client for risk factors for the development of corneal abrasion, including absence of eye closure or blinking and lack of eye moisture.

Interventions. Protect the eye with an eye patch if no blinking is noted. Instill prescribed artificial tears or consult the physician for a prescription if none exists.

Altered Thought Processes. Sometimes it is difficult to make a diagnosis of *Altered Thought Processes* unless you spend some time with the client. Asking simple or common questions may get fixed, yet correct, answers. Often, after spending a morning with a client, you may note difficulty with thought processing that was not evident on first assessment. Changes in behavior may be caused by alterations in body image, sensation, vision, mobility, and perception. Cerebral edema may also increase confusion.

Outcomes. The client will have reduced confusion, as evidenced by recall of information, improved Mini-Mental State examination scores, decreased agitation, cooperation with interventions, and appropriate responses to questions about recent and past events.

Interventions. Try to prevent disorientation by reorienting the client as LOC improves. Continually reorient a confused client. Glasses and hearing aids assist the client in maintaining awareness of the environment and thus improve thought processes. Activity such as sitting up in a chair for meals or at scheduled times throughout the day also improves LOC and orientation. Position a calendar and a clock where the client can see them. Stroke contributes to altered behavioral patterns, including confusion, memory loss, and emotional lability. To decrease agitation, explain all nursing activities before initiating them. Avoid sensory overload.

Visual Sensory/Perceptual Alterations. Ischemia of visual pathways can lead to altered vision. The client may not notice you when you approach from one side or may not eat food from one side of the food tray. A thorough assessment of visual fields is usually needed for this diagnosis.

Outcomes. The client will successfully compensate for altered visual perceptions, as evidenced by safely performing ADL and safely compensating for visual deficit through scanning or other techniques.

Interventions. Approach the client from the side that is not visually impaired. Position the call light and telephone on that side. If possible, position the bed so that the client's side that is not visually impaired is toward the center of the room. Teach clients to position the head to increase the visual field. Warn hemiplegic clients to be very careful when crossing streets because they may not see traffic approaching from the affected side. An eye patch over one eye in clients with diplopia removes the second image and assists vision.

A client with perceptual deficits benefits from simplicity. A busy or noisy environment is difficult to interpret and may increase confusion. Reduce complexity and the need for decision-making. For example:

1. Obtain clothing that is simply designed and easy to put on.
2. Give brief, simple directions.
3. Prepare food trays with a minimum number of utensils, dishes, and foods.

Unilateral Neglect. *Unilateral Neglect* is a pattern of lack of awareness of one side of the body. The client behaves as if that part is simply not there. He or she does not look for the paralyzed limb when moving about. It is caused by damage to portions of the nondominant cerebral hemisphere. Unilateral neglect creates increased risk of injury. It is possible to relearn to look for and to move the limb.

Outcomes. The client will be able to compensate for unilateral neglect, as evidenced by being free from injury and demonstrating an increased awareness of the neglected body side.

Interventions. Initially, adapt the environment to the deficit by focusing on the client's unaffected side. Greet the client as you enter the room, especially if the entrance is toward the neglected side. Keep personal care items and a bedside chair and commode on the unaffected side. Set up the client's food tray toward the unaffected side. Position the client's extremities in correct alignment. Gradually begin to focus the client's attention to the affected side. Move the personal items, bedside chair, and commode to the affected side. Assist the client from the affected side. Have the client groom the affected side first. Cue the client to scan the entire environment and remind the client to keep track of the affected extremities.

Ineffective Individual Coping. Coping strategies are quite varied among people. Any major illness or change in the body challenges a client's or family's coping skills. This process is particularly true after a stroke because of the physiologic changes and frustrations associated with the resulting deficits. The term *coping* refers to the use of all forms of coping strategies: emotional, cognitive, support systems, and risk appraisal.

Outcomes. The client will develop effective coping strategies, as evidenced by appropriate lifestyle modifications, use of the assistance of others, and appropriate social interactions.

Interventions. After a stroke, the client may experience grief over lost mobility, inability to communicate, alterations in sensation and vision, and loss of roles within society. Stroke clients express feelings of profound suffering related to the sudden, devastating changes that accompany stroke.[2, 34] Be understanding and kind. Supportive statements are often helpful, such as "I am sure it's hard for you not to be able to dress alone." The client needs to feel listened to and cared about.

Loss of independence is of particular concern for the stroke client.[45] Care for clients in a way that encourages their independence. Arrange the environment and anticipate needs to reduce frustration. Praise all successes, however small. Break a long-term goal into several short-term goals so the client can experience successes along the way. For example, a long-term goal may be to walk independently, but short-term goals such as sitting on the side of the bed and ambulating with a quad cane will allow the client to have successes and the long-term goal will seem more attainable. Inappropriate behavior may

occur. When necessary, point out the behavior in a matter-of-fact manner and ask them to stop. Significant others often need help to understand that these behaviors may be caused by damage to the inhibitory centers in the brain or they may be a part of the normal grief response. Provide support by helping the client and family to understand this.

Aphasic clients often express their emotional state by irritability and "moodiness." These frustrated clients are often anxious, bewildered, and depressed. Emotional lability may also be present. Accept such behavior in a matter-of-fact but kind manner, without embarrassment. Help families by encouraging short visits by one or two people. If children are allowed to visit, ensure that they are adequately supervised.

Psychosocial Nursing Diagnoses. Various psychosocial nursing diagnoses may be appropriate for clients experiencing stroke, depending on the client and the circumstances. These include *Altered Family Processes* (see Chapter 9), *Diversional Activity Deficit, Anxiety, Fear, Powerlessness, Self-Esteem Disturbance,* and *Social Isolation.* Shift in spousal roles often occurs. The ways in which a couple copes will determine how satisfying their lives are after a stroke.[45] Include significant others in the plan of care. Let them help care for the client if they wish. Provide them with the information they need to understand the client's condition. Many clients with strokes are in ICUs during the acute phase. The complexity of equipment and activity within an ICU may be frightening to the client and to significant others. Explain carefully what is happening, and provide opportunities for questions and discussion. Give frequent reassurance and support.

EVALUATION

Evaluate the degree of outcome attainment on an ongoing basis. After a stroke, some outcomes, such as cerebral perfusion, are achieved early; others, such as self-care deficit, may require long-term rehabilitation. Monitor progress toward outcomes, working with both the client and the family.

Surgical Management

Several criteria are used to identify candidates for rapid evacuation of the hematoma in hemorrhagic stroke. The clients most likely to benefit from surgery are those who are younger than 70 years of age, can open their eyes and follow commands, have elevated ICP (>30 mm Hg), or are rapidly deteriorating neurologically. Clients who have large blood clots removed often can recover a substantial portion of speech. Surgery is usually not performed in clients with bleeding in deep cerebral structures such as the basal ganglia or thalamus.

Most therapies are aimed at reducing increased ICP.[22] Surgery is also performed on some intracranial aneurysms and on the carotid arteries to reduce the risk for stroke.

Modifications for Elderly Clients

Because stroke affects older people more than others, the nursing care discussed here does not have to be significantly altered for older clients. Older people often have multiple medical problems that must be monitored and treated simultaneously.

Self-Care

Clients who have experienced a stroke often are transferred to a rehabilitation unit after they are medically stable. The client is evaluated for rehabilitation potential, and plans are made for ongoing therapy. The plan of care established during acute care can continue. The major nursing diagnoses and collaborative problems include *Impaired Physical Mobility, Self-Care Deficit, Impaired Verbal Communication, Risk for Contracture, Altered Nutrition: Less Than Body Requirements,* and *Ineffective Individual Coping.*

Three adjuncts to discharge from rehabilitation settings to home are:

• Self-medication
• Use of therapeutic passes
• Rehabilitation home visits

Self-medication means that clients can manage their own medications. Goals are to help the client learn about the medications, including dosage, action, and side effects. Provide a supervised trial to evaluate the client's knowledge and compliance and to enable clients to develop increased responsibility for their own care. A clear and accurate medication chart is helpful.

Therapeutic passes allow the client to return to home or family for short stays. They facilitate discharge planning and improve the transition into the community. Passes help the stroke survivor adjust to the home environment and to practice self-care activities at home and help the family adjust to living with the stroke survivor and to any alterations in physical, cognitive, and emotional functioning. Clients and family members can practice problem-solving and can perform some physical care skills needed after discharge from the facility. Much effort goes into planning for the passes and preparing the client and family. Passes are usually for 8 hours at first and then are increased to a weekend. When the client returns to the facility, the client and family discuss any difficulties they had during the pass interval. Team members intervene with information, retraining, or procurement of needed supplies.

For the *rehabilitation home visit,* team members, including the nurse, social worker, and physical and occupational therapists, visit the client's home. The purpose is to evaluate the accessibility of the home and the safety of the home environment based on the client's level of functioning, specifically, the client's ability (1) to get in and out of the house; (2) to perform specific tasks in each room; (3) to transfer onto and off of the toilet, bed, and chair; and (4) to move about from room to room. The client's ability to safely use the telephone and various appliances is also evaluated. On the basis of findings from the visit, the team recommends home modifications, further teaching, or adaptive equipment.

The family needs a clear understanding of the client's residual deficits. If spatial or perceptual deficits or unilateral neglect is present, emphasize the need for assistance with daily activities and the need for adherence to safety precautions to prevent injury. Writing lists of tasks or activities may help clients with impaired memory. Reinforce measures to improve mobility and the ability to perform ADL. The client should have a plan for exercises. Of equal importance, the family and client need to have realistic expectations about the client's abilities, so they can encourage independence when and where the client is able.

Provide written documentation of any anticoagulant schedule as well as a list of warning signs of bleeding. Reinforce the need for caution when the client is using sharp instruments and tools. If appropriate, contact sports must be curtailed while the client is receiving anticoagulants. The INR is closely monitored, and medications are adjusted as needed. The client should be taught to carry Medic-Alert identification.

Provide information about community resources that can assist the client and family with home management and adjustments to residual deficits. These resources include Meals-on-Wheels, the American Heart Association, stroke support groups, social services, local service groups to assist with the purchase of equipment, and individual and family counselors.

At times, the stroke client may not be able to tolerate the intensive therapy of a rehabilitation setting, and placement in an extended care facility may be necessary. This is usually very stressful for the client and family, particularly an older spouse. In some cases, care by nurses and allied health professionals in the home may prevent placement in an extended care facility. If both partners are older or in poor health, placement in an extended care facility may be the only option. This can create feelings of guilt and abandonment. Emotional support must be provided to both the client and family members. Education in how to choose a facility and how to monitor care can be helpful.

TRANSIENT ISCHEMIC ATTACKS

Transient ischemic attacks (TIAs) are sudden, brief episodes of neurologic dysfunction caused by temporary, focal cerebral ischemia. Recovery is complete. By definition, a TIA lasts less than 24 hours, and most TIAs last only 5 to 20 minutes. TIAs lasting greater than 1 hour are often caused by small infarcts.[4] TIAs often serve as warning signs of an impending stroke. In fact, one third of people with untreated TIAs experience a stroke within 5 years.[4]

Etiology and Risk Factors

During a TIA, a transient decrease in blood supply to a focal area of the cerebrum or brain stem occurs. Many factors can cause this ischemia. Thromboembolism from ulcerated plaque on the carotid arteries is the most common cause of TIAs, accounting for 80% of cases. Thromboemboli may originate in the vertebrobasilar system. Other sources of emboli include blood clots forming on diseased or prosthetic heart valves, atrial fibrillation, or breakdown of plaque.

Pathophysiology

The pathophysiology of a TIA is similar to that of a stroke. The major differences are the short duration of ischemia and the lack of permanent deficits.

Clinical Manifestations

Manifestations of TIAs vary, depending on which area of the brain is affected. Common manifestations of a TIA in the carotid artery circulation include a rapid onset of weakness or numbness in an arm or leg, aphasia, and visual field cuts. Manifestations of a TIA in the vertebrobasilar circulation include two or more of the following: vertigo, diplopia, dysphagia, dysarthria, and ataxia.

TIAs are often recurrent; however, some clients have only one or two episodes before having a complete stroke. TIAs may occur for 2 to 6 years before cerebral infarction, or clusters of TIAs may first appear only a few hours or days before a cerebral infarction. Between episodes, neurologic assessment findings are normal.

The diagnosis of TIA is confirmed by the client's reported clinical manifestations. The causes of the TIA and potential risk for stroke are diagnosed by the following examinations:

1. Auscultation for a carotid bruit.
2. CT to rule out stroke or other causes of neurologic deficit.
3. Doppler, computed tomographic angiography (CTA), or magnetic resonance angiography (MRA) studies of the carotid arteries.
4. Cerebral angiogram.
5. ECG to assess for atrial fibrillation.
6. Transthoracic or transesophageal echocardiography (TTE and TEE, respectively) to rule out mural thrombosis and valvular disorders.

The results of the noninvasive carotid artery studies, which include the Doppler, CTA, and MRA, determine whether the more invasive cerebral angiogram is performed. The TTE is often performed before the TEE as it is less invasive; however, the TEE may better visualize prosthetic valves and the left atrium.

Conditions that mimic a TIA include intracranial hemorrhage, seizures, hypoglycemia, migraine, and inner ear disorders.

Outcome Management

■ Medical Management

Preventing the progression of a TIA to a stroke is the goal of medical management. Every effort is made to determine the cause of the TIAs. Another important medical intervention is to identify and decrease the client's modifiable risk factors for stroke.[7] Antihypertensives or antiplatelet drugs may be prescribed. Warfarin may be administered for emboli of cardiac origin.

Teach the client and family about the manifestations of stroke, risk factors for stroke, and emergency care if a stroke occurs at home. If the client is hospitalized, assess neurologic status frequently for progressive ischemia.

Clients experiencing TIAs are often afraid that they are having a stroke. They need emotional support and education during this stressful time. The diagnostic work-up as well as the manifestations themselves can produce anxiety. Thorough, simple explanations of upcoming events can help. Stress the importance of completing the work-up. Baseline neurologic status must be recorded for postoperative comparison.

■ Surgical Management

Clients who are considered for surgery are those who have a low risk for postoperative morbidity and mortality and one of the following: (1) asymptomatic carotid artery disease with greater than 60% stenosis or (2) symptomatic carotid artery disease with greater than 70% stenosis.[21, 28] In these clients, the incidence of stroke with surgical management is significantly reduced compared with those with medical management. Clients considered at increased risk for postoperative morbidity and mortality include those with coronary artery disease, pulmonary disease, and moderate to severe stroke on the ipsilateral side.[21, 28] Surgery is usually performed only on stenotic arteries, not on those that are totally occluded. A client may require bilateral endarterectomy. The interval between surgeries is determined by the client's tolerance of the procedure and the likelihood of symptom progression from the remaining stenotic vessel.

Most surgeons perform cerebral angiography before carotid artery surgery to accurately quantitate the degree of carotid stenosis.[21] The risk for stroke or death from cerebral angiography is 1%.[21] Vast improvements in technology of noninvasive carotid artery studies allow surgeons to use the data to guide the planning for surgery.[28] Preoperative aspirin is often administered to decrease the formation of embolism at the carotid suture line. If the client is receiving heparin, it is usually stopped on arrival to the operating room.

CAROTID ENDARTERECTOMY

Carotid endarterectomy is useful in preventing stroke. Carotid endarterectomy is the opening of the carotid artery to remove obstructing and embolizing plaque (Fig. 70–5). After coronary artery bypass, it is the second most common vascular surgical procedure. An incision is made on the anterior border of the sternocleidomastoid muscle. The vessel is clamped, and the plaque or atheroma is removed. There is a potential for decreased cerebral perfusion during the operation because the artery must be clamped during the procedure. Some surgeons use intraoperative electroencephalogram (EEG) and transcranial Doppler monitoring to detect decreased cerebral perfusion while the carotid artery is clamped. In addition, some surgeons shunt blood from below the targeted carotid artery incision to above it to provide a temporary blood supply to the brain. The client is admitted to the ICU for monitoring of neurologic and vital signs and is usually discharged the following day.

PROGNOSIS. Follow-up Doppler studies are performed at 3 months postoperatively to assess for artery patency and again at 6 months to 1 year to detect restenosis on the operated side and disease on the nonoperated side. Restenosis occurs in approximately 5% of clients after carotid endarterectomy.[21]

COMPLICATIONS. Neurologic complications of carotid endarterectomy include:

- Embolization during surgery, causing cerebral vessel occlusion and ischemia
- Thrombosis of the artery at the endarterectomy site, causing cerebral ischemia
- Inadequate cerebral perfusion from intolerance of the temporary artery clamping during surgery

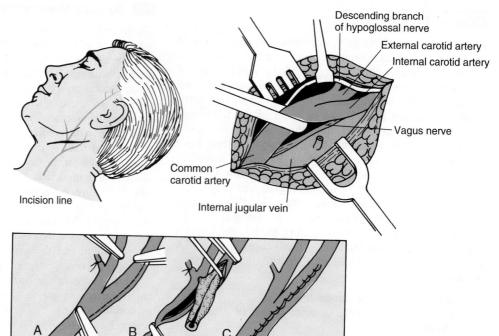

FIGURE 70–5 Carotid endarterectomy. *A,* The common carotid artery is clamped, and an incision is made along the carotid bifurcation. *B,* Plaque is removed. Sometimes portions of the artery are also removed and reconstructed with vein grafts or polyester, such as Dacron. *C,* The artery is sutured closed, and the clamps are removed.

OTHER TECHNIQUES

Recent advances in microcatheter and microballoon technology have lead to the investigational use of interventional neurovascular procedures to treat and prevent cerebrovascular disorders.[10] Results of studies in the use of carotid angioplasty and stenting have been promising. The less invasive procedures would treat severe carotid stenosis in a less invasive way than traditional surgery.[8]

Cerebral angioplasty is similar to coronary angioplasty. A balloon catheter is threaded through the arterial system via the femoral artery to the area of carotid stenosis. A small balloon is inflated to dilate the lesion. A stent catheter can also be used to further open the area of stenosis. The Food and Drug Administration (FDA) views both of these procedures to be experimental. The complications and complication rate are comparable to those of carotid endarterectomy.

▬ Nursing Management of the Surgical Client

Postoperative care after carotid endarterectomy includes neurologic assessments every 1 to 2 hours. Immediately report indications of deterioration of neurologic status. In addition, several cranial nerves are in close proximity to the operative site. The function of the following cranial nerves is assessed: facial (VII), vagus (X), spinal accessory (XI), and hypoglossal (XII). Cranial nerve dysfunction is usually temporary but may last for months. The most common cranial nerve damage causes vocal cord paralysis, difficulty managing saliva, or tongue deviation.

Keep the client's head aligned in a straight position to help maintain airway patency and to minimize stress on the operative site. Antiplatelet agents are often administered. The client can lie supine or on the side, as long as the neck is not flexed.

Elevate the head of the bed when vital signs are stable. Local applications of cold to the operative site may be prescribed.

Frequently assess the client's breathing pattern, pulse, and blood pressure. Maintain the client's blood pressure within 20 mm Hg of the preoperative normal values. Hypertension or hypotension may lead to hemorrhage, ischemia, or occlusion of the anastomosis. Labile blood pressure is a common problem after surgery. Baroreceptors located in the lining of the carotid sinus are one of the primary mechanisms of maintaining normotension. Manipulation of the baroreceptors during surgery causes a short-term disruption in blood pressure regulation.

Observe the operative site. Airway obstruction can occur from excessive swelling of the neck or hematoma formation. Bleeding and hemorrhage are a concern because anticoagulation from intraoperative heparin is not yet reversed. Risk factor modification is essential to the long-term success of the surgery and the general health of the client.[24]

▬ Client and Public Education

The general public has limited knowledge of the manifestations of stroke. In one study, only slightly more than half of the respondents could name at least one stroke manifestation.[33] In addition, only 68% could name a risk factor for stroke.[33] A public education campaign is under way to promote awareness of the manifestations of a stroke. In this campaign, stroke is referred to as "brain attack" to indicate the need for emergency care with the same intensity as a heart attack. Prompt recognition allows for early treatment of a stroke, which may lessen residual deficits and decrease disability. Recognition and modification of risk factors for stroke is the most important prevention available.

CONCLUSIONS

Stroke is being managed today as a treatable problem if it is recognized early. However, because of the limited knowledge of the public about early warning signs, many clients still suffer the consequences of stroke. Treatment of the client with stroke is aimed at maximizing function and preventing disability.

THINKING CRITICALLY

1. **A 70-year-old man had a left-sided stroke 2 days ago. While obtaining his assessment, you note that his blood pressure is elevated at 200 mm Hg systolic; his usual systolic blood pressure is 140 to 160 mm Hg. He is receiving oxygen at 5 L, but his oxygen saturation has dropped from 95% to 88% in the last hour. The client was oriented to person, place, and time an hour ago but has become increasingly restless and slightly confused. The confusion has led him to pull out a nasogastric tube that had been placed for nutritional maintenance. What other neurologic assessments should you do? What is the first priority? Is the suddenness of this change significant?**

Factors to Consider. How has the client's assessment changed from baseline values? Is there any relationship between the increased blood pressure and the hypoxia? Is the removal of the nasogastric tube an immediate problem?

BIBLIOGRAPHY

1. Barch, C., et al., and the NINDS rt-PA Stroke Study Group. (1997). Nursing management of acute complications following rt-PA in acute ischemic stroke. *Journal of Neuroscience Nursing, 29*(6), 367–372.
2. Berquist, W. H., McLean, R., & Kobylinski, B. A. (1994). *Stroke survivors.* San Francisco: Jossey-Bass Publishers.
3. Bernardine, G. L., & Mayer, S. A. (1999). Cardiac and pulmonary complications of cerebrovascular disease. *The Neurologist 5*(1), 24–32.
4. Biller, J., & Love, B. B. (2000). Ischemic cerebrovascular disease. In W. G. Bradley (Ed.), *Neurology in clinical practice: Principles of diagnosis and management* (3rd ed.). Boston: Butterworth-Heinemann.
5. Braimah, J., et al., and the NINDS rt-PA Stroke Study Group. (1997). Nursing care of acute stroke patients after receiving rt-PA therapy. *Journal of Neuroscience Nursing, 29*(6), 373–383.
6. Broderick, J., et al. (1998). The Greater Cincinnati/Northern Kentucky stroke study: Preliminary first-ever and total incidence rates of stroke among blacks. *Stroke, 29*(2), 415–421.
7. Caplan, L. R. (1998). 10 most commonly asked questions about stroke. *The Neurologist, 4*(4), 227–231.
8. Cates, C. (2000). 10 most commonly asked questions about carotid angioplasty and stenting. *The Neurologist, 6*(1), 58–62.
9. Chan, H. (1997). Bladder management in acute care of stroke patients: A quality improvement project. *Journal of Neuroscience Nursing, 29*(3), 187–190.
10. Clark, W. M., Barnwell, S. L., & Nesbit, G. M. (1997). Potential role of interventional neurovascular therapy for cerebrovascular disease. *The Neurologist, 3*(2), 95–103.
11. Counsell, C., et al. (1995). Nimodipine: A drug therapy for treatment of vasospasm. *Journal of Neuroscience Nursing, 27*(1), 53–55.
12. Daley, S., et al., and the NINDS rt-PA Stroke Study Group. (1997). Education to improve stroke awareness and emergent response. *Journal of Neuroscience Nursing, 29*(6), 393–398.
13. Deibert, E., & Diringer, M. N. (1999). The intensive care management of acute ischemic stroke. *The Neurologist, 5*(6), 313–325.
14. Donnarumma, R., et al., and the NINDS rt-PA Stroke Study Group. (1997). Overview: Hyperacute rt-PA stroke treatment. *Journal of Neuroscience Nursing, 29*(6), 351–355.
15. Fisher, M., & Albers, G. W. (1999). Applications of diffusion-perfusion magnetic resonance imaging in acute ischemic stroke. *Neurology, 52,* 1750–1756.
16. Gelber, D. A., & Callahan, G. D. (1999). Neurorehabilitation. *The Neurologist, 5*(5), 271–278.
17. Hershey, L. (1999). 10 most commonly asked questions about stroke in women. *The Neurologist, 5*(3), 166–168.
18. Hinkle, J. L. (1998). Biological and behavioral correlates of stroke and depression. *Journal of Neuroscience Nursing, 30*(1), 25–31.
19. Hock, N. (1998). Neuroprotective and thrombolytic agents: Advances in stroke treatment. *Journal of Neuroscience Nursing, 30*(3), 175–184.
20. Jeffrey, S. (1998). Managing the "dynamic process" of hemorrhagic stroke. *Neurology Reviews,* 28–29.
21. Johnson, C. J., & Jones, C. E. (1997). Carotid artery surgery. *The Neurologist, 3*(3), 146–154.
22. Kase, C. S. (2000). Intracerebral hemorrhage. In W. G. Bradley (Ed.), *Neurology in clinical practice: Principles of diagnosis and management* (3rd ed.). Boston: Butterworth-Heinemann.
23. Kelly-Hayes, M., & Paige, C. (1995). Assessment and psychologic factors in stroke rehabilitation. *Neurology, 45*(suppl. 1), S29–S32.
24. Leonard, A. (1996). Carotid endarterectomy: A nursing perspective. *Journal of Neuroscience Nursing, 28*(2), 99.
25. Liskay, A. M. (1999). Stroke: Are you at risk? *The Neurologist, 5*(1), 53–54.
26. Lyden, P. D., et al. (1997). Intravenous thrombolysis for acute stroke. *Neurology, 49,* 14–29.
27. Macabasco, A. C., & Hickman, J. L. (1995). Thrombolytic therapy for brain attack. *Journal of Neuroscience Nursing, 27*(3), 138–149.
28. Macdonald, R. L. (1996). Controversies in the management of carotid stenosis. *Journal of Neuroscience Nursing, 28*(2), 93–98.
29. Manno, E. M., et al. (1999). The effects of mannitol on cerebral edema after large hemispheric cerebral infarct. *Neurology, 52,* 583–587.
30. Mayer, S. A., & Dennis, L. J. (1998). Management of increased intracranial pressure. *The Neurologist, 4*(1), 2–12.
31. Mayo, N. E., et al. (2000). There's no place like home: An evaluation of early supported discharge for stroke. *Stroke, 31*(5), 1016–1023.
32. National Institute of Neurological Disorders and Stroke rt-PA Stroke Study Group. (1995). Tissue plasminogen activator for acute ischemic stroke. *New England Journal of Medicine, 333*(24), 1581–1587.
33. Pancioli, A., et al. (1998). Public perception of stroke warning signs and knowledge of potential risk factors. *Journal of the American Medical Association, 279*(16), 1288–1292.
34. Pilkington, F. B. (1999). A qualitative study of life after stroke. *Journal of Neuroscience Nursing, 31*(6), 336–347.
35. Post-stroke Rehabilitation Guideline Panel. (1995). *Post-stroke rehabilitation: Assessment, referral and patient management. Quick reference guide for clinicians. No. 16.* Rockville, MD: U.S. Department of Health and Human Services, Agency for Health Care Policy and Research Pub. No. 95-0663.
36. Post-stroke Rehabilitation Guideline Panel. (1995). Post-stroke rehabilitation: Clinical practice guidelines. *American Family Physician, 52*(2), 461–470.
37. Prichard, J. W., & Grossman, R. I. (1999). New reasons for early use of MRI in stroke. *Neurology, 52,* 1733–1736.
38. Quality Standards Subcommittee of the American Academy of Neurology. (1996). Practice advisory: Thrombolytic therapy for acute ischemic stroke. Summary statement. *Neurology, 47,* 835–839.
39. Rapp, K., et al., and the NINDS rt-PA Stroke Study Group. (1997). Code stroke: Rapid transport, triage and treatment using rt-PA therapy. *Journal of Neuroscience Nursing, 29*(6), 361–366.
40. Raps, E. C., & Galetta, S. L. (1995). Stroke prevention therapies and management of patient subgroups. *Neurology, 45*(suppl. 1), S19–S24.
41. Sacco, R. L. (1995). Risk factors and outcomes for ischemic stroke. *Neurology, 45*(2 suppl. 1):S10–S14.
42. Selman, W. R., Tarr, R., & Landis, D. M. D. (1997). Brain attack: Emergency treatment of ischemic stroke. *American Family Physician, 55*(8), 2655–2662.
43. Shepard, T. J., & Fox, S. W. (1996). Assessment and management of hypertension in the acute ischemic stroke patient. *Journal of Neuroscience Nursing, 28*(1), 5–12.

44. Simmons, B. J. (1997). Management of intracranial hemodynamics in the adult: A research analysis of head positioning and recommendations for clinical practice and further research. *Journal of Neuroscience Nursing, 29*(1), 44–49.

45. Smith, G. R., & Mahoney, C. (1995). Coping and marital equilibrium after stroke. *Journal of Neuroscience Nursing, 27*(2), 83–89.

46. Spilker, J., et al., and the NINDS rt-PA Stroke Study Group. (1997). Using the NIH Stroke Scale to assess stroke patients. *Journal of Neuroscience Nursing, 29*(6), 384–392.

47. Suarez, J. L., et al. (1999). Predictors of clinical improvement, angiographic recanalization, and intracranial hemorrhage after intra-arterial thrombolysis for acute ischemic stroke. *Stroke, 30*, 2094–2100.

48. Swanson, R. A. (1999). Intravenous heparin for acute stroke: What can we learn from the megatrials? *Neurology, 52*, 1746–1750.

49. Testani-Dufour, L., & Marano Morrison, C. A. (1997). Brain attack: Correlative anatomy. *Journal of Neuroscience Nursing, 29*(4), 213–222.

50. Toni, D., et al. (1996). Hemorrhagic transformation of brain infarct: Predictability in the first 5 hours from stroke onset and influence on clinical outcome. *Neurology, 46*, 341–345.

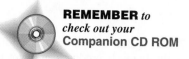

REMEMBER *to*
check out your
Companion CD ROM

Management of Clients with Peripheral Nervous System Disorders

Anne Marie Johnson Fredrichs

NURSING OUTCOME CLASSIFICATION (NOC)
for Nursing Diagnoses—Clients with Peripheral Nerve Disorders

Activity Intolerance	**Altered Urinary Elimination**	**Chronic Pain**
Ambulation: Walking	Urinary Continence	Body Image
Activity Tolerance	Urinary Elimination	Hope
Pain: Disruptive Effects	**Anxiety**	Role Performance
Altered Role Performance	Psychosocial Adjustment: Life Change	Self-Esteem
Role Performance	Symptom Control	Social Interaction Skills
Psychosocial Adjustment: Life Change	**Body Image Disturbance**	**Impaired Physical Mobility**
Altered Tissue Perfusion: Peripheral	Acceptance: Health Status	Mobility Level
Sensory Function: Cutaneous	Self-Esteem	Pain Level
Tissue Perfusion: Peripheral		**Pain**
		Comfort Level
		Pain Level

This chapter examines disorders of the peripheral nerves and cranial nerves. The autonomic disorders are discussed in Chapter 72. Disorders of the spinal cord, apart from spinal cord injury, also are presented. Spinal cord injury is discussed in Chapter 73.

LOWER BACK PAIN

The spine is a mechanical organ that has been described as a crane with the ability to support weight, maintain balance, and counter numerous daily strains during normal work and recreational activities. Although it has tremendous ability to withstand most mechanical stresses, it can be stressed beyond its limits. Forces that exceed the capacity of the tissues to stretch can lead to injury and pain. Low back pain is the second most common reason for visits to a physician. The treatment of low back costs $70 to $100 billion yearly.

Etiology

The origin of back pain is not well known and has never been fully described. Many groups have given up trying to describe the cause of lower back pain and instead have listed several *red flag* conditions that are asso-

ciated with the problem. Three groups of problems lead to back pain:

1. *Biomechanical* origins include compression of the discs, herniation of the disc, torsion injury, or vibration. These problems are seen when clients have occupations that require strenuous or repetitive lifting in a stooped position or occupations that require operating vibrating machinery.
2. *Destructive* origins include infection, tumors, and rheumatoid disorders.
3. *Degenerative* problems include osteoporosis and spinal stenosis.

Vertebrae can also be affected by osteoporosis. Osteoporotic vertebrae can collapse and lead to compression of the nerve roots. The spinal canal can narrow and compress the nerves; this problem is called *spinal stenosis.* It usually occurs in older people. Severity can range from entrapment of one nerve root to compression of the entire cord.

Other disorders include those that have no clear physiologic cause, yet lead to loss of income and pain. There is a growing body of data that show strong psychological influences on the response of clients to lower back pain. The primary determining factors for disability from low back pain appear to be based on whether the client is depressed, unhappy in a work setting, or involved in litigation. These psychosocial issues do not mean the pain is not real. The manner in which the brain processes pain may be implicated. The psychosocial aspects may suppress the serotoninergic pathways and limit the secretion of endorphins.

BACK STRAIN

Back strain is an acute injury leading to lower back pain. Back strain occurs when the client flexes the back without bending the knees or makes rotating movements, creating significant stress on the intervertebral disc and muscles of the lower back.

DISC HERNIATION

An intervertebral disc is a pad that rests between the centers of two adjacent vertebrae. Discs provide cushions for spinal movement. The intervertebral disc is composed of three parts:

1. *Cartilaginous plates* act as the superior and inferior limits of the disc. These plates are composed of hyaline cartilage and cover the top and bottom of the vertebrae.
2. The *annulus fibrosus* is a ring of tissue that gives size and shape to the disc and holds the nucleus pulposus in place.
3. The *nucleus pulposus* is a semigelatinous material that forms the center of the disc and provides the cushioning effect.

Strenuous activity or degeneration of the disc or vertebrae can allow the disc to move from its normal location. Displacement of intervertebral disc material may be referred to as *prolapse, herniation, rupture,* or *extrusion.* Ruptured intervertebral discs may occur at any level of the spine. Lumbar discs are more likely to rupture than cervical discs because of the force of gravity; continual movement in this region; and improper movements of the spine, as with lifting or turning. As in spinal cord injury, thoracic disc disorders are the least common.

More than half of people with clinical manifestations of a herniated disc give a history of a previous back injury. Heavy physical labor, strenuous exercise, and weak abdominal and back muscles increase the risk of herniated disc. Repeated stress progressively weakens the disc, resulting in bulging and herniation.

LORDOSIS

Lordosis is an excessive backward concavity in the lumbar spine. It is commonly associated with sagging shoulders, medial rotation of the legs, and an exaggerated pelvic angle. Excessive lordosis may result in swayback and kyphosis. Back pain is common.

SPONDYLOLISTHESIS

Spondylolisthesis is the forward slipping of one vertebra. It commonly occurs at L4–L5, where the upper vertebra slips forward out of alignment. Spondylolisthesis is graded from 1 to 4. Grades 1 and 2 are managed conservatively; for grades 3 and 4, surgery with fusion is usually required for stabilization (Fig. 71–1).

SPONDYLOLYSIS

Spondylolysis is a structural defect in the lamina or neural arch of the spine. The vertebral arch slips forward. The lumbar spine is most commonly involved.

SPINAL STENOSIS

Spinal stenosis (Fig. 71–2) is due to ligamentous infolding and hypertrophy of the bone. It produces pressure on the entire spinal cord. If compression remains untreated, weakness or paralysis of the innervated muscle groups may result.

Pathophysiology

The pathophysiology of lower back pain is a source of fascination, frustration, and often confusion by clinicians and scientists who attempt to treat and study clients with this problem. The spine is the only organ that consists of bones, joints, ligaments, fatty tissue, multiple layers of muscles, peripheral nerves, sensory ganglia, autonomic ganglia, and the spinal cord. These structures, in turn, are fed by an intricate system of arteries and veins. The movement of the spine is complex and injury to the spine and other structures leads to unique patterns of pain.

Compressive loads have different effects on the intervertebral disc, body of the vertebrae, facets, and spinal ligaments. Under compressive loads, the annular fibers of the discs are stretched. The vertebrae are also compressed and may fracture at the end-plates. Spinal ligaments tend to buckle easily, and the facet joints offer little resistance to compression.

The result is that the disc can herniate. When the disc only bulges, the annulus remains intact. With herniation, the annulus usually is torn, allowing extrusion of the nucleus pulposus (see Fig. 71–2). Compression of spinal nerve roots may result from herniation of the disc. The discs that separate and pad the vertebrae are innervated with fine nerve endings. When a lumbar disc impinges on the sciatic nerve, the condition with its resulting pain is called *sciatica.* Sciatica is a severe, usually activity-dependent, intermittent pain in the leg that occurs along the course of the sciatic nerve and its branches.

Clinical Manifestations

Rupture or herniation of a lumbar disc leads to lower back pain that radiates down the sciatic nerve into the posterior thigh as a result of compression of the spinal nerve roots. Typically, the pain of sciatica begins in the

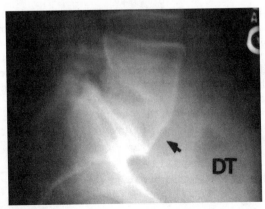

FIGURE 71–1 Preoperative radiograph of spondylolisthesis. Note the slippage of the vertebrae. (Courtesy of James Manz, M.D., Mayo Clinic, Eau Claire, WI.)

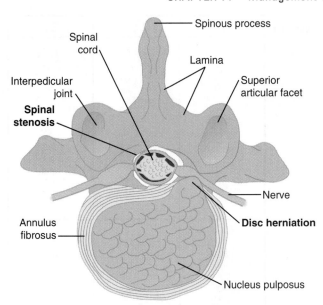

FIGURE 71–2 The usual causes of low back pain are disc herniation and spinal stenosis.

buttocks and extends down the back of the thigh and leg to the ankle. Disc herniation can also lead to groin pain. The client also has muscle spasms and hyperesthesia (numbness and tingling) in the area of distribution of affected nerve roots. The pain is exacerbated by straining (coughing, sneezing, defecation, bending, lifting, and straight-leg raising) or prolonged sitting and is relieved by side-lying with the knees flexed. Any movement of the lower extremities that stretches the nerve causes pain and involuntary resistance. Straight-leg raising on the affected side is limited. Complete extension of the leg is not possible when the thigh is flexed on the abdomen (Lasègue sign). There may be depression of deep tendon reflexes.

Manifestations of spinal stenosis usually begin slowly and are due to pressure placed on nerve roots as they exit the vertebrae. The most common manifestations are aching pain with standing and walking, paresthesias, and heaviness in the legs that progresses as the client walks. There is rapid improvement in manifestations with trunk flexion, stooping, or sitting. The manifestations of spinal stenosis must be differentiated from claudication.

Diagnostic Findings

X-ray studies may show spinal degenerative changes (at any level) that may indicate disc problems but usually do not show a ruptured disc. Osteophytes and narrowed disc interspaces are degenerative changes visible on radiographs. Other spinal disorders (e.g., spinal tumors, vertebral fracture, rheumatoid arthritis, and osteoarthritis) can lead to the same manifestations.

Magnetic resonance imaging (MRI) may show spinal stenosis (narrowing of the spinal canal), extrusion of disc material into the spinal canal, and impingement of a spinal nerve root (Fig. 71–3).

Myelography may show narrowing of the disc space and impingement of a spinal nerve root. This modality can identify the level of herniation and may be used to rule out other spinal diseases. It is typically performed if MRI is not conclusive.

A computed tomography (CT) scan usually is done after myelography. This sequence allows better imaging with only one administration of contrast material. CT scanning may show spinal stenosis or other changes associated with degenerative disc disease. CT scans are more useful at the thoracic or lumbar level than the cervical level.

Discography is the injection of a water-soluble imaging material into the nucleus pulposus. It is used to determine internal changes in the disc. During the injection, information is recorded about the amount of dye accepted and the pressure needed to inject the material. Clients can have allergic responses to the contrast agent and develop disc space infections from the injection. Electromyography of the peripheral nerves also may be used to localize the site of the ruptured disc. Paraspinal mapping and somatosensory evoked potentials may be used for diagnosis.

Outcome Management

◼ Medical Management

Goals of medical care include reducing pain and spasms, improving mobility, and repairing any structural problems in the spine or discs.

Initial assessment of the client with lower back pain is designed to help pinpoint the cause. The client's medical history is obtained to help determine whether a serious underlying condition is responsible for the pain, such as a fracture, tumor, or infection. The client's psychological and socioeconomic history is obtained because such prob-

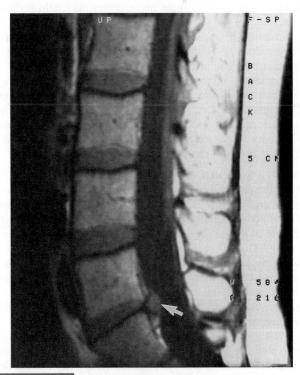

FIGURE 71–3 Magnetic resonance image of the lumbar spine shows herniation of the disc between L5 and S1.

lems can complicate assessment and management. The client also is asked to rate the pain. Physical examination is used to determine whether lumbar nerve roots are involved by testing for reflexes, muscle strength, and the presence of neurologic deficits (Fig. 71–4).

CONTROL PAIN AND SPASMS

Initial care of acute lower back pain is directed at managing the client's pain and directing activities. Pain usually is managed with nonsteroidal anti-inflammatory drugs (NSAIDs) or COX-2 inhibitors, muscle relaxants, and, at times, narcotics. Ice may be used to reduce pain with acute disc herniation for the first 48 hours. After that time, heat usually is a better analgesic. A semi-sitting position (in a recliner chair) usually is comfortable and promotes forward lumbar spine flexion and reduces back strain. Other positions of comfort include (1) the supine position with pillows under the legs and (2) the lateral position, in which the client lies on the unaffected side with a thin pillow between the knees with the painful leg flexed to reduce tension on the sciatic nerve. Lying in a prone position and sleeping with thick pillows under the head should be avoided. Physical therapists may be able to relieve pain and spasm with stretching exercises and ultrasonic heat treatments. Work space or equipment modifications may also be necessary.

If the client has nonspecific lower back pain, manipulation may be used by a physical therapist or chiropractor. *Spinal manipulation* is the use of the hands on the spine to stretch, mobilize, or manipulate the spine and paravertebral tissues. It usually is performed for clients with manifestations that last more than 1 month. The Agent for Health Care Policy and Research (AHCPR)[1] review panel found no evidence that spinal traction with weights was effective in reducing lower back pain. Although unproven, deep ultrasonic heat treatment and moist local heat applications may help reduce pain.

Progressive muscle relaxation exercises and other stress reduction techniques can be helpful. Muscle stretching also has been effective for fascial pain.

For severe lumbar disc problems with leg pain, conservative intervention involves 2 to 4 days of bed rest on a firm mattress. Bed rest relieves back pain by relieving the back muscles and vertebrae of the stresses. The forces of gravity (e.g., weight of the head with cervical problems) and motion can increase back pain during activity.

IMPROVE MOBILITY

Activity modifications are prescribed to reduce back irritation and to prevent debilitation from inactivity. Most clients do not require bed rest; in fact, more than 4 days of bed rest can be debilitating and actually slow recovery. The client is taught to minimize the stress of lifting by keeping objects close to the body and to avoid twisting when lifting. Sitting may worsen leg pain, and clients who sit at work should change positions often. Aerobic activities should be prescribed to help avoid debilitation.

Walking, stationary bicycling, and back strengthening exercises can be performed. Exercise may begin within the first 2 weeks after injury, and each activity should be performed for 20 to 30 minutes, two or three times a week, for best aerobic conditioning.

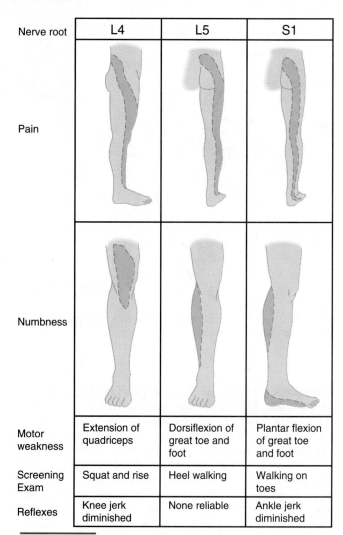

Nerve root	L4	L5	S1
Pain			
Numbness			
Motor weakness	Extension of quadriceps	Dorsiflexion of great toe and foot	Plantar flexion of great toe and foot
Screening Exam	Squat and rise	Heel walking	Walking on toes
Reflexes	Knee jerk diminished	None reliable	Ankle jerk diminished

FIGURE 71–4 Assessment of lumbar nerve root compromise includes testing for motor weakness and reflexes and eliciting pain (screening examination). (Redrawn from Agency for Health Care Policy and Research. [1994]. *Acute low back problems in adults: Assessment and treatment. Quick reference guide for clinicians,* No. 14. Rockville, MD: Author.)

Work activities need to be individualized for each client based on job requirements. See the Client Education Guide on lower back care.

A back brace or corset may be prescribed for a client with a ruptured lumbar disc. Back supports usually are not recommended once clinical manifestations are relieved, however, because restricted back motion progressively weakens muscles and causes further degeneration of spinal structures. Exercise to strengthen the back and abdominal muscles helps prevent further problems if the exercises are done daily throughout life.

■ Nursing Care of the Medical Client

Nursing care focuses on assisting the client to adjust his or her lifestyle to reduce the risk of further back injuries. Many clients are frustrated with the lack of cure of their back pain. Clients have become accustomed to having a well-defined cause of a problem and a well-researched approach for management. Many clients with lower back pain have pain for years without relief. This level of chronic pain can lead to depression and personality or relationship difficulties. Nurses remain sensitive to the exasperation felt by the clients as well as the health care team.

Nurses are actively involved in teaching the client safe methods to lift and bend, how to lie down and how to rise from bed to avoid twisting, and how to take NSAIDs correctly to reduce the risk of gastric ulceration. If the client requires narcotics for pain, instruct the client to eat high-fiber foods to reduce constipation and not to operate machinery or drive. The Client Education Guide on lower back care can be used to teach clients.

■ Surgical Management

Surgery is indicated in clients with spinal disc problems when (1) sciatica is severe and disabling, (2) manifestations of sciatica persist without improvement or worsen, and (3) physiologic evidence of specific nerve root dysfunction is present. Surgery also is used to stabilize spinal fractures and to correct scoliosis and kyphoscoliosis. Some surgeons use other criteria.

CHEMONUCLEOLYSIS

Chymopapain is a proteolytic enzyme isolated from papaya latex that is used as a meat tenderizer. Injected into the disc, chymopapain digests the protein in the disc and shrinks it. It is contraindicated in people with multiple allergies and in people allergic to papaya. Immediate and delayed (after 15 days) allergic responses have been reported. Its use has been abandoned by most practitioners.

PERCUTANEOUS DISCECTOMY

Herniated disc material can be excised with a trocar to remove the center of the disc. The laser also is used to destroy the damaged disc.

MICRODISCECTOMY

Microdiscectomy is the use of microsurgical instruments to remove the herniated fragment of disc. Use of this technique results in less trauma to the surgical site compared with standard surgery, and more tissue integrity is preserved. Advantages of microsurgery include (1) minimal nerve root retraction, (2) preservation of an intact joint capsule (no bone is removed), (3) improved hemo-

stasis, and (4) minimal stripping of the muscle and fascia from the spine.

DECOMPRESSIVE LAMINECTOMY

The term *laminectomy* is confusing and is used loosely. The term *laminectomy* means complete removal of the bone between the spinous process and the facet; this seldom is necessary. The more correct term for what is done is a *laminotomy,* or the creation of a hole in the lamina.

Decompressive laminectomy is surgical removal of the posterior arch of a vertebra, exposing the spinal cord (Fig. 71–5). This procedure gives access to the spinal canal for (1) removing a spinal cord tumor, (2) removing portions of the facets, or (3) decompressing bone infringement on the spinal cord. Sometimes foraminotomy is performed to enlarge the intervertebral foramen if it is narrowed and osteophytic processes (overgrowth of bone) entrap the nerve root and impinge on neural structures.

SPINAL FUSION/ARTHRODESIS

Spinal fusion is the placement of bone grafts (bone chips) between vertebrae (Fig. 71–6). The new bone that grows fuses the two vertebrae and immobilizes them to reduce the pain. Usually no more than five vertebrae are fused; fusing more than five vertebrae causes considerable loss of movement in the spine. The bone graft may be obtained from a bone bank or the anterior-superior iliac crest. During healing, the graft gradually grows onto the vertebrae and forms a bone union. This bone union causes permanent stiffness in the area. The stiffness is hardly noticed in the lumbar area after a while but is noticeable in the cervical area. The client cannot be guaranteed that back pain will be relieved permanently or that further surgery will not be required.

SPINAL FUSION WITH INSTRUMENTATION

Metal rods may be used to straighten and fuse the spine in disorders such as scoliosis or multiple vertebral fractures. Other devices also can be used to provide additional support while the bones heal in a fused manner (Fig. 71–7).

COMPLICATIONS

General potential complications after spinal disc surgery at any level include infection and inflammation, injury to nerve roots, dural tears, cauda equina syndrome, and hematoma. Non-union of the surgical area also is a risk and

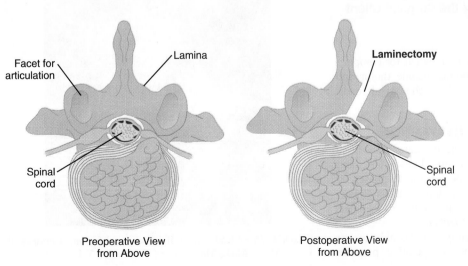

Facet for articulation

Lamina

Spinal cord

Preoperative View from Above

Laminectomy

Spinal cord

Postoperative View from Above

FIGURE 71–5 Laminectomy for the interlaminal removal of a herniated disc.

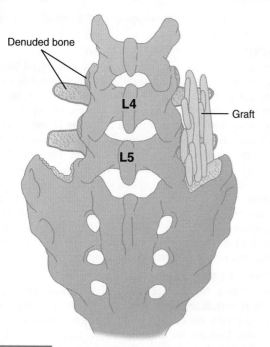

FIGURE 71–6 Lumbar interbody spinal fusion. Bone grafts are taken from the iliac crest and inserted between the vertebrae. The bed of raw bone is shown on the left, and the graft material is shown in place on the right.

is associated with smoking. Some surgeons assess serum nicotine levels prior to surgery to reduce the risk of nonunion and validate statements of smoking cessation.

PROGNOSIS

The AHCPR reviewed outcomes of surgery for lower back problems.[1] In general, lumbar discectomy often relieved manifestations of pain faster than continued medical management in people with severe and disabling leg pain. In other people with no leg pain, however, there appeared to be little difference in outcome between discectomy and conservative care. Most clients who had chymopapain injections required eventual discectomy for permanent pain relief. More study is needed to determine who is best served by the various techniques; client preference also plays a big role in the technique chosen.

■ Nursing Management of the Surgical Client

PREOPERATIVE CARE
ASSESSMENT

A baseline neurologic assessment is obtained for comparison after surgery. Assessment should include motor and sensory function of extremities and psychological readiness for surgery.

DIAGNOSIS, OUTCOMES, INTERVENTION

Knowledge Deficit. Perioperative care of a client having spinal surgery includes providing knowledge about the preoperative, operative, and postoperative phases. It also includes evaluating the client and family's understanding of the experience. A common nursing diagnosis in this circumstance is *Knowledge Deficit*.

Outcomes. The client and family will be able to explain the surgical procedure, the preoperative prepara-

tions, and the postoperative precautions and needs. The client will demonstrate safe mobility, including logrolling and transfer to and from the bed.

Interventions. Include the family in preoperative education. Explain to the client that frequent turning follows surgery and that correct turning protects the back and helps the recovery process. Explain the logrolling method of turning, the necessity for limitations on activity to prevent damage (flexion, extension, or twisting) to the surgical site, and the importance of not straining. Advise the client to ask for help rather than stretch to reach for objects. Stool softeners are given daily while the client is in the hospital to minimize straining with bowel movements. Clients with a recent injury may not be permitted to ambulate before surgery. For these clients, explain and demonstrate.

Encourage clients who smoke to stop smoking. Smoking increases cardiovascular complications and increases the risk of poor wound healing and non-union if a fusion is performed.

If a fusion is to be done, clients need to be evaluated for autologous blood donations. Two to 3 units should be donated, the last one at least 1 week before the surgery. Elderly clients may require more time for blood donation. A fusion also necessitates informing the client of the bone graft site and the additional pain associated with the autograft bone donor site.

The client may also need changes in the home setting. These changes should be considered before surgery and include location of bathroom, devices needed for ambulation, ability to use the shower, and toilet seat risers.

Fear and Anxiety. Many people fear postoperative problems such as paralysis and chronic pain. *Fear and Anxiety* is a common nursing diagnosis in this situation.

Outcomes. The client will express a low level of fear or anxiety related to the upcoming surgery and will use positive coping strategies to decrease fear or anxiety.

Interventions. Encourage the client and family to express their concerns and fears about the spinal surgery. Concerns and fears should be allayed whenever possible. For example, clients need to be aware that some edema is

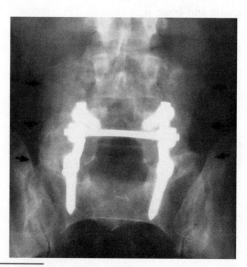

FIGURE 71–7 Radiograph of a multilevel fusion. (Courtesy of James Manz, M.D., Mayo Clinic, Eau Claire, WI.)

expected at the surgical site, and some of the preoperative deficit may still exist after surgery but should improve as the edema lessens.

EVALUATION

Preoperative education should allay some of the concerns of the client and family. Do not expect all anxiety to be relieved; in fact, some new areas of concern may arise. If questions come up about the operation, ask the surgeon to answer them. Do not attempt to provide information outside of your area of expertise.

POSTOPERATIVE CARE
ASSESSMENT

After spinal surgery, assessment is similar to that performed for other surgical clients. A head-to-toe assessment is done. Dressings and drains are checked. Evaluate the level of pain and the response to analgesia. Assess neurologic function by asking the client to move his or her legs and feet and comparing the results with those of the baseline evaluation.

Question the client about the presence of numbness or tingling and changes in sensation or pain. These paresthesias are a consequence of the edema from the surgery but should improve. If progressive weakness or paralysis of the lower extremities, loss of sphincter control, anal numbness, or urinary retention (called the *cauda equina syndrome*) occur, notify the physician immediately. Emergency surgical decompression may be required.

Clients who have had fusions are on bed rest longer and are at higher risk for deep venous thrombosis. Compression devices may be used to improve venous return. Observe for and report any manifestations of deep venous thrombosis: positive Homans' sign, redness or swelling in the leg, or sudden chest pain or dyspnea. Assess the wound for bulging or clear drainage, which may indicate cerebrospinal fluid leakage. If the client has had an anterior approach, usual care for abdominal surgery is required (e.g., assessment of ileus).

Disc problems often create fears and concerns related to pain, treatments, sexual activity, possible length of illness, and possible lifestyle changes. Provide psychosocial support to the client and family. Impaired mobility and altered urinary or bowel elimination also are common problems experienced after disc surgery. Considerations about employment and finances should be referred to a social worker.

DIAGNOSIS, OUTCOMES, INTERVENTIONS

Pain. Pain secondary to incisional trauma and edema is an expected response after spinal surgery. Write this common postoperative nursing diagnosis as *Pain related to tissue trauma secondary to back (and/or abdominal) incision.*

Outcomes. The client will express comfort, such as level 3 on a scale of 0 to 10.

Interventions. Although acute incisional pain is present, often the pain in an extremity is significantly less after herniated disc surgery. Many surgeons inject long-acting local anesthetics into disc spaces during surgery. This injection gives the client immediate relief from pain and promotes a positive attitude toward the outcome of surgery. Often the pain recurs on the second postoperative

day. This recurrence is due to the increase in swelling and the fact that the local anesthetic is wearing off.

Acute postoperative pain can be managed by using a basal dose of a narcotic with an intravenous (IV) pump in combination with a patient-controlled analgesia (PCA) dose for pain peaks (breakthrough pain) not controlled by the continuous dose. Another method of providing basal (continuous) pain medication is by intravenous drip or epidural catheter. If the client is on as-needed (prn) pain management, teach the client to keep pain levels tolerable by asking for narcotics before the pain is too great. Ice may be applied to the incision using an abdominal wrap that holds sheets of ice along the lumbar area and reduces the risk of ice burns.

Impaired Physical Mobility. Clients who have spinal surgery have varying degrees of mobility limitations. The diagnosis can be written as *Impaired Physical Mobility related to pain, leg weakness, prolonged immobility, or fear of pain and spasms.* Choose the etiologic mechanism that best fits your client.

Outcomes. The client will resume a maximal level of progressive activity, starting with logrolling on the day of surgery, progressing to independent movement from the bed to a standing position, followed by independent ambulation before discharge.

Interventions. Encourage the client to move the legs and feet while on bed rest to promote venous return. Alternating compression stockings may be used to promote venous return. Keep the bed linens loose at the foot of the bed to promote movement. If the client requires assistance to turn or when turning to place a bedpan, turn the client in the logrolling manner. A fracture bedpan is used to reduce back arching and strain.

When the client is being transferred to bed postoperatively, at least four people should assist. Transfer devices, such as a sliding board, may be used with adequate help. Transfer the client gently and smoothly, with the spine supported and properly aligned at all times.

Immediately after lumbar discectomy, the client typically is not turned for an hour or so but remains flat to aid hemostasis. Begin side-to-side logrolling, and repeat every 2 hours. If a dural tear was repaired, the surgeon may order the client to remain flat longer to minimize the risk of cerebrospinal fluid leak or a tear in the dural sutures. While clients are immobile and supine, elevate the heels from the bed.

After lumbar fusion, the bed generally is kept flat. The client logrolls from side to side, usually beginning about 4 hours after surgery, then every 2 to 4 hours thereafter. Twisting the client's spine or twisting at the hips must be avoided. Ensure safety during turning to prevent straining of the spine or rolling off the bed. It is beneficial to have extra help in turning a client the first few times after spinal surgery. Spinal bone grafts are delicate and heal slowly. Eventually, turning is permitted without help, while keeping the spine rigid.

It is common for the client to have spasms and pain with turning, and pain medication should be administered before moving. If the client is receiving medication by PCA administer the medication about 10 minutes before moving the client. The advanced dose provides pain control without the immediate nausea and flushing that many clients develop. Once the client is turned, tilt the client back onto pillows to reduce pressure on the iliac crest. Back strain may then be reduced by (1) keeping the client's spine straight, (2) flexing the upper leg and placing a pillow between the legs, and (3) placing a pillow to support the upper arm and prevent the upper shoulder from sagging. If the iliac crest has been used as a donor site, the client may not be able to turn onto that side because of pain. Abdominal incisions should be splinted to reduce pain.

Follow the surgeon's orders on how high the head of the bed can be elevated. Use a pressure-reduction mattress to reduce the risk of pressure ulcers if the client had spinal surgery for fracture stabilization or will be in bed for a long time. Use of a trapeze over the bed is contraindicated because it promotes twisting. The call light and PCA control are placed so that the client can touch them without straining. Once the client is allowed to reach for things, objects should be placed conveniently.

If a client is supine after spinal surgery (e.g., is using a bedpan), the lower back muscles may be relaxed somewhat if pillows are placed under the entire length of the legs. This placement may also prevent thrombophlebitis in the femoral vessels. Do not flex the client's knees by placing anything under the popliteal space; this is hazardous because it increases the risk of deep venous thrombosis. A sign is placed on the bed describing the prescribed position for the bed. Instruct the client clearly about contraindicated activities and positions.

To assist the client into a chair, keep the bed flat, and teach the client to roll onto the side (Fig. 71-8). Then push the torso from the bed with the arms to rise from the bed. This technique has often been used by clients with long-standing back pain and may be familiar to the client. If the client has had long-standing back pain before surgery, review the client's technique for rising from the bed. Usually the client is assisted to a chair the

morning after surgery. Be sure to follow the physician's activity prescriptions.

After spinal surgery, a brace or corset may be required temporarily to support the spine. Clients who have lumbar or thoracic spinal fusions may wear a fiberglass brace. Initially, back braces or corsets may be worn all the time, whether the client is in or out of bed. As the client's muscles strengthen, the use of braces or corsets usually is decreased. Casts may be used for a while after any thoracic spinal surgery for clients with unstable thoracic spines (e.g., thoracic spinal cord trauma).

Altered Urinary Elimination. After spinal surgery, urinary retention may occur. Most commonly, it occurs because of pain and spasms when resting supine and as a side effect of narcotics. Retention also occurs when the cauda equina is affected. Write the nursing diagnosis as *Risk for Altered Urinary Elimination related to pain and spasms with movement, inability to void in a supine position, and side effects from narcotics.*

Outcomes. The client will resume normal bladder emptying by the time he or she is ambulating.

Interventions. Assess for bladder distention and pain 8 hours after surgery. If the client's bladder is distended and painful on palpation, noninvasive measures should be tried first. The client is commonly catheterized with an in-and-out catheter (straight catheterization) twice, after which an indwelling catheter is placed. It may be used for the first few days until the client is ambulating and using less pain medication. When the catheter is removed, generally clients can urinate when sitting or standing rather than lying supine. If the bladder is full or cannot be emptied completely, the physician may order straight catheterization to check for residual urine.

Risk for Paralytic Ileus. The most common bowel problem after laminectomy and spinal fusion is

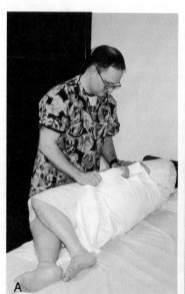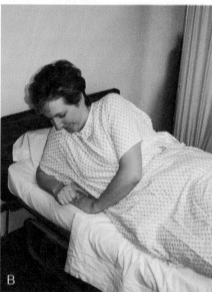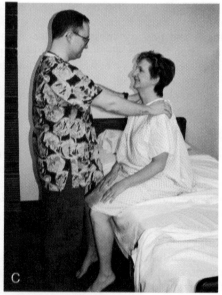

FIGURE 71-8 Helping the client stand after lumbar fusion. *A,* Logroll the client to the edge of the bed using a turning sheet if needed. Leave the bed in that position. *B,* The client pushes off the bed with the hand and the other elbow to sit up without twisting. The client drops her legs off the side of the bed at the same time. *C,* With the client seated on the edge of the bed, the nurse assesses for orthostatic hypotension. The client stands from the bed without flexing the back.

paralytic ileus. This loss of bowel sounds and abdominal distention is due to lack of peristalsis from a sudden loss of parasympathetic function innervating the bowels and manipulation of the intestines in anterior approaches to spinal surgery.

Outcomes. The nurse can expect return of normal bowel function, including normal bowel sound patterns, and evacuation without straining, by the time the client is ambulating. This problem is expressed as a collaborative situation; therefore, the outcome is written in terms of the nurse's actions. The nurse's actions cannot independently alter the outcome, as occurs with nursing diagnoses.

Interventions. Assessment findings with paralytic ileus include nausea, vomiting, a hard abdomen, and absence of bowel sounds. The client is assessed every 4 hours postoperatively for bowel distention.

If the client has paralytic ileus or if ileus is expected to develop as a result of extensive manipulation during surgery, a nasogastric tube connected to low intermittent suction is inserted and the client takes no fluid or food by mouth (NPO status). When a client's gag reflex and bowel sounds have returned and the client passes gas or has a bowel movement, a clear liquid diet is prescribed and the client progresses to a regular diet.

Bowel dysfunction may occur for several days postoperatively. Inactivity often causes problems with bowel elimination. Bowel movements are documented. Fluids are forced as ordered; a regular time for bowel movements and bowel care is encouraged; fiber is provided in the diet (when allowed), and prescribed medications and enemas (e.g., stool softeners, mild bulk laxatives, or a suppository) are administered. Instruct the client not to strain for a bowel movement because this increases pain and cerebrospinal fluid pressure. Often, clients find it difficult or impossible to defecate when lying flat. A bowel movement may not occur until sitting up is possible.

Evaluation. Expect pain to be controlled with mild to moderate narcotic analgesics, bowel and bladder function to be intact, the client to be able to walk steadily for several yards, and the client to be able to eat before discharge.

■ Self-Care

Approximately 80% of the population experience lower back pain at some point in their lives. About 10% of clients who seek medical attention for back pain have herniated discs. Because of the frequency of herniated disc problems, health promotion is an essential activity for health care providers. The Client Education Guide provides suggestions for lower back care.

CERVICAL DISC DISORDERS

Discs may become entrapped in the cervical spine. The process is similar to that with herniated lumbar discs.

CLIENT EDUCATION GUIDE

Lower Back Care

- Get out of bed by rolling onto one side near the edge of the mattress. Push up to a straight position by pushing off the bed with your arms, while keeping your spine straight, and swing your legs over the edge. Avoid twisting while getting up.
- Do not sleep while partially reclined or sitting in a chair. Sleep on a bed with a firm (not hard) mattress.
- Avoid riding in or driving a car for a long distance or time. Sit erect without slouching.
- Avoid low couches and chairs, and use your leg muscles when rising from a chair; a recliner chair is usually comfortable.
- When you must stand for a long time, bend one knee to reduce stress on your lower back by elevating one foot on a stool.
- Maintain a body weight that is close to ideal.
- Exercise and walk or swim to strengthen your back and abdominal muscles. Wear low-heeled shoes.
- Eat a diet high in fiber and fluids to soften bowel movements and reduce strain. When adding fiber to your diet, add it slowly over days.
- Use proper body mechanics when lifting. Get adequate help if the object is heavy. Use the muscles of your legs, not your back, by bending at the knees to get close to the object being lifted. Never turn and lift at the same time.

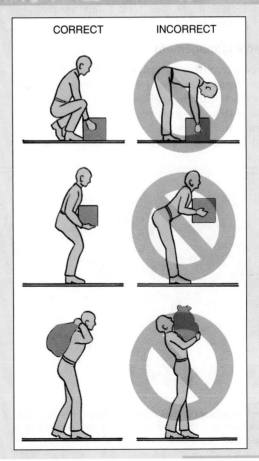

CORRECT   INCORRECT

Manifestations include arm pain, neck pain and spasms, and loss of function (grip strength) and changes in sensation in the hands.

Outcome Management

▰ Medical Management

Initial treatment is with NSAIDs, muscle stretching, and teaching proper body mechanics. Opinions differ concerning the advisability of performing head and neck range-of-motion exercises in the presence of significant cervical disease. Tell the client to avoid activities that increase cervical disc pain. To prevent neck extension when in bed, only one flat pillow (to prevent neck flexion) is recommended. The neck should not be hyperextended. Intermittent traction may be applied for cervical disc herniation (5 to 8 pound weight) to relieve pain. The head of the bed may be elevated slightly with cervical traction. Otherwise, it is best kept flat when cervical pain is present. A review of posture at work is important for clients who work at computer terminals. Keyboards, screens, and written materials should be kept at a height that reduces strain on the neck and shoulders.

A soft cervical collar may be prescribed for mild to moderate cervical disc problems to keep the head slightly flexed. After fracture of a cervical vertebra, cervical disc rupture, or whiplash injury, the client may wear a neck brace (fitted so that the chin rests on a cup and the neck is kept hyperextended), a hard collar (which extends up under the chin and prevents flexion of the neck), or a soft collar. Neck braces tend to limit vision; people wearing them cannot look down at their feet. Safety awareness is important to prevent falls.

▰ Surgical Management

Sometimes conservative treatment does not work, and clients require surgery. Surgery to stabilize bone fragments is necessary if a neck injury involves a bone fracture. Cervical fusion (Fig. 71–9) is performed most commonly through an anterior approach. Immediately after a posterior cervical discectomy, a cervical collar is worn (Fig.

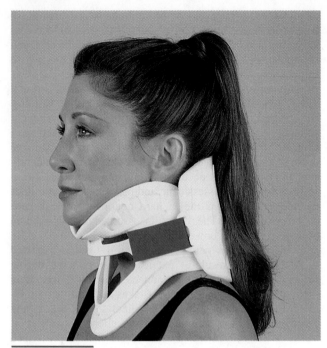

FIGURE 71–10 A cervical collar with a chin piece. This orthosis provides additional support for the head and some restriction of cervical spine motion. (Courtesy of Zimmer, Inc., Dover, OH.)

71–10). A hard cervical collar usually is prescribed after fusion. Complications after posterior cervical surgery include soft tissue hematoma, air embolism, and subcutaneous wound dehiscence. Complications after anterior cervical surgeries include laryngeal nerve damage and injury to neck structures, such as the carotid arteries, trachea, esophagus, and soft tissue.

After microdiscectomy, the client may have the head of the bed elevated to whatever position is comfortable. After cervical spine fusion, the surgeon indicates the degree of head elevation for comfort and to reduce edema. Make sure the spine is in anatomic alignment. The client's head may be elevated, and a folded small towel, bath blanket, or small pillow is placed under the head to maintain spinal alignment while the client lies supine or on the side.

Assess and document the client's neurologic status frequently. The development or worsening of a neurologic deficit must be reported promptly to the surgeon. During the first 24 hours after an anterior cervical discectomy, assess the client's ability to breathe, check the operative site for excessive swelling, and look for shifting of the trachea and changes in the client's voice. Laryngeal nerve damage during surgery may cause permanent vocal impairment, such as hoarseness. If a spinal fusion was performed with the anterior cervical discectomy, the surgeon is notified if radicular pain recurs suddenly. This pain could mean that the bone graft has moved out of place and surgery needs to be repeated. Assess the client for indications of postoperative improvement, such as absence of paresthesias.

After surgery on the cervical spine, watch for indications of respiratory paralysis resulting from cord edema. Emergency tracheostomy equipment is kept at hand.

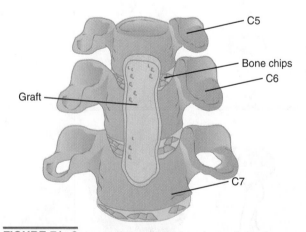

FIGURE 71–9 Anterior cervical fusion. A trough has been cut into the anterior cervical spine for insertion of an iliac graft as a splint. The intervertebral spaces have been filled with bone chips.

Tell the client that it is not unusual for preoperative manifestations to persist for a few days secondary to edema at the operative site, although these manifestations are usually less uncomfortable. Difficulty swallowing and throat discomfort are usually present for several days and usually are due to local irritation from the endotracheal tube. A soft diet, throat lozenges, a viscous lidocaine (Xylocaine) solution, humidified air, minimal talking, and other comfort measures lessen the discomfort.

A wound drain may be present and is usually removed by the surgeon on the second postoperative day, after drainage has decreased. Bladder and bowel management are the same as for clients after lumbar surgery. Cervical surgery may affect the parasympathetic chain, causing urinary retention.

■ Self-Care

With shorter postoperative hospital stays, most clients are discharged before suture or staple removal. Instruction for care of the incision includes keeping the sutures or staples clean and dry and noting any increased redness or drainage from the wound. Clients need clear instructions on walking, lifting, driving, and returning to work. Most clients can resume activity 6 weeks after surgery. Specific physician instructions need to be followed.

Prolonged sitting or standing in one position strains the healing back. Contraindicated activities vary. Instruct the client to ask the surgeon when it will be safe to perform activities that could damage the back (e.g., climbing stairs, lifting a weight heavier than 5 pounds, prolonged travel, sexual activity, sports, exercise, and driving a car). Clients must not smoke. Smoking reduces blood supply to the tissues and delays healing. The Client Education Guide lists other suggestions for home care after a cervical laminectomy or fusion.

CLIENT EDUCATION GUIDE

Home Care After Cervical Laminectomy or Fusion

- Keep the incision clear and dry. Change dressings when damp or soiled.
- Report redness, swelling, odor, or pain in the incision.
- Wear the collar at all times for 6 weeks or until your physician gives you permission to stop.
- You may wash under the collar with mild soap. Dry the skin well.
- If the collar is hard and needs cleaning, you should lie flat, remove the front of the collar, and wash the front first, using the back of the collar for neck support. Then replace the front of the collar and turn onto a pillow for support. Open one side of the collar and wash the back of your neck, then repeat on the other side.
- If the collar itches, a small silk scarf between the neck and the collar may provide some comfort.
- If a soft collar is prescribed, stockinettes made of soft fiber that fit over the collar can be purchased. Purchase two stockinettes so that when one is soiled, it can be removed, laundered, and replaced when dry.
- Riding in a car is permissible, but driving is not allowed until your physician has given you permission.

POST-POLIO SYNDROME

Poliomyelitis is an acute form of paralysis characterized by destruction of motor cells in the spinal cord and brain stem. The disease has been controlled since the 1950s, when mass immunization was used. Post-polio syndrome can develop in polio survivors 30 years after the original disease, however.

Post-polio syndrome is a new onset of progressive weakness, fatigue, decreased temperature tolerance, emotional distress, dysphagia, pain in the joints and muscles, and respiratory problems. The onset is insidious, and weakness occasionally extends to muscles that were not involved during the initial illness. The prognosis generally is good; progression to further weakness is usually slow, with plateau periods of 1 to 10 years. The syndrome is thought to be due to progressive dysfunction and loss of motor neurons that compensated for the neurons lost during the original infection and not to persistent or reactivated poliovirus infection.

The fatigue from post-polio syndrome is treated with pyridostigmine (Mestinon). Side effects of increased muscle twitching, nausea, diarrhea and frequency are common. The weakness is treated with strengthening exercises, steroids to reduce inflammation, and electrical stimulation. Other manifestations also are treated symptomatically.

Post-polio syndrome can be discouraging for clients who have successfully adapted to their disease and disability. Respiratory distress may bring back memories of the initial disease and treatment in an iron lung (an early form of a respirator in which the client's entire body was cocooned in a metal tube). Further restrictions are difficult to accept. Emotional support is vital. Teach the client to balance rest and activity.

SYRINGOMYELIA

Syringomyelia is often associated with the Arnold-Chiari malformation (an abnormal protrusion of the medulla into the spinal canal) or spina bifida. Syringomyelia consists of abnormal cavities filled with dense, glue-like tissue in the spinal cord substance, especially the cervical cord. Scar tissue surrounds the cysts. Syringomyelia is characterized by (1) muscular weakness and wasting; (2) sensory defects; and (3) indications of injury to the long tracts of the spinal cord, such as hyperreflexia.

These disturbances may begin at any age but most often occur between ages 30 and 40. Syringomyelia often occurs with other developmental defects. Kyphosis (abnormal increased convexity in curvature of the thoracic spine when viewed from the side), scoliosis (lateral deviation in the normally straight vertical line of the spine), and clubfoot often occur with syringomyelia.

Early manifestations of cervical syringomyelia often include:

- Atrophy, weakness, and fibrillations of the small muscles of the hands
- Loss of pain sensation in the fingers or forearms
- Weakness and atrophy of the shoulder girdle muscles
- Horner's syndrome, characterized by upper eyelid ptosis, pupil constriction, anhidrosis (absence of sweating), and flushing of the affected side of the face

- Nystagmus
- Vasomotor and trophic disturbances of the upper extremities

Although there is segmental loss or impairment of pain and temperature sensation, sensation for light touch remains. Segments of sensory loss may be separated by zones of normal sensation. Spasticity, ataxia, or paralysis of the lower extremities may occur as well as disturbed bladder control if the lumbosacral region of the spinal cord is involved. Cranial nerve involvement may produce additional problems, such as impairment of facial pain and temperature sensation, loss of the corneal reflex (necessitating protection of the eye), dysphagia, dysarthria, laryngeal stridor (possibly necessitating tracheostomy), nystagmus, and atrophy and fibrillation of the tongue muscles.

Syringomyelia may progress rapidly at first, then become quiescent for many years. Some people live 40 years after onset. Others become incapacitated (from paralysis or sensory defects) or die within a few years.

Treatment includes relieving increased pressure on the cord from the fluid content of the cavities within the spinal canal. The fluid buildup can be removed and cerebrospinal fluid outflow restored by direct surgical drainage or by shunt placement.

SPINAL TUMORS

Spinal tumors are similar in nature and origin to intracranial tumors but occur much less often. They are most common in young or middle-aged adults and most commonly involve the thoracic region. Spinal tumors may occur outside of the spinal cord, such as in the meninges, nerve roots, or vertebrae (extramedullary), or within the substance of the spinal cord (intramedullary). Neurofibromas and meningiomas are the most common spinal cord tumors. Both are benign and operable and may not produce permanent damage if removed early.

Clinical Manifestations

Clinical manifestations of spinal tumors vary according to their location. Extramedullary tumors cause manifestations by compressing the spinal cord or some of its nerve roots or by occluding blood vessels supplying the cord. Early characteristics of spinal cord compression include pain, sensory loss, muscle weakness, and muscle wasting. Progressive cord compression is manifested by spastic weakness below the level of the lesion, decreased sensation, and increased reflexes. Severe cord compression at the cervical level destroys cord function and produces quadriplegia; compression at the thoracic or lumbar level results in paraplegia.

Intramedullary tumors produce more variable clinical manifestations. High cervical cord involvement causes spastic quadriplegia and sensory changes. Tumors in descending areas of the spinal cord produce motor and sensory changes appropriate to functions at that level.

Medical diagnosis is made after a complete general neurologic examination. Diagnostic testing includes a spinal radiograph, CT scan, MRI, and a myelogram, individually or serially.

Outcome Management

Intervention for spinal tumors usually is surgery, radiation therapy, or both. Immediate surgery is indicated if compression of the cord or nerve roots is evident. Often, surgery results in marked improvement or complete restoration of function, especially if the tumor is benign and encapsulated (e.g., meningioma or lipoma). Functional improvement is less common if cord necrosis has developed, however. Complete surgical removal of an intramedullary tumor is rare. Partial resection followed by radiation may improve the client's condition. Usually, the course of the condition is gradually progressive.

VASCULAR SPINAL CORD LESIONS

As with stroke, spinal cord vascular lesions may be caused by rupture, thrombosis, or embolism. Trauma is the usual cause of hemorrhage into the spinal cord. Thrombosis of the spinal vessels usually is secondary to meningitis or to compression of the vessels by tumors, granulomas, or abscesses in the epidural space.

MYELOMALACIA

Myelomalacia is softening or infarction of the spinal cord from spinal artery occlusion. Prognosis is poor. There is little or no return of normal function to the involved areas. Myelomalacia is suspected when indications of transverse myelitis develop suddenly.

Assessment findings in myelomalacia depend on the level of the lesion in the cord. There is always motor paralysis and dissociated sensory loss below the level of the lesion, accompanied by paralysis of bladder and bowel sphincters. Paralysis usually is bilateral but rarely complete. Initially the limbs are flaccid, and no deep tendon or superficial reflexes are elicited, as in spinal shock. After several weeks, spasticity, hyperreflexia, and clonus develop.

Intervention focuses on maintaining body functions, preventing complications of immobility, and providing pain relief. The client usually begins intensive rehabilitation 12 to 14 hours after onset of manifestations.

HEMATOMYELIA

Hematomyelia is hemorrhage into the substance of the spinal cord. It almost always follows trauma but may be caused by vascular malformation or a bleeding disorder.

Clinical manifestations usually develop suddenly, immediately after spinal injury, and depend on the size of the hemorrhage. After trauma, it is important to differentiate between hematomyelia and a vertebral fracture-dislocation. Immediate surgery to relieve cord compression is indicated if fracture-dislocation is evident on radiograph. Spinal angiography, spinal CT scans, and MRI enable visualization of vascular lesions. Some of these lesions are treated by ligating their feeding vessels, others by excising the entire malformation.

Management is the same as for myelomalacia. If surgery is needed, postoperative care is similar to that given to clients with other forms of spinal surgery.

NEUROSYPHILIS

Neurosyphilis is a chronic or late stage of syphilis involving infection of the brain, spinal cord, or both. The oculomotor nerves may be affected, leading to an inability of the pupil to react to light, called an *Argyll Robertson pupil*. The posterior columns and nerve roots of the spinal cord may be affected, which is called *tabes dorsalis*.

Clinical Manifestations

Because these are sensory nerves, the most common manifestation is pain. The pain can occur almost anywhere in the body, although abdominal pain is most common. The pain is severe enough to be confused with gastric ulcers and gallbladder disease. In addition to pain, areas of paresthesias may be noted. A common finding in tabes dorsalis is the loss of position sense in the feet and legs. As a result, clients walk with a slapping step. They are at increased risk for falls when walking in the dark because they must rely on visual cues for placement of their feet with each step. Because the gait is abnormal, bone alignment with walking is altered. Eventually the foot is abnormally shaped (called *Charcot's joint*). This alteration in foot structure can lead to foot ulcerations because the client bears the body weight on abnormal areas. The brain also can be involved in later stages of syphilis. A general deterioration of mental status can develop.

Outcome Management

With improved case finding and the use of penicillin to treat syphilis in its early stages, the management of syphilis is improving. With development of resistant strains of organisms and a rise in the incidence of sexually transmitted diseases, however, problems may recur in the future.

DISORDERS OF THE CRANIAL NERVES

Cranial nerves can be affected in many ways by various nervous system disorders. For example, they may be affected secondarily by compression resulting from increased intracranial pressure, or they may be damaged directly as a result of head injuries. Only the two most common disorders specific to the cranial nerves, not those associated with other disorders, are discussed here. Other cranial nerve disorders exist. Regeneration of the cranial nerves can occur except for the first (olfactory) or second (optic) cranial nerve because these nerves are actually part of the central nervous system.

TRIGEMINAL NEURALGIA

Chronic irritation of the fifth cranial nerve results in trigeminal neuralgia. Approximately 15,000 cases are diagnosed each year in the United States. Although most commonly occurring in people 50 to 70 years old, trigeminal neuralgia can occur in adults of any age. Approximately 60% of clients are women. The trigeminal nerve has three divisions: ophthalmic, maxillary, and mandibular (Fig. 71–11). Trigeminal neuralgia may occur in any one or more of these divisions.

Etiology

Causes of trigeminal neuralgia can be *intrinsic* or *extrinsic* lesions within the nerve itself, such as gross abnormalities of the axon or myelin, as may occur with multiple sclerosis. Extrinsic lesions are outside the trigeminal root and include mechanical compression by tumors, vascular anomalies, dental abscesses, or jaw malformation.

Clinical Manifestations

Trigeminal neuralgia is characterized by intermittent episodes of intense pain of sudden onset. The pain rarely is relieved by analgesics. Tactile stimulation, such as touch and facial hygiene, and talking may trigger an attack. Trigeminal neuralgia is more prevalent in the maxillary and mandibular distributions and on the right side of the face. Bilateral trigeminal neuralgia is rare but does occur. The pain from trigeminal neuralgia can become so intense that the client ponders suicide.

None of the current diagnostic studies identify trigeminal neuralgia. A CT scan, MRI, and angiography can identify a causative lesion. The diagnosis is made on the basis of an in-depth history, with attention paid to triggering stimuli and the nature and site of the pain.

A careful history is obtained from the client regarding stimuli that trigger an attack. This information is used to plan care so as to minimize triggering events. The client's dental hygiene and nutritional intake are evaluated. These clients often do not eat enough to meet their daily nutritional needs and neglect their teeth because of the pain.

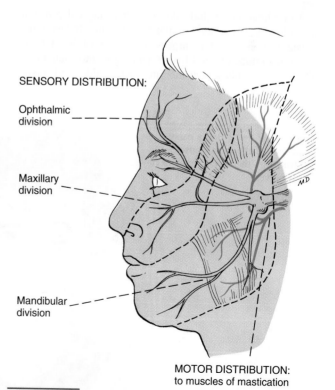

SENSORY DISTRIBUTION:

Ophthalmic division

Maxillary division

Mandibular division

MOTOR DISTRIBUTION: to muscles of mastication

Figure 71–11 Distribution of the trigeminal nerve. Trigeminal neuralgia develops along the course of this nerve.

Outcome Management

Anticonvulsant agents such as carbamazepine (Tegretol) are often prescribed as the initial treatment of trigeminal neuralgia. These drugs may dampen the reactivity of the neurons within the trigeminal nerve. For some clients, these medications are all the treatment that is needed. Liver impairment may result from administration of carbamazepine and phenytoin. Liver enzymes must be monitored before and during therapy. If the client cannot tolerate the dose needed for pain control, phenytoin can be used. These medications should be used cautiously in clients with a history of alcohol abuse. Baclofen (Lioresal) is an antispasmodic that may be used alone or in conjunction with anticonvulsants. Narcotics are not particularly effective in relieving trigeminal neuralgia pain.

Help clients use and improve any pain control strategies they have developed. Clients with trigeminal neuralgia need emotional support to help them deal with pain that has often been present for a long time.

Surgery includes nerve blocks with alcohol and glycerol; peripheral neurectomy; and percutaneous radiofrequency wave forms, which create lesions that alter pain transmission. The relief obtained with these procedures is not always permanent. Complications include development of facial paresthesias and muscular weakness. These procedures, being less invasive, often are tolerated better by elderly or debilitated clients.

More invasive techniques involve major surgical procedures. Microvascular decompression involves removing the vessel from the posterior trigeminal root. A rhizotomy is the actual resection of the root of the nerve. With these procedures, craniotomy is required to allow access to the nerve.

Complications include those of any surgical procedure as well as facial weakness and paresthesias. If facial anesthesia is present after surgery, clients must learn to test the temperature of food before putting it into their mouth. They should chew on the unaffected side and inspect mucous membranes for irritation. Assess for aspiration and advance the diet slowly. Teach clients to use a water jet device instead of a toothbrush for dental hygiene, and advise them to visit the dentist as soon as possible after surgery.

If the corneal reflex has been impaired, the client needs to be taught eye care. During the acute postoperative period, apply eye drops and a protective shield. The client assumes these tasks with supervision, then independently.

BELL'S PALSY

Pathophysiology and Etiology

Bell's palsy affects the motor aspects of the facial nerve, the seventh cranial nerve (Fig. 71–12). Bell's palsy is the most common type of peripheral facial paralysis. It affects women and men in all age groups. It is most common between ages 20 and 40 years.

Bell's palsy results in a unilateral paralysis of the facial muscles of expression. There is no evidence of a pathologic cause. Facial paralysis may be central or peripheral in origin. Central facial palsy is an upper motor neuron paralysis or paresis. Sometimes it produces dissociation of motor function. In this situation, the client cannot voluntarily show his or her teeth on the paralyzed side but can show them with emotional stimulation, such as that causing smiles or laughter. This phenomenon is called *voluntary emotional dissociation.*

Clinical Manifestations

Typical assessment findings on the affected side include (1) upward movement of the eyeball on closing the eye (Bell's phenomenon), (2) drooping of the mouth, (3) flattening of the nasolabial fold, (4) widening of the palpebral fissure, and (5) a slight lag in closing the eye. Eating may be difficult.

FIGURE 71–12 Bell's palsy is paralysis of the facial muscles innervated by the seventh cranial (facial) nerve.

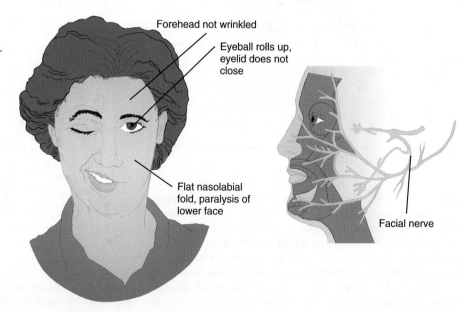

Forehead not wrinkled

Eyeball rolls up, eyelid does not close

Flat nasolabial fold, paralysis of lower face

Facial nerve

Outcome Management

There is no known cure for Bell's palsy. Palliative measures include:

- Analgesics if discomfort occurs from herpetic lesions
- Corticosteroids to decrease nerve tissue edema
- Physiotherapy, moist heat, gentle massage, and stimulation of the facial nerve with faradic current
- Corneal protection with an artificial tears solution, sunglasses, an eye patch at night, and periodic gentle closure of the eye

Clients experiencing Bell's palsy often think they have had a stroke. Reassure the client that this is not the case. Most clients recover from Bell's palsy within a few weeks without residual manifestations. If permanent complete facial paralysis occurs, surgery may be necessary. Anastomosis of the peripheral end of the facial nerve with the spinal accessory or hypoglossal nerve may allow closure of the eye during sleep and restores tone to the facial musculature.

UPPER MOTOR NEURON LESIONS

Because the lower motor neurons (LMNs) send instructions for the muscles to contract, it follows that certain pathways in the central nervous system influence the activity of the LMNs that facilitates and inhibits muscle contractions. Several known pathways that arise from the higher brain centers influence the activity of the LMNs. These pathways constitute the upper motor neurons (UMNs). The UMNs originate in the motor strip of the cerebral cortex and in multiple brain stem nuclei. From the cortex, these axons pass through the internal capsule; most of them cross over in the medulla and descend in the spinal cord through the corticospinal tracts. A few do not cross in the brain but cross later in the spinal cord.

The corticospinal tracts are responsible primarily for precise, fine, voluntary motor movements. They also assist in modulating muscle tone and reflexes to some degree. Any lesion that destroys the UMNs results in contralateral paralysis, such as is seen with cerebrovascular accident (stroke). Initially the involved area is flaccid and hyporeflexic. The flaccidity gradually recedes, and the reflex arc becomes hyperactive because of the lack of inhibition by the UMNs. Muscle tone is hypertonic, and the extremity becomes spastic. Despite the spasms, the muscle becomes atrophied from disuse. The atrophy seen with UMN lesions occurs later than that seen with LMN problems. The Babinski reflex is present.

LOWER MOTOR NEURON LESIONS

LMNs consist of the anterior horn cells located in the anterior gray matter of the spinal cord. They also are located in the motor cranial nuclei of the brain stem. Each anterior horn cell has a long axon that leaves the cord by the anterior spinal root and extends out the peripheral nerve, eventually synapsing at the motor endplate of a neuromuscular junction. These structures form a motor unit that controls skeletal muscle activity, both voluntary and reflex activity. They are the last cells to carry information from the nervous system out to the muscles.

LMN lesions often are associated with spinal cord injury or tumors and surgery on the aorta, which alters blood flow to the spinal cord. When a lesion develops in the LMNs, flaccid muscle weakness or paralysis, loss of reflexes, loss of muscle tone, and atrophy of the involved muscles develop. The degree to which these clinical manifestations develop depends on the extent of the lesion. Each anterior horn cell innervates several separate muscle fibers, and because several anterior horn cells exist at each spinal level, a lesion confined to one spinal segment may not damage all of the anterior horn cells innervating an entire muscle. This type of lesion would cause muscle weakness rather than paralysis.

Paralysis occurs when a lesion involves the column or anterior horn cells in several spinal segments. If all the peripheral motor nerves are involved, the entire muscle becomes flaccid. The muscles atrophy early because of lack of innervation.

DISORDERS OF THE PERIPHERAL NERVES

Peripheral nerves can be injured in many ways—from bone fractures, stretching of the nerves, infections, vascular or metabolic disturbances, constriction by fascial bands, pressure from tumors, trauma associated with perforating wounds, injection of drugs, and exposure to chemicals or toxins. *Neuropathy* is nerve damage from any cause. *Mononeuropathy* is injury to a single nerve as a result of localized injury. *Polyneuropathy* is diffuse damage to many nerves as a result of toxic agents or metabolic disturbances. The peripheral nerves subjected most commonly to external pressure are the median, radial, ulnar, sciatic, common peroneal, tibial, and long thoracic nerves. The common peroneal nerve (a terminal branch of the sciatic) is injured more frequently than any other nerve. Because of its course and distribution, the sciatic nerve is exposed to internal and external trauma and inflammation more than any other nerve. The median nerve most often is injured by constriction from fascial bands. The axillary nerve may be injured as the result of an allergic reaction to serum injections or secondary to improper crutch walking. The sciatic nerve may be injured directly during medication injections. It may also be secondarily injured from diffusion of injected solutions. Any peripheral nerve can be injured by bone fractures or perforating wounds.

Assessment findings with nerve damage depend on the type of nerve injured and the extent of damage. Damaged motor nerves cause clinical manifestations, such as flaccid paralysis, muscle wasting, and reflex loss in the muscle innervated by the injured nerve. Damaged mixed nerves or sensory nerves cause vasomotor and trophic disturbances after partial or complete interruption of the nerve. After partial injury or incomplete division of a nerve, the person may experience stabbing pains, paresthesias (pins-and-needles sensation), and occasionally the burning pains of causalgia. Damaged sensory nerves cause loss of sensation in the nerves' area of anatomic distribution.

PERIPHERAL NEUROPATHIES

■ CUMULATIVE TRAUMA DISORDERS

Cumulative trauma disorders (CTDs) include a group of overuse syndromes that predominantly affect the wrist and hand. They are also often called *repetitive strain injuries* because some repetitive work activities seem to cause or exacerbate manifestations. There are several forms, and some are listed in Table 71–1. The client often describes fatigue, with aching and tiredness during the activity. Rest generally relieves manifestations in this first clinical stage. Later the client reports manifestations that persist into the next day. Finally the client complains of chronic aching, fatigue, and weakness despite rest. In attempts to minimize the incidence and effects of cumulative trauma disorders, health specialists in business and industry have modified work tasks, work stations, tools or equipment, and the work environment (see Table 71–1).

■ CARPAL TUNNEL SYNDROME

Carpal tunnel syndrome (CTS) is an entrapment neuropathy that occurs when the median nerve is compressed as it passes through the wrist along a pathway to the hand. The tunnel, called the *carpal tunnel,* is bordered by the flexor retinaculum, a band of fibrous tissue that prevents the wrist tendons from bowing when the wrist is flexed. Compression causes sensory and motor changes in the thumb, index finger, middle finger, and radial aspect of the ring finger. CTS also leads to atrophy of the radial half of the thenar eminence.

Etiology

CTS may develop spontaneously without a known cause or may result from disease or injury. The most commonly reported cause of CTS is repetitive motion of the wrist, with the wrist in constant flexion. A higher incidence of CTS is reported among homemakers, factory workers, bricklayers, cashiers, musicians, secretaries, and computer operators. Pregnancy, hypothyroidism, gout, and rheumatoid arthritis are other conditions associated with CTS.

Clinical Manifestations

Initially the client may be awakened at night by pain and paresthesia. Although these initial manifestations are temporary and relieved by shaking the hand, later stages may be accompanied by motor loss (e.g., progressive weakness, inability to perform fine motor activities), burning or numbness in the thumb, index finger, or middle finger, and daytime pain.

Assessment of the client begins with a thorough history, including occupational tasks. Diagnostic assessment for CTS includes assessing for Tinel's and Phalen's signs (Fig. 71–13A and B). Tinel's sign is the development of tingling in the hands and fingers when the wrist is tapped. Phalen's test is assessing for the development of numbness and tingling after forceful flexion of the wrists for 20 to 30 seconds (see Fig. 71–13B).

Finally the wrist compression test is done. The test involves manual application of 30 seconds of pressure over the flexor retinaculum (Fig. 71–13C). If paresthesias develop after compression, the result is positive. The wrist compression test is 87% accurate in the diagnosis of CTS. Electromyography procedure also may be used in differential diagnosis to rule out other possible causes.

Outcome Management

Initially, the wrist is splinted in a neutral position to prevent mechanical irritation of the nerve. Injection of steroids into the flexor tendons is done less frequently now because of reported problems with scarring, median nerve damage, and infection. In addition to rest, pyridoxine HCl (vitamin B$_6$) has been helpful. For some clients, pain can be relieved by gently squeezing the distal metacarpal heads together with the affected hand, palm up; in some instances, stretch of digits III and IV also is required. This maneuver also may help in the clinical diagnosis of CTS.

Surgery is indicated with (1) severe manifestations of long duration, (2) muscle atrophy, or (3) progressive sensory loss in the fingers and hand. Regional anesthesia is used for carpal tunnel release (decompression of the median nerve by transecting the transverse carpal ligament). Carpal tunnel release can be performed by opening the wrist or through an endoscope. The transverse ligament is divided to relieve pressure.

After surgery, blood flow is assessed hourly by checking the color, capillary refill, and warmth of the finger tips. When the anesthetic has worn off, assess the fingers for sensation.

Initially, postoperative care centers on wrist immobilization using bulky dressings and a wrist splint. The arm is elevated on pillows to reduce edema. Encourage the client to try to move the fingers, even though they are splinted. After the dressings are removed, progressive exercises, including flexion, extension, and gripping, are begun. The client often returns to the same type of work, so that recovery of strength and flexibility are imperative. Work site analysis should also be completed to avoid reinjury.

The client and family are the care providers beyond the immediate postoperative period. Because this surgery usually is performed on an outpatient basis, provide detailed instructions on home care. The Client Education Guide lists suggestions for home care after carpal tunnel release.

■ ULNAR NERVE SYNDROME

Lying within a bony groove at the elbow, the ulnar nerve is susceptible to compression from direct trauma to the elbow (e.g., hitting the funny bone) or from changes within the groove that gradually squeeze the nerve. Repeated mild trauma (e.g., habitual leaning of the elbows on a hard surface such as experienced by truck drivers) can injure the ulnar nerve. Sensory changes occur in the ulnar aspect of the hand and wrist. The usual treatment for ulnar nerve compression at the elbow is surgical transplantation of the ulnar nerve.

■ TARSAL TUNNEL SYNDROME

Tarsal tunnel syndrome is the counterpart of CTS in the lower extremity. In this syndrome, the posterior tibial nerve is trapped beneath the flexor retinaculum and deep fascia along the foot's medial border.

TABLE 71–1	REPETITIVE MOTION INJURIES		
Condition	Manifestations	People/Occupations at Risk	Usual Treatment
NECK			
Tension neck syndrome	Stiff, aching neck; headache	Typists, keypunch operators, cashiers, and others who must maintain a restricted posture	Prevention is key: (1) pause frequently when typing or keying to stretch about 30 sec every 30 min; (2) place screen directly in front of typist, avoid twisting; (3) place material to be typed at eye level if possible; avoid having materials to be typed consistently on one side of typist; conservative*
Cervical syndrome	Pain on flexion or extension of the neck with radiation down the arm	Common in people who assume awkward positions for a long time, such as painters, dentists	Conservative,* cervical collar, surgery
SHOULDER			
Thoracic outlet syndrome	Numbness, pain, ischemia, and weakened pulse in upper extremity with hyperextension of the shoulder	Overhead assembly workers, automobile repair mechanics, letter carriers	Conservative,* transcutaneous nerve stimulation, surgery
Supraspinatus tendinitis	Pain on elevating arm above 70 degrees at the shoulder	People who must maintain abduction with elbow extended—painters, construction workers	Conservative,* physical therapy, steroid injections
Bicipital tendinitis	Pain over the bicipital tendon in bicipital groove	Window washers, construction workers, shipping clerks	Conservative,* physical therapy, steroid injections
ELBOW, HAND, AND WRIST			
Lateral or medial epicondylitis (tennis elbow)	Local pain and pain on resisted hand motion	Repeated and forceful rotation of the forearm with the wrist bent; can be seen in bowlers, tennis players, and pitchers	Conservative,* steroid injections, surgery
de Quervain's tenosynovitis (inflammation of the extensor pollicus brevis tendons)	Gradual onset of pain, and sometimes swelling of the radial styloid; popping sensation on extension of the thumb	Middle-aged women and those subject to repetitive stress of the thumb	Conservative,* steroid injections, surgery
Carpal tunnel syndrome	Pain and paresthesias on percussion over the median nerve at the wrist (Tinel's sign) or with flexed wrists pressed together (positive Phalen's maneuver); night pain after 3–4 hr of sleep, morning stiffness, daytime numbness	Repetitive forced hand movements, keypunch operators, cashiers, typists, people with degenerative joint disease	Prevention is key: (1) while typing pause frequently at least 30 sec every 30 min; (2) adjust keyboard so the elbows are at 90 degree angle and wrists are straight; (3) do not rest wrists on a hard surface or restpad; wrists should "float" above keyboard; (4) use a light touch when striking the keys; conservative,* steroid injections, surgery
Ulnar nerve entrapment	Pain and paresthesias on percussion of the ulnar nerve over the epicondyle (Tinel's sign); local swelling and tissue hypertrophy around elbow	Rheumatoid arthritis clients, occupational stress on elbow	Conservative,* surgery

*Conservative treatment consists of restriction of the harmful motion, splinting (if appropriate and only for short periods of time or at night), application of ice or heat, mild analgesics and nonsteroidal anti-inflammatory drugs, and gentle stretching exercises.

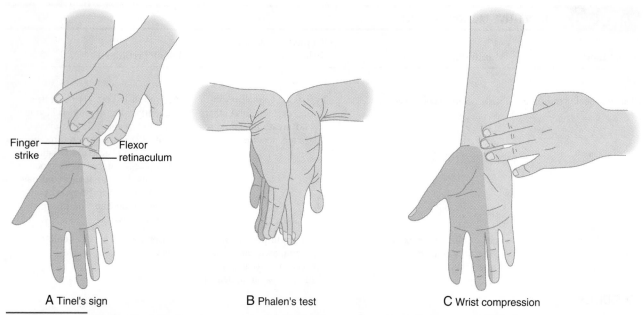

A Tinel's sign   B Phalen's test   C Wrist compression

FIGURE 71–13 Clinical examination of carpal tunnel syndrome includes tests for Tinel's sign (*A*), Phalen's sign (*B*), and wrist compression (*C*). Each of these maneuvers elicits numbness and pain in the thumb, the index and middle fingers, and the radial aspect of the ring finger if carpal tunnel syndrome is present.

DUPUYTREN'S CONTRACTURE

Dupuytren's contracture, a permanent flexor contracture of the fourth and fifth fingers, is inherited as an autosomal dominant trait. It is common in people of Northern European descent and is more common in alcoholics and diabetics.

In severe forms of contracture, a longitudinal fibrous cord forms, which extends from the fingers to the palm and pulls the fingers into a locked position. Milder forms are characterized by less contracture and fewer nodules in the palmar fascia.

Ten years or more may pass before surgery is necessary. The decision to operate is usually made when the client can no longer lay the hand outstretched on a table.

CLIENT EDUCATION GUIDE

Home Care After Carpal Tunnel Release

- Check the circulation in your hand; notify the physician if you notice: increased swelling that results in the hand or fingers becoming pale, tingly, or cold; rings too tight to remove; or if any of these manifestations are present even without swelling.
- Keep the affected wrist elevated as much as possible, using the splint to immobilize the wrist area.
- Flex and extend your fingers hourly during waking hours.
- Observe for signs of infection: odorous dressing, fever, or increased pain at the incisional site.
- Use analgesia as directed for pain relief.
- Restrict lifting for 2 months.
- Wear a splint for 7 to 14 days after surgery or until the sutures are removed.
- Avoid getting the incision site wet until after the sutures are removed.

The operation consists of excision of part of the palmar fascia. After surgery, the hand is dressed in a large compression dressing. Range-of-motion movements are encouraged. Frequent assessments of capillary refill and finger color are needed. Splints may be used at night to promote extension. Many months of physical therapy may be needed, and full function may not be achievable.

GANGLION

The most common soft tissue mass found in the hand or wrist is a ganglion, a firm cystic lesion that often is located deep in the tissues. Trauma or degenerative changes in the fibrous joint capsule are thought to contribute to development of a ganglion. Depending on its location, the ganglion can compress the median nerve, leading to CTS. The benign cyst, which consists of clear mucinous fluid enclosed in a fibrous capsule, is found most often on the dorsum of the wrist.

To relieve pain or numbness, the ganglion may be aspirated or the cyst surgically excised. The area may then be injected with a corticosteroid before a pressure dressing and splint are applied. NSAIDs are commonly used for pain or discomfort. Wrist ganglions may recur in 30% of affected clients.[16]

PERIPHERAL NERVE INJURIES

Nerves can be injured in common household accidents (cut on glass) or in severe motor vehicle accidents. Assessment includes full examination of the hand, a discussion of the client's occupation, and documentation of the dominant hand.

Conservative management may include splinting, ice, elevation of the limb, or administration of NSAIDs and analgesic agents, or a combination of these. If a peripheral nerve is traumatically severed, the ends should be surgically anastomosed to enable healing. The nearer the site of injury occurs to the central nervous system, the less chance of regeneration. When nerves are damaged only slightly, mild edema occurs at the injury site. This edema may cause temporary manifestations of motor and/ or sensory loss that recede in a few days or possibly weeks.

Postoperative care of clients having nerve repair or grafting includes elevation of the extremity. Elevation is critical to reducing edema and improving venous return. The procedure usually is performed with local anesthesia; therefore, assessment of neurovascular status is not conclusive until the anesthesia has worn off. Color, warmth, movement, sensation, capillary refill, and strength are assessed. Some of these assessments can be hampered by dressings, but as many as possible should be performed.

Monitor the finger tips for blood flow with Doppler laser or standard Doppler ultrasonography and temperature probes. The temperature of the hand is usually less than the core temperature, and the surgeon indicates acceptable ranges of temperature. Physical therapy begins within a few days to promote movement after severe injuries.

If the injury is severe, the client may have recurring dreams about the accident and the injury. These dreams are generally normal post-traumatic responses, but if they are bothersome to the client, a psychiatric consultant may be helpful.

PERIPHERAL NERVE TUMORS

Although solitary tumors (generally neurofibromas) may develop on any peripheral nerve, multiple tumors occur most often and are part of a syndrome known as *neurofibromatosis (von Recklinghausen's disease)*. This hereditary disorder is characterized by multiple tumors of the spinal and cranial nerves along with involvement of many other systems. The disease usually is not life-threatening, and lesions are excised only when they interfere with normal activity. Intracranial and intraspinal tumors usually are removed.

Surgery for peripheral nerve tumors is generally performed on an outpatient basis. In the recovery room, the dressings are checked for drainage; circulation, motion, and sensation in the extremity are assessed. Clients are encouraged to perform range-of-motion exercises. Clients and family members are taught the manifestations of circulatory compromise and infection, medication management, and care of the dressing and incision.

CONCLUSIONS

Physical and psychological impairments vary with the degree of damage as well as the client's response and ability to cope with body changes. The coping response is not always related to the degree of physiologic damage. A client can have facial paralysis or trigeminal neuralgia and be more compromised psychologically than a client with spinal cord injury who has strong coping skills. It is imperative that nurses comprehend the severity of the client's dysfunction as it relates to quality of life as well as the impact it has on family dynamics.

THINKING CRITICALLY

1. The client, a 34-year-old woman, had undergone a lumbar laminectomy done earlier today. A previous assessment showed that movement and sensation of both lower extremities were intact. During the current postoperative assessment, she stated that her right toes felt numb, and the dorsiflexion and plantiflexion of the right foot are a little weaker than earlier. She has requested an analgesic because she is starting to get a headache. What are the priorities for her care? What assessments and interventions might be used?

Factors to Consider. What assessment methods can be used to determine the extent of vascular insufficiency? What type of neurologic checks should be done?

BIBLIOGRAPHY

1. Agency for Health Care Policy and Research (AHCPR). (1994). *Acute low back problems in adults: Assessment and treatment.* No. 95-0642. Rockville, MD: U.S. Department of Health and Human Services: Public Health Service, AHCPR.
2. Atroshi, I., et al. (1999). Symptoms, disability, and quality of life in patients with carpal tunnel syndrome. *Journal of Hand Surgery, 24*(2), 398–404.
3. Burge, P., et al. (1997). Smoking, alcohol and the risk of Dupuytren's contracture. *Journal of Bone and Joint Surgery (Br), 79*(2), 206–210.
4. Chen, T. Y. (2000). The clinical presentation of uppermost cervical disc protrusion. *Spine, 25*(4), 439–442.
5. Freidman, R. A. (2000). The surgical management of Bell's palsy: A review. *American Journal of Otolaryngology, 21*(1), 139–144.
6. Geary, S. (1996). Nursing management of cranial nerve dysfunction. *Journal of Neuroscience, Nursing, 27*(2), 102–108.
7. Halderman, S. (1999). Low back pain: Current physiological concepts. *Neurological Clinics, 17*(1), 1–16.
8. Hall, H. (1999). Surgery: Indications and options. *Neurological Clinics, 17*(1), 113–130.
9. Kloen, P. (1999). New insights in the development of Dupuytren's contracture: A review. *British Journal of Plastic Surgery, 52*(8), 629–635.
10. Kuric, J. (1995). Spinal cord tumors. *Critical Care Nursing Clinics of North America, 7*(1), 151–157.
11. Laine, D. E. (1999). Low back pain and carpal tunnel syndrome: Two troublesome presentations in the workplace. *Advances in Nurse Practitioners, 7*(6) 49–50, 74.
12. LeCompte, C. M. (1997). Post polio syndrome: An update for the primary health care provider. *The Nurse Practitioner, 22*(6), 133–154.
13. Maksud, D. (1993). Psychological adjustments to hand injuries: Nursing management. *Plastic Surgical Nursing, 13*(4), 72–76.
14. Manente, G., et al. (1999). A relief maneuver in carpal tunnel syndrome. *Muscle and Nerve, 22*(11), 1587–1589.
15. Massy-Westropp, N., Grimmer, K., & Bain, G. (2000). A systematic review of the clinical diagnostic tests for carpal tunnel syndrome. *Journal of Hand Surgery, 25*(1), 120–127.
16. McConaghy, D. J. (1994). Trigeminal neuralgia: A personal review and nursing implications. *Journal of Neuroscience Nursing, 26*(2), 85–89.
17. Neatherlin, J. S., & Brillhart, B. (1996). Body image in preoperative and postoperative lumbar laminectomy patients. *Journal of Neuroscience Nursing, 27*(1), 43–46.
18. Postacchini, F. (1999). Management of herniation of the lumbar disc. *Journal of Bone and Joint Surgery (Br), 81*(4), 567–574.
19. Swenson, R. (1999). Differential diagnosis: A reasonable clinical approach. *Neurological Clinics, 17*(1), 43–64.
20. Thorsteinsson, G. (1997). Management of post-polio syndrome. *Mayo Clinic Proceedings, 72,* 627–638.

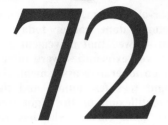

CHAPTER 72

REMEMBER *to check out your* **Companion CD ROM**

Management of Clients with Degenerative Neurologic Disorders

Amy Perrin Ross

NURSING OUTCOMES CLASSIFICATION (NOC)
for Nursing Diagnoses—Clients with Degenerative Neurologic Disorders

Activity Intolerance	Knowledge: Health Resources	Risk Detection
Activity Tolerance	**Constipation**	Safety Behavior: Fall Prevention
Energy Conservation	Bowel Elimination	Safety Behavior: Home Physical
Self-Care: Activities of Daily Living (ADL)	Hydration	Environment
Altered Thought Processes	**Impaired Physical Mobility**	Safety Status: Falls Occurrence
Cognitive Ability	Body Positioning: Self-Initiated	**Risk for Self Care Deficit**
Cognitive Orientation	Joint Movement: Active	Self-Care: Activities of Daily Living (ADL)
Information Processing	Mobility Level	Mobility Level
Memory	**Impaired Verbal Communication**	**Self Care Deficit**
Altered Urinary Elimination	Communication Ability	Self-Care: Activities of Daily Living
Urinary Continence	Communication: Expressive Ability	**Urge Incontinence**
Urinary Elimination	Communication: Receptive Ability	Tissue Integrity: Skin and Mucous
Caregiver Role Strain	Cognitive Orientation	Membranes
Caregiver Emotional Health	Distorted Thought Control	Urinary Continence
Caregiver Performance: Direct Care	**Knowledge Deficit**	Urinary Elimination
Caregiver Performance: Indirect Care	Knowledge: Disease Process	**Self-Esteem Disturbance**
Caregiver Physical Health	Knowledge: Health Resources	Self-Esteem
Caregiver Stressors	Knowledge: Medication	Body Image
Caregiver Well-Being	**Risk for Injury**	Social Support
Depression Control	Neurological Status	

Degenerative neurologic disorders pose a great challenge to the client, the family, and the caregiver, whether it is the nurse, a family member, or a significant other. By their very nature, these disorders cause progressive decline in neurologic function. Some progress relatively quickly (over months to 1 or 2 years) whereas others progress more gradually, sometimes over decades. Common nursing diagnoses for clients with these disorders are *Altered Thought Processes, Memory Deficit, Visual-Perceptual Alteration, Impaired Physical Mobility, Incontinence, Self-Care Deficit,* and *Impaired Individual and Family Coping.* A major goal of intervention is to help the client achieve an optimal level of functioning in light of chronic neurologic deficits.

The diagnosis of degenerative neurologic disease is most often made in an outpatient setting. However, hospital admission may be necessary when acute relapses or life-threatening events occur. Many clients return to their homes and have regular follow-up in outpatient clinics; however, some may require rehabilitation, in either inpatient or outpatient settings, for newly acquired deficits. Other clients may require transfer to long-term care facilities because of significant decline in ability to provide self-care. Still other clients may not survive their acute illness.

ALZHEIMER'S DISEASE

Alzheimer's disease (AD) is the most common form of dementia among people 65 years of age and older. Dementia is intellectual deterioration severe enough to interfere with occupational or social performance. It involves progressive decline in two or more areas of cognition, usually memory and language, calculation, visuospatial perception, constructional praxis, judgment, abstraction, or personality. AD constitutes at least half of all dementias (see Chapter 68 for a general discussion of dementia).

AD affects about 4 million Americans. Slightly more than half of these people receive care at home, and the remainder receive institutional nursing care. The prevalence of AD doubles every 5 years after the age of 65. In fact, some estimates indicate that nearly half of all people over age 85 years have AD.

Etiology and Risk Factors

The cause of AD has not been found, although several risk factors have been identified. As can be seen by the statistics listed earlier, increasing age is a risk factor. Genetic factors can influence AD. At least five chromosomes (1, 12, 14, 19, 21) are involved in some forms of familial AD. Four genetic loci have also been identified as contributing to AD, including the amyloid precursor gene, the presenillin 1 gene, the presenillin 2 gene, and the apolipoprotein E gene. However, these loci do not account for all of the genetic risk. Further, the lack of 100% concordance in studies of identical twins implies that environmental, metabolic, and other factors also may play a role.

Nearly all people with Down's syndrome develop dementia and the pathologic features of AD. Current research is investigating the role of vascular disease and the onset of the clinical manifestations of AD. Female sex, head trauma, lack of education, and myocardial infarction have been linked to AD, but these associations are weak.[6] Some have postulated that aluminum intoxication, disordered immune function, and viral infection may be etiologic, but these factors have not been proven. A role for genetic testing is yet to be defined.

Although the major risk factors for AD (age, family history) cannot be controlled, efforts to reduce the incidence of head trauma and cardiovascular disease may help reduce the incidence of AD and other types of dementia.

Pathophysiology

Alois Alzheimer first described presenile dementia in 1907. He used a new staining technique of human brain tissue to demonstrate the pathologic changes. The changes he noted are now termed *neurofibrillary tangles* and *neuritic (amloid) plaques* (Fig. 72–1). The neuritic plaque is a cluster of degenerating nerve terminals, both dendritic and axonal, that contain amyloid protein. During metabolism, the amyloid precursor protein becomes embedded in the membrane of the neuron. Its effect on the neuron is being studied. These plaques develop first in neocortex and the hippocampus areas of the brain used for memory and other cognitive functions. Neurofibrillary tangles are abnormal neurons in which the cytoplasm is filled with bundles of abnormal protein called *paired helical filaments*. The term "association" is used to describe all the intellectual activities of the cerebral cortex. These functions include learning and reasoning, memory storage and recall, language abilities, and even consciousness.

Gross brain changes evident in clients with AD include thickening of the leptomeninges, shrunken gyri, widened sulci, enlarged ventricles, hippocampal shrinkage, and generalized atrophy.

In addition to structural changes, neurotransmitter changes are evident in the brain of clients with AD. A decline in cholinergic neurons in the basal nucleus leads to loss of choline acetyltransferase in the neocortex and hippocampus. Also affected are neuronal systems that project to the neocortex: the noradrenergic locus ceruleus and the serotonergic dorsal raphe nucleus in the brain stem. These two areas also contain neurofibrillary tangles. Involved neurons in the neocortex include those using corticotropin-releasing factor, somatostatin, and glutamate. Some of the changes are also due to oxidation.

Clinical Manifestations

Clinically, AD is characterized by a relentless impairment of decision-making that generally begins insidiously and can progress for a decade or so. The onset of AD typically occurs in late middle age (age 65 years and older), although some familial cases occur in a person's 40s and 50s.

FIRST STAGE
The sequence of loss of higher cognitive functions is a helpful clue in establishing the clinical diagnosis. The clinical progression of manifestations is usually divided into three stages (Box 72–1).

Memory disturbance is usually the first feature of the disease. Family members or co-workers often notice the

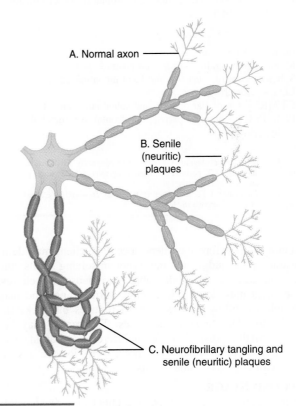

A. Normal axon

B. Senile (neuritic) plaques

C. Neurofibrillary tangling and senile (neuritic) plaques

FIGURE 72–1 Neurofibrillary tangles. In clients with Alzheimer's disease and some other neurologic disorders, these tangles replace the normal neuronal cytoplasm. The tangles are often seen with senile plaques and appear throughout the cortex, hippocampus, and amygdala. The number of plaques and tangles correlates roughly with the severity of the dementia. *A,* Normal axon. *B,* Senile plaques on ends of axon. *C,* Neurofibrillary tangles and senile plaques replacing normal axon.

BOX 72-1   Common Clinical Manifestations in Each Stage of Dementia of the Alzheimer's Type

Stage I (duration of disease 1–3 years)

Memory—new learning defective, remote recall mildly impaired
Visuospatial skills—topographic disorientation, poor complex constructions
Language—poor wordlist generation, anomia
Personality—indifference, occasional irritability
Psychiatric features—depression or delusions in some
Motor system—normal
EEG—normal
CT/MRI—normal
PET/SPECT—bilateral posterior parietal hypometabolism/hyperperfusion

Stage II (duration of disease 2–10 years)

Memory—recent and remote recall more severely impaired
Visuospatial skills—poor constructions, spatial disorientation
Language—fluent aphasia
Calculation—acalculia
Praxis—ideomotor apraxia
Personality—indifference or irritability
Psychiatric features—delusions in some
Motor system—restlessness, pacing
EEG—slowing of background rhythm
CT/MRI—normal or ventricular dilation and sulcal enlargement
PET/SPECT—bilateral parietal and frontal hypometabolism/hypoperfusion

Stage III (duration of disease 8–12 years)

Intellectual functions—severely deteriorated
Motor—limb rigidity and flexion posture
Sphincter control—urinary and fecal incontinence
EEG—diffusely slow
CT/MRI—ventricular dilation and sulcal enlargement
PET/SPECT—bilateral parietal and frontal hypometabolism/hypoperfusion

EEG, electroencephalogram; CT, computed tomography; MRI, magnetic resonance imaging; PET, positron emission tomography; SPECT, single photon emission computed tomography.
From Cummings, J. L., & Benson, D. F. (1992). *Dementia: A clinical approach.* Boston: Butterworth-Heinemann.

---

memory loss before the client does. The client may demonstrate poor judgment and problem-solving skills and become careless in work habits and household chores. The client may do well in familiar surroundings and may be able to follow well-established routines but lacks the ability to adapt to new challenges. The person may become irritable, suspicious, or indifferent. Agitation, apathy, dysphoria, and aberrant motor behavior are associated with cognitive impairments.

SECOND STAGE

In the second stage of illness, the client may demonstrate *language disturbance,* characterized by impaired word-finding and circumlocution (talking around a subject rather than about it directly). Later, spontaneous speech becomes increasingly empty, and paraphasias (words used in the wrong context) are used. Clients may repeat words and phrases just spoken by themselves (*palilalia*) or by others (*echolalia*). Motor disturbance (*apraxia*) is charac-

terized by difficulty in using everyday objects such as a toothbrush, comb, razor, and utensils. Apraxia combined with forgetfulness can create serious safety problems. The person may leave a stove burner on in the kitchen or forget to extinguish a cigarette. Indifference worsens, and restlessness with frequent pacing appears. *Hyperorality* (the desire to take everything into the mouth to suck, chew, or taste) may develop. Swallowing may become difficult.

Depression and irritability may worsen, and delusions and psychosis may appear. The person fears personal harm, theft of property, or infidelity of the spouse. Clients may see bugs crawling on the bed or throughout the house. Wandering at night is common. Occasional incontinence may occur.

THIRD STAGE

In the final stage, virtually all *mental* and *speech abilities* are lost. Voluntary movement is minimal, and the limbs become rigid with flexor posturing. Urinary and fecal incontinence are frequent. The person has lost all ability for self-care.

Diagnostic Findings

Because there is no definitive test for AD, the diagnosis is made by exclusion of known causes of dementia (e.g., toxic or metabolic alterations, drug side effects, cerebrovascular disease, neoplasm, and infection). The diagnosis is confirmed with (1) the presence of dementia involving two or more areas of cognition, (2) insidious onset, steady progression, and (3) loss of normal alertness.[14] When these criteria are applied, nine of 10 people given this diagnosis have AD confirmed at autopsy. Postmortem examination of the brain is the only way an AD diagnosis can be confirmed. The brain is viewed under the microscope for the presence of neuritic plaques and neurofibrillary tangles.

Diagnostic assessments such as electroencephalogram (EEG), computed tomography (CT), and magnetic resonance imaging (MRI) are frequently used in the diagnosis of AD. Position emission tomography (PET) has also been used. In general, these studies rule out other causes of dementia, such as seizures and cerebral bleeding, but do not identify AD. EEG changes may not appear until the later stages. CT and MRI usually reveal atrophy that is greater than what would be considered normal for age.

Finally, laboratory studies are performed to rule out metabolic and drug-related causes of dementia. These studies include urinalysis, complete blood count (CBC), erythrocyte sedimentation rate (ESR), electrolytes, blood urea nitrogen (BUN) and creatinine values, thyroid and liver function tests, calcium, serum B_{12} levels, syphilis serology, and human immunodeficiency virus (HIV) testing.

Outcome Management

There is no cure for AD. Results of studies in which acetylcholine (ACh) precursors (choline, lecithin, and deanol) and anticholinesterase agents (physostigmine and tetrahydroaminoacridine) are used to enhance memory and cognitive function have been disappointing. Tacrine (Cognex) inhibits breakdown of acetylcholinesterase in the brain, allowing more ACh to be available for nerve impulse transmission. Because of potential liver toxicity, liver function test results must be checked weekly for 18 weeks. Donepezil (Aricept), another cholinesterase inhibitor, is a reversible, selective anticholinesterase that produces minimal peripheral side effects. Donepezil is given only once a day, which is helpful for people in the early stages who are responsible for managing their own medications. Rivastigmine, a relatively selective pseudo-irreversible inhibitor of acetylcholinesterase, which is used in Europe, recently received an approval letter from the Food and Drug Administration (FDA). In an effort to combat the effect of oxygen free radicals, alpha-tocopherol (vitamin E) and selegiline have been studied. Both agents have been reported to delay the development of the later stages of AD[36] and show some improvement in levels of independent and behavioral manifestations. An extract of Ginkgo biloba may improve cognitive function for 6 to 12 months.[20] Propentofylline has been effective in the management of AD.

Most pharmacologic therapy is primarily aimed at treating behavioral problems, although behavioral and environmental manipulations are often more effective. Low-dose antipsychotic agents such as haloperidol (Haldol) can be effective for agitation and confusion. The lowest effective dose should be used and should be given just before bedtime. Sometimes twice-a-day dosing is required. Adverse side effects such as akathisia (motor restlessness), parkinsonian symptoms, tardive dyskinesia, orthostatic hypotension, anticholinergic symptoms (urinary retention and confusion), and sedation should be monitored. Antidepressants (e.g., nortriptyline and desipramine) that carry few anticholinergic side effects, fluoxetine, and trazodone are helpful for depression (Table 72–1).

■ Nursing Management of the Medical Client

ASSESSMENT

When AD is suspected, a complete history should be taken to assess for other causes of dementia. Data should be obtained from the client, family, and co-workers (if possible). Secondary sources are used because the client is often unaware of a problem with thought processing and minimizes it. Ask specific questions about difficulties with activities of daily living (ADL), increasing forgetfulness, and changes in personality. Assess past medical history for previous head injury or surgery, recent falls, headache, and a family history of AD. A Mini-Mental State examination may provide objective data for ongoing evaluation of the client (see Chapter 67).

AD has a profound impact on psychosocial behaviors. Ask about the client's reactions to changes in routine or in the environment. It is not uncommon for a client with AD to become very agitated over small changes, and apathy, social isolation, and irritability may be noted. As the brain continues to atrophy and the limbic system becomes dysfunctional, the client may become paranoid, use abusive language, and become suspicious of others.

AD has a profound impact on the family. Assess the family for strengths and weaknesses, their ability to provide care for the client, and their financial concerns. In large centers, the assessment of the client and family is performed through a team approach. The Client Education Guide provides instructions and resources for caregivers of people with AD.

DIAGNOSIS, OUTCOMES, INTERVENTION

Impaired Verbal Communication. Use the nursing diagnosis *Impaired Verbal Communication related to neuronal degeneration* to describe the client with AD.

Outcomes. The client's needs will be communicated effectively, as evidenced by making his or her needs

TABLE 72–1	PHARMACOLOGIC TREATMENT OF BEHAVIORAL PROBLEMS IN DEMENTIA OF THE ALZHEIMER'S TYPE
Problem	**Treatment Options**

Suspiciousness, paranoia, sun-downing	Behavioral
	Environmental
	Correct sensory impairment
	Low-dose antipsychotics
	  Loxapine (5–25 mg/day)
	    Causes fewer EPS
	    More sedative
	    Low-potency antipsychotic
	  Risperidone (1–4 mg/day)
	    Observe for EPS
	  Haloperidol (0.25–1.0 mg/day)

Anxiety	Treat underlying physical problems (pain, dyspnea, urinary urgency, sensory impairment) If acute, offer reassurance If related to confusion, use antipsychotics If diffuse or chronic, use short-acting benzodiazepine (e.g., oxazepam) Avoid non-benzodiazepine sedative-hypnotics, especially barbiturates Role of buspirone unclear
Acute catastrophic reactions	Lorazepam 1–4 mg IM Haloperidol 2–5 mg IM

Insomnia	Environmental, behavioral
	If associated confusion, use low-dose antipsychotics
	If associated depression, use:
	  Nortriptyline
	  Doxepin
	If associated restlessness with antipsychotic treatments:
	  Lorazepam
	  Observe for disinhibition or increased confusion
	  Ambien

Angry or violent outbursts	Very difficult to control
	Behavior log is key to determine relationship to stimuli such as:
	  Pain from arthritis or other chronic illness
	  Urinary problems
	  Constipation
	Low-dose antipsychotic
	  Risperidone, loxapine, clozapine
	Carbamazepine
	Lithium

EPS, extrapyramidal symptoms such as restlessness, drooling, stiffness, shuffling, cogwheel rigidity (like Parkinson's disease); IM, intramuscularly.

CLIENT EDUCATION GUIDE

Caring for Family Members with Alzheimer's Disease

Client Instructions

Be sure that you have verbal and written information about the disease, the results of diagnostic testing (including the results of neuropsychological testing), legal and financial resources, and social support resources such as support groups.

Meet regularly with your health care providers to discuss the demands of caring for people with Alzheimer's, strategies for reducing stress, and resources for support.

Contact the local branches of national and regional Alzheimer's groups. A good place to start for information is the National Alzheimer's Association, 919 Michigan Ave., Suite 1000, Chicago, IL 60661. Call 1-800-272-3900.

Many caregivers have also found it helpful to read various publications.

---

known and interacting meaningfully with others. This outcome is often possible only in the early stages. In later stages, a more appropriate outcome might be expressed as the client's needs are interpreted appropriately.

Interventions. In the initial stage of AD, the client's receptive and expressive language skills are relatively intact. You must be prepared to adapt to the communication level of the client. If the client speaks only single words or short phrases, you should do likewise. It is best to speak slowly and simply, with a firm volume and low pitch. The tone of voice should always be calm and reassuring and project control of the situation. However, when language becomes impaired in the second stage of the illness, be prepared to apply new techniques for communicating with the client.

Nonverbal behavior can provide you with clues. Clients with AD often avert their eyes, look down, back away, and increase hand gesturing when they do not understand. If they are frustrated, angry, or hostile, they may increase motor activity by pacing, rattling doorknobs, waving their arms or shaking their fists, frowning, raising their voice volume and pitch, or tightening their facial muscles. These behaviors should signal staff to increase their alertness, search for the cause of the distress, and prepare to intervene.

Interventions can include the following:

- Decreasing environmental stimuli
- Approaching the client calmly and with assurance
- Taking care not to place any demands on the client
- Gently distracting the client
- Making sure that all verbal and nonverbal communication cues are concordant
- Using multiple sensory modalities (visual, auditory, and tactile) to send the message but not all forms at the same time

The client's memory loss can be an advantage in distracting him or her from the stressful situation. If removed from the situation and provided with a calm, nonthreatening environment, clients may forget why they are

upset. Elicit listening behavior by reaching out and touching, holding a hand, putting an arm around the waist, or in some way maintaining physical contact with the client. Dementia sufferers can perceive nonverbal behavior of others and can become agitated or upset if they sense negative nonverbal behavior from them.

The identification of pain or discomfort in clients with advanced AD is also difficult. Behavioral indicators of discomfort include noisy breathing, negative vocalization (constant muttering, making sounds with a negative quality), a sad or frightened facial expression, frowning, tense body language, and fidgeting.

Altered Thought Processes. Neuronal degeneration also affects thought processing. State this diagnosis as *Altered Thought Processes related to neuronal degeneration.*

Outcomes. The client will have appropriate thought processing, as evidenced by retention of information to maximal capacity, maintaining orientation to maximal capacity, and sharing meaningful life experiences.

Intervention. Because memory deficit occurs in all stages of AD, you must continually apply interventions to enhance memory. Reorient the client as necessary by placing a calendar and clock in obvious places. Because the client's long-term memory is retained longer than short-term memory, allow clients to reminisce. Become aware of a client's past experiences so that they can be shared meaningfully. Repetition is useful for ensuring maximal retention of information by the client.

Risk for Injury. Altered thought processes lead to impaired judgment and forgetfulness. These changes increase risk for injury. State this common diagnosis as *Risk for Injury related to impaired judgment, forgetfulness, and motor impairments* (specify).

Outcomes. The client's physical and environmental safety will be maintained, as evidenced by the absence of physical injury and the existence of a safe living environment.

Interventions. Impaired judgment, forgetfulness, and motor impairment can make any environment unsafe for the client with AD. In the home, electrical devices, toxic substances, loose rugs, hot tap water, inadequate lighting, and unlocked doors can be sources of injury. Teach family members how to eliminate these safety hazards. In the inpatient setting, ensure that clients cannot leave the premises without being noticed, that they wear an identification badge in case they become lost, and that doors and windows are secured. Dangerous objects should be kept out of reach, and potentially dangerous activities, such as cooking, should be supervised. The client's driving skill should be evaluated at regular intervals. See Bridge to Home Health Care on safety solutions.

Self-Care Deficit. State the diagnosis of self-care problems as *Self-Care Deficit related to loss of memory and motor impairments.*

Outcomes. Clients will maintain self-care ability, as evidenced by completing the tasks they are capable of performing and receiving assistance with ADL they are incapable of performing.

Interventions. Encourage the client with AD to do as much as possible, as long as it is safe and appropriate. Carefully balance helping the client with maintaining his or her autonomy; this can boost the client's confidence

BRIDGE TO HOME HEALTH CARE

Safety Solutions for People with Alzheimer's Disease

To live with damaged thinking and judgment is to live at risk. People with Alzheimer's disease cannot take responsibility for their own safety. They are unable to evaluate the potential consequences of their actions and they forget quickly. Verbal reminders and written notes have little value, but there are many other ways to promote safety.

Older people love to live surrounded by their treasures. Although a neat home is always safer than a cluttered one, anticipate that only small changes can be made. Suggest moving knickknacks so that the edges of surfaces can be used for balance. Retain the existing furniture arrangements, but consider removing or altering furniture with sharp corners, rocking chairs that tip easily, coffee tables, and fragile antiques. Block off unsafe areas by placing a sturdy chair in front of them. Eliminate hazards such as trailing wires, extension cords, or telephone cords. Caution caregivers to watch for paper or wooden objects that are tossed into gas fireplaces.

Most accidents happen in the kitchen and the bathroom. Therefore, it is important to thoroughly assess how the person with Alzheimer's disease uses those areas. Disable stoves by removing knobs, installing a special switch behind the stove, removing a fuse, or turning the stove off at the breaker. Because people may retain over-learned food preparation skills, they may be able to safely use sharp utensils and hot surfaces but do need to be supervised. Encourage them to participate in meal preparation by doing single steps of a task, such as tearing lettuce for a salad or putting plates on the table.

Remove rugs and runners that tend to slide, especially those in the bathroom. Install grab bars to help prevent falls during transfers into or out of the tub or shower. Bars should be attached to structural supports rather than drywall or plaster. Consider using a raised toilet seat if rising is difficult and a bedside commode at night if urgency is a problem. Bath benches with non-skid feet are best, and hand-held showers minimize the need for the person to move about. Lower the temperature on the water heater to 120° F so that the water cannot become hot enough to scald anyone. If hot pipes are exposed, cover them with insulation.

While walking is good exercise and can reduce stress, wandering can become a safety issue. If the environment is secured with a fence, camouflaged doors, or locks, people with dementia may move freely within a relatively safe area, reducing the stress of caregivers who are afraid to let them out of sight. It is important to balance freedom, safety, and client rights. If wandering away from home is a potential hazard, the Alzheimer's Association has an excellent program called "Safe Return." More information about this low-cost program is available by calling 1-800-272-3900.

Tammi G. Hardiman, RN, BSN, *Nurse Consultant, Community Services Quality Assurance, Department of Social and Health Services, State of Washington, Arlington, Washington*

and self-respect, which can be very fragile during the early and middle stages of the disease. Give the client plenty of time to complete a task. Constantly encouraging, urging, and reminding the client in a step-by-step approach are necessary.

Urge Incontinence. AD clients develop urge incontinence as cortical neurons degenerate and no longer provide inhibition of the micturition and defecation responses. State this diagnosis as *Urge Incontinence related to neuronal degeneration and forgetfulness.*

Outcomes. The client will have optimal continence of bladder and bowel, as evidenced by having clean, dry clothing and bedding as much as possible; having intact skin; and voiding appropriately in the bathroom.

Interventions. Anticipation of elimination needs and scheduled voiding and defecation times can help in the initial stages. The client may show nonverbal signs of needing to void or defecate, like restlessness, grasping the genital area, or picking at clothing. Sometimes the client forgets where the bathroom is located. Having clear, bright signs indicating where the bathroom is and frequently taking the client there may help control incontinence. Fluid intake after the dinner meal can be restricted to help maintain continence during the night.

Try to arrange a bowel program to coincide with the client's usual pattern. In the later stages of AD, clients may need to wear incontinence pads during the day and external urinary drainage devices at night. Indwelling catheters should be avoided because of the risk of infection and injury.

Caregiver Role Strain. Family members and especially caregivers (usually a spouse or adult child) of clients with AD face a great deal of emotional and physical burden. State this diagnosis as *Caregiver Role Strain related to grieving the loss of a family member to AD, change in social role, and intense demands for time commitment and provision of care.*

Outcomes. The family will demonstrate decreased role strain, as evidenced by voicing their emotional concerns, seeking appropriate assistance, and providing adequate care for the client.

Interventions. Family members grieve the loss of the person they used to know. Each decline in cognitive function becomes another source of grief. Two stages of grief in the family have been described.

The process of grief begins during the caregiving stage and continues after the client's death. Normal family routines are lost, and the relationship between the family member and the dementia sufferer changes. Factors that have the most profound effect on the emotional well-being of caregivers include incontinence, overdemanding behavior, and the need for constant supervision.

Wives tend to experience a higher degree of emotional burden as caregivers than husbands do. Paradoxically, the closer the emotional bond between caregiver and dementia sufferer, the less the strain for the caregiver. Conversely, a low past level of intimacy is associated with an increased level of both perceived strain and depression in the spouse caregiver. Caregivers are most likely to be depressed if they feel a loss of control over their spouse's behavior, if they feel unable to cope with the impact of caregiving, and if they perceive the situation to be stable and to affect everything.

Studies have not determined that formal support of the caregiver (home visits by special practitioners, chore workers, and day care workers) relieves the caregiver's burden more than informal support (family member visits and support groups). The Alzheimer's Disease and Related Disorders Association has local chapters that offer support groups in many major cities in the United States (Phone: 1-800-272-3900).

Interview family members to determine their understanding of the diagnosis and prognosis of AD and to allow them to discuss their concerns about caring for the client.

- Do they know about community resources?
- Do they have someone to call when they can no longer cope with caregiving?

The home environment should be evaluated for safety before the client is sent home from the hospital.

- Is the home on a busy street?
- Can doors be secured so that the client cannot get out without supervision?
- Are potentially dangerous appliances out of reach?

A variety of options are available to caregivers. Chore service workers can help with household chores and relieve the caregiver of these duties. Other paid help can provide in-home respite care by observing the dementia sufferer while the caregiver tends to business outside the home, seeks social interaction, or meets recreational needs.

Adult day care provides time away from home for the dementia sufferer. Day care usually offers a lunchtime meal as well as several hours of scheduled activities that are tailored to the client's abilities. These activities may include games, crafts, music, and exercise.

Respite care involves admission to an extended care facility for a few days to a few weeks to allow the caregiver time to recover from the demands of providing 24-hour care (See the Bridge to Home Health Care on respite for caregivers).

BRIDGE TO HOME HEALTH CARE

Respite Care for Caregivers of People with Alzheimer's Disease

When providing home care for people with Alzheimer's disease, be alert to how well the caregivers themselves are managing their own health. If *their* health fails as a result of the stress of caregiving, the person with Alzheimer's may need to be placed in a nursing home much sooner than expected.

You can help caregivers find physical and emotional respite by following these suggestions:

- Encourage caregivers to be realistic about what needs they can meet for their loved ones and what needs they cannot meet.
- Suggest that caregivers make a list of all the tasks they perform for the person with Alzheimer's. Next to each task, have them write down who else could do the job. (Caregivers may find that they are performing some tasks that their loved ones could still do for themselves.) This exercise will help caregivers identify tasks that they could delegate to someone else.
- Help caregivers identify friends and neighbors who can offer them support, take the caregiver out for dinner, or stay with the person with Alzheimer's while the caregiver gets some precious time alone. Often, friends of caregivers are more supportive than family members, because friends can maintain more objectivity.
- Know the community resources that provide in-home day care for people with Alzheimer's.
- Encourage caregivers to share their knowledge and experience with newly assigned health care staff to foster a team approach in care. Caregivers often fear that "no one will care for my loved one like I do." They are right.
- Know the community centers that provide day care outside the home. Find out about the qualifications of the staff, cost of services, eligibility criteria, availability of financial assistance, daily activities at the centers, and

environment of the centers. Having firsthand knowledge of the centers will help you guide families as they make choices.
- Encourage caregivers to try a day care community center for at least 2 to 3 weeks, knowing that it is normal when their loved one does not like the new experience at first. Sometimes caregivers are more likely to accept assistance if they know they are "just having a trial period for a few weeks."
- Encourage caregivers to make use of support groups offered by the local chapter of the Alzheimer's Disease and Related Disorders Association.
- Validate the caregiver's feelings of anger, guilt, exhaustion, and frustration. Let caregivers know that you understand how bad things can get at home, even though people with Alzheimer's may appear alert and pleasant when company visits.
- Caregivers may complain about "going crazy" as they watch their loved ones perform tedious, repetitive tasks. For example, when they pick up fallen leaves one leaf at a time rather than raking up the leaves. Help caregivers analyze activities in terms of safety. Does the activity harm the person with Alzheimer's? If not, caregivers can reframe their perceptions of the activity and accept it as harmless.
- Know the assisted living facilities that offer extended care for caregivers who want to go away for trips. Use these times to help the caregiver begin planning for long-term care in an assisted living facility or nursing home. Caregivers may consider long-term care when the person with Alzheimer's begins to wander at night, stops eating, becomes incontinent, or becomes belligerent or violent with the caregiver.
- Laugh with caregivers. Help them realize that finding humor in the absurdities of life can make it possible to deal with a situation that might otherwise be unbearable.

Cyndy Hunt Luzinski, RN MS, *Community Nurse Case Manager, Poudre Valley Health System, Fort Collins, Colorado*

Nursing home care is usually the final and most difficult and trying option for a caregiver. This decision creates guilt, self-doubt, and anxiety; however, it may be the only option when the caregiver suffers burnout and becomes unable to provide adequate care. Table 72–2 lists nursing guidelines for meeting family needs.

When the person with AD reaches the terminal stage of illness, questions about end-of-life treatments arise.

- Should a feeding tube be used to provide nourishment?
- Should antibiotics be used to treat pneumonias or other infections?
- Should cardiopulmonary resuscitation be used?

Ideally, decisions about these questions are raised and discussed with the client and family members before the person loses the capacity to make decisions.

Two forms of *advance directives* (means of expressing one's wishes about life-sustaining treatment after losing the mental capacity to make informed decisions) are available. One is the *living will,* a written document signed by the individual (while he or she is still mentally capable of making informed decisions) in the presence of a witness. The living will lists conditions under which the person wishes life-sustaining treatments to be withheld or withdrawn. The other advance directive is a *durable power of attorney for health care.* This is a legal document in which the person (while still mentally capable) assigns someone to act on his or her behalf in matters of health care decisions if the person loses decisional capacity (e.g., becomes demented).

EVALUATION

Continually evaluate the degree of expected outcome attainment. You should expect progress toward outcomes to be slow. If the client is transferred to a new center (e.g., hospital), some regression can be expected. Family evaluation should be completed on regular intervals.

CREUTZFELDT-JAKOB DISEASE

Etiology

Creutzfeldt-Jakob disease (CJD) is a subacute CNS disorder that produces progressive dementia, myoclonus, and distinctive EEG changes. CJD is a unique disease that can apparently arise from two separate mechanisms, genetic and infectious. People with the genetic form have a mutated gene. The infectious form does not develop from a known virus or other pathogen; therefore, words like *virion, slow virus,* and *prion* are sometimes used to describe the etiologic agent. Several reports document human-to-human spread of CJD from cornea transplants, dural allografts, human pituitary growth hormone injections, and reuse of stereotactic EEG electrodes that had been previously implanted in a person with CJD. Apparently, a group of infected cadavers were used for growth hormone replacement. Incubation periods have ranged from 4 to 21 years, which indicates the enormous difficulty of tracing the infection. Additional cases may still appear in people who received the hormone before its discontinuation in 1985. In 1996, CJD was associated

with ingestion of infected beef. This led to the popular term "mad cow disease."

The incidence of CJD peaks in the age group 40 to 70 years. It affects both sexes equally. A higher incidence has been noted in Libyan-born Jewish people and in some groups from Chile and the former Czechoslovakia.

Clinical Manifestations

Manifestations include vague psychiatric or behavior changes suggesting a personality change. About one third of clients report weight loss, anorexia, insomnia, malaise, and dizziness for a period of weeks to months. In the early stages, there is progressive memory loss, visual impairment, and dysphagia. Within a few weeks or months, a relentlessly progressive dementia develops and marked deterioration is noted from week to week. Myoclonus (twitching) is usually present. Deterioration is rapid, with 90% of clients dying within 1 year.

A definitive diagnosis attempts to differentiate CJD from AD. AD has a more protracted course and no myoclonus or EEG changes. Lithium toxicity can mimic the manifestations, but they clear within about 2 weeks after discontinuation of the drug. Brain biopsy during hospitalization or on autopsy is the usual method of establishing a definitive diagnosis.

Outcome Management

No effective treatment is available, and CJD appears to be uniformly fatal. Nursing care is directed at supportive care, preventing skin breakdown, furnishing nutrition, and providing emotional support to the client and family. Families require much support, care, and concern as they try to cope with the sudden onset of this debilitating disease and with managing the day-to-day care of the client.

Although CJD can be transmitted, the risk to health care workers and others having contact with the client is no more than that to the general population. Isolation of clients is not indicated, but personnel should wear gloves when handling tissues, blood, and spinal fluid. Accidental skin contact with possibly infected material should be followed by washing in 10 normal sodium hydroxide or a solution of 5% household chlorine bleach. The agent can be inactivated on surfaces by using a 10% bleach solution for 1 hour. Surgical and pathologic instruments should be steam-autoclaved for 1 hour at 132° C. No organs, tissue, or tissue products from clients with CJD or any other ill-defined neurologic disorders should be used for transplantation or replacement therapy.

HUNTINGTON'S DISEASE

Huntington's disease (HD), also known as *Huntington's chorea,* is a genetically transmitted degenerative neurologic disease. It is characterized by abnormal movements (chorea), intellectual decline, and emotional disturbance. Clinical manifestations usually begin in the 30s and 40s, although occasionally they begin in young adulthood or even in children. Women and men are equally affected. The disease is relentlessly progressive, leading to disabil-

TABLE 72-2	NURSING GUIDELINES FOR MEETING THE NEEDS OF THE FAMILY OF THE CLIENT WITH DEMENTIA OF THE ALZHEIMER'S TYPE

Goals	Selected Interventions
PHYSICAL	
Monitor chronic health problems or physical limitations of family caregiver	Obtain health history of family caregiver to identify past and new health problems
Identify development of new health problems	Support family in following through with routine health examinations
	Refer family members to physician when health problems are observed
	Assess family's understanding of medical management of own health problems
	Teach family members to preserve own health in order to continue caring for patient with Alzheimer's disease
Identify cues for stress	Emphasize family's need for adequate nutrition, hydration, exercise, and rest
Examine somatic health problems	Help family members to be alert to signs of caregiver stress
PSYCHOSOCIAL	
Assist family in coping positively with stress	Instruct family to get respite regularly for rest and relaxation
	Teach stress management techniques (i.e., relaxation, supportive relationships, goal setting, time management, diversion)
Identify destructive methods of coping (i.e., alcohol, drugs, tobacco, overeating or undereating, physical abuse of patient)	Refer family to physician, therapist when stress remains unmanageable even with social or psychological resources
Assess family dynamics	Refer signs of physical abuse to adult protective services
Assist family members in dealing with role change and conflict	Recognize the family's role, discuss capacity to provide care, and give reinforcement for care provided
	Counsel family in dealing with role conflicts, unmet expectations, or interpersonal conflicts
	Teach family the need to maintain roles and social activities outside caregiving experience
	Administer burden interview
	Reinforce family's attempt to cope
	Acknowledge family fears of being unable to continue with caregiving
If need for support identified, direct family members to sources	Refer family to a support group to share with others in similar situations
	Refer family to nearest office on aging or Alzheimer's Disease and Related Disorders Association, Inc. (ADRDA) to identify benefits in community available to Alzheimer's disease clients
Identify family's mixed emotions (i.e., depression, anger, resentment, pity, embarrassment, guilt)	Listen to family and facilitate sharing of emotions and feelings in supportive, empathic environment
Identify alternative plans for care if family members or social support systems become unable to provide care or are ineffective	Counsel and support family if patient placed in care of others (i.e., day care, respite service, home care, nursing home); allay feelings of guilt
	Facilitate family meeting to identify time for socialization
Identify financial limitations	Encourage family to be specific about financial limitations
	Offer family referrals (legal, financial, or social service) for information on eligibility for private, county, state, or federal financial support for home services, and advise and counsel regarding power of attorney or guardianship, trust or estate planning
Assess family's ability to make funeral plans	Help family anticipate and cope with grief process
	Assist family in making prefuneral arrangements
	Address family's fear regarding the possible role of heredity in development of Alzheimer's disease and assist in making decision regarding autopsy

TABLE 72-2	NURSING GUIDELINES FOR MEETING THE NEEDS OF THE FAMILY OF THE CLIENT WITH DEMENTIA OF THE ALZHEIMER'S TYPE *Continued*

Goals	Selected Interventions
ENVIRONMENTAL	
Identify compatibility of environment with family and client	Conduct a family meeting to discuss relationship of family, patient, and environment
Assess learning needs regarding client care tasks	Teach management of concurrent physical health problems of the client with Alzheimer's disease
	Include family in development of patient care plan
	Teach family to encourage the client to continue daily habits to extent possible
	Complete behavior problems checklist
	Anticipate likely problems and teach how to manage them
	Teach environmental modification (consistent, simple, calm routines) to maximize family endurance and enhance safety
	Teach family to relate to patient with creative connectedness (touch, humor, flexibility, reminiscence, music, planned activities)
Assess family need and desire for information about Alzheimer's disease and how it affects the client's behavior	Assist family in understanding symptoms related to memory loss, nature of the illness, symptoms, stages of disease progression, and behavior manifestations
	Provide written material to reinforce education and understanding (i.e., *The 36-Hour Day, Coping and Caring: Living with Alzheimer's Disease;* literature from local, state, or national ADRDA chapters)
	Supply ADRDA 24-hour hotline number: 1-800-621-0379

Adapted from Stevenson, J. P. (1990). Family stress to home care of Alzheimer's disease patients and implications for support. *Journal of Neuroscience Nursing, 22*(3), 185.

ity and death within 15 to 20 years. Death usually results from respiratory complications caused by aspiration.

The disease is autosomal dominant; offspring of an affected person have a 50% chance of inheriting the disease. Because HD does not skip generations, offspring who have not inherited the disease will not pass it on to their offspring. The abnormal gene has been isolated on chromosome 4.

Pathophysiology

The pathologic changes of HD involve degeneration of the striatum (caudate and putamen) in the basal ganglia. Other subtle changes occur in the cortex and cerebellum, namely, loss of neurons and an increased number of glial cells (gliosis). The degeneration of the caudate nucleus leads to a reduction in several neurotransmitters, including gamma-aminobutyric acid, ACh, substance P, and metenkephalin, and their synthetic enzymes. This change leaves relatively higher concentrations of the other neurotransmitters, dopamine and norepinephrine. The relative excess of dopamine in HD, a disorder of excessive movement, can be contrasted to the lack of dopamine in Parkinson's disease (PD), a disorder of lack of movement.

Clinical Manifestations

Emotional disturbances and mental deterioration may precede the abnormal movements. The person may become negative, suspicious, and irritable. This condition may progress to depression and psychosis. Temper outbursts and sexual promiscuity may also occur. Severe mood swings are common. Cognitive decline progresses, and eventually the person becomes demented, incontinent, and completely unable to care for himself or herself.

The abnormal movements in HD are subtle at first. The person may appear restless or fidgety. The person may be aware of these movements and try to mask them by making them seem to be parts of intentional movements, such as head scratching or leg crossing. As the disease progresses, the rapid, jerky choreiform movements become more pronounced and involve all muscles. The person is constantly in motion. Stress, emotional situations, and attempts to perform voluntary movement can aggravate the abnormal movements. During sleep, the movements diminish or disappear.

The diagnosis of HD is made on the basis of clinical manifestations and family history, because there is no specific diagnostic test for the disease itself. CT or MRI imaging of the brain may show atrophy of the head of the caudate, but this factor alone is not diagnostic of HD.

Outcome Management

There is no known treatment to cure or alter the course of HD. Haloperidol, a dopamine blocker, can control the abnormal movements and some behavioral manifestations.

Diazepam can be used to lower anxiety, aiding in control of movements. Antidepressants can help depression.

LATE-STAGE DYSPHAGIA

One of the most common and dangerous problems in the middle to late stages is dysphagia. Several interventions should be tried. Medications need to be evaluated for their anticholinergic and sedative effects, which may impair swallowing. Mealtimes should be free of stress and clutter and have an unhurried atmosphere. Use of adaptive eating utensils can encourage and extend independence in eating. The diet should include foods that are easy to swallow and form a bolus in the mouth (e.g., canned peaches, chopped meat in gravy and mashed potatoes, custards). Many clients with HD require high caloric intake because of excessive movements and should try eating frequent, small meals containing high-calorie foods. Clients should sit upright when eating. While swallowing, they should keep the chin down toward the chest. They can be trained to hold their breath before swallowing and cough after each mouthful is swallowed to clear the throat of any residual food.

■ Nursing Management

If the client continues to have difficulty eating and loses weight despite dietary and environmental modifications, a feeding tube may become necessary. However, artificial feeding methods often frighten families, and they pose ethical dilemmas about prolonging life. Nurses can help clients and their families make these difficult decisions by clarifying the issues and providing information on the types, risks, benefits, and long-term effects of artificial feeding methods.

Poor control of oral and respiratory muscles can make communication difficult. The nurse can assist the family to develop signals such as raising a hand or keeping the eyes open or closed for yes and no responses. If physical signals are not an option, cards with printed words may be helpful. Keep communication simple and unstrained. Repeat words that are understood to let the client know that communication has been successful.

Excessive movements and falls may cause physical injury and can restrict independence. Pads on wheelchairs and beds, shin guards, and walking belts can prevent injury. Aids for ambulation (e.g., walking behind a wheelchair) can extend independence. Clothing should be light and simple to don and doff.

HD has a major impact on the family, not only because of the burden of caregiving but also because of the risk to offspring of inheriting the disease. Many ethical dilemmas surrounding the issue of privacy can surface in cases of HD. Whether test results are positive or negative, the results are of interest to the spouse, other family members, employers, and insurers. However, principles of confidentiality forbid disclosure of medical information to anyone unless the client consents. Be sensitive to the client's desire for confidentiality but use this opportunity to teach the client about the effect the disease may have on other family members. Because a blood test is now available to check for the presence of the abnormal gene, family members face difficult choices about whether to find out if they have the Huntington gene.

MULTIPLE SCLEROSIS

Multiple sclerosis (MS) is a chronic demyelinating disease that affects the myelin sheath of neurons in the CNS. The myelin sheath is essential for normal conduction of nerve impulses. Patches of myelin deteriorate at irregular intervals along the nerve axon, causing slowing of nerve conduction. Axonal destruction also occurs in MS.

The onset of MS usually occurs between ages 20 and 40, and it affects women twice as often as men. Whites are affected more often than Hispanics, blacks, or Asians. The disease is most prevalent in the colder climates of North America and Europe. If someone is born in an area of high risk for MS and moves to an area of low risk after age 15, the person carries the risk of the area of origin.

Etiology and Risk Factors

The exact cause of MS is unknown. Most theories suggest that MS is an immunogenetic-viral disease, that is, an immune-mediated demyelination triggered by a viral infection. A genetic susceptibility apparently alters the body's immune response to viral infection. Multiple genes are probably involved. However, the only consistently identified disease locus is on the HLA gene complex on chromosome 6.

A variety of precipitating factors can precede the onset or an exacerbation of MS, such as infection, physical injury, emotional stress, pregnancy, and fatigue. Most pregnancy-related exacerbations occur 3 months post partum and may relate more to the stress of labor and fatigue during the puerperium than to the pregnancy itself.

Pathophysiology

Myelin is a highly conductive fatty material that surrounds the axon and speeds conduction of nerve impulses along the axon. In MS, *plaques* form along the myelin sheath, causing inflammation, edema, and eventually scarring and destruction (Fig. 72–2). Plaques are characterized by primary demyelination and death of oligodendrocytes in the center of the lesion. Initially, perivascular inflammatory cells (autoreactive T cells) invade the myelin-covered axons in the CNS. This is followed by extensive gliosis or scarring by astrocytes and aberrant attempts at remyelination, with oligodendrocytes proliferating at the edges of the plaque. When edema and inflammation subside, some remyelination occurs but is often incomplete.

Although plaques may occur anywhere in the white matter of the CNS, the areas most commonly involved are the optic nerves, cerebrum, and cervical spinal cord.

Clinical Manifestations

The wide variety of manifestations possible with MS and the unpredictable nature of the disease pose many challenges to the client and family. The course of illness varies from person to person. Four clinical patterns have been identified (Fig. 72–3). The most common initial pattern is *relapsing-remitting* MS. Clients experience manifestations that eventually remit with little or no progression of disability.

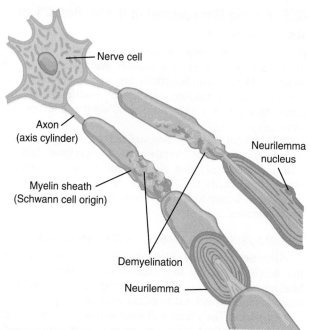

FIGURE 72-2 Changes in the nerve sheath, as seen in multiple sclerosis. Myelin is made by the oligodendrocyte and coats peripheral nerves, facilitating nervous impulse. In clients with multiple sclerosis, the myelin degenerates in patches, causing nerve transmission to become erratic.

The random distribution of MS plaques leads to several clinical manifestations:

- Weakness or tingling sensations (paresthesias) of one or more extremities caused by involvement of the cerebrum or spinal cord
- Vision loss from optic neuritis
- Incoordination that is due to cerebellar involvement
- Bowel and bladder dysfunction as a result of spinal cord involvement

Bladder dysfunction can take several forms, depending on which neural pathways are affected. Dysfunction may involve hesitancy, frequency, loss of sensation, incontinence, and retention. There may be increased or decreased detrusor, bladder neck, or external sphincter tone,

or a combination of these problems. The ultimate bladder dysfunction, however, is usually hyperreflexia in association with sphincter dyssynergia (sphincter contraction during detrusor contraction).[3] Proper diagnosis of the type of bladder dysfunction requires a thorough history, laboratory assessment of kidney function, and identification of possible infection. If bladder emptying is defective, further investigation with urography, cystoscopy, and urodynamic studies should be performed.

Constipation is commonly experienced by clients with MS. Dysfunction can result from one or more of the following factors: spinal cord lesion, immobility, dehydration, medications, and nutritional deficiencies. Stool incontinence, although more rare, is also possible. Sexual dysfunction can also occur as a result of lesions in the ascending or descending autonomic and sensory fibers in the spinal cord.

Fatigue is a common manifestation of MS and usually one of the most disabling. Spasticity can reduce energy, inhibit motor control, and interfere with self-care, sexuality, vocational responsibilities, and recreation.

Because MS strikes young adults during their years of establishing a family and an occupation, the impact of the disease can be devastating. Depression often occurs in clients, but it is not clear whether depression is a reaction to disability or a function of the disease itself. Others may experience euphoria, emotional instability, or apathy.

Because there is no definitive test for MS, clinicians rely on a detailed history, clinical findings, and a variety of diagnostic tests. The history often reveals several episodes of neurologic dysfunction, separated by time and by different locations in the CNS. Current research looking at clients who experience only one manifestation such as optic neuritis is changing the way clinicians diagnose MS.

Diagnostic tests include:

- CSF evaluation for the presence of oligoclonal banding
- Evoked potentials of the optic pathways and auditory system to assess the presence of slowed nerve conduction
- MRI of the brain and spinal cord to determine the presence of MS plaques

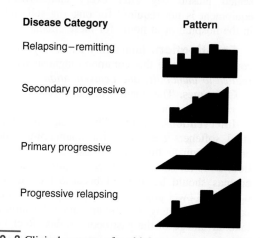

Disease Category	Pattern	Definition
Relapsing–remitting		Episodes of acute worsening with recovery and a stable course between relapses
Secondary progressive		Gradual neurologic deterioration with or without superimposed acute relapses in a client who previously had relapsing–remitting multiple sclerosis
Primary progressive		Gradual, nearly continuous neurologic deterioration from the onset of manifestations
Progressive relapsing		Gradual neurologic deterioration from the onset of manifestations but with subsequent superimposed relapses

FIGURE 72-3 Clinical patterns of multiple sclerosis. (Modified from Lublin, F. D., & Reingold, S. C. [1996]. Defining the clinical course of multiple sclerosis: Results of an international survey. *Neurology, 46,* 907–911.)

Outcome Management

Treatment generally falls into one of three categories: (1) treatment of acute relapses, (2) treatment aimed at disease management, and (3) symptomatic treatment.

TREATING ACUTE RELAPSES

Treatment of acute relapses usually involves the use of intravenous (IV) or oral corticosteroids, which have both anti-inflammatory and immunosuppressive properties. They are often used to enhance recovery from an exacerbation. Methylprednisolone is standard therapy for acute exacerbations sometimes followed by an oral prednisone taper. Azathioprine (Imuran) and cyclophosphamide (Cytoxan), other immunosuppressive agents, may be used for more severe exacerbations or progressive MS.

TREATING EXACERBATIONS

Interferon β_{1b} (Betaseron) is used for ambulatory clients with relapsing-remitting MS. Interferon β_{1b} is a genetically engineered complex protein with both antiviral and immunoregulatory properties that can reduce the number of MS exacerbations. The drug is injected subcutaneously every other day. Interferon β_{1a} (Avonex) is also available for the treatment of relapsing forms of MS. In addition to reducing the number and severity of relapses, interferon β_{1a} provides a delay in disability in placebo-controlled studies.

The third disease-modifying agent avaliable for use in the United States is glatiramer acetate (Copaxone), a synthetic polypeptide approved for use in relapsing-remitting MS. It is not an interferon but is believed to work by mimicking myelin basic protein and interrupting the inflammatory cascade to prevent damage to myelin.

Side effects of the interferons include fever, fatigue, and flu-like manifestations. Clients on interferon β_{1a} have also reported increased depression and injection site reactions. Copaxone does not produce the interferon-type side effects of fever and flu-like manifestations, but rare episodes of face flushing, chest tightness, and shortness of breath lasting less than 15 minutes have been reported. Numerous other therapeutic agents are undergoing clinical trials.

SYMPTOMATIC TREATMENT

Several strategies are available for symptomatic management in MS. Pharmacologic interventions can be used for bladder dysfunction (oxybutynin, propantheline); constipation (psyllium hydromucilloid, bisacodyl pills or suppositories); fatigue (amantadine, modafinil); spasticity (baclofen, diazepam, dantrolene); tremor (propranolol, phenobarbital, clonazepam); and dysesthesias and trigeminal neuralgia (carbamazepine, phenytoin, amitriptyline).

Transcutaneous electrical nerve stimulation (TENS) is also helpful for dysesthesias. Areas of numbness should be inspected regularly to prevent injury and development of pressure ulcers. Skin should be kept dry and free of urine and feces. A seat cushion that distributes pressure should be used for wheelchair-bound clients with insensate buttock skin. Blindness or severely impaired vision may occur. In this case, refer the client to Services for the Blind for rehabilitation. Cognitive and perceptual impairment necessitates psychometric and functional testing for accurate assessment and rehabilitation services.

■ Nursing Management of the Medical Client

ASSESSMENT

If the client is being assessed for possible MS, you should assess the client for clinical manifestations of the disorder. Ocular manifestations are very common. As a result of the fluctuations of clinical manifestations, the client may report a past history of similar findings that went away.

If the client is being hospitalized for an exacerbation of MS, focus on the client's ability to perform ADL as well as other areas that require fine motor movements. Gross motor activities, such as walking, may also be impaired and may lead to problems with bowel and bladder continence.

DIAGNOSIS, OUTCOMES, INTERVENTIONS

Altered Urinary Elimination. Demyelination of the nerves supplying the bladder may result in altered bladder function. This diagnosis is stated as *Altered Urinary Elimination related to bladder dysfunction.*

Outcomes. The client will maintain urinary continence and normal bladder filling, as evidenced by residual volumes of less than 100 ml, application of appropriate bladder elimination procedures, and verbalization of personal satisfaction with urinary elimination status.

Interventions. The following interventions are for neurogenic bladder, the most common type of bladder dysfunction in MS.

Fluid intake should be maintained at 2000 ml/24 hours, ideally, 400 to 500 ml with each meal and 200 ml at midmorning, midafternoon, and late afternoon. Avoiding fluid intake after the evening meal reduces the need for emptying the bladder during the night.

Voiding should be attempted every 3 hours during waking hours. If voiding is not successful, a catheter should be inserted into the bladder and then removed once emptying is complete. This is called *intermittent catheterization.* If the volume of catheterized urine exceeds 500 ml, catheterization may need to be scheduled more frequently.

Instruct the client on how to do self-catheterization if he or she is capable. A clean red rubber catheter can be reused for up to 1 week, as long as it is washed thoroughly with soap and water and placed in a clean, tightly sealed plastic bag after every catheterization. Sterile equipment is not required for ongoing self-catheterization in the hospital or at home for these clients.

Constipation. Immobility and demyelination lead to constipation. State this common diagnosis as *Constipation related to immobility and demyelination.*

Outcomes. The client will have bowel movements of normal consistency and frequency.

Interventions. A high-fiber diet, bulk formers, and stool softeners are useful for maintaining stool consistency. Adequate fluid intake also assists bowel elimination; 2000 ml should be taken. Explain that laxatives and enemas should be avoided because they lead to dependence. A bowel program should be performed every other day, approximately 45 minutes after the largest meal, to take advantage of the gastrocolic reflex. Rectal evacuation may be augmented by the use of glycerin or bisacodyl suppositories or digital stimulation.

Activity Intolerance. State this common diagnosis as *Activity Intolerance related to fatigue and muscle weakness.*

Outcomes. The client will demonstrate improved activity tolerance, as evidenced by (1) maintaining a balance between work, rest, and exercise and recreation; (2) performing ADL without excessive fatigue; (3) using energy-saving devices and techniques; (4) avoiding elevations in environmental and body temperatures; and (5) consuming a diet adequate in calories and protein for body size, frame, and age.

Intervention. Because fatigue can be precipitated by warm temperatures, the environment should be kept cool. If air conditioning is unavailable, cool baths and ice packs may help lower body temperature.

Assist the client to plan activities at his or her peak energy level, which is usually in the morning. This schedule promotes optimal synchrony between circadian rhythms and the client's physical demands. The client should plan for periods of rest throughout the day. Collaboration with the physical and occupational therapist can reveal methods to reduce energy consumption with repeated tasks and apply adaptive devices for ambulation and toileting. The drugs amantadine (Symmetrel) and modafinil (Provigil) may alleviate fatigue in some clients.

Impaired Physical Mobility. Several problems lead to difficulties with mobility. State this diagnosis as *Impaired Physical Mobility related to weakness, contractures, spasticity, and ataxia.*

Outcomes. The client will achieve optimal physical mobility, as evidenced by improved or maintained range of motion in all joints, optimal control of spasticity, and effective use of adaptive aids.

Interventions. Although some clients are bothered by painful muscle spasms, others may rely on spasticity to stabilize weak limbs during transfers and ambulation. Spastic muscles must be stretched at least twice daily through their full range of motion. The drug baclofen (Lioresal) provides synaptic inhibition of spinal reflexes, which can reduce spasticity, although it may increase weakness and fatigue in some clients. Diazepam (Valium), tizanidine (Zanaflex), and dantrolene (Dantrium) are other antispasmotic drugs. Surgical intervention or nerve blocks may be necessary if contractures develop. Monitor the effect of medications on spasticity, promote activity to decrease spasms, and utilize spasms for muscle strength when transferring.

Advise that strengthening exercises for muscle weakness (paresis) must be done with caution because they can exacerbate paresis by causing muscle fatigue. However, selective strengthening of nonaffected or less affected muscles can enhance physical function and well-being. Range-of-motion exercises should be performed at least twice daily. Active movement is preferable to passive movement. Correct body alignment should be maintained to reduce the risk of contractures. Splints may help maintain position and provide support for weak hands and ankles. Ataxia and tremor of the extremities can be lessened by the use of small weights applied to the distal extremities or the use of weighted utensils. Weakness and fatigue can worsen ataxia. Ambulation aids such as a cane or a walker may be necessary.

Risk for Self-Care Deficit. Clients with MS may experience a decline in self-care abilities. State this diagnosis as *Risk for Self-Care Deficit related to muscle weakness.*

Outcomes. The client will reduce the risk for self-care deficits by using ADL aids.

Interventions. Clients may require aids, such as wheelchairs or canes, to perform ADL and ambulate. The performance of ADL may be enhanced if counters and tabletops are adjusted to a comfortable working height. Work in combination with the physical therapist, occupational therapist, social worker, and home health nurse to identify, purchase, and teach the client how to use ADL aids.

Knowledge Deficit. The client with a new diagnosis of MS often lacks knowledge about MS, its unpredictable course, and the role of stress in MS. State this diagnosis as *Knowledge Deficit related to new diagnosis of MS.*

Outcomes. The client will have more knowledge about MS, as evidenced by stating facts about the course of MS and the role of stress in MS.

Interventions. The client with MS needs to have a clear understanding of the unpredictability of this disorder. The client may be free of manifestations for many weeks to months, even years, and then experience them. If the client can identify stressors that exacerbate the clinical manifestations, sometimes these stressors can be avoided. The National Multiple Sclerosis Society can be an excellent resource for education and support. For clients on one of the three disease-modifying agents, each company has a support program to offer education, financial information, and support for people with MS and their families.

Self-Esteem Disturbance. Because of the age of the client, loss of independence and fear of disability can be devastating. Psychosocial diagnosis is important in providing holistic care. State this diagnosis as *Self Esteem Disturbance related to loss of independence and fear of disability.*

Outcomes. The client will achieve improved self-esteem, as evidenced by verbalizing awareness that personal goals and body image will need to be adjusted, willingness to maintain appropriate independence, and positive thoughts and statements about self.

Intervention. Regardless of the cause of disturbance in self-esteem, carefully assess the individual and family history for the presence and type of depressive episodes and the clinical manifestations. Identify previous treatment for depression, including psychotherapy and drug therapy. By assessing the client's problem-solving strategies, you can identify coping behavior strengths and defense mechanisms such as denial, avoidance, or intellectualization that the client may use to mask depression.

Evaluate the client's social support system, which contributes to a sense of well-being. Grieving the loss of function in MS can lead to a reactive depression and require provision of support group therapy for both the client and family. Some clients may not benefit from this kind of therapy, however, because they may see people whose condition is much worse than their own and may fear developing that level of disability. On-line computer services for MS clients can provide a means of social support.

EVALUATION

The degree of expected outcome attainment should be evaluated on an ongoing basis. Most outcomes are long-term and may require weeks to months to attain.

GUILLAIN-BARRÉ SYNDROME

Etiology

Guillain-Barré syndrome (GBS) is an inflammatory disease of unknown origin that involves degeneration of the myelin sheath of peripheral nerves. GBS is seen worldwide and affects people of all ages and races. Since the virtual elimination of poliomyelitis, GBS has become the most common cause of acute generalized paralysis, with an annual incidence of 0.75 to 2.0/100,000 population. In one half to two thirds of cases, an upper respiratory or gastrointestinal infection precedes the onset of the syndrome by 1 to 4 weeks.

Although many organisms have been suspected, including *Cytomegalovirus* and Epstein-Barr virus, *Campylobacter jejuni* is the organism most often implicated. This gram-negative rod is found in poultry, pets, raw milk, and contaminated water. *C. jejuni* targets the myelin sheath. Macrophages penetrate the basal lamina surrounding the axon, displace the Schwann cell from the myelin sheath, and phagocytose the myelin lamellae. An association between HIV and GBS has also been reported, and clients with GBS should be tested for HIV.

Clinical Manifestations

A characteristic feature is ascending weakness, usually beginning in the lower extremities and spreading, sometimes rapidly, to the trunk, upper extremities, and even the face. The weakness evolves over hours to days, with maximal deficit by 4 weeks in 90% of cases. Deep tendon reflexes are lost. Paresthesias (tingling sensation) in the limbs may occur early in the course of the illness.

This *initial phase* is usually followed by a *plateau phase* during which the disease no longer seems to progress but the client does not recover functions initially lost. Deep, aching muscle pain in the shoulder girdle and thighs is common. The two most dangerous features of the disease are respiratory muscle weakness and autonomic neuropathy involving both the sympathetic and parasympathetic systems. The latter feature can involve orthostatic hypotension, hypertension, pupillary disturbances, sweating dysfunction, cardiac dysrhythmias, paralytic ileus, and urinary retention.

The third phase of the disease is the *recovery phase.* Improvement and recovery occur with remyelination. However, if nerve axons are damaged, some residual deficits may remain. Remyelination occurs in a descending pattern; the functions lost last are thus the first to be regained. Recovery is usually maximal at 6 months, although severe cases may take up to 2 years for maximal recovery. Fortunately, 85% to 90% of clients with GBS recover completely.

Diagnosis of GBS is based on history and physical examination, cerebrospinal fluid (CSF) examination, and electrophysiologic studies. The CSF contains increased protein, with few or no white blood cells. Nerve conduction velocity is slowed, although it may be normal in the early stage of the illness. Conduction block, a diminution in amplitude or an absence of elicited muscle action potentials from stimulation of a peripheral nerve, also occurs.

Outcome Management

The focus of therapy is supportive care. Monitor respiratory or cardiovascular status carefully: vital signs, serial measurement of vital capacity, peripheral oxygen saturation, and electrocardiography. When vital capacity falls to 15 ml/kg of body weight, intubation and artificial ventilation are usually necessary. Early treatment with plasmapheresis may accelerate recovery, although the exact mechanism for this effect is not known (hypotheses include the removal of circulating antibodies or other humoral myelinotoxic or immunopathogenic factors). Intravenous immunoglobulin G (IVIG) therapy may prove to be the treatment of choice because it can be administered easily and can be given with other drugs simultaneously (plasmapheresis removes co-medication jointly with adverse disease factors).

During the first several days after hospital admission, it is crucial to assess the client's respiratory, swallowing, and autonomic function (see the Critical Monitoring feature). Assess the following at least every 4 hours: vital signs, forced vital capacity, swallowing, strength in the extremities, and intake and output balance. If ascending

---

CRITICAL MONITORING

Respiratory Distress with Guillain-Barré Syndrome

Monitor the client for:

- Complaints of headache
- Myoclonic jerks
- Drowsiness
- Confusion
- Restlessness
- Reduced cough
- Decreased ability to move pulmonary secretions

Assess pulmonary function studies for:

- Decreased forced vital capacity (<15 ml/kg)
- Decreased tidal volume (<3–4 ml/kg)
- Decreased maximum inspiratory pressure (<10–20 cm H_2O)
- Decreased maximum expiratory pressure (<40 cm H_2O)

Assess arterial blood gases for:

- Decreased PaO_2 (<80 mm Hg on 50% FIO_2 with normal PCO_2)
- Alveolar-arterial gradient > 300 on 50% FIO_2
- $PaCO_2$ > 50 mm Hg
- Vd/Vt > 0.6

FIO_2, fraction of inspired oxygen; $PaCO_2$, partial pressure of arterial carbon dioxide; PaO_2, partial pressure of arterial oxygen; Vd/Vt, ratio of dead space volume to tidal volume.

weakness is noted, increase the frequency of assessment to every 2 hours or even more often. Cardiac monitoring and supplemental oxygen are often needed. Common complications include bladder infection, deep vein thrombosis, pulmonary emboli, pneumonia, and syndrome of inappropriate antidiuretic hormone (SIADH).

Interventions to control infection and prevent complications of immobility are vital. Proper body alignment should be maintained to prevent deformities and injury to paralyzed limbs. Once the client's condition is stabilized, rehabilitative interventions can be implemented.

Assist the client in coping with the progressive nature of GBS. During the early stages, clients are frightened because their paralysis can ascend rapidly. They are often admitted to an acute care agency with progressive weakness and within days are completely paralyzed. Clients fear they will never recover. Help clients in verbalizing their fears, and offer support and encouragement that although the disorder is progressive, most clients gain full recovery. Encouragement is not hollow, however. The client is not taught to expect immediate resolution but is assisted to realize the usual time frames for recovery.

PARKINSON'S DISEASE

Classification

PD is an idiopathic syndrome characterized by disability from tremor and rigidity. Various other forms of parkinsonism cause similar clinical manifestations but have known causes. They include:

- *Postencephalitic* parkinsonism, which occurred after the large epidemic of encephalitis in 1919
- *Drug-induced* parkinsonism, occurring after long-term use of phenothiazines
- *Toxin-induced* parkinsonism, sometimes resulting from carbon monoxide, mercury, or manganese exposure
- Exposure to agricultural herbicides and pesticides (being studied)
- Trauma injury to the midbrain

PD is the most common form of parkinsonism. PD involves degeneration of dopamine-producing cells in the substantia nigra, which leads to degeneration of dopaminergic neurons in the basal ganglia. Once cell loss in the substantia nigra reaches 80%, manifestations appear. The cause of nigral cell degeneration is not known. The net result of the loss of dopaminergic neurons is an imbalance of dopamine in relation to ACh in the basal ganglia, which leads to the clinical characteristics of PD.

Clinical Manifestations

PD most often develops in people in their 60s, although it can strike much younger people as well. It occurs worldwide. About 1% of people over age 50 have PD. The disease has six cardinal features: (1) tremor at rest; (2) rigidity; (3) bradykinesia (slow movement); (4) flexed posture of the neck, trunk, and limbs; (5) loss of postural reflexes; and (6) freezing movement.

Early in the disease, the client may notice a slight slowing in the ability to perform ADL (*bradykinesia*). A general feeling of stiffness (rigidity) may be noticed,

along with mild diffuse muscular pain. *Tremor* is a common early sign that usually occurs in one of the upper limbs. It occurs at rest and involves a coarse "pill-rolling" movement of the thumb against the fingers that can vary in intensity and distribution. Voluntary movement stops or reduces the tremor in some people; however, others may have tremor during voluntary movement (intention tremor) as well.

Bradykinesia makes voluntary movements difficult to execute. When manifestations are severe, total lack of movement (*akinesia*) may occur and the client is literally frozen in one spot. Bradykinesia also affects gait. Initially, there may be a slight stiffness of one leg while walking, and the ipsilateral arm may be held flexed at the elbow and abducted at the shoulder. The person may catch or drag one foot. Later, when both sides of the body are involved, the typical shuffling gait with short steps may develop. There is lack of associated swinging of the arms while walking. In advanced PD, the client stands with head, shoulders, and spine flexed forward, giving the appearance of a stooped posture (Fig. 72–4).

The face of someone with advanced PD appears stiff, mask-like, and without expression. The speech is low in volume, monotonous in tone, and slow. Words are poorly articulated (dysarthria). Saliva may flow involuntarily from the mouth because of the lack of spontaneous swallowing.

PD does not usually affect intellectual ability; however, a dementia similar to that of AD develops in 15% to 20% of clients with PD. Mood disturbance can occur, and emotional stress may intensify clinical manifestations.

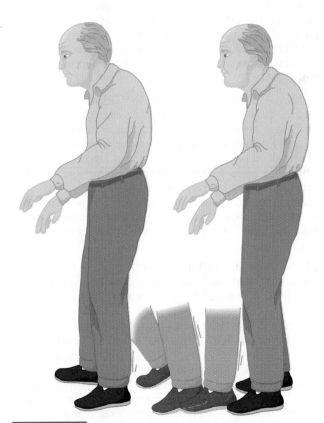

FIGURE 72–4 Gait changes seen in Parkinson's disease. Some of the clinical manifestations of Parkinson's disease are stooped posture, bradykinesia, and a festinant gait.

The course of the disease is slowly progressive. The person becomes more rigid and more disabled, eventually requiring full assistance with ADL.

Outcome Management

The manifestations of PD can be relieved by various medications, particularly levodopa and anticholinergic drugs. The purpose of levodopa is to provide dopamine to the basal ganglia. The purpose of anticholinergic drugs is to block release of acetylcholine, thereby creating a better balance between acetylcholine and dopamine. The most common levodopa drug is carbidopa-levodopa (Sinemet). Levodopa is a synthetic metabolic precursor of dopamine. Dopamine itself cannot be used because it cannot cross the blood-brain barrier. Carbidopa must be given with levodopa because it prevents peripheral metabolism of levodopa, allowing levodopa to reach the brain.

The benefit of the drug seems to decline with prolonged use. The therapy is more effective in treating bradykinesia and rigidity than tremor. The dosage of levodopa is gradually increased until the optimal therapeutic response is achieved. This process may take several months. When the daily dose of levodopa approaches the desired level, the client often has involuntary dyskinesias (jerky, writhing movements), especially of the face, mouth, and tongue. Some clients prefer this stage to being severely bradykinetic, because at least they can be mobile and perform voluntary movements more easily.

In 1998, a new class of drug treatment for PD was approved by the Food and Drug Administration. This class of drugs is called catechol *O*-methyltransferase (COMT) inhibitors. COMT inhibitors are given with levodopa-carbidopa to increase the available dopamine in the brain. Table 72–3 lists drugs used to treat PD.

MANAGE THE PARKINSONIAN CRISIS

Occasionally, clients with PD experience a parkinsonian crisis as a result of emotional trauma or sudden or inadvertent withdrawal of antiparkinsonian medication. Severe exacerbation of tremor, rigidity, and bradykinesia, accompanied by acute anxiety, sweating, tachycardia, and hyperpnea, occur. Intervention for parkinsonian crisis includes respiratory and cardiac support. The person should be placed in a quiet room with subdued lighting. Barbiturates may be prescribed, as well as antiparkinsonian drugs.

MANAGE THE ON/OFF RESPONSE

An "on/off response" (rapid fluctuation of clinical manifestations) may occur in clients with PD; the client may be mobile and active ("on") one moment and akinetic and rigid ("off") the next. This transition may happen quickly, within 1 to 2 minutes. Initially, the off periods tend to occur 3 to 4 hours after a dose of antiparkinsonian medication. Later, the transition may happen at any time and be unrelated to medication ingestion. Apparently, off periods are due to dopamine deficit, but this factor is not clear. A person experiencing on/off response may be temporarily helped by shortening the interval between medication doses or by gradually increasing the total dosage.

Medications such as ropinirole may be given in addition to other PD medications to help smooth out the fluctuations.

■ Nursing Management of the Medical Client

Nursing care of the PD client includes health assessment, medication instruction and monitoring, liaison with other members of the health care team, and client and family education. Case managers are often used to guide transitions from one facility to the next (see Case Management: The Older Adult).

Advise the client to maintain fluid intake of 2L/24 hours and to increase intake of dietary fiber. Stool softeners and mild laxatives can be used. A regular time for bowel movements should be established, usually a half-hour after the morning or evening meal.

Teach the client various techniques to enhance voluntary movement. Clients often need to try different strategies on their own to find what helps most. Some clients grasp coins in their pocket to reduce embarrassing hand tremor. Others grip the arms of a chair. Mental thoughts, such as walking over imaginary lines, can aid ambulation. One client finds that tossing small scraps of paper in front of him aids his walking; another finds that rocking back and forth helps initiate movement. Encourage daily range of motion exercises to avoid rigidity and contractures. Remind the client to maintain good posture and to avoid flexion of the neck and shoulders. The client should sleep on a firm mattress. When resting, the client should avoid using a pillow to prevent flexion of the spine. Periodically lying prone also helps.

Because self-care activities are performed more slowly by the client with PD, extra time should be allowed for completion of tasks such as dressing, bathing, and eating. Warming trays can keep food hot. Recommend rest periods during meals to avoid aspiration.

As PD progresses, clients become rigid and unresponsive to verbal stimuli. During these stages, continue to treat clients with dignity, speaking to the clients rather than ignoring them.

Teach the client about home safety. Loose carpeting should be removed. Grab bars should be placed in the bathroom. An elevated toilet seat should be installed. Clients with severe tremor should avoid carrying hot liquids. Walking aids such as a cane or walker can provide added stability (see the Client Education Guide).

The client and family need emotional support. Support groups are available in most major cities. Refer the client and family to the American Parkinson Disease Association.

■ Surgical Management

Surgical interventions are used for PD. Intractable tremor may be ameliorated by thalamotomy or pallidotomy. Autologous transplantation of adrenal medullary tissue into the brains of PD clients, in the hope that these cells will produce dopamine, has yielded disappointing results. Fetal tissue transplantation has produced better results, although no cases resulted in complete reversal of parkinsonian symptoms.[2] Transplantation of genetically engineered cell lines or vector-mediated gene transfection might ultimately prove to be the most effective strategy for the surgical treatment of PD.[2]

| TABLE 72-3 | PHARMACOLOGIC MANAGEMENT OF PARKINSON'S DISEASE |

Drug Classification and Example	Action	Indications	Common Side Effects	Nursing Implications
ANTICHOLINERGICS				
Trihexyphenidyl (Artane) Benztropine (Cogentin) Procyclidine (Kemadrin) Ethopropazine (Parsidol)	Inhibit action of endogenous acetylcholine and muscarine agonists to block the excitatory effect of the cholinergic system	Tremor, rigidity, drooling	Dry mouth, constipation, blurred vision, confusion, hallucinations	Usually contraindicated in clients with acute-angle glaucoma and tachycardia; monitor pulse and blood pressure during periods of dosage adjustment; administer with meals; do not withdraw medication suddenly
ANTIHISTAMINES				
Diphenhydramine (Benadryl)	Mild anticholinergic	Tremor, rigidity, insomnia	Dry mouth, lethargy, confusion	Use with caution in clients with seizures, hypertension, hyperthyroidism, heart and renal disease, and diabetes; administer with meals or antacids
DOPAMINERGICS				
Amantadine (Symmetrel)	Cause release of dopamine in central nervous system	Rigidity, bradykinesia	Dizziness, ataxia, insomnia, leg edema	Monitor client for postural hypotension, do not administer at bedtime
Carbidopa-levadopa (Sinemet)		Tremor, rigidity, bradykinesia	Orthostatic hypotension, nausea, hallucinations, dystonia, dyskinesias	Monitor blood pressure; use elastic stockings to increase venous return; monitor client for urinary retention
DOPAMINE AGONISTS				
Bromocriptine (Parlodel)	Activate dopamine receptors in the central nervous system	Fluctuation of manifestations, dyskinesia, dystonia	Hallucinations, mental fogginess, orthostatic hypotension, confusion	Monitor blood pressure and mental status
Pergolide (Permax)			Orthostatic hypotension, nausea, insomnia	Monitor blood pressure; do not administer at bedtime
COMT INHIBITORS				
Tolcapone	Enhance effect of dopamine	Adjuvant treatment	Diarrhea, elevated liver enzymes	Monitor liver enzymes
Encapone	Enhance effect of dopamine	Adjuvant treatment	Nausea, headache	Monitor for levodopa side effects
MAO INHIBITORS				
Selegiline (Deprenyl)*	Inhibit monoamine oxidase B, an enzyme that converts chemical byproducts in the brain into neurotoxins that prevent substantia nigra cell death	Adjuvant treatment	Nausea, dizziness, confusion, hallucinations, dry mouth	Monitor for levodopa side effects, as selegiline may increase effect of levodopa

*One study showed that levodopa in combination with selegiline provided no clinical benefit over levodopa alone in treating early, mild Parkinson's disease. Moreover, mortality was significantly higher when these two drugs were used together. (See Lees, A. J. [1995]. *British Journal of Medicine, 311,* 1602–1607.[23])

COMT, catechol-O-methyltransferase; MAO, monoamine oxidase.

CASE MANAGEMENT

The Older Adult

As technology and medication advances have increased the human life span, nurses will frequently be challenged to care for older adult clients experiencing an exacerbation of a chronic condition (such as chronic obstructive pulmonary disease) or who have an acute medical-surgical problem (such as a myocardial infarction) accompanied by multiple co-morbidities (e.g., hypertension, diabetes). You can assist these clients by using case management principles.

Assess

Avoid stereotyping as you perform your assessment, remembering that a client's cognitive changes may result from unfamiliarity with the environment or acute illness, such as an infection or electrolyte imbalance.

- Why has this client entered the health care system (Lack of caregiver or support services? Change in care needs or medications? Sensory changes? Pain management? Recent loss or depression? Poor nutrition or lack of education? Not understanding the care regimen?)
- Is there evidence of physical or psychological abuse or neglect?
- Are there environmental or safety barriers at home?
- Are there financial or insurance concerns, or does this older client need help to apply for assistance?
- Is there a pattern of frequent readmissions?

Work with the case manager, social worker and other team members to resolve these issues before discharge.

Advocate

Consider assignment to a primary nurse.

Allow extra time to explain procedures and treatments; help older adult clients participate in planning care and decision-making rather than deferring to family members. Even cognitively impaired clients can make some choices.

Decisions about advance directives and limitation of treatment may not always coincide with what you believe should be done, but respect such judgments when the client is informed and capable of making decisions. Encourage clients to select health proxies and make wishes known.

Clinical pathway time frames may need to be modified because of age and co-morbidities. Complete documentation of progress toward expected outcomes can ensure reimbursement and appropriate length of stay.

Prevent Readmission

Maintaining or improving baseline nutrition, hydration, mobility and ambulation are paramount to success after hospital discharge. Complicated medication regimens necessitate that you provide a good explanation as well as a written schedule for the client to follow. Changes in lifestyle or place of residence may be necessary and unexpected.

Observe the client's ability to perform the treatments needed; obtain equipment, nursing services, and prescriptions.

Teach preventive measures, such as flu shots and when to call the physician. If possible, follow up by phone after discharge to see that the care plan is being followed and to answer questions.

Cheryl Noetscher, RN, MS, *Director of Case Management, Crouse Hospital and Community–General Hospital, Syracuse, New York*

MYASTHENIA GRAVIS

Etiology

Myasthenia gravis (MG) is an autoimmune disease that presents as muscular weakness and fatigue that worsens with exercise and improves with rest. The manifestations result from a loss of ACh receptors in the postsynaptic neurons of the neuromuscular junction. The cause of MG is unknown, but 80% of people with the generalized form of the disease have elevated titers of antibodies to the ACh receptor in their serum. MG may appear at any age, although there are two peaks of onset. In early-onset MG, at age 20 to 30 years, women are more often affected than men. In late-onset MG, after age 50, men are more often affected. The overall incidence of MG is 0.4 per 100,000 and the prevalence is 0.5 to 5.0 per 100,000.

Clinical Manifestations

The primary feature of MG is increasing weakness with sustained muscle contraction. For instance, if the person is asked to hold the arms up, the power of muscle contraction diminishes and the arms gradually drift downward. After a period of rest, the muscles regain their strength. Muscle weakness is greatest after exertion or at the end of the day.

Ocular manifestations are most common, with *ptosis* (drooping of the upper eyelid) or *diplopia* (double vision) occurring in many clients. Ptosis is due to weakness of the levator palpebrae muscles of the eye. If not present at the time of examination, ptosis can be elicited by prolonged upward gaze, which creates fatigue of the muscle.

Diplopia is a result of weakness or fatigue of the extraocular muscles. Other manifestations are weakness of the orbicularis oculi muscles (which help close the eye), the facial muscles, the muscles of chewing and swallowing, and the limbs. Weakness of the facial and levator palpebrae muscles produces an expressionless face, with droopy eyelids, smoothed features, and a tendency for the mouth to hang open.

An attempt to smile often turns into a snarl because of the weakness. A person may hold a hand under the jaw to keep it closed. Dysphagia and a nasal quality to speech occur when the muscles of chewing and swallowing are involved. In severe cases, respiratory muscle weakness may occur, which may necessitate intubation and mechanical ventilation (see myasthenic crisis).

The course of MG varies, and there may be remissions and exacerbations. Clinical manifestations may progress quickly or slowly and may fluctuate from day to day. The severity of the disease varies greatly from person to person.

Diagnostic Findings

The diagnosis of MG is based on the clinical presentation and can be confirmed by testing the client's response to anticholinesterase drugs. These drugs inhibit cholinesterase, an enzyme that breaks down ACh in the neuromuscular junction, thereby allowing more ACh to bind to the remaining ACh receptors. Edrophonium (Tensilon) is a short-acting drug that is given intravenously *(Tensilon test)*. A test dose of 2 mg (for adults) is injected first. If no untoward reaction occurs (such as increased weakness, change in heart rate or rhythm, nausea, or abdominal cramps), the remaining 8 mg is injected. The client is then observed for objective signs of improvement in muscle strength. The effect is transitory, wearing off after 3 to 5 minutes. Another drug, neostigmine methylsulfate (Prostigmin), may be used because of its longer duration of effect on muscle strength (1 to 2 hours), which allows better analysis of its effect.

When either drug is used, IV atropine sulfate should be available to inject as an antidote. This medication counteracts any severe cholinergic reactions (cardiac dysrhythmias or abdominal cramping). Electromyography (EMG) helps confirm the diagnosis. Repetitive stimulation of the nerve with recording from the involved muscle shows a characteristic decrementing response of the muscle action potential.

Outcome Management

There is no cure for MG. Pharmacologic intervention consists of two groups of medications: (1) short-acting anticholinesterase compounds and (2) corticosteroids. The most effective anticholinesterase drugs are pyridostigmine (Mestinon) and neostigmine (Prostigmin). Dosages are highly individualized, based on physiologic response to the medication. The goal is to achieve the maximum benefit (muscle strength and endurance) with the fewest

---

CLIENT EDUCATION GUIDE

Parkinson's Disease

Client Instructions

Make sure that you understand how to take your medications, the importance of following the correct diet, and what side effects you can expect from your medications.

To avoid rigidity and the development of contractures:

- Exercise and stretch regularly.
- Perform the exercises recommended in your self-help booklets.
- Exercise first thing in the morning, when your energy levels are highest.
- Exercise in bed if getting to the floor is difficult.
- Get out of a chair by bending over slowly so that your head is over your toes; avoid soft, deep chairs.

If your health care provider has told you that you have bradykinesia (slow movements):

- Rock back and forth to get going.
- Imagine that you are stepping over an imaginary line when you walk.
- Throw small objects (e.g., small scraps of paper) in front of you to practice fine motor movements.
- Count to yourself while walking.
- Visualize your intended movement.

If you have a tremor:

- Hold change in your pocket or squeeze a small rubber ball.
- Use both hands to accomplish tasks.
- Lie face down on the floor and relax your entire body.
- Sleep on the side that has the tremor.

If you have trouble getting dressed:

- Dress and undress in front of a mirror.
- Use adaptive devices such as long-handled shoehorns and button fasteners.
- Buy clothes with self-fasteners (e.g., Velcro) and slide-locking buckles.

To ensure safety:

- Wear good, sturdy shoes.
- Use a cane or walker.
- Concentrate on standing upright.
- Consciously pick up your feet to take steps.
- Remove all throw rugs, electrical cords, and clutter from the floor.
- Make sure that you have adequate lighting.
- Arrange essential items so that they are within easy reach.
- Use a bath chair and a handheld shower nozzle.
- Have grab bars installed in the bathroom.
- Have a raised toilet seat installed

To ensure good communication:

- Pause between every few words.
- Exaggerate the pronunciation of words.
- Finish saying the final consonant of a word before starting to say the next word.
- Express ideas in short, concise phrases.
- Plan what to say.
- Face the listener.

To ensure adequate swallowing and prevent aspiration:

- Think through the steps of swallowing:
  - Keep your lips closed.
  - Keep your teeth together.
  - Put food on your tongue.
  - Lift your tongue up and back.
  - Swallow.
- Eat slowly, taking small bites.
- Chew hard and move food around with your tongue.
- Finish one bite before taking another.

To keep saliva from building up in your mouth:

- Make a conscious effort to swallow saliva often.
- Keep your head in an upright position so saliva will collect in the back of your throat and stimulate automatic swallowing.
- Swallow excess saliva before attempting to speak.

side effects (excessive salivation, sweating, nausea, diarrhea, abdominal cramps, or tachycardia). Corticosteroids (usually prednisone) are directed toward reducing the levels of serum ACh receptor antibodies. Corticosteroids may temporarily worsen symptoms; however, this is followed by gradual improvement in muscle strength.

After a peak of improvement is reached and maintained for several weeks, the dosage of both prednisone and anticholinesterase medication may be gradually decreased. A low maintenance dose of alternate-day prednisone may be effective for many months or years. Precautions with any steroid therapy are important, including potassium supplements if indicated and liberal use of antacids.

Potential complications of steroid use are cataracts, hypertension, diabetes, fluid retention, delayed wound healing, insomnia, and osteoporosis. Other treatments include azathioprine (Imuran) and cyclosporine (Sandimmune), which reduce the level of circulating ACh receptor antibodies, and plasmapheresis and IVIG.

PLASMAPHERESIS

Plasmapheresis is an adjunctive therapy for clients with refractory MG. It is a process by which plasma is separated from formed elements of blood. The plasma is discarded and the packed red blood cells are joined with albumin, normal saline, and electrolytes and returned to the client. The purpose is to remove plasma proteins containing antibodies that are believed to cause MG. Plasmapheresis may produce transient improvement in clients who have actual or pending respiratory failure.

Usually, three to five treatments given once daily over 5 to 7 days are required. Potential complications include myasthenic or cholinergic crisis and, rarely, hypovolemia. Muscle strength should be assessed before and after the procedure, with particular attention paid to vital capacity, swallowing ability, diplopia, and ptosis, to evaluate the effectiveness of the treatment.

COMPLICATIONS

Two major complications of MG may occur: *myasthenic crisis* and *cholinergic crisis* (Box 72–2).

MYASTHENIC CRISIS. Clients with moderate or severe generalized MG, especially those who have difficulty swallowing or breathing, may experience a sudden worsening of their condition. This is usually precipitated by an intercurrent infection or sudden withdrawal of anticholinesterase drugs, but it may occur spontaneously. If an increase in the dosage of the anticholinesterase drug does not improve the weakness, endotracheal intubation and mechanical ventilation may be required. In many instances, drug responsiveness returns in 24 to 48 hours, and weaning from the respirator can proceed.

CHOLINERGIC CRISIS. Cholinergic crisis occurs as a result of overmedication. The muscarinic effect of a toxic level of anticholinesterase medication causes abdominal cramps, diarrhea, and excessive pulmonary secretions. The nicotinic effect paradoxically worsens weakness and can cause bronchial spasm. If respiratory status is compromised, the client may need intubation and mechanical ventilation.

▪ Nursing Management of the Medical Client

Clients with MG are usually managed in an outpatient setting. When clients are hospitalized for diagnosis or during a crisis, the following nursing management procedure may be pertinent.

Because MG may involve the muscles of respiration, the client may experience dyspnea and ineffective cough and swallow mechanisms. This may lead to aspiration and pneumonia. Encourage deep breathing and coughing. Have suction equipment available at the bedside; instruct the client on how to use it. Instruct the client to sit upright when eating, to swallow only when the chin is tipped downward toward the chest, and never to speak while food is in the mouth. Oxygen and, in severe cases, mechanical ventilation may be required.

In MG, weakness is usually greatest following exertion and at the end of the day. Activities should be carefully planned to include rest periods so that energy is conserved and the muscles have a chance to regain their strength. Rearrangement of the home environment may help prevent unnecessary energy expenditure. Vocational retraining may be indicated for those who can no longer meet the physical demands of their jobs. Clients with severe disease or an acute exacerbation will be totally dependent on nursing care for ADL. This level of care requires that complications of immobility be avoided.

BOX 72–2   Myasthenic and Cholinergic Crises in Clients with Myasthenia Gravis

Myasthenic Crisis Is Caused by Undermedication

Clinical Manifestations

Sudden marked rise in blood pressure due to hypoxia
Increased heart rate
Severe respiratory distress and cyanosis
Absent cough and swallow reflex
Increased secretions, increased diaphoresis, and increased lacrimation
Restlessness, dysarthria
Bowel and bladder incontinence

Intervention

Increased doses of cholinergic drugs as long as the client responds positively to edrophonium treatment
Possible mechanical ventilation if respiratory muscle paralysis is acute

Cholinergic Crisis Is Caused by Depolarization Block Resulting from Excessive Medications

Clinical Manifestations

Weakness with difficulty swallowing, chewing, speaking, and breathing
Apprehension, nausea, and vomiting
Abdominal cramps and diarrhea
Increased secretions and saliva
Sweating, lacrimation, fasciculations, and blurred vision

Intervention

Discontinue all cholinergic drugs until cholinergic effects decrease
Provide adequate ventilatory support
1 mg intravenous atropine may be necessary to counteract severe cholinergic reactions

Provide the client and family with information about MG and its treatment (see end of chapter). They should be aware of adverse reactions of both anticholinesterase drugs and steroids. Explain how to recognize myasthenic and cholinergic crises and how to have a plan to seek medical intervention, if necessary.

■ Surgical Management

Thymectomy can be used for treatment. The thymus gland, located in the superior mediastinum, is important during fetal growth for development of the immune system. It is usually atrophied and nonfunctioning in adulthood. The effect of thymectomy is not fully understood. It may alter some immunologic control mechanism that affects the production of antibodies to the ACh receptor, or it may eliminate a trigger to antibody production. Thymectomy is indicated for clients with thymoma, selected clients with generalized MG without thymoma, and selected clients with disabling ocular MG.[14] The procedure is recommended early in the course of the disease. Nursing management is similar to care following thoracic surgery.

Eaton-Lambert (Myasthenic) Syndrome

Eaton-Lambert syndrome (also called *myasthenic syndrome*) is a myasthenia-like condition in which weakness is noted in the limbs. It is characterized by defective release of ACh possibly caused by autoantibodies (IgG). Eaton-Lambert syndrome is found almost exclusively in people with oat cell carcinoma of the lung and has been noted less often in people with cancers of the prostate, stomach, rectum, and breast.

The onset is insidious, and clinical manifestations are progressive. In comparison with MG, diplopia is less common and there is proximal weakness of the legs, arms, and pelvic girdle. There is reduced muscle action potential when muscle is stimulated, but repetitive stimulation augments muscle action. Weakness tends to develop with exertion, although some clients have a temporary increase in power when muscles are repeatedly stimulated. Autonomic dysfunction is common, presenting as dry mouth, impotence, and peripheral paresthesias.

Treatment is directed at the primary cancer. Guanidine HCl may improve manifestations by increasing ACh release. Plasmapheresis and immunotherapy have also been used. Calcium-channel blockers can worsen the transmission defect. Because MG can precede the development of cancer by many years, clients with Eaton-Lambert syndrome should be assessed yearly for the development of cancer.

Amyotrophic Lateral Sclerosis

Amyotrophic lateral sclerosis (ALS) is the most common of the motor neuron diseases. It is an age-dependent, fatal paralytic disorder also known as *Charcot's disease* and *Lou Gehrig's disease.* Onset is usually in middle age. Men are affected more often than women. The overall incidence of ALS is 0.4 to 1.8 per 100,000, and the prevalence is 4 to 6 per 100,000.

Clinical Manifestations

ALS involves degeneration of both the anterior horn cells and the corticospinal tracts. Consequently, both upper and lower motor neuron clinical manifestations are seen. Lower motor neuron clinical manifestations include weakness, atrophy, cramps, and fasciculations (irregular twitchings of muscle fibers or bundles). Upper motor neuron signs include spasticity and hyperreflexia. Involvement of the corticobulbar tracts causes dysphagia (difficulty swallowing) and dysarthria (slurred speech). The sensory system is not involved, and cognition is not affected. The client remains alert and mentally intact throughout the course of the disease.

The course of the disease is relentlessly progressive. Death usually results from pneumonia caused by respiratory compromise within 2 to 5 years.

Weakness typically begins in the upper extremities and progressively involves the upper arms and shoulders and then the muscles of the neck and throat. The trunk and lower extremities are usually not affected until late in the disease. When the intercostal muscles and diaphragm become involved, respirations are shallow and coughing is ineffective. Cognition, as well as bowel and bladder sphincters, remains intact, even when the client is totally debilitated. In some cases, weakness begins in the brain stem, causing problems with speech and swallowing. This is called *bulbar ALS.*

Diagnosis of ALS is made by the clinical presentation and EMG. EMG criteria for the diagnosis of ALS include the presence of widespread anterior horn cell dysfunction with fibrillations, positive waves, fasciculations, and chronic neurogenic motor unit potential changes in multiple nerve root distribution in at least three limbs and the paraspinal muscles in the presence of normal sensory responses.

Outcome Management

Supportive therapy was the only intervention for ALS until riluzole (Rilutek) was approved in 1996. Its mechanism of action is unknown, but it is thought to have a neuroprotective effect. The drug extends the life of ALS clients by a few months. Clients with ALS are usually admitted to health care facilities only twice in their illness, first for diagnosis and later in the final stage of debilitation.

Supportive nursing care is an important aspect of managing the ALS client. In the outpatient arena, the nurse can provide ongoing assessment of daily living needs and make suggestions for modifications in activity level, clothing, and diet. Often, just allowing the client or family to talk about problems reduces anxiety and helps them find solutions to problems.[19] Interventions should be aimed at conserving energy. Activities should be spaced during the day. Muscle stress, strenuous activity, and extremes of hot and cold should be avoided. Leg braces, canes, and walkers can prolong independence in ambulation. Hand braces, special utensils, and adaptive devices such as buttonhooks can help with dressing and self-feeding. Pressure ulcers are not usually a problem because the sensory system remains intact and the client can feel when pressure on a body part is too great.

In the acute care setting, gather information from the client and family about communication needs and which positions are best for respiration, handling secretions, eating, and turning routines.

Encourage fluid intake regularly, when the client is not fatigued. Proper positioning is imperative. Providing a cup with a spout may prevent liquid from running out of the corners of the mouth. Give liquids by using a large syringe with short tubing on the tip. The tube is placed on the anterior portion of the tongue, and gentle force is used to deliver small amounts of liquid.

Encourage small, frequent, high-nutrient feedings. Tell the client to sit upright, with the head slightly flexed forward while eating. Papase tablets placed under the tongue 10 minutes before meals can make thick saliva less sticky. Plenty of time should be allowed for eating, and the client should not attempt to speak while food is in the mouth. Have suction equipment available during meals to reduce the risk of aspiration of food and secretions that become lodged in the mouth and pharynx. The head may need to be stabilized with a soft cervical collar. Consult the dietitian for special diet recommendations.

Although speech remains intelligible, the client can be trained to slow the rate of speech and exaggerate articulation. As manifestations progress, the client may need to repeat words or have an interpreter (usually the spouse). At this stage, it is important to eliminate extraneous noise, face the client when he or she is talking, and maintain eye contact. When the client's speech contains only one-word phrases or is no longer possible, writing can be an effective means of communicating and should be encouraged. When writing is no longer possible, a speech pathologist can provide communication devices such as alphabet boards and portable memo writers.[9]

If the client is a smoker, encourage him or her to stop. Exposure to people with respiratory infections should be avoided. Remind the client to use good posture. Pulmonary function tests should be performed regularly to assess ventilatory status. Clients generally experience respiratory fatigue when vital capacity is less than 1.5 L. Some clients can be taught to use their abdominal muscles to enhance respirations when the intercostal muscles and diaphragm become weak. A sign of pending respiratory insufficiency is shortness of breath while eating.

Encourage the client and family to talk about the losses they are experiencing and the feelings associated with them. Family members should be encouraged to take time for rest and activities away from the client. Refer the client and family to an ALS support group.

Eventually, clients face the difficult choice of deciding whether they will accept artificial ventilation. Encourage them to discuss this with family and friends and to seek input from ALS support groups. Encourage clients to complete advance directives to indicate whether they desire life-sustaining treatments such as cardiopulmonary resuscitation, but this should be reassessed at regular intervals. Clients may change their minds on the basis of their experience with their illness, changes in their subjective appreciation of their quality of life, or changes in their evaluation of the benefits and burdens of life-sustaining measures as they come to terms with the imminence of death.[21]

CONCLUSIONS

Degenerative neurologic disorders have many causes, including viruses, autoimmune responses, and heredity. Some have no known cause. In general, they are relentlessly progressive, slowly taking away both physical and mental ability. Nurses should focus care on the management of clinical manifestations and prevention of complications. Family support throughout the process of care is essential.

THINKING CRITICALLY

1. **A 52-year-old man with multiple sclerosis is wheelchair-bound and has a neurogenic bladder. He complains of a sudden onset of generalized weakness, fever, and chills and is admitted to the hospital. What priorities should be set for his care?**

Factors to Consider. What do generalized weakness, fever, and chills suggest in *any* client? If your client has not been following good bladder management, how can you intervene?

2. **A 70-year-old man with Parkinson's disease is admitted to the hospital after experiencing severe nightmares and periods of confusion. During lucid periods, he is very disturbed by these manifestations. At other times, he believes that his wife is participating in a conspiracy to harm him. What assessments and interventions should you consider?**

Factors to Consider. Are hallucinations and paranoia typical manifestations of Parkinson's disease? Might the client's manifestations be related to treatment or to some cause other than Parkinson's disease?

3. **A 41-year-old woman with myasthenia gravis is taking pyridostigmine and prednisone. She is complaining of increased fatigue and weakness and has difficulty breathing. What concerns should you have?**

Factors to Consider. Might the client's difficult breathing be related to her fatigue and weakness? Could these manifestations be related to myasthenia gravis or its treatment?

BIBLIOGRAPHY

1. Acorn, S., & Andersen, S. (1990). Depression in multiple sclerosis: Critique of the research literature. *Journal of Neuroscience Nursing,* 22(4), 209–214.
2. Ahlskog, J. E. (1993). Cerebral transplantation for Parkinson's disease: Current progress and future prospects. *Mayo Clinic Proceedings, 68,* 578–591.
3. Andrews, K. L., & Husmann, D. A. (1997). Bladder dysfunction and management in multiple sclerosis. *Mayo Clinic Proceedings, 72,* 1176–1183.
4. Bansil, S., Cook, S. D., & Rohowsky-Kochan, C. (1995). Multiple sclerosis: Immune mechanisms and update on current therapies. *Annals of Neurology 37*(suppl. 1), S87–101.
5. Brown, P. (1997). The risk of bovine spongiform encephalopathy ('mad cow disease') to human health. *Journal of the American Medical Association, 278*(12), 1008–1011.

6. Coleman, L. M., Fowler, L. L., & Williams, M. E. (1995). Use of unproven therapies by people with Alzheimer's disease. *Journal of the American Geriatrics Society, 43,* 747–750.

7. Corey-Bloom, J., et al. (1995). Diagnosis and evaluation of dementia. *Neurology, 45,* 211–218.

8. Corey-Bloom, J., Galaski, D., & Thal, L. J. (1994). Clinical features and natural history of Alzheimer's disease. In D.B. Calne (Ed.), *Neurodegenerative diseases* (pp. 631–645). Philadelphia: W. B. Saunders.

9. Cummings, J. L., & Benson, D. F. (1992). *Dementia, a clinical approach.* Boston: Butterworth-Heinemann.

10. Franco, D. A., & Bashir, R. M. (1996, December). Current concepts in Guillain-Barré syndrome. *Nebraska Medical Journal,* 406–411.

11. Hillel, A. D., & Miller, R. (1989). Bulbar amyotrophic lateral sclerosis: Patterns of progression and clinical management. *Head and Neck, 11*(1), 51–59.

12. Hogancamp, W. E., Rodriguez, M., & Weinshenker, B. G. (1997). The epidemiology of multiple sclerosis. *Mayo Clinic Proceedings, 72,* 871–878.

13. Hunt, V. P., & Walker, F. O. (1989). Dysphagia in Huntington's disease. *Journal of Neuroscience Nursing, 21*(2), 92–95.

14. Hurley, A. C., et al. (1992). Assessment of discomfort in advanced Alzheimer patients. *Research in Nursing and Health, 15*(5), 369–378.

15. Jones, P. S., & Martinson, I. M. (1992). The experience of bereavement in care givers of family members with Alzheimer's disease. *Image—The Journal of Nursing Scholarship, 24*(3), 172–176.

16. Kernich, A., & Kaminski, H. J. (1995). Myasthenia gravis: Pathophysiology, diagnosis, and collaborative care. *Journal of Neuroscience Nursing, 27,* 207–215.

17. Khoury, S. J., & Weiner, H. L. (1998). Multiple sclerosis: What have we learned from magnetic resonance imaging studies? *Archives of Internal Medicine, 158,* 565–573.

18. Lang, A. E., & Lozano, A.M. (1998). Parkinson's disease. *New England Journal of Medicine 339*(16), 1130–1143.

19. Lanska, D. J. (1990). Indications for thymectomy in myasthenia gravis. *Neurology, 40*(12), 1828–1829.

20. Le Bars, P. L., et al. (1997). A placebo-controlled, double-blind, randomized trial of an extract of ginkgo biloba for dementia. *Journal of the American Medical Association, 278*(16), 1327–1332.

21. Lees, A. J. (1995). Comparison of therapeutic effects and mortality data of levodopa and levodopa combined with selegiline in patients with early, mild Parkinson's disease. *British Journal of Medicine, 311,* 1602–1607.

22. Lucchinetti, C. F., & Rodriguez, M. (1997). The controversy surrounding pathogenesis of the multiple sclerosis lesion. *Mayo Clinic Proceedings, 72,* 665–678.

23. Mayeux, R., & Chun, M. (1995). Dementias. In L. P. Rowland (Ed.), *Merritt's textbook of neurology* (9th ed.). Baltimore: Williams & Wilkins.

24. Mayo Foundation for Medical Education and Research. (1996, October). Alzheimer's disease: Living with a 'long goodbye.' *Mayo Clinic Health Letter* (suppl.), 1–8.

25. McKhann, G., et al. (1984). Clinical diagnosis of Alzheimer's disease: Report of the NINCDS-ADRDA Work Group under the auspices of Department of Health and Human Services Task Force on Alzheimer's Disease. *Neurology, 34*(7), 939–944.

26. Mega, M., et al. (1996). The spectrum of behavioral changes in Alzheimer's disease. *Neurology, 46*(1), 130–135.

27. Mezey, M., et al. (1996). Life-sustaining treatment decisions by spouses of patients with Alzheimer's disease. *Journal of the American Geriatrics Society, 44*(2), 144–150.

28. Mocsny, N. (1991). Precautions to prevent the spread of Creutzfeldt-Jakob disease. *Journal of Neuroscience Nursing, 23*(2), 116–119.

29. Nowotny, M. L. (1998). My journey with amyotrophic lateral sclerosis. *Journal of Neuroscience Nursing, 30*(1), 68–70.

30. Pericak-Vance, M. A., et al. (1997). Complete genomic screen in late-onset familial Alzheimer disease: Evidence for a new locus on chromosome 12. *Journal of the American Medical Association, 278*(15), 1237–1241.

31. Post, S. G., et al. (1997). The clinical introduction of genetic testing for Alzheimer disease: An ethical perspective. *Journal of the American Medical Association, 277*(10), 832–836.

32. Robinson, B. E. (1997). Guideline for initial evaluation of the patient with memory loss. *Geriatrics, 52*(12), 30–39.

33. Rodriguez, M. (1997). Multiple sclerosis: Insights into molecular pathogenesis and therapy. *Mayo Clinic Proceedings, 72,* 663–664.

34. Ropper, A. H. (1992). The Guillain-Barré syndrome. *New England Journal of Medicine, 326*(17), 1130–1136.

35. Rudick, R. A., et al. (1997). Management of multiple sclerosis. *New England Journal of Medicine, 337*(22), 1604–1611.

36. Sano, M., et al. (1997). A controlled trial of selegiline, alpha-tocopherol, or both as treatment for Alzheimer's disease. *New England Journal of Medicine, 336*(17), 1216–1222.

37. Silverstein, M. D., et al. (1991). Amyotrophic lateral sclerosis and life-sustaining therapy: Patients' desires for information, participation in decision making, and life-sustaining therapy. *Mayo Clinic Proceedings, 66*(9), 906–913.

38. Tienari, P. J. (1994). Multiple sclerosis: Multiple etiologies, multiple genes? *Annals of Medicine, 26,* 259–269.

39. van der Meche, F. G. A. (1994). The Guillain-Barré syndrome: Plasma exchange or immunoglobulin intravenously? *Journal of Neurology, Neurosurgery, and Psychiatry, 57*(suppl.), 33–34.

40. Vrabec, N. J. (1997). Literature review of social support and caregiver burden, 1980 to 1995. *Image—The Journal of Nursing Scholarship, 29*(4), 383–388.

CHAPTER

73

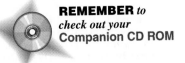

Management of Clients with Neurologic Trauma

Norma D. McNair

NURSING OUTCOMES CLASSIFICATION (NOC)
for Nursing Diagnoses—Clients with Neurologic Trauma

Altered Family Processes
Family Coping
Family Functioning
Psychosocial Adjustment: Life Change
Role Performance
Altered Health Maintenance
Health Belief: Perceived Resources
Knowledge: Health Resources
Risk Detection
Social Support
Altered Nutrition: Less Than Body Requirements
Nutritional Status: Food and Fluid Intake
Altered Oral Mucous Membrane
Oral Health
Tissue Integrity: Skin and Mucous Membrane
Altered Thought Processes
Cognitive Ability
Cognitive Orientation
Information Processing
Neurologic Status: Consciousness
Altered Tissue Perfusion: Cerebral
Cognitive Ability
Neurologic Status: Consciousness
Tissue Perfusion: Cerebral
Anticipatory Grieving
Grief Resolution
Psychosocial Adjustment: Life Change

Chronic Pain
Comfort Level
Depression Control
Pain: Disruptive Effects
Pain: Psychological Response
Constipation
Bowel Elimination
Hydration
Impaired Gas Exchange
Respiratory Status: Ventilation
Vital Signs Status
Impaired Physical Mobility
Ambulation: Wheelchair
Sensory Function: Proprioception
Transfer Performance
Impaired Skin Integrity
Tissue Integrity: Skin and Mucous Membranes
Inability to Sustain Spontaneous Ventilation
Neurologic Status: Central Motor Control
Vital Signs Status
Ineffective Airway Clearance
Aspiration Control
Respiratory Status: Airway Patency
Respiratory Status: Ventilation
Ineffective Family Coping: Compromised
Family Coping
Family Normalization

Ineffective Individual Coping
Coping
Information Processing
Role Performance
Social Support
Ineffective Thermoregulation
Thermoregulation
Post-Trauma Syndrome
Coping
Fear Control
Risk for Aspiration
Cognitive Ability
Immobility Consequences: Physiologic
Neurologic Status
Respiratory Status: Ventilation
Risk for Impaired Skin Integrity
Immobility Consequences: Physiologic
Tissue Integrity: Skin and Mucous Membranes
Risk for Injury
Neurologic Status
Risk Control
Sexual Dysfunction
Sexual Functioning
Role Performance
Total Incontinence
Neurological Status
Tissue Integrity: Skin and Mucous Membranes
Urinary Continence

The complexity of the central nervous system (CNS) allows the human organism to evaluate information about the outside world. Failure of the brain or the spinal cord to accurately process information prevents the affected person from accurately performing tasks and may impair interactions with others as well as self-appraisal.

Admission of a client with CNS trauma to the emergency department requires rapid mobilization of a trauma team. The team provides initial assessment and resuscitation of the trauma victim and performs triage to the appropriate radiologic studies and surgical service. Ulti-

mately, the management of a client with a head injury, spinal cord injury, or combination of neurologic injuries is directed by the neurosurgical service. This chapter examines the needs of clients with CNS trauma, including head and spinal cord injuries.

INCREASED INTRACRANIAL PRESSURE

Intracranial pressure (ICP) is the pressure exerted in the cranium by its contents: the brain, blood, and cerebrospinal fluid (CSF) (Fig. 73–1). ICP is measured with a

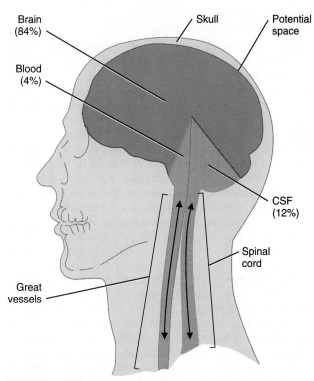

FIGURE 73–1 Components of the intracranial vault.

monitor in either the ventricle, the brain parenchyma, or the subarachnoid space. The normal ICP is 5 to 15 mm Hg. Pressures over 20 mm Hg are considered to represent *increased ICP,* which seriously impairs cerebral perfusion. Recognition of increased ICP is one of the most important assessments made by nurses caring for clients with neurologic disorders.

Cerebral perfusion pressure (CPP) is the amount of blood flow from the systemic circulation that is required to provide adequate oxygen and glucose for brain metabolism. *Mean arterial pressure* (MAP) represents the average pressure during the cardiac cycle. It is calculated by adding the systolic pressure to twice the diastolic pressure and dividing by 3. (Diastole is twice as long as systole.) The formula for calculating cerebral perfusion pressure is as follows:

$$CPP = MAP - ICP$$

When MAP and ICP are equal, there is no CPP and brain perfusion ceases. Therefore, it is crucial to keep ICP and MAP controlled.

Etiology and Risk Factors

Increased ICP is most often associated with a space-occupying lesion, a cerebral infarction, an obstruction to the outflow of CSF, an abscess, an ingested or accumulated toxin, impaired blood flow to or from the brain, vasodilation from increased carbon dioxide ($PaCO_2$) or decreased partial pressure of oxygen (PaO_2), systemic hypertension, or increased intrathoracic pressure. Risk factors include head injury, brain tumors, cerebral bleeding, hydrocephalus, and edema from surgery or injury.

Pathophysiology

The skull is a hard, bony vault filled with brain tissue, blood, and CSF. A balance between these three components maintains the pressure within the cranium. The modified Munro-Kellie hypothesis, a theory for understanding ICP, states that because the bony skull cannot expand, when one of the three components expands, the other two must compensate by decreasing in volume in order for the total brain volume and pressure to remain constant.

As an intracranial mass enlarges, initial compensation occurs through *displacement of CSF* into the spinal canal. The ability of the brain to adapt to increasing pressure without increasing ICP is called *compliance.* The movement of CSF out of the cranium is the first and major compensatory mechanism, but it can accommodate increasing intracranial volume only to a point. When the compliance of the brain is exceeded, the ICP rises, clinical manifestations develop, and other compensatory efforts to reduce pressure begin.

The second form of compensation is *reduction of blood volume* in the brain. When blood flow is reduced by 40%, cerebral tissue becomes acidotic. When 60% of blood flow is lost, the electroencephalogram (EEG) begins to change. This stage of compensation alters cerebral metabolism, eventually leading to brain tissue hypoxia and areas of brain tissue ischemia.

The last stage of compensation and the most lethal is *displacement of brain tissue* across the tentorium, under the falx cerebri, or through the foramen magnum into the spinal canal. This process is called *herniation* and often results in death from brain stem compression. The brain is supported within various intracranial compartments (Fig. 73–2). The supratentorial compartment contains all of the brain tissue from the top of the midbrain upward. This section is divided into right and left chambers by the tough, inelastic fibers of the falx cerebri. The supratentorial compartment is separated from the infratentorial compartment (containing the brain stem and cerebellum) by the tentorium cerebelli. The brain is capable of some movement within these compartments. Pressure increases in one compartment affect surrounding areas of lower pressure.

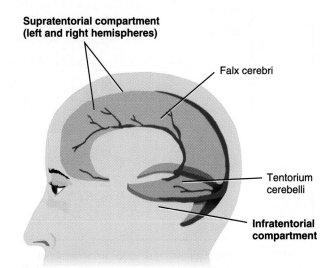

FIGURE 73–2 The intracranial compartments.

With regard to ICP maintenance, *autoregulation* is the occurrence of compensatory changes in the diameter of the intracranial blood vessels designed to maintain a constant blood flow during changes in cerebral perfusion pressure. Autoregulation is lost with increasing ICP. Small increases in brain volume can then cause dramatic increases in ICP, with a longer time required to return to baseline level. When ICP approaches systemic blood pressure, cerebral perfusion decreases and the brain suffers severe hypoxia and acidosis.

CEREBRAL EDEMA

The terms *cerebral edema, brain swelling,* and *increased ICP* are sometimes used interchangeably, but they are not the same. Cerebral edema and brain swelling are causes of increased ICP. An increase in brain bulk caused by an increase in cerebral blood volume is called *brain swelling. Brain edema,* in contrast, is an increase in the fluid content surrounding the tissues of the brain, such as in the extracellular spaces or the white matter, or within the cells themselves. The distinction between these two conditions is important because the interventions differ.

After head injury, edema develops as a result of a disruption of the blood-brain barrier. This type of edema is similar to other forms of edema, such as that seen in a sprained ankle. The fluid contains electrolytes, proteins, and blood. Edema reaches its maximum within 48 to 72 hours after brain surgery or injury. The fluid returns to the systemic circulation via the CSF or the venous system. This form of edema is usually treated with osmotic diuretics.

Brain swelling is also caused by increased blood volume resulting from dilated cerebral blood vessels. Brain swelling appears to be the major mechanism responsible for increasing ICP and for decreasing the size of the ventricles when compensation occurs. This form of swelling may be treated with therapeutic hyperventilation using mechanical ventilation to cause vasoconstriction.

Clinical Manifestations

Manifestations of increased ICP are caused by traction on the cerebral blood vessels from swelling tissues and by pressure on the pain-sensitive dura mater and various structures within the brain and eye. The pathologic process of increased ICP actually comprises several entities that occur at the same time. No single set of clinical manifestations occurs in all clients. Indications of increased ICP relate to the location and cause of the raised pressure and to the speed and extent of its development.

The manifestations of increased ICP are subtle, and diligent observation for changes in the client's condition is necessary. Clinical manifestations include *any* alteration in level of consciousness (restlessness, irritability, confusion), and a decrease in the Glasgow Coma Scale (GCS) score. In addition, the client may have changes in speech, pupillary reactivity, motor or sensory ability, or cardiac rate and rhythm. Headache, nausea, vomiting, or blurred or double vision (diplopia) may be reported. The optic nerve is an extension of the brain, and increased tension in the skull is transmitted to the optic nerve to cause papilledema. Papilledema is swelling and hyperemia of the optic disc and can be observed only through an ophthalmoscope. Early detection (i.e., before clinical manifestations develop) by means of periodic ophthalmologic examination and ICP monitoring in the critical care unit can greatly improve a client's outcome.

Cushing's triad—increased systolic blood pressure with widened pulse pressure and bradycardia—is a late response and indicates severe increased ICP with failure of autoregulation. Respiratory patterns progress from Cheyne-Stokes respiration to central neurogenic hyperventilation to apneustic breathing and ataxic breathing as ICP increases (see Chapter 68). Hyperthermia is typically present when the hypothalamus is first affected by the increase in pressure, followed by hypothermia as ICP increases (Fig. 73–3).

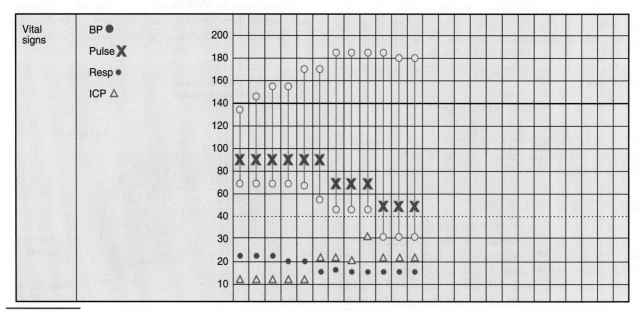

FIGURE 73–3 A late response to increased intracranial pressure is Cushing's triad (also called Cushing's response): bradycardia, systolic hypertension, and a wide pulse pressure, which result from pressure on the medulla. These manifestations can occur with intracranial hypertension or herniation. Alterations in the respiratory pattern also accompany Cushing's triad.

Common diagnostic studies that are performed to determine the source of increased ICP include skull radiography, computed tomography (CT) scanning, and magnetic resonance imaging (MRI). A lumbar puncture is not usually performed because of the risk of causing herniation of the brain stem when the pressure of the CSF in the spinal cord is lower than in the cranium. In addition, the CSF pressure at the lumbar level is not always an accurate reflection of the intracranial CSF pressure.

HERNIATION SYNDROMES

Herniation syndromes have been classified into five types (Fig. 73–4). These conditions occur late in the course of increased ICP and represent the body's last attempt to restore normal brain volume and pressure through displacement of blood, brain tissue, or CSF.

Herniation, regardless of the type, always constitutes an emergency. *Notify the physician immediately of any manifestations that indicate a worsening of the client's condition due to increasing ICP.*

SUPRATENTORIAL HERNIATION SYNDROMES

TRANSCALVARIAL HERNIATION. Transcalvarial herniation occurs with open head injuries when brain tissue is extruded through an unstable skull fracture. Clinical manifestations vary greatly depending on the location and extent of the open skull fracture.

CENTRAL TRANSTENTORIAL HERNIATION. Central transtentorial herniation is the end result of the downward displacement of the diencephalon through the tentorial notch. It is caused by injuries or masses located in the cerebral cortex or on the outward perimeter of the cerebrum.[73] An early indication of central transtentorial herniation is a rapid change in the level of consciousness. As the pressure increases, changes in respiratory patterns are seen: first, Cheyne-Stokes respirations and then central neurogenic hyperventilation; later, apneustic breathing and also ataxic breathing (Biot's respiration); and, finally, apnea (see Chapter 68). Pupils become small but at first remain reactive, with progression to a dilated and fixed state. Pathologic reflexes begin with Babinski's sign (see Chapter 67) and then progress from abnormal flexion to abnormal extensor posturing. Doll's eye reflex and a positive response to caloric testing are noted when brain stem function is still intact but are absent if the brain stem dies (see Chapter 68). The Critical Monitoring feature in Chapter 68 lists the specific areas of brain involvement that are correlated with pathologic manifestation.

LATERAL TRANSTENTORIAL HERNIATION. Lateral transtentorial herniation occurs from displacement by masses in or along the temporal lobe. It is also called *uncal herniation,* because as the temporal lobe is compressed, the uncus (the anteromedial portion of the hippocampus) and/or the hippocampal gyrus shift from the middle fossa through the tentorial notch into the posterior fossa.[73] As the herniation progresses, the pupils first become sluggish in response to light and then become unresponsive; lack of response is seen first in the ipsilateral pupil and then in the contralateral pupil, secondary to third cranial nerve compression at the midbrain level. Other progressive clinical manifestations include a decreasing level of consciousness (stupor to coma), Cheyne-Stokes respirations followed by central neurogenic hyperventilation, and abnormal flexor posturing that progresses to abnormal extensor posturing.

CINGULATE HERNIATION. Cingulate herniation occurs when the frontal lobes of the cerebrum are compressed, resulting in compression of the cingulate gyrus (an arch-shaped convolution situated just above the corpus callosum) under the falx cerebri.[73] Manifestations are related to cerebral artery compression resulting in ischemia and congestion, edema, and increasing ICP.

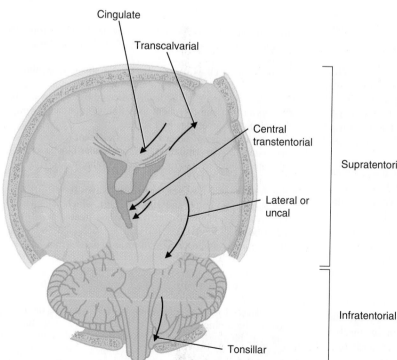

Cingulate

Transcalvarial

Central transtentorial

Lateral or uncal

Supratentorial

Infratentorial

Tonsillar

FIGURE 73–4 Types of intracranial herniation. In *transcalvarial* herniation, edematous brain tissue is extruded through the skull. In *central* transtentorial herniation, the lesion is located centrally or superiorly in the cranium, and compression of central and midbrain structures may result. In *lateral,* or *uncal,* herniation the lesion is located laterally within the cranium and can cause pressure on the midbrain. *Cingulate* herniation occurs between the two frontal lobes; the brain is pressed under the falx cerebri. In *tonsillar* herniation, the cerebellar tonsils are driven between the posterior arch of the atlas and the medulla and may be compressed.

INFRATENTORIAL (TONSILLAR) HERNIATION SYNDROME

Tonsillar herniation, also known as *cerebellar herniation*, occurs when the cerebellar tonsil shifts through the foramen magnum, compressing the medulla and upper portion of the spinal cord. Increasing pressure in the posterior fossa, often secondary to cerebellar bleeding, is the usual underlying problem. Manifestations often progress rapidly and include erratic changes in blood pressure, pulse rate, and breathing; decreased level of consciousness; an arched, stiff neck; and quadriparesis.

Outcome Management

The goals of medical management are to decrease ICP, to maintain optimal neurologic function, and to ready the client for rehabilitation.

DECREASE INTRACRANIAL PRESSURE

Emergency care of the client at high risk for development of increased ICP focuses on maintaining the airway, improving breathing, and promoting circulation. Immediate interventions may include intubation followed by hyperventilation, osmotic diuretics, and elevation of the head to promote venous drainage.

HYPERVENTILATION. Carbon dioxide causes cerebral blood vessels to dilate. By increasing the ventilator settings to cause hyperventilation, a hypocarbic (low carbon dioxide) blood level is created. A partial pressure of CO_2 ($PaCO_2$) level between 30 and 35 mm Hg results in vasoconstriction of the cerebral blood vessels, leading to decreased blood flow and thus decreased ICP. It is also important to maintain oxygenation. The swollen or bruised brain has an increased need for oxygen and glucose because of an increased metabolic rate. The PaO_2 must be kept between 90 and 100 mm Hg.

MANNITOL. Mannitol, a hyperosmotic agent, is the preferred agent for treating increased ICP because it does not cross an intact blood-brain barrier and has fewer rebound effects.[15] It is given in doses of 0.25 g to 1.0 g/kg intravenously. Hyperosmotic agents increase intravascular pressure by drawing fluid from the interstitial spaces and from the brain cells. If the blood-brain barrier is damaged, the medication enters the brain and increases swelling. Renal function, electrolytes, and serum osmolality need to be monitored when the client is receiving mannitol. Diuresis is expected, and the client may become dehydrated with the excessive use of mannitol. Dehydration is manifested by increased serum sodium and osmolality values.

CEREBRAL PERFUSION. Vasoactive medication, given either to raise or lower blood pressure, may be required to maintain CPP at a normal level. CPP is a result of the relationship between blood pressure and ICP. If the physician has not left orders to treat blood pressure changes, notification must occur if the blood pressure range is below 100 or above 150 mm Hg systolic. Often, physician orders specify titration of medication to maintain the CPP at greater than 70 mm Hg.

PREVENTION OF COMPLICATIONS. Antibiotics may be prescribed, especially with an open head injury, the placement of an ICP monitor, or an infection in another body system. Infections increase metabolism and thus also raise ICP.

Anti-seizure medication (e.g., phenytoin, phenobarbital, diazepam) may be given prophylactically to reduce the risk of seizures. Seizures significantly increase metabolic requirements and cerebral blood flow and volume and thus increase ICP. Chapter 69 describes the care of the client with seizures.

Intravenous (IV) fluids are given by IV pump to help monitor the amount of fluids given. The client is maintained in an euvolemic state. Hypertonic IV solutions are avoided because of the risk of promoting cerebral edema.

Temperature reduction decreases metabolism and cerebral blood flow and thus ICP. Antipyretics may be used, but a hypothermic blanket is more commonly the intervention of choice. Muscle relaxants are given to prevent shivering.

MONITOR INTRACRANIAL PRESSURE

Continuous ICP monitoring is used for clients experiencing conditions associated with potentially elevated ICP (e.g., head trauma, preoperative and postoperative aneurysms, tumors, posterior fossa lesions). Use of ICP monitors has several benefits (Box 73–1). However, ICP monitoring devices never replace serial clinical observations of the client's condition.

Several methods of ICP monitoring are available. The most common types measure CSF pressure in the ventricles, brain parenchyma, or subarachnoid space. Intraventricular catheters, parenchymal catheters, and subarachnoid bolts give more accurate results than the epidural catheters, but their use carries a higher incidence of infection. The intraventricular catheter is the most accurate type of intracranial monitor, and it can be used to drain CSF, but it has the highest risk of infection. The screw (bolt) is placed into the subarachnoid space, which allows pressure readings but not removal of fluid. The third

---

BOX 73–1 **Benefits of Intracranial Pressure Monitoring**

- Pressure increases can often be recognized and appropriate treatment started before the onset of clinical manifestations.
- Some systems allow ventricular fluid drainage (e.g., three-way stopcock device) when the intracranial pressure (ICP) has risen above a specific level indicated by the physician.
- Delays in bringing the client to definitive treatment (e.g., surgery) can sometimes be avoided.
- The effectiveness of other types of treatment (such as mechanical hyperventilation, neuromuscular blockade, barbiturate-induced coma, or induced hypothermia) can be monitored.
- Sustained pressure waves, or plateau waves (occurring at pressures between 50 and 100 mm Hg), which can cause brain damage, can be detected early and treatment can be adjusted accordingly.
- Intracranial compliance can be measured.
- The level of ICP elevation can provide prognostic information.
- Cerebral perfusion pressure can be calculated and treatment can be adjusted.
- The effect of nursing interventions on ICP can be monitored. The timing of procedures that raise ICP (e.g., turning) can be altered to coincide with periods of "lower" pressure.

common type is an intraparenchymal monitor. It measures pressure in brain tissue. All of the monitoring devices carry a risk of infection owing to their invasive nature. Most surgeons prescribe antibiotics, limit the length of time for which the ICP monitor remains in place, and monitor CSF samples on a regular basis. The accompanying Bridge to Critical Care describes the nurse's role in caring for clients with these devices.

Monitoring ICP also allows the measurement of intracranial compliance. Introducing a known volume of fluid into the ventricle and measuring its effect on ICP tests compliance. Detecting a change in the critical relationship between volume and pressure allows early treatment before the onset of clinical manifestations or sustained elevated ICP. Measurements of cerebral perfusion pressure (CPP) can be made with ICP monitors. Ideally, CPP should be maintained at greater than 70 mm Hg.

PREVENT COMPLICATIONS
Intracranial Hypertension

Intracranial hypertension is defined as an ICP of 20 to 25 mm Hg and can lead to a fatal herniation of the brain. When the herniation occurs at the level of the medulla, death is imminent. Mannitol administration, hyperventilation, sedation, and CSF drainage constitute the usual steps in management of intracranial hypertension.

BARBITURATES. Some clients require large doses of barbiturates to treat uncontrolled ICP. Barbiturate therapy requires sophisticated monitoring and special training, but its use has been associated with increased survival outcomes. The client is intubated and placed on ventilatory support, and a pulmonary artery catheter is inserted.

Pentobarbital, 5 to 10 mg/kg by slow IV injection over 60 minutes, is given in a loading dose, followed by a maintenance dose of 1 mg/kg per hour until the ICP is under control or until the EEG shows a burst suppression pattern 6 to 10 seconds' duration. Pentobarbital may cause a decrease in the blood pressure, so the MAP should not be allowed to fall below 80 mm Hg.

Monitor serum drug levels daily; the dose should be reduced if serum levels exceed 5 mg/dl or if the burst suppression pattern on the EEG lasts longer than 10 seconds. Monitor temperature because barbiturates reduce metabolism, thereby cooling the body. If the temperature falls below 36° C, active warming is indicated.

Continue pupillary assessment. Even when a client is in a coma, the pupils dilate if the brain stem becomes compressed. Notify the physician of this change. Barbiturate therapy eliminates the client's normal protective functions. The client is completely dependent on nursing care for all basic needs (see Chapter 68). Wean clients slowly from barbiturate therapy to prevent rebound intracranial hypertension.

NEUROMUSCULAR BLOCKING AGENTS. Nondepolarizing neuromuscular blocking agents are sometimes used to induce skeletal muscle relaxation and to promote synchronous breathing during mechanical ventilation. Decreasing muscle activity may be necessary to control ICP. Nurses use a peripheral nerve stimulator to monitor for adequacy of drug dosage as well as for the risk of overdose (see Chapter 63). Pentobarbital and neuromuscular blocking agents usually are not given concomitantly. If the client is receiving a neuromuscular blocking agent,

sedation and analgesia must be given, as the neuromuscular blocking agents do not provide it.

Other Complications

Other complications of increased ICP include Cushing's stress ulcer (which results from decreased mucosal blood flow and hypersecretion of acid from overstimulation of the vagal nuclei), neurogenic pulmonary edema, diabetes insipidus, and syndrome of inappropriate secretion of antidiuretic hormone (SIADH). These complications are described in Table 73–1.

■ Nursing Management Assessment
ASSESSMENT

GLASGOW COMA SCALE. The Glasgow Coma Scale (GCS) is the most commonly used neurologic assessment tool in clinical care (Box 73–2). This scale provides objective measurement of three essential components of the neurologic examination: spontaneity of eye opening, best verbal response, and best motor response. The total of the three scores can range from 3 to 15. The client who is unresponsive to painful stimuli, does not open the eyes, and has complete muscular flaccidity has a score of 3. The client who is oriented, opens the eyes spontaneously, and follows commands scores 15. A score of 8 or less indicates coma. Because the scoring of the GCS is based on the client's ability to respond and to communicate, the following criteria may render the GCS invalid:

- The client is intubated and cannot speak.
- Eyes are swollen closed.
- The client is unable to communicate in English.
- The client has a hearing loss.
- The client is blind.
- The client is aphasic.
- The client is paralyzed or hemiplegic.

The first GCS score recorded for the client becomes the baseline score. Subsequent scores allow assessment of trends or changes in neurologic status. The GCS also can be used to recognize disorders as well as to predict outcomes. The use of consistent criteria for client assessment is more important than the specific tool used. Specific behaviors dictating a given score should be indicated. If variations occur in scoring criteria, the value of the scale is lost, and serious changes in the client's condition can be overlooked or treated unnecessarily (Fig. 73–5). More detailed neurologic assessments are conducted to identify specific trends in responses.

LEVEL OF CONSCIOUSNESS. The first change in a client who presents with altered cerebral tissue perfusion is a change in the level of consciousness (LOC). When decreased LOC is noted, serial and detailed assessments are required until the client has achieved maximum recovery. To eliminate the subjectivity associated with use of terms such as "lethargy," "obtundation," "semi-coma," or "coma," the GCS both objectifies the client's LOC and assists in identifying very subtle changes.

PUPIL RESPONSE. A pupil check includes assessing pupil appearance and physiologic response. The affected pupil is usually on the same (ipsilateral) side as the brain lesion, whereas the motor and sensory deficits are usually on the opposite (contralateral) side. Be careful not to mistake a prosthetic eye for a fixed pupil.

BRIDGE TO CRITICAL CARE

Intracranial Pressure Monitoring

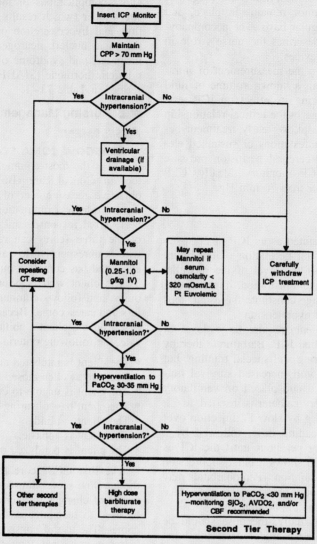

Intracranial Pressure Waveforms

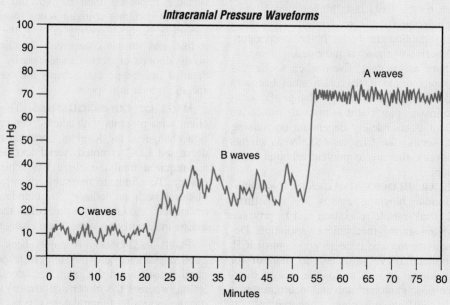

BRIDGE TO CRITICAL CARE *Continued*

The shape of the waves is influenced by cardiac pulsations and respirations as well as by intracranial pressure (ICP).

- *C waves* occur four to eight times per minute and reflect fluctuations in arterial pressure. C waves are not considered significant.
- *B waves* occur at intervals of 30 seconds to 2 minutes and represent increases in ICP to 50 mm Hg. They may be precursors to A waves.

- *A waves* are most pronounced when the amount of cranial contents is increased. Also called *plateau waves,* A waves represent recurrent ICP elevations to 100 mm Hg. An A wave may be caused by coughing or straining but, if recurrent or sustained, may indicate a reduced ability of the brain to compensate. The client may also show other manifestations of increasing ICP.

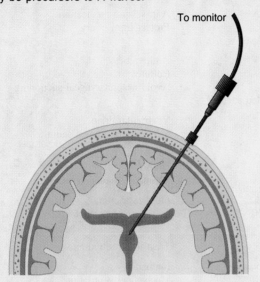

Ventricular catheter (ventriculostomy)

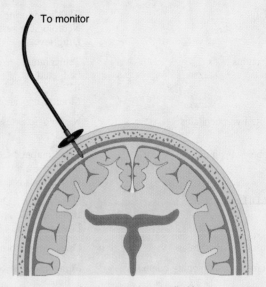

Subarachnoid screw (bolt)

General Interventions for Monitoring Intracranial Pressure

- Ensure that the tubing is long enough to allow the client to be moved in bed but that it is no longer than 14 feet. Use of tubing longer than 14 feet may cause inaccurate readings.
- Be careful to prevent kinks in the tubing.
- Place the catheter at the preset level of the transducer to take a reading.
- Use sterile technique when setting up the device.
- Monitor for manifestations of infection.
- Notify the physician if the readings show damping (lessening of amplitude) of the waves. The catheter may need to be flushed by the physician.
- If inaccurate readings occur, check for:

    - Leaks in the system
    - Differences in the height of the transducer and the device
    - Kinks in the tubing
    - Client activity or behavior involving performance of the Valsalva maneuver
    - Obstruction in the system

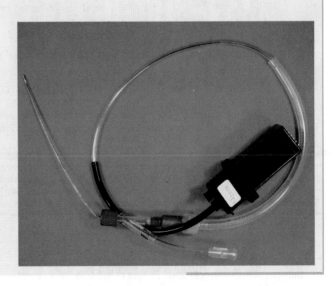

Pupil Equality. Document pupil equality, noting the relative size of each pupil.

Pupil Size. Estimate the size of each pupil in millimeters (mm) before and after light stimulation. A penlight provides more accurate data than obtainable with a flashlight owing to the smaller size of the light and the ability to focus the beam directly at the pupil.

Pupil Position. Note whether the pupil is positioned in the midline or deviated from midline.

Pupil Reaction to Light. Bring the penlight from the lateral aspect of the client's head toward the eye. Observe for constriction in that eye as well as in the opposite eye. Then test the opposite eye in the same way. The detection of subtle change may require four ap-

TABLE 73–1	COMPLICATIONS OF HEAD INJURY	
Condition	**Assessment**	**Treatment**
Cerebral edema	ICP monitor Neurologic assessment	CSF drainage Diuresis Sedation
Stress ulcers	NPO status Monitor nasogastric drainage output for blood	Histamine blockers
Seizures	EEG monitoring Neurologic assessment Drug levels	Anti-seizure medication Protect from injury
Infections	Temperature CSF studies ICP Monitor appearance of affected site(s)	Antipyretics Cultures Avoid nasopharyngeal suctioning
Acute hydrocephalus	Neurologic assessment	Ventricular drain Ventriculoperitoneal shunt
Diabetes insipidus	Urine output >200 ml/hr Specific gravity <1.005 High serum Na$^+$ level	Free water replacement DDAVP Maintain euvolemia
SIADH	Urine output <30 ml/hr Urine specific gravity >1.020 Low serum Na$^+$ level	Fluid restriction Sodium replacement
Cardiac dysrhythmias	Cardiac monitoring	Treat the dysrhythmia
Neurogenic pulmonary edema	Monitor ABGs, SpO$_2$, pulmonary secretions	Intubation Mechanical ventilation Treatment similar to that for ARDS (see Chapter 63)
Subarachnoid hemorrhage/aneurysms	Monitor for exopthalmos, cranial nerve paralysis, distended orbital and periorbital veins Monitor CSF for blood	Notify physician of changes in neurologic examination or of other signs of subarachnoid hemorrhage
Altered behavior	Monitor orientation and memory	Reorient client Educate family regarding behavior
Post-trauma response	Monitor for headache, poor concentration, dizziness, irritability, sensitivity to noise, restlessness, depression, easy fatigability, anxiety, impaired memory	Educate client and family about possible sequelae of head injury Request physician visit if symptoms persist Encourage cognitive rehabilitation if symptoms persist

ABG, arterial blood gas; ARDS, adult respiratory distress syndrome; CSF, cerebrospinal fluid; DDAVP, 1-deamino(8-D-arginine) vasopressin; EEG, electroencephalogram; ICP, intracranial pressure; Na$^+$, sodium ion; NPO, nothing by mouth; SIADH, syndrome of inappropriate secretion of antidiuretic hormone; SpO$_2$, oxygen saturation (as measured by pulse oximetry).

proaches with the penlight. Brisk and equal constriction of the pupils to direct and indirect light is a normal response. Sluggish or unequal direct or indirect (consensual) response is abnormal. Anisocoria, or unequal pupils, occurs normally in about 17% of the population, with one pupil being about 1 mm larger. It is important to ascertain information about pupil inequality from the client or family members so that an unnecessary procedure is not performed.

Pupil Shape. Normally, pupils are round. Describe abnormal shapes with a drawing. Pupils may be oddly shaped owing to previous eye surgery. A pupil that looks oval may be early evidence of increasing ICP.

Pupil Accommodation. Normally, the size of the pupil and the lens (which is not visible to the naked eye) accommodate (adjust) to varying focal lengths. Having the client focus on a distant object and then quickly focus on a close object tests accommodation. Pupils should become smaller as the object is brought nearer the eye and should dilate when the object is moved away from the eye. Accommodation is often not tested in the acute care setting owing to the inability of the client to cooperate.

The acronym PERRLA is often used in practice and indicates that the *p*upils are *e*qual, *r*ound, and *r*eactive to *l*ight and *a*ccommodation. Notify the physician immediately if any change occurs in the pupillary response.

BOX 73-2   Assessment of Clients Using the Glasgow Coma Scale

The Glasgow Coma Scale (GCS) is a numeric expression of cognition, behavior, and neurologic function. It is the most commonly used scale and was designed to measure level of consciousness and severity of injury through eye opening, verbal responsiveness, and motor response. The total of the three scores ranges from 3 to 15, with 3 the most severe and 15 normal. Assessments of abstract thought and problem-solving should be combined with the GCS to give a more complete picture of neurologic status.

Documentation should contain specific descriptive terms. For example, instead of just indicating that the client is "stuporous," record the evidence of stupor that you observe: "no response to verbal commands, responded only to tracheal suctioning with abnormal flexor posturing." Words such as "lethargic," "stuporous," or "comatose" are open to individual interpretation, and a clear description of behavior is less likely to be misunderstood.

Scale Components

Eye Opening

Observe eye opening without speaking to the client. Does the client open the eyes and look around? If the eyes are closed, call the client's name. If no response is noted, raise your voice. If there is still no response, use a mildly painful stimulus, given in the central part of the body, such as squeezing the trapezius muscle or rubbing the sternum.

Avoid supraorbital pressure, as it can cause damage to the eyes. Pinching of the body can cause severe bruising and is unnecessary in a neurologic examination.

Motor Response

Asking the client to follow specific commands such as "Raise your right arm" or "Wiggle your toes" assesses motor responses. Do not ask the client to squeeze your hand because grasp is a reflexive response that can occur with head injury. If agency protocol lists grasp as a neurologic assessment component, ask the client to "let go" after grasping, to measure cognitive ability to control movement.

In a client who is unable to follow commands, observe the response to a painful stimulus. Responses may include (1) localizing (trying to remove the stimulus), (2) withdrawing, and (3) posturing. In addition, a response may not be elicited and the client may remain motionless.

Compare the right and left sides and the upper and lower extremities. Record the best response while also recording any abnormality that indicates decreased movement in a particular extremity.

Motor Activity

Motor activity assessment is the measure of strength of voluntary movement of the arms and legs. If a client cannot cooperate with testing, paralysis may be difficult to detect. Observe the client carefully. If a client is restless, paralysis may

become obvious because the paralyzed part does not move as other body parts move. Additional information may be obtained by:

1. Comparing the tone of one side of the body with that of the other.
2. Lifting the arms or legs on both sides, releasing them, and watching them drop to the bed.
3. Observing the position of the limbs at rest.

If a client can cooperate, assessing "drift" may demonstrate subtle tone and strength alterations. For this assessment, have the client hold both arms up in front of the body with palms upward and eyes closed. Muscles are weak if one arm "drifts" (gradually moves) downward or if the hand pronates (turns over). This maneuver is often referred to as the *pronator drift test.*

Posturing

Review posturing in Chapter 68. As the client's intracranial pressure increases at the cortical level, abnormal flexor posturing occurs. As pressure reaches the pons level, abnormal extensor posturing occurs. When the pressure reaches further to the medullary level, flaccidity is noted, or response is totally lacking—the gravest of all signs.

Verbal Response

Verbal responses assess the client's orientation to self, environment, and time. Ask appropriate questions such as the following: "What is your name? Where are you? What is the month, year, season, nearest holiday?" Avoid asking questions about the date or day of the week.

Being hospitalized can alter accuracy of that response even in a person with normal cognitive function. Structure the conversation to elicit information that can be verified by family members, such as home address or employer's name. In many cases, a slight degree of confusion is not noticeable until some time is spent with the client. An apparently oriented client may ask the same question a few minutes after it was originally asked and answered, or the client may have "learned" the answers to common questions such as "What is your name?" and "What hospital are you in?" Therefore, it is helpful to reassess the client regularly to check memory or to challenge cognitive integrity with various questions. In addition, observing the course of a normal conversation may give evidence of confusion or disorientation.

Scoring

After obtaining the data for all three parts of the GCS, total the points for each part and compare the score obtained with the client's baseline score. If a decrease in the score of even 1 point occurs, complete a detailed neurologic assessment, including pupillary responses, and notify the physician.

EYE MOVEMENT. Document eye movement changes. Observe the position of the eyes when assessing the pupils. The eyes should move together. If dysconjugate (not together) movement is noted, the physician should be notified.

VITAL SIGNS. Initially, vital signs should be assessed every 15 minutes until they are stable. Body temperature should be monitored every 2 hours. If hypothermia or

hyperthermia occurs, continuous temperature monitoring should be used. Trends in vital signs and respiratory patterns should be analyzed. As ICP increases and herniation occurs at the level of the medulla, Cushing's response occurs (see Fig. 73-3).

Vital sign changes are *late* changes. See the following discussion of altered cerebral tissue perfusion for care of a client with increasing ICP. Once the vital signs begin to

MISSION HOSPITAL
REGIONAL MEDICAL CENTER

ADULT NEURO FLOW SHEET

TIME

GLASGOW COMA SCALE		
	Eyes Open	
	Best Motor	
	Best Verbal	
	TOTAL	

VOLUNTARY MOTOR	Right	upper extremity
		lower extremity
	Left	upper extremity
		lower extremity

CRANIAL NERVES	PUPILS	Right	Size
			Reaction
		Left	Size
			Reaction
	EOMS	Conjugate	
		Dysconjugate	
		Tracking Right	
		Left	
	Blink Reflex		
	Gag Reflex		
	Facial Symmetry		

TIME

KEY
MOTOR
5+ Normal Power
4+ Weakness
3+ Anti-gravity
2+ Not anti-gravity
1+ Trace
0 No movement

Pupil   B = Brisk
Size   S = Sluggish
A = Absent

2mm 3mm 4mm 5mm
6mm 7mm 8mm

✓ = Present
O = Absent
S = Symmetrical
A = Asymmetrical

Date

Speech Patterns: _____

Comments: _____

GLASGOW COMA SCALE	Eyes Open	4	Spontaneously
		3	To verbal command
		2	To Pain
		1	No Response
	Best Motor Response	6	Obeys Commands
		5	Localize Pain
		4	Flexion to pain withdraw
		3	Flexion Decorticate
		2	Extension to pain (decerebrate)
		1	No Response to pain
	Best Verbal Response	5	Oriented
		4	Confused
		3	Inappropriate words
		2	Incomprehensible sounds
		1	No Response

Unit _____

R.N. Signature _____ Shift: _____

R.N. Signature _____ Shift: _____

R.N. Signature _____ Shift: _____

ADDRESSOGRAPH

Adult Neuro Flow Sheet

#408 10 89

A

FIGURE 73–5 *A*, A neurologic observation chart. (Courtesy of Mission Hospital Regional Medical Center, Mission Viejo, CA.)

NEUROLOGIC FLOW SHEET

1. Glasgow Coma Scale (GCS). Three areas are assessed: Best eye opening, Best motor response, and Best verbal response. Assign the appropriate numerical score for each category (1st box—best eye, 2nd box—best motor, and 3rd box—best verbal). Place the total score in the fourth box (total score 3-15).

2. Voluntary Motor is evaluated by assessing each extremity on both the right and left side. Note **symmetry vs. asymmetry.** In the cooperative patient, voluntary motor strength is assessed by asking the patient to close their eyes and hold their arms straight ahead with palms up for about 30 seconds. The leg strength is evaluated by asking the patient to push downward against the examiner's hands.

Scoring: Normal power (5+) is the score given if the patient's arms stay in the same position and/or if the legs have equal strong power.

Weakness (4+) is the score given if one of the pt.'s arm drifts downward (hands may pronate) or if the leg strength is diminished. Some resistance to force is noted.

Anti-gravity (3+) is the score given if the patient is able to move an extremity above the plane of gravity (ie flexing & extending a hand up/down against gravity).

Not anti-gravity (2+) is the score given to a patient who can move the extremity back and forth on the bed but not against the forces of gravity.

Trace movement (1+) is the score given to a patient who can move an extremity slightly.

No movement (0) is the score given if a patient cannot move the extremity.

3. **Cranial Nerve Exam:**

Pupillary response: Each pupil is assessed individually. Note the size of the pupil prior to shining the light into the eye. Place your hand at the bridge of the nose to block light to the opposite eye. Using the penlight, shine the light from outside the right eye to midpoint across the eye to assess the direct light reflex. Note the pupillary constriction (Brisk, sluggish, or non-reactive) in the right eye. Also, observe for constriction in the left pupil (consensual light reflex). Repeat the above steps for the left eye observing the direct light reflex in the left eye and the consensual reflex in the right eye. Document the pupil size (prior to light in the eye) and the reaction on the flow sheet.

Extra-ocular movements (EOMS's) are tested on patients who are awake enough to follow instructions. Ask the patient to follow your fingers with his eyes without moving the head. Move your fingers in a figure H and observe both eyes as they move across/up/down. **Conjugate eye movements** occur when both eyes move in parallel motion. **Dysconjugate eye movements** occur when the eyes do not move in a lateral direction together (one eye may move laterally while the other is fixed or moves in another direction). **Tracking** occurs when the patient is consciously following someone's or something's movement around the room. Place a check for present or a 0 for absent.

The Blink reflex is elicited by lightly stroking the patient's eyelashes. When the eyelids are closed, the eyelids will flutter slightly if the reflex is present. In the conscious alert patient, observe for blinking. Place a check for present or a 0 for absent.

The Gag reflex is evaluated by asking the alert, cooperative patient to cough or swallow. If the patient is unable to do so or is unconscious, take a long cotton tipped swab and stroke the back of the patient's throat. Note if the reflex is present (place a check) or absent (place a 0).

Muscles of the face: Note the muscle symmetry of the facial muscles. Note the ability of the eyelids to open spontaneously and equally. Ask the patient to close their eyes as tightly as possible. Note asymmetry. Ask the patient to smile—note the corners of the mouth to identify symmetrical patterns. Ask the patient to frown/wrinkle his forehead—note the symmetry of the muscles. Place a S for symmetrical and an A for asymmetrical.

Speech patterns: Note if speech is clear, slurred, rambling, or aphasic.

Comments: Utilize this section to elaborate on any abnormal findings or document other pertinent data.

Sign your name and document shift worked. Complete the date/unit and addressograph. The neurological flow sheet is for a 24 hour period. Each day at 7 am, obtain a new flow sheet. Document your findings in the appropriate time box.

B

FIGURE 73–5 *Continued B*, Neurologic flow sheet.

deteriorate, many other changes have already occurred, such as a decrease in LOC. Ongoing monitoring for such changes is imperative; do not wait for vital signs to change, as the delay may prove fatal for the client. Any changes in neurologic status may be very significant and must be reported to the physician, no matter how minor they may seem.

DIAGNOSIS, OUTCOMES, INTERVENTIONS

Altered Cerebral Tissue Perfusion. If your patient is in a coma because of increased ICP, use this diagnosis to reflect the risk to cerebral tissue perfusion. Write the diagnosis as *Altered Cerebral Tissue Perfusion related to increased ICP*. The term *patient* is used to refer to a person in a coma. The *client* in this case is the patient's family, who serves as his or her advocate.

Outcomes. The patient will maintain normal cerebral perfusion, as evidenced by (1) stable or improving levels of consciousness; (2) stable or improving GCS score; (3) ICP of 15 mm Hg or less; (4) no restlessness, irritability, or headache; and (5) no pupillary changes, no seizures, no widening pulse pressure, no respiratory irregularity, and no hypertension or bradycardia.

Interventions. Administer the medications ordered to reduce cerebral edema (e.g., osmotic diuretics) and to decrease the risk of seizure (e.g., anticonvulsants), and monitor the patient's response to these medications. If the patient's baseline manifestations of increased ICP are not improving, if the patient's status deteriorates, or if seizures develop, notify the physician. Also, consult the physician for medication to promote bowel evacuation without straining, as straining increases ICP. Disimpaction is not advised because of the vasovagal response that occurs.

Position the Patient. Place the patient supine with the head elevated 30 degrees unless contraindicated (e.g., with some spinal injuries, some aneurysms). Keep the patient's head in a neutral position to facilitate venous drainage from the brain. Avoid extreme rotation and flexion of the neck because these positions compress the jugular veins and increase ICP. Also avoid extreme hip flexion because this position increases intra-abdominal and intrathoracic pressure, which increases ICP.[75] As coma lightens, the patient may become disoriented and combative, making it difficult to maintain proper positioning. If restraints must be used, remember that they often increase agitation, which increases ICP.

Maintain a Patent Airway. Patients need to maintain a patent airway even in the presence of increased ICP. Suctioning assists in preventing buildup of secretions and CO_2 and a resultant elevation of ICP. Adequately oxygenate intubated patients before initiating suctioning, between suctioning efforts, and after suctioning. Try to limit suctioning to three passes, and limit each pass to 10 seconds. Recall that nasal drainage may indicate a dural tear; therefore, suctioning of the nares is contraindicated because of the risk of meningitis.

Balance Fluid Levels. In the past, only small amounts of fluids were administered to clients with head injury, in an effort to decrease cerebral edema. Current data indicate that fluid restriction may actually reduce blood volume and decrease cerebral circulation. The lack of volume causes the blood to be thick and sluggish and may

also decrease the mobilization of nutrition and toxins into and out of the circulation. Evidently, patients should be maintained in a euvolemic state rather than a fluid-restricted state. Fluid restriction may be appropriate for certain conditions (such as SIADH) but otherwise is contraindicated. Strict intake and output measurement is still necessary to assess fluid balance.

Control Body Temperature. Hyperthermia increases ICP because of the increased metabolic demand. Therefore, notify the physician immediately if hyperthermia occurs. If a patient's ICP is being managed with a hypothermia blanket, notify the physician if the patient's response is not within the prescribed parameters. Observe for shivering because this phenomenon also increases metabolism and ICP. Assess for skin breakdown if cooling blankets are used for extended periods, and especially in patients who are thin.

Monitor Intracranial Pressure. The ICP reading should be less than 15 mm Hg, the MAP reading 80 mm Hg or above, and the CPP reading above 70 mm Hg.

Plateau waves (A waves) are noted when ICP goes above 50 mm Hg and can be sustained for longer than 5 minutes. Whenever these sustained pressures are present, assess for contributing factors and intervene appropriately. For example, neck flexion, excessive hip flexion, airway secretions, excess water in the ventilator tubing, taping the endotracheal tube tightly over the jugular veins, and discussing the patient's condition at the bedside all have been known to increase ICP. Spacing and planning of nonessential nursing interventions (e.g., turning the patient) for when the patient's ICP is not elevated help to prevent plateau waves. Plateau waves may not be obvious on the ICP monitor screen; a printout generated at a slow rate may be required for accurate observation of these waves. Whenever ICP is over 20 mm Hg, interventions to decrease ICP should begin.

Assessing the ICP monitor site for infection and leakage, using sterile technique for dressing and drainage bag changes, and maintaining a closed system are helpful in preventing infection or in promoting early intervention if infection occurs. If CSF drainage is required, most systems have a stopcock for attaching the tubing and drainage bag that maintains the closed system, decreasing the likelihood of infection. The system is opened only to change the drainage bag. The drainage bag is changed with strict sterile technique.

EVALUATION

Evaluate the client's response to treatment as often as every 15 minutes, progressing to hourly, then every 2 to 4 hours, and every 8 hours as the client improves. Once the physician has determined that the client's clinical condition has been optimized, the frequency and extent of evaluation can diminish even further. In the immediate and acute stages, anticipate ongoing modification in the care plan to help the client reach maximum recovery.

▇ Surgical Management

Various surgical techniques are used to treat increased ICP. Optimally, the cause of increased ICP is located and removed. Other techniques include surgical placement of a ventriculoperitoneal shunt to allow drainage if CSF circulation is blocked (Fig. 73–6) and decompressive sur-

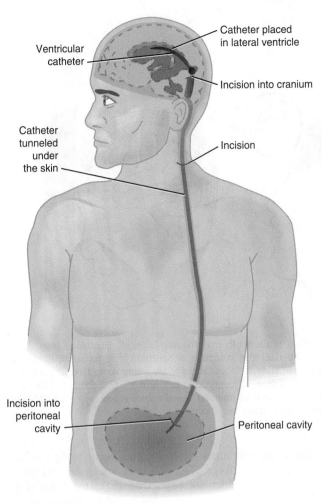

FIGURE 73–6 Ventriculoperitoneal shunt placed for chronic hydrocephalus.

gery. The latter is done by removing some brain tissue (e.g., part of the temporal lobe) to give the remaining structures room to expand. If compliance is low during surgery, the bone flap removed to gain access to the brain is not replaced, or the dura may not be closed. Subsequent surgery is then required to repair the defect. Postoperative care is the same as that required after craniotomy (see Chapter 69).

TRAUMATIC BRAIN INJURY

Traumatic brain injury is an insult to the brain capable of producing physical, intellectual, emotional, social, and vocational changes. In the United States, a head injury is experienced approximately every 15 seconds. Head injuries occur in about 7 million Americans every year. Among these head-injured people, more than 500,000 are hospitalized, 100,000 experience chronic disability, and approximately 2000 are left in a persistent vegetative state.[40]

Head injuries are fatal in more than 30% of cases before the injured person arrives at the hospital owing to the seriousness of the injury. An additional 20% of people die later because of secondary brain injury.[30] Secondary brain events include ischemia from hypoxia and hypotension, secondary hemorrhage, and cerebral edema.

Clients with traumatic head injuries often have other major injuries, including injury to the facial structures, lungs, heart, cervical spine, abdomen, and bones. Facial fractures and lung injuries may contribute to respiratory insufficiency. Airway obstruction and decreased ability to breathe (e.g., from pulmonary contusion, flail chest, pneumothorax) contribute to respiratory insufficiency and poor oxygenation of the brain and other tissues. Ischemia of brain tissue may result.

Hemorrhagic shock in clients with multiple trauma is rarely caused by head injury alone. Frequently, shock is due to ruptured abdominal organs or musculoskeletal injuries (e.g., fractured femur and pelvis). Circulation may be further compromised by cardiac contusion and associated dysrhythmias.

Etiology and Risk Factors

Of clients admitted to the emergency room, 50% have evidence of ingestion of alcohol or other substances of abuse. Most are males younger than 30 years of age. Peak occurrence is during evenings, nights, and weekends. Motor vehicle accidents are the leading cause of head injuries. Other causes are assaults, falls, and sports-related injuries.

A major risk factor for head injury is alcohol consumption. Alcohol slows reflexes and alters cognitive processes and perception. These physiologic changes increase the chances of being involved in an accident or altercation. A second risk factor is driving without seat belts.

MECHANISMS OF INJURY

Head injuries are caused by a sudden force to the head (Fig. 73–7). The results are complex. Three mechanisms contribute to head trauma:

An *acceleration* injury occurs when the immobile head is struck by a moving object (Fig. 73–7A).

Deformation refers to injuries in which the force results in deformation and disruption of the integrity of the impacted body part, as in a skull fracture (Fig. 73–7B).

If the head is moving and hits an immobile object, a *deceleration* injury occurs (Fig. 73–7C). An example is an automobile accident in which the head hits the steering wheel.

In an *acceleration-deceleration* injury, a moving object hits the immobile head and the head then hits an immobile object. Acceleration-deceleration injuries are also associated with *rotation injury,* in which the brain is twisted within the skull.

Blunt Trauma

Blunt trauma occurs when the head strikes an immobile object. Acceleration and deceleration injuries often result from blunt trauma. These are complex injuries involving several cranial structures, including brain parenchyma and vessels. Because the brain is able to move within the skull, movement of the brain can result in injuries at different locations. The brain is partially tethered (at its base) and is also suspended in CSF. Therefore, a blow to the skull can cause the hemispheres to twist on the fixed brain stem.

As the brain moves, it scrapes over the skull's irregular inner prominences, which bruise and lacerate brain

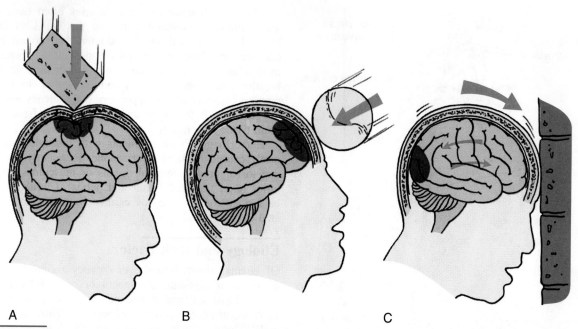

FIGURE 73–7 Some mechanisms of head injury. *A,* Direct injury (a blow to the skull) may fracture the skull. Contusion and laceration of the brain may result from fractures. Depressed portions of the skull may compress or penetrate brain tissue. *B,* Even if a blow to the skull does not result in fracture, it may cause the brain to move enough to tear some of the veins going from the cortical surface to the dura. Subdural hematoma may then develop. Note the areas of cerebral contusion (dark brown). *C,* Rebound of the cranial contents may result in an area of injury opposite the point of impact. Such an injury is called a *contrecoup* injury. In addition to the direct damage sustained in the three injuries depicted, additional brain damage may occur.

tissue. Disruption of the brain's small surface blood vessels may occur. Changes in capillary integrity lead to fluid shifts and petechial hemorrhages. Cranial nerves, nerve tracts, larger blood vessels, and other structures may be stretched, twisted, or rotated, and their functions disrupted.

Penetrating Trauma

Penetrating injuries include those made by foreign bodies (e.g., knives or bullets) or those made by bone fragments from a skull fracture. The damage caused by a penetrating injury often relates to the velocity with which a penetrating object pierces the skull and brain. Bone fragments from a skull fracture may cause local brain injury by lacerating brain tissue and damaging other structures (e.g., nerves, blood vessels). If a major blood vessel is severed or ruptured, a large clot (hematoma) may form, with resultant damage to adjacent or remote structures (e.g., brain compression as in a herniation syndrome). Thus, a hematoma can itself cause extensive brain tissue damage.

High-velocity objects (e.g., bullets) produce shock waves in the skull and brain. The shock waves may significantly damage brain structures beyond those in the object's path. Frequently, penetrating wounds create an open communication between the external environment and the cranial cavity. Thus, infection is a possible complication.

Coup-Contrecoup Injuries

A *coup* (French for "blow") injury occurs immediately at the point of impact. Because of movement within the skull, the same blow may cause injury on the opposite side of the brain, that is, a contrecoup injury (see Fig. 73–7C). *Contrecoup* is French for "counterblow." In ad-

dition, multiple areas of injury often occur along the line of the blow's force. Tissue around major injured areas often swells, which increases damage to the brain (Fig. 73–8).

PRIMARY INJURIES

Primary injury results directly from the impact itself. It is contrasted with secondary injury, which is caused by hypoxia, hypercapnia, hypotension, and intracranial hypertension. The secondary problems occur hours to days after the initial impact.

Scalp Injuries

Scalp injuries can cause lacerations, hematomas, and contusions or abrasions to the skin. These injuries may be unsightly and bleed profusely. Clients with minor scalp injuries not accompanied by damage to other areas do not require hospitalization. The care of these injuries is discussed in Chapter 82.

Skull Fractures

Skull fractures are often caused by a force sufficient to fracture the skull and cause brain injury. The fractures themselves do not signal that brain injury is also present. However, skull fractures often cause serious brain damage. Depressed skull fractures injure the brain by bruising it (resulting in a contusion) or by driving bone fragments into it (causing lacerations). The site of a fracture and the extent of brain injury may not correlate.

The three types of skull fractures are as follows:

- *Linear skull fractures* appear as thin lines radiographically and do not require treatment; they are important only if there is significant underlying brain damage.
- *Depressed skull fractures* may be palpated and are seen radiographically.

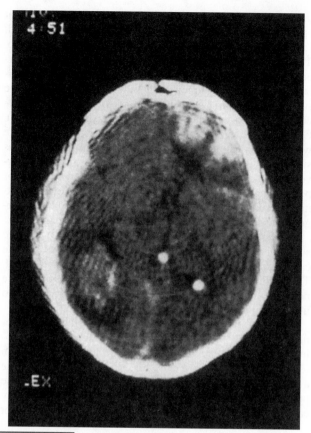

FIGURE 73-8 A magnetic resonance imaging scan showing coup-contrecoup injury after head injury.

- *Basilar skull fractures* occur in bones over the base of the frontal and temporal lobes. These are not observable on plain radiographs but may be manifested as ecchymosis around the eyes or behind the ears.

Brain Injuries

A single classification of brain injuries does not exist. However, the terms *open, closed, contusion,* and *concussion* are often applied to brain injuries. Open head injuries are those that penetrate the skull. Closed injuries are from blunt trauma.

CONCUSSIONS. A concussion is head trauma that may result in loss of consciousness for 5 minutes or less and retrograde amnesia. There is no break in the skull or dura, and no visible damage on a CT or MRI scan.

CONTUSIONS. Contusions are associated with more extensive damage than that from concussions. With contusions, the brain itself is damaged, often with multiple areas of petechial and punctate hemorrhage and bruised areas in brain tissue. Diffuse axonal injury resulting in anatomic disruption of the white matter may result from serious contusions. Microscopic nerve fiber lesions also occur. Abnormalities may be located primarily in one area of the brain, but other areas may also be injured. This is particularly true of brain stem contusions, which are a very serious type of lesion.

DIFFUSE AXONAL INJURY. Diffuse axonal injury is the most severe form of head injury because there is no focal lesion to remove. The injury involves the tissue of the entire brain and occurs at the microscopic level. Diffuse axonal injury is classified as mild, moderate, or severe. With mild diffuse axonal injury, loss of consciousness lasting 6 to 24 hours is characteristic, and there may be short-term disability associated with it. With moderate diffuse axonal injury, coma lasting less than 24 hours is the predominant clinical feature, with incomplete recovery on awakening. Severe diffuse axonal injury involves primary injury to the brain stem. The patient may present with abnormal posturing and in coma, but there is no evidence of cerebral edema or increased ICP. Diffuse axonal injury begins with immediate loss of consciousness, prolonged coma, abnormal flexion or extension posturing, hypertension, and fever.

Focal Injuries

EPIDURAL HEMATOMA. An epidural hematoma, also called an *extradural hematoma,* forms between the skull and the dura mater (see Fig. 73-9). It occurs in about 10% of severe head injuries and is usually associated with a skull fracture. An epidural hematoma occurs from injury to the extracerebral blood vessels, most often the middle meningeal artery. Bleeding is almost always continuous, and a large clot forms, which separates the dura from the skull.

Manifestations are usually acute in onset because the bleeding is often arterial. With an epidural hematoma, the following sequence of events may occur:

1. The client is unconscious immediately after head trauma.
2. The client awakens and is quite lucid.

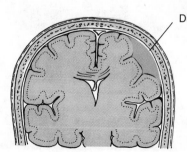
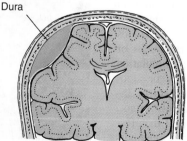
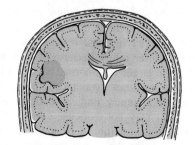

Dura

A. Subdural hematoma   B. Epidural hematoma   C. Intracerebral hematoma

FIGURE 73-9 Formation of a hematoma after head injury.

3. LOC occurs and pupil dilation response rapidly deteriorates, with onset of eye movement paralysis, on the same side as that of the hematoma.
4. The client lapses into a coma.

Although these manifestations are often described as "classic" for an epidural hematoma, few clients present with such classic manifestations, and astute assessment is necessary to prevent death.

Skull radiography and CT scanning confirm the diagnosis. Rapid diagnosis and prompt intervention are essential with an epidural hematoma. Careful, ongoing assessment of neurologic status is also necessary.

SUBDURAL HEMATOMA. Subdural hematoma is a collection of blood in the subdural space (i.e., between the dura mater and arachnoid mater). The tearing of the bridging veins over the brain causes most subdural hematomas.

Subdural hematomas may be classified as acute, subacute, or chronic, depending on how rapidly clinical manifestations develop. Another classification recognizes only acute and chronic, combining the acute and subacute categories.

Acute and Subacute Subdural Hematoma. Acute subdural hematoma usually results from brain or blood vessel laceration. Acute subdural hematomas are a serious complication requiring prompt treatment, because they compress and distort an already damaged, edematous brain. Acute subdural hematoma is symptomatic within 24 to 48 hours of injury. Acute subdural hematoma is seen in approximately 24% of clients with severe head injuries.

Clinical manifestations of acute subdural hematoma are similar to those of acute epidural hematoma. The onset and development of the clinical manifestations may be somewhat slower because the bleeding is more often venous, rather than arterial. Symptom recognition may be difficult because subdural hematoma is often associated with moderate or severe brain injury. A patient developing an acute subdural hematoma may remain unconscious after injury or may have a variable LOC (depending on the extent of injury). A conscious client usually has a headache. The client may become irritable and confused and lapse into a coma or show a fluctuating LOC. Manifestations of increasing ICP appear. Subtle changes in LOC and development of lateralizing changes (i.e., on one side) such as hemiparesis, pupillary dilation, or extraocular eye movement paralysis may be the only findings.

Chronic Subdural Hematoma. Chronic subdural hematoma is most common in older and alcoholic clients (Fig. 73–10). These clients experience atrophy of the brain, which results in stretching of the bridging veins and an increase in the size of the subdural space. These stretched veins are easily ruptured in a fall, even if the fall does not result in other injuries. It develops several weeks or even months after injury because of a slow accumulation of fluid in a larger-than-normal space. Elderly or alcoholic clients may not even recall the mechanism of injury. The initial injury may have been relatively minor, and the client may not associate current clinical manifestations with the past injury. In addition, family members may not recognize the subtle neurologic changes or may not give credence to them because of the client's age.

Gradually, the enlarging blood clot creates pressure on the brain. There is an interval during which the client appears to be recovering or seems completely recovered. Later, manifestations of neurologic deterioration develop. The client may become drowsy, inattentive, and incoherent and display personality changes. Headaches are another prominent symptom. These indications of chronic subdural hematoma may be overlooked until focal or lateralizing signs appear (e.g., hemiparesis, pupil signs). Changes in LOC continue, and LOC may fluctuate widely. Clinical assessment with subdural hematoma is similar to that with epidural hematomas. Surgical intervention usually consists of placing several burr holes or performing a craniotomy to remove the hematoma. Treatment results depend on the client's condition before surgery and the degree of primary brain tissue damage.

A client who has undergone evacuation of a chronic subdural hematoma usually has a drain placed in the cavity to prevent reaccumulation of the fluid and blood. These clients are typically kept flat during the immediate postoperative period. This allows the brain to reexpand to fill the cranial cavity.

INTRACEREBRAL HEMATOMA. Intracerebral hematomas occur less often than epidural or subdural hematomas. They are caused by bleeding directly into brain tissue and may occur at the area of injury, some distance away, or deep within the brain. These hematomas cause problems with increased ICP. Surgical resection may cause as much damage as the clot itself and is usually not

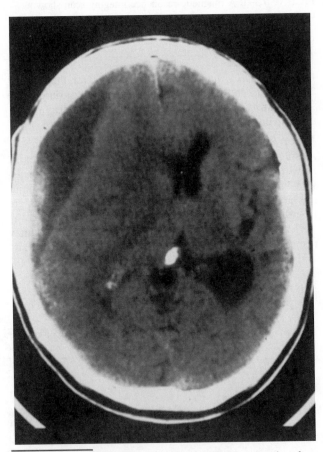

FIGURE 73–10 Magnetic resonance image of a chronic subdural hematoma with an area of acute bleeding, causing a severe midline shift.

performed unless the clot is easily accessible. Clinical manifestations are similar to those that occur with epidural or subdural hematomas, although hemiplegia is more common than hemiparesis. Many assessment findings relate to the lesion's mass effect. Various other clinical manifestations may also be present, depending on the location of the intracerebral hematoma. A diagnosis is established as with other types of hematomas. One form of hematoma, called *delayed traumatic intracerebral hematoma*, occurs after a few days. It is most common in persons with disseminated intravascular coagulation, hypertension, a history of alcohol abuse, or hypoxia. It carries a poor prognosis.

Pathophysiology

A concussion usually causes injury to the brain that is reversible. Some biochemical and ultrastructural damage, such as depletion in mitochondrial adenosine triphosphate and changes in vascular permeability, also can occur.[82]

Major head injuries cause direct damage to the parenchyma of the brain. Kinetic energy is transmitted to the brain, and bruising analogous to that seen in soft tissue injuries results. A blow to the surface of the brain leads to rapid brain tissue displacement and disruption of blood vessels, leading to bleeding, tissue injury, and edema.

Clients with diffuse axonal damage have microscopic injury to the axons in the cerebrum, the corpus callosum, and the brain stem. Widespread white matter injury, white matter degeneration, neuronal dysfunction, and global cerebral edema are characteristic features.

Studies have noted a significantly increased mortality rate in the client who experiences hypotension especially early in the post-injury time frame. When autoregulation is disrupted, as in head injury, cerebral hypoperfusion leads to brain tissue ischemia. Hypoxia has a lesser effect on mortality so long as cerebral perfusion is adequate, because the brain can extract extra oxygen for short periods of time. The combination of arterial hypotension and hypoxemia is significant in the progression of secondary injury. Other causes of secondary brain injury include increased ICP, respiratory problems, electrolyte imbalance, and infection.

Reperfusion injury occurs when ischemia is reversed and blood flow is reestablished; it also leads to secondary injury. Reperfusion injury is probably caused by oxygen free radicals, which are normal byproducts of aerobic metabolism that usually break down into oxygen and water. In cell injury, breakdown of these radicals is impaired so that they accumulate, causing destruction of nucleic acids, proteins, carbohydrates, and lipids and, eventually, cell membranes in the brain tissue. Currently, research is targeted at developing neuroprotective agents that prevent delayed injury progression.[30]

Clinical Manifestations

SKULL FRACTURES

Other than a history of skull fracture, clients may not have clear manifestations of the injury. Therefore, they need careful ongoing assessment. They may develop other clinical signs, including the following:

- CSF or other fluid draining from the ear or nose
- Evidence of various cranial nerve injuries
- Blood behind the tympanic membrane
- Periorbital ecchymoses (bruises around the eyes)
- Later, a bruise over the mastoid process (Battle's sign)

Indications of cranial nerve and inner ear damage may be noted at the time of the initial injury or may not appear until later. They include the following:

- Vision changes from optic nerve damage
- Hearing loss from auditory nerve damage
- Loss of the sense of smell from olfactory nerve damage
- Squint or fixed, dilated pupil and loss of some eye movements from oculomotor nerve damage
- Facial paresis or paralysis (unilateral) from facial nerve damage
- Vertigo caused by damage from otoliths in the inner ear
- Nystagmus from damage to the vestibular system

Basilar skull fractures, depressed fractures, and other open (compound) fractures allow communication between the external environment and the brain. Infection is therefore a possible complication. See Chapter 69 for a discussion of brain abscess and meningitis. Increasing ICP with basilar skull fractures can be difficult to assess because the pressure is not exerted on the motor strip of the frontal lobes, which means that there will be no weakness in the contralateral extremities. Assess for subtle changes in vital signs, especially heart rate and rhythm and breathing patterns.

CONCUSSIONS

After concussion, observers report a loss of consciousness for 5 minutes or less. Retrograde amnesia, post-traumatic amnesia, or both may be present. The duration of amnesia may directly correlate with the severity of the concussion. The client usually presents with headache and dizziness and may complain of nausea and vomiting. There is no break in the skull or dura, and no visible damage is seen on CT or MRI scans.

CONTUSIONS

The clinical manifestations of contusions are varied, partly because any area of the brain can suffer contusion. Contusions are often associated with other serious injuries, including cervical fractures. Secondary effects (e.g., brain swelling and edema) accompany serious contusions. Increased ICP and herniation syndromes may result. Contusions may be divided into cerebral contusions and brain stem contusions.

CEREBRAL CONTUSIONS. Manifestations of cerebral contusions vary, depending on which areas of the cerebral hemispheres are damaged. An agitated, confused head-injured client who remains alert may have a temporal lobe contusion. Hemiparesis in an alert head-injured client may indicate a frontal contusion. An aphasic head-injured client may have a frontotemporal contusion. Other findings indicate contusions in other areas. Although these findings correlate with cerebral contusion, they do not rule out other abnormalities, such as a developing mass lesion. Adverse changes in the client's condition require immediate medical attention. If treated early, these complications may be reversible.

BRAIN STEM CONTUSIONS. Brain stem contusions render a client immediately unresponsive or partially comatose, because of significant brain stem disruption. Typically, an altered LOC continues for at least several hours and usually days or weeks. The client may regain partial consciousness within hours or remain in a coma.

Damage to the reticular activating system may render the client permanently comatose. Other neurologic abnormalities are present and are usually symmetrical (i.e., evenly distributed on both sides of the body). Some may be lateralized (asymmetrical, or on one side of the body only), indicating development of a secondary event, such as a hematoma.

In addition to the altered LOC that is always present with brain stem contusion, respiratory, pupillary, eye movement, and motor abnormalities may occur.

- Respirations may be normal, periodic, very rapid, or ataxic.
- Pupils are usually small, equal, and reactive. Damage to the upper brain stem (third cranial nerve) may cause pupillary abnormalities.
- Loss of normal eye movements may occur because pathways controlling eye movements traverse the midbrain and pons.
- The client may respond to light or noxious stimuli by purposeful movements, such as pushing the stimulus away, or the client may have no response to stimuli (i.e, may be in a flaccid state). In the presence of profound alteration in LOC, flexion and extension posturing may be elicited with or without noxious stimuli (see Chapter 68).

Brain stem contusions do not usually injure the brain stem alone. Localized swelling or direct injury to the hypothalamus may produce autonomic nervous system effects. The client may have a high temperature and a rapid pulse and respirations and may perspire profusely. These effects may wax and wane but, if sustained, can lead to serious complications.

These clinical manifestations often vary from one observation to another, whereas findings with a developing hematoma are more consistent. Careful documentation of assessment findings to identify patterns or trends in the client's condition is important.

Diagnostic assessments such as CT or MRI scanning may reveal fractures and areas of bleeding or brain shift (see Fig. 73-10). Lumbar puncture can also be used to assess for bleeding within the subarachnoid space, provided that any possibility of increased ICP has been ruled out. Currently, CT scans can identify blood in the subarachnoid space, and lumbar punctures are rarely done for this purpose.

Outcome Management

Major goals in the care of severely head-injured clients are as follows:

- Prompt recognition and treatment of hypoxia and acid-base disorders that can contribute to cerebral edema
- Control of increasing ICP resulting from factors such as cerebral edema or expanding hematoma
- Stabilization of other conditions

▰ Medical Management

The medical management of severely head-injured clients focuses on supporting all organ systems while recovery

from the injuries takes place. This involves (1) ventilatory support, (2) management of fluid balance and elimination, and (3) management of nutrition and gastrointestinal function. Head trauma affects all systems of the body, and managing its effects requires a holistic perspective. Clinical manifestations may be the result of the initial head injury or may arise from a complicating process.

INITIAL MANAGEMENT. The initial management of clients with head injury is the same as for any other injured client: airway, breathing, and circulation. There is a high association of cervical fracture with head injury; therefore, the client must be immobilized at the scene of the injury. Lateral cervical spine x-ray films are obtained before the client's head is moved, or the immobilization devices are removed for these studies. The client with head injury is protected from possible complications of cord injury by immobilizing the head and neck immediately, using a cervical collar or sandbags until a collar can be obtained.

If intubation is necessary, a jaw thrust maneuver must be used. A baseline assessment of the client's motor and sensory function is obtained at the scene of the accident. Interventions include lowering the ICP with hyperventilation by mechanical ventilation or by manually ventilating the client with a bag-valve-mask device.

An IV line is placed and fluids are given to stabilize the blood pressure. Head injury alone does not cause major loss of blood. If substantial blood loss is suspected, look for other injuries (e.g., fractures, abdominal injury, severe scalp laceration).

A complete history including the mechanism of injury is important. These data allow the physician to determine the probable extent of injury and allow the emergency department personnel to prepare for the client's arrival. Open head wounds should be covered and pressure applied to control bleeding unless there appears to be an underlying depressed or compound skull fracture.

Do not attempt to remove foreign objects or any penetrating objects from the wound. Uncomplicated scalp wounds (that do not lie over depressed or compound skull fractures) are anesthetized with a local anesthetic agent, cleansed, and sutured. In the emergency department, primary and secondary surveys of the client's injuries are performed. Resuscitation continues with fluid administration.

Laboratory studies are performed, as are necessary radiologic studies. If any identified injuries require emergency surgery, the client is taken directly to the operating room (OR) before admission to the intensive care unit (ICU). Once the client is stabilized enough for transfer to the ICU, the neurosurgical and trauma teams and the nursing staff maintain ongoing care.

ONGOING MANAGEMENT. Ongoing care to reduce ICP is the focus of critical care. Osmotic diuretics, hyperventilation, and adequate oxygenation continue. The cerebral metabolic rate is reduced with sedatives, paralytic agents, antipyretics, barbiturates, and hypothermia. Morphine is a frequently used narcotic for the head-injured client. It reduces pain and can be given intravenously. Respiratory depression is controlled in the client who is intubated and ventilated. Paralytic agents may be used to promote adequate ventilation and should be administered in conjunction with a sedative and an analgesic, because paralytic agents have no sedative or analgesic effect.

PROGNOSIS. Not many clients die instantly from head injury. However, many head-injured clients die within the first few minutes after injury from shock or impaired respiration. Early death may also result from brain stem damage. According to the results of several studies, coma duration is the best predictor of damage severity because it correlates highly with probability of death, intellectual deficit, and social skill impairment. These studies classified a *mild* head injury as loss of consciousness for 20 minutes or less, a *moderate* head injury as 21 to 59 minutes of unconsciousness, and *severe* head injury as coma for 1 hour or more.[12]

Nursing Management

A description of the mechanism of injury is helpful in understanding the nature of a head injury. Whenever there are witnesses to the accident, information obtained can be valuable in determining the extent of the injury. Information about the client's activity and LOC before and after the injury is also helpful. Also important is whether the client was conscious at all or unconscious after injury.

As soon as possible after head injury, assess and document the client's vital signs and neurologic status. This initial assessment and the data obtained from witnesses at the accident scene establish a baseline for later observations. Carefully document all assessment findings. Assessment data collection is described earlier in this chapter.

The physician should be promptly notified of any findings that indicate the possible development of complications. It is particularly difficult to assess the condition of a head-injured client who has ingested large amounts of alcohol or other drugs before injury, because the effects of these substances may obscure significant clinical abnormalities.

DIAGNOSIS, OUTCOMES, INTERVENTIONS

Many nursing and collaborative problems are present in the client with a head injury, such as risk for *Ineffective Airway Clearance, Altered Tissue Perfusion,* seizures, paralysis, infection, diabetes insipidus, and *Post-trauma Syndrome.* Other problems that a client with a head injury may experience include the following:

- Risk for Contractures
- Impaired Skin Integrity
- Altered Oral Mucous Membranes
- Altered Nutrition
- Altered Fluid Volume
- Risk for Injury
- Risk for Increased ICP
- Altered Thought Processes
- Altered Family Processes

Nursing diagnoses for these problems are discussed in Chapters 68 and 69. Investigation of the underlying cause of these problems and the interventions for them must be individualized according to the client's needs.

Risk for Ineffective Airway Clearance. The client with traumatic brain injury may have an altered state of consciousness and may not be able to expectorate secretions. The client is also at increased risk for aspiration.

Outcomes. The client will have effective airway clearance. The upper airway should be free of secretions. Res-

pirations should be of a regular rate (16 to 22 respirations per minute), rhythm, and depth. Breath sounds should be clear in both lungs, and the chest should have symmetrical movement. The trachea should be in a midline position, and there should be no dyspnea or accessory muscle use. Aspiration should be prevented. The PaO_2 should be maintained greater than 90 mm Hg and $PaCO_2$ between 30 and 35 mm Hg initially. The chest film should be clear.

Interventions. Nursing actions aimed at maintaining adequate airway clearance include clearing the mouth and oral pharynx of foreign bodies (e.g., broken teeth) and suctioning the oropharynx and trachea every 1 or 2 hours and as needed. Avoid suctioning the nasopharynx until after a basilar fracture or meningeal tear is ruled out. A semiprone, lateral position may facilitate drainage of secretions and prevent aspiration but is contraindicated with increased ICP or a cervical fracture. Humidified oxygen, endotracheal intubation, mechanical ventilation, or a tracheostomy may be required to maintain the client's PaO_2 and $PaCO_2$ within set parameters.

Altered Cerebral Tissue Perfusion. In clients who suffer from traumatic brain injuries, another appropriate nursing diagnosis is *Risk for Altered Cerebral Tissue Perfusion secondary to hypotension, hypertension, intracranial hemorrhage, hematoma, or other injuries.*

Outcomes. The client will have adequate cerebral tissue perfusion. The client will have a stable or improving LOC with a stable GCS score and an ICP of less than 15 mm Hg. Temperature will be maintained at less than 38.5° C. The client's blood pressure will be maintained within established parameters. Urinary output will be at a minimum of 30 ml per hour and not greater than 200 ml per hour. Laboratory values will remain within normal limits.

Interventions. Although anticipatory, prudent monitoring is key to early detection of altered cerebral tissue perfusion; nursing interventions can actually prevent, delay, or minimize altered cerebral perfusion. These interventions are discussed earlier in this chapter. Briefly, they include maintaining all physiologic parameters within normal limits, positioning the client for optimal venous return, and monitoring extracerebral systems for complications. Communicating a client's neurologic status accurately and completely through verbal reporting and documentation is essential to early identification of change and early intervention. ICP monitoring may be required (see earlier).

Surgical Management

Conditions that may require surgery include subdural and epidural hematomas, depressed skull fractures, and penetrating foreign bodies. An epidural clot may be surgically evacuated through burr holes (Fig. 73–11) or a craniotomy. During surgery, the wound may be drained and bleeding vessels ligated. After surgery, nursing care is the same as for any client recovering from a craniotomy. Simple skull depressions are treated electively by surgically elevating the depressed bone tissue, removing fragments, and repairing lacerated dura. Compound depressed skull fractures are immediately treated surgically. The scalp, skull, and devitalized brain are debrided, and the

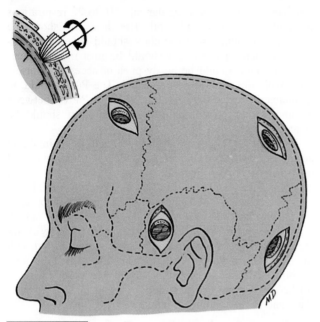

FIGURE 73–11 Placement of burr holes in the skull.

wound is cleaned thoroughly. Unless all foreign material is removed, a brain abscess or seizures may develop. Debridement of a penetrating wound or depressed skull fracture frequently leaves a cranial defect that is cosmetically unsightly. The defect may be surgically corrected by cranioplasty at a later time.

ICP is reduced as much as possible before surgery. Baseline neurologic data are documented. Informed consent needs to be obtained from the family if the patient is unconscious or confused. After surgery, provide nursing care for the client following the guidelines for craniotomy (see Chapter 69).

Self-Care

Clients with possible head injury or mild head injury were previously hospitalized for observation for a minimum of 6 hours (ideally for 48 hours) because of the risk of extradural hemorrhage. If the client is sent home, give clear instructions to help the client's caregiver assess for complications (see the accompanying Client Education Guide).

Rehabilitation

Most clients hospitalized for more than 48 hours because of a head injury ultimately require some rehabilitation. Clients with mild head injury may be overlooked in the population of people who need follow-up care. Mild head injuries can cause headache, memory difficulties, difficulty performing simple tasks, and irritability. These clinical manifestations may persist for a month or longer.

Rehabilitation may take place in an inpatient or outpatient setting, depending on the client's condition. Rehabilitation may include physical, occupational, speech, and cognitive therapy and is essential in returning the client to maximal function. Nurses play a major role in the rehabilitation of the head-injured client and in the education of significant others.

More severely injured clients may be sent to rehabilitation facilities with feeding tubes or tracheostomy tubes in place. Clients and families need assistance in choosing a new health care facility that can deliver the level of care needed. If recovery is unlikely, the client may need to be transferred to an extended-care facility. Because many head-injured clients are young, previously healthy people, placement in a nursing home may be a very difficult reality for family members to accept. Teaching and support can greatly improve coping. Involvement of disciplines such as social services, pastoral care, or discharge planning can increase the family members' understanding of the next phase of care.

The rehabilitation of clients with brain injuries is challenging. In some cases, community reintegration is unsuccessful. Studies have reported improvement in the client's ability to lead a productive life with the use of interdisciplinary techniques that include rehabilitation in cognition, compensatory techniques, social skills, emotional adjustment, leisure skills, physical fitness, and health maintenance. Most clients require 6 months in a rehabilitation program.[52]

Modifications for Elderly Clients

Although most head injuries do not occur in the elderly population, diagnosis is often more difficult in older adults because of an atypical presentation. These clients also experience more complications. An older client may be less able to tolerate respiratory problems or cardiac dysrhythmias. The presence of chronic diseases such as chronic obstructive pulmonary disease or heart failure can make managing ventilation and fluid balance more difficult. If any type of mental impairment was present before the injury, recovery to full independence is less likely. Poor stamina and medical complications may impede rehabilitation.

SPINAL CORD INJURY

Injury to the spinal cord can range in severity from mild flexion-extension "whiplash" injuries to complete transection of the cord with permanent quadriplegia. Trauma to

---

CLIENT EDUCATION GUIDE

Monitoring Family Members After Head Injury

Family Instructions

- Observe your family member for 24 hours.
- Take him or her to the hospital immediately if you notice any of the following:

  - Increased drowsiness or confusion
  - Inability to be awakened
  - Vomiting
  - Convulsions
  - Bleeding or drainage from the nose or ears
  - Weakness in either arm or leg
  - Loss of feeling in either arm or either leg
  - Blurring of vision
  - Slurring of speech
  - Enlargement or shrinkage of one pupil

the cord can occur at any level but most commonly occurs in the cervical and lower thoracic–upper lumbar vertebrae. This finding is due in part to the support given by the ribs to the thoracic spine and the flexibility of the cervical and lumbar spinal segments.

Although this discussion focuses on nursing management of *acute* spinal cord injury (SCI), it should be remembered that there are approximately 200,000 spinal cord–injured people living in the United States.

Etiology and Risk Factors

Trauma is the most common cause of SCI. Each year about 10,000 people sustain such injury. Most are males between the ages of 16 and 30 years. Nine per cent of injuries occur in people over the age of 60. Traumatic spinal cord injuries are most often caused by automobile or motorcycle accidents, gunshot or knife wounds, falls, and sports mishaps. Over half of all SCIs involve the cervical spine, and the rest occur in the thoracic, lumbar, and sacral spinal segments.

The feeling of immortality often experienced by adolescents and young adults contributes strongly to their risk of SCI. Young people may believe they can engage in dangerous behavior without being injured. The use of alcohol and illicit drugs can reinforce this belief in immortality. A young person who has experienced the devastation of SCI may best deliver the message of primary prevention. In several nationwide programs, head-injured and spinal cord–injured people are available to speak at school-sponsored educational programs.

Nontraumatic disorders may also result in SCI. These problems include the following:

- Cervical spondylosis with myelopathy (spinal canal narrowing with progressive injury to the cord and roots)
- Myelitis (infective or noninfective)
- Osteoporosis, causing vertebral compression fractures
- Syringomyelia (central cavitation of the cord)
- Tumors, both infiltrative and compressive
- Vascular diseases, usually infarction or hemorrhage

Whatever the cause, SCI produces distinctive and debilitating damage. Nowhere else in the body can a local insult produce such devastation in proportion to the extent of tissue involved.

FLEXION-ROTATION, DISLOCATION, AND FRACTURE-DISLOCATION INJURIES

By far the most common spinal cord injuries are flexion injuries. When a person strikes the head against the steering wheel or windshield, the spine is forced into acute hyperflexion (Fig. 73–12). Rupture of the posterior ligaments results in forward dislocation of the vertebrae. Blood vessels may be damaged, leading to ischemia of the spinal cord. The cervical spine, usually at the C5–6 level, is most commonly affected by a flexion injury. In the thoracic-lumbar spine, this type of injury is most frequently seen at the T12–L1 level.

HYPEREXTENSION INJURIES

Hyperextension injuries result after a fall in which the chin hits an object and the head is thrown back (see Fig. 73–12). The anterior ligament is ruptured, with fracture of the posterior elements of the vertebral body. Hyperex-

tension of the spinal cord against the ligamentum flavum can lead to dorsal column contusion and posterior dislocation of the vertebrae. Complete transection of the cord can follow a hyperextension injury, although transection of the cord is rare. Clients who present with complete lesions of the spinal cord do not necessarily have transection of the cord. Complete lesions of the cord result in loss of all voluntary movement and sensation below the lesion and loss of reflex function in isolated segments of the cord.

COMPRESSION INJURIES

Compression injuries are often caused by falls or jumps in which the person lands directly on the head, sacrum, or feet (see Fig. 73–12). The force of impact fractures the vertebrae, and the fragments compress the cord. Disc and bone fragments may be propelled into the spinal cord upon impact. The lumbar and the lower thoracic vertebrae are the most commonly injured regions after a compression impact when the person lands on the feet. If the person lands on the head (as in diving into shallow water), the injury is to the cervical spine. About 50% of these injuries result in incomplete lesions. Incomplete lesions occur when some of the spinal tracts remain intact.

UNIQUE CERVICAL INJURIES

Three types of fractures are unique to the cervical spine (Fig. 73–13):

1. *Fractures of the odontoid process* (the odontoid process is the superior projection of the bone on C2) may be intact, with no detectable movement, or may be displaced, with movement and entrapment of the spinal cord.
2. A *hangman's fracture* is a bilateral fracture through the pedicles of C2, separating the posterior elements from the body of the vertebra.
3. The *Jefferson fracture* involves bursting of the ring of C1. The spinal canal usually widens.

These injuries are usually associated with other spinal injuries. Clients with these cervical fractures either die of the injury immediately or are stable and may walk into the emergency department reporting only neck pain.

Pathophysiology

SCIs most often occur as a result of injury to the vertebrae. The most common sites of injury are at the C1–2, C4–6, and T11–L2 vertebrae. These segments of the spine are the most mobile and therefore most easily injured.

The cord is injured as the result of acceleration, deceleration, or another force (e.g., impact) applied to the spine. The forces injure the spinal cord by compressing, pulling, or tearing the tissues. Microscopic bleeding occurs immediately after injury, primarily in the gray matter of the cord. Within the first hour, edema develops and often spreads along segments of the spinal cord. Arachidonic acid and its metabolites (prostaglandins, thromboxanes, and leukotrienes) cause edema. Cord edema peaks within 2 to 3 days and subsides within the first 7 days after injury. Although the site of the initial injury has the most edema and bleeding, some edema and bleeding extend at least for two cord segments on either side of the

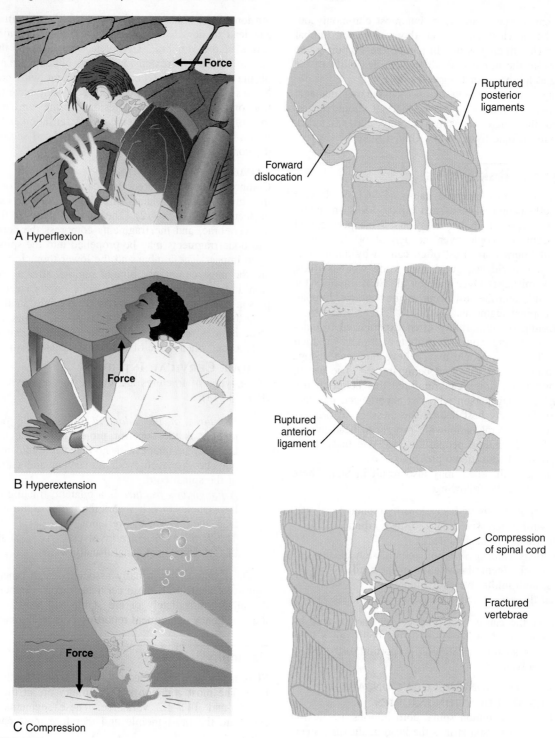

FIGURE 73–12 Patterns of cervical spine injury. *A,* Flexion injury of the cervical spine ruptures the posterior ligaments. *B,* Hyperextension injury of the cervical spine ruptures the anterior ligaments. *C,* Compression fractures crush the vertebrae and force bony fragments into the spinal canal.

injury. The edema of the cord leads to temporary loss of sensation and function. Spinal cord tissue injury is related to the initial insult, biochemical changes, and hemodynamic instability. Therefore, immediately after injury, it is not easy to determine the ultimate degree of permanent impairment.

Further changes include fragmentation of the axonal covering and loss of myelin. Phagocytic cells can injure

surviving axons as they scavenge cellular debris. Chemotactic and inflammatory mediators further extend tissue necrosis. Macrophages engulf the spinal cord tissue and may cause a central cavity (called post-traumatic syringomyelia) to develop as early as 9 days after injury.

In addition, the oligodendroglial cells that support the cord are lost. Injury to the cord leads to rapid loss of axonal conduction from ion changes, such as very rapid

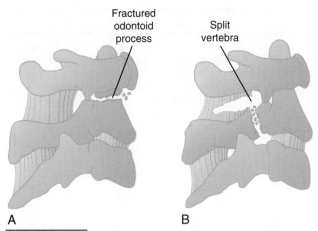

FIGURE 73-13 Fractures of the cervical spine. *A,* Odontoid fractures are fractures of the superior projection of C2 that normally projects into C1. Stabilization is required for healing. *B,* Hangman's fractures are of the pedicle of C2. The vertebra is split in half. These fractures are usually treated with a halo brace. A third type of cervical spine fracture called Jefferson's fracture is described in the text.

increases in extracellular potassium and influx of calcium into the cell. Finally, free radicals are produced. Free radicals are normally found in the body but are quickly controlled by antioxidant enzyme systems. When the antioxidant systems are overwhelmed, the free radicals damage tissues.

The physiologic response to SCI extends beyond changes within the spinal cord. For example, the sympathetic nervous system stress response results in reduced perfusion of the gastrointestinal tract and reduced production of gastric mucus to protect the lining. Ulceration and bleeding may develop.

Spasticity is the increased tone or contraction of muscles, producing stiff movements. Various CNS injuries or diseases such as SCI, cerebrovascular accidents, and cerebral palsy may result in spasticity. After SCI, the brain can no longer influence reflex movements through the spinal cord. Eventually, the lower part of the cord, using spinal reflexes, begins to work automatically. Spinal reflex activities include the flexor withdrawal reflex and reflex emptying of the bladder and bowel. These primitive spinal mechanisms, normally kept inactive by higher centers, are "released" when the normal inhibitions of the higher centers are destroyed. As recovery progresses, flexor responses are interspersed with extensor spasms. These movements ultimately develop into predominantly extensor activity. The client's limbs spasm into extension with movement. Spasticity may remain indefinitely or may gradually decrease over time.

Clinical Manifestations

LEVEL OF INJURY

The initial clinical manifestations of acute SCI depend on the level and extent of injury to the cord. Below the level of injury or lesion, the following functions are lost:

- Voluntary movement
- Sensation of pain, temperature, pressure, and proprioception (ability to know where the body is in space)
- Bowel and bladder function
- Spinal and autonomic reflexes

The level of injury may be described in terms of (1) skeletal injury and (2) neurologic level of injury. Skeletal injury refers to the vertebral damage demonstrated by x-ray study. The criterion of the American Spinal Injury Association (ASIA) is useful in describing the level of spinal cord involvement: *The neurologic level of injury is the lowest segment of the spinal cord with bilateral intact sensory and motor function.* Assess sensory function according to dermatomes to identify the areas of skin with normal sensation. Motor function is measured by testing myotomes to identify muscles with active movement and full range of motion (ROM) against gravity. The ASIA Impairment Scale is:

- Normal with sensory and motor function preserved
- Incomplete with the majority of motor function preserved
- Incomplete with nonfunctional motor function preserved
- Incomplete with only sensation preserved
- Complete with loss of sensation and motor function

Injury to the cervical cord produces quadriplegia. Injuries above the C4 level may be fatal because of loss of innervation to the diaphragm and intercostal muscles. Without immediate rescue breathing after the accident, the injured person will die of respiratory failure. Today, with the general public's knowledge of cardiopulmonary resuscitation, many people survive this injury to the cervical spine. Injuries to the remainder of the cervical spine create specific patterns of motor loss (Table 73-2). Note that a person with a C7 injury is able to lift the shoulders, elbows, and wrists and has some hand function, but below C7 there remains no motor function or sensation.

Injuries to the thoracic or lumbar spinal segment produce paraplegia. People with such injuries have function in their upper extremities and can be mobile in a wheelchair or with crutches and braces. People with L5 injury can extend the great toe and dorsiflex the ankle. They have no sensation in the perianal area, calf, heel, or small toe.

CHANGES IN REFLEXES

Reflexes, which normally cross the spinal cord and return to the stimulated limb, are absent in early SCI because of spinal cord edema. Blood pressure and temperature in denervated (without nervous function or innervation) areas fall markedly and respond poorly to reflex stimuli.

After cord edema subsides, some body functions may return by reflex (e.g., control of the urinary bladder), but they lack integration with other visceral activities. Visceral activities may be initiated by atypical stimuli. For example, scratching the skin may cause vasodilation, sweating, and urination. Nervous system lesions may produce a type of defective urinary bladder function known as *cord bladder.* For example, stimulation of the skin on the lower abdomen or thighs may cause reflex urination. This form of cord bladder is called an *automatic bladder.* Such stimulation may also cause reflex ejaculation and priapism (persistent abnormal penile erection without sexual desire) in paralyzed men.

TABLE 73–2	SPINAL CORD INJURY AND IMPAIRMENT

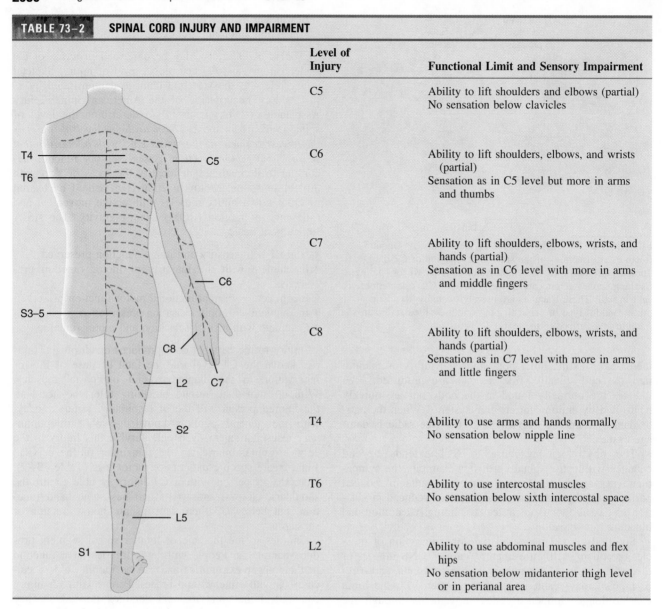

Level of Injury	Functional Limit and Sensory Impairment
C5	Ability to lift shoulders and elbows (partial) No sensation below clavicles
C6	Ability to lift shoulders, elbows, and wrists (partial) Sensation as in C5 level but more in arms and thumbs
C7	Ability to lift shoulders, elbows, wrists, and hands (partial) Sensation as in C6 level with more in arms and middle fingers
C8	Ability to lift shoulders, elbows, wrists, and hands (partial) Sensation as in C7 level with more in arms and little fingers
T4	Ability to use arms and hands normally No sensation below nipple line
T6	Ability to use intercostal muscles No sensation below sixth intercostal space
L2	Ability to use abdominal muscles and flex hips No sensation below midanterior thigh level or in perianal area

MUSCLE SPASMS

Intense and painful muscular spasms of the lower extremities occur following a traumatic complete transverse spinal cord lesion. In assisting the client and the family members to understand these movements, it should be explained that these muscle spasms are involuntary and do not mean that voluntary movement is returning. This information, although disappointing, is essential.

Muscle spasms range in intensity from mild muscular twitching to vigorous mass reflexogenic states. Extreme, involuntary muscle spasms can actually throw a client out of bed or wheelchair. Bed side rails are kept up and restraining straps are comfortably secured over the client lying on a stretcher. Muscle spasms, often aggravated by cold weather, prolonged periods of sitting, or emotionally upsetting events, may become intolerable. Reflex spasms may be triggered by extrinsic or visceral stimuli, such as a distended bladder.

Emotion (e.g., anxiety, crying, anger, laughing) or cutaneous stimulation (e.g., tickling, stroking, pinching) may initiate spastic movements. By learning to recognize events that trigger such reflex spasms, the client may use these potentially annoying movements to achieve functional activities such as urination.

AUTONOMIC DYSREFLEXIA

Autonomic dysreflexia, also known as autonomic hyperreflexia, is a life-threatening syndrome. It is a cluster of clinical manifestations that results when multiple spinal cord autonomic responses discharge simultaneously. This syndrome, observed in as many as 85% of clients with cord injury above the T6 level, can occur anytime after spinal shock has resolved. Dysreflexia often resolves 3 years after injury, but it may recur. The manifestations of autonomic dysreflexia result from an exaggerated sympathetic response to a noxious stimulus below the level of the cord lesion. Common stimuli are bladder and bowel distention but may also be pressure ulcers, spasms, pain, pressure on the penis, excessive rectal stimulation, bladder stones, ingrown toenails, abdominal abnormalities, or uterine contractions.

Exaggerated sympathetic responses cause the blood vessels below the level of injury to constrict. As a result, the client develops hypertension (with pressures possibly as high as 300 mm Hg), a pounding headache, flushing above the level of the lesion, nasal stuffiness, diaphoresis, piloerection ("gooseflesh"), dilated pupils with blurred vision, bradycardia (30 to 40 beats per minute [BPM]), restlessness, and nausea. The manifestations are a result of compensatory efforts to overcome the severe hypertension. Initially, baroreceptors sense the hypertensive stimuli and stimulate the parasympathetic nervous system, which results in vasodilation above the level of cord injury (headache, flushing) and bradycardia. The problem is that the visceral and peripheral vessels do not dilate because the efferent impulses cannot pass through the damaged cord. Thus, the overall effect is one of extreme hypertension. Seizures and cerebral hemorrhage occur in approximately 10% to 15% of cases. See the later discussion on Risk for Autonomic Dysreflexia for interventions.

CLINICAL SYNDROMES CAUSING PARTIAL PARALYSIS

Five spinal cord syndromes cause partial paralysis (Fig. 73–14): central cord syndrome, anterior cord syndrome, Brown-Séquard syndrome, conus medullaris syndrome, and cauda equina syndrome. Each has distinctive neurologic features.

CENTRAL CORD SYNDROME. Central cord syndrome (most common with hyperextension-hyperflexion injuries) produces more weakness in the upper extremities than in the lower. This type of injury occurs most often in the older adult who has a pre-existing spinal stenosis. This injury may also occur in a person who lands on the head such as when diving into shallow water and hitting the bottom. The common mechanism of injury is a fall forward. The weakness is caused by edema and hemorrhage in the central area of the cord, which is predominantly occupied by nerve tracts to the hands and arms.

ANTERIOR CORD SYNDROME. A lesion in the anterior spinal cord causes anterior cord syndrome, with complete motor function loss and decreased pain sensation. Deep pressure, position sense, and two-point discrimination sensations remain intact. Often the anterior spinal artery is affected, causing an infarction of spinal cord tissue. Cervical cord concussion may produce various degrees of motor and sensory deficit, which completely resolve within hours. Occasionally, cervical cord trauma produces only root injuries, which may paralyze isolated muscles or muscle groups in the arms and shoulders. These deficits are usually permanent.

BROWN-SÉQUARD SYNDROME. Brown-Séquard syndrome is caused by lateral hemisection of the cord (i.e., when half the cord is cut or otherwise damaged), as a bullet wound or knife wound. This injury results in ipsilateral motor paralysis, loss of vibratory and position sense, and contralateral loss of pain and temperature sensation.

CONUS MEDULLARIS SYNDROME. Conus medullaris syndrome follows damage to the lumbar nerve roots and the conus medullaris in the spinal cord. The client usually has bowel and bladder areflexia and flaccid lower extremities. The bulbospongiosis penile (erection) and micturition reflexes may be preserved when damage is limited to the upper sacral segments of the spinal cord.

CAUDA EQUINA SYNDROME. Injury to the lumbosacral nerve roots below the conus medullaris results in the cauda equina syndrome. The client experiences areflexia of the bowel, bladder, and lower extremities.

SPINAL SHOCK

The immediate response to cord transection is called *spinal shock*. The client with SCI experiences complete loss of skeletal muscle function, bowel and bladder tone, sexual function, and autonomic reflexes. Loss of venous return and hypotension also occur. The hypothalamus cannot control temperature by vasoconstriction and increased metabolism; therefore, the client's body assumes the environmental temperature. Spinal shock is most severe in clients with higher levels of SCI. Clients with thoracic or lumbar injuries are often unaffected owing to the sparing of the sympathetic nervous system with these levels of injury.

Spinal shock may last for 1 to 6 weeks. Indications that spinal shock is resolving include return of reflexes, development of hyperreflexia rather than flaccidity, and return of reflex emptying of the bladder. The earliest reflexes recovered are the flexor reflexes evoked by noxious cutaneous stimulation. The return of the bulbospongiosus reflex in male patients is also an early indicator of recovery from spinal shock. Babinski's reflex (dorsiflexion of the great toe with fanning of the other toes when the sole of the foot is stroked) is an early-returning reflex.

Diagnostic Findings

Initially, full spinal x-ray films are obtained. If a high-level cervical lesion is suspected, films of the odontoid bone viewed through the open mouth may be required. CT scans may be obtained after the client has achieved hemodynamic and ventilatory stabilization. These studies provide more information regarding the nature of fractures and the status of the spinal cord. They are also useful when a fracture is not seen on x-ray films but neurologic deficit is present. MRI may also be used to locate the level of the lesion. Although controversial, myelography may be used if SCI is suspected and the degree of deficit is increasing. Somatosensory evoked potentials (SSEPs) are used to establish the extent of injury and are often performed within 48 hours of admission.

Outcome Management

Both the initial (especially during the first hour after injury) and long-term interventions provided for a client who has sustained an SCI significantly influence the following:

- The extent of the injury and associated deficits
- How well the person survives the acute phase of injury
- The success of recovery and rehabilitation

People with SCI can lead productive and, in many cases, independent lives. As with head injury, information

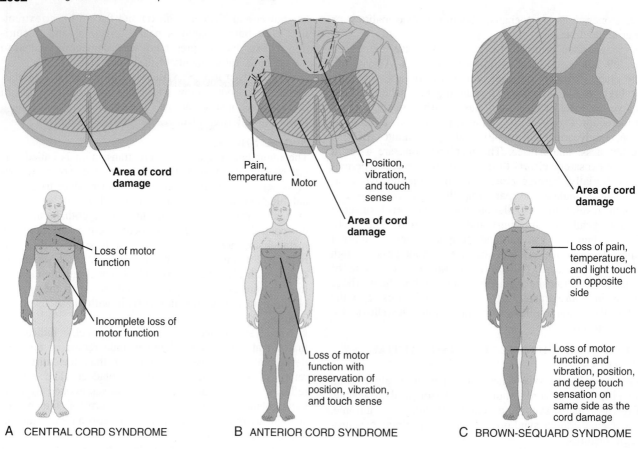

Pain, temperature Motor

Position, vibration, and touch sense

Area of cord damage

Area of cord damage

Loss of motor function

Incomplete loss of motor function

Loss of motor function with preservation of position, vibration, and touch sense

Area of cord damage

Loss of pain, temperature, and light touch on opposite side

Loss of motor function and vibration, position, and deep touch sensation on same side as the cord damage

A CENTRAL CORD SYNDROME

B ANTERIOR CORD SYNDROME

C BROWN-SÉQUARD SYNDROME

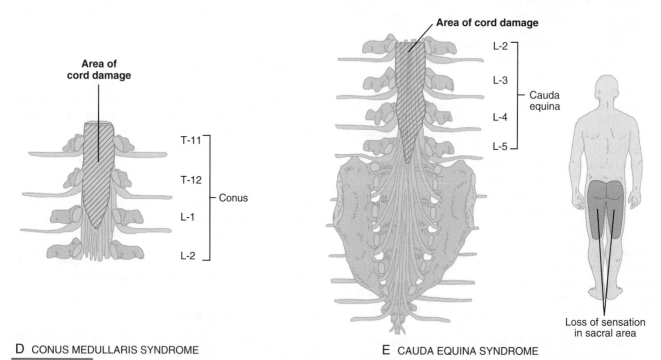

Area of cord damage

T-11

T-12

L-1

L-2

Conus

Area of cord damage

L-2

L-3

L-4

L-5

Cauda equina

Loss of sensation in sacral area

D CONUS MEDULLARIS SYNDROME

E CAUDA EQUINA SYNDROME

FIGURE 73–14 Patterns of injury leading to paralysis. *A,* Central cord syndrome. *B,* Anterior cord syndrome. *C,* Brown-Séquard syndrome. *D,* Conus medullaris syndrome. *E,* Cauda equina syndrome.

obtained from witnesses to the accident can assist in diagnosis and treatment. Information from witnesses or the client should include mechanism of injury, presence and duration of loss of consciousness, and impairment of motor function. It is also important to diagnose SCI correctly. Delays in diagnosis can be attributed to alcohol intoxication, concomitant head injury, or other multiple injuries.

Initial Care

At the scene of the accident, the injured person should be moved only when there are adequate numbers of people to accomplish this with immobilization of the spine. The neck should be stabilized in a neutral position without flexion or extension until a fixed immobilizing device can be applied. Cervical traction should not be applied. Without x-ray films to guide movements, the spinal cord can be injured. The simplest method of immobilizing the spine is to place the affected person on a spine board and to secure the spine with a hard collar around the neck and self-fastening ties across the torso and legs. Transparent stiff collars have become popular because they allow visualization of the carotid arteries and trachea. Excellent on-the-scene care has increased the number of persons who are neurologically intact despite vertebral column fractures.[28] Accurate reporting of the person's baseline deficits is essential to help the physician plan the aggressiveness of treatment interventions.

Spinal trauma is often associated with other injuries such as head injury, chest trauma, extremity fractures, and abdominal injury. Anyone who has sustained multiple trauma should be handled as if spinal injuries were present until assessment proves otherwise. In handling a client suspected of having a cervical spine injury, the spine is kept in neutral alignment and flexion is prevented.

If turning is required, a *logrolling* maneuver is used. The client is placed in a supine position on a firm surface. The head is supported in alignment with the body and is immobilized with a firm, padded cervical collar. Some physicians use halter traction immediately to keep the cervical spine aligned and prevent movement. Clothing is cut off rather than removed. The client is transported on a flat, firm stretcher with the neck immobilized. SCI-trained personnel should remain with the client while x-ray studies are taken to ensure that the cervical spine is not moved.

Cervical spine injury may produce respiratory distress. When difficulty breathing is noted, immediate action is taken to maintain a patent airway and to provide adequate oxygenation. It is important that the client's neck not be hyperextended during intubation; therefore, the jaw thrust technique is used. Suctioning is performed as necessary to maintain a patent airway. Mechanically assisted ventilation is required when definite loss or impairment of respiratory muscle function occurs. Respiratory parameters can be used to guide a decision to mechanically ventilate the client. Serial decreases in vital capacity along with an increase in partial pressure of arterial carbon dioxide ($PaCO_2$) constitute a good predictor of impending pulmonary failure. A vital capacity of less than 15 ml/kg is cause for serious concern.

In the emergency department, a client who has sustained a severe cervical injury should be placed immediately in skeletal traction to immobilize the cervical spine and reduce the fracture and dislocation. Gardner-Wells tongs are inserted through the outer table of the skull (Fig. 73–15). Traction is applied to the tongs via rope, pulleys, and weights. Traction weight is begun with 10 to 20 pounds (4.5 to 9.1 kg) and is gradually increased to accomplish bone reduction. When proper alignment is obtained and verified by x-ray examination, the traction weight may be lessened to maintain the reduction. Traction is not used to stabilize and immobilize thoracic or lumbar spinal fractures or fracture-dislocations because there is no effective way to provide it. Therefore, the spine is kept in alignment, and logrolling is used as needed, until surgical stabilization can be performed.

A cross-table lateral x-ray film of the cervical spine is obtained before transport of the injured person. Lateral and anteroposterior x-ray studies are not usually sufficient. To visualize lower cervical fractures, it is necessary to either apply downward traction to the arms or have the arms in the swimmer's position during x-ray examination.

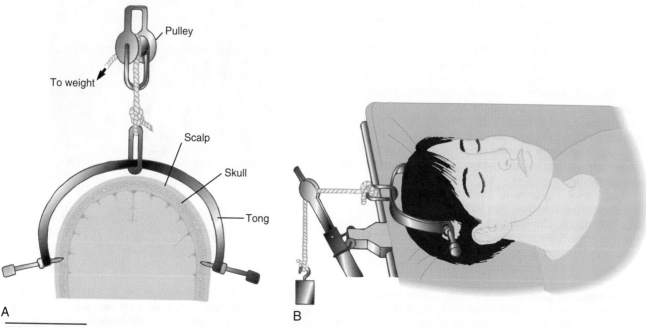

A   B

FIGURE 73–15 Skeletal traction for cervical injuries. *A,* Crutchfield tongs. *B,* Gardner-Wells tongs.

If a high-level cervical lesion is suspected, a view of the odontoid bone through the open mouth may be required. A brief but thorough neurologic examination is made to assess the extent of injury and to establish a baseline of function and involvement for later comparison.

Common emergency interventions include insertion of an IV line and infusion of normal saline, insertion of an indwelling catheter, administration of high-dose steroids, administration of vasoactive medications to maintain systolic blood pressure, insertion of a nasogastric tube, and provision of oxygen if oxygen saturation is low.

Once orthopedic and medical stabilization of the fracture has been achieved, the client is transferred to an ICU or to an SCI center. It is important that the client be appropriately immobilized before transport.

Medical Management

Once the client's spine and emergency medical conditions have been stabilized, a complete neurologic assessment is performed. Several associated injuries are commonly seen with SCI. These include orthopedic injury to the spine, head injury, chest injury, abdominal injury, and genitourinary injury. Some of these injuries may not be immediately evident in the emergency department, and ongoing assessments are made until the problem is ruled out.

The client is monitored for spinal shock and the effects of hypotension, bradycardia, and decreased cardiac output. Respiratory compromise may occur if the client develops diaphragmatic fatigue; mechanical ventilation may be needed. Arterial blood gases are monitored closely. The client may be transferred to a kinetic treatment bed to reduce the risk of pressure ulcer development, improve pulmonary function, and minimize complications of immobility. These beds are shown in Chapter 68, Figure 68–5.

Potential complications include atelectasis, pneumonia, bradycardia, hypotension, deep vein thrombosis, gastrointestinal bleeding, pressure ulcers, joint contractures, and psychological dysfunction such as denial and depression.

Vasoactive agents are commonly used to support blood pressure immediately after injury. Short-term high-dose methylprednisolone therapy is started in people with SCI less than 8 hours old. A bolus dose of 30 mg/kg infused over 1 hour followed by 5.4 mg/kg infused over 23 hours is usual. Other therapies may include the use of neuropeptides and thyrotropin-releasing hormone, which may induce some reversal of lesions by decreasing post-traumatic ischemia. Histamine-2 (H_2) receptor-blocking agents are often given to reduce the risk of gastric and intestinal bleeding. Long-term pharmacologic management may include urinary antiseptics, anticoagulants, laxatives, and antispasmodics.

Respiratory impairment, position, emotional status, or gastrointestinal function may compromise nutritional intake. Intubation eliminates the possibility of oral intake, whereas a tracheostomy does not. Clients with a tracheostomy require time to adjust to swallowing with the tube in place and must be carefully monitored to prevent aspiration.

Aspiration is also a risk for clients who must remain flat while in tongs and traction. Although these clients may be capable of swallowing, it is unlikely that they will be able to safely consume enough food to meet

their metabolic needs. Clients wearing a halo jacket (Fig. 73–16) often experience difficulty eating because the halo jacket immobilizes the head. They should be encouraged to take small bites, eat slowly, and concentrate on swallowing.

Depression is a common reaction to SCI and may be associated with inhibition of the appetite. Choosing when and what to eat may be one of the few areas of control left to the person with SCI. As much free choice of dietary intake as is feasible should be encouraged.

Any of these conditions can severely limit a spinal injury client's oral intake at a time when a high-calorie, high-protein diet is needed. Enteral feeding or total parenteral hyperalimentation is often prescribed until oral intake is sufficient to meet the body's needs.

Initial Nursing Management of the Client with Spinal Cord Injury

ASSESSMENT

A holistic assessment approach is essential in planning for nursing care of clients with SCI. Every system of the body is affected with these injuries. A complete baseline assessment is obtained initially. The results of subsequent assessments are then compared with the baseline results. Specific components in the assessment of the client with an SCI depend on the client's phase of treatment. Therefore, assessment is addressed within the following sections.

Careful monitoring of hemodynamic parameters is essential. Heart rate, blood pressure, temperature, respirations, fluid balance, and peripheral oxygen saturation (as determined by pulse oximetry) should be monitored continuously.

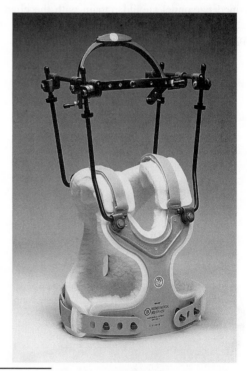

FIGURE 73–16 Halo traction. This form of traction immobilizes the cervical spine so that the client can move without risk of further injury. (Courtesy of Bremer Medical, Jacksonville, FL.)

If the client is conscious, ask whether there is any pain. Determining whether the client can feel a touch or a pinprick in the feet, legs, trunk, hands, and arms tests sensation. Levels of sensation are documented according to dermatomes. To assess motor function, ask the client to wiggle toes, move ankles, flex knees, and move hands and arms. The location, symmetry, and strength of muscle movement are documented (Table 73–3). The major reflexes—that is, the Achilles, patellar, biceps, and triceps tendon reflexes—are briefly tested. Assessment for intact sensation in areas such as the perineum is also necessary. If the patient is unresponsive, assessment is more limited. Assess respiratory status by observing for spontaneous movement and thorax expansion. Sensation and movement of extremities are assessed by watching the client for a few moments or by applying a painful stimulus (nail bed pressure) and observing for withdrawal.

Usually the client is awake and may be concerned about obtaining pain relief, the chances of survival, and the safety of any other people in the accident. Once these issues are addressed, the client may begin to appraise the severity of his or her own injury.

Rehabilitation begins when the client is admitted to the acute health care facility. During the acute stage, nursing and medical attention is appropriately focused on immediate needs. However, it is also imperative to remember that the client probably will have severe residual disabilities and must make major lifestyle changes. Care provided in the acute period can significantly affect the client's later life. Prevention of complications such as infection, pressure sores, and contractures facilitates rehabilitation and reduces suffering, disability, and expense. Challenges in care of clients with SCI is presented in the Case Study.

DIAGNOSIS, OUTCOMES, INTERVENTIONS

Risk for Hypotension. Clients suffering from SCI are at risk for the development of hypotension. The collaborative problem of *Risk for Hypotension* is related to vasodilation and the inability to vasoconstrict, rather than to volume depletion.

Outcomes. Expected outcomes for collaborative problems address actions of the nurse, rather than client outcomes. The problem is within the physician's domain; therefore, nurses monitor for it.

The nurse will monitor for hypotension. The client will have no manifestations of pulmonary fluid overload. The client's systolic blood pressure will remain greater than 90 mm Hg. The heart rate will be maintained at more than 60 BPM.

Interventions. Hypotension associated with spinal shock is initially treated with IV fluid. It is important to remember that fluid depletion is not the cause of hypotension; rather, lack of reflexes is the cause. Therefore, fluid resuscitation should be carefully monitored to avoid fluid overload, which can lead to pulmonary edema. Vasopressor agents are often given in the acute phase of SCI to maintain blood pressure.

Inability to Sustain Spontaneous Ventilation, Ineffective Airway Clearance, Impaired Gas Exchange. Cervical-level SCI carries a high risk of respiratory compromise. Any or all three of these nursing diagnoses may be appropriate.

Outcomes. The client will show no signs of respiratory compromise, as evidenced by clear lung sounds; PaO_2, PCO_2, pH, and oxygen saturation values within normal limits; unlabored respirations; and normal vital capacity.

Interventions. Chest physical therapy can help mobilize secretions and prevent pneumonia, as can suctioning and assisted coughing. When spinal cord edema has temporarily impaired respiratory function, mechanical ventilation is used to support respiration. Intubation and ventilation can be frightening to a person who has been able to breathe independently. Provide reassurance that mechanical ventilation will probably not be permanent. Clients may also be placed on a kinetic bed in order to maximize pulmonary function. Sedation is administered as needed after intubation.

For extended airway management, a tracheostomy may be required to allow for long-term controlled ventilation, to facilitate the removal of tracheobronchial secretions, and to seal off the esophagus from the trachea for the prevention of aspiration. An abdominal binder is often used to provide abdominal support, to facilitate diaphragmatic breathing, and to increase venous return.

Risk for Aspiration. Clients with a tracheostomy or ineffective airway clearance or in whom the gag reflex is absent are at higher risk for aspiration. Aspiration is a common cause of morbidity in spinal cord–injured clients.

Outcomes. The client will exhibit no signs of aspiration, as evidenced by clear lung sounds; absence of stridor and fever; minimal amounts of clear mucus upon suctioning; and PaO_2, $PaCO_2$, pH, and oxygen saturation values within normal limits.

Interventions. Suctioning equipment should be kept available and breath sounds assessed every 1 or 2 hours in acutely ill clients. The results of arterial blood gas analysis and pulse oximetry are monitored to determine the degree of oxygenation provided with mechanical ven-

TABLE 73–3	MOTOR ASSESSMENT AFTER SPINAL CORD INJURY
Spinal Nerve(s)	**Assessment Technique**
C4–5	Shoulders are shrugged against downward pressure of examiner's hands
C5–6	Arm is pulled up from resting position against resistance
C7	From the flexed position, arm is straightened out against resistance
C7	Index finger is held firmly to thumb against resistance to pull it away
C8	Hand grasp strength is evaluated
L2–4	Leg is lifted from the bed against resistance
L2–4	From flexed position, knee is extended against resistance
L5–S1	Knee is flexed against resistance
L5	Foot is pulled up toward nose against resistance
S1	Foot is pushed down (as in stepping on automobile gas pedal) against resistance

Ben Brown is a 21-year-old college junior who was admitted to the intensive care unit (ICU) via the emergency department for evaluation and treatment of a spinal cord injury (SCI) sustained in a diving accident. Consider the type of fracture most typical from this kind of accident. He is accompanied by his fiancée and his parents.

Admission Orders

Admit to ICU
Routine vital signs
Neurologic checks every hour for 24 hours
Bed rest; may logroll side to side
Maintain position of hard cervical collar
NPO status
Foley catheter with dependent drainage
IV Decadron 10 mg now and 4 mg every 4 hours
No sedation
CT scan of head and neck without contrast agent

Skeletal tongs are applied at the bedside, and cervical traction is instituted.

Nursing Admission Assessment

Ben is awake, alert, and cooperative. He has no known allergies. He states that he is an engineering major in college and is planning to be married this spring. His fiancée is an elementary education major. During the assessment, Ben makes several jokes and does not talk about or ask about his lack of sensation or movement below the nipple line. Consider the level of spinal injury that would be reflected by these manifestations.

Nursing Physical Assessment

Height: 6'2"   Weight: 170 lb (77.3 kg)
Vital signs: BP 150/90   TPR 97.6 90 22
LOC: Alert and oriented ×3
EENT: PERRLA
Cardiac: Sinus rhythm without ectopic beats, S_1 and S_2 readily audible without rubs or murmur
Pulmonary: Lung sounds clear bilaterally, diminished from the mid-lung fields to the bases
Abdominal: Abdomen is flat with active bowel sounds in all four quadrants
Genitourinary: Foley catheter in place and draining clear straw-colored urine
Peripheral pulses: 2/2, without edema noted

The CT scan reveals a compression fracture at C6 with multiple bone fragments in the spinal canal. There is no evidence of transection of the spinal cord. Consider the alternatives available to Ben for treatment of this type of injury. Ben continues to display lack of sensation and movement below the nipple line. Yesterday, Ben pushed his lunch tray on the floor and threw a flower vase at the wall. Ben's fiancée left the room in tears and stated: "The wedding is off." Consider the stage of grieving in which these manifestations might occur.

Ben is fitted for a halo brace and is scheduled to be transferred to a regional rehabilitation facility at the end of the week: "Oh, great—I'm being turfed to the freak ward." Consider the possible responses to this remark that Ben's nurse could make.

Discharge and Post-treatment Considerations

Average length of stay: 4.6 days in acute care facility followed by rehabilitation stay dictated by client's rehabilitation potential
Client transfer sheet: include most current assessment, medical treatment plan and previous laboratory work, and radiology reports
Community referrals: SCI support group, social services referral for home care or assisted living arrangements after discharge

Questions to Be Considered

1. This morning Ben complained of an excruciating headache, and BP was 210/110. Identify the etiologic factors that might cause these manifestations and the nursing interventions.
2. Compare and contrast the sensory and motor deficits expected for various levels of SCI. Include C1–2, C4–6, T4–6, L1–5, and S1–5 in your discussion. Identify the rehabilitation potential and priority nursing actions for each of these categories.
3. Identify the teaching on sexual function that is necessary for clients with SCI. When should this teaching begin?
4. Identify the key nursing actions for clients in skeletal traction for cervical injuries. Compare these nursing actions with those given after treatment for these injuries.
5. Consider the risks and benefits of halo traction versus spinal fusion for the treatment of cervical injuries.
6. Compare and contrast the nursing roles and priorities of the acute or critical care nurse and the rehabilitation nurse in caring for clients with SCI.
7. Compare and contrast the traumatic and nontraumatic disorders that may result in SCI. Consider how the source of the injury may influence nursing care.

BP, blood pressure; CT, computed tomography; EENT, eye-ear-nose-throat; IV, intravenous; LOC, level of consciousness; LOS, length of stay; NPO, nothing by mouth; PERRLA, pupils equal, round, and reactive to light and accommodation; TPR, temperature, pulse, respirations.

tilation or supplemental oxygen administration. Tracheo-bronchial suctioning is performed frequently to prevent or reduce the accumulation of secretions from immobility, lack of a cough reflex, or pneumonia. Monitor the electrocardiogram for dysrhythmias (e.g., premature ventricular contractions) due to hypoxia during suctioning.

Ineffective Thermoregulation. Thermoregulation may be altered because of loss of hypothalamic control of the sympathetic nervous system in clients with SCI above the T6 level.

Outcome. The client will maintain normothermic status.

Interventions. Rectal or core temperature is monitored every 4 hours during the first 72 hours after injury. Skin surfaces are palpated for areas of warmth, coolness, and moisture. Control the environmental temperature by using bed linens as needed to warm the client, eliminating drafts in the room, and using hypothermia blankets cautiously.

EVALUATION

The problems identified in the early period of SCI care should resolve within 72 hours, especially if there are no other serious injuries or medical problems. If the client remains in an ICU for a prolonged time, implement other aspects of SCI care as discussed later on.

◼ Surgical Management

Surgical intervention for progressive neurologic deficit is indicated for any of the following:

- Compound fractures and penetrating wounds of the spine
- Presence of bone fragments in the spinal canal
- Syndrome of acute anterior spinal cord trauma[37]

Some neurosurgeons and orthopedic surgeons recommend decompressive laminectomy for complete SCIs. In this type of surgery, the laminae of the vertebrae are removed to minimize pressure on the spinal cord. Others believe that laminectomy should not be used routinely to treat SCI. Similarly, some surgeons recommend stabilization by surgical fusion within the first few days after trauma, whereas others do not. Insertion of metal plates and screws or the use of bone grafts or a combination of these accomplishes fusion.

Cervical fractures can also be allowed to heal with stabilization of bone fragments achieved by immobilization in a brace or halo jacket (see Fig. 73–16). The halo jacket has a ring that is fixed to the skull with pins. This ring is then attached to the jacket by rods. This system provides the traction required to maintain cervical alignment. A halo jacket allows early mobilization and rehabilitation. The wrench that comes with the brace should always be taped to the front of the jacket, to allow quick removal in case of emergency. Never grasp the rods to help reposition the client. If the client has some mobility remaining, always assist during the client's first attempt at any activity. The halo jacket changes the client's center of gravity, making falls a constant risk. Perform pin site care around the pin insertion sites daily. Refer to your agency's policy manual for guidelines.

Burst fractures of the thoracic and lumbar spinal segments can be treated with body casts, Harrington rods, or other devices for spine stabilization. Spine stabilization devices are commonly inserted through a posterior incision (Fig. 73–17). After the operation, perform the usual postoperative assessments, including an assessment of the neurovascular status of the legs. Chest tubes and nasogastric tubes are inserted during surgery. The client is log-rolled to facilitate maintenance of respiration and skin perfusion. Pain is managed with continuous-infusion or injected narcotics. The client usually is fitted for a body brace, and mobilization begins on the fourth day.

Complications of surgery include infection and poor wound healing, as well as those related to anesthesia. Both infection and impaired wound healing are more likely to occur in a malnourished client.

◼ Spinal Cord Injury Rehabilitation

In 1970, the United States Rehabilitation Service Administration adopted a model system for rehabilitation of spinal cord–injured people. The key to the system is the use of multidisciplinary teams of physicians, nurses, and allied health care providers (physical therapists, occupational therapists, speech and language pathologists) to reduce morbidity, maximize functional recovery, and promote independence.

ESTABLISH FUNCTIONAL GOALS

Prediction of functional ability after SCI can generally be guided by the degree of residual muscle function (Table 73–4). Clients with all levels of injury and of all ages benefit from rehabilitation. The client and family are involved in all phases. The client delegates needed skills to another caregiver so that care can be provided at home. The skills learned in a rehabilitation setting must be adapted to the home environment and community setting before hospital discharge. This process can be accomplished by use of therapeutic weekend passes and partici-

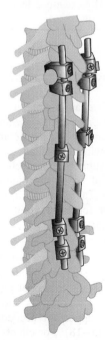

FIGURE 73–17 Fractures of the spine are often stabilized with internal fixation devices.

TABLE 73-4	FUNCTIONAL GOALS IN REHABILITATION AFTER SPINAL CORD INJURY	

Spinal Cord Level	Muscle Function	Functional Goals
C1-2	No phrenic nerve function	Respirations managed with phrenic pacemaker
C3-4	Neck control; scapular elevators; diaphragm function may be weak or absent	Manipulate electric wheelchair with breath control, chin control, or voice activation
C5	Fair to good shoulder control; functional deltoids/biceps; elbow flexion	Dress upper trunk; turn self in bed with or without arm slings Propel wheelchair with hand splints or after tenodesis Assist in getting into and out of bed May learn to write or type
C6	Good shoulder control; wrist extension; supinators	Dress upper trunk; sometimes dress lower trunk Propel wheelchair with hand rim projections Self-feeding with hand splints Transfer from wheelchair to bed with or without minimal assistance (e.g., sliding board) Assist in getting to and from bedside commode; self-catheterization
C7	Possibly weak shoulder depression; weak elbow extension; some hand function; triceps	Independent in transfer to bed, car, and toilet Total dressing independence Propel wheelchair with standard hand rims Self-feeding with no assistive devices
T1-4	Good to normal upper extremity muscle function; intrinsic muscles of the hand; no trunk control	Independent in transfer to bed, car, and toilet Total dressing independence Propel wheelchair with standard hand rims Self-feeding with no assistive devices Transfer from wheelchair to floor and return Propel wheelchair up and down curb Transfer from wheelchair to tub and return
T5-L2	Partial to good trunk stability	Total wheelchair independence Limited ambulation with bilateral long leg braces and crutches (injury at T12 or below)
L3-4	All trunk-pelvic stabilizers intact; hip flexors, adductors, quadriceps	Ambulation with short leg braces with or without crutches, depending on level of injury
L5-S3	Hip extensors, abductors; knee flexors; ankle control	No equipment needed if plantiflexion is strong enough for push-off at end of stance

pation in community activities as a part of the rehabilitation process.

In all phases of rehabilitation, it is imperative that a motivated client be given the opportunity to perform any skill, even if the nurse or the physician can accomplish it more quickly. Allowing the client to attempt a complex skill demonstrates support of the client's self-care abilities. A description of functional outcomes for rehabilitation is provided in Table 73-4. It is intended to be a guide and may not represent ability in all clients with various levels of injury.

Promote Mobility

Wheelchairs provide mobility, and having the proper wheelchair is crucial. The wheelchair design must provide the client with the ability to propel the chair and prevent development of spinal deformities and pressure ulcers. A high back and head support are needed for clients without arm function (Fig. 73-18). For clients who can use their arms, the back of the wheelchair should be at the level of the scapula and the wheelchair should be lower than normal to facilitate transfers. Cushions help reduce pressure and the risk of pressure ulcers. However, cushions do not prevent pressure ulcers, and weight shifts are still needed every 10 to 15 minutes of time spent in the wheelchair. Physical therapists work with the client to teach how to transfer from bed to a wheelchair, from a wheelchair into and out of a car, and from the wheelchair onto a toilet.

Current emphasis is on strengthening muscles rather than using braces. However, back braces may be prescribed after lumbar spinal injury or for intervertebral disc problems. More frequently, a thoracolumbosacral orthosis is used. This device is a custom-made plastic brace with front and back pieces that attach together with self-fastening straps. This brace provides stability for the healing spine. The nurse is responsible for supervising the unlicensed professional whenever he or she is assisting with positioning transfers for a client with a spinal abnormality.

Reduce Spasticity

Spasticity often interferes with positioning and functional activities. Spasticity does serve to maintain muscle bulk

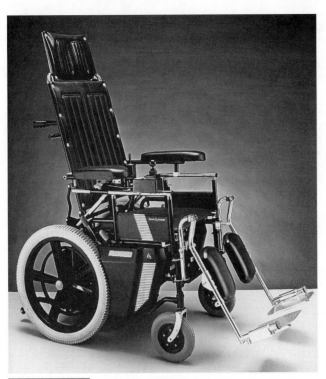

FIGURE 73–18 A wheelchair with power hand controls for clients with C1–3 cervical spine injury. A respirator can be attached to the wheelchair. (Courtesy of Everett and Jennings, St. Louis, MO.)

and venous return and can aid in transfers. Treatment includes range-of-motion (ROM) exercises and antispasmotic medications such as baclofen, dantrolene sodium, and clonidine. Medications for the treatment of spasms are given only when the spasms cause discomfort or safety concerns.

Improve Bladder and Bowel Control

The term *neurogenic bladder* is used to describe bladder control changes that occur with both upper and lower motor neuron disorders. Upper motor neuron disorders produce a spastic or reflex bladder. Lower motor neuron disorders produce a flaccid bladder. There are many ways to manage the bladder, and treatment options must be tailored to fit the client's preferences and lifestyle as well as his or her functional abilities.

Most clients with arm function are taught to empty their bladder using the Credé maneuver over the bladder to relax the sphincter and express urine (see Bladder Retraining in the nursing management section later on). To ensure complete emptying, this method is often combined with other techniques such as catheterization and use of external catheters. Intermittent catheterization reduces the risk of infection and bladder stone formation caused by indwelling catheters. Clients with injuries at the C6 level and lower can perform self-catheterization, although the technique requires adequate hand function and the ability to manage lower extremity clothing. External catheters are used for men who void between catheterizations or for those who leak urine during bladder spasms.

Suprapubic catheters seem to offer the advantages of less infection and urethral injury over indwelling cathe-

ters. Indwelling catheters are not ideal from a medical standpoint but are preferred by many clients because of the ease of management. Complications include infection, bladder stones, urethral damage, and a reported increased incidence of bladder cancer. A neurogenic bladder may also be managed pharmacologically with medications such as bethanechol (Urecholine) to stimulate bladder contraction. Urine-acidifying agents may also be prescribed to reduce the risk of infection.

A neurogenic bowel is similar to a neurogenic bladder in that the client cannot control defecation. The goal is to develop a bowel elimination method that is convenient, effective, and least expensive for the client. Sufficient fluid and fiber intake is essential. When fiber is added to or increased in the diet, it must be done slowly to avoid cramping and diarrhea. Stool softeners and bulk laxatives may also be used.

Bowel movements of clients with upper motor neuron damage are generally regulated with suppositories or digital stimulation every day, or every other day to reduce the risk of autonomic dysreflexia. A lower motor neuron neurogenic bowel is more difficult to regulate, and often the client requires manual removal of impacted material.

Prevent Pressure Ulcers

Anesthetic skin is associated with any increased frequency of pressure ulcers. During the acute care period, the risk of pressure ulcer development is related to the level of injury, completeness of the injury, and duration of immobilization. Guidelines based on many studies recommend that clients be turned or have their weight shifted at least every 2 hours. The Agency for Health Care Policy and Research (AHCPR) guidelines for prevention of skin injury include completing a daily systematic skin inspection, using proper positioning techniques (to minimize shearing and friction effects), maintaining adequate nutritional support, minimizing environmental exposure (i.e., excessive moisture or dryness), and avoiding massage over bony prominences. Prevention of pressure ulcers should include use of pressure-relieving devices (such as cushions or specialty bed). Wheelchair-bound clients are taught to relieve pressure every 15 minutes.

Reduce Respiratory Dysfunction

Respiratory dysfunction is a significant cause of morbidity and mortality after SCI. The diaphragm may be the only functional muscle active in respiration because the intercostal and abdominal muscles are often paralyzed. Vital capacity and inspiratory reserve volume are markedly diminished. The client should be taught to use incentive spirometry and diaphragmatic breathing to enhance vital capacity. Glossopharyngeal breathing uses the tongue and muscles of the pharynx to force air into the lungs. This technique enhances vital capacity and promotes chest expansion.

Promote Expression of Sexuality

Sexual function in spinal cord–injured men depends on the location of the lesion (Table 73–5). Reflex erection is possible in some clients with upper motor neuron lesions and also with some lower motor neuron lesions. Ejaculation is possible with lower motor neuron lesions and if the lesion is more caudal. Unfortunately, the fertility rate is about 5%, but it is hoped that this rate will improve

TABLE 73–5	SEXUAL FUNCTION IN CLIENTS WITH SPINAL CORD INJURY	
Sexuality	**Reproductive Functioning**	**Special Considerations for Contraceptive Methods**
FEMALES		
Lesions at C1–3: Reflex lubrication is probable; erogenous areas may develop above injury; libido is intact **Lesions at C4–6:** Psychogenic lubrication is unlikely; nongenital orgasm may be experienced **Lesions at C7:** Able to use hands for holding and caressing **Lesions at T12–L5:** Psychogenic stimulation of the clitoris, lubrication, labial swelling, and skin flush are possible but unlikely	Menstruation and fertility unaffected Pregnancy is not affected Incidence of bladder infection during pregnancy increases Risk of autonomic hyperreflexia during labor and delivery increases	Birth control pills are contraindicated when circulatory problems are present Thrombophlebitis and other problems could go undetected owing to lack of sensation in extremities Intrauterine devices may be contraindicated because of pelvic inflammatory disease Client must be able to assess for vaginal bleeding
MALES		
Lesions at C1–3: Reflex erection is caused by genital stimulation psychogenic erection is not possible; erogenous zones above injury site may develop; libido is intact **Lesions at C4–6:** Reflex erection is possible; nongenital orgasm may be experienced; no ejaculation; oral sex is possible; libido is intact **Lesions at C7:** Holding and caressing with hands is possible **Lesions at T12–L6:** Psychogenic stimulation and erection are possible; no reflex erection **Lesions at S2–4:** Reflex erection is possible; ejaculation is possible but may be retrograde	Semen can be obtained from the bladder of clients who have retrograde ejaculation For clients who cannot ejaculate, semen can be obtained through glandular vibratory stimulation In general, semen quality is impaired, with poor motility the most common abnormality Some clients are candidates for penile prosthesis	Client or partner may apply condom

with advances in technology. It is becoming a common practice for semen to be collected and frozen for later in vivo fertilization. Sexual dysfunction is approached from two avenues: psychological counseling and education about technological advances in the facilitation of sexual activity. Erection can be restored with external aids, an implantable penile prosthesis, or medications.

Female clients retain fertility after SCI. Problems with sexual function generally relate to positioning and the lack of vaginal lubrication. These problems can usually be addressed through client education.

Control Pain

Long-term pain occurs in almost all spinal cord–injured clients with intact sensation. Dysesthetic pain, which is distal to the site of injury, is extremely disabling. It is similar to the phantom pain experienced after amputation. It is described as cutting, burning, piercing, radiating, or tightening. The usual treatment is with non-narcotic analgesics and transcutaneous nerve stimulators. A prn (as-needed) approach to pain management is not recommended for chronic pain. However, routine analgesics may need to be supplemented with other pain-relieving medications given prn during a client's pain peaks.

Reduce Abnormal Bone Growth

Heterotopic ossification is the formation of bone in abnormal locations, occurring most often around the hips and knees after SCI. The client may develop swelling in the joint or loss of ROM. Heterotopic ossification is diagnosed by x-ray study or bone scan. Treatment includes the use of etidronate disodium (Didronel) and ROM exercises of the affected joints. Sometimes the bone is removed surgically.

Promote Psychological Adjustment

Psychological counseling is ongoing. Commonly, spinal cord–injured clients participate in peer group counseling sessions in which experiences and solutions are shared to help newly injured clients to cope better with their losses. Vocational rehabilitation may help clients reach their maximum rehabilitation potential.

■ Ongoing Nursing Management of the Client with Spinal Cord Injury

ASSESSMENT

The client usually is transferred from the ICU after becoming hemodynamically stable. Clients with high cervical injuries may remain on ventilators. The care of the ventilator-dependent client is discussed in Chapter 63. Some of the nursing diagnoses that applied in the critical care unit may still apply after transfer. The client remains at risk for skin impairment and may still have difficulty swallowing, with attendant risk for aspiration. A baseline assessment should be completed upon transfer.

DIAGNOSIS, OUTCOMES, INTERVENTIONS

Impaired Physical Mobility. SCI causing permanent impaired physical mobility produces problems with ambulation and potential complications arising from immobility. The relevant diagnosis is *Impaired Physical Mobility related to inability to move upper and/or lower extremities secondary to paralysis.*

Outcomes. The client will have maximal physical mobility, as evidenced by absence of tendon contractures, joint ankylosis, and muscle shortening and will demonstrate effective use of adaptive devices.

Interventions. Throughout the acute and rehabilitative phases of nursing care, make every effort to maximize functional abilities and independence by encouraging the client to perform independently any activities of daily living (ADL) for which capability remains.

Provide Positioning and Adaptive Equipment. Improper positioning of the client in the bed or chair and lack of joint movements (e.g., related to spasticity or immobility) lead to tendon contractures, joint ankylosis, and muscle shortening. Interventions to prevent such problems include the following:

- Frequent position changes
- Proper positioning of joints
- Use of splints and removable casts
- Intermittent turning to a prone position
- Positioning of upper extremities away from the body
- Draping of bed linen over frames to keep pressure off the feet
- Keeping knee joints flexed 15 degrees when the client is supine
- Use of active and passive conditioning exercises (see Risk for Contractures later on)

Wristdrop and footdrop are inevitable sequelae in paralyzed extremities unless specific preventive measures are used. Footdrop may be prevented by keeping the client's feet firmly supported in dorsiflexion at right angles to the hips to counteract the force of gravity on weakened muscles. Many devices are available to prevent footdrop. Skin must be frequently assessed to prevent associated skin breakdown. Support a paralyzed arm in a sling when the client is out of bed and in a cock-up splint when the client is in bed. Usually, the hand end of the splint is elevated 2 inches to support the wrist, and the fingers are maintained in a position of function. Posterior molded casts may be used instead of splints to support a paralyzed wrist while the client is in bed. For some clients, pillows and a hand roll are adequate.

Assist with Transfers and Ambulation. Rehabilitative programs often require strength and endurance. To prepare a client for ambulation, the unaffected parts of the body must be strengthened and suitable exercises started early. Tolerance for activity gradually increases. Take care not to fatigue the client. Periods of planned rest and recreation are important.

Physical therapy is essential for all clients with SCI. Paraplegic clients need to learn various transfers in order to become self-sufficient. One transfer method is illustrated in Figure 73–19. Learning to sit up precedes learning to transfer. Many paralyzed clients become mobile by using a wheelchair. Many types of wheelchairs are available, and selection needs to be made carefully, according to individual needs.

The brace or corset should be applied before the client is assisted to get out of bed. A thin, knitted undershirt is worn under the brace or corset to protect the skin and to keep the appliance clean. To apply the brace or corset, turn the client to one side, place the appliance against the back, and then roll the client back into it. The brace or corset is secured while the client lies supine. As recovery and rehabilitation progress, many clients learn to apply their own brace or corset while in bed. Others continue to need help. The degree of arm and hand function determines the client's ability to apply a brace.

Weight-bearing begins as early as possible after SCI. Weight-bearing stimulates osteoblastic activity and thus decreases demineralization of bone *(osteoporosis)* that develops with prolonged immobilization. Use of a standing board or tilt table assists the person to gradually tolerate a standing position. Having the client assume a standing position periodically each day also helps prevent contrac-

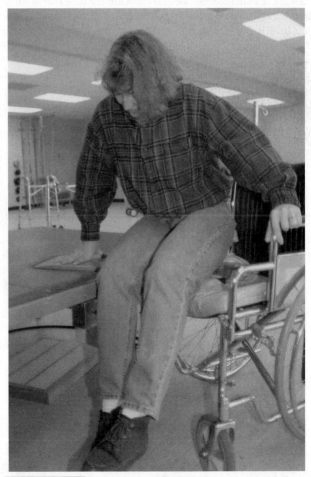

FIGURE 73–19 Bed-to-wheelchair lateral transfer using a sliding board.

tures (e.g., hip contractures resulting from long periods of sitting).

Take care in helping clients to stand or sit in a chair for the first time. Because of the effects of loss of muscular activity on the peripheral venous system, these clients are prone to orthostatic hypotension. Always check blood pressure before and after transfers. Syncope during a wheelchair transfer may be avoided in the quadriplegic client by use of an abdominal binder, thigh-high support hose, and slowly elevating the head of the bed to 90 degrees. Using a recliner or a wheelchair with an adjustable back will help achieve gradual elevations.

Clients easily lose balance when wearing braces, particularly the halo brace, and must be very careful to avoid falling. The accompanying Client Education Guide describes the use of a halo vest. A brace feels surprisingly heavy at first, especially if the client is weak. For safety, shoes, rather than slippers or just stockings or socks, should be worn during ambulation. Shoes should tie or have self-fastening straps for firm support and have a low heel. High-top athletic shoes give added support. Slick soles, high or narrow heels, and stockinged feet are hazardous. Wearing shoes also helps prevent footdrop when the client lies down.

The fit, comfort, and appearance of braces, corsets, and shoes are important to the client. Try to accommodate the preferences of clients who want to be as stylish as possible as well as benefit from therapeutic garments. Disabled clients are helped by being encouraged to express their feelings concerning their self-image and by having their desires taken into consideration when being fitted for therapeutic garments. Some garments can be painful when

first worn. The pain worsens if the garments do not fit properly. The client's skin should be inspected frequently, especially at first, because pressure sores can develop very quickly.

Ineffective Airway Clearance. Airway clearance may be impaired because of paralysis of the abdominal and intercostal muscles. The relevant nursing diagnosis is *Ineffective Airway Clearance related to inability to cough.*

Outcomes. The client will participate in "quad-assisted" coughing, remain afebrile, and have normal blood gas or pulse oximetry values and clear sputum.

Interventions. Use the "quad-assisted" cough manuever to promote airway clearance. As for the Heimlich maneuver, place a fist or heel of the hand between the umbilicus and the xiphoid process. Press inward and upward during the client's cough. Other interventions, such as turning, hydration, and chest physical therapy, may also be used.

Risk for Contractures. Active ROM is severely limited or nonexistent in the upper extremities and nonexistent in the lower extremities in a client with cervical cord damage; it is also nonexistent in the lower extremities in a client with thoracic or lumbar cord damage. This deficit increases the risk for contractures. The nursing diagnosis is *Risk for Contractures related to inability to move purposefully.*

Outcomes. Monitor the client for changes in ROM in all joints. The client will have no change in ROM compared with the level before injury.

Interventions. Passive exercises prevent contractures and painful reflex dystrophies of the hand and shoulder.

CLIENT EDUCATION GUIDE

Use of a Halo Vest

- The vest or the halo ring bolts are to be adjusted only by the neurosurgeon or by someone designated to do so. If the bolts become loose, tell your physician.
- Use fleece or foam inserts to relieve discomfort at pressure points.
- Keep the vest lining dry. If the fleece gets wet, dry it with a hair dryer (on a cool setting); do not allow the fleece to become matted.
- Clean the pins at least once a day; cleaning agents include soap and water applied using cotton-tipped swabs, alcohol swabs, or shampoo soap if hair is being washed. Crusts can be removed using hydrogen peroxide or alcohol. Ointments and antiseptics are not recommended for routine care. Use a separate sterile swab for each pin site.
- Report redness, swelling, drainage, open areas around the pin (tracking), pain, tenderness, or a clicking noise from the pin site. Retightening is usually necessary during the first 24 to 48 hours for the first week.
- Recheck the pins every 2 to 3 weeks.
- Wash the skin under the vest. Use a bath towel wrung out in hot water (alcohol is permitted) and pull it back and forth. Do not use soap, lotion, or powder because it cannot be removed adequately. Assess daily for skin breakdown under the vest using a flashlight. Showering is prohibited. A sponge bath or tub bath with minimal water to prevent the vest liner from getting wet may be

permitted. When the hair is shampooed, the shoulders and neck of the vest must be protected with plastic. Do not use any products other than shampoo on your hair (no dyes, tints, sprays, or conditioners).
- When getting out of bed, roll onto your side and push on the mattress with your arm; sitting straight up puts too much stress on the front pins. *Never use the metal frame for turning or lifting!*
- A rolled towel or pillowcase between the back of your neck and the bed or next to your cheek when lying on your side and raising the head of the bed will increase sleeping comfort.
- Adapt your clothing to fit over the halo, or select clothing with button, self-fastening, or zipper closures. The vest will be needed for about 3 months, followed by a hard collar.
- Eat food products high in protein and calcium to promote bone healing.
- Have the correct size of wrench with you in case of an emergency. The anterior portion of the vest including the anterior bolts can then be loosened as necessary; the posterior portion of the vest should remain in place to provide stability for the spine during cardiopulmonary resuscitation.

Adapted from Reid, B., & Marr, J. (1990). *Health professional's guide to caring for the client with a halo vest* (pp. 1–12). Jacksonville, FL: Bremer Medical.

Such exercises may be prescribed as soon as 48 to 72 hours after injury. Active exercises, massage, and electrical stimulation may also be prescribed. Begin shoulder and arm exercises early. Strength in these areas and in the chest and back is essential for effective self-transfers and ambulation when the lower spine is stable enough to permit mobilization.

Self-Care Deficit. The client who has suffered an SCI is often unable to perform many self-care activities.

Outcomes. The client will independently perform as many ADL tasks as possible. If unable to independently perform an activity, the client will be able to direct a caregiver's performance. These goals will be evaluated by observing successful performance of ADL by the client or under the client's direction.

Interventions. Self-care deficit can lead to a feeling of powerlessness. Assisting the client to maximize independence can lessen this feeling. The client is assisted with muscle-strengthening exercises and the use of adaptive devices. Clients with high cervical injuries are able to perform very few activities independently. Allow them adequate time to accomplish whatever tasks they can. If help with ADL is needed, adapt nursing care to the client's routine. In collaborating to maintain intact oral mucous membranes, a schedule is established for brushing teeth at least twice daily and cleaning the tongue, roof of the mouth, and gums with agents not containing lemon or alcohol.

Risk for Altered Nutrition: Less Than Body Requirements. After traumatic injury there is increased metabolic demand because of the response to stress and the body's requirements for healing. The relevant nursing diagnosis is written *Risk for Altered Nutrition: Less Than Body Requirements related to increased metabolic demand and inability to access nutrients.* Anorexia related to depression may be another etiologic factor.

Outcomes. The client will not experience excessive weight loss (more than 10 lb) during hospitalization.

Interventions. The client should be weighed on admission to obtain a baseline measurement. Nutrient supplementation should begin by 72 hours after injury if the client is not eating. Enteral feeding can be used if the client has bowel sounds. If the client still has paralytic ileus, hyperalimentation is commonly used. Weigh the client at least once a week to monitor progress.

Total Incontinence. Observe the client carefully for indications of faulty bladder control and infection, including incontinence, retention, urgency, dribbling, frequency, enuresis, and precipitate micturition. Document such observations and inform the physician. The relevant nursing diagnosis is written *Total Incontinence related to paralysis.*

Outcomes. The client will have improved bladder control, as evidenced by no infection and emptying of the bladder every 4 to 6 hours.

Interventions. Nursing intervention is planned to prevent urinary tract infection, to preserve existing bladder capacity and muscle tone, and to establish and maintain a routine pattern of elimination requiring minimal artificial assistance.

Urinary bladder atony (absence of tone) may last several weeks or months after SCI. In clients with upper motor neuron lesions, when spinal shock subsides and the reflexes return, as evidenced by an increase in rectal tone, a reflex contraction will empty the bladder. During the period of atony, a retention catheter may be inserted to prevent bladder distention and keep the client dry and comfortable. Bladder overdistention causes stretching and fissure formation—a predisposing factor for infection—and may result in bladder rupture. When sensory pathways are damaged, the client does not feel the discomfort of bladder distention. However, prolonged catheter use also predisposes to infection. Therefore, catheterization every 6 hours is preferred over a retention catheter.

Urinary complications may be avoided by periodically examining the client for bladder distention, accurately documenting fluid intake and output, using aseptic technique when handling urinary catheters, and observing for signs of bladder infection. Encourage the client to drink water to keep the urine diluted, which lessens the possibility of infection. Urine acidifiers may be prescribed.

Urinary complications occur because of incomplete emptying of the bladder, necessitating catheterization. Catheterization may predispose the client to infection and vesicoureteral reflux, which may lead to kidney complications. Renal calculi, pyelonephritis, and hydronephrosis are major causes of considerable disability and even death in paralyzed clients.

To prevent development of renal calculi, encourage the client to drink about 3000 ml of fluid per day, unless contraindicated by other medical conditions. This is sufficient to maintain a minimal urinary output of 2000 ml per day. Drinking this much fluid may increase incontinence but is necessary to prevent renal calculi.

Bowel Incontinence or Constipation. Bowel dysfunction is a common but manageable problem in a client with SCI. This common nursing diagnosis is written as *Constipation related to paralysis.*

Outcomes. The client will have reduced risk of bowel incontinence or constipation, as evidenced by a bowel movement every 1 to 2 days, no signs of fecal impaction, no incontinence, and no signs of hyperreflexia.

Interventions. Nursing intervention is planned to prevent constipation, distention, and impaction; to detect and treat these conditions if they occur; and to reestablish habitual, controlled bowel movements by conditioned reflex activity. Paralytic ileus is common after SCI. By frequently assessing bowel sounds and documenting the passage of stool, return of peristalsis can be determined, and the client can resume oral intake. The client is observed carefully for indications of constipation, diarrhea, or tenesmus (straining at stool). If the bowel becomes impacted, a cleansing enema may be prescribed to initially empty the lower bowel. However, enemas should be avoided for long-term bowel management. A paraplegic or quadriplegic client cannot retain an enema solution, nor can the degree of intestinal distention be felt. Therefore, enemas must be administered carefully to avoid overdistending the intestine with excessive fluid; 500 ml or less is usually given.

The client's intake of fluid and food and elimination patterns are documented. The routine daily pattern of bowel elimination is established, with the client using suppositories and other means of stimulating evacuation until reflex evacuation occurs.

A daily fluid intake of 3000 ml per day is important for proper bowel function as well as bladder function. Also, the diet must be high in bulk and roughage such as bran, whole grains, fresh and dried fruits, and leafy green and raw vegetables. A stool softener such as docusate sodium (Colace) may be taken daily, but laxatives should be carefully administered. Bulk-forming medications (e.g., psyllium hydrophilic mucilloid [Metamucil]) are very effective for spinal cord–injured clients so long as adequate hydration is maintained.

Risk for Impaired Skin Integrity. Clients with SCI are at higher risk of impairment of skin integrity because of immobility and loss of protective functions.

Outcomes. The client will have intact skin, as evidenced by no reddened areas over bony prominences and no areas or signs of skin irritation or dryness.

Interventions. The spinal cord–injured client cannot respond to the sensory cues to local tissue hypoxia resulting from being in one position for an extended period of time. Impaired skin sensation occurring with quadriplegia and paraplegia predisposes the client to the development of pressure ulcers and other injuries. Spinal cord–injured clients should be placed on pressure-reducing beds or mattresses. However, the use of these special beds does not eliminate the need to assess the skin every 2 to 4 hours and does not eliminate the risk of pressure ulcers. In addition, the client's nutritional needs must be met to reduce the risk of pressure ulcers.

A client with spinal fractures may be placed on a Roto-Rest bed. A Roto-Rest bed is currently popular for management of clients with SCI or other disorders requiring prolonged immobilization (see Chapter 68, Fig. 68–5). It is equipped with supportive packs and straps that keep the body in neutral alignment while it continuously oscillates from side to side. If rotation is greater than 35 degrees, the continuous motion helps prevent skin breakdown, reduce urinary stasis, and promote lung aeration. Unfortunately, the constant movement may also stimulate peristalsis, resulting in severe diarrhea. Some clients also experience disorientation from the constant movement and have reported fear of falling. Staff members should remain with the client initially to provide emotional support and reassurance. Also, it is important to pull window curtains at night, as a client in a Roto-Rest bed who can see himself or herself "floating" in the window reflection can become disoriented or frightened.

Chronic Pain. Clients with SCI may experience pain at the level of the injury and radiating along spinal nerves originating in the area. Phantom pain may also be experienced. The onset of pain is usually later than for muscle spasms. Some paraplegic and quadriplegic clients experience both pain and spasm. Pain most often occurs in the lower extremities.

Outcomes. The client will experience adequate pain relief, as evidenced by verbalization of improvement in comfort, ability to rest without interruption by pain, and ability to participate in therapies without hindrance by pain.

Interventions. Analgesics such as aspirin and nonsteroidal anti-inflammatory drugs (NSAIDs) may be prescribed. Narcotics are seldom used after the initial injury and are contraindicated in clients with high cervical-level injuries because of the risk of respiratory depression.

Clients with thoracic pulmonary injuries tend to breathe more shallowly to avoid pain. Inadequate depth of respirations can lead to complications. Give prescribed pain medication and encourage deep-breathing and coughing to aerate the lungs and remove secretions from the respiratory tract.

Antispasmodics, NSAIDs, and non-narcotic analgesics are prescribed for pain associated with spasticity. Surgery (e.g., neurectomy, chordotomy) is sometimes required for pain relief.

Risk for Autonomic Dysreflexia. Autonomic dysreflexia/hyperreflexia is a serious complication of SCI when injury is above the T6 level. This collaborative problem is documented as *Risk for Autonomic Dysreflexia related to spinal cord injury.*

Outcomes. The nurse will monitor for clinical manifestations of autonomic dysreflexia and respond to them quickly.

Interventions. Assess the client for sudden onset of severe hypertension, severe throbbing headache, profuse diaphoresis, flushing of the skin above the level of the lesion, nasal stuffiness, pilomotor spasm, blurred vision, nausea, and bradycardia. (See the Critical Monitoring feature.)

Educate the client about early warning signs and symptoms of autonomic dysreflexia and the importance of calling for a nurse immediately should any occur. Adaptive call lights are available to facilitate calling for assistance. If autonomic dysreflexia does occur, institute the following measures:

1. Elevate the head of the bed to a sitting position immediately.
2. Check blood pressure.
3. Check for possible sources of irritation (e.g., kinked or clogged catheter or distended bladder or lower bowel).
4. Remove the stimulus if it can be done quickly. Once the source of irritation is removed, manifestations of autonomic dysreflexia usually subside.
5. If blood pressure remains elevated, antihypertensive medication (nitrates, hydralazine, guanethidine, or diazoxide) may be administered according to pre-

---

CRITICAL MONITORING

Features of Autonomic Dysreflexia

- Severe hypertension (up to 300 mm Hg)
- Pounding headache
- Flushing (above the level of the lesion)
- Piloerection
- Diaphoresis
- Dilated pupils, blurred vision
- Nasal stuffiness
- Bradycardia (pulse < 60 BPM)
- Restlessness
- Nausea

scription or procedural policy (intravenously, intranasally, or sublingually).

6. If there is no order or policy or if these measures do not correct the problem, notify the physician.

Once manifestations have subsided, observe the client's vital signs and neurologic status closely for 3 to 4 hours. If an antihypertensive medication has been given, the client may become hypotensive after the stimulus is removed. Autonomic dysreflexia may recur if the stimulus is not completely removed. If the identified source is bladder distention, use caution when emptying the bladder. Remove 500 ml every 5 to 15 minutes. If the identified source of irritation is bowel distention, be very careful when removing the impacted material from the bowel. An anesthetic lubricant is used, and another nurse must monitor the client's blood pressure every few minutes. The stimulation of trying to remove the impacted material can increase the severity of the autonomic response. When a quadriplegic client complains of a headache, *do not automatically give analgesics without first checking the blood pressure.*

Risk for Injury. In clients with SCI, another appropriate nursing diagnosis is *Risk for Injury related to abnormal reflexes, spasms, and corneal drying.* Corneal abrasions may result unless proper interventions are instituted.

Outcomes. The client will sustain no injuries due to spasms, as evidenced by no abrasions or bruising. Corneal abrasions will not occur.

Interventions. Injections should be avoided whenever possible. Medications should be given orally or IV if needed. When injections are unavoidable, give above the level of the cord lesion whenever possible. Absorption may be compromised in denervated areas of the body with impaired capillary and precapillary circulation. Moisten the cornea with natural tears every 4 hours for a client with altered blinking reflexes.

Clients can also be injured from involuntary spasms. Avoid unnecessary stimulation of areas that elicit reflex spinal automatisms. When such reactions do occur, an unembarrassed, accepting response helps relieve the client's anxiety and embarrassment. Gentle, slow hyperextension of a limb in spasm can often override the trigger points and interrupt the spasm. Abnormal spinal reflexes make people respond to stimuli in ways that may be puzzling to them and others unless the origin of such responses is explained. For example, stimulation of the limbs (perhaps toe flexion while the person's foot is being dried) may cause mass flexion of the upper and lower extremities. Mass flexion reactions may be accompanied by massive contractions of the abdominal wall, evacuation of the urinary bladder and bowel, and automatic response such as sweating, flushing, penile erection, or pilomotor reactions below the level of the lesion.

Risk for Thrombophlebitis. Muscular activity is a major factor in venous circulation. A paralyzed client experiences slowed venous return and pooling of blood in dependent limbs. These phenomena constitute the basis for the diagnosis *Risk for Thrombophlebitis.*

Outcomes. Monitor for thrombophlebitis, as evidenced by unilateral leg edema, erythema, and warmth.

Interventions. In the acute phase of SCI, antiembolism stockings, sequential compression devices, and subcutaneous heparin may be used prophylactically.

Education is vital to preventing vascular complications and minimizing their impact. Teach the client the importance of all preventive activities. During assessment of the legs for signs of clot formation (i.e., redness and unilateral swelling and warmth), explain the components of assessment, and emphasize the importance of incorporating this activity into daily routines. Measuring calf diameter on both legs daily to detect any changes is a more objective way of assessing swelling. Clients also learn not to cross their legs while sitting in a wheelchair.

Ineffective Individual Coping. When the reality of the injury and the permanence of deficit are understood, coping skills may need to be taught. The nursing diagnosis can be written as *Ineffective Individual Coping related to paralysis.*

Outcomes. The client will use adaptive coping strategies and resources appropriately.

Interventions. Clients need to find appropriate methods for coping with new approaches to performing ADL and managing bodily functions. The learning needs of spinal cord–injured clients and their family members are complex and ongoing. In the acute phase, education about spinal anatomy and physiology is needed. This teaching begins in the acute phase of hospitalization and should be incorporated into all aspects of care. Successful learning in this stage affects the client's entire life.

Anticipatory Grieving. Clients with SCI experience many changes (e.g., functional ability, role definition, body image, and financial security). Grief is a normal response to these losses. Write the diagnosis as *Anticipatory Grieving related to multiple losses.*

Outcomes. The client will progress through the grieving process and develop adaptive coping strategies, as evidenced by verbalizing his or her feelings about the injury and the future, participating in community activities, and expressing positive thoughts about the future.

Intervention. Adjusting to paralysis is difficult physically and psychosocially for the client and family. Family members may experience the same reactions as those experienced by the disabled client, and may need the same kind of help. Sudden paralysis in a previously healthy, active person can be devastating. Typically, the sudden lifestyle changes brought about by serious SCI produce a grief reaction. The reaction may involve initial shock and denial, leading to depression and anger. Crying and talking about the injury may be helpful. Social services or pastoral care may also be of assistance during this time of grief.

It takes time to adjust to disability and to develop ways of coping. Psychological adjustment occurs when the client can function appropriately in the real world.

A client may use psychological defense mechanisms in adjusting to paralysis. When caring for such a client, assess the possible reasons for observed behavior. Hostility, depression, anger, or withdrawal may be upsetting to staff and family. These emotions and behaviors represent coping mechanisms and should not be taken personally.

Paralysis may cause complex changes in self-concept and body image. In the acute phase, immobilization can contribute to sensory deprivation and its consequences (e.g., hallucinations). Providing visual, auditory, and tactile stimulation as desired by the client may minimize the experience of deprivation.

Paralyzed clients are often helped initially by being with others who are experiencing similar problems. Clients should be allowed to wear their own clothing as soon as possible and encouraged to be out of bed and out of the hospital room. Planned social activities may reduce feelings of social isolation and may help clients regain self-confidence. Peer counseling, in which newly disabled clients are provided with opportunities to talk with others who have adjusted to similar disabilities, may be helpful.

A sense of security is particularly important for a newly paralyzed client adjusting to enforced dependency. A paralyzed client should always have a means of summoning help, yet needs to learn that it is safe to be alone at times. Blow lights, minimal-pressure call lights, pads, and voice-activated call lights are now available in many settings.

Gradually, the client develops trust in his or her abilities and resources and relinquishes some reliance on others. These feelings and attitudes develop slowly as the client experiences genuinely trustworthy relationships.

To avoid unnecessary frustrations, try to keep the client's environment comfortable, with necessary items conveniently placed. It is difficult and depressing for the client to have to ask for help repeatedly. Although recent advances have been made in the rehabilitation prognosis of paraplegic and quadriplegic clients, it is important to be realistic as well as optimistic. Nurses need to understand the tremendous lifestyle changes disabled clients must make. Some people can be rehabilitated to a level of near-independence: walking (perhaps with braces or other appliances), driving a car, and coping with full-time employment outside the home. Quadriplegic clients usually rely on a wheelchair and other devices and appliances.

Most paralyzed clients can become productive and happy. One well-known SCI victim, the actor Christopher Reeve, has been serving as a positive role model regarding *abilities* that remain after SCI. Even if some clients are unable to be "productive," all disabled clients have a right to a satisfying, happy life. Although many paralyzed clients achieve complete rehabilitation, others lead lives that are difficult, frustrating, and psychophysiologically complex. At times, severe mental depression develops. Depression is assessed, and professional counseling is offered as indicated. Unfortunately, ideations of suicide are frequent.

Ineffective Family Coping: Compromised. A family is a unit. A trauma as devastating as SCI to one of the members of the family unit affects the entire family. The relevant nursing diagnosis can be written *Ineffective Family Coping: Compromised related to multiple changes in the family roles.*

Outcomes. The client and family members will identify areas of significant or potential loss and changes in family roles, work together to overcome obstacles, seek appropriate support services, and be able to restore a supportive family structure.

Interventions. The injury affects not only physical functioning but also the psychological, vocational, educa-

tional, and social aspects of life. An organized team approach is vital to helping the injured client and family cope with lifestyle changes. Nurses are often the first health care professionals to assess client and family coping. An open, empathetic manner can allow the people involved to express their grief and uncertainty and to ask questions. Educate the family about the normal grief response. Also carefully probe into persistent denial of grief or lack of progression through grieving. Encouraging as much optimism as possible while remaining truthful and realistic may help SCI survivors to face the future.

Assess the previous roles of the client and other family members and how they have handled stressful situations or losses. Identify the family's sources of strength. Assess patterns of interaction between family members; their spiritual, social, and economic status, their lifestyle, and cultural or ethnic influences should also be noted. These variables often influence how the family responds to grief. Sometimes the nurse can play a valuable role simply by giving family members permission to have a day off from visiting.

Ineffective Management of Therapeutic Regimen (Individual). Clients with SCI have bladder function changes. Bladder emptying has to be learned using a different approach, and bowel retraining is often necessary. A common nursing diagnosis in this circumstance is *Ineffective Management of Therapeutic Regimen (Individual).*

Outcomes. The client will be able to manage his or her bowel and bladder or instruct others how to do so.

Interventions. One of the most common stimuli for autonomic dysreflexia, a life-threatening complication in people with SCI, is bladder distention. Therefore, intervention leading to bladder management is crucial.

Promote Bladder Retraining. When the initial indwelling catheter is removed, a program of intermittent catheterization is commonly prescribed to empty the bladder regularly every 4 to 6 hours for several weeks. During this time, the client is taught methods of emptying the bladder without catheterization. Such methods promote urination by increasing intra-abdominal pressure on the bladder. For some clients with SCI, urinary flow can be initiated by using the Credé maneuver, the Valsalva maneuver, or the rectal stretch.

The *Credé maneuver* involves placing the fist or fingers directly over the bladder and pressing down toward the pubic bone with a kneading motion. This motion is continued until the bladder is empty.

The *Valsalva maneuver* involves inhaling deeply, holding the breath, and bearing down as hard as possible, as if for a bowel movement.

The *rectal stretch* involves inserting a lubricated, gloved finger into the rectum. When the anal sphincter is relaxed, the client maintains the relaxation by gently pulling on the sphincter. This relaxes the perineal floor. The Valsalva maneuver is performed at the same time.

Urination may also be prompted by reflex stimulation. The following stimuli may be successful: tapping the suprapubic area; stroking the glans penis, thigh, or vulva; tugging pubic hairs; or flexing the toes. The client or caregiver may apply the stimulation. As training continues, less stimulation is needed to initiate urination.

Catheterization may be required at home. Teach the client and caregiver clean, rather than sterile, technique. This technique has the same infection rate as for sterile insertion methods used for home catheterization. Suprapubic catheters may be inserted for long-term bladder management.

Occasionally, a surgical procedure such as sphincterotomy may be necessary. The bladder then empties continuously. An external, condom-type catheter connected to a closed drainage bag may be used to collect urine in men. External appliances for females are not consistently effective.

Teach Bowel Retraining. Bowel retraining is possible for most paraplegic and quadriplegic clients. It involves developing controlled bowel movements by conditioned reflex activity. Begin bowel retraining as soon as feasible. Ensure privacy during the daily bowel routine, and if possible, have the client sitting upright. When possible, include appropriate family members in the bowel retraining program, as they may be involved in this aspect of long-term management. Always assess the family members' willingness to participate in such care. If the sexual partner is also responsible for hygiene and personal care, problems in role separation and intimacy may result. These issues should be openly discussed between partners.

With an effective bowel program, a client has a bowel movement once a day or every other day and is not incontinent at other times. Attaining continence may influence a paralyzed client's vocational future and positively affect ability to have satisfying social relationships. It can also give the client the confidence to cope with other problems.

Sexual Dysfunction. Spinal cord–injured clients are often concerned about sexuality and their ability to achieve sexual fulfillment. They often worry about such concerns long before they express them to others. Nurses are often asked about sexuality issues before other professionals are approached, perhaps because nurses provide intimate care. Such care can promote a high degree of trust.

Outcomes. The client will develop personally satisfying and socially acceptable means of expressing sexuality, as evidenced by interacting appropriately in social situations, verbalizing the effects of the injury on sexual function, discussing sexual issues with a health care team member, verbalizing methods of sexual expression, and verbalizing understanding of contraceptive implications.

Interventions. Some clients discuss their own sexual potential directly. Others refer to it subtly or appear crude in the way they introduce the topic, such as making inappropriate sexual comments or gestures. Such behaviors are attempts to acknowledge sexuality. Try to look beyond the behavior to the underlying emotional concerns. Acknowledge the client's concerns and offer to open a discussion, by saying, for example, "You seem concerned about your sexuality, James. This is a common concern that others with spinal cord injury have had. Sometimes talking about it helps. If you like, we can talk about how this has affected you, and when you are ready, I can share with you interventions that have helped others who have had similar problems."

To be helpful, nurses need to be able to talk about sexuality without embarrassment. They also need accurate information about "normal" sexuality and how physiologic changes that occur because of the injury affect sexual function.

The client can be referred to another person or an agency if appropriate. Referral should not be made too hastily, however. If a client talks with a nurse about this subject, it is probably because the client feels most comfortable speaking with that nurse at that time. Allow the client to lead the conversation, which may be difficult. Professionals must be aware that they do not always know what a client needs and wants and should listen carefully to the client's voiced concerns.

Generally, a physiologic sexual response requires an intact nervous system. For example, psychogenic erection requires an intact spinal cord with preservation of S2–4 nerve roots and spinal reflexes; ejaculation is a function of skeletal muscle controlled by the somatic center in the pudendal nerve originating in the S2–4 roots; and orgasm involves contraction of both smooth and skeletal muscle. It should be remembered, however, that there is more involved in sexual expression than physiologic response.

To some extent, sexual function can be predicted by the level of the spinal cord lesion (see Table 73–5). For example, psychogenic erection is often difficult or impossible after SCI. However, although physical limitations certainly exist, every person is different. Many men do have reflex erections after SCI. Many disabled people enjoy "paraorgasm" (phantom orgasm) by developing alternative erogenous zones. The genitals are not the only body areas in which sexual stimulation is possible, and intercourse is not the only means of sexual expression.

Some people find it disappointing, perhaps devastating, that they can no longer function sexually as they did before the injury. However, they can be helped to learn new ways of giving and receiving sexual pleasure. Sex and relationship counseling is sometimes helpful. Some form of sexual expression is possible for anyone, regardless of disability. Before making specific suggestions for alternative expressions of sexuality, discussion with the client should occur to identify past sexual behavior and cultural taboos. Some clients may find some methods of giving and receiving sexual pleasure unacceptable. Lack of a sexual partner may be a deterrent but should not preclude discussion of sexuality. Society as a whole is becoming progressively more open about sexuality.

Increasingly, the parenting potential of disabled people is receiving societal attention. Physical assessment is needed to determine a client's ability to reproduce. Male infertility is a frequent complication of SCI because of testicular atrophy, decreased sperm formation, and infrequent ejaculation. Most men are unable to ejaculate after SCI. Women usually remain fertile and can conceive and deliver a child. Adoption is a viable option, and conception by artificial insemination is possible.

Disabled people may have contraception concerns. Little is known about the effects of various kinds of contraceptives on disabled people. Oral contraceptives may be contraindicated. Paralyzed women often have slowed circulation, increasing the potential circulatory complications of oral contraceptives. To use an intrauterine device, a woman must have feeling in her pelvis to be able to recognize early manifestations of pelvic inflammatory disease. Many paralyzed women do not have such sensation. Barrier devices, such as a diaphragm, a condom, or foam, may be used if at least one partner has enough manual dexterity to insert the diaphragm or foam or put on the condom.

Risk for Injury. Sensory loss poses serious problems for paralyzed clients because they cannot feel the pain or pressure that normally warns of tissue damage.

Outcomes. The client will be free of injury, as evidenced by absence of abrasions, reddened areas, ulcerations, or burns.

Interventions. Spinal cord–injured clients should not wear tight, restrictive clothing or ill-fitting shoes or braces. They need to develop the habit of preventive thinking to avoid potential danger. Dangerous situations include getting too close to heaters, radiators, and fireplaces and using heating pads or hot-water bottles. Burns can be a serious problem because impaired circulation delays healing. External heat should not be applied if there is a loss of sensation, and the bath water should not be too hot.

Regular foot and nail care is required to prevent overgrown nails from rubbing or cutting the skin and to prevent ingrown nails. Instruct the client not to cut corns or calluses; cutting too deep is easy to do and may lead to a foot infection. Cocoa butter or oils without alcohol may be used to soften calluses and reduce cracking.

Altered Health Maintenance. SCI results in many alterations in physiologic functioning that place the client at risk for maintaining normal health status. A possible nursing diagnosis is *Altered Health Maintenance.*

Outcomes. The client and family members will be able to meet the client's needs, as evidenced by intact skin, bowel and bladder continence, ability to transfer into and out of a wheelchair, absence of infection, maintenance of appropriate weight, and satisfaction with personal relationships.

Interventions. Teaching should be conducted in short sessions, using easily understood terms. For example, teach the caregiver the importance of providing good skin care on the hands and skinfolds to prevent *Candida* overgrowth. Complex tasks should be taught in steps, with return demonstrations provided by the client or caregiver.

Most spinal cord–injured people are transferred from an acute care hospital to a rehabilitation facility. After functional capabilities have been maximized, the person is then discharged from the rehabilitation facility. The accompanying Bridge to Home Health Care feature provides suggestions for helping caregivers support the client with SCI who lives at home.

EVALUATION

Spinal cord–injured clients are hospitalized for a long time. Therefore, certain functions important to expected outcomes need to be evaluated frequently, such as respiratory and cardiac function. Other expected outcomes will not be achieved for months, such as independence in ADL. The plan of care must reflect these individual needs of the client.

◼ Modifications for Elderly Clients

For older adults with SCI, the most important modification of the nursing care plan is increased vigilance. Older people are more prone to the complications of immobility. A person with heart failure may have difficulty breathing when lying flat. Before initiation of halo traction in this age group, some neurosurgeons perform a temporary prophylactic tracheostomy, because the older client has difficulty swallowing oral secretions and eating. Older people are also more susceptible to sensory deprivation. The nurse must make sure the client has his or her eyeglasses and hearing aid. If a window or clock is not within range of vision, the client should be reoriented as needed. Discharge plans for elderly clients may be complicated if the caregiver is also elderly. The spouse of an older spinal cord–injured person may not have the physical strength to provide the needed care. Learning to provide home care may also be problematic.

◼ Self-Care

Paraplegic clients can usually live independently. Most quadriplegic clients need assistance with daily activities. Depending on the amount of assistance needed and the specific situation, this care may be provided by family members or by a part-time or full-time paid attendant. By using a wheelchair, clients may become completely independent in ADL, with minimal help of social services personnel, a home health aide, or family members. Many clients drive and hold outside jobs.

Ventilator-dependent people who cannot obtain in-home care and others who do not have the personal or financial resources for in-home care may have no option except institutional living. The problem of limited government resources for all clients requiring rehabilitative care remains an important ethical issue in nursing. Group living situations, especially for young adults, are becoming more available, however.

CONCLUSIONS

Disorders of the spinal cord and peripheral nervous system range from life-threatening SCIs to temporary peripheral nerve compressions. The physical and psychological impairments vary with the degree of damage as well as the client's response to and ability to cope with the body changes. The coping response is not always related to the degree of physiologic damage. A client who has facial paralysis or trigeminal neuralgia can be more compromised psychologically than a client with SCI who has developed strong coping skills. It is imperative that nurses comprehend the severity of the client's dysfunction as it relates to quality of life, as well as the impact it has on family dynamics.

Management of the client with SCI is complex and multidisciplinary. Successful rehabilitation provides the client with the opportunity to be productive in society in spite of severe neurologic deficit.

THINKING CRITICALLY

1. **A 23-year-old man was admitted from the emergency department (ED) after a car accident in**

which he sustained a concussion and thoracic injuries with thoracic spinal cord involvement. The client's baseline data included loss of consciousness for 15 minutes, headache, nausea, and inability to move or feel any sensation from his thorax down. One hour after this man arrived in the intensive care unit (ICU), additional assessment changes included inability to move fingers and hands and to flex or extend the arms. Shoulder movement was still intact. He was fully conscious and his vital signs were stable. What critical interventions initiated in the ED need to be continued in the ICU? What do these changes in data indicate? What nursing interventions are appropriate both initially and as precautions?

Factors to Consider. What are the implications when a high thoracic injury occurs? What changes indicate ascending cord dysfunction?

2. A 22-year-old man was admitted 4 hours after sustaining a C6 spinal cord compression injury. No neurologic deficits were found, but his blood alcohol level was very high on admission. Initially, he kept falling asleep after you completed your assessments. Gardner-Wells tongs with 10 pounds of traction were placed. Now that the client is more awake, he has begun thrashing his arms and attempting to roll over in bed. What are the priorities for his care? What nursing interventions should be used?

Factors to Consider. What is the purpose of the Gardner-Wells tongs? How would edema and microscopic bleeding compromise recovery in this client?

3. The client, a 34-year-old woman, had a lumbar laminectomy done earlier in the day. An earlier assessment showed that movement and sensation of both lower extremities were intact. During the current postoperative assessment she states that her right toes feel numb, and the dorsiflexion and plantiflexion of the right foot are a little weaker than earlier. She has requested an analgesic because she is starting to get a headache. What are the priorities for her care? What assessments and interventions might be used?

Factors to Consider. What assessment methods can be used to determine the extent of vascular insufficiency? What type of neurologic checks should be done?

BIBLIOGRAPHY

1. American Association of Neuroscience Nurses. (1997). *Clinical guideline series: Intracranial pressure monitoring.* Chicago: Author.
2. American Spinal Injury Association (ASIA). (1992). *Standards for neurological and functional classification of spinal cord injury.* Chicago: Author.
3. Bauman, W. A., & Spungen, A. M. (2000). Metabolic changes in persons after spinal cord injury. *Physical Medicine and Rehabilitation Clinics of North America, 11*(1), 109–140.
4. Bell, G. B. (1999). Spinal cord injury, pressure ulcers, support surfaces. *Ostomy and Wound Management, 45*(6), 48–50, 52–53.
5. Brain Trauma Foundation. (1995). *Guidelines for the management of severe head injury.* Chicago: Author.
6. Bryce, T. N., & Ragnarsson, K. T. (2000). Pain after spinal cord injury. *Physical Medicine and Rehabilitation Clinics of North America, 11*(1), 157–168.
7. Buckley, D. A., & Guanci, M. M. (1999). Spinal cord trauma. *Nursing Clinics of North America, 34*(3), 661–687.
8. Cantella, D. (1999). Sports-related spinal cord injuries. *Critical Care Nursing Quarterly, 22*(2), 14–19.
9. Chen, D., & Nussbaum, S. B. (2000). The gastrointestinal system and bowel management following spinal cord injury. *Physical Medicine and Rehabilitation Clinics of North America, 11*(1), 45–56, viii.
10. Clear, D., & Chadwick, D. W. (2000). Seizures provoked by blows to the head. *Epilepsia, 41*(2), 243–244.
11. Cruz, J. (1996). Adverse effects of pentobarbital on cerebral venous oxygenation of comatose patients with acute traumatic brain swelling: Relationship to outcome. *Journal of Neurosurgery, 85,* 758–761.
12. Cruz, J., et al. (1998). Severe acute brain trauma. In J. Cruz (Ed.), *Neurological and neurosurgical emergencies* (pp. 405–436). Philadelphia: W. B. Saunders.
13. Davis, B., & Handy, C. (1996). Cellulitis: An unreported complication of long-term SCI patients. *SCI Nursing, 13*(2), 35–38.
14. Dennis, G. C., et al. (2000). Somatosensory evoked potentials, neurologic examination and MRI for assessment of spinal cord decompression. *Life Science, 66*(5), 389–397.
15. Dubendorf, P. (1999). Spinal cord injury pathophysiology. *Critical Care Nursing Quarterly, 22*(2), 31–35.
16. Fortune, J. B., et al. (1995). Effect of hyperventilation, mannitol and ventriculostomy drainage on cerebral blood flow after head injury. *Journal of Trauma, 39,* 1091–1097.
17. Fowler, S. B., et al. (1995). Pharmacological interventions for agitation in head-injured patients in the acute care setting. *Journal of Neuroscience Nursing, 27*(2), 119–123.
18. Geary, S. (1996). Nursing management of cranial nerve dysfunction. *Journal of Neuroscience Nursing, 27*(2), 102–108.
19. Germon, K. (1994). Intracranial pressure monitoring in the 1990s. *Critical Care Nursing Quarterly, 17*(1), 21–32.
20. Goldstein, B. (2000). Musculoskeletal conditions after spinal cord injury. *Physical Medicine and Rehabilitation Clinics of North America, 11*(1), 91–108, viii–ix.
21. Gregory, R. J. (1995). Understanding and coping with neurological impairment. *Rehabilitation Nursing, 20*(2), 74–78.
22. Guerra, W. K. W., Piek, J, & Gaab, M. R. (1999). Decompressive craniectomy to treat intracranial hypertension in head injured patients. *Intensive and Critical Care Medicine, 25*(11), 1327–1329.
23. Gupta, A. K., & Bullock, M. R. (1998). Monitoring the injured brain in intensive care: present and future. Hospital Medicine 59(9), 704–713.
24. Hanson, C. W. (1998). Acute respiratory failure in neuroemergencies. In J. Cruz (Ed.), *Neurological and neurosurgical emergencies* (pp. 21–38). Philadelphia: W. B. Saunders.
25. Hickey, J. V. (1997). Craniocerebral injuries. In J. V. Hickey (Ed.), *The clinical practice of neurological and neurosurgical nursing* (4th ed., pp. 385–417). Philadelphia: J. B. Lippincott.
26. Hickey, J. V. (1997). Intracranial pressure: Theory and management of increased intracranial pressure. In J. V. Hickey (Ed.), *The clinical practice of neurological and neurosurgical nursing* (4th ed., pp. 295–328). Philadelphia: J. B. Lippincott.
27. Hickey, J. V. (1997). Vertebral and spinal cord injuries. In J. V. Hickey (Ed.), *The clinical practice of neurological and neurosurgical nursing* (4th ed., pp. 419–465). Philadelphia: J. B. Lippincott.
28. Hilton, G. (1994). Secondary brain injury and the role of neuroprotective agents. *Journal of Neuroscience Nursing, 26*(4), 251–255.
29. Jacobs, D. G., & Westerbrand, A. (1998). Antibiotic prophylaxis for intracranial pressure monitors. *Journal of the National Medical Association, 90*(7), 417–423.
30. Kavchak-Keyes, M. A. (2000). Autonomic hyperreflexia. *Rehabilitation Nursing, 25*(1), 31–35.
31. Kelly, D. F. (1995). Alcohol and head injury: An issue revisited. *Journal of Neurotrauma, 12,* 883–890.
32. Kirshblum, S. (1999). Treatment alternatives for spinal cord injury related spasticity. *Journal of Spinal Cord Medicine, 22*(3), 199–217.
33. Kirshblum, S. C., & O'Connor, K. C. (2000). Levels of spinal cord injury and predictors for neurologic recovery. *Physical Medicine and Rehabilitation Clinics of North America, 11*(1), 1–27, vii.

34. Lanig, I. S., & Peterson, W. P. (2000). The respiratory system in spinal cord injury. *Physical Medicine and Rehabilitation Clinics of North America, 11*(1), 29–43, vii.

35. Linsenmeyer, T. A. (2000). Sexual function and infertility following spinal cord injury. *Physical Medicine and Rehabilitation Clinics of North America, 11*(1), 141–156, ix.

36. Little, J. W., et al. (2000). Neurologic recovery and neurologic decline after spinal cord injury. *Physical Medicine and Rehabilitation Clinics of North America, 11*(1), 73–89.

37. Lovasik, D. (1999). The older patient with a spinal cord injury. *Critical Care Nursing Quarterly, 22*(2), 20–30.

38. Marcotte, P. J., Shaver, E. G., & Weil, R. J. (1998). Acute spinal disorders. In J. Cruz (Ed.), *Neurological and neurosurgical emergencies* (pp. 363–403). Philadelphia: W. B. Saunders.

39. Marion, D. W., & Speigel, T. P. (2000). Changes in the management of severe traumatic brain injury: 1991–1997. *Critical Care Medicine, 28*(1): 16–8.

40. McNair, N. D. (1996). Intracranial pressure monitoring. In J. M. Clouchesy, et al. (Eds.), *Critical Care Nursing* (2nd ed., pp. 289–307). Philadelphia: W. B. Saunders.

41. McNair, N. D. (1999). Traumatic brain injury. *Nursing Clinics of North America, 34*(3), 637–659.

42. Mitcho, K., & Yanko, J. R. (1999). Acute care management of spinal cord injuries. *Critical Care Nursing Quarterly, 22*(2), 60–79.

43. Nayduch, D., Lee, A., & Butler, D. (1994). High-dose methylprednisolone after acute spinal cord injury. *Critical Care Nurse, 14*(4), 69–78.

44. Neatherlin, J. S., & Brillhart, B. (1996). Body image in preoperative and postoperative lumbar laminectomy patients. *Journal of Neuroscience Nursing, 27*(1), 43–46.

45. Neatherlin, J. S. (1999). Foundation for practice: Neuroassessment for neuroscience nurses. *Nursing Clinics of North America, 34*(3), 573–592.

46. Peterson, P. L., et al. (1998). Initial evaluation and management of neuroemergencies. In J. Cruz (Ed.), *Neurological and neurosurgical emergencies* (pp. 1–20). Philadelphia: W. B. Saunders.

47. Quint, D. J. (2000). Indications for emergent MRI of the central nervous system. *Journal of the American Medical Association, 283*(7), 853–855.

48. Ramson, K. P., et al. (1998). Neuroemergency nursing. In J. Cruz (Ed.), *Neurological and neurosurgical emergencies* (pp. 467–501). Philadelphia: W. B. Saunders.

49. Richmond, T., Metcalf, J., & Daly, M. (1995). Requirements for nursing care services and associated costs in acute spinal cord injury. *Journal of Neuroscience Nursing, 27*(1), 47–52.

50. Rosner, M. J., Rosner, S. D., & Johnson, A. H. (1995). Cerebral perfusion pressure: Management protocol and clinical results. *Journal of Neurosurgery, 83,* 949–1062.

51. Rovlias, A., & Kotson, S. (2000). The influence of hyperglycemia on neurologic outcome in patients with severe head injury. *Neurosurgery, 46*(2), 335–342.

52. Sandel, M. E., et al. (1998). Neurorehabilitation. In J. Cruz (Ed.), *Neurological and neurosurgical emergencies* (pp. 503–546). Philadelphia: W. B. Saunders.

53. Segatore, M. (1999). Corticosteroids and traumatic brain injury: Status at the end of the decade of the brain. *Journal of Neuroscience Nursing, 31*(4), 239–250.

54. Seidl, E. C. (1999). Promising pharmacological agents in the management of acute spinal cord injury. *Critical Care Nursing Quarterly, 22*(2), 44–50.

55. Shaddinger, D. E. (1996). An acute spinal cord injury: My family's perspective. *Journal of Neuroscience Nursing, 27*(4), 236–239.

56. Shpritz, D. W. (1999). Neurodiagnostic studies. *Nursing Clinics of North America, 34*(3), 593–606.

57. Stewart-Amidei, C. (1998). Neurologic monitoring in the ICU. *Critical Care Nursing Quarterly, 21*(3), 47–60.

58. Thurman, D. J., et al. (1999). Traumatic brain injury in the United States: A public health perspective. *Journal of Head Trauma Rehabilitation, 14*(6), 602–615.

59. Veltman, R. H., et al. (1993). Cognitive screening in mild brain injury. *Journal of Neuroscience Nursing, 25*(6), 367–372.

60. Winemuller, M. K., et al. (1999). Prevention of venous thromboembolism in patients with spinal cord injury: Effects of sequential pneumatic compression and heparin. *Journal of Spinal Cord Medicine, 23*(3), 182–191.

61. Yundt, K. D., & Diringer, M. N. (1997). The use of hyperventilation and its impact on cerebral ischemia in the treatment of traumatic brain injury. *Critical Care Clinics, 13*(1), 163–184.

62. Zasler, N. D. (1994). Mild traumatic brain injury and post-concussive disorders: Neuromedical and medicolegal caveats. *Network, 5*(3), 3–5.

UNIT
16

Protective Disorders

Anatomy and Physiology Review
The Hematopoietic System
Joyce M. Black

Enemies of many kinds and in great numbers assault the body during a lifetime. Injury can lead to bleeding, and wounds are common. The body is also threatened by hordes of microorganisms. The body defends itself against attack by viruses, bacteria, and other parasites by using two sets of separate but interrelated functions: (1) *resistance* (called by some innate immunity) and (2) *immunity*. Both of these systems must be present and operating properly in order to block establishment of infectious agents, to minimize damage caused by disease in progress, and to expel, destroy, or isolate infectious agents that gain access to inner tissues.

Through time, the old and new defenses merged together to form a sort of three-layered approach providing both *surveillance* ("inside" threats) and *defense* ("outside" threats) functions. The importance of these mechanisms to our health and well-being becomes apparent when the defenses of a healthy body are compromised by infection or suppressed by medication or chemotherapy. Parts of the defense system in a healthy body may function inappropriately to reject organ and tissue transplants and may produce autoimmune disease or hypersensitivity states that cause pathologic changes and sometimes death.

RESISTANCE: A FORM OF NONSPECIFIC DEFENSE

The first line of defense in the body is the aspect of resistance that stops a threatening agent or condition. Defenses provide a form of resistance against disease by combatting anything not recognized as *self*. Resistance components are usually the first to encounter infectious agents or parasites. Many of these functions operate independently of the immune system but, as shown later, some of the components and features participate in or amplify acquired immune responses.

SURFACE DEFENSES

Intact skin and mucous membranes are sufficient to provide barriers that prevent penetration to underlying tissues by many pathogens. Lysozyme in tears and bile in the gut inhibit gram-positive bacteria; hydrochloric acid in the stomach is lethal to all pathogens; and fatty acids help protect the skin from infectious agents. Surface-clearing mechanisms (such as washing of oral surfaces by saliva, tear-washing, urine-flushing, the mucociliary escalator in the trachea), mucoperistaltic propulsion in the small intestine, and the cough reflex prevent attachment of invading organisms. Autochthonous (natural) flora interfere with colonization of pathogens by both *niche* (function) and *habitat* (location) *competition*.

The *reticuloendothelia system* (RES) includes mononuclear phagocytic cells (macrophages). Fixed (attached) macrophages in the sinusoids of the liver, spleen, and bone marrow monitor the circulating blood and remove all foreign particulates and any moribund self cells. Resident mobile macrophages in lymph nodes remove foreign particulate matter. Macrophages in the alveolar spaces are the most active of the RES cells and help remove inspired particulates that reach the lower recesses of the lung.

ORGANS OF THE IMMUNE AND HEMATOLOGIC SYSTEMS

The organs of the immune and hematologic systems are shown in Figure U16–1. There are both peripheral and central organs.

■ PERIPHERAL LYMPHOID TISSUE

Peripheral lymphoid tissues are sites for antigen processing and presentation and for T-cell and B-cell activation. These are the only locales for the production of the molecules and cells that serve as effector units of the immune response.

LYMPH NODES

Lymph nodes are mostly small organs (many are less than 5 mm in diameter) that are present throughout the body interconnected by means of lymph vessels. Their structure is fairly complex and provides both RES and immune functions. The lymph node receives fluid, particulates, and solutes that are taken up by lymphatic capillaries from distal tissue sites. Resident macrophages within the node monitor the lymph fluid passing through for the presence of foreign particulates and remove them by phagocytic action. Antigenic substances, either particulates or solutes, are taken up by the macrophages or dendritic cells serving as antigen-presenting cells (APCs). Immunocompetent cells in the lymph node can give rise to either a humoral immune response or a cell-mediated immune response. The masses of cells called lymph or medullary cords also exist as a site of secondary humoral immune responses.

Lymph nodes are found in large numbers in the thoracic and abdominal cavities. Those lying close to the body surface are called *superficial nodes*. Cervical nodes lie alongside the neck, axillary nodes in the armpit, and inguinal nodes in the crease between the upper thigh and the trunk. When inflamed, these nodes become swollen and may be palpated, serving as diagnostic signs.

LYMPH NODULES

The structure of the lymph nodules is much less organized than that of the lymph nodes. The nodules occur in the mucosal epithelium lining the respiratory, gastrointestinal (GI), and urogenital tracts. Antigenic materials are translocated across a dome epithelium through a special

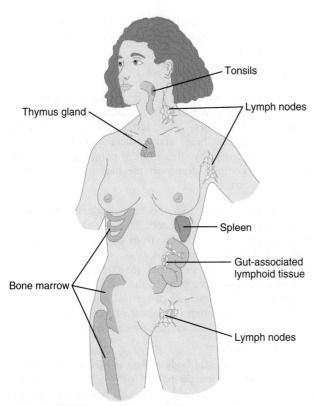

white zones. The white zones are accumulations of lymphocytes and APCs. Loss of the spleen or diminished function due to injury or infection greatly increases the risk of infection with extracellular bacteria.

Other functions of the spleen include (1) assisting in recycling iron by capturing hemoglobin released from destroyed red blood cells (RBCs) and (2) performing pitting (removal of particles from RBCs without destroying the cell itself).

THYMUS

The thymus is a lymphoepithelial organ located in the mediastinum, the thoracic cavity between the lungs and above the heart. The thymus reaches peak development during childhood. After puberty, it begins to atrophy but remnants persist into old age. The thymus is an endocrine organ that secretes hormones that contribute to the maintenance and function of peripheral T-cell populations. The interior of the early thymus is filled with thymocytes from the bone marrow and from a high rate of cell replication within the organ.

A fundamental paradigm in immunology is the rearrangement of germ line genes during differentiation of lymphocytes in the central lymphoid tissues, leading to the production of molecules for the recognition of antigen. In both cell types, the antigen recognition unit is inserted into the membrane with the antigen-reactive ends extending out into the extracellular environment. The T cell uses the T-cell antigen receptor, and the B cell has a tetrapeptide monomer called *surface immunoglobulin* (SIg). The individual cells each have a unique receptor capable of reacting only with a single antigenic determinant (Fig. U16–2). Each specifically reacting cell is called a *clonotype*; when properly stimulated by antigen, the clonotype produces effector units (either antibody molecules or specially reactive cells) and a memory cell clone, both of which have the identical specificity of the original clonotype.

The positive and negative selection processes acting on cells in the thymus make it possible for the mechanism to discriminate between *self* and *non-self* in immune function. This distinction is accomplished by making antigen recognition absolutely dependent on the variable but individually unique composition of the transcription products of gene loci located in the major histocompatibility region of the genome.

Class I major histocompatibility complex (MHC) molecules are found on nearly all nucleated cells in the body and represent a major antigenic distinction between individuals of a given species with different genotypes. This

FIGURE U16–1 Organs of the immune system. The bone marrow, spleen, lymph nodes, tonsils, and gut-associated lymphoid tissue (GALT) function in both specific and nonspecific immunity, whereas the thymus functions primarily in specific immunity.

cell (M cell). The translocated material is deposited directly into the nodule structure where it is taken up by APCs. Immunocompetent B cells in lymph nodules produce either immunoglobulin E (IgE) or IgA. These two classes of immunoglobulins provide for the development either of allergy of the immediate hypersensitivity type (atopy) or of a mucosal immune response.

■ CENTRAL LYMPHOID ORGANS

SPLEEN

The spleen is the largest lymphoid organ in the body. Its defensive functions include the blood-clearing process via fixed macrophages in sinusoids as well as serving as a major site of humoral immune responses to blood-borne antigens. The splenic pulp is divided into red zones and

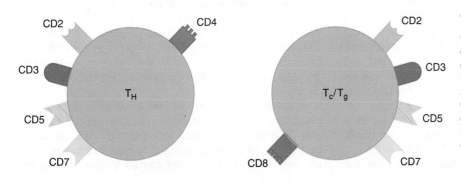

FIGURE U16–2 T cells can be distinguished by distinctive molecules located on their cell surfaces. They are called cluster designations (CDs). All mature T cells carry markers known as T2 (or CD2), T3 (or CD3), T5 (or CD5), and T7 (or CD7). T helper (T_H) cells carry a T4 (CD4) marker, and suppressor and cytotoxic T (T_c/T_g) cells carry a T8 (CD8) marker.

molecule is necessary for antigen recognition by T cells with CD8 surface markers. Class II MHC molecules are found on some APCs, on all B cells, and on antigen-activated T cells. This molecule is necessary for antigen recognition by T cells with CD4 surface markers. MHC antigens in humans were intitially discovered on leukocyte membranes and are thus called *human leukocyte antigens* (HLAs). It is this recognition system that forms the basis for the rejection of foreign or transplanted tissue. The cells in the recipient's immune system recognize the surface HLA proteins of the donor's tissue as being nonself.

BONE MARROW

Bone marrow constitutes one of the largest organs in the body, with an aggregate weight in adults of about 3000 g (comparable in mass to the liver). Based on visual appearance, the marrow mass was originally described as being either red or yellow. *Red marrow* consists of a mass of supporting cells surrounding aggregates of hematopoietic cells and interspaced with sinusoidal capillaries.

Yellow marrow has a large number of adipose cells, which accounts for its characteristic light color. This portion, or compartment, of the marrow is generally not active in hematopoiesis in a normal healthy person. However, following severe blood loss or the development of a sustained state of hypoxia, the yellow marrow can be converted into a red marrow state and production of blood cells initiated.

Function of Bone Marrow

Bone marrow provides for the following:

- Maintenance of a self-renewing pluripotent stem cell population from which all blood cells are derived
- An environment for the differentiation and maturation of blood cells
- A storage site for large numbers of neutrophils and erythrocytes
- Transformation of undifferentiated lymphocytes into mature B cells
- A site of antibody production in a secondary immune response to thymic-dependent antigens administered intravenously

Sinusoids bearing fixed macrophages serve an RES function in blood clearing. This is a defensive action based on the phagocytic activity of the macrophages attached to the luminal side of the marrow sinuses. These phagocytes, part of the RES or mononuclear phagocytic system, monitor the blood for the presence of foreign particulate matter, remove it, and destroy it.

FORMATION OF BLOOD CELLS. *Hematopoiesis*, the important process of formation and development of blood cells, begins very early in the development of the human embryo and must persist unabated throughout one's lifetime. The demands made on this function are enormous. Cells in the peripheral blood have a finite life span and must be continuously renewed at a rate probably greater than 10 billion cells/day. For a 100-year-old person, this would amount to more than 10^{14} cells.

During childhood, all blood cells are essentially produced in marrow sites of the flat bones of the skull, clavicle, sternum, ribs, vertebrae, and pelvis. After puberty, hematopoiesis becomes localized within the flat bones of the sternum, ilium, ribs, and vertebrae, sometimes occurring in the proximal ends of long bones (humerus and femur).

■ BLOOD

Blood is much more than the simple liquid it appears to be. Blood is a mixture of cells—RBCs, white blood cells (WBCs), and platelets—and plasma. It circulates continuously through the heart and vascular system. Propelled through the body by the heart's pumping action, the blood is a complex transport mechanism that performs many functions, such as:

- Supplying oxygen from the lungs and absorbed nutrients from the GI tract to cells
- Removing waste products from tissues to the kidney, skin, and lungs for excretion
- Transporting hormones from their origin in the endocrine glands to other parts of the body
- Protecting the body from dangerous microorganisms
- Promoting *hemostasis* (the arrest of bleeding)
- Regulating body temperature by heat transfer

COMPOSITION

About 8% of our total body weight is blood; for example, a healthy young female has 4 to 5 L and a male has about 5 to 6 L. Blood volume also varies by age and body composition. There is an inverse relationship between blood volume and kilograms of body weight. The less body fat, the more blood per kilogram of body weight is present.

Arterial blood is bright red because of the oxygen bound to hemoglobin and oxygen within RBCs. Venous blood is dark red because of its lower oxygen content. Blood is three to four times more viscous (thick) than water. Specific gravity is 1.048 to 1.066. Blood is slightly alkaline, with a pH of 7.35 to 7.45 (neutral pH is 7.0).

PLASMA

Plasma, the liquid portion of the blood, is one of the three major blood fluids (along with interstitial and intracellular fluids). Plasma makes up about 55% of the blood, and solid suspended particles (blood cells and platelets) compose the other 45%. The major function of plasma is to maintain the blood volume within the vascular compartment.

A straw-colored, watery substance, plasma is composed of 92% water, 7% proteins, and less than 1% nutrients, metabolic wastes, respiratory gases, enzymes, hormones, clotting factors, and inorganic salts. The proteins include serum albumin (alpha-globulin, and alpha$_2$-globulin, beta-globulin, and gamma-globulin) as well as fibrinogen, prothrombin, and proteins essential for blood coagulation. Serum albumin and gamma globulin are necessary for maintaining colloidal osmotic pressure (see Chapter 12). Gamma globulin also contains the antibodies (immunoglobulins) IgM, IgG, IgA, IgD, and IgE, which are essential in the body's defense against microorganisms.

If a tube of blood is allowed to stand or is spun in a centrifuge, the cells separate. The term *packed cell volume* or *hematocrit* is used to express the volume or percent of the RBCs in the sample. Normal hematocrit levels are 35% to 45%. Hematocrit can be increased from loss of plasma (e.g., dehydration) or increased production of RBCs (polycythemia). Low hematocrit levels are seen in overyhydration and low numbers of RBCs (Fig. U16–3). The WBCs and platelets make up less than 1% of the blood volume. These cells form a buffy coat or white layer and are seen at the interface of the RBCs and plasma.

HEMATOPOIESIS

Stem cells are poorly characterized, undifferentiated cells that exist within the red marrow. These totipotent, or pluripotent, stem cells are self-replicating and maintain a small population throughout the lifetime of the individual. Following stimulation by one or more signal molecules called *poietins,* the stem cells can undergo differentiation into erythrocytes (RBCs), megakaryocytes, and leukocytes. The steps of hematopiesis and the divisions of each cell, once it takes a committed path, are shown in Figure U16–4.

Control of Hematopoiesis

Much of the mechanism of hematopoietic regulation that stimulates the initial differentiation of stem cells and controls the early differentiation of the expanding cell lines is either not known or is poorly characterized. The so-called *hematopoietic inductive environment* is provided mainly by growth factors. These growth factors (*cytokines*) control cell growth, proliferation, and differentiation. Growth factors are usually identified by using acronyms that are a legacy from original studies of colony-forming cells. The suffix "-CSF" (colony-stimulating factor) describes the growth factor that stimulates or regulates the development of the corresponding cell type identified by the prefix "CFU-." For example, G-CSF is the growth factor for CFU-G (colony-forming unit–granulocytic series), and M-CSF is the growth factor regulating the development

of monocytes (CFU-M). Other growth factors, interleukins (ILs), are given numbers to distinguish between different molecules; IL-1 is derived from macrophages, IL-3 from activated T cells, and so forth.

RED BLOOD CELLS

RBCs (erythrocytes) carry oxygen or hemoglobin to the cells and carbon dioxide back to the lungs. RBCs also assist with acid-base balance. They contain carbonic anhydrase, an enzyme that joins carbon dioxide to water to form carbonic acid. The acid dissociates to form bicarbonate and hydrogen ions, which diffuse out of the RBC.

The mature RBC has no nucleus and is only 7.5 μm in diameter. Each RBC has a depression on the flat surface which provides a thin center and thicker edges. The RBC's unique structure supplies a very large surface area relative to its volume and allows the cell to change shape passively as it is transported through capillaries that are smaller than 7.5 μm. The average RBC count is 5,500,000 cells/mm³ of blood.

Packed within each RBC are about 200 to 300 million molecules of hemoglobin. Each hemoglobin molecule is composed of four protein chains (globin). The globin is bound to a heme group that contains one iron atom. In healthy men, 100 ml of blood contains 14 to 16 g of hemoglobin. Women have slightly less, about 12 to 14 g. When hemoglobin levels fall to less than 10 g, anemia exists.

Erythrocyte Production

The production of erythrocytes is termed *erythropoiesis.* Everyday RBCs are produced at a very rapid rate. Normally, every minute of the day, more than 100 million RBCs are formed to replace an equal number of destroyed cells. The rate of RBC production increases when oxygen levels decrease, during pregnancy and under the influence of erythropoietin. Healthy bone marrow has the capacity to increase its production of erythrocytes six to eight times over the normal rate and is thus able to keep pace with increased destruction or loss of RBCs. This response mechanism can maintain a remarkably constant number of erythrocytes within each of us.

Erythrocytes are produced in the red bone marrow. Required for this process are (1) precursor cells, (2) a proper microenvironment, and (3) adequate supplies of iron, vitamin B$_{12}$, folic acid, protein, pyridoxine, and traces of copper. If any of these factors is missing, the resultant erythrocytes will be fragile, misshapen, abnormally large or small, deficient in hemoglobin, or too few in number. Erythrocytes arise from nucleated cells called *hematopoietic stem cells. Stem cells* can maintain a constant population of newly differentiating cells. Differentiation takes about 7 days and involves about six stages (Fig. U16–5).

Immature erythrocytes leave the bone marrow via veins in the marrow and enter the general circulation as reticulocytes. After their release from the marrow sites, the reticulocytes travel to the spleen, where they undergo conditioning and evolve into mature erythrocytes before being released into the general circulation.

The life span of RBCs is about 105 to 120 days. As erythrocytes age, they become increasingly fragile and eventually rupture. The released hemoglobin and the empty membranes ("ghost cells") are taken up by macro-

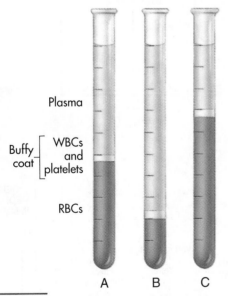

FIGURE U16–3 Tubes showing hematocrit levels of normal blood, anemia, and polycythemia. Note the buffy coat located between the packed red blood cells (RBCs) and the plasma. *A,* A normal percentage of RBCs. *B,* Anemia (a low percentage of RBCs). *C,* Polycythemia (a high percentage of RBCs). WBCs, white blood cells. (From Thibodeau, G., & Patton, K. [1999]. *Anatomy and physiology* [4th ed., p. 529]. St. Louis: Mosby.)

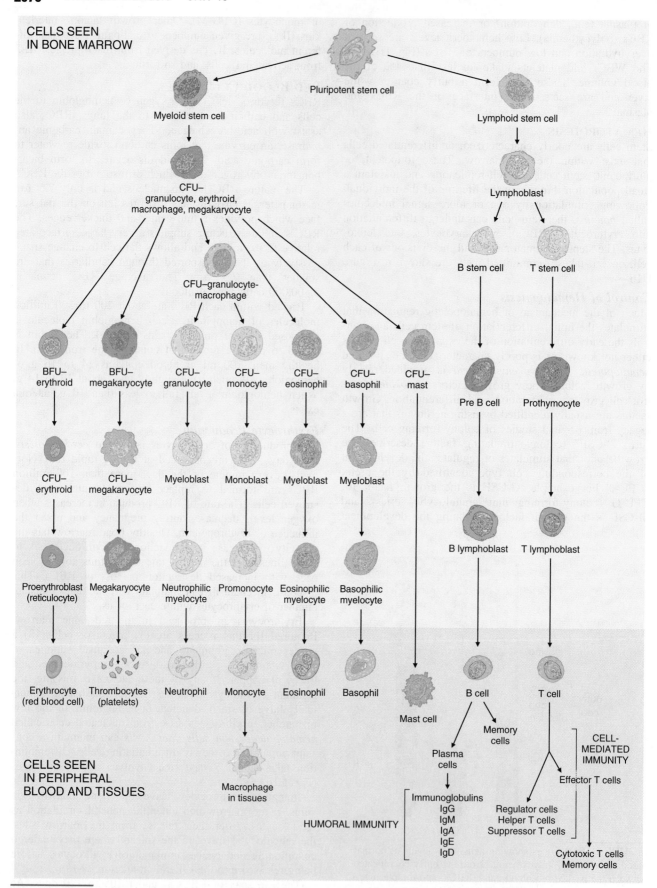

FIGURE U16–4 Hematopoietic cascade. The pluripotent stem cell is the origin of all cells. Once a pathway is chosen, the cell is committed to the final cell type.

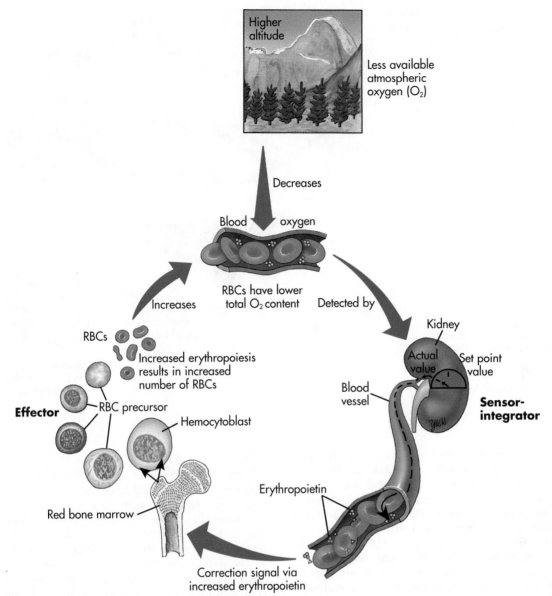

FIGURE U16–5 Erythropoiesis. In response to decreased blood oxygen, the kidneys release erythropoietin, which stimulates erythrocyte production in the red bone marrow. (From Thibodeau, G., & Patton, K. [1999]. *Anatomy and physiology* [4th ed., p. 533]. St. Louis: Mosby.)

phages within the liver, spleen, lymph nodes, and bone marrow. The hemoglobin is broken down into heme (iron and porphyrin) and globin (polypeptide chain) fractions. The iron of the heme fraction is returned to the liver, spleen, and bone marrow to be reused in making hemoglobin. The liver converts the porphyrin of the heme fraction into bilirubin, an orange pigment, and secretes it into the bile to be excreted from the body in the feces and urine (Fig. U16–6). During periods of increased RBC destruction (e.g., in hemolytic anemia), excessive amounts of bilirubin are formed and may accumulate in the body's tissues.

Nutritional Influences on Red Blood Cell Production

Vitamin B_{12} is essential for normal RBC maturation and nervous system functions. Because it is not synthesized in the body, vitamin B_{12} must be a component of the daily diet. Animal products such as meat and dairy products are the only sources of this vitamin. In this context, vitamin B_{12} is called *extrinsic factor* (meaning outside the body). When released from food during gastric digestion, vitamin B_{12} binds with an autogenous glycoprotein called *intrinsic factor* (inside the body) present in the duodenum, and the complex is transported to the distal ileum, where specific receptors in the mucosa bind vitamin B_{12} for absorption into the blood.

Folic acid, a B-group vitamin, is necessary for RBC formation and maturation; unlike vitamin B_{12}, however folic acid does not play a role in nervous system function. The molecule is synthesized by many plants and bacteria. Major dietary sources of folic acid are vegetables and fruits. Cooking destroys some forms of folic acid.

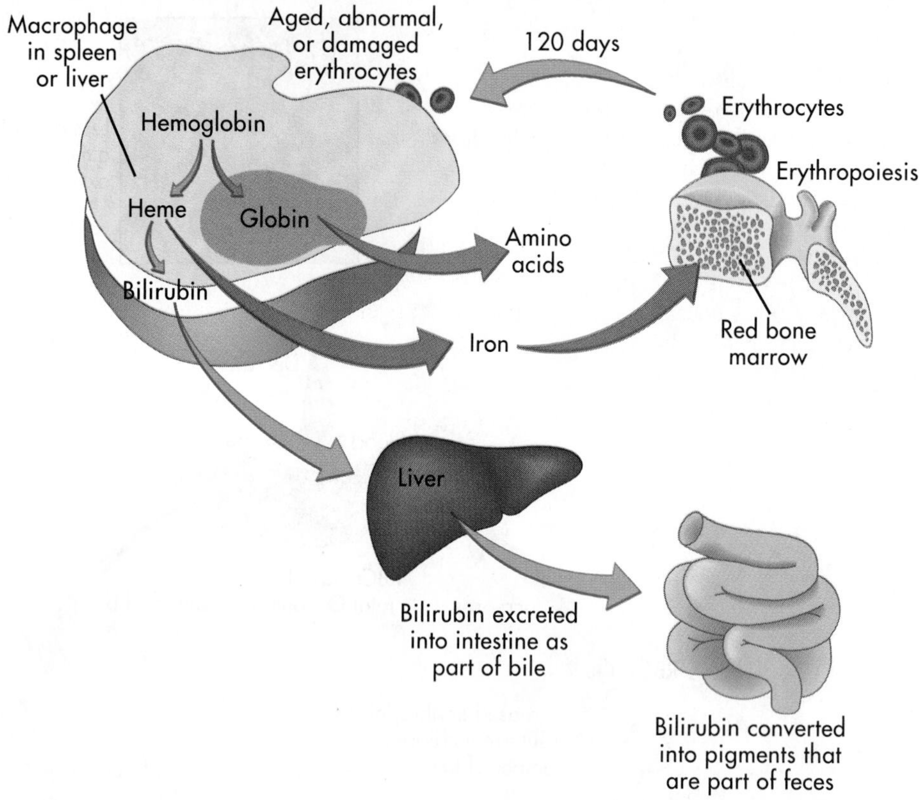

FIGURE U16–6 Destruction of red blood cells. (From Thibodeau, G., & Patton, K. [1999]. *Anatomy and physiology* [4th ed., p. 534]. St. Louis: Mosby.)

Iron is essential to hemoglobin production. The adult human body contains about 50 mg of iron per 100 ml of blood. Total body iron ranges between 2 and 6 g, depending on the size of the person and the amount of hemoglobin sequestered within the cellular compartment. Hemoglobin accounts for about two thirds of the total iron (called *essential iron*). The other third resides in the bone marrow, spleen, liver, and muscle. When an iron deficiency develops, the latter iron stores are depleted first, followed by a gradual loss of the iron contained in hemoglobin.

MEGAKARYOCYTES AND PLATELETS

Platelets *(thrombocytes)* have two essential roles in hemostasis: (1) occlusion of small openings in blood vessels (a hemostatic function) and (2) provision of chemical components in the molecular cascade leading to coagulation (a thromboplastic function).

Individual platelets are produced by a fragmentation process from giant multinucleated cells in the red bone marrow called *megakaryoctes* (see Fig. U16–4). The earliest percursor in this transformation sequence, a megakaryoblast, is large (~30 mm in diameter), has a basophilic cytoplasm, and, when mature, contains multiple nuclear equivalents. The time required for the formation of human platelets is about 5 days. Cytoplasmic extensions from megakaryoblasts are extruded into sinusoids, and platelets are formed by fragmentation at the terminal ends of the filaments. Normal human marrow may have up to 6 million megakaryocytes per kilogram of body weight, with each megakaryocyte being able to give rise to a thousand or more individual platelets. Platelet production in a normal person appears to be under tight control and is remarkably consistent, since the numbers in a healthy person often remain constant for years.

Roles of the Liver and Spleen

The spleen and liver both have important roles in the hematopoietic system. The spleen sequesters some of the peripheral blood erythrocytes, providing a ready reserve supply whenever the RBC count drops significantly.

The liver is also important in the blood-clearing process. Fixed macrophages *(Kupffer cells)* remove inanimate particulates and bacterial cells that appear in the peripheral blood. The roles of the liver in hematopoiesis are mostly indirect and consist of:

- Production of small quantities of erythropoietin
- Synthesis of plasma proteins and clotting factors
- Decomposition of hemoglobin into bilirubin
- Storage of iron in the form of *ferritin*

Hemostasis

Normal hemostasis is a process that repairs vascular breaks to reduce blood loss from blood vessels while maintaining the flow of blood through the vascular system. The three components of the hemostatic mechanism are (1) the blood vessels, (2) the platelets (or thrombocytes), and (3) coagulation factors. These components accomplish hemostatis in three stages (Fig. U16–7):

1. The vascular phase, in which *vasoconstriction* of the vessels occurs.
2. Formation of a platelet plug.
3. Coagulation or formation of a fibrin clot. Once the fibrin clot has served its purpose, it is balanced by *fibrinolysis* (clot dissolution), thus preventing thrombosis.

Whenever bleeding results from injury or disease, the blood vessels that supply the damaged site constrict. Vasoconstriction slows the flow of blood to the injured area, decreasing blood loss. Vasoconstriction results from muscular tissue and reflex nervous system reactions. *Serotonin,* a potent local vasoconstrictor, is secreted by cells in the small intestine and promotes blood vessel constriction on injury.

Adequate numbers of cells (150,000 to 400,000/mm³) are required in the peripheral blood for hemostasis. When platelets come into contact with an alteration of the endothelial cell lining of a blood vessel, they become sticky and adhere to one another, thus sealing the surface of the vessel lining. Platelets also release intracellular storage granules, which include substances that can stimulate circulating platelets and cause them to acquire new adhesive properties. These platelet constituents can activate additional platelets that aggregate to form a *thrombus.*

Platelets control hemostasis unless large blood vessels

have been damaged. If bleeding is severe, coagulation factors must join with platelets to form a permanent clot. The coagulation system consists of a series of interactions that result in the formation of a fibrin clot. The system consists of clotting proteins (except factor IV), that is, factors that circulate in the plasma (except factor III, which is released from damaged cells) in an inactive state.

The formation of a fibrin clot can result from activation of one of two pathways: *intrinsic* or *extrinsic.* Various factors are needed by these two pathways for completion of a final common pathway that results in a fibrin clot.

The *extrinsic pathway* is initiated when tissue injury occurs outside the vessels, such as a burn. Damaged tissues release factor III (tissue thromboplastin), which initiates the clotting cascade to form activated factor X, which leads to the final common pathway of clot formation.

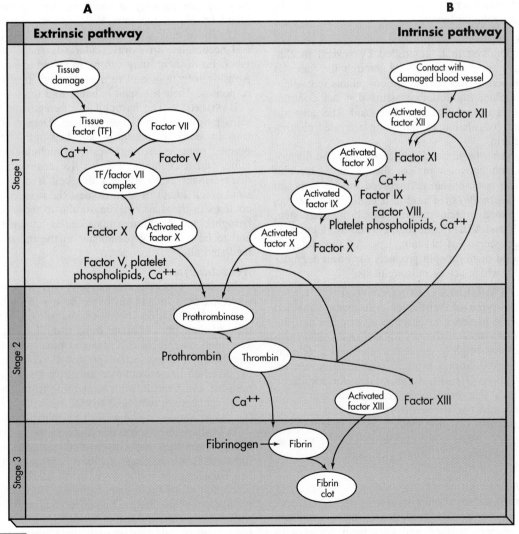

FIGURE U16–7 Clot formation. *A,* Extrinsic clotting pathway. *Stage 1:* Damaged tissue releases tissue factor (TF), which with factor VII and calcium ions activates factor X. Activated factor X, factor V, phospholipids, and calcium ions form prothrombinase. *Stage 2:* Prothrombin is converted to thrombin by prothrombinase. *Stage 3:* Fibrinogen is converted to fibrin by thrombin. Fibrin forms a clot. *B,* Intrinsic clotting pathway. *Stage 1:* Damaged vessels cause activation of factor XII. Activated factor XII activates factor XI, which activates factor IX. Factor IX, along with factor VIII and platelet phospholipids, activates factor X. Activated factor X, factor V, phospholipids, and calcium ions form prothrombinase. *Stages 2* and *3* take the same course as in the extrinsic clotting pathway. (From Thibodeau, G., & Patton, K. [1999]. *Anatomy and physiology* [4th ed., p. 543]. St. Louis: Mosby.)

The *intrinsic pathway* involves the blood itself (i.e., antigen-antibody reactions and endotoxins) or damage to the blood vessels. All factors for the intrinsic system are present in the plasma. This pathway is initiated when factor XII is exposed to a foreign surface, which initiates a cascade of enzymatic reactions to activate factor X, leading to the common pathway.

Activated factor X is responsible for the conversion of prothrombin to thrombin and of soluble fibrinogen to an insoluble fibrin clot. The protein fibrin forms dense interlacing threads that entrap erythrocytes and platelets. The platelets then release a contractile protein, which causes shrinkage and retraction of the clot into a firm, insoluble fibrin mass. The process of retraction squeezes out the clear yellow serum. Serum differs from plasma, in that it does not contain clotting factors.

In some cases, formation of a fibrin clot is unnecessary because hemostasis occurs at an early stage. Temporary clots are sometimes insufficient. For example, bleeding from a small pinprick can normally be ended by a platelet plug, whereas more serious cuts require the interaction of the various coagulation factors.

Fibrinolysis and Anticoagulants

The coagulation system is controlled by several mechanisms to maintain a flow of blood through the vascular space. The blood carries natural anticoagulants (e.g., heparin, antithrombin, antithromboplastin) that act continuously to inhibit coagulation. The liver and RES also aid in controlling coagulation by removing activated clotting factors and fibrin.

In fibrinolysis, the fibrin clot is dissolved. The fibrinolytic mechanism activates in less than a day after clot formation. The two substances involved in clot lysis are *plasmin* and *plasminogen.* Plasmin, a proteolytic enzyme, can dissolve such protein material as fibrin, fibrinogen, and factors V and VIII. Plasminogen, a serum globulin, is the inactive precursor of plasmin. Lysis of the clot produces formation of fibrin split products (or fibrin degradation products), which act as anticoagulants.

WHITE BLOOD CELLS (LEUKOCYTES)

There are five types of WBCs, or *leukocytes,* classified according to the presence or absence of granules and the staining characteristics of their cytoplasm. As a group, the leukocytes appear brightly colored when stained. *Granulocytes* are derived from a myeloid stem cell that differentiates (see Fig. U16–4). Granulocytes include three types of WBCs that have large granules in their cytoplasm. Their names are derived from the staining properties: (1) *neutrophils,* (2) *eosinophils,* and (3) *basophils.*

There are two types of agranulocytes (WBCs without cytoplasmic granules): (1) *monocytes* and (2) *lymphocytes.*

Granulocytes

NEUTROPHILS. Neutrophils stain very light pink-purple with netural dyes. The granules in their cytoplasm make them appear "coarse," and they have nuclei with many lobes. Because of the appearance of their nuclei, they are also called polymorphonuclear leukocytes ("polys").

The neutrophil is the primary cell to respond during an acute inflammatory response (see Fig. U16–4). About 90% of mature neutrophils remain in the bone marrow, a storage arrangement that enables the body to quickly release large numbers of these cells when inflammation occurs in perimeter tissues. The remaining 10% of neutrophils in the peripheral blood are subdivided, about half and half, into a circulating cell group and a cell group that adheres to endothelial linings in small blood vessels.

Thus, a complete blood count (CBC) for a healthy person accounts for only about 5% of the total number of mature neutrophils actually present in the body at that time. The increases seen in peripheral WBC counts during episodes of inflammation are the result of large numbers of neutrophils being released from the bone marrow reserve. If the inflamed state is prolonged, the supply of mature cells with lobed nuclei will be exhausted, and immature neutrophils with a banded nucleus will appear in the circulating blood (shift to the left). The neutrophil's life span is hours to 3 days.

EOSINOPHILS. Eosinophils contain numerous large granules that stain orange. Under normal circumstances, mature eosinophils do not remain long in the marrow; they are present only in small numbers in the peripheral blood (<3% of the total WBC count in a healthy person). These cells exit the peripheral blood compartment and accumulate in extravascular sites near epthelial surfaces. From there, they can be recruited to protect against parasitic infections and to modulate IgE-mediated allergic responses. Their life span is hours to 3 days.

BASOPHILS. The basophil is an enigmatic cell type. It sains purple and has large granules. Details of its normal role in body homeostasis are lacking. The intracytoplasmic granules (storage vesicles) include heparin, histamine, and a chemotactic factor for eosinophils. There is disagreement as to whether this cell is a precursor to a similar cell found in solid tissues: the mast cell. Vesicular contents in the mast cell are similar to those found in the basophil, and the human mast cell is known to bind IgE and to be a primary participant in the induction of IgE-mediated allergic cascades.

Agranulocytes

MONOCYTES. The monocyte is derived from a precursor cell that is indistinguishable from a myeloblast. Subsequent differentiation, however, leads to a cell structure that is markedly different from that of the granulocyte. The monocyte released from the bone marrow into the circulation is a hypoactive phagocytic cell. After becoming attached to sinusoidal endothelium in the spleen, bone marrow, and liver, or after emigrating from the blood into lung, connective, lymphoid tissue, this cell becomes transformed into a *macrophage* with full phagocytic function.

In earlier times some macrophages were given special names when they were discovered: alveolar macrophages (dust cells) in the lungs, histiocytes in connective tissues, and Kupffer cells in the liver. In the 1920s, it was recognized that all of these cells formed a large, dispersed cell population whose major functional feature was phagocytosis. These cells constitute the RES and are responsible for removing all foreign particulate material that enters the body.

The macrophage is attracted secondarily to acute inflamed sites and is the characteristic cell in chronic and in many secretory T cell–orchestrated inflammatory lesions. Some macrophages also have immune functions by serving as antigen-processing cells and APCs.

LYMPHOCYTES. In their mature form, lymphocytes are assigned to one of three groups according to the presence of characteristic surface markers and cell function (see Fig. U16–2): (1) Some lymphocytes are programmed in the thymus to become *T cells;* (2) others are programmed in the bone marrow become *B cells;* and (3) some lymphocytes, not identifiable as either T or B cells, are *null cells.*

B cells function in antibody-mediated immune responses helping to defend the body against invasive types of bacteria, bacterial toxins, and some viruses.

T cells are the basis of cell-mediated immune functions that defend against facultative and obligate intracellular pathogens, fungi, and viruses.

Null lymphocytes, sometimes called *natural killer cells,* defend against some viral infections and are able to destroy some tumor cells.

The Natural Killer Cell System. Natural killer (NK) cells are a poorly understood group of lymphoid cells that make up about 5% to 10% of the circulating lymphoctes. They are involved in killing some tumor cells and some virally infected cells. Their cytotoxicity can be enhanced by exposure to cytokines, which convert a naive NK cell into a lymphokine-activated cell. After binding to a target cell, the NK cell secretes special protein molecules called *perforins* into the intercellular space. The perforins cause holes to form in the target cell membrane in a manner analogous to the membrane attack complex (MAC) of complement. Interestingly, people who have normal T-cell and B-cell populations but who are deficient in NK cells experience repetitive life-threatening infections by viruses such as varicella and cytomegalovirus.

Inflammation

Inflammation is a complex response to sublethal injury to a tissue, having both local and systemic consequences. The process can be initiated by products released from damaged cells, by components from microbial cells, and by the interaction of effector units and antigen. Within the injured tissue site, the first indication is a transient constriction followed by a sustained dilation of small blood vessels. Swelling at the site is caused by the escape of plasma (with its solutes: complement, fibrinogen, immunoglobulins). At about the same time that the vessels are responding, WBCs begin to stick to the vascular endothelium, a process called *margination.* Neutrophils are the first to escape from the vessels *(diapedesis)* and, in response to a chemotactic gradient, accumulate at the site of injury.

After a few hours, monocytes from the local circulation and macrophages present in local connective tissues begin to infiltrate the site of injury and soon replace the neutrophils as the dominant cell type. In a limited type of injury, the healing and resolution begin shortly afterward (see Chapter 16). Some cytokines produced by stimulated macrophages act locally to stimulate vascular changes and to activate fibroblasts and other cells. The same or other cytokines are distributed systemically and help to initiate the *acute phase response.* This systemic response accompanies a strong local inflammatory response. Many aspects of the acute phase response are initiated by the action of cytokines produced by stimulated macrophages.

These stimulatory molecules include IL-1, tumor necrosis factor (TNF), and IL-6. The systemic responses of the host include (1) elevation of serum cortisol; (2) induction of fever; (3) leukocytosis; (4) the de novo appearance of C-reactive protein, an opsonizing protein that aids in phagocytosis; (5) increased production of complement components; and (6) increased production of siderophores (iron-binding proteins).

IMMUNITY

We can become immunized by *direct* (active) or *indirect* (passive) means as follows:

1. *Active* immunity; we produce effector units following stimulation by an antigen.
2. *Natural* immunity is produced by disease and environmentally acquired allergies.
3. *Artifical* immunity is produced via vaccinations and allergies from therapeutic drugs.
4. *Passive* immunity; we receive effector units produced by an animal, another human, or by gene-engineering procedures.

Natural immunity is produced via colostrum (topological protection in humans) and across the placenta (systemic protection in humans). Artificial immunity is produced through pooled gamma (immune)-globulin, $RH_0(D)$ immune globulin (RhoGAM), and genetically engineered human antibody.

ACQUIRED IMMUNITY

Four types (or compartments) of active immunity are identified based on the type and body location of the effector units:

1. *Humoral immunity.* The effector units are immunoglobulins (IgM, IgG, and IgA) present in the peripheral blood.
2. *Mucosal immunity.* The effector unit is an immunoglobulin (secretory IgA) present in mucous secretions of the respiratory tract, GI tract, and urogenital tract.
3. *Cell-mediated immunity.* The effector units are cytotoxic T cells that circulate in peripheral blood and are present in peripheral lymphoid tissues.
4. *Atopic hypersensitivity (type I hypersensitivity).* The effector unit is IgE, which is attached to surface receptors on mast cells found in connective tissues and subsurface tissues of the respiratory and GI tract.

THE PRIMARY IMMUNE RESPONSE AND THE IMMUNE CASCADE

A primary immune response arguably occurs only once (Fig. U16–8). The quality and quantity of the primary immune response depend on many factors, some of which are host-related whereas others depend on the composition of the antigen and how it is presented to the recipient. The primary immune response can be divided into three stages (the immune cascade).

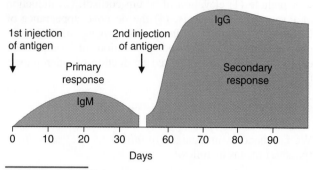

■ Antibody concentration in serum

FIGURE U16–8 Primary and secondary antibody response. The second exposure of an antigen to the host causes a more rapid, stronger, and longer-acting response than the first exposure, owing to the presence of memory cells. Immunoglobin M (IgM) is most often produced in the primary response, whereas IgG is more likely to be produced predominantly in the secondary response.

■ PHASE I: AFFERENT PHASE

APPLICATION OR EXPOSURE TO THE ANTIGEN

Topical (skin) exposure is successful only with certain materials called *proantigens*. Examples of these substances include plant secretions (poison oak, poison ivy), salts of nickel and chromium, and formaldehyde. Mucosal exposure, through epithelia in the respiratory, GI, or urogenital tract, is triggered by foods (strawberries, peanuts), drugs (aspirin), pollens, or house dust. Parenteral (subcutaneous, intradermal, intravenous) exposure is via vaccines, allergens for testing, and so forth.

TRANSPORT OF ANTIGEN

Lymph nodules lie immediately under modified mucosal epithelium (bearing M cells in the gut). No transport of antigen is required. Antigen deposited into solid tissues gains access to draining lymphatics and is then carried to the nearest regional lymph node. Antigen introduced intravenously localizes in the white pulp of the spleen. Proantigens applied to the skin are absorbed and, in conjunction with Langerhans cells in the subepithelial tissues, are coupled with an autogenous protein. The resultant complex is transported to a regional lymph node.

ARRIVAL OF ANTIGEN

Arrival of antigen in peripheral lymphoid tissue is followed by its uptake by APCs.

Any exogenous molecule or any cell that does not have the self-markers of the recipient can serve as an antigen. Antigens may be natural, artificial, or synthetic.

Natural antigens include unmodified bacteria, fungi, viruses, parasites, foreign tissue cells, and large individual molecules such as proteins.

Artificial antigens are natural antigens that have been altered, usually to produce a vaccine: killed or attenuated bacteria, inactivated viruses, and toxoids.

Synthetic antigens are not found in nature but are produced in the laboratory (e.g., molecules genetically engineered to improve current or proposed immunization protocols).

The reactive sites of antigens are called determinant sites (or *epitopes*) and consist of three to five monosac-

charide or amino acid residues that act together as a unit. The determinant sites are complementary to the reactive sites of the T cell antigen receptor (on T cells) and the serum immune globulin (SIg) (on B cells). Each natural antigen has many different epitopes, each of which is capable of stimulating a specific B-cell or T-cell clonotype (Fig. U16–9).

■ PHASE 2: CENTRAL PHASE

In phase 2, the central phase, antigen is taken up by or becomes affiliated with processing and presenting cells. Protein antigens are processed intracellularly by the APCs into peptide fragments, and the fragments, in association with the major histocompatibility molecules. They are placed on the surface of the APCs for presentation to T cells or to B cells that react to antigen in solute form, or they are adsorbed to the surfaces of follicular dendritic cells. T and B lymphocytes become activated and produce effector units and memory clonotypes.

■ PHASE 3: EFFERENT PHASE

Effector units and memory clonotypes are exported to all body sites. If residual antigen remains in the tissues, effector units may combine with it, causing manifestations until the antigen is neutralized or removed. Residual antigen is most often seen with obligate or facultative intracellular parasites or pathogens. This condition is not likely to occur with an extracellular pathogen.

THE SECONDARY IMMUNE RESPONSE

The secondary immune response occurs when a person who has been previously immunized with an antigen is rechallenged later with the same substance. This second (and any subsequent) response is characterized by several features that distinguish it from the primary immune response. Effector units are generally produced in greater quantity for a longer period of time, and antibody molecules may exhibit a higher affinity for antigen (see Fig. U16–8).

■ ANTIGEN PROCESSING AND PRESENTATION

T-cell recognition of antigen is limited to peptide fragments presented by an APC in conjunction with an MHC molecule. The recognition process is assisted by CD4 or CD8 molecules on the T cell surface. Class I MHC mole-

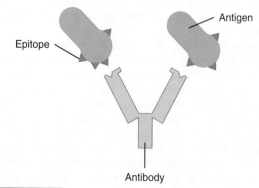

FIGURE U16–9 Epitopes protrude from the surface of an antigen and combine with the appropriate receptor of an antibody, much as a key fits into a lock.

cules are used to present peptides to CD8 cells, and class II molecules present peptides to CD4 cells. This recognition process is said to be self-MHC–restricted; that is, the APC and the T cell both must have the same MHC molecules (each must recognize the other as self). The cells that can function as APCs in peripheral lymphoid tissue sites are B cells, dendritic cells, and some macrophages. Other locations include endothelial cells in peripheral vasculature (in humans) and Langerhans cells in the skin.

■ B CELLS AND THE ANTIBODY RESPONSE

B cells recognize antigen in one of two forms:

1. When free, unprocessed antigen, characteristically carbohydrate is encountered, the response is limited; only IgM is produced, and there are no memory B clonotypes developed.
2. When proteins or protein conjugates are used as antigens, the APCs must first process the molecules to produce peptide fragments, which are combined with MHC molecules and then presented to T helper cells (Fig. U16–10).

The activated T cells secrete cytokines, which assist the B cell in responding to its own set of determinant sites present on the protein antigen. The cytokines stimulate growth and maturation in B cells, induce isotype switching, and make possible the development of memory clonotypes in both T and B cell lines.

After being activated by antigen and stimulated by cytokines, the B cell is transformed morphologically and physiologically into a distinct cell type: the *plasma cell*. Plasma cells are highly differentiated and specialized cells that are capable of producing large quantities of secreted immunoglobulin.

■ IMMUNOGLOBULINS

Antibodies, or immunoglobulins, are a family of glycoprotein molecules that are present in the body as solutes in body fluids (plasma and mucous secretions) and attached to a group of cells in solid tissues. Once attached, they inactivate and bind to antigens to facilitate phagocytosis and initiate inflammation by activating the complement cascade (Fig. U16–11). The terminal amino acid residues react with receptors on the surface of macrophages, neutrophils, B cells, and mast cells. There are five types (Table U16–1).

IGG. IgG is available to react with any antigen that gains access to the circulating blood, either by opsonizing it for accelerated uptake by RES cells or by activating complement via the classic pathway. When inflammation occurs in extravascular tissues, IgG is carried out of the vascular compartment to the septic site. IgG is the immunoglobulin that crosses the placenta and protects the newborn during the first few months of life. There are four subclasses of IgG based on variation in amino acid composition in the heavy chain.

IGA. IgA is the predominant immunoglobulin in saliva, tears, colostrum, breast milk, and intestinal and bronchial secretions. The secretory (or mucosal) form of IgA serves to prevent the adherence of microorganisms to mucosal epithelium and thus supplements resistance mechanisms

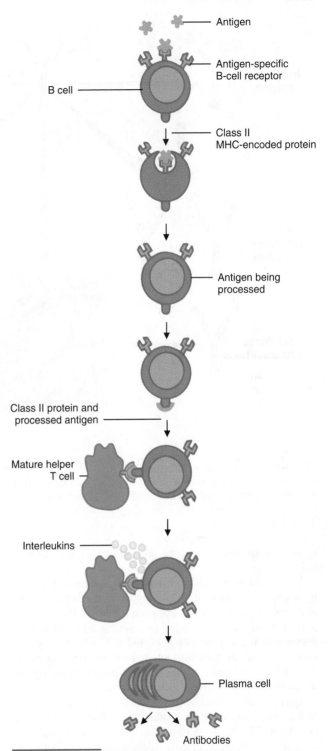

FIGURE U16–10 Activation of B cells to make antibody. The B cell uses its receptor to bind matching antigen, which it engulfs and processes. The B cell then presents a piece of antigen, bound to class II protein, on its surface. The complex binds to the mature T helper cell, which releases interleukins that transform the B cell into an antibody-secreting plasma cell. (Redrawn from Schindler, L. W. [1991]. *Understanding the immune system.* Washington, DC: National Institutes of Health.)

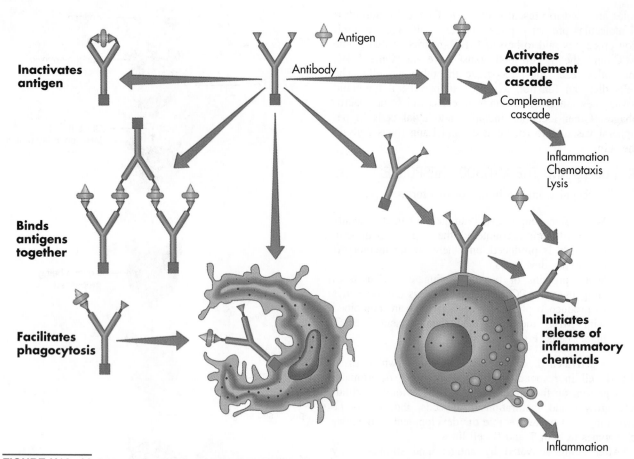

FIGURE U16–11 Actions of antibodies. Antibodies act on antigens by inactivating and binding them together to faciliate phagocytosis and by initiating inflammation and activating the complement cascade. (From Thibodeau, G., & Patton, K. [1999]. *Anatomy and physiology* [4th ed., p. 652]. St. Louis: Mosby.)

against local infections in the respiratory, GI, and urogenital tracts.

IGM. IgM is normally present as a pentamer stabilized by a peptide J chain. It is the largest of the immunoglobulin molecules and is the class identified by the designation "natural." It is produced in response to challenge by bacteria in the normal gut flora and not only acts against these and similar bacteria that may infect tissue sites but also is the main immunoglobulin composing the isoagglutinins reacting with blood group antigens.

IgM is more effective than IgG in activating complement, since only a single pentameric molecule bound to a cell is sufficient to initiate the cascade sequence (IgG requires the presence of two adjacent molecules bound to the cell surface). IgM is the early antibody seen in response to a thymic-dependent antigen and is the sole antibody produced against a thymic-independent antigen.

IGE. In most people, IgE is normally present only in trace amounts within the blood. Exceptions are people who have active atopic allergies or who are infected with parasitic worms. In humans, IgE is normally bound to a surface receptor on mast cells, where, following antigen binding, it triggers the release of chemical mediators such as histamine, which helps initiate the cascade of events leading to the expression of atopic allergy.

IGD. IgD contributes fewer than 1% of the total circu-

TABLE U16–1	CLASSES AND CHARACTERISTICS OF IMMUNOGLOBULINS (Ig)	
Class	**% of Total**	**Characteristics**
IgG	75	Present in circulation and tissue spaces Opsonizes antigen Activates complement Transferred transplacentally The first Ig synthesized in secondary immune response
IgA	15	Present in the circulation and seromucous secretions Prevents adherence of microorganisms to mucosal surface
IgM	10	Present primarily in the circulation Powerful agglutinating antibody The first Ig of the primary immune response Activates complement
IgE	<1.0	Mediates hypersensitivity reactions Binds to mast cells and triggers mediator release
IgD	<1.0	Lymphocyte differentiation Full function unknown

lating immunoglobulins. The physiologic function of IgD is unknown. It is present in large numbers on the cell membrane of naive B lymphocytes, and its only role is thought to be for antigen recognition.

MONOCLONAL ANTIBODIES

Monoclonal antibodies are immunoglobulins that can be synthesized by fusing a normal plasma cell (for antibody) with a myeloma cell (for longevity). The products of such a hybrid cell are immunoglobulins with an identical specificity. Current technology enables large quantities of immunoglobulins with almost any specificity to be produced at reasonable cost. Because they have a single specificity, they are widely used in research and for diagnostic and therapeutic regimens. Some of the applications include leukocyte identification, parasite and pathogen identification, quantitative estimation of peptide hormones, antitumor therapy, immunosuppression, and fertility control.

COMPLEMENT AND AMPLIFICATION OF ANTIBODY FUNCTION

Complement refers to a group of proteins existing as solutes in plasma. When activated, the various components react in a cascade fashion. Complement activated by antibodies form holes in a bacterium's plasma membrane. Sodium and water diffuse into the cells and cause them to swell and burst (Fig. U16–12). Plasma complement can be activated by either of two methods: (1) a classic pathway requiring the participation of antibody and (2) an alternative pathway that is independent of antibody.

The alternative pathway is the older from an evolutionary standpoint and is a major contributor to defense against pathogens. Surface molecules of many bacterial species can initiate the complement cascade, leading to the destruction of the bacterial cell either indirectly by opsonization or by direct cell lysis.

Activation of complement by the classic pathway must be preceded by the interaction of antigen with antibody (either IgG or IgM). The advantage of this pathway is that complement can be recruited to assist in the removal of any solute or of any cell against which antibody can be produced.

T LYMPHOCYTES AND CELL-MEDIATED IMMUNITY

Cell-mediated immunity (CMI) includes immune responses in which antibodies are not involved. CMI is vital in protecting the body against infection by viruses, slow-growing bacteria, and fungal infections. It also has a major role in immunosurveillance, reacting to abnormal clones of self cells, some of which are malignant. Such altered self cells can be destroyed in early stages by cytotoxic T cells or by NK cells, preventing them from becoming established tumors. Other CMI functions include primary rejection of allografts and development of delayed hypersensitivity reactions such as contact derma-

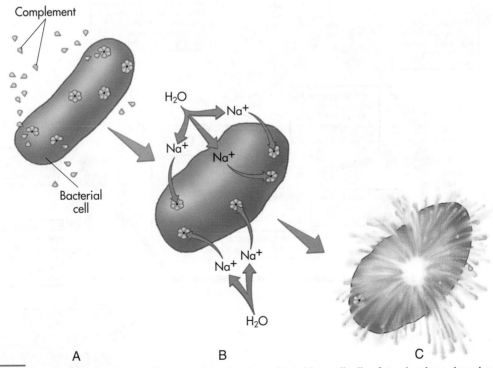

FIGURE U16–12 Complement fixation. *A,* Complement molecules activated by antibodies form doughnut-shaped complexes in a bacterium's plasma membrane. *B,* Holes in the complement complex allow sodium (Na^+) and then water (H_2O) to diffuse into the bacterium. *C,* After enough water has entered, the swollen bacterium bursts. (From Thibodeau, G., & Patton, K. [1999]. *Anatomy and physiology* [4th ed., p. 653]. St. Louis: Mosby.)

titis (poison oak) and hypersensitivity to products of the tubercle bacillus. Many, if not all, of the biologic actions of T lymphocytes are mediated through the secretion of factors called lymphokines (cytokines). Although humoral and cell-mediated responses are often discussed separately, these two arms of the immune system work together (Fig. U16–13), sometimes inseparably, and failure or malfunction in one part of the system frequently alter the effectiveness of the other.

The T lymphocytes that play a predominant role in CMI belong to a variety of T cell subsets. Some have a regulatory function and are designated as *T helper cells* or *T suppressor cells;* others act as effector cells. Cytokines from antigen-activated T helper cells assist B cells to mature and produce antibody and also modulate the maturation and function of cytotoxic T cells (see Fig. U16–13). The importance of T helper cell function is reflected by the severe consequences seen when it is suppressed by physical or chemical means or depleted during infection with human immunodeficiency virus (HIV); the T helper cell is a primary target of HIV. The decline of T

helper cells in infected people is almost inevitably followed by recurrent episodes of opportunistic infections and the development of malignancy in people with acquired immunodeficiency syndrome (AIDS).

The homeostatic reduction or suppression of B and T cell responses to antigen is no longer considered to be restricted to a single suppressor cell population (once thought to be a subset of T cells bearing the CD8 marker). It is now hypothesized that this type of negative regulation may be a function of essentially all T cells. Whether a given cell will act to produce a positive immune response (produce effector units) or will mediate a negative response (tolerance) may be a function of the mechanism by which an individual T cell is activated by antigen.

The cytotoxic T lymphocyte reacts individually with target cells to establish a contact boundary that is required for target cell destruction. The intimate contact between the target cell and the cytotoxic T lymphocyte is mediated by an antigen-specific process and allows the cytotoxic T lymphocyte to release lytic molecules (*porins*)

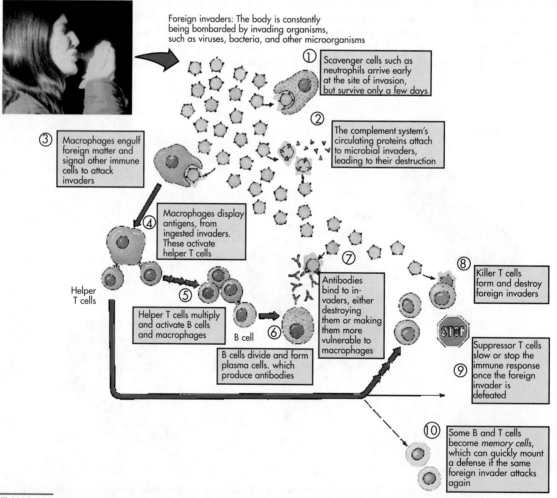

FIGURE U16–13 The protective systems include both arms of defense. Sneezing decreases exposure to the virus. Humoral immunity is shown in steps 1 and 2, cell-mediated immunity in steps 3 and 10. (From Thibodeau, G., & Patton, K. [1999]. *Anatomy and physiology* [4th ed., p. 657]. St. Louis: Mosby.)

directly into the membrane of the target cell. Cytokines produced and released by the cytotoxic T lymphocyte during the cell contact phase enhance the action of porins. The cytotoxic T lymphocyte function is to kill viral-infected host cells, malignant cells, and cells in allograft transplants.

CYTOKINES

The *cytokine* is a general term for cell-derived factors that mediate interactions between cells. Cytokines produced by lymphocytes are called *lymphokines;* those produced by monocyte-macrophage cells are called *monokines.* Some of these factors are called interleukins, indicating service as regulatory signals between various leukocytes (Table U16–2).

Cytokines are a diverse group of proteins with four areas of function:

1. Enhancement of mononuclear phagocytes.
2. Regulation of lymphocyte growth, differentiation, maturation, and secretory activities.
3. Inflammation.
4. Systemic effects such as fever induction and induction of hemopoietic activity in the bone marrow.

One of the best known cytokines is *IL-1,* originally described in the early 1960s. Produced by macrophages, it plays a role in induction of fever, acts as a coactivator of T cells, assists in activation of B cells and NK cells, and initiates the acute phase response.

TABLE U16–2	MAJOR CYTOKINES
Cytokine	**Principal Effects**
Interleukin-1 (IL-1)	Lymphocyte activation Macrophage and neutrophil stimulation Stimulation of acute phase proteins Fever and sleep Pituitary hormone regulation
Interleukin-2 (IL-2)	Enhances T cell growth and function
Interleukin-3 (IL-3)	Stimulates differentiation of hematopoietic cells (colony-stimulating factor)
Interleukin-4 (IL-4)	B cell growth factor
Interleukin-5 (IL-5)	B cell growth and differentiation
Interleukin-6 (IL-6)	B cell growth and differentiation Stimulates the acute phase response
Colony-stimulating factor	Stimulates division and differentiation of bone marrow stem cells
Interferon	Antiviral factor
Tumor necrosis factor	Activates macrophages, granulocytes, and cytotoxic cells Cachexia Mediates septic shock Increases leukocyte adhesion Enhances antigen presentation

IL-2 is also well known from its first identification as a T-cell growth factor. The growth-enhancing function was crucial in the original studies of some of the retroviruses. Current research efforts are directed toward finding an application for IL-2 for treatment of malignant conditions.

IL-3 and *IL-4* are necessary for inducing antigen-stimulated B cells to undergo isotype switching to change from synthesis and secretion of IgM to IgG (or IgA or IgE). IL-3 also stimulates bone marrow stem cells to differentiate into monocytic and granulocytic precursors.

Interferons (IFNs) are another group of molecules that serve as intercellular messengers. There are three major types:

1. IFN-α, produced by many cells.
2. INF-β, produced by fibroblasts.
3. IFN-γ, produced by T lymphocytes.

All interferons have antiviral activity and have a down-regulating effect on proliferation of both normal and malignant cells.

Tumor necrosis factor acts as a growth factor for fibroblasts and has a necrotizing effect on tumor cells. TNF participates in inducing the acute phase response, and is apparently one of the major factors in inducing endotoxic shock (sometimes seen in infections with gram-negative bacteria). This cytokine is thought to be a major cause of infection-related cachexia.

BLOOD GROUPS AND BLOOD TYPING

Human RBCs display antigens that are either glycoproteins or glycolipids on the surface of the membrane. Together the various blood group systems contribute more than 400 characterized antigens. Antigens are inherited from the parents. Fewer than a dozen of these blood group antigens attract frequent clinical notice, and of these only the ABO and rhesus (Rh) systems are major determinants of compatibility testing.

■ THE ABO BLOOD GROUP SYSTEM

The ABO blood type is inherited as an autosomal trait. The four major blood types of clinical importance in this genetic system are A, B, AB, and O. Blood is typed according to the antigens found on the RBC and the antibodies found in the serum.

For the antibodies to be formed, usually there must be exposure to foreign or homologous RBC antigens through pregnancy or transfusion. The major exceptions are the A and B antigens, for which there are structurally similar proteins in the environment, resulting in antibody formation against the missing A or B or AB antigen by the age of 3 months.

The two major antigens within the blood group system are antigens A and B. We may have one (type A or type B), both (type AB), or neither (type O) antigen on our RBCs. There also are two major antibodies found in the serum: anti-A and anti-B. A client with type A blood would have anti-B antibodies; a client with type B blood, anti-A antibodies; a client with type O blood, anti-A and anti-B antibodies; and a client with type AB blood, neither antibody (Table U16–3).

TABLE U16-3	THE ABO BLOOD GROUP SYSTEM		
Blood Type	Agglutinogens on RBCs	Agglutinins in Plasma	Frequency in United States
A	A	Anti-B	41%
B	B	Anti-A	10%
AB	A and B	None	4%
O	None	Anti-A and anti-B	45%

RBCs, red blood cells.

■ THE Rh SYSTEM

The Rh blood groups are nearly equal in clinical importance to the ABO groups. Although Rh serology involves more than 20 different antigens, the D antigen has the most clinical significance because of the high risk of formation of an anti-D in an Rh-negative recipient. The term *Rh-positive* means that the client has the D antigen; the *Rh-negative* client has no D antigen.

The most striking difference between the ABO and Rh systems is that in the ABO system, there is spontaneous development of antibodies directed against A and B antigens not present on the RBC. In the Rh system, antibody formation is never spontaneous. Instead, a client must first be exposed to the Rh antigen, for example, through a blood transfusion or pregnancy. Thus, clients with Rh-negative blood, transfused for the first time with Rh-positive blood, do not experience a reaction because their blood does not yet contain anti-Rh antibodies (anti-D). About 50% of people, however, develop sensitivity and form antibodies against the D antigen as a result of exposure to it from transfusion or pregnancy. Should a sensitized client receive a second transfusion or have a second pregnancy with exposure to the D antigen, some degree of RBC destruction will occur. However, it is usually possible to prevent sensitization from occurring the first time by administering a single dose of anti-Rh antibodies in the form of $Rh_0(D)$ immune globulin (RhoGAM) immediately following exposure to the D antigen.

THE HLA SYSTEM

HLAs are also called *histocompatibility antigens* because the antigens (glycoproteins) are found on the surface of most cells in the body except RBCs (including circulating and tissue cells). The HLA system is a series of closely linked genes located on the short arm of chromosome 6. The major function of the HLA antigen is regulation of the immune response, distinguishing self from non-self. This plays a major role in the rejection of transplanted tissues when donor and recipient HLA antigens do not match. There also is an association between HLA antigens and some diseases. For example, in ankylosing spondylitis, the association with HLA factor is so strong that HLA typing can be used diagnostically.

CONCLUSIONS

The immune system is extremely complex. It has evolved through the years to become a pervasive and highly structured group of complex functions that defend the body against pathogens and parasites from the outside and are able to detect and attack altered self cells that pose threats to organismal homeostasis.

BIBLIOGRAPHY

1. Ader, R., & Cohen, N. (1993). Psychoneuroimmunology: Conditioning and stress. *Annual Review of Psychology, 44,* 53.
2. Arai, K., et al. (1990). Cytokines: Coordinators of immunity and inflammatory responses. *Annual Review of Biochemistry, 59,* 783.
3. Hedrick, S. M. (1992). Dawn of the hunt for nonclassical MHC function. *Cell, 70,* 177.
4. Knight, S. C., & Stagg, A. J. (1993). Antigen-presenting cell types. *Current Opinion in Immunology, 5,* 374.
5. Lanzavecchia, A. (1993). Identifying strategies for immune intervention. *Science, 260,* 937.
6. Ogawa, M. (1993). Review: Differentiation and proliferation of hematopoietic stem cells. *Blood, 81,* 2844–2854.
7. Spivak, J., et al. (1996). Cell cycle–specific behavior of erythropoietin. *Experimental Hematology, 24*(2), 141–150.
8. Springer, T. A. (1990). Adhesion receptors in the immune system. *Nature, 346,* 425.
9. Tomlinson, S. (1993). Complement defense mechanisms. *Current Opinion in Immunology, 5,* 83.
10. Virella, G. Patrick, C. C., & Goust, J. M. (1993). Diagnostic evaluation of lymphocyte functions of cell-mediated immunity. *Immunology Series, 58,* 291.
11. von Boehmer, H., & Kisielow, P. (1991). How the immune system learns about self. *Scientific American, 265*(4), 74.
12. Williams, W. J., et al. (1995). *Hematology* (5th ed.). New York: McGraw-Hill.
13. Young, J. D. E., & Cohn, Z. A. (1988). How killer T cells kill. *Scientific American, 258*(1), 38.

CHAPTER

74

Assessment of the Hematopoietic System

Mary A. Allen

HISTORY

The nature of the presenting problem determines the focus of the health history for the hematopoietic system. Clients may present with manifestations suggesting a hematologic or an immunologic problem.

■ BIOGRAPHICAL AND DEMOGRAPHIC DATA

When assessing the hematopoietic system, note the client's age, sex, race, ethnicity, and family health history. The immune response is diminished in both very young and older people. Some hematologic and immunologic disorders occur more frequently at certain ages, in women or men, and in those of a particular race or ethnic background. In addition, the normal values of some hematologic tests have age-specific and sex-specific norms. For example, hemoglobin and hematocrit levels are lower in women, particularly during the menstrual years, than in men. Hemoglobin values in blacks are approximately 0.5 g/dl lower than in whites.

Collect family health history data because several hematologic and immunologic disorders are inherited. Note occupations, housing, and hobbies to identify possible exposure to chemicals, radiation, and allergens. Inquire about residence and work locations to determine environmental triggers of allergic responses.

■ CURRENT HEALTH

Chief Complaint

Disorders of the hematopoietic system often affect all organs and tissues of the body, resulting in widespread pathophysiologic manifestations. Manifestations may be vague and nonspecific, such as fatigue, malaise, fever, anorexia, weight loss, and chronic diarrhea. In general, anemias often manifest with fatigue, paleness, and weakness; bleeding disorders with bruising, petechiae, epistaxis, and bleeding gums; and immunodeficiencies with recurrent infections, fever, and chronic diarrhea. Allergic manifestations range from mild to severe and can be systemic or organ-specific such as integumentary, respiratory, gastrointestinal, or cardiovascular reactions. Conduct

a symptom analysis (see Chapter 9). The Review of Systems outlines the body systems, their common hematopoietic findings, and the possible pathophysiologic bases.

Symptom Analysis

TIMING. Ask the client when the manifestations began and whether the onset was abrupt or gradual. Manifestations of anemias and immunodeficiencies can develop over time. Bleeding disorders may be present since childhood or may have a recent onset. Some allergic manifestations begin in childhood, whereas others develop later in life. Ask which allergens trigger a response and whether allergies are seasonal in appearance. Determine how long the allergic manifestations last and whether they are relieved or persist once the allergen is removed.

QUALITY AND QUANTITY. How long do bleeding episodes last and how severe are they? Does blood ooze from a site or does sudden, massive bleeding occur? (Sudden bleeding is less common than prolonged, slow hemorrhage.) How often do bleeding episodes occur and how long do they last? What does the client do to stop them? Ask about injury or physical trauma resulting in a break in the skin's integrity. Does the client report associated manifestations, such as lymph node swelling, edema, fever, pain, tenderness, pruritus, redness, or drainage?

Note allergic manifestations such as rhinitis, sneezing, nasal stuffiness, postnasal drip, sore throat, voice changes, hoarseness, wheezing, persistent cough, dyspnea, malaise, fatigue, tearing, or altered hearing acuity. Manifestations vary, depending on the nature of the allergen and individual sensitivity patterns. A symptom analysis for each reported manifestation assists in identifying the allergen.

SEVERITY AND LOCATION. Fatigue is the most common manifestation of anemia. Is more rest than usual needed? Is endurance affected? Ask the client to compare how activities and activity tolerance have changed over time (e.g., in the past month compared to a year ago).

Attempt to quantify the severity of bleeding tendency. Does the client bruise easily? Has bleeding into the joints occurred? For menstruating women, ask whether the number and saturation of sanitary products used during a recent cycle has increased from the usual pattern.

Do allergic manifestations present as simple skin rashes, nasal stuffiness, and cough, or are they more severe such as wheezing and respiratory distress? Do different allergens trigger different responses? Has the client ever experienced an anaphylactic reaction?

PRECIPITATING FACTORS. Hepatic, splenic, or renal diseases may manifest as hematologic or hemorrhagic problems. Anticoagulant medications can precipitate bleeding episodes. Bone marrow suppression can lead to anemia, leukopenia, and thrombocytopenia. Causative agents include antineoplastic drugs, some antibiotics, and radiation. Other hematologic effects from certain drugs include hemolysis and disruption of platelet aggregation.

Has the client recently been exposed to infectious agents? Does the client take corticosteroids or other immunosuppressive drugs, thus increasing the risk of infection? Systemic and local infections can result from broken skin integrity, ingrown nails, or puncture wounds. Altered lymph vessel structure (from surgical disruption, trauma, neoplasm, or scarring from radiation) can lead to edema, particularly in an extremity.

The major types of allergic triggers include (1) inhalants (pollens, molds, spores, dust mites, trees, grasses, animal dander), (2) contact agents (dyes in clothing, fibers, cosmetics, metals in jewelry, plant oils and secretions, topical drugs, numerous chemicals), (3) ingested agents (foods, food additives, drugs), (4) injectable agents (drugs, vaccines, insect venom).

AGGRAVATING AND RELIEVING FACTORS. Medications containing salicylates, including many over-the-counter (OTC) drugs, can aggravate bleeding tendencies (see later). Is the client's edema aggravated by dependent positioning or tight, restrictive clothing? Does elevation of the affected body part reduce or relieve swelling? Are elastic support garments worn to reduce or prevent edema?

What relieves allergic manifestations (antihistamines, antipruritic agents)? What does the client use for relief from a rash? Is an inhaled medication needed for respiratory manifestations?

■ PAST HEALTH HISTORY

Assess for hematologic disorders by asking whether there is a history of anemia; concurrent disorders, such as renal, liver, or autoimmune disease; cancer; or organ transplantation.

Assess for bleeding disorders. Ask whether the disorder may be related to genetic factors, exposure to toxins, or liver disease. Cirrhosis, hepatitis, and other liver diseases can result in reduced production of clotting factors as well as reduced clearance of factors that inhibit clotting or promote fibrinolysis.

When assessing the client with a bleeding disorder, ask the following: How long has there been a bleeding problem? Was it present in childhood, or has it appeared recently? Do any family members have a history of bleeding disorders? Is the bleeding linked to any specific event or procedure? For example, does severe bleeding occur with menses or following minor trauma, a tooth extraction, minor surgery (including circumcision), shaving, or participation in contact sports? Does the client have frequent nosebleeds (epistaxis)? Is there a history of bleeding into the joints or cavities? Does the client bruise easily or report petechiae? How severe are bleeding epi-

sodes, and how long do they last? Is bleeding slow and prolonged or sudden and massive?

Immunodeficiencies may be present at birth or may develop later in life and may be iatrogenic (i.e., a result of treatment with cytotoxic agents, corticosteroids or other immunosuppressants, or radiation). Immunodeficiencies may also result from protein-deficiency malnutrition, protein-losing enteropathy, nephrotic syndrome, or hypercatabolic states (major trauma, severe thermal injury) Immunodeficiencies may be related to loss of anatomic integrity from instrumentation (catheters), impaired dermatologic barrier function (burns, psoriasis, atopic dermatitis), mucosal inflammation (atopic diseases, irritants such as cigarette smoke), or mucociliary elevator dysfunction (cystic fibrosis or the immotile cilia syndrome).

Ask the client about indications of a possible immunodeficiency: poor or delayed wound healing; chronic diarrhea; unusually frequent bacterial infections; unusually severe viral infections; development of an infection with an unusual microorganism (fungus or protozoa); exposure to human immunodeficiency virus (HIV) through sexual activity, injection drug use, transfusion of blood or blood products, or other source; or family history of recurrent infection.

When assessing lymphatic problems, inquire about trauma or other injury, especially to an extremity. Has the client had a recent infection or neoplasm? Edema may be related to altered anatomy or disorders affecting the vascular system, such as heart failure, deep vein thrombosis, or renal disease.

Ask whether allergic manifestations have been present since childhood. Can the client identify triggers? Is there a seasonal pattern associated with the manifestations? Has hospitalization or emergency treatment been necessary for a severe allergic reaction? Was desensitization therapy (allergy shots) undertaken, and was it effective?

Childhood and Infectious Diseases

Did the client experience an unusually severe course of measles, mumps, or other infectious diseases of childhood? Were there severe reactions to vaccinations, especially immunizations with live virus vaccines such as measles and mumps? Are vaccinations current? (See Chapter 9.)

Major Illnesses and Hospitalizations

Ask about major illnesses and hospitalizations. Has the client received a blood or blood product transfusion, and for what reason? Have there been retroperitoneal, intracranial, or paratracheal hemorrhages? Were there problems or reactions to the blood or blood products? Does the client know his or her blood type, including Rh factor? This information is important for the pregnant client who is Rh-negative (see Chapter 37).

Has the client recently donated blood or blood components? Donating whole blood, erythrocytes, leukocytes, platelets, or plasma may affect laboratory values for days or weeks.

Ask the client about the occurrence of any major illnesses, including (1) cancer, (2) lymphoproliferative diseases (lymphoma, leukemia, multiple myeloma), (3) infection (HIV-1, HIV-2, rubella, cytomegalovirus, influenza, varicella zoster), (4) systemic inflammatory diseases (rheumatoid arthritis, systemic lupus erythematosus, sarcoidosis, vasculitis), (5) diabetes mellitus, (6) renal or liver disease, and (7) sickle cell disease.

Is there a history of diseases involving the terminal ileum, Crohn's disease, tropical sprue, ulcers, or severe atrophic gastritis? Ask the client to describe the disorder and its treatment.

Operations

Surgical procedures can influence the development of hematologic disorders or immunodeficiency. For example, cardiac valve replacement may cause erythrocyte hemolysis and subsequent anemia. Anemia may also occur following partial or total gastrectomy or removal of the terminal portion of the ileum because of the consequent reduction in absorption of vitamin B_{12}. Surgical removal of duodenal tissue can decrease iron absorption and thus produce iron deficiency anemia. Splenectomy increases the risk of overwhelming infections with encapsulated bacteria such as *Streptococcus pneumoniae*. Surgical instrumentation and loss of anatomic integrity increase the risk of infection.

Medications

Note the client's past and current use of both prescription and over-the-counter drugs as well as herbal or complementary remedies. Many medications can prolong bleeding, cause hemolysis of red blood cells, or through selective or general bone marrow suppression, produce anemia, thrombocytopenia, or leukopenia. Medications can also inhibit folic acid absorption from the intestine, leading to folic acid deficiency and anemia.

Inquire whether the client takes medications that can cause hemolysis: (1) antihypoglycemic (antidiabetic) agents, such as chlorpropamide, glyburide, and tolbutamide; (2) cardiovascular medications, such as mefenamic acid, methyldopa, and procainamide; and (3) antibiotics, including sulfonamides and penicillins.

Ask about current or recent anticoagulant therapy or antithrombolytic treatment. The anticoagulants heparin and warfarin prolong bleeding, and heparin may also cause immune-mediated thrombocytopenia. The thrombolytic agents streptokinase, tissue plasminogen activator (t-PA), and urokinase also prolong bleeding.

A wide range of medications can affect platelet function or cause thrombocytopenia. Ask about over-the-counter medications containing aspirin or other nonsteroidal anti-inflammatory drugs (NSAIDs) that can interfere with platelet aggregation and prolong bleeding.

Has the client taken corticosteroids, antineoplastic agents (cyclophosphamide, chlorambucil, cisplatin, etoposide), other immunosuppressants (gold salts, NSAIDs), or therapies (irradiation) for the treatment of cancer or autoimmune diseases? These agents may suppress bone marrow production of blood cells or the immune response. Effects may continue long after the medications have been stopped. Treatment with cytotoxic agents or high doses of corticosteroids can mask fever and other manifestations until an infection is serious and widespread.

Has the client received other medications for which myelosuppression is an adverse effect? These include chloramphenicol, cephalosporins, penicillin, tetracycline, sulfonamides, d-penicillamine, amphotericin B, antimalarials, captopril, phenothiazines, or antithyroid drugs.

Determine whether the client has received intravenous immune globulin (IGIV) or intramuscular immune globulin (IMIG) to treat an immunoglobulin deficiency or other condition.

Herbal preparations to ask the client about include comfrey (*Symphylum officinale*), echinacea (*Echinacea angustifolia, E. pallida, E. purpura*), evening primrose (*Oenothera biennis*), ginseng (*Panax ginseng, P. quinquefolius, Eleutherococcus senticosus*), goldenseal (*Hydrastis canadensis*), licorice (*Glycyrrhiza glabra, G. uralensis*), maitake (*Grifola frondosa*), St. John's wort (*Hypericum perforatum*), and stinging nettle (*Urtica dioica*). Topical comfrey acts as an anti-inflammatory on wounds. Herbs used to boost the immune system include echinacea, evening primrose, ginseng, goldenseal, and maitake. St. John's wort has antiviral actions. Licorice is used to reduce inflammation, fight viruses and bacteria, and reduce asthma and allergy manifestations. Stinging nettle is used as a hay fever remedy. Products associated with anticancer properties include vitamins E and C, beta-carotene, selenium, garlic (*Allium sativum*), and green tea. Folic acid (vitamin B_6) and cobalamin (vitamin B_{12}) are necessary to prevent pernicious anemia.

Allergies

If there is a history of transfusions with blood or blood products, ask about complications. Reactions to blood products include fever, chills, back or flank pain, wheezing, headache, vomiting, urticaria (hives), and shock.

Ask the client about past episodes of allergic reactions. Is there a seasonal pattern to the episodes? What manifestations developed? What treatment was given, and was it effective? Inquire about food and drug allergies or sensitivities. Has the client ever had an anaphylactic reaction or been hospitalized for an allergic reaction? Has the client had desensitization treatment with allergy injections. If so, was it effective?

Has the client undergone procedures requiring administration of radiopaque contrast medium, or is this likely in the future? Clients with a history of allergies or asthma may be at higher risk of a reaction to these media and may be candidates for low-ionic-contrast media or pretreatment with medications to reduce the risk of serious reaction. Previously, clients often were asked about allergies to shellfish or iodine before administration of radiopaque contrast media because it was thought that iodine-based cross-reactions could occur. However, seafood allergies are immunoglobin E (IgE)–mediated reactions to the muscle protein tropomyosin that is present in shellfish and mollusks and do not involve reactions to iodine. Conversely, most reactions to radiopaque contrast media do not appear to be IgE-mediated and are unrelated to allergies to tropomyosin or iodine.

■ FAMILY HEALTH HISTORY

Explore the family history for (1) anemia; (2) thrombocytopenia; (3) bleeding disorders, such as hemophilia or von

Willebrand's disease; (4) congenital blood disorders, such as sickle cell anemia; (5) jaundice; (6) infections that are unusually frequent, unusually severe, or caused by an unusual organism; (7) delayed healing; (8) cancer; or (9) autoimmune disease. A family history of neonatal jaundice or early cholecystectomy (gallbladder removal) may indicate a genetic hematologic disorder.

Ask the client to identify allergies and sensitivities in family members, particularly atopic reactions. Hay fever tends to occur among family members.

■ PSYCHOSOCIAL HISTORY

Hematopoietic disorders can result in physiologic changes that affect the client's psychosocial status and ability to perform activities of daily living (ADL). Assess for work-related problems, sexual dysfunction, and fatigue that may interfere with role performance. Encourage the client to discuss current levels of stress and whether they seem to relate to the appearance of allergic manifestations. How does the client react to allergic manifestations? For example, some people break out in hives when under emotional stress. Their appearance triggers more emotional distress and can lead to further outbreaks. A cycle may develop that is difficult to interrupt.

Occupation

Ask about occupational exposure to agents that might predispose the client to the development of hematopoietic disorders: radiation, aromatic hydrocarbons (kerosene, gasoline), benzene (used in manufacture of pharmaceuticals, rubber, leather, and explosives), inorganic arsenics, trinitrotoluene, insecticides, weed killers, lead, and phenylbutazone. Exposure to toxic chemicals and ionizing radiation may occur in several industries (chemicals, plastics, ceramics, steel, metal refinery); in the manufacturing of rubber tires, shoes, incandescent lamps, vacuum tubes, glue, and varnish; in nuclear reactors, uranium mines, research laboratories, hospital radiology, or sterile supplies; and in farming and horticulture.

Does the client have sufficient energy to perform normal activities and occupational tasks? Do fatigue, dyspnea, or other manifestations interfere with a productive lifestyle? Has the client missed time from work or school, resulting in financial loss or other economic concerns, such as health or life insurance eligibility?

Exposure to allergens at work may trigger reactions. Ask about the heating and cooling systems if airborne allergens are suspected.

Geographical Location and Environment

Geographical location may be associated with exposure to possible health hazards. Living at altitudes above 10,000 feet may result in increased hemoglobin levels and other physiologic adaptations. Immunologic disorders may be more prevalent in certain geographical areas. High levels of air pollution can increase the incidence of allergy-related respiratory problems. Ask about home and work environments. Are pets, house plants, or fresh-cut flowers present? What type of vegetation is in the immediate vicinity?

Nutrition

The hematopoietic system depends on the adequate intake of protein, calories, vitamins (A, B_{12}, folic acid), minerals, and trace elements such as iron and zinc. Inadequate intake of any of these substances can lead to anemia or immunodeficiency. Assess for conditions that increase nutritional needs, such as pregnancy, lactation, and hypercatabolic states that occur with thermal injuries. When assessing anemia, obtain a dietary history focusing on the intake of foods such as meat, fish, eggs, dairy products, whole grains, dark green vegetables, legumes, and nuts. Strict vegetarians who do not eat foods of animal origin may be at higher risk for a deficiency anemia, especially related to inadequate intake of vitamin B_{12} (see Chapter 28).

Does the client have allergies to foods or food additives? Do these allergies limit the intake of specific nutrients as previously identified? A food diary is useful to help identify food-related allergic reactions. See Chapter 28 for further discussion.

Habits

Assess the client's current and past use of tobacco (including exposure to second-hand smoke that can aggravate allergies), alcohol, and illicit drugs. Excessive use of alcohol in particular often results in poor nutrition, folic acid deficiency, and decreased immunity as well as acute or chronic loss of blood from gastritis and esophageal varices. Many substances, most notably alcohol, damage the structure and function of liver cells, decreasing the production of clotting factors and reducing the clearance of factors that promote clot dissolution; the result is a bleeding tendency.

■ REVIEW OF SYSTEMS

General manifestations of hematopoietic disorders include fatigue, malaise, weakness, and fever. Specific manifestations can vary if the disorder is related to anemia, bleeding, or immunodeficiency. Allergic manifestations can be general or specific.

Anemia is characterized by pallor, weakness, and light-headedness; severe anemia manifests with chronic severe fatigue, exertional dyspnea, headache, or vertigo. Clients with bleeding disorders manifest petechiae, purpura, and ecchymoses (bruises); spontaneous bleeding from the nose, gingiva, vagina, and rectum; oozing of blood from cuts and venipuncture sites; jaundice; conjunctival or retinal hemorrhage; hemoptysis, hematemesis, hematuria, and back and flank pain.

Clients with hemophilia and other congenital coagulation disorders have a history of lifelong bleeding tendencies, such as (1) excessive or prolonged bleeding after circumcision or dental extraction; (2) repeated episodes of spontaneous bleeding into joints (hemarthrosis), and (3) life-threatening hemorrhages (retroperitoneal, intracranial, paratracheal).

Clients with immunodeficiencies have a history of recurrent infections, especially of mucous membranes (e.g., oral cavity, anorectal area, genitourinary tract, respiratory tract); poor wound healing; diarrhea; and manifestations of systemic activation of the inflammatory response (fever, malaise, fatigue, anorexia, unexplained weight loss, headache, and irritability). Clients with allergies may have rhinitis, sinusitis, urticaria, and pruritus.

Skin

Integumentary manifestations may be pallor (anemia); pruritus and ruddy skin (polycythemia vera); jaundice (bile pigment accumulation from hemolytic anemia), dry skin, dry hair, brittle nails, and spoon-shaped concave nails with longitudinal ridges (iron deficiency anemia); petechiae, especially of the lower legs and hard palate (thrombocytopenia), purpura, and ecchymoses (thrombocytopenia and bleeding disorders); delayed wound healing, lymphadenopathy, and severe acne or acne scars (immunodeficiency); and rashes, urticaria, pruritus, dryness, and scaling (allergies).

Assess for local inflammation (redness, heat, swelling, pain). Clients with severe neutropenia or immunosuppression may be unable to mount the inflammatory response of fever, redness, and pus formation.

Eyes

Ocular manifestations include visual disturbances (anemia, polycythemia), blindness (retinal hemorrhage related to thrombocytopenia or bleeding disorder), scleral jaundice (hemolytic anemia) and conjunctivitis, tearing, eye rubbing, styes, and dark circles or "allergic shiners," or "raccoon eyes" (allergies).

Ears

Aural manifestations are vertigo or tinnitus (severe anemia). Bleeding disorders may manifest as blood in the external auditory canal or as a bluish tympanic membrane, suggesting blood in the middle ear. Immunodeficiencies can manifest as chronic otitis media, mastoiditis, and hearing impairment related to chronic infections (eardrum rupture, scarring, perforated tympanic membrane) or treatment with ototoxic drugs.

Nose

Nasal manifestations include epistaxis (thrombocytopenia and bleeding disorders); crusting around nares, sinopulmonary drainage, and indications of chronic sinusitis (immunodeficiency); and sneezing, sniffling, rhinitis, nasal polyps, nasal voice quality, a crease across the bridge of the nose from chronic rubbing, and stuffiness (allergies).

Mouth

Oral manifestations include a smooth, glossy, bright red, and sore tongue (pernicious anemia, iron deficiency anemia); gingival bleeding (thrombocytopenia, bleeding disorders); and oral ulcers (aphthous, herpetic), candidiasis, gingivitis, periodontitis, dental caries, and tooth loss (immunodeficiencies). The tonsils may be absent without a history of tonsillectomy, or they may be enlarged, inflamed, or pustular. Lip and tongue swelling, frequent throat clearing from postnasal drip, sore throat, itching of the palate, throat, or neck, and hoarseness can occur (allergies).

Lungs

Respiratory manifestations include dyspnea and orthopnea (anemia, sickle cell crisis), wheezing, frequent cough, ineffective cough, and respiratory arrest (allergies).

Cardiovascular System

Cardiovascular manifestations include tachycardia, palpitations (compensatory mechanism to increase cardiac output secondary to anemia), murmurs, particularly systolic (increased volume and velocity of blood through valves related to anemia), and angina (decreased oxygen supply to the heart related to rapid-onset anemia).

Gastrointestinal Tract

The gastrointestinal system may be affected by dysphagia (mucous membrane atrophy related to iron deficiency anemia), abdominal pain (sickle cell disease, retroperitoneal bleeding, acute hemolysis), hepatomegaly, splenomegaly (hemolytic anemia resulting in increased need for removal of erythrocytes), hematemesis and melena (thrombocytopenia and bleeding disorders), vomiting, cramping, and diarrhea (allergies).

Genitourinary Tract

Urinary manifestations include hematuria (hemolysis and bleeding disorders). Reproductive manifestations are amenorrhea and menorrhagia (iron deficiency and bleeding disorders) and decreased fertility (severe anemia).

Musculoskeletal System

Musculoskeletal manifestations are back pain (hemolysis), sternal tenderness and excruciating bone pain (sickle cell crises), and joint pain (hemarthroses or bleeding into joints, often related to hemophilia).

Nervous System

Neurologic manifestations are headache and confusion (anemia, polycythemia); brain hemorrhage (thrombocytopenia or a bleeding disorder); and peripheral neuropathy, paresthesias, and loss of balance (pernicious anemia). The client may experience mental depression (hematopoietic disorders that cause fatigue, discomfort, and acute and chronic problems related to a disease process) or coping difficulties related to a diagnosis of life-threatening illness.

PHYSICAL EXAMINATION

The physical examination of the hematopoietic system can entail both a complete head-to-toe examination and examinations of specific systems, depending on the nature of the client's problem. For example, anemia or fever can cause tachycardia and systolic ejection murmur; immunodeficiency manifested by repeated episodes of pulmonary infections may result in adventitious breath sounds. (See Chapters 54 and 59 for discussions of cardiac and respiratory assessment, respectively.) The Physical Assessment Findings in the Healthy Adult feature outlines expected findings.

The portions of the lymphatic system accessible for a physical examination are the superficial lymph nodes, liver, and spleen (see Chapter 42). Note the presence of a surgical splenectomy scar. Assess the superficial lymph nodes using inspection and palpation. Supplement the findings from the history and physical examination with results from laboratory tests and specific diagnostic studies.

Inspection

Inspect surfaces overlying the lymph nodes for masses, scars, swelling, and redness. Note extremity swelling or edema. Look for symmetry and compare with the contralateral side.

Palpation

Use a methodical approach to examine the lymph nodes; do not overlook single nodes or chains of nodes. Palpate nodes for location, size, shape, consistency, symmetry, discreteness, mobility, tenderness, temperature, overlying edema, or red streaks. Avoid excessive pressure to discern small, yet palpable nodes. Chapter 10 describes the palpation technique.

Lymph nodes are generally nonpalpable. However, small (≤ 1 cm in diameter), single, round, soft, mobile, nontender nodes are common, particularly in the head, neck, and inguinal areas, and are usually not significant. Nodes that are inflamed, tender, large (>1 cm in diameter), hard, matted together, or fixed to underlying structures are abnormal. Describe their characteristics thoroughly. If you see a mass, palpate the area and compare with the contralateral side. The supraclavicular area is a frequent site of metastatic disease; investigate palpable nodes in this site.

PHYSICAL ASSESSMENT FINDINGS IN THE HEALTHY ADULT

Hematopoietic System

Inspection

Alert and oriented; febrile. Skin color even, without pallor, flushing, jaundice, bruises, or petechiae. Lumps or masses absent, no draining lesions. Sclerae white. Lingual papillae visible; oral lesions absent. Eupneic. Joints not swollen; full range of motion

Palpation

Lumps, masses absent. Lymph nodes, liver, and spleen nonpalpable and nontender. Joints nontender. Several round, small (<0.5 cm), discrete, soft, mobile nodes palpable in submandibular area

Auscultation

Heart sounds regular, without murmurs or palpitations

The nodes of the head and neck and the clavicular and epitrochlear areas are most easily palpated while the client is sitting. Palpate inguinal and popliteal nodes when the client is lying down. Axillary nodes may be palpated with the client sitting or lying. Specific guidelines for palpating the lymph nodes are presented in Table 74-1. Palpation techniques are shown in Chapter 10, Figure 10-3.

DIAGNOSTIC TESTS

Diagnosis of hematologic, bleeding, or immunologic disorders depends primarily on laboratory analysis. There is no particular preprocedure or postprocedure care associated with the simple blood tests that are involved in most hematopoietic assessments.

Although dozens of specific tests are used to diagnose individual disorders, all cases generally call for (1) a complete blood count (CBC) to determine the number of leukocytes, erythrocytes, and platelets; (2) a white blood cell (WBC) differential count to indicate the relative percentages of the different leukocytes; (3) coagulation studies such as prothrombin time (PT), partial thromboplastin time (PTT), and bleeding time; and (4) a peripheral blood smear for red blood cell morphology to differentiate various anemias and blood dyscrasias.

The diagnosis of deficiency anemias may require measuring serum levels of iron, total iron-binding capacity (TIBC), transferrin saturation, ferritin, folic acid, and vitamin B_{12} (Table 74-2). Bone marrow aspiration and biopsy are performed to determine both the cellularity of the bone marrow and the morphology of the cells present. The diagnosis of particular hematologic disorders requires specialized blood tests, such as the Schilling test, hemoglobin electrophoresis, and measurement of levels of specific clotting factors. These specialized tests are discussed in Chapter 75.

■ HEMATOLOGIC TESTS

Complete Blood Count

The CBC includes the red blood cell (RBC) count, hemoglobin, hematocrit, RBC indices, WBC count with or without differential, and platelet count. Table 74-3 presents reference values for the CBC. Table 74-4 reviews the effects of diseases, disorders, and conditions on the CBC and the RBC indices.

RED BLOOD CELL COUNT. The RBC count measures the number of RBCs per cubic millimeter (mm^3) of blood. This value is useful in verifying findings from other hematopoietic tests for diagnosis of anemia and polycythemia. Normal values vary with age and sex.

HEMOGLOBIN LEVEL. A hemoglobin determination is used to evaluate the hemoglobin content (and thus the iron status and oxygen-carrying capacity) of erythrocytes by measuring the number of grams of hemoglobin per deciliter (100 ml) of blood. This measurement helps to indicate anemias and polycythemia. Normal hemoglobin levels vary with age and sex.

HEMATOCRIT LEVEL. Often used in place of the RBC count, the hematocrit is a measure of the volume of RBCs in whole blood expressed as a percentage. This test is useful in the diagnosis of anemia, polycythemia, and

TABLE 74-1	SEQUENCE AND PALPATION TECHNIQUE FOR LYMPH NODES	
Nodes	**Location**	**Palpation Technique**
Occipital	Posterior at base of skull and lateral to cervical spine	Flex the client's neck forward slightly to relax the trapezius. Palpate right and left node centers simultaneously.
Posterior auricular (mastoid)	Behind auricle of ear, over outer surface of mastoid process	Palpate over both mastoid processes simultaneously.
Preauricular (anterior auricular)	In front of tragus of ear	Palpate right and left sides simultaneously, anterior to the tragus and posterior to the temporomandibular joint.
Retropharyngeal (tonsillar)	Near angle of jaw at jaw margin	Flex the client's neck slightly in the midline. Palpate behind both jaw angles simultaneously.
Submandibular (submaxillary)	Along medial border of mandible, between angle of jaw and chin	Palpate along the medial borders of the mandible from the angle of the jaw toward the chin. Palpate right and left node centers simultaneously.
Submental	At the midline, posterior to tip of mandible under chin	Palpate with one hand under the client's chin just behind the tip of the mandible. Steady the client's head with the free hand if necessary.
Anterior superficial cervical chain	Along and over (anterior to) sternocleidomastoid, in anterior triangle	Flex the client's neck forward to relax the sternocleidomastoid. Palpate one side at a time. Palpate slowly against the sternocleidomastoid, progressing from the clavicle toward the jaw.
Posterior superficial cervical chain	Along anterior edge of trapezius, in posterior triangle	Flex the client's neck to relax the trapezius muscles. Palpate slowly against the trapezius muscles, progressing from the mastoid processes toward the clavicles.
Deep cervical chain	Under sternocleidomastoid	Flex the client's neck laterally toward the side being examined to relax the muscles and soft tissue. Palpate one side at a time. Hook the thumb (on one side) and fingers (on the other side) around the sternocleidomastoid muscle to feel deep to the muscle. Progress from the jaw toward the sternum.
	Along anterior edge of sternocleidomastoid, in anterior triangle	With the client's neck still flexed laterally, palpate along the anterior edge of the sternocleidomastoid from the sternum to the jaw angle. Repeat on the opposite side of the neck.
Supraclavicular (scalene)	Above clavicle, in angle formed by clavicle and sternocleidomastoid	Flex the client's neck sharply with one hand and encourage the client to relax the shoulders so that clavicles drop. Palpate one side at a time with fingers over the client's right clavicle lateral to the sternocleidomastoid. Ask the client to inhale deeply while pressing in and behind the clavicle. Repeat using the right hand to palpate the client's left node centers.
Infraclavicular	Below the clavicle, in midclavicular area	Palpate the right and left sides simultaneously, pushing in and up, under the clavicles.
Axillary (anterior pectoral, midaxillary, and posterior subscapular)	In the axilla (performed during breast examination)	Palpate one side at a time, anteriorly, centrally, and posteriorly. If the client is sitting, support the client's right forearm with your right hand and use the finger tips of your left hand to palpate, starting low in the anterior axilla, advancing higher to the central nodes, then to the posterior nodes. If nodes are palpable, try to slide fingers beneath to evaluate. Repeat on the other side (see Chapter 37).
Epitrochlear (cubital)	Medial surface of upper arm in groove between the biceps and triceps muscles (included in breast examination)	Flex the client's elbow about 90 degrees, support the elbow with one hand and palpate with the other. Feel for nodes in the fossa, about 3 cm proximal to the medial epicondyle of the humerus (see Chapter 37).
Inguinal	Superior (horizontal) chain, just below inguinal ligament	Have the client lie supine with knee slightly flexed. Palpate one side at a time, rolling fingers along the inguinal ligament.
	Inferior (vertical) chain: close to upper portion of great saphenous vein	
Popliteal	In popliteal fossae on lateral aspect of the knee	Have the client lie supine with the knee slightly flexed. Palpate one side at a time.

abnormal hydration states. The hematocrit value is roughly three times the hemoglobin concentration. Normal values vary with age and sex.

RED BLOOD CELL INDICES. RBC indices are measures of erythrocyte size and hemoglobin content. These values derive from the RBC count and hemoglobin level. Table 74–5 describes the three RBC indices: mean corpuscular volume, mean corpuscular hemoglobin, and mean corpuscular hemoglobin concentration. The indices are helpful in assessing the various anemias.

TABLE 74–2	LABORATORY TESTS USED IN THE DIAGNOSIS OF ANEMIA
Test	**Normal Value**
Iron	50–150 μg/dl
Total iron-binding capacity (TIBC)	250–350 μg/dl
Transferrin	250–430 mg/dl
Transferrin saturation	20%–55%
Ferritin	Men: 15–200 μg/ml
	Women: 11–200 μg/ml
Folate	7–20 μg/ml
Vitamin B$_{12}$	200–800 pg/ml
Schilling test (vitamin B$_{12}$ absorption)	8.5%–28% excretion in 24–48 hr

dl, deciliter; ml, milliliter; μg, microgram; pg, picogram.

PLATELET COUNT. The platelet count measures the number of platelets (thrombocytes) per cubic millimeter of blood. Platelets have a key role in blood clotting. The count is valuable in assessing the severity of thrombocytopenia (abnormally low platelet count), which can result in spontaneous bleeding, as well as thrombocytosis (abnormally high platelet count).

WHITE BLOOD CELL COUNT. The WBC count measures the number of WBCs in a cubic millimeter (mm^3) of blood. It is used to detect infection or inflammation and to monitor a client's response to or adverse effects of chemotherapy or radiation therapy.

WHITE BLOOD CELL DIFFERENTIAL. The WBC differential determines the proportion of each of the five types of WBCs in a sample of 100 WBCs. To determine the actual (absolute) count of a specific WBC type, multiply the total WBC count by the cell percentage reported in the differential. The differential helps in evaluating the body's capacity to resist and overcome infections, in detecting and classifying leukemias and other disorders, and in detecting allergies and helminthic infections.

Peripheral Blood Smear

A peripheral blood smear is obtained to determine variations and abnormalities in erythrocytes, leukocytes, and platelets. Cells of normal size and shape are termed *normocytes;* cells of normal color are *normochromic.* Abnormalities of erythrocyte size, shape, and color usually indicate some form of anemia (Table 74–6).

Reticulocyte Count

A reflection of RBC production, the reticulocyte count measures the responsiveness of the bone marrow to a diminished number of circulating erythrocytes. Specifically, this test measures the number of reticulocytes released from the bone marrow into the blood. An increased reticulocyte count indicates increased erythrocyte production, probably because of excessive RBC destruction (hemolytic anemia) or loss (hemorrhage). A decrease in the reticulocyte count may indicate bone marrow failure or pernicious anemia. The reticulocyte count is also used to evaluate the effectiveness of treatment of pernicious anemia and bone marrow failure.

Antiglobulin Tests

The *direct* antiglobulin test (Coombs' test) is used to (1) detect certain antigen-antibody reactions between serum antibodies and RBC antigens, (2) differentiate between various forms of hemolytic anemia, (3) determine unusual blood types, and (4) identify hemolytic disease in newborns. This test examines erythrocytes for the presence of antibodies (agglutinins) that damage erythrocytes without causing clumping or hemolysis. It is used to crossmatch blood for blood transfusions, test umbilical cord blood for erythroblastosis fetalis, and diagnose acquired hemolytic anemia.

The *indirect* antiglobulin test identifies antibodies to erythrocyte antigens in the serum of clients who have a greater than normal chance of developing transfusion reactions. Both the direct and the indirect tests are agglutination procedures that use a suspension of RBCs.

Coagulation Screening Tests

Laboratory studies are the most crucial for pinpointing the type and cause of bleeding disorders (Table 74–7). Initially, four basic laboratory tests are performed to discern whether the bleeding problem is related to a platelet, coagulation, or vascular defect: (1) platelet count, (2) PT, (3) PTT, and (4) bleeding time. Most bleeding disorders are diagnosed by the PT and PTT.

TABLE 74–3	NORMAL VALUES FOR COMPLETE BLOOD COUNTS IN ADULTS
Measure	**Value***
ERYTHROCYTES	
RBC count (number of cells/mm^3 of blood)	Women: 4.2–5.4 million/mm^3
	Men: 4.7–6.1 million/mm^3
Hemoglobin (oxygen-carrying pigment of RBC)	Women: 12–16.0 g/dl
	Men: 13.5–18.0 g/dl
Hematocrit (% volume of RBCs in whole blood)	Women: 37%–47% (pregnancy >33%)
	Men: 42%–52%
Reticulocytes	0.5%–2% of total erythrocytes
LEUKOCYTES	
WBC count (number of cells/mm^3 of blood)	4000–9000/mm^3
WBC differential	
Granulocytes	
Neutrophils	55%–70%
Eosinophils	1%–4%
Basophils	0.5%–1.0%
Agranulocytes	
Lymphocytes	20%–40%
Monocytes	2%–8%
PLATELETS	
Platelet (thrombocyte) count (number of cells/mm^3 of blood)	150,000–450,000/mm^3

*Normal values may differ significantly among laboratories. g/dl, grams per deciliter; mm^3, cubic millimeter; RBC, red blood cell; WBC, white blood cell

TABLE 74–4 DISEASES, DISORDERS, AND CONDITIONS AFFECTING THE COMPLETE BLOOD COUNT (CBC), AND RED BLOOD CELL (RBC) INDICES

CBC, RBC Index	Increased by	Decreased by
RBC count	Polycythemia vera, cardiac and pulmonary disorders characterized by cyanosis, dehydration, acute poisoning	Anemia, fluid overload, recent hemorrhage, leukemia
Reticulocyte count	Hemolytic anemia, hemorrhage, following effective treatment for pernicious anemia	Bone marrow failure, pernicious anemia
Hemoglobin	Hemoconcentration from polycythemia or dehydration	Hemodilution (fluid overload), anemia, recent hemorrhage
Hematocrit	Hemoconcentration from loss of fluid, dehydration, polycythemia	Hemodilution, anemia, acute massive blood loss
Mean corpuscular volume	Pernicious anemia, macrocytic anemia, folic acid or vitamin B_{12} deficiency anemias	Microcytic anemia, iron deficiency anemia, hypochromic anemia, thalassemia, lead poisoning
Mean corpuscular hemoglobin	Macrocytic anemia	Microcytic anemia
Mean corpuscular hemoglobin concentration	Spherocytosis	Microcytic anemia, hypochromic anemia, thalassemia, iron deficiency anemia
WBC count	Infection, leukemia, tissue necrosis	Bone marrow depression
Neutrophils	Inflammatory disease or response, tissue necrosis (burns, myocardial infarction), granulocytic leukemia and other malignancies, acute stress response, bacterial infection	Bone marrow depression, viral diseases, drugs (chemotherapy, some antibiotics, psychotropics)
Eosinophils	Allergic reactions, parasitic infections, skin diseases, neoplasms, pernicious anemia	Stress response, Cushing's syndrome
Basophils	Leukemia, some hemolytic anemias, polycythemia vera	Corticosteroids, allergic reactions, acute infections (*Note:* decline is unlikely to be detected because normal count is 0%–2%)
Lymphocytes	Infectious mononucleosis, chronic bacterial infections, tuberculosis, pertussis, lymphocytic leukemia	AIDS, corticosteroids, immunosuppressive drugs
Monocytes	Infections (tuberculosis, malaria, Rocky Mountain spotted fever), collagen-vascular diseases, monocytic leukemia	Drug therapy, prednisone
Platelet count	Malignancies, polycythemia vera, splenectomy (rebound thrombocytosis)	Idiopathic thrombocytopenia purpura, aplastic anemia, hemolytic disorders, chemotherapeutic drugs or radiation, hypersplenism or splenomegaly, infiltrative bone marrow disease, disseminated intravascular coagulation, viral infections, AIDS

RBC, red blood cell; WBC, white blood cell; AIDS, acquired immunodeficiency syndrome.

TABLE 74–5 RED BLOOD CELL INDICES

Mean Corpuscular Volume (MCV)	Mean Corpuscular Hemoglobin (MCH)	Mean Corpuscular Hemoglobin Concentration (MCHC)
Measures average size or volume of individual RBC; differentiates anemias into microcytic, normocytic, and macrocytic	Measures hemoglobin content within one RBC of average size	Measures average hemoglobin concentration within 100 ml (1 dl) of packed RBCs
Formula: $\dfrac{Hct}{RBC}$	Formula: $\dfrac{Hb}{RBC}$	Formula: $\dfrac{Hb}{Hct}$
Normal value: 80–95 μm	Normal value: 27–31 pg	Normal value: 32–36 g/dl of packed RBCs
MCV <80 μm means abnormally small (i.e., *microcytic*) RBCs	MCH <27 pg indicates hemoglobin deficiency, hypochromic RBCs	MCHC <32 g/dl indicates hemoglobin deficiency
MCV >94 μm means abnormally large (i.e., *macrocytic*) RBCs	MCH >32 pg indicates macrocytic cells with abnormally large volume of hemoglobin	MCHC remains normal when MCH >32 g/dl because cells are oversized (i.e., fewer cells can be packed together within 1 dl)
	MCH >35.5 suggests spherocytosis	

Hb, hemoglobin; Hct, hematocrit; RBC, red blood cell; μm, micrometer; pg, picogram; g/dl, grams per deciliter.

TABLE 74-6	ABNORMALITIES OF THE ERYTHROCYTE	
Abnormality	Characteristics of Abnormal Cell	Conditions Characterized by Abnormality
Anisocytes	Vary from normal in size	Any of the anemias
Poikilocytes	Abnormally shaped (e.g., tear- or club-shaped)	Any of the anemias; most bizarre shapes seen in the severe anemias
Microcytes	Abnormally small (<6 mm)	Microcytic anemias (e.g., iron deficiency anemia, thalassemia major)
Macrocytes	Abnormally large (>9 mm)	Macrocytic anemias (e.g., pernicious anemia, folic acid deficiency anemia)
Hypochromic cells	Pale appearance because of abnormally low hemoglobin content	Any of the anemias
Spherocytes	Relatively small and round rather than biconcave	Hereditary spherocytosis, warm antibody-induced immunohemolytic disease
Schistocytes	Fragmented, with bizarre shapes (e.g., triangles, spirals)	Hemolytic anemia, thrombotic thrombocytopenic purpura
Sickle cells	Crescent- or sickle-shaped from presence of abnormal hemoglobin (Hb S)	Sickle cell anemia
Target cells	Thin, with small amount of hemoglobin in center	Hemoglobin C diseases, thalassemia major, sickle cell anemia
Metarubricytes	Nucleated	Severe anemia

Because the normal and therapeutic ranges for PT vary according to the type of reagent used in the assay, the PT is standardized by conversion to the International Normalized Ratio (INR). For most clinical conditions that necessitate anticoagulation, the recommended INR is 2 to 3.5. Clients with mechanical prosthetic valves or recurrent systemic embolism need higher INR levels. PT may be performed with a finger stick sample at the point of care via a portable laser photodetector.

Additional coagulation screening tests are (1) the D-dimer, which confirms diagnosis of disseminated intravascular coagulation (DIC), (2) the fibrinogen level, which is low in DIC, and (3) fibrin degradation products (FDP) which are elevated in DIC.

Bone Marrow Aspiration and Biopsy

Bone marrow aspiration and biopsy are used to assess and identify most blood dyscrasias (e.g., aplastic anemia, leukemias, pernicious anemia, thrombocytopenia). Examination of the bone marrow reveals the number, size, and shape of the RBCs, WBCs, and platelet precursors. Hematologists examine marrow cells for various maturational abnormalities. Bone marrow aspiration and biopsy may be performed by a physician or a specially trained nurse. The practitioner may elect to perform the biopsy first and the aspiration second. Bone marrow samples are most commonly taken from the posterior iliac crests. An alternative site for specimens is the sternum.

PREPROCEDURE CARE

Prepare the client for the test. Explain the purpose of the procedure and what to expect. Advise the client that there will be pain during the procedure. Verify that the client has signed an informed consent form. Provide sedation as prescribed. Some protocols use conscious sedation or anesthesia (see Chapter 15).

PROCEDURE

Help the client assume the lateral decubitus position, with the side from where the biopsy will be taken uppermost.

Clean the client's skin with an antiseptic solution such as povidone-iodine. A local anesthetic is administered to numb the skin and subcutaneous tissue to the level of the periosteum. Applying ice to the contralateral side reduces pain.

BONE MARROW ASPIRATION. The skin is incised with a scalpel. The bone marrow aspiration needle containing an obturator is inserted through the incision to the bone cortex and into the marrow space. Once the needle is in place, the obturator is removed. A syringe is then attached to the needle, and about 1 ml of marrow is withdrawn. Because the marrow space itself cannot be anesthetized, removal of the marrow usually produces moderate to severe pain of short duration. The pain usually stops as soon as suction on the marrow space is stopped. The marrow is ejected onto labeled slides. The needle is withdrawn. Specimens should be sent to the laboratory immediately.

BONE MARROW BIOPSY. The bone marrow biopsy needle is advanced through the soft tissue to the periosteum of the biopsy site. The obturator is removed, and the biopsy needle is advanced into the cortex. After the cortex is penetrated, the biopsy needle is advanced another 2 to 3 cm through the bony trabeculae. The needle is rotated several times in a circular back-and-forth motion to cut the core sample and then is withdrawn. A small probe is used to remove the core sample from the end of the biopsy needle, and the sample is placed in formalin. Specimens are labeled and sent to the laboratory immediately.

POSTPROCEDURE CARE

After the procedure, apply pressure until bleeding stops. Most clients require only a small bandage over the site because bleeding is usually minimal. However, many clients who require bone marrow aspiration are thrombocytopenic and may need a longer period of pressure to stop bleeding. A pressure dressing and sandbag may be applied in these cases. Instruct the family to observe the site frequently on the day of the procedure and for several

TABLE 74-7	LABORATORY TESTS USED IN THE DIAGNOSIS OF HEMORRHAGIC DISORDERS		
Name of Test	**Purpose**	**Normal Values**	**Interpretation of Findings**
Platelet count	Measures number of circulating platelets in venous or arterial blood	150,000–450,000/mm^3	Low count results in prolonged bleeding time and impaired clot retraction; diagnostic of thrombocytopenia
Prothrombin time (PT)	Determines activity and interaction of factors V, VII, and X, prothrombin, and fibrinogen; determines dosages of oral anticoagulant drugs	11–15 sec (one-stage) INR: 2–3.5	Prolonged PT is seen in clients receiving anticoagulant therapy; with low levels or deficiencies of fibrinogen, clotting factors II, V, VII, and X; impaired prothrombin activity; in the presence of circulating anticoagulants as seen in SLE
Partial thromboplastin time (PTT, aPTT)	Complex method for testing the normalcy of intrinsic coagulation process; employed to identify deficiencies of coagulation factors, prothrombin, and fibrinogen; used to monitor heparin therapy	25–38 sec	Prolongation of time indicates coagulation disorder that is related to deficiency of a coagulation factor; not diagnostic for platelet disorders
Thrombin time	Measures functional fibrinogen available, as shown by the time needed to form fibrin clot after thrombin is added	10–15 sec	Prolonged time indicates DIC or hypofibrinogenemia; presence in blood of excess heparin or other anticoagulants
Thromboplastin generation test (TGT)	Measures generation of thromboplastin; if result abnormal, second stage is done to identify missing coagulation factor	<12 sec (100%)	Abnormal values found in hemophilia
Fibrinogen level	Measures level of fibrinogen	200–400 mg/dl	Abnormally low values may indicate DIC, liver disease, congenital or acquired afibrinogenemia
Fibrin split products (FSPs), fibrin degradation products (FDPs) test	Measures products that result from breakdown of fibrin	Less than 10 μg/ml	Abnormally high levels are seen in DIC; helpful in monitoring fibrinolytic therapy
D-dimer	Measures a specific product resulting from breakdown of fibrin	Less than 0.5 μg/ml	Abnormally high levels confirm the diagnosis of DIC; screen for abruptio placentae (placental abruption)
Activated clotting time	Crude measure of coagulation process in venous blood; used to control heparin therapy; commonly used during cardiovascular surgery and in the ICU	7–120 sec (depends on type of activator used)	Prolonged time occurs in severe coagulation problems and therapeutic administration of heparin
Bleeding time	Measures ability to stop bleeding after a small puncture wound	3–8 min in adults (varies with test method)	Prolonged bleeding time occurs in vascular maladies and after aspirin ingestion
Capillary fragility test (tourniquet test, Rumpel-Leede test)	Crude test of vascular resistance and platelet number and function; a BP cuff is placed on the arm and inflated to a pressure midway between systolic and diastolic BP for 5 min; petechiae in area are counted	No petechiae	Petechiae (five or more) are seen in thrombocytopenia and vascular purpura
Clot retraction	Indicates function and number of platelets; measures time needed for contraction of an undisturbed clot	50%–100% in 24 hr	Clot retraction is retarded in thrombocytopenia; clot is small and soft in thrombasthenia (functional disturbance of platelets)

BP, blood pressure; DIC, disseminated intravascular coagulation; ICU, intensive care unit; INR, International Normalized Ratio; mg/dl, milligrams per deciliter; μg, microgram; SLE, systemic lupus erythematosis.

TABLE 74–8	LYMPHOCYTE IMMUNOPHENOTYPING			
Cell	Total Lymphocyte Count (%)	Absolute Count	Decreased	Increased
CD3 (mature T cells)	56%–77%	860–1880/mm³	AIDS, chronic lymphocytic leukemia, SCID, immunosuppressive therapy	Acute lymphocytic leukemia, infectious mononucleosis, multiple myleoma
CD19 (total B cells)	7%–17%	140–370/mm³	Acute lymphocytic leukemia, SCID	Chronic lymphocytic leukemia, multiple myeloma, SLE
CD4 (T helper cells)	32%–54%	530–1190/mm³	AIDS	—
CD8 (T killer/suppressor cells)	24%–37%	430–1060/mm³	AIDS	—

mm³, cubic millimeter; AIDS, acquired immunodeficiency syndrome; SLE, systemic lupus erythematosus; SCID, severe combined immunodeficiency disease.

days thereafter for clients with an increased risk for bleeding. Clients may experience some discomfort or pain and may require a mild analgesic.

■ IMMUNOLOGIC STATUS TESTS

Most immunodeficiencies can be identified through three blood tests requiring no preprocedure or postprocedure care: (1) WBC and differential, (2) immunoglobulin levels, and (3) total serum complement. Additional immunodeficiencies can be determined through more complex tests, including lymphocyte immunophenotyping, measures of immunoglobulin subclasses, complement assays, and the presence of specific antibodies (after immunizations or exposure to antigens as with communicable diseases).

Lymphocyte Immunophenotyping

Lymphocyte subpopulation analysis by flow cytometry measures total numbers and percentages of B lymphocytes, T lymphocytes, and T lymphocyte subsets (CD4, CD8) in a peripheral blood sample. Table 74–8 lists normal levels of T and B lymphocytes and conditions in which abnormal levels of T and B cells occur.

Advanced lymphocyte assays (not detailed here) include

- Mixed lymphocyte culture reaction with the client as stimulator and the client as responder
- Lymphoproliferation assays using chemicals such as phytohemagglutinin (PHA) or concanavalin A (ConA) to stimulate T cells and pokeweed mitogen to stimulate B cells
- Tests of natural killer cell activity
- Tests for deficiencies of adenosine deaminase and purine nucleoside phosphorylase

Immunoglobulin Isotypes

The immunoglobulin isotype examination measures the serum level of the various immunoglobulins: IgG, IgA, IgM, IgD, and IgE (Table 74–9). Subclasses of IgG may also be measured (IgG1, IgG2, IgG3, IgG4).

Complement Assays

Immunodeficiencies or disorders that are related to a lack of normal levels of complement components may be detected by the level of the total serum complement (CH50) or may require measuring levels of specific complement components such as C3 and C4. In rare cases, functional complement assays are required to diagnose complement disorders. Table 74–10 provides normal complement levels.

Radiography

Congenital absence of thymic tissue (diagnostic of certain immunodeficiencies) or tumor of the thymus gland (associated with myasthenia gravis) can be detected by a chest radiograph (see Chapter 11).

Other radiographic procedures may be performed to assist the diagnosis of allergy-related disorders. X-ray films and computed tomography (CT) may be ordered to assess the integrity of the sinuses (see Chapter 11).

Lymphangiography allows visualization of the lymphatic system to assess malignancy, metastases, or obstruction. Following local anesthesia administration, blue dye is injected into the dorsa of the feet and is taken up

TABLE 74–9	IMMUNOGLOBULIN (Ig) ISOTOPES
Immunoglobulin	Normal Range (mg/dl)
IgG	550–1990
IgG1	280–1020
IgG2	60–790
IgG3	14–240
IgG4	11–330
IgM	45–145
IgA	70–310
IgE	0.01–0.04
IgD	0–8

mg/dl, milligrams per deciliter.

TABLE 74–10	COMPLEMENT ASSAYS	
Test		**Normal Range**
Total serum complement (CH50)		75–160 U/ml
C3		55–177 mg/dl
C4		15–50 mg/dl

mg/dl, milligrams per deciliter; U/ml, units per millilter.

by the lymphatics. When a lymphatic channel is located, a surgical incision into the channel allows insertion of a catheter. An oil-based dye is injected, and its progress through the lymphatic system is monitored with x-rays taken over 1 to 2 days.

Postprocedure care and complications are similar to those for angiography (see Chapter 11). Explain that the dye colors the urine blue until it is completely excreted. The dorsa may also remain blue for months.

Skin Tests

Skin tests confirm sensitivity to a specific allergen. A known antigen is placed on or directly beneath the skin to detect the presence of antibodies. Antigens are applied by one of three methods:

1. *Patch tests* (see Chapter 48).
2. *Scratch tests* (also known as *tine tests* or *prick tests*). Antigens are applied to superficial scratches that cut the outer layer of skin. The skin is then covered with gauze.
3. Intradermal allergy tests involve injecting a small amount (usually 0.1 ml) into the intradermal layer of the skin. Intradermal testing is the most accurate method but carries a higher risk of severe allergic reaction.

Take a thorough client history of allergies, and explain the purpose of the test and the procedure. Verify the specific antigens prescribed by the physician for testing, and ensure the availability of emergency resuscitation equipment in the event of an anaphylactic reaction.

Nurses often administer skin tests and interpret test results. Observe the client for the following. An immediate, positive reaction can appear within 10 to 20 minutes after antigen application, marked by erythema and wheal formation. Positive reactions indicate an antibody (B cell) response to a previous exposure to the antigen; they also suggest that the client is allergic to the substance causing the reaction. Negative reactions may be inconclusive, indicating the need for further assessment. Negative results may indicate that (1) antibodies have not formed to the specific antigen, (2) the antigen was deposited too deeply into the skin (subcutaneously rather than intradermally), or (3) the client is immunosuppressed as a result of disease or therapy (chemotherapy, corticosteroids, radiation therapy, or long-acting antihistamines that can mute an allergic response).

Problems following skin testing range from minor itching and discomfort at the injection site (common) to anaphylaxis (rare). Relieve itching and minor discomfort with the application of cool compresses and topical corticosteroids. If ulceration of the injection site occurs, keep the area clean and dry. Anaphylaxis is potentially lethal. Clients who have known anaphylactic reactions to specific antigens should never be tested for allergy to that substance. Anaphylaxis is treated with the administration of oxygen and subcutaneous epinephrine and by establishing intravenous access for administration of corticosteroids, antihistamines, and other medications, such as bronchodilators.

DELAYED-TYPE HYPERSENSITIVITY SKIN TESTING. T-cell responsiveness may be evaluated by DTH skin testing. Antigens to which people have been immunized (mumps, tetanus) or to which they commonly have been exposed (*Candida albicans*) are injected intradermally into the ventral forearm. After 24 to 72 hours, people with normal T-cell immunity exhibit an area of hard, reddened swelling (*induration*) at the injection site. The localized thickening and redness indicate accumulation of sensitized T lymphocytes at the site of antigen administration. Absence of induration may indicate *anergy* (a state of immunologic hyporesponsiveness) and an inability to react to common antigens. Anergy is associated with congenital T-cell immunodeficiency, malnutrition, cancer, HIV infection, immunosuppressant therapy, and, in the elderly, aging of the immune system.

DTH antigens are most accurately administered by separate intradermal injections of mumps antigen, *C. albicans* antigen, and tetanus toxoid fluid (1:5 dilution). Other antigens such as streptokinase, streptodornase, or trichophytin may be used but may be less reliable in assessment of T-cell immunity.

A commercial kit (CMI Multitest, Merieux, France) permits the simultaneous administration of several DTH antigens as well as a positive and a negative control. However, the kit may be less reliable for tuberculosis screening because it contains *old tuberculin* rather than *purified protein derivative* (PPD). For consistency, it is best if the same person administers and reads the skin test.

PROCEDURE

Use a 1-ml syringe with a 1/2-inch 26 to 27 gauge needle to administer the antigen. Select a site on the ventral surface of the forearm, avoiding veins or bruises. Clean the skin with alcohol, and allow it to dry. Stretch the skin taut. Inject 0.1 ml of the antigen intradermally, producing a wheal 6 to 10 mm in diameter. Circle the area with a marking pen. If more than one antigen is administered, administer each antigen 5 cm apart. Document the site of administration of each antigen using a schematic drawing.

POSTPROCEDURE CARE

After 48 to 72 hours, palpate the site for induration. Use a flexible ruler to measure the area of induration; redness alone is not significant. Induration of 5 mm or more with erythema indicates a positive response to the antigen and probable intact cell-mediated immunity. Record the results.

Food Allergy Testing

Food allergies are evaluated by skin testing or by either a *challenge diet* or *elimination diet*. In the challenge diet, the suspected food is eaten by the client in increasingly larger amounts until a reaction occurs. Reactions range from erythema, itching, and rash to vomiting or diarrhea. Manifestations such as fatigue, depression, or restlessness are not conclusive. In the elimination diet, foods are eliminated from the diet, one by one, until manifestations are relieved. Reactions may indicate an allergy to food additives or the food itself.

CONCLUSIONS

The hematopoietic system is extremely complex. Understanding the structure, function, and assessment of the hematopoietic system will help you care for clients with any of the wide variety of disorders that affect this highly complex system.

BIBLIOGRAPHY

1. Anderson, K. N. (Ed.). (1998). *Mosby's medical, nursing, and allied health dictionary.* St. Louis: Mosby–Year Book.
2. Bates, B. (1995). *A guide to physical examination and history taking* (6th ed.) Philadelphia: J. B. Lippincott.
3. Bennett, J. C., & Plum, F. (Eds.). (1996). *Cecil textbook of medicine* (20th ed.). Philadelphia: W. B. Saunders.
4. Chernecky, C. C., & Berger, B. J. (Eds.). (1997). *Laboratory tests and diagnostic procedures* (2nd ed.). Philadelphia: W. B. Saunders.
5. Coakley, F. V., & Panicek, D. M. (1997). Iodine allergy: An oyster without a pearl? *American Journal of Roentgenology, 169*(4), 951–952.
6. Conn, H. F., Clohency, R. J., & Conn, R. B. (Eds.). (1997). *Current diagnosis.* Philadelphia: W. B. Saunders.
7. Corbett, J. (1996). *Laboratory tests and diagnostic procedures with nursing diagnoses* (4th ed.). Stamford, CT: Appleton & Lange.
8. Freeman, T. M. (1998). Anaphylaxis: Diagnosis and treatment. *Primary Care, 25*(4), 809–817.
9. Gibbar-Clements, T., Shirrell, D., & Free, C. (1997). PT and APTT: Seeing beyond the numbers. *Nursing, 27*(7), 49–51.
10. Goyette, R. E. (1997). *Hematology: A comprehensive guide to the diagnosis and treatment of blood disorders.* Los Angeles: Practice Management Information Corporation (PMIC).
11. Gruchalla, R. S. (1998). Drug allergies. *Primary Care, 25*(4), 791–807.
12. Guyton, A. C., & Hall, J. E. (1996). *Textbook of medical physiology* (9th ed.). Philadelphia: W. B. Saunders.
13. Hash, R. B. (1999). Intravascular radiographic contrast media: Issues for family physicians. *Journal of American Family Practice, 12*(1), 32–42.
14. Henry, J. B. (Ed.). (1996). *Clinical diagnosis and management by laboratory methods* (19th ed.). Philadelphia: W. B. Saunders.
15. Jarvis, C. (2000). *Physical examination and health assessment* (3rd ed.). Philadelphia: W. B. Saunders.
16. Kee, J. L. (1995). *Laboratory and diagnostic tests with nursing implications* (4th ed.). Norwalk, CT: Appleton & Lange.
17. Kurt J., et al. (Eds.). (1998). *Harrison's principles of internal medicine* (13th ed.). New York: McGraw-Hill.
18. Mandell, G. L., Douglas, R. G., & Bennett, J. E. (1995). *Principles and practice of infectious diseases* (4th ed.). New York: Churchill Livingstone.
19. Metcalfe, D. D. (1998). Food allergy. *Primary Care, 25*(4), 819–829.
20. Pagana, K. D., & Pagana, T. J. (1997). *Mosby's diagnostic and laboratory reference* (3rd ed.). St. Louis: Mosby–Year Book.
21. Seidel, H. M., et al. (1995). *Mosby's guide to physical examination* (3rd ed.). St. Louis: Mosby–Year Book.
22. Stellato, C., & Adkinson, N. F. (1998). Pathophysiology of contrast media anaphylactoid reactions: New perspectives on an old problem. *Allergy, 53*(12), 1111–1113.
23. Stevens, M. L. (1997). *Fundamentals of clinical hematology.* Philadelphia: W. B. Saunders.
24. Tierney, L. M., McPhee, S. J., & Papadakis, M. A. (Eds.). (1998). *Current medical diagnosis and treatment 1998* (36th ed.). Stamford, CT: Appleton & Lange.
25. Treseler, K. M. (1995). *Clinical laboratory and diagnostic tests: Significance and nursing implications* (3rd ed.). Stamford, CT: Appleton & Lange.
26. Watson, J., & Jaffee, M. S. (1995). *Nurse's manual of laboratory and diagnostic tests* (2nd ed.). Philadelphia: F. A. Davis.

REMEMBER *to*
check out your
Companion CD ROM

Management of Clients with Hematologic Disorders

Linda Yoder

This chapter discusses disorders affecting red blood cells (erythrocytes), the spleen, platelets, and clotting factors. Priorities of nursing care center around lack of oxygenated blood flow and risk of hemorrhage. Leukemia and lymphoma are discussed in Chapter 78.

DISORDERS AFFECTING RED BLOOD CELLS

THE ANEMIAS

Anemia is a reduction in red blood cells (RBCs), which in turn decreases the oxygen-carrying capacity of the blood. Not a disease in itself, anemia reflects an abnormality in RBC number, structure, or function. The prevalence of anemia increases with age; an estimated 20% of older adults are anemic. However, anemia cannot be assumed to be caused simply by aging without the exclusion of reversible causes. The elderly client should be fully assessed for an underlying cause of anemia.

Etiology

Major causes of anemia are deficiencies and abnormalities of RBC production or excessive blood loss or destruction of RBCs.

Hematopoiesis is reviewed in the Anatomy and Physiology review preceding this unit. RBCs are produced in bone marrow. The requirements for RBC production, called *erythropoiesis,* include precursor cells (*reticulocytes*), adequate supplies of iron, vitamin B_{12}, folic acid, protein, pyridoxine, and traces of copper. If any of these factors is missing, the RBCs will be fragile, misshapen, of abnormal size, lacking hemoglobin, or too few in number.

Anemia may be due to acute or chronic blood loss. Increased destruction of RBCs can result from extrinsic sources, physical causes such as prosthetic heart valves, or thrombotic thrombocytopenic purpura. It also can result from antibodies, as in transfusion mismatch; from infectious agents and toxins; or from other causes, such as hypersplenism or osmotic and physical injury to the cell seen in sickle cell disease.

Classification

Anemias are classified according to the size of the RBC. Normal RBCs are shown in Figure 75–1A. *Normocytic anemia* is anemia with normal RBC size and shape. This form of anemia is commonly due to blood loss, chronic disease, and bone marrow suppression with chemotherapy. *Microcytic anemia* is defined as anemia with small RBCs and low levels of hemoglobin in each RBC. Common causes of microcytic anemia include iron deficiency due to protein malnutrition and occult gastrointestinal (GI) bleeding with gastritis or colon cancer. *Macrocytic anemia* is characterized by large RBCs. Common causes include vitamin B_{12} and folic acid deficiency. Anemias can also be due to defective hemoglobin in which case, the condition is called *sickle cell anemia* (Fig. 75–1B).

Pathophysiology

Transport of oxygen is impaired with anemia. Hemoglobin is lacking or the number of RBCs is too low to carry adequate oxygen to tissues, and hypoxia develops.

Clinical Manifestations

Manifestations accompanying anemia differ, depending on the severity and speed of blood loss, the chronicity of the anemia, the age of the person, and the presence of other disorders. Tissue hypoxia is the underlying cause of all manifestations accompanying anemia. Other manifestations listed below are due to the underlying problem.

Clients often appear pale, particularly of palm lines, nail beds, conjunctivae, and circumoral area. Because of tissue hypoxia, clients are fatigued. There may be shortness of breath, dyspnea on exertion, or palpitations. Hypotension is common, especially if the client has lost blood. If the client has GI bleeding, tarry stools may be present. If heart failure develops, orthopnea, angina, tachycardia, dependent edema, bruits, and tachypnea may occur.

Clients with mild anemia (hemoglobin of 10–12 g/dl) are usually asymptomatic. If manifestations do occur, they typically follow strenuous exertion. Clients with moderate anemia may suffer from dyspnea, palpitations, diaphoresis with exertion, and chronic fatigue. Some clients with se-

vere anemia, such as those with chronic renal failure, may be asymptomatic because their anemia develops gradually.

The RBC count, hemoglobin level, and hematocrit confirm the presence of anemia. A bone marrow specimen may be required to confirm the type of anemia. A peripheral blood smear (RBC indices) is needed to determine the size of the RBC.

Outcome Management

▆ Medical Management

The goals of care for clients with anemia include (1) alleviating or controlling the causes, (2) relieving the manifestations, and (3) preventing complications. Management of the anemias ranges from specific treatments to symptomatic care. Treatment also varies in intensity and duration because some anemias resolve after blood transfusion, others resolve within a few weeks or months, and still other forms require lifelong intervention.

ALLEVIATE AND CONTROL THE CAUSES

Four common forms of anemia along with specific interventions are discussed next.

RELIEVE MANIFESTATIONS

Oxygen Therapy

Oxygen therapy may be prescribed for clients with severe anemia because their blood has a reduced capacity for oxygen. Oxygen helps prevent tissue hypoxia and lessens the workload of the heart as it struggles to compensate for the lower hemoglobin levels.

Erythropoietin

Subcutaneous injections of erythropoietin can be given to treat anemias of chronic disease. For this drug to be effective, the client must have bone marrow capable of producing RBCs and sufficient nutrients to produce RBCs.

Iron Replacement

Iron can be given to augment oral intake. Oral forms of iron are usually given for mild forms of anemia. The medications of choice are ferrous sulfate (Feosol), 0.325 g orally three times a day with meals; ferrous gluconate (Fergon), 0.3 g orally twice a day; and intramuscular (IM) iron dextran (Imferon), 100 to 250 mg. Clients usu-

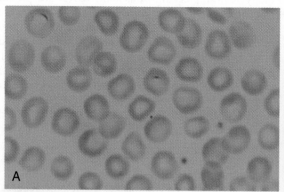 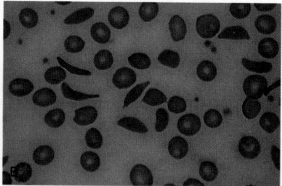

FIGURE 75–1 *A*, Normal red blood cells. *B*, Sickle cell anemia. (Magnification ×875.) Note the elongated and sickle-shaped cells. (From Rodak, B. [1995]. *Diagnostic hematology* [pp. 83, 257]. Philadelphia: W. B. Saunders.)

ally receive iron supplements for at least 6 months for repletion of the body stores. Parenteral iron therapy is administered to clients who (1) have an intolerance to oral iron preparations, (2) habitually forget to take their medications, or (3) continue to suffer blood losses. Iron dextran is the parenteral drug of choice. The client typically feels more energetic and has an increased appetite within 48 hours. Peak reticulocytosis occurs at about day 10. RBC indices and hemoglobin content gradually return to normal. Because of the high risk of allergic reaction, if iron is to be given intravenously, the physician usually administers the first dose.

Blood Transfusions

Blood transfusions are valuable in treating anemia resulting from acute blood loss and also may benefit clients with severe chronic anemia (hemoglobin < 6 g/dl) who have responded poorly to other forms of therapy. Packed RBCs may be given to clients who have lost blood in surgery or due to trauma. The Joint Commission on Accreditation of Healthcare Organizations (JCAHO) requires that all blood transfusions be evaluated to confirm that clear medical indications for the transfusion exist and that the client responds as expected. The physician's order for transfusion should specify blood component, volume, and rate of infusion. Table 75–1 describes blood components.

Blood is administered after informed consent is obtained. Consent includes an explanation of medical indications for homologous transfusion and its benefits, risks, and alternatives. Documentation of informed consent may consist of a form in the medical record stating that this information was presented in a manner understandable to the client (e.g., "Risks of and alternatives to blood transfusion were explained, and the client consented"). If the client is clinically unable to consent to transfusion, a reasonable effort should be made to secure consent from a family member. If no family member is available or time does not allow, place a note to this effect in the chart. Assess the client's understanding of the transfusion, and accurately respond to questions and concerns.

Two alternatives to homologous (random) blood transfusion should be considered: *autologous* and *directed* (designated) donation. Clients who do not have leukemia or bacteremia should be offered the option of donating their own blood before a scheduled surgical procedure when there is a reasonable expectation that blood will be required. Although the risk-benefit ratio should be evaluated, experience to date indicates that even clients with heart disease and other high-risk conditions tolerate donating blood well. The elimination of disease transmission, alloimmunization, and other potential transfusion complications makes this a reasonable option for many surgical clients.

Autologous donations can be made every 3 days if the donor's hemoglobin remains at or above 11 g/dl. For the blood to be maintained in a liquid state, donations should begin within 5 weeks of the transfusion date. RBCs can be stored frozen for 10 years, but the expense involved and time required for final preparation limit this practice to those who have extremely rare blood types. Donations should cease at least 3 days before the date of transfusion.

Another commonly used method of autologous blood collection is intraoperative, postoperative, or post-traumatic blood salvage. Blood is suctioned from body cavities, joint spaces, and other closed operative or trauma sites. Tissue debris and other sterile contaminants may necessitate special processing such as washing. Salvaged blood must be reinfused within 6 hours of collection.

A second option is for transfusion recipients to designate their own donors. Directed donations have not decreased the risk of contracting human immunodeficiency virus (HIV) infection. In fact, directed donors appear to have a higher incidence of hepatitis. This is probably due to the fact that a large percentage of directed donors are giving blood for the first time, and first-time donors commonly test positive for hepatitis surrogate markers. Despite this evidence, clients frequently feel more comfortable identifying their donors. Discuss all of these options with the client in sufficient time to permit donation and blood testing.

PRETRANSFUSION TESTING. The client's major concern is likely to be the safety of the transfusion, specifically the risk of contracting acquired immunodeficiency syndrome (AIDS). Provide accurate information for the client, and begin efforts to ensure a safe and effective transfusion before the blood or component is collected. For many decades, prospective donors have been asked two categories of questions: (1) those intended to protect the donor from possible risks of donation, and (2) those intended to protect the recipient from risks of transfusion.

To reduce the risk of HIV transmission to blood recipients, there has been a marked increase in the second group of questions. In addition, donors are required to read information about behaviors known to increase the risk of HIV infection; in most collection centers, they are questioned directly about their involvement in such activities.

Finally, a method must be made available for donors to indicate anonymously that their unit is or is not safe for transfusion. In addition to obtaining a thorough donor history, many diagnostic tests for serologic and infectious disease are routinely performed on the donor's blood.

When a need for blood is identified, several tests are done to confirm that the client's blood is compatible with that of the donor. First, the recipient's ABO and Rh type are identified. To determine the presence of antibody other than anti-A or anti-B, an antibody screen is performed. This test (the "indirect antiglobulin test") is done by adding the recipient's serum to donor RBCs known to have a certain set of minor blood group antigens. Coombs' serum (antihuman globulin) is added to facilitate visibility of cellular agglutination, an indicator of antigen-antibody complex formation. The results are viewed macroscopically and microscopically. More than 400 minor RBC antigens have been identified in RBCs, each of which can stimulate the production of an antibody. However, only the few (~30) that are of sufficiently potent antigenicity to be clinically significant are included in the routine antibody screen.

It is not uncommon for chronically transfused clients to develop multiple antibodies. Identifying the antibodies and obtaining blood from donors who do not possess the antigens can significantly complicate the testing procedure and lengthen the time required for blood preparation.

Blood products containing RBCs may be further tested for compatibility to crossmatch testing. For this procedure, donor RBCs are combined with the recipient's se-

TABLE 75-1   BLOOD COMPONENTS

	Whole Blood	Red Blood Cells	Platelet Concentrates	Fresh Frozen Plasma	Cryoprecipitate	Granulocyte Concentrates	Plasma Derivatives	Coagulation Factor Concentrates
COMPOSITION	RBC, plasma, plasma proteins (globulins, antibodies), 63 ml of anticoagulant-preservative	RBC with CPDA-1 solution (anticoagulant-preservative only), final hematocrit no higher than 80% (80% RBC, 20% plasma) RBC with 100 ml additive solution, final hematocrit about 55%–60%	Single-unit platelets contain a minimum of 5.5×10^{10} (1 unit) platelets in 50–70 ml of plasma obtained by separating platelet-rich plasma from 1 unit of fresh whole blood; 6–10 units may be pooled for 1 transfusion Single-donor platelets contain a minimum of 3.0×10^{11} platelets (6 units) obtained from single donor by use of automated cell separator during apheresis; recipient exposed to fewer donors, which decreases complications	91% water, 7% protein (globulin, antibodies, clotting factors), and 2% carbohydrates Freezing within 8 hr of collection preserves all clotting factors	Each unit contains about 80–120 units of factor VIII (antihemophilic factor) that represents 50% of antihemophilic factor originally present in unit, vWF, 250 mg of fibrinogen, and 20%–30% of factor XIII present in a unit of whole blood, suspended in 10–20 ml of plasma	Unit obtained by granulocytaphresis contains a minimum of 1.0×10^{10} granulocytes, variable amounts of lymphocytes (usually <10%), 30–50 ml of RBC and 100–400 ml of plasma, and 6–10 units of platelets; the platelets can be separated from the unit if the granulocyte recipient is not thrombocytopenic	*Albumin:* 96% albumin, 4% globulin and other proteins extracted from plasma; available as a 5% solution, oncotically equivalent to plasma, and also a concentrated 25% solution *Plasma protein fraction:* 83% albumin and 17% globulins extracted from plasma; less pure than albumin and has higher degree of contamination with other plasma proteins; in 5% solution only	*Factor VIII:* Lyophilized concentrate containing large quantities of factor VIII; prepared from large pools of donor plasma, but heat treatment during fractionation process significantly reduces risk of transmitting viral disease *Factor IX:* Lyophilized concentrate containing large quantities of factor IX; also contains factors II, VII, and X; product prepared from large pools of donor plasma, but heat treatment during fractionation process significantly reduces risk of transmitting viral disease
VOLUME	500 ml/unit	250–350 ml/unit 350–400 ml/unit	50–70 ml/unit 200–400 ml/unit	200–250 ml	5–10 ml/unit	200–400 ml with platelets 100–200 ml without platelets	Albumin: 250 and 500 ml (5%); 50 and 100 ml (25%)	Multiple-dose vial

ABO/Rh COMPATIBILITY	The ABO type of the donor should be identical with the recipient's; Rh– blood can be given to an Rh– or Rh+ recipient	A can match with A or O; B can match with B or O; O can match only with O; AB can match with A, B, or O; Rh– blood can be given to either Rh+ or Rh– recipient	Whereas platelets have no ABO or Rh antigens, they are suspended in 200–400 ml of plasma containing donor antibodies and a small number of RBC; ABO and Rh compatibility is recommended	A can match with A or AB; B can match with B or AB; AB can match only with AB; O can match with A, B, AB, or O; Rh– and Rh+ blood can be given to either Rh+ or Rh– recipient	Cryoprecipitate contains no RBC and a small volume of plasma; ABO crossmatching not needed, and plasma compatibility preferred but not required	Granulocytes contain a significant number of RBC and plasma; therefore, ABO of donor should be identical with recipient's; Rh– components may be transfused to an Rh+ recipient	Antibodies destroyed during processing; therefore, compatibility not a factor	Antibodies destroyed during processing, so compatibility not a factor
SPECIAL CONSIDERATIONS	Whole blood transfusion is rarely indicated; Treatment with specific blood components is usually recommended	RBC may be viscous, thus 0.9% saline may be added to achieve optimal flow rates; For some clients, a leukocyte depletion filter may be used to prevent complications	Because platelet concentrates contain few RBC, crossmatch testing is not required; Plasma ABO and Rh compatibility is recommended, especially when the total volume of the transfusion exceeds 150–200 ml; Only filters specially designed for platelet transfusion should be used	Plasma carries same risk of disease transmission as does whole blood; If only volume expansion is required, products of choice are crystalloid or colloid solutions, such as saline or albumin; Plasma contains no RBC, and Rh compatibility and crossmatching are not required; ABO compatibility must be confirmed before administration	Single units of cryoprecipitate may be pooled into 1 container by the blood collection center; If individual bags are issued, 0.9% saline may need to be added to rinse residual cryoprecipitate from bags and tubing	Granulocytes have short survival (<24 hr); infuse as soon as possible; Granulocyte concentrates contain a significant number of RBC; pretransfusion testing recommended; Increased incidence of febrile, nonhemolytic reactions with granulocyte transfusions; infuse slowly, observe client closely; premedication with an antihistamine, acetaminophen, steroids advised; Do *not* administer amphotericin B within 4 hr of granulocyte transfusion to avoid pulmonary insufficiency	PPF and albumin cannot transmit hepatitis or HIV infection; the pasteurization process used to prepare the products destroys such viruses; Hypotension has been associated with rapid infusion of PPF; 25% albumin can cause a significantly increased blood pressure because of its ability to draw fluid into the intravascular space	Factor VIII and factor IX assays should be performed at appropriate intervals to assess response; Factor VIII concentration lacks vWF and should not be used in treatment of von Willebrand's disease

Table continued on following page

2107

TABLE 75–1   BLOOD COMPONENTS Continued

Whole Blood	Red Blood Cells	Platelet Concentrates	Fresh Frozen Plasma	Cryoprecipitate	Granulocyte Concentrates	Plasma Derivatives	Coagulation Factor Concentrates
OUTCOMES							
Prevention or resolution of hypovolemic shock and anemia In a nonbleeding adult, 1 unit of whole blood should increase hematocrit by 3% and hemoglobin by 1 g/dl	Resolution of manifestations of anemia In a nonbleeding adult, 1 unit of RBC should increase hematocrit by 3% and hemoglobin by 1 g/dl	Prevention or resolution of bleeding due to thrombocytopenia or platelet dysfunction 1 unit should raise peripheral platelet count 5000–10,000/mm^3 if underlying cause is resolved or controlled Efficacy of platelet transfusion can be determined by obtaining platelet counts at 1 hr and 18–24 hr after infusion	Treatment effectiveness is assessed by monitoring coagulation function, specifically, PT and PTT, or by specific factor assays	Correction of factor VIII, vWF, factor XIII, and fibrinogen deficiency; cessation of bleeding in uremic clients Laboratory values required to assess effectiveness of treatment	Improvement in or resolution of infection No increase in peripheral WBC count usually seen after granulocyte transfusion in adults, although increase may be seen in children An improvement in clinical condition because of resolving infection is the only measure of treatment effectiveness	The client will acquire and maintain adequate blood pressure and volume support	The client will develop hemostasis because of increased levels of factor VIII and factor IX activity

CPDA-1, citrate-phosphate-dextrose-adenine; FFP, fresh-frozen plasma; HIV, human immunodeficiency virus; IV, intravenous; PPF, plasma protein fraction; PT, prothrombin time; PTT, partial thromboplastin time; RBC, red blood cells; vWF, von Willebrand's factor; WBC, white blood cells.

rum and Coombs' serum. After an inoculation period, the results are viewed microscopically. If no RBC agglutination has occurred, the crossmatch is compatible. Crossmatching adds very little to the safety of transfusion (0.01% to 0.1%) if a negative antibody screen is initially obtained. In these situations, the Coombs' phase can be eliminated to shorten the procedure and reduce cost.

Routine serologic testing requires a 10-ml clotted sample and a 7-ml citrated sample. Approximately 1 hour is required for testing in routine situations. In the event of a medical emergency, O-negative RBCs and AB plasma can be safely administered to most clients without serologic testing.

Failure to correctly label the samples used for blood bank testing may lead to fatal errors. Several precautionary measures should be taken to reduce this risk. Label the sample at the bedside after asking the client to state his or her name and comparing it with the name on the identification bracelet. If the client cannot state his or her name, identity should be confirmed by a family member or other person familiar with the client whenever possible. The date and initials of the phlebotomist must be written on the sample label. Many institutions have adopted a secondary identification system. Several commercial systems are available; each is designed to ensure that the sample used for crossmatch has been drawn from the client who receives the transfusion.

DELAYED TRANSFUSION COMPLICATIONS. Complications can occur days to years after a transfusion. Fever, mild jaundice, and decreased hematocrit may indicate a delayed hemolytic reaction. Hemolysis of RBCs may occur 3 days to several months after the transfusion if an antibody was undetected during crossmatch testing and RBCs containing that antigen were transfused. Usually no medical treatment is required.

Iron overload may occur in clients receiving more than 100 units of blood over a period of time, such as clients with aplastic anemia. The normal iron level of 2 to 3 g usually remains constant because iron is metabolized at a fixed rate. Each unit of RBCs contains an additional 200 mg of iron. In clients who receive more than 100 units of RBCs, excess iron stores in major organs often develop. Complications of iron overload include cardiac myopathies (pericarditis, arrhythmias, heart failure), thyroid insufficiency, endocrine and pancreas malfunction (glucose intolerance), liver fibrosis, profound anemia, and skin discoloration. Cardiomyopathies related to iron overload are a frequent cause of death in the chronically transfused client. Deferoxamine, which chelates and removes accumulated iron via the kidneys, may be administered intravenously or subcutaneously to prevent this potentially fatal complication.

Post-transfusion graft-versus-host disease (GVHD) can occur if donor lymphocytes engraft and divide in the marrow spaces of an immunocompromised recipient. Manifestations are fever, rash, diarrhea, and hepatitis. This frequently fatal complication can be prevented by irradiation of all cellular components before administration to high-risk clients.

Many diseases can be transmitted through blood transfusion. The most common is hepatitis C. Although manifestations are milder than those seen with hepatitis B, chronic liver disease and cirrhosis may develop. Hepatitis

B should be considered if the recipient experiences anorexia, malaise, nausea, vomiting, dark urine, and jaundice within 4 to 6 weeks of transfusion. Elevated alanine aminotransferase (ALT) and aspartate aminotransferase (AST) levels are frequently seen, indicating liver damage that may be permanent. Hepatitis B and C are treated symptomatically. With advances in donor testing and screening in the United States, the risk of hepatitis has decreased to about 3%.

On rare occasions, HIV-1 is transmitted from an infected donor to a blood recipient. The client may be asymptomatic for several years or may have flu-like manifestations in 2 to 4 weeks. Whereas more than 25,000 cases of transfusion-associated AIDS were reported before routine donor testing in 1985, the incidence has decreased to 1 in 100,000 to 150,000 as a result of careful donor screening and testing.

■ Nursing Management
ASSESSMENT
The general nursing care of clients with anemia includes adequate assessment by the nurse to help identify the cause of the anemia and client education. You can help in diagnosis by taking a complete health history focusing on the elements outlined in Chapter 74. Client teaching is extremely important in treating the anemias because most of the care takes place in an outpatient clinic or the client's home. Help the client and family become knowledgeable about self-care in both preventing and treating anemia.

DIAGNOSIS, OUTCOMES, INTERVENTIONS
Activity Intolerance. Write the diagnosis as *Activity Intolerance related to decreased blood supply or low hemoglobin levels, as evidenced by fatigue, dyspnea, pallor, and tachycardia.*

Outcomes. The client will tolerate activity, as evidenced by walking increasing distances, or sitting up without fatigue, dyspnea, pallor, or tachycardia.

Interventions. A unit of packed RBCs may be administered to improve overall blood volume or increase hematocrit (see blood transfusion earlier).

Obtain Venous Access. The gauge of the needle used for transfusion varies with the product being infused. When packed RBCs weighing less than 300 g are infused, a 20-gauge or larger needle is needed to achieve maximal flow rate. If a smaller-gauge needle must be used, the RBCs can be diluted with 0.9% saline. To prevent hemolysis, add no solution other than normal saline to blood components.

Components containing a significant volume of plasma or other diluent can be safely infused at a rapid rate through smaller-gauge needles or catheters. A central venous catheter is an acceptable access option for blood transfusion. However, a large volume of refrigerated blood infused rapidly into the ventricle of the heart may cause cardiac dysrhythmias. Warming the blood can reduce the risk of this complication.

Another issue of concern is the use of multilumen catheters, which may allow blood to mix with incompatible solutions and medications as they exit the catheter tips. Experience indicates that the circulation achieved through a blood vessel suitable for central line placement results in rapid mixing of fluids. As a result, no harmful effects have been reported.

Request Blood Release. Blood bank regulations state that refrigerated components may not be returned to inventory if they have been warmed to more than 10° C (50° F). To meet this requirement, most transfusion medicine services consider 30 minutes to be the maximal allowable time out of monitored storage. To avoid wasting a scarce commodity, certain procedures should be performed before blood is requested.

An IV catheter appropriate for transfusing the requested component should be functional, flushed with normal saline, and maintained at a keep-vein-open (KVO) rate. Vital signs should then be taken and recorded. Fever may be a reason for delaying the transfusion. In addition to masking a possible manifestation of an acute transfusion reaction, fever can also compromise the efficacy of platelet transfusions.

Premedication also may be required if the client has a history of adverse reactions. In many cases, febrile reactions can be prevented by administering acetaminophen. A history of allergic reactions may warrant prophylactic administration of antihistamines (e.g., diphenhydramine HCl). To ensure effectiveness, administer oral medication 30 minutes before the transfusion is started. IV medication may be given immediately before the transfusion is initiated.

Blood should be released from the blood bank only to adequately trained personnel. The name and identification number of the recipient must be provided and a permanent record of this information maintained in the blood bank. So that delivery to the wrong client is avoided, blood should be transported to only one client at a time.

Confirm Blood Acceptability. The most crucial phase of transfusion is confirming product compatibility and verifying the client's identity. Before going to the client's bedside, verify ABO and Rh compatibility, usually by comparing the bag label with the medical record and forms issued from the blood bank. Also check the bag label to ensure that the correct component has been issued and for date of expiration. Components expire at midnight of the day marked on the bag unless otherwise specified.

Inspect the unit for leaks, abnormal color, clots, excessive air, and bubbles. Check carefully for important labels (such as "autologous," "directed") or instructions (such as "use leukocyte-depleting filter"). Cellular components (whole blood, RBCs, and platelets) for an immunosuppressed client should be clearly marked *irradiated.* Clients with Hodgkin's or non-Hodgkin's lymphoma, acute leukemia, or congenital immunodeficiency disorders and bone marrow transplant recipients may develop posttransfusion GVHD if lymphocytes contaminating cellular components engraft and divide. Transfusions from firstdegree family members may also cause fatal GVHD. A small dose of radiation delivered to the component before release from the blood bank renders the lymphocytes incapable of mitotic action.

At the bedside, compare the name and number on the identification bracelet with the tag on the blood bag. If applicable, check the secondary identification system. The American Association of Blood Banks recommends that two qualified people perform this critical step.

Infuse Blood. Most blood products should be infused through administration sets designed specifically for this use. The set usually contains a 170-mm filter designed to trap fibrin clots and other debris that accumulates during blood storage. Most standard filters can filter 4 units of blood.

Tubing is available in two basic configurations: straight or Y-type. The use of Y-type tubing simplifies the process of adding normal saline to RBCs and provides ready access to a saline flush if the transfusion must be interrupted. Straight tubing usually has a medication injection site a few inches from the needle. If an adverse reaction develops, a keep-vein-open saline drip initiated at this site maintains patency of the IV line but avoids exposure to the 30 to 50 ml of blood remaining in the tubing and filter. Change the administration set every 4 to 6 hours, or according to institution policy, to reduce the risk of septicemia.

Several types of infusion devices are available to regulate and monitor the flow of IV solutions. There are basically two types:

- Infusion controllers, which regulate flow by gravity
- Infusion pumps, which deliver solutions under pressure

Infusion controllers may be used with all blood products if they are designed to function with opaque solutions. However, the negative pressure exerted by the peristaltic or syringe-like cassette action of infusion pumps may cause RBC hemolysis. If the transfusion product contains a significant number of RBCs, consult the manufacturer before a pump designed for crystalloid and colloid solutions is used.

If manual pressure cuffs are used to increase RBC flow rate, the pressure should not exceed 300 mm Hg. Do not use standard sphygmomanometers for this purpose because they do not exert uniform pressure against all parts of the bag.

Blood warmers may be used to prevent hypothermia, which can be induced by rapid infusion of large volumes of refrigerated blood. Neonatal exchange transfusion, plasma exchange, surgery, and trauma are all clinical situations that may require the use of a blood warmer. Other clients of concern are those with cold agglutinin disease. These clients have antibodies that react at temperatures under 37° C (98.6° F). Systemic circulatory cooling can cause intravascular agglutination. This condition may be detected during serologic testing. Once this client has been identified, the transfusion service may recommend the use of a blood warmer for all transfusions.

Two types of devices are approved by blood bank regulatory agencies for warming blood. For dry heating, a bag is placed between two aluminum heating plates or a disposable cuff-style bag is wrapped around a cylindrical aluminum heating element. A second type uses warm water to increase the temperature of the blood. Water baths containing water warmed to 37° C (98.6° F) may be used only if they have been specifically designed for warming blood. The blood bag should never be fully immersed in water.

Monitor During the Transfusion. The first 10 to 15 minutes of any transfusion are the most critical. If a major ABO incompatibility exists or a severe allergic reaction such as anaphylaxis occurs, it is usually evident within the first 50 ml of the transfusion. Therefore, it is recommended that the transfusion begin slowly and that the client be closely monitored. If no evidence of a reaction is noted within the first 15 minutes, flow can be increased to the prescribed rate.

Before leaving the client unattended, instruct the client to report anything unusual immediately. Take and record vital signs before the transfusion begins, after the first 15 minutes, and every hour until 1 hour after the transfusion has been discontinued. Check vital signs immediately if the client displays any untoward manifestations.

The recommended rate of infusion varies with the blood component being transfused. Components such as platelets, plasma, and cryoprecipitate may be infused rapidly, but take care to avoid circulatory overload, especially with geriatric clients and clients with cardiac disease. For avoiding the risk of septicemia, infusions should not exceed 4 hours. If the client's size or medical condition does not allow infusion within 4 hours, the unit may be split into smaller aliquots in the blood bank.

Regulatory agencies require complete documentation of the transfusion, including identification of personnel starting and ending the transfusion, unique product number, and outcome (e.g., "no reaction noted"). If an adverse reaction does occur, document the manifestations, actions taken, and future recommendations in the client's medical record.

Watch for Transfusion Reaction. Exposure to foreign blood elements may mediate immunologic and nonimmunologic reactions affecting all major body systems. Consider any unusual manifestation occurring during or immediately after a transfusion a potential reaction. Monitor unconscious patients closely because manifestations of a reaction may be inhibited in the unconscious state. The acute reactions most frequently seen are described in Table 75–2.

Whereas treatment may vary depending on the manifestations, follow certain standard procedures when a reaction is suspected. In all cases, stop the transfusion and keep the intravenous line open with normal saline. Treat life-threatening manifestations such as respiratory or circulatory failure immediately. Contact the client's physician and the blood bank. According to institutional policy, obtain appropriate laboratory samples. Samples used to evaluate a reaction include blood and urine. Free hemoglobin found in either indicates that RBCs have hemolyzed, the most serious serologic finding.

To avoid clouding the diagnostic picture by venous trauma, obtain blood samples from a large peripheral vein using at least a 19-gauge needle. The blood sample is also used to repeat ABO and Rh typing, antibody screening, and direct antiglobulin testing. A discrepancy in results between initial and repeat testing may indicate that incompatible blood was transfused. When future transfusions are required, special processing (e.g., washing) may then be performed in the blood bank to reduce the risks of another adverse reaction.

Altered Tissue Perfusion. The lack of circulating blood volume can create tissue hypoxia. State this diagnosis as *Altered Tissue Perfusion related to loss of blood volume.*

Outcomes. The client will have adequate tissue perfusion, as evidenced by normotension, warm extremities, heart rate between 60 and 100 beats/min, ability to perform activities of daily living or walk without dyspnea or tachycardia.

Interventions. Monitor vital signs and peripheral pulses, peripheral skin temperature, and activity tolerance. Clients should receive adequate food and fluids to assist with blood volume and provide protein for hemoglobin manufacturing. Keep the client warm, adding blankets to the feet for additional comfort.

Altered Nutrition: Less Than Body Requirements. Write the nursing diagnosis as *Altered Nutrition: Less than Body Requirements related to disease, treatment, or lack of knowledge of adequate nutrition.*

Outcomes. The client will have nutritional deficiencies corrected and optimal nutrition will be achieved, as evidenced by blood test results reaching normal range, improved tolerance for activity, and anemia resolved.

Interventions. Teach the basics of good nutrition; encourage a diet high in protein, iron, and vitamins with frequent small meals. Encourage foods cooked in iron pots and ingestion of foods such as liver (the richest source), oysters, lean meats, kidney beans, whole wheat bread, kale, spinach, egg yolks, turnip tops, beet greens, carrots, apricots, and raisins. Document the client's weight. Encourage good oral hygiene.

Risk for Ineffective Management of Therapeutic Regimen (Individuals). This nursing diagnosis is related to the client's self-care ability and the ability to take iron preparations.

Outcomes. The client will verbalize correct dosage of, route of, and indications for iron preparations, as evidenced by correct administration of iron medications and an absence of complications.

Interventions. Inform the client that iron salts are gastric irritants and should always be taken after meals. Liquid iron preparations should be well diluted and taken through a straw (undiluted liquid iron stains teeth). Constipation, commonly seen during iron therapy, can be avoided by a high-fiber diet and use of stool softeners or laxatives as required. Avoid consumption of coffee and tea with iron; absorption is hampered by the tannates. To administer parenteral iron medications, use Z track methods (see Fundamentals textbooks for a review).

EVALUATION

Resolution of anemia requires time. When packed RBCs are used, anemia will be corrected immediately. When oral iron preparations are used, it takes weeks for anemia to resolve and the client will thus need assessments at intervals to monitor the progress of therapy.

▪ Modifications for Elderly Clients

Older clients are at risk for iron deficiency anemia because of poor nutritional intake and a decreased absorption of iron in the intestine. These clients also require complete assessment for diagnosis of the cause of the anemia. They often experience chronic blood loss from a variety of diseases that also may cause anemia, and differential diagnosis is thus required.

TABLE 75-2	ACUTE TRANSFUSION REACTIONS

Reaction	Cause	Clinical Manifestations	Management	Prevention
IMMUNOGENIC				
Allergic Incidence: 1%	Sensitivity to foreign proteins in plasma	Urticaria, flushing, itching (no fever)	Administer antihistamines as directed. If manifestations mild and transient, transfusion may resume	Treat prophylactically with antihistamines
Febrile, nonhemolytic Incidence: 0.5%–1.0%	Sensitization to donor white blood cells, platelets, or plasma proteins	Sudden chills and fever (rise in temperature > 1° C [1.8° F]), headache, flushing, anxiety, muscle pain	Give antipyretics as prescribed; avoid aspirin in thrombocytopenic clients	Consider leukocyte-poor blood products (filtered, washed, or frozen) if fever occurs more than once
Acute hemolytic Incidence: 1:25,000 Fatal: 2:1 × 10⁶	Infusion of ABO-incompatible red blood cells	Chills, fever, low back pain, flushing, tachycardia, tachypnea, hemoglobinuria, hemoglobinemia, hypotension, vascular collapse, bleeding, acute renal failure, shock, cardiac arrest, death	Treat shock. Maintain blood pressure. Give diuretics as prescribed to maintain urine flow. Insert indwelling catheter or measure hourly output. Dialysis may be needed	Meticulously verify recipient from sample collection to transfusion
Anaphylactic Incidence: 1:150,000	Infusion of IgA proteins to IgA-deficient recipient who has developed anti-IgA antibodies	Anxiety, urticaria, wheezing progressing to cyanosis, shock, and possible cardiac arrest	Initiate CPR if indicated. Have epinephrine ready for injection (0.4 ml of a 1:1000 solution SC)	Give blood components from IgA-deficient donors or remove *all* plasma by washing
NONIMMUNOGENIC				
Circulatory overload Estimated Incidence: 1:10,000 (not usually reported to blood bank)	Infusion of blood at a rate too rapid for size, cardiac status, or clinical condition of recipient	Cough, dyspnea, pulmonary congestion (rales), headache, hypertension, tachycardia, distended neck veins	Place client in upright position with feet in dependent position. Administer diuretics, oxygen, and morphine as prescribed. Phlebotomy may be required	Adjust transfusion volume and flow rate on basis of client size and clinical status. If slow transfusion will exceed 4 hr, request that unit be aliquoted into smaller volumes
Septicemia Incidence: very rare	Transfusion of component contaminated with microorganism	Rapid onset of chills, high fever, vomiting, diarrhea, marked hypotension, and shock	Treat manifestations and administer antibiotics, IV fluids, vasopressors, and steroids as directed. Obtain culture of client and blood containers	Collect, process, store, and transfuse blood according to industry standards. Infuse within 4 hr of starting time

CPR, cardiopulmonary resuscitation; IG, immunoglobulin; IV, intravenous; SC, subcutaneously.

IRON DEFICIENCY ANEMIA

Etiology and Risk Factors

Iron deficiency anemia is associated with either inadequate absorption or excessive loss of iron; it is a chronic, microcytic, hypochromic anemia (see Fig. 75–1B). Iron deficiency anemia is caused by an inadequate supply of iron needed to synthesize hemoglobin. Iron is essential to the oxygen-carrying function of heme; without it, the marrow produces RBCs that are deficient in hemoglobin concentration.

The major risk factors for iron deficiency anemia are (1) chronic blood loss, (2) insufficient intake of iron, (3) impaired absorption of iron, and (4) excessive demands for RBC production. An average diet supplies the body with about 12 to 15 mg/day of iron, of which only 5% to 10% (0.6 to 1.5 mg) is absorbed. The amount of iron normally absorbed daily is sufficient for meeting the needs of women past childbearing age and healthy men, but it does not meet the greater needs of menstruating and pregnant women, adolescents, children, and infants. These five groups must have a higher daily intake of iron. Economic constraints, poor dentition, and lack of interest in food preparation commonly lead to iron deficiency in older people. Fortunately, the GI tract can increase its absorption of iron from 10% daily to about 20% to 30% daily. In this way, the body often compensates for diminishing iron stores due to inadequate iron intake or excessive iron loss.

Iron is stored in the form of ferritin, an iron-phosphorus-protein complex that contains about 23% iron. It is formed in the intestinal mucosa when ferric iron joins with the protein apoferritin. Ferritin is stored in the tissues, primarily in the reticuloendothelial cells of the liver, spleen, and bone marrow.

Normal iron excretion is less than 1 mg/day. Iron is excreted in urine, sweat, bile, and feces and from the skin in desquamated cells. The average woman loses another 15 mg monthly during menses. Menstruation is the most common cause of iron deficiency in women. GI tract bleeding is a common etiologic factor in men; it may result from peptic ulcers, hiatal hernia, gastritis, cancer, hemorrhoids, diverticula, ulcerative colitis, or salicylate poisoning. It may also be associated with gastritis from the use of aspirin, steroids, or nonsteroidal anti-inflammatory drugs (NSAIDs). Bleeding from the GI tract is usually chronic and occult (too small to be seen). A chronic blood loss of as little as 2 to 4 ml/day can result in iron deficiency anemia, because every 2 ml of blood contains 1 mg of iron. The body can compensate for such losses to some degree by excreting less than 0.5 mg of iron daily rather than the normal 1 mg.

Alteration in the mucosa of the duodenum and proximal jejunum (as in chronic diarrhea, malabsorption syndromes such as celiac disease, and gastrectomy) affects iron absorption, predisposing to iron deficiency states. Tannates (in tea and coffee), carbonates, the chelating agent ethylenediaminetetraacetic acid (EDTA), and the medicinal antacid magnesium trisilicate all hinder non-heme iron absorption.

Clinical Manifestations

In mild cases of iron deficiency anemia, the client is asymptomatic; in more severe cases, assessment reveals the general manifestations of anemia, including:

- Peripheral blood smears revealing microcytic and pale (hypochromic) RBCs
- A hemoglobin level decreased to as low as 6 to 9 g/dl
- Moderately reduced total RBC count, rarely dropping below 3 million cells/mm³
- Reduced mean corpuscular volume, mean corpuscular hemoglobin, and mean corpuscular hemoglobin concentration
- Serum iron level (normally 50 to 150 mg/dl) decreased to 10 mg/dl

- Total iron-binding capacity elevated to 350 to 500 mg/dl (normal is 250 to 350 mg/dl)
- Complete absence of hemosiderin (an insoluble form of storage iron) from bone marrow
- Immunoradiometric serum ferritin level below normal

Outcome Management

Management of iron deficiency anemia focuses on (1) diagnosis of and correction of the underlying cause and (2) treatment through diet and supplemental iron preparations. Once the diagnosis of iron deficiency anemia is confirmed, studies are conducted to find the cause. Radiographic studies (GI tract series), stool examination for occult blood, esophagoscopy, gastroscopy, and sigmoidoscopy are commonly done to identify the site of blood loss.

Supplemental iron is administered to increase iron available in the blood. Oral and injectable forms of iron are available (see earlier).

MEGALOBLASTIC ANEMIA

Anemias caused by deficiencies of vitamin B12 and folic acid are called megaloblastic anemias because they are characterized by the appearance of megaloblasts (large, primitive RBCs) in blood and bone marrow. Other common features are:

- Leukopenia, a decreased number of white blood cells (WBCs)
- Thrombocytopenia, a decreased number of platelets
- Oral, GI, and neurologic manifestations
- A favorable response to injections of either vitamin B12 or folic acid

PERNICIOUS ANEMIA

Etiology and Risk Factors

Pernicious anemia is a type of macrocytic anemia caused by failure of absorption of vitamin B12 (cobalamin). It is the most prevalent form of vitamin B12 deficiency in the United States and Canada. Cobalamin is released from its protein-bound state by an acidic gastric environment. Lack of gastric acid may lead to pernicious anemia, however; the most common cause is lack of intrinsic factor, a glucoprotein produced by parietal cells of the gastric lining. Vitamin B12 is absorbed in the terminal ileum; if that portion of the bowel is surgically resected, absorption cannot occur. The cause of pernicious anemia may also be from an autoimmune response. Ninety per cent of people with pernicious anemia have autoantibodies that react specifically against parietal gastric cells, and 60% have anti-intrinsic factor antibody.

Without vitamin B12, deoxyribonucleic acid (DNA) synthesis and cell replication are impaired. RBC precursors do not divide normally, and large, poorly functioning RBCs are created. Erythropoiesis (from impaired folic acid from the lack of vitamin B12) and production of myelin on nerves (from vitamin B12 directly) are greatly affected.

Clinical Manifestations

The major manifestations of pernicious anemia are low hemoglobin, hematocrit, and RBC levels. The diagnosis is based on the presence of anemia, GI manifestations, and neurologic disorders; laboratory blood and bone marrow tests; absence of gastric hydrochloric acid (HCl) and a favorable response to a vitamin B_{12} "therapeutic trial." The Schilling test measures the absorption of orally administered radioactive vitamin B_{12} (tagged with cobalt 60) before and after parenteral administration of intrinsic factor. This procedure detects lack of intrinsic factor and is the definitive test for pernicious anemia.

Gastric secretion analysis to check for the presence of free HCl is another important test; most clients with pernicious anemia have low-volume gastric secretions with a high pH and free hydrochloric acid. Furthermore, these findings do not change, even after the administration of histamine, which normally stimulates gastric secretion.

Outcome Management

VITAMIN B_{12}

Clients with pernicious anemia need both immediate treatment and lifelong therapy with maintenance vitamin B_{12}. During the acute phase of illness, the client may be given vitamin B_{12} injections. The response to the injections is usually quick and dramatic, often occurring within 24 to 48 hours. Within 72 hours, reticulocytes begin to increase; by the end of the first week, the total RBC count rises significantly. Cardiovascular involvement usually lessens with improved erythropoiesis. Peripheral nerve function may improve with treatment.

IRON SUPPLEMENTS

Additionally, the client may need oral iron supplementation if the hemoglobin level fails to rise in proportion to an increased RBC count. As stated earlier, iron deficiency may be an etiologic factor in pernicious anemia and must be corrected if it is present. Iron deficiency anemia can also develop during treatment of pernicious anemia. Injections of vitamin B_{12} may cause a rapid regeneration of RBC that depletes iron. As a result, the hemoglobin level remains low, although the total RBC count rises. Once the acute stage of the illness is past, the client with pernicious anemia must undertake a lifelong program of maintenance therapy. Monthly injections of vitamin B_{12} are needed to avoid relapse. The nurse plays a vital role in educating clients with this disorder on the importance of continuous care.

Encourage the client to eat a diet high in folic acid and iron to supplement the medication used to treat the anemia. If the cause involves altered absorption of vitamin B_{12}, nutritional supplements are useless. If the disease is related to decreased intake of the vitamin, a diet high in vitamin B_{12} is encouraged.

FOLIC ACID

Folic acid is sometimes given with vitamin B_{12} to clients with a history of poor nutrition. Folic acid can be dangerous, however, because it may intensify neurologic problems, and large doses of folate may obscure a vitamin B_{12} deficiency. Therefore, a therapeutic trial of folate should never be given before pernicious anemia is ruled out.

DIGESTANTS

Digestants to enhance the metabolism of vitamins, such as HCl diluted in water and given with meals, are often used during the first few weeks of vitamin B_{12} therapy.

ANEMIA CAUSED BY FOLIC ACID DEFICIENCY

Etiology and Risk Factors

Anemia associated with folic acid deficiency is very common. There are many causes, most of which are the same as those of vitamin B_{12} deficiency. Usually, folic acid deficiency results from a diet lacking in such foods as green leafy vegetables, liver, citrus fruits, and yeast. Clients with chronic alcoholism, because of their typically inadequate diets, are particularly at risk. High levels of alcohol in the blood also partially block the response of the bone marrow to folic acid, which thereby interferes with erythropoiesis.

Folic acid deficiency, like vitamin B_{12} deficiency, can develop with malabsorption syndromes (e.g., sprue, celiac disease, steatorrhea). Certain medications can also impede folic acid absorption and utilization. For example, a serious anemia may develop under the following conditions:

- Long-term use of anticonvulsant medications (e.g., primidone, phenytoin, phenobarbital)
- Administration of antimetabolites (e.g., folic acid antagonists, purine, pyrimidine analogs) to clients with cancer and leukemia
- Use of certain oral contraceptives

Finally, folic acid deficiency may occur with increased demands for folate, such as during the growth spurts of infancy and adolescence.

Folic acid, like vitamin B_{12}, is necessary for DNA synthesis; unlike pernicious anemia, however, folic acid deficiency does not cause neurologic manifestations. Anemia due to folic acid deficiency has a slow and insidious onset. The client, often thin and emaciated, usually appears quite ill. The client's malnourished and debilitated state frequently leads to other deficiencies, for example, of iron, protein, minerals, and other vitamins. Some clients may also have an electrolyte imbalance and neurologic manifestations may develop as a result of thiamine, calcium, or magnesium deficiency (commonly linked with alcoholism). Cirrhosis of the liver and bleeding varices further complicate anemia for the alcoholic client.

The megaloblastic anemia caused by folic acid deficiency is the same as that seen in pernicious anemia. The diagnosis is confirmed by blood smear and bone marrow examinations. With folic acid deficiency, the serum folate level is less than 4 ng/ml (normal, 7 to 20 ng/ml): the Schilling test finding is normal; HCl is probably present in the gastric juice; neurologic manifestations are absent; and the client responds favorably to a therapeutic trial of 50 to 100 mg folic acid administered intramuscularly daily for 10 days.

Outcome Management

For correction of anemia caused by folate deficiency, the client receives oral doses of folic acid 0.1 to 5.0 mg/day until the blood profile improves or until the cause of intestinal malabsorption is corrected. Clients with malabsorption syndromes may need parenteral folic acid initially, followed by maintenance therapy with oral doses. Folic acid is administered intramuscularly in the form of folinic acid (leucovorin calcium injection). Additionally, vitamin C is sometimes prescribed because it increases the role of folic acid in promoting erythropoiesis.

APLASTIC ANEMIAS

Aplastic anemia is caused by bone marrow that is severely hypoplastic (underdeveloped), that is, devoid of erythroid, myeloid, and megakaryocytic cell lines. Hypoplastic bone marrow results in anemia, leukopenia, and thrombocytopenia. When all three cellular elements are suppressed, the condition is known as *pancytopenia*. Aplastic anemia affects people of all ages, and men and women are equally susceptible. The incidence of aplastic anemia is about 4 per million population. *Congenital aplastic anemia (Fanconi's anemia)* usually occurs in childhood.

Etiology and Risk Factors

Acquired aplastic anemia may result from either an autoimmune mechanism or a direct injury by *myelotoxins*. Three groups of myelotoxins are:

1. Agents that always cause marrow damage when received in sufficiently large doses, such as radiant energy (x-rays, radium, and radioactive isotopes of gold or phosphorus), benzene and its derivatives, alkylating agents, and antimetabolites used to treat malignant tumors. Radiation causes the bone marrow to stop producing blood cells by inhibiting mitosis, or cell division, and antimetabolites used in cancer therapy block the synthesis of purines or nucleic acids.
2. Agents that occasionally cause marrow failure, such as chloramphenicol (Chloromycetin, the drug most commonly linked with aplastic anemia), sulfonamides, quinacrine, phenylbutazone, the anticonvulsants phenytoin and mephenytoin, and gold compounds.
3. Agents that have been linked with aplastic anemia in only a few cases, such as streptomycin, tripelennamine, DDT, meprobamate, hair and aniline dyes, and carbon tetrachloride.

The onset of aplastic anemia may be insidious or rapid. In idiopathic or hereditary cases, the onset is usually gradual. When bone marrow failure results from a myelotoxin, however, the onset may be explosive, with quickly developing manifestations. If the condition does not reverse itself when the offending agent is removed, it can be fatal.

Clinical Manifestations

Manifestations of pancytopenia are particularly severe. The RBC count and leukocyte and platelet counts all decline. The three conditions then develop: (1) normocytic anemia, (2) neutropenia, and (3) thrombocytopenia.

The RBC count is usually below 1 million/mm³, with a low reticulocyte count. The client reports progressive fatigue, lassitude, and dyspnea. The leukocyte count may be less than 1000/mm³ (normal range, 5000 to 10,000/mm³). The client, therefore, suffers from an increased susceptibility to infection, because without leukocytes the body cannot adequately battle bacteria and other invading organisms. If the absolute neutrophil count drops below 500/mm³, a fulminating bacterial infection may develop, often from the client's own normal flora. The platelet count may fall below 30,000 to 15,000/mm³ (normal range, 150,000 to 450,000/mm³), which usually causes bleeding into the skin and mucous membranes. The client is also at risk for retinal hemorrhage and intracranial hemorrhage. If the platelet count is severely reduced, the client may hemorrhage spontaneously.

The diagnosis of aplastic anemia and pancytopenia is based on the differential blood count, the client's manifestations, history of exposure to a myelotoxin, and bone marrow examination.

Outcome Management

The client with pancytopenia is often critically ill. Prompt medical attention and skillful nursing care are necessary. The first step in halting the process of aplastic anemia is immediate withdrawal of the offending agent or drug.

Monitor any client undergoing radiotherapy or receiving a medication that is a suspected myelotoxin for marrow failure by frequent complete blood counts (CBCs). A significant drop in the RBC, leukocyte, or platelet count signals the need to stop the drug. Usually, stopping a suspected agent is followed by a rise in the CBC. Unfortunately, marrow failure due to chloramphenicol may progress despite discontinuation of the drug. If aplastic anemia develops from a suspected myelotoxic agent, blood transfusions are the mainstay of therapy until bone marrow activity signals recovery. Because the marrow of the aplastic client is severely depressed, cellular blood components should be irradiated before transfusion to inactivate lymphocytes and to prevent transfusion-associated GVHD (see Chapter 78). If the marrow does not recover and long-term RBC support is required, iron overload often results. Before iron chelating therapy became available, this complication was a leading cause of death.

Bone marrow transplantation is now the treatment of choice in aplastic anemia when (1) an autoimmune phenomenon is suspected or (2) the bone marrow fails to regenerate after discontinuation of myelotoxic agents. Currently, transplantation can take place only if the client has a human leukocyte antigen (HLA)–matched donor. Comparing the results of clients treated by bone marrow transplantation with conventional therapy of steroids and androgens reveals a 2-year survival rate of 60% to 80% with bone marrow transplantation versus 25% for those treated conventionally.

HEMOLYTIC ANEMIA

Hemolytic anemias are due to a shortening of the RBC life span, abnormal destruction of RBCs by macrophages or a hyperactive spleen, or failure of the bone marrow to replace destroyed RBCs.

The client with hemolytic anemia suffers from all the general manifestations of anemia discussed earlier (lassitude, fatigue, etc.). Renal failure may be a complication of severe hemolysis. It is caused by excretion of an increased load of RBC degradation products.

Laboratory findings indicative of hemolytic anemia usually include normocytic anemia, reticulocytosis due to increased efforts of the bone marrow to compensate for excessive erythrocyte destruction, increased RBC fragility, shortened erythrocyte life span, hyperbilirubinemia, increased fecal and urinary urobilinogen, and (in cases of massive intravascular hemolysis) hemoglobinemia.

Treatment includes removal of the offending agent. Adequate fluids are given to flush the kidneys. In addition, sodium bicarbonate or sodium lactate are administered to alkalize the urine, which decreases the likelihood of precipitation in the renal tubules. Splenectomy may be required.

SICKLE CELL ANEMIA AND SICKLE CELL TRAIT

Sickle cell anemia is an inherited disorder of hemoglobin synthesis resulting in tissue hypoxia and obstruction of blood vessels. It primarily affects the world's black population (Fig. 75–2). Worldwide, sickle cell anemia is the most common form of anemia. Sickle cell trait is a milder form of the disorder. The trait is prevalent in Africa, possibly because the abnormal hemoglobin is more resistant to the parasite that causes malaria, which is endemic in some areas.

Etiology and Risk Factors

The genetic defect results in substitution of the amino acid valine for glutamine on one of the globin chains of the hemoglobin molecule. This sickle cell hemoglobin (Hb S) is less soluble than the normal adult hemoglobin (Hb A). Hb S also assumes a sickle or crescent shape when deoxygenated. As shown in Figure 75–2, whether a client will have sickle cell anemia, sickle cell trait, or neither depends on the genes for hemoglobin inherited from each parent.

Pathophysiology

Sickle cell anemia is named for the appearance of the RBC when blood oxygen decreases. The cell assumes a sickle, or crescent, shape (Fig. 75–1D). Once the RBC sickles, it becomes rigid, and the blood becomes more viscous and may obstruct capillary blood flow, causing further hypoxia and, consequently, more sickling. Thus, a vicious circle ensues. The organs most vulnerable to infarction and necrosis are the brain and kidneys, because of their constant demand for oxygen, and the bone marrow and spleen, because of their normally sluggish circulation.

The mechanisms that precipitate the various forms of sickling crises remain unclear. However, two major factors are definitely linked with the sickling of cells: (1) hypoxia, due to low oxygen tension, and (2) an increased blood viscosity, due to an increased concentration of sickled cells. Exposure to low oxygen tensions (e.g., at high

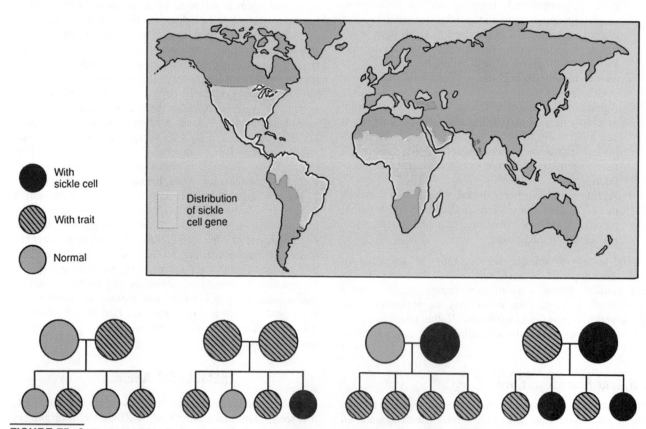

FIGURE 75–2 Geographic distribution and inheritance pattern of sickle cell gene. (Redrawn from Page, J., et al. [1981]. *Blood: The river of life.* Washington, DC: Torstar Books.)

altitudes, flying in nonpressurized planes, exercising strenuously, or undergoing anesthesia without receiving adequate oxygenation) results in hypoxia. Although both Hb S and Hb A have the same solubility when oxygenated, deoxygenation of the blood drastically affects Hb S.

Sickle cell crisis is an acute exacerbation of the disorder due to respiratory infections or other stressors that reduce blood oxygen levels. Five causes have been described:

1. Vaso-occlusive or pain crisis: Pain originating from an area of vascular occlusion. This type shows no change on hematologic examination.
2. Aplastic crisis: in bone marrow hypoplasia with decreased hemoglobin and RBCs; pain may be present.
3. Hemolytic crisis: RBC destruction and fever.
4. Sequestration crisis: a result of sudden and massive trapping of RBCs by visceral organs, such as the spleen.
5. Mixed crisis: manifestations of more than one type.

Clinical Manifestations

Sickle cell anemia is usually manifested after a child is 6 months old, when fetal hemoglobin is no longer present. Occasionally, clinical manifestations do not appear until adulthood. Young children who have the disease do not grow properly because of anemia. Weakness and fatigue are also present. Developmental delays in sexual maturity and retarded growth may be seen.

Sluggish circulation leads to edema of the hands and feet. Jaundice or pallor may be present. Infarctions in the spleen are so common that, after childhood, the spleen of most sickle cell anemia clients is small and scarred. Leg ulcers are found in about 75% of older children and adults with the disease. Other manifestations include necrosis of the head of the femur, possibly leading to osteomyelitis and necrotic bone marrow with development of infection, joint pain, renal medullary ischemia resulting in diminished capacity to concentrate urine, priapism, pulmonary infarctions, myocardial infarctions, and cerebrovascular accidents. Hyperactivity of the bone marrow leads to spindly legs, a short trunk, and a tower-shaped skull.

Sickle cell crisis is characterized by:

- Cardiac systolic murmurs, dysrhythmias, heart enlargement
- Dyspnea, chest pain, cyanosis
- Sensorimotor manifestations of increased intracranial pressure due to cerebral hemorrhaging
- Renal manifestations of uremia, such as decreased urinary output and edema

Diagnostic Findings

Hemolytic anemia develops from the destruction of sickle cells; hemoglobin values usually lie in a range of 12 to 18 g/dl, depending on age and sex. An elevated bilirubin level from the released hemoglobin may result in gallstone formation (cholelithiasis). Four laboratory procedures demonstrate the presence of Hb S in either homozygous or heterozygous carriers:

- Stained blood smear
- Sickle cell slide preparation
- Sickle-turbidity tube test
- Hemoglobin electrophoresis

STAINED BLOOD SMEAR
A stained blood smear is examined for the presence of sickle cells.

SICKLE CELL SLIDE PREPARATION
A blood specimen is observed for the sickling phenomenon after deoxygenation of the blood. This test is accurate but time-consuming.

SICKLE-TURBIDITY TUBE TEST
The sickle-turbidity tube test is an excellent mass screening test to detect Hb S. After a finger prick, blood is mixed with Sickledex solution in a test tube. Five minutes later, the specimen is observed for cloudiness, which indicates the presence of Hb S. Solutions mixed with normal hemoglobin remain clear. Although the test demonstrates Hb S, it does not differentiate sickle cell disease from the trait.

HEMOGLOBIN ELECTROPHORESIS
Hemoglobin electrophoresis differentiates sickle cell anemia from sickle cell trait. By means of an applied electric field, the various types of hemoglobin within a blood specimen are separated. If a blood specimen contains both Hb S and Hb A, the client is heterozygous—has sickle cell trait. If Hb S is 75% to 100% of the total and the rest Hb F or Hb A_2, the client is homozygous—has sickle cell anemia.

Many African Americans are unaware that they carry the sickle cell trait and that they can transmit this trait to their offspring. Consequently, researchers are perfecting mass screening tests for the detection of Hb S among the black population. Clients having only the sickle cell trait may never be detected unless they are exposed to extremely low oxygen tension (e.g., mountain climbing, flying in a nonpressurized plane), extremely hard work or exercise, or pregnancy. When exposed to extreme stressors, the client with the trait may experience manifestations of sickle cell disease.

Outcome Management

▬ Medical Management

Treatment of sickle cell anemia consists chiefly of supportive care (e.g., rest, oxygen, IV administration of fluids and electrolytes to ensure adequate hydration, sedation, and analgesics).

In some cases, the slow administration of packed RBCs or partial exchange transfusion helps relieve severe anemic manifestations. During episodes of increased risk (e.g., surgery, pregnancy), some clients benefit from *hypertransfusion* (or transfusions until more than 50% of the circulating RBCs are of donor origin).

Anticoagulants, steroids, and cobalt treatments have all been used without success to reverse the sickling process. Clients with sickle cell disease have an increased need for folic acid and, therefore, usually receive a daily oral supplement to prevent increased anemia from folate deficiency. Prophylactic penicillin may also be ordered. Hydroxyurea and erythropoietin are being used in clinical trials in an attempt to increase fetal hemoglobin in clients with a diagnosis of sickle cell disease.

■ Nursing Management

ASSESSMENT

Assess the client for the pattern of data that may indicate sickle cell crisis. Assess for the ability of the family and client to cope with the disorder and understanding of the disease and the triggers of crisis.

DIAGNOSIS, OUTCOMES, INTERVENTIONS

Pain. Because of the joint swelling secondary to sickling crisis, one nursing diagnosis is *Pain related to joint swelling.*

Outcomes. The client will experience diminished pain, relieved, as evidenced by verbalization of pain relief and reliance on less opiates for control of pain.

Intervention. Assess for pain every 2 to 4 hours, and administer analgesics as needed according to orders; monitor for effectiveness of analgesia. Apply heat to joints as ordered. Provide rest periods. Administer fluids to prevent dehydration and recurrence of pain crisis. Increase oral fluid intake, and monitor intake and output.

Knowledge Deficit. Another nursing diagnosis is *Knowledge Deficit related to disease, treatment, and prevention of crises.*

Outcomes. The client will understand the disease, treatment, and prevention of crises, as evidenced by the client's statements and the absence of crises.

Interventions. When educating clients about sickle cell anemia or sickle cell trait, remember to:

1. Explain the nature of the disease, and give the client a chance to express feelings and ask questions.
2. Encourage African American parents to have themselves and their children tested for the presence of Hb S.
3. Advise the client to have routine medical examinations that include an RBC count.
4. Encourage young adults who carry Hb S to ask their physician for genetic counseling before marrying or having children.
5. Alert young women with sickle cell anemia that pregnancy carries a very high risk for them.
6. Explain that pulmonary or renal complications, or both, may develop.
7. Explain how to prevent crises, such as (a) avoiding high altitudes and flying in nonpressurized planes (because oxygen tension is lowered under these conditions) and (b) taking caution against becoming dehydrated and to call a physician if vomiting, diarrhea, high fever, or any other cause of water loss develops.

EVALUATION

An appropriate outcome for the client with sickle cell disease is that the disease will remain in remission as long as possible. It is impossible to prevent every crisis;

however, with education and an effort by the client, the number of attacks can be reduced.

POLYCYTHEMIA VERA

Polycythemia vera, the excessive bone marrow production of erythrocytes, leukocytes, and platelets, is caused by excessive activation of pluripotent stem cells. The inordinate mass production of these three cell lines results in (1) an increase in blood viscosity; (2) an increase in the total blood volume, which may be twice or even three times greater than normal; and (3) severe blood congestion of all tissues and organs. Because of these problems, the client suffers many manifestations, including an increased risk of clot formation.

Clinical Manifestations

In its early stages, polycythemia usually remains asymptomatic (an increased hematocrit level may be an incidental finding). However, hypervolemia and hyperviscosity may lead to dizziness, headache, tinnitus, visual disturbances, and other manifestations, depending on the body system affected. The client may also have a ruddy complexion (plethora) and dusky, red mucosa; cardiovascular hypertension (with dizziness, headache, and a sense of fullness in the head) and heart failure (shortness of breath, orthopnea); increased clotting leading to cerebrovascular accident, myocardial infarction, or peripheral gangrene; and bleeding (hemorrhage in capillaries, venules, and arterioles), which causes rupture of vessels; GI peptic ulcers, enlargement of liver and spleen; and skeletal gout (painful swollen joints, usually the big toe) characterized by an increased uric acid level.

Diagnostic findings include (1) an RBC count as high as 8 to 12 million/mm^3; (2) hemoglobin level of 18 to 25 g/dl; (3) hematocrit greater than 54% in men and 49% in women; (4) platelet count usually increased; (5) normal arterial blood gases (ABG) values; (6) hyperplastic bone marrow; and (7) a serum uric acid level three to four times normal.

Outcome Management

The goals of care in polycythemia vera are twofold: reduction of (1) blood volume and viscosity and (2) bone marrow activity. These decreases are accomplished through phlebotomy, administration of myelosuppressive agents, and radiation therapy. Emergency phlebotomy can be used to remove 500 to 2000 ml of blood until the hematocrit reaches 45%. Subsequent phlebotomies should be carried out as frequently (monthly) as necessary to maintain the hematocrit at about 45%. As iron deficiency supervenes, RBC production will be retarded, so that clients managed by phlebotomy alone may require as few as two or three phlebotomies a year.

Myelosuppressive agents can be used to retard the bone marrow. Radioactive phosphorus sometimes produces remissions that last from 6 months to 2 years. Other drugs include chlorambucil, busulfan, and hydroxyurea. Radiation therapy may be used to reduce the production of RBCs in the marrow.

DISORDERS AFFECTING WHITE BLOOD CELLS

White blood cells (WBCs), also called *leukocytes,* are divided into two groups:

- *Granulocytes* (polymorphonuclear leukocytes)
- *Agranulocytes* (mononuclear cells)

Granulocytes, in turn, are divided into three groups: (1) neutrophils, (2) basophils, and (3) eosinophils. The names denote affinity for the dyes used in staining. Agranulocytes include lymphocytes (B and T) and monocytes.

Plasmacytes (plasma cells) are derived from B lymphocytes. Plasmacytes are formed within the bone marrow and lymph nodes and are active in producing immunoglobulins (antibodies). Leukemia and lymphoma are discussed in Chapter 78.

AGRANULOCYTOSIS

Agranulocytosis (granulocytopenia, malignant neutropenia) is an acute, potentially fatal blood dyscrasia characterized by profound *neutropenia* (a reduced number of circulating neutrophils). Because neutrophils make up roughly 93% of all granulocytes, the terms *neutropenia* and *agranulocytosis* are often used interchangeably. Agranulocytosis is a fairly rare condition. For unknown reasons, females are much more susceptible to this condition than males, although even among females, agranulocytosis is relatively rare.

Etiology and Risk Factors

Agranulocytosis results either from the failure of neutrophil production to keep pace with destruction of the cells or from increased destruction of neutrophils, which removes them from circulation. Chemotherapy, radiation, and aplastic anemia all reduce or stop neutrophil production through interference with granulopoiesis. The most common cause of agranulocytosis is drug toxicity or hypersensitivity. Two groups of agents are capable of suppressing granulocyte production:

1. Agents that always produce neutropenia when given in sufficiently large doses over time, such as many cancer chemotherapeutic agents, ionizing radiation, and benzene.
2. Agents that produce neutropenia only in clients particularly sensitive to the drug, such as tranquilizers (chlorpromazine), antithyroid agents (propylthiouracil), anticonvulsants (phenytoin), antibiotics (chloramphenicol), and phenylbutazone.

Agranulocytosis can occur in clients with anemias related to diminished erythropoiesis (e.g., aplastic and megaloblastic anemias). It may also accompany certain diseases (e.g., tuberculosis, typhoid fever, malaria, uremia).

Accelerated destruction of neutrophils can result from infection, autoimmune disease, and idiosyncratic reactions to many drugs. The destruction may be so rapid that production cannot keep up with it. If agranulocytosis is not reversed when the cause is removed, the client will require an allogeneic bone marrow transplant for survival.

Pathophysiology

Failure to produce adequate numbers of white blood cells prevents normal surveillance and phagocytosis; infection from the neutropenia is a common sequela. Neutrophils constitute a swift and powerful defense against invading microorganisms. Consequently, decreases in their number result in a greater susceptibility to bacterial invasion, especially when the client's absolute neutrophil count (ANC) drops below 500/mm^3.

Clinical Manifestations

The manifestations of agranulocytosis are a result of the neutropenia. Typically, the onset of this acute disease is rapid. For the first 2 or 3 days, severe fatigue and weakness occur, next followed by a sore throat, ulcerations of the pharyngeal and buccal mucosa, dysphagia, high fever, weak and rapid pulse, and severe chills. Without prompt antibiotic treatment, the disorder usually causes death within a week. The mucous membranes of the throat and mouth are particularly vulnerable.

The diagnosis of agranulocytosis rests on the following:

- Leukopenia, evidenced by WBC counts of 500 to 3000/mm^3 with extreme reduction in polymorphonuclear cells (0 to 2%)
- Bone marrow examination revealing an absence of granulocytes, a maturational arrest of young developing cells, or an increased number of myeloid precursors (signifying peripheral granulocyte destruction)
- Cultures of urine, blood, and ulcerative lesions in the throat and mouth that are positive for bacteria, usually gram-positive cocci
- A history of exposure to an offending agent as well as all the aforementioned findings (with many clients medicating themselves with potentially dangerous drugs; all drugs taken within the past 6 to 12 months need to be investigated)

Outcome Management

Treatment of clients with agranulocytosis involves eliminating potentially toxic agents that may be responsible for marrow suppression. Agranulocytosis caused by toxic substances is usually reversed within 2 to 3 weeks after their elimination.

Surveillance cultures of blood, throat, sputum, urine, and stool should be taken at frequent intervals to monitor the status of infections. Combinations of broad-spectrum antibiotics are usually administered until the offending organism is identified. Untreated infectious processes in this situation carry a mortality rate of 80%.

Treatment of agranulocytosis includes various *colony-stimulating factors,* such as granulocyte colony-stimulating factor (G-CSF), granulocyte macrophage colony-stimulating factor (GM-CSF), and erythropoietin (EPO). These are given after the offending agent has been eliminated.

MULTIPLE MYELOMA

Multiple myeloma is a B-cell neoplastic condition characterized by abnormal malignant proliferation of plasma cells secreting a monoclonal paraprotein, accumulation of mature plasma cells in the bone marrow, and complications throughout the body as a result of dissemination of the disease (e.g., lytic bone lesions and osteoporosis, hematopoietic suppression, hypercalcemia, proteinuria, and renal failure). Risk factors include an increased incidence in some families, ionizing radiation, and occupational chemical exposures.

Pathophysiology

Multiple myeloma is characterized by an abnormal proliferation of plasma cells. With this overproduction of plasma cells, bone destruction also occurs. In addition to bone destruction, multiple myeloma is characterized by disruption of RBC, leukocyte, and platelet production, which results from plasma cells crowding the bone marrow. Impaired production of these cell forms causes anemia, increased vulnerability to infection and bleeding tendencies, respectively.

Clinical Manifestations

Once manifestations appear, they typically involve the skeletal system, particularly the pelvis, spine, and ribs. Some clients have backache or bone pain that worsens with movement. Others suffer sudden pathologic fractures accompanied by severe pain. In time, skeletal destruction increases and the client may develop sternum and rib cage deformities. Diffuse osteoporosis usually appears, accompanied by a negative calcium balance. The skull shows multiple osteolytic lesions. Loss of calcium and phosphorus from damaged bones eventually leads to the development of renal stones, particularly in immobilized clients.

Diagnostic Findings

Diagnosis of multiple myeloma rests on radiographic studies, bone marrow biopsy, and blood and urine examination. Radiographic studies reveal diffuse lesions in the bone, widespread demineralization, and osteoporosis. The bone marrow contains large numbers of immature plasma cells. Normally, plasma cells constitute 5% of the bone marrow cell population. Because of the abnormal number of plasma cells producing immunoglobulins, peripheral blood samples sent for plasma electrophoresis reveal a large amount of abnormal immunoglobulins. Another diagnostic manifestation of multiple myeloma is the appearance of Bence-Jones protein in the urine, consisting of monoclonal immunoglobulin light chains.

Outcome Management

Management is aimed at early recognition and treatment of complications of the disease. Clients with hypercalcemia often become anorectic, nauseated, drowsy, confused, and disoriented and may require hospitalization. Not all clients with multiple myeloma should be treated.

Manifestations, physical findings, and laboratory data must be considered. In some cases, treatment might be withheld and the client re-evaluated in 2 to 3 months. If overt manifestations are present, chemotherapy is the preferred initial treatment. Palliative radiation should be limited to clients with disabling pain from a well-defined location that has not been responsive to chemotherapy. Autologous or allogeneic bone marrow transplantation is also an option.

SUPPRESS THE BONE MARROW

There is some controversy over the most effective chemotherapy regimen. Therapy with melphalan and prednisone or a combination of alkylating agents can be effective. Prednisone and melphalan given orally for a period of 4 to 7 days and repeated at 4- to 6-week intervals produces positive results in 50% to 60% of clients. Leukocyte and platelet counts are monitored regularly and doses adjusted until modest cytopenia occurs. Combination chemotherapy, commonly melphalan, cyclophosphamide, carmustine (BCNU), vincristine (Oncovin), and prednisone, has shown a 70% to 75% response rate. This therapy may continue for 1 to 2 years, but relapse almost always occurs when chemotherapy is discontinued. Interferon-alfa appears to be beneficial in prolonging the duration of remission.

REDUCE SERUM CALCIUM LEVELS

In the past, corticosteroids such as high-dose dexamethasone, mithramycin, furosemide, and IV hydration were commonly prescribed for hypercalcemia; however, newer agents now exist. Etidronate disodium (Didronel) or gallium nitrate (Ganite) and IV hydration are effective. The newest and most effective agent is pamidronate sodium (Aredia).

Administer fluids in adequate amounts to maintain an output of 1.5 to 2.0 L/day. Clients with multiple myeloma usually require about 3 L of fluid per day. The client needs sufficient fluid not only to dilute the calcium overload but also to prevent protein from precipitating in the renal tubules, even after effective treatment with chemotherapy. Administer medications to increase calcium excretion and to decrease calcium loss from bone, such as furosemide (Lasix), steroids, and plicamycin, etidronate, gallium, or pamidronate.

If the client is able, encourage activity that places stress on the long bones to increase calcium resorption. Antiemetics may be required for relief of nausea and vomiting. Small, frequent feedings may be better tolerated, and stool softeners may be routinely required. Closely monitor intake, output, and blood studies to determine effectiveness of treatment. Weigh the client daily so that any significant loss can be noted and corrected.

Closely monitor the client's mental status. If disorientation or confusion occurs, remove sharp objects and other potentially hazardous items from the environment. The side rails should be raised, and light restraints may be required.

Teach significant others the manifestations of hypercalcemia and to report them immediately to the physician. Instruct family members or significant others on how to institute safety measures to prevent falls and injuries. The client may need some assistive devices at home, such as a toilet riser and handhold bars in the bathroom. Measure the client's calcium level at regular intervals for assessment of the development of hypercalcemia.

INFECTIOUS MONONUCLEOSIS

Pathophysiology and Etiology

Infectious mononucleosis, also known as glandular disease or the "kissing disease," is a self-limiting condition characterized by painful enlargement of the lymph nodes, lymphocytosis, sore throat, and fever. Primarily a disease of the young, it usually strikes children between the ages of 3 and 5 years and young adults between the ages of 15 and 25 years. The greatest incidence occurs among college students, medical students, and nurses. Although this disease usually occurs sporadically, epidemic forms may sweep through colleges and children's homes.

The cause of infectious mononucleosis is Epstein-Barr virus (EBV), a herpesvirus. Although the mode of transmission remains unknown, the disease may be transmitted through the oropharyngeal route during close contact, as with kissing.

Clinical Manifestations

The onset of infectious mononucleosis follows an incubation period of 2 to 6 weeks. Before frank clinical manifestations present, the person may experience fatigue, headaches, malaise, and myalgias. Subsequently, assessment reveals temperatures up to 39° C (102.2° F), pharyngitis, and lymphadenopathy that is more pronounced in the cervical regions. In 10% to 15% of those affected, a maculopapular rash develops, closely resembling the rash of rubella. Splenic enlargement causes left upper quadrant pain. Nervous system involvement may lead to severe headache. In rare cases, liver involvement may develop into a hepatitis-like syndrome.

When infectious mononucleosis is severe, two complications may develop: (1) splenic rupture resulting from the infiltration of the spleen by massive numbers of lymphocytes and (2) streptococcal pharyngitis (Vincent's angina) secondary to bacterial invasion of the throat.

The diagnosis of infectious mononucleosis is based on three criteria: (1) physical assessment, (2) laboratory tests, and (3) the Paul-Bunnel test.

The WBC count usually ranges from 12,000 to 20,000/mm^3, of which 50% are lymphocytes and monocytes and 10% to 20% are large, atypical lymphocytes. The *mono spot test* is also performed with a throat swab. It detects anti-EBV antibodies and is positive in 50% of cases within the first week and 90% of cases in the fourth week.

Outcome Management

No specific intervention either mitigates or shortens the disease process. Because infectious mononucleosis must simply run its course, treatments are directed at control of manifestations. Bed rest is recommended until fever is resolved. Acetaminophen, cool sponge baths, and a large fluid intake help control fever. Warm saline throat irrigation may relieve the sore throat. Aspirin is avoided because of the risk of Reye's syndrome. Contact sports must be avoided to reduce the risk of splenic rupture.

Although complications sometimes develop, the prognosis for clients with infectious mononucleosis is generally excellent. The febrile phase of this disorder typically lasts 2 to 4 weeks. During the long convalescence, the client slowly regains strength and energy.

SPLENIC RUPTURE AND HYPERSPLENISM

Etiology

The most frequent indication for splenectomy is rupture of the spleen complicated by severe hemorrhage. Causes of splenic rupture include:

- Trauma (e.g., automobile accidents, bullet or knife wounds, severe blows to the spleen).
- Accidental tearing of the splenic capsule during surgery on neighboring organs
- Disease of the spleen that causes softening or damage (e.g., infectious mononucleosis and malaria)

In hypersplenism, a second important indication for splenectomy, the spleen destroys, in excessive numbers, one of the blood cell types (i.e., erythrocytes, leukocytes, or platelets). Primary hypersplenism occurs in idiopathic thrombocytopenic purpura and congenital spherocytosis. Some etiologic factors associated with secondary hypersplenism include lymphomas (including Hodgkin's disease), leukemia, polycythemia vera, acute infections (including infectious mononucleosis), chronic infections, malaria, syphilis, hemoglobinopathy, and cirrhosis of the liver.

Clinical Manifestations

Manifestations of hypersplenism include moderate to massive splenomegaly, anemia, leukopenia, or thrombocytopenia, and a compensatory increase in the production of the affected cell line by the bone marrow. Overactivity of the spleen develops either as a primary condition of unknown origin or as a condition secondary to another disease.

Laboratory indications for splenectomy include granulocytopenia of less than 500/mm^3 and thrombocytopenia of less than 20,000/mm^3.

Outcome Management

Primary hypersplenism can be alleviated by splenectomy. Splenectomy is palliative only for clients with secondary hypersplenism because the surgery has little or no effect on the course of the primary illness. When the diagnosis is confirmed, it is important to teach the client to prevent complications associated with the specific cytopenia.

The spleen has an important role in the phagocytosis of circulating opsonized organisms. After splenectomy, young children are at high risk for fulminant infections due to *Streptococcus pneumoniae, Haemophilus influenzae, Neisseria meningitidis,* and other encapsulated organisms. Continuous prophylactic antibiotics may be advisable during the early years or indefinitely. Adults are also at increased risk for infection, especially during the first 3 years after surgery. The splenectomized client should be advised to seek medical treatment at the earliest manifestations of infection.

The unique functions performed by the spleen are eventually taken over by other organs. However, the loss of the spleen due to cessation of function or splenectomy does require the client to be monitored for potentially serious complications. The nursing care of the client undergoing splenectomy is generally the same as that discussed in Chapter 15 for any client undergoing surgery.

DISORDERS OF PLATELETS AND CLOTTING FACTORS

Disorders of hemostasis affecting platelets and clotting factors include (1) hemorrhagic disorders, (2) purpura, and (3) coagulation disorders.

HEMORRHAGIC DISORDERS

Normal clot formation and lysis depend on (1) intact blood vessels, (2) an adequate number of functioning platelets, (3) sufficient amounts of the 12 clotting factors, and (4) a well-controlled fibrinolytic system. Consequently, the four basic problems underlying hemorrhagic (bleeding) disorders are as follows:

- Weak, damaged vessels that rupture easily or spontaneously
- Platelet deficiency (*thrombocytopenia*) due to hypoproliferation, excessive pooling of platelets in the spleen, or excessive platelet destruction
- Deficiency or total lack of one of the clotting factors
- Excessive or insufficient fibrinolysis

Disorders of hemostasis fall into two major categories: *purpura* and *coagulation* (Box 75–1).

The diagnosis of a hemorrhagic disorder depends on a complete health and family history, physical examination, and laboratory tests for platelet and clotting defects. The history usually offers numerous clues to the type of bleeding problem and its cause.

If the history indicates a bleeding disorder, examine the client for overt manifestations of bleeding. Petechiae

(tiny hemorrhagic spots caused by intradermal or submucosal bleeding) are usually present in vascular and thrombocytopenic purpuras. The presence of *ecchymoses* (large, blotchy, subcutaneous hemorrhagic areas), *hematomas* (subdermal hemorrhage), and *hemarthrosis* (blood within the joints) points to *hemophilia*. However, ecchymoses may develop in any hemorrhagic disorder. Clients who hemorrhage severely from several areas during childbirth or a major surgical procedure may have a fibrinogen deficiency. In addition to any evidence of bleeding, search for manifestations of hepatic cirrhosis (e.g., hepatomegaly, jaundice) and splenomegaly. Laboratory studies provide the most crucial evidence for pinpointing the type and cause of a bleeding disorder.

Clients with hemorrhagic disorders need to understand (1) why they are at risk for bleeding, (2) the manifestations of bleeding, and (3) preventive measures to avoid bleeding. Those who can be managed by home health care should be referred to appropriate health care agencies. Clients with bleeding disorders should carry an identification card at all times that indicates their diagnosis, name of physician or health care agency, and blood type. Assess each client before even minor invasive procedures, such as dental extractions, to rule out a history of bleeding disorders.

IDIOPATHIC THROMBOCYTOPENIC PURPURA

Idiopathic thrombocytopenic purpura (ITP) is an autoimmune bleeding disorder characterized by the development of autoantibodies to one's own platelets, the binding of autoantibodies to antigens, and the destruction of platelets in the spleen and, to a lesser extent, in the liver. Normally, platelets survive 8 to 10 days within the circulation; in ITP, however, platelet survival is as brief as 1 to 3 days or less. In most cases, ITP takes a course of remissions and exacerbations that, in untreated cases, may continue for years.

Clinical Manifestations

Clinical manifestations include petechiae, ecchymosis, epistaxis, bleeding from the gums, and easy bruising. Women may have extremely heavy menses or bleeding between periods.

Diagnostic findings that confirm the presence of ITP include:

- A platelet count below 100,000/mm³
- Prolonged bleeding time with normal coagulation time (all coagulation factors are present and normal)
- Increased capillary fragility, as demonstrated by the tourniquet test
- Positive platelet antibody screening
- Bone marrow aspirate containing normal or increased numbers of megakaryocytes

Complications of ITP include (1) cerebral hemorrhage, which proves fatal in 1% to 5% of clients with ITP; (2) severe hemorrhages from the nose, GI tract, and urinary system; (3) bleeding into the diaphragm, which can result in pulmonary complications; and (4) nerve pain, extremity anesthesia, or paralysis resulting from the pressure of hematomas on nerves or brain tissues.

BOX 75–1 **Classification of Disorders of Hemostasis**

Purpura

Vascular defect purpura
 Familial hemorrhagic telangiectasia
 Anaphylactoid purpura (allergic purpura)
 Toxic purpura
Platelet disorder purpura
 Idiopathic thrombocytopenic purpura
 Secondary thrombocytopenias

Coagulation Disorders

Hemophilia
Hypoprothrombinemia
Disseminated intravascular coagulation (DIC)

Outcome Management

The treatment of choice for clients with ITP is steroids to inhibit the macrophage ingestion of the antibody-coated platelets. Plasmapheresis is sometimes used as short-term therapy until the steroid therapy takes effect. If the client is actively bleeding or requires surgery, IV gamma globulin can be used to increase the platelet count.

If the client does not have a sustained remission, splenectomy may be needed (see earlier). In 60% to 80% of cases, removal of the spleen results in complete and permanent remission. The effectiveness of splenectomy is believed to be related to the removal of the site of premature destruction of the antibody-sensitized platelets.

Danazol (Danocrine) has been used with success in some clients. Immunosuppressive therapy used in refractory cases includes vincristine, vinblastine (Velban), azathioprine (Imuran), and cyclophosphamide.

Nursing care of clients at high risk for bleeding is discussed in Chapter 78.

COAGULATION DISORDERS

The coagulation disorders stem from a defect in the clotting mechanisms. One or more of the clotting factors is depleted or absent. The important coagulation disorders discussed here are (1) hypoprothrombinemia, (2) disseminated intravascular coagulation (DIC), and (3) the hemophilias.

HYPOPROTHROMBINEMIA

Pathophysiology

Hypoprothrombinemia refers to a deficiency in the amount of circulating prothrombin. Prothrombin is a protein produced in the liver and normally found in the blood. For prothrombin synthesis to take place, vitamin K (a fat-soluble vitamin) must be present in the liver to act as a catalyst. Hypoprothrombinemia develops from a vitamin K deficiency or liver disorder or from an overdose of aspirin, coumarin, or coumarin-derivative anticoagulant (such as warfarin), which antagonizes the action of vitamin K.

The fat-soluble vitamin K is largely synthesized by bacteria in the small intestine, a classic example of symbiosis. The bacteria do more than their share, since we excrete large amounts of the vitamin. There is no standard dietary daily allowance. Because vitamin K is fat-soluble, it depends on the presence of bile for absorption. Once absorbed, vitamin K catalyzes prothrombin synthesis within the liver cells. Vitamin K deficiency is seen in newborns, who arrive with a limited supply and a largely sterile digestive tract, and in clients with GI tract disorders that interfere with the absorption of vitamin K, such as (1) malabsorption syndrome and jaundice due to bile duct obstruction; (2) liver damage so extensive that liver cells cannot produce bile or synthesize prothrombin; and (3) prolonged sulfonamide or antibiotic administration that sterilizes the bowel, thereby halting vitamin K manufactured by GI tract bacteria.

Dicumarol is an effective anticoagulant, interfering with vitamin K in prothrombin synthesis. In excessive doses, prothrombin time is prolonged. If the prothrombin time is too long, the danger of bleeding or spontaneous hemorrhage increases.

Clinical Manifestations

The major manifestations of hypoprothrombinemia are ecchymosis after minimal trauma, epistaxis, postoperative hemorrhage from the incision, hematuria, gastrointestinal tract bleeding, and prolonged bleeding from a venipuncture. The outstanding laboratory finding is a prolonged prothrombin time.

Outcome Management

Treatment of hypoprothrombinemia aims at the underlying cause. For example, vitamin K deficiency resulting from malabsorption is corrected through intramuscular or IV administration of vitamin K, such as phytonadione (AquaMEPHYTON) or menadione (Synkayvite). If overdosage with a coumarin anticoagulant is the underlying problem, anticoagulant therapy is stopped. To normalize the prothrombin time, phytonadione is administered orally for minor bleeding problems or intravenously for hemorrhage. Finally, if prothrombin deficiency results from liver disease, concentrates of prothrombin or of prothrombin and factors VII, IX, and X may be transfused.

DISSEMINATED INTRAVASCULAR COAGULATION

DIC is a complex and important coagulation disorder characterized by two apparently conflicting manifestations: (1) diffuse fibrin deposition within arterioles and capillaries, with resultant widespread clotting, and (2) hemorrhage from the kidneys, brain, adrenal glands, heart, and other organs occurs following activation of clotting factors and fibrinolytic enzymes throughout arterioles and capillaries. DIC is often called a "consumptive coagulopathy" because of the depletion of platelets.

Etiology and Risk Factors

The causes of DIC are many, and there is considerable overlap among the syndromes that precede its occurrence. Sepsis is the leading cause; up to 73% of clients with sepsis develop DIC. Four categories of causative factors are:

- Introduction of tissue coagulation factors into the circulation
- Damage to vascular endothelium
- Stagnant blood flow
- Infection

Box 75–2 lists conditions that may precipitate DIC.

Pathophysiology

Two pathways can initiate DIC. An extrinsic pathway of massive tissue damage due to burns or trauma or an intrinsic pathway due to damage to the endothelium release thromboplastic substances that result in activation of

---

BOX 75-2 Conditions That May Precipitate Disseminated Intravascular Coagulation

Shock
Cirrhosis
Purpura fulminans
Glomerulonephritis
Acute fulminant hepatitis
Acute bacterial and viral infections

Conditions that may cause the release of platelet factor III:

- Fat emboli
- Snakebites

Hemolytic processes caused by:

- Infection
- Transfusion reactions
- Immunologic disorders

Tissue damage caused by:

- Trauma
- Heat stroke
- Extensive burns
- Transplant rejections
- Surgery—particularly if extracorporeal circulation was used

Conditions that may cause the release of thromboplastin from tissues:

- Neoplastic growths
  - Acute leukemias
  - Prostatic cancer
  - Bronchogenic cancer
  - Giant cavernous hemangioma
- Obstetric conditions
  - Abruptio placentae (placental abruption)
  - Retained dead fetus
  - Amniotic fluid embolism

---

thrombin, which in turn activates fibrinogen and results in deposition of fibrin throughout the microcirculation. The formation of fibrin results from increased generation of thrombin, suppression of anticoagulation mechanisms, and delayed removal of fibrin due to impaired fibrinolysis (see Understanding DIC and Its Treatment).

Platelet aggregation or adhesiveness is increased; this enables fibrin clots and microthrombi to form in the brain, kidneys, heart, and other organs, causing microinfarcts and tissue necrosis. RBCs become trapped in the fibrin strands and are destroyed (hemolysis). The resultant sluggish circulation of blood reduces the flow of nutrients and oxygen to the cells. Platelets, prothrombin, and other clotting factors are consumed in the process, which compromises coagulation and predisposes to bleeding.

Excessive clotting activates the fibrinolytic mechanism, which causes the production of fibrin degradation products. Fibrin degradation products act to inhibit platelet clotting functions, which causes further bleeding. Ultimately, with lysis of clots and depletion of clotting factors, the blood loses its ability to clot.

Clinical Manifestations

The onset of DIC is usually acute and develops within days to hours after an initial assault to the body system, such as shock. Subacute DIC may not be apparent initially but may become fulminant as the clinical course progresses. Chronic cases of DIC characteristically develop in clients with cancer or in women carrying a dead fetus.

Manifestations may be mild or extremely severe. They include purpura, petechiae, and ecchymoses on the skin, mucous membranes, heart lining, and lungs; prolonged bleeding from venipuncture; severe, uncontrolled hemorrhage during surgery or childbirth; oliguria and acute renal failure; and convulsions and coma. Ischemia of the peripheral tissue leads to coolness and mottling of the extremities.

The prognosis for clients with DIC varies. The condition may be self-limiting. On the other hand, hemorrhage, organ damage (especially acute respiratory distress syndrome), or even death may occur within a few days or even a few hours if associated with gram-negative sepsis. In severe cases, the mortality rate reaches 80%.

Diagnostic Findings

Diagnostic findings in severe cases of DIC indicate that the hemostatic mechanism has failed totally. A prolonged prothrombin time and activated partial thromboplastin time, very low (and falling) platelet count ($<100,000/mm^3$), low plasma levels of coagulation inhibitors, and prolonged clotting times are common findings. Table 75-3 lists the laboratory tests used in the diagnosis of DIC.

Outcome Management

Medical Management

The treatment of DIC is currently under investigation as researchers attempt to validate the most suitable means of managing this syndrome. To treat DIC successfully, clinicians must (1) correct the basic problem (such as infection, delivery of a fetus, surgery, or irradiation for cancer), (2) reverse the pathologic clotting, (3) control bleeding and shock, (4) detect occult bleeding, (5) measure blood loss, (6) administer blood products and medication as prescribed, and (7) observe for and report transfusion reactions and medication side effects.

Manifestations of thrombosis are treated with IV heparin, which interrupts the clotting cascade by blocking thrombi. The use of heparin is controversial and is reserved for clients with thrombosis seen as acute renal failure to skin ischemia. Low doses are given, such as 300 to 500 units per hour by continuous infusion. Antithrombin III, a natural inhibitor of coagulation, such as the drug desirudin, might be more effective than heparin and is being studied. Washed packed RBCs are administered to replace blood volume lost through hemorrhage without administering anticoagulant substances.

Cryoprecipitate is given for depletion of factors V and VIII. Administration of antithrombin III (in fresh frozen

Understanding DIC and Its Treatment

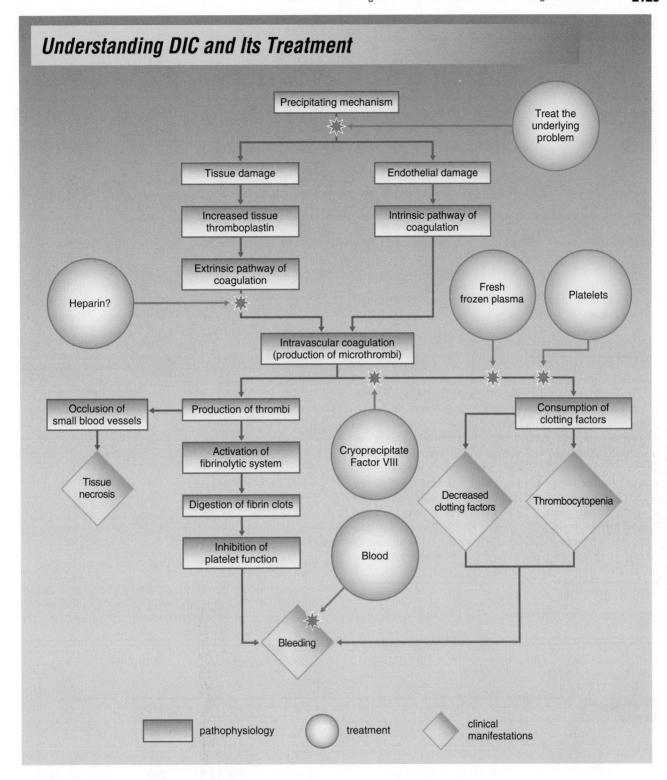

plasma) shortens the course of the disorder and reduces the complications of DIC. When bleeding cannot be controlled with heparin, aminocaproic acid (Amicar) is given. Cardiac, renal, and electrolyte studies should be followed closely during its use.

Several new agents to control bleeding and reverse laboratory manifestations of DIC are being studied. The protease inhibitors gabexate and aprotinin (Trasylol) have been used with some success. These drugs are still considered investigational.

◼ Nursing Management

Assess all body systems for the effects of DIC, including:

- Integumentary bleeding or oozing of blood from venipuncture sites or mucosal surfaces and wounds, pallor, petechiae, ecchymoses, and hematomas
- Respiratory tachypnea, hemoptysis, orthopnea, and basilar rales
- Cardiovascular tachycardia and hypotension

TABLE 75–3	LABORATORY TESTS USED IN DIAGNOSIS OF DISSEMINATED INTRAVASCULAR COAGULATION
Test	**Results**
Prothrombin time	Prolonged
Partial thromboplastin time	Usually prolonged
Thrombin time	Usually prolonged
Fibrinogen level	Usually depressed
Platelet count	Usually depressed
Fibrin degradation products	Elevated
Protamine sulfate test	Strongly positive
Factor assays II, V, VII	Reduced

- GI abdominal distention, guaiac-positive stools or gastric contents
- Genitourinary hematuria and oliguria
- Neurologic vision changes, dizziness, headache, changes in mental status, and irritability

Nursing care of clients with DIC varies, depending on the severity of the process. Generally, the goal is to monitor and quantify blood loss and provide supportive therapy with blood components to resolve manifestations of hemorrhage and control further bleeding. Monitor appropriate laboratory values to determine treatment effectiveness and observe for manifestations of thrombosis. To prevent further complications, avoid injections, apply pressure to bleeding sites, and turn and reposition the client frequently and gently. DIC sometimes results in overt bleeding from body orifices and other clinical manifestations that are very frightening to the client and significant others. They will all require intense emotional support.

THE HEMOPHILIAS

Classification

The hemophilias are characterized by prolonged bleeding, particularly after accidental, surgical, or dental trauma.

There are three major types of hemophilia: (1) hemophilia A (*classic* hemophilia), (2) hemophilia B (*Christmas disease*), and (3) von Willebrand's disease.

Hemophilia A, the most common of the congenital coagulation disorders, is due to a deficiency in the procoagulant protein factor VIII. The major characteristics of the hemophilias are compared in Table 75–4. Because classic hemophilia makes up 80% of all hemophilias, the discussion of manifestations and treatment refers only to this type.

The hemophilias are relatively common disorders. Within the United States alone, an estimated 25,000 clients are afflicted with a form of hemophilia.

Etiology

Hemophilia is genetically transmitted in a sex-linked (X chromosome) recessive pattern. Females usually transmit the defective gene, but males express the bleeding disorder. Females rarely have hemophilia. Female hemophilia carriers transmit the gene to half of their daughters and transmit the disorder to half of their sons. Males with hemophilia transmit the gene to all of their daughters but to none of their sons. Because this is a hereditary disease, the only way to control the risk is through genetic testing and counseling for decreasing the transmission.

Clinical Manifestations

Hemophilia may be mild or severe, depending on the level of factor VIII or IX coagulant activity. Usually diagnosed in childhood, this disorder is manifested in the following ways:

- Slow persistent bleeding from cuts, scratches, and other minor traumas
- Delayed hemorrhage that follows minor injuries; bleeding may not start from a site until hours or even days after the traumatic event
- Severe hemorrhaging from the gums after dental extraction or even brushing the teeth with a hard toothbrush
- Severe, sometimes fatal, epistaxis after injury to the nose
- Overwhelming gastric hemorrhage, which may be linked to gastric disorders such as ulcers

TABLE 75–4	COMPARISON OF THE THREE FORMS OF HEMOPHILIA		
Form of Hemophilia	**Etiology**	**Transmission**	**Major Laboratory Findings**
Hemophilia A (classic hemophilia)	Inherited factor VIII (antihemophilic globulin) deficiency	Transmitted as sex-linked *recessive* trait; transmitted by females; occurs in males and, rarely, homozygous females	Coagulation time prolonged but bleeding time normal; factor VIII missing from plasma
Hemophilia B (Christmas disease)	Inherited factor IX (plasma thromboplastin component) deficiency	Transmitted as sex-linked *recessive* trait; transmitted by females; occurs in males and, rarely, homozygous females	Laboratory findings and symptoms same as in hemophilia A; factor IX missing
von Willebrand's disease	Inherited factor VIII deficiency and defective platelet dysfunction	Transmitted as autosomal *dominant* trait to both sexes; occurs in both males and females	Both coagulation time and bleeding time prolonged; low factor VIII levels; platelet adhesiveness decreased

- Recurrent hematoma formation in the deep subcutaneous tissue, in the intramuscular tissues, and around the peripheral nerves

If nerves are compressed by hematomas, the client suffers severe pain, anesthesia of the innervated part, nerve damage, and paralysis. In addition, muscular atrophy sometimes results.

Finally, recurrent *hemarthrosis* (bleeding into the joints) is common in untreated cases and may result in serious joint deformity and permanent crippling. Hemarthrosis affects the knees, ankles, elbows, wrists, fingers, hips, and shoulders, in that order. All of this bleeding can be controlled with the administration of the missing factor (VIII or IX).

Platelet function, platelet count, bleeding time, and prothrombin time are normal. The activated partial thromboplastin time (a pTT) is prolonged. Quantitative assays for factor VIII determine the severity of the disease.

Outcome Management

The goals of care for clients with hemophilia are as follows:

- Stop topical bleeding as quickly as possible
- Raise the level of antihemophilic factor (AHF) in the plasma, thereby temporarily supplying the missing factor causing hemorrhage;
- Prevent complications leading to and caused by bleeding

Immediate transfusion of factor VIII or IX concentrate is the primary treatment. Although plasma and cryoprecipitate contain factor VIII, concentrates have a known AHF content and carry less risk of blood volume overload. As a result of the volume of blood products required, hepatitis and HIV infection represent the major infectious risks, but improved purification techniques now used routinely in the preparation of concentrated factors have virtually eliminated this threat. Because the procoagulant activity of AHF disappears rapidly, clients need transfusions every 12 hours until bleeding stops.

Transfusion of packed RBCs or WBCs are used only to replace blood volume when there has been severe loss. Prophylactic transfusion of factor VIII to a level of 50% above normal is recommended in cases of minor injury, surgery, and dental extractions.

One major complication is linked to repeated transfusions and AHF therapy. About 5% of persons with hemophilia become sensitized to AHF and develop autoimmune anti-AHF antibodies. In clients with low titers of factor VIII antibodies, major and life-threatening hemorrhages are treated with massive doses of factor VIII from animal sources (bovine and porcine), inactivated prothrombin complex concentrates (Konyne 80, Proplex T), or activated prothrombin complex concentrates (Feiba VH Immuno, Autoplex T). Clinicians are using various experimental treatments such as immunosuppressive therapy to combat this problem. Topical bleeding can usually be temporarily controlled by applying pressure to the injured site, packing the area with a fibrin foam, and applying topical hemostatics such as thrombin.

Hemarthrosis may be controlled if the client receives AHF in the early stages of bleeding. Joint immobilization and local chilling (such as packing ice around the joint) may bring relief. If pain is severe, it may be necessary to aspirate blood from the joint. Once bleeding stops and swelling subsides, the client should perform active range-of-motion exercises without weight-bearing to prevent further complications, such as deformity and muscle atrophy.

The prognosis for clients with hemophilia has greatly improved since the discovery of AHF. Before this, 50% of people with hemophilia died before they reached their 5th year; today, death rarely occurs after minor trauma. Home infusion of AHF ensures that treatment is instituted at the first manifestation of bleeding, with complications thus prevented. Clinicians have developed training programs with strict guidelines. When these guidelines are carefully followed, clients with hemophilia lose less time from work or school and need fewer visits to the emergency department. Fatalities mainly follow the development of autoimmune antibodies (anti-AHF) and retroperitoneal bleeding after internal hemorrhage.

Analgesics and corticosteroids often reduce joint pain and swelling. In mild hemophilia, the use of IV desmopressin may eliminate the need for AHF. Desmopressin acts by causing an increase in plasma factor VIII activity.

Although most clients with hemophilia are successfully maintained with home health care, they may be seen in the hospital during acute bleeding episodes or for nonrelated treatments. If even a minor invasive procedure is planned, it is crucial to assess the factor VIII level and administer a sufficient quantity of factor concentrate before the procedure. During routine medical examinations, these clients should be assessed for frequency of bleeding episodes and effectiveness of home therapy. Examine joints for manifestations of bleeding and related atrophy.

During client teaching, review routine situations that increase the client's risk of bleeding, such as contact sports, minor invasive procedures, falls, and cuts. Teach the client to recognize early manifestations and why it is critical to intervene with treatment immediately. Discuss situations that require medical consultation. Provide teaching about bleeding precautions for prevention of injury or trauma that may precipitate a bleeding episode. Effective and prompt administration of factors to reduce the incidence of bleeding episodes and resultant complications, such as joint atrophy, is a priority. The client will need to learn IV infusion administration techniques to control the bleeding.

CONCLUSIONS

Hematologic diseases are complex disorders that require the nurse to understand the hematopoietic system. The nurse is often involved in the administration of blood and blood products for treatment of these various disorders. Many of the blood disorders are life-threatening; others are easily controlled with proper nutrition or regular medication.

Because blood and blood product transfusions are widely used in the treatment of hematologic disorders, it is vital that you understand this procedure, the implications of these procedures, and the proper techniques of administration so the client will receive safe and effective care.

THINKING CRITICALLY

1. **A 62-year-old client underwent a gastric resection for peptic ulcer disease 3 months ago at a hospital in another state. She comes to the nursing clinic complaining of shortness of breath and fatigue with minimal physical exertion. She currently takes ranitidine (Zantac). What assessments should you make now?**

Factors to Consider. What is the significance of the history of gastric resection? How might this contribute to the client's lethargy? What might be causing the shortness of breath and fatigue? What laboratory results would be appropriate to evaluate? What teaching should you consider with this client?

2. **A 40-year-old client has recently been told that she has multiple myeloma. She has been admitted to the oncology inpatient unit for initial evaluation and treatment. On her 4th day after admission, she becomes confused and difficult to arouse. Bowel sounds are diminished, and she begins to vomit. What priority assessment should you make now?**

Factors to Consider. What might predispose the client to this change in her level of consciousness? What additional assessments would you need to make? What interventions should you anticipate at this time?

BIBLIOGRAPHY

1. Bataille, R., & Harousseau, J. (1997). Multiple myeloma. *New England Journal of Medicine, 336*(23), 1657–1664.
2. Boyland, L., & Gleeson, C. (1999). Clinical management: The management of anemia. *European Journal of Palliative Care, 6*(5), 145–148.
3. Bunn, H. F. (1997). The pathogenesis and treatment of sickle cell disease. *New England Journal of Medicine, 337*(11), 762–769.
4. Cella, D., & Bron, D. (1999). The effect of epoetin alfa on quality of life in anemia cancer patients. *Cancer Practice, 7*(4), 177–182.
5. Charache, S., and Investigators of the Multicenter Study of Hydroxyurea in Sickle Cell Anemia. (1995). Effect of hydroxyurea on the frequency of painful crises in sickle cell anemia. *New England Journal of Medicine, 332*(20), 1317–1322.
6. George, J., et al. (1998). Drug-induced thrombocytopenia: A systemic review of published case reports. *Annals of Internal Medicine, 129*(11), 886–890.
7. Gobel, B. H. (1999). Disseminated intravascular coagulation. *Seminars in Oncology Nursing, 15*(3), 174–182.
8. Goldberg, M., Murphy, S., & Wallach, H. (1998, September 30). Myeloproliferative disorders. *Patient Care,* 37–57.
9. Hawkins, R. (1999). Disseminated intravascular coagulation. *Clinical Journal of Oncology Nursing, 3*(3), 127, 131.
10. Johns, A. (1998). Overview of bone marrow and stem cell transplantation. *Journal of Intravenous Nursing, 21*(6), 356–360.
11. Lee, E. J., Phoenix, D., Brown, W., & Jackson, B. (1997). A comparison study of children with sickle cell disease and their non-disease siblings on hopelessness, depression and perceived competence. *Journal of Advanced Nursing, 25,* 79–86.
12. Levi, M., & Cate, H. T. (1999). Disseminated intravascular coagulation. *New England Journal of Medicine, 341*(8), 586–592.
13. McBrien, N. (1997). Thrombotic thrombocytopenic purpura. *American Journal of Nursing, 97*(2), 28–29.
14. Paquette, R. L., et al. (1995). Long-term outcome of aplastic anemia in adults treated with antithymocyte globulin: Comparison with bone marrow transplantation. *Blood, 85*(1), 283–290.
15. Richer, S. (1997). A practical guide for differentiating between iron deficiency anemia and anemia of chronic disease in children and adult. *The Nurse Practitioner, 22*(4), 82–103.
16. Schilling, R. F., & Williams, W. J. (1995). Vitamin B_{12} deficiency: Underdiagnosed, overtreated? *Hospital Practice (Office Edition), 30*(7), 47–52; discussion 52, 54.
17. Stephan, F., et al. (1999). Thrombocytopenia in a surgical ICU. *Chest, 115*(5), 1363–1370.
18. Vichinsky, E. P., and The Preoperative Transfusion in Sickle Cell Disease Study Group. (1995). A comparison of conservative and aggressive transfusion regimens in the perioperative management of sickle cell disease. *New England Journal of Medicine, 333*(4), 206–213.
19. Worrall, L. M., Thompkins, C. A., & Rust, D. M. (1999). Recognizing and managing anemia. *Clinical Journal of Oncology Nursing, 3*(4), 153–160, 180–182.
20. Young, N. S., & Maciejewski, J. (1997). The pathophysiology of acquired aplastic anemia. *New England Journal of Medicine, 336*(19), 1365–1372.

CHAPTER

76

Management of Clients with Immune Disorders

Linda Ludy Scott

The immune system constitutes the body's defense system against invading foreign substances. A functioning immune system must protect the body from potential pathogens. An immune system that is malfunctioning predisposes an individual to the development of a wide variety of diseases, ranging from severe infection to autoimmune disease, and the resultant tissue injury. The Unit 16 review describes the normally functioning immune system; this chapter looks at alterations in the immune system and how these changes affect the human organism.

HYPERSENSITIVITY DISORDERS

As health care providers, nurses deal with allergic conditions far more often than might be suspected. Allergic rhinitis, asthma, and dermatitis are just a few examples of these immunologic diseases.

The tendency to develop allergies involving immunoglobulin E (IgE) antibody formation is known as *atopy.* The terms *atopic, allergic,* and *hypersensitive* are frequently used interchangeably. *Allergy* (or, more appropriately, hypersensitivity) describes the increased immune response to the presence of an allergen, also known as an *antigen.* Between 10% and 20% of the population has allergies. We cannot exactly predict who will have allergies; however, there is a higher incidence of allergies among children of allergic parents.

People must progress through a two-step process to become allergic. Step 1 starts with *sensitization.* Sensiti-zation occurs when an individual develops IgE antibodies against a substance that is inhaled, ingested, or injected. Newly formed IgE antibodies stick to basophils and mast cells, found in the skin's mucosal surfaces and the respiratory and gastrointestinal (GI) tracts. Hypersensitivity can be claimed only after IgE antibodies against a certain foreign substance have formed and are bound to the surface of tissue mast cells and circulating basophils.

Hypersensitivity does not produce any of the manifestations typically associated with allergic disease. It is not until step 2, *reexposure to the allergen,* that allergic manifestations such as sneezing, asthma, and anaphylaxis occur. Even though the cellular events for all immediate allergic reactions tend to be similar, there are differences in the clinical sequelae that occur, based on the state of the individual's host defenses, the nature of the allergen, the concentration of the allergen, the route by which the allergen enters, the amount of allergen exposure received, and which organ is affected.

Etiology and Risk Factors

HOST DEFENSES. Some people are more susceptible to hypersensitivity than others for reasons that are unclear. Specific IgE formation can be influenced by vital infections, especially those caused by cytomegalovirus (CMV) and mononucleosis. Factors such as air pollution, sex, age, and exposure to second-hand smoke may all influence manifestations of allergies.

NATURE OF THE ALLERGEN. Allergens are proteins capable of inducing IgE antibody, thus triggering an allergic response. Molecules that combine with proteins to produce antibodies are called *haptens.* Haptens, along with other environmental allergens, are carried on vectors that may become airborne (e.g., pollen, dust particles, animal dander). Contact with these allergens causes sensitization and atopy and evokes the acute manifestations of allergy. Some haptens (e.g., penicillin) are highly antigenic.

CONCENTRATION OF THE ALLERGEN. Higher concentrations usually result in hypersensitivity responses of greater intensity. Lower concentrations of the allergen may then cause severe manifestations when reexposure occurs.

ROUTE OF ENTRANCE INTO THE BODY. Routes by which allergens enter the body include inhalation, injection, ingestion, and direct contact. Most allergens are inhaled.

EXPOSURE TO THE ALLERGEN. Sensitization to allergens is necessary in order for hypersensitivity to occur. A few factors that influence the likelihood of development of allergy are a person's age at the time of exposure (exposure early in life), the type of allergen (house dust mite, cockroach, various medications, and pollen), the allergen load (lower levels are capable of inducing specific IgE production), and the month of a person's birth (a greater affinity for allergies is seen in those born in the spring and fall).

Pathophysiology

The key intermediate in allergic disease is the IgE antibody. The production of IgE in response to an allergen renders an individual allergic. There are two general categories of hypersensitivity reactions: (1) *immediate* (humoral or antigen-antibody) and (2) *delayed* (cell-mediated).

IMMEDIATE REACTION. The immediate (antigen-antibody) reaction occurs within minutes after exposure to the allergen. The resultant IgE production mediates the immediate response by activating mast cells and basophils, causing them to degranulate and release mediators such as histamine.

The mediators, whether preformed or newly formed after activation, are able to increase vascular permeability, dilate vessels, cause bronchospasm, contract smooth muscle, and ignite other inflammatory cells. Table 76–1 describes chemical mediators of the allergic reaction, their action, and the associated manifestations.

Manifestations of mediator release vary, depending on the organ where the mediators' receptors are found. For example, histamine is a preformed mast cell mediator that has receptors in various organs, including skin, oral and nasal mucosa, lungs, and the smooth muscle in the GI tract. Once histamine binds to its receptor, it can cause many reactions. Vasodilation causes edema; smooth muscle contraction results in dangerous airway narrowing; and glandular stimulation leads to increased mucus secretion in the nose, lungs, and GI tract.

Newly formed mediators, including lipid mediators and cytokines, are made after the mast cell has been activated and have similar actions to those of histamine, but their effects tend to last much longer. Once released into the blood and after binding to their receptors, these mediators cause more bronchial smooth muscle contraction, vasodilation in the skin, nasal congestion, and edema.

DELAYED REACTION. The delayed (cell-mediated or late-phase) reaction is seen when there is a prolonged response to the initial allergen. T cells govern the delayed inflammatory response that occurs approximately 2 to 8 hours after mast cells have been activated by the initial allergen exposure.

Hypersensitivity reactions are divided into four main types (Table 76–2):

- I, Immediate or anaphylactic
- II, Cytolytic or cytotoxic
- III, Immune complex
- IV, Cell-mediated or delayed

TYPE I (ANAPHYLACTIC) HYPERSENSITIVITY

The anaphylactic response (described previously) is a rapidly occurring reaction mediated by IgE antibodies. The allergen binds to IgE antibodies, which are attracted to the surface of mast cells and basophils, causing release of mediators (see Table 76–1). Examples of type I hypersensitivity reactions include anaphylaxis, allergic rhinitis, asthma, and acute allergic drug reactions.

TYPE II (CYTOLYTIC OR CYTOTOXIC) HYPERSENSITIVITY

Cytolytic or cytotoxic reactions are complement-dependent and thus involve IgG or IgM antibodies. The antigen-antibody binding results in activation of the complement system and destroys the cell upon which the antigen is bound, usually a circulating blood cell, thus causing tissue injury. Examples of tissue injury caused by type II hypersensitivity include hemolytic anemia, Rh hemolytic disease in the newborn, autoimmune hyperthyroidism, myasthenia gravis, and blood transfusion reactions.

During a blood transfusion, blood group incompatibility causes cell lysis, which results in a transfusion reaction. The antigen responsible for initiating the reaction is a part of the donor red blood cell membrane. Manifestations of a transfusion reaction result from intravascular hemolysis of red blood cells. They include headache and back pain (flank), chest pain similar to angina, nausea and vomiting, tachycardia and hypotension, hematuria, and urticaria.

Transfusions of more than 100 ml of incompatible blood can result in severe, permanent renal damage, circulatory shock, and death. Therefore, if manifestations develop, stop the transfusion at once, maintain an open intravenous (IV) line, check the client's vital signs, and notify the physician immediately. For detailed nursing interventions related to transfusion reactions, see Chapter 75.

TYPE III (IMMUNE COMPLEX) HYPERSENSITIVITY

Immune complex reactions result when antigens bind to antibodies leading to tissue injury. The molecular size of the antigen-antibody complexes is an important feature in eliciting immune complex reactions. Larger complexes are rapidly cleared by phagocytic cells. The smaller complexes formed in antigen excess persist longer in the circulation because they are not as easily captured by

TABLE 76–1 **CHEMICAL MEDIATORS OF THE ALLERGIC REACTION**

Mediator	Action	Manifestations
Histamine	Dilates blood vessels and increases vascular permeability	Erythema, tissue swelling, and shock
	Constricts smooth muscles in the bronchial airways	Shortness of breath and wheezing
	Stimulates nerve endings	Itching and painful skin
	Increases mucus production in the airways and GI tract	Congestion, gastric reflux, and heartburn
Platelet-activating factor	Dilates the blood vessels and constricts the bronchial airways	Same as for histamine
	Aids in the secretion and aggregation of platelets	Same as for histamine
Eosinophil chemotactic factor of anaphylaxis (ECF-A)	Increases eosinophil migration	Inflamed airways
Neutrophil chemotactic factor	Increases neutrophil migration	Inflamed airways
Heparin	Anticoagulation	Increased bleeding and bruising
Bradykinin	Slows smooth muscle contraction	Mucous plugging
	Increases vascular permeability	Swelling
	Increases mucus production	Congestion
LIPID MEDIATORS OR SRS-A		
Leukotrienes	Increase vascular permeability	Same as for histamine
	Increase smooth muscle contraction	
Prostaglandin D	Constricts bronchial airways	Wheezing, shortness of breath, and cough
	Vasodilation	Flushing and swelling
Cytokines (IL-4, IL-5, TNF-α)	Allow cells to influence the activity and development of other unrelated cells	Inflammation, edema, and fibrosis
	Aid in eosinophil production	
	Increase vascular permeability	

GI, gastrointestinal; IL, interleukin; SRS, slow-reacting substance of anaphylaxis; TNF, tumor necrosis factor.

phagocytic cells in the spleen and liver. Inflammation results and leads to acute or chronic disease of the organ system in which the immune complexes were deposited.

Immune complex–mediated inflammation is produced by IgG or IgM antibodies, antigen, and complement. The mediators of inflammatory injury include the complement cleavage peptides, which can activate mast cells, neutrophils, monocytes, and other cells. Release of lysosomal

TABLE 76–2 **TYPES OF HYPERSENSITIVITY REACTIONS**

	Type	Causative Component	Pathologic Process	Reaction
I	Immediate/anaphylactic	IgE	Mast cell degranulation ↓ Histamine and leukotriene release	Anaphylaxis Atopic diseases Skin reactions
II	Cytolytic/cytotoxic	IgG IgM Complement	Complement fixation ↓ Cell lysis	ABO incompatibility Drug-induced hemolytic anemia
III	Immune complex	Antigen-antibody complexes	Deposition in vessels and tissue walls ↓ Inflammation	Arthus reaction Serum sickness Systemic lupus erythematosus Acute glomerulonephritis
IV	Cell-mediated/delayed	Sensitized T cells	Lymphokine release	Tuberculosis Contact dermatitis Transplant rejection

Ig, immunoglobulin.

granules from white blood cells and macrophages causes further tissue injury.

The antigen may be tissue-fixed or released locally, as in Goodpasture's syndrome, in which circulating antibodies react with autologous antigens in the glomerular basement membranes of the kidneys, causing inflammation of the glomerulus.

Antigen-antibody complexes are formed in the bloodstream and get trapped in capillaries or deposited in vessel walls, causing urticaria, arthritis, arteritis, or glomerulonephritis.

Alternatively, antigen-antibody complexes may form in the joint space, with resultant synovitis, as in rheumatoid arthritis.

The Arthus reaction is a localized area of tissue necrosis that results from immune complex hypersensitivity.

The antigen may also be circulating, as in serum sickness. Serum sickness develops 6 to 14 days after injection with a foreign serum. Deposition of complexes on vessel walls causes complement activation, with resultant edema, fever, inflammation of blood vessels and joints, and urticaria. Classic serum sickness is rare, because large doses of heterologous sera (e.g., horse antisera to human lymphocytes) are seldom used.

However, a serum sickness–like reaction may occur after administration of such medications as penicillin, sulfonamides, streptomycin, thiouracils, and hydantoin compounds. Rather than being dominated by cutaneous vasculitis, these reactions more often manifest with fever, arthralgias, lymphadenopathy, and urticaria. The illness is usually benign and self-limiting. It resolves after the offending medication is discontinued.

Nursing care of the client with serum sickness depends on the severity of the reaction. For a mild reaction, care includes control of fever and pain with aspirin and antihistamines. For a severe reaction, care may require steroids.

Serum sickness can be prevented by avoiding allergen exposure. Obtain an allergy history and information about any previous reactions to drugs or vaccines. Document findings in the client's chart, care plan, and medication record so that the risk of subsequent exposure will be minimized.

TYPE IV (CELL-MEDIATED, LATE-PHASE OR DELAYED) HYPERSENSITIVITY

In cell-mediated hypersensitivity, sensitized T cells respond to antigens by releasing lymphokines, some of which direct phagocytic cell activity. This reaction occurs 24 to 72 hours after exposure to an allergen. Delayed hypersensitivity is induced by chronic infection (e.g., tuberculosis) or by contact sensitivities, as in contact dermatitis.

Type IV reactions occur after the intradermal injection of tuberculosis antigen or purified protein derivative (PPD). If the client has been sensitized to tuberculosis, sensitized T cells react with the antigen at the injection site. The reaction leads to edema and fibrin deposits, which result in the induration characteristic of a positive tuberculosis reaction.

Graft-versus-host disease (GVHD) and transplant rejection are also type IV reactions. In GVHD, immunocompetent donor bone marrow cells (the graft) react against various antigens in the bone marrow recipient (the host). Various clinical manifestations result, including skin, GI,

and hepatic lesions. Transplant rejection and GVHD are discussed in Chapter 80.

Contact dermatitis is another type IV reaction that occurs after sensitization to an allergen, commonly a cosmetic, adhesive, topical medication, drug additive (such as lanolin added to lotions), or plant toxin (such as poison ivy). With the first exposure, no reaction occurs but antigens are formed. On subsequent exposures, hypersensitivity reactions are triggered, which lead to itching, erythema, and vesicular lesions.

Clinical Manifestations

During an allergic response, mast cell activation and the release of chemical mediators result in increased vascular permeability, edema, dilation of blood vessels, smooth muscle contraction, bronchospasm, and increased mucus secretion in the nose, lungs, and GI tract.

The diagnosis of an allergic disease is based on the client's history, manifestations experienced during or after allergen exposure, and the results from commonly used allergy tests. Common allergy tests include (1) skin testing; (2) radioallergosorbent test (RAST), which is used for measuring IgE levels to certain allergens in vitro; (3) pulmonary function tests (PFTs) to diagnose asthma; and (4) blood assays for IgE levels.

SKIN TESTING. The health care practitioner introduces a small quantity of allergen into the skin by quickly pricking, scratching, or puncturing it or by using intradermal injection. A wheal and flare reaction usually occurs soon after the allergen is introduced into the skin if the client is allergic. Skin testing is generally considered safe, but it always carries a risk of causing a systemic reaction such as anaphylaxis.

Intradermal testing or injecting the known allergen directly below the skin is the most accurate skin test but is linked to a higher incidence of severe allergic reactions. Therefore, it should be used with extreme caution and under close supervision. A patch test can be used to evaluate contact allergies; the allergen is applied directly to the skin and then covered with a gauze dressing.

Nurses often administer skin tests and interpret test results. An *immediate* reaction (i.e., appearing within 10 to 20 minutes after the injection), marked by erythema and wheal formation greater than 3 mm of the positive control (usually histamine), denotes a positive reaction. *Positive* reactions indicate antibody response to previous exposure to this antigen and suggest the person is allergic to the particular substance that causes the reaction. *Negative* reactions may be inconclusive, requiring further assessment. Negative results may indicate the following: (1) antibodies have not formed to this antigen, (2) the antigen was deposited too deeply into the skin (e.g., subcutaneously), (3) the client is immunosuppressed from disease or therapies (e.g., steroids, chemotherapy, radiation therapy), or (4) the client has taken antihistamines within the past 72 hours.

Problems that arise from skin testing range from minor itching to anaphylaxis. Itching and discomfort at the injection site are common and can be relieved by the application of cool compresses, topical steroid or antihistamine creams, and oral antihistamines such as diphenhydramine (Benadryl). Ulceration of the injection site is best treated by keeping the area clean and dry. Anaphylactic shock is a rare but potentially lethal complication of skin testing. A client with a history of an anaphylactic reaction to a substance should never undergo skin testing for an allergy to that substance. This is especially true of allergens such as penicillin, which can produce lethal anaphylaxis in susceptible clients.

RADIOALLERGOSORBENT TEST. RAST uses the principle of immunoabsorption and reveals elevated levels of allergen-specific IgE associated with atopy. The allergen of interest is first bound to some solid surface, usually a paper disc. The client's blood is then incubated with the disc. If the client has antibodies specific to the allergen being tested, they bind to that allergen. The unbound antibodies are washed away, and the level of antigen-specific IgE can be measured. This test is somewhat less sensitive than skin testing and is more time-consuming and costly.

PULMONARY FUNCTION TEST. PFTs are done to confirm the diagnosis or to evaluate the respiratory status in asthmatic disease, to assess the severity of lung obstruction, and to guide the medical treatment of asthma. The principal abnormality associated with asthma is reversible airway obstruction, reflected by a reduction in the forced expiratory volume measured in 1 second (FEV_1). Reversibility is noted if an increase of more than 10% in the FEV_1 is noted after giving a bronchodilator such as albuterol (Ventolin).

BLOOD ASSAYS. Immunometric blood assays measure the total amount of IgE normally present in the circulation. Most studies have shown that blood concentrations of IgE are increased in the presence of allergic disease. However, a normal or even decreased level may occur in IgE-mediated sensitivities. Elevated serum eosinophil levels also may suggest hypersensitivities.

Outcome Management

Medical Management

Allergies are among the most common disorders seen in the medical community. The client often requires a combination of treatments, ranging from avoidance of known allergens to environmental control and immunotherapy.

IDENTIFY ALLERGEN
It is imperative to obtain a detailed history, perform a thorough assessment and examination, and ensure that appropriate diagnostic tests are performed. The clinician must know the times of the year during which manifestations occur in order to determine a correct diagnosis on the basis of the offending allergen. If year-round manifestations are present, find out whether they are worse at any time.

AVOID ALLERGEN
Avoidance of the allergen is often the easiest, cheapest, and safest way of dealing with allergies. However, identification of the specific allergen is sometimes difficult, especially if the client refuses, cannot afford, or cannot locate allergen-testing services. Even if the allergen can be identified, complete avoidance may not be possible, as with pollens and food additives.

CONTROL ENVIRONMENT
Environmental control sometimes helps eliminate airborne allergens. Figure 76-1 illustrates ways to desensitize a room. These environmental controls, combined with air filters that remove small particles from the air, can help eliminate many allergens.

ADMINISTER MEDICATIONS
Atopic clients benefit greatly from selected prescriptions and over-the-counter medications. Usually, clients self-administer these agents, although in some settings the nurse or a family member administers them.

ANTIHISTAMINES.
Antihistamines are the major group of prescription and over-the-counter drugs used to alleviate allergic manifestations. These medications relieve sneezing, rhinitis, itching, and other manifestations of allergic rhinitis. They bind to the H_1 receptor. Traditional antihistamines such as diphenhydramine (Benadryl) pass the blood-brain barrier and can produce significant drowsiness. Because newer agents (cetirizine [Zyrtec], fexofenadine [Allegra], and loratadine [Claritin]) do not cross the blood-brain barrier (or do so poorly), they do not cause the drowsiness that limits the use of older medications.

DECONGESTANTS.
Decongestants (oral sympathomimetics) help relieve nasal congestion by stimulating the alpha-adrenergic receptors that control the capillary sphincters at the entrance to the venous plexuses of the turbinates. Decongestants act primarily on turbinate swelling and are more effective and rapid in onset when used topically rather than orally. However, because the prolonged use of topical nasal sprays can cause rhinitis medicamentosa (recurrence of congestion), it is advisable to limit their use to no more than 1 week. These drugs can be combined with antihistamines to treat the multiple manifestations of allergy.

STEROIDS.
Corticosteroids, anti-inflammatory agents, and immunosuppressants can be used to treat allergic manifestations. Corticosteroids are the most effective drug for the treatment of rhinitis. Oral steroids are in general more effective and rapid in onset than topical forms, but their systemic effects can produce a myriad of complications. Topical steroid creams can be used to treat dermatitis. Beclomethasone dipropionate (Beconase), triamcinolone (Nasacort), flunisolide (Nasarel), budesonide (Rhinocort), and fluticasone (Flonase) are nasal sprays useful in treating allergic rhinitis, and they evoke few systemic side effects.

AEROSOLS.
Cromolyn sodium is a topical or aerosol medication used to treat allergic rhinitis (Nasalcrom) and asthma (Intal). Its mechanism of action is not completely understood, but it helps prevent the release of chemical mediators (e.g., histamine and leukotrienes) from mast cells during both immediate and late-phase reactions. Cromolyn sodium should be administered before allergen exposure. It should be started a week before allergy season to be most effective in the treatment of seasonal allergic rhinitis. It must be used on a regular basis and, unfortunately, dosing is required three to four times a day.

Inhaled steroids are fundamental to the treatment of asthma. New inhaled steroids with a greater topical potency ratio and fewer systemic effects allow greater control in asthma management. Fluticasone (Flovent), triamcinolone (Azmacort), and beclomethasone (Vanceril) are examples of inhaled steroids.

ANTICHOLINERGICS.
Anticholinergics are used primarily to treat allergic rhinitis and rhinorrhea caused by

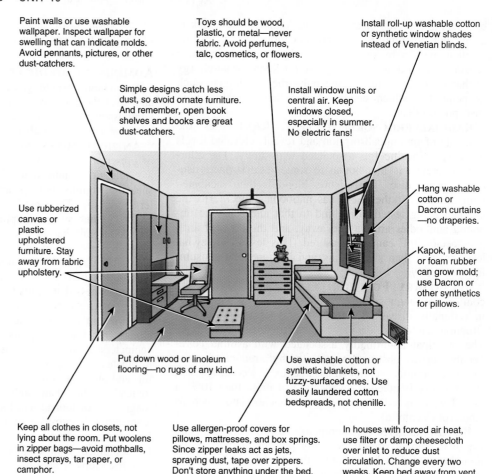

Paint walls or use washable wallpaper. Inspect wallpaper for swelling that can indicate molds. Avoid pennants, pictures, or other dust-catchers.

Simple designs catch less dust, so avoid ornate furniture. And remember, open book shelves and books are great dust-catchers.

Toys should be wood, plastic, or metal—never fabric. Avoid perfumes, talc, cosmetics, or flowers.

Install window units or central air. Keep windows closed, especially in summer. No electric fans!

Install roll-up washable cotton or synthetic window shades instead of Venetian blinds.

Use rubberized canvas or plastic upholstered furniture. Stay away from fabric upholstery.

Hang washable cotton or Dacron curtains —no draperies.

Kapok, feather or foam rubber can grow mold; use Dacron or other synthetics for pillows.

Put down wood or linoleum flooring—no rugs of any kind.

Use washable cotton or synthetic blankets, not fuzzy-surfaced ones. Use easily laundered cotton bedspreads, not chenille.

FIGURE 76–1 Controlling the environment of a room. Dacron is a trade name for polyester. (Courtesy of A. H. Robins Company, Richmond, VA.)

Keep all clothes in closets, not lying about the room. Put woolens in zipper bags—avoid mothballs, insect sprays, tar paper, or camphor.

Use allergen-proof covers for pillows, mattresses, and box springs. Since zipper leaks act as jets, spraying dust, tape over zippers. Don't store anything under the bed.

In houses with forced air heat, use filter or damp cheesecloth over inlet to reduce dust circulation. Change every two weeks. Keep bed away from vent.

the common cold. Ipratropium (Atrovent) was a major advance in the therapeutic regimen for asthma. It does not cross the blood-brain barrier and is relatively free of side effects. Anticholinergics are also available in oral forms in combination with antihistamines and decongestant preparations (Dura-Vent DA, Extendryl SR).

BRONCHODILATORS. Beta$_2$ agonists are commonly used to control bronchospasm in asthma. Albuterol (Ventolin) and other short-acting bronchodilators have proved to be well tolerated. The drawback of the older bronchodilators is their short duration of action (only 4 to 6 hours), which limits their use for manifestations experienced at night. This problem has been addressed with the new generation of long-acting beta$_2$ agonists such as salmeterol (Serevent).

ANTILEUKOTRIENES. Antileukotrienes are used to treat manifestations of asthma and anaphylaxis. They block the synthesis or action of leukotriene mediators, which are known to contribute to airway edema, smooth muscle contraction, and the process of inflammation. These drugs include zafirlukast (Accolate) and zileuton (Zyflo).

PROMOTE DESENSITIZATION

Immunotherapy ("desensitization therapy") is designed for the treatment of type I, IgE-mediated hypersensitivity reactions. Precise doses of allergens are injected at intervals over a prolonged period. The doses are increased gradually over time. Immunotherapy increases IgG antibody levels and may increase suppressor T-cell function. Specific IgG interferes with IgE binding to allergens and thus mitigates the hypersensitivity response. Immunotherapy is widely used in the treatment of allergic rhinitis (hay fever), for which its greatest success has been achieved. It also is used for Hymenoptera sensitivity (bee, yellow jacket, wasp, and hornet stings) with reportable success. There is some controversy regarding the efficacy of this treatment in the management of asthma.

Nurses often administer these injections and assess and treat side effects. Clients are asked to wait at least 30 to 40 minutes after receiving the injections so that immediate reactions can be treated. Side effects are similar to those seen in skin testing.

Nursing Management of the Medical Client

ASSESSMENT

As a nurse, you play a crucial role in obtaining a detailed medical history of the client and ensuring that appropriate diagnostic tests are performed. The most important part of evaluating the allergic client is the history. The history should elicit all of the client's current manifestations. It is important for clinicians to know whether the manifestations are always present or what times of the year they worsen.

Indoor allergens are causing increasing amounts of distress. House dust mites and cockroach and animal allergens are problematic and are present year-round in many homes. Assess whether animals are present in the home and, if so, how many. Is the house filled with plants that may harbor mold spores? Is the client exposed to moist rooms such as a basement that is constantly damp?

Environmental factors such as smoke may exacerbate manifestations. Where these manifestations present is very important to ascertain. Many occupations involve exposure to certain allergens such as smoke, latex, chemicals, and animals. Manifestations may be reported as worse during the workweek versus the weekend. Inquiries such as these help to narrow down possible causes of manifestations.

DIAGNOSIS, OUTCOMES, INTERVENTIONS

Altered Health Maintenance. The key nursing diagnosis for the client with hypersensitivity disorders is *Altered Health Maintenance related to lack of knowledge of disease process, treatment regimen and risk control methods.*

Outcomes. The client will follow a mutually agreed on health maintenance plan that includes stated understanding of disease process, treatment regimen, and control of risk factors.

Interventions

Provide Teaching. Although clients usually self-administer medications, as described under the medical management section, you are responsible for instructing clients and significant others about these medications. The client needs to learn what the medication is, why it is being prescribed, how to take it, when to take it, and what the possible side effects might be. In addition, the client needs to know what to do during an anaphylactic reaction (see Anaphylaxis).

If an inhaler is prescribed, the client must be taught how to use it correctly (see Chapter 61). A spacer (an attachment added to the inhaler that holds the medication in the additional chamber or space until the client inhales) may be recommended to help the client obtain the maximal effect. Some clients are taught to perform desensitization injections themselves. In this case, teach clients the proper injection technique and the signs of any untoward reactions to the medications.

Clients may need to carry medications for anaphylaxis with them at all times. In such instances, clients should also wear a medical-alert bracelet. Other nursing interventions are described in the following sections under specific disorders.

EVALUATION

It is expected that the client will obtain relief from allergic manifestations when the treatment regimen is followed. The client will be able to avoid or control risk factors for allergic manifestations. Ideally, the client will be able to avoid anaphylactic events and obtain treatment before serious problems develop.

ALLERGIC DISORDERS

FOOD ALLERGY

Adverse food reactions can be classified in one of two ways: (1) *food allergies,* which occur by a specific IgE-mediated response to the offending food, such as food-induced anaphylaxis from peanuts, and (2) *food intolerances,* which do not result from an IgE-mediated response but which cause manifestations such as diarrhea and vomiting. The prevalence of food intolerances is much higher than that of food allergies.

A thorough history is the most important factor in the diagnosis of food allergy or intolerance. Food allergies can be determined through skin testing. Food diaries (a record of events, including dietary intake for subsequent episodes) are used to provide insight for the correct diagnosis. The standard of diagnosis in food allergy is the double-blind, placebo-controlled food challenge. The suspected food is eliminated from the diet for 10 to 14 days. Antihistamines are not to be taken for at least 24 hours before the challenge, and a fasting state should be maintained for 12 to 18 hours before testing. The challenge starts with the introduction of a very low dose of the suspected food, and the dose is gradually increased every 20 to 30 minutes until a reaction is noted or the amount of food present in a normal feeding is reached. *Elimination diets* are also used and consist of removing one food at a time until the adverse manifestations are relieved.

Measuring serum blood tryptase levels can also prove helpful, because elevations in tryptase occur and are detectable in the blood for up to 2 hours after a severe systemic reaction. However, negative results do not rule out a positive reaction.

See Bridge to Home Health Care: Immunosuppression and Health.

ATOPIC DERMATITIS

Atopic dermatitis occurs in about 10% of the population. Clients typically have a history of or complaints about itchy skin, in addition to a history of rashes in the area of skin creases. Other common complaints are of generally dry skin initially experienced in children younger than 2 years of age, accompanied by manifestations of asthma, hay fever, or dermatitis. Lesions of atopic dermatitis are red and pruritic, contain exudates, and are maculopapular in younger clients, becoming drier and thicker as clients age. The lesions are typically found on the cheeks, scalp, and forehead; in later years, they may occur on the trunk and extremities.

■ Medical Management

Treatment is aimed at controlling and reducing the manifestations because there is no true cure. Antihistamines are used with good results to help alleviate the itch-scratch cycle that is common to atopic dermatitis. The mainstay of therapy is topical corticosteroids, which control the inflammation in the skin lesions. Gels penetrate more effectively but are drying. Ointments should be used in more severe cases, because they promote hydration; however, some clients do not care for them, because they are oily and become messy in the heat. Creams and lotions are the least penetrating but are preferred by most clients. They are absorbed quickly and promote comfort. Antibiotics may be needed to treat superficial skin infections caused by intense pruritus and scratching.

BRIDGE TO HOME HEALTH CARE

Managing Immunosuppression and Nutrition

The client who is immune-compromised faces numerous challenges related to nutrition, one of the most fundamental human needs. Anorexia, fatigue, weakness, nausea, and vomiting make it difficult to maintain or improve weight and nutritional status. Sometimes as a result of treatments and medications, immune-suppressed clients experience painful mouth sores and an altered sense of taste. Foods that they previously enjoyed no longer "taste right," and the act of eating holds little pleasure.

Conserving energy and enhancing adequate caloric intake are the ways to maintain nutritional status. Clients who have willing family members or friends should let them assist with meal preparation and clean-up. They should eat frequent, small amounts of high-calorie, nutritious foods that are flavorful and easy to prepare, ingest, and digest. Some clients do not like common supplements like canned shakes because of their thick texture. Adding ice to these drinks can make them more palatable and does not alter the calorie content. Homemade shakes can be made using yogurt, ice cream, or whole milk and adding fruit or concentrated fruit juice. Shakes can be prepared in advance and frozen for later use.

Mouth ulcers can be "painted" with a 4:1 mixture of aluminum/magnesium hydroxide (e.g., Maalox) and lidocaine (Xylocaine) to make eating more pleasant. Clients need to avoid constipation because it is likely to affect their appetite adversely. A daily routine of dried prunes or apricots, stool softeners, and gentle abdominal massage can help immensely.

Maximize your client's dietary success by encouraging full use of the senses. For example, caregivers can bake bread or cookies so that the aroma will stimulate appetite. Ask your client to visualize warm bread with melting butter, jam, or peanut butter. Encourage your client to eat meals with healthy family members and friends. Even snacking together can help maintain social interaction and minimize the isolation that many immune-suppressed individuals experience. Isolation breeds depression. Depression can have dire effects on appetite.

Clients who have poorly functioning immune systems need to evaluate the safety of their food choices and preparation. It is essential that all food handlers wash their hands carefully. Thoroughly clean fresh food; avoid other food that may harbor bacteria. Clients may want to avoid dining away from home, because they risk exposure to infection amid large groups of people. Food prepared for restaurants, vendors, picnics, or other social functions may harbor bacteria such as *Escherichia coli* or *Salmonella.* Even people with healthy immune systems can become seriously ill from these organisms; for people with immunosuppression, they can be deadly.

Some clients need total parental nutrition (TPN) in order to achieve adequate caloric intake. Although TPN may be necessary for survival, it provides nutrition in a rather unnatural way. Allow clients to have some degree of control by incorporating the therapy into their usual nighttime routines. Early risers should "hook-up" early in the evening so they can enjoy the morning time, when they usually have the most energy. "Night-owls" may want to use the opposite schedule. Clients whose gastrointestinal systems still function should continue to take some food by mouth. This helps to preserve the ability to taste and swallow and to maintain fundamental social and cultural connections.

Jeannine Mueller Harmon, RN, CS, MSN, FNP, *Family Nurse Practitioner, Metropolitan State University, St. Paul, Minnesota*

Nursing Management of the Medical Client

Teach clients the importance of environmental control. A key strategy is to minimize allergen exposure and physical stimuli that provoke pruritus. Explain that the client can reduce itching by avoiding severe changes in temperature, wearing loose cotton clothing, using gentle detergents, and rinsing clothing completely. Advise them to avoid chemical irritants, emotional stress, aeroallergens such as dust and animal dander, and dietary allergens. Teach the client general skin care measures, such as how to:

1. Maintain good skin hydration by bathing in lukewarm water
2. Use gentle soaps (e.g., Basis, Dove)
3. Apply a lubricant like Alpha Keri, petroleum jelly, Eucerin, or Aquaphor to the skin immediately after bathing
4. Avoid scratching
5. Keep fingernails trimmed to avoid infection

URTICARIA

Urticaria (or hives) is a cutaneous reaction associated with several different causes. It occurs in as many as 25% of all people at some point in time. Hives that are present daily or intermittently over a period of less than 6 weeks are termed *acute* urticaria. Hives present for more than 6 weeks are referred to as *chronic* urticaria.

Lesions of urticaria tend to be papules or plaques that fade within 24 hours. They do not leave areas of hyperpigmentation. Hives are round or oval and range in size from a few millimeters to several centimeters.

Mast cells and their mediators may play a key role in urticaria, causing intense pruritus and vascular changes. A lesional skin biopsy to identify which types of inflammatory cells are present in the lesion is useful in structuring treatment. Some known provoking stimuli of urticaria are medications, foreign substances, foods and food additives, infections, insect bites and stings, contact irritants, inhalants, heat, cold, light, and pressure.

Medical Management

Although management focuses on identifying and eliminating any known causative factors, in approximately 80% of chronic cases no cause of urticaria is found. All clients with urticaria should be cautioned about aspirin and nonsteroidal anti-inflammatory drugs (NSAIDs), which may exacerbate existing hives. Opiates or narcotics should be used cautiously as well, because they are typically mast cell degranulators.

Antihistamines are the mainstay of therapy for urticaria. Nonsedating antihistamines are recommended during the day; more sedating antihistamines may be preferred at night. Doxepin (Sinequan), a tricyclic antidepressant, is sometimes used for treatment because of its actions on both H_1 and H_2 receptors. Corticosteroids should not be used except for short-term therapy.

Nursing Management of the Medical Client

Urticaria tends to evoke anxiety and frustration in both clients and clinicians. The most effective treatment is to eliminate any triggers. Help the client identify factors that may be suspect, and suggest elimination diets and challenges if foods or food additives are thought to provoke manifestations. Encourage clients to avoid initiating physical factors, such as pressure from tight clothing, heat, vibration, sunlight, and rubbing of the skin. Good skin hydration is mandatory; counsel the client to avoid harsh soaps and irritants and to apply moisturizing lotions after bathing while the skin is still damp.

ANAPHYLAXIS, INSECT STING ALLERGY, AND LATEX ALLERGY

The most common causes of anaphylaxis are drugs, foods, latex exposure, and insect bites and stings. Common food offenders in adults are peanuts, tree nuts, and shellfish (Table 76–3). Insect stings cause many deaths in the United States every year. The incidence of anaphylaxis related to latex exposure, especially in health care workers, has dramatically increased since the 1990s with the increased use of latex gloves.

Anaphylactic events commonly present with hives and angioedema and often with dyspnea, wheezing, syncope, hypotension, nausea, vomiting, diarrhea, abdominal pain, flushing, headache, rhinitis, substernal pain, and itching. Cardiovascular collapse, shock, and respiratory obstruction, which can occur immediately and without other manifestations, are the primary cause of death from anaphylaxis. Although manifestations usually begin 5 to 30 minutes after the offending trigger has been encountered, there can be a delay of an hour or more. The more rapid the onset, the more severe the episode.

The incidence of anaphylaxis related to insect stings ranges from 0.3% to 3% in the general population. The sting insects are members of the order Hymenoptera. People may be allergic to one or all of the stinging insects, but the sting of the yellow jacket is the most common cause of allergy. Common reactions to an insect sting include pain, swelling, and redness that may be localized or extend over a large area. The swelling usually peaks in 24 to 48 hours and may last for 7 to 10 days. There are no factors that identify those at potential risk for anaphylaxis from an insect sting other than a prior history. Those who have had severe anaphylaxis have an 80% chance of another reaction.

Health care workers are at particular risk for latex allergy. Workers with allergies to latex also have a high incidence of reactions to certain foods, such as chestnuts, bananas, kiwi, and papaya. Manifestations range from

| TABLE 76–3 | COMMON AGENTS CAUSING ANAPHYLAXIS |

DRUGS

Penicillins (most common)	Vancomycin
Cephalosporins	Amphotericin B
Tetracyclines	Polymyxin
Streptomycin	Bacitracin
Kanamycin	Aspirin, other anti-inflammatory agents
Neomycin	
Heparin	Colchicine
Protamine	Tranquilizers

FOODS

Peanuts	Milk
Seafood	Citrus fruits
Eggs	Strawberries
Nuts	Legumes

INSECT VENOMS

Hymenoptera (honeybees, wasps, yellow jackets, hornets, fire ants)

BIOLOGICALS

Heterologous antisera (especially equine)
Enzymes
Hormones
Vaccines (especially egg-cultured types)

BLOOD PRODUCTS

Plasma
Cryoprecipitate
Whole blood
Gamma globulin

ALLERGEN EXTRACTS

Skin-testing agents
Desensitization

DIAGNOSTIC AGENTS

Sulfobromophthalein
Iodinated contrast media

simple dermatitis to generalized itching, urticaria, sneezing, coughing, wheezing, hypotension, and shock on exposure. The diagnosis of type I hypersensitivity to latex is confirmed by in vivo skin testing with raw latex extracts or in vitro blood assays that measure specific IgE responses to latex.

Medical Management

Anaphylaxis is treated by (1) subcutaneous epinephrine injection, (2) removing or discontinuing the causative agent, (3) administering emergency oxygen, (4) maintaining an open airway, (5) placing the client in the Trendelenburg position, and (6) giving supportive IV fluids, such as 0.9% normal saline or lactated Ringer's solution as necessary.

■ **Nursing Management of the Medical Client**

Nursing Diagnoses. *Risk for Latex Allergy and Latex Allergy Response* are more specific nursing diagnoses for latex allergy reactions. Most of the interventions for these diagnoses have been described under the nursing diagnosis *Altered Health Maintenance*. In addition, the incidence and severity of anaphylactic reactions are decreased by both general and specific measures. Take a thorough history for drug, food, insect, pollen and animal allergies from every client. Counsel all clients with a history of anaphylaxis or anaphylactic-like reactions to carry epinephrine with them at all times in the form of Epi-Pen or Ana-Kit for self-injection. Recommend that they carry a medical-alert bracelet or necklace and an identification card in their wallet or purse and that they register with the proper authorities.

ALLERGIC RHINITIS

Manifestations of allergic rhinitis are persistent and show seasonal variation. Nasal manifestations are often accompanied by eye irritation, which causes pruritus, erythema, and excessive tearing. Numerous allergens may cause these manifestations, such as tree pollens (most common in the spring), grasses (summer), ragweed (fall), or dust mites and animal dander (year-round).

When the nasal mucosa is exposed to an allergen, a series of events is set in motion. Allergen exposure increases the production of IgE, which binds to the receptors on mast cells and basophils and eventually causes a release of mediators. The mediator release leads to increased swelling and blockage of the nose, watery discharge, sneezing, and nasal itching.

■ Medical Management

Nasal glucocorticoid sprays are used with good results for the treatment of allergic rhinitis. The newer, nonsedating antihistamines are beneficial in maintaining control over allergic rhinitis and are a crucial component of therapy.

■ Nursing Management of the Medical Client

Educating the client is the most important component of therapy. Teach clients to avoid allergens and to use air filters and air conditioning. Emphasize that compliance with medication is essential. Explain the reasoning behind daily medication use as well as how to adjust the medication to control minor flare-ups and to prevent progression of the disease.

ASTHMA

Because the diagnosis and treatment of asthma account for a substantial number of outpatient visits in allergy clinics, a heightened awareness and thorough understanding of the disease are warranted. See Chapter 61 for a thorough discussion of asthma management.

CONCLUSIONS

The immune system is a complex, interrelated system that affects the whole body. As a nurse, you must understand immune responses in order to provide clients with complete and individualized care. Because the care of these clients requires multifaceted interventions, you must be able to develop and implement complex care plans to meet their needs.

THINKING CRITICALLY

1. **L. S. is a 41-year-old woman admitted for surgery. After surgery, she was to receive prophylactic IV cephalosporin but received a dose of penicillin by mistake. She has a known allergy to penicillin. With a history of allergy to penicillin, what type of hypersensitivity reaction is L. S. most likely to experience? Using the concepts of hypersensitivity, explain this process.**

Factors to Consider. What reactions might the nurse expect? What should be the nurse's first actions? What medications might the nurse expect the physician to prescribe to treat this reaction? How can such a reaction be prevented from occurring in the future?

2. **A. W. is a 21-year-old college student admitted with an asthmatic attack that has not responded to his usual treatments. He is admitted for a course of IV medications and respiratory treatments. When you enter the room to start the IV line, his wheezing is audible. He is also anxious and gasping for air. What actions should you implement? What problems might you experience when you start the IV line?**

Factors to Consider. After the acute phase is over, what might the nurse assess to determine the cause of the asthma attack and why the typical interventions were unsuccessful? What additional teaching might be required?

3. **R. H. is a newly graduated Registered Nurse on an oncology unit. She has been wearing gloves more than ever during the past 2 weeks following orientation. A rash develops on her hands, and she complains of itching all over her body. What type of allergic reaction might be occurring? What actions to assess the allergy should be taken?**

Factors to Consider. Can R. H. expect to continue in her new job? Does the organization have a responsibility to keep her employed?

BIBLIOGRAPHY

1. Aaronson, D. (1998). Side effects of rhinitis medications. *Journal of Clinical Immunology, 101*(2), S379–S383.
2. Blaylock, B. (1995). Latex allergies: Overview, prevention and implications for nursing care. *Ostomy Wound Management, 41*(5), 10–15.
3. Boguniewicz, M. (1997). Advances in the understanding and treatment of atopic dermatitis. *Current Opinion in Pediatrics, 9*, 577–581.
4. Burks, A., et al. (1998). Atopic dermatitis and food hypersensitivity reactions. *Journal of Pediatrics, 132*(1), 132–136.
5. Costa, J., Weller, P., & Galli, S. (1997). The cells of the allergic response. *Journal of the American Medical Association, 278*(22), 1815–1822.
6. DeShazo, R. (1997). Future trends in allergy and immunology. *Journal of the American Medical Association, 278*(22), 2024–2025.

7. Donohoe, M. (1997). Allergic diseases. *Lippincott's Primary Care Practice, 1*(2), 117–128.
8. Gift, A. G., & Pugh, L. C. (1993). Dyspnea and fatigue. *Nursing Clinics of North America, 28*(2), 373–384.
9. Glaspoli, I. (1997). Stinging insect allergies: Assessing and managing. *Australian Family Physician, 26*(12), 1395–1401.
10. Kaplan, A. (1997). Treatment of chronic urticaria. *Western Journal of Medicine, 167*(5), 348.
11. Kim, K., Safadi, G., & Sheikh, K. (1997). Diagnostic evaluation of type I latex allergy. *Annals of Allergy, Asthma and Immunology, 80,* 66–76.
12. Kumar, A., Busse, W. (1996). Clinical aspects of anti-inflammatory therapy in asthma. *Current Opinion in Pulmonary Medicine, 2*(1), 40–47.
13. Leff, A. (1998). Pharmacologic management of asthma. *Journal of Clinical Immunology, 101,* S397–S399.
14. Lemanske, R. (1998). A review of the current guidelines for allergic rhinitis and asthma. *Journal of Clinical Immunology, 101,* S392–S396.
15. Lemanske, R., & Busse, W. (1997). Asthma. *Journal of the American Medical Association, 278(22),* 1855–1873.
16. Lundeberg, M., et al. (1997). Diagnosis of latex allergy. *Allergy, 52,* 1042–1043.
17. Naclerio, R., & Solomon, W. (1997). Rhinitis and inhalant allergens. *JAMA, 278*(22), 1842–1848.
18. Negro, J., et al. (1997). Leukotrienes and their antagonists in allergic disorders. *Allergy Immunopathology, 25*(2), 104–112.
19. Nettina, S. (1997). Patient with recurrent episodes of hives: Answers and discussion of allergic disorders case study. *Lippincott's Primary Care Practice, 1,* 351–354.
20. Nilsson, G., Metcalfe, D. (1996). Contemporary issues in mast cell biology. *Allergy and Asthma Proceedings, 17*(2), 59–63.
21. Rachelefsky, G. (1998). Pharmacologic management of allergic rhinitis. *Journal of Clinical Immunology, 101,* S367–S369.
22. Rumsaeng, V., & Metcalf, D. (1998). Asthma and food allergy. *Nutrition Reviews, 56*(1), S153–S160.
23. Sabroe, R., & Greaves, M. (1997). Food allergy. *Journal of the American Medical Association, 278*(22), 1888–1894.
24. Schoenwetter, W. (1996). Safe allergen immunotherapy: The correct allergen, the appropriate client, the adequate dose. *Postgraduate Medicine, 100*(2), 123–126, 131–135.
25. Slavin, R. (1998). Complications of allergic rhinitis: Implications for sinusitis and asthma. *Journal of Allergy and Clinical Immunology, 101,* S357–S360.
26. Storms, W. (1998). A comprehensive diagnostic approach to upper airway disease. *Journal of Allergy and Clinical Immunology, 101,* S361–S363.
27. Volcheck, G., & Li, J. (1997). Subspecialty clinics: Allergic diseases. Exercise-induced urticaria and anaphylaxis. *Mayo Clinic Proceedings, 72,* 140–147.
28. Weber, R. (1997). Immunotherapy with allergens. *Journal of the American Medical Association, 278*(22), 1881–1887.
29. Wheeler, A., & Drachenberg, K. (1997). New routes and formulations for allergen-specific immunotherapy. *Allergy, 52*(6), 602–612.
30. Workman, M. L. (1995). Essential concepts of inflammation and immunity. *Critical Care Nursing Clinics of North America, 7*(4), 601–615.

CHAPTER

77

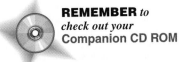

REMEMBER *to* check out your Companion CD ROM

Management of Clients with Autoimmune Disease

Joyce M. Black

NURSING OUTCOMES CLASSIFICATION (NOC)
for Nursing Diagnoses—Clients with Autoimmune Disease

Activity Intolerance
Self-Care: Activities of Daily Living
Endurance
Altered Health Maintenance
Health Promoting Behavior
Knowledge: Health Promotion
Knowledge: Treatment Regimen
Participation: Health Care Decisions
Social Support
Altered Role Performance
Coping
Depression Control
Psychosocial Adjustment: Life Change
Role Performance

Altered Tissue Perfusion: Peripheral
Tissue Perfusion: Peripheral
Sensory Function: Cutaneous
Chronic Pain
Comfort Level
Depression Control
Pain Control
Pain: Psychological Response
Fatigue
Activity Tolerance
Endurance
Energy Conservation
Sleep
Quality of Life

Impaired Social Interaction
Role Performance
Social Involvement
Impaired Physical Mobility
Ambulation: Walking
Mobility
Self-Care: Activities of Daily Living

Imagine trying to wear an antique suit of armor 24 hours a day. Consider how it would limit your movements. Think about how painful it would be if some of the joint hinges were rusty. Walking or even moving would cause you to feel tired and worn out. For many people living with rheumatoid arthritis or one of the other connective tissue disorders referred to as "rheumatic disorders," life is like living in a painful suit of armor.

More than 100 different connective tissue disorders, or collagen disorders, have been identified,[11] and one in every seven persons, more than 37 million people, have evidence of some form of arthritis. The term *rheuma*, meaning "flux," was used in the first century. Early physicians believed that these diseases originated in the brain as viscous fluid, "a bad humor," which flowed down into the body and attacked joints. We use a more common term, *arthritis*, which means inflammation of a joint.

Connective tissue, the most abundant tissue in the body, is found as loose connective tissue, dense connective tissue, elastic connective tissue, hematopoietic tissue, and strong connective tissue (Box 77–1). The primary

functions of connective tissue are to bind cells, organs, and tissues together; to provide warmth; and to permit ease of mechanical movement. Collagen and elastin are the major components of connective tissue. The underlying problem in connective tissue disorders is alteration or disruption of the protein component in the collagen.

The most common disorders are osteoarthritis, osteoporosis, gout, rheumatoid arthritis, systemic lupus erythematosus (SLE), scleroderma, and ankylosing spondylitis. Less common disorders include rheumatic syndromes associated with infectious agents, metabolic and endocrine diseases associated with rheumatic states, connective tissue neoplasms, extra-articular disorders, and miscellaneous disorders associated with joint symptoms. Disorders with an autoimmune cause are discussed in this chapter. Other orthopedic disorders are discussed in Chapter 26. Although the conditions have different clinical patterns, pain and impaired mobility are common problems with these disorders. Many connective tissue diseases are autoimmune disorders without a known cause or cure. Most of these disorders are chronic and follow a course of progressive deterioration. Before the specific disorders can be discussed, an understanding of autoimmunity is important.

This chapter includes material written for the fifth edition by Cleda L. Meyer.

BOX 77-1	Types of Connective Tissue

Loose connective tissue

- Areolar
- Adipose
- Reticular

Dense connective tissue

- Tendons
- Fascia
- Dermis
- Submucosa of gastrointestinal tract
- Fibrous joint capsules

Elastic connective tissue

- Walls of the aorta
- Part of the trachea and bronchi
- Vocal cords
- Some ligaments

Hematopoietic tissue

Strong supportive tissue

- Cartilage
- Bone
- Ligaments

AUTOIMMUNITY

Connective tissue disorders are caused by problems with the immune system. The immune system provides antibodies that recognize and destroy antigens. Antigens can include bacteria, fungi, parasites, viruses, our own damaged tissues, or foreign bodies (e.g., wood splinters). Antibodies can recognize "self" and "non-self" markers. All cells with a nucleus have protein markers on their cell membranes, known as *major histocompatibility complexes* (MHCs). Foreign cells also have cell markers, called *antigenic determinants* or *epitopes.* Properly functioning antibodies recognize both types of markers and either attack them or leave them alone, as appropriate.

Crucial to the process of immunity is the ability to recognize normal tissue and *not* invade or destroy it. When the immune system loses its ability to distinguish normal from abnormal tissue, normal tissue is destroyed. This process is called *autoimmunity;* the disorder arising therefrom is called *autoimmune disease.* There is now compelling evidence that a growing number of disorders are due to autoimmune responses.

Autoimmune disorders form a spectrum; for example:

At one end of the spectrum are conditions in which autoantibodies are directed at a single organ or tissue, resulting in local tissue damage. A classic example is Hashimoto's thyroiditis, in which autoantibodies have absolute specificity for the thyroid tissues (see Chapter 43).

At the other end of the spectrum is SLE (discussed later). In SLE, autoantibodies react with virtually every cell. The result is widespread lesions throughout the body.

In the middle of the spectrum falls Goodpasture's syndrome, in which autoantibodies destroy the basement membrane of the lungs and kidneys, leading to disease in these organs (see Chapter 35).

THEORIES ON AUTOIMMUNITY

Although it would be appealing to explain all autoimmune disorders by a single mechanism, there are a number of ways in which normal tolerance of self is bypassed. More than one defect might be present in a disorders and the defects may vary from one disorder to the next. Furthermore, the development of autoimmune disorders is through the interaction of immunologic, genetic, and environmental components. Not everyone with the same genetic susceptibility will have an autoimmune disorder. Therefore, other factors, such as the environment, probably play a role. Here we can only scratch the surface of a rapidly evolving area of health care.

Normal T helper cell tolerance is crucial to the prevention of autoimmunity. Developing T cells that can recognize normal tissues are usually deleted in the peripheral T cell pools and therefore never reach the tissues. In an autoimmune disorder, this tolerance is bypassed.

Several theories have been proposed to explain the etiology of autoimmune diseases. Genetic predisposition seems to be an important factor. Human leukocyte antigen (HLA) genes are frequently associated with autoimmune disorders. Certain genes appear to increase the risk substantially. The HLA-B27 phenotype is present in 95% of clients with ankylosing spondylitis. However, not everyone with HLA-B27 develops ankylosing spondylitis because of differences in the way the antigen is presented to the immune system.

MODIFICATION OF THE MOLECULE

If a potentially damaging molecule, called an autoantigenic determinant, is attached to a new carrier, part of the new complex may be recognized as foreign. This process can happen with drugs or microorganisms. Some drugs, like the antihypertensive agent methyldopa, alter the surface of the red blood cell (RBC). This change makes the damaged RBC look foreign and it is attacked (Fig. 77–1A).

RELEASE OF SEQUESTERED ANTIGENS

The release theory proposes that the self-antigens are isolated from the immune system within an organ during the neonatal period. When the organ is damaged later in life, these antigens are exposed to the immune system, which does not recognize them as self and therefore destroys the damaged cells. Bacteria, viruses, and parasites can degrade collagen and gamma-globulin. There are specific autoantibodies developed for gamma-globulin called *rheumatoid factors* (RFs), which are described later (Fig. 77–1B).

MOLECULAR MIMICRY

Several infectious agents cross-react with human tissues because of similarities between the molecular segments or epitopes of the foreign antigens and the person's own cells. Rheumatic heart disease sometimes follows streptococcal infection because an antibody to the streptococcal M protein cross-reacts with the M protein in the sarcolemma of the cardiac muscle. Once the infectious agent provokes tissue damage, the process continues because tissue injury releases more self-antigens (Fig. 77–1C).

INTERACTION OF T CELLS AND B CELLS

One of the tolerance mechanisms is inactivation of T lymphocytes when fully competent B lymphocytes are present. This normal process is called *clonal anergy.* Sev-

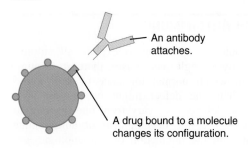

A   Modification of the molecule

An antibody attaches.

A drug bound to a molecule changes its configuration.

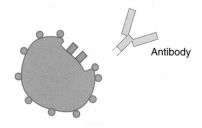

Antibody

B   Release of sequestered antigens

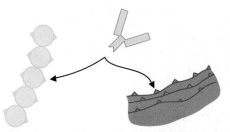

Streptococcus viridans bacteria are attacked.

A sarcolemma with a similar configuration is also attacked.

C   Molecular mimicry

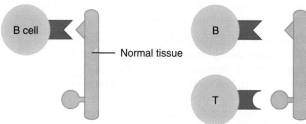

B cell

Normal tissue

Normal state: A B cell is not stimulated without a T cell.

B

T

When a T cell is stimulated, a B cell is also triggered.

D   Interaction of B cells and T cells

FIGURE 77–1 Theories of autoimmunity. *A,* Molecule modification. *B,* Release of antigens. *C,* Molecular mimicry. *D,* B- and T-cell interaction.

eral microorganisms are capable of producing polyclonal (antigen-nonspecific) B cells. Failure of this process leads to the production of nonspecific B lymphocytes. *Epstein-Barr virus* (EBV) is often cited as a cause of autoimmune disorders (Fig. 77–1*D*).

Any loss of T suppressor cell function contributes to autoimmunity. Conversely, excessive T cell help may drive B cells to extremely high levels of autoantibody production. Enhanced T helper cell function is seen in people with SLE.

RHEUMATOID ARTHRITIS

Rheumatoid arthritis (RA) is an autoimmune connective tissue disease that most commonly causes inflammation of the joints and joint deformity. RA affects about 1% of the worldwide population,[11] and more than 3 million people in the United States have RA. The incidence is two to three times higher in women until age 65 years, when men are affected equally. Clinical manifestations are most likely to occur in women during the menopausal years (ages 48–52). A 35-year review of research studies showed that median life expectancy for people with RA was shortened by 7 to 10 years in men and 3 to 7 years in women.[27]

Etiology and Risk Factors

A combination of factors, rather than a single cause, appears to be responsible for the onset of RA. RA occurs in genetically predisposed people, and is probably triggered by an unknown infectious agent. Some evidence shows an association of EBV, parvovirus, and other viruses[11] with RA. Seventy per cent of people with RA have the HLA-D4 and HLA-DR1 genes, a fact that supports a possible genetic predisposition. An initial self-limited infection may trigger an autoimmune attack against synovial membranes.

Pathophysiology

The initial infection induces inflammation of the synovial membranes (synovitis). T lymphocytes migrate into the inflamed area, activating monocyte-macrophage and B lymphocytes. In most clients, the antibodies produced during this activation are autoantibodies in the immunoglobulin M (IgM) class. The altered antibodies (*rheumatoid factors* [RFs]) form immune complexes with IgG that are deposited in the synovial membranes, where they stimulate local inflammation. See Understanding Rheumatoid Arthritis and Its Treatment.

Joint deformity in RA occurs from repeated episodes of inflammation. The damage to the joint occurs in four distinct phases (Fig. 77–2):

1. The mechanism of the first phase, *initiation,* is not understood. Some changes in the synovial lining are present.

2. During the *immune response* phase, large numbers of infiltrating lymphocytes (T cells, most of them CD4 cells) and RFs are present in the synovial fluid. These antibodies trigger the release of complement, which attracts leukocytes and macrophages to the area. RFs also stimulate the release of prostaglandins, which attract more leukocytes to the synovial fluid. Cytokines normally stimulate remodeling and rebuilding of cartilage; however, in RA this process is disrupted and cartilage is destroyed.

3. As the disease process continues during the *inflammatory* phase, the resultant swelling damages tiny blood vessels in the synovial membrane, which contains the synovial fluid. In response to this damage, the body releases arachidonic acid and lysosomal enzymes. Oxygen radicals are also present.

Understanding Rheumatoid Arthritis and Its Treatment

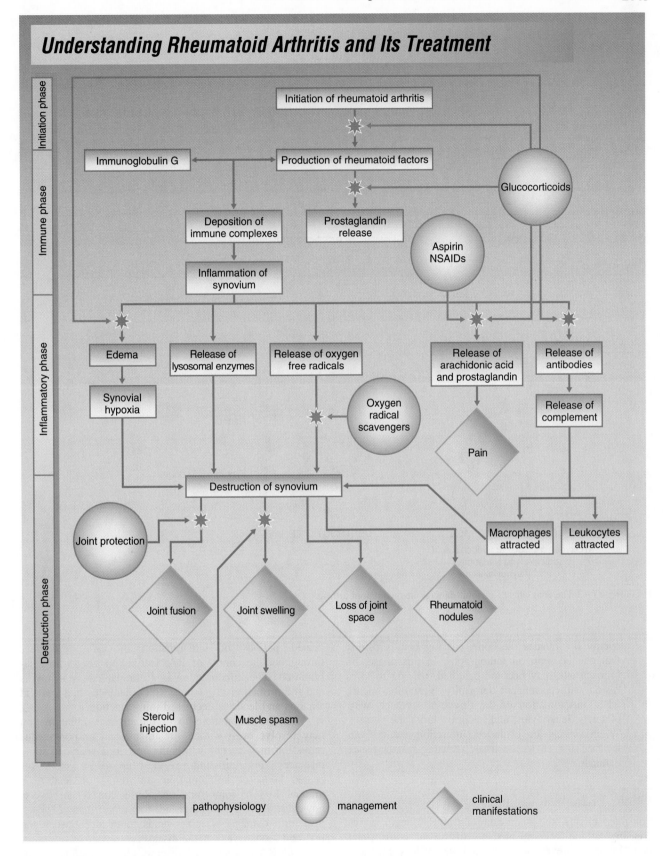

These substances create fissures in the surface of the synovium. They intensify the inflammation, eventually causing cells to enlarge and change into hyperactive stromal cells that thicken the membrane.

4. The *destruction* phase occurs over time. If the inflammatory process is not arrested, a thickened fibrous scar tissue (pannus) is formed. Pannus adheres to the articular surface of the cartilage and

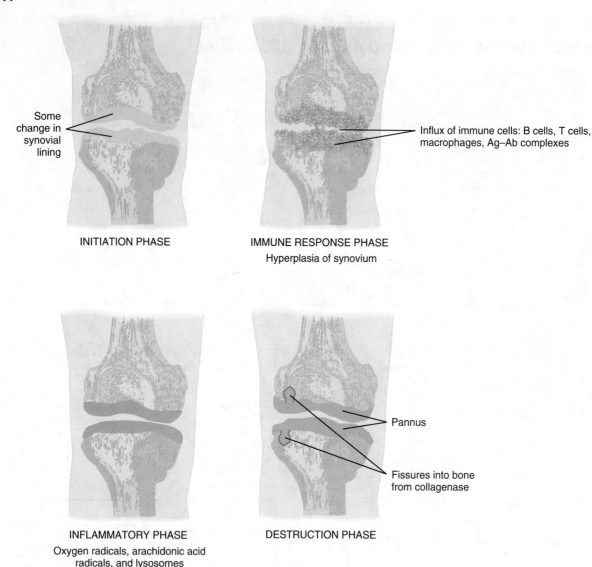

Some change in synovial lining

INITIATION PHASE

Influx of immune cells: B cells, T cells, macrophages, Ag–Ab complexes

IMMUNE RESPONSE PHASE
Hyperplasia of synovium

INFLAMMATORY PHASE
Oxygen radicals, arachidonic acid radicals, and lysosomes destroy synovial tissue

Pannus

Fissures into bone from collagenase

DESTRUCTION PHASE

FIGURE 77–2 The four phases of joint damage in rheumatoid arthritis.

eventually invades the bone, causing bony erosions that can be seen on radiographs. In this phase, fibrous tissue may become calcified, leading to joint fusion with permanent deformity. Vasculitis occurs when inflammation of the tiny blood vessels with platelets, leukocytes, and fibrin occludes the vessels. When vessels are occluded, infarction results from lack of oxygen to the tissue, causing further tissue damage.

Clinical Manifestations

For most clients, the manifestations of RA begin as increasing fatigue, accompanied by diffuse musculoskeletal pain, low-grade fever, anorexia, and weight loss. Stiffness occurs after inactivity, such as sleep or prolonged sitting. In fact, the duration of morning stiffness is one measure of the severity of RA.

With the passage of time, the manifestations become more sustained. The more common course includes re-

peated periods of inflammation of varying degrees throughout the course of RA, leading to progressive debilitation. The inflammation is accompanied by synovitis and the formation of pannus, which damages muscles and tendons and leads to decreased joint function.

After the initial flare-up of the disease, inflammation may resolve even without treatment, and a spontaneous remission may occur for months or 1 to 2 years. In some instances, this remission may last up to 25 years. Repeated bouts of inflammation and remission lead to a gradual loss of joint function. Remission is not likely, however, if RA has persisted for more than 2 years. Structural damage of joints tends to occur between the first and second year of the disease.

Since RA is a systemic disease, clinical manifestations may occur in various parts of the body; however, the joints are generally affected first. Joints tend to be affected symmetrically. For example, if one wrist is affected, the other is likely to be affected also. The wrist, proximal interphalangeal (PIP), and metacarpophalangeal

(MCP) joints are usually involved first. Joint swelling is more apparent in the morning after an accumulation of fluid during the night.

Clinical manifestations of RA are divided into (1) *articular,* or within the joint (e.g., synovitis, hand deformity, muscle spasm and weakness, rheumatoid nodules) and (2) *extra-articular,* or outside the joint (e.g., Sjögren's syndrome, vasculitis, pulmonary fibrosis, pericarditis, nerve compression, Felty's syndrome).

Synovial fluid is a protective cushion that permits free joint articulation. Inflammation inside the synovial capsule, spreading into synovial fluid, results in swelling, warmth, pain, and increased pressure on surrounding tissue. The inflammatory process of synovitis causes the tendons and ligaments to become shortened and less flexible, leading to deformity. The wrist, PIP, and MCP joints are most commonly involved. The result of this involvement is three types of hand deformity (Fig. 77–3):

1. *Ulnar drift* occurs when synovitis stretches and damages the tendons. Eventually, the tendons become shortened and fixed. An imbalance of damaged extensor tendons and intact flexor tendons causes the *subluxation* (drift) of the MCP joint.
2. *Boutonnière deformity* results from flexion of the PIP joint and hyperextension of the distal interphalangeal (DIP) joint extensor tendon, causing it to shift.
3. *Swan-neck deformity* is due to flexion contracture of the MCP joint, hyperextension of the PIP, and flexion of the DIP. Muscle spasm occurs in RA when the muscles are stretched over inflamed joints. The abnormal position of enlarged bone ends and inflamed muscles leads to further deformity. Pain and swelling cause the client to avoid using the joint or to move the joint guardedly, further weakening the muscles.

Rheumatoid nodules are composed of granulation tissue surrounding a central core of fibrous debris. These firm, nontender nodules are usually in subcutaneous tissue, although they have been found in visceral organs, including the lungs and the heart. They tend to develop during exacerbations of the disease. The most common sites are the wrist, carpal, knee, and elbow joints, and MCP and PIP joints of the fingers (Fig. 77–4). Rheumatoid nodules behind the knee may be tender, and this tenderness may be mistaken for a positive Homans' sign.

Extra-articular manifestations of RA may occur at any time in the course of the disorder and may, at times, overshadow the articular manifestations. These systemic manifestations must be treated quickly because they are major predictors of morbidity and even mortality.

Ocular problems are commonly associated with connective tissue disorders. Many of the problems are potentially blinding. The most common ocular problem seen in RA is *Sjögren's syndrome,* (see later). These people usually have scleritis and episcleritis. Episcleritis produces redness in the eye and some discomfort but no pain, and there is seldom a discharge. It rarely, if ever, causes loss of vision. Episcleritis is a benign self-limiting problem that seldom requires treatment. In contrast, scle-

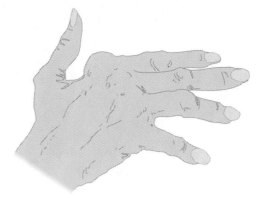

Ulnar drift

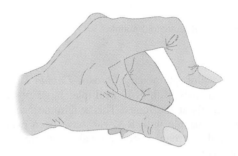

Boutonnière deformity

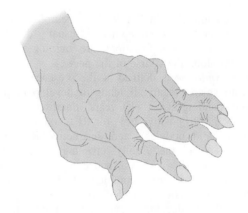

Swan-neck deformity

FIGURE 77–3 Three types of hand deformity characteristic of clients with rheumatoid arthritis.

ritis can lead to blindness and severe ocular pain. Untreated, the problem can lead to ulcers of the cornea and glaucoma.

Vasculitis is actually a group of disorders, including polyarteritis nodosa, systemic necrotizing vasculitis, and allergic granulomatous angiitis. All of these disorders result in necrotizing inflammation of the blood vessels. Circulating immune complexes are deposited in the blood vessels, causing inflammation and damage to large and small vessels. The result is end-stage organ damage. The specific manifestations vary, depending on the organs affected.

Pulmonary fibrosis, a common problem in clients with RA, is caused in part by smoking. Up to 28% of persons

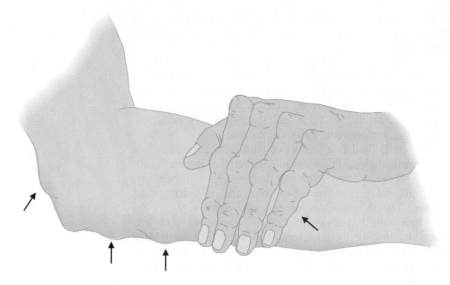

FIGURE 77–4 Rheumatoid nodules.

with RA develop pulmonary fibrosis. *Caplan's syndrome* is pneumoconiosis with RA. Multiple, large nodules are present throughout the lungs. This syndrome occurs most commonly in people with RA who have been exposed to silica, usually through occupational exposure, such as granite workers.

Pericarditis is the most common cardiac disorder in people with RA (~50%). Mitral and aortic valve disease have been noted.

Nerve compression in RA leads to neurologic impairment. Peripheral nerve entrapment is usually due to extensive synovitis. Manifestations are burning pain and paresthesias along the course of the nerve.

Felty's syndrome is defined as the presence of leukopenia with splenomegaly. It tends to develop in people with long-standing RA (>10 years' duration), seropositive RA (RA with positive tests for RF), nodular RA (RA with rheumatoid nodules), and destructive RA. People with Felty's syndrome usually have high levels of RF, antinuclear antibodies (ANAs), and cryoglobulins and diminished levels of serum complement. The neutropenia predisposes to infections, and 60% to 90% of people with Felty's syndrome develop pneumonia or joint infections. Felty's syndrome is usually managed with disease-modifying antirheumatic drugs for RA, such as gold salts or methotrexate.

Clients presenting with manifestations suggestive of RA actually have RA only if the following criteria are met:

- Morning stiffness lasting at least 1 hour
- Swelling of three or more joints
- Swelling of the wrist, PIP, or MCP joints
- Symmetrical joint swelling
- Rheumatoid nodules
- Positive results on tests for RF
- Changes on hand radiographs typical of RA, specifically erosions or bony decalcification

The first four criteria must be present for at least 6 weeks. A definite diagnosis requires that four of these seven features be present at the same time.

Diagnostic Findings

Additional manifestations are visible only on x-ray studies, which are of value in diagnosis and in the evaluation of treatment. High-resolution films, as used in mammography, aid in the early detection of bony erosions. Radiographs are also helpful for identifying narrowing of the joint spaces and loss of cartilage (Fig. 77–5). These ero-

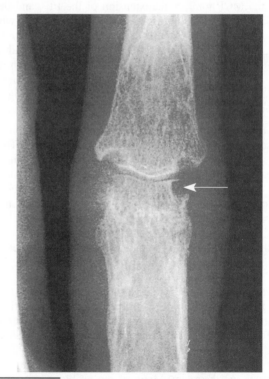

FIGURE 77–5 X-ray of an interphalangeal joint affected by rheumatoid arthritis. Pocket erosion is shown with the arrow. Pocket erosions can spread into trabecular bone and weaken the bone surface. There is also joint space narrowing and soft tissue swelling. (From Resnick, D., Berthiaume, M. J., & Sartoris, D. [1993]: Imaging. In W. N. Kelley, et al. [Eds.], *Textbook of rheumatology* [4th ed., p. 600]. Philadelphia: W. B. Saunders.)

sions may first be detected at the edges of the bone that have direct contact with the inflamed synovium. The formation of pannus and osteoporotic changes may also be detected on x-ray film.

Laboratory tests for the presence of RF aid in definitive diagnosis; however, elevations in RF levels take a while to appear. Within the first 3 months after the onset of clinical manifestations, test results for RF are positive in only 25% of people with RA; after 1 year, however, RF is found in 80% of people with RA. Nevertheless, RF is not specific for RA and may be found in 3% of the population without any clinical manifestations of RA.

Other laboratory findings in RA include an accelerated erythrocyte sedimentation rate (ESR), elevated serum globulins, and a positive test for C-reactive protein. A secondary finding is normochromic, normocytic anemia, which is often found in chronic disease. Synovial fluid may be aspirated for examination. Abnormal findings in the synovial fluid of clients with RA include reduced viscosity and white blood cell (WBC) counts as high as 50,000/mm³.

Outcome Management

■ Medical Management

The goals for clients with RA are to relieve pain, reduce inflammation, protect articular surfaces, maintain function, and control systemic involvement. The management of RA uses a balanced program of pharmacologic therapy with nonsteroidal anti-inflammatory drugs (NSAIDs), education, physical therapy, occupational therapy, and psychosocial therapy. With this balanced program, many clients with RA are able to maintain function and continue active, productive lifestyles. If these measures are unsuccessful, pharmacologic therapy with disease-modifying antirheumatic drugs may be used. Corticosteroid therapy, surgery, and therapy with experimental drugs are reserved for RA resistant to less aggressive approaches.

For most clients with RA, diagnosis and treatment occur in a community setting. Part of the initial and ongoing assessment of people with RA involves determining their degree of functional impairment. The American College of Rheumatology identifies four categories for rating functional ability in people with arthritis:

1 = normal function
2 = adequate function for normal activities
3 = limited function for activities of daily living (ADL)
4 = inability to function independently

RELIEVE PAIN AND INFLAMMATION

Medical management of RA involves four general approaches (Table 71–1):

1. Aspirin and other NSAIDs as well as simple analgesics are used to control the local inflammatory process. Anti-inflammatory medications impair the natural action of the mediators of inflammation (arachidonic acid, prostaglandins, and oxygen radicals). These drugs work on the end process of inflammation, and the client's response to these drugs is usually quick and easily noticed. However, be-

cause these drugs do not reverse the initial arthritic processes in RA, bone edges remain rough and weakened, and inflammation returns once the effects of the drugs subside.
2. Although low-dose oral glucocorticoids have been widely used to suppress inflammation, they may also retard the development and progression of bone erosions.
3. A variety of agents classified as disease-modifying or slow-acting antirheumatic drugs appear to decrease elevated levels of acute-phase reactants in treated clients and are thought to modify the destructive capacity of the disease. Other agents, the immunosuppressive and cytotoxic drugs, ameliorate the disease process in some clients.
4. Intra-articular glucocorticoids can provide transient relief when systemic medical therapy has failed to resolve inflammation.

A "last-resort" approach that can be entertained involves the use of investigational therapies, including combinations of disease-modifying antirheumatic drugs (DMARDs) and other experimental agents. Substituting *omega-3 fatty acids,* such as eicosapentaenoic acid found in certain fish oils, for dietary omega-6 essential fatty acids, found in meat, has provided symptomatic improvement in clients with RA. Some nontraditional approaches also have been claimed to be effective (e.g., diet, plant and animal extracts, vaccines, hormones, topical preparations). Many of these are costly, and none has been shown to be effective. However, belief in their efficacy ensures their continued use by some clients.

Whole-body rest can decrease joint inflammation in RA, and many clients with RA find that an afternoon nap reduces fatigue and helps them cope with the rest of the day. In addition, rest of specific joints with splints protects the joints and facilitates healing. However, the use of rest requires a fine balance; once inflammation subsides, the client should begin activity again to preserve as much joint function as possible. Of interest is that when people with RA have strokes, the joints affected by RA lose their inflammation. Clearly, activity and strain exacerbate the inflammation.

PROTECT ARTICULAR SURFACES

Joint protection and alleviation of discomfort are important aspects of the management of RA. Joint protection techniques and techniques for carrying out tasks without pain are typically taught by an occupational therapist and reinforced by nurses. Table 77–2 lists the principles of joint protection and strategies for lessening discomfort.

MAINTAIN FUNCTION

RANGE OF MOTION EXERCISES. Safe and effective exercises strengthen weakened muscles and improve function. Exercises may be carried out in group activities or independently. Daily range-of-motion (ROM) exercises are an important component of this program and do relieve pain. Isometric exercises help maintain muscle function, even when the client wears splints. Physical therapists also measure clients for orthoses, splints, and assistive devices that may be necessary in advanced disease. A correct fit of such devices is important to preserve a functional joint and maintain skin integrity. Physi-

TABLE 77–1		MEDICATIONS USED IN THE TREATMENT OF RHEUMATOID ARTHRITIS				
Class	Example	Action	Therapeutic Outcomes	Adverse Outcomes	Dosing
Anti-inflammatory	Aspirin (Ecotrin)	Inhibits synthesis of prostaglandin	Reduction in pain and inflammation	Increased bleeding tendencies, gastric ulceration	Take with food, milk, or antacid; toxic levels cause tinnitus; observe for dark stools (occult bleeding)
Nonsteroidal anti-inflammatory drugs (NSAIDs)	Ibuprofen (Motrin, Advil)	Inhibits prostaglandin synthesis by blocking precursor enzymes	Reduction in joint pain and inflammation	GI upset, gastritis, GI bleeding Dizziness Decreased platelet aggregation	Do not crush enteric-coated forms Take with food or milk
Nonsteroidal anti-inflammatory agents (COX-2)	Celecoxib (Celebrex)	Inhibits COX-2 enzymes	Decrease in joint pain, tenderness, and swelling	GI upset No effect on platelet aggregation	Take with food or milk
Glucocorticoids	Prednisone	Decreases inflammation by suppressing the migration of WBCs and the immune response	Marked reduction in pain and inflammation	Delayed wound healing, insomnia, increased appetite Addison's crises if withdrawn suddenly or during periods of intense stress	Take with food or milk Taper dose slowly
Disease-modifying antirheumatic drugs (DMARDs)	Methotrexate	Immunosuppressive	Inhibits DNA synthesis	Bone marrow suppression, nausea and vomiting	Take on an empty stomach Monitor CBC, differential, and platelet counts

CBC, complete blood count; COX, cyclooxygenase; DNA, deoxyribonucleic acid; GI, gastrointestinal; WBC, white blood cell.

cal therapists also help clients learn the correct methods of using walkers and wheelchairs when the lower extremities are severely impaired by RA.

OCCUPATIONAL THERAPY. Occupational therapists teach clients ways to avoid placing strain on weak joints. For example, to protect joints during ADL, they may instruct clients to use both hands to carry items or may teach clients with weak grips how to use jar openers, levers attached to doorknobs, and other adaptive devices. Occupational therapists can also recommend workplace modifications and modifications in clothing to assist in dressing. For example, they might advise wearing clothing with self-fastening fabric (e.g., Velcro) closures rather than zippers. Occupational therapy promotes independence and enhances self-esteem.

CONTROL SYSTEMIC INVOLVEMENT

Anti-inflammatory medications are used to control systemic involvement. Most clients' manifestations can be managed with aspirin, cyclooxygenase (COX-2) inhibitors, and NSAIDs. Sometimes anti-inflammatory treatments call for corticosteroids, slow-acting antirheumatic drugs, and some experimental medications (see Table 77–1).

ASPIRIN. Aspirin (acetylsalicylic acid) is a prostaglandin inhibitor used to decrease inflammation. Aspirin has historically been one of the first drugs used to treat RA.

However, it is used less often today because the high doses required in RA leave the client susceptible to troublesome side effects, such as gastrointestinal (GI) irritation and bleeding, impaired platelet function, and ototoxicity. To achieve anti-inflammatory effects, the therapeutic dose of aspirin is 2.4 to 3.6 g/day. At these high doses, aspirin is frequently toxic. In addition, to sustain therapeutic blood levels, aspirin must be taken four times a day, and such frequent dosing often leads to problems with compliance with the medication regimen. As with the other NSAIDs, clients should be instructed to take aspirin with food and watch for clinical manifestations of GI bleeding, easy bruising, and tinnitus. Few clients tolerate the doses needed to achieve therapeutic benefit.

CYCLOOXYGENASE 2 INHIBITORS. Celecoxib is an anti-inflammatory agent that inhibits COX-2 enzymes while allowing normal activity of COX-1 enzymes. Celecoxib has been shown to be effective at all doses studied in providing pain relief and anti-inflammatory relief while reducing the GI side effects more than naproxen, an anti-inflammatory agent that inhibits both COX-1 and COX-2 enzymes.

OTHER NSAIDs. NSAIDs are used extensively to decrease inflammation and provide pain relief in clients with RA. Many NSAIDs are available over the counter at low doses. The most common NSAIDs are ibuprofen (Motrin, Advil), naproxen (Naprosyn), tolmetin (Tolectin), sulindac (Clinoril), piroxicam (Feldene), diclofenac (Voltaren), and ketoprofen (Orudis). The therapeutic effect of these drugs is to inhibit prostaglandin synthesis, thus decreasing the pain and swelling that accompany the inflammatory response. Unfortunately, because NSAIDs suppress prostaglandin production, they also decrease production of gastric mucus and intestinal bicarbonate. These unwanted changes in the GI mucosa greatly increase the risk of bleeding and ulceration. These drugs are therefore usually taken with food, and a histamine receptor antagonist such as ranitidine (Zantac) is usually prescribed concurrently to reduce secretion of stomach acids.

NSAIDs also decrease platelet adherence ("stickiness") and therefore increase the risk of bleeding. Clients therefore need to be taught to watch for bruising and clinical manifestations of GI bleeding. When about to undergo surgery or dental work, clients should also inform the surgeon or dentist of their current medications.

Most NSAIDs permit simpler dosing schedules and have fewer side effects than aspirin. Nevertheless, clients need to be taught the importance of using the prescribed dosage and the need for continued medical monitoring during therapy.

GLUCOCORTICOIDS. Glucocorticoids, such as prednisone and cortisone, have both anti-inflammatory and immunosuppressive effects; however, they do not directly modify RA. Long-term use of these drugs is accompanied by serious side effects, such as adrenal suppression, osteoporosis, paper-thin skin, delayed healing, and cataracts. The health care provider, therefore, usually tries to control manifestations with other medications first. The lowest possible dose to establish control of pain and inflammation is used. The dose is reduced as soon as possible to keep the client on the smallest dose that keeps the symptoms under control. The dosage must be increased during periods of major physiologic stress, such as illness or surgery, because the suppressed adrenal glands cannot respond with the usual cortisol boost during stress. Careful monitoring of the client taking glucocorticoids is essential because of the serious complications that result from their long-term use.

When inflammation and tenderness are localized to particular joints, intra-articular injections of corticosteroids may be helpful. Reduced pain and improved function may last for weeks or months after these injections. Corticosteroid injections have been useful in delaying surgery for carpal tunnel syndrome, and they can decrease the need for larger oral doses of corticosteroids. Intra-articular injection of corticosteroids is a sterile procedure requiring careful skin preparation. The physician first aspirates excess fluid, then injects the corticosteroids. The client should keep the needle insertion area clean, dry, and covered with a sterile dressing for the first 24 hours after the procedure.

TABLE 77-2 PRINCIPLES OF JOINT PROTECTION AND STRATEGIES FOR LESSENING DISCOMFORT

Principles of Joint Protection	Strategies for Lessening Discomfort
Respect pain (fear of pain can lead to inactivity; ignoring pain can lead to joint damage)	Carry out activities and exercise only to the point of fatigue or discomfort Reduce the time spent in doing painful activities Avoid doing activities (other than gentle ROM) when joints are inflamed
Balance work and rest	Rest 5–10 min periodically when doing tasks that take more time Get sufficient sleep Take a 30-min rest during the afternoon
Reduce effort by joints	Slide objects rather than lift them Store items at convenient heights Avoid stooping, bending, or overreaching Sit to work whenever possible
Avoid positions of stress on joints	Avoid tight pinch or grip: use built-up handles and holders for objects such as toothbrushes and pens Avoid turning fingers toward the little finger: turn fingers toward the thumb Avoid wrist flexion and rotation during stirring (e.g., use spoon like a dagger) Use two hands to lift or carry objects Always consider adaptive devices (jar opener, reachers, built-up keys)
Use larger, stronger joints	Lift with palm and forearm instead of fingers Use a backpack, waist pack, or shoulder bag instead of a handbag
Use joints in most stable positions	Avoid or minimize excessive stretch of joint ligaments (e.g., rise from chair symmetrically and avoid leaning to either side) Maintain good posture
Avoid remaining in one position	Change position (or stretch) every 20 min Balance sitting tasks with those that require moving around
Avoid activities that cannot be stopped	Break activities into defined parts

ROM, range of motion.
From Maher, A., Salmond, S., & Pellino, T. (Eds.). (1994). *Orthopedic nursing.* Philadelphia: W. B. Saunders.

SLOW-ACTING ANTIRHEUMATIC DRUGS. Slow-acting antirheumatic drugs (SAARDs), also called disease-modifying antirheumatic drugs (DMARDs), are gaining acceptance for primary therapy. These medications—gold salts, antimalarials, immunosuppressive agents, and *d*-penicillamine—seem to slow progression of RA by blocking the immunologic aspects of inflammation. However, like other drugs used in the treatment of RA, they do not correct the underlying cause of the disease. Previously used for clients who did not respond adequately to symptomatic therapy, these drugs are being used more aggressively to arrest clinical manifestations and thus decrease joint destruction. They may be used alone or in combination with NSAIDs. Because DMARDs are generally slow-acting, they must be taken for several months before an effective response becomes noticeable. Some of these agents are also used in cancer treatment. Because the doses in RA are much lower than those used in cancer treatment, the side effects are therefore decreased, but careful monitoring for toxicity is still important.

EXPERIMENTAL DRUGS. Experimental drugs are also used in the treatment of RA. Such drugs include biologic response modifiers, immunomodifiers, antioxidants, and inhibitors of cartilage metabolism. Of course, when these drugs are used, clients are monitored closely so that therapy can be adjusted to avoid or decrease side effects.

The stress of living with a chronic disease such as RA, with pain and loss of independent function, can lead to depression. Altered body image, sexual problems, and decreased ability to work outside the home also contribute to depressed mood. Depressed clients report more pain and fatigue and decreased activity, with further loss of independence and function.

Outcomes

Living with a progressive, painful, chronic debilitating condition like RA presents many problems. Current therapeutic regimens enable many people to preserve function and lead productive lives with less pain. The psychosocial problems associated with this disease present additional challenges. The median life expectancy of persons with RA is shortened by 3 to 7 years. The increased mortality rate seems to be limited to clients with more severe articular disease and can be attributed largely to infection and GI bleeding. Drug therapy also may play a role in the increased mortality rate seen in these individuals. Factors correlated with early death include disability, disease duration or severity, glucocorticoid use, age at onset, and low socioeconomic or educational status.

■ Nursing Management of the Medical Client

The primary nursing goal in the management of a client with RA is to promote the healthiest possible life for the client. The nurse's role is to assess, educate, coordinate treatments, facilitate adaptations in the home, reevaluate periodically, and serve as client advocate. Providing information to help the client deal with chronic pain, comply with treatment, and cope with a chronic disease are some of the challenges faced in managing clients with RA. The nurse provides information and encourages the client's self-management by allowing choices about when

to exercise, which adaptive equipment to use, and what other self-care techniques to employ. Clients with RA appreciate caring and empathy by the nurses.

See the Bridge to Home Health Care feature on independent living.

ASSESSMENT

Nursing assessment begins by identifying the client's concerns and needs. The history should include information about the duration of clinical manifestations and ways the client has been managing those manifestations, particularly pain. It is important to identify other conditions that the client may have. The client's current understanding of RA and the coping strategies used for dealing with pain and fatigue are important. Determine the methods that the client is now using to obtain pain relief (and the amount of pain that the client considers tolerable). Find out what methods the client is using for joint protection.

Evaluate the amount of swelling and pain in each joint, and the number of affected joints (to obtain a "joint count"). Recall that disease severity is based on the joint count, laboratory findings, and radiographic changes. In addition, physiologic measures of function such as a timed walk, measures of grip strength, and results of self-report instruments that evaluate flexion and extension enable further evaluation of functional impairment and the impact of the disease on the client's life. Assess for current clinical manifestations in the client's eyes, heart, lungs, and peripheral nerves. It is important to note new manifestations and marked changes in previous clinical manifestations.

RA can be a crippling disorder. After 10 to 15 years with the disorder, less than one half of clients can still perform their own ADL. These physical limitations can greatly alter the client's usual role in the family, ability to work gainfully, ability to participate in family events, and ability to be an active sexual partner. Extreme fatigue and pain usually lead to early bedtimes and a reluctance to socialize. In addition, physical changes in the body can lead to lowered self-esteem. Western society values beauty and youth. Clients may find it psychologically difficult to be seen in public and deal with stares brought on by a hand deformity and other changes. As the client grieves the loss of a healthy, youthful body, thoughts of suicide can occur. Be sensitive to these issues and bring them into the discussion if the client or family hints at suicidal thoughts. Despite these changes, however, RA does not have to be a crippling disorder; with good medical and nursing care, many clients can maintain a healthy, productive, active lifestyle.

In caring for clients with RA, the nurse also acts as a liaison to obtain orders and arrange appointments with physical therapists, occupational therapists, and other providers. In rural settings, where these "extra" services are limited, you may need to provide supplemental information that these specialists would otherwise provide, and you may need to use printed resources to help clients.

DIAGNOSIS, OUTCOMES, INTERVENTION

Chronic Pain. The primary diagnosis of clients with RA is *Chronic Pain related to inflammation and swelling from pressure on surrounding tissues, joint deformity, and joint destruction.* The amount of pain that these clients

BRIDGE TO HOME HEALTH CARE

Increasing Independent Living with Rheumatoid Arthritis

Because the development of rheumatoid arthritis is often insidious, it is important to identify clients who are having difficulty managing in their homes and provide health education and home modification information before their problems become significant. Pain, fatigue, and joint deformities often limit clients' ability to perform normal reach and grasp patterns, and, therefore, limit their ability to perform daily tasks. Examples of such tasks are turning knobs, obtaining items from the refrigerator and cupboard shelves, getting dressed, writing, and using the phone. Mobility may be impaired to the extent that it is difficult to get on and off chairs or the toilet, and to stand long enough to prepare a meal or take a shower.

Clients commonly feel as if they cannot control pain and fatigue because of the dramatic fluctuations they experience. Clients may react by insisting that they perform tasks even during acute inflammatory stages, a decision that may increase joint stress, pain, and deformity. In contrast, other clients may stop performing some activities of daily living (ADL) and may become reliant on others. This latter decision may decrease their overall daily activity level, leading to weakness and dependence. All of these clients need accurate information.

Clients who have rheumatoid arthritis often experience joint pain with activity. For example, pain can occur when they attempt to lift a milk carton. Clients may experience pain long after a task is performed, as when they sustain the pinch needed to use an eating utensil. They need to identify situations that increase their pain so that they and their health care providers can problem-solve and determine the best use of adaptive methods and devices. Without this understanding, clients may become reluctant to use various beneficial approaches. For example, to decrease joint pain, clients should consider using devices such as large-handled eating utensils and using a small pitcher of milk instead of a heavy milk carton.

The disease process and daily, repetitive joint strain can lead to joint stress and deformity. When clients struggle each day to get out of a low recliner chair or obtain heavy dishes from a shelf above shoulder height, they may create further deformity and pain. Use health education to help clients understand this relationship and become more receptive to beneficial changes, such as higher chairs or rearranging the kitchen.

It is critical that clients maintain consistent range of motion and strength activities as well as ADL while using the correct joint protection and energy-conservation methods. Before clients use the assistance of housekeepers and home health aides, or lift-up chairs and other equipment, the potential benefits and disadvantages must be carefully calculated. When introduced at the appropriate times, such assistance may allow clients to remain in their own homes. If assistance is introduced before occupational and physical therapists have completed evaluations, it may lead to further dependence and deterioration.

Health education should incorporate the client's goals and lifestyle. Clients need information about the link between their disease and ADL and how they can positively influence this link. To be successful, clients need to use adaptive methods and devices correctly and balance their rest and activity in addition to taking medications. The home health care team is responsible for providing clients with tools and options that will promote independence and productivity at present and in the future. In this way, clients can make choices about their lifestyles and maintain maximum independence within their homes.

Linda J. Svatora, OTR/L, MBA, *Occupational therapist, Visiting Nurse Association of Omaha, Omaha, Nebraska*

---

experience permeates all aspects of their life. Recall the earlier analogy of living in a rusty armored suit.

Outcomes. The client's pain will be controlled at a level that permits the client to perform ADL.

Interventions. Chronic pain must be managed to allow the client to perform daily activities and function normally, to increase mobility, and to reduce fatigue. Teach the client the purpose and expected action of prescribed analgesics. You can use a handout to describe which side effects the client should report. Other pain relief interventions may include the use of heat or cold, exercise, and massage. Paraffin baths have been used for arthritis of the hands; however, the greatest benefit from this intervention occurs when the client exercises immediately after the treatment. Cold therapy is applied by cold packs, ice massage, immersion, or vapocoolant sprays. Although heat or cold may reduce pain, they may not be effective in decreasing inflammation. Transcutaneous electrical nerve stimulation (TENS) units have been used to reduce pain and local joint inflammation if only one or two joints are involved. Caution should be used when applying topical creams, rubs, or sprays (see the Client Education Guide).

Relaxation techniques, such as guided imagery, help some people cope with pain. Classes to teach coping techniques have been effective in decreasing pain and anxiety. When correctly performed, massage may also help relieve muscular aches and pain; however, it is important to massage only the surrounding muscles. *Never massage acutely inflamed joints;* doing so may aggravate inflammation.

Many clients with RA are perceived as demanding and manipulative. This misconception has stemmed from clients' attempts to control what little of their world they can. Chronic pain and fatigue often push coping skills to the limit. With what little energy is left, these clients attempt to control other parts of their lives. Approach these clients with compassion and appreciation for their problems. Many of their idiosyncrasies, such as statements like "Don't put the covers over my toes," are attempts to reduce pain. There is no such thing as a rheumatoid personality.

Impaired Physical Mobility. Another common nursing diagnosis is *Impaired Physical Mobility related to pain, stiffness, and joint deformity.* Using the armored suit analogy, you can see how movement of any kind is hampered when most or all of the articular joints are inflamed.

Outcomes. The client will maintain mobility at the highest possible level to carry out desired activities.

Interventions. Encourage the client to stay active. In cooperation with a physical therapist or trained exercise physiologist, help the client to develop an exercise program to preserve ROM while protecting joints. Maintaining function and mobility are necessary for the client to manage self-care activities.

Exercise can decrease morning stiffness, pain, and fatigue and enhance the client's self-esteem. Participating in group exercise programs, such as community water exercise programs (Fig. 77–6), provides social support and strengthens coping. Seek programs led by arthritis-certified instructors who monitor movement for adequate joint protection. Each session should include a warm-up period, full ROM exercises, endurance exercises, muscle-strengthening exercises, and cool-down exercises. Clients may use analgesics prior to exercise to permit increased freedom of movement. If a joint becomes painful during the exercise and the pain persists for 2 hours or more after the exercise, the activity should be modified.

Fatigue. Fatigue is a complex physiologic process involving the muscles, heart, lungs, and immune system. Clients with RA often experience fatigue, in part because of their chronic inflammatory process, pain, and depression. The diagnosis you may be working with is *Fatigue related to chronic inflammation, pain, or depression.*

Outcomes. The client will develop methods to balance rest and activity and will express satisfaction with his or her current level of activity and energy.

Interventions. Help the client to explore reasonable options for gaining enough sleep and finding time during the day to rest or nap. This may require changes in job performance or work relationships (if others need to do the client's work while he or she rests). Be sensitive to these concerns, and ask if your suggestions are reasonable in the client's personal setting. Practitioners can find it easy to say "be sure to rest now" without determining the feasibility of this protocol. For example, if the client is a young mother, she may need to send her young children to a neighbor for an hour or two each afternoon or nap while the children nap.

Altered Role Performance, Body Image Disturbance, Self-Esteem Disturbance. Several psychosocial nursing diagnoses may apply to the client with RA. Choose the one that best fits the client. All of these diagnoses may be related to chronic pain, the need for others to perform previous roles, feelings of helplessness,

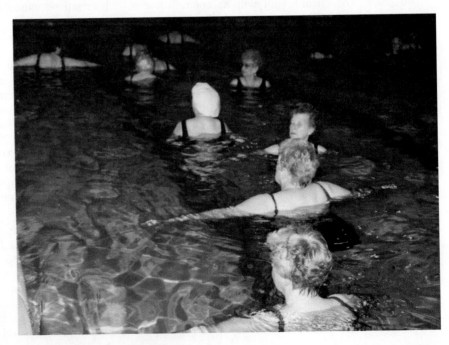

FIGURE 77–6 A community water exercise program. Many clients with rheumatoid arthritis find that water exercise helps to control pain and disability and improves exercise tolerance. The people in this class demonstrate the importance of keeping the shoulders submerged to allow the buoyancy of the water to protect their joints.

and feelings of embarrassment. We next present several avenues of care; select those that apply best to the particular client.

Outcomes. Although the actual outcomes statement depends on the client's particular diagnosis, most outcomes focus on the client's being able to express improved satisfaction with the problem. The problems identified by the three psychosocial diagnoses are usually very closely related, and improvement in one area can lead to improvement in others.

Interventions. The disease itself alters appearance, and in the client given corticosteroids several side effects from these medications can lead to alterations in self-esteem. Corticosteroids cause abnormal deposition of fat in the face (giving the client a "moon face" appearance) and shoulders (causing a "buffalo hump"); other side effects include acne, paper-thin skin that bruises easily, striae, and weight gain. Because of these and other side effects, the prescriber must always consider the risk-benefit ratio when initiating corticosteroid therapy. Also, the client may question the use of corticosteroids because the physical changes caused by them can be humiliating, even though the medications slow the inflammation. Most of these changes are permanent, and the client needs time to work through a new body image. Changes in body image take months to accept. Be sensitive to negative self-talk by the client, and express acceptance of the client's appearance; suggest clothing options to minimize visible changes.

The client and family will need time to plan for and accept the changes in the client's ability to perform previous tasks. Initially, it may seem easy to fill the role of two people in the home, and clients and their families may seem wary of efforts to encourage them to think about this change over the years that follow. Clients may also think initially that they will be able to go back to work full-time and that joint inflammation is only temporary. Be sensitive to this type of denial, and work with the client and family "where they are." Gradually, as the disease progresses, clients and families may need additional help as they try to come to terms with the long-term implications of the disease.

Risk of Ineffective Management of Therapeutic Regimen (Individuals). A final nursing diagnosis for the medically managed client with RA is *Risk for Ineffective Management of Therapeutic Regimen related to complex medications, schedules, high risk of side effects from medications, health maintenance, and self-care.* The management of any chronic disorder is complex, and the management of RA is no exception. Clients often have to take several types of medications with many undesirable side effects. They must plan for exercise and rest, and cope with daily pain and stiffness.

Outcomes. The client will make informed decisions about the management of the disease that will lead to a satisfactory quality of life despite the disease.

Interventions. Education focuses on coping skills, alternative methods of managing pain, joint protection, exercise, and adaptations for retaining functional independence. Inadequate knowledge may contribute to noncompliance with treatment regimens. Also, because of the pattern of remissions and exacerbations characteristic of RA, people tend to become discouraged with their pre-

scribed treatments. Likewise, the medications used in the treatment of RA may provide only moderate pain relief, and many are slow-acting. Clients with RA therefore are susceptible to "quack" cures and unproven remedies (Box 77–2).

Unproven arthritis remedies are treatments that in scientific studies have not been shown to work and to be safe. Proven treatments for arthritis must show in repeated, controlled scientific tests that they work by meeting one or more of the following goals:

- Pain reduction
- Reduction of inflammation
- Safe joint mobility
- Avoidance of stress damage to joints

Proven treatments also must show how safe they are. The benefits of a treatment in controlling arthritis should be greater than the risk of unwanted or harmful effects. Some unproven remedies are harmless, others are harmful, and still others have health effects that are unknown. Even if an unproven remedy is in itself harmless, it can still have a detrimental effect if it causes a person to stop or slow down proven treatments to control arthritis. Nevertheless, despite the many problems that people with RA face daily, many of these people courageously overcome these problems to maintain active, productive lives. There are news groups on America On-Line for arthritis that clients or health care providers can access and World Wide Web browsers can go to *http://www.arthritis.org*.

EVALUATION

The process of RA is slow to improve. It takes several weeks to months for the expected outcomes for most of these diagnoses to be met. When joints are already severely damaged and pain is uncontrollable, joint replacement becomes an option. These and other surgical therapies are discussed under Surgical Management.

Modifications for Elderly Clients

Older adults can slowly succumb to the pain and immobility associated with the disease, becoming complacent and sedentary. Some of these people with RA virtually *never* leave home for fear of pain and embarrassment about being slow to walk and move. Help these clients to find ways of improving mobility by having them work among other clients of their own age and abilities. In addition, elderly clients are often being treated for several other problems, such as lung or heart disease, each with its own treatment regimen. The proper integration of all of these medications and other treatments is important.

Surgical Management

Surgical procedures may be helpful for clients with arthritis. Surgery may be used to relieve pain, improve function, and correct deformities. Previously, surgery was considered only late in the course of arthritis, often after severe joint destruction or deformity had developed. Now, however, early surgery is used to prevent deformities during the early phases or active stages of the disease.

TENDON TRANSFER AND OSTEOTOMY

Tendon transfers can prevent progressive deformity caused by muscle spasm. During these procedures, nod-

BOX 77–2 Unproven Remedies for Arthritis

Harmless

Copper bracelets
Mineral springs
Uranium mines
Vibrators
Vinegar and honey

Harmful

Dimethyl sulfoxide (DMSO)
Large doses of vitamins
Drugs with hidden ingredients such as corticosteroids
Snake venom

Unknown

Biofeedback
Diets
Fish oil
Lasers
Yucca

The Arthritis Foundation estimates that most people with arthritis have tried an unproven arthritis remedy at some point.

One in 10 people who have tried unproven arthritis remedies report harmful side effects, according to a Health and Human Services survey.

An estimated $1 billion is spent yearly on unproven arthritis remedies.

Any unproven remedy, no matter how harmless, can become harmful if it stops or delays someone from seeking a prescribed treatment program from a physician.

How To Determine Whether a Remedy Is Unproven

It may be difficult to spot an unproven remedy at first glance. The only source of information about a remedy may be what is given out by its promoters. People with arthritis should be cautious if the proposed remedy falls into one or more of the following categories:

- *Works for all types of arthritis:* There are more than 100 types of arthritis and treatments vary for each kind.
- *Uses case histories and testimonials:* Claims of individuals helped by a treatment need to be backed up by repeated studies on large numbers of people.
- *Cites only one study:* A single study may obtain results that other studies cannot repeat. A number of scientists must repeat the same study and get similar results for a treatment to be considered proven. A single study may, however, suggest a treatment that may have promise and should be studied further.
- *Cites a study without a control group:* Use of a control group helps show that results are due to the new treatment, not to another factor.
- *Does not list contents:* Some advertisements for a miracle drug for arthritis feature just aspirin at a high price. Other treatments contain corticosteroids and other powerful drugs. These drugs may cause severe side effects and should not be taken without a doctor's supervision.
- *Has no warnings about side effects:* There should be warnings on the label or instructions stating who should not use the treatment.
- *Claims to be based on a secret formula:* Scientists share their discoveries so that other experts in arthritis can review and question their findings.

ules or benign bony tumors (*exostoses*) may be surgically removed and flexion contractures surgically relieved. *Osteotomies* (excising or cutting through bone) may improve the function of deformed joints or limbs. For example, a femoral head osteotomy may give symptomatic relief by changing the position of the head of the femur when it is being subjected to the stress of impact against the acetabulum. Postoperative care varies, depending on the joint treated. In general, joints operated on are immobilized for a short time and then remobilized with physical therapy.

SYNOVECTOMY

Synovectomy (surgical removal of synovia, as in the elbows, wrists, fingers, or knees) may be used in clients with RA to help maintain joint function. With RA, joint destruction begins in the synovial tissue and then proceeds to involve bone, cartilage, and other structures. Early synovectomy helps prevent recurrent inflammation. Short-term immobilization is needed after surgery.

ARTHRODESIS

Arthrodesis is an operation to produce bony fusion of a joint. Most commonly, arthrodesis is used for clients with bone loss after joint infection, with tumors, with musculo-skeletal trauma, and with paralysis. Arthrodesis can also help certain clients with RA or degenerative arthritis to regain some mobility. The surgeon usually uses metal screws and plates to fuse the joint. Although arthrodesis immobilizes the joint, the procedure eliminates much of the pain of the arthritic process and improves the client's functional mobility. The ankle is the joint most commonly treated with arthrodesis, usually to relieve post-traumatic arthritis, although the hip and knee can also be fused.

Despite its limited benefits, arthrodesis also has its drawbacks. It often results in stiffness in adjacent joints and increases the energy required for ambulation. It is possible, at times, to convert some fused joints to arthroplasties later in life. Bone grafts can also be used to stabilize the joint when desired union fails to occur after arthrodesis or when the use of screws or other devices is inadvisable. After surgery, the limb is casted. Nursing care is the same as for clients with casts (see Chapter 27).

JOINT REPLACEMENT

Joint replacement (*arthroplasty*) is the surgical replacement of natural diseased joints or joint components with

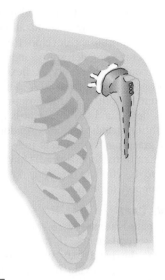

FIGURE 77–7 Total shoulder arthroplasty.

artificial joints or joint components. The operation restores motion to a joint and function to the muscles, ligaments, and other soft tissue structures that control a joint. The concept of joint replacement surgery is actually several hundred years old, but the modern ideas of joint replacement began in the 1960s, with the development of replacement components for the hip joint made of stainless steel and polyethylene (a lightweight plastic). Soon after, replacement joints were designed for the knee, shoulder, elbow, and fingers.

Today, joint prostheses are still a combination of a metal surface articulating with a polyethylene surface. The metal surfaces are made of strong, lightweight alloys such as cobalt-chromium and titanium-aluminum-vanadium. Both surfaces of an arthritic joint are replaced. If only one surface is replaced, the prosthesis would rub against the remaining tissue and not relieve pain or improve function. Arthritic joints can be replaced. Arthroplasty of the shoulder, elbow, and fingers is discussed next; hip and knee replacement is described in Chapter 26 following discussion of osteoarthritis.

Shoulder Arthroplasty

Disorders of the shoulder that require arthroplasty are much less common than those problems in weight-bearing joints. Although the shoulder is classified as a ball-and-socket joint, it permits more mobility than any other joint in the body. The large head of the humerus articulates against, not inside, the small glenoid cavity. This freedom of movement comes at the expense of stability. No inherent stability exists in the shoulder joint. The shoulder relies on soft tissue and ligaments for stability, particularly the rotator cuff muscle-tendon unit.

Four muscles and their tendons compose the rotator cuff, which allows the normal shoulder to move through three planes: flexion and extension, abduction and adduction, and internal rotation and external rotation.

Shoulder pain can have several causes; it is thus important to determine the true cause of the problem before treatment begins. Common manifestations of glenohumeral disorders include difficulty in flexion and extension and increased pain with attempted movement. An increase

in joint stiffness may occur after sleeping. Local injections of steroids and physical therapy can usually delay surgery.

Shoulder arthroplasty is the replacement of the humeral head and glenoid articulating surface with a metal and polyethylene prosthesis (Fig. 77–7). The primary indication for total shoulder replacement is pain caused by incongruity of the glenoid and humeral head. Improvement in function and ROM is a secondary objective of the operation. Usual problems that are treated with total shoulder arthroplasty are RA, osteoarthritis, fractures, and dislocations. There are no specific age limitations, but the client must be well motivated and be a reasonable surgical risk. In many clients with RA, the rotator cuff is thin and diseased. This is a disadvantage for full recovery of shoulder function.

Contraindications include infection and inability to comply with rehabilitation, such as clients with physiologic (e.g., neuropathy) or psychological problems. Complications include brachial nerve palsy, prosthetic loosening, joint dislocation or subluxation, and impingement syndrome.

POSTOPERATIVE CARE

Nursing assessment includes neurovascular examination of the operative arm at least every 4 hours (see the Critical Monitoring feature). A possible complication is development of impingement syndrome because of the proximity of the brachial plexus. Hemovac drainage should be less than 100 ml during the first 12 hours. Elevate the head of the bed 30 degrees to reduce swelling and improve comfort. Aggressive pain management is needed; the shoulder arthroplasty usually causes more pain during the first 24 hours than the other joint replacements.

Patient-controlled analgesia (PCA) works well when supplemented with non-narcotic anti-inflammatory agents

---

CRITICAL MONITORING

Postoperative Brachial Plexus Compromise

- To assess median nerve status, have the client grasp your hand. Note the strength of the first and second fingers. A weak grip may indicate compromise of the median nerve.
- To assess radial nerve status, note the movement of the client's thumb toward the palm, and back to neutral. Problems with this motion may indicate compromise of the radial nerve.
- To assess ulnar nerve status, have the client spread all the fingers wide and resist pressure. Weakness against pressure may indicate compromise of the ulnar nerve.
- To assess cutaneous nerve status, assess for flexion of the biceps by having the client raise the forearm. Poor biceps flexion may indicate compromise of the cutaneous nerve.
- To assess axillary nerve status, have the client push the elbow outward against pressure. Hold the arm still while you palpate the deltoid for contraction. Weak contraction may indicate compromise of the axillary nerve.

(e.g., ketorolac tromethamine [Toradol]). Ice is applied to the shoulder. It may be difficult for the client to find a comfortable position to lie in; position the shoulder for comfort without forcing it into motion. Place the client's personal items within easy reach of the nonoperative arm.

After surgery, the client's arm is placed in a sling or Velpeau bandage. Clients with rotator cuff repair wear a light brace to prevent abduction and external rotation. A shoulder continuous passive motion (CPM) device can be used for all three planes of motion. Initially, the shoulder is placed in forward flexion and external rotation. Shoulder rehabilitation begins quickly after surgery and continues for about 6 weeks. For no other joint is rehabilitation as important as for the shoulder. The shoulder is placed through progressive external and internal ROM, hyperextension, and finally exercises with resistance once the rotator cuff has healed (~6 weeks). Usually, the client can be taught how to use the nonoperative arm to move the operative arm through ROM.

Elbow Arthroplasty

Early forms of elbow arthroplasty were metal-to-metal hinges, replacing the hinge structure of the elbow joint. Few of these prostheses are used today because they loosen after 2 to 3 years. Later, hinge joints were made that contained metal and polyethylene. This metal and plastic joint allows for some medial to lateral and rotational movements. A nonhinged elbow joint contains a metal and polyethylene component.

Indications for elbow arthroplasty are pain, mechanical instability, and bilateral elbow arthrodesis (fusion of the elbow). It is also possible to correct pain in the elbow by resecting the olecranon; this is called a *resection arthroplasty*. Severe RA is the most common indication for total elbow arthroplasty. After surgery, the arm is dressed in compressive dressings or splinted, and wound drains are placed.

POSTOPERATIVE CARE

Postoperative care includes elevating the arm above the shoulder for 4 to 5 days. Assess the client every 4 hours for ulnar nerve entrapment. Check the client's hand strength; especially assess the thumb and index finger's ability to pinch and ability to adduct the fourth and fifth fingers. The ulnar nerve lies close to the posteromedial surface of the elbow. This nerve is called the "funny bone" because of the uncomfortable sensation in the arm and fingers when it is hit.

Assess for radial and ulnar pulses and capillary refill. Some institutions use pulse oximetry to continuously assess tissue perfusion. Pain is managed with PCA narcotics. Elbow flexion and extension are allowed as tolerated. Personal items should be placed within easy reach of the nonoperative arm.

An occupational therapist should guide the client on how to modify ADL. Clients should not lift more than 5 pounds or begin triceps and biceps strengthening exercises for 3 months. The client will never be able to lift heavy items or play sports with the operative arm.

Hand Arthroplasty

Various hand deformities develop from the synovitis of RA (see Fig. 77–4). Synovitis stretches the central portion of the extensor tendon, causing it to shift. Eventually, the tendons become shortened and fixed. *Ulnar drift*

occurs when the imbalance of damaged extensor tendons and intact flexor tendons cause subluxation of the MCP joint. Other hand deformities develop from synovitis of the PIP joint: boutonnière deformity and swan-neck deformity. A boutonnière deformity is flexion of the PIP joint and hyperextension of the DIP joint. There is no loss of MCP joint mobility. In the swan-neck deformity, the DIP joint is flexed and the PIP joint is hyperextended. Surgery of arthritic hands includes tendon transfers to improve pinch grasp and arthrodesis for strength and position of the thumb for opposition. Hinge implants are placed to restore function to the fingers. Fluff dressings are applied to support the hand.

POSTOPERATIVE CARE

After surgery, neurovascular assessments are performed every hour for several hours. If the client has regional block anesthesia, the hand may be numb. The hand is elevated off the bed to prevent ulnar pressure. The hand is usually placed in a stockinette and suspended from the bed. An opening is made to assess the fingers. Encourage the client to exercise the fingers 10 times every hour, attempting full extension and flexion. Finger exercises reduce edema and pain. Place the client's personal items within easy reach of the nonoperative arm. If the opposite hand is equally deformed from RA, the client is quite helpless and will require assistance with most components of ADL.

Encourage the client to use the nonoperative arm as much as possible. Some clients may express great concern about being dependent. Promote independence, and praise actions that foster self-care.

Rehabilitation is a long process. Most clients are fitted with outrigger splints with rubber bands that allow exercise with resistance after 1 week. Therapy continues for several weeks to assist the client to regain strength and control.

■ Modifications for Elderly Clients

Older clients may have adapted to RA very well but often find any further dependency needed after surgery difficult to handle. They tend to be slower in their recovery from total joint replacement. They may require prolonged hospitalization in an extended care facility or subacute care setting until they regain adequate mobility to function independently or with some assistance and safety.

SYSTEMIC LUPUS ERYTHEMATOSUS

SLE is a chronic, inflammatory, autoimmune disorder characterized by a wide array of clinical manifestations in vascular and connective tissue. *Lupus* is the Latin word for wolf, referring to a belief in the 1800s that the rash associated with this disease was caused by a wolf bite. Although this red butterfly rash is distinctive in some clients, it is absent in others.

There are two types of lupus erythematosus (LE): systemic and discoid. There is also a reversible form of lupus that is caused by reactions to various medications. SLE is the most severe form of the disorder; however, if well controlled, it can also be mild. Discoid LE is a mild form of the disorder that involves only the skin. The face, neck, and upper chest are usually affected.

SLE is relatively rare, occurring in 1 in 2000 persons. It most commonly develops in younger women between

BOX 77–3 **Medications Associated with Lupus-Like Syndrome**

Definite

Hydralazine
Procainamide

Possible

Chlorpromazine
Ethosuximide
Hydantoin
Isoniazid
Methyldopa
d-Penicillamine
Oral contraceptives
Practolol
Quinidine

ages 15 and 40 years. It is also more common in African Americans, followed by Asians and then whites. It is almost 10 times more common in women than in men. This suggests a hormonal influence.[13]

Etiology and Risk Factors

The cause of SLE is unknown. Certain factors, such as genetic predisposition, infection, environmental irritants, physical and emotional stress, and exposure to ultraviolet B radiation, have been implicated. It is suggested that the genetic predisposition for the disease is present in some clients and a virus or some other agent triggers it, resulting in disease occurrence. This theory is as yet unsupported. SLE also has a familial tendency; when a twin has the disease, the incidence is 25% to 50% greater in the other twin than in the general population.

Several medications have been implicated in the development of a reversible form of lupus-like syndrome (Box 77–3). These drugs bind to and alter deoxyribonucleic acid (DNA), possibly enhancing the response. There may also be a correlation between the client's ability to metabolize the medication and a predisposition to SLE.

Pathophysiology

People with SLE produce several autoantibodies. The primary autoantibodies produced are directed at the cell nuclei and are called antinuclear antibodies (ANAs). SLE produces autoantibodies against double-stranded (ds) DNA, and the presence of these antibodies in the serum is considered typical of SLE. Normally, the T suppressor cells prevent autoantibody formation. In SLE, a defect in the T suppressor cell prevents this protective process. Natural killer (NK) cell function is also suppressed; NK cells cannot kill abnormal cells as readily. There are inherited defects in complement factors and cell surface receptors that normally assist with clearing immune complexes.

ANAs do not cause much of cellular destruction alone, primarily because ANAs do not come in contact with intact cell nuclei. When cells die, the nuclei are released

and then bind to the ANAs. The immune complex that is formed triggers the inflammatory response, which is the primary cause of tissue damage. In addition, the immune complex is large and is often deposited in tissues. Deposition of this complex causes even more tissue damage by initiating the complement cascade and further increasing inflammation. A common site of deposition is the basement membrane of the kidney, which leads to glomerulonephritis. The complexes can also cause vasculitis, or inflammation of the vessels, resulting in a decrease of oxygen in organs and tissues. The immune complexes can also be deposited in the heart and brain.

Clinical Manifestations

SLE is not a single specific disorder, and therefore manifestations can vary greatly among people. About 90% of clients have polyarthritis and polyarthralgias. Pain is most common in the small joints of the hands, feet, wrists, and knees. Clients also have nonspecific manifestations, such as weight loss, fever, malaise, and lethargy. Many of the manifestations of SLE are due to the deposition of immune complexes in the tissues. The course of SLE also has exacerbations or flares and controlled periods (remissions).

ACUTE FORMS

Manifestations of acute SLE may include fever, musculoskeletal aches and pains, butterfly rash on the face, pleural effusion, basilar pneumonia, generalized lymphadenopathy, pericarditis, tachycardia, hepatosplenomegaly, nephritis, delirium, convulsions, psychosis, and coma.

CHRONIC FORMS

Manifestations of chronic SLE depend on the organs involved but may include fever, malaise, weight loss, cutaneous discoid LE lesions, erythematosus of exposed skin, generalized lymphadenopathy, severe hemolytic anemia, thrombocytopenic purpura, hypersplenism, pericarditis, pleural effusion, tachycardia, peripheral vascular syndromes (e.g., Raynaud's phenomenon, gangrene) (Fig. 77–8), ulcerative mucous membrane lesions, abdominal pains, nausea, vomiting, anorexia, bloody stools, hepatic dysfunction, hepatomegaly, focal glomerulitis progressing

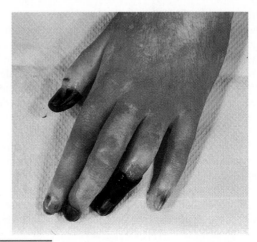

FIGURE 77–8 Vasospasm that occurs with advanced systemic lupus erythematosus can lead to gangrene of the fingers.

to glomerulonephritis, myalgia, arthralgia, neuritis, hemiplegia, psychosis, convulsions, and coma.

Diagnostic Findings

Diagnostic findings include the presence of LE cells (autoantibodies) in the serum, and the severity of SLE usually correlates with the degree of LE cell formation. Clients with SLE also have decreased complement levels; immune antibodies to DNA anti-samarium in the serum; increased gamma-globulin fraction due to increased antibody production; decreased levels of RBCs, WBCs, and platelets; and an elevated ESR.

At some point, abnormalities in the kidneys can be noted on an intravenous pyelogram; a barium enema might reveal colonic ulceration; a magnetic resonance imaging study might reveal central nervous system (CNS) involvement; and an electrocardiogram or echocardiogram might show cardiac changes.

Outcome Management

■ Medical Management

The goals of care for the client with SLE focus on (1) maintenance of skin integrity, (2) promotion of a healthy lifestyle and reduction of stress, (3) maintenance of proper nutrition, (4) promotion of comfort, (5) increase in the client's independence, and (6) maintenance of emotional well-being. The client is examined every 3 months with a complete blood count, determination of creatinine and cholesterol levels, urinalysis, and sometimes serum C3, C4, and anti-ds DNA.

Management of SLE is based on the organ systems involved. For example, if the client has cardiac involvement with either pericarditis or pleural effusion, intravenous pulse methylprednisolone may be used for 3 days, followed by oral prednisone. Cutaneous manifestations are managed with antimalarial agents. Most treatments are with medications; an algorithm has been developed to guide care (Fig. 77–9). Plasmapheresis may also be used to remove circulating autoantibodies and immune complexes from the blood before organ and tissue damage occur. The efficacy of this treatment has not been determined.

Clients with SLE require more than medications for proper management. Advise the client of lifestyle changes needed to reduce the risk of coronary artery disease, including management of hypertension, smoking cessation, and prevention of obesity and hyperlipidemia. Hypertension is aggressively managed with medications because it commonly leads to renal failure and death. Advise the client to reduce salt, fat, and cholesterol intake.

People in the United States have been called sun worshipers because they strive for a "healthy tan." Of course, tanning is dangerous to everyone, but the client with SLE must consider the sun an enemy. Photosensitivity is common; in many clients with SLE a rash develops after sun exposure as a result of stimulation of inflammatory processes.

All SLE clients receiving corticosteroids or immunosuppressants should receive the pneumococcal pneumonia

vaccine and yearly influenza vaccine. Teach clients to report any signs of infection quickly. If possible, sulfa antibiotics should be avoided because of their tendency to cause allergy and flares of SLE. Ongoing dental care is important to avoid a potential source of systemic infection. Yearly ophthalmologic examinations are also important to monitor for side effects of antimalarial therapy and to detect and treat cataracts secondary to long-term corticosteroid use.

Renal disease, such as nephritis leading to renal failure, is a common outcome. Again, high-dose corticosteroids are given initially. If the creatinine level rises above 3 mg/dl, dialysis is considered.

Strides have been made in treating life-threatening SLE with allogeneic stem cell transplantation. This procedure may offer hope to clients with acute forms of SLE who have had a poor response to 3 or more months of high-dose corticosteroids and immunosuppressive agents.

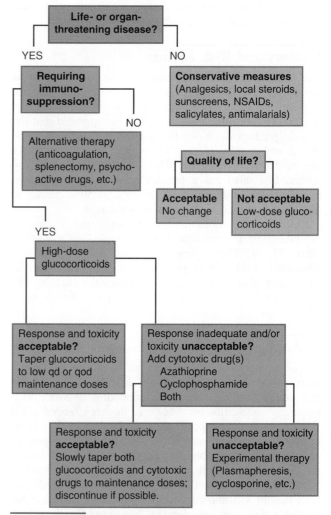

FIGURE 77–9 An algorithm for the management of clients with systemic lupus erythematosus. NSAIDs, nonsteroidal anti-inflammatory drugs. (From Hahn, B. H. [1993]. Management of systemic lupus erythematosus. In W. N. Kelley, et al. [Eds.], *Textbook of rheumatology* [4th ed.]. Philadelphia: W. B. Saunders.)

■ Nursing Management of the Medical Client

Nursing intervention for clients with SLE depends on how the client responds to the condition and on the severity and specific types of clinical manifestations. In a newly diagnosed client, you can expect knowledge deficits with respect to the diagnosis itself, prescribed drug therapies, and the prognosis. Explain how to relieve anxiety and avoid misunderstandings. This is particularly important in terms of the prescribed medications. Advise the client and significant others of the actions, side effects, and potential interactions of prescribed medications, especially corticosteroids.

During follow-up visits, review changes in all body systems. A physical examination is needed, with attention given to skin, muscles, and joints. CNS involvement is common, and a complete psychosocial assessment is important to detect changes in cognition and emotional stability.

During exacerbations, provide physiologic support to prevent skin breakdown, maintain nutritional and metabolic status, and minimize the risk of opportunistic infection. Also, provide emotional support to the client facing a chronic, potentially fatal disease. Clients may experience grief reaction following diagnosis, with exacerbations, or both. Allow for verbalization of these feelings. In such situations, be supportive and understanding; when necessary, refer the client or family members for counseling.

OUTCOMES

In general, the clinical pattern and prognosis of SLE are variable. The illness may develop rapidly with an acute fulminant course. More commonly, it develops insidiously and becomes chronic, with remissions and exacerbations. The course of the disorder is more severe when onset occurs at a young age. The survival rate has improved dramatically in recent years, although the disease is still potentially fatal. More than 95% of clients are alive 5 years after diagnosis. Improvements in treatments mean that clients can now live for many years.

The leading cause of death in clients with SLE is renal failure. There is some degree of kidney involvement causing progressive changes within the glomeruli in most clients with SLE. With progression of SLE nephritis, the glomeruli become increasingly abnormal and accumulate immune complex deposits. Once 75% of the glomeruli have been affected, the client shows manifestations of renal failure. The heart is the other major organ involved in SLE. The immune complexes are deposited in the coronary vessels, myocardium, and pericardium. CNS involvement, usually leading to cerebral infarction, can also occur.

PROGRESSIVE SYSTEMIC SCLEROSIS (SCLERODERMA)

Progressive systemic sclerosis (PSS) is a disorder caused by excessive collagen deposition, microvascular injury, and changes in humoral and cellular immunity. PSS is commonly known as *scleroderma,* although the skin is not the only organ system affected by the progressive sclerosis. Actually, this is a connective tissue disease characterized by fibrosis and degenerative changes of the skin, synovium, digital arteries, and parenchyma and small arteries of the internal organs.

Etiology

The exact etiologic mechanisms of PSS are not fully understood. Excess deposition of collagen is the characteristic feature of PSS, but the cause of excess collagen production is not known. However, the collagen that is produced is normal in other aspects. Vascular changes include fibrosis of the endothelium of small arterioles. Endothelial damage and cell death activate platelets and cause more inflammation. The activated platelets also lead to vasoconstriction and increased capillary permeability and recruit other inflammatory cells (e.g., fibroblasts) into the area. Alterations in humoral immunity are seen in the development of antibodies to type IV collagen found in the basement membranes of tissues. People with PSS have hypergammaglobulinemia, with the greatest increase in immunoglobulin G (IgG). Cellular immunity is also altered. In PSS, T lymphocytes accumulate in involved tissues; therefore, circulating T lymphocytes may be slightly decreased.

Clinical Manifestations

Scleroderma is classified into two categories: localized and generalized.

Localized scleroderma is the less severe form and affects primarily the skin. It may involve muscles and bones but does not affect the internal organs. Localized scleroderma is further divided into *morphea* and *linear* forms. Morphea is the development of skin lesions that are hard, oval, and white with a purple ring around them. Morphea often improves in time. Linear scleroderma is seen as a skin lesion that looks like a thick line of skin. It often begins in childhood and develops on the arms, legs, or forehead. The lesion can extend into the muscle and bone beneath it and alter growth.

Generalized scleroderma (true PSS) involves the skin and many other internal organs such as the kidneys, lungs, joints, muscles, cardiovascular system, and digestive system. Generalized PSS can also be further divided into *limited subcutaneous* and *diffuse subcutaneous* forms, often called CREST:

*C*alcinosis is the development of small white calcium deposits beneath the skin. The lumps may break open and drain a chalky fluid.

*R*aynaud's syndrome, common in most clients with PSS, consists of spasms of the arteries and arterioles. Spasms can occur spontaneously but most often are brought on by exposure to cold or emotional stress.

*E*sophageal motility is decreased from excessive deposits of collagen and muscle atrophy.

*S*clerodactyly is scleroderma of the fingers and toes.

*T*elangiectasia is permanent dilation of the capillaries, arterioles, and venules.

Limited subcutaneous scleroderma usually has a slow onset and may take 10 to 20 years before manifestations appear. Manifestations are usually one of the CREST forms. Prognosis is favorable. Diffuse subcutaneous scleroderma affects the entire body and most of the manifestations of CREST appear.

Progressively fatal PSS is associated with a generalized skin thickening and invasion into internal organs. Common clinical manifestations include subcutaneous edema, fever, and malaise. The skin becomes thickened and hide-like and loses normal skinfolds (Fig. 77–10). Ulcerations around the fingertips and subcutaneous calcification occur. Polyarthritis and polyarthralgias are also present. Dysphagia due to esophageal dysfunction, from abnormalities in motility, and later from fibrosis, occurs in about 90% of clients. Fibrosis and atrophy of the GI tract cause hypermotility and malabsorption. Diffuse pulmonary fibrosis and pulmonary vascular disease are reflected by low oxygen-diffusing capacity and decreased lung compliance. Hypertensive uremic syndrome, resulting from obstruction in small renal vessels, is serious. RF may be present in a small number of clients. Mild anemia is often present. An elevated ESR and hypergammaglobulinemia are also common. PSS typically progresses slowly. When death occurs, it is usually from infection or renal or cardiac failure.

Outcome Management

Treatment of PSS is supportive and symptomatic. The primary goal of medical treatment is to trigger a remission of the disease. Steroids and immunosuppressants are used to treat the disease, often in high doses.

Nursing interventions are directed at control of clinical manifestations. One of the major areas of concern is skin care to prevent breakdown and ulceration. The skin should be carefully inspected daily so any injury or breakdown is noted and treatment begun immediately. Teach the client to use gentle soaps and nonalcohol astringent lotions to maintain skin integrity.

Helping the client control acute pain, which is sometimes associated with Raynaud's phenomenon, polyarthralgia, and polyarthritis, is another important nursing function. The client must learn to avoid activities that might trigger pain. This includes actions such as joint protection behaviors, avoiding extreme cold, wearing gloves when hands are exposed to cold (even when removing food from the freezer), eliminating smoking, and resting the painful part when pain is acute.

If the client is experiencing esophageal dysfunction, modification of the diet may be necessary. Clients usually tolerate small, frequent, bland feedings better than three regular meals a day. The client also should learn to sit up for at least 1 hour after meals to promote digestion and food motility. Histamine receptor antagonists and antacids may be prescribed to decrease the acidity some clients feel.

The client will need continued follow-up care and monitoring. As with SLE, the client also needs psychosocial support to cope with this chronic debilitating disease. Encourage the client to continue to receive psychological support as needed after hospitalization.

ANKYLOSING SPONDYLITIS

Ankylosing spondylitis (AS), or *Marie-Strumpell disease,* is a chronic, progressive inflammation of the spine and sacroiliac joints. It affects 1% of the population, mostly males. The exact cause of AS is not known, but transmission is genetic. The joints of the sacroiliac begin to inflame and then ossify (fuse) as the joints and disc spaces are replaced by bone. The process moves up the spinal column until the spine is stiff and rigid, and then the disorder extends into the hips, knees, and shoulders.

AS begins insidiously in adolescence or young adulthood, usually with morning backache and stiffness in the lumbar area. The pain and stiffness subside with movement but return with inactivity. Other manifestations include iritis, arthritis or arthralgia, weight loss, and malaise. In advanced stages of AS, the client is rigid and stooped forward (Fig. 77–11). The spine is rigid and looks like bamboo shoots on radiographs. Laboratory tests reveal increased HLA-B27. ESR and RF are usually negative.

FIGURE 77–10 *A,* Long-term scleroderma. *B,* Appearance of the hands in a client with scleroderma.

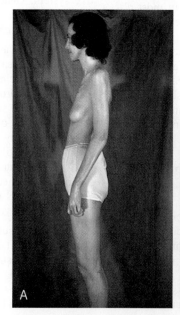
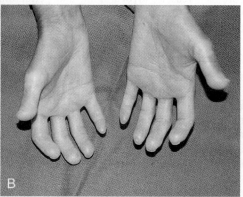

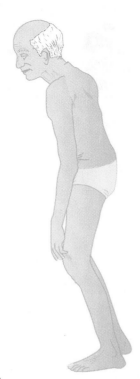

FIGURE 77–11 Posture of a client with advanced ankylosing spondylitis.

Outcome Management

There is no management to prevent or slow the progress of AS. Since stiffening of the spine is inevitable, the goals of management are to relieve pain, maintain optimal posture, and prevent respiratory involvement from minimal chest movements. Pain is usually treated with NSAIDs and heat. Instruct the client to try to maintain an erect posture and to rest frequently throughout the day. Splints and back braces are helpful for support.

Surgical management may include osteotomy for marked deformities of the hip or spine. Occasionally hip or knee arthroplasty is used.

SJÖGREN'S SYNDROME

Sjögren's syndrome, a chronic inflammatory disorder of the eyes, can be a primary problem or secondary to RA. It involves a decrease in lacrimation and salivation caused by obstruction of the secretory ducts by immune complexes. People with Sjögren's syndrome exhibit dry eyes (keratoconjunctivitis sicca) and a dry mouth (xerostomia).

Common manifestations include swelling of the lacrimal ducts and parotid glands and fatigue. This disorder affects mainly women, who experience an additional manifestation of vaginal dryness. Almost half of people with Sjögren's syndrome also exhibit another connective tissue disorder, especially RA.

Diagnostic tests reveal hypergammaglobulinemia and the presence of RF, ANAs, and anti-extractable nuclear antigen. Autoantibodies against salivary duct antigens are also found. If the client also has RA, the treatment is directed at the underlying arthritis. Artificial tears are helpful for keeping the eyes moist and preventing corneal abrasions. Artificial saliva can be used for the xerostomia. If the syndrome is left untreated, the client can develop visual problems, oral ulcerations, dental caries, and dysphagia.

Clients with Sjögren's syndrome have difficulty when going to surgery. Placing these clients on NPO (nothing by mouth) status can cause great oral discomfort because saliva secretion is decreased. Artificial saliva should be used. In addition, these clients are at risk for corneal abrasion because of the low humidity in the surgery suite. Ocular lubricants should be used preoperatively.

FIBROMYALGIA SYNDROME

Not all people complaining of musculoskeletal pain have arthritis. Fibromyalgia syndrome is an increasingly recognized chronic musculoskeletal pain disorder of unknown cause. It occurs in about 2% of the general population, predominately in girls and young women. Active research is being conducted to find the cause; some data indicate that there may be alterations in several hormones (e.g., adrenocorticotropic hormone, growth hormone) and the hypothalamus-pituitary-adrenal axis.

Clinical Manifestations

Clinical manifestations include fatigue, morning stiffness, non-refreshing sleep due to lack of stage 4 sleep, and postexertional muscle pain. About one third of clients have associated problems such as irritable bowel syndrome, tension headaches, premenstrual syndrome, numbness and tingling, and Raynaud's phenomenon. Fatigue is the most common clinical manifestation, and the most common cause of the fatigue is chronic depression. The physical examination is often unremarkable unless attention is paid to the tender points (Fig. 77–12).

Palpate these points with moderate pressure with the pulp of your thumb or forefinger. Intersperse examination of tender points with examination of nontender points to avoid anticipation reactions if every point is associated with pain.

Outcome Management

Management includes L-tryptophan to increase sleep, tricyclic antidepressants to inhibit serotonin uptake, benzodiazepines for the treatment of anxiety associated with depression, and corticosteroids and NSAIDs for pain control. Low-intensity exercise is also important and helps to decrease pain. Biofeedback, acupuncture, and hypnotherapy have also been used to help manage nonmuscular problems such as functional diarrhea, tension headache, and fatigue. The efficacy of these treatments is yet to be fully ascertained.

Many clients with fibromyalgia perceive themselves to be significantly disabled and have a reduced quality of life that rivals conditions such as RA and terminal emphysema. Clients with fibromyalgia have difficulty coping with "daily hassles" and this, in turn, increases the psychological stress. Cognitive behavioral therapy is often effective in providing these clients a sense of control over their lives.

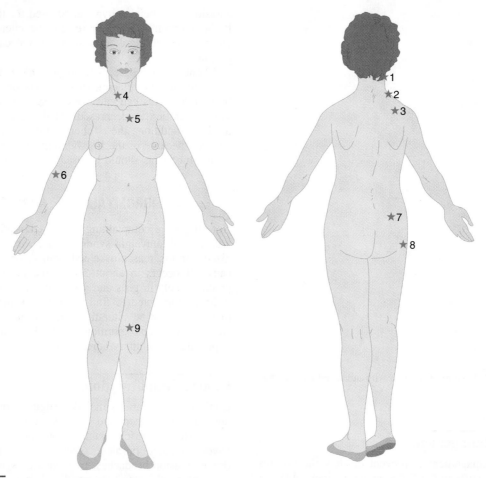

FIGURE 77–12 The nine paired tender points recommended by the 1990 American College of Rheumatology Criteria Committee for establishing a diagnosis of fibromyalgia. 1, Insertion of the nuchal muscles into the occiput. 2, Upper border of the trapezius—midportion. 3, Muscle attachments to the upper medial border of the scapula. 4, Anterior aspects of C5 and C7 intertransverse spaces. 5, Second rib space—about 3 cm lateral to the sternal border. 6, Muscle attachments to the lateral epicondyle—about 2 cm below the bony prominence. 7, Upper outer quadrant of the gluteal muscles. 8, Muscle attachments just posterior to the greater trochanter. 9, Medial fat pad of the knee proximal to the joint line. Eleven or more tender points in conjunction with a history of widespread pain are characteristic of the fibromyalgia syndrome. (From Bennett, R. [1993]: The fibromyalgia syndrome. In W. N. Kelley, et al. [Eds.], *Textbook of rheumatology* [4th ed., p. 472]. Philadelphia: W. B. Saunders.)

POLYMYOSITIS AND DERMATOMYOSITIS

Polymyositis is an acute or chronic inflammatory disorder of the striated muscles causing symmetrical weakness. When there is a rash associated with polymyositis, the condition is referred to as *dermatomyositis*. As with other connective tissue diseases, polymyositis and dermatomyositis are characterized by periods of remission and exacerbation and are chronically progressive. This disorder is twice as common in women as in men and occurs equally among all races. People between ages 30 and 60 are most at risk. Polymyositis may be associated with a malignancy.

Clinical manifestations of the disease, besides the symmetrical muscle weakness and rash, include polyarthralgia, polyarthritis, and Raynaud's phenomenon. Clients with dermatomyositis have characteristic heliotrope B (lilac) rash and periorbital edema. The muscle weakness can lead to problems with speaking and swallowing. Diagnostic tests reveal positive ANAs and focal deposition of complement, IgG, and IgM in vessels of the involved muscles.

These disorders are treated with high-dose corticosteroids and immunosuppressants. Nursing care is mainly supportive. Monitor the client's ability to swallow so that aspiration does not occur.

VASCULITIS

Vasculitis comprises a group of disorders leading to inflammation and necrosis of blood vessel walls. Soluble immune complexes are deposited in blood vessel walls in areas where capillaries have increased permeability. After deposition, the immune system is activated and the complex is destroyed along with the blood vessel wall. These disorders include polyarteritis nodosa, systemic necrotizing vasculitis, and allergic granulomatous angiitis. Inflammation and damage to large and small vessels result in end-stage organ damage.

Specific manifestations vary, depending on the organs affected. Steroids are the treatment of choice for these disorders.

REITER'S SYNDROME

Reiter's syndrome is a triad of arthritis, urethritis, and conjunctivitis. The syndrome is triggered by genitourinary or gastrointestinal infections, especially *Chlamydia*. Other manifestations may include prostatitis, penile or vaginal lesions, and urethral discharge. Achilles tendon and plantar fascia inflammation also occur. HLA-B27 is present in most clients and indicates an immunologic aspect.

The syndrome is treated with steroid therapy and aggressive physical therapy. NSAIDs may be used to treat the joint pain. Antibiotics are not used, since no organism can be obtained for culture.

The major nursing concerns are with pain and stiffness. Most problems are similar to those seen in clients with RA.

POLYMYALGIA RHEUMATICA AND CRANIAL ARTERITIS

Polymyalgia rheumatica is a clinical syndrome occurring more commonly in women than in men. It is a disease of aging, rarely occurring before age 60 years. It is characterized by pain and stiffness in the neck, shoulder, back, and pelvic girdle, especially in the morning. Headaches or painful areas on the head may be present. The client also may have a low-grade fever or temporal arteritis. Laboratory findings include an elevated ESR, mild anemia, and possible elevation of immunoglobulins. Steroids usually produce symptomatic relief within days.

Giant cell arteritis, also known as temporal or cranial arteritis, is also a disease of older people. The client often has manifestations of polymyalgia rheumatica for months, then suddenly experiences the severe headaches associated with temporal arteritis. The onset of this disorder is usually sudden, with severe pain often appearing in the temporal area. The pain also may be felt in the occipital area, face, jaw, or side of the neck. It is usually associated with hyperesthesia, which makes any touch exquisitely painful. The client may experience visual changes, including sudden onset of blindness in one or both eyes.

It is very important to diagnose and treat this disorder before blindness occurs. Because older women are often affected, their complaints of decreased vision and headaches are sometimes ignored as normal aging. Treatment is with corticosteroids, which are highly effective in controlling this disorder.

MIXED CONNECTIVE TISSUE DISEASE

Mixed connective tissue disease is a combination of several connective tissue diseases. Clients have manifestations that are not typical of any one disorder. This diagnosis is applied to about 10% of clients with connective tissue disease. Frequent combinations are SLE and PSS and RA. Mixed connective tissue diseases are managed according to their manifestations. Often clients are managed as if they had SLE. The term mixed connective tissue disease is used less frequently today.

LYME DISEASE

Lyme disease is one form of rheumatic joint disease with a known cause. It is included as a connective tissue disorder because the skin, joints, nervous system, and heart are involved. This complex multisystem disease is caused by the tick-borne spirochete *Borrelia burgdorferi.* Clinical manifestations found from 3 to 32 days after the bite may include a red flat rash that clears in the center, severe headache, stiff neck, fever, chills, myalgias, joint pain, severe malaise, and fatigue.

The disease can be treated with a course of antibiotic therapy. Doxycycline is the most common antibiotic used. Neurologic abnormalities may occur if treatment is ineffective. Intra-articular steroids and NSAIDs may be used to relieve joint inflammation and pain. Long-term effects include fatigue and arthralgia for many years after the initial infection.

SECONDARY ARTHRITIS

WHIPPLE'S DISEASE

Whipple's disease is a secondary arthritis associated with a GI disorder. The disease was first described in the early 1900s as a condition characterized by arthralgias, diarrhea, abdominal pain, and weight loss. Other manifestations include fever, lymphadenopathy, and increased skin pigmentation. The disease can affect almost every organ system in the body. Whipple's disease occurs most commonly in middle-aged white men. Although an organism was described as the cause, it was not isolated until 1992.

Treatment of Whipple's disease consists of broad-spectrum antimicrobial agents.

OTHER DISORDERS CAUSING ARTHRITIS

Other conditions that may produce arthritis-type symptoms include Crohn's disease, ulcerative colitis, tuberculosis, hyperthyroidism, hyperparathyroidism, sickle cell anemia crisis, and psoriasis. Treatment of the primary condition usually leads to a decrease in the severity of the arthritis.

CONCLUSIONS

Autoimmune disorders most often lead to problems of the joints, such as rheumatoid arthritis, and problems with other connective tissues, such as scleroderma. These chronic problems and resulting pain and deformity quickly test the resources of the client. Client education for self-care is critical. Most of these problems have no cure, so the nurse considers the effects of chronic pain, multiple treatments, and progressive deformity on self-concept, role performance, and family systems.

THINKING CRITICALLY

1. **You are working in an outpatient clinic and receive a call from a 66-year-old woman who is**

experiencing a flare-up of rheumatoid arthritis. She was seen 2 days ago in the clinic and given a high dose of prednisone. Now, she reports epigastric abdominal pain. A symptom analysis reveals the following: her pain has a burning quality, is worse between meals, is relieved by food, and is aggravated by coffee. She has taken some over-the-counter ibuprofen for the pain but states, "It didn't help." What other information do you need to collect? What interventions would you advise?

Factors to Consider. Consider the side effects of corticosteroids and NSAIDs.

2. **A 55-year-old woman with a history of joint pain is scheduled for a total hip replacement. She has experienced increasing pain while walking and hopes to be able to walk pain-free so she can resume her job as a waitress. What nursing assessments are pertinent to this type of condition and proposed surgery? How realistic is the client's desire to return to work as a waitress?**

Factors to Consider. How will assessments help in the prevention of postoperative complications? Are clients able to return to an improved level of functioning following joint replacement surgery?

BIBLIOGRAPHY

1. Albert, L. J., & Inman, R. D. (1999). Molecular mimicry and autoimmunity. *New England Journal of Medicine, 341*(27), 2068–2074.
2. Awerbach, M. (1995). Different concepts of chronic musculoskeletal pain. *Annals of Rheumatic Disease, 54*(5), 331–332.
3. Belza, B. L., et al. (1993). Correlates of fatigue in older adults with rheumatoid arthritis. *Nursing Research, 42*, 93–99.
4. Bertsch, C. (1995). CREST syndrome: A variant of systemic sclerosis. *Orthopaedic Nursing, 14*(2), 53–60.
5. Bonafede, R. D., Downey, D. C., & Bennet, R. M. (1995). An association of fibromyalgia with primary Sjögren's syndrome. *Journal of Rheumatology, 22*(1), 133–136.
6. Carson, D. A., & Tan, E. M. (1995). Apoptosis in rheumatic disease. *Bulletin on the Rheumatic Diseases, 44*(1), 1–3.
7. Dav, P. C., & Callahan, J. P. (1994). Immune modulation during treatment of systemic sclerosis with plasmapheresis and immunosuppressive drugs. *Clinical Immunology and Immunopathology, 76*(2), 159–165.
8. Dildy, S. (1996). Suffering in people with rheumatoid arthritis. *Applied Nursing Research, 9*(4), 177–183.
9. Goldenberg, D. (1995). Fatigue in rheumatic disease. *Bulletin on the Rheumatic Diseases, 44*(1), 4–7.
10. Halverson, P. B. (1995). Extraarticular manifestations of rheumatoid arthritis. *Orthopaedic Nursing, 14*(4), 47–50.
11. Harris, E. (1993). Etiology and pathogenesis of rheumatoid arthritis. In W. N. Kelley, et al. (Eds.), *Textbook of rheumatology.* Philadelphia: W. B. Saunders.
12. Johnson, R. L. (1993). Total shoulder arthroplasty. *Orthopaedic Nursing, 12*(1), 14–22.
13. Kuper, B., & Failla, S. (2000). Systemic lupus erythematosus: A multisystem autoimmune disease. *Nursing Clinics of North America, 35*(1), 253–266.
14. Legerton, C. W. (1995). Systemic sclerosis: Clinical management of its major complications. *Rheumatic Disease Clinics of North America, 21*(11), 203–216.
15. Meyer, C. L., & Hawley, D. J. (1994). Characteristics of participants in water exercise programs compared to patients seen in a rheumatic disease clinic. *Arthritis Care and Research, 7*(2), 85–89.
16. Mikanowicz, C., & Leslie, M. (2000). Polymyalgia rheumatica and temporal arteritis: A case presentation. *Nursing Clinics of North America, 35*(1), 245–252.
17. Minor, M. A., & Brown, J. D. (1993). Exercise maintenance of persons with arthritis after participation in a class experience. *Health Education Quarterly, 20*(1), 83–95.
18. Morrow, A. K., Parker, J. C., & Russell, J. L. (1994). Clinical implications of depression in rheumatoid arthritis. *Arthritis Care and Research, 7*(2), 58–63.
19. Neuberger, G. B., et al. (1993). Promoting self-care in clients with arthritis. *Arthritis Care and Research, 6*(3), 141–148.
20. Osial, T. A., Jr., Cash, J. M., & Eisenbeis, C. H., Jr. (1993). Arthritis-associated syndromes. *Primary Care, 20*, 857–879.
21. Parker, J. C., et al. (1992). Psychological factors, immunologic activation, and disease activity in rheumatoid arthritis. *Arthritis Care and Research, 5*(1), 196–201.
22. Rankin, J. A. (1995). Pathophysiology of the rheumatoid joint. *Orthopaedic Nursing, 14*(4), 39–46.
23. Riott, I. M. (1994). Autoimmune disease. In *Essential immunology* (8th ed., pp. 412–418). Cambridge, MA: Blackwell Scientific Publications.
24. Seltzer, E., et al. (2000). Long term outcome of persons with Lyme disease. *Journal of the American Medical Association, 283*(5), 609–616.
25. Sisk, T. D., & Wright, P. E. (1992). Arthroplasty of shoulder and elbow. In A. H. Crenshaw (Ed.), *Campbell's operative orthopaedics* (pp. 627–673). St. Louis: Mosby–Year Book.
26. Vale, D. (2000). Recognition and management of Sjogren's syndrome: Strategies for the advanced practice nurse. *Nursing Clinics of North America, 35*(1), 267–278.
27. Wolfe, F., et al. (1994). The mortality of rheumatoid arthritis. *Arthritis and Rheumatism, 37*, 481–494.
28. Workman, M. L. (2000). Immune mechanisms in rheumatic disease. *Nursing Clinics of North America, 35*(1), 175–188.

REMEMBER *to*
check out your
Companion CD ROM

CHAPTER 78

Management of the Client with Leukemia and Lymphoma

Linda Yoder

NURSING OUTCOMES CLASSIFICATION (NOC)
for Nursing Diagnoses—Clients with Leukemia and Lymphoma

Altered Nutrition: Less Than Body Requirements
Nutritional Status
Nutritional Status: Food and Fluids
Nutritional Status: Nutrient Intake
Sensory Function: Taste and Smell
Altered Oral Mucous Membranes
Immune Status
Infection Status
Oral Health
Self-Care: Oral Hygiene
Pain Level
Swallowing Status
Tissue Integrity: Skin and Mucous
   Membranes
Altered Protection
Coagulation Status
Coping
Immune Status
Infection Status
Nutritional Status
Altered Role Performance
Coping
Depression Level
Family Functioning
Psychosocial Adjustment: Life Change
Anticipatory Grieving
Coping
Family Coping
Grief Resolution
Sleep
Body Image
Acceptance: Health Status
Body Image
Self-Esteem

Death Anxiety
Dignified Dying
Fear Control
Depression Level
Diarrhea
Bowel Elimination
Electrolyte/Acid-Base Balance
Fluid Balance
Hydration
Symptom Severity
Dysfunctional Grieving
Coping
Family Coping
Grief Resolution
Role Performance
Energy Field Disturbance
Spiritual Well-Being
Well-Being
Fatigue
Activity Tolerance
Endurance
Energy Conservation
Nutritional Status: Energy
Psychomotor Energy
Hopelessness
Depression Control
Depression Level
Hope
Quality of Life
Sleep
Impaired Skin Integrity
Tissue Integrity: Skin and Mucous
   Membranes
Ineffective Denial
Acceptance: Health Status

Anxiety Control
Fear Control
Nausea
Comfort Level
Hydration
Nutritional Status: Food and Fluid Intake
Symptom Severity
Pain
Comfort Level
Pain Control
Pain Level
Symptom Control
Well-Being
Risk for Ineffective Management of Therapeutic Regimen
Knowledge Therapeutic Regimen
Risk for Infection
Immune Status
Nutritional Status
Sexual Dysfunction
Acceptance
Sexual Functioning
Spiritual Distress
Anxiety Control
Coping
Dignified Dying
Hope
Quality of Life
Spiritual Well-Being
Well-Being

Cancers of the hematopoietic system are disorders resulting from the proliferation of malignant cells that originate in the bone marrow, thymus, and lymphatic tissue. Blood cells that originate in bone marrow are called *hematopoietic cells;* cells that originate in the lymph are called *lymphoid cells.* Leukemia is cancer of the bone marrow, and lymphoma is cancer of the lymphoid tissue.

LEUKEMIA

Leukemia is a malignant disease of the blood-forming organs. Leukemia accounts for 8% of all human cancers and is the most common malignancy in children and young adults. Half of all leukemias are classified as acute, with rapid onset and progression of disease resulting in 100% mortality within days to months without appropriate therapy. The remaining leukemias, classified as chronic, have a more indolent course. In children, 80% of leukemias are lymphocytic, with 20% nonlymphocytic. In adults, the percentages are reversed, with 80% being nonlymphocytic.

Etiology and Risk Factors

Although the cause of leukemia is unknown, several risk factors are associated with leukemia, including (1) genetic factors, (2) exposure to ionizing radiation and chemicals, (3) congenital abnormalities (i.e., Down's syndrome), and (4) presence of primary immunodeficiency, and infection with the human T-cell leukemia virus type 1 (HTLV-1). Genetic factors increase the risk of leukemia. A high incidence of acute leukemias and *chronic lymphocytic leukemia* (CLL) is reported in certain families. Hereditary abnormalities associated with an increased incidence of leukemia are Down's syndrome, Fanconi's aplastic anemia, Bloom's syndrome, ataxia telangiectasia, trisomy 13 (Patau's syndrome), Wiskott-Aldrich syndrome, and congenital X-linked agammaglobulinemia. Identical twins, fraternal twins, and siblings of children with leukemia are also at increased risk. In *chronic myelogenous leukemia* (CML), more than 90% of clients have the Philadelphia chromosome, an abnormal chromosome (see Chronic Leukemia).

Overexposure to ionizing radiation is a major risk factor for development of leukemia, with the disease developing years after the initial exposure. Alkylating agents used to treat other cancers, especially in combination with radiation therapy, increase a person's risk of leukemia. Workers exposed to chemical agents, such as benzene, an aromatic hydrocarbon, are at a much higher risk.

Causal risk factors acting together with a genetic predisposition can alter nuclear deoxyribonucleic acid (DNA). The leukemic cell is then unable to mature and respond to normal regulatory mechanisms. Abnormal chromosomes are reported in 40% to 50% of clients with acute leukemia, and certain chromosomes are repeatedly more involved than others. It appears that a mutation in a single cell gives rise to some leukemias.

Pathophysiology

In normal bone marrow, efficient regulation ensures that cell proliferation and maturation are adequate to meet a person's needs. Pluripotent stem cells commit to differentiate along the myeloid or lymphoid pathway in the presence of growth factors. In leukemia, control is missing or abnormal. Leukemia is an uncontrolled proliferation of leukocytes. This lack of control causes normal bone marrow to be replaced by immature and undifferentiated leukocytes or *blast cells* (Fig. 78–1). Abnormal, immature leukocytes then circulate in the blood and infiltrate the blood-forming organs (liver, spleen, lymph nodes) and other sites throughout the body.

The French-American-British (FAB) Cooperative Group developed a classification system that is universally accepted. Under this system, acute leukemias are classified on the basis of morphologic characteristics and histochemical staining of blast cells, which indicates the percentage of immature cells in the bone marrow (Table 78–1).

ACUTE LEUKEMIA

For the leukemic process to be termed *acute,* at least 50% of the marrow cells must be immature. *Acute lymphoblastic leukemia* (ALL) is most common in children (median age, 11 years). *Acute nonlymphocytic leukemia* (ANLL) is more common in adults (median age, 67 years). Leukemias are considered clonal disorders, in that a single cell undergoes transformation, and leukemic cells then proliferate. An interesting paradox is that leukemic cells apparently divide more slowly and take longer to synthesize DNA than other blood precursors do. Acute leukemia is not caused by rapid cellular proliferation but instead is caused by the blocking of blood cell precursors. Leukemic cells accumulate relentlessly in most affected individuals, and they compete with normal cellular proliferation. Acute leukemia has also been termed an *accumulation disorder* as well as a *proliferation disorder.*

The development of leukemia occurs in the most primitive blood precursors, pluripotent stem cells, which give rise to all other blood cells (see in the Hematologic A & P review for Unit 16). The leukemia blasts, or precursor cells, literally "crowd out" the marrow and cause cellular proliferation of the other cell lines to cease. Normal granulocytic, monocytic, lymphocytic, erythrocytic, and megakaryocytic stem cells cease to function, causing pancytopenia (a reduction in all cellular components of the blood). Transformation also may occur specifically in the granulocyte-monocyte series and not in the erythrocyte series.

CHRONIC LEUKEMIA

Chronic leukemia is classified as CML or CLL. CML originates in the pluripotent stem cell. Initially, the marrow is hypercellular with most cells normal. Typically, the peripheral blood smear reveals leukocytosis and thrombocytosis with an increased production of granulocytes. In 90% of cases, examination of the bone marrow cells during metaphase shows a translocation called the *Philadelphia chromosome.* After a relatively slow course for a median period of 4 years, the client with CML invariably enters a *blast crisis* that resembles acute leukemia.

Blast crisis results in the death of more than 70% of clients with CML. During this phase, increasing numbers of blasts (immature myeloid precursor cells, especially myeloblasts, the most primitive granulocyte precursors) proliferate in the blood and bone marrow. In blast crisis, the blasts and promyelocytes (another myeloid cell precursor type) exceed 20% in the blood and 30% in the marrow. Increased fibrotic tissue in the marrow is another manifestation of blast crisis. Leukopenia, thrombocytopenia, and anemia also are evident. Without treatment, death usually occurs within 6 months of onset.

CLL is characterized by the proliferation of early B lymphocytes and is an indolent leukemia most often seen

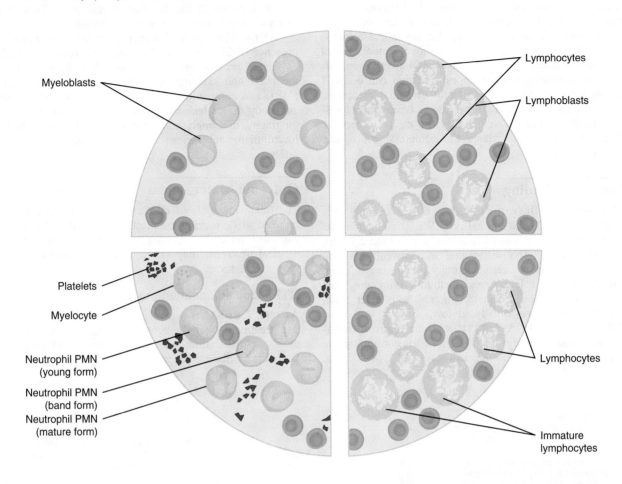

A Acute nonlymphocytic leukemia (ANLL)

B Acute lymphocytic leukemia (ALL)

Myeloblasts

Lymphocytes

Lymphoblasts

Platelets

Myelocyte

Neutrophil PMN (young form)

Neutrophil PMN (band form)

Neutrophil PMN (mature form)

Lymphocytes

Immature lymphocytes

C Chronic myelogenous leukemia (CML)

D Chronic lymphocytic leukemia (CLL)

FIGURE 78–1 Comparison of types of leukemia.

in men older than 50 years of age. It is usually discovered when the complete blood count (CBC) is performed as part of a routine physical examination. A peripheral blood smear reveals increased numbers of mature and slightly immature lymphocytes. As the disease progresses, lymphocytes infiltrate the lymph nodes, liver, spleen, and ultimately the bone marrow. A staging system is based on the extent of lymphocyte infiltration. Progression of the disease may take 15 years.

Clinical Manifestations

The manifestations of all types of leukemia are similar. The clinical history usually reveals anemia, thrombocytopenia, and leukopenia.

Clinical manifestations of bone marrow depression include fatigue caused by anemia, bleeding resulting from thrombocytopenia (reduced numbers of circulating platelets), fever caused by infection, anorexia, headaches, and papilledema. Bleeding can occur in the skin, gums, mucous membranes, and gastrointestinal (GI) and genitourinary tracts. Bleeding also is the underlying cause of petechiae and ecchymosis (discoloration visible through the skin).

Anorexia is associated with weight loss, diminished sensitivity to sour and sweet tastes, wasting away of muscle, and difficulty swallowing. Liver, spleen, and lymph node enlargement are more common in ALL than in

TABLE 78–1	FRENCH-AMERICAN-BRITISH (FAB) CLASSIFICATION OF ACUTE LEUKEMIA

Acute lymphocytic leukemia
  L1 Common childhood leukemia
  L2 Adult acute lymphocytic leukemia
  L3 Rare subtype, blasts resembling those in Burkitt's lymphoma

Acute myeloblastic leukemia
  Granulocytic
    M1 Myeloblastic leukemia without maturation
    M2 Myeloblastic leukemia with maturation
    M3 Hypergranular promyelocytic leukemia

  Monocytic
    M4 Myelomonocytic leukemia
    M5 Monocytic

  Erythroid
    M6 Erythroleukemia

ANLL. Splenomegaly and hepatomegaly usually occur together. The leukemic client commonly experiences abdominal pain and tenderness and breast tenderness.

Headache, vomiting, and papilledema are associated with central nervous system (CNS) involvement. Facial nerve involvement causes facial palsy. Blurred vision, auditory disturbances, and meningeal irritation can occur if leukemic cells infiltrate the cerebral or spinal meninges. Because chemotherapeutic agents do not pass the blood-brain barrier, leukemia cells can grow easily within the CNS. Intracranial hemorrhage and compression also can occur (Fig. 78–2).

Diagnostic Findings

COMPLETE BLOOD COUNT. CBC values vary greatly. The total white blood cell (WBC) count may be normal, abnormally low (<1000/mm³), or extremely high (>200,000/mm³). The differential may reveal that one type of leukocyte is overwhelmingly predominant. There may be abnormal leukocytes, including immature blast forms, noted on the peripheral smear. The platelet count and hemoglobin level usually are low.

BONE MARROW ASPIRATION. Bone marrow aspiration or biopsy is a key diagnostic tool for confirming the diagnosis and identifying the malignant cell type. Typical findings in the bone marrow aspirate and biopsy are an overall increase in the number of marrow cells with an increase in the proportion of earlier forms.

OTHER FINDINGS. Lumbar puncture determines the presence of blast cells in the central nervous system; 5% of clients present with this abnormality. Radiography of the chest and skeleton and magnetic resonance imaging (MRI) and computed tomography (CT) scans of the head and body detect lesions and sites of infection. Lymphangiography or lymph node biopsy may be performed to locate malignant lesions and classify the disease accurately.

Outcome Management

The treatment goals of all classifications of leukemia are targeted at destroying neoplastic cells and maintaining a sustained remission. During each phase of therapy, the medical treatment may vary but the basic nursing principles are the same.

■ Medical Management

ACUTE LEUKEMIA
The treatment plan for acute leukemia is determined by disease classification, presence or absence of prognostic factors, and disease progression. The goal of treatment is

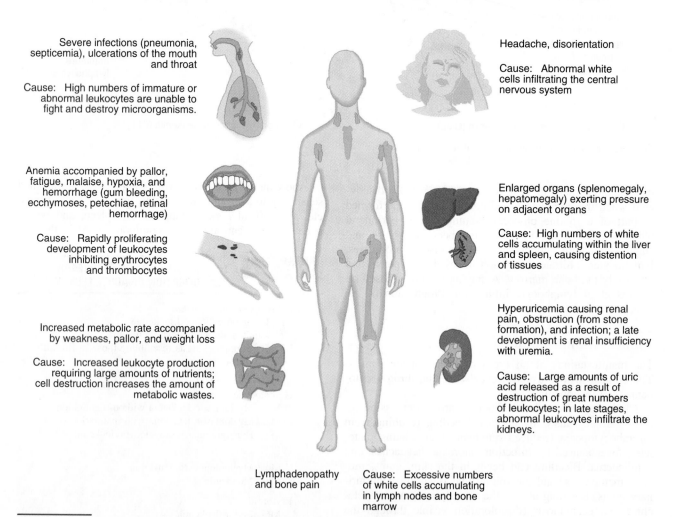

Severe infections (pneumonia, septicemia), ulcerations of the mouth and throat

Cause: High numbers of immature or abnormal leukocytes are unable to fight and destroy microorganisms.

Anemia accompanied by pallor, fatigue, malaise, hypoxia, and hemorrhage (gum bleeding, ecchymoses, petechiae, retinal hemorrhage)

Cause: Rapidly proliferating development of leukocytes inhibiting erythrocytes and thrombocytes

Increased metabolic rate accompanied by weakness, pallor, and weight loss

Cause: Increased leukocyte production requiring large amounts of nutrients; cell destruction increases the amount of metabolic wastes.

Headache, disorientation

Cause: Abnormal white cells infiltrating the central nervous system

Enlarged organs (splenomegaly, hepatomegaly) exerting pressure on adjacent organs

Cause: High numbers of white cells accumulating within the liver and spleen, causing distention of tissues

Hyperuricemia causing renal pain, obstruction (from stone formation), and infection; a late development is renal insufficiency with uremia.

Cause: Large amounts of uric acid released as a result of destruction of great numbers of leukocytes; in late stages, abnormal leukocytes infiltrate the kidneys.

Lymphadenopathy and bone pain

Cause: Excessive numbers of white cells accumulating in lymph nodes and bone marrow

FIGURE 78–2 Clinical manifestations and pathophysiologic bases of leukemia.

complete remission with restoration of normal bone marrow function; this means a level of blast cells in the marrow less than 5%. Approximately 60% to 80% of adults with ALL achieve complete remission, with 35% to 45% surviving 2 years. The cure rate remains low without bone marrow transplantation, however. Of adults with ANLL, 60% to 70% achieve complete remission, with about 25% surviving 5 years or more.

Destruction of Neoplastic Cells

CHEMOTHERAPY. Chemotherapy is given to destroy the malignant cells of the bone marrow. The treatment protocol for acute leukemia involves three phases:

1. *Induction phase.* The client receives an intensive course of chemotherapy designed to induce complete remission. The usual criteria for complete remission are blast cells less than 5% of the bone marrow cells and normal peripheral blood counts. Both conditions must be sustained for at least 1 month. Once remission is achieved, the consolidation phase begins.
2. *Consolidation phase.* Modified courses of intensive chemotherapy are given to eradicate any remaining disease. Usually, a higher dose of one or more chemotherapeutic agents is administered.
3. *Maintenance phase.* Small doses of different combinations of chemotherapeutic agents are given every 3 to 4 weeks. This phase may continue for a year or more and is structured to allow the client to live as normal a life as possible. This phase is used more commonly with ALL.

TUMOR LYSIS SYNDROME. A potentially fatal complication resulting from the treatment of acute leukemia, tumor lysis syndrome is a group of metabolic complications associated with the rapid destruction of a large number of WBCs. If the WBC count is high when chemotherapy is initiated, rapid cell lysis can lead to: (1) increased serum uric acid, phosphate, and potassium levels and (2) decreased serum calcium levels. Manifestations include confusion, weakness, numbness, bradycardia, electrocardiographic (ECG) changes, and dysrhythmias (hyperkalemia); numbness, tingling, muscle cramps, seizures, tetany, and ECG changes (hypocalcemia); and uric acid crystalluria, renal obstruction, and acute renal failure (hyperuricemia). Acute tumor lysis syndrome can be prevented by increasing intravenous (IV) hydration, alkalizing the urine, and administering allopurinol (Zyloprim).

REPLACING CELLS AND CONTROLLING INFECTION. Current treatment modalities for acute leukemia destroy normal and aberrant cells. Therapy is aimed at preventing and resolving the complications of acquired and induced pancytopenia—anemia, bleeding, and infection. Transfusions of red blood cells (RBCs) and platelets may be required until the marrow produces mature cells. If the client requires IV infusions of RBCs and amphotericin B, an antifungal agent, they should be separated by at least 1 hour so that adverse (e.g., allergic) reactions, can be detected.

RADIATION THERAPY. Radiation therapy may be administered as an adjunct to chemotherapy when leukemic cells infiltrate the CNS, skin, rectum, and testes or when a large mediastinal mass is noted upon diagnosis (as may occur in ALL).

CHRONIC MYELOGENOUS LEUKEMIA

The goal of therapy in the chronic phase of CML is to control leukocytosis and thrombocytosis. When unwanted cells accumulate, apheresis is a method of blood collection in which blood is withdrawn. The unwanted component is separated, and the remainder of the blood is returned to the client. *Apheresis* is usually performed with use of automated blood cell separators designed to selectively remove the desired blood element. *Leukapheresis* may be performed to lower an extremely high peripheral leukocyte count quickly and to prevent acute tumor lysis syndrome, but results are temporary (Fig. 78–3). Likewise, for thrombocytosis of 2 million/mm^3, *thrombocytapheresis* may be necessary. If painful splenomegaly develops, irradiating or removing the spleen relieves this manifestation.

The most widely used medications are interferon alfa and hydroxyurea, which are given orally and intravenously. Clients with a blast crisis (Fig. 78–4) require intensive chemotherapy with the same agents as used in acute leukemia. These drugs can destroy leukemic blast cells, transform them into normal granulocytes, or prevent leukemic cells from inhibiting formation of normal granulocytes. Unfortunately, drugs are usually ineffective in achieving long-term remission.

CHRONIC LYMPHOCYTIC LEUKEMIA

The goal of therapy in CLL is palliation or symptom control. Local radiation to the spleen may be given as a palliative treatment to reduce complications. Two complications seen during the later stages are hemolytic anemia resulting from autoimmune disorder, and hypogammaglobulinemia, which further increases susceptibility to infection. Antibiotics, transfusions of RBCs, and injections of gamma-globulin concentrates may be required for these clients. Leukapheresis is performed when the WBCs are great enough to cause vascular thrombosis or embolism, especially in clients who are unresponsive to chemotherapy.

Chemotherapy

Chlorambucil (Leukeran) or cyclophosphamide (Cytoxan) may be given orally to reduce manifestations of CML. Chemotherapy generally is given for 2 weeks of every month. When anemia (stage III) and thrombocytopenia (stage IV) develop, daily oral prednisone is given as an adjunct to the alkylating agents. Prednisone has a marked lymphocytolytic effect and may stimulate the production of RBCs and platelets. Fludarabine is a new chemotherapeutic agent that appears effective in treating CLL.

▇ Nursing Management of the Medical Client

ASSESSMENT

Obtain a thorough health history to aid in diagnosis and treatment. The initial history and physical examination provide baseline data to facilitate assessment of complications of ablative chemotherapy and radiation therapy. Be sure to obtain a thorough health history from the client and family members. The severity and longevity of the manifestations of leukemia are important facts to obtain and document.

Ask the client about risk factors and causative factors. Age is important to note because the incidence of leukemia increases with age. The client's occupation and hob-

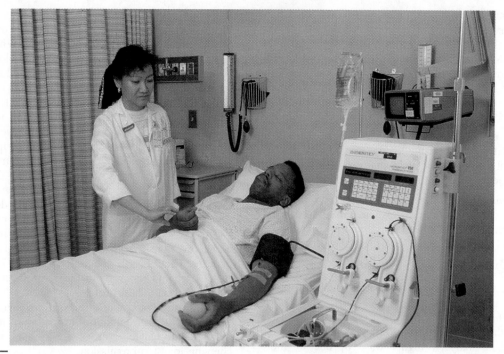

FIGURE 78-3 The white blood cell (WBC) level can be temporarily lowered by leukapheresis. Several automated blood cell separators effectively remove large numbers of WBCs and return red blood cells and plasma to the client. The Haemonetics V50 cell separator is commonly used to perform this procedure.

bies may also give hints about environmental exposures. Previous illnesses and medical history may indicate risk factors.

Because leukemia increases the risk of infection resulting from loss of WBC function, ask about the frequency and severity of infections, such as colds, pneumonia, bronchitis, and unexplained fever, during the past 6 months. Leukemia reduces the production of RBCs. The client may report activity intolerance, headache resulting from cerebral hypoxia, increased sleepiness, decreased attention span, anorexia, and weight loss.

The loss of platelet function increases the risk of bleeding. The client may report a tendency to bleed or bruise easily (e.g., nosebleeds), inability to stop bleeding from small nicks, bleeding in saliva with toothbrushing, increased menstrual flow, or blood in stool or urine.

Physical examination findings may include the manifestations shown in Figure 78-2. A complete head-to-toe assessment is performed. Clients with leukemia or blast crisis may have tachycardia, hypotension, tachypnea, murmurs or bruits, and increased capillary fill time resulting from low RBC counts. Skin and mucous membranes may

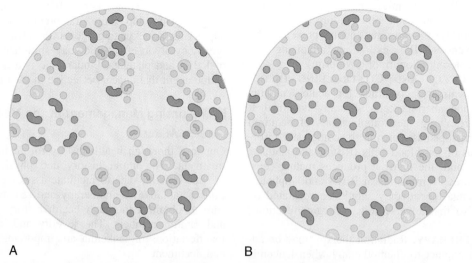

A   B

FIGURE 78-4 *A,* Microscopic view of a normal bone marrow specimen showing a normal distribution of blood cell types and fatty spaces. Blast cells appear as round, dark gray circles. *B,* During blast crisis, the number of blast cells increases and fatty spaces shrink.

show evidence of bruising and bleeding. Petechiae (small raised red spots) may be present. Lymph node enlargement may be present. If the leukemic cells have infiltrated the spleen or liver, abdominal tenderness may be noted. If the leukemic cells have infiltrated the brain, the client may be confused, have seizures, or become comatose.

The therapeutic relationship initiated during assessment is used to support the psychosocial needs of clients and their families. Leukemia is a life-threatening illness, and working with the client and family as a team is beneficial. Educating the client is an ongoing process to increase understanding of the disease and may help in obtaining compliance with treatment.

The nursing role during the acute phases of leukemia is extremely challenging because the client has many physical and psychosocial needs. Modern therapies offer hope for remission and possibly cure for some clients, but leukemia is still a diagnosis equated with pain, expensive long-term therapy, and potential death.

DIAGNOSIS, OUTCOMES, INTERVENTIONS

Risk for Sepsis. The diagnosis is written as *Risk for Sepsis related to neutropenia or leukocytosis secondary to leukemia or treatment.*

Outcomes. Infection will be prevented or will be discovered early and treated effectively, as evidenced by a neutrophil count greater than 1000/mm³, an absence of fever, and no respiratory difficulty.

Interventions. Institute required hand-washing for everyone coming in contact with the client. The client's risk for infection is estimated by calculating the absolute neutrophil count (ANC) (Box 78–1). The client should be in protective isolation if the ANC count is below 500/mm³. Visitors with possible communicable diseases should be screened for the presence of infection, and visitors or staff with colds or respiratory infections should not be allowed near the client. Avoid all live plants, flowers, and stuffed animals in the client's room.

The client should be on a low-bacteria diet that excludes raw fruits and vegetables. Assist the client with a daily bath using antimicrobial soap. Encourage the client to perform meticulous oral hygiene several times a day. Female clients should not douche and should avoid the use of tampons. Daily stool softeners are ordered to reduce the risk of anal fissures. Avoid insertion of rectal suppositories and rectal thermometers. Oral, axillary, or tympanic temperature should be taken every 4 hours and the physician notified if a temperature is higher than 38° C (100.5° to 101° F) or lower than 36° C (97° to 97.5° F). Fever may be the only manifestation in a neutropenic client. Assess the cause of fever before initiation of therapy by obtaining specimens of blood, sputum, urine, central line sites, and other potential sources of infection for culture.

Administer antibiotics as ordered. Therapy usually consists of multiple IV broad-spectrum antibiotics administered on alternating schedules. Administer analgesics as ordered for relief of discomfort, avoiding aspirin if the client is thrombocytopenic. Aspirin or aspirin-containing products also should be avoided because they may mask fever.

Invasive procedures should be avoided if possible. Provide meticulous skin decontamination before venipunc-tures. Maintain sterile occlusion of central venous catheters and perform routine dressing care according to institutional policy. Change IV tubing according to agency policy.

Monitor the client closely for manifestations of fungal or viral infections (i.e., increased respirations, rales, dyspnea, changed oral mucosa). Monitor the respiratory rate and auscultate breath sounds regularly. Viral and fungal pneumonia are common causes of death in the neutropenic client.

Risk for Hemorrhage. The client eventually becomes thrombocytopenic because of the progression of the disease or because of chemotherapy treatment, leading to the nursing diagnosis of *Risk for Hemorrhage related to thrombocytopenia secondary to either leukemia or treatment.*

Outcomes. Bleeding as a result of injuries, such as falls, punctures, cuts, or other environmental hazards, will be prevented or will be diagnosed and treated successfully, as evidenced by absence of bleeding and a platelet count greater than 20,000/mm³.

Interventions. Institute bleeding precautions, as follows:

- Provide soft toothbrushes or nonimpregnated cotton swabs or sponges for oral hygiene; avoid flossing, hard toothbrushes, and commercial mouthwashes.

BOX 78–1   Determining the Absolute Neutrophil Count

A leading complication in oncology clients is infection, and to recognize this risk, the absolute neutrophil count (ANC) is calculated daily. The ANC (or granulocyte count) provides a numeric estimate of the client's immune status, risk for bacterial infection, and need for reverse isolation. For example, the client with leukemia may have a high white blood cell (WBC) count or a normal count. On calculating the ANC, however, you may find that the client is at high risk for infection. For example, if a client had a WBC count of 9000 mm³, composed of 10% segmented neutrophils (segs), 60% blast cells, and 30% other WBCs, this client would have an increased risk of infection because the functional neutrophils are only 900.

Three numbers are required:

- Banded neutrophil count
- Segmented neutrophil count
- Total WBC

Obtain these numbers from the complete blood cell count and differential. The total WBC count is composed of five types of cells; the results from the laboratory show the total count and the percentage of each WBC type. For example, on the differential counts, the value next to monocytes represents the percentage of monocytes among the total number of WBCs.

Then use the following formula to calculate the ANC:

$$(\% \text{ band} + \% \text{ segs}) \times \text{total WBC count} = \text{ANC}$$

Example:

$$(2\% \text{ bands} + 55\% \text{ segs}) \times 1600 = 912$$

When the ANC is less than 1000, the client is at risk for bacterial infection.

When the ANC count is less than 500, the client is at high risk for bacterial infection.

- Instruct the client to avoid blowing or picking the nose, straining at bowel movements, douching or using tampons, or using nonelectric razors. Men and women should use only electric razors to shave with during the neutropenic phase.
- Do not give any injections, intramuscularly or subcutaneously, and do not insert rectal suppositories.
- Do not give medications containing aspirin, and instruct the client to avoid aspirin-containing medications.
- Avoid urinary catheters whenever possible. If a catheter must be inserted, use the smallest size possible, lubricate it well, and insert it gently.
- Avoid mucosal trauma during suctioning. Remove all potential hazards and sharp objects from the environment.
- Use a pressure-reducing mattress, and turn the client frequently to prevent pressure sores. Use bed cradles to protect extremities.
- Avoid overinflation of the blood pressure cuff, and rotate the cuff to different sites. Avoid prolonged use of tourniquets.
- Use only paper tape, and avoid strong adhesives that may cause skin adhesions.

Teach the client and significant others or family members to institute bleeding precautions during periods of thrombocytopenia. Monitor the client at least every 4 hours for manifestations of bleeding, such as ecchymosis, petechiae, epistaxis, gingival bleeding, hematuria, occult blood in stools, enlarged abdominal girth, disorientation, confusion, and changes in level of consciousness. All urine, stools, and emesis should be tested for blood. Take and record vital signs routinely, noting manifestations of altered tissue perfusion related to anemia (increased respirations and pulse, decreased blood pressure).

Check the platelet count, hemoglobin level, and hematocrit daily. Report a hemoglobin level of less than 10 g/dl and a platelet count of less than 20,000/mm³. Administer packed RBCs and platelets as ordered. Keep a current blood sample in the laboratory for crossmatching if needed in an emergency.

Fatigue. Fatigue is a common complaint by clients. It may be cumulative, a gradually worsening response to treatments for cancer, low hematocrit, low hemoglobin, altered blood glucose levels, decreased oxygen saturation levels, abnormal electrolyte levels, or unintentional weight loss. Fatigue is the greatest about 2 to 3 days after IV chemotherapy. The nursing diagnosis is written *Fatigue related to side effects of treatments, low hemoglobin levels, pain, lack of sleep, or other causes* as made evident by the client. A scale to rate fatigue numerically is used, such as the Piper Fatigue Scale (see Chapter 22).

Outcomes. The client will report less fatigue, plan adequate rest periods, and be able to do an increasing amount of usual activities with decreasing assistance from others.

Interventions. Assess the physical, psychological, and treatment-related causes of fatigue. Encourage exercise to maintain strength. Ask a physical therapist to assist with bed and strengthening exercises. An occupational therapist may be able to offer suggestions or devices to conserve energy. If the client has thrombocytopenia or fever or has just received chemotherapy (past 24 hours), exer-

cise is not encouraged to avoid injury. If possible, administer cisplatin and interferon at night to reduce the fatigue. Advocate for adequate pain relief, minimizing interruptions and reducing visitors when rest is needed. Outpatient chemotherapy is best scheduled on Fridays for clients who continue to work allowing them to rest over the weekend.

Altered Nutrition. The client usually experiences decreased appetite and decreased nutritional intake as a result of the effects of radiation therapy and chemotherapy on the GI tract. Write the diagnosis as *Altered Nutrition: Less Than Body Requirements related to anorexia, pain or fatigue.*

Outcomes. The client will maintain adequate nutrition, maintain body weight, as evidenced by stable weight, adequate caloric intake, and maintenance of fluid and electrolyte balance.

Interventions. Administer antiemetics, as ordered, around the clock to prevent nausea and vomiting. Premedicate the client with sufficient antiemetics before meals to encourage food and fluid intake. Administer local and IV analgesics, as ordered, to relieve pain caused by mucositis.

Discuss daily dietary requirements with the client and provide high-carbohydrate meals and oral supplements. Allow the client to make food selections. Cold foods, shakes, and sandwiches are tolerated better than hot or spicy foods. Small, frequent feedings may be tolerated better than three large meals a day. Monitor weight daily. If the client cannot tolerate food for an extended period, begin total parenteral nutrition (TPN), as ordered, and monitor intake. The client's own digestive system should be used as long as possible, with TPN used as a last resort. Use antidiarrheal agents as needed to treat diarrhea. Coordinate and plan rest periods and activities of daily living in increments as needed to minimize fatigue.

Body Image Disturbance. Most clients experience body image disturbance. The nursing diagnosis is written as *Body Image Disturbance due to alopecia, weight loss, and fatigue.*

Outcomes. The client will be able to demonstrate and discuss understanding of the disease condition and the temporary nature of changes in body image and energy.

Interventions. Inform the client before treatment of the potential for hair loss over the entire body. Encourage the use of scarves, hats, or wigs as desired. Explain the temporary nature of alopecia, although the hair may have a different color or texture when it returns.

Encourage the client to balance rest with exercise and activities to maintain muscle tone without developing severe fatigue. Discuss daily dietary requirements with the client, and provide high-carbohydrate meals and oral supplements in an attempt to help clients maintain their body weight and an appearance that is acceptable to them.

Risk for Reproductive or Sexual Dysfunction. Many clients experience reproductive or sexual dysfunction. The nursing diagnosis is written *Reproductive and/or Sexual Dysfunction related to the effects of chemotherapy or radiation therapy on reproductive organs.*

Outcomes. The client will be able to discuss the potential for sterility and decreased libido that may result from therapy.

Interventions. Describe the normal cellular destruction that might lead to temporary or permanent destruction of reproductive function in the client. Inform the client that sexual libido may be altered during and after the acute phase of the illness because of fatigue or other side effects of therapy. Provide the client with emotional support and references to support groups. Provide manuals for alternative sexual positioning and techniques. In appropriate cases, inform the client of reproductive alternatives, such as sperm banking and artificial insemination.

Risk for Ineffective Management of Therapeutic Regimen (Individuals) and Risk for Ineffective Management of Therapeutic Regimen: Families. Because hospital lengths of stay have become shorter and many oncology clients receive their care in outpatient settings, there is *Risk for Ineffective Management of Therapeutic Regimen (Individuals) and Risk for Ineffective Management of Therapeutic Regimen: Families* related to the chronic nature of the disease process and the risk for complications.

Outcomes. The client and family will manage the therapeutic regimen, as evidenced by effective medication administration, an absence of infections, no hemorrhage, and the client's ability to remain independent at home.

Interventions. After the induction phase of therapy is completed successfully, the client frequently returns home to recover and await subsequent courses of therapy that may be given on an outpatient basis, if no serious complications arise. It is common for clients to return home with anemia and thrombocytopenia. They also may suffer from the residual effects of chemotherapy or radiation therapy, such as loss of appetite, nausea, and mucositis. Some clients find it difficult to leave the security of the hospital setting because of significantly altered body image, fatigue, and fear.

Teach the client and significant others how to recognize manifestations of complications as well as appropriate actions to take. Inform them of measures to ensure safety and to reduce risks of bleeding and infection. Provide phone numbers of nursing personnel they can call with questions and for suggestions for interventions. The client and family should be referred to an oncology clinical nurse specialist or case manager as soon as possible after diagnosis. These nurses often assist the client and family concerning the disease process, the planned treatment, and strategies for successful transition from the hospital to home and outpatient care.

EVALUATION

The desired outcome for the client with leukemia is that the disease will become a chronic condition that the client and family can cope with in a positive manner. If acute leukemia does not respond to therapy, the client's life expectancy is short.

■ Surgical Management

BONE MARROW TRANSPLANTATION

To achieve cure with acute leukemia, BMT is the current recommended treatment. Allogeneic BMT presents a treatment option for clients younger than 60 years of age who have a suitable HLA-matched donor. Transplantation performed during the first remission has a higher success rate than transplantation performed during repeated remissions or in the blast phase of chronic leukemia. BMT is discussed later in this chapter.

■ Modifications for Elderly Clients

Older clients are at greater risk for chronic leukemia. The treatment of chronic leukemia in older clients is less vigorous. BMT is an option in the elderly if they are otherwise fit and if their organ systems can endure the stress of the procedure. Some older adults with excellent physical and psychological functioning have done quite well with BMT.

LYMPHOMAS

Primary tumors originating from the lymphatic system were identified in 1932. Lymphoma is the most common tumor of the lymphoid system, with about 55,000 new cases diagnosed annually. Lymphomas are tumors of primary lymphoid tissue (thymus and bone marrow) or secondary tissue (lymph nodes, spleen, tonsils, and intestinal lymphoid tissue). Most lymphomas are neoplasms of secondary lymphoid tissue and involve mostly lymph nodes, the spleen, or both. Malignant lymphoid cells sometimes are found in circulating blood, indicating bone marrow involvement. The major subdivisions of malignant lymphomas are *Hodgkin's lymphoma* (*Hodgkin's disease* [HD]) and *non-Hodgkin's lymphoma* (NHL). Bone marrow involvement occurs more often in non-Hodgkin's lymphoma than in HD.

HODGKIN'S DISEASE

In 1832, Hodgkin described a disease characterized by relentless enlargement of lymph nodes beginning in the neck and spreading throughout the body. He also reported that biopsy tissue showed a distinctive large cell, called a *Reed and Sternberg cell,* for the scientists who named it. Today the disease is called *Hodgkin's disease* and is known to be cancer of the lymph, or a lymphoma. Incidence rates differ with respect to age, gender, geographic locations, and socioeconomic class. Approximately 7500 new cases of HD are diagnosed annually. The male-to-female ratio is 1.4:1.

In economically advantaged countries, the incidence of HD is bimodal, with the first peak occurring in the mid-20s and the second peak occurring after age 50. In economically underdeveloped countries, the overall incidence of HD is lower than in developed countries but the incidence of HD before age 15 is higher, with only a modest increase into young adulthood. The incidence in people older than age 60 is declining, probably because of improved diagnostic techniques that classify NHL more correctly.

Etiology

The exact cause of HD is unknown, although indirect evidence indicates a viral cause. The Epstein-Barr virus (EBV) is believed to be a causative agent. EBV-associated lymphomas are well documented in clients who have received organ transplants or who have an immunodeficiency disease. A two-fold to three-fold increase of HD is seen among clients who have a history of mononucleosis, a disease caused by EBV. Researchers have shown that 30% to 50% of HD specimens contained EBV genome fragments in the diagnostic Reed-Sternberg cells.

Some studies indicate a genetic predisposition for HD. The disease occurs more frequently in Jews and among first-degree relatives. Siblings were shown to have a two-fold to five-fold increased risk, and same-sex siblings have a nine-fold increased risk. An increased risk was found among parent-child pairs but not among spouses, suggesting a genetic rather than infectious cause. Research continues in an attempt to identify the genetic role in the development of HD.

Pathophysiology

Cancerous transformation occurs from a particular site in the lymph node. With continuing growth, the entire node becomes replaced, with zones of necrosis obscuring the normal nodular pattern. The mechanism of growth and spread of Hodgkin's disease remains unknown. Some have suggested that the disease progresses by extension to adjacent structures. It also may disseminate by the lymphatics because lymphoreticular cells inhabit all tissues of the body except the CNS. Hematologic spread also may occur, possibly by means of direct infiltration of blood vessels.

Clinical Manifestations

Clients often are asymptomatic and may present with painless lymphadenopathy. Enlarged lymph nodes most commonly are found in the supraclavicular, cervical, and mediastinal regions (Fig. 78–5). Local manifestations produced by lymphadenopathy usually are caused by pressure or obstruction. Involvement of the extremities can be manifested by pain, nerve irritation, and obliteration of the pulse. Clients may experience a nonproductive cough, with the chest radiograph revealing a mediastinal mass, which is present in 50% of clients.

Pericardial involvement can occur by direct invasion from mediastinal lymph nodes. This involvement can cause pericardial friction rub, pericardial effusion, and engorgement of neck veins. Other manifestations arise when enlarged lymph nodes obstruct or compress an adjacent structure (e.g., edema of the face, neck, and right arm secondary to superior vena cava compression or renal failure secondary to urethral obstruction).

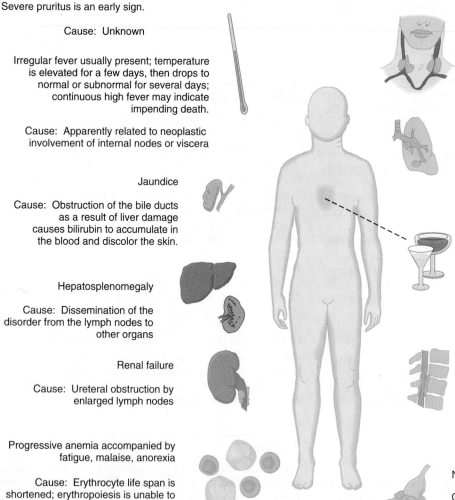

Severe pruritus is an early sign.

Cause: Unknown

Irregular fever usually present; temperature is elevated for a few days, then drops to normal or subnormal for several days; continuous high fever may indicate impending death.

Cause: Apparently related to neoplastic involvement of internal nodes or viscera

Jaundice

Cause: Obstruction of the bile ducts as a result of liver damage causes bilirubin to accumulate in the blood and discolor the skin.

Hepatosplenomegaly

Cause: Dissemination of the disorder from the lymph nodes to other organs

Renal failure

Cause: Ureteral obstruction by enlarged lymph nodes

Progressive anemia accompanied by fatigue, malaise, anorexia

Cause: Erythrocyte life span is shortened; erythropoiesis is unable to keep pace with erythrocyte destruction.

Edema and cyanosis of the face and neck

Cause: Enlarged lymph nodes place pressure on veins, obstructing drainage of this area.

Pulmonary symptoms including nonproductive cough, stridor, dyspnea, chest pain, cyanosis, and pleural effusion

Cause: Mediastinal lymph node enlargement, involvement of the lung parenchyma, and invasion of the pleura

Alcohol-induced pain in the bones, in involved lymph nodes, or around the mediastinum occurs immediately after drinking alcohol and lasts for 30 to 60 minutes.

Cause: Unknown

Bone pain, vertebral compression

Cause: Dissemination of disease from the lymph nodes to the bones

Paraplegia

Cause: Compression of the spinal cord resulting from extradural involvement

Nerve pain

Cause: Compression of the nerve roots of the brachial, lumbar, or sacral plexuses

FIGURE 78–5 Clinical manifestations and pathophysiologic bases of Hodgkin's disease.

If the tumor infiltrates the spine and presses on the spinal cord, manifestations of spinal cord compression can develop. Manifestations range from early back pain with motor weakness and sensory loss to loss of motor function, urinary retention, constipation, and other manifestations of compression of the cord late in the disease.

Associated clinical manifestations of unexplained weight loss of more than 10% of body weight in 6 months, frequent drenching night sweats, and fever above 38° C also may be present. Pruritus is a systemic manifestation that can be significant if it is recurrent. These additional manifestations are known as *B* symptoms for staging purposes; they occur in greater frequency in older clients and are negatively related to the prognosis.

The diagnosis is confirmed by lymph node and bone marrow biopsy. A chest radiograph to evaluate complaints of persistent cough or dyspnea may identify mediastinal involvement. The extent of disease is determined by CT scans of the thoracic, abdominal, and pelvic areas as well as gallium scans of mediastinal or hilar lymph nodes and lymphangiography of the lower extremities. If the extent of the disease cannot be determined by these diagnostic tests and confirmation of abdominal disease is necessary for determining treatment choice, a staging laparotomy may be performed.

STAGING

HD is divided into categories, or stages, according to the microscopic appearance of the involved lymph nodes, the extent and severity of the disorder, and the prognosis. Accurate staging of HD is important for determining treatment options. Table 78–2 shows the Cotswold Staging Classification, which modified the Ann Arbor classification system, primarily to incorporate the newer diagnostic tests and the evidence that bulky disease is an important prognostic indicator.

Outcome Management

Since the advent of combination chemotherapy, adult HD has become one of the most curable malignancies, resulting in a long-term survival rate of about 70%. The goal of therapy for clients with stage I and II disease is to achieve long-term disease-free survival with minimal acute and long-term complications that affect quality of life. Treatment consists of radiation therapy alone or combined with chemotherapy.

ERADICATION OF TUMOR CELLS

Radiation treatment for HD involves three locations: the mantle, the para-aortic region, and the pelvis (Fig. 78–6). The mantle field encompasses the submandibular, cervical, infraclavicular, axillary, mediastinal, subcarinal, and hilar lymph nodes. In clinical stage I and II disease, combined chemotherapy and radiation therapy are recommended for clients with unfavorable prognostic indicators. Most cancer centers classify B symptoms (fever, night sweats, and unexplained weight loss), high erythrocyte sedimentation rate (ESR), or large mediastinal adenopathy as poor prognostic factors. Some centers include large numbers of site involvement and older age as poor prognostic indicators.

Chemotherapy has become the primary treatment strategy, with or without radiation therapy, in stage I and II disease with poor prognostic indicators and in clients with

advanced HD. There are numerous chemotherapy regimens for HD. For years, MOPP (mechlorethamine, vincristine [oncovin], procarbazine, prednisone) was the gold standard of therapy; however, ABVD (doxorubicin [Adriamycin], bleomycin, vinblastine, dacarbazine) has emerged as the best alternative to MOPP. The primary advantages of ABVD are its ease of delivery in full doses, fewer side effects, and less risk of subsequent development of leukemia. With proper treatment, the 20-year disease-free survival rate of HD is 70% to 80% and the overall survival rate, with salvage chemotherapy for clients who relapse, is 80% to 95%.

Research has shown that clients with advanced stage disease (II and IV) may achieve better treatment results with MOPP plus ABVD than with MOPP alone. Other studies showed that ABVD alone can achieve results similar to MOPP plus ABVD. Many physicians recommend ABVD alone given for as many cycles as required to achieve a complete remission, plus two consolidation cycles (usually six cycles total). The use of radiation therapy in advanced disease is individualized to the client, especially those with local-regional disease problems.

Clients who relapse after definitive HD therapy generally require some type of systemic therapy, which depends on the type of initial therapy used. Therapies range from chemotherapy and wide-field radiation to high-dose chemotherapy with autologous or allogeneic stem cell

TABLE 78–2	COTSWOLD STAGING CLASSIFICATION FOR HODGKIN'S DISEASE
Stage I	Involvement of a single lymph node region or a lymphoid structure (e.g., spleen, thymus, Waldeyer's ring)
Stage II	Involvement of two or more lymph node regions on the same side of the diaphragm (i.e., the mediastinum is a single site, hilar lymph nodes are lateralized). The number of anatomic sites should be indicated by a subscript (e.g., II$_2$)
Stage III	Involvement of lymph node regions or structures on both sides of the diaphragm: III$_1$: With or without involvement of splenic, hilar, celiac, or portal nodes III$_2$: With involvement of para-aortic, iliac, or mesenteric nodes.
Stage IV	Involvement of extranodal site(s) beyond that designated E.

DESIGNATION APPLICABLE TO ANY DISEASE STAGE

A	No manifestations
B	Fever, drenching sweats, weight loss (B symptoms)
X	Bulky disease: >$\frac{1}{3}$ the width of the mediastinum <10 cm maximal dimension of nodal mass
E	Involvement of a single extranodal site, contiguous or proximal to a known nodal site.
CS	Clinical stage
PS	Pathologic stage

Data from Bennett, J. C., et al. (1996). *Cecil textbook of medicine* (20th ed.). Philadelphia: W. B. Saunders.

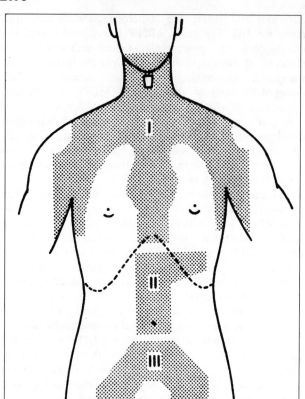

FIGURE 78–6 Radiation fields in therapy for Hodgkin's disease. *Shaded areas* represent the three treatment fields. The *mantle field* is the uppermost field (I). Lungs and vocal cords are protected by lead blocks; the heart and thyroid gland are within the field. The *para-aortic field,* or middle field (II), extends from the diaphragm to just above the bifurcation of the aorta. When the spleen has not been removed, this field is extended to include the entire spleen and splenic hilum. The *pelvic* or *inverted Y field* is the lowest field (III). It encompasses the pelvic and inguinal nodes and includes a large area of bone marrow. (From Murphy G. P., Lawrence, W., & Lenhard, R. E. [1995]. *American Cancer Society textbook of clinical oncology.* [2nd ed.]. Atlanta: American Cancer Society.)

transplant. Of clients with stages I to II HD, 20% to 30% relapse within 5 years after radiation therapy. In these cases, the use of combination chemotherapy produces a 57% to 62% disease-free survival at 10 years. At the National Cancer Institute, a 93% second complete remission rate was seen in clients with initial remissions longer than 12 months after chemotherapy. The positive results of several studies investigating the use of stem cell transplant have provided the basis for recommending bone marrow and stem cell transplantation for all HD clients who relapsed or did not respond to any primary chemotherapy, regardless of the length of the initial remission.

Complications

The complications related to HD are numerous because they are a result of the disease itself, radiation therapy, chemotherapy, or a combination of several of these factors (Table 78–3).

■ Nursing Management of the Medical Client

Obtain a thorough health history from the client and family members. The severity and longevity of the manifestations of lymphoma are important facts to obtain and document. Nurses play an essential role in symptom management associated with therapy. Because of the side effects of chemotherapy, clients may ask for a reduction of the dosage or may want to stop therapy completely. Provide clients with information regarding the effect of reducing or stopping therapy on long-term survival.

Explain to clients that they may have an impaired antibody response to vaccination. Clients who are projected to undergo chemotherapy are given *Haemophilus influenzae* type B, meningococcal, and pneumococcal vaccines before initiating therapy. Nurses are key to ensuring that these vaccines are provided at the appropriate time.

NON-HODGKIN'S LYMPHOMA

NHL comprises a group of malignancies with a common origin in the lymphoid cells. They are heterogeneous in cellular origin, morphologic appearance, and clinical behavior. The American Cancer Society estimates approximately 55,000 new cases of NHL annually and 25,000 related deaths in the United States.

NHL is seven times more common than HD. Between 1973 and 1991, there was a 73% increase in the incidence of NHL. Part of this increase was attributed to

TABLE 78–3	COMPLICATIONS OF HODGKIN'S DISEASE
Problem	**Cause**
Thyroid dysfunction Thymic hyperplasia	Underlying disease, therapy, or both
Hypothyroidism Thyroid cancer	Direct or indirect radiation exposure
Sexual dysfunction Male impotence Male and female infertility Female dyspareunia	Underlying disease, therapy, or both
Herpes zoster or varicella	Underlying disease, therapy, or both
Pulmonary dysfunction Pneumonitis (acute, chronic, or both)	Direct or indirect radiation exposure, bleomycin, nitrosoureas, radiation recall
Cardiac dysfunction Cardiomyopathy	Mediastinal radiation therapy, pericarditis (acute), doxorubicin, radiation recall
Pericarditis (chronic)	Mediastinal radiation therapy
Dental caries	Salivary changes related to radiation therapy
Myelodysplastic syndrome	Therapy, especially if age >40 yr or lymphocytic leukemia
Non-Hodgkin's lymphoma	Therapy
Solid tumors	Direct or indirect radiation exposure

acquired immunodeficiency syndrome (AIDS). NHL is about 60 times more common in people with AIDS than in the general population of the United States. NHL is the sixth most common cause of cancer-related deaths in the United States. Men are affected more often than women, and the incidence is higher in whites than other races. Survival outcomes are better for women than men and for people younger than 65 years of age. NHL can occur in any age group, but an increase in incidence occurs in the 50s and 60s. Because the average age at diagnosis is in the 50s, the number of years of life lost to these malignancies ranks NHL fourth in economic impact among cancers in the United States.

Etiology

No hereditary, ethnic, or dietary risk factors have been associated with NHL. An increased risk is associated with immunodeficiency states, autoimmune disorders, and infectious physical and chemical agents. As with HD, a viral or bacterial cause has been implicated (EBV, HTLV-1, human herpesvirus 8, *Helicobacter pylori*). A greater than expected incidence of NHL is reported in people with ataxia-telangiectasia, Wiskott-Aldrich syndrome, and Chédiak-Higashi syndrome.

Classifications

Terminology describing NHL is complex, inconsistent, and ambiguous, and there are several classifications. Rappaport's widely used classification, developed in 1956, distinguishes two major histopathologic patterns: nodular and diffuse (Table 78-4). These two patterns in NHL illustrate two different pathologic states. The nodular (and diffuse, well-differentiated lymphocytic) pattern involves nodal and extranodal sites. The diffuse pattern does not show the cell aggregates that are evident in the nodular pattern.

Based on expanding knowledge of the lymphatic system physiology, six distinct classification systems emerged worldwide in the 1970s. To standardize terminology, the Revised European-American Lymphoma (REAL) classification system was proposed in 1994. This classification includes all lymphoma types and the extra-nodal lymphomas not included in the other classification systems.

TABLE 78-4	RAPPAPORT STAGING CLASSIFICATION
Grade	**Characteristics**
Low grade	Diffuse, lymphocytic, well differentiated
	Nodular, lymphocytic, poorly differentiated
	Nodular, mixed, lymphocytic and histiocytic
Intermediate grade	Nodular, histiocytic
	Diffuse, lymphocytic
	Diffuse, mixed, lymphocytic and histiocytic
High grade	Diffuse, histiocytic
	Diffuse, lymphoblastic
	Diffuse, undifferentiated

Pathophysiology

In clients with NHL, an abnormal proliferation of neoplastic lymphocytes occurs. The cells remain fixed at one phase of development and continue to proliferate. Both T and B lymphocytes mature in the lymph nodes. Clinical manifestations are due to mechanical obstruction of the enlarged lymph nodes. Lymphocytic infiltration of the abdomen or oropharynx also can occur.

Clinical Manifestations

Clients with NHL present with localized or generalized lymphadenopathy. The cervical, axillary, inguinal, and femoral chains are the most frequent sites of lymph node enlargement. The swelling is generally painless, and the nodes have enlarged and transformed over months or years. Extranodal sites of involvement are the nasopharynx, GI tract, bone, thyroid, testes, and soft tissue. Some clients have retroperitoneal and abdominal masses with abdominal fullness, back pain, ascites (fluid in the peritoneal cavity), and leg swelling.

Several sites of involvement in NHL are not common in HD, such as Waldeyer's ring (lymphoid tissue that encircles the tonsils), the stomach, the small and large bowel, mesenteric lymph nodes, the thyroid, the skin, the pancreas, the kidneys, and the CNS. With diffuse NHL, clinical manifestations are variable and generally involve more systemic findings. Clients also may experience systemic *B* symptoms, including night sweats, fever, and weight loss. Approximately one third of clients have hepatomegaly or splenomegaly.

Certain other clinical conditions mimic the malignant lymphomas, including tuberculosis, syphilis, systemic lupus erythematosus, lung cancer, and bone cancer. A thorough diagnostic evaluation is required.

Diagnostic Findings

Blood work includes a CBC, ESR, and peripheral smear to rule out other causes of lymphadenopathy, such as mononucleosis. Blood cultures and other serologic studies for viral and autoimmune diseases provide important differential information. Elevated lactate dehydrogenase (LDH) levels may be seen in advanced NHL.

A lymph node biopsy is an important diagnostic tool. Indications for biopsy are

- Adenopathy for longer than 3 weeks, which progresses in size or spreads to other areas
- *B* symptoms that cannot be attributed to other causes
- Abnormal blood test results indicative of lymphoma
- Radiographs that suggest possible extranodal involvement

Because of the aggressive nature of AIDS-related NHL, any symptomatic client at increased risk or known to be positive for human immunodeficiency virus (HIV) should have a biopsy to rule out high-grade lymphoma.

Just as in HD, once the diagnosis of NHL is made, disease staging should take place. Noninvasive imaging techniques, such as CT and MRI, are useful tools in the initial staging of NHL. Renal and liver function tests are performed to determine the presence of extranodal involvement. Bilateral bone marrow biopsies are important because metastasis to the bone marrow is common, especially in low-grade disease.

Outcome Management

Many classification systems are used to differentiate NHL according to histologic type and cytologic characteristics. Treatment varies based on the histology and stage of the tumor. The treatment of a low-grade lymphoma is different from that for high-grade disease. Low-grade tumors tend to progress slowly and often are asymptomatic for long periods; the natural course of the disease may fluctuate considerably over 5 to 10 years with or without treatment. Low-grade cells eventually transform into a more aggressive disease process, however, and quickly cause the death of the client. Because of this process, indolent NHL is believed to be incurable, and many controversies exist concerning treatment standards, especially in clients who have disseminated disease.

The progression of intermediate-grade and high-grade lymphomas is similar to that of other cancers. Because of their higher growth fraction, however, these tumors tend to be more sensitive to chemotherapy and radiation therapy; there is a higher response rate when these tumors are treated. Combination chemotherapy is used to produce tumor shrinkage and remission. Cyclophosphamide and doxorubicin are active against lymphoma. Various combination drug regimens that include these two drugs are used in the treatment of NHL. Controversy regarding first-line standard of care therapy still exists. Studies comparing various treatment protocols affirmed the practice of using CHOP (cyclophosphamide, hydroxydaunorubicin [doxorubicin], vincristine [oncovin], prednisone) as first-line therapy in many academic and community settings.

For clients with low-grade NHL in stage I to II, radiation therapy alone may be curative, although there are reports of recurrence past 10 years. Depending on whether the disease is supradiaphragmatic or subdiaphragmatic, single-mode therapy includes mantle and inverted Y field irradiation (see Fig. 78–6). Management of stage III to IV low-grade lymphoma with any therapy is controversial. In clients who are asymptomatic, a watch-and-wait approach may be used. In some studies comparing clients treated with aggressive initial chemotherapy versus those using watchful waiting, the disease-free survival at 4 years was striking (51% in the treatment group versus 12% in the observed clients). There was no difference in the overall survival of the groups, however. Such findings contribute to the ongoing confusion as to the best initial treatment of such clients.

Clients with stage III to IV intermediate-grade lymphoma require combination chemotherapy as an immediate intervention. Clients who are older than 60 years of age and have elevated LDH levels, poor performance status, and stage III to IV intermediate disease are at higher risk and should be offered aggressive regimens that provide higher-dose intensities.

The diagnosis of a high-grade NHL warrants immediate and aggressive treatment. Clients may present with rapidly growing disease that has the potential to double in bulk in days or hours. Treatment includes dose-intense chemotherapy, with or without radiation therapy, and prophylactic CNS therapy. It is necessary to provide prophylaxis for the CNS because the blood-brain barrier prevents chemotherapy from getting into CNS spaces. Without such treatment, lymphoma cells may look for "sanctuary" in the CNS (CNS metastasis). High-grade NHL clients also are excellent candidates for bone marrow or stem cell transplantation because the tumors respond dramatically to high-dose chemotherapy, which is part of the preparative regimen of transplant.

Many clients (30% to 60%) with NHL do not achieve a complete remission and require salvage therapy to control the disease; however, none of the salvage therapies offer the client more than a small likelihood of surviving another 24 months after treatment. Biologic response modifiers (BRMs) and monoclonal antibodies (rituximab) have been used with varied success.

■ Nursing Management of the Medical Client
ASSESSMENT

Although the appearance of an enlarged lymph node in the absence of infection may cause worry, 56% of healthy adults may experience cervical adenopathy. Any enlargement of lymph nodes warrants further evaluation.

The work-up for NHL begins with a thorough history and physical examination. On examination, lymph nodes involved in infectious processes may be tender or painful, whereas lymphomatous nodes tend to be firm and "rubbery" and are found in generalized patterns. Carcinomatous nodes often are hard and sometimes matted to one another or fixed to underlying structures in contiguous or regional patterns. Other hallmarks of lymphoma, such as systemic *B* symptoms (fever, night sweats, unexplained weight loss), are seen in 20% to 30% of clients, but these manifestations also may be seen in other disease states, such as certain infections and connective tissue diseases.

The heterogeneous nature of NHL challenges nurses to meet a variety of physical and psychosocial needs for both clients and their families. The client and family members are confronted with managing a demanding diagnosis and treatment and the effects of the disease on daily routines. Health care professionals often assume that clients with supportive families manage well, but family members do share the strain of the illness, are deeply affected (psychologically, financially, and perhaps physically), and need ongoing support. It is crucial that nurses adapt their plans of care for these clients along the disease trajectory which can wax and wane for many years.

DIAGNOSIS, OUTCOMES, INTERVENTIONS

The nursing diagnosis, outcomes, and interventions for HD and NHL are the same as those for the client with leukemia.

Nursing Diagnoses. These clients are *At Risk for Sepsis, At Risk of Bleeding* (as a result of thrombocytopenia secondary to treatment), *At Risk for Sexual/Reproductive Dysfunction,* prone to *Altered Nutrition,* and *At Risk for Ineffective Management of Therapeutic Regimen* (Individuals and Families).

Outcomes. The desired outcome for the client with lymphoma is that the disease will become a chronic condition that the client and family can cope with in a positive manner. If the disease becomes terminal, the outcome should include a death with dignity, in which comfort measures and psychological support are emphasized.

Interventions. Interventions for these problems were discussed previously for leukemic clients.

EVALUATION

Physiologic problems may resolve quickly with medication. Psychological diagnosis will require prolonged intervention.

BONE MARROW TRANSPLANTATION

Since the 1970s, BMT has progressed from a treatment of last resort to a viable therapeutic modality for a variety of hematologic, malignant, and nonmalignant disorders. Peripheral stem cell transplantation and autologous transplants have further revolutionized the field. The status of the disease to be treated by BMT is an important determinant of the outcome for the client. When BMT is performed in clients with acute leukemia in full relapse, the disease-free survival rates approximate 15%, whereas BMT mortality falls dramatically in clients with chemotherapy-induced remission.

INDICATIONS

Bone marrow transplant may be considered as a treatment for clients with the following:

- Aplastic anemia
- Malignant disorders, specifically myelodysplastic syndromes, leukemia (certain types of acute leukemic, chronic leukemic, and preleukemic states), lymphoma, multiple myeloma, neuroblastoma, and selected solid tumors (breast cancer, ovarian cancer, testicular cancer, poor-risk germ cell tumors)
- Nonmalignant hematologic disorders, such as Fanconi's anemia, thalassemia, and sickle cell anemia
- Immunodeficiency disorders, such as severe combined immunodeficiency disease and Wiskott-Aldrich syndrome

BONE MARROW HARVESTING

Sources of Bone Marrow

There are three types of bone marrow donors: (1) allogeneic, (2) syngeneic, and (3) autologous.

ALLOGENEIC BONE MARROW. Allogeneic bone marrow is obtained from a relative or unrelated donor having a close HLA type. This was the most common type of marrow transplant but it carried the highest rate of morbidity and mortality because of complications of incompatibility such as graft-versus-host disease (GVHD). The rate of allogeneic transplants has dropped with the drop in the birth rate and the increased use of autologous and peripheral stem cell transplants.

SYNGENEIC BONE MARROW. Syngeneic marrow is donated by an identical twin. Although syngeneic marrow is a perfect HLA match, which eliminates the risks of marrow rejection, the incidence of leukemic relapse is higher than when an allogeneic donor is used because GVHD is considered to have an antileukemic effect.

AUTOLOGOUS BONE MARROW. Autologous marrow is removed from the intended recipient during the remission phase to allow another course of ablative therapy to be given if a relapse occurs. Although autologous marrow eliminates the risk of adverse immunologic responses, such as GVHD and graft rejection, relapse after autologous BMT is a frequent occurrence. This relapse may be due to contamination of the harvested bone marrow by malignant cells or to failure of pretransplant chemotherapy to eradicate completely the tumor cells from the body. The role of techniques used to purge residual tumor cells from marrow (chemotherapy, monoclonal antibodies) remains uncertain because of the absence of controlled trials.

Histocompatibility Testing for Allogeneic and Syngeneic Transplantation

Immunologic recognition of the differences in HLA antigens is the first step in host transplant rejection. The HLA system antigens are a complex set of protein structures found on the surface membrane of all human nucleated cells, solid tissues, and circulating blood cells except red blood cells. This genetically inherited mixture of antigens is considered representative of the tissue type of each person.

Siblings have a 1 in 4 chance of having identical sets of HLA antigens. This situation would provide the optimally matched allogeneic bone marrow donor. Because of the complexity of the HLA system, nonrelated clients have less than a 1 in 5000 chance of having identical HLA types. The establishment of the National Bone Marrow Donor Program (NMDP) in 1986 has given hope to many clients who do not have a compatible relative donor. As of June 2000, approximately 1 million donors are listed in the NMDP's registry, with about 25,000 new volunteer donors added to the registry every month. This has increased the use of unrelated donors for allogeneic transplants.

ALLOGENEIC DONOR PREPARATION

An extensive work-up is performed for ensuring compatibility and the mental and physical well-being of the prospective donor. This evaluation includes histocompatibility testing, medical history, physical examination, chest film, ECG, laboratory evaluation (complete blood count, chemistry profile, viral testing, rapid plasma reagin test [syphilis], ABO and Rh blood typing, coagulation studies), and psychological testing (may include psychiatric consultation).

Before marrow harvest, an informed consent, including potential donor complications (pain, fever, hematoma), must be obtained. In rare instances, the donor may experience serious adverse effects from general anesthesia. Because of the potential for significant blood loss during the harvesting process, syngeneic and allogeneic donors are required to donate autologous blood for reinfusion before the procedure.

Newborns currently are being used as potential donors through the use of their cord blood, which is rich in stem cells. Some parents are being encouraged to freeze their newborn's cord blood for future use, especially if there is a history of cancer in the family.

Marrow Collection

When collecting marrow, the client or donor is given general or spinal anesthesia in the operating room. The marrow is obtained in 2- to 5-ml aliquots from the marrow spaces of the posterior and, occasionally, anterior iliac crest and sternum. Numerous skin punctures may be required; the aspiration needle is redirected to various marrow spaces without being withdrawn. A total of 400 to 800 ml of marrow usually is obtained. The blood is placed in heparinized tissue culture media and filtered for removal of fat and bone particles. Marrow can be infused immediately or frozen in a solution containing dimethyl sulfoxide (DMSO), which preserves stem cells in the frozen state.

Peripheral Stem Cell Collection

Peripheral stem (progenitor) cells are harvested by apheresis or leukapheresis, a process that removes blood through a large-bore catheter and runs it through a machine that removes the stem cells before returning the blood to the client. Because stem cell concentration is much lower in peripheral blood compared with bone marrow, a process to increase the concentration in the peripheral blood must be initiated first. To increase the number of circulating stem cells, a stimulus, such as a colony-stimulating factor (CSF), interleukins (ILs), fusion molecules (made from a combination of a CSF and IL-3), or some chemotherapeutic agents, may be given to the donor before the stem cell harvest. As mentioned earlier, the umbilical cord of newborns also is rich in stem cells.

Once the stem cells are harvested, they are preserved in the same manner as bone marrow. The engraftment of stem cells occurs at approximately the same rate as or slightly faster than with marrow transplantation.

ALLOGENEIC TRANSPLANT

Recipient Preparation

The physical and psychological evaluation of the recipient is similar to that of the donor. Additional testing may be required to stage existing disease accurately. The recipient must undergo a preparative regimen before transplantation. Such a regimen serves three purposes:

1. Malignant cells are destroyed.
2. The immune system is inactivated, which reduces the risk of GVHD in allogeneic transplant clients.
3. The marrow cavities are emptied to provide space for implantation of the transfused stem cells.

Common protocols combine total body irradiation and high doses of a single chemotherapeutic agent (cyclophosphamide is one of the most common agents used) or fractionated/high doses of multiple agents. A multilumen central venous catheter is inserted to provide suitable access for marrow infusion as well as for antibiotics, blood products, hyperalimentation, and frequent blood sampling.

Bone Marrow Infusion

The infusion of the marrow is commonly anticlimactic after the client has undergone the rigorous preparatory chemotherapy and radiation therapy (often referred to as the *conditioning regimen*). The marrow usually is administered immediately after the conditioning regimen is complete. Marrow is administered from a large blood infusion bag by a multilumen catheter, using an infusion pump, or small volumes may be prefiltered and given by IV push by a physician.

The BMT client remains pancytopenic until the transplanted stem cells make their way to the medullary cavities, where subsequent growth and reconstitution of the marrow are confirmed. Indications of successful engraftment are an increase in platelets and RBCs in the peripheral blood count. This change may occur 14 days after marrow infusion. Each day that recovery is delayed places the client at added risk. Graft rejection is evident if the bone marrow fails to produce peripheral blood cells after several weeks.

◼ Nursing Management

Nursing management of BMT clients follows the plan of care for any completely immunosuppressed client. Clients receiving allogeneic transplants must be observed closely for manifestations of GVHD. Potential immediate adverse reactions are allergic (urticaria, chills, fever), volume overload, and pulmonary complications secondary to fat emboli. Renal damage may occur from too many erythrocytes. The period immediately after transplant is crucial. Multisystem failure related to ablative therapy is common, as are immune reactions caused by the transplanted cells.

GRAFT-VERSUS-HOST DISEASE

The most common and potentially disastrous complication of allogeneic BMT is GVHD, which may occur 7 to 30 days after infusion of viable lymphocytes. The donor T lymphocytes form an immunologic reaction against the host cells. The clients at highest risk for development of GVHD are those who have had allogeneic BMT. Of those clients, risk is greatest when the donor mismatched two to three antigens and when the client is older than age 30 years. There remains a moderate risk (35% to 50% incidence) in clients who have HLA-identical donors.

ACUTE GRAFT-VERSUS-HOST DISEASE

Acute GVHD is staged according to the organ system affected (Table 78–5). It usually affects the gut, skin, lungs, or liver. *Stage I* GVHD occurs in many allogeneic transplant clients. Skin manifestations may resolve without treatment. Systemic complications may be treated with immunosuppressive drug therapy.

Therapy for GVHD includes high doses of methylprednisolone, antithymocyte globulin, antilymphocyte globulin, cyclosporine, and anti–T cell immunotoxins. These also leave the client immunosuppressed and vulnerable to infection. The prognosis and treatment depend on the severity of the syndrome. Acute GVHD that does not respond to treatment greatly increases the morbidity and mortality of BMT.

Nursing management of clients with stage I GVHD is shown in the Care Plan.

TABLE 78–5	STAGES OF ACUTE GRAFT-VERSUS-HOST DISEASE		
Stage	**Skin Manifestations**	**Liver Manifestations**	**Gastrointestinal Manifestations**
1	Maculopapular rash >25% body surface area	Bilirubin 2–3 mg/dl	Diarrhea 500–1000 ml/day
2	Maculopapular rash 25%–50% body surface area	Bilirubin 3–6 mg/dl	Diarrhea 1000–1500 ml/day
3	Generalized erythroderma	Bilirubin 6–15 mg/dl	Diarrhea >1500 ml/day
4	Desquamation and bullae	Bilirubin >15 mg/dl	Abdominal pain or ileus

■ THE CLIENT WITH STAGE I GRAFT-VERSUS-HOST DISEASE

Nursing Diagnosis: Risk for Injury related to graft-versus-host disease

Outcome: Client exhibits resolution of early graft-versus-host disease (GVHD) as evidenced by healing of skin, return of liver functions to normal, resolution of diarrhea and abdominal cramping, normal serum electrolytes, and control of pain.

Interventions	Rationales
1. Assess client's or significant other's knowledge of GVHD.	1. The client or significant other also can monitor for clinical manifestations and by reporting them early enhance treatment.
2. Teach client or significant other about the early manifestations of GVHD and to report them: a. Erythematosus rash on palms, soles, ears and trunk b. Anorexia, abdominal cramping, diarrhea, nausea, vomiting	2. Client is ambulatory and may not recognize the need to report these data to the nurse.
3. Determine baseline status or skin condition, liver function (alkaline phosphatase, bilirubin), and gastrointestinal function before donor marrow infusion.	3. Baseline data guide assessments of further data.
4. Assess for manifestations of GVHD at day 25 post-transplant.	4. The median onset time of GVHD is 25 days after bone marrow transplant.
5. Administer prescribed preventive agents.	5. Medications such as methotrexate and cyclosporine are used to suppress response.
6. Monitor magnesium levels daily.	6. Cyclosporine can induce seizures in hypomagnesemic clients.
7. Monitor renal function daily.	7. Bilirubin levels rise in GVHD.
8. Irradiate all blood products before infusing.	8. Irradiation prevents the infusion of immunocompetent T lymphocytes.
9. Bathe daily in warm saline or warm Hibiclens solution diluted to 1:8 with sterile water. Pat skin dry.	9. Skin care is important to reduce the risk of infection and avoid injury to the skin.
10. Apply prescribed lotions to the moist skin after bathing.	10. Keeping the skin moist reduces the risk of cracks, which increase the risk of infection.
11. Monitor characteristics of stools. If diarrhea develops, keep the client on NPO (nothing by mouth). Administer antidiarrheal agents, and test all stools for blood.	11. Diarrhea is a manifestation of GVHD. Blood loss through stool may require transfusion for replacement.
12. Monitor intake and output strictly, and record daily weights.	12. GVHD can lead to dehydration. Clients receiving chemotherapeutic agents need ample fluids during administration to prevent renal damage.

CHRONIC GRAFT-VERSUS-HOST DISEASE

Chronic GVHD, a long-term form of the disease with less acute manifestations, may occur even if the client has not experienced acute GVHD. Chronic GVHD appears approximately 100 days after transplantation; it may affect the liver, GI system, oral mucosa, and lungs as well as the skin. Chronic GVHD resembles autoimmune collagen-vascular disorders, such as systemic lupus erythematosus. It is characterized by scleroderma-like skin fibrosis and Sjögren's syndrome, in which the mucosa and lacrimal ducts are abnormally dry.

Diagnosis of chronic GVHD is confirmed by skin and oral mucosal biopsy. Although severe GVHD usually is fatal, researchers believe that a complete absence of this immune reaction increases the risk of leukemic relapse. This situation may be due to a beneficial graft-versus-leukemic reaction that mild GVHD stimulates. In allogeneic BMT recipients with GVHD stages II through IV, the relapse rate is 2.5 times lower than in syngeneic recipients or allogeneic recipients without GVHD.

CONCLUSIONS

Leukemia and lymphoma are complex diseases affecting physiologic and psychological aspects of the client and the family. Nursing care focuses on protecting the client from infection resulting from loss of WBC function, protection from hemorrhage resulting from loss of platelet function, and protection from hypoxia resulting from loss of RBC function.

THINKING CRITICALLY

1. **A 68-year-old woman is admitted with acute nonlymphocytic leukemia (ANLL). She is receiving chemotherapy. Her white blood cell count is 1000; 3% are banded neutrophils, and 54% are segmented neutrophils. What, if any, precautions are needed?**

Factors to Consider. How is her risk of sepsis determined? Why does body temperature serve as one marker of infection? What precautions are followed?

2. **A 34-year-old man with acute myelogenous leukemia comes to the outpatient oncology facility for his second round of chemotherapy. Three days later, the client calls the clinic nurse and is complaining of bleeding gums. What is the priority problem you should address? What instructions should the clinic nurse give the client at this time?**

Factors to Consider. What pathologic process underlies the client's manifestations? Are there laboratory results you would want to check? What other precautions should you institute on the basis of the client's other manifestations and the laboratory data? What other data are significant to collect at this time?

BIBLIOGRAPHY

1. Bean, C. A. (1997). Acute lymphocytic leukemia: Nursing care, psychosocial issues, and discharge education. *Oncology Nursing Forum, 24*(6), 961–962.
2. Bilodeau, B. A., & Fessele, K. L. (1998). Non-Hodgkin's lymphoma. *Seminars in Oncology Nursing, 14*(4), 273–283.
3. Buchsel, P. C., Leum, E. W., & Randolph, S. R. (1996). Delayed complications of bone marrow transplantation: An update. *Oncology Nursing Forum, 23*(8),1267–1291.
4. Coleman, S. (1995). Bone marrow transplantation: Issues for critical care nurses: An overview of the oral complications of adult patients with malignant hematological conditions who have undergone radiotherapy or chemotherapy. *Journal of Advanced Nursing (England), 22*(6), 1085–1091.
5. Courtens, A. M., & Abu-Saad, H. H. (1998). Nursing diagnoses in patients with leukemia. *Nursing Diagnosis, 9*(2), 49–61.
6. De Meyer, E. S., Fletcher, M. A., & Buchsel, P. C. (1997). Management of dermatologic complications of chronic graft versus host disease: A case study. *Clinical Journal of Oncology Nursing, 1*(4), 95–104.
7. Ezzone, S. A. (1999). Tumor lysis syndrome. *Seminars in Oncology Nursing, 15*(3), 202–208.
8. Fernsler, J., & Fanuele, J. S. (1998). Lymphomas: Long-term sequelae and survivorship issues. *Seminars in Oncology Nursing, 14*(4), 321–328.
9. Hays, K., & McCartney, S. (1998). Nursing care of the patient with chronic lymphocytic leukemia. *Seminars in Oncology, 25*(1), 75–79.
10. Hogan, D. K., & Rosenthal, L. D. (1998). Oncologic emergencies in the patient with lymphoma. *Seminars in Oncology Nursing, 14*(4), 312–320.
11. Hurley, C. (1997). Ambulatory care after bone marrow or peripheral blood stem cell transplantation. *Clinical Journal of Oncology Nursing, 1*(1), 19–21.
12. Johns, A. (1998). Overview of bone marrow and stem cell transplantation. *Journal of Intravenous Nursing, 21*(6), 356–360.
13. Kosits, C., & Callaghan, M. (2000). Rituximab: A new monoclonal antibody therapy for non-Hodgkin's lymphoma. *Oncology Nursing Forum, 27*(1), 51–59.
14. McGuire, D. B., et al. (1998). Acute oral pain and mucositis in bone marrow transplant and leukemia patients: Data from a pilot study. *Cancer Nursing, 21*(6), 385–393.
15. Roach, M. (1998). Nurses manage recombinant interleukin-2 side effects in elderly patients with leukemia. *Oncology Nursing Forum, 25*(1), 29–30.
16. Sheely, L. C. (1996). Sleep disturbances in hospitalized patients with cancer. *Oncology Nursing Forum, 23*(1), 109–111.
17. Shelton, B. K., Baker, L., & Stecker, S. (1996). Critical care of the patient with hematologic malignancy. *AACN Clinical Issues 7*(1), 65–78.
18. Skalla, K. (1996). The interferons. *Seminars in Oncology Nursing, 12*(2), 97–105.
19. Stolar, K. (1999). A graft versus host disease prevention and management tool: A mechanism for improving continuity of care. *Oncology Nursing Forum, 26*(6), 977–978.
20. Vogelsang, G. B. (2000). Advances in the treatment of graft-versus-host disease. *Leukemia (England), 14*(3), 509–510.
21. Wagner, N. D., & Quinones, V. W. (1998). Allogeneic peripheral blood stem cell transplantation: Clinical overview and nursing implications. *Oncology Nursing Forum, 25*(6), 1049–1055.
22. Warmkessel, J. H. (1997). Caring for patients with non-Hodgkin's lymphoma. *Nursing, 27*(6), 48–49.
23. Yeager, K. A., et al. (2000). Implementation of an oral care standard for leukemia and transplantation patients. *Cancer Nursing, 23*(1), 40–47.

UNIT
17

Multisystem Disorders

REMEMBER *to*
check out your
Companion CD ROM

Management of Clients with Acquired Immunodeficiency Syndrome

Peter J. Ungvarski

NURSING OUTCOMES CLASSIFICATION (NOC) for Nursing Diagnoses—Clients with HIV/AIDS

Altered Nutrition: Less Than Body Requirements
Nutritional Status
Nutritional Status: Food and Fluid Intake
Nutritional Status: Nutrient Intake
Effective Management of Therapeutic Regimen: Individual
Adherence Behavior
Compliance Behavior

Family Participation in Professional Care
Knowledge: Treatment Regimen
Participation: Health Care Decisions
Risk Control
Symptom Control
Fatigue
Activity Intolerance
Endurance
Energy Conservation

Nutritional Status: Energy
Psychomotor Energy
Hyperthermia
Immune Status
Thermoregulation
Pain
Comfort Level
Pain Control
Pain: Disruptive Effects
Pain Level

The human immunodeficiency virus (HIV) infects people worldwide and results in the destruction of the body's host defenses and immune system. By 1999, HIV infected more than 47 million people throughout the world, with an estimated 6 million people newly infected each year. HIV kills more people than any other infectious disease and ranks fourth among the leading causes of death worldwide.

For many years, because of our lack of understanding and effective treatment, HIV was considered a rapidly progressing fatal disease. Today, HIV infection is viewed more optimistically as a chronic disease that can be controlled with appropriate health care. However, the cost of such health care (~$12,000 yearly per person) limits its accessibility to developed, industrialized nations such as the United States. Because many parts of the world, such as Africa and Asia, lack adequate economic resources to treat this disease, HIV infection continues to be a rapidly progressing fatal illness in these areas.

From both a medical and nursing perspective, clinical management parallels the HIV illness trajectory. Once infected with HIV, a person who receives appropriate treatment can live for many years and continue to func-

tion without major problems. In the latter stages of disease, for a variety of reasons to be discussed, the illness progresses, wearing out the immune system. The person is then given the diagnosis acquired immunodeficiency syndrome (AIDS).

Because of this dual clinical picture, the material presented in this chapter is divided into (1) caring for the person with HIV disease and (2) caring for the person with AIDS. Remember, that advances and breakthroughs occur rapidly in this area of health care; you must seek additional information to stay up to date.

Etiology and Risk Factors

ETIOLOGY

The etiologic agent associated with AIDS was first isolated by French scientists in 1983 and named the *lymphadenopathy-associated virus.* One year later, an American scientist claimed the discovery of the etiologic agent and named it the *human T-cell lymphotropic virus type III.* Although both scientists actually identified the same virus, much confusion took place. In 1986, the International Society on the Taxonomy of Viruses renamed the virus, calling it the human immunodeficiency virus. In that same year, much to everyone's surprise, a second and distinctly different strain of the virus was discovered in Africa. Therefore, since 1986, the scientific names to distinguish between the two viruses are HIV-1 and HIV-2.

This was a major—and alarming—discovery because it was the first clue that HIV could change its appearance, or mutate, very rapidly. The capability of HIV to mutate rapidly is often referred to as *genetic promiscuity,* and it has become the hallmark of this virus, creating a monumental challenge for scientists and researchers alike. HIV-1 is distributed worldwide, but it is most prevalent in Europe and the United States. HIV-2 predominates in west African nations but has been isolated in other parts of the world. By 1999, approximately 79 cases of HIV-2 had been identified in the United States; most of the infected people had been born in Africa. Most worldwide infections are HIV-1.

By 1996, scientists discovered that HIV-1 had also mutated several times. It has two major subtypes, or *clades,* designated (1) HIV-1 major (group M) viruses and (2) HIV-1 outlier (group O) viruses.

HIV-1 Group M

Group M viruses have been assigned to 10 genetic subtypes, designated HIV-1, group M, subtype A, B, C, D, E, F, G, H, I, and J, according to the phylogenetic analysis of their genes. The distribution of subtypes varies worldwide. For example, whereas subtype B predominates in North America and Europe, subtypes A, B, C, and E have been identified in India. There is concern that subtypes other than B will invade the United States, because American service personnel assigned to overseas duty who have become infected with HIV-1 have been found to be infected with subtypes A, D, and E.

It is important to mention these complexities to illustrate the rapidly changing nature of HIV. The virus poses a considerable challenge to researchers investigating new drugs to treat the disease or developing vaccines because their work is usually limited to one specific subtype of HIV-1. Indeed, vaccine trials have demonstrated that a vaccine for one subtype may not work for other subtypes.

HIV-1 Group O

The designation O was deliberate, because this mutation was an outlier and differed from the others, in that it cannot be detected with the routine HIV antibody tests used in the United States. Group O was primarily identified in west and central Africa, with a few isolated cases found through special tests in France and the United States. The Centers for Disease Control and Prevention (CDC) is working with the manufacturers of HIV-1 antibody test kits to ensure that testing methods are reconfigured to detect HIV-1 group O as well as group M.

RISK FACTORS

Modes of transmission have remained constant throughout the course of the HIV pandemic. The virus is spread through certain sexual practices, through exposure to blood, and through perinatal transmission. The patterns in the spread of HIV changed considerably during the first 19 years of the epidemic in the United States. Comparing the 1980s with the 1990s, significant increases have been noted in intravenous (IV) drug users, women, and hetero-

sexuals. Although most Americans infected with HIV continue to be men who have sex with men, the overall number has decreased considerably. This decline, however, has been limited to white men; the number of new HIV infections among racial and ethnic minority men who have sex with men continues to increase, as outlined in the Diversity in Health Care feature. In young adults (ages 19 to 29 years), the number of new infections has been increasing, especially in the South and Midwest. HIV infection and AIDS are the second leading causes of death among adults ages 25 to 44 years.

Perhaps the most overlooked population in the HIV epidemic is adults over age 50 years. By 1999, about 11% of the nation's total number of reported AIDS cases were in this age group. People over age 50 years may not be tested promptly for HIV because they and their health care providers may not perceive them to be at risk for this disease. Women over age 50 years are acquiring HIV infection primarily through heterosexual contact. Although the largest numbers of AIDS and HIV cases have been reported in large cities, such as New York and San Francisco, there has been a shift of newly diagnosed infections to small cities and rural areas, especially in the South and Midwest.

The principal mode of transmission of HIV throughout the world has been through sexual exposure. With the exception of Australia, Europe, and the United States, most HIV transmission has been through heterosexual activities. One important lesson that health care professionals have learned from the HIV epidemic is that sexual *practices,* not sexual *preferences,* place people at risk for sexually transmitted diseases (STDs). Homosexual men who do not engage in unprotected anus-penile sex or expose themselves to another person's body fluids are no more at risk for acquiring HIV infection than anyone else; similarly, heterosexual or homosexual couples in long-term, monogamous relationships are at low risk. The problem of unsafe sexual encounters outside of these relationships does, however, pose a risk.

Sexual practices that are *completely safe* include (1) autosexual activities (such as masturbation), (2) mutually monogamous relationships between noninfected partners, and (3) abstinence. *Very safe* sexual practices include non-insertive activity. Insertive practices with a condom are considered *probably safe* as long as the condom does not break and no contact with body fluids occurs. Everything else is considered risky. Other cofactors, such as engaging in sexual activities while under the influence of drugs or alcohol, having multiple sex partners, and the presence of sores in the genital area, increase the risk of acquiring HIV. Although the number of reported cases is small, oral sexual practices, whether performed on a man or a woman, have been implicated as a possible transmission activity.

Transmission by exposure to blood is a very broad category that encompasses numerous possible routes. The most obvious are through the administration of blood or blood products, transplantation of donated tissue or organs, and implantation of semen contaminated with HIV. Prevention of HIV infection by any of these means is possible by donor exclusion (excluding persons from high-risk groups), routine serologic testing of donated tissues or fluids for HIV antibodies, and heat inactivation of

HIV and AIDS in Minority Populations

Culture is an important variable in understanding the transmission and prevention of the human immunodeficiency virus (HIV) and acquired immunodeficiency syndrome (AIDS) because of the disproportionate occurrence of the disease in minority populations. AIDS affects many aspects of life that have cultural meanings, such as reproduction, birth, death, the roles of women, and sexuality.[2] Health care workers are challenged to understand the complex factors that account for the disproportionate occurrence of HIV and AIDS in minorities. Understanding these factors is the first step in finding interventions to prevent the further escalation of the HIV/AIDS epidemic. Clearly, health care workers must become "culturally competent" if they are to work effectively with their various patient groups in preventing and treating HIV disease.

The Problem

Minorities are disproportionately affected by HIV and AIDS. This is clearly represented by the HIV and AIDS statistics in the United States.[1] Cumulative case reports for people with AIDS through 1998 indicate that 58.6% were black or Hispanic. Specifically, by the end of 1997, the number of African-Americans living with AIDS *increased* from 32.7% of people with AIDS in 1992 to 39.2% in 1997. For Hispanics, the same category of figures *increased* from 17% in 1992 to 19.4% in 1997. For whites, the figures *decreased* from 1992 to 1997. In 1992, the number of whites with AIDS was 49%; this figure declined to 40% in 1997.[6]

The elimination of HIV and AIDS through preventing their spread is, at present, the only viable goal. Culture is an important variable in understanding HIV and AIDS because it is apparent in values, attitudes, and behaviors associated with everyday life. Consequently, health care workers must become *culturally competent*[4]; that is, they must:

- Develop an awareness of one's own sensations and beliefs
- Demonstrate knowledge and understanding of the client's culture
- Accept and respect cultural differences
- Adapt care to be congruent with the client's culture

Cultural competence facilitates assessments and interventions with culturally diverse populations. It includes the recognition that the Western biomedical explanation of HIV and AIDS is viewed as limited by ethnic minorities. One can only speculate how this variable influences the finding that people reported with AIDS increasingly represent those whose diagnosis was too late for them to benefit from treatment, people who did not seek care or did not have access to care, or people for whom treatment failed.[6] Consequently, health care workers should become familiar with alternative lay beliefs and explanations regarding AIDS and appropriate intervention.

An example is provided by the research of Suarez and colleagues.[5] Building on the fact that Hispanics residing in the United States are disproportionately affected by HIV infection and AIDS, these researchers investigated the beliefs and practices of Hispanics who were receiving medical care for their HIV infection. More than three quarters of the study population reported that they engaged in folk, religious, and other alternative healing practices.

Interventions

HIV infection and AIDS have provided an opportunity to focus on prevention and to understand how disease interacts with the complexities of culture. HIV prevention and treatment programs ideally are based on the following goals[2]:

- To use and enhance cultural beliefs, values, and roles as core elements of the intervention process
- To use traditional gender roles as well as the role of the family in health education and care as a starting point
- To enhance beneficial beliefs and practices that relate to HIV disease
- To clarify misperceptions that feed fear and stigma
- To modify harmful beliefs or negative attitudes and practices within the context of positive ethnocultural and community values

There is promising evidence that culturally sensitive theory-based interventions can be successful in reducing the HIV risk-associated sexual behavior of adolescents. For example, Jemmott and associates[3] noted that African American adolescents are at a high risk for contracting HIV and AIDS but that little is known about what interventions to reduce risk are most effective. Their research was designed to evaluate the effects of abstinence and safer sex HIV risk-reduction interventions on the sexual risk behaviors of inner-city African American adolescents. The study interventions were based on cognitive-behavioral theories. The interventions were designed to be educational, entertaining, and culturally sensitive. For example, each intervention incorporated the theme "Be Proud, Be Responsible" for yourself and your community. The interventions involved group discussions, videos, games, brainstorming, experiential exercises, and skill-building activities. The results suggest that both abstinence and safer sex interventions can reduce HIV sexual risk behaviors, but safer sex interventions may be especially effective with sexually experienced adolescents and may have longer-lasting effects.[3]

The elimination of HIV and AIDS through prevention is a viable goal. HIV and AIDS have provided an opportunity to focus on prevention and understand how disease interacts with the complexities of culture. If we continue to ignore the complexities of HIV and AIDS, it will not be long before the next great global epidemic demonstrates that ignorance and prejudice are the greatest human risks.[1]

For further information on HIV/AIDS and minority populations, the following selected resources may be consulted:

African American AIDS Policy and Training Institute
3418 Huxley Street
Los Angeles, CA 90027
Tel: 323-663-4194
Fax: 323-666-8846
e-mail: *info@aaainstitute.org*
Web site: *http://www.aaainstitute.org*

AIDS Education Services for Minorities
http://www.accessatlanta.com/community/groups/aesm

American Red Cross African American AIDS Program
http://www.redcross.org/hss/HIVAIDS/afam/index.html

CDC National Prevention Information Network
http://www.cdcnpin.org

Chart continued on following page

Centers for Disease Control and Prevention
Divisions of HIV/AIDS Prevention
http://www.cdc.gov/nchstp/hiv_aids

Community HIV/AIDS Technical Assistance Network
 (CHATAN)
National Coalition of Hispanic Health and Human Services Organizations (COSSMHO)
1501 Sixteenth Street, NW
Washington, DC 20036
Tel: 202-387-5000
Fax: 202-797-4353
e-mail: *info@cossmho.org*
Web site: *http://www.cossmho.org/hiv.html*

Gay and Lesbian Latino AIDS Education Initiative
 (GALAEI)
1233 Locust Street
Philadelphia, PA 19107
Tel: 215-985-3382
Fax: 215-985-3388
Web site: *http://www.critpath.org/galaei*

Hispanic AIDS Awareness Program (Programa
 de Informacion Sobre el SIDA)
2350 Coral Way, Suite 301
Miami, FL 33145
Tel: 305-860-0780
Fax: 305-860-0580
e-mail: *HAAP@emservices.com*
Web site: *http://www.emservices.com/haap*

Minority AIDS Project
5149 Jefferson Boulevard
Los Angeles, CA 90016-3836
Tel: 213-936-4949
Fax: 213-936-4973
e-mail: *Paul519@aol.com*
Web site: *http//www.geocities.com/Hollywood/9930/map.html*

National Minority AIDS Council
1931 13th Street, N.W
Washington, DC 20009
Tel: 202-483-6622; 800-559-4145
Fax: 202-483-1135
e-mail: *info@nmac.org*
Web site: *http://www.nmac.org*

"Race/Ethnicity and HIV/AIDS," in *The Body: An AIDS and HIV Information Resource*
Web sites: *http://thebody.com/whatis/race.html*
            http://thebody.com/bbs/forums.html

U.S. Department of Health and Human Services,
 Office of Minority Health Resource Center:
"Minority HIV/AIDS Initiative"
Tel: 1-800-444-6472
e-mail: *info@omhrc.gov*
Web site: *http://www.omhrc.gov/omh/aids/aidshome.htm*

University of California, San Francisco:
"HIV InSite: Gateway to AIDS Knowledge"
Web site: *http://HIVInSite.ucsf.edu*

References

1. Bradley-Springer, L. (1999). The complex realities of primary prevention for HIV infection in a "just do it" world. *Nursing Clinics of North America, 34*(1), 49–70.
2. Flaskerud, J. (1999). Culture and ethnicity. In P. Ungvarski, & J. Flaskerud (Eds.), *HIV/AIDS: A guide to primary care management.* Philadelphia: W. B. Saunders.
3. Jemmott, J., Jemmott, L., & Fong, G. (1998). Abstinence and safer sex: HIV risk-reduction interventions for African American adolescents. *Journal of the American Medical Association, 279*(19), 1529–1536.
4. Paulanka, B., & Purnell, L. (1998). *Transcultural health care: A culturally competent approach.* Philadelphia: F. A. Davis.
5. Suarez, M., Raffaelli M., & O'Leary, O. (1996). Use of folk healing practices by HIV-infected Hispanics living in the United States. *AIDS Care, 8*(6), 683–690.
6. U.S. Department of Health and Human Services, Public Health Service, Centers for Disease Control and Prevention. (1998). *HIV/AIDS Surveillance Report,* 10(2).

Joyce Larson-Presswalla, PhD, RN, *President, "Culture Counts," Marketing Coordinator, James A. Haley Veterans Hospital, Tampa, Florida*

certain blood products, such as factor VIII concentrate. Other means of preventing HIV infection related to blood products are autologous (self-donated) blood programs and limiting the administration of any blood product to situations in which it is absolutely necessary.

Use of injected drugs accounts for the largest number of HIV infections through exposure to contaminated blood. The only *absolutely safe* injection drug use behavior is not to inject. *Very safe* practice with injected drugs is to use sterilized injection paraphernalia and never share needles and syringes. A *probably safe* practice is to clean injection paraphernalia with full-strength bleach before injecting, although disposable needles and syringes are difficult to clean. Anything else is considered risky. Other cofactors that increase the chances of acquiring HIV by drug injection include the seroprevalence of HIV in the geographical location of the drug user, the social setting of injection drug use (e.g., "shooting galleries," where injection paraphernalia is shared), and the frequency of injection.

Needle exchange programs provide sterile injection equipment, latex condoms, counseling, and access to social and health programs, including drug detoxification treatment. Numerous studies have shown that needle exchange programs decrease the spread of HIV and hepatitis B and C and do not increase or promote injection drug use. Despite the proven success of this approach to disease prevention, state and federal legislators have been reluctant to appropriate funds to support this model of care. In the United States, because of existing attitudes about IV drug use, needle exchange programs may operate as legal, illegal but tolerated, or illegal or underground programs. In Europe, where the approach to preventing disease has received more favorable support, governments providing national health care services for their citizens have found that needle exchange programs not only have reduced the incidence of disease but also have significantly reduced health care spending for diseases associated with IV drug injection.

Occupational exposure to blood is a potential problem not only for health care workers but also for members of other occupations, such as police and corrections officers. The state of Connecticut legalized the sale of sterile needles and syringes in certain drugstores and found that they not only reduced the incidence of needle sharing in IV drug users but also resulted in a significant decrease in the number of occupationally acquired needle-stick injuries in police officers.

The problem of HIV transmission to health care workers by clients is an ongoing concern of workers, employers, and public health officials. In the United States, by January 1999, the cumulative total number of health care workers with documented, occupationally acquired HIV or AIDS was 54. The number with possible (less clear evidence) transmission was 134. Although most health care workers occupationally infected with HIV acquired the virus after percutaneous exposure, other modes of transmission included mucocutaneous exposure and direct exposure to HIV in the laboratory setting. The actual average risk to a health care worker for exposure to HIV is extremely low (0.3% after a needle-stick or sharp instrument injury and 0.09% after a mucous membrane exposure). The risk, when an exposure occurs, is increased in situations in which a deep injury occurs, when there is visible blood on the device causing the injury, when the device involved was previously placed in a client's artery or vein, and when AIDS was diagnosed in the source client who died within 60 days after the health care worker's exposure (presumably because concentrations of HIV in the blood are very high at this time).

Accidental needle-stick exposure poses the greatest hazard to health care workers. As a health care worker, you should learn and follow Standard Precautions when handling blood and body fluids and when performing procedures that could expose you to blood and body fluids. When any incident reflects potential exposure to blood-borne pathogens, seek medical treatment immediately. The U.S. Public Health Service has issued guidelines for evaluating and treating exposures to HIV. In the case of high-risk exposures, they recommend that combination antiretroviral therapy be given for at least 4 weeks for post-exposure prophylaxis.

In the United States, only one case of HIV transmission from a health care worker to clients has been documented. It was reported in 1990 and involved a Florida dentist. Six clients reportedly became infected with HIV after receiving dental care. The circumstances of this case implied inadequate disinfection and sterilization of instruments in the dental office. Since this incident, retrospective (look-back) studies of possible HIV transmission from infected health care workers to clients have not identified any other cases in the United States. In 1999, one additional case of HIV transmission from a health care worker to a client was reported in France. An HIV-positive physician who was injured during orthopedic surgery transmitted HIV to the client. The surgeon acquired HIV in 1983 when he sustained an injury while operating on an HIV-infected client.

Perinatal HIV exposure can occur during pregnancy, during vaginal delivery, and post partum through breast-feeding. Of all babies born to HIV-infected women worldwide, about 23% are infected. The risk of transmission from mother to child (*vertical transmission*) increases if viral activity is high and the CD4+ titer is low,

which is usually the case in later stages of HIV disease, when the diagnosis is AIDS. Clinical trials were conducted to see whether giving pregnant women antiretroviral therapy for HIV could reduce the risk by controlling HIV activity and raising the CD4+ cell count; administration of zidovudine reduced the rate of vertical HIV infection from 23% to 8%. The CDC has published guidelines for the use of zidovudine and other antiretroviral therapies for pregnant women and their newborn infants. Although no increase in birth defects has been noted in babies born to mothers who took zidovudine during pregnancy, one newer antiretroviral agent (efavirenz) caused birth defects in animal trials and should be avoided during pregnancy.

The only absolute method of preventing perinatal exposure is to avoid pregnancy. All health care workers should discuss HIV infection as part of routine prenatal care with all clients, because many mothers may be unaware that they are infected with HIV. Infected women who carry to term should be advised against breast-feeding, as this has been implicated as a mode of HIV transmission.

Primary prevention of HIV infection for exposed individuals is an emerging concept being applied not only to health care workers but also to the treatment of other accidental exposures. Post-exposure prophylaxis is being used as a health maintenance strategy by some clinicians for people who:

- Have unprotected anal or vaginal intercourse
- Have receptive oral intercourse with ejaculation
- Share needles with an infected partner
- Have a single-event exposure, such as a rape
- Intend to stop high-risk behaviors

Considerable controversy surrounds the use of post-exposure prophylaxis except in cases of rape, and the ethical aspects of providing such treatment continue to be discussed.

Since 1987, about 15 experimental HIV vaccines have been tested on more than 2000 healthy people. Vaccines are being developed to prevent HIV infection (preventive vaccine) and to treat people infected with HIV (therapeutic vaccine). To date, vaccine development has focused on recombinant vaccines structured from HIV envelope glycoproteins gp120 and gp160. Trials have begun with about 5000 volunteers to determine the effectiveness of these vaccines. One major drawback to soliciting volunteers for these trials is the possibility that they will have a false-positive result for HIV after receiving the vaccine because their bodies have developed antibodies to the virus. This may pose a problem for these people when HIV testing is required, such as when they are seeking employment or applying for insurance.

Pathophysiology

HIV-1 is a member of the lentivirus subfamily of human retroviruses. Diseases caused by lentiviruses are characterized by an insidious onset with progressive involvement of the central nervous system (CNS) and may result in disorders of the immune system. HIV-1 is one of five viruses in the lentivirus family (Fig. 79–1). The others are HIV-2 and human T-lymphotropic virus (HTLV) types I, II, and IV.

A retrovirus belongs to the family Retroviridae and

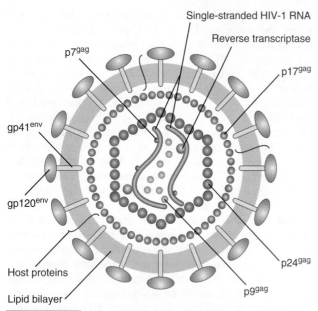

Single-stranded HIV-1 RNA
Reverse transcriptase
p7^{gag}
p17^{gag}
gp41^{env}
gp120^{env}
Host proteins
Lipid bilayer
p24^{gag}
p9^{gag}

FIGURE 79–1 Schematic diagram of the human immunodeficiency virus-1 (HIV-1) virion. RNA, ribonucleic acid. Redrawn from Sande, M., & Volberding, P. [1997]. *The medical management of AIDS* [5th ed.]. Philadelphia: W. B. Saunders, p. 18.)

possesses ribonucleic acid (RNA)-dependent deoxyribonucleic acid (DNA) polymerase (reverse transcriptase). HIV infects T helper cells (T4 lymphocytes), macrophages, and B cells. HIV does not directly affect the central nervous system or peripheral neurons, astrocytes, or oligodendrocytes. HIV infection in the central nervous system is indirectly caused by neurotoxins produced by infected macrophages or chemical substances produced by the dysregulation of cytokines and chemokines.

T helper cells are infected more readily than are other cells. The depletion of T helper cells occurs in the following steps:

1. Once inside the host, HIV attaches to the target cell membrane by way of its receptor molecule, CD4$^+$.
2. The virus is uncoated, and the RNA enters the cell.
3. The enzyme known as reverse transcriptase is released, and viral RNA is transcribed into DNA.
4. This newly created DNA moves into the nucleus and the DNA of the cell.
5. A provirus is created when the viral DNA integrates itself into the cellular DNA or genome of the cell.
6. Once the provirus is in place, its genetic material is no longer pure cell but part virus.
7. The cell may function abnormally.
8. The host cell dies, and viral budding occurs (Fig. 79–2). The new virus proceeds to infect other cells.

The main target for HIV is the T4 helper cell; however, the "glue" to which HIV is attracted is the CD4$^+$ molecule, which acts as the receptor for HIV on the T4 helper cell. Even though the CD4$^+$ molecule is also found on other cells, such as macrophages and monocytes, clinicians usually refer to T4 helper cells as CD4$^+$ cells. Therefore, in articles, research papers, or laboratory reports about HIV the labels *T4, T4 helper, CF4$^+$* and *CD4$^+$ T helper cell* are used synonymously. Other substances known as *chemokines* act as messengers to facilitate entry of HIV into cells. Examples of such chemokines are cysteine-cysteine receptor 3 (CCR3) and CCR5. In 1996, scientists discovered that certain people have a genetic defect in the CCR5 gene and, despite repeated exposure to HIV, never become infected.

The CD4$^+$ T helper cells are the regulating cells in the immune system. They interact with monocytes, macrophages, cytotoxic T cells, natural killer cells, and B cells. In the analogy of an orchestra and a conductor, the T cells are the "conductor" of the immune system, directing all of the activity ("music") produced by the other immune cells ("orchestra"). Therefore, it is apparent that the loss of the CD4$^+$ T helper cells results in chaos. The body loses its basic ability to maintain a consistent state of health. With significant losses of these regulatory cells, the HIV-infected person become highly susceptible to acquired infection and pathogens that have previously caused disease may reactivate and also cause infection. A prime example is the varicella zoster virus, which may have caused chickenpox in an HIV-infected person as a child and may reactivate as shingles when the CD4$^+$ T-cell count drops to low levels.

The average laboratory range for the CD4$^+$ T-cell count is 500 to 1600 mm^3. A gradual physiologic decline occurs in these cells over the life of an individual. In fact, CD4$^+$ T-cell counts in newborns are almost double those of an adult. In the adult, CD4$^+$ cell counts below 200/mm^3 are considered dangerously low and infection is

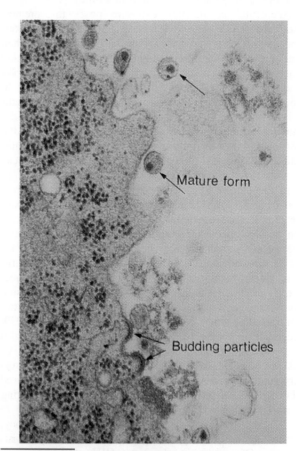

Mature form
Budding particles

FIGURE 79–2 Human immunodeficiency virus. Electron micrograph of the virus budding from a T lymphocyte. (From Friedman-Kien, A., & Cockerell, C. [1996]. *Color atlas of AIDS* [2nd ed.]. Philadelphia: W. B. Saunders, p. 11.)

likely to develop. Other laboratory changes that indicate immune dysfunction include:

- An overall decline in the total numbers of white blood cells
- Decreases in both the total number and percentage of lymphocytes
- Significant changes in the $CD4^+/CD8^+$ ratio
- Decreased $CD4^+$ T-cell test findings
- Absent or decreased skin test reactivity (*anergy*)
- Increased immunoglobulin levels

The cause of all this damage to the immune system is the extensive amount of HIV activity that takes place in the body of an infected person from the time of infection. HIV replicates at a very rapid rate. In fact, it may produce 10 million new *virions* (viral particles) daily. Although a person with HIV may be asymptomatic and $CD4^+$ cell counts may be within the normal range, insidious destruction of the immune system is taking place. Antiretroviral drugs play a key role in interrupting the HIV disease process by inhibiting the ability of the virus to replicate, thus reducing the amount of circulating virus in the body and halting its destructive activity. Once this happens, the immune system begins to heal and restore itself, as noted by rising $CD4^+$ cell counts.

There are numerous challenges to sustaining the beneficial effects of antiretroviral therapy. The biggest problem is the ability of HIV to mutate and to become resistant to antiretroviral drugs. When this happens, the infected person is said to have drug failure manifested by a rise in viral load and a decline in $CD4^+$ cell counts. The combination of drugs must then be changed. Because two to three drugs are usually ordered at one time and fewer than 15 drugs have been approved to treat HIV infection, the number of combinations that can be prescribed is limited. Additionally, although the drugs can contain the disease in plasma, the virus can hide in many other cells in the body. Finally, because most antiretroviral agents do not cross the blood-brain barrier in the CNS, treatment of CNS problems caused by HIV infection can be very difficult.

The course of HIV illness often varies from person to person. Several cofactors may accelerate the immunodeficiency, including malnutrition, continued use of injected drugs and recreational substances, allergic conditions, genetics, age, pregnancy, gender, and presence of infections. In some instances, research has clearly implicated some of these cofactors as contributing to a more rapid decline in $CD4^+$ cell levels; for others, the evidence is less clear. Factors that have been linked to increased mortality and morbidity include lower socioeconomic status, lack of access to adequate care, receiving care in a hospital with limited AIDS experience, and being treated by a physician with little experience in AIDS care.

Overall, comparing the 1980s with the 1990s, survival among clients with AIDS has doubled. Most authors attribute increases in survival to the introduction of drugs to prevent opportunistic infections when the $CD4^+$ count falls below 200 mm^3 and to the use of antiretroviral agents to treat HIV disease.

To illustrate further the differences observed in HIV-infected people, scientists have reported that about 5% of them are perfectly healthy after many years and show no signs of disease progression. These *long-term non-progressors:*

- Have had documented evidence of HIV infection for more than 10 years
- Are asymptomatic
- Have normal, stable immune profiles
- Have never required any treatment for HIV disease

Long-term non-progressors appear to produce vigorous amounts of serum antibodies that keep HIV activity at extremely low levels, thus preventing immune system damage. Do not confuse a long-term non-progressor with a *long-term survivor*, defined as someone who has lived for more than 8 years after an AIDS diagnosis, who shows all clinical and laboratory manifestations of disease, and who continuously requires treatment.

Although the principal target of HIV is the immune system, considerable damage occurs to other parts of the body as a direct result of HIV in body tissues. A few examples of clinical conditions that can be directly attributed to HIV include cranial and peripheral neuropathies, uveitis, cardiomyopathy, pneumonitis, malabsorption in the small intestine, nephritis, cervicitis, arthritis, psoriasis, gonad dysfunction, and adrenalitis. Additionally, damage to the hematologic system, which is due in part to impaired blood cell production, commonly results in anemia, granulocytopenia, and thrombocytopenia throughout the course of disease.

In addition to managing HIV disease, clinicians are challenged with addressing those illnesses that existed before the person acquired HIV infection. These not only require continuing treatment and attention but also may complicate the course of illness. Frequently encountered pre-existing and co-morbid conditions seen in HIV-infected clients include, but are not limited to, alcoholism, drug dependence, liver disease, kidney disease, psychiatric illness, and a history of STDs. As therapy improves and people with HIV disease live longer, they will also require treatment for such illnesses as cancer, coronary artery disease, chronic obstructive lung disease, hypertension, and diabetes, all of which may occur in the aging population not infected with HIV.

Clinical Manifestations

As knowledge has evolved regarding the HIV disease process, the CDC has developed and revised numerous classification systems (Box 79-1). The most recent classification system for HIV disease in adults and adolescents is based on two monitoring parameters used to follow a client: (1) laboratory data ($CD4^+$ cell counts) and (2) clinical presentation (the person's clinical manifestations of diseases). The period in which a person becomes infected is referred to as *primary infection*. If HIV is detected in a client at the time of initial infection, the client is considered to be in category A.

Primary infection is the initial period after a person has acquired HIV, usually through a high-risk behavior (e.g., certain sexual practices or IV drug use). The length of time that primary infection lasts varies from several weeks to a few months. During primary infection, 50% to 70% of people become sick. Many clinicians are unaware of this fact and tend to think that primary infection is

BOX 79-1 Human Immunodeficiency Virus (HIV) Classification System for Adolescents and Adults

The Centers for Disease Control and Prevention (CDC) classification system for HIV-infected adolescents and adults emphasizes the importance of CD4+ lymphocyte testing in clinical management. The classification system is divided into laboratory and clinical categories as follows.

	Clinical Categories		
Laboratory Categories (CD4+ Cell Categories)	A Asymptomatic, Acute (Primary) HIV or PGL	B Symptomatic, Not A or C Conditions	C AIDS-Indicator Conditions
≥500 mm³	A1	B1	C1
200–499 mm³	A2	B2	C2
<200 mm³ AIDS-indicator T-cell count	A3	B3	C3

Shaded areas in the chart are *AIDS-defining* categories. *Laboratory* categories are based on the most recent CD4+ cell count. *Clinical* categories describe the clinical status of the client and the presence or absence of certain diseases.

Category A

One or more of the following conditions occurring in an adolescent or adult with documented HIV infection. Conditions listed in categories B and C must not have occurred.

- Asymptomatic HIV infection
- PGL
- Acute (primary) HIV infection with accompanying illness or history of acute HIV infection

Category B

Symptomatic conditions occurring in an HIV-infected adolescent or adult that are not included among conditions listed in clinical category C and that meet at least one of the following criteria:

- The conditions are attributed to HIV infection or indicate a defect in cell-mediated immunity
- The conditions are considered by physicians to have a clinical course or management that is complicated by HIV infection

Examples of conditions in clinical category B include, but are not limited to, the following:

- Bacterial endocarditis, meningitis, pneumonia, or sepsis
- Candidiasis, vulvovaginal; persistent for more than 1 month, or poorly responsive to therapy
- Candidiasis, oropharyngeal (thrush)
- Cervical dysplasia, severe; or carcinoma
- Constitutional manifestations, such as fever (38.5° C) or diarrhea lasting more than 1 month
- Hairy leukoplakia, oral
- Herpes zoster (shingles), involving at least two distinct episodes or more than one dermatome
- Idiopathic thrombocytopenic purpura
- Listeriosis
- Nocardiosis
- Pelvic inflammatory disease
- Peripheral neuropathy

Category C

Any condition listed in the 1987 surveillance case definition of acquired immunodeficiency syndrome (AIDS) and affecting an adolescent or an adult. The conditions in clinical category C are strongly associated with severe immunodeficiency, occur frequently in HIV-infected clients, and cause serious morbidity or mortality. According to the classification system, HIV-infected clients would be classified on the basis of both the lowest accurate (not necessarily the most recent) CD4+ lymphocyte determination *and* the most severe clinical condition diagnosed, regardless of the client's current clinical condition. Specific diseases that are considered AIDS-defining diagnostic categories include:

- Candidiasis of bronchi, trachea, or lungs
- Candidiasis, esophageal
- Cervical cancer, invasive
- CD4+ T lymphocyte cell count < 200 mm³ (<14%)
- Coccidioidomycosis, disseminated or extrapulmonary
- Cryptococcosis, extrapulmonary
- Cryptosporidiosis, chronic intestinal (more than 1 month duration)
- Cytomegalovirus disease (other than liver, spleen, or nodes)
- Cytomegalovirus retinitis (with loss of vision)
- Encephalopathy, HIV-related
- Herpes simplex: chronic ulcer or ulcers (>1 month duration), bronchitis, pneumonitis, or esophagitis
- Histoplasmosis, disseminated or extrapulmonary
- Isosporiasis, chronic intestinal (>1 month duration)
- Kaposi's sarcoma
- Lymphoma, Burkitt's (or equivalent term)
- Lymphoma, immunoblastic (or equivalent term)
- Lymphoma, primary, of brain
- *Mycobacterium avium* complex or *M. kansasii,* disseminated or extrapulmonary
- *Mycobacterium tuberculosis,* any site (pulmonary or extrapulmonary)
- *Mycobacterium,* other species or unidentified species, disseminated or extrapulmonary
- *Pneumocystis carinii* pneumonia
- Pneumonia, recurrent
- Progressive multifocal leukoencephalopathy
- Salmonella septicemia, recurrent
- Toxoplasmosis of brain
- Wasting syndrome due to HIV

PGL, persistent generalized lymphadenopathy.
Adapted from Centers for Disease Control and Prevention. (1992). 1993 revised classification system for HIV infection and expanded surveillance case definition for AIDS among adolescents and adults. *Morbidity and Mortality Weekly Report, 41*(RR-17), 1–19.

silent. In addition to constitutional manifestations (fever, fatigue, lymphadenopathy, nausea, vomiting), the infected person may experience headache; truncal (torso and arms) rash; ulcers of the mouth, genitals, or both; thrush; pharyngitis; diarrhea; hepatomegaly; myalgia; arthralgia; anemia; thrombocytopenia; and leukopenia. In some people, the manifestations are mild and comparable to those of mononucleosis. Other people have severe manifestations and may need hospitalization.

During primary infection, a sudden and intense burst of HIV activity results in a high viral load and a dramatic drop in the CD4$^+$ cell count. In fact, the CD4$^+$ cell count may drop at the time of primary infection to below 100 mm^3, with the concomitant development of an AIDS-defining illness. This is also the period in which most newly infected people develop antibodies to HIV, which can then be detected through enzyme immunoassay testing. There is a "window" period for *seroconversion* (the time it takes for a newly infected person to develop antibodies to HIV that can be detected in a laboratory specimen). On average, antibodies can be detected in 4 to 12 weeks.

Unfortunately, in most instances the diagnosis is not confirmed at the time of primary infection, either because the person does not seek medical care or because the clinician does not take an adequate history that raises the suspicion of HIV infection. This is quite a serious situation, because preliminary studies have shown that starting antiretroviral therapy at the time of initial infection may prevent damage to the immune system and to other body systems. Table 79–1 lists the parts of the health history needed to detect a client's HIV exposure risk.

Except in certain instances, as when seeking a federal job or when testing infant umbilical cord blood, the decision to seek an enzyme immunoassay test for HIV antibodies is left up to the individual. Testing also involves pretest and post-test counseling. Laws governing the reporting of HIV antibody test results vary from state to state, and testing may be performed either anonymously or confidentially. If the enzyme immunoassay result is positive, a second test, the Western blot, is performed to confirm a positive HIV status.

If testing is performed too early in the initial infection period, a false-negative result may occur. A few cases of outliers also did not test positive for up to 3 years after becoming infected. False-positive results are extremely rare but may occur in clients with autoimmune disorders, such as lupus erythematosus, or in clients who have taken part in HIV vaccine studies.

Other methods for detecting HIV infection include home test kits, salivary tests, and urine tests. The marketability, cost, and popularity have limited the use of home test kits thus far. Saliva test results are as accurate as serologic testing, but the urine test is slightly less accurate.

In general, test results are reported as (1) positive, (2) negative, or (3) indeterminate. A *positive* result means that the person is HIV-infected, but it does not predict the future course of disease. A *negative* result means that HIV antibodies were not detected. Indeterminate results usually mean that the enzyme immunoassay test was positive but the Western blot test did not confirm those findings. Repeated testing on indeterminate results often

shows an HIV-negative antibody test. Repeated testing later is commonly recommended as a means of validating initial test results.

The period following primary infection is one in which the person usually remains asymptomatic for many years. Therefore, clients with HIV disease are commonly categorized in group A for extended periods. Although the clients have no obvious major manifestations they may start to notice recurrent infections of the sinuses or respiratory tract or may feel increasing fatigue. Although no significant disease is apparent, viral destruction takes place throughout the body. A major portion of this destructive activity occurs in lymph tissue and results in a slowly declining CD4$^+$ cell count. The damage to lymphatic structures also has a negative effect on the quality of CD4$^+$ cells that are continuously produced within the body. After a while, although the numbers may be adequate, CD4$^+$ cells lose their ability to contain the destructive nature of HIV.

Since the beginning of the HIV epidemic, the focus of clinical monitoring has been on evaluating the quantity of CD4$^+$ cells. In essence, CD4$^+$ cell counts are an indirect measurement of the clinical course of HIV disease, showing the end result of HIV activity. In 1996, *viral load testing* became available to directly measure how much viral activity was occurring in a person with the disease. Viral load tests measure the amount of HIV RNA in plasma, quantify HIV activity, determine prognosis, indicate the need for treatment, evaluate the biologic response to treatment, and detect treatment failure. CD4$^+$ cell counts should not be a substitute for viral load testing, because the correlation between the two results is weak. High viral loads may not always correlate with clinical manifestations and a low CD4$^+$ cell count, and vice versa. Viral load results may be reported in copies per milliliter (e.g., 10,000 copies/ml). The actual numbers may be reported as follows:

- Decimal numbers, as in 10,000 copies
- Exponents, as in 10^4, where the exponent 4 indicates the number of zeros after the 1
- A logarithm, in this case 4, which indicates 10^4 or 10,000

Thus, a report that sets viral activity at 5 logs would be interpreted as 10^5 or 100,000 copies/ml.

As the disease progresses, manifestations such as thrush or vulvovaginal candidiasis usually appear, which are distinct manifestations of an underlying immunodeficiency. This development is what commonly causes people to seek HIV antibody testing. Those who have symptomatic illness are then classified into group B (see Box 79–1). Eventually, a client with HIV infection develops one or more AIDS-defining diseases and is finally classified into group C. Once again, this may be the first time that HIV infection is discovered.

Outcome Management for HIV Infection

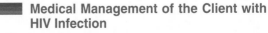
Medical Management of the Client with HIV Infection

The outcomes for medical and nursing management of the client infected with HIV are to maintain the person's

| TABLE 79–1 | ACTUAL OR POTENTIAL RISKS FOR EXPOSURE TO HUMAN IMMUNODEFICIENCY VIRUS (HIV): THE HEALTH HISTORY |

SOCIAL HISTORY

Sexual activities	Sex with men, women, or both
	Preferred sexual activities
	Absolutely safe behavior: abstinence or mutually monogamous with a noninfected partner
	Very safe behavior: noninsertive sexual practices
	Probably safe behavior: insertive sexual practices using condoms and spermicide
	Risky behavior: everything else
	Use of condoms (both male and female), including application, removal, use of lubricants, and difference in condom efficacy
	Engaging in sex with multiple partners
	Use of mood-affecting drugs before or during sexual activities
	Whether HIV infection has been diagnosed in anyone with whom the client has had sexual relations
Needle exposure	Use of drugs via intravenous route
	Sharing of needles, syringes, and other drug paraphernalia
	Other needle-exposure activities, such as tattoos, acupuncture, treatment by unskilled individuals or "folk doctors," or sharing prescribed drugs between friends
	Whether HIV disease has been diagnosed in anyone with whom client has shared needles
Occupational history	Current employment status
	Client's occupation and responsibilities in relation to risk potential for HIV exposure
	Whether client experienced any exposures
	Type of health care follow-up the client has pursued since exposure
	Client's knowledge of signs and symptoms of seroconversion and need for follow-up
Travel	Within the past 10 years
	Sexual activities when traveling in areas with many AIDS cases, such as New York, California, New Jersey, Texas, Florida, Haiti, or Zaire
	Treatment for illnesses or accidents while traveling
	Immigration history and potential exposures in country of origin

FAMILY HISTORY

Medical and mental health problems	Substance use in the home or by other family members
	Tuberculosis
	HIV infection
	Other pertinent data

DRUG HISTORY

Use of mood-altering drugs	Alcohol, marijuana, cocaine, crack, LSD, Quaaludes (methaqualone), amphetamines, barbiturates, tranquilizers, amyl or butyl nitrite ("poppers"), heroin, "crystal meth," or "ecstasy"
	Route of administration: oral, inhalation (including sniffing, snorting, and smoking), intravenous, or subcutaneous ("skin-popping")
	Any current or previous treatment for substance abuse

MEDICAL HISTORY

HIV testing	Whether testing has ever been recommended
	Where testing was done
	Test results
	Whether client has documentation of test and results
Major diseases	Hemophilia
	Treatment with clotting replacements, such as factor VIII
	Other pertinent disorders
Transfusion	Whether client was donor or recipient
Sexually transmitted diseases	Syphilis, gonorrhea, amebiasis, herpes simplex (oral or genital), *Giardia lamblia* enteritis, *Chlamydia,* condylomata, trichomoniasis, or pelvic inflammatory disease
	Other pertinent disorders

AIDS, acquired immunodeficiency syndrome; LSD, lysergic acid diethylamide.

health, initiate and maintain an effective antiretroviral regimen, and prevent infectious complications. This requires health care follow-up at specified intervals and an understanding that, to achieve these outcomes, the client has to make lifestyle changes.

MAINTAIN HEALTH

Initiating a plan of care for any client infected with HIV requires a detailed laboratory and clinical assessment not only for the initial evaluation but also on an ongoing basis. Initial and follow-up laboratory testing provides invaluable information on disease progression, serves as a guide for treatment decisions, and determines the efficacy of treatment prescribed. A complete blood count is needed to identify anemia, thrombocytopenia, leukopenia, and developing infections. Multichannel chemistry panels and urinalysis reveal renal, liver, metabolic, or nutritional disease. Both tests are repeated at 6- to 12-month intervals to detect any abnormalities resulting from disease progression or prescribed drugs. These results are also needed to modify dosages of antiretroviral drugs for clients with impaired kidney or liver function.

An annual tuberculin skin test detects mycobacterial disease, and a chest x-ray identifies pulmonary problems. For women, a pregnancy test and Papanicolaou (Pap) smear are usually performed. Pap smears are performed twice during the first year after a diagnosis of HIV infection and then at least annually. Screening for venereal diseases includes testing for syphilis, gonorrhea, and *Chlamydia*. These are repeated annually if the client is sexually active. Hepatitis A and B antibody testing is performed to identify acute or prior infection and to determine the need for immunization. Although no vaccine is yet available, hepatitis C antibody testing may also be performed because there is a high incidence of hepatitis C in people infected with HIV.

Testing for pathogens known to cause opportunistic infections in people infected with HIV includes serologic tests intended to detect previous exposure to toxoplasmosis, histoplasmosis, cryptococcosis, and cytomegalovirus. For seronegative clients, repeated testing may reveal a primary exposure. For seropositive clients, rising titers of antibodies to these pathogens indicate the need for prophylactic therapy.

Finally, CD4+ cell counts, ratios, and percentages are performed to determine the degree of immunodeficiency, and viral load testing is ordered to calculate the amount of viral activity. Viral load test result interpretations are as follows:

- < 10,000 copies/ml: poses a low risk for AIDS
- 10,000 to 100,000 copies/ml: doubles risk for AIDS
- > 100,000 copies/ml: poses a high risk for AIDS

The initial test, without any treatment, may reveal viral loads of 80,000 to 1 million copies/ml or even higher. These same tests are repeated at intervals determined by the presence or absence of manifestations or disease in the client through the course of illness. Because several viral load tests have been approved for use, clinicians are advised to use the same viral load test when performing serial measurements to control variations in test results. Diseases such as influenza, herpes, or pneumonia, as well as testing immediately after the influenza vaccine is ad-

ministered, can cause a temporary rise in test results. Therefore, testing should be deferred in any of these situations.

INITIATE AND MAINTAIN ANTIRETROVIRAL THERAPY

The decision to treat HIV disease should involve both the primary care provider and the client. Many clients, because of personal experience or preference, may refuse recommended antiretroviral therapy. Clinicians should, in a noncoercive manner, provide as much objective information as possible so that the person with HIV can make an informed choice about taking these drugs. Because of the accumulating data indicating increased survival in people who receive antiretroviral therapy, most clinicians would recommend starting an antiretroviral combination therapy regimen.

Current guidelines recommend that therapy begin when the viral load is 5000 to 10,000 copies/ml and when the client has evidence of clinical or immunologic deterioration (CD4+ cell count <500 mm³) or when the viral load is more than 20,000 copies/ml, regardless of clinical manifestations. Many clinicians also recommend that antiretroviral therapy be started close to primary HIV infection or as soon as HIV infection is identified. They reason that less damage is done to the immune system the sooner therapy is started.

Three classes of antiretroviral agents have been approved in the United States:

- Nucleoside reverse transcriptase inhibitors (NRTIs)
- Protease inhibitors (PIs)
- Non-nucleoside reverse transcriptase inhibitors (NNRTIs)

NRTIs block HIV replication by protecting noninfected cells. PIs render HIV particles noninfectious in cells already infected with HIV. NNRTIs work in a manner similar to that of nucleoside analogs. Table 79–2 presents the three classes of antiretrovirals. The goals of therapy are to inhibit the replication of HIV, reduce the viral load to undetectable levels, and stabilize the disease.

The first NRTI, approved in March 1987, was zidovudine (Retrovir, AZT). The original dosage was 1,200 mg/day taken at specified intervals. The most profound side effect was myelosuppression, resulting in anemia and leukopenia, which often required repeated transfusions. Many people currently infected with HIV remember the difficult experience of a friend or loved one and consequently may be reluctant to try antiretroviral therapy. By 1990, research demonstrated that 600 mg/day of zidovudine (half the original dose) was sufficient to achieve the desired effects. Other NRTIs include didanosine (Videx, ddI, approved in 1991), zalcitabine (Hivid, ddC, approved in 1992), stavudine (Zerit, d4T, approved in 1994), lamivudine (Epivir, 3TC, approved in 1995), a combination of lamivudine and zidovudine (Combivir, approved in 1997), and abacavir (Ziagen, approved in 1998).

Eager anticipation preceded the approval of PIs, a new class of drugs, because large numbers of clients developed resistance to NRTIs. PIs include saquinavir (Invirase or Fortovase, approved in 1995), indinavir (Crixivan, approved in 1996), ritonavir (Norvir, approved in 1996), nelfinavir (Viracept, approved in 1997), and amprenavir (Agenerase, approved in 1999). The newest class of

Drug	Adverse Outcomes	Adult Dosing	Nursing Implications
NUCLEOSIDE REVERSE TRANSCRIPTASE INHIBITORS			
Abacavir (Ziagen)	Fatigue, changes in liver function tests, headache, abdominal pain, constipation, diarrhea, nausea, vomiting, insomnia, skin rash, and dizziness	300 mg PO bid	During the first 4 weeks of therapy, client should stop treatment immediately if flu-like manifestations develop and keep getting worse (fever, rash, malaise, nausea, vomiting, diarrhea) Once a hypersensitivity reaction is noted the drug should not be restarted (rechallenged) May be taken with or without food
Didanosine (Videx, ddI)	Pancreatitis (abdominal pain, nausea, vomiting), peripheral neuropathy (tingling, burning, numbness, or pain in the finger tips or feet), anxiety, headache, irritability, inability to sleep, restlessness, dry mouth, nervousness, and rash	>60 kg—*tablets:* 200 mg PO q 12 h; *powder:* 250 mg PO q 12 h <60 kg—*tablets:* 125 mg PO q 12 h; *powder:* 167 mg PO q 12 h	Give on an empty stomach 30 minutes before or 2 hours after a meal Tablets can be chewed, crushed, or dispersed in water (when dispersed, use within 1 hour); powder should be mixed only in drinking water Pediatric powder is mixed into solution by pharmacist and is stable for 30 days if refrigerated Must be separated by 1 hour from other drugs
Lamivudine (Epivir, 3TC)	Peripheral neuropathy (tingling, burning, numbness, or pain in the hands, arms, feet, or legs), pancreatitis (nausea, vomiting, severe abdominal or stomach pain), unusually tired or weak, fever, chills or sore throat, skin rash, headache, nausea, malaise, diarrhea, cough, insomnia, dizziness, muscle pain, joint pain, abdominal cramps, and dyspepsia	>50 kg—150 mg PO bid <50 kg—2 mg/kg PO bid	Give in combination with other antiretrovirals, never as monotherapy May take without regard to food Store at room temperature Tell client to avoid alcohol Report persistent severe abdominal pain, nausea, vomiting, and numbness or tingling
Lamivudine/zidovudine (Combivir)	Headache, malaise, fever, chills, nausea, vomiting, diarrhea, anorexia, abdominal pain and cramps, neuropathy, insomnia, dizziness, nasal manifestations, musculoskeletal pain, rash, neutropenia, and anemia	1 tablet (contains 150 mg of lamivudine and 300 mg of zidovudine) PO bid	May be taken with or without food
Stavudine (Zerit, d4T)	Numbness, tingling, or pain in the hands or feet, headache, diarrhea, chills and fever, nausea, vomiting, muscle pain, loss of strength or energy, insomnia, anxiety, joint pain, back pain, loss of appetite, nervousness, and dizziness	>60 kg—40 mg PO q 12 h <60 kg—30 mg PO q 12 h	Compounded with lactose; lactose intolerant clients can take LactAid (lactase enzyme) tablets before taking stavudine May take without regard to food Tell client to avoid alcohol Report tingling, burning, pain, or numbness of hands or feet
Zalcitabine (Hivid, ddC)	Numbness, tingling, burning, and pain in lower extremities, abdominal pain, nausea, vomiting, rash, gastrointestinal intolerance, fever, sore throat, headache, fatigue, nausea, pruritus, muscle pain, difficulty swallowing, and arthralgia	0.75 mg PO q 8 h	Store tablets at room temperature Best taken on an empty stomach Swallow tablets whole with plenty of water

Drug	Dosage	Side effects	Nursing considerations
Zidovudine (Retrovir, AZT)	As prophylaxis for vertical transmission of HIV: **maternal use after first trimester**—200 mg PO tid or 300 mg PO bid; **during delivery**—2 mg/kg IV loading dose over 30–60 minutes followed by continuous infusion of 1 mg/kg/hour until the cord is clamped. As treatment: 200 mg PO tid or 300 mg PO bid	Fatigue, muscle pain, headache, nausea, vomiting, insomnia, anemia (pale skin, unusually tired or weak), neutropenia (fever, chills, sore throat), confusion, mental changes, seizures, and bluish-brown bands on fingernails	Store capsules and syrup at room temperature. Protect from light. May take without regard to food. Take with food to decrease nausea, but avoid high-fat meal because it impairs absorption. Infusion should be given over at least 60 minutes. Give in combination with other antiretrovirals except during pregnancy, when it can be given as monotherapy

PROTEASE INHIBITORS

Drug	Dosage	Side effects	Nursing considerations
Amprenavir (Agenerase)	1200 mg PO bid	Nausea, vomiting, rash, diarrhea, flatulence, fatigue, headache, and perioral paresthesia	During the first few weeks of therapy, observe for skin reactions; Stevens-Johnson syndrome has been reported
Indinavir (Crixivan)	800 mg PO q 8 h	Kidney stones (blood in urine, sharp back pain), nausea, diarrhea, vomiting, abdominal pain, headache, insomnia, altered taste, dizziness, generalized weakness, and asymptomatic hyperbilirubinemia. May increase triglycerides. May cause hyperglycemia. May cause fat redistribution in the body	Give in combination with other antiretrovirals, never as monotherapy. Store at room temperature. Take on an empty stomach or with a light meal (high-fat, high-protein meals decrease blood levels by 77%). Give at least 1 hour apart if given with didanosine. Must drink at least 1.5 liters of water daily. Compounded with lactose; lactose intolerant clients can take LactAid tablets before taking indinavir. Extremely moisture sensitive; keep in original container with desiccants; do not pre-pour into medication box; do not keep in bathroom. Blood glucose should be monitored
Nelfinavir (Viracept)	750 mg PO tid or 1250 mg PO bid	Diarrhea, flatulence, nausea, abdominal pain, generalized weakness, and rash. May increase triglycerides. May cause hyperglycemia. May cause fat redistribution in the body	Give in combination with other antiretrovirals, never as monotherapy. Loperamide will control diarrhea. Oral powder may be mixed with a small amount of water, milk, dietary supplement, chocolate milk, or pudding. Do not mix with acidic foods, such as apple sauce, apple juice, or orange juice, because doing so produces a bitter taste. Once mixed, consume entire contents within 6 hours. Take with food for optimal absorption. Blood glucose should be monitored

Table continued on following page

Drug	Adverse Outcomes	Adult Dosing	Nursing Implications
Ritonavir (Norvir)	Nausea, vomiting, diarrhea, loss of appetite, abdominal pain, taste alterations, headache, dizziness, sleepiness, tingling sensation or numbness around the lips, hands, or feet, fatigue, weakness May increase liver enzymes and triglycerides May cause hyperglycemia May cause fat redistribution in the body	Initially, 300 mg PO q 12 h, increasing by 100 mg PO q 12 h to a maximum of 600 mg PO q 12 h	Store capsules and solution in refrigerator and protect from light Refrigeration of solution not necessary if used within 30 days, but store below 77° F Take with food (increases blood levels) Taste of oral solution may be improved by mixing with plain or chocolate milk, pudding, or ice cream within 1 hour of dosing; by dulling the taste buds through chewing on ice, Popsicles (frozen dessert), or spoonfuls of partially frozen orange or grape juice; by eating peanut butter before administration to coat the mouth; or by chewing gum or hard candies after taking the dose Tobacco decreases blood levels Blood glucose should be monitored Alcohol intake can worsen manifestations (ritonavir oral solution contains alcohol)
Saquinavir (Invirase, Fortovase)	Nausea, diarrhea, ulcers in mouth, abdominal discomfort, abdominal pain, burning or prickling sensation, skin rash, weakness, and headache May increase triglycerides May cause hyperglycemia May cause fat redistribution in the body	Invirase, 600 mg PO tid; Fortovase, 1200 mg PO tid	Compounded with lactose; lactose intolerant clients can take LactAid tablets before taking saquinavir Take with a full meal; high-fat meal increases blood levels Photosensitivity can occur; use sunscreen or protective clothing Blood glucose should be monitored
NON-NUCLEOSIDE REVERSE TRANSCRIPTASE INHIBITORS			
Delavirdine (Rescriptor)	Diffuse, itchy, maculopapular rash, nausea, arthralgia, insomnia, changes in dreams, headache, diarrhea, fatigue, and increased liver enzymes	Initially, 200 mg PO tid for 14 days, then 400 mg PO tid	May take without regard to food
Efavirenz (Sustiva)	52% of clients in clinical trials experienced central nervous system and psychiatric manifestations, including dizziness, nightmares, confusion, insomnia, somnolence, cognitive impairment, amnesia, agitation, depersonalization, hallucinations, and euphoria; other side effects include nausea, vomiting, diarrhea, rash, and fatigue	600 mg PO once daily at bedtime	Do not give to pregnant women; birth defects occurred in animal studies Most side effects disappear after 2–4 weeks of therapy
Nevirapine (Viramune)	Rash, fever, nausea, headache, abnormal liver function tests, stomatitis (sores or ulcers in mouth), numbness, muscle pain, hepatitis (yellow skin, diarrhea, nausea, headache)	Initially 200 mg daily PO for 14 days, then 200 mg PO bid or 400 mg PO once daily	May take without regard to food

Note: Except for zidovudine, which may be prescribed as monotherapy for pregnant women, all of the antiretrovirals are prescribed in combinations of three or more at once.
bid, twice a day; h, hour; IV, intravenous; PO, by mouth; q, every; tid, three times a day.

drugs, the NNRTIs, includes nevirapine (Viramune, approved in 1996), delavirdine (Rescriptor, approved in 1997), and efavirenz (Sustiva, approved in 1998).

Perhaps the greatest challenge in treating HIV infection has been the genetic promiscuity of this virus. As stated earlier, HIV mutates rapidly. In the presence of an antiretroviral drug, it can develop resistance to the drug and continue to grow in the presence of the drug. Three types of drug resistance are of concern:

• *Genotype resistance,* in which the virus mutates
• *Phenotype resistance,* in which the virus shows a decrease in sensitivity to the drug
• *Cross-resistance,* in which the virus, having developed resistance to one drug, becomes resistant to other drugs in that class

Monotherapy (prescription of one antiretroviral agent at a time) is more likely to result in drug resistance than combination therapy. *Subtherapeutic* levels of a drug also lead to drug resistance. Subtherapeutic levels can occur when the client does not take the prescribed dosage, does not take doses at specified intervals, or both, and can also occur when other prescribed drugs interact with the antiretroviral drug and cause lower blood levels.

In an attempt to prevent drug resistance, clinicians order combination therapy, believing that combinations of drugs "confuse" the virus, thus interfering with its ability to develop resistance. Unfortunately, preliminary data show that even in combinations of three drugs at once, resistance develops to one or more of the agents being taken. Combination therapy includes two or more drugs given simultaneously from the NRTI group either exclusively or in combination with a PI or an NNRTI. The goal is to find combinations that are the least toxic and that produce the largest and most long-lasting viral response (lowest viral load) and the best immune response (highest CD4$^+$ cell counts).

Evaluation of the efficacy of antiretroviral therapy is based on the client's clinical manifestations and on laboratory tests of viral load and CD4$^+$ cell counts. The most reliable objective determinant is viral load testing, which is performed 3 to 4 weeks after initiating or changing therapy. If the decrease in viral load is not at least three times the original laboratory reports, or decreased by at least 0.5 log, the therapy is usually changed. Repeated testing to make sure that the drugs are working is usually performed at 3- to 4-month intervals.

Drug failure, in which the ordered combination is no longer effective, can occur after trying several standard combinations or antiretrovirals. The challenge to the clinician at that point is to try combinations of four to six drugs in an effort to suppress HIV activity once again. This approach to therapeutic intervention is commonly called *salvage therapy.* In many instances, salvage therapy fails because the HIV-infected person has developed drug resistance to most of the available drugs.

Studies are also being conducted to identify other chemotherapeutic strategies to control HIV infection. Scientists are looking at the use of HIV vaccines as a therapeutic strategy to stimulate host responses and control viral replication. Research continues to investigate the development of *immunomodulators,* drugs designed to modulate or reconstitute the immune system. Drugs being studied include tumor necrosis factor alpha (TNF-α), interleukin-2 (IL-2), IV immune globulin, and interferon alfa. IL-2 used in adults and IV immune globulin used in children have shown some promising effects.

PREVENT INFECTION

By 1986, surveillance data indicated that in more than 80% of people with HIV disease, *Pneumocystis carinii* pneumonia occurred at least once before death. Studies eventually showed that morbidity and mortality could be significantly reduced by giving a drug prophylactically for *P. carinii* pneumonia. Since 1989, the U.S. Public Health Service has recommended that all HIV-infected clients with a CD4$^+$ cell count below 200 mm^3 receive prophylaxis for *P. carinii* pneumonia. Drugs include trimethoprim-sulfamethoxazole (TMP-SMX); dapsone; dapsone, pyrimethamine, and leucovorin; aerosolized pentamidine; or atovaquone. Alternatives include intermittent parenteral pentamidine, pyrimethamine-sulfadoxine, clindamycin plus primaquine, atovaquone, and IV trimetrexate. TMP-SMX and dapsone also provide protection against toxoplasmosis.

Although surveillance data alone do not reflect the true incidence of infection with *Mycobacterium avium-intracellulare* complex, postmortem examinations revealed that more than 60% of HIV-infected people had an active infection. Since 1993, the U.S. Public Health Service has recommended that all HIV-infected clients with a CD4$^+$ cell count below 50 mm^3 receive prophylaxis for *M. avium-intracellulare* complex. Recommended drugs include clarithromycin, azithromycin, and rifabutin. However, these drugs may interact with antiretrovirals.

All HIV-infected clients with a positive result to a tuberculin skin test that have no evidence of active tuberculosis should receive 9 months of preventive therapy with isoniazid. Pyridoxine should be added to reduce the potential for peripheral neuropathy. An alternative regimen is rifabutin and pyrazinamide for 2 months. However, these drugs may interact with antiretrovirals.

Other recommended prophylactic measures include prevention of respiratory infections using pneumococcal vaccine and influenza vaccine and prevention of traveler's diarrhea, when traveling to countries where diarrhea is common, using antimicrobials such as ciprofloxacin. Finally, prophylactic medication may be ordered to prevent cytomegalovirus infection, recurrent candidiasis, cryptococcosis, or histoplasmosis.

Nursing Management of the Client with HIV Infection

ASSESSMENT

To help a client with health maintenance behaviors, do not restrict your nursing assessment to the client's immediate clinical status. Instead, focus on potential problems that may be encountered during the illness trajectory. For example, federal legislation passed in 1996 barred states from providing Medicaid to illegal immigrants to the United States. It is of no value to tell people that they need regular health care follow-up if they have no insurance and no money to pay for it. Social work intervention is needed to find an alternative source of health care services, such as the federally funded AIDS Drug Assistance Program, which provides more than just drugs. If the client lives alone and has no one willing to assist, he or she may need to be placed in an institution when the illness progresses. As a coordinator of care, you should have information readily available to identify problems and plan ahead.

Before performing any teaching, evaluate the client's existing level of knowledge about HIV infection. Some clients may know very little. Others may be very knowledgeable and may have even suspected they were infected but avoided being tested. Try to assess exactly what the client does or does not know about transmission and health-promoting behaviors before you make any assumptions.

The psychological burden of HIV disease can be overwhelming. Crisis points at which you can anticipate anxiety, fear, or depression include the following:

- Time of the initial HIV-positive diagnosis
- Time of the initial AIDS diagnosis
- Changes in treatment
- Development of new manifestations
- Recurrence of problems or relapse
- Terminal illness

Psychological conflicts that clients commonly experience include fear of transmitting HIV to others, constant worry about developing an infection, guilt about a previous lifestyle, and changes in personal relationships. Social stressors may include disclosure of one's HIV status, stigma conferred by that status, insecurity about employment and insurance, and loneliness and social isolation.

DIAGNOSIS, OUTCOMES, INTERVENTIONS

Effective Management of Therapeutic Regimen: Individual. The primary nursing diagnosis encountered with newly diagnosed HIV infection is *Effective Management of Therapeutic Regimen: Individual, related to behaviors that will improve the level of health and prevent complications.* Although some clients may know about HIV disease, it is unlikely that they know all that can be done to improve their health.

Outcomes. The client will know about HIV disease, how to prevent transmission, how to manage the disease, and how to prevent complications.

Interventions

Provide Education. Health teaching should be ongoing and repeated at frequent intervals. An HIV-infected person can adopt several behaviors that not only improve immune function but also increase a sense of well-being. The content outline for teaching health maintenance includes stress management, exercise, safe sex practices, procreation and HIV infection, nutrition (with emphasis on a high-protein, high-calorie, low-fat diet), food and water safety, skin care, hair care, routine mouth care, proper hand-washing, environmental cleaning and safety, pet care, limiting alcohol consumption, use of injected drugs, travel safety and avoiding exposure to infectious pathogens, importance of health care follow-up, and understanding and interpreting viral load tests and CD4+ cell counts.

Carefully explain viral load test results to your clients because many people misunderstand the results. When successful therapy begins, the viral load drops from very high levels, such as 750,000 copies/ml, down to what are called "undetectable" levels. However, most laboratory personnel can detect HIV copies down to only 400 copies/ml. Because anything lower cannot be measured, the laboratory report reads "undetectable levels." Although this is great news and indicates the success of the prescribed regimen, it does not mean that the person no longer has HIV infection. Some clients with HIV infection leave their primary care provider thinking that they are disease free and no longer at risk of spreading HIV. This must be clarified whenever you report laboratory results to a client; emphasize that the client must still practice safer sex, avoid sharing needles, and so on.

Encourage clients to tell their health care providers about any self-prescribed therapies they may be taking, because they may have a positive or negative influence on the outcomes of care. Keep track of over-the-counter medications because they may interact with prescribed therapies. Some clients may also obtain drugs through buyers' clubs or underground pharmacies. This may not only be detrimental to the effectiveness of prescribed treatments but may also have an adverse effect on observations made during a drug trial.

Some clients may opt to try alternative or complementary treatments, including (1) spiritual or psychological interventions (e.g., guided imagery, meditation, faith healing); (2) nutritional alternatives (e.g., a Macrobiotic diet; (3) drug and biologic therapies, (e.g., homeopathy, oxygen, ozone therapy); and (4) physical forces (e.g., acupuncture, acupressure, massage therapy). In most cases, these choices can have a positive effect on the person's emotional well-being but may also have a negative effect. For example, a Macrobiotic diet can lead to vitamin and mineral deficiencies as well as weight loss. Herbal remedies may cause nausea, vomiting, diarrhea, or CNS depression. Despite these effects, some clients may continue to use these methods.

Initiate and Maintain Antiretroviral Therapy. One of the most important aspects of providing nursing care to the HIV-infected client is helping with the antiretroviral regimen. Studies suggest that clients with chronic diseases such as hypertension and diabetes take their prescribed drugs about 50% of the time. In contrast, to sustain the durability and efficacy of antiretroviral therapy, clients must maintain about a 90% compliance rate. This places high expectations on both the HIV-infected client and the physicians and nurses. Because therapy is now recommended early in the course of HIV infection, within weeks after the initial infection, you should discuss the potential benefits and risks of antiretroviral therapy. Potential benefits include:

- Control of HIV replication and mutation, with reduction in viral load
- Prevention of destruction of the immune system and loss of CD4+ T helper cells
- Delayed progression to AIDS-defining illnesses
- Decreased risk for development of HIV resistance to drugs
- Decreased risk drug toxicity (drugs are started when the client is healthier)
- Increased survival with HIV disease (the most important benefit)

Potential risks include:

- Reduced quality of life from adverse drug effects and the inconvenience of a complex regimen
- Earlier development of drug resistance
- A limited number of drugs available to respond to drug resistance
- Unknown long-term toxicity of antiretroviral therapy
- Unknown duration of the effectiveness of current antiretroviral therapies

The decision of whether to take antiretrovirals is ultimately up to the client. The regimens ordered are commonly complex and require the client to take large numbers of pills daily, often at exactly spaced intervals, such as every 8 hours rather than simply three times a day. Didanosine must be taken on an empty stomach and separated by time from all other medications. Saquinavir must be taken with a high-fat meal. Indinavir must be taken with a low-fat meal. Liquid preparations often taste horrible, and the client must try various strategies to mask the taste. All of the drugs have side effects to which the person must learn to adjust and control. They also interact with numerous other drugs. These drug-drug interactions are usually not life-threatening, but they may interfere with antiretroviral blood levels, causing subtherapeutic effects, drug resistance, and drug failure. Instruct all clients taking antiretrovirals as follows:

- Take the drug at specified intervals.
- Do not skip a dose.
- Do not increase or decrease the number of pills you take.
- Follow meal and fluid requirements.
- If side effects occur, tell your physician or nurse. If side effects are significant, ask your primary care provider for information or medication to help manage them.
- Store all drugs as instructed.
- If you do not want to take the drugs, tell your primary care provider.

- If you take the drugs only periodically, it would be better not to take them at all. Discuss this with your physician or nurse.
- Remember, the treatment plan is yours. If you do not agree with it, discuss it with your physician or nurse.

Because of the concern over the development of drug resistance and drug failure, several studies have been started on methods to help people infected with HIV adhere to their drug regimens. Several strategies have proved very helpful, especially when used together:

1. Write out the client's drug and meal schedule, explaining when to eat and when to take which drugs (Table 79-3).
2. Provide the client with an electronic reminder. Research suggests that the main reason why people with HIV miss a drug dose is because they "forget." An alarm set to go off at the next dosing time can keep the client from forgetting.
3. Provide a large pill box with removable sleeves so that the client can conveniently carry the day's supply of drugs.

This combination of interventions can be used for any client with a chronic condition who must take medications daily.

Other strategies that enhance drug adherence behaviors include (1) ongoing supervision (telephone follow-up or home visits), (2) providing the client with written information about drugs and how to take them, and (3) interactive teaching sessions in which the client provides return demonstrations. Primary care providers also need to incorporate cultural and religious beliefs when addressing drug adherence behaviors. Meal planning because of fat content requirements or dietary restrictions or preferences, as well as the need to abstain from food and water on certain days because of religious practices, may be necessary.

Prevent Infection. Nursing strategies to prevent infection include health teaching and helping the client take

TABLE 79-3	SAMPLE MEDICATION AND MEAL SCHEDULE		
Time	Comments	Medicine to Take	Box Label to Use
7 AM	Eat *breakfast* and drink a full glass (8 oz) of fluid	Zerit, Epivir, LactAid, Fortovase, Norvir, multivitamin, Biaxin, Bactrim, sulfadiazine, pyrimethamine, leucovorin	AM
12 noon	Eat *lunch,* and drink a full glass (8 oz) of fluid	Sulfadiazine	Noon
7 PM	Eat *supper,* and drink a full glass (8 oz) of fluid	Zerit, Epivir, LactAid, Fortovase, Norvir, Biaxin, sulfadiazine	PM
10 PM	Eat a snack, and drink a full glass (8 oz) of fluid	Sulfadiazine	Bed
During the night	If you get up during the night, drink a full glass (8 oz) of fluid		

Note: Take Fortovase and Norvir with food. These drugs are not absorbed well if taken on an empty stomach.

drugs properly to prevent opportunistic infections. Health teaching focuses on safer sex practices not only to prevent HIV transmission but also to keep from acquiring STDs. Practicing food and water safety can prevent such diseases as salmonellosis, cryptosporidiosis, and toxoplasmosis. Maintaining skin and mucous membrane integrity with good skin and mouth hygiene can reduce the incidence of candidiasis.

EVALUATION

Evaluation includes the client's understanding of teaching that has been provided and the choices that each person may make. If a client chooses not to adopt a recommended behavior, it does not mean that the client is noncompliant. People with HIV who smoke may find that their stress level rises too high when they try to quit, even when using a nicotine patch or gum. Such clients may choose to continue to smoke. Health care providers can have a difficult time evaluating the outcomes of teaching and weighing them against the client's free choice. Remember, the ultimate decision about following a health care provider's advice belongs to the client. The client's decisions do not reflect failure on the part of the health care professional.

Evaluation of a client's ability to adhere to a prescribed drug regimen includes both subjective and objective techniques. *Subjective* evaluation is by self-report; clients and their care partner describe the client's ability to take all prescribed medications. *Objective* analysis of the success of the plan of care is by laboratory evaluation of CD4+ cell counts and viral load. Avoid "pill counting" as a way to evaluate whether a client is taking drugs as prescribed. This should be performed only if the client wants this intervention and participates. Pill counts have been used for many years by nurses as a sort of policing activity when they find a client is not following a drug regimen properly. Today, pill counts are considered by many nurse experts to be a waste of time because clients often simply discard leftover pills if they know that a nurse will be performing a pill count.

A totally different situation exists when minimal learning takes place because of cognitive impairment. It is well documented that problems with thinking or memory may exist and go unidentified if they are not obvious. This is more likely to occur in clients with less than a 12th grade education and in clients over age 50. In such a situation, a care partner should be designated, who receives all information when it is provided to the client. Whenever the care partner cannot make a clinic or office visit, provide telephone teaching and document that you accomplished this.

Outcome Management for AIDS

As both the quantity and quality of CD4+ cells diminish, "AIDS-indicator" diseases occur. The categories of AIDS-defining illnesses include opportunistic infections, cancers, and other conditions specific to HIV disease. The four main types of opportunistic infections are (1) bacterial, (2) fungal, (3) protozoal, and (4) viral. Bacterial infections are the easiest to treat, and viruses are the most difficult. Neoplasms associated with AIDS include Kaposi's sarcoma, non-Hodgkin's lymphoma, and invasive cervical cancer. Two other conditions that are unique to AIDS are (1) HIV encephalopathy and (2) HIV wasting syndrome. Since the introduction of combination anti-retroviral therapy in 1996, the onset of AIDS-defining illness has been delayed and treating these diseases has become easier.

■ Medical Management of the AIDS Client

PREVENT AND TREAT OPPORTUNISTIC INFECTIONS

Most of the pathogens responsible for opportunistic infections are ubiquitous; that is, they are all around us. *P. carinii* is in the air we breathe. The reason most people do not become sick from this organism is that their immune systems are intact. Once the regulators of the immune system (CD4+ cells) are destroyed by HIV, however, infection occurs. Most opportunistic infections result from secondary reactivation of previously acquired pathogens rather than from a new or primary infection. For example, most people are infected with *P. carinii* in the early preschool years, when it causes respiratory manifestations and is probably dismissed as a common cold. The child's intact immune system brings the infection under control. However, the organism remains dormant in the person's body. The potential then exists that if an immunodeficiency occurs, the organism can reactivate, causing disease again. This concept applies to any person with an immunodeficiency, regardless of the cause. To illustrate further, clients with cancer who receive chemotherapy and become immunodeficient may also develop infection from *P. carinii*.

Single opportunistic infections are rare, and clients may have multiple infections. Many of the opportunistic infections that occur in people with HIV are not curable. Because the immune system no longer has the strength to contain the infection, it becomes chronic and requires lifetime suppressive therapy. Helping the client comply with the antibiotic regimen to keep opportunistic infections under control is an essential part of the care planning process. Because the client must take antibiotics for extended periods, drug resistance may develop, and both physicians and nurses must constantly observe the client for recurrence of manifestations that may indicate the infection is reactivating and the drugs no longer work.

Bacterial Infections

MYCOBACTERIUM TUBERCULOSIS INFECTION. Co-infection with *M. tuberculosis* (TB) and HIV is common, especially in large metropolitan areas. Because the bacterium is airborne, the presence of an immunodeficiency makes the person with HIV very susceptible to TB. All HIV-infected people should be tested annually to detect new or active infection. Nosocomial spread of TB among clients hospitalized and placed on AIDS units has been a problem. Manifestations of active infection are categorized as constitutional, pulmonary, or extrapulmonary. Constitutional manifestations include fever, chills, weight loss, night sweats, lymphadenopathy, and fatigue. Pulmonary manifestations may include cough, dyspnea, chest pain, and hemoptysis. Extrapulmonary presentation may involve lymph nodes, bones, joints, liver, spleen, central nervous system, skin, gastrointestinal tract, mass lesions, urine, and blood.

The recommended therapy includes a combination of drugs that may include isoniazid, rifampin, pyrazinamide, and either ethambutol or streptomycin. Drug selection is based on culture and sensitivity reports and potential drug-drug interactions with antiretrovirals already being taken.

Multi-drug–resistant TB was identified as an emerging problem in the United States around 1987. By 1990, significant numbers of cases were identified, especially among people with HIV infection. Studies attributed the development of multi-drug–resistant TB to physicians prescribing insufficient numbers of drugs to treat new cases of TB and once again the development of TB strains resistant to the most widely prescribed agents, isoniazid and rifampin. Based on drug sensitivity reports, second-line therapy for multi-drug–resistant TB includes ciprofloxacin, ofloxacin, kanamycin, amikacin, capreomycin, ethionamide, cycloserine, aminosalicylic acid, or clofazimine as single drug or combination therapy.

In institutional settings, clients are placed in respiratory isolation until sputum tests reveal that they are no longer infectious. In many cases of multi-drug–resistant TB, despite therapy, sputum results indicate the presence of organisms; it is not uncommon to have clients remain in respiratory isolation until discharge. TB is a reportable communicable disease, and health care professionals are required to report new cases to local health authorities.

Follow-up care focuses on management of clinical manifestations. Monitoring drug compliance is essential to ensure effective treatment and to prevent recurrent active disease. In cities where multi-drug–resistant TB has become a significant problem, local health departments have established monitoring programs (known as *directly observed therapy*), in which health care workers travel to client locations and watch them take their medications. Psychological stressors for the client include coping with the stigma of both HIV and TB.

MYCOBACTERIUM AVIUM COMPLEX. *M. avium* complex is also sometimes called *M. avium-intracellulare.* The organism exists in soil, water, animals, eggs, and unpasteurized dairy products. Not all members of the *Mycobacterium* family of bacteria are communicable. *M. avium* complex is referred to as an atypical, noncommunicable mycobacterial disease. Because most people with HIV develop active disease and the risk of infection increases with CD4$^+$ cell counts below 50 mm^3, prophylaxis to prevent infection is recommended. Additionally, *M. avium* complex infection is much easier to prevent than to treat.

The clinical presentation of *M. avium* complex infection includes fever, night sweats, fatigue, anorexia, weight loss, abdominal pain, and diarrhea. Because the disease is difficult to treat and side effects of the medications are numerous, the decision whether to treat *M. avium* complex infection depends on the severity of manifestations and the presence of renal or hepatic disease. Two to six drugs may be used at one time, including some combination of azithromycin, clarithromycin, clofazimine, ethambutol, ciprofloxacin, rifabutin, and amikacin.

Follow-up care focuses on managing clinical manifestations because they may persist despite drug therapy. It is important to evaluate the client's ability to comply with the prescribed therapy because some clients may decrease the dosage of prescribed pills on their own to minimize side effects. Both clients and their care providers need to be taught that this is not a communicable disease.

SALMONELLOSIS. *Salmonella* infection can be prevented by teaching the client about food and water safety and proper food handling. Infection occurs after ingestion of contaminated food, including (1) beef, pork, poultry, and eggs; (2) drinking contaminated water; (3) ingesting contaminated drugs or diagnostic agents; (4) directly handling contaminated feces; or (5) sexual activity involving oral-anal contact. Food handlers may be asymptomatic carriers, and pets, especially turtles, may be a source of exposure. Presenting clinical manifestations include fever, night sweats, fatigue, anorexia, weight loss, abdominal pain, and diarrhea. Treatment includes ampicillin, chloramphenicol, trimethoprim-sulfamethoxazole, ciprofloxacin, or norfloxacin. Follow-up care focuses on management of manifestations, including preventing and managing skin breakdown in the perianal region.

BACTERIAL PNEUMONIA. Recurrent bacterial pneumonia is common among IV drug users. Predisposing factors include needle sharing, environmental exposure, heavy alcohol use, smoking, and inadequate nutrition. Pathogens most often associated with bacterial pneumonia, seen in people infected with HIV, are *Streptococcus pneumoniae* and *Haemophilus influenzae.* The risk of bacterial pneumonia increases when the CD4$^+$ cell count is below 200 mm^3. Antibiotic treatment is based on culture and sensitivity reports. Follow-up care includes focusing on behavioral changes that decrease the possibility of recurrence (such as smoking cessation, adequate nutrition, and using clean needles to inject drugs).

Pneumococcal vaccination should be given at 5-year intervals. Prophylactic therapy prescribed to prevent *P. carinii* pneumonia or *M. avium* complex may provide some protection against recurrent bacterial pneumonia.

Fungal Infections

CANDIDIASIS. *Candida albicans* not only is ubiquitous (in soil and food, on fomites) but also is a commensal organism normally found on the skin and in the mouth, vagina, and large intestine. Most infections are *endogenous;* that is, the person's own organism is the source of the infection. *Nosocomial* spread in hospitals and nursing homes can also occur. Human-to-human transmission can occur from mother to infant during vaginal delivery and between sexual partners. Clinical presentation is related to the site of infection: dysphagia with esophagitis, oral lesions with thrush, cutaneous lesions with intertrigo, vulvovaginal irritation and discharge with vaginitis, and constitutional symptoms with disseminated disease. Treatment is also site-dependent:

- For *oral/esophageal candidiasis,* clotrimazole troches, nystatin suspension, ketoconazole, fluconazole, and amphotericin B oral suspension (for esophagitis only)
- For *intertrigo* and *vaginitis,* clotrimazole, miconazole, ketoconazole, fluconazole, imidazole, and itraconazole (for nail infection)
- For *disseminated disease,* amphotericin B, with or without flucytosine

Follow-up care includes teaching routine skin and mouth care. Encourage the client to eat 8 ounces of yogurt made from live cultures (*Lactobacillus acidophi-*

lus) to help control recurrent infection with *Candida.* For recurrent, frequent episodes or after a severe episode, prophylactic therapy with fluconazole, ketoconazole, or itraconazole may be ordered.

CRYPTOCOCCOSIS. *Cryptococcus neoformans* is ubiquitous and found in pigeon droppings, nesting places, soil, fruit, and unpasteurized fruit juices. The organism is aerosolized and inhaled. As an AIDS-indicator disease, it causes lung and brain infection. HIV-infected smokers are more prone to development of cryptococcosis. Clinical manifestations primarily involve the CNS but can also include the lungs, skin, and mouth.

CNS manifestations include low-grade fever, fatigue, headaches, nausea, vomiting, and altered mental status. Pulmonary manifestations include cough, dyspnea, and pleuritic chest pain. Cutaneous and oral manifestations include painless lesions that may mimic Kaposi's sarcoma or molluscum contagiosum. Treatment includes amphotericin B, with or without flucytosine, fluconazole, or itraconazole. Maintenance lifetime suppressive therapy is required with fluconazole, itraconazole, or amphotericin B, and follow-up care focuses on assisting with medication compliance and monitoring for recurrence of symptoms that indicate resistance to maintenance drug therapy.

HISTOPLASMOSIS. *Histoplasma capsulatum,* a fungus endemic to certain regions of the United States, is most prevalent in the middle, central, and south central states and Puerto Rico. Therefore, people with HIV disease and living in these areas are susceptible to the disease. When diagnosed in other parts of the country (e.g., New York, California), the disease usually appears in a client who either grew up in or traveled to the endemic regions. Manifestations include fever; weight loss; enlarged lymph nodes, liver, and spleen; abdominal pain; oral and skin lesions; anemia; leukopenia; and thrombocytopenia.

Treatment includes amphotericin B, itraconazole, or fluconazole. Maintenance lifetime suppressive therapy (itraconazole or amphotericin B) is required. Follow-up care focuses on helping with drug compliance and monitoring for recurrence of manifestations that indicate resistance to maintenance drug therapy.

COCCIDIOIDOMYCOSIS. *Coccidioides immitis* is a fungus endemic to the southwestern United States. It was originally discovered in the San Joaquin Valley in southern California and is also referred to as *valley fever.* As an AIDS-defining diagnosis, it is commonly seen in people infected with HIV residing in Arizona, California, Nevada, New Mexico, Texas, and Utah. When diagnosed in other parts of the United States, the disease usually appears in a client who either grew up in or traveled to the endemic regions. Clinical presentation includes fever, dyspnea, fatigue, weight loss, and cough.

Treatment includes amphotericin B, ketoconazole, itraconazole, or fluconazole. Maintenance lifetime suppressive therapy is required using fluconazole, itraconazole, or amphotericin B. Follow-up care focuses on helping with drug compliance and monitoring for recurrence of manifestations that indicate resistance to maintenance drug therapy.

Protozoal Infections

PNEUMOCYSTOSIS. *P. carinii* is a ubiquitous organism that is airborne and can be found in the lungs of humans and animals. Most healthy people have had a primary infection by 4 years of age. Although most of the literature suggests that *P. carinii* infection in people with HIV is a secondary appearance of a previously acquired pathogen (reactivation), more recent information has revealed that some clients have different strains of the organism, which may indicate that reinfection is possible through airborne transmission.

Clinical presentation can be elusive, and about 7% of clients with the infection are asymptomatic. With *P. carinii* pneumonia, coughing is a frequent first manifestation. The pneumonia begins with a nonproductive cough and progresses to a productive cough. Eventually, the client has fever and dyspnea on exertion and then dyspnea at rest. Extrapulmonary *P. carinii* infection can occur in the eyes, ears, lymph nodes, heart, spleen, liver, and pleural space and on the skin.

Clients who are receiving prophylaxis for *P. carinii* pneumonia sometimes also go on to have infection because of poor drug compliance, unusual or erratic pharmacokinetics, or development of drug resistance. Treatment may be with trimethoprim-sulfamethoxazole, pentamidine, atovaquone, trimethoprim-dapsone, clindamycin-primaquine, or trimetrexate. Maintenance lifetime suppressive therapy is required with trimethoprim-sulfamethoxazole, pentamidine aerosol, atovaquone, dapsone, or clindamycin-primaquine. Follow-up care focuses on helping with drug compliance and monitoring for recurrence of manifestations that indicate resistance to maintenance drug therapy.

TOXOPLASMOSIS. *Toxoplasma gondii* is ubiquitous in nature and is acquired through ingestion of contaminated meat (lamb and pork), vegetables, eggs, and unpasteurized dairy products. The only documented human-to-human transmission noted is from mother to fetus, if the mother acquires primary infection during pregnancy. Toxoplasmosis can also be acquired through direct handling of contaminated cat feces. However, fewer than 1% of domestic cats are infected with *T. gondii.* A veterinarian can perform a simple blood test to determine whether a cat is infected. Studies of cat owners infected with HIV have not shown any increased risk for the development of toxoplasmosis. The potential for the development of toxoplasmosis increases when the CD4+ cell count is below 100 mm^3. If trimethoprim-sulfamethoxazole or dapsone is prescribed for *P. carinii* pneumonia prophylaxis, the drug would provide prophylaxis against toxoplasmosis as well.

Clinical manifestations of CNS infection include headache, impaired cognition, hemiparesis, aphasia, ataxia, vision loss, cranial nerve palsies, motor problems, and seizures. Infection can also involve the heart, lungs, skin, stomach, abdomen, and testes. Treatment includes pyrimethamine plus sulfadiazine, dexamethasone, phenytoin, leucovorin, clindamycin plus pyrimethamine, clarithromycin, or azithromycin. Maintenance lifetime suppressive therapy calls for pyrimethamine plus sulfadiazine plus leucovorin or clindamycin plus pyrimethamine plus leucovorin. Follow-up care focuses on helping with drug compliance and monitoring for recurrence of manifestations that indicate resistance to maintenance drug therapy.

CRYPTOSPORIDIOSIS. *Cryptosporidium* is found in mammals, birds, reptiles, and fish. The primary mode of transmission in people infected with HIV is through the ingestion of contaminated food or water. Water-borne transmission can occur when drinking supplies become contaminated, including municipal water supplies, because chlorine does not destroy the organism. Boiling water for 1 minute destroys this organism.

Cryptosporidial disease can also be acquired from contaminated swimming pools, from handling infected animals, and through anal-oral sexual contact with an infected person. When cryptosporidiosis occurs in immunocompetent people, the disease is self-limiting. In an immunodeficient person with HIV, the disease is chronic and causes malabsorption, dehydration, and malnutrition. It can lead to death. Clinical presentation includes profuse diarrhea, steatorrhea (1 to 25 L/day), flatulence, abdominal cramping and pain, anorexia, nausea, vomiting, profound weight loss, fever, fatigue, myalgia, and electrolyte imbalance.

There is no effective treatment for cryptosporidiosis. Drugs that may be tried include paromomycin, letrazuril, azithromycin, clarithromycin, nitazoxanide, and symptomatic therapy to decrease peristalsis and control pain. Spontaneous remission has occurred once combination antiretroviral therapy was started, presumably because the immune system restores itself and controls the disease. Special attention is also needed to manage skin breakdown in the perianal region. Clients with cryptosporidiosis are vulnerable to depression and social isolation.

ISOSPORIASIS. *Isospora belli* is a parasite that is transmitted through contact with infected animals or humans or contaminated water. The disease is often seen in immigrants from Mexico, Haiti, and Central America. Clinical manifestations of the disease include diarrhea, anorexia, nausea, vomiting, weight loss, abdominal pain, and fever. Drug therapy includes trimethoprim-sulfamethoxazole or pyrimethamine plus leucovorin. Treatment is usually successful, and lifetime suppressive therapy is not usually required.

Viral Infections

CYTOMEGALOVIRUS DISEASE. Cytomegalovirus (CMV) is ubiquitous in humans throughout the world. Almost everyone eventually becomes infected with CMV, which is transmitted through direct contact with infected secretions, including saliva, cervical fluid, urine, semen, breast milk, feces, and blood. In people infected with HIV, CMV infection can be asymptomatic or can cause chorioretinitis, pneumonitis, encephalitis, adrenalitis, colitis, esophagitis, hepatitis, or cholangitis.

Drugs used to treat CMV infection systemically include ganciclovir, foscarnet, and cidofovir. Treatment also may involve intraocular ganciclovir implants or intravitreal injection of ganciclovir, foscarnet, or cidofovir. Maintenance lifetime suppressive therapy is required using any of these drugs. Follow-up care focuses on helping with drug compliance and monitoring for recurrence of manifestations that indicate resistance to maintenance drug therapy.

HERPES SIMPLEX. Herpes simplex virus (HSV) is ubiquitous and is spread by direct contact with infected secretions. HSV-1 is present in oral secretions, and HSV-2 is present in genital secretions. Transmission also takes place with "symptom-free excretors" (people previously infected with HSV and with no apparent lesions). Clinical presentation includes painful vesicular lesions that coalesce and rupture. Lesions usually occur in the oral, genital, or perianal region. HSV can also cause encephali-

tis, esophagitis, bronchitis, keratitis, pericarditis, and hand infection.

Treatment includes acyclovir, foscarnet, or famciclovir. Topical acyclovir also relieves pain and itching associated with skin lesions. Follow-up care focuses on monitoring the client for recurrent disease. Chronic disease requires lifetime suppressive therapy with acyclovir.

PROGRESSIVE MULTIFOCAL LEUKOENCEPHALOPATHY. Progressive multifocal leukoencephalopathy is caused by the JC virus (initials of the first client in whom it was discovered). The JC virus is ubiquitous in nature and appears to infect most middle-aged people. Active disease in people infected with HIV results in limb weakness, ataxia, cognitive impairment, vision loss, speech impairment, and headache. In the latter stages of illness, it progresses to dementia, blindness, paralysis, and death.

There is no effective therapy, but drugs that may be used include acyclovir, foscarnet, adenine arabinoside, cytosine arabinoside, and interferon alfa. There have been reports of spontaneous remission of this disease once combination antiretroviral therapy is started, presumably because the immune system restores itself and controls the disease. Follow-up care focuses on palliative therapy, safety measures, and preventing complications from immobility.

TREAT NEOPLASMS

Kaposi's Sarcoma

Four types of Kaposi's sarcoma may be encountered in clinical practice:

- Classic Kaposi's sarcoma, which tends to occur in older men who are black, of Mediterranean descent, or from certain Jewish populations
- African Kaposi's sarcoma, seen in Africa
- Transplant Kaposi's sarcoma, seen in people who receive organ transplants
- HIV-related Kaposi's sarcoma, which differs from the others in that it runs a fulminant course, is disseminated throughout the body, and results in shorter survival

HIV-related Kaposi's sarcoma is the only form associated with HIV disease. It has been diagnosed predominantly in men who have sex with men and is thought to be associated with a sexually transmitted pathogen that then predisposes the person to development. A new type of herpesvirus, named human herpesvirus type 8 (HHV-8), is suspected. Kaposi's sarcoma differs from most AIDS-defining diseases, in that it is unrelated to low $CD4^+$ cell counts and can occur early in HIV infection.

Clinical presentation typically starts with an initial "patch" that is flat and pink, looks like a bruise, and is symmetrical on both sides of the body. Later, it turns into dark violet or black plaques (see Fig. 49–19). Clinical presentation of the lesions can include the mouth, skin, mucous membranes, head, neck, torso, limbs (soles of feet), genitals, lung, brain, intestines, testes, liver, spleen, pancreas, adrenal gland, and lymph nodes. They can be painful.

Treatment depends on the extent of tumors (tumor burden), $CD4^+$ cell count, associated manifestations and diseases, and the client's functional ability. Local therapy includes radiation, localized chemotherapy, and cryotherapy. Systemic therapy includes vincristine, vinblastine, etoposide, doxorubicin, daunorubicin, bleomycin, and interferon alfa, with or without an HIV-specific antiretroviral agent. Experimental therapies under investigation include possible treatment of the underlying viral cause of Kaposi's sarcoma with foscarnet or ganciclovir. Initially, several therapies may be tried, which may be effective in suppressing the course of Kaposi's sarcoma; eventually, however, the clinical decline in the client's condition makes continued treatment impossible.

Non-Hodgkin's Lymphoma

Non-Hodgkin's lymphoma tends to occur late in the course of HIV disease and is related to low CD4+ cell counts. The primary sites of occurrence are the brain, gastrointestinal tract, bone marrow, and liver. The initial clinical presentation may be nonspecific and include fever, night sweats, and weight loss, all of which are associated with *M. avium* complex infection, TB, and CMV infection.

Treatment includes methotrexate, bleomycin, doxorubicin, cyclophosphamide, vincristine, and dexamethasone. Despite aggressive treatment, the prognosis is poor except in clients on combination antiretroviral therapy, who tend to survive longer.

Invasive Cervical Cancer

Cervical intraepithelial neoplasia (CIN), the precursor to cervical cancer, occurs at a high rate in women infected with HIV, progresses more rapidly, is less responsive to therapy, and is related to low CD4+ cell counts. In early stages of disease, the client is asymptomatic. Cervical dysplasia is usually detected by Pap smear. Early clinical manifestations include postcoital bleeding, metrorrhagia, and a blood-tinged vaginal discharge. Manifestations of more extensive disease include back, pelvic, and leg pain; weight loss; vaginal bleeding; anemia; lymphadenopathy; and edema of the legs.

Treatment of CIN can include conization, laser therapy, cryosurgery, electrocautery, or hysterectomy. For invasive cancer, treatment may involve surgery, radiation, and chemotherapy with cisplatin, vincristine, bleomycin, or mitomycin. Follow-up care focuses on recurrent disease and control of manifestations and metastasis.

TREAT CONDITIONS SPECIFIC TO AIDS

AIDS Dementia

HIV encephalopathy, also referred to as *AIDS dementia complex,* appears to affect the very young and older HIV-infected clients and clients with anemia and weight loss. In addition, HIV-infected people with less than a 12th grade education may be more likely to show clinical manifestations. Manifestations include cognitive dysfunction, motor problems, and behavioral changes. Cognitive manifestations include an inability to concentrate, decreased memory, impaired judgment, and slowed thinking. Motor impairment may be manifested as leg weakness, ataxia, and clumsiness. Behavioral changes can range from apathy, reduced spontaneity, and social withdrawal to irritability, hyperactivity, anxiety, mania, and delirium.

The staging system for AIDS dementia complex is as follows:

* Stage 0: normal
* Stage 0.5: minimal
* Stage 1: mild
* Stage 2: moderate
* Stage 3: severe
* Stage 4: end stage

Some studies have shown a favorable response to combination antiretroviral therapy. Delirium with agitation can be treated with haloperidol, lorazepam, or molindone. Follow-up monitoring focuses on detecting the progression of AIDS dementia complex and on evaluating the client's ability to safely maintain independent living and comply with prescribed therapies.

HIV Wasting Syndrome

Weight loss occurs at some point in more than 90% of people with HIV-infected infection. *HIV wasting* is defined as profound involuntary weight loss (>10% of total body baseline weight) and either chronic diarrhea or chronic weakness and fever. The primary causes of HIV wasting syndrome are reduced food intake, malabsorption of nutrients, and altered metabolism of nutrients. The clinical evaluation of a client with HIV wasting syndrome includes an attempt to determine the cause. For example, if the origin is a gastrointestinal (GI) infection (e.g., salmonellosis), treating the underlying infection usually alleviates the progressive weight loss. In men with HIV infection, low testosterone levels lead to weight loss, a trend that can be reversed with testosterone replacement.

Once wasting has begun, treatment usually results in only partial recovery. The goal of drug therapy is to stimulate appetite, produce weight gain, and increase lean muscle mass. Weight gain that results in increased body fat is of little benefit. Drugs used to treat HIV wasting syndrome include oxandrolone, thalidomide, megestrol acetate, and dronabinol. The latter two drugs usually result in weight gain that is primarily fat. The drug used most successfully to treat wasting is human growth hormone. Follow-up therapy includes constant assessment for factors that may interfere with the plan of care (cognitive impairment, severe fatigue, or a lack of resources to buy or prepare food).

▄▄ Nursing Management of the AIDS Client

In advanced HIV disease, the goal of nursing care is to diagnose and treat human responses to actual or potential health problems related to the development of clinical manifestations and the diagnosis of AIDS. All efforts are directed at controlling manifestations. Actual or potential problems seen in people with AIDS include fever, fatigue, weight loss, nausea, diarrhea, dry and painful mouth, dry skin, skin lesions, pain, dyspnea, cough, impaired cognition, impaired vision, insomnia, and sexual dysfunction. Common nursing diagnoses that have been identified through nursing research associated with the diagnosis of AIDS are presented in Box 79–2. Four problems that affect most AIDS clients are described here. Also see the HIV Case Study and Bridge to Home Care Health.

ASSESSMENT

Assessment of clinical manifestations should include both subjective and objective data. All clinical manifestations should be quantified. The easiest way to measure the severity of a clinical manifestation is by asking the client to rate it on a scale from 0 to 10, with 0 being no

Human Immunodeficiency Virus (HIV)

Edith Jones is a white woman, age 50 years, who presents to an outpatient clinic with complaints of fever, fatigue, "swollen glands," and a sore throat. She is an elementary school teacher and states that she believes she has been exposed to some virus in her classroom. She is concerned because the manifestations have not resolved as quickly as they usually do when she catches a "classroom bug."

Nursing Assessment

Mrs. Jones is alert and cooperative. She says that she has had these manifestations for the past 2 weeks. She has a 17-year-old daughter. Mrs. Jones relates that her husband was killed in a car accident 5 years ago and that she has recently begun dating again. She fears that the stresses of a new relationship and raising a teenager are catching up with her. She states, "Dating has changed so much since before I was married. Maybe I'm just too old to start dating again." Consider the factors that place Mrs. Jones at risk for contracting HIV.

Nursing Physical Assessment

Height: 5'6"
Weight: 140 lb (63.6 kg)
Vital signs: blood pressure, 120/80; TPR, 99.0, 90, 20
LOC: alert and cooperative
EENT: mouth and pharynx are reddened, submaxillary and tonsillar lymph nodes are readily palpable
Cardiac: heart tones are regular, S_1 and S_2 are readily audible with no murmurs or rubs noted
Pulmonary: lung sounds are clear bilaterally
Abdominal: abdomen is flat with hyperactive bowel tones
Genitourinary: deferred
Peripheral pulses: 2/2, without edema

A complete blood count (CBC) is ordered.

CBC Results	
RBC	4.0 μl
Hb	12.0 g/dl
Hct	36%
WBC	2500 μl
Neutrophils	80%
Basophils	2%
Lymphocytes	14%
Monocytes	4%
Platelets	100 × 10⁹/L

Consider the patholophysiologic factors that might cause the alterations noted in these results. A more detailed dating history obtained from Mrs. Jones reveals that she has had sexual intercourse with three different men during the past 12 months and did not use condoms. When questioned further, she insists that these men told her that she was the only woman they were dating and that she did not realize she needed to get a more detailed sexual history from them. She is reluctant to contact these men now because she is no longer seeing any of them.

An enzyme immunoassay and a CD4$^+$ cell count are ordered. Mrs. Jones is instructed to call the clinic in 5 days to obtain her results. Her enzyme immunoassay is positive for antibodies to HIV, and her CD4$^+$ cell count is 75/mm³. Mrs. Jones is instructed to return to the clinic for follow-up tests and treatment. A Western blot, HIV RNA viral load test, and purified protein derivative (PPD) skin test by Mantoux method are performed. The Western blot confirms the diagnosis of HIV, and the initial HIV RNA viral load is 11,000 copies/ml. Mrs. Jones' PPD result is negative.

Mrs. Jones remains reluctant to talk about her prior sexual activities, but she does agree to contact her three recent sexual partners and tell them about her diagnosis. She is more concerned about what to tell her daughter and her parents. "I certainly haven't set a very good example for my daughter. I wonder if I'll live long enough to see her married," she states.

Her primary care provider explains that she could consider initiating antiretroviral therapy because her viral load is above 10,000 copies/ml and her CD4$^+$ cell count is low. However, considering the fact that variations may occur with these test results, the primary care provider schedules her for a second HIV RNA viral load and CD4$^+$ count. In the meantime, teaching is begun regarding the basics of HIV infection and prevention of transmission.

More tests reveal an HIV RNA viral load of 13,500 copies/ml and a CD4$^+$ count of 64 mm³. After discussing treatment options with her primary care provider, Mrs. Jones agrees to start antiretroviral therapy.

Initial Antiretroviral	Therapy Orders
Combivir	1 tablet orally twice a day
Sustiva	600 mg orally at bedtime

Consider other teaching and referrals that should be made at this time.

Mrs. Jones returns to the clinic in 3 weeks for follow-up laboratory work. Her HIV RNA viral load is now reported as being undetectable, and her CD4$^+$ is now 90/mm³. Mrs. Jones exclaims "Maybe I don't really have AIDS after all." Consider appropriate responses that could be made to this remark. Mrs. Jones is instructed to continue the same drug regimen and to return to the clinic on a regular basis for follow-up.

Case Study continued on following page

Discharge and Post-treatment Considerations

Average length of stay: outpatient only
Complete client instruction (including diet, medications, safe sexual practices, infection prevention, support groups, and follow-up appointments)
Community referral: HIV support group

Questions to Be Considered

1. Compare and contrast the practical and ethical considerations of treatment options for clients with and without health insurance coverage. Identify alternate sources of funding for clients without private health insurance.
2. Identify the precautions that Mrs. Jones should take to protect herself from secondary infections and to protect others from becoming infected with HIV. Considering her CD4$^+$ count, should she receive any prophylactic therapy to prevent an opportunistic infection?
3. Discuss the medication teaching necessary for the various antiretroviral drugs. What implications do these drugs have for nursing practice?
4. Identify the assessment and laboratory findings that would indicate Mrs. Jones had progressed to acquired immunodeficiency syndrome (AIDS).
5. Compare and contrast the nursing care required for the HIV client versus the AIDS client.
6. Discuss safe sexual practice and how this information might be most effectively conveyed to the various at-risk populations. Include age, race, marital status, socio-economic, and geographical factors in your discussion.
7. Compare and contrast the assessment data that would indicate a client with HIV is coping positively with the illness. Identify measures to promote effective coping.

EENT, eyes, ears, nose, throat; Hb, hemoglobin; Hct, hematocrit; μl, microliters; LOC, level of consciousness; RBC, red blood cell count; RNA, ribonucleic acid; TPR, temperature, pulse, respirations; WBC, white blood cell count.

problem at all and 10 being the worst possible. This method works very well for most manifestations, such as fatigue and pain. Fever assessment can be made easy if the client is willing to keep a fever diary (writing down his temperature whenever he takes it). For clients who have no scale at home, you will have to rely on their self-report about how they look and how their clothes fit to detect trends in weight.

Pain is a subjective experience. The single most reliable indicator of the existence and intensity of acute pain and any related discomfort or distress is the client's self-report. Neither behavior nor vital signs can substitute for

BRIDGE TO HOME HEALTH CARE

Living with HIV/AIDS

People who have a diagnosis of HIV or AIDS face a very different future today than even 5 years ago because of recently developed medications and treatments. They have new and complex challenges because they are living longer. If you provide care in community settings such as homes or clinics, expect to work as a team member with clients, other health care providers, clients' partners, significant others, children, extended family members, and the community to deal with the challenges and help provide the highest quality care possible. Become familiar with community resources that are available to clients and their families. Transportation to health care facilities, the location of the pharmacy and grocery store, availability of volunteers and respite programs, financial assistance, and career counseling or job retraining are examples of needed resources.

Because the client's immune system is compromised, it is important to teach the client and caregivers how to prevent infections and use standard precautions. Instruct about proper food handling, water and sanitation, linens, and dressings. Find out about the health status of others in the home, especially those who have or are at high risk for acute or chronic health problems. Such information will help you develop a successful plan of care.

Become comfortable discussing sexual issues and family planning or contraception with clients. If you are not able to do this, refer your clients to someone who is knowledgeable and who can deal with these issues in a confidential manner.

The spiritual and emotional health needs of people who live with HIV and AIDS must be addressed. The stress of living with a serious illness can take its toll on the clients and those near to them. Encourage the client and others to express their feelings and listen to them; you may hear many significant and difficult issues. Allow clients and family members to deal with the issues, and help them achieve resolution and closure. Consider a referral to a mental health expert, a spiritual counselor, or a social worker when appropriate.

Be alert for signs of family violence, spouse abuse, or child abuse. Stress, cognitive impairment, loss of work, expenses, and difficulties related to illegal drug use and sales can contribute to these problems. Know related regulations, and contact proper authorities when needed.

Clients who have HIV and AIDS usually need to take many medications to be administered on a specific schedule. Determine whether clients can manage their medications themselves or need assistance and whether they have adequate knowledge about the medications. Make sure the medication schedule is reasonable and encourages compliance. Assess for drug allergies and for potential drug interactions that can occur when various physicians prescribe many drugs.

Considering your own safety is essential when you provide community-focused services to any clients. If you are visiting areas with high crime rates or known drug use, talk to your clients and their families and ask for their assistance. It may be safer to schedule your visits in the mornings. You may need to be accompanied by a volunteer or agency escort who is familiar with the area and neighborhood. Always try to blend into the neighborhood, be alert for signs of trouble, and leave immediately if you sense trouble.

Pamela J. Nelson, RN, MS, *Assistant Professor of Nursing, Bethel College, St. Paul, Minnesota*

BOX 79-2 **Common Nursing Diagnoses for Clients with Human Immunodeficiency Virus and Acquired Immunodeficiency Syndrome**

Altered Oral Mucous Membrane
Altered Thought Processes
Altered Nutrition: Less Than Body Requirements
Altered Health Maintenance
Altered Protection
Anxiety
Bathing/Hygiene Self-Care Deficit
Body Image Disturbance
Diarrhea
Death Anxiety
Dressing/Grooming Self-Care Deficit
Fatigue
Fluid Volume Deficit
Hyperthermia
Impaired Physical Mobility
Impaired Skin Integrity
Impaired Tissue Integrity
Ineffective Management of Therapeutic Regimen
Ineffective Breathing Pattern
Knowledge Deficit
Nausea
Pain
Powerlessness
Risk for Altered Body Temperature
Risk for Caregiver Role Strain
Risk for Ineffective Individual Coping
Risk for Injury
Sensory/Perceptual Alterations
Sleep Pattern Disturbance
Toileting Self-Care Deficit

that self-report. A client may be in excruciating pain even while smiling or laughing to cope with it. Trying to figure out whether a client has pain when the client is actually reporting pain is a waste of time.

DIAGNOSIS, OUTCOMES, INTERVENTIONS

Hyperthermia. An important nursing diagnosis for a client with AIDS is *Hyperthermia related to chronic HIV infection, secondary opportunistic infection, malignancy, autoimmune disorders, diarrhea, dehydration, allergic response to medications, or infection at IV sites, catheters, drains, and incisions.*

Outcomes. After discussing the finding of assessment and the nursing diagnosis, select interventions in concert with the client, care partner, or both to control fever and replace fluid loss.

Interventions. Because of the underlying immunodeficiency and impaired inflammatory response, clinical manifestations of infection, including fever, may be greatly muted. Nonpharmacologic interventions include keeping the client in a warm room to avert shivering and applying a sheet and a loosely woven blanket. Avoid fanning the bed covers, exposing skin, or rapidly removing clothing that might cause chilling.

Avoid counterproductive treatments, such as tepid water sponge bathing, which causes defensive vasoconstric- tion and has not been shown to be an effective coolant in fever. Indeed, sponge baths can cause shivering and can be distressing. Avoid alcohol sponging as well, which also causes vasoconstriction, shivering, and toxic fumes. The alcohol also can be absorbed cutaneously, causing hypoglycemia.

Increase caloric and fluid intake by providing a plan for six feedings distributed over 24 hours and high-protein, high-calorie nutritional supplements, especially if the client has anorexia. Provide 2 to 2.5 L of fluid to drink daily.

Maintain comfort and safety by providing dry clothes and bed linens made out of cotton rather than synthetics. Use emollient creams for dry skin. Monitor mental status frequently, especially when the client has a fever. Evaluate the client's need for assistance with all activities of daily living. Teach the client how to manage chronic recurrent night fever and night sweats by:

- Taking the antipyretic agent of choice before going to sleep
- Having a change of bedclothes nearby in case a change is necessary
- Keeping a plastic cover on the pillow
- Placing a towel over the pillow in case of profuse diaphoresis
- Keeping liquids at the bedside to drink

Pharmacologic treatment can include aspirin, nonsteroidal anti-inflammatory drugs (NSAIDs), or acetaminophen. Follow-up should include comparing patterns of use of these agents with laboratory evaluation of hepatic and hematologic abnormalities, as well as interactions with other agents.

Fatigue. Another common nursing diagnosis is *Fatigue related to chronic HIV infection, anemia, secondary opportunistic infection, malnutrition, dehydration, prolonged immobility, and psychological and situational factors.*

Outcomes. After discussing and validating the findings of assessment and nursing diagnosis, select interventions in concert with the client, care partner, or both to increase self-awareness of fatigue, associated clinical manifestations, environmental factors affecting fatigue, and activity tolerance. Identify interventions to highlight the importance of resting when needed and accepting assistance when needed. Develop a plan for a lifestyle that keeps the client independent, socially active, and involved in activities of daily living.

Interventions. Promote self-care and self-awareness by having the client keep a daily fatigue diary for at least 1 week to identify sources of fatigue and appropriate interventions, as well as patterns of peak fitness. Advise the client to avoid coffee, tobacco, and alcohol, any of which may increase fatigue in some people. Promote adequate sleep by increasing the amount of sleep each day. Reduce the amount of sleep-cycle interruptions by preparing for sleep and keeping needed items at the bedside (e.g., ice water, a urinal, and a towel to absorb perspiration).

Promote rest and activity by developing a written 24-hour schedule of daily activities that alternates short activities with rest periods. Identify activity priorities, such as eating breakfast and then resting before bathing in the morning, as opposed to the reverse. Evaluate the client's needs and point out ways to conserve energy, such as sitting down while dressing, shaving, or preparing food; sitting on a shower chair while bathing; or using disposable items for eating so that no cleanup is needed. Help the client write up a plan for rest and activities that progresses from daily to weekly. Encourage the client to always plan activities ahead of time.

Prepare an exercise schedule (immobilization may lead to decreased endurance and increased fatigue) and plan exercises at peak energy times (after a rest period). Follow the exercises with rest. Aerobic exercise, which increases endurance, can reduce fatigue. Additional natural techniques that may be of benefit include progressive muscle relaxation, acupressure, massage, reflexology, imagery and visualization, autogenic relaxation, reframing and positive affirmations, therapeutic touch, and social support and support groups

Altered Nutrition: Less Than Body Requirements.

A frequently encountered nursing diagnosis is *Altered Nutrition: Less Than Body Requirements related to increased nutrient requirements, decreased food intake secondary to side effects of medications and infection such as an anorexia, nausea, vomiting, altered taste, or impaired swallowing or chewing, diarrhea, fatigue, depression, or impaired cognition.*

Outcomes. After discussing and validating the findings of assessment and the nursing diagnosis, select interventions in concert with the client, care partner, or both to increase food intake, preserve lean body mass, and provide adequate levels of all nutrients.

Interventions

Minimize Anorexia. Minimize factors contributing to anorexia. For *hyperosmia* (an increased sense of smell), avoid cooking odors by keeping windows open and the home well aerated. Encourage meals that include cold foods. For *hyposmia* (a decreased sense of smell), use spices such as basil, oregano, rosemary, thyme, cloves, mint, cinnamon, or lemon juice to enhance smell. For alterations in sense of taste (especially related to distaste for red meat), marinate meat in a commercial marinade, wine, or vinegar before cooking it, and use substitutes for red meat, such as eggs, peanut butter, tofu, cheeses, poultry, and fish.

Prevent Weight Loss. Weight loss can be a significant problem for clients who live alone or who have fatigue or depression. Interventions include:

* Eating small meals frequently throughout the day
* Eating high-calorie snacks or commercially prepared supplements (liquids or bars)
* Indulging in favorite foods
* Consuming more nutrient-dense foods and beverages rather than filling up on low-calorie items
* Drinking liquids 30 minutes before eating instead of with meals
* Preparing meals (such as soups or casseroles) ahead of time so they can be divided into individual servings and frozen until ready to use
* Keeping easy-to-prepare foods on hand, such as frozen dinners, canned foods, and eggs
* Encouraging the client to dine with friends or family

* Getting family members and friends involved in meal preparation; the pleasant atmosphere they can provide may stimulate the client's appetite

Many communities have home food delivery service for people with AIDS as well.

Improve Food Intake. Minimize factors related to difficulty in chewing, dysphagia (difficulty in swallowing), or odynophagia (painful swallowing) by advising clients to avoid rough foods, such as (1) raw fruits and vegetables; spicy, acidic, or salty foods; (2) alcohol or tobacco; (3) excessively hot or cold foods; and (4) sticky foods, such as peanut butter; and (5) slippery foods, such as gelatin, bologna, and elbow macaroni. Encourage the client to:

* Eat foods at room temperature
* Choose mild foods and drinks, such as apple juice rather than orange juice
* Eat dry grain foods (such as breads, crackers, and cookies) after softening them in milk, tea, or another mild beverage
* Eat nonabrasive foods that are easy to swallow, such as ice cream, pudding, well-cooked eggs, noodle dishes, baked fish, and soft cheese
* Eat Popsicles (frozen dessert) to numb pain
* Use a straw when drinking
* Tilt the head forward or back to make swallowing easier

Increase the Availability of Food. Minimize factors related to the client's inability to obtain food by evaluating his or her financial resources and the need for referral for Medicaid, food stamps, or other services. Evaluate the client's home and ability to prepare and obtain food. Look for such problems as an absence of cooking facilities and the need for alternative housing arrangements. Explore community resources that provide free meals.

Teach Nutritional Requirements. If the client has no metabolic condition that requires a special diet, the prescribed diet for people with HIV disease should include high-protein, high-calorie, low-fat foods. Help the client plan a 24-hour menu, and review the essential elements of a low-microbe diet and food safety and preparation. Nutritional teaching should, as much as possible, follow the client's usual pattern of food intake rather than expect the client to follow a totally new, unfamiliar prescription for meal planning.

Pain. A common nursing diagnosis is *Pain related to arthralgia, myalgia, or neuropathy associated with HIV disease, mass lesions associated with opportunistic infection(s) or cancer, side effects of medications, co-morbid disease such as diabetic neuropathy, or interventions such as surgery.*

Outcomes. After discussing and validating the findings of assessment, select interventions in concert with the client, care partner, or both to reduce the incidence and severity of pain, communicate effectively about pain experiences, and enhance comfort and satisfaction.

Interventions

Provide Comfort Measures. Non-drug interventions include identifying activities of daily living that seem to increase the intensity and severity of pain. Provide additional comfort measures, such as using a pressure-relieving mattress, positioning and supporting limbs comfortably when in bed or a chair, and using a "pull sheet" to move clients or help them change positions. For institutionalized clients, encourage family members or significant others to bring in familiar objects, such as pillows and blankets, favorite photographs, religious articles, personal clothing, cologne, make-up, face powder, and other cosmetics.

Provide Physical Therapy. Physical therapy can be very helpful in managing pain. The physical therapist can provide:

- Exercise to maintain or increase physical activity levels and endurance
- Ultrasound and physical treatments, such as application of heat or cold, to reduce musculoskeletal pain
- Therapeutic massage
- Instruction and supervision in using a transcutaneous electrical nerve stimulation (TENS) device, commonly called a *TENS unit*

Administer Pain Medications. Pharmacologic treatments usually include *non-opioid analgesics,* such as aspirin and acetaminophen for mild pain, (2) *weak opioids,* such as codeine and oxycodone for moderate pain, and (3) *strong opioids,* such as morphine for severe pain. For neuropathic pain (such as HIV-associated polyneuropathy, acute and postherpetic neuralgia, and nucleoside toxicity with didanosine, zalcitabine, and stavudine), adjuvants such as ibuprofen may be used as well as amitriptyline, desipramine, nortriptyline, doxepin, carbamazepine, divalproex, phenytoin, gabapentin, or mexiletine.

Primary care providers should anticipate several changes in prescriptions for analgesics when starting the client with a pain control regimen. A major error in initial pain management occurs when a clinician prescribes a 2-week supply of an analgesic, assumes that the prescription works, and has no further contact until the client returns 2 weeks later for follow-up. On the contrary, during the initial phase of pain control, the clinician should have daily contact with the client, even if by telephone, and should anticipate schedule changes. Dosage frequency should be adjusted to prevent pain from recurring once the duration of analgesic action is determined. Similarly, it is a waste of money to prescribe large amounts of an analgesic, such as a 30-day supply, knowing that the orders will change. Orders for opioid analgesics should include "rescue" doses for breakthrough pain when regularly scheduled doses are insufficient.

Orders for analgesics as needed (prn) result in delays in administration and intervals of inadequate pain control. Tell clients and their care partners that the client may sleep for extended periods and may appear very drowsy during the first few days of a pain control regimen. Although this may result in part from the initial effects of the drug, it probably also reflects exhaustion and the need for rest as a result of sleep deprivation caused by pain. This situation usually reverses itself within a few days after a scheduled pain management regimen is begun.

Clients may refuse an analgesic if they are not in pain or may forgo it when they are asleep. Explain that this decision may lower blood analgesia levels and cause a resurgence of pain and failure of the pain control plan.

Although the anti-inflammatory effects of aspirin are highly effective as an analgesic adjuvant, because aspirin inhibits platelet function, it may be contraindicated if the client has a low platelet count.

Helpful guidelines for managing pain in the injecting drug user include (1) having a single practitioner prescribe medications, (2) refusing to refill lost prescriptions, (3) carefully rationing narcotic prescriptions, and (4) limiting rescue doses of narcotic analgesics on a monthly basis. Clients who are in recovery for narcotic addiction and are being treated with methadone maintenance still experience pain and in most instances require higher and more frequent doses of analgesia than a narcotic-naive client would. Some antiretroviral drugs, such as nevirapine and ritonavir, interfere with the half-life of methadone and may decrease its blood levels. The client will experience mild withdrawal symptoms. Increasing the daily dose of methadone usually resolves the problem.

Because diarrhea is common in clients with HIV disease, especially when protease inhibitors are prescribed, the constipating effects of analgesics may actually be beneficial. Evaluate each client's response to therapy instead of automatically using stool softeners when initiating the pain control plan.

Encourage Complementary Therapies. Complementary therapies that may be used include cognitive-behavioral interventions, such as education and instruction in pain control, relaxation exercises, imagery, music distraction, biofeedback, and therapeutic touch.

EVALUATION

It is expected that the client, care partner, or both will be able to (1) identify appropriate measures to take for a fever, (2) initiate and maintain adequate hydration and nutrition, and (3) demonstrate the ability to take and record the client's temperature accurately. Although infection-related fever can be controlled with appropriate antibiotic therapy, this problem can be expected to recur throughout the illness.

It is expected that the client, care partner, or both will be able to (1) identify causative factors that increase fatigue, (2) plan a schedule of paced activity for a 24-hour period, (3) demonstrate the ability to participate in a program of exercise, and (4) verbalize a decrease in the client's fatigue for a 24-hour period. Fatigue is a manifestation that can be expected to recur throughout HIV disease, especially because it is a side effect of some antiretroviral medications, such as zidovudine and ritonavir.

It is expected that the client will maintain or increase weight. It is expected that the client, care partner, or both will (1) identify factors related to anorexia, difficulty in chewing, dysphagia, or odynophagia; (2) identify sufficient resources to obtain and prepare food or make use of social work interventions employed to obtain food stamps or public assistance; (3) identify ways to increase protein and calorie intake; (4) identify key concepts in planning a low-microbial diet; and (5) select a balanced 24-hour menu. The client's weight will fluctuate during the course of HIV disease related to the development of new disease processes and the side effects of prescribed medications.

It is expected that the client, care partner, or both will (1) identify aggravating factors or precipitating factors related to the pain experienced, (2) identify measures to control pain, and (3) verbalize a decrease in the amount and type of pain experienced over 24 hours. Pain may be either chronic or acute, depending on the cause. In most instances, it can be managed effectively, as with any client with another diagnosis.

CONCLUSIONS

HIV continues to be a major threat to human health worldwide. At one time or another, you will care for a person with HIV infection or AIDS. To provide adequate care for a person with HIV infection, you must understand the illness trajectory and the therapeutic interventions needed to maintain health. Always seek expert guidance when starting to care for a client with HIV infection or AIDS. The nature of care is very complex, and the client's clinical needs are numerous.

THINKING CRITICALLY

1. **A 30-year-old woman presents with fever, fatigue, lymphadenopathy, thrush, diarrhea, and pain in her muscles and joints. She has a rash on her torso and arms. What questions would you ask to determine her possible exposure to HIV? How will the client be evaluated and treated?**

Factors to Consider. What tests confirm the diagnosis of AIDS? How is the $CD4^+$ cell count used? What is the purpose of the viral load test? What treatment may be used?

2. **You are working in a homeless shelter and are scheduled to present a 20-minute program on AIDS prevention. A small class of four men and three women have gathered. They are all known to you, and you suspect that one couple may be infected with HIV. What should you plan to teach?**

Factors to Consider. What main areas of HIV education should be addressed? What is an effective method of communicating this information?

3. **Your HIV-infected female client leaves the physician's office and comes over to you and says, "I don't have HIV anymore. The doctor just told me that my viral load was undetectable." How would you respond?**

Factors to Consider. What does an undetectable viral load test result mean? What would you tell this client about safer sex practices and becoming pregnant?

4. **Your 40-year-old male client with AIDS and *P. carinii* pneumonia is about to be discharged from the hospital. His $CD4^+$ cell count is 35. He asks you what he should do now. What teaching would you provide?**

Factors to Consider. When does a person with HIV infection get an AIDS diagnosis? Does this client need any medication for his pneumonia? Given the fact that the $CD4^+$ cell count is 35, does he need any medication to prevent any other opportunistic infections?

BIBLIOGRAPHY

1. American Dietetic Association. (1994). Position of the American Dietetic Association and the Canadian Dietetic Association: Nutrition intervention in the care of persons with human immunodeficiency virus infection. *Journal of the American Dietetic Association, 94,* 1042–1045.
2. Anastasi, J. K., & Sun Lee, V. (1994). HIV wasting: How to stop the cycle. *American Journal of Nursing, 94,* 18–24.
3. Bartlett, J. (1997). *Medical management of HIV infection.* Available: *http://www.hopkins-aids.edu.*
4. Breitbart, W., & McDonald, M. V. (1996). Pharmacologic pain management in HIV/AIDS. *Journal of the International Association of Physicians in AIDS Care, 2*(7), 17–26.
5. Centers for Disease Control. (1992). 1993 Revised classification system for HIV infection and expanded surveillance case definition for AIDS among adolescents and adults. *Morbidity and Mortality Weekly Report, 41* (RR-17), 1–19.
6. Centers for Disease Control and Prevention. (1998). *HIV/AIDS Surveillance Report, 10*(2), 1–39.
7. Centers for Disease Control and Prevention. (1999). *1999 USPHS/IDSA guidelines for the prevention of opportunistic infections in persons infected with human immunodeficiency virus.* Atlanta: Author.
8. Centers for Disease Control and Prevention. (1999). *Guidelines for the use of antiretroviral agents in HIV-infected adults and adolescents.* Atlanta: Author.
9. Dolin, R., Masur, H., & Saag, M. (Eds.). (1999). *AIDS therapy.* New York: Churchill Livingstone.
10. Ferris, F. D., et al. (1995). *A comprehensive guide for the care of persons with HIV disease: Module 4 palliative care.* Toronto, Canada: Mount Sinai Hospital and Casey House Hospice.
11. Friedman-Kien, A., & Cockerell, C. (1996). *Color atlas of AIDS* (2nd ed.). Philadelphia: W. B. Saunders.
12. Gorbach, S., Bartlett, J., & Blacklow, N. (1998). *Infectious diseases* (2nd ed.). Philadelphia: W. B. Saunders.
13. Hinkle, K. (1991). A literature review: HIV seropositivity in the elderly. *Journal of Gerontological Nursing, 7*(10), 12–17.
14. Jewitt, J. F., & Hecht, F. M. (1993). Preventive health care for adults with HIV infection. *Journal of the American Medical Association, 269*(9), 1144–1153.
15. Katsufrakis, P. (Ed.). (1997). HIV/AIDS management in office practice. *Primary Care Clinics in Office Practice. 24*(3), 469–690.
16. Lipsky, J. J. (1996). Antiretroviral drugs for AIDS. *Lancet, 348,* 800–803.
17. Mellors, J. W., et al. (1996). Prognosis in HIV-1 infection predicted by the quantity of virus in plasma. *Science, 272*(5265), 1167–1170.
18. National Institute of Allergy and Infectious Diseases. (1997). HIV persists and can replicate despite prolonged combination therapy. *NIAD News.*
19. Rosenberg, E., & Cotton, D. (1997). Primary HIV infection and the acute retroviral syndrome: The urgent need for recognition. *AIDS Clinical Care, 9*(3), 19, 23–25.
20. Sande, M., & Volberding, P. (1997). *The medical management of AIDS* (5th ed.). Philadelphia: W. B. Saunders.
21. Sherman, D. (Ed.). (1999). HIV/AIDS update. *Nursing Clinics of North America, 34*(1), 1–256.
22. Ungvarski, P. J. (1995). Meeting the challenge of AIDS. *Imprint, 42*(4), 51–54.
23. Ungvarski, P. J. (1996). Waging war on HIV wasting. *RN, 59*(2), 26–32.
24. Ungvarski, P. J. (1996). Challenges for the urban home care provider: The New York experience. *Nursing Clinics of North America, 31*(1), 81–95.
25. Ungvarski, P. J. (1997). Update on HIV infection. *American Journal of Nursing, 97*(1), 4–52.
26. Ungvarski, P. J. (1997). Adherence to prescribed HIV-1 protease inhibitors in the home setting. *Journal of the Association of Nurses in AIDS Care, 8*(Suppl.), 37–45.
27. Ungvarski, P. J., & Flaskerud, J. H. (Eds.). (1999). *HIV/AIDS: A guide to primary care management* (4th ed.). Philadelphia: W. B. Saunders.
28. Zeller, J. M., Swanson, B., & Cohen, F. L. (1993). Suggestions for clinical nursing research: Symptom management in AIDS patients. *Journal of the Association of Nurses in AIDS Care, 4*(3), 13–17.

CHAPTER 80

Management of Clients Requiring Transplantation

Connie White-Williams

NURSING OUTCOMES CLASSIFICATION (NOC)
for Nursing Diagnoses—Clients Requiring Transplantation

Altered Nutrition: More Than Body Requirements	**Effective Management of Therapeutic Regimen: Individual**	**Risk for Ineffective Individual Coping**
Nutritional Status: Food and Fluid Intake	Adherence Behavior	Coping
Nutritional Status: Nutrient Intake	Compliance Behavior	Decision Making
Weight Control	Family Participation in Professional Care	Impulse Control
Altered Protection/Risk for Infection	Knowledge: Treatment Regimen	Information Processing
Immune Status	Participation: Health Care Decisions	Role Performance
Knowledge: Infection Control	Risk Control	Social Support
Risk Control	Symptom Control	**Risk for Injury**
Treatment Behavior: Illness or Injury	**Pain**	Knowledge: Personal Safety
Tissue Integrity: Skin/Mucous Membrane	Comfort Level	Risk Control
Wound Healing: Primary Intention	Pain Control	Risk Detection
Wound Healing: Secondary Intention	Pain: Disruptive Effects	Safety Behavior: Personal
	Pain Level	Symptom Control

The field of organ transplantation has evolved from the early beginnings of experimental kidney transplantation to the current practice of multiple organ transplantation. The advances made have been due largely to the increased knowledge in the areas of immunology and organ preservation, recipient and donor selection, and management of postoperative complications.

Organ transplantation is needed when an organ is irreversibly diseased or injured, leading to end-stage organ failure. Transplantation offers people with end-stage organ failure a chance to live longer and to overcome conditions that were once considered hopeless. Thus, nurses have an increasing opportunity to care for clients with end-stage disease who are awaiting transplantation or who have undergone organ transplantation. In addition, nurses may also play a vital role in identification of potential donors and their management during the donor maintenance period.

HISTORICAL PERSPECTIVE

Transplantation had its beginnings in the 17th century with blood transfusions; however, the era of modern transplantation originated with a tooth replacement by John Hunter in the 18th century.[19] In 1912, Alexis Carrel developed the techniques for surgical suturing and vascular anastomosis that opened the pathway to solid organ transplantation.[25] Much of the work during the succeeding years focused on immunology, the importance of ABO and Rh blood group compatibility, and, later, the development of histocompatibility testing, all of which are crucial to organ transplantation today.[26, 33] In 1943, Medawar[39] described the immune response of acute rejection, and by 1970 the relationship between donor and recipient histocompatibility in the role of acute rejection was recognized.[56]

Although many attempts at kidney transplantation were

made in the early 1900s, it was not until 1954 that Merrell and Murray performed the first successful kidney transplantation, between identical twin brothers.[19] Experimental heart transplantation took place in the early 1900s. Hardy transplanted a chimpanzee heart (xenograft) into a 68-year-old man in 1964. In 1967, Barnard performed the first human-to-human heart transplant.[5, 19] The first lung transplantation was performed by Hardy in 1963.[11] Experimental liver transplantation began in the 1950s. The first human liver transplantation was performed in 1963 by Starzl.[53] Figure 80–1 presents a summary of the number of transplantation procedures reported by the United Network of Organ Sharing (UNOS).[61]

With current success and survival statistics, these procedures are no longer deemed experimental. Organ transplantation is clearly an option for clients with end-stage organ disease. Much of the success is due to the availability of new immunosuppressive therapies, advances in organ preservation, improved surgical techniques, and the

recognition of risk factors that affect survival after transplantation. Because transplant recipients now live longer, however, numerous social, economic, ethical, and quality of life (QOL) issues have arisen.

RELATED ISSUES

■ COST

Average costs for the surgical procedure plus 5-year posttransplantation expenses are approximately $172,000 for kidney transplantation, $317,000 for heart transplantation, $312,000 for lung transplantation, and $394,000 for liver transplantation.[60] The Social Security Act was amended in 1972 to cover the cost of dialysis and transplantation for end-stage renal disease. Although coverage by private insurance companies, health maintenance organizations, (HMOs), preferred provider organizations (PPOs), and Medicare/Medicaid has increased, the high

Number of U.S. Transplants: 1988 to December 31, 1998 by Organ and Donor Type*

ORGAN	DONOR TYPE	YEAR OF TRANSPLANT PROCEDURE										
		1988	1989	1990	1991	1992	1993	1994	1995	1996	1997	1998
KIDNEY*	CADAVER	7231	7087	7782	7733	7696	8171	8384	8602	8571	8613	8938
	LIVING	1812	1903	2094	2393	2536	2850	3008	3347	3605	3797	4017
	TOTAL	9043	8990	9876	10126	10232	11021	11949	12176	12410	12955
LIVER	CADAVER	1713	2199	2677	2931	3031	3404	3592	3879	4013	4101	4384
	LIVING	0	2	14	22	33	36	60	46	53	69	66
	TOTAL	1713	2201	2691	2953	3064	3440	3652	3925	4066	1470	4450
PANCREAS*	CADAVER	244	413	526	529	554	772	840	1018	1013	1056	1216
	LIVING	5	4	2	1	3	2	2	7	11	6	2
	TOTAL	249	417	528	530	557	774	842	1025	1024	1062	1218
HEART	CADAVER	1670	1696	2095	2122	2170	2295	2338	2361	2342	2294	2340
	LIVING†	7	9	12	4	1	2	3	0	1	0	0
	TOTAL	1677	1705	2107	2126	2171	2297	2341	2361	2343	2294	2340
LUNG	CADAVER	33	93	202	401	535	660	708	849	790	912	829
	LIVING	0	0	1	4	0	7	15	23	20	18	20
	TOTAL	33	93	203	405	535	667	723	872	810	930	849
HEART-LUNG	CADAVER	74	67	52	51	48	60	70	69	39	61	45
	LIVING	0	0	0	0	0	0	0	0	0	0	0
	TOTAL	74	67	52	51	48	60	70	69	39	61	45
INTESTINE‡	CADAVER			5	12	22	34	23	44	43	65	68
	LIVING			0	0	0	0	0	1	2	2	1
	TOTAL			5	12	22	34	23	45	45	67	69
TOTAL*	CADAVER	10965	11555	13339	13779	14056	15396	15955	16822	16811	17102	17820
	LIVING	1824	1918	2123	2424	2573	2897	3088	3424	3692	3892	4106
	TOTAL	12789	13473	15462	16203	16629	18293	19043	20246	20503	20994	21926

* In this table, Simultaneous Kidney-Pancreas transplants are counted *twice*, both in Kidney Transplants and in Pancreas Transplants. The number of Simultaneous Kidney-Pancreas transplants performed in each year were: 1988–170, 1989–334, 1990–459, 1991–452, 1992–493, 1993–661, 1994–748, 1995–918, 1996–859, 1997–853, 1998–965.

† Living heart donors donate their healthy heart when they become heart-lung recipients. This is called a domino transplant.

‡ Data on Intestine transplants were not collected prior to April 1994. At that time, information was collected retrospectively for transplantations performed January 1990–March 1994.

Note: Double kidney, double lung, and heart-lung transplants are counted as one transplant. All other multiorgan transplants are being included in the total for each individual organ transplanted.

Based on UNOS Scientific Registry data as of April 19, 1999. Data subject to change based on future data submission or correction.

FIGURE 80–1 Number of transplant procedures in the United States, 1988–1998. (Modified from United Network of Organ Sharing [UNOS], Richmond, VA.)

cost remains a factor for clients who wish to undergo transplantation. In 1996, Medicare extended the coverage of immunosuppressive medications to 3 years after transplantation, which was a positive step toward helping clients financially.

■ SHORTAGE OF ORGAN DONORS

The shortage of organ donors is the most significant limitation to transplantation. There are simply not enough organs for the thousands of clients waiting for transplantation. As of the year 1999, the number of clients with end-stage disease waiting for an organ were as follows: 41,135 for a kidney; 4203 for a heart; 3195 for a lung; 12,618 for a liver; and 444 for a pancreas.[61] Required request/referral and presumed consent programs are being implemented to increase organ donation. Also, the transplantation community is investigating methods to increase donor organ supply. For example, redefining brain death to include cerebral death and anencephaly, use of xenotransplantation (transplanting organs from one species to another), and expanding the donor criteria to include older donors and living extrarenal donors (as in lobar transplantation of lung or liver) all are methods to increase donor organ supply.

■ ETHICAL CONSIDERATIONS

Many moral and ethical issues surround transplantation. Religious and cultural customs and beliefs related to death and organ donation and transplantation create challenges for health care professionals (Table 80–1). As ways to increase the organ donor pool are explored, additional ethical dilemmas may be encountered. The future trends for transplantation include more living-related donation and new experimentation such as cell transplantation. As nurses, it is important to be knowledgeable about these issues and communicate and discuss dilemmas with peers and professionals.

DEFINITION OF DEATH. There continues to be debate on the issue of death and how it is defined. The Uniform Determination of Death Act states that "an individual is considered dead if sustaining either (1) irreversible cessation of circulatory and respiratory function or (2) irreversible cessation of all functions of the entire brain, including the brain stem."[55] Different criteria are recognized for children and infants. In clients in chronic vegetative states or in anencephalic infants, brain stem function is intact but body and mental functions are not. Should death be redefined to include these people as donors? In transplantation, there will always be the dilemma of too few organs available in the face of the need to respect the life of people in a vegetative state who may be potential donors.

BUYING AND SELLING OF ORGANS. The National Organ Transplant Act of 1984 prohibits the sale of human organs and tissues. In addition, the Uniform Anatomical Gift Act of 1968 prohibits the sale or purchase of body parts or organs.[55] The conflict arises with respect to property rights. Supporters of organ sales believe that people own their bodies and have the right to do what they wish with their bodies—including the sale of their organs. The legal sale of blood plasma and sperm, which are body fluids, fuels the debate. The sale of organs in the United States is unlawful. A change in the law would alter the existing practice of free, altruistic donation.

PRISONERS AS DONORS OR RECIPIENTS. A number of concerns arise in exploring solutions to the organ donor shortage. Once again, payment for organs enters the picture. Should prisoners be allowed to donate a kidney or bone marrow for a reduced sentence? This practice would not comply with current altruistic donation. In the same context, should a convicted criminal be allowed to be a transplant recipient? Some authorities believe that being a convicted criminal should not be an exclusion criterion, whereas others argue that it should be an exclusion criterion because of the prisoner's limited life expectancy outside prison.

NON–HEART-BEATING DONORS. Other potential organ donors are people who have experienced a respiratory or circulatory death. The hearts of these potential donors have stopped beating at the time of organ recovery. Ethical issues arise with the brain death definition and when death occurs after asystole.

XENOTRANSPLANTATION. Xenotransplantation, the transplantation of organs, tissues, or cells from one species to another (e.g., transplantation of a baboon heart into a human body), has been proposed as one answer to the organ donor shortage. Many medical and ethical issues become considerations with this concept. Medical issues include organ rejection, new modes of infection transmission, and incompatible immune system responses. Ethical considerations include informed consent, the use of animals as donors, potential benefits versus risks, and public health issues.

OUTCOME MANAGEMENT

■ CLIENTS WITH END-STAGE ORGAN DISEASE

REFERRAL AND RECIPIENT SELECTION

A primary responsibility of the transplantation team is to transplant organs into clients who have the best chance for a long-term successful outcome. It is expected that the transplant recipient will experience an improvement in functional status, maintain long-term graft function, and enjoy improved QOL. This result is accomplished by the selection of an appropriate candidate. The transplantation evaluation is a complex, multidisciplinary process that is usually initiated after a referral by the primary physician. The evaluation begins with an initial assessment of medical records and an examination of the client by the transplantation team. On the basis of findings from the client's history and physical examination, the transplantation team determines whether the client should undergo further evaluation for transplantation. A depiction of the referral and evaluation process can be seen in Figure 80–2.

The goals of the evaluation process are to determine:

- The medical necessity for transplantation
- The surgical feasibility of the procedure
- Risk factors and the proper timing of transplantation
- Psychosocial suitability
- Immunologic status

The evaluation can be performed on either an inpatient or outpatient basis and usually takes 3 to 5 days. During this period, extensive testing is completed, client education is provided, and the client and family members meet the members of the transplantation team. Tests and proce-

TABLE 80-1	RELIGIOUS AND CULTURAL CUSTOMS AND BELIEFS RELATED TO DEATH AND ORGAN DONATION/TRANSPLANTATION	
Religious or Cultural Group	**Death**	**Organ Donation/Transplantation**
Religious Groups		
Adventist	Dead are asleep until return of Jesus Christ	Individual and family may receive or donate organs
Baha'i	No official rituals	Both permitted
Baptist	Desire clergy present	Both approved if donor not endangered
Buddhist	"Last rite" chanting may be practiced at bedside	Matter of individual conscience
Church of Christ	No official rituals	No official position
Church of God	"Home-going ritual"	No conflict
Church of Jesus Christ of Latter Day Saints (Mormons)	Proper to bury dead in ground; cremation is discouraged	Personal choice; reflection encouraged
Eastern Orthodox Church	"Last rites"; cremation discouraged	No conflict; both are permitted
Episcopalian	"Last rites" not mandatory; desirable—Litany at the Time of Death read	No conflict if donor is not violated
Friends (Quakers)	Do not believe in life after this life	Both are permitted
Grace Brethren	No "last rites"; burial or cremation permitted	No conflict; they encourage both
Greek Orthodox	"Last rites"	Organ transplantation has always been acceptable
Hindu	Certain prescribed rites followed by priest; bodies cremated	No conflict
Islamic (Muslim, Moslem)	Patient must confess sins and beg forgiveness before death; family present	Organ donation provided that donors consent in advance in writing; not stored in organ banks
Jehovah's Witness	No official "last rites"	Do not encourage organ donation; a matter for the individual conscience; all organs drained of blood before transplantation
Judaism	Relatives and close friends remain with the deceased; no cremation	Donation or transplantation of organs requires rabbinical consultation
Lutheran	"Last rites" are optional	Both are acceptable and encouraged
Mennonite	No formal prescribed action	No conflict; both acceptable
Methodist, United	Believe in divine punishment after death; good rewarded, evil punished	Encourages both
Pentecostal (Assembly of God, Foursquare Church)	No official "last rites"	No official position
Presbyterian	Read scripture and pray	Encourage and endorse organ donation
Roman Catholic	"Last rites"	Transplantation and organ donation permissible
Russian Orthodox	Do not believe in autopsies, embalming, or cremation	Donation/transplantation of kidneys, eyes and tissues permitted; heart donation/transplantation not allowed
Cultural Groups		
African American	Funeral attendance symbolizes respect; "sticking together"; cultural rituals and quick "pulling together" by the family facilitates this process	No conflict with organ donation/transplantation
American Indian	Burial practices vary among tribal groups	Information not available
Black Muslim	Carefully prescribed procedure for washing and shrouding and funeral rites	Will accept a transplant if needed to live

TABLE 80–1	RELIGIOUS AND CULTURAL CUSTOMS AND BELIEFS RELATED TO DEATH AND ORGAN DONATION/TRANSPLANTATION *Continued*	
Religious or Cultural Group	**Death**	**Organ Donation/Transplantation**
Chinese American	Chinese have an aversion to death and to anything concerning it; funeral rituals crucial to the well-being of descendants	Information not available
Hispanics (Puerto Rican, Mexican, Latino)	Spirit of the dying person needs reassurance from the living; a wake held 1 day prior to funeral; use of funeral home popular; "luto" (or mourning) is marked by wearing black and subdued behavior	No conflicts; whole family participates in the decision
Japanese American	Among Buddhists death is considered a passage; rituals: body of a dead loved one is prepared by close family member and given a bath of warm water, purification rites before the body is wrapped in a white kimono	Organ donation a matter of individual conscience
Southeast Asian Americans (Vietnamese, Cambodian, Laotian, Hmong)	Oldest male makes decisions; death of an infant is deeply mourned; expressions of grief vary	Information not available
West Indian (Haitian, Jamaican, Dominican Republican)	Death arrangements are usually made by the male kinsman of the deceased; death caused by angry voodoo spirits can give rise to conflicting feelings of guilt and anger	Permitted according to the specific religious beliefs of the individual

Data from McQuay, J. E. (1994). Cross-cultural customs and beliefs related to health crises, death, and organ donation/transplantation: A guide to assist health care professionals understand different responses and provide cross-cultural assistance. *Critical Care Nursing Clinics of North America, 7*(3), 581–594, an appendix adapted from Turner, J. W. (1987). Appendix: Attitudes and requirements of various religious groups. In DeGroot, K. D., & Damato, M. B. *Critical care skills* (pp. 389–395). Norwalk, CT: Appleton & Lange.

dures performed during the evaluation are listed in Table 80–2. These tests provide the transplantation team with information regarding the status of all organ systems, infections, coexisting medical conditions, organ-matching, and the psychosocial issues that may affect the client and family. Psychosocial factors include neurocognitive status, coping skills, compliance history, availability of support systems, financial status, and extent of resources (Table 80–3). An example of an evaluation summary sheet to be completed for transplantation candidates is depicted in Figure 80–3.

The details of the evaluation process may vary between transplantation centers and with the organs being evaluated. It is important for you to understand the evaluation process and to know the indications for and contraindications to transplantation. In addition, preoperative education is an important responsibility of the nurse. The goal of education of the potential organ recipient is to provide the client and family with factual information regarding the waiting time for an organ, the surgical procedure, and the post-transplant regimens, including diet, exercise, medication, routine follow-up, complications and return to "normal" life expectations (return to work). Many centers provide this education using several teaching skills such as one-to-one teaching, group classes and/or written information. The client uses this information to make an informed decision to undergo transplantation.

If contraindications are found during the transplanta-tion evaluation (Box 80–1), the transplantation team reviews treatment options with the client and family. If no contraindications are found, the client can then be listed on the national waiting list according to criteria established by UNOS, a nationwide system dedicated to the equitable sharing and distribution of donor organs.

LISTING FOR TRANSPLANTATION AND WAITING FOR A DONOR ORGAN

The criteria for listing a client for transplantation are governed by UNOS and vary according to the organ to be transplanted. These criteria include urgency, blood type, and recipient weight and height.

Stable clients wait at home or near the transplantation center. Many clients choose local housing such as an apartment. A few centers provide hospital-owned housing dedicated to use by pre- and post-transplantation clients and their families. Cellular telephones or beeper systems must be available to allow the transplantation team to contact the client at any time. Usually, a client who lives at a distance from the transplantation center requiring more than 2 hours' travel time must relocate or arrange air transportation to arrive at the center within an acceptable time.

Unstable clients wait in the hospital, often in an intensive care unit. Some clients, particularly those awaiting heart transplantation, may live outside the hospital with continuous inotropic support. Intermittent hospitalization

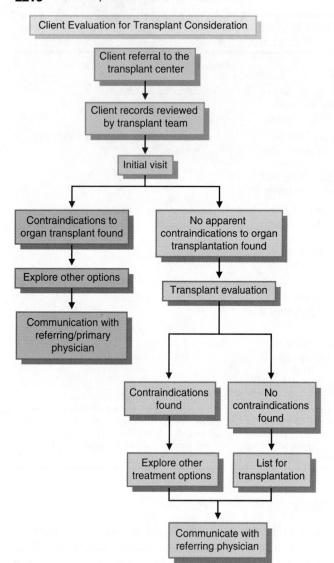

Client Evaluation for Transplant Consideration

Client referral to the transplant center

Client records reviewed by transplant team

Initial visit

Contraindications to organ transplant found

No apparent contraindications to organ transplantation found

Explore other options

Transplant evaluation

Communication with referring/primary physician

Contraindications found

No contraindications found

Explore other treatment options

List for transplantation

Communicate with referring physician

FIGURE 80–2 Client evaluation for transplantation.

may be needed throughout the waiting period. In heart transplantation candidates who become hemodynamically unstable, the use of an intra-aortic balloon pump or a ventricular-assist device may be necessary. Clients waiting for renal transplantation may be receiving dialysis, and those waiting for lung transplantation may require ventilator assistance. In liver transplantation candidates, mechanical assistance devices are not used during the wait for the transplant. Cardiac or pulmonary rehabilitation before transplantation is beneficial to optimize the client's strength and aerobic capacity.

Waiting for transplantation is perhaps the most stressful time for clients and families as they cope with terminal illness, altered lifestyles, financial strain, and impending surgery. Both the client and family members may experience feelings of anxiety, depression, and helplessness.[23, 46] An often forgotten but important component of transplantation nursing is the care of clients with end-stage organ disease who are waiting for transplantation. The transplantation nurse may care for clients while they wait in the hospital for a donor organ, in the clinic setting, or in the home. This wait may be days, months or

even years, and it is natural for the nurse to develop strong personal and professional relationships with these clients.

Along with the intense nursing that is involved in keeping the client alive during the waiting period, emotional stress may develop in nurses caring for these clients. It is important for nurses to have periodic meetings to discuss their feelings and difficult cases and to develop plans of care for the clients. More than 80,000 people in the United States die from end-stage renal disease, while 30,000 receive dialysis each year.[2, 4] Approximately 1.1 million Americans were expected to experience a new or recurrent heart failure by year 2000.[1] Cirrhosis is the fourth leading cause of death, accounting for 25,000 deaths yearly.[3, 22] It is important for transplantation nurses to understand that while there may be many happy moments when an organ becomes available for the clients, there will also be tragedies when death occurs before an organ is located. Working with transplantation clients can be both emotionally draining and frustrating during the waiting period for organ availability. Nurses can strive to provide excellent care for the client but have little control over the availability of organs. It is important that emotional support be provided not only for health care staff members and their families but also for transplantation clients and their families. Many centers have established support groups vital to the emotional well-being of the people involved.

During the waiting time, the nurse, as part of the transplantation team, and the client with end-stage organ disease begin to establish a trusting relationship, participate in the client's education, and work together to grasp the realities of life after transplantation. Many clients and their families unrealistically expect that transplantation will cure all life's problems. The problems of end-stage organ disease may be resolved, but new problems associated with transplantation, including medication side effects, rejection, infections, and financial limitations, are frequently encountered. Help the client understand the post-transplantation regimen, and explain what to expect once the client is discharged from the hospital.

ORGAN DONATION AND RECOVERY

The gifts of organ and tissue by donation are a vital part of transplantation. Without the gracious decision of the donor or donor family to give the "gift of life" by donation, there would be no post-transplantation miracles.

If the potential donor is a living relative, careful physical and psychosocial assessment is necessary. Potential donors must be psychologically evaluated as to their real desire to donate an organ, usually a kidney, and the ability to make a lifelong adjustment to having one kidney. To avoid conflict of interest, evaluation of the donor is commonly done by a team different from that caring for the recipient. Discussions with the donor should be held in strict confidence; if the potential donor decides not to donate, the medical team frequently cites a physical contraindication, in order to allow continued acceptance of that person by the other family members.

Several legislative initiatives have advanced issues of donation and transplantation. In 1968, the Uniform Anatomical Gift Act, aimed at increasing volunteer organ donation, became law. Included in this law were the specifications for notifying legal next of kin of donation wishes, uniform donor cards, and designation of donation

TABLE 80–2	EVALUATION FOR ORGAN TRANSPLANTATION

GENERAL

Complete medical history and physical examination
Psychiatric and social evaluation
Laboratory studies
  Electrolyte and metabolic profile
  Liver function tests
  Hematologic profile
  Fasting cholesterol/lipid profile
  Arterial blood gas analysis
  Urinalysis, urine specific gravity determination
  Creatinine clearance determination
  ABO blood typing
  Antibody screen
  Human leukocyte antigen (HLA) tissue typing
  Lymphocyte cytotoxicity screen (assay for preformed reactive antibodies)
Virologic and microbiologic profile testing for the following:
  Cytomegalovirus (CMV)
  Toxoplasmosis
  Human immunodeficiency virus (HIV)
  Hepatitis B surface antigen (HBsAg)
  Hepatitis C antibody
  Epstein-Barr virus (EBV)
  Syphilis: Veneral Disease Research Laboratory (VDRL) assay
  Tuberculosis: Purified protein derivative (PPD) testing with controls

KIDNEY

Laboratory studies
Glomerular filtration rate determination
Radiographic and radionuclide scanning studies
  Renal ultrasound examination
  Kidney-urethra-bladder radiographic series
  Renal radionuclide scanning
  Renal angiography
  Magnetic resonance imaging
  Renal biopsy
  Cystourethrography

HEART

Radiographic and radionuclide scanning studies
  Posteroanterior (PA) and lateral chest radiographs
  Sinus and panoramic films
  Resting radionuclide angiography
  Pulmonary function tests
  Ventilation-perfusion lung scan
  Nuclear magnetic resonance imaging when indicated
  CT studies when indicated
  Resting and exercise gas exchange studies
Cardiac catheterization
Two-dimensional echocardiography
Electrocardiography

LIVER

Laboratory studies: additional blood work for diagnosis of specific liver disease may be indicated
Radiographic and radionuclide scanning studies
  Ultrasound examination of liver and biliary tree
  CT scan of head
  CT scan of abdomen with liver volumes
  Endoscopic retrograde cholangiopancreatography
  Percutaneous transhepatic cholangiogram
  Pulmonary and cardiac evaluation

LUNG

Radiographic and radionuclide scanning studies
  CT scan of chest
  Ventilation-perfusion scan
  Pulmonary function tests
  Cardiac evaluation

CT, computed tomography.

---

preference on the driver's license. The National Transplant Act of 1984 addressed medical, legal, ethical, and social issues of donation such as requiring national scientific registries for assessment by the federal government and declaring it illegal to buy and sell human organs.[55]

TABLE 80–3	CONSIDERATIONS IN THE PSYCHOSOCIAL EVALUATION FOR TRANSPLANTATION

Demographics	**Health maintenance**
Age	Oxygen requirements
Marital status	Dialysis
Support systems	Compliance with medication regimen
Financial	Compliance with clinical appointments
Insurance	**Transportation**
Savings	Ability to get to clinic or hospital
Social habits	Travel time to transplantation center
Smoking	**Home environment**
Drinking	Telephone
Illicit drugs	Running water
Coping skills	Trailer/home (e.g., financial? steps? cleanliness?)
	Heating and air conditioning

Also, the Organ Procurement and Transplant Network (OPTN) was established to create a national client registry and to coordinate organ allocation and distribution. UNOS is under contract from the U.S. Department of Health and Human Services to operate OPTN.[43]

The Omnibus Budget Reconciliation Act (OBRA) of 1986 requires hospitals to have written policies and procedures for identification and referral of potential donors. Under the 1987 Organ Donation Request Act, consideration of the donor's religious beliefs is mandated, and guidelines are set forth to guide the health care team's approach to next of kin for donor consent, attainment of consent, and notification of the organ procurement organization (OPO).

OBRA also requires transplantation centers and OPOs to be members of OPTN. OPOs are nonprofit organ recovery services in the United States that constitute an integral link in the identification, acceptance, and management of the potential organ donor. In addition to the coordination of organ recovery, transplant procurement coordinators within the OPO provide professional and public education, assist hospitals during donor evaluation, and offer family counseling. Other responsibilities of the procurement coordinators are assisting in donor manage-

PRINT IN BLACK INK   CONFIDENTIAL

ORGAN EVALUATION SUMMARY SHEET

Name: (Last, First, Middle) | Sex

Date of Birth (M/D/Y) | Age | Race (UNOS def) | Hospital Number

SS Number | Phone: Home | Phone: Work | Stamp Patient Keyplate Here

Address | Occupation | Number living children: | Admit Date:

☐ Spouse, or… ☐ Companion (check one) | Name | Years Married/Together | Discharge Date:

Travel Distance from UAB (miles) | Travel Time by Auto to UAB (miles) | Spouse/Companion Occupation | Number Pregnancies: | UAB MD:

Referring MD: | Med Hx (check all that apply) ☐ Hepatitis: Dt:____ | ☐ TIA: Dt Last:____ ☐ Peripheral Embolus: yr___ | ☐ Peripheral Vas Disease | ☐ Peptic Ulcer:
☐ Gout: Dt:___ Last:___ ☐ Diverticulitis: DtDx:___ | ☐ Carotid Bruit: ☐ L ☐ R ☐ Pul. Emb: mo/yr___ | ☐ Renal Insufficiency | Dt:___
Referring MD Address: | ☐ Hypertension: Dt:____ ☐ Prior Transfusions: #___ | ☐ CEA: ☐ L yr__ ☐ R yr__ ☐ Nephrolithiasis: Yr.Last___ | ☐ Perm Pacemaker: | ☐ G.I. Bleed:
☐ Pancreatitis: Dt:___ ☐ CVA: Dt Last:___ | ☐ Diabetes; Insl: ☐ Y ☐ N ☐ Asthma/COPD/Emphysema | mo/yr 1st___ mo/yr last___

Cardiac History: | ☐ Angina History: Class at present____(I–IV) | ☐ CABG: #:___ year(s):___ | Other Medical Problems (specify):
Primary Cardiac Diagnosis, check one (reason for tx): | ☐ CHF History. Onset:___/___; Class now:___ | ☐ V. Tach:(☐ Stable ☐ Arrest) ☐ V. Fib |
☐ Ischemic ☐ Idiopathic ☐ Myocarditis | ☐ Congenital Heart Disease Surgery: #:___ | ☐ EP Study: ☐ + inducible: (☐ VT ☐ VF) Dt:___ |
☐ Congenital (& congen valvular) ☐ Post partum | ☐ Valvular Heart Disease Surgery: #:___ | ☐ A Fib/A Flutr: (☐ Parox. ☐ Chronic) Dt:___ |
☐ Acquired valvular (not isch) ☐ Alcoholic | TypeSurg:___ yr: | ☐ Cardiac Arrest? Date(s):___ | Non-cardiac Surgical History (specify, with dates):
☐ Other:___ | TypeSurg:___ yr: | ☐ ICD Placed: Date:___/___ Location:___ |
Comments:___ | TypeSurg:___ yr: | *Manufacturer:___ Model:___ |
☐ Chronic anticoagulation (Coumadin), yr started:___ | TypeSurg:___ yr: | ☐ LV thrombus (documented) |

Allergies/Intolerences (specify, with sign/symptom):

Habits | Tobacco: | Alcohol: | Drug:

Social: | Insurance: | Covers Transplant? | Psychiatric:

Neuropsychology: Grade 1–5, 1=poor, 5=excellent | Neurophology: | Psychiatric: | Compliance: | Support: | Knowledge: | Planning: | Coping:

Comments:

Dental Evaluation:

Significant Physical Exam | Height: | Weight: | HEENT:

Lungs: | Cardiovascular:

Abdomen: | Extremities:

Neuro: | Rectal: | Hemacult x 3:

D/C Meds: | RN:

Laboratory Tests

Chemistry Date:	Na	K	Cl	Mag	HCO3	Glucose	BUN	Creat	Uric Acid	Calcium	Phospho	T Bili	Ind Bili	Dir Bili
	Alk Phos	LDH	GOT	GGT	CPK		T Choles	Triglycer	HDL	CAD Risk	Alk Phos	Creatinine Clearance: = ____ml/mr ___mg(T.Vol)/14.4/ ___mg/dl(SerCreat)		

Hematology Date:	Hct	Hg	WBC	Segs	Bands	Eosino	Lymphs	Other	PT	INR	PTT	Platelets	TProt	Albu

Allotype Data Date:	PRA, flow		PRA, Specificity:	AB Screen	H L A	A	A	B	B	Bw	Bw	Cw	Cw
	ABO Blood Type & Rh		Coomb's Test			DR	DR	DR	DR	DQ	DQ	DPw	DPw

Infectious Dis. Screening Date:	General	HIV:	IFA Toxo:	RPR:	Hepatitis	HBs Ag	HBs Ab	HB core Ab	TB	24 hr	48 hr	72 hr
		CMV:	Herpes:	EBV:		HepA IgM	HepA IGG	Hep C Ab	PPD Controls			

CHF Eval Date:	Free T4	T4	T3RIA	TSH	Sed Rate	RA Latex	Ferritin	Serum Iron	TIBC		

Other Tests	UA: Date:						If Female: HCG		If Male: Prostate Spec. Ag

Electrocardiogram Date: | If Female: Mammograms: Date:

Chest X-Ray Date: | Sinus X-Rays Date:

24 Hour Holter: Date: | Abdominal Ultrasound:: Date:

Echocardiogram: Description: Date: ( ): LVd___mm MR:___ TR:___ AI:___ PI:___ Est. PA systolic pressure:___mmHg | Echo: LV EF:___% RV EF:___%

VQ Lung Scan Date: | Radionuclide Ventriculogram (MUGA) | MUGA LV EF = ___%

Pulmonary Function Testing Date: | FVC (value/%) | FEV1 (value/%) | FEF 25%–75% (value/%) | MaxVC (value/%) | DLCO (value/%)

Interpretation: | ABGs on | Ph | PO2 | PCO2 | Saturation | COHb

Rest/Exercise Gas Exchange Data Date: | Total Exercise Time | Anaerobic Threshold | VO2 Max (peak)

Cardiac Cath Data

Coronary Angiograms Date: Location:

Date	H.R.	AoSyst	AoDiast	RAm	PAs	PAd	PAm	PCWP	C.O.	C.I.	PVR	SVR	IV Meds & dose/NTG During Cath

Other Tests:

Final Disposition: ☐ Listed for Tx: date___ Status @ listing:___ ☐ Not listed due to:___

☐ **If checked, explanted heart should be sent to pathology as diagnosis not confirmed prior to transplant**

FIGURE 80–3 Transplantation evaluation summary sheet. (Courtesy of University of Alabama–Birmingham Heart and Lung Program.)

> ### BOX 80–1   General Contraindications to Organ Transplantation
>
> - Presence of active systemic infection (bacteremia, fungemia, viremia)
> - Malignant disease (except skin cancer and some primary tumors of the diseased organ)
> - Active peptic ulcer disease
> - Active abuse of alcohol or other substances
> - Severe damage to organ system(s) other than that to be transplanted (such as severe cardiovascular dysfunction in the potential liver transplant recipient)
> - Severe psychiatric disease
> - Demonstration of past or current inability to comply with a prescribed medical regimen
> - Lack of a functional social support system
> - Lack of sufficient financial resources to pay for surgery, hospitalization, medication, and follow-up care

ment, arranging transportation to and from the donor hospital, and assisting surgical personnel in the operating room. The procurement coordinator provides information to the clinical transplantation coordinator and the transplantation surgeon throughout the recovery process.

OPOs are either hospital-based or independent. They must meet criteria mandated by the Health Care Finance Administration (HCFA), which includes (1) arranging for appropriate tissue typing, (2) demonstrating a working relationship with 75% of hospitals within the OPO area, (3) discussing accounting procedures, (4) providing a method of transport of donated organs, (5) submitting center-specific data, (6) cooperating with local tissue banks, and (7) having a governing board of directors.

ROLE OF THE NURSE IN ORGAN DONATION

The nurse plays an important role in organ donation and recovery with early identification of potential donors, referral to the OPO, and assisting in the medical management of the organ donor.[16] The nurse may act as a liaison with donor families or may be involved in the clinical management of the donor. This nursing role can be a very emotional experience. A nurse involved in this process must acknowledge the personal loss incurred when faced with the brain death of a donor client. The nurse then begins to focus on managing that client's vital systems until donation is completed.

The nurse's identification of a potential organ donor is a vital link to transplantation. To be a donor, a person must meet certain criteria, including sustaining an injury resulting in brain death. According to the Uniform Determination of Death Act, "An individual is dead if he has sustained either irreversible cessation of circulatory and respiratory functions or irreversible cessation of all functions of the brain, including the brain stem, as determined in accordance with accepted medical standards."[55]

The nurse may be the first to recognize the manifestations of brain death, including lack of responsiveness; absence of cough, gag, or corneal reflexes; and lack of response to painful stimuli. These findings should be reported to the physician. Refer all clients who meet brain death criteria to the local OPO. It is most often a nurse who notifies the OPO of the potential donor. Notification

should occur when brain death is imminent, to allow the procurement coordinator to become familiar with the potential donor's case. Figure 80–4 depicts the organ donor referral and triage procedure.

The first step in the donation process is awareness of potential organ donors. Organ donors are people who have suffered an injury leading to brain death. The most common causes of injury are head trauma, cerebrovascular accidents (CVAs), subarachnoid hemorrhage, and primary brain tumors. Once a potential donor is identified, the organ procurement agency should be notified. The next steps are documentation of brain death and family consent of donation.

Next, medical management of the potential donor begins. The goal of donor management is to maintain optimal conditions ensuring functional and infection-free organs for transplantation. This goal is accomplished by the diligent management of hydration and tissue perfusion, oxygenation, infection control, diuresis, and temperature regulation. Common problems encountered in management of the potential donor are hypotension, shock, electrolyte imbalances, disseminated intravascular coagulation (DIC), and loss of thermoregulation. The ideal organ donor is a person who unfortunately has suffered a fatal injury resulting in brain death who was otherwise healthy

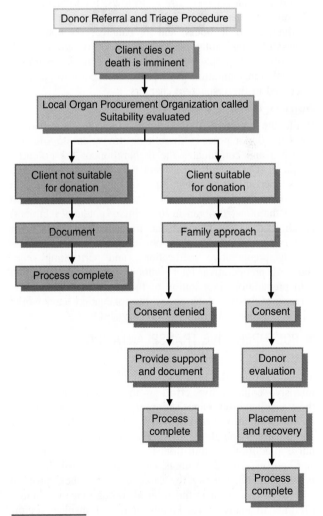

FIGURE 80–4 Organ recovery process.

and infection-free. Criteria for organ donation are listed in Table 80–4.

Initiation of the organ donor process should proceed according to hospital policy. Organ recovery occurs in the operating room only after (1) identifying a potential donor, (2) notifying an OPO, (3) diagnosing brain death, (4) obtaining family consent, and (5) managing the donor until organ removal is complete.

ORGAN RECOVERY

Multiple organ procurement, or recovery of more than one type of organ from a single donor, is standard practice. As many as four separate surgical teams may be present in the operating room, each focusing on recovery of one organ. Usually, a separate surgical team prepares the recipient for the new organ. After a midline incision is made, dissection of organs occurs. Once cross-clamping of the aorta is done and cardioplegia is begun, the heart is removed. Then lungs, liver, and finally kidneys are procured.

The organs are preserved in a cold storage solution selected by the transplantation center. Examples of such solutions are University of Wisconsin solution (UW solution), Euro-Collins solution, Belzer's solution, and other, institution-specific solutions. Organs are preserved in a sterile storage solution, packed in ice, and transported to the recipient in a cooler.

Viability times for donated organs vary. Standard periods after organ recovery are as follows: for kidney, 48 to 72 hours; for heart, 4 to 5 hours; for lung, 4 to 6 hours; for liver, 24 to 30 hours; and for pancreas, 24 hours. For successful transplantation, the timing of organ removal, transport, and preparation of the recipient is essential. Surgical transplantation procedures for specific organs are discussed in the respective chapters.

PREPARATION OF RECIPIENT

While the procurement coordinator manages and coordinates the donor process, the clinical transplant coordinator manages and coordinates the preparation of the potential recipient. The potential recipient (or recipients—in many cases a second client is also told to come to the hospital in case the transplantation team encounters a problem with use of the donated organ in the primary potential recipient) is admitted to the hospital and immediately prepared for surgery. Preparation involves obtaining blood work, administering preoperative medications, and performing other standard preoperative interventions such as shaving and skin preparation. Preparation of the recipient may become a race against the clock as the transplantation team works within the time constraints of organ viability.

■ POSTOPERATIVE TRANSPLANTATION CLIENTS

Management of the post-transplantation client involves an intensive collaborative effort of the various members of the transplantation team. The transplantation team consists of transplantation surgeons and other physicians, nurse coordinators, social workers, pharmacists, psychologists, nurse practitioners, nutritionists, members of the clergy, staff nurses, and consultants. Depending on which organ is transplanted, usually the same team members provide care to clients from initial referral throughout the client's lifetime. In many cases, kidney or liver transplant recipients return to their referring physicians for long-term

---

TABLE 80–4   **CONDITIONS OF PARTICIPATION FOR ORGAN DONATION**

CONDITIONS OF PARTICIPATION

The Department of Health and Human Services (HHS), in an attempt to optimize donor potential and abate the critical shortage of organs for transplantation, issued the Hospital Conditions of Participation (COP) for Medicare and Medicaid on June 22, 1998. This rule took effect on August 21, 1998, and requires all U.S. hospitals to adopt a "routine notification" policy or mandates that hospitals have and implement written protocols to ensure that the organ procurement organization (OPO) is notified of all deaths. According to the COP, the hospital must, "in a timely fashion," notify the OPO of individuals who die or whose death is imminent," thus eliminating the need for hospital staff to identify a potential donor.* All patients who die should be considered a potential organ and/or tissue donor.

Routine notification ensures that an individual who is most familiar with the current criteria on donation, specifically the OPO, evaluates every individual who dies to determine suitability for donation. If the policy were consistently followed, routine notification would make it virtually impossible for the hospital not to refer all potential organ donors. Thus, routine notification places the decision-making and determination of medical suitability for a person to be a donor in the hands of the procurement and transplant community, not in the hands of hospital staff.

This rule is designed not to exclude hospital professionals from the process but, rather, to ensure that the procurement professionals are included.

Five stipulations are contained in the COP:

- A hospital must have an agreement with an OPO and must contact the OPO in a timely manner about all individuals who die or whose death is imminent. The OPO will then determine medical suitability for donation.

- Every hospital must have an agreement with a designated eye and tissue bank to cooperate in the recovery of eyes and tissues.

- Every hospital must ensure that the family of every potential donor is offered the option to donate organs and/or tissues or not to donate.

- Every hospital must work in collaboration with the OPO and tissue or eye bank in educating their staff, participating in death records to identify potential donors and maintain potential donors during the donor management period while necessary testing and the placement of organs and tissues take place.

- Every hospital must provide organ-transplant–related data, as requested by the national Organ Procurement and Transplantation Network and the U.S. Scientific Registry of Transplant Recipients and the OPOs.†

*Final Rule: *Federal Register,* Vol. 63, No. 119, June 22, 1998. 42 CFR Part 482.4.5. Department of Health and Human Services: Health Care Financing Administration. Medicare and Medicaid Programs; Hospital Conditions of Participation; Identification of Potential Organ, Tissue and Eye Donors and Transplant Hospitals, Provision of Transplant Related Data.

† From Chabalewski, F. L. et al. *Donation and transplantation: Into the new millennium.* Available: www.medscape.com, October 5, 2000.

Source: United Network for Organ Sharing.

care. Nursing care should be designed to recognize life-threatening clinical problems, to prevent complications, and to promote the client's return to normal activities with improved QOL.

BASIC IMMUNOLOGY RELATED TO TRANSPLANTATION

To effectively care for the transplant client, you must understand basic immunology concepts related to transplantation (see Chapters 74 and 76). The immune response elicits mechanisms that direct the body to recognize transplanted organs as foreign (non-self). Although this immune response is normal, it is the goal of immunosuppressive agents to alter this immune response in transplanted clients.

The innate or nonspecific immune responses consist of natural mechanisms for the protection of the client against foreign antigens. These natural defenses are present at birth, lack memory, and do not need prior exposure for antigens to develop. Innate immunity mechanisms include physical barriers, chemical barriers, and leukocyte reactions, all of which play a role in the body's immune response.

Acquired or specific immunity involves mechanisms elicited by the lymphoid system. Lymphoid cells include plasma cells and lymphocytes. Lymphocytes constitute 30% of the white blood cells (WBCs) and are responsible for the recognition of antigens. These lymphocyte defense mechanisms recognize foreign antigens and can elicit rejection of transplanted organs. Two types of lymphocytes can elicit a response: B lymphocytes, which mediate a humoral immune response through the production of antibodies, and T lymphocytes, which are derived from maturing stems cells in the thymus and act to defend the body by interaction with an antigen with a sensitized T lymphocyte.[8, 48] There are regulator (T helper and T suppressor) and effector (cytoxic and memory) T lymphocytes.

In humans, the genetic factor used to determine specific antigen recognition is called the major histocompatibility complex (MHC). The MHC is the human leukocyte antigen (HLA) gene complex, located on chromosome 6. Antigens of the HLA complex are divided into two classes: class I comprises HLA types, A, B, and C; class II consists of HLA types DR, DQ, and DP. Histocompatibility testing is used to minimize specific immune responses to the transplanted organ. The type of histocompatibility testing varies according to the organ transplanted and with time limitations. Before transplantation, the potential recipient undergoes ABO typing, Rh typing, and HLA tissue typing. An assay for preformed reactive antibodies (PRAs) determines the presence of preformed antibodies to HLA antigens. Results range from zero to 100%. If a potential recipient is found to have antibodies against specific HLA antigens, a donor organ with those antigens is not suitable for transplantation.

Several types of cross-matching procedures can be performed to identify the presence of antibodies in the potential recipient to antigens located on the lymphocytes of the potential donor. A positive result on cross-matching means that antibodies are present, and transplantation is usually inadvisable because of the associated higher risk of rejection. A negative result on cross-matching means that no antibodies are present, with a reduced risk of rejection.

IMMUNOSUPPRESSION

The goal of immunosuppressive therapy involves the delicate balance of adequately suppressing the immune response to prevent organ rejection without developing complications from the therapy itself. This intricate balance of the immunosuppressive medication regimen is individualized for each client. The transplantation team aims to keep the dose of each drug within the therapeutic range. Management of the immunosuppressive regimen is crucial to long-term outcomes in post-transplantation clients; for example, excessive immunosuppression may lead to increased risk of infection, liver or kidney insufficiency, joint necrosis, cataracts, or malignancies, whereas inadequate immunosuppression may lead to rejection of the transplanted organ. Although in many cases long-term graft acceptance can be maintained with less drug as time goes by, most clients require immunosuppression for life to prevent rejection of the transplanted organ.

Immunosuppressive agents are utilized in the post-transplantation population in three categories of use: induction, maintenance, and anti-rejection. Specific agents and dosages vary according to category of use. Protocols are dependent on the type of organ(s) transplanted, transplantation center–specific practices, and the client's history and current health status. See Table 80–5 for nursing implications for the major immunosuppressive agents.[6, 21, 50, 51, 62] Most transplantation centers use multiple-drug regimens containing agents that act on various functions of the immune system and also minimize side effects. Many new immunosuppressant medications are currently being developed and tested in the United States and Europe.

COMPLICATIONS

Rejection

Transplantation of allografts (organs transplanted between genetically different individuals in the same species) elicits an immune response in which the antigens in tissue of the transplanted organ are recognized as foreign; hence, a series of events occur, resulting in rejection of the organ. Rejection is classified into three types: (1) hyperacute, (2) acute, and (3) chronic (Fig. 80–5).

HYPERACUTE REJECTION. Hyperacute rejection can occur within minutes to hours of implantation of the organ. It is caused by the presence of antibodies. Usually, a destructive humoral or B-cell reaction to antigens on the vascular endothelium results in organ necrosis. Most hyperacute rejection episodes can be prevented by previous PRA assay, histocompatibility testing, and cross-matching. If hyperacute rejection occurs, treatment options are limited. Clients who have received kidney or kidney-pancreas transplants may need to return to dialysis. Clients who have received other organ transplants may receive plasmapheresis, which is a procedure utilized to remove circulating antibodies from the blood. If this measure fails, re-transplantation is indicated.

ACUTE REJECTION. Acute rejection usually occurs in the first 3 months after transplantation; however, it can occur at any time, particularly if the immunosuppression regimen is altered or if an infection develops. Acute rejection can be either a purely cellular immune response mediated by T cells or an antibody-mediated response, or a combination of the two.[31] Diagnosis is based on clinical

TABLE 80–5	NURSING IMPLICATIONS FOR IMMUNOSUPPRESSIVE AGENTS USED IN TRANSPLANTATION				
Agent	**Action(s)**	**Indication**	**Potential Effects**	**Dosing Considerations**	
Cyclosporine (Neoral, Sandimmune)	Inhibits production of T lymphocytes Suppresses activity of T lymphocytes Inhibits IL-2 production	Prevention and treatment of organ rejection	Hypertension Renal dysfunction Tremor Hirsutism Gum hyperplasia	Gelatin capsules Oral solution IV solution Brand-name and generic preparation available Monitor trough levels and drug interactions	
Tacrolimus (FK506)	Prevents synthesis of IL-2	Prevention and treatment of organ rejection	Tremor Diabetes Renal dysfunction Hypertension Nausea	Capsules Pediatric suspension IV solution Monitor trough levels and drug interactions	
Corticosteroids—anti-inflammatory agents Methyloprednisolone (Solu-Medrol)	Inhibits IL-1 Inhibits production of T lymphocytes	Adjunctive immunosuppressive agent for prevention and treatment of organ rejection	Diabetes Cataracts Obesity Muscle weakness GI bleeding Cushingoid state Osteoporosis	Tablets IV solution Give with anti-ulcer medications for high doses	
Immunosuppressive antimetabolites Azathioprine (Imuran)	Interferes with DNA and RNA synthesis Inhibits proliferation of T and B lymphocytes	Prevention of organ rejection	Leukopenia Anemia Hepatoxicity Nausea Neoplasia	Tablets IV solution Allopurinol potentiates action	
Mycophenolate mofetil (CellCept)	Selectively inhibits de novo purine synthesis of activated T and B lymphocytes	Prevention of organ rejection	Diarrhea Leukopenia Vomiting Sepsis	Capsules Tablets IV solution	
Monoclonal Antibodies Muromonab-CD3 (Orthoclone OKT3)	Blocks function of CD3 molecule and inhibits T lymphocyte function	Treatment of organ rejection	Flu-like syndrome Anaphylactic response	IV solution; give via filter Chest film, vital signs should be monitored	
Daclizumab (Zenapax), basiliximab (Simulect)	IL-2 antagonist that inhibits activation of lymphocytes	Prevention of organ rejection	Fever Fatigue GI distress	IV solution	
Polyclonal Antibodies Antithymocyte globulin (ATG) Antilymphocyte globulin (ALG)	Depletes number of circulating T lymphocytes	Treatment of organ rejection	Fever Chills Leukopenia Thrombocytopenia Fatigue	IV solution; give via filter	

GI, gastrointestinal; IL, interleukin.

manifestations, laboratory data, or results of tests such as organ biopsy. Clinical manifestations of rejection are listed in Box 80–2.

Treatment usually consists of high-dose steroids; if recurrent episodes occur, muromonab-CD3 (Orthoclone OKT3) may be administered.

CHRONIC REJECTION. Chronic rejection evolves gradually, usually after the first 3 months after transplantation. It may be the result of frequent episodes of acute rejection, increased ischemic time, or cytomegalovirus (CMV) infection. Chronic rejection results in progressive loss of graft function. The transplanted organ develops a persistent, perivascular inflammation associated with focal myocyte necrosis. Chronic rejection is treated in similar fashion to test for acute rejection; however, re-transplantation may be required as a result of the progressive deterioration of organ function.

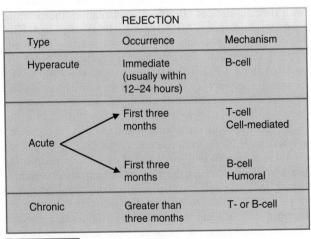

FIGURE 80–5 Transplant rejection.

BOX 80–2	Clinical Manifestations of Graft Rejection

- Fever
- Graft tenderness
- Fatigue
- Heart: shortness of breath, irregular heart beat
- Lung: shortness of breath
- Abnormal laboratory test results

  - Kidney: ↑ serum creatinine, blood urea nitrogen levels
  - Liver: ↑ total bilirubin, liver enzyme levels
  - Pancreas: ↑ urine amylase

Infection

Infection is the leading cause of morbidity and mortality after transplantation. Many factors contribute to the potential risk of infection, including the client's age, nutritional status, medical condition before transplantation, infection history and exposure, and the immunosuppressive regimen. Infections seen in transplant recipients are usually the result of immunosuppression or altered immune defenses.[15, 47] During the first month after transplantation, nosocomial infections are common; then, between 1 and 6 months, opportunistic infections such as *Pneumocystis carinii* pneumonia, candidiasis, and CMV infection occur.[40, 57] The lungs are the most common site for infection, followed by blood, urine, and the gastrointestinal tract. Common infections seen in transplant recipients are listed in Table 80–6. Infection is the most common indication for hospital readmission after transplantation.[30]

Malignancy

The development of post-transplantation malignancies caused by the immunodeficient state is well documented.[45] Types of malignancies seen in the post-transplantation population include basal cell and squamous cell carcinomas of the skin and lip, seen most commonly, followed by the lymphoproliferative disorders and cancers of the vulva, perineum, and lungs.[45] Reduction in the level of immunosuppression, surgical resection, chemotherapy, and radiation therapy are treatment options.

All clients should be screened for development of cancer after transplantation. Routine gynecologic examinations, including mammography and cervical smear in women; annual prostate-specific antigen (PSA) testing in men; and regular physical examination of neck and groin lymph nodes should be performed to detect any problems. Report any unusual lesions to the transplantation team. In addition, monitor clients who are seronegative for Epstein-Barr virus for conversion to seropositivity, which may place them at higher risk for lymphoproliferative disease after transplantation.[65] Clients need to be educated to use sun screen products with a sun protection factor (SPF) of 15 or greater and to wear protective clothing to help prevent skin malignancies.

■ CLIENTS RECEIVING A SPECIFIC ORGAN TRANSPLANT

RENAL TRANSPLANTATION

The potential renal transplant recipient has end-stage renal disease, most commonly the result of hypertension, dia-

betic nephropathy, or a hereditary or congenital disorder.[49] In most cases the renal transplant candidate is anemic and fatigued and has been maintained on chronic hemodialysis (see Chapter 36). Contraindications to renal transplantation include seropositivity for the human immunodeficiency virus (HIV), active infection, severe coronary artery disease with left ventricular dysfunction, malignancy, severe peripheral vascular disease, severe carotid artery disease, and chronic active hepatitis.

Unlike the heart, lung, liver, or pancreas transplantation candidate, the kidney transplantation candidate has several potential donors: living related, living non-related, and cadaver. Eighty-five per cent of all renal transplants are from cadaveric donors.

Extensive histocompatibility testing is completed for renal transplantation, because evidence now indicates that six antigen matches are necessary for long-term graft survival. Six-antigen-matching means that six antigens recognized on recipient HLA tissue typing match six antigens found on donor HLA tissue typing. A negative

TABLE 80–6	COMMON INFECTIONS AFTER TRANSPLANTATION	
Infecting Organism	**Site(s) Affected**	**Therapeutic Agent of Choice**
Bacteria		
Gram-negative bacilli		Ticarcillin-clavulanate (Timentin)
Klebsiella	Lung	
Pseudomonas	Blood	Gentamicin
Escherichia coli	CNS	
Legionella	Lung	
Enterobacter		
Gram-positive cocci		Vancomycin
Enterococci		
Staphylococci		
Streptococci		
Viruses		
Cytomegalovirus	Lung Blood GI tract	Ganciclovir
Varicella-zoster virus	Skin Blood	Acyclovir
Protozoa		
Toxoplasma gondii	Transplanted organ Lung Liver	Pyrimethamine Sulfadiazine Folinic acid
Pneumocystis	Lung	Trimethoprim-sulfamethoxazole
Fungi		
Aspergillus	Lung CNS	Amphotericin B
Candida	Oral mucosa	Nystatin Fluconazole Amphotericin B

CNS, central nervous system; GI, gastrointestinal.

result on cross-matching is required for transplantation to occur.

NURSING CARE. Nursing care of the renal transplant recipient is focused on the recognition and prevention of complications. Ongoing assessment of renal function—by determination of blood urea nitrogen (BUN), serum creatinine, glomerular filtration rate (GFR), fluid intake and output, weight, and serum electrolytes—is routine in these clients. If indicated, a renal scan or ultrasound study may be used to detect complications. Renal biopsy may be performed to make a definitive diagnosis, as rejection, acute tubular necrosis (ATN), and obstructive complications have similar manifestations.

Goals are to maintain hydration, promote diuresis, avoid fluid overload, and prevent infection. Complications after renal transplantation include fluid and electrolyte imbalances, ATN, obstructive or vascular complications, rejection, and infection. Clinical manifestations of potential complications in the renal transplantation client are decreased urine output, graft tenderness or pain, rising serum creatinine level, fever, and weight gain.

PANCREAS AND PANCREAS-KIDNEY TRANSPLANTATION

Pancreas transplantation is indicated for the client with type 1 diabetes mellitus to restore normal glucose metabolism.[54] Pancreas-kidney transplantation is performed in the diabetic client with end-stage renal disease (see Chapter 45).[20, 59] Contraindications are the same as in renal transplantation.

NURSING CARE. Nursing care includes monitoring for fluid and electrolyte imbalances, especially BUN, serum creatinine, bicarbonate, and CO_2. Urine amylase is also monitored to assess pancreatic function. Clinical manifestations of graft thrombosis are a sudden rise in serum glucose, severe graft pain, and increased serum creatinine with combined kidney-pancreas transplantation.

HEART TRANSPLANTATION

Potential candidates for heart transplantation are usually New York Heart Association class III or IV and younger than 65 years of age and have a life expectancy of less than 12 months. The most common diseases treated by heart transplantation are coronary artery disease and cardiomyopathy.[12] Contraindications to heart transplantation include malignancy; active infection; autoimmune disorders; irreversible kidney, lung, or liver disease; and severely elevated pulmonary vascular resistance. Relative contraindications, which vary between transplantation centers, are peptic ulcer disease, CVA, peripheral vascular disease, diabetes mellitus, and obesity.[42]

When listed for transplantation, candidates are evaluated periodically, usually every 4 to 6 weeks, to monitor their overall condition. Stable clients wait at home or near the hospital, and clients who are hemodynamically unstable wait at the hospital. Clients who become critically ill may need continuous inotropic infusions or ventricular-assist devices.

CARDIAC TRANSPLANTATION PHYSIOLOGY ALTERATIONS

Unique to the cardiac transplant recipient is cardiac transplant denervation. Denervation occurs after orthotopic transplantation, in which the vagus nerve is severed. The resultant lack of vagal nerve stimulation results in (1) a higher resting heart rate, (2) a gradual increase in heart rate with exercise and delayed return to baseline, (3) absence of angina, and (4) enhanced response to certain drugs (e.g., adrenaline, adenosine) and decreased response to other drugs (e.g., atropine, digoxin).[7] Finally, two P waves may be detected on the electrocardiogram resulting from the presence of both donor and recipient heart sinoatrial (SA) nodes. It is important to note that only the donor heart SA node regulates the electrical conduction of the heart.

NURSING CARE. The nursing assessment is a vital component in the care of the cardiac transplant recipient. The physical assessment should include auscultation of heart and breath sounds and assessment of pedal pulses and of the jugular vein for distention. Ongoing assessment of renal and liver function and monitoring of immunosuppressant drug levels and the complete blood count (CBC) are important in the overall care of the client. Complications seen after heart transplantation include organ dysfunction, rejection, infection, coronary vasculopathy, and malignancy.[10, 13, 38] Chest radiography is used to monitor possible lung infection, whereas echocardiography and endomyocardial biopsy are utilized to detect rejection. Clinical manifestations of rejection include fever, shortness of breath, fatigue, presence of S_3 or S_4 heart sound, decreased blood pressure, decreased ejection fraction, and jugular vein distention.

LIVER TRANSPLANTATION

Indications for liver transplantation include chronic irreversible liver disease due to a number of underlying disorders. In adults, the most common indications are cirrhosis secondary to chronic hepatitis, cryptogenic cirrhosis, primary biliary cirrhosis, and primary sclerosing cholangitis (see Chapter 47).[9, 41] Contraindications to liver transplantation are center-specific and may include portal vein thrombosis, active alcoholism, active infection, malignancy outside the hepatobiliary system, and advanced cardiopulmonary disease. The client evaluation takes into account technical feasibility and optimal timing of surgery in addition to the usual physical and psychosocial indications.

NURSING CARE. The postoperative care of the liver transplant client is complex. Nursing care focuses on monitoring graft function, managing fluid and electrolyte imbalances, preventing problems with other organ systems, and assessing for signs of rejection or infection. Clinical manifestations of rejection include fever, elevation of liver enzymes, and change in color, amount, and consistency of bile drainage through the T tube.

Diagnosis of rejection is confirmed by liver biopsy. In addition, a sudden increase in the International Normalized Ratio (INR) (a system for reporting prothrombin values), serum bilirubin, or liver enzymes may indicate a complication such as hepatic artery thrombosis or biliary obstruction. If neurologic status is affected, serum ammonia levels may be monitored. Finally, as in all organ transplantation procedures, renal function, immunosuppressant drug levels, and white blood cell (WBC) count should be closely monitored.

LUNG TRANSPLANTATION

The lung transplantation candidate has end-stage pulmonary disease; is generally younger than 65 years of age for single-lung transplantation, 60 years for two-lung transplantation, or 55 years for heart-lung transplantation; and is able to participate in pulmonary rehabilitation (i.e., is not wheelchair-dependent).[32, 58] The decision on whether to perform a single-lung or double-lung procedure varies among transplantation centers but is based on the likelihood of achieving the best outcome and most improvement in QOL.

Contraindications to lung transplantation are active malignancy, positive results on hepatitis B antigen assay, hepatitis C, autoimmune disorders, and dysfunction of organ(s) other than the lungs. Risk factors that affect eligibility include symptomatic osteoporosis, the need for steroid therapy in doses greater than 20 mg/day, severe musculoskeletal disease, impaired nutritional status (malnutrition or obesity), the need for mechanical ventilation, and colonization with fungi or atypical mycobacteria.[37]

LUNG TRANSPLANTATION PHYSIOLOGY ALTERATIONS. Removal of native lung and lung replacement entail denervation of the transplanted lung. Denervation interferes with autonomic nervous system communication, resulting in dysfunctional ciliary movement, loss of cough reflex, and changes in mucus production, which lead to ineffective clearance of airway secretions. Health maintenance interventions to maintain patent airways are chest vibropercussion, postural drainage, and use of an incentive spirometer.

NURSING CARE. The postoperative care of the lung transplant recipient is gratifying. It is a pleasure to watch a pre-transplantation oxygen-dependent client gasping for breath become an active person requiring no oxygen after transplantation. Immunosuppressant drug levels, electrolyte determinations, liver function tests, CBC, chest radiography, and pulmonary function tests are important monitoring tests in this population.

Complications include surgical side effects, graft dysfunction, rejection, infection, and bronchiolitis obliterans, or obliterating bronchiolitis (OB). OB is the greatest limiting factor to long-term survival after lung transplantation. OB is progressive in nature, resulting in severe shortness of breath, and must be treated aggressively. Usual medical management may include administration of intravenous steroids, cytolytic therapy (with OKT3), administration of thymoglobulin, photopheresis, and retransplantation. Goals in nursing management are to prevent and recognize complications and to promote return to a functional lifestyle.

SELF-CARE

Before discharge from the hospital, pertinent information is discussed with the client and family members. Postoperative education after transplantation can be quite challenging, because many clients are discharged between 1 and 2 weeks after surgery. Many institutions provide client education booklets. Information discussed with the client and family is presented in Box 80–3.

Of special importance are knowledge of the clinical manifestations of rejection and infection and indications for contacting the transplantation team. A schedule of return appointments is usually given at discharge. Most clients reside close to the transplantation center for 2 to 8 weeks before going home. This proximity allows for frequent medical visits, ongoing education, and familiariza-

---

BOX 80–3   Client and Family Education After Transplantation

- Members of transplantation team
- When to call the transplant coordinator
- Immunosuppression
  - Administration of medications
  - Side effects of medications
- Rejection
  - Definition, manifestations, diagnosis, treatment
- Infection
  - Definition, manifestations, diagnosis, treatment
- Routine care
  - Temperature
  - Weight
  - Skin care
  - Incision care
  - Fluid intake and output
  - Pedal pulses
  - Incentive spirometry
  - Clinic schedule
- Diet after transplantation
- Activities after transplantation
  - Precautions
  - Exercise
  - Physical therapy

- Self-care
  - Blood pressure
  - Blood glucose levels
  - Medical identification bracelet and card
  - Sun exposure
  - Sexual activity
  - Sending specimens for laboratory monitoring tests
  - Vacations
  - Over-the-counter medicines to be avoided
  - Driving
  - Birth control
- Psychosocial issues
  - Physical appearance
  - Family participation and support
  - Writing to the donor family
  - Cost of transplantation
- Health maintenance
  - Dental care
  - Ophthalmologic examinations
  - Gynecologic examinations
  - Yearly evaluations of transplant

tion of the client with the postoperative regimen. It also allows the client to become more independent and resume self-care responsibilities. Often it is the nurse who is best able to monitor compliance with the medical regimen and to identify difficulty coping with the post-transplantation regimen. Once the client returns home, it may be necessary for a home health nurse to provide wound care, perform intravenous infusions, or perform other nursing care measures. Findings on home visits are communicated to the transplantation coordinator.[44] Box 80–4 lists nursing diagnoses related to care of the post-transplantation client.

Meticulous follow-up evaluation (assessing for manifestations of rejection, infection, or other complications) is essential to the long-term well-being of the post-transplantation client. Long-term care of the transplant recipient requires communication between the client and transplantation team. Each client should be assessed for infection, rejection, malignancy, organ dysfunction, and adverse signs of immunosuppression such as diabetes, hypertension, abnormalities on liver function testing, and gastrointestinal distress.

Psychosocial issues that should be investigated are financial status, family dynamics, and return to work. The social worker at the transplantation center can assist the client with insurance questions, medication assistance programs, and ways of dealing with the financial stresses of transplantation.

Health maintenance areas to evaluate are screening by mammography and Papanicolaou (Pap) smears in women, colon cancer screening, and immunizations such as with the influenza vaccine and pneumococcal vaccine (Pneumovax). Routine dental and ophthalmologic examinations should be scheduled. Communication with the referring physician or the primary health care provider is also important. Constant relaying of information including laboratory findings, clinic visit results, and follow-up plans should occur between the transplantation center and the client's primary health care provider.

QUALITY OF LIFE AFTER TRANSPLANTATION

Examining quality of life (QOL) before and after transplantation is becoming a common practice in all areas of organ transplantation. Not only the traditional factors of survival and morbidity but also how the client functions, copes, and lives after the transplantation operation are now perceived as important. The diabetic client who is no longer insulin-dependent or the client who had end-stage renal disease who no longer requires dialysis has experienced a major change in lifestyle. Although there are challenges related to immunosuppressive therapy, most clients who undergo successful transplantation report improved QOL. Research studies may evaluate QOL at a specific period either before or after transplantation.[17, 23] Differences in the effects of drug treatment, device intervention, or medical therapy on QOL may be examined also.[29]

Hathaway reported improved QOL in renal transplant recipients regardless of race or gender of the client.[27] Hathaway also completed a longitudinal study of 91 kidney transplant recipients who underwent QOL testing before transplantation and at 6 and 12 months after transplantation. The Sickness Impact Profile, the Adult Self-Image Scale, and the Personal Resource Questionnaire were used for this study. Variables that predicted post-transplantation QOL were employment status, the number of transplantation-related hospitalizations, and available social support.[28] White-Williams and colleagues found that males reported better QOL than that described by females both before heart transplantation and at 6 months after transplantation.[63]

Grady and colleagues reported on compliance at 1 year and at 2 years after heart transplantation in 120 recipients. Compliance was measured with the Heart Transplant Compliance Instrument developed for this study. The heart transplant recipients had no difficulty following medication regimens but did have difficulty with diet, exercise, and taking their vital signs.[24]

De Geest and associates also examined compliance with taking medications in heart transplant recipients. They found that compliance with immunosuppressive medication was high; however, clients who were considered "moderate noncompliers" had a higher incidence of late acute rejection episodes. The findings in this study suggest that client compliance plays a pivotal role in long-term outcome after transplantation.[14]

Limbos and colleagues studied QOL in women before and after lung transplantation. Overall QOL improved after transplantation; however, the women reported impairments with sexuality and body satisfaction.[34] Manzetti reported that a health maintenance program of education and exercise improved QOL in clients awaiting lung transplantation.[36] Similarly, LoBiondo-Wood and colleagues reported improved QOL over time in 41-post–liver transplantation clients.[35] Long-term studies of QOL should enable nurses to understand and appreciate the impact of chronic illnesses and transplantation on clients and families.

CONCLUSIONS

Nursing care of the transplantation client is both challenging and extremely rewarding. With thorough understanding of the end-stage disease process and its manifestations, the organ donation and recovery process, and postoperative management, the nurse has the unique abil-

---

BOX 80–4   **Nursing Diagnoses for the Post-Transplantation Client**

- *Altered Nutrition: Risk for More Than Body Requirements* related to side effects of immunosuppressant agents/*Risk for Less Than Body Requirements* related to increased caloric needs after transplantation
- *Altered Protection and Risk for Infection* related to immunosuppression required after organ transplantation
- *Effective Management of Therapeutic Regimen* related to post-transplantation regimen
- *Pain* related to transplantation surgery
- *Risk for Ineffective Individual Coping* after transplantation related to increased stress, anxiety, fear, and lifestyle changes
- *Risk for Injury:* rejection of transplanted organ related to impaired immunocompetence; malignancy/diabetes/hypertension related to immunosuppression

ity to work as a member of the interdisciplinary team caring for this group of clients. The nurse may serve as primary care provider, client advocate, and liaison with other team members. To maximize QOL, caring for the client and family must focus on both the physical and psychosocial aspects of transplantation, including not only medical treatments but also nursing interventions that address the client's specific QOL issues. If psychosocial issues are not fully explored, the client is likely to experience poorer satisfaction with the post-transplantation outcome. Meticulous medical care, long-term follow-up, and addressing physical and psychosocial QOL issues all are important components of management to improve both survival and QOL in the population of clients who have undergone organ transplantation.

THINKING CRITICALLY

1. **A client has been receiving dialysis for several years awaiting kidney transplantation. She is notified that a kidney donor has been found and that she should proceed to the hospital. What teaching will be completed before she goes to surgery? What psychosocial care should be offered?**

Factors to Consider. What teaching and support will the family require? What are the ramifications if the donor kidney is found to be an unsuitable match for the client?

2. **A client has recently undergone heart transplantation and is to be discharged from the hospital in 2 days. What client education should be completed? What education should be completed for the family?**

Factors to Consider. What living arrangements are required for the client after discharge? What are the long-term concerns related to financial factors, QOL issues, and long-term immunosuppressive therapy?

3. **At a pre-transplantation support group, a client makes the following statement: "I think I may need to buy my new organ." How should the nurse react to this statement? What ethical issues are raised by this statement?**

Factors to Consider. What other ethical considerations regarding organ donation should the transplantation nurse be aware of?

BIBLIOGRPHY

1. American Heart Association. Available: *http://www. american-heart.org.*
2. American Kidney Foundation. Available: *http://www.kidney.org.*
3. American Liver Foundation. Available: *http://www.liverfoundation. org.*
4. Baily, M. A. (1988). Economic issues in organ substitution technology. In D. Mathieu (Ed.), *Organ substitution technology: Ethical, legal and public policy issues.* Boulder, CO: Westview.
5. Barnard, C. N. (1967). A human cardiac transplant. *South African Medical Journal, 41,* 1271–1274.
6. Beniaminovitz, S., et al. (1999). Use of daclizumab decreases the frequency of early allograft rejection: De novo heart transplant recipients. *Journal of Heart and Lung Transplantation, 18,* 47.
7. Britow, M. R. (1990). The surgically denervated transplanted human heart. *Circulation, 82,* 658–660.
8. Campbell, P., & Halloran, P. F. (1996). Antibody-mediated rejection. In K. Solz, L. Racusen, & M. Billingham (Eds.), *Solid organ transplant rejection.* New York: Marcel Dekker.
9. Coleman, J., Mendoza, M., & Bindon-Peiler, P. (1991). Liver disease that leads to transplantation. *Critical Care Nurse, 13,* 41–50.
10. Constanzo-Nordin, M., et al. (1992). Cardiac allograft vasculopathy: Relationship with acute cellular rejection and histocompatibility. *Journal of Heart and Lung Transplantation 11,* S90.
11. Cooper, J. D. (1995). Historical perspective lung transplantation. In G. Patterson & L. Couraud (Eds.), *Lung transplantation.* New York: Elsevier.
12. Costanzo, M., et al. (1995). Selection and treatment of candidates for heart transplantation. *Circulation, 92,* 3593–3612.
13. Costanzo, M., et. al., & The Cardiac Transplant Research Database Group. (1996). Heart transplant coronary artery disease detected by angiography: A multi-institutional study. *Journal of Heart and Lung Transplantation, 15,* S39.
14. De Geest, S., et al. (1998). Late acute rejection and subclinical noncompliance with cyclosporine therapy in heart transplant recipients. *Journal of Heart and Lung Transplantation, 17,* 854–863.
15. Dummer, J. (1990). Infection complications of transplantation. In M. Thompson & A. Brest (Eds.), *Cardiac transplantation* (pp. 163–178). Philadelphia: F. A. Davis.
16. Ehrle, R., Shafer, T., & Nelson, K. (1999). Referral, request, and consent for organ donation: Best practice—a blueprint for success. *Critical Care Nurse, 19*(2), 21–33.
17. Evans R. W., et al. (1985). The quality of life of clients with end stage renal disease. *New England Journal of Medicine, 312,* 553–559.
18. Fishman, J., & Rubin, R. (1998). Medical progress: Infection in organ transplant recipients. *New England Journal of Medicine, 338,* 1741–1751.
19. Flye, M. (Ed.). (1989). History of transplantation. In *Principles of organ transplantation.* Philadelphia: W. B. Saunders.
20. Freise, C, et al. (1999). Simultaneous pancreas-kidney transplantation: An overview of indications, complications and outcomes. *Western Journal of Medicine, 170,* 11–18.
21. Gaber, A., et al. (1998). Results of the double-blind randomized, multicenter phase II clinical trial of Thymoglobulin versus Atgam in the treatment of acute graft rejection episodes after renal transplantation. *Transplantation, 66,* 29–37.
22. Galamobos, J. (1979). *Cirrhosis.* (*Major problems in internal medicine* series [Vol. 17]). Philadelphia: W. B. Saunders.
23. Grady, K., Jalowiec, A., & White-Williams, C. (1995). Predictors of quality of life in patients with advanced heart failure awaiting transplantation. *Journal of Heart and Lung Transplantation, 14,* 2–10.
24. Grady, K., et al. (1998). Patient compliance at one year and two years after heart transplantation. *Journal of Heart and Lung Transplantation, 17,* 383–394.
25. Guthrie, C. (Ed.). (1912). Applications of blood vessel surgery. In *Blood vessel surgery.* New York: Longmans, Green.
26. Hansen, T., Carreno, B., & Sachs, D. (1993). The major histocompatibility complex. In W. Paul (Ed.), *Fundamental immunology* (3rd ed., pp. 577–628). New York: Raven Press.
27. Hathaway, D., et al. (1996). Racial and gender differences in quality of life prior to and following kidney transplantation. *Proceedings of the Tenth Annual Southern Nursing Research Society Conference.*
28. Hathaway, D., et al. (1998). Post kidney transplantation quality of life prediction models. *Clinical Transplantation, 12,* 168–174.
29. Hilbrands, L., Hoitsma, A., & Koene, R. (1995). The effect of immunosuppressive drugs on quality of life after renal transplantation. *Transplantation, 59,* 1263–1270.
30. Hosendpud, J., et al.(1998). *The Registry of the International Society for Heart and Lung Transplantation: 15th Official Report—1998, 17,* 656–668.
31. Hruban, R. H., Baldwin, W. M., & Sanfilippo, F. (1996). Immunopathology of rejection. In K. Solz, L. Racusen, & M. Billingham (Eds.), *Solid organ transplant rejection.* New York: Marcel Dekker.
32. Kaiser, L., & Cooper, J. D. (1992). The current status of lung transplantation. *Advances in Surgery, 25,* 259–307.
33. Landsteiner, K. (1928). Cell antigens and individual specificity. *Journal of Immunology, 15,* 589–600.

34. Limbos, M., Chan, C., & Kesten, S. (1997). Quality of life in female lung transplant candidates and recipients. *Chest, 112,* 1165–1174.

35. LoBiondo-Wood, G., et al. (1997). Impact of liver transplantation on quality of life: A longitudinal perspective. *Applied Nursing Research, 10*(1), 27–32.

36. Manzetti, J., et al. (1994). Exercise, education and quality of life in lung transplant candidates. *Journal of Heart and Lung Transplantation, 13,* 297–305.

37. Maurer, J., et al. (1998). International guidelines for the selection of lung transplant candidates. *Journal of Heart and Lung Transplantation, 17,* 703–709.

38. McGiffin, D., et al. (1995). Cardiac transplant coronary artery disease: A multivariable analysis of disease development and morbid events. *Journal of Thoracic and Cardiovascular Surgery, 108*(6), 1081–1089.

39. Medawar, P. B. (1945). A second study of the behavior and fate of skin homografts in rabbits: A report to the War Wounds Committee of the Medical Research Council. *Journal of Anatomy, 69,* 157–176.

40. Miller, L., et al. (1994). Infection after heart transplantation: A multiinstitutional study. *Journal of Heart and Lung Transplantation, 13,* 353.

41. National Digestive Disease Advisory Board. (1990). Conference on Liver Transplantation, Arlington, VA.

42. O'Connell, J., et al. (1992). Cardiac transplantation: Recipient selection, donor procurement, and medical follow-up: A statement for health professionals from the Committee on Cardiac Transplantation of the Council on Clinical Cardiology, American Heart Association. *Circulation, 86,* 1061–1079.

43. Office of Organ Transplantation. (1987). *The status of organ donation and coordination serves: Report to Congress for fiscal year 1987.* Washington, DC: U.S. Department of Health and Human Services.

44. Olesen, M., Leum, E., & Randolph, S. (1999). *Heart failure, transplantation and the role of the home care.* Resources.

45. Penn, I. (1991). Cancer in the immunosuppressed organ recipient. *Transplantation Proceedings, 23,* 1771–1772.

46. Reither, A. M. (1990). Psychiatric aspects of transplantation. In S. L. Smith (Ed.), *Tissue and organ transplantation: Implications for professional nursing practice.* St. Louis: Mosby-Year Book.

47. Rubin, R. (1988). Infection in the renal and liver transplant client. In R. Rubin & L. Young (Ed.), *Clinical approach to infection in the compromised host* (2nd ed., pp. 557–621). New York: Plenum Press.

48. Sabatine, M., & Auchincluss, H. (1996). Cell-mediated rejection. In K. Solz, L. Racusen, & M. Billingham (Eds.), *Solid organ transplant rejection.* New York: Marcel Dekker.

49. Shapiro, R., & Simmons, R. L. (1992). Renal transplantation. In T. Starzl, et al. (Eds.), *Atlas of organ transplantation.* New York: Gower.

50. Shumway, S. J., & Frist, W. H. (1995). Immunosuppressants. In S. J. Shumway & N. E. Shumway (Eds.), *Thoracic transplantation.* Cambridge: Blackwell Science.

51. Simulect. Novartis Product Insert. East Hanover, NJ.

52. Spector, N., Connolly, M., & Garrity, E. (1996). Lung transplant rejection: Obliterative bronchiolitis. *American Journal of Critical Care, 5,* 366–372.

53. Starzl, T. E., et al. (1963). Homotransplantation of the liver in humans. *Surgery, Gynecology and Obstetrics, 117,* 659–676.

54. Sutherland, D. E. R., Gruessner, R. W. G., & Gores, P. F. (1994). Pancreas and islet transplantation: An update. *Transplantation Reviews, 8*(4), 185–206.

55. Task Force on Organ Transplantation. (1986). *Organ transplantation: Issues and recommendations.* (HRP-0906976.) Rockville, MD: Health Resources and Services Administration.

56. Terasaki, P. I., Marchioro, P. L., & Starzl, T. E. (1965). *Histocompatibility testing.* Washington, DC: National Academy of Sciences.

57. Tolkoff-Rubin, N. E., & Rubin, R. H. (1992). Infection in organ transplant recipients. In S. Gorback, J. Bartlett, & N. Blacklon (Eds.), *Infectious diseases.* Philadelphia: W. B. Saunders.

58. Trulock, E. (1993). Recipient selection. *Chest Surgery Clinics of North America, 3*(1), 1–18.

59. Trusler, L. A. (1991). Simultaneous kidney-pancreas transplantation. *ANNA Journal, 18*(5), 487–491.

60. United Network of Organ Sharing (UNOS). (1997). *Annual report of the U.S. Scientific Registry for Transplant Recipients and Organ Procurement and Transplantation Network—Transplant data.* Richmond, VA: Author.

61. United Network of Organ Sharing (UNOS) OPTN and Scientific Registry Data, April 19, 1999.

62. White-Williams, C. (1993). Immunosuppressive therapy after cardiac transplantation. *Critical Care Nurse Quarterly, 16*(2), 1–10.

63. White-Williams, C., Jalowic, A., & Grady, K. (1997). Gender differences in quality of life outcomes before and 6 months after heart transplantation. *Journal of Heart and Lung Transplantation, 16,* 100.

64. Williams, T. (1995). Rejection in lung transplantation. In G. Paterson (Ed.), *Lung transplantation.* New York: Elsevier.

65. Zangwill, S., et al. (1998). Incidence and outcome of primary Epstein-Barr virus infection and lymphoproliferative disease in pediatric heart transplant recipients. *Journal of Heart and Lung Transplantation, 17,* 116–120.

REMEMBER *to*
check out your
Companion CD ROM

C H A P T E R

81

Management of Clients with Shock and Multisystem Disorders

Louise Nelson LaFramboise

SHOCK

Shock is a complex clinical syndrome that may occur at any time and in any place. It is a life-threatening condition often requiring team action by many health care providers, including nurses, physicians, laboratory technicians, pharmacists, and respiratory therapists. Shock causes thousands of deaths and unknown numbers of permanent injuries each year. The economic impact of shock is staggering, with health care costs for treatment of shock in the billions of dollars each year. Because shock is potentially lethal, debilitating, and costly, it is essential that nurses identify clients at risk for shock, recognize the early assessment findings indicating shock, and initiate appropriate interventions before shock ensues.

Shock is defined as failure of the circulatory system to maintain adequate perfusion of vital organs. Disorders leading to inadequate tissue perfusion result in decreased oxygenation at the cellular level. Inadequate oxygenation results in anaerobic cellular metabolism and accumulated waste products in cells. If this condition is untreated, cell and organ death occur.

Shock is commonly divided into three major classifications:

- Hypovolemic
- Cardiogenic
- Distributive

Hypovolemic shock is due to inadequate circulating blood volume resulting from hemorrhage with actual blood loss, burns with a loss of plasma proteins and fluid shifts, or dehydration with a loss of fluid volume. It is the most common type of shock and develops when the intravascular volume decreases to the point where compensatory mechanisms are unable to maintain organ and tissue perfusion.

Cardiogenic shock is due to inadequate pumping action of the heart because of primary cardiac muscle dysfunction or mechanical obstruction of blood flow caused by myocardial infarction (MI), valvular insufficiency caused by disease or trauma, cardiac dysrhythmias, or an obstructive condition, such as pericardial tamponade or pulmonary embolus. Cardiogenic shock occurs in 10% to 15% of all clients following MI and carries an associated mortality rate of up to 80%. Cardiogenic shock after an MI usually occurs when 40% or more of the myocardium has been damaged.

Sometimes the term *obstructive shock* is used to include conditions that lead to a sudden obstruction of blood flow (i.e., cardiac tamponade, tension pneumothorax, pulmonary embolism). Obstructive causes are discussed within the topic of cardiogenic shock because the ability of the heart to pump effectively is the primary problem.

Distributive shock (also called *vasogenic shock*) is due

to changes in blood vessel tone that increase the size of the vascular space without an increase in the circulating blood volume. The result is a relative hypovolemia (total fluid volume remains the same but is redistributed). Distributive shock is further divided into three types:

- *Anaphylactic shock,* a severe hypersensitivity reaction resulting in massive systemic vasodilation
- *Neurogenic shock,* or interference with nervous system control of the blood vessels, such as with spinal cord injury (especially cervical spine injury), spinal anesthesia, or severe vasovagal reactions caused by pain or psychic trauma
- *Septic shock,* caused by a release of vasoactive substances

Some amount of neurogenic shock is seen with all spinal cord injuries. More dramatic cases of neurogenic shock are seen with cervical spine injuries. The duration of neurogenic shock is usually 1 to 6 weeks, provided there has been no irreparable cord injury. The incidence of septic and anaphylactic shock is variable. Clients who are at risk for either type of shock should be monitored closely.

Etiology and Risk Factors

All causes of shock focus on some component of blood distribution throughout the body. There can be an insufficient quantity of blood (hypovolemic shock), an incompetent pump (cardiogenic shock), or an ineffective delivery of blood (distributive shock).

HYPOVOLEMIC SHOCK

The primary event precipitating hypovolemic shock is a large reduction in the circulating blood volume so that the body's metabolic needs cannot be met. Hypovolemic shock may be due to a loss of plasma or blood. Conditions that may cause a reduction in the circulating volume include hemorrhage, burns, and dehydration.

Health promotion activities to prevent hypovolemic shock include client education to avoid injuries that would put someone at risk for hypovolemic shock (see Client Education Guide later). Health maintenance activities are the use of oxygen and maintenance of fluid and electrolyte balance. To restore health, monitor the client with telemetry and hemodynamic monitoring, and give vasoactive medications and blood and fluid replacements as ordered.

Hemorrhage

Hemorrhage is the loss of blood. Clinical manifestations may begin to appear with a blood volume deficit of 15% to 25%, or about 500 to 1500 ml in an adult with a normal circulating volume. Shock fully develops if a previously healthy client loses about one third of the normal circulating blood volume of 5 L.

The loss of smaller amounts of blood may cause shock in clients less able to compensate rapidly (e.g., older people with decreased vascular tone and impaired cardiac function). The extent to which shock develops after blood loss also depends on the length of time over which the blood loss occurs. Clients experiencing slow blood loss over a period of days or weeks tolerate their blood loss better than clients whose blood loss occurs rapidly over minutes or hours. Hypovolemic shock following trauma is typically the result of hemorrhage. The classes of hemorrhage and the associated assessment findings are listed in Table 81–1.

Burns

Hypovolemic shock produced by burns occurs most often in people with large partial-thickness or full-thickness burns. It is caused primarily by a shift of plasma from the vascular space into the interstitial space. In addition to these fluid losses or shifts, the client may have cardiac dysfunction that is due to the presence of *myocardial depressant factor* (MDF), a polypeptide (see later). MDF affects the contractility of cardiac muscle by depressing myocardial muscle function. The result is impaired cardiac output, even in the presence of a normal circulating volume. Shock related to burns is discussed in Chapter 50.

TABLE 81–1	ASSESSMENT FINDINGS AND CLASSIFICATIONS OF ACUTE HEMORRHAGE*			
Assessment Finding	**Class I**	**Class II**	**Class III**	**Class IV**
Blood loss (%)	<15	15–30	30–40	>40
Blood loss (ml)	<750	750–1500	1500–2000	>2000
Pulse rate/min	<100	>100	>120	>140
Respiratory rate/min	Normal (14–20)	20–30	30–40	>35
Blood pressure	Normal	Normal	Decreased	Decreased
Pulse pressure	Normal or increased	Decreased	Decreased	Decreased
Central nervous system/ mental status	Slightly anxious	Mildly anxious	Anxious, confused	Confused, lethargic
Urinary output (ml/hr)	>30	20–30	5–15	Negligible
Intravenous fluid replacement	Crystalloid at 3 ml/1 ml of blood loss	Crystalloid at 3 ml/1 ml of blood loss	Crystalloid plus blood at 3 ml/1 ml of blood loss	Crystalloid plus blood at 3 ml/1 ml of blood loss

*Assumes a normal 70-kg man.
Data from American College of Surgeons Committee on Trauma. (1997). *Advanced trauma life support student manual* (p. 98). Chicago: Author.

Other causes of hypovolemic shock that may produce fluid shifts similar to those in burns include nephrotic syndrome, severe crush injuries, starvation, surgery, and conditions causing plasma fluids to accumulate in the abdominal cavity (e.g., cirrhosis of the liver, pancreatitis, and bowel obstruction).

Dehydration

Shock may also occur from either reduced oral fluid intake or significant fluid losses (e.g., rigorous exercise causing fluid loss from sweating and insensible fluid loss through the respiratory tract and hot environments). Loss of fluid, leading to dehydration-induced hypovolemic shock, may occur in people with excessive urine output or prolonged vomiting or diarrhea. Clients with chronic illnesses, especially older people, may be at increased risk because of impaired recognition of thirst or an inability to obtain fluids, inadequate maintenance of chronic conditions (i.e., increased blood glucose levels with diabetes), or inadequate monitoring of therapeutic regimens (i.e., diuretic-induced dehydration). With prolonged fluid deficit, all compartments—intravascular, interstitial, and intracellular—are depleted.

Cardiogenic Shock

Cardiogenic shock results primarily from an inability of heart muscle to function adequately or mechanical obstructions of blood flow to or from the heart. As with other causes of shock, the lack of blood flow decreases tissue and organ perfusion.

Myocardial Infarction

Impaired heart muscle action is most often caused by MI (see Chapter 58). The area of dead or dying tissue that occurs with infarction impairs contractility of the myocardium, and the cardiac output decreases. Impaired myocardial contractility may also occur with blunt cardiac trauma, cardiomyopathy, and heart failure.

Prevention of cardiogenic shock related to MI begins with health promotion activities directed at client education for decreasing the risk factors associated with coronary artery disease (e.g., increasing exercise and modifying dietary intake). Supportive oxygenation and administration of inotropic agents and vasodilators are health maintenance activities. An intra-aortic balloon pump (IABP) may be needed for health restoration.

Clients in cardiogenic shock may also develop some degree of hypovolemic shock. This is most often due to the therapeutic use of diuretics or to edema in the extremities or other dependent areas (caused by inadequate cardiac pumping activity and venous congestion).

Obstructive Conditions

Several types of mechanical obstructions to blood flow may cause cardiogenic shock:

1. *Large pulmonary embolism.* An *embolus* is usually the result of a blood clot that breaks loose in a person with deep vein thrombosis (DVT). This embolus travels through the venous system to the right side of the heart and into the pulmonary artery. The size of the embolus determines at what point it lodges in the pulmonary artery. A large embolus can inhibit perfusion of a major portion of the lung field, resulting in an increased workload for the right ventricle.

2. *Pericardial tamponade* is an accumulation of blood or fluid in the pericardial space that compresses the myocardium and interferes with the myocardium's ability to expand.

3. A *tension pneumothorax* is a significant amount of air in the pleural space compressing the heart and great vessels, thus interfering with venous return to the heart.

Other Causes of Cardiogenic Shock

Additional causes of cardiogenic shock include (1) cardiac valvular insufficiency from trauma or disease, (2) myocardial aneurysms (usually due to previous MI or congenital abnormalities), (3) rupture of a valvular papillary muscle, (4) ventricle rupture, (5) aortic stenosis, (6) mitral regurgitation, and (7) cardiac dysrhythmias.

Clients with hypovolemic shock are also at risk for cardiogenic shock. The myocardium normally receives its blood supply during diastole. When the heart rate increases to compensate for the decreased volume and to increase cardiac output, diastole is shortened, leading to insufficient time for the coronary arteries to fill with blood. Because these arteries supply blood to the myocardium, the myocardial oxygen supply is impaired. The increased heart rate also increases the myocardium's need for oxygen, predisposing the myocardium to injury because of the decreased blood flow and resultant decreased oxygen supply. In addition, the decreased venous return associated with hypovolemia results in decreased coronary artery perfusion and inadequate oxygenation of the myocardium.

Finally, shock results in the release of MDF and lactic acid, which depresses myocardial function.

DISTRIBUTIVE (VASOGENIC) SHOCK

Distributive shock results from inadequate vascular tone. Blood volume remains normal, but the size of the vascular space increases dramatically because of massive vasodilation. The result is maldistribution of the blood because of decreased blood pressure (BP) and lack of blood returning to the heart, which is why it is often referred to as "relative" hypovolemia. The volume of blood remains constant, but the blood has pooled because of increased capacity of the vascular system.

After extensive vasodilation, the BP, return of venous blood to the heart, and cardiac output are decreased. As with other forms of shock, tissue anoxia and cell destruction result. The massive vasodilation present with distributive shock has several major causes.

Acute Allergic Reaction (Anaphylactic Shock)

Anaphylactic shock occurs as a result of an acute allergic reaction from exposure to a substance to which the client has been sensitized. Common sensitizing agents are penicillin, penicillin derivatives, bee stings, chocolate, strawberries, peanuts, snake venom, iodine-based contrast for x-rays, foods, and nonsteroidal anti-inflammatory drugs (NSAIDs).

Reexposure to the foreign substance results in the offending antigen binding to previously made immunoglobulins (i.e., IgE) located on the mast cell. This binding causes the release of several chemical mediators from the cell, such as histamine, platelet-activating factor, leukotrienes, and prostaglandins (see Chapter 76). Manifestations include massive vasodilation, urticaria (hives), laryngeal edema, and bronchial constriction. Without prompt treatment, a person with anaphylactic shock will die of cardiovascular collapse and respiratory failure.

To help prevent the onset of anaphylactic shock, teach clients to avoid precipitators and to use an epinephrine injection (e.g., Epi-Pen). Encouraging clients to wear medical alert bracelets and to seek allergy desensitization also decreases their potential for anaphylactic shock.

Spinal Cord Injury (Neurogenic Shock)

With injury to the cervical spine, the autonomic nervous system is affected. Below the level of injury, there is blocking of sympathetic nervous stimulation and the parasympathetic system goes unopposed. This unopposed stimulation causes vasodilation, decreased venous return, decreased cardiac output, and decreased tissue perfusion. Teaching clients safety measures may help prevent spinal cord injury and neurogenic shock.

Health maintenance actions are to protect the client's spine, maintain the client's airway and breathing, provide circulatory support, and provide for thermoregulation. Health restoration involves rehabilitation when the client is stable.

Infection (Septic Shock)

Sepsis is the systemic response to infection. The process begins with the growth of various microorganisms at the site of infection. Organisms may invade the bloodstream directly (leading to positive blood cultures) or may remain in one area. The organisms release various substances into the bloodstream. These substances include structural parts of the organism, such as endotoxins and elements synthesized by them called *exotoxins*. Once these substances are released into the body, they activate the complement cascade. A complex shock picture occurs (see later). Septic shock is lethal, with a mortality rate of up to 50%.

Encouraging clients to treat infections immediately and completely may help reduce the incidence of septic shock. Older and immunocompromised clients should be monitored closely for infection, and treatment should begin immediately when infection is diagnosed. Shock is a serious development. Identify high-risk clients, and implement measures to prevent shock whenever possible.

Pathophysiology

Remember, adequate circulating volume is dependent on three interrelated components of the cardiovascular system: (1) the heart, (2) vascular tone, and (3) blood volume. A minor impairment in one component is compensated for by the other two. Prolonged or severe impairments lead to shock. Some of the problems with decreased organ and tissue perfusion in shock are due to failure of the normal mechanisms.

Blood flows throughout the body because of its driving pressure as it leaves the left ventricle (LV). Nowhere else in the cardiovascular system is blood under as high a pressure as it is in the LV. About 100 ml of blood (called *stroke volume*) leaves the LV at systolic BP about 80 times a minute. Because the metabolic demands are continuous rather than intermittent, blood is delivered into muscular walled arterioles, where it can be stored and released more consistently into the capillaries. From here,

blood flows slowly through the capillaries that have greatest demand. (For example, when you run, more blood flows to your legs and lungs and less flows to your gastrointestinal (GI) tract. After you eat, the opposite is true.)

The microcirculation has the potential capacity to hold a great volume of blood. Nonetheless, the capillaries normally are relatively ischemic, containing only about 5% of the body's volume of blood. Typically, blood flow through the capillary bed is influenced by the varying needs of the cells located near the vessel. The capillaries open on demand of the cells adjacent to them. The size of the body's larger blood vessels is regulated by the autonomic nervous system, but this is not true for the microcirculation. Arteriole and capillary sphincters are separate mechanisms governed by different controls.

The microcirculation is relatively autonomous as a functional entity. Its patterns of behavior (in both normal and abnormal situations) are highly independent of the vasomotor influences affecting the systemic circulation lying next to it. The systemic circulatory bed and the microcirculatory bed apparently do not have sensing devices that would allow a unified, coordinated response throughout the entire circulation. Thus, events occurring within one bed do not influence events in the other. The relative autonomy of the microcirculation and the lack of coordination between it and the systemic circulation are important in determining the course of events in shock.

In the capillaries, nutrients in the blood are delivered to interstitial spaces to be picked up by the cells and wastes are transported to the capillary. The microcirculation is governed locally by vasoactive substances released into the area by the actions of various types of cells. This local regulation is a sensitive mechanism that can adjust blood flow from moment to moment according to tissue needs. The capillaries eventually join and meet veins that deliver blood to the heart. Veins have no muscle and are very low-pressure systems in which blood returns to the heart by using one-way valves. Veins can also store very large amounts of blood.

Two major receptors sense blood flow and volume and help the body make needed adjustments. The *arterial baroreceptor,* located in the aortic arch, senses how full the system is. If pressure in the muscular arterioles is low because of increased demand, the baroreceptor stimulates the sympathetic nervous system. This stimulation results in increased cardiac output, by increasing rate and stroke volume, and through increased muscle tension on the arteriole walls (*systemic* or *peripheral vascular resistance*). If BP was low to begin with, there is insufficient pressure for perfusion at the capillary end.

On the right side of the heart is the *atrial baroreceptor,* which measures the fluid volume returning to the heart. It also stimulates the sympathetic nervous system and constricts vessels storing blood in areas that are not considered vital to survival. The heart and brain are the organs considered most vital to survival. All other areas are considered less essential to survival.

Chemoreceptors are also located in the aortic arch and carotid bodies. These receptors sense decreased pH and increased partial pressure of arterial carbon dioxide ($PaCO_2$). When tissues do not receive adequate blood, they maintain their metabolism using an anaerobic pathway. A product of this pathway is lactic acid. When there is inadequate perfusion, carbon dioxide (CO_2) accumulates in the tissues. If breathing is also impaired, CO_2 is not exhaled. When these changes are sensed by chemoreceptors, respiratory rate and depth increase and cardiac output increases to correct the imbalance.

A juxtaglomerular receptor in the kidney measures blood flow to the kidney. When blood volume falls, the cells in the receptor release renin. Renin begins a cascade of response (angiotensin I, angiotensin II) that eventually produces potent peripheral vasoconstriction. In addition, antidiuretic hormone (ADH) is released when osmoreceptors in the hypothalamus are triggered. Osmoreceptors sense the osmolality, that is, how "concentrated" the blood is. When osmolality is increased, ADH release prevents diuresis, increases water returned to the body from the kidney and thus increases total blood volume.

All of these receptors and hormones maintain volume and thus arterial pressure. When the circulatory system is functioning properly, mean arterial pressure (MAP) is maintained at normal levels (70 to 105 mm Hg):

$$MAP = \frac{(\text{systolic} + [2 \times \text{diastolic}])}{3}$$

MAP is the average effective pressure that drives blood through the systemic organs. If MAP is not maintained at normal or near-normal levels, tissues are inadequately perfused.

If one of the three components of circulation fails, other parts of the system initiate compensatory mechanisms. For example, vasoconstriction and increased cardiac output may be used to compensate for decreased volume. As long as two of these factors can maintain a satisfactory compensatory action, adequate blood circulation can be maintained even though the third factor is not functioning normally. If compensatory mechanisms fail or if more than one of the three factors necessary for adequate circulation malfunction, circulatory failure results and shock develops.

STAGES OF SHOCK
Early Compensation Stage
During the initial or compensated stage of shock, cardiac output is slightly decreased because of loss of actual or relative blood volume. During this stage, the body's compensatory mechanisms can maintain BP within a normal to low-normal range and can maintain tissue perfusion to the vital organs. During the compensatory phase, the systemic circulation and microcirculation work together. Both undergo a major readjustment in which their activities are coordinated to preserve the entire system. Figure 81–1 illustrates these readjustments.

Decompensation Stage
If shock and the compensatory vasoconstriction persist, the body begins to decompensate and the systemic circulation and microcirculation no longer work in unison. As vasoconstriction continues, the supply of oxygenated blood to the tissues is reduced. This results in anaerobic metabolism and lactic acidosis. Acidosis and the increasing $PaCO_2$ cause the microcirculation to dilate. This dilation causes decreased venous return and decreased circulation of reoxygenated blood.

Lactic acidosis also causes increased capillary permeability and relaxation of the capillary sphincters. Relaxation of the sphincters allows increased blood in the capillaries and increased capillary pressure. This increased pressure along with the increased capillary permeability allows fluid to move out of the vascular space and back into the tissues. In doing so, the microcirculation has reversed its pattern and is trying to secure for itself (and the tissue it supplies) more of the limited supply of available blood. Thus, the blood supply is progressively retained in the capillary bed and blood pools in the microcirculation. Because the cells demand greater perfusion time, many or most of the capillaries remain open at any one time, increasing the vascular space in the microcirculation.

Increased vascular capacity, decreased blood volume, or decreased heart action reduces the MAP. In turn, the pressure gradient for the venous return of blood decreases. This also contributes to venous pooling of blood, decreased venous return to the heart, and decreased cardiac output.

Because there are no feedback systems within the body to change this pattern, the cycle of events becomes progressively more severe. Eventually, the circulation is totally disrupted. Once the vascular space enlarges (because of vasodilation of the microcirculation), even a normal blood volume cannot fill all these small vessels and the larger ones as well. The result is a low central venous pressure (CVP), except in cardiogenic shock, and inadequate venous return to the right side of the heart, with a further decrease in cardiac output.

This resultant decrease in circulating volume and capillary flow does not allow adequate perfusion and oxygenation of the vital organs. With the prolonged decrease in capillary blood flow, the tissues become hypoxic. This cycle of events is illustrated in Figure 81–2.

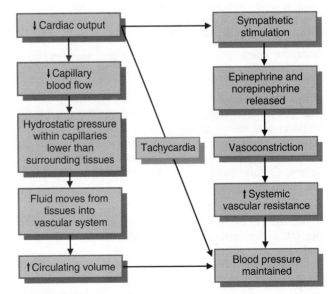

FIGURE 81–1 Compensated stage of shock. Regardless of the cause, a decreased cardiac output is generally the stimulus that precipitates the body's response to compensate for the hypovolemia (relative or actual) to maintain blood pressure.

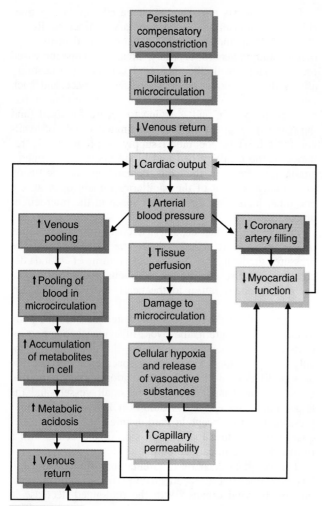

FIGURE 81–2 Vicious cycle of events occurring in shock. The shock syndrome can be initiated anywhere in the cycle, depending on the precipitating cause (e.g., impaired myocardial function due to myocardial infarction, blood loss due to trauma, or the release of vasoactive toxins due to sepsis). Hypovolemic shock resulting from blood loss, for example, results in decreased arterial blood pressure, setting in motion a cascade of events that worsen the shock state.

Progressive Stage

The progressive stage of shock occurs if the cycle of inadequate tissue perfusion is not interrupted. The shock state becomes progressively more severe, even though the initial cause of the shock is not itself becoming more severe. Cellular ischemia and necrosis lead to organ failure and death.

SYSTEMIC EFFECTS OF SHOCK

Shock affects every system within the body. Equally important to understanding the cellular level of shock is understanding what happens to the various organs. Figure 81–3 depicts the systemic effects of shock.

Respiratory System

Getting oxygen in (*ventilation*) and delivering oxygenated blood to the tissues (*perfusion*) are crucial for survival. Shock produces prolonged circulatory insufficiency. This leads to variable and inadequate perfusion of certain or-

gans and tissues, particularly at the microcirculation level. Such circulatory deprivation results in tissue hypoxia and anoxia. Hypoxia and anoxia can be tolerated for a short time. As the time lengthens, the chances of recovery diminish. A lack of oxygen appears to initiate the progressive stage of shock. The greater the difference between the amount of oxygen available and the amount needed, the more rapidly progressive shock develops. If sufficient oxygen is available to the cells to meet the body's needs, progressive shock is less likely to occur.

Despite many advances in shock prevention, early recognition, and management, respiratory failure continues to be a major cause of death in shock. The magnitude of this problem surfaced during the Vietnam War when soldiers sustaining massive injuries and profound blood loss were successfully resuscitated only to die several days later of acute respiratory distress syndrome (ARDS) (see Chapter 63). Although ARDS remains the greatest contributing factor to respiratory failure, other causes of respiratory failure during shock include aspiration and loss of neurologic control of breathing.

ACID-BASE BALANCE. To function properly, cells depend on adequate circulation to receive nutrients, electrolytes, and oxygen and to remove waste products. Oxygen and nutrients are essential to life because they make possible chemical transformations resulting in the synthesis of adenosine triphosphate (ATP). ATP is the ultimate source of energy for life processes.

When oxygen is not present, ATP is produced through a different set of reactions called *anaerobic metabolism*. Although production of ATP in this manner is a useful emergency measure, it is inefficient compared with the normal process of *aerobic (oxidative) metabolism*. Anaerobic metabolism produces anaerobic metabolites, such as lactic acid (which causes intracellular acidity with consequent cellular damage) and substrates of the adenylic acid system (which depress the heart) (Fig. 81–4).

In response to the chemoreceptors sensing decreased pH, the rate and depth of respirations are increased to "blow off" (exhale) CO_2 in an attempt to compensate for the metabolic acidosis. This results in respiratory alkalosis. However, the cellular hypoxia is caused not by inadequate ventilation but by inadequate tissue perfusion. Therefore, the increased respiratory effort does little to correct the problem.

Because lactic acid is not exhaled, it accumulates in tissue fluids, which thus become increasingly acidic. Eventually, metabolic acidosis is produced. During metabolic acidosis, blood pH and bicarbonate levels fall. Pyruvate, lactate, phosphate, and sulfate levels rise. Unless circulation is restored, the acidotic reaction resulting from metabolic acidosis ultimately kills the cells. The buildup of lactic acid causes such a severe local acidosis that cellular enzymes are inactivated. As a result, the cells soon die.

Respiratory alkalosis or *respiratory acidosis* (induced by pulmonary ventilatory or diffusion changes) may be superimposed on the metabolic acidosis. As perfusion and oxygen delivery to the tissues decrease, cellular energy production decreases. To compensate, cells increase anaerobic metabolism, which results in the buildup of lactic acid in the cell. As the pH of the cells decreases, lysosomes within the cell explode, releasing powerful, de-

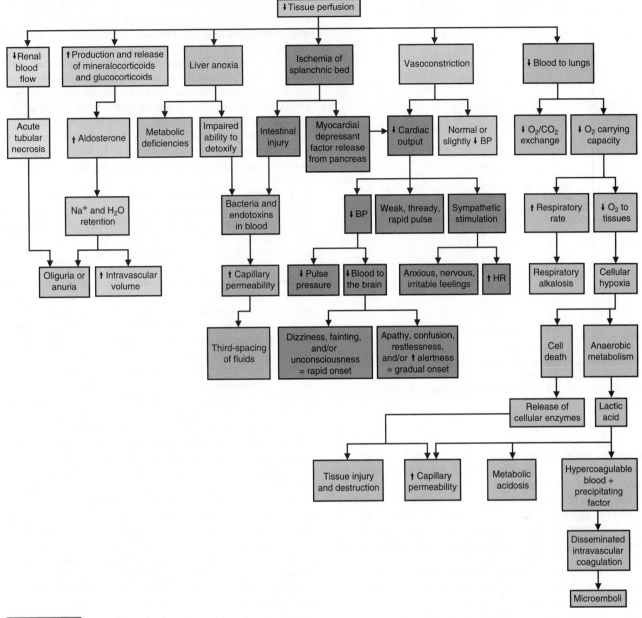

FIGURE 81–3 Systemic effects of shock.

structive enzymes. These enzymes destroy the cellular membrane and digest the cell contents. Once this process begins, the cellular changes are irreversible. The final result is cellular death (Fig. 81–5).

Cardiovascular System

MYOCARDIAL DETERIORATION. As shock progresses, the heart deteriorates. Cardiac deterioration is one of the major causes of death in shock. Although the exact cause of myocardial depression is unclear, much attention has been directed at MDF. MDF, a polypeptide with vasoactive properties, is released in response to ischemia of the GI tract. It causes a significant reduction in cardiac output, even in the presence of a normal circulating volume of blood. Another factor contributing to cardiac deterioration may be myocardial zonal lesions, which appear in the myocardium after ischemia or infarction. Cells in

these areas do not fully repolarize and thus interfere with the usual efficient electrical conduction in the heart, which results in impaired contraction and possibly cardiac failure.

Cardiac depression is often compensated for by the large cardiac reserve of a normal person. Because of this reserve, the heart can deteriorate to less than one third (sometimes less than one fifth) of its normal pumping strength without measurable evidence of cardiac failure.

DISSEMINATED INTRAVASCULAR COAGULATION. During shock, tissue hypoxia results from the sluggish movement of blood in the capillaries. Anaerobic metabolism begins, increasing the production of lactic acid. The slow-moving acidic blood is hypercoagulable; however, it does not coagulate unless a clot-initiating factor is present. Such factors include bacterial endotoxins and

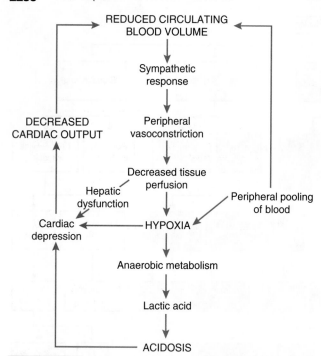

REDUCED CIRCULATING
BLOOD VOLUME

Sympathetic
response

DECREASED
CARDIAC OUTPUT

Peripheral
vasoconstriction

Decreased tissue
perfusion

Hepatic
dysfunction

Peripheral pooling
of blood

Cardiac
depression

HYPOXIA

Anaerobic metabolism

Lactic acid

ACIDOSIS

FIGURE 81–4 Shock leads to tissue hypoxia, with blockage of normal aerobic metabolism. Lactic acid accumulates, resulting in tissue acidosis. (Modified from Condon, R. E., & Nyhus, L. M. [1978]. *Manual of surgical therapeutics* [4th ed.]. Boston: Little, Brown.)

thromboplastin of red blood cells (liberated by hemolysis). Hemolysis (destruction of red blood cells with the liberation of hemoglobin) accompanies trauma, especially when massive crushing injury occurs. When any of these factors is present, along with the stagnant, acidic blood of shock, widespread intravascular clotting may occur in the vessels. This disorder is called disseminated intravascular coagulation (DIC) (see Chapter 75).

DIC is associated with multiple thrombi or emboli that are deposited in the microvascular circulation, with resultant organ obstruction and increased tissue ischemia. As blood attempts to flow through partially obstructed vessels, widespread hemolysis may occur. When red blood cells are destroyed, again hemoglobin is liberated. Anemia occurs because the liberated hemoglobin is excreted by the kidneys.

Because of the inappropriate clotting that occurs with DIC, the body attempts to reverse the process by breaking down clots. However, clots are destroyed throughout the body, not just the inappropriately formed clots. This results in bleeding in areas previously sealed by clots (i.e., venipuncture sites, vascular leaks in the brain). As DIC progresses, clotting factors are depleted, causing an inability for normal clot formation in the presence of bleeding.

Treatment of the precipitating cause, anticoagulant therapy, and replacement of clotting factors must be started as soon as possible for maximal effectiveness. DIC is a serious complication that occurs in almost 40% of clients in septic shock and is often fatal.

VASOCONSTRICTION. Sluggish circulation also results in decreased removal of CO_2 from the tissues. Increased CO_2 dilates arterioles located in active tissues and constricts those in nonactive tissues. Because of the heart's increased activity, excessive CO_2 is produced in the myocardium. Increased CO_2 directly dilates the coronary arteries leading to the myocardium, which allows the myocardium to receive more arterial blood. CO_2 is also a powerful stimulant of the vasoconstrictor center in the sympathetic nervous system. With vasoconstriction of nonactive tissues, blood is shunted to the more active tissues, which have a greater immediate need.

RELEASE OF LYSOSOMAL ENZYMES. Lysosomal enzymes are released from dead cells undergoing autolysis. They are also released just before cell death produced by cellular anoxia or some other form of injury. For example, these enzymes may be liberated as a result of trauma and endotoxins. During shock, the disruption of lysosomes and the release of their enzymes seem to occur in the liver. This is one mechanism of cell destruction resulting from prolonged shock. The presence of hepatic lysosomal active enzymes in the bloodstream, along with blocking of the *reticuloendothelial system* (RES), may contribute to death from shock. Blockade of the RES drastically reduces its capacity to clear bacteria from the bloodstream.

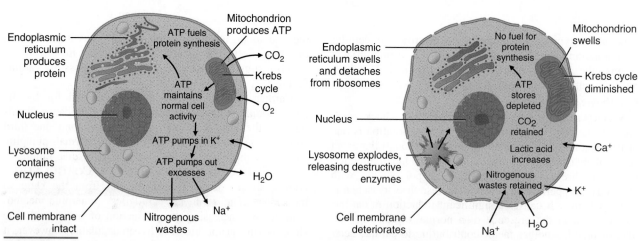

FIGURE 81–5 *Left,* Normal cell. *Right,* Alterations in cell function during late shock. ATP, adenosine triphosphate; Ca^+, calcium; CO_2, carbon dioxide; H_2O, water; Na^+, sodium; O_2, oxygen.

Lysosomal enzymes become most active in an acid pH range. Thus, as long as normal acid-base balance is maintained within the body, these enzymes are repressed within normal cells. During shock, however, the accompanying metabolic acidosis accelerates the activation of these enzymes in hypoxic tissues. The activation of lysosomal hydrolases within the cells and their release into the circulation markedly exacerbate the tissue injury that occurs during shock. The release of active lysosomal proteases and other enzymes from damaged tissue into the bloodstream and their action on extracellular and intracellular structures probably contribute to the progression of injury from cell to cell.

Vasoactive Substances. Vasoactive substances are highly variable in promoting vasoconstriction or vasodilation in a person experiencing shock. The influence they exert may be altered by factors such as pH, the specific tissue (e.g., heart, lung), the presence of drugs or other substances, serum electrolyte levels, and the sensitivity of the end organ.

Catecholamines. Catecholamines, such as epinephrine and norepinephrine, are present early in shock and are related to the fight-or-flight response. Their general effects are to increase blood flow to the brain, heart, and striated (skeletal) muscle and to decrease blood flow to the skin, kidneys, and splanchnic bed. Although the initial effect of vasoconstriction in the skin, kidneys, and splanchnic bed (GI tract) serves to increase the intravascular volume, sustained vasoconstriction contributes to stagnant hypoxia and cellular death.

Histamine. Histamine causes vasodilation, increased capillary permeability, bronchoconstriction, coronary vasodilation, and cutaneous reactions (flares, wheals). The effects of histamine are especially obvious in anaphylactic and septic shock.

Vasoactive Polypeptides. Among the more important vasoactive polypeptides that appear to play significant roles in shock are:

1. *Bradykinin.* A kinin peptide, bradykinin is known to produce vasodilation, increased capillary permeability, smooth muscle relaxation, pain, and infiltration of an area with leukocytes. Kinins appear to be most active in late shock. They may be a factor in the development of pulmonary insufficiency associated with shock.
2. *Angiotensin.* Angiotensin results from the action of renal renin on angiotensinogen. This potent substance causes vasoconstriction and increased vascular resistance. Although similar to norepinephrine in effect, angiotensin may produce fewer negative effects. Its role in sodium and water retention (through the stimulation of aldosterone secretion) is discussed under the adrenal response.
3. *MDF.* MDF is a vasoactive polypeptide that contributes to cardiac failure in clients in shock by depressing cardiac muscle contraction.

Neuroendocrine System

GENERAL ADAPTATION SYSTEM (GAS) RESPONSE.
Neuroendocrine responses during shock are defensive reactions that occur during the body's stage of resistance in the general adaptation syndrome (GAS). Recall that the length of the stage of resistance varies among people and is determined by a body's ability to compensate for its deficiencies. Hence, one person may be able to combat shock longer than another. For example, a previously healthy person may have a longer stage of resistance against shock compared with a client who is debilitated before shock develops.

ADRENAL RESPONSE. Some basic features of the neuroendocrine responses include (1) the release of epinephrine and norepinephrine from the adrenal medulla (which results in increased respiratory and heart rates, increased BP, increased blood flow to organs, decreased blood flow to peripheral tissues) and (2) the release of mineralocorticoids (which control fluid and electrolyte balance) and glucocorticoids (which affect energy and tissue resistance) from the adrenal cortex.

Increased production of adrenocortical mineralocorticoid hormones occurs. The main mineralocorticoids—aldosterone and desoxycorticosterone—help to increase intravascular fluid volume by stimulating the kidneys to retain sodium and hence water. The renal tubular conservation of sodium occurs with any type of fluid loss or blood volume depletion. Aldosterone is essential to conservation of sodium. Because water is retained in the body along with sodium, urine excretion is diminished during shock. This fluid is retained in the bloodstream in an effort to increase blood volume. Increasing the volume of blood in this way is aimed at increasing venous return, cardiac output, and BP.

PITUITARY RESPONSE. Of major importance in regulating water and sodium balance are aldosterone and ADH, also called *vasopressin.* ADH is produced by the posterior pituitary gland. The blood's osmolality (osmotic concentration) increases with dehydration. This stimulates osmoreceptors in the hypothalamus to release ADH from the posterior pituitary gland. Via the blood, the ADH is carried to the kidneys. There it causes the body to retain water.

Various components of the sympathoadrenal (sympathetic part of the autonomic nervous system and adrenal medulla) response to a major stressor are shown in Figure 81–6.

Metabolic Response. Generally, the hormonal response to stress rapidly provides fuel for the body's various tissues, organs, and systems. These fuels (e.g., amino acids, fatty acids, and glucose) are produced by the breakdown of food. These substances are then chemically converted into energy, resulting in the formation of ATP. ATP is the main source of energy produced and used inside the body's cells.

The glucocorticoids, particularly hydrocortisone, mobilize energy stores. During the initial phase of shock, the body's small stores of available carbohydrate are rapidly depleted. It then becomes necessary to mobilize protein and fat stores to meet the body's energy requirements. Protein catabolism and negative nitrogen balance occur as part of the metabolic response, because of gluconeogenesis (resulting from glucocorticoid action) and starvation.

NEUROLOGIC RESPONSE. With shock, cerebral blood flow and cerebral metabolism may become insufficient to maintain normal mental functioning and level of consciousness. Brain cells are highly sensitive to a shortage of oxygen and glucose and to fluid imbalances. When the brain becomes hypoxic, the cerebral vessels dilate to re-

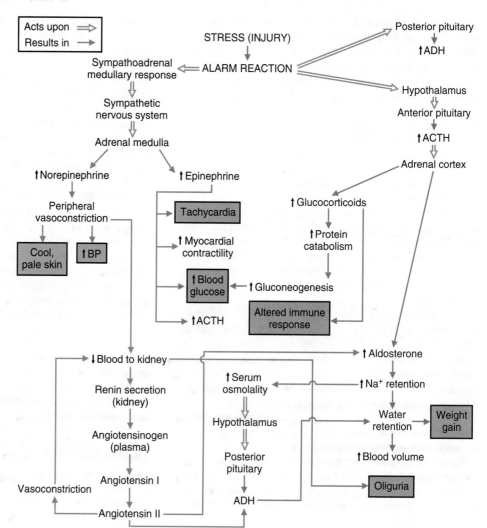

FIGURE 81–6 Components of the neuroendocrine response to a major stressor. Readily observed clinical signs as well as laboratory values are indicated by the boxes. ACTH, adrenocorticotropic hormone; ADH, antidiuretic hormone; BP, blood pressure.

store blood flow. Likewise, blood is diverted to the brain from the other, less vital organs.

Immune System

All forms of shock severely depress macrophages, which are located in both the blood and tissues. The capacity of macrophages to remove bacteria and the constantly formed endotoxins from the bloodstream is greatly reduced. Alterations in the blood itself are partially due to tissue hypoxia and impairment of monitoring activities of the macrophage. The stasis, sludging, tendency for venular thrombosis, impaired capillary permeability, and subnormal vascular reactivity that occur during shock can all be traced to macrophage dysfunction.

The impaired ability of macrophages to ward off toxic agents is critical. Reduced blood flow through the intestines during shock extensively impairs the integrity of intestinal tissue. This results in the movement of normal GI flora across the impaired intestinal tissue into the bloodstream, leading to a possible bacteremic state. The person in a state of shock is more susceptible than normal to bacterial products, particularly bacterial endotoxins, because of alterations in macrophage function.

Gastrointestinal System

Under sympathetic stimulation, vagal stimulation to the GI tract slows or stops, resulting in ileus with an absence of peristalsis. A lack of nutrient blood supply to the intestines increases the risk of tissue necrosis and sepsis.

GI changes appear to have a more important role in the progression of shock than previously thought. The submucosa of the intestine becomes ischemic early in shock. If ischemia is prolonged, actual tissue necrosis of intestinal mucosa occurs. The intestinal arterioles and venules seem highly susceptible to the extensive vasoconstriction that occurs during shock. The massive amount of tissue destruction within the intestines that results from vasoconstriction and tissue anoxia is sufficient to cause death even if bacteria are not present. Bacteria and their toxins contribute to shock by escaping into the systemic circulation following destruction of the intestinal mucosa barrier.

Shock causes serious changes in the functions of the liver, the major organ of detoxification. The liver also suffers from this impaired circulation and appears to be a source of toxic materials. Normally, the liver protectively traps and disposes of toxic materials (released from the bowel contents) that are products of bacterial enzyme actions. During shock, the anoxic liver develops metabolic deficiencies, has an impaired ability to detoxify, and may release vasoactive substances. In addition, enhanced bacterial invasion of the liver from the intestine apparently occurs.

Finally, during shock, pooling of blood occurs in the viscera. Pooling of blood in the liver and portal bed may result from masses of agglutinated (clotted) blood plugging numerous small hepatic vessels, sinusoids, and intrahepatic radicles of the portal vein and hepatic artery.

Renal System

The rate of urinary production reflects visceral blood flow and body fluid balance. Thus, urinary output indicates the status of circulation through the vital organs. Adequate urinary output indicates adequate circulation even if the arterial blood pressure is below normal.

ALTERED CAPILLARY BLOOD PRESSURE AND GLOMERULAR FILTRATION. Glomerular filtration within the kidneys depends on the pressure at which the blood is circulating through the glomerular capillaries. Usually, the average capillary pressure of blood is much higher in the glomeruli than in other capillaries. Interestingly, under usual circumstances, the kidneys can maintain this heightened capillary pressure in the glomeruli in spite of changes in systemic BP. Afferent arterioles supplying the glomeruli dilate as the BP falls and constrict as it rises. However, eventually this adaptive mechanism cannot protect the kidneys against damage from a falling systemic BP.

During shock, when blood volume and BP decline steadily, glomerular filtration is progressively reduced, which leads to an inability of the kidneys to excrete sodium and water. To compensate, the body excretes some sodium and water through the sweat glands. Damaged kidneys also lose their crucial ability to regulate electrolyte and acid-base balance.

Inadequate perfusion of renal capillaries is believed to be the cause of early renal failure in shock. The afferent and efferent arterioles constrict, shunting blood away from the glomeruli. Later, if shock persists, actual renal shutdown occurs from focal tubular necrosis. Unfortunately, vasoconstriction in the kidneys may continue for a prolonged period of time after the systemic BP is restored to normal levels.

RENAL ISCHEMIA. During shock, the kidneys may experience renal ischemia. Because the kidneys have a high rate of metabolism, they are highly susceptible to injury of the tubule cells when the blood supply is deficient. When injury to the kidneys is extensive and renal failure ensues, acute tubular necrosis (ATN) occurs. With appropriate intervention, including careful fluid administration, the kidneys can heal. Normal kidney function usually returns after 10 to 14 days.

Clinical Manifestations

SYSTEMIC MANIFESTATIONS OF SHOCK

Because shock affects every system within the body, there are numerous clinical manifestations. The body is made up of many cells, which may function or malfunction at different stages of metabolic impairment. Subjective complaints are usually nonspecific and may not be particularly helpful to the clinician attempting to diagnose shock and treat the client. The client may report feeling sick, weak, cold, hot, nauseated, dizzy, confused, frightened, thirsty, or short of breath. Observable and measurable manifestations (Fig. 81–7) are often conflicting. BP, cardiac output, and urinary output are usually (but not always) decreased. Respiratory rate is usually increased. Variable indicators of shock include alterations in heart rate, core body temperature, skin temperature, systemic vascular resistance, and skin color. Dyspnea, altered sensorium, and diaphoresis may be present. The manifestations discussed in the sections that follow are usually present in people with shock of any type.

Respiratory System

Rapid, shallow respirations (tachypnea) typically occur during shock because of decreased tissue perfusion. The

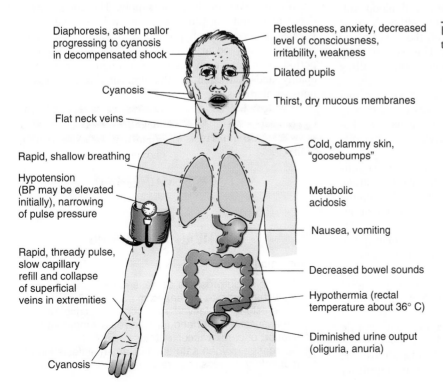

Diaphoresis, ashen pallor progressing to cyanosis in decompensated shock

Cyanosis

Flat neck veins

Rapid, shallow breathing

Hypotension (BP may be elevated initially), narrowing of pulse pressure

Rapid, thready pulse, slow capillary refill and collapse of superficial veins in extremities

Cyanosis

Restlessness, anxiety, decreased level of consciousness, irritability, weakness

Dilated pupils

Thirst, dry mucous membranes

Cold, clammy skin, "goosebumps"

Metabolic acidosis

Nausea, vomiting

Decreased bowel sounds

Hypothermia (rectal temperature about 36° C)

Diminished urine output (oliguria, anuria)

FIGURE 81–7 Clinical manifestations of the client with hypovolemic shock.

respiratory rate increases as the blood's oxygen-carrying capacity decreases. These changes may signal the development of hypoxemia and respiratory alkalosis.

Cardiovascular System

TACHYCARDIA. During shock, the pulse rate usually increases as a result of increased sympathetic stimulation. Tachycardia (rapid heartbeat) occurs in an attempt to maintain adequate cardiac output when the blood's circulating volume is declining. With increased rate, the pulse becomes typically weak and thready. At the onset of shock, the pulse rate does not relate as directly to the severity of shock as does BP. This is because in the early stage of shock, worry, excitement, and fear may influence the heart rate out of proportion to the underlying conditions. However, when emotional factors are no longer significant, serial observations of the pulse rate over a period of time are highly useful to assess the client's condition and the direction of the shock state and to evaluate the effectiveness of intervention.

Older clients (with and without various degrees of heart block) and clients taking beta-blockers are exceptions to this event. Their heart rates may show little change despite the presence of conditions causing circulatory failure (e.g., hemorrhage). The pulse rate may become extremely slow in the terminal stages of shock and is usually slow in neurogenic shock.

HYPOTENSION. The systolic BP indicates the integrity of the heart, arteries, and arterioles. The diastolic BP indicates the resistance (*systemic vascular resistance* [SVR] or *vasoconstriction*) of blood vessels. For example, an increasing diastolic BP indicates increasing systemic blood vessel resistance. Conversely, a declining diastolic BP indicates decreasing SVR. When the diastolic BP falls significantly, vasoconstriction is being lost as a compensatory mechanism. When vasoconstriction is replaced by marked vasodilation, there is no resistance to blood flow and an adequate BP is difficult to maintain.

Usually, the BP begins to fall when total blood volume is decreased by about 15% to 20%; although some people may lose as much as 25% of the total blood volume without having a fall in BP. This is especially true in young adults; therefore, in young adults, falling BP is a *very* late manifestation of shock.

Typically, as shock progresses, both the systolic and diastolic BPs drop, with the systolic pressure dropping more than the diastolic. The pulse pressure narrows because it is equal to the difference between the systolic and diastolic BPs.

During shock, pulse pressure is actually more significant than BP because it tends to parallel cardiac stroke volume. The pulse pressure is affected by stroke volume (amount of blood ejected by the LV during contraction) and by peripheral resistance. If stroke volume is decreased from a decreased circulating blood volume, pulse pressure decreases. In shock, pulse pressure may decrease even in the presence of an acceptable systolic BP. This may provide a clue to worsening shock. In shock, pulse pressure is often less than 20 mm Hg. See the Critical Monitoring feature.

To maintain coronary circulation, a minimal systolic BP of 60 to 70 mm Hg is necessary. In interpreting BP readings, it is important to know what the client's BP has been. A systolic BP of 100 mm Hg or less is significant for clients whose systolic BP usually ranges from 110 to 140 mm Hg. When a client is supine, a decline in BP may be a late finding. Hypotension by itself is not shock. Healthy clients often have BP readings lower than textbook normal values.

Additional problems need to be considered in assessment of BP that make BP an unreliable criterion for assessing the presence and severity of shock. In the early, compensated stages of shock, BP changes are generally unreliable because the arterial pressure may actually be normal or slightly elevated even though shock is present. In fact, blood volume deficits of 1 L or more may occur even though arterial and venous pressures are normal or elevated. When severe vasoconstriction is present, BP may be normal even though the circulation is actually highly inadequate. Conversely, the blood flow may be adequate even though BP is decreased (e.g., because of mechanisms such as vasodilation).

Valuable information about the level of arterial pressure in clients with vasoconstriction can be gained by assessing the strength of the femoral pulses. Doppler study may also be appropriate to obtain an accurate peripheral BP. With displaced or depleted blood volume, it is important to consider adequate venous filling. Hypovolemia, whether actual or relative, causes superficial veins to flatten. This change may hamper attempts to insert intravenous (IV) catheters for fluid replacement.

NEUROENDOCRINE SYSTEM. Early in shock, hyperactivity of the sympathetic nervous system with increased secretion of epinephrine usually causes the client to feel anxious, nervous, and irritable. Anxiety and worry are seen in the client's facial expressions.

Assessment findings associated with lack of blood to the brain are determined by the suddenness with which the shock develops and by its severity. With sudden, severe shock, the body may not have time to initiate its compensatory adjustment mechanisms. Consequently, the brain is deprived of its blood supply. The client may feel dizzy and faint on sitting up from a horizontal position because of postural hypotension. Fainting and unconsciousness may occur. If shock develops gradually over a period of hours, early assessment findings may include apathy and confusion or the opposite, restlessness and unusual alertness.

The systolic BP is important in maintaining blood flow to the brain. A cerebral perfusion pressure (CPP) of at least 50 mm Hg is required to deliver blood to the brain

$$CPP = MAP - ICP$$

CRITICAL MONITORING

Worsening Shock

- Systolic blood pressure decreased more than 20 mm Hg with heart rate increased more than 20 beats indicates actual or relative hypovolemia requiring immediate assessment of need for fluid replacement and support of cardiovascular status.
- Decreased oxygen saturation or any manifestations of respiratory distress require immediate intervention.

where ICP is intracranial pressure. Usually, a decrease in systolic BP is accompanied by a reduced flow of blood to the brain. The brain's vessels, like those of the heart, however, are not constricted by the vasoconstrictor center in the medulla oblongata. Thus, blood from the peripheral vessels can be shifted to the brain as an emergency compensatory measure.

A client's level of consciousness decreases as circulation to brain tissue becomes increasingly impaired. Confusion, agitation, and restlessness may occur. In trauma situations, restlessness can be mistaken for pain. If narcotics are given, the client's situation may be worsened or it may be difficult to detect worsening hypoxia. Drowsiness and stupor are more likely in shock related to severe infection than in shock caused by trauma and hemorrhage. As compensatory mechanisms fail, apathy may ensue. Ultimately, a comatose condition may be reached.

Renal System
A fall in urinary volume, often the earliest manifestation of developing shock, may occur even while arterial BP and pulse remain stable. Although urinary output is one of the most sensitive indices in shock, any form of shock that develops very rapidly shows other manifestations before decreased urinary output is noticed.

Urinary output should be kept above 0.5 ml/kg/hr. If the hourly output diminishes significantly, treatment must be instituted to prevent renal failure. Urinary flow of less than 20 ml/hour can cause ATN from inadequate renal circulation.

CLINICAL MANIFESTATIONS OF SPECIFIC TYPES OF SHOCK
Hypovolemic Shock
Initially, urine osmolality and specific gravity increase because of sodium and water reabsorption, which attempts to support circulating volume. As altered tissue perfusion and the hypovolemic shock progress, urine osmolality and specific gravity decrease because of the kidneys' inability to reabsorb sodium and water.

Sympathetic nervous system stimulation of the skin leads to marked diaphoresis. Clients sweat profusely, which increases insensible fluid loss, leading to further hypovolemia and temperature instability. Sympathetic stimulation also results in increased pulse and respirations and decreased tissue perfusion to the skin, causing the skin to feel cool and clammy and to appear pale.

Cyanosis may indicate either decreased tissue perfusion or decreased oxygenation or both. Cyanosis is a late manifestation of decreased oxygenation.

Cardiogenic Shock
Because of the impaired muscle action or mechanical obstruction that caused the cardiogenic shock, blood is inadequately pumped through the heart. This results in a back-up of blood. When the shock is due to right-sided heart failure, this back-up is evidenced as jugular venous distention and increased CVP. (See Chapters 55 and 62 for discussions of cardiac tamponade and tension pneumothorax.) When the shock is due to left-sided failure, blood backs up into the pulmonary circulation, resulting in pulmonary edema, crackles in the lungs, and increased pulmonary capillary wedge pressure (PCWP). As in hypovolemic shock, there is stimulation of the sympathetic

nervous system because of decreased cardiac output and decreased BP and all of its resultant clinical manifestations.

Distributive Shock
ANAPHYLACTIC SHOCK. Initially, the client may complain of a vague feeling of uneasiness or a feeling of impending doom. The massive vasodilation that occurs with anaphylaxis may cause complaints of headache as well. This may be followed by severe anxiety, dizziness, disorientation, and loss of consciousness.

Respiratory involvement may be apparent through a variety of manifestations. The initial complaint may be a feeling as though there were a lump in the throat. This is due to laryngeal edema and is followed by hoarseness, coughing, dyspnea, and stridor. Diffuse wheezes and a prolonged expiratory phase are heard on auscultation. If a pulse oximeter is in use, there may be a rapid decline in oxygen saturation.

Additional complaints may include pruritus and urticaria. Direct observation may also demonstrate edema of the eyelids, lips, or tongue (angioedema).

NEUROGENIC SHOCK. In neurogenic shock, abnormal distribution of fluid volume occurs from interruption or loss of innervation. Exceptions to the usual clinical manifestations are bradycardia and hypotension (which cannot be corrected because of loss of the ability of vasoconstriction). Below the level of injury, skin temperature takes on the same temperature as the room (poikilothermia). Skin is dry to the touch because of an inability to sweat.

SEPTIC SHOCK. In the early stages of septic shock, the body experiences massive vasodilation. Warm, dry, flushed skin is apparent during this hyperdynamic stage of septic shock. The compensatory increase in cardiac output and resultant increased perfusion of the skin give this stage the name "warm shock." During later stages, when compensatory mechanisms fail, the release of MDF and decreased venous return result in decreased perfusion and "cold shock," or the hypodynamic stage. At this point, the skin becomes pale, cold, clammy, and mottled. Body temperature drops to subnormal levels. Auscultation of the lungs reveals crackles and wheezes, which develop secondary to pulmonary congestion as ARDS ensues. In addition to the clinical manifestations seen with shock in general, changes in the level of consciousness may include drowsiness and stupor progressing to coma.

DIAGNOSTIC ASSESSMENT
Diagnostic assessments of clients in shock should include oxygenation, organ perfusion, and fluid balance. Assessment of respiratory status can be accomplished to some degree by noninvasive procedures such as spirometry, pulse oximeter, or arterial blood gases (ABGs).

ABG analysis may also be done to determine whether the metabolic acidosis that occurs with shock is being effectively combated by hyperventilation. A low $PaCO_2$, along with low pH and bicarbonate levels (metabolic acidosis), indicates that hyperventilation is trying to compensate. However, a rising $PaCO_2$ in the presence of a persistently low pH indicates that respiratory assistance is needed. It is also important to monitor PaO_2 levels to determine whether the client is being adequately oxygenated. (See Critical Monitoring and Chapter 63 for discussions of respiratory interventions.)

CVP measurement is one of the first invasive assessments made in the presence of shock to estimate fluid loss. A pulmonary artery or Swan-Ganz catheter may also be inserted to assist with assessments of fluid status, cardiac function, and tissue oxygen consumption.

Other noninvasive assessment and monitoring tools are the cardiac monitor and the 12-lead electrocardiogram (ECG). Laboratory studies include a complete blood count, blood chemistry, and blood and body fluid cultures for certain clients.

Outcome Management

Treatment should generally be instituted for shock whenever at least two of the following three conditions occur: systolic BP of 80 mm Hg or less, pulse pressure of 20 mm Hg or less, and pulse rate of 120 or more. Pulse pressure is calculated by subtracting diastolic BP from systolic BP and normally is between 30 and 50 mm Hg.

The therapeutic management of shock has changed markedly over recent years. Lowering the head, raising the feet, and administering potent vasoconstrictor drugs were once the foundation of treatment for a client in shock. Now, emphasis is placed on maintaining adequate circulating volume, positions that do not interfere with pulmonary ventilation, and the use of medications having both vasoconstrictor and vasodilator effects.

◼ Medical Management

CORRECT THE CAUSATIVE FACTOR

Assessment and an accurate differential medical diagnosis, which establish the specific cause of the shock state, form the basis for treatment. The differential medical diagnosis is usually readily made unless the shock is in an advanced stage, in which several specific forms of shock may exist at the same time. Some forms of shock more easily recognized are hypovolemic shock that is due to extensive burns or trauma and cardiogenic shock with severe chest pain and acute MI. Septic shock is probably the most difficult shock state to diagnose because of its insidious onset and complex manifestations.

IMPROVE OXYGENATION

Maintaining the client's airway is vital to the treatment of shock. In all types of shock, supplemental oxygen is administered to protect against hypoxemia. Oxygen can be delivered via a nasal cannula, a mask, a high-flow non-rebreathing mask, an endotracheal tube, or a tracheostomy tube.

Endotracheal intubation, or tracheostomy, may be performed to rest an exhausted client during severe or prolonged shock and to correct respiratory failure. By increasing the rate of pulmonary ventilation (through spontaneous or mechanical hyperventilation), it is possible to compensate for minor degrees of metabolic acidosis. This increased "blowing off" of carbon with hyperventilation begins to compensate for acid-base imbalance. Positive end-expiratory pressure (PEEP) may be added when the client is being mechanically ventilated. This assists in preventing atelectasis and may provide a higher PaO_2 for the client at a lower oxygen concentration setting. The goal of therapy is to maintain a PaO_2 greater than 50 mm Hg and an SaO_2 greater than 90% to avoid anaerobic metabolism. If the chest is congested, chest physical therapy, including vibration, percussion, and postural drainage, may be required.

Sometimes the interventions discussed cannot establish optimal tissue oxygenation. In these instances, hyperbaric oxygenation (HBO) or extracorporeal membrane oxygenation may be used. HBO involves the administration of 100% oxygen under 2 to 3 atm of pressure. This raises tissue oxygen tension to normal or above-normal levels. HBO requires the use of special chambers, which usually are available only in highly specialized institutions.

Extracorporeal membrane oxygenation is most commonly used in adults as a temporary intervention for refractory ARDS. Arterial and venous catheters are inserted, and some of the client's blood is diverted through them into a machine that artificially oxygenates the blood. This is a relatively expensive form of therapy and is usually done only in large medical centers.

RESTORE AND MAINTAIN ADEQUATE PERFUSION

The primary aim in treating shock is to maintain an adequate circulating blood volume. Unless this is accomplished early, subsequent therapeutic measures are of no avail, and death can be anticipated. In addition, other treatment adjuncts are necessary, which are discussed in the sections that follow. The adjuncts facilitate the distribution of blood to the body and enhance perfusion and oxygenation of the tissues with the circulating blood.

Administer Vasoactive Medications

Table 81–2 lists vasoactive medications commonly used to treat shock.

VASOCONSTRICTORS. Vasoconstrictors elevate the systemic BP by constricting peripheral arterioles. Vasoconstrictor agents may be used briefly in shock if compensatory vasoconstriction is unable to maintain blood flow to vital organs. They may also be used to correct hypotension secondary to vasoconstrictor nerve paralysis, as in spinal anesthesia or conditions associated with massive vasodilation. However, vasoconstrictors should not

TABLE 81–2	VASOACTIVE MEDICATIONS USED IN SHOCK MANAGEMENT
Medication	**Action**
High-dosage dopamine (Intropin); norepinephrine (Levophed); phenylephrine (Neo-Synephrine)	Systemic vasoconstriction, especially in the gastrointestinal tract, skin, and kidney
Amrinone (Inocor); epinephrine (Adrenalin); dobutamine (Dobutrex); isoproterenol (Isuprel)	Increased heart rate, increased contractility
Amrinone; dobutamine; epinephrine; isoproterenol; nitroprusside (Nipride)	Vasodilation of blood vessels in heart and skeletal muscle
Low-dosage dopamine	Vasodilation of renal and mesenteric blood vessels
Amrinone; nitroglycerin (Tridil); nitroprusside	Relaxation of vascular smooth muscle

be used exclusively but should be given concomitantly with IV fluids in an attempt to restore adequate circulation and perfusion.

Perfusion of vital organs with blood is impossible when systolic BP is below 50 mm Hg. Usually, the goal of using vasoconstrictors is to achieve and maintain a mean BP of 70 to 80 mm Hg, which is sufficient to perfuse tissues. Generally, attempts to increase the BP beyond this level are not advisable because vasoconstrictors increase the heart's oxygen demand and may cause fatal dysrhythmias. Vasoconstrictors are used with extreme caution in cardiogenic shock. Other major adverse effects of vasoconstrictors include decreased renal and splanchnic blood flow, excessive or sudden rise in arterial BP (which may precipitate heart failure), pulmonary edema or LV decompensation, and gangrene of the fingers and toes from prolonged vasoconstriction.

Although the use of vasoconstrictors during shock is being critically evaluated, they do favorably increase blood flow to the brain and heart in severely hypotensive clients. Reduced tissue perfusion when systolic pressures are below 60 to 70 mm Hg may precipitate MI or a cerebrovascular accident.

VASODILATORS. Agents that induce vasodilation or inhibit vasoconstriction may promote recovery from shock in which intensive vasoconstriction is contributing to the problem. These include adrenergic blocking agents, ganglionic blocking agents, and direct-acting peripheral vasodilators.

Adrenergic blockade prevents harmful effects of prolonged vasoconstriction such as increased pressure in capillaries, promoting fluid loss from the vascular to the interstitial compartment, and altered blood flow, especially in the splanchnic area. Prolonged vasoconstriction also impairs cellular nutrition and allows accumulation of waste products. Adrenergic blockade prevents these changes in circulation and may also induce opposite beneficial changes.

Vasodilators may be helpful during shock when vasoconstriction is severe and persists even though fluids have been infused in what should be adequate amounts for fluid replacement. Vasodilators may be administered to try to inhibit vasoconstriction of peripheral blood vessels (the result of norepinephrine from sympathetic stimulation) so that blood can be redistributed to enhance tissue perfusion and increase vascular volume.

When shock is caused by hypovolemia, rapid and adequate fluid replacement is essential before vasodilators are used. Vasodilators are dangerous because they lower arterial blood pressure if they are given while circulating blood volume is deficient. When the circulating blood volume is inadequate, the body depends on vasoconstriction to try to maintain arterial pressure. However, when the vascular space is full and cardiac venous return is adequate, vasodilation should open arterioles in the lungs and elsewhere. This lets blood circulate, increasing cardiac output and capillary perfusion without lowering systemic BP. In fact, a vasodilator may produce a dramatic, sustained rise in the systemic arterial pressure.

Keep clients who are receiving vasodilators lying relatively flat. Elevation of the head can produce dangerous orthostatic hypotension. Older clients may have sclerotic blood vessels and may not tolerate the hypotension that

may accompany administration of vasodilators. In this situation, a cardiotonic drug (such as dobutamine) may be given with the vasodilator to increase cardiac output.

Vasoconstrictor medications are sometimes given in combination with vasodilator medications. This may be done to offset the profound effects that may occur with some vasoconstrictors and to provide the benefits both types of drugs have to offer.

Characteristically, impaired tissue perfusion is correctable during early shock. However, it may be fatal if treatment is not received or is inadequate. In the later stages of shock, impaired tissue perfusion becomes "irreversible," leading to death in spite of treatment. However, treatment for "irreversible" shock is never abandoned while the client remains alive. Before a client's shock state is viewed as probably irreversible, restoration of circulating volume and identification and treatment of occult bleeding, any factors interfering with cardiopulmonary function, and overwhelming infection must be attempted.

During shock intervention, all of the basic pathophysiologic changes associated with the development of shock must be corrected. Some problems that must often be treated are the vascular problem of vasoconstriction, with the diminished tissue perfusion it causes; the intravascular problem of coagulation and sludging of blood cells; and the extravascular problem of extravasation of fluid into the extravascular space.

Assist Circulation

Mechanical devices that assist circulation or decrease the heart's workload may be used as temporary measures in managing clients in shock. Examples of these include the military or medical antishock trousers (MAST), IABP, and external counterpulsation device. (See Chapter 56 for more information.)

MAST GARMENT. MAST, also called pneumatic antishock garment (Fig. 81-8), encases the lower part of the body in a one-piece, three-chambered (one abdominal and two leg chambers) suit from the lower costal margin to the ankles. The external pressure provided by the MAST garment causes increased vascular resistance and reduces the diameter of blood vessels in the abdomen and legs. This results in impedance of blood flow and may decrease leakage into the tissues, resulting in increased perfusion of vital organs. Cardiac output and arterial BP increase.

MAST garments are most often used in trauma situations occurring outside the hospital setting for management of massive blood loss with no obtainable BP, fluid loss other than hemorrhage, and cardiac arrest caused by severe fluid or blood loss. They also help further reduce bleeding in areas being compressed, immobilize fractures of the femur and pelvis, and facilitate insertion of the IV line by increasing upper extremity cardiac output and vein filling. The use of MAST garments continues to be controversial because the decreased perfusion in the lower extremities leads to acidosis in the compressed tissues. MAST garments may be contraindicated in cardiogenic shock.

INTRA-AORTIC BALLOON PUMP. An IABP is used primarily in clients with cardiogenic shock and after open heart surgery. The heart's ability to adequately pump blood is augmented by a balloon-tipped catheter placed in

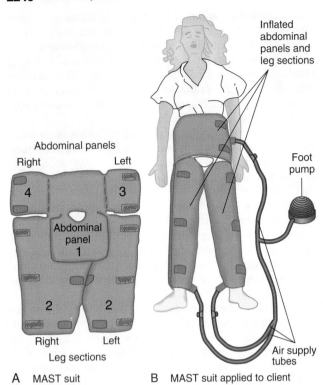

FIGURE 81–8 MAST suit, or pneumatic antishock garment. *A,* The suit is composed of two leg compartments and an abdominal compartment. *B,* MAST suit in place. Abdominal and leg compartments are attached to air tubes and a foot pump for inflation. MAST, *Military Antishock Trousers.*

the descending thoracic aorta. The catheter is attached to a unit that inflates during diastole and deflates just before systole. This counterpulsation displaces blood back into the aorta and improves coronary artery circulation. In cardiogenic shock, use of the IABP reduces preload, allowing the heart to more efficiently empty, thereby increasing cardiac output. Details of the IABP are found in the Bridge to Critical Care feature on IABP in Chapter 56.

EXTERNAL COUNTERPULSATION DEVICE. This device uses the same general principles as an IABP but is applied externally to the legs. The legs are encased in air- or water-filled tubular bags connected to a pumping unit. Pressure is applied to the legs during diastole and is released in systole.

MODIFIED TRENDELENBURG POSITION. A client in shock is usually placed in a modified Trendelenburg position with the lower extremities elevated 30 to 45 degrees, the knees straight, the trunk horizontal or very slightly raised, and the neck comfortably positioned with the head level with the chest or slightly higher (Fig. 81–9). This position promotes increased venous return from the lower extremities without compressing the abdominal organs against the diaphragm.

Elevating the legs mobilizes blood that has pooled in the lower extremities. As a result of gravity, the additional circulating blood increases venous return to the heart, thus improving cardiac output. The position is of temporary value in moderate hypovolemia. However, it does not help in severe hypovolemia, because the extrem-

ities have very little blood in them in such a state. Generally, the modified shock position is not used with cardiogenic shock, when there is already circulatory overload.

The traditional Trendelenburg position (head down, with legs elevated at least 30 degrees above the head) was once the classic shock position but is no longer used for shock management because it compresses the abdominal contents against the diaphragm, interfering with pulmonary excursion, and promotes congestion of blood in the brain, possibly contributing to cerebral edema.

Replace Fluid Volume

The mainstay of hypovolemic shock therapy is expansion of circulating blood volume by IV administration of blood or other appropriate fluids. Fluid replacement should be administered through large-bore peripheral lines, central venous lines, or both.

Various fluids are given to correct specific problems, such as electrolyte or protein deficiencies or other defects of the blood, including acidosis and hyponatremia. However, in treating hypovolemic shock, the immediate results of therapy seem to depend less on the type of fluid administered for fluid replacement than on the amount of fluid administered. Generally, enough fluid is given to exceed the normal blood volume. In part, this "extra" fluid is required because the vascular space is expanded as a result of dilation of the microcirculation. Additional fluid is also administered to replace intracellular fluid that was mobilized into the circulation as an early response to the hypovolemia.

In replacing fluids, enough volume must be administered to fill the capillaries and run through into the veins. Such fluid replacement maintains CVP and provides an adequate venous return to the heart. This promotes additional cardiac output. In addition, adequate fluid replacement decreases the blood catecholamine level and thus produces a vasodilation that promotes capillary flow. Adequate flow of fluids in the capillaries in turn perfuses tissues and prevents sludging and coagulation of blood within the vessels. Carefully monitor IV fluid replacement therapy to prevent circulatory overload. Hypervolemia can be lethal; thus aggressive fluid replacement should be tapered off when urinary output is at least 60 ml/hour, BP is greater than 100 mm Hg, or the heart rate is 60 to 100 beats per minute.

IV fluids used in shock management may include warmed crystalloids or balanced salt solutions, colloids,

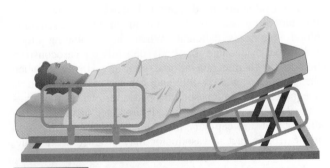

FIGURE 81–9 Positioning of the person in shock. This position is a modification of Trendelenburg's position and includes elevating the legs, leaving the trunk flat, and elevating the head and shoulders slightly.

and blood. Dextrose and water should not be used to resuscitate a client; once the dextrose is metabolized, only hypotonic water remains, which leads to greater fluid shifts.

CRYSTALLOID OR BALANCED SALT SOLUTIONS. During hypovolemic shock, the loss of circulating blood volume is also associated with redistribution of extravascular fluid. A sizable amount of fluid (about 4 L in moderately severe shock) leaves the interstitial space. This is in addition to fluid lost from the circulating volume. Thus, fluid replacement therapy must replace both blood lost from the circulation and fluid lost from the interstitial space. About two thirds of the crystalloid solution administered moves out of the vascular space into the tissues. To assist with fluid administration, a three-to-one rule has been developed. For a client's estimated blood loss, three times as much crystalloid solution must be administered for adequate volume resuscitation. Crystalloid solutions that may be administered include normal saline, Ringer's lactate, or half-normal saline.

Electrolyte solutions such as Ringer's lactate help expand extracellular volume, reduce viscosity, and prevent sludging. In a client with impaired liver function, a solution containing lactate could further compound the problem of lactic acidosis because lactate is converted to bicarbonate by the liver. If the liver is functioning normally, lactate does not accumulate. Because the liver is not an organ of primary perfusion during times of stress for the body, other solutions should be considered before Ringer's lactate.

Abnormalities of electrolyte and acid-base balance are corrected with the specific substance needed rather than with a solution that administers multiple electrolytes and acid-base components. Therapy is gauged by serial ABG and electrolyte determinations.

COLLOID SOLUTIONS. Colloid solutions contain proteins normally too large to exit at the capillary; thus they remain in the vascular compartment and increase osmotic pressure of the capillaries. This increased osmotic pressure helps retain fluid in the vascular compartment and maintain circulating volume. These solutions may be used in conjunction with crystalloid solutions in treating hypovolemic shock in an attempt to maintain an adequate circulating volume. The most commonly used colloid solutions include plasma and its components, plasma substitutes (e.g., dextran), oxygen-carrying solutions other than blood (e.g., perfluorochemicals), and hetastarch. (See discussions of blood and blood transfusions, Chapter 75.) Colloid solutions are often not used in initial fluid resuscitation after major burn injury. The capillary leakage is large enough that even the proteins escape.

Plasma is sometimes used in treating clients with low serum protein levels in an effort to control fluid escape from the vascular system. Fresh frozen plasma (FFP) is the form commonly used to improve serum protein levels. FFP may be administered after massive transfusions to restore some clotting factors deficient in "banked" blood. Because FFP requires 15 to 30 minutes to thaw, it is not used in initial fluid resuscitation with shock.

Albumin may also be used to achieve adequate osmotic pressure. Occasionally, it is administered when sufficient amounts of other fluids fail to restore an adequate circulating volume. Use of albumin is controversial because it may move into the pulmonary interstitial space, drawing water along with it. Thus, albumin may contribute to the development of ARDS.

Dextran may be used in both high- and low-molecular-weight forms. By initiating therapy with low-molecular-weight dextran and then progressing to high-molecular-weight forms, the incidence of hypersensitivity reactions to dextran can be lowered. The advantage in using dextran is that it contains large molecules that should effectively and rapidly expand the intravascular volume. Dextran can interfere with blood type and crossmatch procedures and with clotting factors. It should therefore be used only after type and crossmatch have been done and until blood is available for transfusion.

Although the administration of crystalloids, albumin, and blood has been the standard treatment of hypovolemic shock for many years, several new substances have been introduced for shock management. Perfluorochemicals such as Fluosol are non-blood, oxygen-carrying solutions that remain in the circulation for about 12 to 24 hours. Major limitations associated with the use of perfluorochemicals relate to limited immediate availability (the product must be stored frozen), administration of 80% to 100% O_2 for the solution to be effective, and accumulation of the chemicals in the body. Advantages include the high solubility of perfluorochemicals, making them readily available to the tissues, and their acceptability to clients whose religious beliefs prohibit the use of blood products. Perfluorochemicals have been researched since the 1970s and are still considered experimental at this time. Hetastarch is a glycogen-like synthetic colloid that has been used to treat hypovolemic shock and also may provide alternatives to blood administration.

BLOOD. When hemorrhage is the primary cause of shock, the rapid administration of large volumes of packed cells or whole blood may be necessary. Type-specific, crossmatched blood is the most desirable form of blood replacement. However, if the client is hemorrhaging, it may be necessary to administer type-specific, uncrossmatched blood: O-negative blood or O-positive, low–antibody titer blood. Women should receive Rh-negative blood.

When shock resulting from hemorrhage is treated, crystalloid is usually given as an initial emergency treatment to sustain blood pressure. Later, the acute anemia resulting from hemorrhage must be corrected by administration of packed cells for the prevention of hypoxemia.

During fluid replacement, a normal red blood cell mass should be maintained. Fluids given in excess of normal volume should be fluids other than blood so that they can be easily removed from the circulation by the kidneys once the shock is corrected. If the normal red blood cell mass is exceeded, it is difficult for the body to get rid of the excess red blood cells after the vascular volume contracts to normal (after adequate perfusion of tissues with blood is achieved). Because dangers also are involved in blood transfusions, blood should not be used if another fluid can satisfactorily maintain an adequate oxygen-carrying capacity and can sufficiently increase blood volume. Clients can become so dilute that there are relatively few blood cells as the result of up to 8 to 12 L of fluid being administered in only a few hours.

Provide Autotransfusion

Autotransfusion involves collecting and retransfusing blood into the same client. Autotransfusion is used in the prevention or treatment of existing hypovolemic shock caused by hemorrhage. It is common in the treatment of chest injuries.

Evaluate Fluid Replacement

Often, fluid replacement is the only treatment required for shock. However, it is difficult to evaluate whether fluid replacement is adequate. Internal losses of circulating fluid volume, including whole blood, into areas of traumatized tissue, infection, and so forth are difficult to estimate. If a vasoconstrictor drug has been administered or if prolonged vasoconstriction occurs, an additional considerable loss of circulating volume may also occur because of vasoconstriction. Large volumes of IV fluid may be administered either until systemic BP, urinary volume, and lactate levels become relatively normal or until central venous or pulmonary artery pressures, or both, become elevated.

Infusion of blood or other fluids usually continues only as long as the CVP is low, that is, below 4 cm H_2O or 2 mm Hg. When the CVP is higher than normal (e.g., above 15 cm H_2O or 11 mm Hg), benefit cannot be expected from the continued infusion of fluids or blood beyond maintenance amounts. When the CVP is low and the lungs are clear, with no indications of congestive heart failure, fluids are administered to improve the return of blood to the heart. However, some clients have a normal or low CVP in spite of faulty LV function. They readily develop congestive failure or pulmonary edema. Thus, a low or normal CVP does not always mean that fluid administration is advisable.

IV fluid administration should be stopped before extremely high elevations of pulmonary artery pressure occur if there is an adequate systemic response. An adequate volume of circulating fluid causes an ample venous return to the right side of the heart and increases the right-sided output. Pulmonary artery hypertension may develop if continued pulmonary obstruction is present because of coagulation in the microcirculation or vasoconstriction. This appears as increased pulmonary artery pressure. In the presence of right-sided heart failure, this increased pressure may back up through the right side of the heart, causing an abnormal elevation in CVP. Vasodilators may help open this partially blocked pulmonary microcirculation.

PREVENT COMPLICATIONS

Prevent Renal Impairment

Impaired kidney function and ATN may result from inadequate renal tissue perfusion, as discussed earlier. In an attempt to prevent acute renal damage, the urinary output is monitored with an indwelling catheter, and diuretics (e.g., furosemide) may be given. Correcting metabolic acidosis (see Chapter 14) and using other measures to increase blood volume and improve cardiac output also benefit the kidney as well as other tissues. If tubular necrosis is present, peritoneal dialysis or hemodialysis may be needed until regeneration of functioning renal tubular epithelium occurs. (See also Chapter 36.)

During shock, urinary output should be measured and compared with normal urinary production. The normal rate of urinary excretion from the kidneys is 1 ml/minute or 60 ml/hour. A client who becomes acutely hypovolemic or is experiencing a redistribution of circulating volume cannot maintain an hourly output of 40 to 60 ml of urine. Decreased urinary output (oliguria) typically occurs in shock. Often during shock, the urinary output may stop completely (anuria). When this occurs, the client is said to be in renal shutdown or renal failure.

Oliguria does not contraindicate the administration of large volumes of fluid in the treatment of shock. In fact, restoring renal capillary perfusion along with that of other vital capillaries restores urine volume production as long as tubular necrosis is not already present. Fluid administration may prevent ATN in the kidneys.

A large amount of tissue damage (e.g., crush injuries) may cause a release of myoglobin from muscle tissue. Because the myoglobin molecule is large, a type of mechanical renal failure may result from attempts to excrete large amounts of myoglobin. Fluid administration is again important to decrease damage to the tubules.

Prevent Gastrointestinal Bleeding

An early physiologic response to shock is a decrease in splanchnic circulation. This reduces the blood supply to the stomach and bowel, causing inadequate gastrointestinal tissue perfusion and delayed gastric emptying; thus, vomiting with aspiration of gastric contents into the lung may occur. For this reason and for diagnostic purposes, nasogastric (NG) suction is often used during treatment of shock. A double-lumen, 16 Fr. NG tube is usually used in adults.

Assess gastric aspirate periodically for blood. Guaiac solution or Hemoccult tablets and reagent can be used to check for blood; litmus paper checks the pH to determine the acidity of the stomach. Promptly report new findings of blood or increases in the amount of blood. Histamine blockers and proton pump inhibitors are used to reduce gastric acid in the stomach. Antacids may also be instilled through the tube when the pH is acidic.

When shock is caused by gastrointestinal bleeding, other NG tubes may be used. If the suspected cause of bleeding is a gastric ulcer, a 36 Fr. Ewald tube may be used. This tube's many large holes facilitate saline lavage and removal of blood clots. If esophageal varices are suspected or present, a Sengstaken-Blakemore tube is often used. This triple-lumen tube exerts pressure on the lower portion of the esophagus and the upper portion of the stomach, where varices are most prominent. Pressure is created by esophageal and gastric balloons inflated with air. Gentle traction is applied to keep the balloons in proper position (see Chapter 47).

The medical management of shock has been discussed in general. Tables 81–3, 81–4, and 81–5 give some of the specific interventions for hypovolemic, cardiogenic, and distributive shock, respectively.

PROVIDE PHARMACOLOGIC MANAGEMENT

Antibiotics

Antibiotics are essential when shock is due to infection. If septic shock is suspected, a blood specimen for culture and sensitivity is taken at once, and broad-spectrum antibiotics are started even though the specific infectious organism has not yet been identified. When the blood sample is drawn, samples of urine, sputum, and fluid from

TABLE 81–3	SUMMARY OF THE MANAGEMENT OF HYPOVOLEMIC SHOCK	
Etiology	**Clinical Situation**	**Intervention***
Blood loss	Massive trauma Gastrointestinal bleeding Ruptured aortic aneurysm Surgery Erosion of vessel from lesion, tubes, or other devices DIC	Stop external bleeding with direct pressure, pressure dressing, tourniquet (as last resort) Reduce intra-abdominal or retroperitoneal bleeding by applying MAST garment or prepare for emergency surgery Administer lactated Ringer's solution or normal saline Transfuse with fresh whole blood, packed cells, fresh frozen plasma, platelets, or other clotting factors, if significant improvement does not occur with crystalloid administration Use non-blood plasma expanders (albumin, hetastarch, dextran) until blood is available Conduct autotransfusion if appropriate
Plasma loss	Burns Accumulation of intra-abdominal fluid Malnutrition Severe dermatitis DIC	Administer low-dose cardiotonics (dopamine, dobutamine) Administer lactated Ringer's solution or normal saline Administer albumin, fresh frozen plasma, hetastarch, or dextran if cardiac output is still low
Crystalloid loss	Dehydration (e.g., diabetic ketoacidosis, heat exhaustion) Protracted vomiting, diarrhea Nasogastric suction	Administer isotonic or hypotonic saline with electrolytes as needed to maintain normal circulating volume and electrolyte balance

*Assumes that airway management and cardiac monitoring are ongoing.
DIC, disseminated intravascular coagulation; MAST, *military* or *medical antishock trousers.*

TABLE 81–4	SUMMARY OF THE MANAGEMENT OF CARDIOGENIC SHOCK	
Etiology	**Clinical Situation**	**Intervention***
Myocardial disease or injury	Acute myocardial infarction Myocardial contusion Cardiomyopathies	Fluid-challenge with up to 300 ml of normal saline solution or Ringer's lactate to rule out hypovolemia, unless heart failure or pulmonary edema is present Insert CVP or pulmonary artery catheter; monitor cardiac output, pulmonary artery pressure, and PCWP; administer IV fluids to maintain left ventricular filling pressure of 15–20 mm Hg Administer inotropics (e.g., dopamine or dobutamine) Vasodilators (e.g., sodium nitroprusside, nitroglycerin, calcium-channel blockers, morphine) Diuretics (e.g., mannitol or furosemide) Cardiotonics (e.g., digitalis) Beta-blockers (propranolol) Glucocorticosteroids† Intra-aortic balloon pump or external counterpulsation device if unresponsive to other therapies
Valvular disease or injury	Ruptured aortic cusp Ruptured papillary muscle Ball thrombus	Same as above: if rapid response does not occur, prepare for prompt cardiac surgery
External pressure on the heart interferes with heart filling or emptying	Pericardial tamponade due to trauma, aneurysm, cardiac surgery, pericarditis Massive pulmonary embolus Tension pneumothorax Ascites Hemoperitoneum Mechanical ventilation	Relieve tamponade with ECG-assisted pericardiocentesis; repair surgically if it recurs Thrombolytic (streptokinase) or anticoagulant (heparin) therapy; surgery for removal of clot Relieve air accumulation with needle thoracostomy or chest tube insertion Relieve fluid accumulation with paracentesis Reduce inspiratory pressure
Cardiac dysrhythmias	Tachydysrhythmias Bradydysrhythmias Pulseless electrical activity	Treat dysrhythmias; be prepared to initiate CPR, cardiac pacing

*Assumes that airway management and cardiac monitoring are ongoing.
†Controversial.
CPR, cardiopulmonary resuscitation; CVP, central venous pressure; ECG, electrocardiogram; IV, intravenous; PCWP, pulmonary capillary wedge pressure.

TABLE 81-5	SUMMARY OF THE MANAGEMENT OF DISTRIBUTIVE SHOCK	
Etiology	**Clinical Situation**	**Intervention***
Anaphylactic shock	Allergy to food, medicines, dyes, insect bites, stings, or latex	Prepare for surgical management of the airway Decrease further absorption of antigen (e.g., stop IV fluid, place tourniquet between injection or sting site and heart if feasible) Epinephrine (1:100) 2 inhalations every 3 hours, *or* Epinephrine (1:1000) 0.2–0.5 ml every 5–15 min given subcutaneously, *or* Epinephrine (1:10,000) 0.5–1.0 ml every 5–15 min given at a rate of 1 mg/min IV fluid resuscitation with isotonic solution Diphenhydramine HCl or H$_1$-receptor antagonist IV Theophylline IV drip for bronchospasm Steroids IV Vasopressors (e.g., norepinephrine, metaraminol bitartrate, high-dosage dopamine) Gastric lavage for ingested antigen Ice pack to injection or sting site Meat tenderizer paste to sting site
Septic shock	Often gram-negative septicemia but also caused by other organisms in debilitated, immunodeficient, or chronically ill clients	Identify origin of sepsis; culture all suspected sources Vigorous IV fluid resuscitation with normal saline Empirical antibiotic therapy: until sensitivities are reported If suspected organism is gram-positive, vancomycin is used; if suspected organism is gram-negative, give expanded-spectrum penicillin or a cephalosporin and aminoglycoside Administer cardiotonic agents (e.g., dopamine or dobutamine, norepinephrine, isoproterenol, digitalis, calcium) Naloxone (narcotic antagonist) Prostaglandins Monoclonal antibodies Temperature control (both hypothermia and hyperthermia are noted) Heparin, clotting factors, blood products if DIC develops
Neurogenic (spinal) shock	Spinal anesthesia Spinal cord injury	Normal saline to restore volume Treat bradycardia with atropine Vasopressors (e.g., norepinephrine, metaraminol bitartrate, high-dosage dopamine, and phenylephrine) may be given Place client in modified Trendelenburg's position
Vasovagal reaction	Severe pain Severe emotional stress	Place client in a head-down or recumbent position Give atropine if bradycardia and profound hypotension; eliminate pain

*Assumes airway management and cardiac monitoring are ongoing.
DIC, disseminated intravascular coagulation; IV, intravenous.

draining wounds, sinuses, and so forth are also taken for culture. The antibiotic selected depends on the cause of the infection and should not be initiated until after all cultures have been taken. However, once cultures have been obtained, treatment with empirical broad-spectrum antibiotics should be initiated. Cephalosporins, gentamicin, and aminoglycosides may be used in combination until specific culture and sensitivity information is available. Antibiotics may also be administered along with appropriate surgical management to clients with open or potentially contaminated wounds who are experiencing hypovolemic shock.

Monoclonal Technology
Multiple therapies that specifically target the mediators of septic shock are currently being researched. Monoclonal antiendotoxin (e.g., HA-1A and E5) neutralizes the endotoxin or toxicity of the offending pathogen or the immune response itself. Interleukin-1 receptor agonists, anti-tumor necrosing factor antibodies, and platelet activating factor

inhibitors are also in research trials for their effectiveness in reducing the morbidity and mortality from septic shock. Research results to date on these three therapies are mixed, but researchers continue to search for the solution in preventing the significant negative outcomes of septic shock.

Heparin

The anticoagulant effect of heparin may help prevent complications or treat DIC. The dosage is usually adjusted according to clotting studies. Heparin is also used because of the prolonged immobility often associated with shock. Immobility predisposes clients to venous thrombosis and pulmonary emboli. The treatment of DIC may include heparin administration to minimize consumption of clotting factors. Heparin also may be appropriate for clients with ARDS if the primary cause of the respiratory insufficiency is suspected to be DIC or massive microembolism.

Steroids

Steroids have several effects that may assist the client in neurogenic shock after spinal cord injury. They are given to reduce edema in the cord and have been shown to improve recovery. They assist in treatment by stabilizing lysosomal membrane and preventing intracellular release of enzymes. Complications from high-dose steroid therapy include acute gastrointestinal bleeding, aggravation of diabetes, and immunosuppression. Steroids used to be given to treat septic shock, but mortality was not reduced and the practice was abandoned.

Naloxone

Naloxone (Narcan), an opiate antagonist, is commonly used to treat narcotic and synthetic narcotic overdosages. During stress, opiate-like substances known as enkephalins and endorphins are released from the brain. Although the mechanisms of action are not clear, endorphins may play a role in capillary bed vasodilation found in all forms of shock. Studies indicate that when naloxone is administered to animals not in shock, no significant cardiovascular effects are noted. However, when administered during shock, naloxone reverses the hypotension and decreases cardiac contractility. It is believed that naloxone blocks the effects of endorphins and enkephalins.

Epinephrine

Epinephrine is the drug of choice for emergency treatment of allergic reactions (anaphylaxis). Epinephrine inhibits histamine release and antagonizes its effects on end organs, resulting in reversal of the bronchial constriction, increased capillary permeability, and vasodilation, which occur with acute anaphylactic reactions. The overall effect is improved respiratory status and cardiovascular stability.

Diphenhydramine

Anaphylaxis can also be treated with antihistamines, like diphenhydramine (Benadryl). This medication acts primarily to relieve clinical manifestations associated with anaphylaxis rather than to stop the release of histamine. Therefore, epinephrine is always administered first in treating anaphylaxis.

Histamine H_2-Receptor Antagonists

Histamine H_2-receptor antagonists, which inhibit gastric acid secretion, may be administered intravenously to a client experiencing shock to prevent stress ulcers. They may be prescribed in combination with oral antacids. Stress ulcers are often lethal complications of severe illness or injury produced by continuous shunting of blood from the gastrointestinal tract from extended sympathetic nervous system stimulation.

Narcotics

The need for pain relief may be obvious in clients experiencing different types of shock. However, the use of narcotics for pain management may, unfortunately, be dangerous. Narcotics interfere with vasoconstriction, and vasoconstriction may be the mechanism by which the client's BP is maintained. Morphine sulfate, however, causes pooling of blood in the extremities and contributes to a decrease in anxiety. These effects may prove useful for the client in cardiogenic shock.

Cardiotonic Medications

Medications that improve myocardial contraction are basic in treating those forms of shock that decrease cardiac output (e.g., hypovolemic shock and cardiogenic shock):

- Digitalis is often used if there is evidence of cardiac failure. By strengthening and slowing the heart beat, digitalis supports a weakened heart and may reduce the heart rate to a more normal level.
- Lidocaine, bretylium, quinidine, and procainamide may treat dysrhythmias that tend to reduce cardiac efficiency. However, these medications reduce myocardial contractility.
- Atropine may treat bradycardia, which predisposes clients to cardiogenic shock.

Calcium

Calcium is needed for normal functioning of the nervous and cardiovascular systems and for blood clotting. The value and dosages of calcium in treating shock are not clear. However, calcium may be administered if impaired cardiac function is evident. Calcium may precipitate toxic effects in a person who has received digitalis. It is given only with extreme caution to such a person. Monitor for evidence of digitalis toxicity (e.g., bradyarrhythmias or tachyarrhythmias, ST-segment depression).

Calcium chloride should be given intravenously only. Calcium gluconate may be given intramuscularly but is very irritating to tissues. Although calcium chloride and calcium gluconate are both available as 10% solutions, they are not identical in concentration. Do not substitute one for the other. Indications of hypocalcemia may be subtle. Careful assessment is essential. (See discussions of calcium in Chapter 13.)

▬ Nursing Management of the Medical Client

Nursing outcomes are similar to medical outcomes in that the overall goals of care are to correct the causative factor if possible, improve oxygenation, restore and maintain adequate tissue perfusion, and prevent complications. However, a majority of the interventions provided for clients in shock require a physician's order and are not independent nursing actions. The nurse's major responsibilities in shock include assessment of the client's condition and timely and accurate performance of dependent interventions.

ASSESSMENT

Because a client's condition can change rapidly in shock, frequent nursing assessment is essential. Documentation of the progress and response to interventions needs to be concise, yet convey the client's status minute by minute.

Initiate a flow sheet containing all pertinent data in an easily read format. This flow sheet must accompany the assessments are essential in treating shock. Blood chemistries, blood gases, oxygen saturations, and electrolytes need to be determined frequently and reported promptly so therapy can be adjusted to the client's rapidly changing physiologic status.

The first step in assessing a person in shock is a general overview, giving attention to airway, breathing, and circulation (ABC). Once the airway is patent, air exchange is adequate, a pulse is present, and the cervical spine is immobilized (if it is a trauma situation), perform a rapid, cursory initial head-to-toe physical assessment. The initial assessment goal is to identify major problems and gross abnormalities. Give further detailed attention to specific injuries or problems after shock is stabilized.

IMPROVE OXYGENATION.

Several assessments should be performed to determine that no airway or breathing problems exist. To determine airway patency, assess for the presence of noisy respirations and check for obstructions. Listen to lung sounds to determine adequate air movement. Assess the respiratory rate and effort to evaluate the adequacy of breathing. Evaluate chest wall expansion and assess for chest wall bulges or defects. Monitor for tracheal deviation, which could indicate tension pneumothorax.

When caring for clients experiencing shock, carefully differentiate nursing diagnoses concerning pain and impaired gas exchange. Restlessness is an assessment finding common to both and can thus be easily misinterpreted. Too often, clients who are restless, especially trauma victims, are given narcotics because their behavior is incorrectly interpreted as resulting from pain. However, the restlessness frequently is actually due to hypoxia, and narcotics worsen the problem. The decision to administer narcotics is often a nursing decision. It is important to assess the need for these medications carefully. Attention to positioning, splinting of injured areas, breathing techniques, and comfort measures may provide safer and more effective pain relief than narcotics. (Pain is discussed in detail in Chapter 23.)

RESTORE AND MAINTAIN ADEQUATE PERFUSION.

To complete the critical assessment of ABCs, circulation must be evaluated. Assess the client's pulse, blood pressure, skin color, temperature, heart sounds, peripheral pulses, state of hydration, and skin perfusion (e.g., capillary refill time <3 seconds). Check the condition of the mucous membranes, sclera, and conjunctivae; the presence of pallor or cyanosis; and fullness of the neck veins (jugular venous distention, which may suggest right heart failure and cardiogenic shock).

It is imperative that the adequacy of blood volume be determined prior to administration of narcotics to a client suffering from acute, multiple trauma. Narcotic administration causes vasodilation, which results in severe hypotension or shock. If a narcotic is administered intramuscularly to a client in shock, it also may not be completely absorbed because of the vasoconstriction that is present. Because the client experiences little or no pain relief, then a second injection may be given. Once fluid resuscitation is complete and the circulating volume is restored, the client may absorb both doses of the narcotic. No one in shock should be given intramuscular medications.

When narcotics are appropriate for a client in shock, they are most effective if administered intravenously in small doses. When caring for trauma victims, especially those with massive injury, remember that the extent of the injury does not necessarily coincide with the amount of pain being experienced. Careful assessment is necessary once narcotic administration seems safe (in terms of the client's hemodynamic status). Assess the client's blood pressure more closely after IV administration of narcotics to watch for hypotension.

Even though a person in shock may feel cold and may be hypothermic, do not apply heat to the skin. Heat application dilates peripheral blood vessels and draws blood away from the vital organs (where it is life-sustaining) into the vessels of the skin. This interferes with the body's initial compensatory mechanism of peripheral vasoconstriction. Heat also increases the body's metabolism. In turn, this increases the need for oxygen and puts an added strain on the heart.

This does not mean that the person is kept in a cold environment. The environment is kept warm because it is important that the person not become chilled. Chilling and shivering require energy expenditure needed to maintain vital functions. Chilling also contributes to sludging of blood in the microcirculation. Hypothermia slows the heart, increases the likelihood of ventricular fibrillation, and inhibits the body's reparative processes.

After potentially life-threatening problems are treated, take complete vital signs, with BP taken in both arms to rule out other causes of hypovolemic shock (i.e., thoracic dissection, aneurysm). It is important to take postural vital signs if applicable and if it is safe to do so. Do not take postural vital signs if the client has multiple traumatic injuries; if there is evidence of vertebral, pelvic, or femoral fracture; or if hypotension already exists. Clients with postural hypotension should not be sent to the x-ray department for upright films until they are adequately volume-resuscitated. If x-rays must be taken, clients require constant attendance by a nurse who monitors vital signs, administers IV fluids if necessary, and provides guidance to x-ray department personnel regarding movement, positioning, and timing of studies.

Measurement of postural vital signs is taken when there is a history or presence of significant blood loss, unexplained tachycardia, a history of fluid loss (e.g., diarrhea, vomiting, diuretic therapy, or third-space loss), unexplained syncope, blunt chest or abdominal trauma, or abdominal pain.

Alternative Methods of Blood Pressure Monitoring.

Often when a client is in shock, it is difficult to hear the BP with a standard stethoscope. Two commonly used techniques to obtain BP measurements are palpation of the radial or brachial pulse during deflation of the BP cuff and use of a Doppler instrument. When palpation is used, the first palpable pulse noted during deflation of the cuff is the systolic BP. Document the BP as such (e.g., 90/palp). A Doppler amplifies arterial and venous pulsations by ultrasonography. Various Doppler probes are available and are used instead of a stethoscope to measure BP. Systolic BP is easily heard by placing the probe over the brachial artery after applying transmission gel. The diastolic BP is not obtainable when the Doppler is used.

For clarity and accuracy, document the method by which BP readings are taken (in addition to the readings themselves) and whether palpation or a Doppler monitor is used. This is important because these readings may be higher or lower than those obtained in the standard way with a cuff and stethoscope. Likewise, document whether readings are obtained by automatic BP machines even though readings from these machines may not differ from those taken in the standard way.

Direct measurement of arterial BP by use of an arterial line often is done during shock. Discussion of arterial lines is found in Chapter 55.

Temperature Monitoring.
An accurate core temperature measurement is important in assessing a client in shock. Sometimes an indwelling flexible rectal probe connected to a continuous display monitor is more accurate and less traumatic than intermittent rectal temperature measurements with a standard thermometer. Core temperature can also be measured with a thermometer inserted by the manufacturer into an indwelling urinary catheter. Tympanic temperatures are commonly used in critical care settings and provide core temperature measurements. Core temperature can also be obtained if the client has a thermodilution (Swan-Ganz) catheter in place.

Oral temperature measurement is neither accurate nor safe. During shock, the buccal mucosa is poorly perfused, and the client should be receiving oxygen by mask or nasal prongs. (Because clients in shock are hypoxemic, the procedure of removing the oxygen long enough to obtain an oral temperature is not routinely recommended.)

Cardiac Monitoring.
For assessment and evaluation purposes, the electrical activity of the heart needs to be continuously monitored in all clients in shock, regardless of age. Nurses caring for clients experiencing shock need to be able to initiate cardiac monitoring, recognize cardiac dysrhythmias, and initiate treatment for any potentially lethal dysrhythmias that occur (see Chapter 57).

During the initial resuscitation period, it may be more appropriate to place the ECG monitor electrodes on the client's shoulders rather than on the chest. This placement does not interfere with chest film findings. It also allows better access to the chest for thoracic procedures such as insertion of chest tubes, pericardiocentesis, and CVP line placement. Once the client is stabilized, the electrodes may be moved to the chest.

Hemodynamic Monitoring.
Measurement of CVP is one hemodynamic technique that may be used in initial shock management, especially with hypovolemic shock. However, because CVP only provides information regarding preload, peripheral intra-arterial lines or a pulmonary artery catheter is inserted as soon as possible. Blood volume needs to be expanded as the vascular space enlarges, and CVP measurements are used to determine the amount of fluid needed to fill the enlarging vascular space. The rate of fluid replacement is adjusted to maintain the desired CVP. It is serious if the CVP continues

to fall in spite of fluid replacement. This means that the rate and volume of fluid replacement are not sufficient to meet the client's physiologic needs.

Peripheral arterial catheters are commonly used in shock to measure arterial BP and MAP and to obtain blood samples for chemical and blood gas analysis. These catheters are usually placed in the radial artery but may also be placed in the femoral or brachial arteries. Pulmonary artery and PCWP measurements are monitored to assess left-sided heart function and to guide fluid administration. These pressures are measured through a Swan-Ganz catheter. The PCWP corresponds to the LV end-diastolic pressure. This is the pressure in the LV just before contraction. A rise in this pressure in a client with cardiogenic shock may indicate left-sided heart failure. A low value in a client with hypovolemic shock may indicate that volume replacement is needed. In a client with septic shock, lower values would be expected during the warm phase and higher values during the cold phase.

Depending on the type of Swan-Ganz catheter used, additional measurements may be obtained. Some catheters have a fiberoptic tip that allows measurement of oxygen saturation of hemoglobin in the venous blood (SvO_2). SvO_2 is measured in the pulmonary artery, just before the blood's reoxygenation in the lungs. This reading gives an average of the tissue's uptake or use of oxygen in the body. The normal range for SvO_2 is 60% to 80%. When the SvO_2 falls below 60%, it may indicate either decreased arterial oxygenation or increased tissue oxygen demand. If the SvO_2 is greater than 80%, the indication, in relation to shock, is that the oxygen is unable either to reach the tissues or to be extracted by the tissues.

Most Swan-Ganz catheters also have a thermistor bead just proximal to the balloon. This may be used to determine cardiac output by a thermodilution technique. A fourth lumen opens at the level of the right atrium, and CVP measurements (preload) can be obtained through this lumen.

Monitoring Cardiac Output.
Cardiac output, measured in liters per minute, is the amount of blood pumped by the LV into the aorta each minute. During shock, cardiac output may be decreased because of myocardial damage resulting from an MI or, in hypovolemic shock, from inadequate volume replacement.

Because of the widespread use of Swan-Ganz catheters and the ease of performing measurements, cardiac output monitoring is used in managing all types of shock. These measurements assess overall cardiac function and the function of the LV. Factors that may alter cardiac output include heart rate, SVR, age, body size, exercise, and (in persons with cardiac problems) decreased filling or emptying of the LV.

Cardiac index is the cardiac output divided by the body surface area. Cardiac output as a separate reading does not take into account the amount of tissue that needs to be perfused. By figuring body size into the calculation, a more accurate assessment is obtained.

SVR can be determined by using the cardiac output and the MAP. SVR measures afterload and provides information regarding vasoconstriction or vasodilation. Decreased SVR indicates systemic vasodilation and may indicate the need for administration of vasoconstrictors. Increased SVR indicates systemic vasoconstriction and the potential need for vasodilators. Arterial BP and cardiac function should always be taken into consideration before administering vasoconstrictors or vasodilators.

PREVENT COMPLICATIONS. Although it is important to begin assessments and interventions with the ABCs, additional assessments are necessary to evaluate the client's overall condition and prevent complications. Additional assessments important in preventing complications include evaluation of:

- Level of consciousness and orientation ×3 (i.e., person, place, time)
- Ability to move extremities
- Sensation in all extremities
- Hand grasps
- Response to verbal and painful stimuli
- Pupil size and reaction to light
- Presence of abnormal posturing; presence, location, intensity, and duration of pain and what relieves the pain
- Bowel sounds
- Abdominal distention or rigidity
- Circumference of abdomen or extremities
- Presence of lacerations, contusions, ecchymoses, petechiae, and purpura (also check for bruising over flank area)
- Bone deformities
- Presence of medical alert tags or bracelets

RENAL IMPAIRMENT. An indwelling urinary catheter is a simple means of monitoring a client during shock. Continuously measuring urinary flow provides important information about peripheral blood flow and kidney function. Because the amount of urine excreted during shock is often very small, it is important to have an accurate, calibrated urine collector. In some settings, the catheter may be attached to a urimeter collector or to a more complex electric urimeter.

Urinary volume changes can be highly important as an index of the success or failure of therapy. Minimal (<0.5 ml/kg/hr) or absent urinary output indicates treatment is not successful. Increasing urinary output is a favorable sign. Assess the client's urinary output routinely and record it at least every hour.

DIAGNOSIS, OUTCOMES, INTERVENTIONS

Altered Tissue Perfusion. The nursing diagnosis *Altered Peripheral Tissue Perfusion* can be used to describe the reduced tissue perfusion and inadequate effective circulating intravascular blood volume. This diagnosis does not describe the oxygen-carrying capacity of the blood, but rather the volume of circulating blood and its ability to reach the tissues. The diagnosis can be written *Altered Peripheral Tissue Perfusion related to actual or relative (specify type) hypovolemia secondary to shock (specify type).* Other potential nursing diagnoses for the client in shock are listed in Box 81–1.

Outcomes. Nursing care of the client with shock is complex. Specific nursing and medical interventions vary according to individual needs and the setting in which care is delivered (e.g., emergency department versus intensive care unit). However, four major outcomes of care are desired:

1. Adequate blood flow (tissue perfusion) and cellular oxygenation are achieved to maintain the integrity of the tissue or organ.
2. The metabolic needs of the tissue or organ are reduced or maintained.
3. The client and family will cope effectively during the acute stage of shock.
4. The client and significant others will understand the cause of the problem and will modify their lifestyle to minimize or eliminate the causative factor.

Interventions. In caring for clients with altered tissue perfusion, your responsibilities are as follows:

- Provide continuous assessment of the client. Cardiovascular and respiratory changes can occur rapidly, and interventions must be adjusted promptly. Document observations clearly and concisely.
- Help decrease tissue oxygen demand. Because shock states can double the body's O_2 consumption, promote factors that decrease tissue oxygen need. Interventions aimed at decreasing total body work, pain, anxiety, and temperature will decrease tissue oxygen demand.
- Help the client (and family) to feel physically and emotionally comfortable.
- Facilitate expression of concerns and questions by the client and family. For example, try to reduce the client's fears and anxieties about what is happening and about the equipment being used.
- Keep equipment and supplies (e.g., suction, emergency drugs) available and in working order.

BOX 81–1   Potential Nursing Diagnoses for the Client in Shock

Activity Intolerance
Altered Family Processes
Altered Nutrition: Less than Body Requirements
Altered Role Performance
Altered Thought Processes
Altered Tissue Perfusion: Cerebral, Cardiopulmonary, Renal, Gastrointestinal, Peripheral
Anticipatory Grieving
Anxiety
Body Image Disturbance
Constipation
Decreased Cardiac Output
Fear
Fluid Volume Deficit
Impaired Gas Exchange
Impaired Physical Mobility
Impaired or Risk for Impaired Skin Integrity
Impaired Verbal Communication
Ineffective Airway Clearance
Ineffective Breathing Pattern
Ineffective Family Coping: Compromised
Pain
Personal Identity Disturbance
Self-Esteem Disturbance
Self-Care Deficit: Feeding, Bathing/Hygiene, Dressing/Grooming, Toileting
Sensory/Perceptual Alterations: Visual, Auditory, Kinesthetic, Gustatory, Tactile
Sleep Pattern Disturbance
Spiritual Distress

- Implement appropriate, planned nursing interventions to prevent complications that can develop from enforced immobilization.
- Provide adequate pain relief, because pain intensifies shock. Base this intervention on careful assessment.
- Provide care to the family.

A client in shock is extremely ill and may die. In addition, the stress of the situation is compounded by emergency medical treatment, with all the people, equipment, and movement this entails. During shock management, nurses have to attend to numerous delegated medical care activities. However, there must be sufficient nursing resources to provide psychosocial care (e.g., reassurance, emotional support) to the client and family. All of these people involved may be frightened, anxious, confused, and very dependent.

Keep the client's family informed of what is happening. They need information on which to base decisions. Because of the family's anxiety, the nurse may need to calmly repeat information several times. See the Client Education Guide for information to be conveyed. Remember that the client and significant others may be experiencing "psychological shock." They often need (and greatly appreciate) opportunities to discuss with care providers their important concerns.

Do not keep loved ones away from the client unnecessarily. Because of limited space, there may be times when they have to wait in another room for a period of time. However, they should not be kept away long and should be given a reasonable explanation of why it is necessary to leave their loved one.

A client experiencing shock requires emotional support. When caught up in the sudden drama of an emergency or critical care, health professionals sometimes forget that the experience and setting are often new and very frightening for the client. Unfortunately, "dehumanization" of the client may occasionally occur during the rush of emergency treatment. Whether a client appears to be conscious or not, always explain what is happening. Keep the atmosphere as quiet and orderly as possible. Eliminate unnecessary chatter. Commonly, recovered clients remember hearing what was said and were aware of what happened to them even though they appeared to be unconscious.

Among a nurse's greatest responsibilities are providing support, comfort, and advocacy to clients receiving care and to their significant others. In nursing clients who are critically ill and experiencing shock, this is very important.

EVALUATION

It is expected that the client will achieve adequate tissue perfusion and make a full recovery without complications from the type of shock being experienced, be transferred to a medical unit, and eventually be dismissed to home. Recovery from the cause of the shock may be delayed because of the complications created from the shock episode (e.g., wound healing).

Surgical Management

Although surgical interventions that can help in shock states are limited, they may be very useful in trauma situations. In hypovolemic shock caused by trauma, surgery can be performed in an attempt to control sources of bleeding. Once bleeding has been controlled, interventions aimed at restoring adequate fluid volume are more effective.

Self-Care

Shock must be fully resolved before a client is transferred or discharged (unless the client is being transported for the treatment of shock). Clients who survive shock find that recovery from the precipitating problem is delayed. They may also experience some feelings of confusion, depression, or grief when they realize that they lived through a very critical illness.

MULTIPLE ORGAN DYSFUNCTION SYNDROME

Single organ failure (e.g., heart failure, renal failure) has long been recognized as a cause of mortality and morbidity in critically ill clients. In trauma centers in the late 1960s, a new form of organ failure was recognized, that of sequential failure of the lungs, liver, and kidneys usually followed by death. By the 1970s, the syndrome of sequential organ failure was well described. Today, this problem is named *multiple organ dysfunction syndrome* (MODS), *multiple organ system failure,* or *multiorgan system failure* and is considered to be present when two or more organs fail. More recently, the precursor to MODS has been labeled as *systemic inflammatory response syndrome* (SIRS).

Etiology and Risk Factors

There are several causes of MODS, including dead tissue, injured tissue, infection, perfusion deficits, and persistent sources of inflammation such as pancreatitis or pneumonitis. Acute lung injury is usually present in some form. People known to be at high risk for developing MODS include those with impaired immune responses such as the elderly, clients with chronic illnesses, clients with malnutrition, and clients with cancer. In addition, clients with prolonged or exaggerated inflammatory responses are

CLIENT EDUCATION GUIDE

Shock

- It is difficult to prevent the occurrence of shock because the causes are often unpredictable. If your family member is in shock, obtain precise, consistent information about his or her current status and prognosis.
- Learn about the monitoring equipment in use.
- Learn how to communicate with the client who is intubated or unconscious.
- Learn how to demonstrate love and caring to someone surrounded by equipment.
- Participate in your family member's care during the hospital stay; this increases your ability to provide care at home.
- Learn how to prevent recurrence if the cause was avoidable.

at risk, including victims of severe trauma and clients with sepsis.

Prevention is a primary direction of current therapy. Source control is a major emphasis. Whenever possible, the potential source of sepsis or inflammation is excised or removed (e.g., full-thickness burn wound). Unfortunately, the source cannot be removed in many cases, such as pneumonia, pancreatitis, soft tissue injury, and hematoma. When the source cannot be removed, empirical antimicrobial agents are used to reduce risk.

It would be helpful to clinicians to be able to predict which clients are at the highest risk, but accurate prediction remains elusive. The most predictive variables appear to be the ratio of arterial oxygen tension (PaO_2) to the fraction of inspired oxygen (FiO_2) on day 1; the plasma lactate on day 2; the serum bilirubin on day 6; and the serum creatinine of day 12 postinjury. When nurses note these predictors, increased surveillance should begin.

Pathophysiology

In the healthy person, the normal integrated inflammatory immune response (IIR) functions to protect tissue from microbial invasion and rid the body of cellular debris and foreign material. The IIR is a continual process of responses until the insult slows and the client's condition stabilizes. The IIR stops once it is no longer needed. SIRS is a case of unchecked inflammatory responses. MODS is the end result of the prolonged response.

Most inciting events start with a local injury from trauma, infection, or lack of perfusion. Bacteria introduced into the wound or allowed to grow in necrotic tissues because of a decreased immune response activate the systemic inflammatory responses. Bacteria release toxins that activate systemic mediators of inflammation. Activation of the systemic response is an effort to "recruit help" to battle the invasion of microorganisms.

Once the inflammatory response becomes systemic, it is controlled by chemical mediators of inflammation. Mediators include bradykinin, complement, histamine, interleukin-1, prekallikrein, prostaglandins, and tumor necrosis factor. These powerful mediators of inflammation induce a systemic response. Endothelial cells are a common target for some mediators. The endothelium is destroyed, and blood flow is reduced to the tissues. Endothelial damage is produced by endotoxins from bacteria, tumor necrosis factor, interleukin-1, platelet activating factors, and many others. When this inflammatory response is unchecked, it produces damage to organs and tissues by altering perfusion, disturbing oxygen supply or demand, or changing metabolic dysfunctions. Metabolism increases under the direction of mediators such as cortisol and the catecholamines.

Many organs "respond" to MODS. The lungs are usually the first to malfunction, because of the large surface area of pulmonary epithelium combined with the presence of bacterial contamination from systemic blood return. The GI tract is the second system to malfunction, and it propagates conditions for further deterioration of other organs. Once the GI tract is malfunctioning, bacteria quickly relocate from tract to other organs. Additionally, the hypermetabolic state increases gastric acid production, increasing the risk of ulceration and bleeding. The most

serious metabolic problem is hypermetabolism. The hypermetabolic state is continued by cell-to-cell communication and the sympathetic nervous system responding in its usual "fight-or-flight" response.

Classification

There are two types of MODS. *Primary* MODS results directly from "a well-defined insult in which organ dysfunction occurs early and is directly attributed to the insult itself."[1] The direct insult initially causes a localized inflammatory response that may or may not progress to SIRS. An example of primary MODS is a primary pulmonary injury, such as aspiration. Only a small percentage of clients develop primary MODS.

Secondary MODS is a consequence of widespread systemic inflammation, which develops after a variety of insults, and results in dysfunction of organs not involved in the initial insult.[1] The client enters a hypermetabolic state that lasts for 14 to 21 days. During this time, the body engages in autocatabolism that causes profound changes in the body's metabolic processes. Unless the process can be stopped, the outcome for the client is death. Secondary MODS occurs with conditions such as septic shock and ARDS.

Clinical Manifestations

There is usually a precipitating event to MODS, including aspiration, ruptured aneurysm, or septic shock, which is associated with resultant hypotension. The client is resuscitated; the cause is treated; and the client appears to do well for a few days. The following possible sequence of events often develops.

The client experiences SIRS before MODS develops. Within a few days, there is an insidious onset of a low-grade fever, tachycardia, increased numbers of banded and segmented neutrophils on the differential count (called a left shift), and dyspnea with the appearance of diffuse patchy infiltrates on the chest x-ray. The client often has some deterioration in mental status, with reasonably normal renal and hepatic laboratory results. Dyspnea progresses, and intubation and mechanical ventilation are required. Some evidence of consumptive coagulopathy (DIC) is usually present. The client is usually stable hemodynamically and has relative polyuria, an increased cardiac index (>4.5 L/min), and systemic vascular resistance of under 600 dynes cm^{-5}. Clients often have increased serum glucose levels in the absence of diabetes. Some physicians use the criteria presented in Table 81–6 to make the diagnosis of MODS.

Between 7 and 10 days, the bilirubin level rises and continues to rise, followed by an increase in serum creatinine. Blood glucose and lactate levels continue to rise because of the hypermetabolic state. Other progressive changes include excretion of urinary nitrogen and protein combined with decreased levels of serum albumin, prealbumin, and retinol binding protein. Bacteremia with enteric organisms is also common. In addition, infections from *Candida* and viruses such as herpes and cytomegalovirus are common. Surgical wounds display delayed healing, and pressure ulcers may develop. During this time, the client needs increasing amounts of fluids and inotropic medications to keep blood volume and cardiac

TABLE 81–6	MODIFIED APACHE II CRITERIA FOR DIAGNOSIS OF MULTIPLE ORGAN DYSFUNCTION SYNDROME

CARDIOVASCULAR FAILURE (PRESENCE OF ONE OR MORE OF THE FOLLOWING)

Heart rate <54 beats/min
Mean arterial pressure ≤49 mm Hg (systolic pressure ≤60 mm Hg)
Occurrence of ventricular tachycardia or ventricular fibrillation
Serum pH ≤7.24 with a $PaCO_2$ of ≤40 mm Hg

RESPIRATORY FAILURE (PRESENCE OF ONE OR MORE OF THE FOLLOWING)

Respiratory rate ≤5 breaths/min or ≥49 breaths/min
$PaCO_2$ ≥50 mm Hg
Alveolar-arterial oxygen difference ≥350 mm Hg (calculate as follows, at sea level: (713 × % oxygen in inspired gas) − $PaCO_2$ − PaO_2)
Dependent on ventilator or CPAP on the second day

RENAL FAILURE (PRESENCE OF ONE OR MORE OF THE FOLLOWING)

Urine output ≤479 ml/24 hr or ≤159 ml/8 hr
Serum BUN ≥100 mg/dl (35.7 mmol/L)
Serum creatinine ≥3.5 mg/dl (309 μmol/L)

HEMATOLOGIC FAILURE (PRESENCE OF ONE OR MORE OF THE FOLLOWING)

WBC count ≤1000/μl (1 × 10^9/L)
Platelets ≤20,000/μl (20 × 10^9/L)
Hematocrit ≤20%

NEUROLOGIC FAILURE

Glasgow Coma Scale score ≤6 (in absence of sedation)

HEPATIC FAILURE (PRESENCE OF BOTH OF THE FOLLOWING)

Serum bilirubin ≥6 mg%
Prothrombin time ≥4 sec over control in the absence of systemic anticoagulation

CPAP, continuous positive airway pressure; BUN, blood urea nitrogen; WBC, white blood cell.
From Knaus, W. A., & Wagner, D. P. (1989). Multiple systems organ failure: Epidemiology and prognosis. *Critical Care Clinics, 5*(2), 221.

preload near normal and to replace fluids lost through polyuria.

Between day 14 and day 21, the client is unstable and appears close to death. The client may lose consciousness. Renal failure worsens to the point of considering dialysis. Edema may be present because of low serum protein levels. Mixed venous oxygen levels may rise because of problems with tissue uptake of oxygen caused by mitochondrial dysfunction. Lactic acidosis worsens, liver enzymes continue to rise, and coagulation disorders become impossible to correct.

Prognosis

If the process of MODS is not reversed by day 21, it is usually evident that the client will die. Death usually occurs between days 21 and 28 after the injury or precipitating event. Not all clients with MODS die; however, MODS remains the leading cause of death in the intensive care unit (ICU), with mortality rates from 50% to 90% despite the development of better antibiotics, better resuscitation, and more sophisticated means of organ support. For those clients who survive, the average duration of ICU stay is about 21 days. The rehabilitation, which is directed at recovery of muscle mass and neuromuscular function, lasts about 10 months.

Outcome Management

Medical Management

RESTRAIN THE ACTIVATORS

Manifestations of potential infection must be quickly treated to restrain the activators of MODS. If the agent is known, antibiotics to which the organism is sensitive should be administered. If the organism is not known, broad-spectrum antibiotics are given. Antibiotics are sometimes directed at the probable organism (an empirical treatment). Early aggressive management of sources of infection should be carried out. For example, the client may need to have a large infected wound incised and drained or necrotic tissue excised. Extreme caution must be taken to avoid infecting the client. These clients have many invasive monitors and may have open wounds. Unfortunately, clients in critical care units exist in a paradox. The ICU is the only environment with sophisticated equipment and health care professionals to provide safe care, yet it is an environment where the risk of infection is higher. In addition, there is a high prevalence of multi-resistant organisms, such as vancomycin-resistant *enterococci* (VRE) and methicillin-resistant *Staphylococcus aureus* (MRSA).

Because the lungs are often the first organs to fail, they require special attention. Aggressive pulmonary care is needed in all clients who are at risk of MODS. Interventions may be as simple as coughing and deep breathing to ambulation. The client's oxygen saturation should be monitored.

Because malnutrition develops from the hypermetabolism and the GI tract often seeds other areas with bacteria, some clinicians require the client to be fed enterally. They believe that feeding enhances perfusion and decreases the bacterial load and the effects of endotoxins. Nutrient intake is usually 30 to 35 kcal/kg/day of carbohydrates. Fats are restricted to 0.5 to 1 g/kg/day. Proteins are given to the client via modified amino acids. Some practitioners administer protein until a rise in plasma transferrin or prealbumin is noted. Increases in these values indicate hepatic protein synthesis rather than a breakdown of body stores. Decontamination of the GI tract and pharynx has been found to decrease infection but has shown no effect on the death rate from MODS.

CONTROL THE MEDIATORS

Controlling the mediators of inflammation is directed at (1) general levels of care and (2) specific treatments targeted at the problem cells. Maintenance of a positive nitrogen balance via nutrition, promotion of sleep and rest, and management of pain are important general care areas. Specific treatments include monoclonal antibodies to control mediators such as interleukin-1, endotoxins, and tumor necrosis factors. These therapies are shown in Table 81–7. Outcomes from research in these treatments are conflicting, and it appears that there is no "magic bullet" to cure the problem. Development of more specific monoclonal antibodies is ongoing.

PROTECT THE AFFECTED ORGANS

Care is directed toward maintaining the function of organs that fail with MODS. The client is intubated and mechanically ventilated in order to maintain adequate oxygenation. Oxygen is given to the client until blood levels of lactate decrease toward normal. Elevated serum lactate levels indicate the use of anaerobic metabolism. Nurses must recognize that certain clinical problems further increase the need for oxygen. Problems such as fever, seizures, and shivering increase oxygen demands. These problems should be controlled with medications or environmental changes (e.g., warming).

Fluids and inotropic drugs are used to support hemodynamic parameters. The client often becomes more unstable and needs continuous monitoring. Nutritional support is also critical to reduce the catabolism that accompanies hypermetabolism. Dialysis is often used to reduce azotemia from renal failure.

■ Nursing Management of the Medical Client

Care of the client with MODS is multifaceted, balancing the needs of one system against the needs of another while trying to maintain optimal functioning of each system. Nursing diagnoses appropriate for the client with

TABLE 81–7	SUMMARY OF POTENTIALLY USEFUL THERAPIES FOR MULTIPLE ORGAN DYSFUNCTION SYNDROME
Rationale	**Therapy**
Treatment of infection	Monoclonal antibodies Passive antibody protection Gut decontamination regimens
Support of gut function	Mucosal trophic agents: e.g., glutamine, bombesin, ketone bodies Early enteral feeding Regulation of gut microbial flora
Improved resuscitation	Hypertonic saline In-line sensors Tissue-specific sensors Noninvasive monitoring
Endothelial cell protection	PAF inhibitors WBC adherence inhibition Antioxidant therapy Eicosanoid modulation
Modulation of macrophage function	n3 polyunsaturated fatty acids Signal transduction modulation
Stimulation of lymphocyte function	Arginine w3 polyunsaturated fatty acids

PAF, platelet activating factor; WBC, white blood cell.
From Lekander, B. J., & Cerra, F. B. (1990). The syndrome of multiple organ failure. *Critical Care Clinics of North America* 2(2), 338.

MODS are determined by the system involved and the clinical manifestations identified.

The number of independent nursing interventions for the client with MODS is very limited. The overall goal for nursing is effective client and family coping. This complex disorder taxes the client and family. Nurses must remain sensitive to the needs of the family. Caring for the family of critically ill clients is a challenge in that understanding, predicting, and intervening with families in crisis is less exact than the calculation of oxygen needs. There are no easy formulas to use to provide hope, courage, coping, and caring. Nurses must remain alert to the needs of the family as well as the client during this stressful time.

CONCLUSIONS

This chapter has discussed shock under three major classifications: hypovolemic, cardiogenic, and distributive. The pathophysiology, clinical manifestations, and medical and nursing management have been presented. Shock is a critical condition with a high mortality rate. Early diagnosis and intervention are necessary for the best possible outcomes. Multiple organ dysfunction syndrome is a syndrome of multiple organs progressively failing because of prolonged inflammatory responses.

THINKING CRITICALLY

1. **The client is a 20-year-old man with a gunshot wound to the right chest and massive hemorrhage. His BP is 60 (palpated), heart rate is 130, and respiratory rate is 36. The skin is pale, cold, and clammy; capillary refill is greater than 3 seconds; pulses are weak and thready. What priority assessments should be done? What interventions might be performed?**

Factors to Consider. What do his vital signs tell you? What injuries might have occurred with a major chest trauma? How can his need for fluid and blood replacement best be met?

2. **A 69-year-old man was brought to the emergency department by a rescue squad. He had undergone a colon resection 2 weeks ago. His wife said that he was having increased difficulty breathing and he could feel his heart beating in his chest. He also has seemed "slower" to her. He is not moving as fast as usual and gets very dizzy when he stands up. He almost passed out, which is why she called the rescue squad. What priority assessments should be done? What interventions might be performed?**

Factors to Consider. What might be happening that could lead to all of the problems with breathing, dizziness, and confusion? What risk might be present as a result of the surgery?

3. **A 65-year-old man in the coronary care unit had an acute myocardial infarction (MI) 3 days ago. The monitor alarms and assessments reveal that his BP is 76/50; respiratory rate is 20. His pulse**

is rapid (128) and thready. His skin is cool and diaphoretic, with a slight ashen color; the capillary refill is greater than 3 seconds. The client is restless and confused. What priority assessments should be done? What interventions might be performed?

Factors to Consider. What form of shock can quickly develop in a client after an MI? Does he need fluid resuscitation to increase his blood pressure? Why or why not? What medications are commonly used to support a heart in distress? Are special forms of monitoring needed while these medications are used?

BIBLIOGRAPHY

1. American College of Chest Physicians/Society of Critical Care Medicine Consensus Conference Committee. (1992). Definitions for sepsis and organ failure and guidelines for the use of innovative therapies in sepsis. *Critical Care Medicine, 20*(6), 864–874.
2. Astiz, M. E., & Rackow, E. C. (1998). Septic shock. *The Lancet, 351,* 1501–1505.
3. Biro, G. P., et al. (1995). Oxyradical generation after resuscitation of hemorrhagic shock with blood or stroma-free hemoglobin solution. *Artificial Cells, Blood Substitutes, and Immobilization Biotechnology, 23*(6), 631–645.
4. Bone, R. C., et al. (1995). A second large controlled clinical study of E5, a monoclonal antibody to endotoxin: Results of a prospective, multicenter, randomized, controlled trial. *Critical Care Medicine, 23*(6), 994–1005.
5. Bone, R. C., Sprung, C. L., & Sibbald, W. J. (1992). Definitions for sepsis and organ failure. *Critical Care Medicine, 20*(6), 724–726.
6. Brass, N. J. (1994). Predisposition to multiple organ dysfunction. *Critical Care Nursing Quarterly, 16*(4), 1–7.
7. Bunn, H. F. (1995). The role of hemoglobin based blood substitutes in transfusion medicine. *Transfusion Clinique et Biologique, 2*(6), 433–439.
8. Campbell, J. (1997). Anaphylaxis. *Professional Nurse, 12*(6), 429–432.
9. Cashin, S. (1996). Is there a role for prehospital intramuscular adrenaline in anaphylaxis? *Australian Journal of Emergency Care, 3*(1), 11–15.
10. Crowley, S. R. (1996). The pathogenesis of shock. *Heart and Lung, 25*(2), 124–134.
11. DeJong, M. J. (1997). Clinical snapshot: Cardiogenic shock. *American Journal of Nursing, 97*(6), 40–41.
12. Evangelisto, M. (1997). Latex allergy: The downside of standard precautions. *Today's Surgical Nurse, 19*(5), 28–33.
13. Fehlings, M. G., & Louw, D. (1996). Initial stabilization and medical management of acute spinal cord injury. *American Family Physician, 54*(1), 155–162.
14. Fisher, D., & Sawin, K. (1998). Pearls for practice: Latex allergy in the primary care setting. *Journal of the American Academy of Nurse Practitioners, 10*(5), 203–208.
15. Graham, P., & Brass, N. J. (1994). Multiple organ dysfunction: Pathophysiology and therapeutic modalities. *Critical Care Nursing Quarterly, 16*(4), 8–15.
16. Green, T. (1997). Systems and diseases. The immune system. Part I. Anaphylaxis. *Nursing Times, 93*(42), 60–63.
17. Kavanagh, R. J., Radhakrishnan, D., & Park, G. R. (1995). *Care of the Critically Ill, 11*(3), 114–119.
18. Kellum J. A., & Decker, J. M. (1996). The immune system: Relation to sepsis and multiple organ failure. *AACN Clinical Issues: Advanced Practice in Acute and Critical Care, 7*(3), 339–350, 459–460.
19. Kimmings, A. N., Gouma, D. J., & van Deventer, S. J. H. (1994). Endotoxin in the pathogenesis of gram-negative sepsis. *Care of the Critically Ill, 10*(4), 170–173.
20. Levins, T. T., & Brown, K. K. (1995). Hemodynamic puzzle: Critical interventions in septic shock. *American Journal of Nursing, 95*(1), 20–21.
21. Livingston, D. H., Mosenthal, A. C., & Deitch, E. A. (1995). Sepsis and multiple organ dysfunction syndrome: A clinical-mechanistic overview. *New Horizons, 3*(2), 257–266.
22. Maier, R. V., & Bulger, E. M. (1996). Endothelial changes after shock and injury. *New Horizons, 4*(2), 211–223.
23. McCloskey, R. V., et al. (1994). Treatment of septic shock with human monoclonal antibody HA-1A. *Annals of Internal Medicine, 121*(1), 1–5.
24. McMahon, K. (1995). Multiple organ failure: The final complication of critical illness. *Critical Care Nurse, 15*(6), 23–30.
25. Monchik, K. O. (1998). Prehospital management of acute pulmonary edema with accompanying cardiogenic shock. *Emergency Medical Services, 27*(8), 35–36, 39–41, 56.
26. O'Donnell, L. (1996). Complications of MI: Beyond the acute stage. *American Journal of Nursing, 96*(9), 25–30.
27. O'Neal, P. V. (1994). How to spot early signs of cardiogenic shock. *American Journal of Nursing, 94*(5), 36–41.
28. Nose, Y. (1998). Oxygen-carrying macromolecules: Therapeutic agents for the treatment of hypoxia. *Artificial Organs, 22*(7), 618–622.
29. Ostrow, C. L., Hupp, E., & Topjian, D. (1994). The effect of Trendelenburg and modified Trendelenburg positions on cardiac output, blood pressure, and oxygenation: A preliminary study. *American Journal of Critical Care, 3*(5), 382–386.
30. Shoemaker, W. C., et al. (1996). Resuscitation from severe hemorrhage. *Critical Care Medicine, 24* (suppl. 2), S12–S23.
31. Smail, N., et al. (1995). Role of systemic inflammatory response syndrome and infection in the occurrence of early multiple organ dysfunction syndrome following severe trauma. *Intensive Care Medicine, 21*(10), 813–816.
32. Stapczynski, J. S. (1999, June). *Septic shock* [On-line]. Available: *www.emedicine.com/emerg/topic533.htm.*
33. Talan, D. A. (1997). Sepsis and septic shock. *Emergency Medicine Clinics of North America, 29*(3), 54–56, 61, 65–68.
34. Wardle, E. N. (1997). New research findings in septic shock/endotoxaemia. *Care of the Critically Ill, 13*(6), 222–224, 226.
35. Wiessner, W. H., Casey, L. C., & Zbilut, J. P. (1995). Treatment of sepsis and septic shock: A review. *Heart and Lung, 24*(5), 380–392.
36. Williams, J. G., Bernstein, S., & Prager, M. (1998). Effect of melatonin on activated macrophage TNF, IL-6, and reactive oxygen intermediates. *Shock, 9*(6), 406–411.
37. Young, J. S., Fernandez, M., & Meredith, J. W. (1997). The effect of oxygen delivery-directed resuscitation on splanchnic and hepatic oxygen transport after hemorrhagic shock. *Journal of Surgical Research, 71*(1), 87–92.

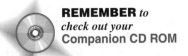

REMEMBER *to*
check out your
Companion CD ROM

CHAPTER

82

Management of Clients in the Emergency Department

Judy Selfridge-Thomas

NURSING OUTCOMES CLASSIFICATION (NOC)
for Nursing Diagnoses—Clients in the Emergency Department

Acute Confusion
Cognitive Ability
Distorted Thought Control
Information Processing
Memory
Neurologic Status: Consciousness
Sleep
Decreased Cardiac Output
Cardiac Pump Effectiveness
Circulation Status
Tissue Perfusion: Abdominal Organs
Tissue Perfusion: Peripheral
Vital Signs Status
Fluid Volume Excess
Electrolyte and Acid-Base Balance
Fluid Balance
Hydration
Fluid Volume Deficit
Electrolyte and Acid-Base Balance
Fluid Balance
Hydration
Nutritional Status: Food and Fluid Intake
Hypothermia
Thermoregulation
Impaired Gas Exchange
Electrolyte and Acid-Base Balance
Respiratory Status: Gas Exchange
Respiratory Status: Ventilation
Tissue Perfusion: Pulmonary
Vital Signs Status
Impaired Physical Mobility
Ambulation: Walking
Ambulation: Wheelchair
Body Positioning: Self-Initiated

Joint Movement: Active
Mobility Level
Sensory Function: Proprioception
Transfer Performance
Impaired Skin Integrity
Tissue Integrity: Skin and Mucous
  Membranes
Wound Healing: Primary Intention
Wound Healing: Secondary Intention
Ineffective Airway Clearance
Aspiration Control
Respiratory Status: Airway Patency
Respiratory Status: Gas Exchange
Respiratory Status: Ventilation
Ineffective Breathing Patterns
Respiratory Status: Airway Patency
Respiratory Status: Ventilation
Vital Signs Status
Ineffective Individual Coping
Aggression Control
Coping
Decision Making
Impulse Control
Information Processing
Role Performance
Social Support
Pain
Comfort Level
Pain Control
Pain: Disruptive Effects
Pain Level
Risk for Infection
Dialysis Access Integrity
Immobility Consequences: Physiologic

Immune Status
Immunization Behavior
Knowledge: Infection Control
Nutritional Status
Risk Control
Risk Control: Sexually Transmitted
  Diseases (STDs)
Risk Detection
Tissue Integrity: Skin and Mucous
  Membranes
Treatment Behavior: Illness or Injury
Wound Healing: Primary Intention
Wound Healing: Secondary Intention
Risk for Poisoning
Knowledge: Medicine
Medication Response
Risk Control
Risk Control: Drug Use
Risk Detection
Safety Behavior: Home Physical
  Environment
Self-Care: Nonparenteral Education
Self-Care: Parenteral Medication
Suicide: Self-Restraint
Sensory Perceptual Alterations
Anxiety Control
Body Image
Cognitive Ability
Cognitive Orientation
Distorted Thought Process
Energy Conservation
Hearing Compensation Behavior
Vision Compensation Behavior

During the mid-1960s, the need for the specialization of emergency services throughout the United States was identified as a national priority in order to reduce the associated morbidity and mortality resulting from catastrophic illness or injury. Since then, the specialties of emergency medicine, emergency nursing, and prehospital care services have grown. In the United States, more than 100 million clients use emergency departments (EDs) for health care services each year.[41] The scope of these services ranges from treatment of acute conditions that threaten the loss of life, limb, or vision to management of non-urgent, chronic conditions.

EMERGENCY MEDICAL SERVICES

The Emergency Medical Services (EMS) system encompasses all aspects of emergency care. Federal, state, and county EMS systems are designed to complement each other. The systems are responsible for establishing, regulating, and monitoring the components involved in the provision of emergency care. These components include such entities as 911 telephone access systems, Emergency Medical Technician (EMT) and paramedical personnel scopes of practice, ground and air ambulance services, dispatch communication between points of incident and responding personnel, and telecommunications between paramedical personnel and specialty-designated EDs known as *base station hospitals*. EMS systems are also instrumental in the coordination of activities for management of disaster situations.

Two goals of the EMS system are (1) to provide emergency care to a client as quickly as possible and (2) to assure that the "right client arrives at the right hospital in the least amount of time." Consequently, EMS systems are involved with specialty-designated hospital departments and EDs such as local or state trauma centers, burn centers, and pediatric care centers.

EMERGENCY NURSING

Emergency nursing was officially recognized as a specialty in 1970. The national association representing these nurses is the Emergency Nurses Association (ENA). Its current membership comprises more than 25,000 nurses who have chosen this area of professional nursing.

According to the ENA, the definition of emergency nursing involves

. . . the assessment, diagnosis, and treatment of perceived, actual or potential, sudden or urgent, physical or psychosocial problems that are primarily episodic or acute. These may require minimal care or life-support measures, education of patient and significant others, appropriate referral and knowledge of legal implications.[13]

In addition to provision of direct client care, other multifaceted roles exist within emergency nursing. The emergency nurse may be involved in the initial triaging of clients according to illness severity, may perform as a mobile intensive care nurse (MICN) by directing prehospital care personnel via telecommunication, and frequently may provide client care in the prehospital environment. Community clinics utilize ED nurses, and many emergency nurses have become active in injury prevention programs at both national and local levels. Advanced practice roles such as clinical nurse specialists and nurse practitioners are used in many EDs throughout the United States. Nurses in these advanced practice roles often have a master's degree–level of education or higher in addition to specialty certification.

Nurses employed in an ED must be prepared to provide care to clients of all age groups who may have any possible illness or injury. It is often cited that emergency nurses must have an understanding of almost all disease processes specific to any age group. Unfortunately, ED nursing is not usually addressed in depth in generic nursing programs. The education of ED nurses frequently occurs through hospital orientation programs, post-employment internship courses, and continuing education programs. ED nurses can obtain national specialty certification through an examination process. A certified ED nurse can use the credential of Certified Emergency Nurse (CEN).

LEGAL ISSUES

Nurses deal with a variety of legal issues in whatever specialty area they practice. The ED is no exception; however, certain issues are of paramount importance in this setting.

FEDERAL LEGISLATION

Past federal legislation has mandated that any client who presents to an ED seeking treatment must be rendered aid regardless of financial ability to pay for services. Since the mid-1980s, additional specific legislation was enacted requiring ED personnel to stabilize any client considered medically unstable before transfer to another health care facility—the Consolidated Omnibus Budget Reconciliation Act (COBRA) of 1986 and the Omnibus Budget Reconciliation Act (OBRA) of 1990.[2] This stabilization must occur regardless of the client's financial ability to pay for services. ED personnel who transfer clients to another institution without first providing this initial stabilization can incur substantial fines and penalties, as can the hospital administration.

Clients with various illnesses seek health care services in the ED, even with the proliferation of managed health care plans and gatekeeping policies.[41] Financial reimbursement for rendered services has been denied to EDs from managed health care plans after retrospective determinations that the client's problem did not constitute a true emergency. Again, legislation has been enacted (Emergency Medical Treatment and Active Labor Act [EMTALA] legislation of 1988, 1989, 1990, and 1994)[2] requiring that a medical screening examination be performed on all ED clients before solicitation of information about ability to pay. This medical screening examination must be inclusive enough to determine whether the client requires emergency medical treatment or is in active labor. Violations of this legislation can again result in fines and penalties. Every congressional year, new legislation is proposed in an attempt to provide appropriate emergency medical treatment to the public while continuing to acknowledge cost-containment issues.

CONSENT TO TREAT

Most adult clients who receive treatment in the ED give voluntary consent to the standard and usual treatment performed in this setting. In some instances, however, a client is deemed unable to give consent for treatment. This inability may be due to the critical nature of the client's illness or injury or to other conditions, such as an altered level of consciousness. In these instances, emergency care may be rendered to the client under the implied emergency doctrine.[1] This doctrine assumes that the client would consent to treatment to prevent death or disability if the client were so able.

Children under the age of legal majority must have the consent of their parent or legal guardian for medical care to be rendered. Exceptions include (1) emancipated minors; (2) minors seeking treatment for communicable diseases, including sexually transmitted diseases, injuries from abuse, and alcohol or drug rehabilitation; and (3) minor-aged females requiring treatment for pregnancy or pregnancy-related concerns. Some states also allow the adult caregiver with whom the child resides to give treatment authorization even though that caregiver may not be the parent.

The issue of informed consent in the ED is the same as in any other health care setting. Adult clients must be informed about the necessity of required treatments, expected outcomes, and potential complications. Clients must also be mentally competent and understand the information being explained. As in any other setting, a mentally competent adult client always maintains the right to refuse treatment or withdraw previously given consent.

RESTRAINTS

Restraining a client while he or she is in the ED may at times become necessary. The need for restraint usually arises because the client is becoming agitated or possibly violent. Hard leather or chemical restraints are used if the client is in danger of injuring self or others. If restraints are required, departmental guidelines for their use must be followed.[1] A physician's order for applying restraints along with the client's behavior mandating the use of restraints must be documented. The client must be periodically reevaluated both for the continued need for restraints and for integrity of distal circulation, motor movement, and sensory level of the restrained extremities. The findings must be documented. Offering water to the client and providing opportunities to urinate or relieve other body needs are required, as is documentation of this nursing care. No client may be kept in restraints against his or her will unless the client's behavior indicates the existence of safety issues.[1]

Clients in the ED who have psychological conditions that render them a danger to themselves or to others, or who are unable to provide food or shelter for themselves, can be held on a legal psychiatric restraining order. This order mandates that such clients be placed in a locked psychiatric facility for their protection for a maximum of 72 hours. Within that 72-hour period, the client must be evaluated by a psychiatrist to determine whether the legal order needs to be extended or whether the client can be released back into society.

MANDATORY REPORTING

Every state has mandatory reporting regulations that affect emergency nurses. Incidents and conditions may need to be reported to federal, state, or local authorities or to the Department of Public Health, Department of Motor Vehicles, coroner's offices, or animal control agencies.

The types of incidents requiring reporting are suspected child, sexual, domestic, and elder abuse; assaults; motor vehicle crashes; communicable diseases such as hepatitis, sexually transmitted diseases, chicken pox, measles, mumps, meningitis, tuberculosis, and food poisoning; seizure activity; death; and animal bites. Every ED has written policies regarding these mandatory reports.

EVIDENCE COLLECTION AND PRESERVATION

Recognition of unusual circumstances surrounding a client's injury or death is an important aspect of ED nursing because of the associated legal implications. Not only must the legal authorities be notified; in many instances, the ED nurse may be required to collect and preserve evidence taken from the client. This evidence can include bullets, weapons, clothing, and body fluid specimens.

All collected evidence must be identified by the client's name, hospital identification number, date and time of evidence collection, type of evidence and source (e.g., venipuncture, hematoma, aspiration vomitus, swab), and the initials and/or signature of the person collecting the evidence. Once the evidence has been collected, its preservation and the maintenance of the "chain of custody" is extremely important. Tables 82–1 to 82–3 relate to evidence collection.

VIOLENCE

Violence directed against ED personnel has become an issue of concern during the past decade.[24, 35] The environment inherent in the ED, the emotional circumstances often surrounding the illness or injury that affect both clients and family members, and the increasingly violent

TABLE 82–1	EVIDENCE COLLECTION IN THE EMERGENCY DEPARTMENT
Evidence	**Collection/Container**
Glass fragments, bullets, broken fingernails, paint chips, loose hair follicles, fibers, or trace evidence such as soil	Place each item in a paper envelope or specimen container.
Head or pubic hair samples	Collected samples from combings and cuttings are each placed in a paper envelope.
Blood (from both venipuncture and possible hematoma evacuation), urine, gastric washings, or vomitus	A 20- to 30-ml sample placed in a sealed container.
Swabs from wounds, membranes, or orifices	Air-dry before placing in a collection container or paper envelope.

From Selfridge-Thomas, J. (1995). *Manual of emergency nursing* (p. 382). Philadelphia: W. B. Saunders.

TABLE 82-2	TIPS FOR PRESERVING EVIDENCE IN THE EMERGENCY DEPARTMENT

1. Minimally handle the body of a deceased person.
2. Place paper bags on the hands and feet and possibly over the head of a deceased person to protect trace evidence or residue.
3. Place wet clothing in individual paper bags. Do not use plastic bags, as wet clothes can "sweat," thereby destroying evidence.
4. Photograph inflicted wounds or injury before cleansing or repair.
5. Do not insert invasive tubes through pre-existing wounds or holes (e.g., do not place chest tubes through chest wounds or intravenous catheters through needle track marks).
6. Do not cut clothing through evidence holes such as stab wounds or bullet wounds.
7. Collect the client's personal items such as written notes, drugs or medications, and items from clothing pockets.
8. Do not allow family members, significant others, or friends to be alone with the client.

From Selfridge-Thomas, J. (1995). *Manual of emergency nursing* (p. 382). Philadelphia: W. B. Saunders.

trends in the United States all play a role in this unfortunate phenomenon. Administrative changes have been made in some EDs to enhance both public and health care worker safety. These measures have included the installation of items such as metal detectors, "panic buttons," bullet-proof glass, and lock-down doors at public entrances; increasing the visibility of security guards; utilizing patrol guard dogs; and instituting visitor control policies.[35]

Education of ED personnel in violence prevention is also of paramount importance. The following areas are crucial to address:

- Recognizing potentially violent clients and situations
- Identifying verbally and physically abusive signs from clients, family members, or friends
- Understanding the importance of instinct or "gut reactions"
- Using simple communication strategies to defuse potentially problematic situations

TABLE 82-3	MAINTAINING "CHAIN OF CUSTODY" OF EVIDENCE IN THE EMERGENCY DEPARTMENT

1. Label all collected evidence with client information data.
2. Document all collected evidence with the date and time and the initials of the person collecting evidence.
3. Document all transfers of evidence from one person to another and include the reason for transfer of evidence.
4. Obtain signatures of the person releasing evidence and of the person receiving evidence.
5. *Never* leave collected evidence unattended.

From Selfridge-Thomas, J. (1995). *Manual of emergency nursing* (p. 383). Philadelphia: W. B. Saunders.

- Requiring clients to completely undress before physical examination
- Minimizing the presence of "potential weapons" in client care areas such as scalpels, needles, excess tubing attached to oxygen flow meters, scissors, stethoscopes worn around the neck, and personal jewelry
- Restraining clients, when necessary, using a team approach
- Avoiding becoming a hostage in a volatile situation

Once a violent situation has erupted, the protection of ED personnel and others in the department is of utmost concern. Any means necessary to ensure their safety must be undertaken.

ETHICAL ISSUES

The ethical issues confronting ED nurses usually concern end-of-life concerns. Initial resuscitation and stabilization of clients in critical condition constitutes universal standard practice in the ED. At times, however, the desired outcome of client survivability is not achievable.

UNEXPECTED DEATH

When death occurs in the ED setting, it is usually sudden and unexpected, even if the client has had a prolonged illness. The unexpected nature of the death, or impending death, can present ethical dilemmas for both the survivors and the ED personnel. One such issue deals with the length to which resuscitation is performed. This is usually a physician's decision; however, family members may at times have input. Allowing family members or significant others to be present during client resuscitation is becoming more common. This practice is not necessarily disruptive to the resuscitation process, and it can be of comfort to the survivors and the involved ED personnel.[4, 23]

When death does occur, the ED nurse and the ED physician have important roles in informing the family:

- Inform the family of the client's death, and refer to the deceased client by name.
- Provide the family with an explanation of the course of events related to the death; use simple explanations.
- Offer the family an opportunity to view the body if desired. If a child has died, allow the parent to hold the child if they so desire. Providing the parent with a lock of the child's hair may be comforting.
- Help the family to focus on decisions requiring immediate attention such as taking possession of the deceased person's valuables, postmortem examination if desired or required, possible organ or tissue donation, and funeral home selection.
- Inform family members when they can leave the ED setting.
- Provide community agency referral as needed.

ADVANCE DIRECTIVES

In 1991, Congress enacted the Patient Self-Determination Act (PSDA). This act allows a client, or the client's health care proxy, to make determinations related to end-of-life measures.[9] Emergency care personnel are obligated to abide by the client's advance directive decisions, if that information is available and provided in writing. When this written information is not available, ED personnel have a responsibility to stabilize and/or resuscitate any client according to standard treatment guidelines regardless of a family member's expressed wishes.

ORGAN AND TISSUE DONATION

Issues related to potential organ or tissue donation often arise in the ED setting. Once a potential donor is identified, the surviving family members need to be approached. A team approach involving a physician, a nurse, and possibly an organ procurement coordinator is optimal. Utmost dignity and professionalism must be maintained. (Chapter 80 reviews religious and cultural customs and beliefs related to death and organ transplantation.) Remember, whatever decision the family makes regarding organ or tissue donation, that decision must be supported by health care personnel.

COMPONENTS OF EMERGENCY CARE

Even though treatment decisions in the ED may at first appear to occur in a chaotic fashion, there is an inherent order in the timing and choice of interventions performed throughout a client's stay. The organizational flow of events involves client triage (prioritizing), nursing assessment of the client, diagnostic testing, formulation of diagnoses, outcome management, evaluation, disposition, and documentation.

TRIAGE

Whether clients arrive via ambulance or are ambulatory, they are triaged at some point by either an ED physician or an ED nurse. The purpose of this triage process is to expediently determine the severity of a client's problem or condition. The acuity level of the presenting problem is rated according to predetermined categories; the most frequently used ratings are *emergent, urgent,* and *non-urgent.* Table 82–4 provides a definition for each of these categories.

Once an initial determination is made about the sever-

TABLE 82–4	THREE-CATEGORY TRIAGE RATING IN THE EMERGENCY DEPARTMENT

Emergent category: Client must be treated immediately; otherwise, life/limb/vision is threatened.

Urgent category: Client requires treatment, but life/limb/vision is not threatened if care cannot be provided within 1 to 2 hours.

Non-urgent category: Client requires evaluation and possible treatment, but time is not a critical factor.

ity of the client's condition, a more in-depth nursing and medical assessment is completed. Appropriate diagnostic testing and specific interventions are performed using a team approach as emergency physicians and nurses work collaboratively to provide appropriate and expeditious management of the client's problem.

NURSING ASSESSMENT

The nursing assessment process for any client entering the ED is divided into the *primary* assessment and the *secondary* assessment (Fig. 82–1).

The purpose of the *primary assessment* is to immediately identify any client problem that poses a threat, immediate or potential, to life, limb, or vision. Information is gathered primarily through objective data. If any abnormalities are found during the primary assessment, immediate interventions such as cardiopulmonary resuscitation (CPR) and Advanced Life Support (ALS) must be instituted to aid in preserving the client's life, limb, or vision. The primary assessment is made using the ABC mnemonic:

A   Airway patency
B   Breathing effectiveness
C   Circulation (both peripheral and organ-specific)

For any client arriving in the ED who has been involved in a major traumatic injury, the primary assessment must also include an evaluation of the cervical spine area for any potential injury.

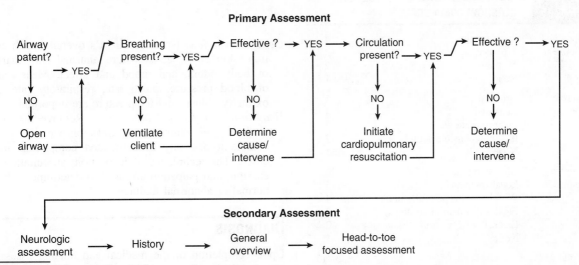

FIGURE 82–1 Primary and secondary assessment process.

Once it is determined that a client's ABC status is satisfactory, the *secondary assessment* is performed to identify any other non–life-threatening problems the client may be experiencing. Both subjective information and objective data are obtained. The secondary assessment includes the following elements.

Neurologic assessment. Determine the client's (1) level of consciousness; (2) orientation to person, place, time, and event; (3) Glasgow Coma Scale (GCS) score (Table 82–5); (4) pupillary size, equality, and reaction to light and accommodation; and (5) motor movement and strength of hand grips and pedal pushes.

History. Elicit the nature of the client's chief complaint, duration of the problem, mechanism of injury from blunt or penetrating forces (Table 82–6), associated manifestations related to the primary problem, past pertinent medical history, current medications and compliance, use of over-the-counter (OTC) medications or herbs, routine use of alcohol or illicit drugs, known medication allergies, and immunization history. Women of childbearing age may need to be questioned about the date of the last normal menstrual period (LNMP), number of pregnancies and outcomes, and age at onset or at end of menstruation.

Pain. The most frequent complaint for which clients seek emergency care is related to pain. Obtaining specific information regarding pain patterns can be extremely helpful. Asking questions according to the PQRST mnemonic often provides useful information:

P Provokes: Are there any specific factors that cause the pain to increase or decrease?

Q Quality: What descriptive terminology identifies the type of pain—dull, sharp, colicky, pressure?

R Region/Radiation: Where is the pain located? Does it move to other areas?

S Severity: Use a rating scale of 1 to 10 to describe pain severity, with 1 indicating no or minimal pain and 10 representing severe pain.

T Timing: How long has the pain been present? Are there cycles related to when the pain is present or absent?

TABLE 82–6	HISTORY QUESTIONS RELATED TO INJURY

MOTOR VEHICLE CRASHES

- Were you the driver or passenger?
- Were you wearing a seatbelt or shoulder harness (or both) correctly?
- Did the airbag deploy?
- Did you hit the steering wheel or the dashboard? If so, with what part of your body?
- Did you lose consciousness? If so, for how long?
- How fast was the vehicle going?
- What did the vehicle hit?
- Did the vehicle hit a moving object or a nonmoving object? (Paramedical personnel may provide information describing the condition of the car.)
- Where is your pain?
- How far were you thrown from the car?
- What is the condition of the other passengers?

BLUNT INJURY FROM FALLS

- How far did you fall?
- What precipitated the fall?
- What did you land on?
- Where is your pain?
- Did you lose consciousness?

GUNSHOT WOUNDS

- How long ago did the incident occur?
- How many shots did you hear?
- What type of gun was it?
- From what direction do you think the bullet entered your body?
- How far away was the assailant?
- Where is your pain?

PENETRATING WOUNDS OR STAB WOUNDS

- How long ago did the injury occur?
- How many times were you stabbed?
- How long was the knife or sharp object?
- How far in did the sharp object go?
- From what direction were you stabbed?
- Where is your pain?

From Kitt S., et al. (Eds.). (1995). *Emergency nursing: A physiologic and clinical perspective* (2nd ed.). Philadelphia: W. B. Saunders.

TABLE 82–5	GLASGOW COMA SCALE	
Eye-opening response	Spontaneous	4
	To voice	3
	To pain	2
	None	1
Best verbal response	Oriented	5
	Confused	4
	Inappropriate words	3
	Incomprehensible sounds	2
	None	1
Best motor response	Obeys command	6
	Localizes pain	5
	Withdraws (to painful stimulus)	4
	Flexion (to painful stimulus)	3
	Extension (to painful stimulus)	2
	None	1
Total		3–15

General overview. Note the client's overall health condition, skin color, gait, posture, unusual skin markings or body odors, and mood and affect. Measurements of blood pressure, pulse rate, respiratory rate, pulse oximetry values, and temperature are important.

Head-to-toe or focused assessment. Remove the client's clothing and examine the areas on which the chief complaint and any or associated complaints are focused. The techniques of inspection, auscultation, percussion, and palpation are used to determine additional normal or abnormal findings.

DIAGNOSIS

Upon completion of the medical and nursing assessment process, diagnostic tests (radiographic, cardiology, laboratory, special studies) may be initiated. Once all pertinent information has been collected, a working diagnosis is formulated. The physician provides a medical diagnosis; in addition, the ED nurse may incorporate a variety of nursing diagnoses. These diagnoses provide a framework on which to build a plan of appropriate client care.

OUTCOME MANAGEMENT

Necessary client care interventions may be initiated by the ED nurse, the ED physician, or other health care providers. There is frequent collaboration among all health care providers involved, and interventions are assigned priority according to the severity of the client's condition.

EVALUATION

The desired goal in client care is to achieve positive client outcomes after medical or nursing management. This is an integral component of ED nursing care. If the client's condition does not improve with initial interventions, the plan of care must be reexamined and additional interventions may be required.

CLIENT DISPOSITION

All clients entering the ED are eventually discharged from the ED. They may be transferred to another healthcare facility, admitted to the hospital, or released to home or another facility. Most clients are released to home following treatment. Before being discharged from the ED, a client and/or family members must be given both oral and written instructions concerning follow-up care. These instructions should identify the client's diagnosed problem, explain necessary continued treatments, describe potential complications, and specify time frames for rechecks and the name of the physician to whom the client is being referred. These instructions should be presented in both oral and written form in the client's primary language. At times, a hospital or family interpreter may be required to accomplish this outcome.

NURSING DOCUMENTATION

Because ED nurses frequently are responsible for an assigned area, zone, or "pod" within the department and clients enter and exit those areas on a continual basis, nursing documentation is of paramount importance. Include the recording of all assessment findings, diagnostic tests, interventions and management, responses to treatment, achieved outcomes, and client education. Documentation needs to be complete but concise. It provides an ongoing record of the client's condition and responses. The format may be a flow sheet, narrative, or computer-generated format or a combination of these.

EMERGENCY CONDITIONS

INEFFECTIVE AIRWAY CLEARANCE

A compromised or ineffective airway may be due to either complete or partial airway obstruction. Common

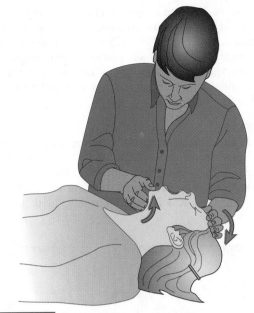

FIGURE 82–2 Chin lift maneuver to open the airway.

causes of airway compromise include the presence of a foreign object in the airway, airway edema, airway infection, facial or airway injury, and tongue obstruction.[37, 38]

Clinical Manifestations

The clinical manifestations of airway compromise include absence of respirations, drooling, stridor, intercostal or substernal retractions, cyanosis, and agitation. A decreased level of consciousness may lead to airway compromise as a result of obstruction of the posterior pharynx by the relaxed tongue.

Outcome Management

REMOVE OBSTRUCTION

If an obstruction is present, the airway should be opened by a chin lift or jaw thrust maneuver (Figs. 82–2 and 82–3). If either of these maneuvers opens the client's airway, patency is maintained via the insertion of a nasopharyngeal tube or oral airway device. If these maneuvers fail to relieve the obstruction, more aggressive interven-

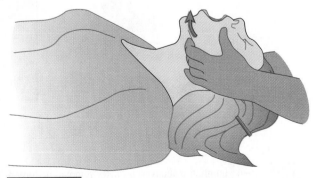

FIGURE 82–3 The jaw thrust maneuver to open the airway is the preferred method for use in clients with head or cervical neck injury.

tions must be instituted, such as (1) performing abdominal or chest thrusts if an aspirated foreign object is the suspected cause (Fig. 82–4), (2) suctioning the oral cavity to remove secretions or visible foreign objects, (3) intubating via the nasal or oral route, and (4) assisting with creating a surgical airway via a cricothyroidotomy (Fig. 82–5).

INTUBATE

In some cases, oral or nasal intubation may require the use of *rapid-sequence induction* (RSI). This procedure is used in awake clients who require intubation either to maintain the airway or as a mechanism to provide adequate ventilation. RSI is most frequently used in clients who have sustained a head or spinal injury and in clients who are rapidly tiring from the effort of maintaining respirations. RSI involves (1) establishing venous access; (2) hyperventilating the client with 100% oxygen; and (3) administering an intravenous (IV) general barbiturate or anesthetic medication such as thiopental 3 to 5 mg/kg, fentanyl (Sublimaze) 3 to 15 μg/kg, ketamine (Ketalar) 1 to 2 mg/kg, etomidate (Amidate) 0.3 mg/kg, or propofol (Diprivan) 2.0 mg/kg, followed immediately by the administration of an IV muscle-paralyzing agent such as succinylcholine (Anectine) 1.5 to 2.0 mg/kg.[12] Once the client loses consciousness and adequate muscle relaxation and paralysis have been obtained, intubation with ventilation using 100% oxygen is implemented.

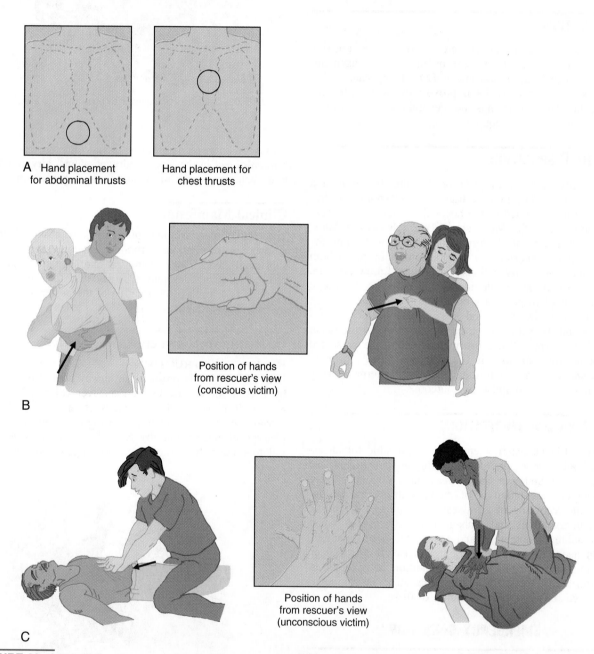

FIGURE 82–4 Heimlich maneuver, used for removal of foreign bodies blocking the upper airway. Vigorous upward chest or abdominal thrusts produce a rush of air that expels the foreign body. The abdominal thrust is the original Heimlich maneuver. The chest thrust is an adaptation that is useful for obese or pregnant victims. Use four quick thrusts in the positions shown. *A,* Hand placement. *B,* Maneuver for conscious victims. *C,* Maneuver for unconscious victims.

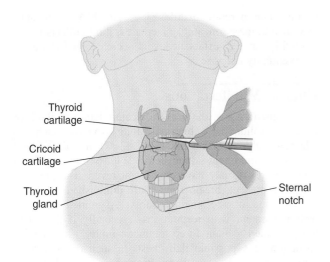

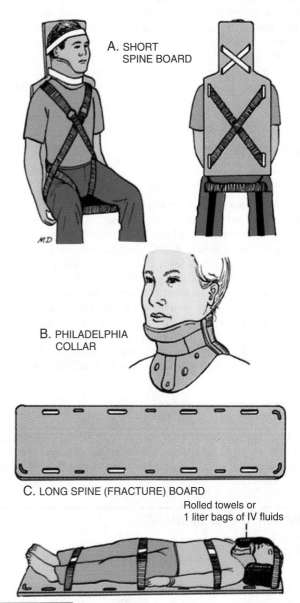

FIGURE 82–5 A cricothyrotomy procedure is performed to create a temporary airway. An opening is made into the trachea and is maintained with a small plastic tube.

VERIFY ENDOTRACHEAL TUBE PLACEMENT

After an oral intubation procedure, the ED nurse is immediately responsible for auscultation of the client's chest during assisted ventilation to confirm the presence of equal bilateral breath sounds. If breath sounds are heard over the epigastric area, the endotracheal tube must be removed, the client hyperventilated, and the procedure reattempted. Breath sounds heard more prominently over the upper right chest indicate that the endotracheal tube has advanced too far into the right main bronchus. The tube needs to be pulled back and breath sounds reassessed. Once the presence of equal and bilateral breath sounds is confirmed, the tube is secured in place, and a chest film is obtained to document correct tube placement.

Securing and maintaining a patent airway constitute the first priority in any ED client. Other treatments directed at the cause of airway compromise will then be instituted. These measures may include administration of IV medications if infection or local edema is present.

IMMOBILIZE THE SPINE

If the client with an actual or potential airway problem has had a traumatic injury, simultaneous stabilization of the client's cervical, thoracic, and lumbar spine must be instituted and maintained to prevent any further possible spinal injury. Stabilization is accomplished utilizing a team approach and involves the following steps: (1) manually stabilizing the client's head and cervical spine; (2) applying a hard cervical collar around the client's nuchal area; (3) placing the client on a long, rigid backboard; (4) securing the client to the backboard; (5) placing immobilization devices, such as rolled towels, at the side of the client's head/neck; and finally (6) placing a strip of adhesive tape across the client's forehead and immobilization devices and then onto the back board (see Fig. 82–6).

INEFFECTIVE BREATHING PATTERNS

Breathing patterns are affected if a client is either hyperventilating or hypoventilating. The normal respiratory rate for an adult is between 12 and 20 breaths/minute; children normally have faster respiratory rates until approximately the age of 10 years.

■ HYPERVENTILATION

Clinical Manifestations

Respiratory rates faster than normal constitute tachypnea and, in many cases, hyperventilation. Common causes for hyperventilation include anxiety reactions, pulmonary infections, and metabolic deviations.[37, 38] With excessive and prolonged hyperventilation, carbon dioxide levels de-

FIGURE 82–6 Spine-immobilizing devices. A, The short spine board is applied to a client who is seated (e.g., in an automobile) and is applied along with a cervical collar before extrication of the person from the vehicle. B, The Philadelphia collar, a two-piece, hard, molded plastic device, can be applied without manipulating the neck and provides good immobilization of the cervical spine. C, The long spine (fracture) board is made of wood and contains cut-out sections along the sides for securing restraining straps and for lifting the injured client.

crease, and respiratory alkalosis can result. The client may report numbness and tingling sensations in the distal extremities or around the lips, along with carpal or pedal spasms. A sensation of chest pain may also be present. Frequently this condition is caused by client anxiety, but it is important to also investigate other possible causes, such as pain, aspirin toxicity, diabetic ketoacidosis, fluid loss, central nervous system (CNS) lesions, and pulmonary embolism.

Outcome Management

The goals of treatment are to return the client's breathing pattern and rate to normal and to restore normal gas exchange.[37, 38] If anxiety is the cause of the hyperventilation, the client needs to be instructed to take slow, deep breaths through the nose and slowly exhale through the mouth. Having clients breathe into a paper bag and rebreathe their own carbon dioxide may be helpful. If another cause is identified as the reason for the client's altered breathing pattern, specific treatments such as administration of oxygen and inhaled, intravenous, or oral medications are initiated to reverse the process.

■ HYPOVENTILATION

Clinical Manifestations

Hypoventilation occurs when an adult client's respiratory rate falls below 12 breaths/minute. At this rate, not enough oxygen is available to maintain adequate tissue oxygenation. Clinical manifestations may include a decrease in the client's level of consciousness, pallor, cyanosis, and pulse oximetry readings of less than 96%. Carbon dioxide is retained, and respiratory acidosis develops. Causes of hypoventilation include brain stem lesions, head injury, drug-induced depression of the respiratory center, impaired respiratory muscle innervation from spinal cord injury, and the presence of neuromuscular diseases such as muscular dystrophy or Guillain-Barré syndrome.[37, 38]

Outcome Management

Administering high-flow oxygen via a bag-valve-mask device is often required to reduce the systemic hypoxemia and to return oxygen levels to between 80 and 100 mm Hg.

IMPAIRED GAS EXCHANGE

Etiology

Obstructions, infections, and injury within the pulmonary system can lead to the development of gas exchange abnormalities. Common causative disorders include asthma, reactive airway disease, chronic obstructive pulmonary disease, pulmonary embolism, bronchitis, pneumonia, tuberculosis, pneumothorax, and chest injuries such as a flail chest.[6, 8, 14, 20, 37, 38]

A less common cause of a gas exchange problem is noncardiac pulmonary edema, which results from acute damage to the alveolocapillary membrane. This damage can occur from inhalation injury, near-drowning, sepsis, trauma, and narcotic overdose.[37, 38] As the alveolocapillary membrane permeability increases, fluid collects in the interstitial space, surfactant levels decrease, and the alveoli eventually collapse.

Clinical Manifestations

With constriction of the bronchi, accumulation of fluid, or lung consolidation, abnormal lung sounds such as wheezes, rales, or rhonchi (Table 82–7) are often heard throughout the client's lung fields. With pulmonary infections, the client may have concurrent fever. If a pneumothorax is present, breath sounds are diminished or absent on the side of the pneumothorax. Asymmetrical chest wall movement with respirations, especially if the client has sustained a blunt force traumatic injury, should raise suspicion of a possible flail chest. In such cases a chest film provides valuable diagnostic information about the cause of the client's problem. A ventilation-perfusion (V/Q) scan can aid in the diagnosis of pulmonary embolism.

Outcome Management

ADMINISTER OXYGEN
Oxygen therapy with a flow rate of between 2 and 10 L/min via nasal cannula or face mask is the priority intervention for clients with an obstructive or infectious cause of ineffective gas exchange.

ADMINISTER MEDICATIONS TO OPEN AIRWAYS
Oxygen administration is frequently followed by administering aerosolized bronchodilator medications such as metaproterenol (Alupent) or albuterol (Ventolin) in order to open constricted upper or lower bronchi.[28] Subcutaneous epinephrine 1 : 1000 may be administered to relax constricted bronchi and to reduce the degree of airway or bronchial edema.[16] Administration of steroid medications, either intravenously or orally, is a frequent therapy.[20] A client with a suspected pulmonary embolus may be given IV thrombolytic medications, such as tissue-type plasminogen activator (t-PA [Activase]), to lyse the offending embolus and also heparin to prevent the formation of new emboli.

MINIMIZE SPREAD OF INFECTION
Infectious diseases that are the cause of impaired gas exchange are treated with IV or oral antibiotic medications. A client thought to have a highly contagious pulmonary disease such as tuberculosis must be isolated

TABLE 82–7	RESPIRATORY SOUNDS ASSOCIATED WITH ILLNESS
Illness	**Lung Sounds**
Asthma	Wheezes
COPD	Rales, rhonchi, wheezes
Bronchitis	Rhonchi
Pneumonia	Rhonchi, abnormal bronchial sounds
Tuberculosis	Rhonchi, abnormal bronchial sounds
Bronchiolitis	Wheezes

COPD, chronic obstructive pulmonary disease.

from the general ED client population. The use of a high-efficiency particulate air (HEPA) filter mask placed over the nose and mouth is indicated to prevent spreading of aerosol droplets.[29] ED personnel caring for the client may also need to wear this type of mask to decrease exposure risks.

■ TRAUMATIC PNEUMOTHORAX

A pneumothorax can be classified as a simple pneumothorax, open pneumothorax, or tension pneumothorax (Fig. 82–7).[26] In a *simple pneumothorax,* air from the bronchus, bronchioles, or alveoli escapes into the pleural space and diminishes lung expansion capacity. With an *open pneumothorax,* a traumatically created opening in the client's chest wall allows air to move freely into and out of the thoracic cavity during inspiration and exhalation. A tension pneumothorax occurs when air continues to become trapped in the pleural cavity with no mechanism of escape during the exhalation process. This type of pneumothorax is an emergent condition.

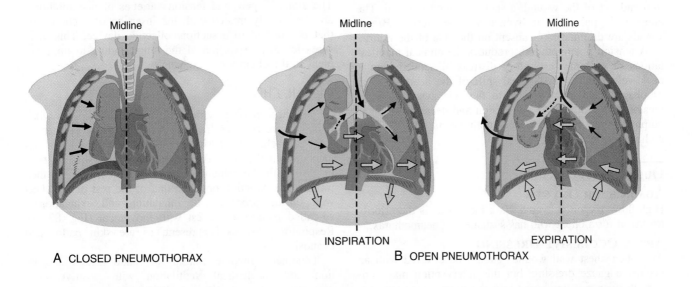

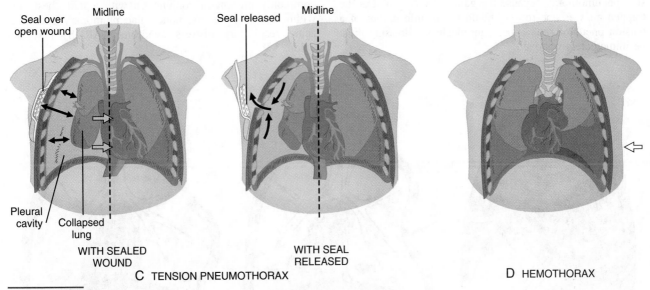

FIGURE 82–7 Pneumothorax.

A, Closed pneumothorax. The lung collapses as air gathers in the pleural space.

B, Open pneumothorax (sucking chest wound). *Solid arrows* indicate air movement; *open arrows,* structural movement. A chest wall wound connects the pleural space with atmospheric air. During inspiration, atmospheric air is sucked into the pleural space through the chest wall wound. Positive pressure in the pleural space collapses the lung on the affected side and pushes the mediastinal contents toward the unaffected side. This reduces the volume of air in the unaffected side considerably. During expiration, air escapes through the chest wall wound, lessening positive pressure in the affected side and allowing the mediastinal contents to swing back toward the affected side. Movement of mediastinal structures from side to side is called mediastinal flutter.

C, Tension pneumothorax. *Left,* If an open pneumothorax is covered (e.g., with a dressing), it forms a seal, and tension pneumothorax with a mediastinal shift develops. A tear in lung structure continues to allow air into the pleural space. As positive pressure builds in the pleural space, the affected lung collapses, and the mediastinal contents shift to the unaffected side. *Right,* Tension pneumothorax is corrected by removing the seal (e.g., dressing), allowing air trapped in the pleural space to escape.

D, Hemothorax. Massive hemothorax *(arrow)* below the left lung causes collapse of lung tissue.

Clinical Manifestations

A simple pneumothorax can occur spontaneously but is frequently associated with penetrating injury forces delivered to the chest or with blunt forces causing a rib fracture. Pain with respirations is present, as is the auscultative finding of unequal breath sounds. Pulse oximetry readings are less than 94%.

An obvious chest wound is present with an open pneumothorax, as this type of pneumothorax is most commonly caused by penetrating injury forces. As air moves into and out of the wound, a sucking sound is heard. The client is in pain, and tachypnea will be present. Breath sounds are diminished or absent on the side of the injury.

A tension pneumothorax produces the clinical manifestations of extreme respiratory distress, distended jugular neck veins, and a mediastinal shift of the heart, trachea, esophagus, and great vessels to the side away from the tension pneumothorax. Hypotension and decreased cardiac output are other findings. Pneumothorax is diagnosed by a chest radiograph.

Outcome Management

ADMINISTER OXYGEN

High-flow oxygen delivered via a face mask is the priority treatment for a client who has sustained a pneumothorax.

APPLY OCCLUSIVE DRESSING

Any open chest wall wounds should be covered with an occlusive gauze dressing, but this intervention may convert an open pneumothorax into the more dangerous tension pneumothorax because the gauze covering blocks the trapped air's escape route. Should the manifestations of a tension pneumothorax appear, the occlusive dressing must be immediately removed.

RELEASE TRAPPED AIR

If a tension pneumothorax is thought to be the cause of respiratory distress and if it has not been iatrogenically produced by covering an open chest wound, a 14- to 16-gauge catheter needle is immediately inserted into the client's anterior chest wall on the affected side at the second midclavicular intercostal space.[25] This life-saving intervention allows the immediate release of trapped air and decompresses the pleural cavity.

PLACE CHEST TUBE

The simple, open, and tension varieties of pneumothorax are definitively treated with the insertion of a chest tube that is attached to a suction/collection device. This measure aids in reexpansion of the lung, leading to improvement in the client's gas exchange.

■ FLAIL CHEST

A flail chest involves serious rib fractures. It occurs when two or more ribs are fractured in two or more places on the same chest wall side or when the sternum is detached from the ribs. The fractured segment has no connection with the remaining rib cage. This segment then moves in a direction opposite that of the rest of the chest wall during processes of inhalation and exhalation—so-called paradoxical chest wall movement (Fig. 82–8). Respiratory distress is present, as are skin pallor and cyanosis.

Treatment involves nasal or endotracheal intubation and mechanical ventilation with positive end-expiratory pressure (PEEP). Pulmonary contusions are commonly present in conjunction with a flail chest, and within 24 to 48 hours, noncardiac pulmonary edema or acute respiratory distress syndrome (ARDS) may develop.[19, 25]

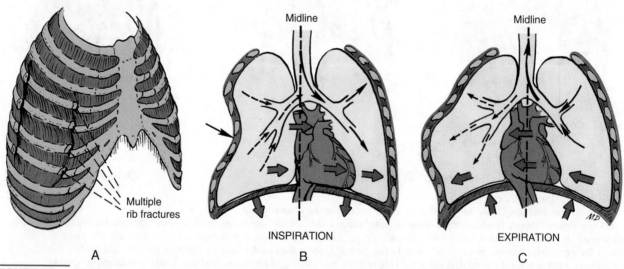

FIGURE 82–8 Flail chest. *Dashed arrows* indicate air movement; *solid arrows,* structural movement. *A,* A flail chest consists of fractured rib segments that are unattached (free-floating) to the rest of the chest wall. *B,* On inspiration, the flail segment of ribs is sucked inward. The affected lung and mediastinal structures shift to the unaffected side. This compromises the amount of inspired air in the unaffected lung. *C,* On expiration, the flail segment of ribs bellows outward. The affected lung and mediastinal structures shift to the affected side. Some air within the lungs is shunted back and forth between the lungs instead of passing through the upper airway.

FLUID VOLUME DEFICIT

A decrease in circulating blood volume leads to fluid volume deficit and, subsequently, to decreased tissue perfusion. Therefore, any condition producing a profound volume deficit necessitates immediate intervention. The more common causes of volume loss include shock due to acute hypovolemia, dehydration, and major burn injuries.[37, 38] Clients can lose blood volume through either internal or external active bleeding. The internal bleeding sites usually associated with large volume loss include the posterior nasal passages, aortic vessel injury or dissecting aneurysm, pulmonary vasculature, stomach, liver, spleen, uterus or fallopian tube, and fractures of the pelvis and femur. Illness leading to prolonged vomiting or diarrhea can also produce large fluid losses. "Third-spacing" volume loss or interstitial volume sequestering associated with major burn injury occurs approximately 12 hours after injury (see Chapter 50).

As volume loss occurs, various compensatory mechanisms act to produce vasoconstriction of the vasculature, retain fluid via the renal tubules, and increase cardiac output.[36] These compensatory mechanisms—such as stimulation of the sympathetic nervous system; the release of renin, angiotensin, aldosterone, and antidiuretic hormones; and fluid shifts—continue in an effort to restore tissue perfusion, thus ensuring cell survival. However, these mechanisms are limited in scope, and if the lost volume is not restored, eventually cellular structures incur irreversible damage from the oxygen debt, and death ensues.[36]

Clinical Manifestations

The client often provides a history of recent injury or illness with associated volume loss. Clinical manifestations may include agitation or decreasing level of consciousness, pale and diaphoretic skin, delayed capillary refill time of longer than 2 seconds, tachycardia, tachypnea, decreased urinary output, and hypotension.[36–39] Positive orthostatic vital signs (a decrease in systolic blood pressure by 20 mm Hg and an increase in pulse rate by 20 beats/min associated with the client changing from a lying to an upright position) may be present in clients with a mild to moderate volume loss. If blood has accumulated in the thoracic cavity (hemothorax) or abdominal cavity, percussion over the area elicits a dull sound. A collection of blood under the thoracic diaphragm or in the peritoneal cavity can produce Kehr's sign (referred shoulder pain unrelated to injury) or a rigid, hard abdomen with increased rebound tenderness upon palpation.

Diagnostic testing is directed at locating the source of any internal bleeding. Tests may include radiography, ultrasonography, and computed tomography (CT) scans of the chest, pelvis, extremities, or abdomen. The laboratory tests of blood typing, complete blood count (CBC), hemoglobin concentration and hematocrit, and electrolyte panel are performed on collected blood samples. A urine specimen should be tested for specific gravity and the presence of blood and leukocytes and, in females, for pregnancy. If gastrointestinal bleeding is suspected, a nasogastric tube is passed and the aspirate tested for the presence of blood. Stool is tested for blood.

A diagnostic peritoneal lavage (DPL) procedure is occasionally performed in unstable clients who have sustained abdominal injury. A peritoneal catheter is inserted into the client's peritoneal cavity, and 1 L of normal saline is infused. The fluid is then drained, via gravity, from the peritoneal cavity back into the emptied fluid bag. The fluid is examined for the presence of blood, bile, feces, amylase, and white blood cells to determine whether organs within the peritoneal cavity have been injured (Fig. 82–9).

Diagnostic testing not only helps in identifying the source and severity of volume loss but also aids in determining whether the client requires immediate surgery or hospital admission.

Outcome Management

Treatment is directed at preventing further volume loss and replacing fluid volume.[36–38]

MAINTAIN BLOOD FLOW TO VITAL ORGANS

High-flow oxygen is delivered via face mask to provide additional oxygen to tissues. Positioning the client in a supine position with the legs elevated is appropriate.

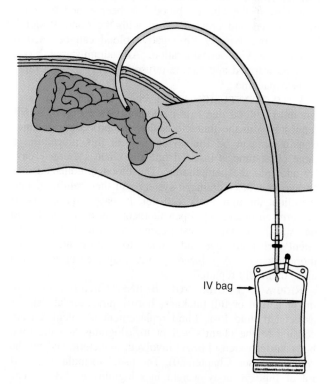

IV bag

INTERPRETATION OF RESULTS

Positive result	Free-flowing blood on aspiration
	Grossly bloody lavage return
	>100,000 RBC/mm3
	>500 WBC/mm3
	Exit of lavage fluid from urinary or thoracic catheters
Equivocal result	50,000–100,000 RBC/mm3
	100–500 WBC/mm3
Negative result	<50,000 RBC/mm3
	<100 WBC/mm3

FIGURE 82–9 Diagnostic peritoneal lavage.

STOP OR DECREASE BLEEDING

If external bleeding is present, direct pressure should be applied to control further blood loss. The application of tourniquets and clamping of exposed vessels should be avoided if possible. If the bleeding source is the posterior nasal passages, the client needs to be seated and leaning forward in a high Fowler position. Nasal packing is required.

REPLACE FLUIDS

Venous access must be obtained using a large-bore catheter (14 to 16 gauge). Usually two IV sites are required for fluid replacement. At the time of vein cannulation, blood samples should also be obtained for laboratory testing.

CRYSTALLOIDS. Crystalloid fluids (normal saline, lactated Ringer's solution) are the replacement fluids of choice. They should be warmed and administered at a ratio of 3:1 (3 L of solution for every 1 L of volume loss) in an adult.

COLLOIDS. Colloid fluids (e.g., blood, hetastarch, albumin) may also be given fluid resuscitation. These fluids contain proteins and are infused at a 1:1 ratio (1 unit of solution for every 1 unit of blood loss). Blood can be administered as whole blood or as packed red blood cells. It is best if the client's blood has been typed or, optimally, typed and cross-matched with the donor's blood, but universal type O Rh-negative blood can be used if speed is a vital consideration. All administered blood must be warmed and can be infused quickly using a rapid infuser machine.

AUTOTRANSFUSION. After chest trauma, if a large amount of blood due to a hemothorax (see Fig. 82–7) is sequestered in the thoracic cavity, the procedure of auto-transfusion can be life-saving.[31] With this procedure, a large chest tube is inserted into the client's thoracic cavity and into the hemothorax. The blood is collected into an autotransfuser drainage system and then reinfused into the client through an IV catheter. It may be necessary to perform an emergency open thoracotomy on a client who has sustained major chest trauma and is near death. The client's ribs are cut and spread to expose the internal thoracic cavity. Any bleeding sites may then be identified and potentially repaired.

REPLACE FLUIDS FOR BURNS. Clients who have major partial or full-thickness burn injuries are at risk for associated fluid loss. Fluid replacement is calculated according to the client's weight in kilograms and the total body surface area (TBSA) involved, as determined by the *rule of 9s* (see Chapter 50). The usual formula is 2 to 4 ml of fluid × body weight in kilograms × TBSA. The calculated amount of fluid is used as the total fluid replacement volume required over the 24-hour period from the time of injury. One half of the total fluid amount is infused in the first 8-hour period, one fourth of the fluid amount in the second 8-hour period, and the remaining one fourth amount in the last 8-hour period.

INSTITUTE OTHER MEASURES

Once fluid resuscitation is begun, other interventions can be instituted. A nasogastric tube is passed to prevent vomiting and possible aspiration. In clients with gastrointestinal bleeding, gastric lavage is performed using room-temperature normal saline instilled and aspirated through the nasogastric tube. An indwelling urinary catheter is inserted for the purpose of measuring urinary output. The client with volume loss is prone to the development of mild hypothermia. Keeping the client warm with blankets, warming lights, and infusion of warmed fluids aids in maintaining a normal body temperature. Continual monitoring of cardiac rate and rhythm, blood pressure, pulse oximetry readings, respiratory rate, and temperature is indicated.

FLUID VOLUME EXCESS

Clients who have an excess of fluid volume can concurrently have pulmonary congestion, leading to respiratory distress. Although clients with renal failure experience fluid volume excess, the disorder most commonly associated with fluid overload in the ED is heart failure. Heart failure results in fluid excess because of the inability of the cardiac muscle to function effectively. Ejection fraction decreases, pressure in the left ventricle increases, and eventually pressure increases affect the left atrium and right ventricle and atrium.[30]

Clinical Manifestations

The clinical manifestations of heart failure include agitation or restlessness, tachypnea and increased respiratory effort, respiratory rales, distended jugular neck veins, tachycardia, skin pallor, diaphoresis, ascites, and pitting dependent edema. Pulse oximetry readings are less than 94%, and the client may also cough up excessive, frothy sputum. Cardiac dysrhythmias, such as atrial fibrillation, may be noted with cardiac monitoring.[30]

Because these clients often have a chronic history of heart failure, their daily medication regimen usually includes digoxin, furosemide (Lasix), and potassium. Electrolyte imbalances are common, and serum levels of digoxin must be assessed via laboratory studies. Chest films provide information about the severity of the heart failure.

Outcome Management

IMPROVE OXYGENATION

Treatment is directed at improving the client's ability to breathe. Positioning the client in a high Fowler position facilitates the ability to breathe. Oxygen is administered at a high flow rate via face mask, although this intervention may be difficult for the client to tolerate. If respiratory fatigue develops, the client must be intubated in order to provide adequate ventilation. The use of rapid-sequence induction (RSI) before intubation may be indicated. A newer method of treating respiratory failure associated with heart failure involves the use of a tight-fitting mask placed over the client's nose and mouth and then connected to a mechanical ventilator.[34]

ADMINISTER MEDICATIONS

Establishing venous access for medication administration is necessary. The common medications include nitroglycerin 5 to 10 μg/minute given by IV infusion, furosemide (Lasix) 40 to 100 mg given intravenously, and morphine sulfate 2 to 10 mg given intravenously. If serum digoxin levels are subtherapeutic and the client is not hypokalemic, then digoxin may be administered 0.6 to 1 mg intravenously. Dobutamine, angiotensin-converting enzyme (ACE) inhibitor, and beta-blocker medications may be administered cautiously in some settings to reduce cardiac preload and to produce inotropic effects.[16]

MONITOR RESPONSE TO TREATMENT

Continual monitoring of the client's response to treatment is of paramount importance. Assessment should include level of consciousness, cardiac status, blood pressure, respiratory rate and effort, pulse oximetry, and urinary output.

DECREASED CARDIAC OUTPUT

Any illness or injury that has a direct effect on the heart can produce a decrease in cardiac output. Such disorders include cardiac dysrhythmias, acute myocardial infarction, cardiac injury, cardiac tamponade, and cardiac infection or myopathy.[37, 38]

When cardiac output decreases, tissue perfusion is adversely affected. Cardiac output (CO) is determined by stroke volume (SV) and heart rate (HR):

$$CO = SV \times HR$$

Therefore, a reduction in stroke volume or an alteration in heart rate has a direct effect on cardiac output. Cardiac dysrhythmias and acute myocardial infarction directly affect heart rate. Acute myocardial infarction also reduces stroke volume as a result of the death of cardiac muscle. Cardiac tamponade results in compression of the cardiac muscle by the collection of blood or fluid in the pericardial sac. This effect produces a decrease in stroke volume. Infection and cardiac myopathy also affect the cardiac muscle structures, thereby reducing stroke volume.

Clinical Manifestations

Depending on the cause of the reduced cardiac output, clients may present with differing clinical manifestations. Dysrhythmias are self-evident on cardiac monitoring. The most prominent manifestations include chest pain, skin pallor, diaphoresis, hypotension, nausea, and agitation or a decrease in level of consciousness. External chest wall injury may be evident with cardiac contusions. Cardiac tamponade produces the additional manifestations of distended jugular neck veins and muffled heart sounds. Fever may be present with cardiac infections.

Diagnostic tests include cardiac monitoring, chest radiography or ultrasonography, and laboratory studies. Levels of the cardiac enzymes creatine kinase (CK) and the CK-MB fraction and of the cardiac markers myoglobin and troponin T and troponin I are especially important in diagnosing the occurrences of a myocardial infarction.[17] Treadmill stress testing and dobutamine stress echocardiography (DSE) may also be performed to aid in the evaluation of chest pain.[43]

Outcome Management

IMPROVE CARDIAC OUTPUT

The goal of treatment is to improve cardiac output.[40, 41] High-flow oxygen should be administered via face mask, and venous access should be secured for the administra-

tion of medications. Supraventricular tachycardic dysrhythmias are frequently treated with the IV adenosine (Adenocar) 6 mg, whereas bradycardic rhythms may be treated with IV atropine 0.5 to 2 mg or with the insertion of a cardiac pacemaker. Lidocaine 1 mg/kg is administered to clients with premature ventricular contractions provided that they are not associated with a bradycardic rhythm. Clients who have sustained a cardiac contusion from traumatic injury may also develop cardiac dysrhythmias. For further discussion of dysrhythmia treatment, see Chapter 57.

INCREASE CORONARY ARTERY BLOOD FLOW

An acute myocardial infarction is often caused by an embolus or thrombus that occludes a coronary artery. Initially, nitroglycerin, administered sublingually or intravenously, and morphine sulfate are given to reduce pain and to produce vasodilation of the coronary arteries. Treatment may then involve the administration of oral aspirin, thrombolytic IV medications, and IV heparin or the more invasive procedure of percutaneous transluminal coronary angioplasty (PTCA). Beta-blocker therapy is also instituted in clients who do not have concurrent heart failure or cardiogenic shock.[7, 17]

Clients who have received thrombolytic medications must be continuously monitored for the presence of active bleeding. Other monitoring parameters include pain relief, cardiac rate and rhythm, blood pressure, pulse oximetry readings, and respiratory rate.

REMOVE PERICARDIAL FLUID

Blunt or penetrating force injury to the left chest can cause cardiac tamponade. If this injury is suspected or diagnosed, treatment involves pericardiocentesis (Fig. 82–10). A long spinal needle attached to a 60-ml syringe is inserted beneath the xiphoid into the pericardial sac. The accumulated blood is removed, compression of the ventricles is relieved, and cardiac output is restored.

TREAT INFECTIOUS CAUSES

Infections of the heart structures, such as pericarditis or endocarditis, may be treated with pain-relieving medications and/or antibiotics. Pericarditis is frequently caused by a viral organism, whereas endocarditis is of bacterial origin and requires antibiotic therapy.

PAIN

Pain is the most common complaint of clients seeking emergency care. Pain can be caused by almost any entity; therefore, identifying the source of pain is of paramount importance. The sensation of pain may be the only complaint, or pain may be associated with other clinical evidence of illness or injury. Pain is assessed as described earlier in the chapter.

Outcome Management

PROMOTE COMFORT

Pain relief is the goal of treatment and may be provided by administering oral, intramuscular, or IV analgesic or narcotic medications.[42] With isolated orthopedic injuries, such as digit injuries, pain relief may be obtained by injecting affected nerves with anesthetizing medications.

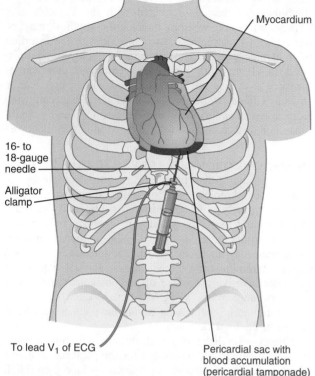

Myocardium

16- to
18-gauge
needle

Alligator
clamp

To lead V₁ of ECG

Pericardial sac with
blood accumulation
(pericardial tamponade)

FIGURE 82–10 Pericardiocentesis procedure. (Modified from Kosmos, C. A. [1995]. In Kitt, S., et al. [Eds.], *Emergency nursing: A physiologic and clinical perspective* [2nd ed., p. 66]. Philadelphia: W. B. Saunders.)

Client comfort measures should also be instituted. Measures may include client positioning to ease stress on painful areas, elevating injured extremities, applying ice or cool compresses to injured areas, and attempting to make the room environment comfortable for the client.

INDUCE CONSCIOUS SEDATION

Instituting conscious sedation is a routine practice in many EDs. This procedure involves controlled pharmacologic depression of the level of consciousness that nevertheless allows maintenance of the client's reflexes to protect the airway as well as spontaneous ventilation.[40] Conscious sedation is most commonly induced with medications such as midazolam (Versed), ketamine (Ketalar), or fentanyl (Sublimaze).[40] Dose and route of administration vary with the agent used. The most common routes are intramuscular (IM), IV, and nasal. The ED nurse's responsibility is to continually monitor the client for airway patency, oxygen saturation levels, cardiac activity, and response to physical or verbal stimulation until recovery from the anesthesia has occurred. The duration of sedation may be anywhere from 30 to 60 minutes. The only two absolute contraindications to conscious sedation are (1) hemodynamic instability and (2) refusal by a competent client or a parent.

ACUTE CONFUSION

Clients can have an altered level of consciousness from many causes. Underlying disorders such as cerebrovascu-

lar accident (CVA), metabolic abnormalities, seizure, intoxication, or injury need to be considered.[37, 38] A helpful guide to use in attempting to determine the cause is the "vowels-TIPS" mnemonic: A, alcohol; E, epilepsy, encephalopathy, endocrine; I, insulin; O, overdose; U, underdose or uremia; T, trauma; I, infection; P, psychogenic; S, stroke or shock.

The normal state of wakefulness and consciousness is controlled by the reticular activating system (RAS) and the brain's cerebral hemispheres. Various factors can produce a decreased state of wakefulness: impairment of the CNS from lesions or hemorrhage; a decreased supply of oxygen, blood, or glucose to cerebral tissues; and exposure to, ingestion of, or withdrawal from substances toxic to cerebral tissue.

Family members or prehospital personnel may be the only sources for obtaining historical information. It is extremely important to determine any known illnesses of the client, current medications, recent injury, known alcohol or drug use, and duration of the client's altered mental state.

Clinical Manifestations

Clinical manifestations vary according to the cause of the client's illness or injury. The Glasgow Coma Scale score is less than 15. Pupil size and equality may be altered. Unequal pupil size and reaction may indicate compression of the third cranial nerve caused by increased intracranial pressure. Small, pinpoint pupils may signify opiate overdose, pontine hemorrhage, cholinesterase poisoning, or recent use of miotic eye drops. Cranial nerve abnormalities and unilateral decreased muscle strength may be present with a recent CVA. Tongue lacerations can indicate recent seizure activity. Pale, cool, clammy skin can occur with shock or hypoglycemia. Fresh needle marks on the skin indicate recent IV drug use. A petechial rash on the skin can be an indication of a lethal bacterial meningitis. Bruising of the face, eyes (raccoon eyes), or mastoid process (Battle's sign) or a bluish hue to the tympanic membrane can indicate recent head injury and an associated basilar skull fracture.[37, 38]

Diagnostic testing involves first obtaining a bedside serum glucose level. Other laboratory studies may be indicated, including serum levels of specific medications, serum and urine toxicology screening tests, CBC, blood cultures, electrolyte panel, arterial blood gas analysis, and urinalysis. Urine specimens should also be tested for the presence of myoglobin, as clients who have been comatose for a prolonged time can develop rhabdomyolysis, resulting from ischemia and damage to large muscle groups. Other diagnostic studies include electrocardiogram (ECG), chest film, and brain CT scan. Occasionally a lumbar puncture may need to be performed.

Outcome Management

ESTABLISH AND MAINTAIN AIRWAY

The first treatment priority in a client with an altered level of consciousness is establishing and maintaining the airway. If required, oral or nasal airway devices should be inserted, or preparations for intubation should be undertaken. During interventions directed at maintaining airway patency, spinal immobilization should also be considered if there is any suspicion that a traumatic injury may have occurred. High-flow oxygen via a face mask must be administered to provide supplemental oxygen to brain tissue.

ESTABLISH VASCULAR ACCESS FOR APPROPRIATE MEDICATIONS

Venous access must be secured for possible IV fluid or medication administration. If a bedside glucose level reading is less than 45 mg/dl, 50% dextrose (D_{50}) is administered intravenously. If the bedside glucose level reading indicates a high level of glucose, therapy should be instituted for treatment of diabetic ketoacidosis or hyperglycemic hyperosmolar nonketotic coma (Chapter 45).

Naloxone (Narcan) 2 to 4 mg intravenously may also be administered. If the cause of the alteration in consciousness is an opiate overdose, naloxone reverses the process.

If a CVA is considered to be the cause of the client's altered level of consciousness, treatment may involve administering an IV thrombolytic medication.[5] The thrombolytic drug can be administered only after the brain CT scan has been obtained and examined by a radiologist to rule out a nonhemorrhage cause of the stroke. Research is currently being conducted on the early administration of brain-protective medications for the treatment of a CVA.[33]

If tonic-clonic seizure activity begins, the client is medicated with diazepam (Valium) 5 to 10 mg intravenously to terminate the seizure. This intervention may need to be followed by IV administration of phenytoin (Dilantin). Phenytoin must be diluted in normal saline solution and infused at a rate of less than 50 mg/minute.

IV antibiotic medications are administered in any client with known or suspected bacterial infection within the brain tissue or cerebrospinal fluid. In clients with bacterial meningitis, this can be a life-saving intervention.

MONITOR INTOXICATED CLIENTS AND TREAT TOXICITY STATES

Intoxicated clients with an altered level of consciousness must be monitored in the ED for a minimum of 4 to 6 hours. Treatment involves IV fluid support and nutritional supplementation with thiamine, multivitamins, and occasionally folic acid. If the level of consciousness does not improve within 4 to 6 hours, a brain CT scan should be done. It is not unusual for these clients to have suffered minor head trauma during their intoxicated state, with subsequent development of a subdural hematoma.

MONITOR CLIENTS WITH HEAD TRAUMA AND TREAT THE INJURIES

Neurologic trauma can result in minor disturbances such as a concussion (Table 82–8). The majority of head-injured clients are released to home without any definitive treatment. Before leaving the ED, the client and or family members must be given instructions on manifestations that indicate worsening of the client's condition.

Other types of neurologic trauma, such as skull fractures, cerebral edema, subdural hematomas, epidural hematomas, and cerebral contusions, may require operative intervention. The client must be closely monitored in the ED for any manifestations of increasing intracranial pressure. Diuretic medications such as mannitol may be ad-

TABLE 82–8	CLASSIFICATION OF CONCUSSION
Grade	Clinical Manifestations
I	No loss of consciousness; transient confusion (lasting a few minutes); rapid return to normal functioning; no amnesia
II	Brief loss of consciousness; mild confusion; some amnesia, usually anterograde
III	Loss of consciousness for less than 6 hours; profound confusion; anterograde and retrograde amnesia
IV	Loss of consciousness for more than 6 hours; confusion; anterograde and retrograde amnesia

ministered intravenously to prevent or diminish cerebral edema.[26]

PREVENT INJURY

Safety is an important issue in a client with an altered level of consciousness. The client may need to be positioned on the left side, and frequent oral suctioning may be necessary. If in place, spinal immobilization must be maintained. Bed side rails must be up and locked in position at all times. Clients are monitored for changes in level of consciousness along with cardiac rate and rhythm, blood pressure, pulse oximetry, and respiratory rates.

SENSORY PERCEPTUAL ALTERATIONS

Altered vision is the most common complaint associated with sensory perceptual changes. Such alterations can be caused by infection, inflammation, or trauma.[18, 37, 38]

Clinical Manifestations

The client may be able to provide information related to the visual changes and the circumstances surrounding the onset of the changes. The affected eye should be assessed for discharge from the eye, excessive tearing, redness of the conjunctiva, presence of a ciliary flush (a ring of inflammation surrounding the corneal-scleral junction), obvious foreign objects, presence of a cloudy cornea, extruded globe contents, and obvious ecchymosis, laceration, or trauma to the eye and surrounding structures. A baseline visual acuity test must be performed in any client with a complaint related to the eye.

Changes in vision can be present with non-urgent conditions such as conjunctivitis. This infection of the conjunctival tissue is highly contagious. Foreign objects or chemicals in the eye, corneal abrasions, and deep structure infections or injury are more significant problems, and the client usually presents with a complaint of pain as well as visual changes.

Outcome Management

Anesthetizing ophthalmic drops can be placed in the affected eye to diminish pain and allow for a more thorough examination of the eye. Superficial conjunctival infections are treated with topical ophthalmic antibiotic drops or ointments. Small superficial foreign objects are removed by the ED physician. For exposure to harmful chemicals, the eye must be irrigated with a minimum of 1 L of normal saline. After irrigation, the pH of the eye is checked; if it has not returned to normal (pH 6 to 7), irrigation may need to be continued. If corneal abrasions are present, the client is given oral pain relief medications and topical ophthalmic antibiotic medication. Patching of the affected eye is not recommended.

More serious problems associated with the eye necessitate an immediate consultation with or referral to an ophthalmologist.[11] These problems include complaints of sudden changes in or loss of vision with or without pain, impaled foreign objects, extensive injury, and globe rupture. Any client who receives treatment from the ED physician for an eye problem should be instructed to be rechecked within 24 hours by his or her primary physician or an ophthalmologist.

INFECTION

Clients frequently present to the ED because of an infectious process. The infection may be caused by either viral or bacterial organisms. The source of the infection may be localized, or the infection may have spread to surrounding tissues or be systemic. It also may be contagious.

Clinical Manifestations

The type of clinical manifestations depends upon the organism causing the infection, the extent of the infection, and the location of the infection.[37, 38] Bacterial infections usually produce more obvious and severe manifestations than those seen in viral infections. With bacterial infections, the client may have a fever. Older adults and neonates frequently have subnormal temperatures with an infectious process. The client may have pain at the site of the infection, such as the ear, throat, abdomen, genitourinary tract, or an area of skin. Meningeal infections can also produce headache, vomiting, neck pain, and occasionally petechiae. Pulmonary infections are frequently accompanied by productive cough and sputum. Erythema, edema, lymphadenopathy, and observable discharge or pus may be present with ear, throat, or skin infections. A skin rash may also be the presenting problem.

A systemic infectious process can lead to septic shock, in which endotoxins from bacterial organisms are released into the circulation. The client is acutely ill and may have clinical manifestations of fever, tachycardia, hypotension, and decreased urinary output. In later stages of sepsis, the client may become hypothermic, the skin may have a mottled appearance, and the level of consciousness becomes diminished.[36] These findings are usually associated with a high mortality rate.

A primary decision must be made about whether the infection is considered contagious to other clients in the ED. If the infection is thought to be contagious, the client must be isolated as quickly as possible from other clients. It then becomes important to identify the primary source of the infection. The ears, throat, lungs, skin, and genital and pelvic areas must be assessed for evidence of infec-

tion. A chest film is obtained, in addition to possible abdominal and pelvic ultrasound studies. Laboratory studies include a urinalysis, CBC, and culture of discharge and blood specimens. If the source of the infection has not been identified, a lumbar puncture may be required.

Outcome Management

ADMINISTER MEDICATIONS

Treatment involves administering antibiotic medications selected according to the identified or probable source of the infection. These agents may be administered orally, intramuscularly, or intravenously. The antipyretic medications acetaminophen (Tylenol) and ibuprofen can be administered orally to reduce fever. Other treatments to reduce fever involve undressing the client and allowing heat to dissipate into the environment. Cooling the client using tepid bath water is not routinely performed. Abscesses due to skin infections may need to be incised, drained, and packed.

MONITOR AND TREAT SEPSIS

If sepsis is suspected, it is important to also administer high-flow oxygen to the client, infuse IV fluids of normal saline, and insert a nasogastric tube and an indwelling urinary catheter. Additional infused medications, after antibiotic administration, may include dopamine and corticosteroids. The client must be closely monitored for changes in blood pressure, heart rate, respiratory rate, oxygen saturation, cardiac rhythm, urinary output, level of conscious changes, and prolonged bleeding times. These clients are at risk for disseminated intravascular coagulopathy (DIC).

IMPAIRED PHYSICAL MOBILITY

Any injury to the musculoskeletal system can lead to a decrease in the client's mobility.[32] Other causes of impaired mobility are injuries to the vertebral bodies and possibly the spinal cord. Sprains of ligaments, fractures to bones, dislocated joints, muscle strains, and amputated extremities or digits are the majority of problems for which clients seek emergency care related to mobility deficits.

Spinal cord injury can involve edema of the cord, with transitory or minimal deficits; cord edema can be marked; or the cord can actually be severed. With marked edema or cord severance, deficits are usually devastating and permanent. Neurogenic shock can develop with loss of the sympathetic component of the autonomic nervous system. With only the parasympathetic nervous system functioning, massive vasodilation occurs, and tissue perfusion is decreased.

Clinical Manifestations

Clinical manifestations with the majority of musculoskeletal injuries include swelling around the injured area, presence of ecchymosis, obvious deformity of the area, palpable tenderness, and limited movement of the area. Amputations are self-evident, and depending upon whether a complete or partial amputation has occurred, active bleeding may be minimal or profuse. With a complete amputation, active bleeding is minimal as a result of constriction of the severed vessels. It is important that the ED nurse assess the effectiveness of circulation, motor movement, and presence and degree of sensation distal to any musculoskeletal injury.

An injury to the spinal cord produces either or both motor and sensory deficits below the level of injury. If the injury is in the upper thoracic or cervical area, the diaphragm and thoracic intercostal muscles can be affected, leading to respiratory compromise.[22, 37, 38] A client with neurogenic shock has warm and dry skin, hypotension, and bradycardia, with no movement or sensation below the level of injury.

Radiographic films of the injured area are obtained to aid in identifying fractures. Depending upon the extent of the injury, additional laboratory tests or other diagnostic studies may be performed.

Outcome Management

TREAT SPRAINS, STRAINS, AND FRACTURES

Treatment of extremity sprains and fractures consists of immediately elevating the extremity above the level of the client's heart, applying ice to the area, and immobilizing the extremity with pillows or cardboard splints.[22] Oral, intramuscular, or IV pain medication may also need to be administered. More definitive immobilization of the area with the application of splints, molds, or immobilizers is accomplished before the client leaves the ED. Lower extremity injuries may require the client to use crutches. Detailed crutch-walking instructions must be provided (Table 82–9), and the client should be able to demonstrate adequate use of the crutches to the ED nurse.

Pain-relieving medication is also administered to clients with muscle strains.[21, 27] Once clients achieve relief of pain, they are usually discharged to home with instructions to rest and to apply alternating ice and heat to the injured area for the next 24 hours.[21]

REDUCE DISLOCATIONS

A joint dislocation requires reduction in the ED. This procedure is performed by the ED physician. Pain-reliev-

TABLE 82–9	CRUTCH-WALKING INSTRUCTIONS

1. Measure for correct size of crutches—with client standing, measure from 3.75–5.0 cm below the axillary fold to a point on the floor 10 cm in front of the client and 15 cm lateral to the small toe.
2. With client standing, shoulders and back are straight, elbows flexed at 30 degrees, wrists extended, and hands dorsiflexed. Do not bear weight on axilla.
3. Three-point gait sequence involves movement of the weaker leg with both crutches simultaneously.
4. To go down stairs, place crutches on affected side, place weight on unaffected leg, place crutches on next lower step, and bring unaffected leg down to share the work of lowering the body with the support of the crutches.
5. To walk up stairs, place crutches on affected side a half-step width from the lowest step, place weight on hands, and lift the stronger leg to the step.

From Kitt S., et al. (Eds.). (1995). *Emergency nursing: A physiologic and clinical perspective* (2nd ed.). Philadelphia: W. B. Saunders.

ing and muscle-relaxant medications may need to be administered before the reduction procedure. Once joint reduction has been achieved, a post-reduction radiographic film must be obtained. After successful reduction, the joint is immobilized with the required orthopedic device.

TREAT AMPUTATION

The goal in the management of a client who has sustained an amputation is to attempt to salvage the part so that possible replantation can occur.[21, 37, 38] Any profuse bleeding from the stump should be controlled with direct pressure. The use of tourniquets and clamps is discouraged, as these measures can further damage the injured tissue. If the client has sustained significant blood loss, high-flow oxygen is administered, venous access is established, and replacement fluids are given.

The stump is then gently cleansed with normal saline. The amputated part is wrapped in sterile gauze moistened with normal saline. It is then placed in a plastic bag or container, and the plastic bag or container is placed on ice. The amputated part should *never* be placed directly on ice, as freezing of the tissues will result, making replantation impossible. The client is given pain-relieving medications and possible tetanus prophylaxis with tetanus and diphtheria toxoids (Td) 0.5 ml if more than 5 years have elapsed since the last tetanus immunization.

TREAT SPINAL CORD INJURY

Clients with a spinal cord injury must be maintained in complete spinal immobilization. At a minimum, a cross-table lateral cervical spine radiograph is required, and this study may be followed by more extensive spinal films or a CT scan. When a high thoracic or cervical injury is present, the client may become fatigued with the effort of maintaining respirations. The need for nasal intubation and assisted ventilation must be considered. IV fluids are necessary to maintain perfusion. Administration of high-dose IV steroids such as methylprednisolone (Solu-Medrol), 30 mg/kg over 15 minutes and then 5.4 mg/kg by infusion over the following 23 hours, may be considered to reduce cord edema.[23, 40, 41] IV administration of high-dose dopamine to counteract parasympathetic nervous system effects is another treatment consideration. This therapy, however, must be instituted cautiously, as the vasoconstrictive effect may decrease perfusion to the injured cord. A nasogastric tube and indwelling urinary catheter are inserted.

The client must be kept warm with blankets and heating lights as necessary, because often the ability to regulate internal body temperature has been lost. Stabilization of cervical fractures may involve applying Gardner-Wells tongs with traction or a halo traction device. Monitoring of body temperature, cardiac rate and rhythm, blood pressure, respiratory rate and effort, pulse oximetry, urinary output, and changes in sensory and motor movement is vital.

IMPAIRED SKIN INTEGRITY

Skin and soft tissue injury is a common problem encountered in the ED. Injury to the skin and surrounding soft tissue can occur from sharp objects, blunt force injury, scraping mechanisms, or bites resulting in lacerations, contusions, abrasions, avulsions, or puncture wounds.[37, 38]

Clinical Manifestations

Once the skin barrier has been interrupted, the potential for infection is increased. Skin flora and other bacteria now have access to the underlying structures. After injury to the skin, natural, or secondary, healing processes occur, resulting in skin closure and scarring. Primary closure, or suturing, of skin wounds also closes the skin and reduces the amount of scarring. Wounds caused by forces in which bacteria were deeply embedded in the tissues, or that are older than approximately 12 hours, are not routinely managed by primary closure. Diagnostic tests may involve radiographic films of the wound area. Such studies are important if there is any suspicion that a foreign object may be embedded in the wound.

Outcome Management

Skin and soft tissue wounds can occur anywhere on the body. Scalp and facial lacerations often bleed profusely because of the high vascularity of these areas. Direct pressure over the wound is usually sufficient to control bleeding.

CLEANSE THE WOUND

Cleansing of wounds is best achieved using high-pressure irrigation and normal saline solution. Directing the stream flow from a 20- to 30-ml syringe directly into the wound adequately cleanses most wounds.[39] A minimum of 100 ml of solution should be used. Shaving an area around a wound to remove hair is controversial. In most instances, shaving is not necessary and absolutely should NEVER be performed on a wound located in a client's eyebrow.

Open wounds often need to be anesthetized before cleansing and most definitely must be anesthetized before primary repair is attempted. A cotton ball can be saturated with a topical solution of tetracaine-adrenaline-cocaine (TAC) or lidocaine-epinephrine-tetracaine (LET) and then applied directly to a face or scalp wound, so long as it is not used near mucous membranes. Other anesthetic agents include lidocaine 1% or 2%, with or without epinephrine, and bupivacaine (Marcaine) 0.25% or 0.5%, with or without epinephrine. Anesthetic agents with epinephrine should never be injected into wounds located on the fingers, toes, ears, nose, or penis because of the vasoconstricting effects of epinephrine. Bupivacaine provides a longer anesthetic effect than that obtained with lidocaine.

CLOSE THE WOUND

Small, superficial wounds may be closed with adhesive paper strips or Dermabond glue. It is important to evert and bring the wound edges close together and then apply the paper strips or glue.[39]

Larger wounds that are gaping, involve injury to deeper structures, and are located in high-tension areas or over joints need to be sutured for optimal healing. The type of suture material required varies depending upon the size and location of the open wound (Table 82-10).

Abrasion injuries are not sutured. Abrasion injuries need to be thoroughly cleansed in order to remove any particles or debris left in the wound. If particles do remain in the wound, a tattooing effect results with the healing process. Human and animal bites are not routinely sutured because of the highly contaminated nature of the

TABLE 82-10	SUTURE MATERIAL
Suture Size	**Indicated Use: Body Area(s)**
2-0, 3-0	Tissue subjected to strong tensile forces (e.g., knees, elbows, over joints)
3-0, 4-0	Epidermal and dermal layers, except for face
5-0, 6-0	Facial area

wound. The wound is thoroughly irrigated, and prophylactic antibiotic medications are frequently administered. Animal bites should be reported to the local animal control authorities.

APPLY A DRESSING

Protective dressings must be applied to wounds before the client leaves the ED. The majority of dressings involve first applying a thin layer of antibacterial ointment or gauze impregnated with petrolatum (Vaseline) or other occlusive substance. Then dry, sterile gauze is applied for padding, followed by a wrap of woven gauze (Kling or Kerlix). Adhesive tape is used to hold the dressing in place.

ADMINISTER TETANUS AND RABIES PROPHYLAXIS

Clients must be questioned about their tetanus immunization status. Table 82-11 presents current recommendations for tetanus prophylaxis. Td 0.5 ml is the preferred agent for active immunization in adults. Should passive immunization be necessary, human tetanus immune globulin (TIG) 250 units is administered. If both preparations must be administered, separate sites for injection should be selected.

Rabies prophylaxis should be considered in clients who have been bitten by dogs, cats, skunks, raccoons, bats, squirrels, or opossums, even though the incidence of rabies is low in the United States.[16] Prophylaxis is especially important if the animal cannot be located and placed under quarantine for an observation period. The

TABLE 82-11	TETANUS PROPHYLAXIS IN WOUND MANAGEMENT			
Immunization History (No. of Doses)	**Clean Minor Wounds**		**All Other Wounds**	
	Td*	**TIG†**	**Td**	**TIG**
Uncertain	Yes	No	Yes	Yes
0-2	Yes	No	Yes	Yes
3 or more	No (Yes, if >10 yr since last dose)	No	No (Yes, if >5 yr since last dose)	No

Modified from Centers for Disease Control and Prevention: *MMWR Morbidity and Mortality Weekly Report*, 1989-1990.

*Td, tetanus and diphtheria toxoids: used for persons 7 years of age or older. For children younger than 7 years, diphtheria-pertussis-tetanus (DPT).

† TIG, tetanus immune globulin (Hypertet).

dose of human rabies immune globulin (RIG) for passive immunization is 20 units/kg, with as much as possible injected into and around the wound site and the remainder of the dose injected intramuscularly in the buttocks. For active immunization with human diploid cell vaccine (HDCV), the dose is 1 ml initially and again on days 3, 7, 14, and 28 following the bite incident.

INSTRUCT ON WOUND CARE

Instructions related to the care of the wound are given to the client and/or family member before they leave the ED. These instructions should identify the manifestations of infection and explain care of the wound and timing for a follow-up appointment with the appropriate physician for a recheck of the wound and for another appointment for removal of sutures.

POISONING

◼ ACCIDENTAL AND INTENTIONAL POISONINGS

Poisonings are either accidental or intentional. Accidental poisonings occur more commonly in the pediatric age group, whereas intentional poisonings are more frequent in the adolescent and adult population. Poisoning can also occur from injected venom, such as snake or insect bites.

Obtaining accurate information about the offending substance, amount, and time of ingestion or exposure can be difficult. Details may be available from family or friends. Other important information to obtain is whether the client has vomited since the exposure, whether the client has been depressed or had any previous episodes of intentional poisoning, and any other associated details.

Clinical Manifestations

Assessment must be directed toward the intactness of the client's ABCs (airway, breathing, and circulation). There may be very few outward clinical manifestations that aid in determining the substance that was was ingested, inhaled, or injected.

Diagnostic tests may include electrocardiography and continual cardiac monitoring. Blood and urine specimens need to be obtained for toxicology screening and testing. In many cases the results of these tests are not rapidly available. Chest films may aid in diagnosing possible aspiration. If envenomation is the source of poisoning, bleeding and coagulation studies must be performed.

Outcome Management

MAINTAIN AIRWAY

If the client demonstrates a decrease in level of consciousness, initial interventions include establishing and maintaining a patent airway, possibly with airway adjunct devices. Oxygen should be administered, and venous access should be obtained.

REMOVE OFFENDING SUBSTANCE

Treatment is directed at removing or absorbing the offending substance. If the substance was injected, naloxone 2 to 4 mg may be administered intravenously. If the client's level of consciousness is decreased and the substance was ingested, a large nasogastric (Ewald) tube is passed either nasally or orally and gastric lavage performed. This procedure involves instilling approximately 250–500 ml normal saline solution through the tube and then removing the solution either with a syringe or gravity drainage into a collection bag. This process is repeated until the returned contents are clear. Then liquid-activated charcoal and a cathartic are instilled through the Ewald tube and allowed to remain in the stomach. The charcoal aids in absorbing any other remaining particles of the toxic substance.

Awake and alert clients are given liquid-activated charcoal to drink. Occasionally, the charcoal slurry may cause the client to vomit, and an additional dose of the charcoal may be required. The purpose of activated charcoal is again to quickly absorb the ingested toxic substance to minimize its harmful effects. Syrup of ipecac is not routinely administered[3]; it is not effective in removing the toxic substance, unless the ingestion has occurred within the previous 30 minutes, as its emetic effect prolongs the time until activated charcoal can be administered. Clients who have ingested an alkaline-based substance are not given syrup of ipecac, charcoal, or any substance that can cause emesis.

If a specific toxic substance exposure is known and an antidote is available, the antidote is administered. Table 82–12 provides a list of the more common poisoning substances and antidotes.

TABLE 82–12	POISONINGS AND ANTIDOTES
Toxic Substance	**Treatment**
Beta-blocker medications	Treat hypotension initially with fluids; if unsuccessful, administer glucagon 100–150 μg/kg IV followed by 2–5 mg/hr by infusion
Calcium channel-blocker medications	Calcium chloride 5–10 ml IV, or calcium gluconate 10–20 ml IV
Carbon monoxide	100% oxygen; possibly use of hyperbaric chamber
Iron	Deferoxamine (Desferal) 80 mg/kg IV or IM and repeated q 8 hr
Isoniazid (INH)	Pyridoxine (vitamin B$_6$) IV in a dose equivalent to amount ingested (gram for gram); if ingested amount is unknown, administer 5 g IV over 3–5 min, then repeat q 3–5 min until seizures are controlled
Methanol, ethylene glycol	50% ethanol 0.7 g/kg, or 7 ml/kg of 10% ethanol IV; continuous IV infusion of 0.07 to 0.1 g/kg/hr to maintain blood ethanol concentration between 100 and 200 mg/dl
Phenothiazine medications	Diphenhydramine (Benadryl) 0.5–1 mg/kg IV or benztropine (Cogentin) 1–2 mg IM

PROVIDE PSYCHIATRIC EVALUATION AS NEEDED

Any client who is in the ED because of an intentional poisoning must have a psychiatric evaluation before discharge and release from the ED. Many communities have psychiatric evaluation teams (PETs) that provide this service.

■ SNAKE BITE

Snake antivenin is available for clients who have been envenomated by a pit viper (a poisonous snake). The area of the envenomation may be swollen and ecchymotic, and pain may be present at the site. Pit viper venom produces both proteolytic and hemotoxic effects. Massive swelling producing a compartment syndrome may develop, and a coagulation disorder such as DIC may result. The wound area should be gently cleansed. Ice should not be applied to reduce swelling. Antivenin is administered intravenously, but skin or conjunctival testing must be performed before administering the antivenin.[10]

HYPERTHERMIA

Hyperthermic emergencies are usually the result of environmental exposure. The geriatric population is at the greatest risk for developing hyperthermia. The types of hyperthermic problems are heat cramps, heat exhaustion, and heat stroke.[37, 38] Heat stroke is the most severe.

Clinical Manifestations

Muscle spasms of the arms and legs are evident with heat cramps. Often there is a depletion of sodium because the client has been perspiring excessively. Excessive sweating can lead to dehydration and heat exhaustion. The client may complain of headache, dizziness, nausea, and weakness. Mild hypotension can be present, and the skin is frequently cool and clammy to the touch.

Heat stroke is an emergent condition. The client is often comatose. Other clinical manifestations include hypotension, tachycardia, hot and flushed-appearing skin, and a core temperature of greater than 105° F (40.5° C).

Outcome Management

ADMINISTER FLUIDS AND ELECTROLYTES

For the client with mild heat cramps, administering oral fluids with electrolytes and removal from the hot environment are usually the only necessary treatments. Treatment of a client with heat exhaustion also involves removal from the hot environment and administering either oral or IV fluids to correct the problem.

RESOLVE HEAT STROKE

Heat stroke treatment involves establishing and maintaining a patent airway, administering high-flow oxygen, and establishing venous access. IV normal saline is administered to restore fluid volume. Cooling measures must be instituted quickly. These measures include removing all clothing from the client; spraying tepid mist over the client's body and using a fan to increase air flow; placing ice packs on the scalp and neck and in the axillae and groin; and using a cooling blanket. Gastric lavage with cool saline and peritoneal dialysis may be necessary.

Cooling measures should continue until the client's body temperature is 101° F (38.4° C).[37, 38] As the temperature decreases, administering chlorpromazine (Thorazine) or diazepam (Valium) may be required to reduce shivering.

A nasogastric tube and indwelling urinary catheter must be inserted. Continual cardiac, pulse oximetry, blood pressure, respiratory rate, and temperature monitoring are performed.

HYPOTHERMIA

Clinical Manifestations

A body temperature of below 94° F (34.4° C) indicates the condition of hypothermia. The development of hypothermia is usually unintentional and involves accidental and prolonged exposure to cold temperatures.

Hypothermia severity can be divided into stages depending upon the client's core temperature. Different clinical manifestations are present with each stage (see Table 82–13).

Outcome Management

REWARM THE CLIENT

After the establishment and maintenance of a patent airway, heated high-flow oxygen administration, and venous access with warmed fluid replacement, treatment is then directed at rewarming the client. Rewarming must be done slowly, as the hypothermic client is especially prone to the development of ventricular fibrillation and cardiovascular collapse if blood is returned too rapidly to a cold heart. Rewarming methods include the following[37, 38]:

1. *Passive warming*
   a. Removing wet clothing
   b. Covering the client with warm blankets
   c. Placing the client in a warm room

TABLE 82–13	STAGES OF HYPOTHERMIA
Stage	Clinical Manifestations
Mild: 93° to 95° F (34.0°–35° C)	Person is conscious and alert but may have lethargy and confusion Shivering Bradycardia or tachycardia
Moderate: 86° to 93° F (30°–34° C)	Decreased level of consciousness or coma Hypoventilation Bradycardia Atrial fibrillation Hypovolemia Cessation of shivering Possible hyperglycemia due to underutilization of glucose
Severe: <86° F (<30° C)	Coma Fixed and dilated pupils Bradycardia Apnea Hypotension Ventricular fibrillation Asystole

2. *Active warming*
   a. Immersing the client in a warm bath (104° F [40° C])
   b. Placing the client on a warming blanket
   c. Placing radiant lamps over the client
3. *Active core warming*
   a. Infusing warmed IV fluids
   b. Providing heated, humidified supplemental oxygen
   c. Performing warm fluid lavage (peritoneal, gastric, bladder, or colonic lavage)
   d. Performing continuous arteriovenous rewarming (CAVR), hemodialysis, or cardiopulmonary bypass

Insertion of a nasogastric tube and indwelling urinary catheter is an additional component of care. Continual cardiac, pulse oximetry, blood pressure, respiratory rate, and temperature monitoring must be instituted.

■ FROSTBITE

Hypothermia to the extremities can lead to frostbite injury. The feet, hands, nose, ears, and cheeks are most commonly affected.[37, 38] Damage to the tissues occurs, and peripheral blood flow is reduced. The area may appear red and swollen or may be pale in color. Formation of blisters containing either clear or purple bloody fluid may be seen. Rewarming of the frostbitten area should begin once the client is removed from the cold environment. The frostbitten part should be immersed in heated water at 105° to 115° F (40.6° to 46.1° C). The frostbitten area needs to be handled gently so that blood-filled blisters remain intact. Loose, sterile, bulky dressings are then applied and changed daily. The rewarming process is painful; therefore, pain-relieving medications must be administered.

INEFFECTIVE INDIVIDUAL COPING

Clients present to the ED not only with medical and traumatically induced problems but with psychological issues as well. Psychological disorders can range from mild anxiety to psychosis to deep depression. It is important that clients with psychological problems be taken as seriously as clients seeking treatment for medical problems.

A brief mental status examination needs to be conducted to assess the client's behavior, speech patterns, mood and affect, thought processes, and judgment and insight. Has the client recently experienced a crisis-producing situation? Is the client experiencing auditory or visual hallucinations? A physical examination must be performed to identify any concurrent medical condition that may be compounding the problem.

It is important to communicate with the client in a calm, nonjudgmental, and accepting manner. Focusing the client on reality and explaining expected behaviors constitute part of the therapeutic communication process. In some cases, involuntary psychiatric hospitalization may be required. Should the client be discharged from the ED, providing outside agency assistance and referral can be helpful.

CONCLUSIONS

Providing care to clients in the ED setting can be challenging and rewarding. An understanding of the principles of emergency care is the cornerstone of the specialty of emergency nursing. The majority of clients present to the ED without a working diagnosis but only a cadre of clinical manifestations. Therefore, assessing each client using an organized approach is paramount for the ED nurse in order to be able to establish care priorities and to institute appropriate interventions. The nursing process from assessment to evaluation is continually utilized. The scope of ED nursing is constantly changing and expanding beyond the hospital walls into the areas of community practice and community education.

THINKING CRITICALLY

1. **A 23-year-old man walks into the emergency department. He tells you that he was in a motor vehicle accident about 4 hours ago. The police were at the scene, but he refused to be transported to the emergency department because he felt fine; he went home. At home, however, the client started to experience worsening shoulder and posterior neck pain. His mother urged him to come to the emergency department. He tells you that he has "numbness" in his fingers and a "tingling" feeling in his right elbow. If you were the triage nurse, what potential problems would you consider that this client might have? Would you classify the client as emergent, urgent, or nonurgent? What measures should you take to ensure the client's safety?**

Factors to Consider. What injuries sustained in a motor vehicle accident might account for the client's manifestations?

2. **A 35-year-old man was brought in to the emergency department by the city police, who were arresting him for drunk and disorderly conduct. He had been involved in a barroom brawl, during which he acquired several small lacerations about the face and arms from broken glass, a hit to the head, and kicks to his ribs. He is conscious, verbally abusive, and threatening to fight his way out of the emergency department because he wants "to go home and be left alone." He has twice threatened you with bodily harm if you persist in preventing him from leaving. How would you proceed with this case?**

Factors to Consider. Whom should you call? Would it be appropriate to sedate this client? What should you do if the client actually harms you physically?

3. **A 60-year-old man has arrived at the emergency department with a complaint of headache. He states that he never had headaches until about 2 weeks ago, when he began awakening in the morning with head pain. The headache would go away each day after he had been up and around for a few hours and had taken aspirin. In the last few days, however, neither aspirin nor acetaminophen has helped and the headache has become nearly continuous. His wife states that his speech and balance have been "off" a little. He**

wonders whether there can be any connection between his headaches and a recent fall or a recent elevation in blood pressure. Describe how you would proceed with an evaluation of this client. What further information should you elicit from him? What is your assessment priority? What triage classification would be best for this client? What interventions should you anticipate?

Factors to Consider. What diagnostic assessments should you anticipate? What should you include in your physical examination and nursing history?

4. The client, a 70-year-old man, has been brought to the emergency department by ambulance. His wife states that he has become increasingly confused over the past few months. Within the past few days, he has become worse, is difficult to awaken in the morning, and is "sleepy" all day. This situation progressed until today, when the client's wife could not keep him awake at all; she called an ambulance and had him brought in. The client has a long history of hypertension, coronary artery disease, diabetes mellitus, and depression. Ambulance records show evidence that the client is difficult to arouse, but upon aggressive stimulation he "wakes up" and can follow basic commands. His vital signs are stable, but his pulse is slow and irregular. Blood pressure is now lower than his "norm." His wife has brought his medications with her in a large paper bag. What is your priority assessment? What should you include in your physical assessment? What interventions should you anticipate?

Factors to Consider. What body systems should you assess? What diagnostic studies should you anticipate?

BIBLIOGRAPHY

1. Andrews, M., Goldberg, K., & Kaplan, H. (1996). *Nurses' legal handbook* (3rd ed.). Springhouse, PA: Springhouse Corporation.
2. Baier, F. E. (1993). Implications of the Consolidated Omnibus Budget Reconciliation "antidumping" legislation for emergency nurses. *Journal of Emergency Nursing, 19*(2), 115–120.
3. Bartscherer, D. J. (1997). Syrup of ipecac: Appropriate use in the emergency Department. *Journal of Emergency Nursing, 23*(3), 251–253.
4. Belanger, M. A., & Reed, S. (1997). A rural community hospital's experience with family-witnessed resuscitation. *Journal of Emergency Nursing, 23*(3), 238–239.
5. Bethel, S. A. (1997). Intravenous thrombolytic therapy for stroke emergencies. *Journal of Emergency Nursing, 23*(4), 344–346.
6. Brucker, J. M. (1998). Respiratory syncytial virus. *ADVANCE for Nurse Practitioners, 6*(2), 61–65.
7. Buhse, M. (1998). Quick thinking needed: Early management of acute myocardial infarction. *ADVANCE for Nurse Practitioners, 6*(8), 29–35.
8. Coakley-Maller, C., & Shea, M. (1997). Respiratory infections in children. *ADVANCE for Nurse Practitioners, 5*(9), 21–27.
9. Cornell, S. (1998). Advance directives: Whose death is it, anyway? *ADVANCE for Nurse Practitioners, 6*(7), 68–70.
10. Deer, P. J. (1997). Elapid envenomation: A medical emergency. *Journal of Emergency Nursing, 23*(6), 574–577.
11. DelGross, C., & Smally A. J. (1997). A 24-year-old male with eye trauma. *Clinical Reviews, 7*(10), 142–144.
12. Dronen, S. C. (1998). Pharmacologic adjuncts to intubation. In J. R. Roberts & J. R. Hedges (Eds.), *Clinical procedures in emergency medicine* (3rd ed.). Philadelphia: W. B. Saunders.
13. Emergency Nurses Association (1999). In J. Dains, et al. (Eds.), *Standards of emergency nursing practice* (4th ed., pp. 59–64). St. Louis: Mosby–Year Book.
14. Frakes, M. A. (1997). Asthma in the emergency department. *Journal of Emergency Nursing, 23*(5), 429–435.
15. Gerchufsky, M. (1996). Collaring a killer: What you need to know about rabies. *ADVANCE for Nurse Practitioners, 4*(9), 49–52
16. Dambro, M. R., & Griffith, J. A. (1996, September). Griffith's 5-minute clinical consult: Congestive heart failure. *Clinical Reviews,* 138–139.
17. Hahn, M. S. (1995). Matters of the heart. *ADVANCE for Nurse Practitioners, 3*(9), 13–17.
18. Hahn, M. S. (1996). Common eye problems in primary care. *ADVANCE for Nurse Practitioners, 4*(3), 27–31.
19. Harrahill, M. (1998). Flail chest: A nursing challenge. *Journal of Emergency Nursing, 24*(3), 288–289.
20. Higgins, B., & Barrow, S. (1998). Asthma in adolescents. *ADVANCE for Nurse Practitioners, 6*(2), 28–37.
21. Jagmin, M. G. (1995). Musculoskeletal emergencies. In S. Kitt, et al. (Eds.), *Emergency nursing: A physiologic and clinical perspective* (2nd ed.). Philadelphia: W. B. Saunders.
22. Jaworski, M. A. (1995). Spinal trauma. In S. Kitt, et al. (Eds.), *Emergency nursing: A physiologic and clinical perspective* (2nd ed.). Philadelphia: W. B. Saunders.
23. Jezierski, M. (1993). Foote Hospital Emergency Department: Shattering a paradigm. *Journal of Emergency Nursing, 19*(3), 266–267.
24. Keep, N., et al. (1992). California Emergency Nurses Association's informal survey of violence in California emergency departments. *Journal of Emergency Nursing, 18*(5), 433–439.
25. Kosmos, C. A. (1995). Multiple trauma. In S. Kitt, et al. (Eds.), *Emergency nursing: A physiologic and clinical perspective* (2nd ed). Philadelphia: W. B. Saunders.
26. Leccese, C. (1997). Reducing the toll of brain injury: New guidelines offer principles for intervention. *ADVANCE for Nurse Practitioners, 5*(6), 57–60.
27. McIntosh, E. (1997). Low back pain in adults. Guidelines for the history and physical exam. *ADVANCE for Nurse Practitioners, 5*(8), 16–25.
28. Maller, C. C. (1995). Adult asthma management: All things considered. *ADVANCE for Nurse Practitioners, 3*(9), 20–26.
29. Mathias, S., & Hodgdon, A. K. (1997). Resurgence of tuberculosis: Implications for emergency nurses. *Journal of Emergency Nursing, 23*(5), 425–428.
30. Miller, S. K. (1997). Congestive heart failure: Clinical assessment and pharmacologic management. *ADVANCE for Nurse Practitioners, 5*(6), 17–27.
31. Murdock, M. A., & Roberson, M. L. (1993). Reported use of autotransfusion systems in initial resuscitation areas by one hundred thirty-six United States hospitals. *Journal of Emergency Nursing, 19*(6), 486–490.
32. O'Hanlon-Nichols, T. (1998). A review of the adult musculoskeletal system. *American Journal of Nursing, 98*(6), 48–52.
33. Richman, E. (1996). Acute stroke interventions: Proactive strategies to preserve brain tissue. *ADVANCE for Nurse Practitioners, 4*(4), 79–97.
34. Reynolds, J. E. (1997). Noninvasive ventilation for acute respiratory failure. *Journal of Emergency Nursing, 23*(6), 608–610.
35. Sarnese, P. M. (1997). Assessing security in the emergency department: An overview. *Journal of Emergency Nursing, 23*(1), 23–26.
36. Selfridge-Thomas, J. (1995). Shock. In S. Kitt, et al. (Eds.), *Emergency nursing: A physiologic and clinical perspective* (2nd ed.). Philadelphia: W. B. Saunders.
37. Selfridge-Thomas, J. (1997). *Emergency nursing: An essential guide for patient care.* Philadelphia: W. B. Saunders.
38. Selfridge-Thomas, J. (1995). *Manual of emergency nursing.* Philadelphia: W. B. Saunders.
39. Walters, G. K. (1996). Managing soft tissue wounds: Caveats for everyday practice. *ADVANCE for Nurse Practitioners, 4*(3), 37–54.
40. Ward, K. R., & Yealy, D. M. (1998). Systemic analgesia and sedation for procedures. In J. R. Roberts & J. R. Hedges (Eds.), *Clinical procedures in emergency medicine* (4th ed.). Philadelphia: W. B. Saunders.
41. Williams, R. M. (1997). Are emergency departments really the most expensive place of all? *Journal of Emergency Nursing, 23*(4), 292–294.
42. Winslow, E. H. (1998). Effective pain management. *American Journal of Nursing, 98*(7), 16HH–16II.
43. Zielinski, S., Pavey, S., & Dunham, S. (1998). Dobutamine stress echocardiogram: Emergency department evaluation of chest pain. *Journal of Emergency Nursing, 24*(3), 240–246.

Fever-Related Interventions

QUESTIONS

When are interventions to control fever most beneficial to a critically ill client?
How is fever most effectively managed in the critically ill?

CITATION

Henker, R. (1999). Evidence-based practice: Fever-related interventions. *American Journal of Critical Care, 8*, 481–487.

STUDIES

Approximately 30 research reports from biologic, critical care, nursing, and medical journals were reviewed and integrated. Four animal studies were included. The method of assembling the studies was not described, and tables summarizing the studies cited were not provided. The author rated the strength of the evidence for each recommendation using the levels of the American Association of Critical-Care Nurses (AACN) Research-Based Practice Protocols.*

Summary of Findings

When Should Fever Be Treated in the Critically Ill?
(p. 481)

Physiologic Responses Associated with Fever (p. 482)

Four animal studies demonstrating that fever is a beneficial host defense response were cited. Although fever may be beneficial to survival, in treating humans other factors such as the client's comfort and demands that fever makes on cardiopulmonary physiology must be considered. Fever, possibly in association with bacterial endotoxins, causes increased oxygen consumption, heart rate, serum levels of norepinephrine and epinephrine, and cardiac output.[23, 28] In a clinical study,[2] the heart rate of critically ill patients with temperatures greater than 37.8° C (100° F) was significantly higher than those with temperatures less than that level (average of 111 beats per minute for the first group, 94 for the latter).

Elevated Body Temperature in Clients with Head Injuries
(p. 483)

The use of moderate hypothermia for treatment of clients with traumatic brain injury may improve outcomes. Two studies have found that hypothermia decreased intracranial pressure (ICP),[17, 25] and three studies found that clients treated with hypothermia had higher Glasgow Coma Scale scores.[6, 16, 17] Two studies indicated that in patients with head injuries the brain temperature tends to be higher than the core temperature.[9, 24]

Fever in Clients with Sepsis (p. 483)

Studies of the effects of fever in clients with sepsis are difficult to interpret because of the multiple factors that can affect out-

comes. However, these clients are an interesting group to study because altered thermoregulation causes some of them to be hypothermic and others to be febrile. In a study of 500 clients with bacteremia or fungemia, the survival rate of 405 in whom fever developed was higher than in the relatively hypothermic clients.[29] In a large clinical trial,[5] the 9% of the septic population with hypothermia had a much worse prognosis than the febrile clients with sepsis. Compared with febrile clients, hypothermic clients had a higher incidence of central nervous system (CNS) dysfunction, shock, clotting abnormalities, inability to recover from shock, and death. The authors concluded that hypothermia associated with sepsis syndrome is related to poor clinical outcomes. In a randomized, double-blind clinical trial of 455 clients, treating sepsis with ibuprofen decreased fever, tachycardia, oxygen consumption, and lactic acidosis but did not reduce the incidence or duration of shock or respiratory distress syndrome, nor did this treatment improve survival.[1]

How Is Fever Most Effectively Treated in the Critically Ill?

Clinical Comparison of Antipyretic Agents and Physical Cooling

Antipyretic agents, tepid sponging, iced cloths, and cooling blankets are often used to reduce fever. Two important issues of concern when these interventions are used are the effect on core body temperature and the associated cardiovascular responses. In a study of 21 clients with neurologic dysfunction, these three methods were compared in terms of time required to return to 100° F and shivering.[19] No difference was found in the time required; however, the small size of each group may have made a difference impossible to detect even if it existed. Clients cooled by acetaminophen and a hypothermia blanket demonstrated significantly more shivering compared with clients cooled by acetaminophen alone or by acetaminophen and sponging. Another small study of 14 patients[10] compared acetaminophen alone (n = 5), acetaminophen and cooling blanket (n = 3), and cooling blanket alone (n = 6); after 3 hours, the mean pulmonary artery temperature of the first group increased 0.2 of a degree, whereas it decreased on average 0.4 and 0.3 of a degree in the other two groups. These were the only studies found by the reviewer comparing treatments of fever in critically ill clients.

Physical Cooling

In a study of the care of critically ill clients, cooling blankets were used to treat fever in clients whose body temperature was above 39.7° C; most were receiving mechanical ventilation or had acute disease of the CNS[21]; 41% of the 94 episodes of fever in this study were treated with cooling blankets. Four

---

*Recommendation levels of the AACN Research-Based Practice Protocols[4]: level 1, manufacturer's recommendation only; level 2, theory-based, no research data to support the recommendation; level 3, laboratory data but not clinical data to support the recommendation; level 4, limited clinical studies to support the recommendation; level 5, clinical studies in more than one or two different populations or situations; and level 6, clinical studies in a variety of populations and situations.

Bridge continued on the following page

Fever-Related Interventions *Continued*

cooling blanket temperatures (7.2° C, 12.8° C, 18.3° C, 23.9° C) were evaluated in a random assignment study of 89 febrile, critically ill clients.[3] The clients were placed between two cooling blankets and were also given acetaminophen. No statistically significant difference was found among the four groups in terms of amount of time required to decrease temperature, but clients were more comfortable at the higher temperatures. Although there was no difference in the average time in which clients started shivering, less shivering occurred with warmer blanket temperatures. These findings were interpreted as meaning that warmer blanket temperatures provide similar rates of cooling, possibly less shivering, and greater comfort to patients. No reports were found evaluating the effectiveness of one versus two blankets or anterior versus posterior placement of cooling blankets.

The effectiveness of cooling with tepid water sponging, ice packs, and exposure of more body surface to room air has received surprisingly little attention. A study comparing acetaminophen, external cooling, and metamizole (an analgesic) in 20 critically ill adults found external cooling with cloths soaked in ice water was the most effective method of decreasing core body temperature; the administration of acetaminophen was the least effective.[22] A chart review study examined the temperature responses of 88 febrile medical-surgical patients to administration of acetaminophen alone and acetaminophen in combination with physical cooling.[7] Temperatures decreased in 82 (92%) of the clients, with an average decrease of 2.4° C. Ice packs were the most commonly used means of physical cooling; of five patients treated with acetaminophen and ice packs, three experienced a decrease in temperature, whereas two experienced a small increase.

In summary, physical cooling is effective but the relative benefits of various methods of physical cooling have not been studied, nor has the extent to which physical cooling interventions other than the cooling blanket induce shivering.

Antipyretic Agents (p. 485)

In one study of critically ill adults[15] a combination of acetaminophen and paralytic agents was found to decrease oxygen consumption, cardiac output, and heart rate. As mentioned earlier, in the critically ill, acetaminophen was less effective than external cooling[10, 22] and less effective than metamizole in decreasing body temperature.[22] The extent to which acetaminophen is absorbed in the gastrointestinal tract of the critically ill may be a factor in its effectiveness, although one study comparing burn patients with healthy volunteers found no difference in drug absorption in the two groups.[20]

Another study of 27 critically ill clients with a variety of problems[26] documented wide variations in drug level 60 minutes after administration. No studies compared oral administration with rectal administration in critically ill persons. Two studies of young children after surgery[13, 18] suggest that absorption of acetaminophen is faster and better via the upper gastric route than via the rectal route.

No studies were found comparing the effects of various antipyretics on fever in critically ill clients. In two studies of febrile children, peak levels of oral acetaminophen were reached in 0.5 to 1.0 hour after administration, whereas peak levels of oral ibuprofen occurred from 1.0 to 1.5 hours.[2, 14] A comparison of oral acetaminophen (650 mg) to three doses of intramuscular

ketorolac (15, 30, and 60 mg), a nonsteroidal anti-inflammatory drug, in healthy adult volunteers found that those who received 60 mg of ketorolac had the smallest increase in temperature after injection with an endotoxin; those who received 30 mg of ketorolac had increases similar to those who were given acetaminophen.[27]

"Other Methods of Treating Fever" (p. 486)

Cooling by blowing cold air across the skin surface (convective cooling) has not been studied as extensively as rewarming with warm air. Another approach involving the wrapping of extremities over peripheral skin sensors has been used to decrease shivering. In a randomized study of clients receiving amphotericin B, the responses of 20 subjects whose extremities were wrapped were compared to those of the control group.[11] The duration of shivering episodes in the control group was longer than what was experienced by the extremity-wrapped group.

Limitations/Reservations. Critically ill clients are a widely diverse group and many have multisystem dysfunctions. As a result, separating the effects of fever from those of underlying disease and dysfunction is difficult. CNS dysfunctions and variations in blood flow in particular make evaluation of fever interventions difficult to study. Hence, the body of research is affected by multiple uncontrolled variables.

An important uncontrolled variable is the manner in which the interventions were delivered. Many of the studies did nothing to ensure that the interventions were delivered in a consistent manner or that temperatures were measured in the same way; such lack of control decreases the likelihood of detecting an effect of the interventions on fever.

In addition, many of the studies are small, suggesting that the lack of difference in intervention effectiveness found in some of these studies might be the result of an inadequate sample size, not a true difference in intervention effectiveness. Hence, this body of research lacks findings from high quality studies in which clinicians can have confidence, and many questions remain regarding whether, how, and when to intervene to manage fever.

Research-Based Practice

The benefits of fever as a host defense mechanism and an indicator of disease must always be weighed against the metabolic, cardiovascular, and pulmonary demands (i.e., energy expenditures) imposed by fever. These demands may not be tolerated by older or debilitated persons, infants, and those with coronary heart disease, heart failure, or pulmonary disease. When a person is at risk to not tolerate fever, intervention to reduce temperature is indicated.

If the fever is determined to be of infectious origin, antibiotic treatment of the underlying infection will be started. In fever of a noninfectious or an infectious basis, interventions may need to be instituted to control the fever itself until the underlying disorder can be brought under control. A common form of intervention is to administer antipyretic medication (e.g., aspirin, acetaminophen, paracetamol, metamizole). However, the benefits of these medications alone in critically ill clients are not well supported by the research findings of this review; in several studies, acetaminophen or metamizole when used alone either did not reduce temperature or was not as effective as physical cooling.

Some form of physical cooling should be considered as a means of reducing temperature in critically ill clients; options include removing bed linens, tepid water sponging, placement of ice water–cooled cloths on the client, or the use of a circulating cooling blanket. Physical cooling may be most effective when used in combination with an antipyretic medication. However, the high incidence of shivering associated with the use of cooling blankets must be kept in mind. From the findings of one study, cooling blanket temperatures in the range of 23.9° C should be used to avoid shivering and to promote comfort. Wrapping of extremities, using the method suggested by Holtzclaw,[12] may prevent shivering and its associated costs in some cases. Every attempt should be made to prevent shivering, and when it does occur, it should not be allowed to continue because it can drive temperatures higher while imposing metabolic and cardiovascular burdens.

Regarding client outcomes, the evidence regarding reducing the fever of patients with sepsis is inconclusive. There are more advantages associated with reducing fever in clients with head injury.

From the evidence assembled for this review, one can only conclude that there are many gaps in the research base regarding management of fever in the critically ill. The literature does not address all the decisions clinicians make in managing fever. Until more research is available, clinicians must combine the little research-based knowledge that is available with considerable experience-based knowledge and close observation of how individual clients respond to antipyretic medications, physical cooling, or both. Also, nurses and physicians who treat particular critically ill populations on a regular basis may have additional insights regarding what works best.

References

1. Bernard, G. R., et al. (1997). The effects of ibuprofen on the physiology and survival of patients with sepsis. *New England Journal of Medicine, 336,* 912–918.
2. Brown, R. D., et al. (1992). Single-dose pharmacokinetics of ibuprofen and acetaminophen in febrile children. *Journal of Clinical Pharmacology, 32,* 231–241.
3. Caruso, C. C., et al. (1992). Cooling effects and comfort of four cooling blanket temperatures in humans with fever. *Nursing Research, 41,* 68–72.
4. Chulay, M. (1998). Information for contributors. *AACN Research-Based Practice Protocols.* Aliso Viejo, CA: American Association of Critical-Care Nurses.
5. Clemmer, T. P., et al. (1992). The Methylprednisonolone Severe Sepsis Study Group: Hypothemia in the sepsis syndrome and clincial outcome. *Critical Care Medicine, 20,* 1395–1401.
6. Clifton, G. L., et al. (1993). A phase II study of moderate hypothermia in severe brain injury. *Journal of Neurotrauma, 10,* 263–271.
7. Grossman, et al. (1995). Current practices in fever management. *Journal of Medical-Surgical Nursing, 4,* 193–198.
8. Haupt, M. T., & Rackow, E. (1983). Adverse effects of febrile state on cardiac performance. *American Heart Journal, 105,* 763–768.
9. Henker, R. A., Brown, S. D., & Marion, D. W. (1998). Comparison of brain temperature with bladder and rectal temperatures in adults with severe head injury. *Neurosurgery, 42,* 1071–1075.
10. Henker, R., et al. (1997). Core temperature and cardiovascular responses to antipyretics in febrile critically ill adults [Abstract]. *Critical Care Medicine, 25,* A23.
11. Holtzclaw, B. J. (1990). Control of febrile shivering during amphotericin B therapy. *Oncology Nursing Forum, 17,* 521–524.
12. Holtzclaw, B. (1993). The shivering response. *Annual Review of Nursing Research, 11,* 31–55.
13. Hopkins, G. S., Underhill, S., & Booker, P. D. (1990). Pharmacokinetics of paracetamol after cardiac surgery. *Archives of Disease in Childhood, 65,* 971–976.
14. Kelley, M. T., et al. (1992). Pharmacokinetics and pharmacodynamics of ibuprofen isomers and acetaminophen in febrile children. *Clinical Pharmacology and Therapeutics, 52,* 181–189.
15. Manthous, C. A., et al. (1995). Effect of cooling on oxygen consumption in febrile critically ill patients. *American Journal of Respiratory and Critical Care Medicine, 151,* 10–14.
16. Marion, D. W., et al. (1993). The use of moderate therapeutic hypothermia for patients with severe head injuries: A preliminary report. *Journal of Neurosurgery, 79,* 354–362.
17. Marion, D. W., et al. (1997). Treatment of traumatic brain injury with moderate hypothermia. *New England Journal of Medicine, 336,* 540–546.
18. Montgomery, C. J., et al. (1995). Plasma concentrations after high-dose (45 mg*kg⁻¹) rectal acetaminophen in children. *Canadian Journal of Anaesthesia, 42,* 982–986.
19. Morgan, S. P. (1990). A comparison of three methods of managing fever in the neurological patient. *Journal of Neuroscience Nursing, 22,* 19–24.
20. Oliver, Y.-P. H., et al. Evaluation of gastric emptying in severe, burn-injured patients. *Critical Care Medicine, 21,* 527–531.
21. O'Donnell, J., et al. (1997). Use and effectiveness of hypothermia blankets for febrile patients in the intensive care unit. *Clinical Infectious Diseases, 24,* 1208–1213.
22. Poblete, B., et al. (1997). Metabolic effects of IV propacetamol, metamizol, or external cooling in critically ill febrile sedate patients. *British Journal of Anaesthesia, 78,* 123–127.
23. Revhaug, A., et al. (1988). Inhibition of cyclo-oxygenase attenuates the metabolic response to endotoxin in humans. *Archives of Surgery, 123,* 162–170.
24. Rumana, C. S., et al. (1998). Brain temperature exceeds systemic temperature in head-injured patients. *Critical Care Medicine, 26,* 562–567.
25. Shiozaki, T., et al. (1993). Effect of mild hypothermia on uncontrollable intracranial hypertension after severe head injury. *Journal of Neuorsurgery, 79,* 363–368.
26. Tarling, M. M., et al. (1997). A model of gastric emptying using paracetamol absorption in intensive care patients. *Intensive Care Medicine, 23,* 256–260.
27. Vargas, R., et al. (1994). Evaluation of the antipyretic effect of ketorolac, acetaminophen, and placebo in endotoxin-induced fever. *Journal of Clinical Pharmacology, 34,* 848–853.
28. Weinberg, J. R., et al. (1989). Studies on the circulation in normotensive febrile patients. *Quarterly Journal of Experimental Physiology, 74,* 301–310.
29. Weinstein, M. P., et al. (1983). The clinical significance of positive blood cultures: A comprehensive analysis of 500 episodes of bacteremia and fungemia in adults. II: Clinical observations with special reference to factors influencing prognosis. *Reviews of Infectious Diseases, 5,* 54–70.

Sarah Jo Brown, PhD, RN, *Principal and Consultant, Practice-Research Integrations, Norwich, Vermont*

Quality of Life After Organ Transplantation

QUESTIONS

Does quality of life (QOL) improve from the pre-transplantation to the post-transplantation period?
Is QOL in transplant recipients better than QOL in other similarly ill comparison groups?
Is QOL in transplant recipients similar to or better than QOL in healthy people?

CITATION

Dew, M. A., Switzer, G. E., Goycoolea, J. M., Allen, A. A., DiMartini, A., Kormos, R. L., and Griffith, B. P. (1997).
   Does transplantation produce quality of life benefits? A quantitative analysis. *Transplantation, 64,* 1261–1273.

"Quality of life" was defined as well-being in three areas of well-being: (1) physical functioning, (2) mental/cognitive health, and (3) social functioning. Within each of these functional areas, several variables were analyzed. For example, in physical functioning the following seven variables were analyzed: ambulation, mobility, pain, fatigue, sleep, activities of daily living, and perceived physical status.

STUDIES

Published studies conducted from 1972 through 1996 were located; 218 were included in the analysis. Studies of kidney recipients were most prevalent, followed by studies of heart, liver, and bone marrow recipients. Studies of pancreas/kidney-pancreas and lung/heart-lung recipients were considerably less common. The 218 studies included almost 15,000 recipients and varied widely in sample size and study design. Most studies assessed recipients just once, most often within the year after surgery, but 36% of the studies observed recipients from 1 to 3 years. Only 9% of the studies followed recipients more than 3 years after surgery.

Summary of Findings

Does Quality of Life Improve From Before to After Transplantation? (p. 1267)

Seventy-six studies evaluated clients before and then again after transplantation. In general, QOL improved with the procedure, but variations by area of functioning and by transplant type occurred. Across transplant types, 86% of the studies documented improvement in physical functioning, 67% in social functioning, and 62% in mental/cognitive functioning.

Physical functioning was improved, according to all (100%) studies involving pancreas/kidney-pancreas recipients and all studies involving lung/heart-lung recipients. In contrast, 67% of the studies involving bone marrow recipients found improvement. The proportion of studies finding improvement in the other transplant types fell between these two levels. Within the mental/cognitive area, more than 80% of the studies involving kidney recipients found improvement, whereas only 32% of studies involving pancreas/kidney-pancreas recipients did. For social functioning, all (100%) studies involving lung/heart-lung recipients found improvement; in contrast, only 50% of bone marrow transplant studies found improvement. Thus, despite the considerable variation among the transplant types and across the three functional areas, in most studies recipients experienced improved QOL after transplantation.

Is Quality of Life in Transplant Recipients Better Than Quality of Life in Other Similarly Ill Comparison Groups? (p. 1268)

Eighty-four studies addressed this issue, typically comparing recipients to people with similar conditions who did not receive transplants. The majority of studies (58%) found that physical functioning for transplant recipients was better than that of ill comparison groups. Although some studies examining mental/cognitive and social functioning found advantages for transplant recipient over comparison groups, most *did not* find advantages; instead, the majority of studies noted that mental/cognitive and social functioning in recipients were the same or poorer than in comparison groups.

Studies of lung/heart-lung recipients found the greatest advantage for transplant recipients over similarly ill comparison groups; the group with the least documented improvement, when compared with a similar ill group, were bone marrow recipients. Again, each group of recipients (i.e., by transplant type) varied somewhat across the three areas of functioning.

Is Quality of Life in Transplant Recipients Similar to or Better Than Quality of Life in Healthy Samples? (p. 1270)

Although a few of the 67 studies that addressed this issue found that QOL in recipients was equal to or better than that in healthy people, the majority of the studies noted a poorer quality of life in all three areas of functioning. Heart and lung/heart-lung recipients compared most favorably, whereas no studies of bone marrow recipients or pancreas/kidney-pancreas found QOL in recipients to be at least as good as that in healthy persons.

In summary, although transplantation may not restore QOL to previous levels, the evidence has established clear QOL benefits. The specific nature and degree of benefits depend on the type of transplantation procedure.

Other Issues

Recipients rated their overall QOL as "high." This high rating is somewhat at odds with the more modest improvements in the specific areas of functioning. The researchers who conducted the meta-analysis suggest that this is because transplant clients feel that they have been given the gift of an extended life. This perception probably leads to a redefinition of "normal" life and an increased valuing of life even when their daily lives have difficulties. Importantly, the longitudinal studies found QOL either to be stable or to improve over the first 1 to 7 years after transplantation.

Limitations/Reservations These findings do not mean that every transplant client will realize an improved QOL, although the research evidence regarding the change in QOL from before to after surgery on average is impressive. All studies considered averaged experiences of all those in the sample. For this question, an average result means that most recipients experienced a higher QOL. For others, QOL stayed the same; however, a few recipients may have even experienced a decline in QOL. The authors note that most of the studies in this analysis were conducted in the pre-cyclosporine or pre-FK506 era. These

Quality of Life After Organ Transplantation *Continued*

two medications have been found to improve QOL in some recipients.

Research-Based Practice

Because the benefits in QOL vary from one type of transplantative procedure to another, nurses caring for clients who have undergone a particular type of procedure should look at the findings of this meta-analysis that specifically pertain to that population. Only some of those specific findings have been presented in this synopsis.

The fact that most recipients rated their overall QOL as high, even though they admitted having problems and difficulties in specific areas of functioning, indicates that a person's perception of QOL is a very personal and subjective assessment—"personal" in that QOL depends on personal values and priorities. For example, physical functioning may be most important determinant of QOL for some people because it affects independence and the ability to get out in the world. Other people may not view independence and mobility as this important and may say instead, "I can't do what I use to do, but as long as I can take care of most of my own bodily functions, I'm okay. The important thing is that I have my wits about me and can make my own decisions."

Rating one's QOL is relative because the experience of having a life-threatening illness changes how one thinks about life in general and about one's own life in particular. From the outside, someone's life may look as if it is shaped by medication schedules, treatment procedures, side effects, and limitations; To the person living that life, however, there may be sufficient joys to make it worthwhile, even rich. Health providers often focus on the problems and difficulties, neglecting to take the time to talk with clients about what is going on in their lives that brings meaning, enjoyment, and social connectedness. Nurses must be careful to not make any assumptions about an individual client's QOL, particularly if they do not know the client well.

Nurses must also be aware that when clients rate their overall QOL, they are using some kind of standard. For some people, that standard may be their QOL before they became ill; others may evaluate their QOL as it is in the present; and others still may base their rating on how they think their QOL will be or would have been had they not undergone the transplantation surgery. Still others may look at another person who they think has a life that is more constrained and difficult than their own and may compare their QOL to that person's QOL. Most people have an amazing capacity to adapt to difficult circumstances and to continue to find meaning in life. This analysis of QOL studies speaks to that capacity just as much as it documents the objective benefits of organ transplantation technology.

Nurses working with a particular population of transplant clients acquire insights into the post-transplant issues that clients may encounter. This knowledge can be combined with the findings of this meta-analysis to help clients and families who are considering transplantation to think through the effects a transplant is likely to have on their lives. The information in this meta-analysis regarding the experiences of the recipients of a particular type of transplant can be used as long as the nurse remains aware that these findings are based on the average experience and are not a guarantee of how things will be for any one client.

Sarah Jo Brown, PhD, RN, *Principal and Consultant, Practice-Research Integrations, Norwich, Vermont*

Religious Beliefs and Practices Affecting Health Care

Religious Group	Beliefs and Practices
WESTERN RELIGIONS	
Judaism Orthodox and some Conservative Jewish groups	*Care of women:* A woman is considered to be in a ritual state of impurity whenever blood is coming from her uterus, such as during menstrual periods and after the birth of a child. During this time, her husband does not have physical contact with her. When this time is completed, she will bathe herself in a pool called a *mikvah.* Be aware of this practice, and be sensitive to the husband and wife because the husband will not touch his wife. He cannot assist her in moving in the bed; the nurse must do this. An Orthodox Jewish man will not touch any women other than his wife, daughters, and mother. *Dietary rules:* (1) Kosher dietary laws include the following: no mixing of milk and meat at a meal; no consumption of food or any derivative thereof from animals not slaughtered in accordance with Jewish law; use of separate cooking utensils for milk and milk products; if a client requires milk and meat products for a meal, the dairy foods should be served first, followed later by the meat. (2) During Yom Kippur (Day of Atonement), a 24-hour fast is required, but exceptions are made for those who cannot fast because of medical reasons. (3) During Passover, no leavened products are eaten. (4) The client may say benediction of thanksgiving before meals and grace at the end of the meal. Time and a quiet environment should be provided for this. *Sabbath:* Observed from sunset Friday until sunset Saturday. Orthodox law prohibits riding in a car, smoking, turning lights on and off, handling money, and using television and telephone. Nurses need to be aware of these customs when caring for observant Jews at home and in the hospital. Medical or surgical treatments should be postponed if possible. *Death:* Judaism defines death as occurring when respiration and circulation are irreversibly stopped and no movement is apparent. (1) Euthanasia is strictly forbidden by Orthodox Jews, who advocate the strict use of life support measures. (2) Prior to death, Jewish faith indicates that visiting of the person by family and friends is a religious duty. The Torah and Psalms may be read and prayers recited. A witness needs to be present when a person prays for health so that if death occurs, God will protect the family and the spirit will be committed to God. Extraneous talking and conversation about death are not encouraged unless initiated by the client or visitors. In Judaism, the belief is that people should have someone with them when the soul leaves the body; thus, family and/or friends should be allowed to stay with the client. After death, the body should not be left alone until buried, usually within 24 hours. (3) When death occurs, the body should be untouched for 8 to 30 minutes. Medical personnel should not touch or wash the body but should allow only an Orthodox person or the Jewish Burial Society to care for the body. Handling of a corpse on the Sabbath is forbidden to Jewish persons. If need be, the nursing staff may provide routine care of the body, wearing gloves. Water in the room should be emptied, and the family may request that mirrors be covered to symbolize that a death has occurred. (4) Orthodox Jews and some Conservative Jews do not approve of autopsies. If an autopsy must be done, all body parts must remain with the body. (5) For Orthodox Jews, the body must be buried within 24 hours. No flowers are permitted. A fetus must be buried. (6) A 7-day mourning period is required by the immediate family. Family members must stay at home except for Sabbath worship. (7) Organs or other body parts such as amputated limbs must be made available for burial for Orthodox Jews, who believe that all of the body must be returned to earth. *Birth control and abortion:* Artificial methods of birth control are not encouraged. Vasectomy is not allowed. Abortion may be performed only to save the mother's life.

Table continued on following page

Religious Group	Beliefs and Practices

WESTERN RELIGIONS *(Continued)*

Organ transplantation: Although it has been assumed that donor organ transplantation is not permitted by Orthodox Jews but is allowed with rabbinic consent, using an organ to save a life is encouraged.*

Shaving: The beard is regarded as a mark of piety among observant Jews. For the very Orthodox, shaving should not be done with a razor but with scissors or electric razor, because a blade should not contact the skin.

Head covering: Orthodox men wear skull caps at all times, and women cover their hair after marriage. Some Orthodox women wear wigs as a mark of piety. Conservative Jews cover their heads only during acts of worship and prayer.

Prayer: Praying directly to God, including a prayer of confession, is required for Orthodox Jews. Provide quiet time for prayer.

Reform Jews

Care of women: Reform Jews do not observe the rules against touching.

Dietary rules: Reform Jews usually do not observe kosher dietary restriction.

Sabbath: Usual custom is to worship in temples on Friday evenings. No strict rules.

Death: Reform Jews advocate use of life support without heroic measures. They allow cremation but suggest that ashes be buried in a Jewish cemetery.

Organ transplantation: Donation or transplantation of organs allowed with permission of a rabbi.

Head covering: Men usually pray without wearing skull caps.

Christianity
Roman Catholic

Holy Eucharist: For clients and health care providers who are to receive communion, abstinence from solid food and alcohol is required for 15 minutes (if possible) prior to reception of the consecrated wafer. Medicine, water, and nonalcoholic drinks are permitted at any time. If a client is in danger of death, the fast is waived because the reception of the Eucharist at this time is very important.

Anointing of the sick: The priest uses oil to anoint the forehead and hands and, if desired, the affected area. The rite may be performed on any who are ill and desire it. Clients receiving the sacrament seek complete healing and strength to endure suffering. Prior to 1963, this sacrament was given only to clients at time of imminent death; be sensitive to the meaning this has for the client. If possible, call a priest before the client is unconscious but you may also call when there is sudden death, because the sacrament may also be given shortly after death. Record on the care plan that this sacrament has been administered.

Dietary habits: Obligatory fasting is excused during hospitalization. However, if there are no health restrictions, some Catholics may still observe the following guidelines: (1) Anyone 14 years or older must abstain from eating meat on Ash Wednesday and all Fridays during Lent. Some older Catholics may still abstain from meat on all Fridays of the year. (2) In addition to abstinence from meat, persons 21 to 59 years of age must limit themselves to one full meal and two light meals on Ash Wednesday and Good Friday. (3) Eastern Rite Catholics are stricter about fasting and fast more frequently than Western Rite Catholics, and it is important for you to know if a client is Eastern or Western.

Death: Each Roman Catholic should participate in the anointing of the sick as well as the Eucharist and penance before death. The body should not be shrouded until after these sacraments are performed. All body parts that retain human quality must be appropriately buried or cremated.

Birth control: Contraception is prohibited except for abstinence or natural family planning. Referral to a priest for questions about this can be of great help. You can teach the techniques of natural family planning if you are familiar with them; otherwise, this should be referred to the physician or to a support group of the church that instructs couples in this method of birth control. Sterilization is prohibited unless there is an overriding medical reason.

Organ donation: Donation and transplantation of organs are acceptable as long as the donor is not harmed and is not deprived of life.

Religious objects: Rosary prayers are said using rosary beads. Medals bearing the images of saints, relics, statues, and scapulars are important objects that may be pinned to a hospital gown or pillow or may be at the bedside. Take extreme care not to lose these objects, because they have special meaning to the client.

Eastern Orthodox

Holy Eucharist: The priest is notified if the client desires this sacrament.

Anointing of the sick: The priest conducts this rite in the hospital room.

Religious Group	Beliefs and Practices
WESTERN RELIGIONS *(Continued)*	
	Dietary habits: Fasting from meat and dairy products is required on Wednesday and Friday during Lent and on other holy days. Hospital clients are exempt if fasting is detrimental to health.
	Special days: Christmas is celebrated on January 7 and New Year's Day on January 14. This is important to know when you are caring for a client who is hospitalized on these days.
	Death: Last rites are obligatory. This is handled by an ordained priest who is notified by the nurse while the client is conscious. The Russian Orthodox Church does not encourage autopsy or organ donation. Euthanasia, even for the terminally ill, is discouraged, as is cremation.
	Birth control: Contraception as well as abortion is not permitted.
Protestant	*Holy Communion:* Notify clergy if the client desires.
Assemblies of God (Pentecostal)	*Anointing of the sick:* Members believe in divine healing through prayer and the laying on of hands. Clergy is notified if client or family desires this.
	Dietary habits: Abstinence from alcohol, tobacco, and all illegal drugs is strongly encouraged.
	Death: No special practices.
	Other practices: Faith in God and in the health care providers is encouraged. Members pray for divine intervention in health matters. Encourage and allow time for prayer. Members may speak in "tongues" during prayer.
Baptist (over 27 different groups in the United States)	*Holy Communion:* Clergy should be notified if the client desires.
	Dietary habits: Total abstinence from alcohol is expected.
	Death: No general service is provided, but the clergy does minister through counseling, prayer, and Scripture as requested by the client or family, and the client is encouraged to believe in Jesus Christ as Savior and Lord.
	Other practices: The Bible is held to be the word of God. Either allow quiet time for Scripture reading, or offer to read to the client.
Christian Church (Disciples of Christ)	*Holy Communion:* Open communion is celebrated each Sunday and is a central part of worship services. Notify the clergy if the client desires it, or the clergy may suggest it.
	Death: No special practices.
	Other practices: Church elders as well as clergy may be notified to assist with meeting the client's spiritual needs.
Church of the Brethren	*Holy Communion:* Is usually received within church, but clergy may give it in the hospital when requested.
	Anointing of the sick: Practices for physical healing as well as spiritual uplift are held in high regard by the church. The clergy is notified if the client or family desire.
	Death: The clergy is notified for counsel and prayer.
Church of the Nazarene	*Holy Communion:* Pastor will administer if the client wishes.
	Dietary habits: The use of alcohol and tobacco is forbidden.
	Death: Cremation is permitted, and term stillborn infants are buried.
	Other practices: A belief in divine healing but not to the exclusion of medical treatment. Clients may desire quiet time for prayer.
Episcopal (Anglican)	*Holy Communion:* The priest is notified if the client wishes to receive this sacrament.
	Anointing of the sick: Priest may administer this rite when death is imminent, but it is not considered mandatory.
	Dietary habits: Some clients may abstain from meat on Fridays. Others may fast before receiving the Eucharist, but fasting is not mandatory.
	Death: No special practices.
	Other practices: Confession of sins to a priest is optional; if the client desires this, the clergy should be notified.
Lutheran (18 different branches)	*Holy Communion:* Notify the clergy if the client desires this sacrament. Clergy may also inquire about the client's desire.
	Anointing of the sick: The client may request an anointing and blessing from the minister when the prognosis is poor.
	Death: A service of Commendation of the Dying is used at the client's or family's request.

Table continued on following page

Religious Group	Beliefs and Practices

WESTERN RELIGIONS *(Continued)*

Religious Group	Beliefs and Practices
Mennonite (12 different groups)	*Holy Communion:* Served twice a year, with foot-washing a part of the ceremony. *Dietary habits:* Abstinence from alcohol is urged for all. *Death:* Prayer is important at time of crisis, and contacting a minister is important. *Other practices:* Women may wear head coverings during hospitalization. Anointing with oil is administered in harmony with James 5:14 when requested.
Methodist (over 20 different groups)	*Holy Communion:* Notify the clergy if a client requests it prior to surgery or another health crisis. *Anointing of the sick:* If requested, the clergy will come to pray and sprinkle the client with olive oil. *Death:* Scripture reading and prayer are important at this time. *Other practices:* Donation of one's body or part of the body at death is encouraged.
Presbyterian (10 different groups)	*Holy Communion:* Given when appropriate and convenient, at the hospitalized client's request. *Death:* Notify a local pastor or elder for prayer and Scripture reading if desired by the family or client.
Quaker (Friends)	*Holy Communion:* Because Friends have no creed, there is a diversity of personal beliefs. One belief is that outward sacraments are usually not necessary because there is the ministry of the Spirit inwardly in such areas as baptism and communion. *Death:* Believe that the present life is part of God's kingdom and generally have no ceremony as a rite of passage from this life to the next. Personal beliefs and wishes need to be ascertained, and you can then act on the client's wishes.
Salvation Army	*Holy Communion:* No particular ceremony. *Death:* Notify the local officer in charge of the Army Corps for any soldier (member) who needs assistance. *Other practices:* The Bible is seen as the only rule for one's faith, and the Scriptures should be made available to a client. The Army has many of its own social welfare centers, with hospitals and homes where unwed mothers are cared for and outpatient services provided. No medical or surgical procedures are opposed, except for abortion on demand.
Seventh-day Adventist	*Holy Communion:* Although this sacrament is not required of hospitalized clients, the clergy are notified if the client desires. *Anointing of the sick:* The clergy are contacted for prayer and anointing with oil. *Dietary habits:* Because the body is viewed as the temple of the Holy Spirit, healthy living is essential. Therefore, the use of alcohol, tobacco, coffee, and tea and the promiscuous use of drugs are prohibited. Some are vegetarians, and most avoid pork. *Special days:* The Sabbath is observed on Saturday. *Death:* No special procedures. *Other related practices:* Use of hypnotism is opposed by some. Persons of homosexual or lesbian orientation are ministered to in the hope of correction of these practices, which are believed to be wrong. A Bible should always be available for Scripture reading.
United Church of Christ	*Holy Communion:* Clergy are notified if the client desires to receive this sacrament. *Death:* If the client desires counsel or prayer, notify the clergy.

Other
Christian Science	*Dietary habits:* Because alcohol and tobacco are considered drugs, they are not used. Coffee and tea are often declined. *Death:* Autopsy is usually declined unless required by law. Donation of organs is unlikely, but is an individual decision. *Other practices:* Adherents do not normally seek medical care, because they approach health care in a different, primarily spiritual, framework. They commonly utilize the services of a surgeon to set a bone but decline drugs and, in general, other medical or surgical procedures. Hypnotism and psychotherapy are also declined. Family planning is left to the family. They seek exemption from vaccinations but obey legal requirements (e.g., report infectious diseases and obey public health quarantines). Nonmedical care facilities are maintained for those needing nursing assistance in the course of a healing. *The Christian Science Journal* lists available Christian Science nurses. When a Christian Science believer is in the hospital, allow and encourage time for prayer and study. Clients may request that a Christian Science practitioner be notified to come.

Religious Group	Beliefs and Practices
WESTERN RELIGIONS (*Continued*)	

Religious Group	Beliefs and Practices
Jehovah's Witnesses	*Dietary habits:* Use of alcohol and tobacco is discouraged, because these harm the physical body. *Death:* Autopsy is a private matter to be decided by the persons involved. Burial and cremation are acceptable. *Birth control and abortion:* Use of birth control is a personal decision. Abortion is opposed on the basis of Exodus 21:22–23. *Organ transplantation:* Use of organ transplants is a private decision. If an organ is transplanted, it must be cleansed with a nonblood solution. *Blood transfusions:* Blood transfusions violate God's laws and are therefore not allowed. Clients do respect physicians and will accept alternatives to blood transfusions. These might include use of nonblood plasma expanders, careful surgical techniques to decrease blood loss, use of autologous transfusions, and autotransfusion through use of a heart-lung machine. Nurses should check unconscious patients for medical alert cards that state that the person does not want a transfusion. Since Jehovah's Witnesses are prepared to die rather than break God's law, you need to be sensitive to the spiritual as well as the physical needs of the client.
Church of Jesus Christ of Latter-day Saints	*Holy Communion:* A hospitalized client may desire to have a member of the church priesthood administer this sacrament. *Anointing of the sick:* Mormons commonly are anointed and given a blessing by laying on of hands before going to the hospital and after admission. *Dietary habits:* Abstinence from the use of tobacco; beverages with caffeine such as cola, coffee, and tea; alcohol and other substances considered injurious. Mormons eat meat but encourage the intake of fruits, grains, and herbs. *Death:* Burial of the body is preferred. A church elder should be notified to assist the family. If need be, the elder will assist the funeral director in dressing the body in special clothes and will give other help as needed. *Birth control and abortion:* Abortion is opposed except when the life of the mother is in danger. Only natural means of birth control are recommended. Artificial means can be used when the health of the woman is at stake (including emotional health). *Personal care:* Cleanliness is very important to Mormons. A sacred undergarment may be worn at all times by Mormons and should be removed only in emergency situations. *Other practices:* Allowing quiet time for prayer and the reading of the sacred writings is important. The church maintains a welfare system to assist those in need. Families are of great importance, and visiting should be encouraged.
Unitarian Universalist Association	*Death:* Cremation is often preferred to burial. *Other practices:* Use of birth control is advocated as part of responsible parenting. Strong support for a woman's right to choice regarding abortion is maintained. Unitarian Universalists advocate donation of body parts for research and transplants.
Unification Church	*Baptism:* No baptism. *Special days:* Sunday mornings are used to honor Reverend and Mrs. Moon as the true parents, and members get up at 5:00 AM, bow before a picture of the Moons three times, and vow to do what is needed to help the Reverend accomplish his mission on earth. *Death:* Adherents believe that after death one's place of destiny will depend on his or her spirit's quality of life and goodness while on earth. In the afterlife, one will have the same aspirations and feelings as before, when on earth. Hell is not a concern, because it will not be a place as heaven grows in size. Persons who leave the Unification Church are warned that Satan may try to possess them. *Other practices:* All marriages must be solemnized by Reverend Moon in order to be part of the perfect family and have salvation. The church supplies its faithful members with life's necessities. Members may use occult practices to have spiritual and psychic experiences.
Islam	*Dietary habits:* No pork or alcoholic beverages allowed. All halal (permissible) meat must be blessed and killed in a special way. This is called *zabihah* (correctly slaughtered).

Table continued on following page

Religious Group	Beliefs and Practices
WESTERN RELIGIONS *(Continued)*	

	Death: Prior to death, family members ask to be present so that they can read the Koran and pray with the client. An Imam may come if requested by the client or family but is not required. Clients must face Mecca and confess their sins and beg forgiveness in the presence of their family. If the family is unavailable, any practicing Muslim can provide support to the client. After death, Muslims prefer that the family wash, prepare, and place the body in a position facing Mecca. If necessary, the health care providers may perform these procedures as long as they wear gloves. Burial is performed as soon as possible. Cremation is forbidden. Autopsy is also prohibited except for legal reasons, and then no body part is to be removed. Donation of body parts or organs is not allowed, because according to culturally developed law, persons do not own their bodies. *Abortion and birth control:* Abortion is forbidden, and many conservative Muslims do not encourage the use of contraceptives because this interferes with God's purpose. Others feel that a woman should only have as many children as her husband can afford. Contraception is permitted by Islamic law. *Personal devotions:* At prayer time, washing is required, even by those who are sick. A client on bed rest may require assistance with this task before prayer. Provision of privacy is important during prayer. *Religious objects:* The Koran must not be touched by anyone ritually unclean, and nothing should be placed on top of it. Some Muslims wear *taviz,* a black string on which words of the Koran are attached. These should not be removed and must remain dry. Certain items of jewelry, such as bangles, may have religious significance and should not be removed unnecessarily. *Care of women:* Because women are not allowed to sign consent forms or make a decision regarding family planning, the husband needs to be present. Women are very modest and frequently wear clothes that cover all of the body. During a medical examination, the woman's modesty should be respected as much as possible. Muslim women prefer female physicians. For 40 days after giving birth and also during menstruation, a woman is exempt from prayer because this is a time of cleansing for her.
American Muslim Mission	*Dietary habits:* In addition to refusing pork, many will not eat traditional African American foods, such as corn bread and collard greens. *Death:* The family is contacted before any care of the deceased is performed. There are special procedures for washing and shrouding the body. *Other practices:* Quiet time is necessary to permit prayer. Members are encouraged to use African American physicians for health care. Because these clients do not smoke, their request for a nonsmoking roommate should be honored.
EASTERN RELIGIONS	
Hinduism	*Dietary habits:* Some sects are vegetarian, believing meats and intoxicants to be too stimulating to the senses. *Belief about illness:* Hindus view illnesses as a result of misuse of the body or a consequence of sins committed in a previous life. They do not oppose medical treatment, but they view its effect as transitory. They believe that praying for health is the lowest form of prayer. *Death:* See death as a union with Brahman (God) achieved through prayers, ritual, purity, self-control, detachment, truth, nonviolence, charity, and compassion toward all creatures. Following death, one will be reborn (reincarnated) into a future life based on the behavior in this life. The record of behavior is called *karma.* Eventually, the process of rebirth stops, which is called *moksha.* A priest may be called at the time of death, and may tie a thread around the neck or waist as a blessing. The family washes the body, and it is cremated. *Other practices:* Offer daily worship at a shrine in the home. Daily offering to god, and morning and evening rites. Society is organized into castes, or strata. People are born into a caste, and the caste shapes one's entire life. Hindus practice a discipline of the mind and body, called yoga, to reach God. In the highest state, a meditating yogi does not see, hear, taste, feel, or smell. Beyond good and evil, time and space, he is one with God.

Religious Group	Beliefs and Practices
EASTERN RELIGIONS *(Continued)*	
Buddhism	*Death:* Buddhists believe that salvation depends on one's own right living; they believe in reincarnation. Buddhists can speed the process toward Nirvana, the goal of all humanity's striving, through acts of merit. Meditation, worship, and prayer are some of the acts of merit. Buddhists may drive themselves into more and more ritual or contemplation in the hope that their last moments of consciousness may be filled with thoughts worthy enough to elevate them to a higher existence. Last rites of chanting may be performed at bedside. *Renunciation:* The most important Buddhist feasts. Young boys are taught to despise the world's vanity, and the boy spends a night in a nearby monastery.
Taoism/Confucianism	*General beliefs:* Founded on ethical principles of Confucius. God is not clearly defined as in other religions. Taoism is a mixture of magic and religion. Believers hold that humans and nature are inseparable, and that if heaven is upset, earth does not prosper. This relationship is described as *yin* and *yang,* which are two interplaying forces. When *yin* and *yang* are in balance, good occurs. *Death:* The dead are remembered in all festivals. The fate of the dead in the afterworld depends not only on the life they led but also on being properly honored after death. Otherwise they may become demons. Graves are mounds like those dedicated to the gifts of the soil. Graves and houses must be in harmony with the universe, otherwise evil will befall the occupants.

*The American Scene. (2000). *Hadassah* (suppl, Summer), 4.
Modified from Carson, V. B. (1989). *Spiritual dimensions of nursing practice.* Philadelphia: W. B. Saunders.

A Health History Format That Integrates the Assessment of Functional Health Patterns

Functional Health Pattern	Assessment
Health perception–health management	Quality of usual and current health rated on a scale of 1 to 10
	Self-rating of the importance of health on a scale of 1 to 10
	Perceived ability to control and manage health
	Resources used in health management including primary health care provider
	Self-care measures to maintain or prevent disruption of health status
	Health habits (e.g., seat belt use, diet, alcohol consumption, tobacco use)
	Complete description of present health problem (i.e., chief complaint)
	Expectations for outcome of current health problem
	Expectations for care givers
	Previous illnesses or hospitalizations, reaction to these events, and their outcomes
	Developmental history, including childhood illnesses and immunizations
	Ability to manage and comply with recommended treatment of health problems
	Current medications, including over-the-counter and recreational (street) drugs
	Allergies
	Environmental factors affecting health (e.g., occupation, home, leisure)
	Socioeconomic factors affecting health (e.g., financial concerns, health care insurance, living conditions)
	Knowledge and use of community resources to manage health
	Family history
Nutritional-metabolic	Recall of usual food and fluid intake for the past 24 hours
	Comparison of the 24-hour recall diet to typical pattern of diet intake
	Quality of appetite
	Dietary restrictions (medical order)
	Food preferences and dislikes
	Use of food supplements (e.g., vitamins)
	Knowledge level of dietary recommendations (e.g., Food Guide Pyramid, recommended dietary allowances, special dietary guidelines)
	Past alterations in dietary habits (e.g., bulimia nervosa, anorexia nervosa)
	Usual weight
	Minimum and maximum weight range
	Recent weight gain or loss (how much? time span? intentional?)
	Social significance of food
	Who shops for food items?
	Who usually prepares meals?
	Religious or cultural beliefs affecting diet or meal preparation
	Ability to swallow and chew
	Are there any feeding problems?
Elimination	
Bowel	Usual bowel habits, including frequency, time of day, color, consistency, assistive devices used (e.g., laxatives, suppositories, enemas), constipation, diarrhea
	Change in bowel habits; describe
Bladder	Usual frequency, amount, color of voiding
	Assistive devices used (e.g., self-catheterization)
	Problems with frequency, urgency, burning, retention, incontinence, dribbling, dysuria, polyuria, nocturia
Skin	Condition, color, temperature, turgor, lesions, edema, pruritus
Activity-exercise	Description of usual daily activities
	Weekend schedule, if different from daily
	Occupation-related activities
	Leisure activities including hobbies
	Description of exercise regimen
	Limitation in ambulation, bathing, dressing, toileting, and feeding
	Dyspnea with exertion
	Fatigue

Functional Health Pattern	Assessment
Sleep-rest	Usual sleep habits including bedtime, hours of sleep obtained, wake-up time Problems falling asleep or staying asleep Sleep aids used, including medications, food, beverages, and sexual intercourse Rating of quality of sleep obtained (does client feel rested?) Periods of decreased wakefulness during the day Naps or rest periods
Cognitive-perceptual	Ability to understand Educational level obtained Self-rating of intelligence level Ability to communicate with others Ability to make decisions and the relative ease or difficulty experienced with decision-making Ability to see, hear, feel, taste, smell Compensations made for sensory deficits and their effectiveness Problems with vertigo, heat or cold intolerance Pain (including a symptom analysis) Desire to learn
Self-perception–self-concept	Description of self, including strengths and weaknesses Major concerns Health goals Body image and feelings about self Level of satisfaction with current age Perceived developmental level Emotional status Effect of illness on self-perception Personal factors contributing to illness, recovery, health maintenance
Role relationship	Language, quality of speech and relevancy Ability to express self Family life, including family members and their relationships to client Roles client and family members fill Interpersonal relationships within family Support systems within family, including person client feels closest to Family-related problems including living arrangements, parenting, marital problems, abuse Occupation and job-related role expectations Problems at work Societal relationships beyond family or work Most important person to client Type of neighborhood or community in which client lives Participation in social groups (e.g., church, synagogue, clubs) Perceived contributions to society
Sexuality-reproductive	Level of satisfaction with role as male or female Anticipated changes related to health problem (e.g., fertility, libido, impotence, pregnancy, contraception, menstruation) Sexual activity, including how long client has been sexually active, number of partners, use of contraceptives Known exposure to venereal diseases, including human immunodeficiency virus infection Level of satisfaction with intercourse Problems with intercourse (e.g., premature ejaculation, impotence, pain, bleeding)
Female	Menstrual history including age at menarche, description of typical cycle, last menstrual period, age at menopause, or manifestations of menopause Obstetric history including number of pregnancies, number of births, problems during pregnancy or labor and delivery Practice of breast self-examination, knowledge of technique, compliance Last Pap test and results, frequency of pelvic examinations and Pap tests
Male	Circumcision Age at climacteric and description of manifestations experienced Practice of testicular self-examination, knowledge of technique, compliance Prostate examination, prostate-specific antigen test and results

Table continued on following page

Functional Health Pattern	Assessment
Coping–stress tolerance	Coping strategies used and their effectiveness
	Personal loss or major changes in past year
	Comfort and security needs
	Most stressful event in life and reaction to it
	Use of stress management techniques and their effectiveness (e.g., eating, sleeping, self-medication, counseling, exercise, biofeedback)
	Effect of stress on lifestyle and ability to function, including decision-making
Value-belief	Most important value to client
	Sources of strength and hope
	Importance of religion, type, and frequency of worship
	Life goals
	Values influencing decision-making and ability to resolve moral questions
	Recent changes in values or beliefs
	Conflict in values or beliefs with those of significant others
	Spirituality needs, particularly during time of illness or hospitalization

Laboratory Values of Clinical Importance in Medical-Surgical Nursing

Reference laboratory values can provide guidelines for the clinician to use when assessing clients with a wide variety of problems. The laboratory values given here are for reference only and are not absolute normal values. Remember, there is no sharp dividing line between normal and abnormal. Clients with only slightly elevated values may have apparent disease, whereas those with more elevated values may not. Trends in laboratory values are often much more important than the single value.

When analyzing laboratory values, consider the following questions:

- Is the value an expected abnormal finding? For example, creatinine is normally elevated in clients with renal failure.
- Is the value an unexpected abnormal finding? For example, elevated blood glucose levels in a client without diabetes may signal a disease.
- Is the value an unexpected normal finding? For example, a client with angina and probable myocardial infarction would be expected to have elevated isoenzymes. Normal levels may mean that the client has another cause of chest pain.
- Is the value an expected normal finding? For example, a healthy client should have a normal complete blood count.

Use the analytic technique as a guide to determine when to call the physician. Remember, the laboratory only reports findings; nurses help interpret their significance.

Appendix C summarizes the common laboratory diagnostic studies for use as a quick reference. A complete explanation of the diagnostic study and its meaning is covered in the appropriate section (such as liver function studies in Chapter 47). This Appendix simply provides a convenient way to check the normal values for the most common diagnostic studies. For details concerning the meaning of the value, see the appropriate section in the text.

The following abbreviations are used throughout the laboratory studies:

g = gram
kg = kilogram
mg = milligram (10^{-3})
μg = microgram (10^{-6})
ng = nanogram (10^{-9})
pg = picogram (10^{-12})
L = liter
ml = milliliter
dl = deciliter (100 ml)
fL = femtoliter
mm = millimeter
mm^3 = cubic millimeter
U = unit
mU = milliunit
μU = microunit
mOsm = milliosmole
mol = mole
μmol = micromole
nmol = nanomole
pmol = picomole
fmol = femtomole (10^{-15})
mEq = milliequivalent
μm = micrometer

REFERENCE VALUES IN HEMATOLOGY*

Test		Conventional Units	SI Units
Acid hemolysis test (Ham)		No hemolysis	No hemolysis
Alkaline phosphatase, leukocyte		Total score 14 to 100	Total score 14 to 100
Cell counts			
Erythrocytes			
Males		4.6 to 6.2 million/mm³	4.6 to 6.2 × 10¹²/L
Females		4.2 to 5.4 million/mm³	4.2 to 5.2 × 10¹²/L
Children (varies with age)		4.5 to 5.1 million/mm³	4.5 to 5.1 × 10¹²/L
Leukocytes, total		4500 to 11,000/mm³	4.5 to 11.0 × 10⁹/L
Leukocytes, differential	*Percentage*	*Absolute*	*Absolute*
Myelocytes	0	0/mm³	0/L
Band neutrophils	3 to 5	150 to 400/mm³	150 to 400 × 10⁶/L
Segmented neutrophils	54 to 62	3000 to 5800/mm³	3000 to 5800 × 10⁶/L
Lymphocytes	25 to 33	1500 to 3000/mm³	1500 to 3000 × 10⁶/L
Monocytes	3 to 7	300 to 500/mm³	300 to 500 × 10⁶/L
Eosinophils	1 to 3	50 to 250/mm³	50 to 250 × 10⁶/L
Basophils	0 to 1	15 to 50/mm³	15 to 50 × 10⁶/L
Platelets		150,000 to 400,000/mm³	150 to 400 × 10⁹/L
Reticulocytes		25,000 to 75,000/mm³ (0.5% to 1.5% of erythrocytes)	25 to 75 × 10⁹/L
Coagulation tests			
Bleeding time (template)		2.75 to 8.0 min	2.75 to 8.0 min
Coagulation time (glass tubes)		5 to 15 min	5 to 15 min
D-Dimer		<0.5 μg/ml	<0.5 mg/L
Factor VIII and other coagulation factors		50% to 150% of normal	0.5 to 1.5 of normal
Fibrin split products (Thrombo-Welco test)		<10 μg/ml	<10 mg/L
Fibrinogen		200 to 400 mg/dl	2.0 to 4.0 g/L
Partial thromboplastin time (PTT)		20 to 35 sec	20 to 35 sec
Prothrombin time (PT)		12.0 to 14.0 sec	12.0 to 14.0 sec
Coombs' test			
Direct		Negative	Negative
Indirect		Negative	Negative
Corpuscular values of erythrocytes			
Mean corpuscular hemoglobin (MCH)		26 to 34 pg/cell	26 to 34 pg/cell
Mean corpuscular volume (MCV)		80 to 96 μm³	80 to 96 fL
Mean corpuscular hemoglobin concentration (MCHC)		32 to 36 g/dl	320 to 360 g/L
Haptoglobin		20 to 165 mg/dl	0.20 to 1.65 g/L
Hematocrit			
Males		40 to 54 ml/dl	0.40 to 0.54 volume fraction
Females		37 to 47 ml/dl	0.37 to 0.47 volume fraction
Newborns		49 to 54 ml/dl	0.49 to 0.54 volume fraction
Children (varies with age)		35 to 49 ml/dl	0.35 to 0.49 volume fraction
Hemoglobin			
Males		13.0 to 18.0 g/dl	8.1 to 11.2 mmol/L
Females		12.0 to 16.0 g/dl	7.4 to 9.9 mmol/L
Newborns		16.5 to 19.5 g/dl	10.2 to 12.1 mmol/L
Children (varies with age)		11.2 to 16.5 g/dl	7.0 to 10.2 mmol/L
Hemoglobin, fetal		<1.0% of total	<0.01 of total
Hemoglobin A₁C		3% to 5% of total	0.03 to 0.05 of total
Hemoglobin A₂		1.5% to 3.0% of total	0.015 to 0.03 of total
Hemoglobin, plasma		0 to 5.0 mg/dl	0 to 3.2 μmol/L
Methemoglobin		30 to 130 mg/dl	19 to 80 μmol/L
Sedimentation rate (ESR)			
Wintrobe			
Males		0 to 5 mm/hr	0 to 5 mm/hr
Females		0 to 15 mm/hr	0 to 15 mm/hr
Westergren			
Males		0 to 15 mm/hr	0 to 15 mm/hr
Females		0 to 20 mm/hr	0 to 20 mm/hr

*For some procedures, reference values may vary, depending on the method used.

Modified from Conn, R. B., Borer, W. Z., & Snyder, J. W. (1997). *Current diagnosis* (9th ed., pp. 1235–1241). Philadelphia: W. B. Saunders; and data from Malarkey, L. M., & McMorrow, M. E. (2000). *Nurses' manual of laboratory tests and diagnostic procedures* (2nd ed.). Philadelphia: W. B. Saunders.

REFERENCE VALUES FOR BLOOD, PLASMA, AND SERUM*

Test	Conventional Units	SI Units
Acetoacetate plus acetone		
Qualitative	Negative	Negative
Quantitative	0.3 to 2.0 mg/dl	3 to 20 mg/L
Acid phosphatase, serum (thymolphthalein monophosphate substrate)	0.11 to 0.60 U/L	0.11 to 0.60 U/L
Adrenocorticotropin, plasma (ACTH)		
8:00 AM	10 to 80 pg/ml	2–18 pmol/L
Alanine aminotransferase, serum (ALT, SGPT)	1 to 45 U/L	1 to 45 U/L
Albumin, serum	3.3 to 5.2 g/dl	33 to 52 g/L
Aldolase, serum	0.0 to 7.0 U/L	0.0 to 7.0 U/L
Aldosterone, plasma		
Standing	5 to 30 ng/dl	140 to 830 pmol/L
Recumbent	3 to 10 ng/dl	80 to 275 pmol/L
Alkaline phosphatase, serum (ALP)		
Adult	35 to 150 U/L	35 to 150 U/L
Adolescent	100 to 500 U/L	100 to 500 U/L
Child	100 to 350 U/L	100 to 350 U/L
Ammonia nitrogen, plasma	10 to 50 μmol/L	10 to 50 μmol/L
Amylase, serum	25 to 125 U/L	25 to 125 U/L
Anion gap, serum, calculated	8 to 16 mEq/L	8 to 16 mmol/L
Ascorbic acid, blood	0.4 to 1.5 mg/dl	23 to 85 μmol/L
Aspartate aminotransferase, serum (AST, SGOT)	1 to 36 U/L	1 to 36 U/L
Base excess, arterial blood, calculated	0 ± 2 mEq/L	0 ± 2 mmol/L
Bicarbonate		
Venous plasma	23 to 29 mEq/L	23 to 29 mmol/L
Arterial blood	21 to 27 mEq/L	21 to 27 mmol/L
Bile acids, serum	0.3 to 3.0 mg/dl	0.8 to 7.6 μmol/L
Bilirubin, serum		
Conjugated	0.1 to 0.4 mg/dl	1.7 to 6.8 μmol/L
Total	0.3 to 1.1 mg/dl	5.1 to 19 μmol/L
Calcium, serum	8.4 to 10.6 mg/dl	2.10 to 2.65 mmol/L
Calcium, ionized, serum	4.25 to 5.25 mg/dl	1.05 to 1.30 mmol/L
Carbon dioxide, total, serum or plasma	24 to 31 mEq/L	24 to 31 mmol/L
Carbon dioxide tension, blood (P_{CO_2})	35 to 45 mm Hg	35 to 45 mm Hg
β-Carotene serum	60 to 260 μg/dl	1.1 to 8.6 μmol/L
Catecholamines, plasma		
Epinephrine (supine)	<50 pg/ml	<273 pmol/L
Norepinephrine (supine)	110 to 410 pg/ml	650 to 2,423 pmol/L
Ceruloplasmin, serum	23 to 44 mg/dl	230 to 440 mg/L
Chloride, serum or plasma	96 to 106 mEq/L	96 to 106 mmol/L
Cholesterol, serum or EDTA plasma		
Desirable range	<200 mg/dl	<5.20 mmol/L
LDL Cholesterol	60 to 180 mg/dl	1.55 to 4.65 mmol/L
HDL Cholesterol	30 to 80 mg/dl	0.80 to 2.05 mmol/L
Copper	70 to 140 μg/dl	11 to 22 μmol/L
Cortisol, plasma		
8:00 AM	6 to 23 μg/dl	170 to 630 nmol/L
4:00 PM	3 to 15 μg/dl	80 to 410 nmol/L
10:00 PM	<50% of 8 AM value	<0.5 of 8 AM value
Creatine, serum		
Males	0.2 to 0.5 mg/dl	15 to 40 μmol/L
Females	0.3 to 0.9 mg/dl	25 to 70 μmol/L

Table continued on following page

REFERENCE VALUES FOR BLOOD, PLASMA, AND SERUM* *Continued*

Test	Conventional Units	SI Units
Creatine kinase, serum (CK, CPK)		
Males	55 to 170 U/L	55 to 170 U/L
Females	30 to 135 U/L	30 to 135 U/L
Creatine kinase MB isozyme, serum	<5% of total CK activity	<5% of total CK activity
	<5% ng/ml by immunoassay	<5% ng/ml by immunoassay
Creatinine, serum	0.6 to 1.2 mg/dl	50 to 110 μmol/L
Ferritin, serum	20 to 200 ng/ml	20 to 200 μg/L
Fibrinogen, plasma	200 to 400 mg/dl	2.0 to 4.0 g/L
Folate		
Serum	3.0 to 18.0 ng/ml	6.8 to 41.0 nmol/L
Erythrocytes	145 to 540 ng/ml	330 to 1220 nmol/L
Follicle-stimulating hormone, plasma (FSH)		
Males	4 to 25 mU/ml	4 to 25 U/L
Females	4 to 30 mU/ml	4 to 30 U/L
Postmenopausal	40 to 250 mU/ml	40 to 250 U/L
γ-Glutamyltransferase, serum	5 to 40 U/L	5 to 40 U/L
Gastrin, (fasting) serum	0 to 110 pg/ml	0 to 110 ng/L
Glucose (fasting), plasma or serum	70 to 115 mg/dl	3.9 to 6.4 nmol/L
Growth hormone, plasma (HGH)	0 to 6 ng/ml	0 to 6 μg/L
Haptoglobin, serum	26 to 165 mg/dl	0.20 to 1.65 g/L
Immunoglobulins, serum		
IgG	640 to 1350 mg/dl	6.4 to 13.5 g/L
IgA	70 to 310 mg/dl	0.70 to 3.1 g/L
IgM	90 to 350 mg/dl	0.90 to 3.5 g/L
IgD	0.0 to 6.0 mg/dl	0.0 to 60 mg/L
IgE	0.0 to 430 ng/ml	0.0 to 430 μg/L
Insulin (fasting), plasma	5 to 25 μU/ml	36 to 179 pmol/L
Iron, serum	75 to 175 μg/dl	13 to 31 μmol/L
Iron-binding capacity, serum		
Total	250 to 410 μg/dl	45 to 73 μmol/L
Saturation	20% to 55%	0.20 to 0.55
Lactate		
Venous blood	5.0 to 20.0 mg/dl	0.6 to 2.2 mmol/L
Arterial blood	5.0 to 15.0 mg/dl	0.6 to 1.7 mmol/L
Lactate dehydrogenase, serum (LD, LDH)	110 to 220 U/L	110 to 220 U/L
Lipase, serum	10 to 140 U/L	10 to 140 U/L
Lipids, total, serum	400 to 800 mg/dl	4.0 to 8.0 g/L
Luteinizing hormone, serum (LH)		
Males	1 to 9 mU/ml	1 to 9 U/L
Females		
Follicular phase	2 to 10 U/L	2 to 10 U/L
Midcycle peak	15 to 65 U/L	15 to 65 U/L
Luteal phase	1 to 12 U/L	1 to 12 U/L
Postmenopausal	12 to 65 U/L	12 to 65 U/L
Magnesium, serum	1.3 to 2.1 mg/dl	0.65 to 1.05 mmol/L
Osmolality	275 to 295 mOsm/kg H_2O	275 to 295 mOsm/kg H_2O
Oxygen, blood, arterial, room air		
Saturation (SaO$_2$)	95% to 98%	95% to 98%
Partial pressure (PaO$_2$)	80 to 100 mm Hg	80 to 100 mm Hg
pH, arterial blood	7.35 to 7.45	7.35 to 7.45
Phenylalanine, serum (Guthrie test)	<2 mg/dl	121 μmol/L
Phosphate, inorganic, serum	3.0 to 4.5 mg/dl	1.0 to 1.5 mmol/L
Potassium, serum	3.5 to 5.0 mEq/L	3.5 to 5.0 mmol/L

REFERENCE VALUES FOR BLOOD, PLASMA, AND SERUM* *Continued*

Test	Conventional Units	SI Units
Prolactin, serum		
Males	1 to 15 ng/ml	1 to 15 μg/L
Females	1 to 20 ng/ml	1 to 20 μg/L
Protein, serum		
Total	6.0 to 8.0 g/dl	60 to 80 g/L
Albumin	3.5 to 5.5 g/dl	35 to 55 g/L
α_1-Globulin	0.2 to 0.4 g/dl	2 to 4 g/L
α_2-Globulin	0.5 to 0.9 g/dl	5 to 9 g/L
β-Globulin	0.6 to 1.1 g/dl	6 to 11 g/L
γ-Globulin	0.7 to 1.7 g/dl	7 to 17 g/L
Pyruvate, blood	0.3 to 0.9 mg/dl	0.03 to 0.10 mmol/L
Sodium, serum or plasma	135 to 145 mEq/L	135 to 145 mmol/L
Testosterone, plasma		
Males	300 to 1200 ng/dl	10.4 to 41.6 nmol/L
Females	20 to 75 ng/dl	0.7 to 2.6 nmol/L
Pregnant	40 to 200 ng/dl	1.4 to 6.9 nmol/L
Thyroglobulin	3 to 42 ng/ml	3 to 42 μg/L
Thyroid-stimulating hormone, serum (TSH)	0.4 to 4.8 μIU/ml	0.4 to 4.8 mIU/L
Thyroxine, free, serum (FT$_4$)	0.9 to 2.1 ng/dl	12 to 27 pmol/L
Thyroxine, serum (T$_4$)	4.5 to 12.0 μg/dl	58 to 154 nmol/L
Triglycerides, serum, after 12 hr fast	40 to 150 mg/dl	0.4 to 1.5 g/L
Triiodothyronine, serum (T$_3$)	70 to 190 ng/dl	1.1 to 2.9 nmol/L
Triiodothyronine uptake, resin (T$_3$RU)	25% to 38% uptake	0.25 to 0.38 uptake
Urate		
Males	2.5 to 8.0 mg/dl	150 to 480 μmol/L
Females	2.2 to 7.0 mg/dl	130 to 420 μmol/L
Urea, serum or plasma	24 to 49 mg/dl	4.0 to 8.2 nmol/L
Urea nitrogen, serum or plasma	11 to 23 mg/dl	8.0 to 16.4 nmol/L
Viscosity, serum	1.4 to 1.8 $\times$ water	1.4 to 1.8 $\times$ water
Vitamin A, serum	20 to 80 μg/dl	0.70 to 2.80 μmol/L
Vitamin B$_{12}$, serum	180 to 900 pg/ml	133 to 664 pmol/L

*For some procedures, reference values may vary, depending on the method used.

Modified from Conn, R. B., Borer, W. Z., & Snyder, J. W. (1997). *Current diagnosis* (9th ed., pp. 1235–1241). Philadelphia: W. B. Saunders; and data from Malarkey, L. M., & McMorrow, M. E. (2000). *Nurses' manual of laboratory tests and diagnostic procedures* (2nd ed.). Philadelphia: W. B. Saunders.

REFERENCE VALUES FOR URINE*

Test	Conventional Units	SI Units
Acetone and acetoacetate, qualitative	Negative	Negative
Albumin		
Qualitative	Negative	Negative
Quantitative	10 to 100 mg/24 hr	0.15 to 1.5 μmol/24 hr
Aldosterone	3 to 20 μg/24 hr	8.3 to 55 nmol/24 hr
δ-Aminolevulinic acid	1.3 to 7.0 mg/24 hr	10 to 53 μmol/24 hr
Amylase	<17 U/hr	<17 U/hr
Amylase/creatinine clearance ratio	0.01 to 0.04	0.01 to 0.04
Bilirubin, qualitative	Negative	Negative
Calcium (usual diet)	<250 mg/24 hr	<6.3 nmol/24 hr
Catecholamines		
Epinephrine	<10 μg/24 hr	<55 nmol/24 hr
Norepinephrine	<100 μg/24 hr	<590 nmol/24 hr
Total free catecholamines	4 to 126 μg/24 hr	24 to 745 nmol/24 hr
Total metanephrines	0.1 to 1.6 mg/24 hr	0.5 to 8.1 μmol/24 hr
Chloride (varies with intake)	110 to 250 mEq/24 hr	110 to 250 nmol/24 hr
Copper	0 to 50 μg/24 hr	0 to 0.80 μmol/24 hr
Cortisol, free	10 to 100 μg/24 hr	27.6 to 276 nmol/24 hr
Creatine		
Males	0 to 40 mg/24 hr	0.0 to 0.30 mmol/24 hr
Females	0 to 80 mg/24 hr	0.0 to 0.60 mmol/24 hr
Creatinine	15 to 25 mg/kg/24 hr	0.13–0.22 mmol/kg/24 hr
Creatinine clearance (corrected to 1.73 m² body surface area)		
Males	110 to 150 ml/min/1.73 m²	110 to 150 ml/min/1.73 m²
Females	105 to 132 ml/min/1.73 m²	105 to 132 ml/min/1.73 m²
Dehydroepiandrosterone		
Males	0.2 to 2.0 mg/24 hr	0.7 to 6.9 μmol/24 hr
Females	0.2 to 1.8 mg/24 hr	0.7 to 6.2 μmol/24 hr
Estrogens, total		
Males	4 to 25 μg/24 hr	14 to 90 nmol/24 hr
Females	5 to 100 μg/24 hr	18 to 360 nmol/24 hr
Glucose (as reducing substance)	<250 mg/24 hr	<250 mg/24 hr
Hemoglobin and myoglobin, qualitative	Negative	Negative
17-Hydroxycorticosteroids		
Males	3 to 9 mg/24 hr	8.3 to 25 μmol/24 hr
Females	2 to 8 mg/24 hr	5.5 to 22 μmol/24 hr
5-Hydroxyindoleacetic acid		
Qualitative	Negative	Negative
Quantitative	2 to 6 mg/24 hr	10 to 31 μmol/24 hr
17-Ketosteroids		
Males	8 to 22 mg/24 hr	28 to 76 μmol/24 hr
Females	6 to 15 mg/24 hr	21 to 52 μmol/24 hr
Magnesium	6.0 to 10 mEq/24 hr	3.0 to 5.0 mmol/24 hr
Metanephrines (see Catecholamines)		
Osmolality	38 to 1,400 mOsm/kg H_2O	38 to 1,400 mOsm/kg H_2O
pH	4.6 to 8.0	4.6 to 8.0
Phenylpyruvic acid, qualitative	Negative	Negative
Phosphate	0.4 to 1.3 g/24 hr	13 to 42 mmol/24 hr
Porphobilinogen		
Qualitative	Negative	Negative
Quantitative	<2.0 mg/24 hr	<9 μmol/24 hr

REFERENCE VALUES FOR URINE* Continued

Test	Conventional Units	SI Units
Porphyrins		
Coproporphyrin	50 to 250 µg/24 hr	77 to 380 nmol/24 hr
Uroporphyrin	10 to 30 µg/24 hr	12 to 36 nmol/24 hr
Potassium	25 to 125 mEq/24 hr	25 to 125 mmol/24 hr
Pregnanediol		
Males	0.0 to 1.9 mg/24 hr	0.0 to 6.0 µmol/24 hr
Females		
Proliferative phase	0.0 to 2.6 mg/24 hr	0.0 to 8.0 µmol/24 hr
Luteal phase	2.6 to 10.6 mg/24 hr	8 to 33 µmol/24 hr
Postmenopausal	0.2 to 1.0 mg/24 hr	0.6 to 3.1 µmol/24 hr
Pregnanetriol	<2.5 mg/24 hr	<7.4 µmol/24 hr
Protein		
Qualitative	Negative	Negative
Quantitative	10 to 150 mg/24 hr	10 to 150 mg/24 hr
Protein-creatinine ratio	<0.2	<0.2
Sodium (usual diet)	60 to 260 mEq/24 hr	60 to 260 mmol/24 hr
Specific gravity, random	1.003 to 1.030	1.003 to 1.030
Urate (usual diet)	250 to 750 mg/24 hr	1.5 to 4.4 mmol/24 hr
Urobilinogen	0.5 to 4.0 mg/24 hr	0.6 to 6.8 µmol/24 hr
Vanillylmandelic acid (VMA) (4-hydroxy-3-methoxy-mandelic acid)	1 to 8 mg/24 hr	5 to 40 µmol/24 hr

*For some procedures, reference values may vary, depending on the method used.
Modified from Conn, R. B., Borer, W. Z., & Snyder, J. W. (1997). *Current diagnosis* (9th ed., pp. 1235–1241). Philadelphia: W. B. Saunders; and data from Malarkey, L. M., & McMorrow, M. E. (2000). *Nurses' manual of laboratory tests and diagnostic procedures* (2nd ed.). Philadelphia: W. B. Saunders.

REFERENCE VALUES FOR THERAPEUTIC DRUG MONITORING (Serum)

	Therapeutic Range	Toxic Levels	Proprietary Names
Antibiotics			
Amikacin	25 to 30 µg/ml	Peak > 35 µg/ml Trough > 10 µg/ml	Amikin
Chloramphenicol	10 to 20 µg/ml	>25 µg/ml	Chloromycetin
Gentamicin	5 to 10 µg/ml	Peak > 12 µg/ml Trough > 2 µg/ml	Garamycin
Tobramycin	5 to 10 µg/ml	Peak > 10 µg/ml Trough > 2 µg/ml	Nebcin
Vancomycin	5 to 10 µg/ml	Peak > 40 µg/ml Trough > 10 µg/ml	Vancocin
Anticonvulsants			
Carbamazepine	5 to 12 µg/ml	>15 µg/ml	Tegretol
Ethosuximide	40 to 100 µg/ml	>150 µg/ml	Zarontin
Phenobarbital	15 to 40 µg/ml	Vary widely because of developed tolerance	Luminal
Phenytoin	10 to 20 µg/ml	>20 µg/ml	Dilantin
Primidone	5 to 12 µg/ml	>15 µg/ml	Mysoline
Valproic acid	50 to 100 µg/ml	>100 µg/ml	Depakene
Analgesics			
Acetaminophen	10 to 20 µg/ml	>250 µg/ml	Tylenol Datril
Salicylate	100 to 250 µg/ml	>300 µg/ml	Aspirin Bufferin

Table continued on following page

REFERENCE VALUES FOR THERAPEUTIC DRUG MONITORING (Serum) *Continued*

	Therapeutic Range	Toxic Levels	Proprietary Names
Bronchodilator			
Theophylline (aminophylline)	10 to 20 μg/ml	>20 μg/ml	Theo-Dur
Cardiovascular Drugs			
Amiodarone (specimen must be obtained more than 8 hr after last dose	1 to 2 μg/ml	>2 μg/ml	Cordarone
Digitoxin (specimen must be obtained 12 to 24 hr after last dose)	15 to 25 ng/ml	>35 ng/ml	Crystodigin
Digoxin (specimen must be obtained more than 6 hr after last dose)	0.8 to 2.0 ng/ml	>2.4 ng/ml	Lanoxin
Disopyramide	2 to 5 μg/ml	>7 μg/ml	Norpace
Flecainide	0.2 to 1.0 ng/ml	>1 ng/ml	Tambocor
Lidocaine	1.5 to 5.0 μg/ml	>6 to 8 μg/ml	Xylocaine
Mexiletine	0.7 to 2.0 ng/ml	>2 ng/ml	Mexitil
Procainamide (measured as procainamide + *N*-acetyl procainamide)	4 to 10 μg/ml 8 to 30 μg/ml	>12 μg/ml >30 μg/ml	Pronestyl
Propranolol	50 to 100 ng/ml	Variable	Inderal
Quinidine	2 to 5 μg/ml	>6 μg/ml	Cardioquin Quinaglute Quinidex
Tocainide	4 to 10 ng/ml	>10 ng/ml	Tonocard
Psychopharmacologic Drugs			
Amitriptyline (measured as amitriptyline + nortriptyline)	120 to 150 ng/ml	>500 ng/ml	Elavil Endep Limbitrol Triavil
Bupropion	25 to 100 ng/ml	Not applicable	Wellbutrin
Desipramine (measured as desipramine + imipramine)	150 to 300 ng/ml	>500 ng/ml	Norpramin Pertofrane
Imipramine (measured as imipramine + desipramine)	125 to 250 ng/ml	>400 ng/ml	Janimine Tofranil
Lithium (obtain specimen 12 hr after last dose)	0.6 to 1.5 mEq/L	>1.5 mEq/L	Lithobid
Nortriptyline	50 to 150 ng/ml	500 ng/ml	Aventyl Pamelor

Modified from Conn, R. B., Borer, W. Z., & Snyder, J. W. (1997). *Current diagnosis* (9th ed., pp. 1235–1241). Philadelphia: W. B. Saunders; and data from Malarkey, L. M., & McMorrow, M. E. (2000). *Nurses' manual of laboratory tests and diagnostic procedures* (2nd ed.). Philadelphia: W. B. Saunders.

REFERENCE VALUES IN TOXICOLOGY

	Conventional Units	SI Units
Arsenic, blood	3.5 to 7.2 μg/dl	0.47 to 0.96 μmol/L
Arsenic, urine	<130 μg/24 hr	<1.7 μmol/24 hr
Bromides, serum, inorganic	<100 mg/dl Toxic above 140 to 1000 mg/dl	14 to 100 mmol/L Toxic above 14 to 100 mmol/L
Carboxyhemoglobin, blood Symptoms occur	<5% saturation >15% saturation	<0.05 saturation >0.15 saturation
Ethanol, blood	<0.05 mg/dl <0.005%	<1.0 mmol/L
Marked intoxication	300 to 400 mg/dl 0.3% to 0.4%	65 to 87 mmol/L
Alcoholic stupor	400 to 500 mg/dl 0.4% to 0.5%	87 to 109 mmol/L
Coma	>500 mg/dl >0.5%	>109 mmol/L
Lead, blood	<25 μg/dl	1.2 μmol/L
Lead, urine	<80 μg/24 hr	<0.4 μmol/24 hr
Mercury, urine	<30 μg/24 hr	<150 nmol/24 hr

Modified from Conn, R. B., Borer, W. Z., & Snyder, J. W. (1997). *Current diagnosis* (9th ed., pp. 1235–1241). Philadelphia: W. B. Saunders; and data from Malarkey, L. M., & McMorrow, M. E. (2000). *Nurses' manual of laboratory tests and diagnostic procedures* (2nd ed.). Philadelphia: W. B. Saunders.

REFERENCE VALUES FOR CEREBROSPINAL FLUID

	Conventional Units	SI Units
Cells	<5/mm^3 All mononuclear	<5 $\times$ 10^6/L All mononuclear
Electrophoresis	Predominantly albumin	Predominantly albumin
Glucose	50 to 75 mg/dl (20 mg/dl less than serum)	2.8 to 4.2 mmol/L (1.1 mmol/L less than serum)

IgG
  Children <14 yr
  Adults
	
	<8% of total protein
	<14% of total protein
		
		<0.08 of total protein
		<0.14 of total protein

IgG index	0.3 to 0.6	0.3 to 0.6
$\quad$ CSF/serum IgG ratio CSF/serum albumin ratio		
Oligoclonal banding on electrophoresis	Absent	Absent
Pressure, opening	70 to 180 mm H$_2$O	70 to 180 mm H$_2$O
Protein, total	15 to 45 mg/dl	150 to 450 mg/L

Modified from Conn, R. B., Borer, W. Z., & Snyder, J. W. (1997). *Current diagnosis* (9th ed., pp. 1235–1241). Philadelphia: W. B. Saunders; and data from Malarkey, L. M., & McMorrow, M. E. (2000). *Nurses' manual of laboratory tests and diagnostic procedures* (2nd ed.). Philadelphia: W. B. Saunders.

REFERENCE VALUES FOR SEMEN ANALYSIS

	Conventional Units	SI Units
Volume	2 to 5 ml	2 to 5 ml
Liquefaction	Complete in 15 min	Complete in 15 min
Leukocytes	Occasional or absent	Occasional or absent
Count	60 to 150 million/ml	60 to 150 $\times$ 10^6/ml
Motility	>80% motile	>0.80 motile
Morphology	80% to 90% normal forms	0.80 to 0.90 normal forms
Fructose	>150 mg/dl	>8.33 mmol/L

Modified from Conn, R. B., Borer, W. Z., & Snyder, J. W. (1997). *Current diagnosis* (9th ed., pp. 1235–1241). Philadelphia: W. B. Saunders; and data from Malarkey, L. M., & McMorrow, M. E. (2000). *Nurses' manual of laboratory tests and diagnostic procedures* (2nd ed.). Philadelphia: W. B. Saunders.

REFERENCE VALUES FOR TESTS OF GASTROINTESTINAL FUNCTION

Test Name	Conventional Units	Test Name	Conventional Units
Bentiromide	6-hr urinary arylamine excretion > 57% excludes pancreatic insufficiency	Gastric acid output *(continued)* Maximum (after histamine or pentagastrin)	
β-Carotene, serum	60–250 ng/dl	Males	9.0–48.0 mmol/hr
Fecal fat estimation		Females	6.0–31.0 mmol/hr
Qualitative	No fat globules seen by high-power microscope	Ratio: basal/maximum	
		Males	0.0–0.31
Quantitative	<6 g/24 hr (>95% coefficient of fat absorption)	Females	0.0–0.29
		Secretin test, pancreatic fluid	
Gastric acid output		Volume	>1.8 ml/kg/hr
Basal		Bicarbonate	>80 mEq/L
Males	0.0–10.5 mmol/hr		
Females	0.0–5.6 mmol/hr	D-Xylose absorption test, urine	>20% of ingested dose excreted in 5 hr

Modified from Conn, R. B., Borer, W. Z., & Snyder, J. W. (1997). *Current diagnosis* (9th ed., pp. 1235–1241). Philadelphia: W. B. Saunders.

Index

Note: Page numbers in *italics* indicate illustrations; those followed by t indicate tables; and those followed by b indicate boxed material.

STANDARD AND TRANSMISSION-BASED PRECAUTIONS

STANDARD PRECAUTIONS FOR THE CARE OF ALL PATIENTS

Hand-washing	Wash your hands immediately after removing gloves, between client contacts, and after contact with blood, body fluids, secretions, excretions, and contaminated equipment or articles.
Gloves	Wear gloves when touching mucous membranes or nonintact skin, and when touching blood, body fluids, secretions, excretions, and contaminated items.
Mask, eye protection, face shield	Wear a mask, an eye protector, or a face shield during procedures that are likely to generate splashes or sprays of blood, body fluids, secretions, and excretions.
Gown	Wear a gown during procedures that are likely to generate splashes or sprays of blood, body fluids, secretions, and excretions.
Client care equipment	Handle soiled client care equipment in a manner that prevents skin and mucous membrane exposure, contamination of clothing, and transfer of microorganisms to other clients and environments. Reusable equipment must be cleaned and reprocessed appropriately.
Environmental control	Ensure adequate procedures for the routine care, cleaning, and disinfection of client furniture, equipment, and environmental surfaces.
Linen	Handle soiled linen in a manner that prevents skin and mucous membrane exposure, contamination of clothing, and transfer of microorganisms to other clients and environments.
Sharps	Do not recap used needles. Do not bend, break, or manipulate used needles by hand. Place used needles, scalpels, and other sharps in puncture-resistant, labeled sharps containers.
Client resuscitation	Use a mouthpiece, resuscitation bag, or other ventilation device to avoid mouth-to-mouth resuscitation.
Client placement	Use a private room for a client who contaminates the environment or cannot assist in maintaining appropriate hygiene.

ADDITIONAL TRANSMISSION-BASED PRECAUTIONS

Contact precautions[3]	1. Place client in a private room or with another client who is infected with the same organism. The client should remain in the room unless it is essential to leave.
	2. Wear gloves when entering the room, and change them after contact with infective material such as feces or wound drainage.
	3. Wash your hands with an antimicrobial agent immediately after removing gloves while still in the client's room.
	4. Wear a gown if you anticipate contact with infected material.
	5. Do not share client care equipment if possible. If you must share equipment, clean and disinfect it between client contacts.
	6. Take additional precautions to prevent the spread of vancomycin-resistant organisms.[2]
Droplet precautions[3]	1. Place client in a private room or with another client who is infected with the same organism. The door to the room may remain open. The client should remain in the room unless it is essential to leave.
	2. Wear a mask when working within 3 feet of the client. Have the client wear a mask during transport outside the room.
Airborne precautions[3]	1. Place client in a negative-pressure isolation room with at least six air exchanges per hour. Air from the room must be discharged to the outdoors or through a high-efficiency filter before the air is circulated to the other areas in the hospital. The room door must remain closed.
	2. Wear a mask when entering the room. Have the client wear a mask during transport outside the room. All persons entering the room should wear a mask.
	3. Follow additional CDC guidelines for preventing the transmission of tuberculosis.[1]

Data from Centers for Disease Control and Prevention (CDC). (1994). Guidelines for preventing the transmission of *Mycobacterium tuberculosis* in health-care facilities. *Morbidity and Mortality Weekly Report, 43*(RR-13), 1–132[1]; Centers for Disease Control and Prevention (CDC). (1995). Recommendations for preventing the spread of vancomycin resistance: Recommendations of the Hospital Infection Control Practices Advisory Committee (HICPAC). *Morbidity and Mortality Weekly Report, 44*(RR-12), 1–13[2]; and Garner J. S., & Hospital Infection Control Practices Advisory Committee. (1996). Guidelines for isolation precautions in hospitals. *Infection Control and Hospital Epidemiology, 17,* 54–80.[3]